1972 The AVMA House of Delegates votes to accredit training programs for animal technicians. The Committee on Accreditation of Training for Animal Technicians (CATAT) is formed and takes on this responsibility.

The first national continuing education meeting for animal technicians in the United States is held at the Western States Veterinary Conference in Las Vegas, Nevada.

1973 The first two programs to be accredited by the AVMA are those at Michigan State University and Nebraska College of Technical Agriculture.

The Association of Animal Technician Educators (AATE) is formed at the Third Symposium on Animal Technician Training.

The AVMA House of Delegates passes a resolution proposing "registration" but not "licensing" of animal technicians. The Committee on Accreditation for Training of Animal Technicians changes its name to the Committee on Animal Technician Activities and Training.

1975 The Washington State Association of Veterinary Technicians (WSAVT) is established.

The AATE constitution is adopted and the first officers are elected.

1976 CATAT is recognized by the U.S. Office of Education as the accrediting body for animal technician training programs.

The first professional journal for veterinary technicians, *Methods: The Journal for Animal Health Technicians,* is published.

The Veterinary Technicians and Assistants Association of Pennsylvania (VTAAP) is created.

1977 The first written state examination for animal health technicians in the state of New York is administered.

1978 The Virginia Association of Licensed Veterinary Technicians is established.

1978 The AVMA adds a continuing education section for veterinary technicians to its program at the annual convention in Dallas, Texas.

The Alberta Association of Animal Health Technologist is formed.

1980 *The Compendium on Continuing Education for the Animal Health Technician* (later called *Veterinary Technician*) is first published.

At the annual AVMA convention, members of an ad hoc committee composed of representatives from the United States and Canada discuss the idea of forming a United States–Canadian veterinary technicians' association.

Association Technicien Sante Animal du Quebec (ATSAQ) begins, with 25 members.

1981 The North American Veterinary Technician Association (NAVTA) is organized.

The Association of Zoo Veterinary Technicians is formed.

The Veterinary Hospital Managers Association is formed.

1982 CALAS creates a plan for the voluntary registration of laboratory animal technicians.

NAVTA adopts *The Compendium on Continuing Education for the Animal Health Technician* (later called *Veterinary Technician*) as its first official journal.

1984 *The Compendium on Continuing Education for the Animal Health Technician* is changed to *Veterinary Technician.*

NAVTA adopts a national code of ethics for veterinary technicians.

1985 The AVMA Executive Board establishes the Animal Technician Testing Committee, which generates the Animal Technician National Examination (ATNE) in conjunction with Professional Education Services (PES).

The Association of Animal Technician Educators (AATE) changes its name to the Association of Veterinary Technician Educators (AVTE).

1986 The first ATNE is given in Maine.

1988 In Canada, the Eastern Veterinary Technician Association (EVTA) is established, with 30 members.

CALAS implements a testing and registration plan for laboratory animal technicians.

The AVMA votes no to a resolution that would change terminology from "animal technician" to "veterinary technician."

CLINICAL TEXTBOOK *for* VETERINARY TECHNICIANS

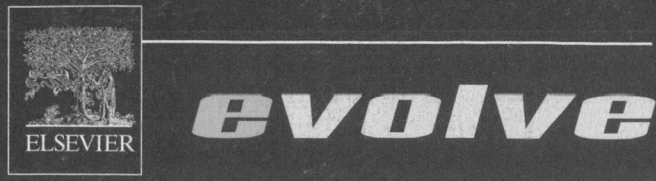

ELSEVIER

evolve

To access your Student Resources, visit the web address below:

http://evolve.elsevier.com/McCurnin/vettech/

- **Crossword Puzzles**
  Crossword puzzles have been created for each chapter using Key Words from the text. These provide you with an easy way to test your knowledge of terminology.

- **Picture-it Exercises**
  Drag-and-drop activities help you identify labels on critical illustrations.

- **Hangman Games**
  Another interactive activity helps build vocabulary.

- **Quiz Shows**
  May be played as group activities or solitaire.

- **WebLinks**
  This exciting resource lets you link to hundreds of websites carefully chosen to supplement the content of the textbook. The WebLinks are regularly updated, with new ones added as they are developed.

CLINICAL TEXTBOOK *for* VETERINARY TECHNICIANS

— SIXTH EDITION —

DENNIS M. MCCURNIN, DVM, MS, Dipl ACVS

Professor, Department of Veterinary Clinical Sciences
Hospital Director, Veterinary Teaching Hospital and Clinics
School of Veterinary Medicine
Louisiana State University, Baton Rouge, Louisiana

JOANNA M. BASSERT, VMD

Professor and Director
Program of Veterinary Technology
Manor College, Jenkintown, Pennsylvania

With 1330 illustrations, more than 1200 in full color

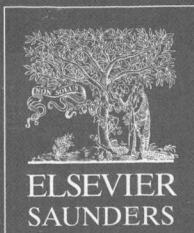

ELSEVIER
SAUNDERS

**ELSEVIER
SAUNDERS**

11830 Westline Industrial Drive
St. Louis, Missouri 63146

Notice

Knowledge and best practice in this field are constantly changing. As new research and experience broaden our knowledge, changes in practice, treatment and drug therapy may become necessary or appropriate. Readers are advised to check the most current information provided (i) on procedures featured or (ii) by the manufacturer of each product to be administered, to verify the recommended dose or formula, the method and duration of administration, and contraindications. It is the responsibility of the practitioner, relying on their own experience and knowledge of the patient, to make diagnoses, to determine dosages and the best treatment for each individual patient, and to take all appropriate safety precautions. To the fullest extent of the law, neither the Publisher nor the Authors assume any liability for any injury and/or damage to persons or property arising out of or related to any use of the material contained in this book.

The Publisher

Previous editions copyrighted 2002, 1998, 1994, 1990, 1985

International Standard Book Number 0-7216-0612-1

Publishing Director: Linda L. Duncan
Managing Editor: Teri Merchant
Publishing Services Manager: John Rogers
Senior Project Manager: Beth Hayes
Senior Designer: Julia Dummitt

Printed in the United States of America

Last digit is the print number: 9 8 7 6 5 4 3 2 1

This book will always be dedicated
to the profession of veterinary technology
and all technicians.

To my grandson, Evan Michael McCurnin,
who is the light of my life.
DMM

To the wise and brilliant Gertrude P. Marshall,
with love and gratitude.
JMB

Contributors

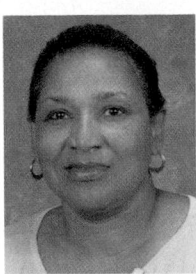

Marvene Augustus, BS, Doctor of Pharmacy
Pharmacy Manager
Veterinary Teaching Hospital and Clinics
School of Veterinary Medicine
Louisiana State University
Baton Rouge, Louisiana

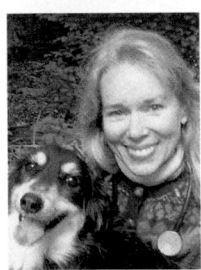

Joanna M. Bassert, VMD
Professor and Director
Program of Veterinary Technology
Manor College
Jenkintown, Pennsylvania

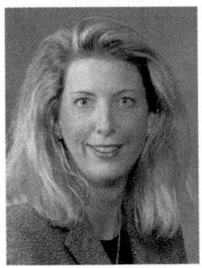

Susan A. Berryhill, BS, RVT
Veterinary Nursing Specialist
Veterinary Specialty Team
Pfizer Animal Health Group
Olathe, Kansas

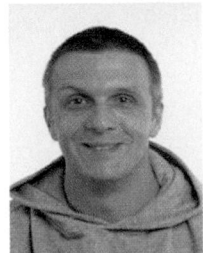

David M. Bolt, DrVetMed, MS
Department of Veterinary Clinical Science
School of Veterinary Medicine
Louisiana State University
Baton Rouge, Louisiana

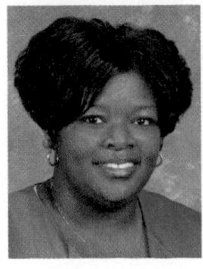

Sonja Bremer Boss, RPh
Assistant Pharmacy Manager
Veterinary Teaching Hospital and Clinics
School of Veterinary Medicine
Louisiana State University
Baton Rouge, Louisiana

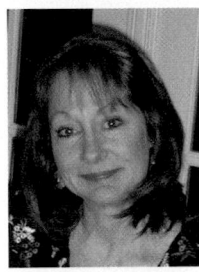

Sandra Brackenridge, MSW
Assistant Professor, Social Work
Idaho State University
Pocatello, Idaho

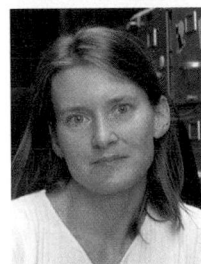

Loretta J. Bubenik, DVM, MS, Dipl ACVS
Assistant Professor, Companion Animal Surgery
Department of Veterinary Clinical Studies
School of Veterinary Medicine
Louisiana State University
Baton Rouge, Louisiana

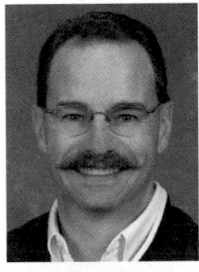

Daniel J. Burba, DVM, Dipl ACVS
Associate Professor, Equine Surgery
Department of Veterinary Clinical Sciences
School of Veterinary Medicine
Louisiana State University
Baton Rouge, Louisiana

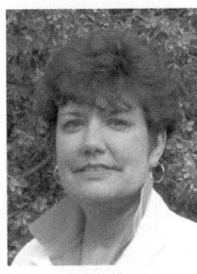

Vickie Byard, CVT
President-Elect, Acadamy of Veterinary Dental Technicians
In-Patient Supervisor
Rau Animal Hospital
Glenside, Pennsylvania

Ann M. Chapman, DVM
Resident, Equine Internal Medicine
Department of Veterinary Clinical Sciences
School of Veterinary Medicine
Louisiana State University
Baton Rouge, Louisiana

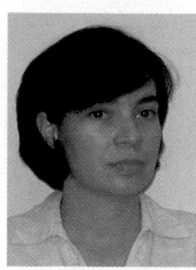

Lais R. R. Costa, MV, PhD, MS, Dipl ACVIM
Clinical Fellow, Equine Medicine
Department of Veterinary Clinical Sciences
School of Veterinary Medicine
Louisiana State University
Baton Rouge, Louisiana

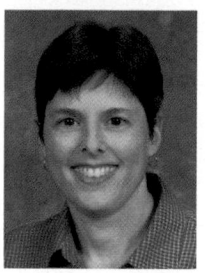

Jacqueline R. Davidson, DVM, MS, Dipl ACVS
Associate Professor, Companion Animal Surgery
Department of Veterinary Clinical Sciences
School of Veterinary Medicine
Louisiana State University
Baton Rouge, Louisiana

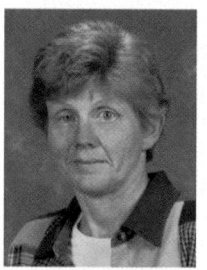

Susan C. Eades, DVM, PhD, Dipl ACVIM
Professor, Equine Medicine
Department of Veterinary Clinical Studies
School of Veterinary Medicine
Louisiana State University
Baton Rouge, Louisiana

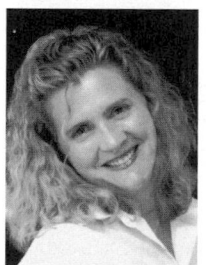

Lee Ann Eddleman, CVT
Associate Clinical Specialist
School of Veterinary Medicine
Louisiana State University
Baton Rouge, Louisiana

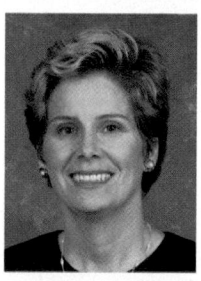

Susan M. Eddlestone, DVM, Dipl ACVIM
Assistant Professor, Small Animal Medicine
Department of Veterinary Clinical Studies
School of Veterinary Medicine
Louisiana State University
Baton Rouge, Louisiana

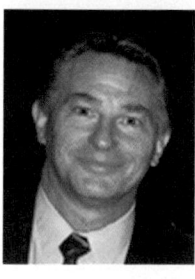

Bruce E. Eilts, DVM, MS, Dipl ACT
Professor, Theriogenology
Department of Veterinary Clinical Studies
School of Veterinary Medicine
Louisiana State University
Baton Rouge, Louisiana

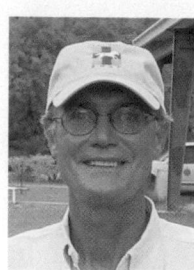

Dennis D. French, BS, DVM, Dipl ABVP
Professor, Farm Animal Health Management
Department of Veterinary Clinical Studies
School of Veterinary Medicine and AgCenter
Louisiana State University
Baton Rouge, Louisiana

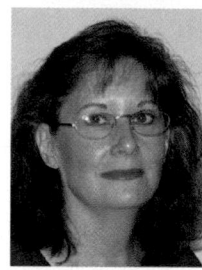

Marjorie S. Gill, DVM, MS, Dipl ABVP
Associate Professor
Food Animal Medicine and Surgery
Department of Clinical Sciences
School of Veterinary Medicine
Louisiana State University
Baton Rouge, Louisiana

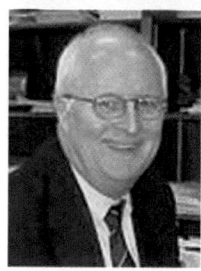

Michael G. Groves, DVM, MPH, PhD, Dipl ACVM and ACVPM
Dean, School of Veterinary Medicine
Louisiana State University
Baton Rouge, Louisiana

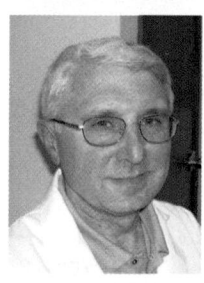

Perry L. Habecker, VMD, Dipl ACVP
Staff Pathologist; Chief, Large Animal Pathology Service
New Bolton Center
School of Veterinary Medicine
University of Pennsylvania
Kennett Square, Pennsylvania

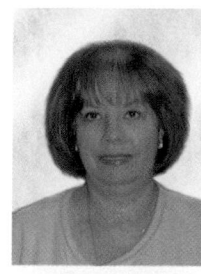

Kathleen Story Harrington, MS
Instructor, Department of Pathobiological Sciences
School of Veterinary Medicine
Louisiana State University
Baton Rouge, Louisiana

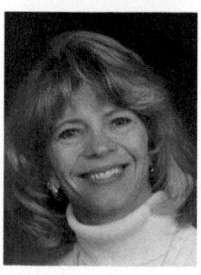

Suzanne Hetts, PhD, Certified Applied Animal Behaviorist
President, Animal Behavior Associates, Inc.
Littleton, Colorado

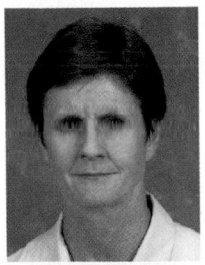

Giselle Hosgood, BVSc, MS, PhD, FACVSc, Dipl ACVS
Professor, Veterinary Surgery
Department of Veterinary Clinical Sciences
School of Veterinary Medicine
Louisiana State University
Baton Rouge, Louisiana

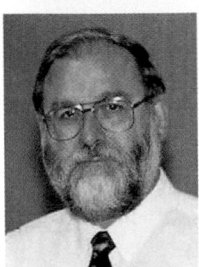

Johnny D. Hoskins, DVM, PhD, Dipl ACVIM
Small Animal Consultant
DocuTech Services, Inc.
Choudran, Louisiana

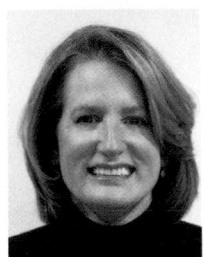

Tracey J. Jaffe, BA, BS, DVM
Detroit Metro Veterinary Services
Senior Year Guest Lecturer
Veterinary Technology Program
Wayne County Community College
Wayne State University
Detroit, Michigan

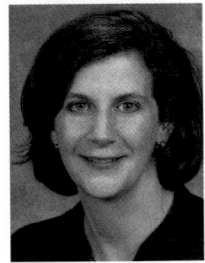

Stephanie W. Johnson, BA, MSW
Instructor, Department of Veterinary Clinical Sciences
School of Veterinary Medicine
Louisiana State University
Baton Rouge, Louisiana

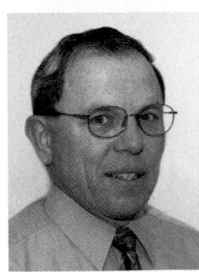

Robert L. Jones, DVM, PhD, Dipl ACVM
Professor
Department of Microbiology, Immunology and Pathology
College of Veterinary Medicine
Colorado State University
Fort Collins, Colorado

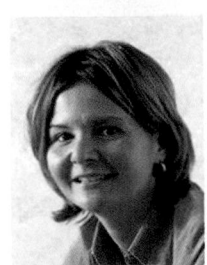

Christine Jurek, DVM
TOPS Veterinary Rehabilitation
Grayslake, Illinois

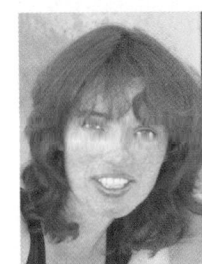

Susanne K. Lauer, DrMedVet, Dipl ACVS
Assistant Professor, Companion Animal Surgery
Department of Veterinary Clinical Sciences
School of Veterinary Medicine
Louisiana State University
Baton Rouge, Louisiana

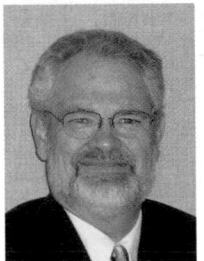

Roger L. Lukens, MS, DVM
Professor, Veterinary Technology
Veterinary Administration
School of Veterinary Medicine
Purdue University
West Lafayette, Indiana

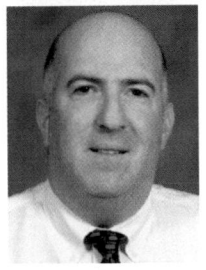

Steven L. Marks, DVM, Dipl ACVIM
Associate Professor, Department of Veterinary Clinical Medicine
College of Veterinary Medicine
University of Illinois
Urbana, Illinois

G. Neal Mauldin, DVM, Dipl ACVIM, ACVR
Associate Professor, Veterinary Oncology
Department of Veterinary Clinical Sciences
School of Veterinary Medicine
Louisiana State University
Baton Rouge, Louisiana

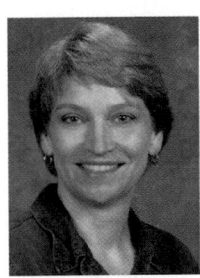

Glenna E. Mauldin, DVM, MS, Dipl ACVIM (Oncology)
Associate Professor, Veterinary Oncology
Department of Veterinary Clinical Sciences
School of Veterinary Medicine
Louisiana State University
Baton Rouge, Louisiana

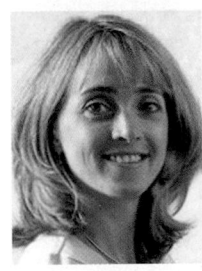

Laurie McCauley, DVM
Medical Director
TOPS Veterinary Rehabilitation
Grayslake, Illinois

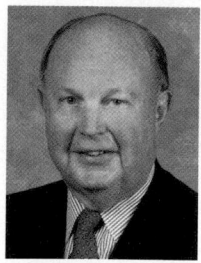

Dennis M. McCurnin, DVM, MS, Dipl ACVS
Professor, Department of Veterinary Clinical Sciences
Hospital Director, Veterinary Teaching Hospital and Clinics
School of Veterinary Medicine
Louisiana State University
Baton Rouge, Louisiana

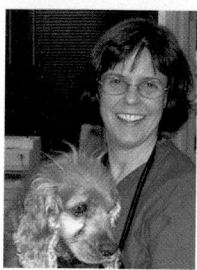

Ellen Miller, DVM, MS, Dipl ACVIM
Internal Medicine
Parker, Colorado

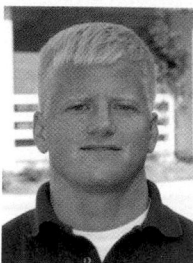

Rustin M. Moore, DVM, PhD, Dipl ACVS
Service Chief, Equine Medicine and Surgery
Director, Equine Health Studies Program
Department of Veterinary Clinical Sciences
School of Veterinary Medicine
Louisiana State University
Baton Rouge, Louisiana

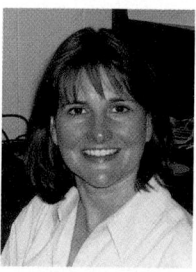

Ashley B. Oakes, DVM, Dipl AVDC
Veterinary Dentist
Clearwater, Florida

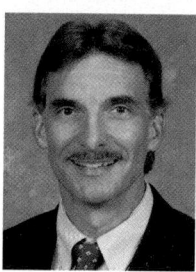

Dale L. Paccamonti, DVM, MS, Dipl ACT
Professor, Theriogenology
Department of Veterinary Clinical Sciences
School of Veterinary Medicine
Louisiana State University
Baton Rouge, Louisiana

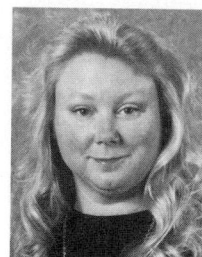

Beth Paugh Partington, DVM, MS, Dipl ACVR
Adjunct Associate Professor, Veterinary Radiology
Department of Veterinary of Clinical Sciences
School of Veterinary Medicine
Louisiana State University
Baton Rouge, Louisiana

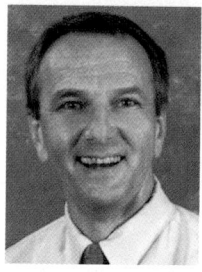

Glenn R. Pettifer, BA (Hons), BSc, DVM, DVSc, Dipl ACVA
Associate Professor, Veterinary Anesthesiology and Pain Management
Department of Veterinary Clinical Sciences
School of Veterinary Medicine
Louisiana State University
Baton Rouge, Louisiana

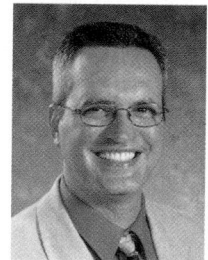

Carlos R. F. Pinto, MedVet, PhD, Dipl ACT
Assistant Professor, Theriogenology
Department of Population Health & Pathobiology
College of Veterinary Medicine
North Carolina State University
Raleigh, North Carolina

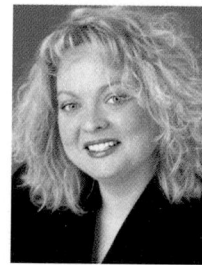

Jill A. Richardson, DVM
Associate Director, Technical Services
The Hartz Mountain Corporation
Consultant in Toxicology, Veterinary Information Network
Secaucus, New Jersey

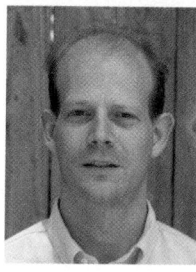

Kirk Ryan, DVM, Dipl ACVIM
Staff Internist Louisiana
Veterinary Referral Center
Mandeviller, Louisiana

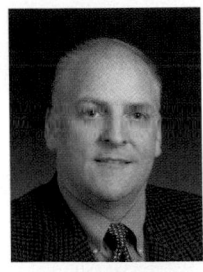

William D. Schoenherr, PhD
Principal Nutritionist
Science and Technology Center
Hill's Pet Nutrition
Topeka, Kansas

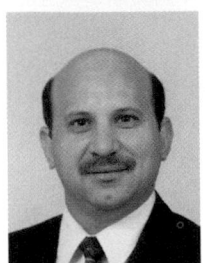

Philip J. Siebert, Jr., CVT
Veterinary Practice Consultants
Calhoun, Tennessee

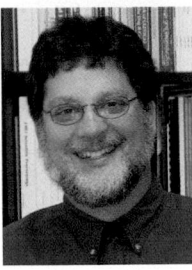

Joseph Taboada, DVM, Dipl ACVIM
Professor, Small Animal Internal
  Medicine
Department of Veterinary of Clinical
  Sciences
Associate Dean, School of Veterinary
  Medicine
Louisiana State University
Baton Rouge, Louisiana

Leslie A. Talley, LAT
Supervisor, Equine Technicians
Veterinary Teaching Hospital and Clinics
School of Veterinary Medicine
Louisiana State University
Baton Rouge, Louisiana

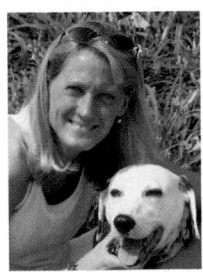

Mary Tefend, LVT, MS
Hill's Instructor of Veterinary Critical
  Care Nursing
Department of Clinical Sciences
College of Veterinary Medicine
Auburn University
Auburn, Alabama

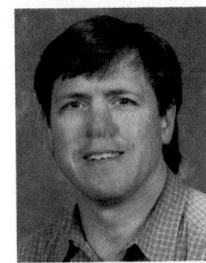

**Thomas N. Tully, Jr., DVM, MS, Dipl
  ABVP (avian) and ECAMS**
Professor, Zoological Medicine
Department of Veterinary Clinical
  Sciences
School of Veterinary Medicine
Louisiana State University
Baton Rouge, Louisiana

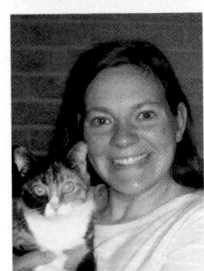

Katie Underwood, BS, MSW
Social Worker
Denham Springs, Louisiana

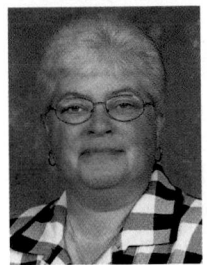

**Jan L. Van Steenhouse, DVM, PhD,
  Dipl ACVP**
Director, Clinical Pathology
MPI Research
Mattawan, Michigan

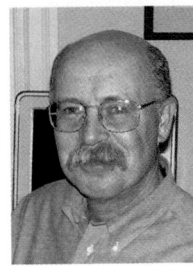

**Thomas J. Van Winkle, VMD, Dipl
  ACVP**
Professor, Laboratory of Pathology and
  Toxicology
Chief, Small Animal Necropsy Service
School of Veterinary Medicine
University of Pennsylvania
Philadelphia, Pennsylvania

Preface

The Profession of Veterinary Technology is moving forward with strength and confidence in the fifth decade of its existence. What began in the 1960s, with the graduation of a few veterinary technicians, has grown to include more than 116 AVMA-accredited programs and thousands of alumni. Through its many editions, *Clinical Textbook for Veterinary Technicians* has supported the growth and maturity of the profession. Now in its sixth edition, it is fitting for it to be the first all-curriculum textbook in veterinary technology to be published in full color!

The extensive use of figures and illustrations has become a hallmark of the publication. This edition includes more than 1200 new color illustrations. Restraint, behavior, surgical instruments, medical and surgical nursing of all species, practice management, and medical records are some of the topics enhanced by all-new illustrations.

The sixth edition continues to provide the latest techniques in veterinary clinical practice and covers a wide range of topics written by experts in their specialty. New to this textbook are chapters on geriatrics, alternative medicine, and toxicology. Almost a fourth of the chapters have been completely rewritten, specifically, Animal Behavior, Companion Animal Nutrition, Anesthesia, Emergency Nursing, Small Animal Surgical Nursing, Food Animal Medical and Surgical Nursing, Medical Records, Computer Applications, and Occupational Health and Safety. In addition, all the drug information throughout the chapters has been thoroughly updated and expanded, including chemotherapy drugs in the Oncology chapter, vaccinations in the Preventive Health Programs, anesthesia protocols in the Anesthesia chapter, transdermal fentanyl administration in Pain Management, and ivermectin toxicities in Pharmacology.

We are pleased to offer with the sixth edition an Instructor's Resource Manual and Test Bank that includes teaching/learning objectives, key terms, chapter outlines with teaching strategies, critical thinking challenges, practical situations, and chapter quizzes. The Test Bank contains more than 1600 test questions in a variety of formats. These ancillaries are free to instructors using the text in their programs. The CD in the back of the Instructor's Resource Manual contains an image bank of the images in the book.

The CD in the back of this book contains student exercises, including crossword puzzles to help study key terms, picture-it exercises to test knowledge of key illustrations, quiz shows and hangman exercises to make self-study fun, and WebLinks, an exciting resource that lets you link to hundreds of websites carefully chosen to supplement the content of the textbook.

In keeping with the rapid pace of advancements in veterinary medicine and veterinary technology, we are committed to providing a new edition every 4 years. In addition, we hope that this text will be so useful that it will be used daily and worn out in 4 years.

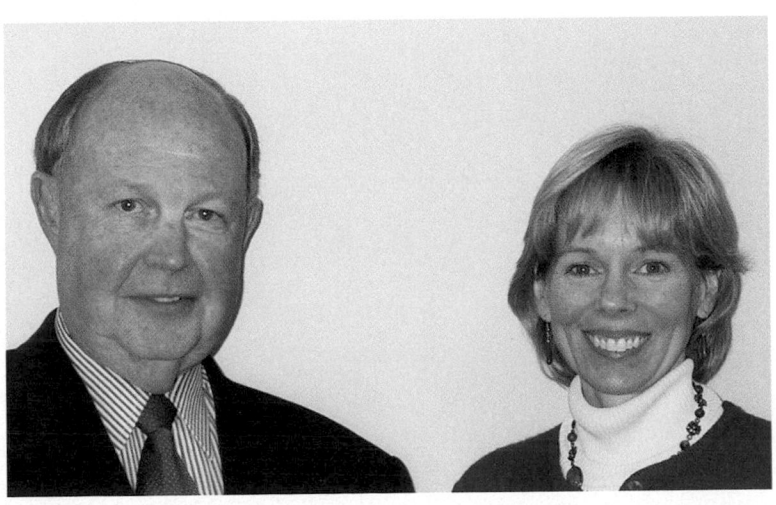

Acknowledgment

We are indebted to Harry Cowgill, our photographer,
for his expertise in producing many of the beautiful color photographs.

Dennis M. McCurnin
Joanna M. Bassert

Contents

PART TWO
Clinical Sciences, 184

Part Four
Anesthesia and Pharmacology, 573

Part Five
Surgical and Medical Nursing, 670

Part Six
Topics in Practice Management, 1027

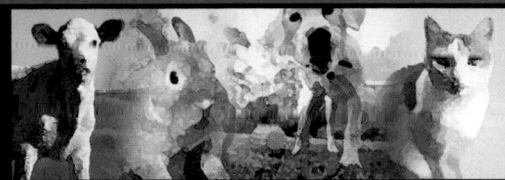

An Introduction to the Profession of Veterinary Technology

JOANNA M. BASSERT

I solemnly dedicate myself to aiding animals and society by providing excellent care and services for animals, by alleviating animal suffering, and by promoting public health.

I accept my obligations to practice my profession conscientiously and with sensitivity, adhering to the profession's Code of Ethics, and furthering my knowledge and competence through a commitment to lifelong learning.

Veterinary Technician Oath

The veterinary technician has emerged as a critical component of the veterinary health care team. Like the registered nurse in the human health care field, the veterinary technician supports the clinical activities of the supervising doctor. However, unlike registered nurses, veterinary technicians are expected to perform the duties of a radiology and laboratory technician as well as those of a medical and surgical nurse. In addition, veterinary technicians must be prepared to work with multiple species rather than just one. Thus the veterinary technician has a surprisingly broad range of clinical responsibilities.

Over the past 45 years, veterinary medicine has become highly sophisticated. Many veterinarians find they can no longer meet their practice goals, in terms of both providing a high level of medical care and attaining acceptable profit margins, without the skilled assistance of veterinary technicians. In addition, the development of veterinary-centered television programs has given the public a look into the inner workings of the animal hospital. For the first time, the public is able to see the important role veterinary technicians play in the real-life drama of saving animal lives. Thus there is heightened awareness of veterinary technology and an increased expectation, for both the practitioner and the pet owner, that animal patients will receive excellent veterinary nursing care. This introduction presents an overview of the profession of veterinary technology. It discusses the profession's history, laws, and ethics and presents job-related opportunities, duties, salaries, and professional organizations.

HISTORY OF VETERINARY TECHNOLOGY

Historically, many veterinarians practiced independently and performed many of the laboratory and nursing duties themselves. Often, spouses and other laypersons served as veterinary assistants, receptionists, and office managers. Today, many practices employ multiple veterinarians and require a staff of veterinary technicians, assistants, receptionists, and kennel workers to carry out the many duties required in running a successful practice. This team approach is a fundamental part of veterinary practice management today, and the veterinary technician often serves as an important link between the veterinarian and support personnel.

The profession of veterinary technology began to take form in the early 1960s with the establishment of the first formal university-level program for the education of animal health technicians. The period that followed 1960 is rich with the accomplishments of dedicated veterinarians and veterinary technicians whose professional developments are listed on the inside cover of this book. Of particular importance are the accomplishments of Dr. Walter E. Collins (Box 1), who is now considered the Father of Veterinary Technology. Veterinary technicians were first called "animal health technicians." The adjective "veterinary" referred exclusively to veterinarians until 1989 when the term "veterinary technician" was approved for use by the American Veterinary Medical Association's House of Delegates. As of this printing, more than 119 programs of veterinary technology are accredited by the American Veterinary Medical Association (AVMA), including four distance learning programs. Thousands of individuals have graduated from these programs, and the number of veterinary technology programs continues to grow as the demand for educated, skilled personnel increases.

THE VETERINARY TECHNICIAN TODAY

Veterinary technicians work in a wide range of facilities, perform many different kinds of tasks, and may encounter all manner of animal species (Figure 1). For example,

---

Box 1 WALTER EMMETT COLLINS, DVM, THE FATHER OF VETERINARY TECHNOLOGY

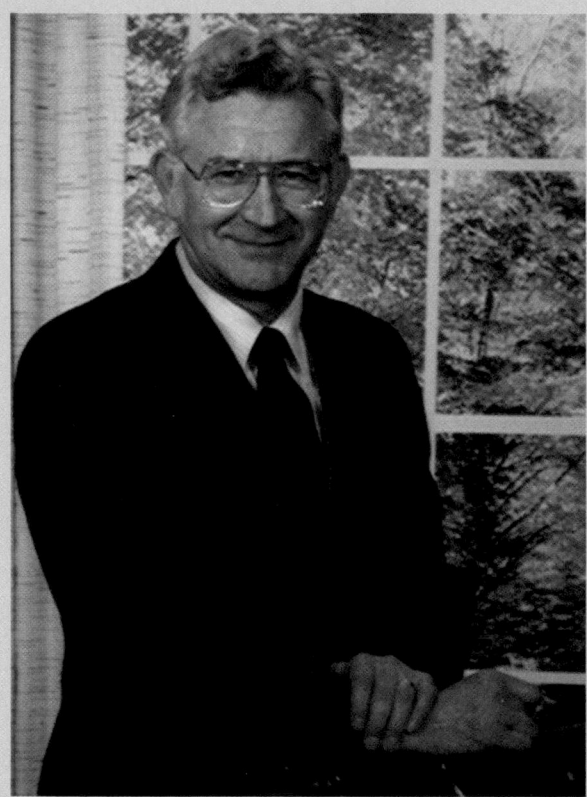

On November 19, 1930, Dr. Walter Collins was born on a small farm in Milford, New York. Like many children reared in a bucolic setting, Dr. Collins grew to love the expansive fields of crops and the many farm animals that were part of his young life. In 1948, after graduating from high school, his interest in agriculture led him to the State University of New York (SUNY) at Delhi, where he studied general agriculture for 2 years. Afterward, he served as a dairy herd improvement supervisor for 2 years before entering the United States Air Force. Dr. Collins felt fortunate to be assigned to the Veterinary Department at Webb Air Force Base in Big Spring, Texas, where he worked under the direction of three "understanding and stimulating" veterinarian–commanding officers who encouraged him to pursue a career in veterinary medicine. When his tour ended in the spring of 1956, Dr. Collins moved to Ithaca, New York, where he studied pre-veterinary science and subsequently attended New York State College of Veterinary Medicine at Cornell University. He graduated and received a doctor of veterinary medicine (DVM) degree in June 1961 and later returned to Delhi, New York, where he joined a large animal practice. After one year, he opted to establish his own private veterinary practice in Delhi.

In the fall of 1964, while still practicing part-time in Delhi, Dr. Collins became a teacher for the first time by joining the faculty of the Animal Science Technology Program. He was hired by Dr. Winfield Stone, the director of the program, who soon became an important mentor and friend. Several years later, in 1967, after Dr. Stone accepted another position on campus, Dr. Collins became the new program director at Delhi. During his tenure as director, Dr. Collins was awarded, as administrator, a grant from the U.S. Department of Health, Education, and Welfare to develop a model curriculum guide for training animal health technicians. From 1969 to 1975, Dr. Collins authored or co-authored several significant publications as well as the model curriculum.

In the early 1970s, Delhi's faculty was anxious to prove that the program was meeting real needs of New York practitioners. Dr. Collins decided to survey veterinarians and presented his findings at the 62nd New York State Conference for Veterinarians. Dr. Collins wrote "For myself, I had felt the veterinary practitioner employer could use his/her new technician employee to relieve them of many non-professional duties as was already being accomplished similarly in human medicine. Both, my staff and I were very gratified at the time by this small sampling survey which certainly hinted that we were on the right track!"

After leaving Delhi, Dr. Collins served as program director for one year at Mountain View College in Dallas, Texas. He subsequently became an associate professor and coordinator of the Veterinary Technology Program at Michigan State University, where he stayed from 1977 until his retirement in 1990. In Michigan, he served on the Michigan Veterinary Medical Association (MVMA) Veterinary Technician Committee, which assisted in the development of legislation that defined veterinary technology for Michigan.

When asked about the important events occurring in his professional life, Dr. Collins readily recalled his involvement in the formation of the Association of Animal Technician Educators (now the Association of Veterinary Technician Educators). In addition, he remembered well his service during the formative years on AVMA's Committee on Animal Technician Activities and Training (now called the Committee on Veterinary Technician Education and Activities) and on the National Veterinary Technician Testing Committee, which was charged with developing the Veterinary Technician National Examination. Finally, Dr. Collins was proud to host the 1981 AVTE Symposium at Michigan State University, which gave rise to the first professional organization for veterinary technicians, the North American Veterinary Technician Association (now known as the National Association of Veterinary Technicians in America).

For these efforts and a lifetime of commitment to the development of the profession, Dr. Collins is considered to be the "father of veterinary technology in the United States."

Dickinson K: Unpublished data. Comparative Oncology Unit, Colorado State University Veterinary Teaching Hospital, May 1996.

veterinary technicians may work in private veterinary practices, such as companion animal, equine, food animal, or mixed practices. (A mixed practice is one that treats both farm and companion animals.) Veterinary technicians may also work in zoos, aquariums, wildlife rehabilitation centers, and research facilities. In addition, they may work for pharmaceutical companies as sales representatives of veterinary products, or they may become entrepreneurs by establishing their own kennel facility or pet-sitting businesses. Qualified veterinary technicians may also become instructors in veterinary technology programs or other academic programs. The range of job opportunities for the veterinary technician today is broader than ever before. (Table 1 shows the distribution of career paths selected by recent graduates of AVMA-accredited programs.)

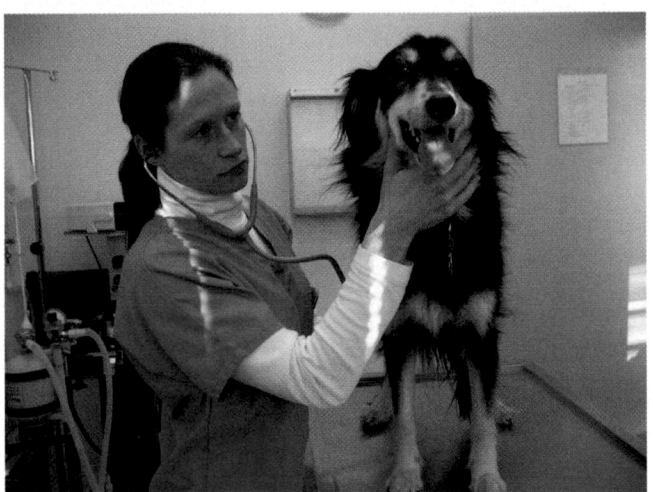

Figure 1 Veterinary technicians work in a wide variety of facilities and with a diverse array of species. This technician works primarily with companion animals. (Courtesy Dr. Joanna Bassert.)

Within this diverse array of opportunities, veterinary technicians may also narrow their field of work and concentrate on specific areas. For example, a technician working in a practice that treats exotic species, such as birds and reptiles, will develop skills and knowledge particular to that aspect of veterinary medicine. In addition, some veterinary practices are called "specialty" or "referral" practices because they employ veterinarians who have completed special training in a particular aspect of veterinary medicine, such as dermatology, surgery, internal medicine, radiology, or ophthalmology. The veterinary hospitals associated with schools of veterinary medicine are examples of very large specialty practices. They are also the hospitals where most veterinary specialists complete their specialty training. Veterinarians who are general practitioners and not specialists may refer particularly challenging or difficult cases to specialty practices. Veterinary technicians who work in specialty practices see unusual cases and become skilled in addressing the particular needs of these critically ill patients. It is not uncommon for specialty practices to share their facility with an emergency and trauma practice. Some veterinary technicians prefer the challenge and excitement of emergency practice, rather than general practice, and have dedicated their careers to this aspect of veterinary technology.

Recently, veterinary technicians have also been given the opportunity to become specialists as defined by the National Association of Veterinary Technicians in America (NAVTA). Refer to the discussion of veterinary technician specialists in this chapter for additional information.

JOB PROSPECTS, SALARIES, AND ATTRITION

Presently there are widespread shortages of veterinary technicians nationwide, and graduates of veterinary technology programs are therefore finding ample job opportunities. Although job opportunities are bright, salaries vary

Table 1 DISTRIBUTION OF EMPLOYMENT AND SALARIES FOR RECENT VETERINARY TECHNICIAN GRADUATES

Employment Setting or Field	Percentage (%) of Recent Graduates Working in this Field	Salary Range ($)	Average Starting Salary ($)
Companion animal practice	73	10,717-40,000	18,755
Food animal practice	2	14,560-24,000	15,968
Equine practice	2	15,000-30,000	20,906
Mixed animal practice	12	10,717-27,560	17,238
Specialty practice	4	15,000-30,000	20,256
Industry/sales	1	20,000-28,000	21,000
Veterinary technician education	0.2	N/A	N/A
Government	0.4	20,000-28,000	23,625
Diagnostic/research laboratories	2	10,717-30,000	22,807
Other	3	12,480-25,000	20,896
Overall average salary			20,161

From the 1999 AVMA survey results of accredited programs in veterinary technology at www.avma.org.
N/A, Not available.

Box 2 TYPES OF COURSES REQUIRED IN VETERINARY TECHNOLOGY PROGRAMS

BASIC MATH AND SCIENCE
Technical math
Biology
Chemistry
Microbiology
Comparative anatomy and physiology
Medical terminology
Computer science

VETERINARY TECHNOLOGY
Introduction to veterinary technology
Veterinary practice management

Animal management and nutrition
Farm animal clinical procedures
Companion animal clinical procedures
Laboratory animal science
Animal medicine
Veterinary radiology
Animal parasitology
Veterinary hematology
Veterinary clinical chemistry and urinalysis
Veterinary surgical assisting
Veterinary pharmacology and anesthesiology

depending on the field of interest and the level of experience (see Table 1). For example, in 1999 the AVMA reported that the average salary for new graduates in companion animal practice was $18,755, and for experienced graduates in the same field, the average salary was $21,860. Similarly, the average salary in diagnostic and research laboratories was $22,807 for recent graduates and $26,635 for experienced graduates. The salaries within a particular field can vary greatly. For example, salaries for experienced technicians in industry/sales ranged from $13,000 to $81,000, and in mixed animal practice they ranged from $11,000 to $32,000. Overall, however, from 1998 to 2002 the U.S. Bureau of Labor Statistics reported a 17.2% increase in the average salary of the veterinary technician (from $20,520 to $24,050). One can extrapolate a 4.3% annual increase since 2002 to estimate the average salary of veterinary technicians today.

In addition to salary compensation, many employers offer a range of benefits, including health care coverage, retirement plans, and payment of continuing education and professional membership fees. Large companies or practices are generally better equipped to provide more complete benefit packages than small private businesses.

The profession of veterinary technology has a high rate of attrition, estimated to be about 50% to 65% after only 4 years of employment. Graduate technicians report leaving the profession because of lack of appreciation and underutilization by their employer, low pay, and lack of advancement opportunities. Attrition from the profession is a critical part of the current shortage problem. Many states have shortages of veterinarians and veterinary assistants as well as technicians.

EDUCATION

Like nursing schools in the human health care field, programs of veterinary technology may include 2, 3, or 4 years of undergraduate study and may result in either an associate of science degree (2 or 3 years) or a bachelor of science degree (4 years). Programs in the United States are accredited by the Committee on Veterinary Technician Education and Activities (CVTEA), which is under the

auspices of the AVMA. For accreditation, a program must meet 11 essential criteria for curricula, faculty, facility, and admissions requirements. Each program must submit reports to CVTEA for review semiannually, annually, or biannually depending on the age and stability of the program. In addition, the CVTEA carries out on-site visits of each program. Based on the on-site evaluation, recommendations by the CVTEA are classified into three categories: critical, major, and minor recommendations. Programs must document in reports to the CVTEA progress made in addressing the deficits cited by the on-site review committee.

The curriculum of veterinary technology programs includes general college-level courses, such as biology and chemistry, as well as courses specific to clinical practice, such as veterinary parasitology, medicine, and clinical chemistry. In addition, there are approximately 200 "essential" and 84 "recommended" tasks listed in the Accreditation Policies and Procedures Handbook of the CVTEA, which constitutes the foundation of the hands-on curriculum for laboratories and practical training. Refer to Box 2 for a list of courses typically offered in veterinary technology programs.

Distance Education
Although most veterinary technology programs are offered to students in the traditional on-campus fashion, some programs have begun to offer an exciting new type of veterinary technology course by using the Internet or teleconferencing. These institutions have made an entire program of veterinary technology available to distance-education students around the world.

As of this printing, the following distance programs have been accredited by the AVMA:

- St. Petersburg College in Florida
- Cedar Valley College in Texas
- Blue Ridge Community College in Virginia
- Purdue University in Indiana

Continuing Education
Most states require veterinary technicians to attend continuing education lectures and workshops to maintain

licensure, certification, or registration. These lectures are available at various national, regional, and local professional conferences and workshops throughout the United States and through AVMA-accredited programs of veterinary technology. As veterinary medicine progresses and changes, it is particularly important for veterinary technicians to commit themselves to a career of life-long learning.

Responsibilities of the Veterinary Technician

Veterinary technicians perform a myriad of animal care–related duties, but they may also be involved in non-clinical tasks, such as office management, client education, and inventory control. Veterinary practices are organized into distinct working areas. A veterinary technician, depending on his or her job description and the size of the practice, may work in all, a few, or only one of the areas discussed in the following sections.

Reception Area

Although many practices hire receptionists, and not veterinary technicians, to work in the reception area, it is important for the clinical staff to be cross-trained in this aspect of the practice so that important information can be accessed easily when the receptionist is not available. The veterinary technician should be familiar with the computer network system and practice management software used by the practice. This will facilitate obtaining existing records, creating new patient records, and accessing medical histories and billing information during emergencies that may occur after hours.

Examination Rooms and Outpatients

The veterinary technician ensures that office visits are handled in an efficient and professional manner. This involves directing clients to the appropriate examination room or treatment area, obtaining a brief history, weighing the patient, and acquiring the necessary vaccines, instruments, and materials needed for the visit. The veterinary technician may also draw blood at this time and obtain skin scrapings and fecal, urine, and cytology samples for laboratory testing. In addition, the veterinary technician provides important information to clients regarding preventive care, diet, behavior modification, medication, discharge instructions, and spay and neutering procedures for their animals.

Because pet owners often feel more at ease talking to the veterinary technician than to the doctor, the technician can be a valuable support person for bereaved or worried pet owners. In addition, the veterinary technician answers clients' questions both in person and over the telephone and occasionally must address difficult or angry pet owners.

Laboratory and Pharmacy

The veterinary technician has the skills to perform all of the routine laboratory tests used in practice (Figure 2). The number of the laboratory tests actually performed on site varies from practice to practice. In veterinary hospitals

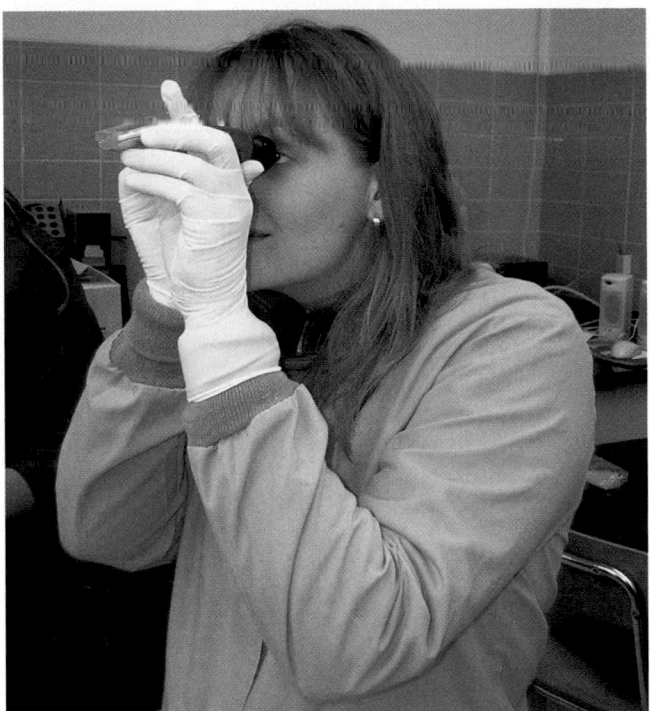

Figure 2 In college, veterinary technicians study clinical chemistry, hematology, immunology, cytology, and parasitology. This important education enables them to perform all of the routine laboratory tests used in practice. (Courtesy Dr. Joanna Bassert.)

that make full use of these skills, veterinary technicians perform complete blood counts, differential counts, and morphologic examinations of blood. They perform urinalysis, including examination of urine sediment, and fecal analysis for evidence of parasites. Veterinary technicians are skilled in the use of enzyme-linked immunosorbent assay (ELISA) test kits, dextrometers, refractometers, and dry chemistry analyzers. In addition, veterinary technicians are familiar with interpreting common cytologic preparations, such as ear swabs and vaginal smears.

> **✎ TECHNICIAN NOTE**
>
> Being able to take initiative and think quickly during unexpected events is an important quality of the veterinary technician.

Once a diagnosis is made, the veterinarian prescribes, either in writing or orally, a treatment for the animal patient. The veterinary technician interprets the prescription language, then fills and dispenses the medication to the pet owner with instructions for its use. In addition, veterinary technicians are often responsible for ensuring that the pharmacy is well stocked, that expired drugs are discarded, and that controlled substances are handled appropriately.

Radiology

The x-ray film (also known as a radiograph) is an important diagnostic tool for veterinarians. Veterinary technicians are skilled in radiographic techniques, including positioning of the patient, making the proper settings, and taking exposures at the appropriate times (Figure 3). In addition, veterinary technicians are skilled in both manual and automatic development techniques and in trouble-shooting technical errors. If an x-ray service is not employed by the practice, veterinary technicians may be responsible for maintaining the development and fixative solutions and for keeping the x-ray screens and other equipment clean and in good working order. In addition, technicians ensure that the hospital staff members protect themselves from harmful radiation by wearing appropriate protective clothing, such as lead aprons, gloves, and thyroid shields, and that dosimeters are used routinely to monitor x-ray exposure. Often, technicians are responsible for managing the ordering and mailing of the dosimeters. Finally, veterinary technicians may also assist with special imaging and contrast studies, such as ultrasound studies and those in which gas, barium sulfate, or other contrast agents are used.

Treatment Room

Most veterinary hospitals have a treatment room where patients are brought for various procedures and where animals are prepped for surgery. In more contemporary hospital designs, the treatment area is a large central room that may include a bank of cages for the postoperative and critical care patients. This arrangement facilitates the monitoring of in-house patients and enables the technical staff to be more efficient in completing important treatment duties. Dental operatories and procedure sinks may also be part of the main treatment room where dentistry and minor surgical procedures are completed.

Veterinary technicians are responsible for carrying out treatment orders given by the supervising veterinarian (Figure 4). This involves giving medications by all routes (e.g., orally, intramuscularly, intravenously). It may also involve setting up and monitoring intravenous fluids. Small amounts of blood may be collected every few hours, and the animal may be routinely checked for alertness, temperature, pulse, respiration, urination, and defecation. For critical cases, treatment may include changing bandages; lavaging open wounds; placing and monitoring nasal oxygen; and maintaining chest, tracheal, urethral, or abdominal tubes. Veterinary technicians are responsible for recording all treatments, data, and physical findings in the patient's record. The patient record is an important legal document as well as a means of ensuring that errors in treatment are not made.

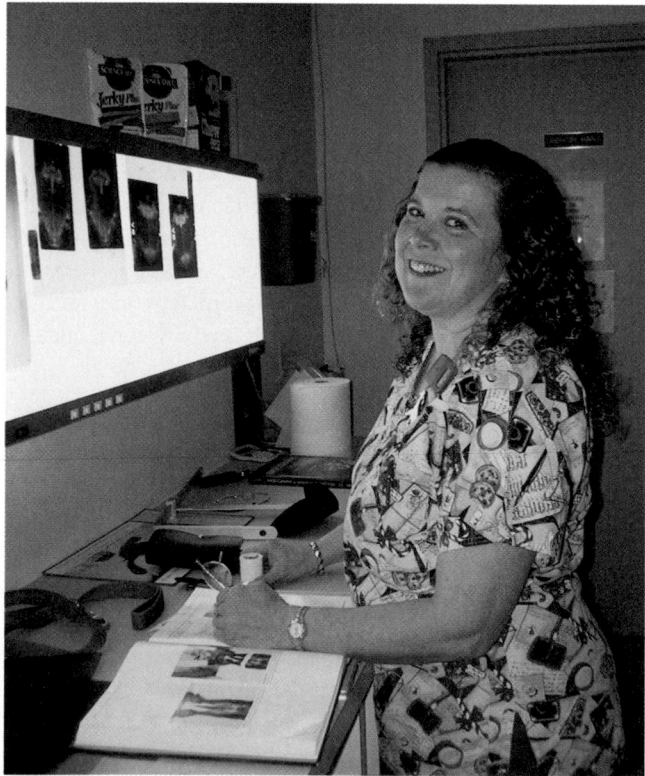

Figure 3 Veterinary technicians are skilled in the use of radiographic equipment. Not only do they position the animals and obtain x-ray films, they also develop the x-ray films and trouble-shoot any exposure problems. (Courtesy Dr. Joanna Bassert.)

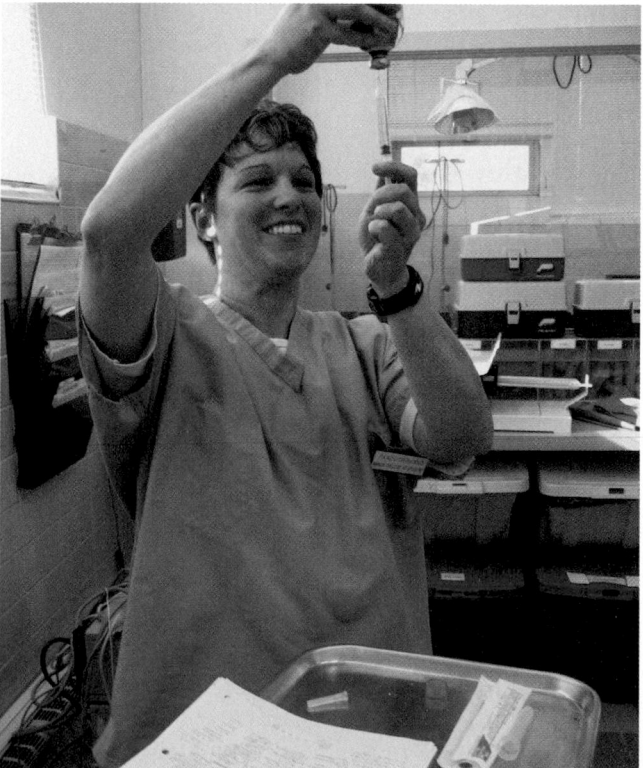

Figure 4 Carrying out the treatment orders of the veterinarian is an important part of the veterinary technician's many responsibilities. (Courtesy Dr. Joanna Bassert.)

The veterinary technician prepares the patient before it enters the operating room. This involves ensuring that the animal has not had anything to eat or drink and that the animal urinates before surgery. The technician is responsible for weighing the animal and then calculating and administering preoperative anesthetic agents. In many veterinary practices, the veterinary technician is responsible for induction and maintenance of anesthesia. Although there are many ways to anesthetize an animal, this usually involves placing an intravenous catheter, setting up fluids, placing an endotracheal tube, and administering intravenous and/or gas anesthetic agents. Monitoring equipment, such as a pulse oximeter, esophageal stethoscope, Dinamap monitor, Doppler ultrasonography machine, or oscilloscope, may be used by the technician to assist in monitoring the anesthetized patient. Before moving the patient to the operating room, the technician clips hair from the region of the animal that will undergo surgery and performs an initial cleansing of the area.

Often, a technician is responsible for performing routine dental prophylaxis procedures, which must be done while the animal is anesthetized. In this situation, the technician must perform two important jobs at once, namely, monitor the patient under anesthesia and clean and polish the animal's teeth. The veterinary technician must be prepared for an anesthetic emergency and should be familiar with the emergency drugs and procedures needed to resuscitate animals in crisis.

✎ TECHNICIAN NOTE

NAVTA has designated the third week in October as National Veterinary Technician Week! Mark your calendars! For more information, check NAVTA's website at http://www.navta.net.

Operating Room

The operating room technician, or circulating nurse, positions the animal patient on the operating table and completes the final surgical scrub. Instruments, equipment, and materials needed by the surgeon are made available.

In addition, the technician retrieves additional materials requested during the procedure. In some practices, the technician acts simultaneously as both anesthetist and circulating nurse. Occasionally, technicians are asked to assist during a particularly challenging operation and must be skilled in proper sterile techniques, including gloving and gowning. After the procedure, the technician washes and dries the surgical instruments and reorganizes them into surgical packs for sterilization. The technician may also perform the duties of the postoperative care nurse for the recovering patient.

Wards

Veterinary technicians can play an important role on the wards, not only in ensuring that treatments are given correctly and in a timely manner, but also in providing animals with compassion and a gentle touch. Nurturing animals when they are sick is an important part of their recovery. Even healthy animals that are being boarded benefit from special care and reassurance from the technical staff.

Hospital Management

Veterinary technicians, particularly those with a background in business, may act as hospital managers. They may oversee the veterinary staff and assist with scheduling, hiring, bookkeeping, and inventory control. Increasingly, veterinary technicians, particularly in large practices, are drawn into some management duties, such as personnel management and ordering supplies. Some veterinary technicians are practice owners as well as managers.

TERMINOLOGY AND THE VETERINARY HEALTH CARE TEAM

A productive and efficiently managed veterinary practice depends on the dedication of a team of veterinary professionals and support personnel (Box 3). As described the following sections, each member of the team plays a collaborative role in helping to provide quality health care for the animal patient.

Box 3 AMERICAN VETERINARY MEDICAL ASSOCIATION NOMENCLATURE

NOMENCLATURE

Veterinary technology is the science and art of providing professional support to veterinarians. AVMA accredits programs in veterinary technology that graduate veterinary technicians and/or veterinary technologists.

A veterinary technician is a graduate of a two- or three-year AVMA-accredited program in veterinary technology. In most cases the graduate is granted an associate degree or certificate.

A veterinary technologist is a graduate of a four-year baccalaureate AVMA-accredited program in veterinary technology.

Veterinary assistant: The adjectives animal, veterinary, ward, or hospital combined with the nouns attendant, caretaker, or assistant are titles sometimes used for individuals where training, knowledge, and skills are less than that required for identification as a veterinary technician or veterinary technologist.

From Committee on Veterinary Technician Education and Activities: *Accreditation policies and procedures*, 2004, The Committee.

VETERINARIAN

A veterinarian typically completes 4 years of study at an AVMA-accredited school of veterinary medicine after completing 4 years of undergraduate study. Graduates of veterinary medical schools are distinguished by the initials DVM after their names, unless they have graduated from the University of Pennsylvania, in which case they will have the initials VMD after their name. To practice, veterinarians must be licensed by the state in which they work. Typically, this requires successful completion of national and state examinations and the payment of a licensing fee. In addition, graduates of foreign veterinary medical colleges that are not accredited by the AVMA are eligible to apply for licensure in most states following certification by the Educational Commission of Foreign Veterinary Graduates (ECFVG). There are 27 American and 4 Canadian colleges of veterinary medicine.

In some states, exceptions for licensure are made to veterinarians who are employed in university veterinary teaching hospitals.

VETERINARY TECHNICIAN SPECIALIST

Recently, veterinary technicians have also been given the opportunity to become specialists. In February 1994, NAVTA formed the Committee on Veterinary Technician Specialties (CVTS) to address a growing interest among veterinary technicians who wanted to attain higher levels of skill and knowledge in a particular aspect of veterinary technology. For this reason, CVTS established a process and a list of criteria for the formation of academies in specialized fields of veterinary technology.

The first step in this process is for a group of veterinary technicians who share an interest in a particular field of

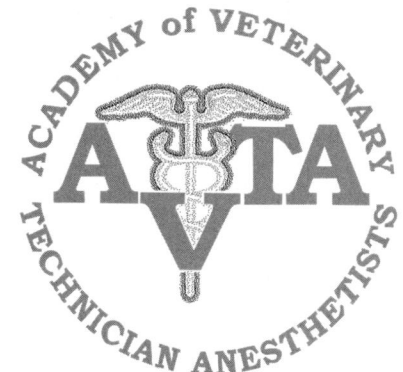

The Academy of Veterinary Technician Anesthetists
Presents this
Achievement Certificate To

Susan Barbour, AS, CVT

For having complied with the specialized training, experience and examination requirements, the above named is recognized as a

Veterinary Technician Specialist, Anesthesia
VTS (Anesthesia) *

Charter Member Number 001

The above named is likewise elected a
Member of the Academy of Veterinary Technician Anesthetists (AVTA).

Dated this 16th day of February, 2003

A NAVTA Technician
Specialty Certification

_____   _____
      President   *Executive Secretary*

Figure 5 The first certificate awarded by the Academy of Veterinary Technician Anesthetists was given to Susan Barbour, AS, CVT, in February 2003.

veterinary technology to establish a professional society or association. After the society has grown in size, it may then petition CVTS for recognition as an academy. The organizing committee of the proposed academy, together with CVTS, establishes the advanced requirements and examination process for becoming a veterinary technician specialist. As of this printing, NAVTA has recognized three specialties in veterinary technology. These fall under the auspices of the following academies:

- The Academy of Veterinary Emergency and Critical Care Technicians
- The Academy of Veterinary Technician Anesthetists
- The Academy of Veterinary Dental Technicians

Thus the veterinary technician specialist is a veterinary technician who has reached a higher level of skill and understanding in a particular field of veterinary technology. The veterinary technician specialist must meet the following criteria:

- Be a graduate of an AVMA-accredited program of veterinary technology and/or be legally credentialed to practice veterinary technology in his or her respective state, province, or country.

- Successfully complete the education, training, and experience requirements established by the respective academy of specialists.
- Be reviewed and approved for specialist status by the academy.

Veterinary technicians who have achieved specialty status are signified by the initials *VTS* (and their field of specialty in parentheses) after their names. For example, the technician Mary Jones, CVT, VTS (ECC), is a specialist in emergency and critical care.

The veterinary technician specialist often works in specialty and referral veterinary hospitals and in teaching hospitals associated with universities. In these environments the veterinary technician specialist can concentrate on his or her field of interest and share knowledge with veterinary medical and veterinary technology students.

VETERINARY TECHNOLOGIST

The veterinary technologist holds a bachelor of science (BS) degree in veterinary technology from a 4-year, AVMA-accredited program. The veterinary technologist works in positions that may require a greater level of education than the veterinary technician, such as project leader, practice supervisor, or teacher in a veterinary technology program. Some veterinary technologists, particularly those employed in teaching hospitals of veterinary medical schools, may become highly skilled in a particular aspect of veterinary technology. Some institutions and practices use the term *veterinary technologist* to refer to a veterinary technician who holds a BS degree in any field.

VETERINARY TECHNICIAN

A veterinary technician is a person who has earned an associate of science (AS) degree in veterinary technology from a 2-year or 3-year, AVMA-accredited program of veterinary technology. In many states, veterinary technicians are required to complete national and state examinations before they can be licensed, registered, or certified. Frequently, veterinary technicians are required to pay a fee to the state or state veterinary association in order to receive a license, certification, or registration.

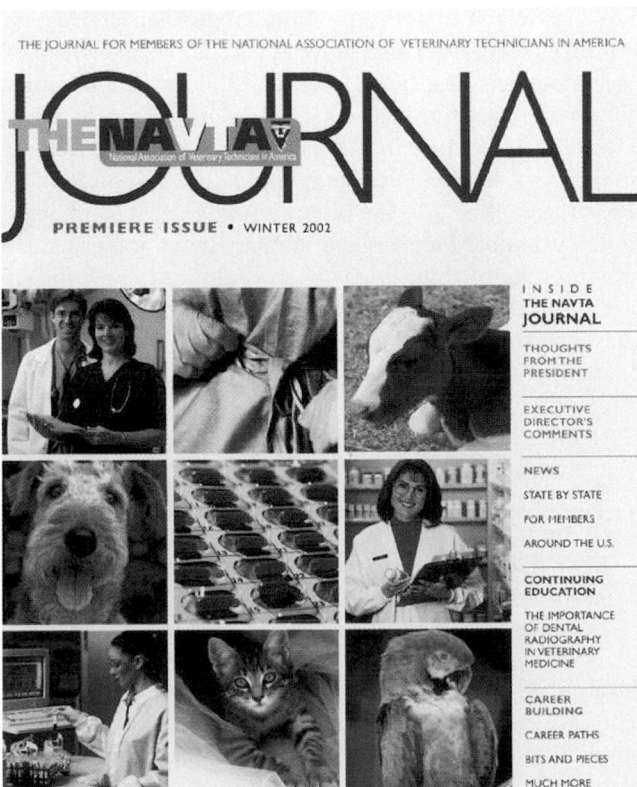

THE JOURNAL FOR MEMBERS OF THE NATIONAL ASSOCIATION OF VETERINARY TECHNICIANS IN AMERICA

JOURNAL

THE NAVTA
National Association of Veterinary Technicians in America

PREMIERE ISSUE • WINTER 2002

INSIDE
THE NAVTA
JOURNAL

THOUGHTS
FROM THE
PRESIDENT

EXECUTIVE
DIRECTOR'S
COMMENTS

NEWS
STATE BY STATE
FOR MEMBERS
AROUND THE U.S.

CONTINUING
EDUCATION

THE IMPORTANCE
OF DENTAL
RADIOGRAPHY
IN VETERINARY
MEDICINE

CAREER
BUILDING
CAREER PATHS
BITS AND PIECES
MUCH MORE

Figure 6 The cover of the premier issue of *The NAVTA Journal* (Winter 2002).

TECHNICIAN NOTE

Veterinary technicians must take responsibility for their own safety. The first step involves having personal health care coverage and always staying up-to-date with rabies and tetanus immunizations.

VETERINARY ASSISTANT

The term *veterinary assistant* is used to describe those individuals involved in the care of animals who are not veterinary technicians, laboratory animal technicians, or veterinarians. Typically, veterinary assistants are responsible for assisting the veterinary technician and the veterinarian by restraining animals, setting up equipment and supplies, cleaning and maintaining clinic and laboratory facilities, and feeding and exercising patients. Most veterinary assistants are trained on the job by a supervising veterinary technician or veterinarian, but some assistants complete 4 to 6 months of training in a formal course of study.

The profession of veterinary technology started to take form in the early 1960s. Before this time, veterinary technicians, as defined today, did not exist, and veterinary practices depended exclusively on the skill of on-the-job–trained veterinary assistants. Today, veterinary assistants continue to constitute a large and important portion of the work force in veterinary practices nationwide. Veterinary technicians and veterinary assistants work together in many veterinary practices, and although the AVMA and NAVTA make clear distinctions between the two groups, some states have confused these distinctions.

As the number of traditional and distance AVMA-accredited programs grows, education in the field of veterinary technology becomes increasingly more accessible to veterinary support staff members who wish to become veterinary technicians.

VETERINARY NURSE

The term *veterinary nurse*, rather than *veterinary technician*, is used in European countries.

LABORATORY ANIMAL TECHNICIANS

The American Association for Laboratory Animal Science (AALAS) has established a certification program that certifies the following three levels of animal technicians:

- Assistant laboratory animal technician (ALAT)
- Laboratory animal technician (LAT)
- Laboratory animal technologist (LATG)

AALAS-certified animal technicians care for the laboratory animals used in research facilities and teaching institutions. These facilities are registered by the U.S. Department of Agriculture (USDA) and may be located in pharmaceutical companies, universities, and colleges. A technician does not need to be a graduate of an AVMA-accredited program of veterinary technology to be eligible for AALAS certification; however, many are. Graduates of AVMA-accredited programs must complete 6 months of additional training in a USDA-registered facility before they are eligible for the level one ALAT examination.

Like the Veterinary Technician National Examination (VTNE), AALAS certification examinations are developed and administered by the Professional Examination Service (PES), but they fall under the auspices of AALAS rather than the American Association of Veterinary State Boards (AAVSB). All three levels of examinations are multiple choice, but each level becomes more rigorous and asks more questions. For example, the ALAT examination is composed of 100 questions; the LAT examination, 125 questions; and the LATG examination, 150 questions. Candidates must complete a specified amount of on-the-job experience to qualify for the next level of AALAS certification.

THE VETERINARY TECHNICIAN NATIONAL EXAMINATION

The VTNE is developed under a contractual agreement between the AAVSB and the PES. The AAVSB is represented by the Veterinary Technician Testing Committee (VTTC), which is composed of veterinarians and veterinary technicians who are engaged in clinical practice or academia. Members of the committee are appointed by the executive boards of AVMA, NAVTA, AVTE, and the Canadian Association of Animal Health Technologists and Technicians (CAAHTT). The PES provides the committee with two draft examinations for their review and validation. These drafts are developed from a computerized bank of questions, originally written by veterinarians and veterinary technicians from all aspects of the veterinary medical profession. The questions are reviewed independently for accuracy, relevance to the field of veterinary technology, and level of difficulty. In addition, the questions are further screened for grammar, style, and conformity to psychometric principles. Each state licensing board is responsible for the administration of the examination and establishes the location, date, and time when it is offered. Although PES provides test scoring services, the state boards are responsible for reporting the scores to the veterinary technician candidates.

The examination is offered in many states and Canadian provinces on the third Friday in June and the third Friday in January of every year. It is composed of 200 multiple-choice questions that cover the following seven primary areas or domains within the profession of veterinary technology:

1. Pharmacy and pharmacology
2. Surgical preparation and assisting
3. Laboratory procedures
4. Animal nursing
5. Radiology, ultrasound, and other electronic imaging
6. Anesthesia
7. Office and hospital procedures

On a scale from 200 to 800, each state determines the passing score, which can be found in the "data resource" section of the website of the AAVSB at http://www.aavsb.org. A total score and a locally derived scale score may also accompany the test results report that is sent to each candidate. Candidates who need to have their VTNE scores sent to multiple state boards must register with the Interstate Reporting Service. There is a fee for registration with the Interstate Reporting Service and a second fee for each transfer.

> ### ✎ TECHNICIAN NOTE
>
> Candidates have 4 hours to complete the VTNE. Because candidates receive no additional penalties for incorrect responses, test takers are encouraged to answer all the questions, even if it means guessing.

LAWS GOVERNING VETERINARY TECHNOLOGY

CERTIFICATION, REGISTRATION, AND LICENSURE

Each state defines the profession of veterinary technology in its own way, through its own state laws. Some states use the term *certify*, whereas others use *register* or *license*. These terms are effectively synonymous. This is to say that *certified*, *registered*, and *licensed* veterinary technicians are all considered to be "credentialed," and all enjoy the benefits of practicing within the profession of veterinary technology. However, each state has a different set of requirements for becoming credentialed, so it is important for an applicant to be familiar with the laws of the state in which he or she works. For example, most states, but not all, require that to be credentialed, an applicant must be a graduate of an AVMA-accredited program of veterinary technology. In addition, most states but not all require successful completion of the VTNE. Some states require successful completion of their own state examination, whereas others may require completion of a clinical competency examination. The specific requirements for credentialing in each state can be found on the AVMA website at http://www.avma.org/carefor animals/animatedjourneys/aboutvets/vtstregs.asp.

Now, having said that "licensing," "registered," and "certified" are effectively the same, let's examine some differences among the three terms (but don't let this confuse you).

License

As its name implies, a "licensed" technician receives a license to practice veterinary technology. Licenses are distributed to veterinary technicians by the state's Board of Veterinary Medical Examiners. This group may also be called the "Licensing Board of Veterinary Medicine" or the "Veterinary Medical Board," depending on the state in which you live, so it is often referred to simply as "the Board." Members of the Board are primarily veterinarians, nominated by the state veterinary medical association but officially appointed by the governor. Because veterinary technicians do not have their own state boards, as do nurses in the human health care field, it is recommended that each state appoint at least one veterinary technician to the state Board of Veterinary Medical Examiners.

There is a "board" that oversees every profession that is licensed. However, not every profession is licensed. In most licensed professions, it would be *illegal* to practice without a license. This is called mandatory licensing. An architect, for example, must acquire a license before he or she can work as an architect. Most licensed professions have mandatory licensing. Through affiliation, the term *licensed* has come to imply that the veterinary technician must have a license to legally work in practice and be known as a veterinary technician. However this is not always the case.

Typically, the Board charges a licensing fee and an annual or biannual licensing renewal fee. In addition, technicians who hold licenses are often required to complete continuing education classes before the licenses can be renewed. Therefore licensed technicians may be subject to random audits by the Board to ensure that the continuing education requirement is met. In addition, a technician's license can be suspended by the Board when disciplinary action is taken. Similarly, the Board may fine a veterinary technician for practicing without a license.

Certified

Despite the title "certified," veterinary technicians may or may not receive a certificate. In Pennsylvania, for example, certified veterinary technicians receive a license from the state board, and therefore must meet all of the requirements for licensure described previously. In many professions, however, the term *certified* is typically used when a non-governmental body or professional association verifies that specific professional standards were achieved and a certificate is awarded to acknowledge this accomplishment. Certification may be voluntary. In veterinary technology, there are some states, such as Connecticut and Colorado, that provide voluntary certification by a private organization (the state technician association), but there are equally, if not more states, such as Pennsylvania, that mandate certification under the auspices of the state board and award licenses.

Registered

The term *registered* implies that a list of individuals, eligible to practice within a profession, is maintained by a governmental organization. In veterinary technology, states such as California and Idaho mandate registration through the state board. However, there are also states such as Texas and New Jersey where veterinary technicians are registered by the state veterinary medical association, which is a private group, not a governmental body. Registration in New Jersey is voluntary, whereas in many states, registration is mandatory.

There is a great deal of variability among states regarding the requirements to become a credentialed veterinary technician. Notice that the term *registered* does not mean that the credentialing process is the same in all of the states that register veterinary technicians. Similarly, the process is not the same in all states that certify technicians. Each state dictates its own approach toward credentialing and determines the terminology to be used. This can be particularly confusing to veterinary technicians who are relocating to another state.

RECIPROCITY

What happens when a credentialed veterinary technician moves to another state? Can he or she automatically practice as a veterinary technician? The answer is "It depends." A credentialed veterinary technician in one state may or may not be able to be credentialed in another state. Some states offer reciprocity to any technician who is credentialed in any other state. Other states, however, credential only those technicians that meet their own state requirements for credentialing. For example, Pennsylvania gives reciprocity to and licenses only those technicians who have completed Pennsylvania's requirements for licensure. Thus a registered veterinary technician from California may be licensed in Pennsylvania ONLY if he or she is a graduate of an AVMA-accredited program of veterinary technology AND has successfully completed the VTNE. Because California has its own state examination and recognizes programs of veterinary technology that are not accredited by the AVMA, there are registered veterinary technicians in California who would not be given reciprocity to practice veterinary technology in Pennsylvania.

TECHNICIAN NOTE

In a well-managed practice, veterinary technicians perform all the duties associated with the care and treatment of animal patients except those tasks that by law can only be performed by the veterinarian. In addition, they are empowered to delegate appropriate tasks to the veterinary assistant and kennel staff.

SCOPE OF PRACTICE

As the sophistication of veterinary medicine has increased, the responsibilities of the veterinary technician in clinical practice have broadened. Veterinarians are rapidly moving away from doing the nursing and laboratory tasks themselves and are delegating these tasks to veterinary technicians. However, there is much variability among veterinary practices in the way in which veterinary technicians are employed. In a well-managed practice, veterinary technicians perform all the duties associated with the care and treatment of animal patients except those tasks that by law can only be performed by the veterinarian. In addition, they are empowered to delegate appropriate tasks to veterinary assistants. Although the state laws that define veterinary medicine differ, it is widely accepted and proposed by both the AVMA and the AAVSB that ONLY veterinarians may do the following:

1. Prescribe
2. Diagnose
3. Prognose
4. Perform surgery

Veterinary technology typically includes the remaining scope of practice (i.e., all tasks other than the four in the list). Restrictions for the veterinary technician may vary from state to state. For example, some states prohibit a veterinary technician from extracting teeth (because it is considered surgery), whereas other states may permit it.

Where the Confusion Lies . . .

Remarkably, there are still some states that do not define veterinary technology in the law. Because these states have no laws to guide the profession in the use of veterinary technicians, much is left to the interpretation and judgment of the supervising veterinarian. In addition, state legislation that defines only the profession of veterinary medicine and ignores the profession of veterinary technology may unintentionally create a confusing situation in which veterinary support personnel, while carrying out their routine clinical duties, are in fact practicing veterinary medicine. For example, this would occur if the state's definition of veterinary medicine includes nursing duties such as administering medication and placing and intravenous catheter. Clearly, the need for unambiguous laws (such as those suggested by the AVMA, NAVTA, and AAVSB) that delineate the role of the veterinary technician as well as that of the veterinarian are necessary to protect the practitioner and his or her employees against potential disciplinary action from the state board (and/or litigation) and to protect the public against acts of malpractice.

PRACTICE ACTS

The "umbrella" law that governs the practice of veterinary medicine within a state is called a practice act. Each state writes its own practice act. In an effort to standardize technician utilization from state to state and to help eliminate confusion regarding the roles of the veterinarian, the veterinary technician, and the veterinary assistant, the AAVSB, AVMA, and NAVTA have all developed model practice acts (see Boxes 4 and 5). Periodically, the practice act is changed and updated to stay current with the changes in veterinary medicine and veterinary technology. A change in the law is called an amendment, and the document that includes the specific changes to be made is called a bill. A bill must be approved by both the State House of Representatives and the State Senate. Ultimately, it is signed into law by the governor. Although the House and the Senate are permitted to make additional changes or amendments to a bill, the governor (in most states) is not "allowed" to change a bill. The governor can only veto (reject) a bill or sign a bill into law (approve it).

The process of writing, proposing, and getting a law passed can be a long and expensive one, particularly if the proposed changes are controversial and if there is much disagreement. Typically, amendments to the practice act are written by a task force committee that is made up of veterinarians and veterinary technicians in the state. After

Box 4 AMERICAN VETERINARY MEDICAL ASSOCIATION MODEL VETERINARY PRACTICE ACT

SECTION 1. TITLE

This act shall be known as the [name of state] Veterinary Practice Act. Except where otherwise indicated by context, in this act the present tense includes the past and future tenses and the future tense includes the present, each gender includes both genders, and the singular includes the plural, and the plural the singular.

SECTION 2. DEFINITIONS

When used in this act these words and phrases shall be defined as follows:

1. "Abandoned" means to forsake entirely, to neglect or refuse to provide or perform legal obligations for the care and support of an animal, or to refuse to pay for treatment or other services without an assertion of good cause. Such abandonment shall constitute the relinquishment of all rights and claims by the client to such an animal.

2. "Accredited college of veterinary medicine" means any veterinary college, school, or division of a university or college that offers the degree of Doctor of Veterinary Medicine or its equivalent and that is accredited by the Council on Education of the American Veterinary Medical Association (AVMA).

3. "Accredited program in veterinary technology" means any postsecondary educational program that is accredited by the Committee on Veterinary Technician Education and Activities of the AVMA.

4. "Animal" means any animal other than a human.

5. "Board" means the [State Board of Veterinary Medicine].

6. "Client" means the patient's owner, owner's agent, or other person responsible for the patient.

7. "Complementary, alternative, and integrative therapies" means a heterogeneous group of preventive, diagnostic, and therapeutic philosophies and practices, which at the time they are performed may differ from current scientific knowledge, or whose theoretical basis and techniques may diverge from veterinary medicine routinely taught in accredited veterinary medical colleges, or both. These therapies include, but are not limited to, veterinary acupuncture, acutherapy, and acupressure; veterinary homeopathy; veterinary manual or manipulative therapy (ie, therapies based on techniques practiced in osteopathy, chiropractic medicine, or physical medicine and therapy); veterinary nutraceutical therapy; and veterinary phytotherapy.

8. "Consultation" means when a licensed veterinarian receives advice in person, telephonically, electronically, or by any other method of communication, from a veterinarian licensed in this or any other state or other person whose expertise, in the opinion of the licensed veterinarian, would benefit a patient. Under any circumstance, the responsibility for the welfare of the patient remains with the licensed veterinarian receiving consultation.

9. "Credentialed veterinary technician or technologist" means a veterinary technician or veterinary technologist who is validly and currently registered, certified, or licensed by the Board.

10. "Direct supervision" means a licensed veterinarian is readily available on the premises where the patient is being treated.

11. "ECFVG® certificate" means the certificate issued by the Educational Commission for Foreign Veterinary Graduates® of the AVMA indicating that the holder has demonstrated knowledge and skill equivalent to that possessed by a graduate of an accredited college of veterinary medicine.

12. "Extralabel use" means actual use or intended use of a drug in an animal in a manner that is not in accordance with the approved labeling. This includes, but is not limited to, use in species not listed in the labeling, use for indications (disease or other conditions) not listed in the labeling, use at dosage levels, frequencies, or routes of administration other than those stated in the labeling, and deviation from the labeled withdrawal time based on these different uses.

13. "Impaired veterinarian" means a veterinarian who is unable to practice veterinary medicine with reasonable skill and safety because of a physical or mental disability as evidenced by a written determination from a competent authority or written consent based on clinical evidence, including deterioration of mental capacity, loss of motor skills, or abuse of drugs or alcohol of sufficient degree to diminish the person's ability to deliver competent patient care.

14. "Indirect supervision" means a veterinarian has given either written or oral instructions for treatment of the patient and is readily available by telephone or other form of communication.

15. "Informed consent" means the veterinarian has informed the client, in a manner that would be understood by a reasonable person, of the diagnostic and treatment options, risk assessment, and prognosis, and has provided the client with an estimate of the charges for veterinary services to be rendered and the client has consented to the recommended treatment.

16. "Licensed veterinarian" means a person who is validly and currently licensed to practice veterinary medicine in this state.

17. "Patient" means an animal that is examined or treated by a veterinarian.

18. "Person" means any individual, firm, partnership (general, limited, or limited liability), association, joint venture, co-operative, corporation, limited liability company, or any other group or combination acting in concert; and whether or not acting as a principal, partner, member, trustee, fiduciary, receiver, or as any other kind of legal or personal representative, or as the successor in interest, assignee, agent, factor, servant, employee, director, officer, or any other representative of such person.

19. "Practice of veterinary medicine" means:
    a. To diagnose, treat, correct, change, alleviate, or prevent animal disease, illness, pain, deformity, defect, injury, or other physical, dental, or mental conditions by any method or mode; including:
       i. the prescription, dispensing, administration, or application of any drug, medicine, biologic, apparatus, anesthetic, or other therapeutic or diagnostic substance or medical or surgical technique, or
       ii. the use of complementary, alternative, and integrative therapies, or
       iii. the use of any manual or mechanical procedure for reproductive management, or
       iv. the rendering of advice or recommendation by any means including telephonic and other electronic communications with regard to any of the above.

Continued

b. To represent, directly or indirectly, publicly or privately, an ability and willingness to do an act described in subsection 19(a).

c. To use any title, words, abbreviation, or letters in a manner or under circumstances that induce the belief that the person using them is qualified to do any act described in subsection 19(a).

20. "Practice of veterinary technology" means:

a. To perform patient care or other services that require a technical understanding of veterinary medicine on the basis of written or oral instruction of a veterinarian, excluding diagnosing, prognosing, surgery, or prescribing drugs, medicine, or appliances.

b. To represent, directly or indirectly, publicly or privately, an ability and willingness to do an act described in subsection 20(a).

c. To use any title, words, abbreviation, or letters in a manner or under circumstances that induce the belief that the person using them is qualified to do any act described in subsection 20(a).

21. "Veterinarian" means a person who has received a professional veterinary medical degree from a college of veterinary medicine.

22. "Veterinarian-client-patient relationship" means that all of the following are required:

a. The veterinarian has assumed the responsibility for making clinical judgments regarding the health of the animal and the need for medical treatment, and the client has agreed to follow the veterinarian's instructions.

b. The veterinarian has sufficient knowledge of the animal to initiate at least a general or preliminary diagnosis of the medical condition of the animal. This means that the veterinarian has recently seen and is personally acquainted with the keeping and care of the animal either by virtue of an examination of the animal, or by medically appropriate and timely visits to the premises where the animals are kept.

c. The veterinarian is readily available or has arranged for emergency coverage for follow-up evaluation in the event of adverse reactions or the failure of the treatment regimen.

23. "Veterinary medicine" means all branches and specialties included within the practice of veterinary medicine.

24. "Veterinary premises" means any premises or facility where the practice of veterinary medicine occurs, including but not limited to a mobile clinic, outpatient clinic, satellite clinic, or veterinary hospital or clinic, but shall not include the premises of a veterinary client, research facility, a federal military base, or an accredited college of veterinary medicine.

25. "Veterinary prescription drug" means a drug that may not be dispensed without the prescription of a veterinarian and that bears the label statement: "CAUTION: Federal law restricts this drug to use by or on the order of a licensed veterinarian."

26. "Veterinary specialist" means that a veterinarian has completed all of the requirements to become a Diplomate within an AVMA-recognized veterinary specialty organization.

27. "Veterinary technician" means a graduate of a two- or three-year accredited program in veterinary technology.

28. "Veterinary technologist" means a graduate of a four-year accredited program in veterinary technology.

SECTION 3. BOARD OF VETERINARY MEDICINE

1. A Board of Veterinary Medicine shall be appointed by the governor and shall consist of five licensed veterinarians, one credentialed veterinary technician or technologist, and one member of the public who is not a veterinarian or veterinary technician or technologist. All persons appointed to the Board shall have been residents of this state for at least the two years immediately preceding appointment. Each member shall be appointed for a term of five years or until a successor is appointed, except that the terms of the first appointees may be for shorter periods to permit a staggering of terms. Members of the Board appointed under the chapter that this act replaces may continue as members of the Board until the expiration of the term for which they were appointed. Vacancies due to death, resignation, or removal shall be filled for the remainder of the unexpired term in the same manner as regular appointments. No person shall serve more than two consecutive full terms.

a. A licensed veterinarian shall be qualified to serve as a member of the Board if he has been licensed to practice veterinary medicine in this state for the five years immediately preceding the time of his appointment. A credentialed veterinary technician or technologist shall be qualified to serve as a member of the Board if he has been credentialed in this state for the five years immediately preceding his appointment.

b. Each member of the Board shall be paid for each day or substantial portion thereof if he is engaged in the work of the Board, in addition to such reimbursement for travel and other expenses as is normally allowed to state employees.

c. Any member of the Board may be removed in accordance with the Administrative Procedures Act of this state or other applicable laws.

2. The Board shall meet at least once each year at the time and place fixed by rule of the Board. Other necessary meetings may be called by the Board by giving notice as may be required by rule. Except as may otherwise be provided, a majority of the Board constitutes a quorum. Meetings shall be open and public except that the Board may meet in closed session to prepare, approve, administer, or grade examinations, or to deliberate the qualification of an applicant for license or the disposition of a proceeding to discipline a licensed veterinarian.

3. The Board shall annually elect officers from its membership as may be prescribed by rule. Officers of the Board serve for terms of 1 year and until a successor is elected, without limitation on the number of terms an officer may serve. The duties of officers shall be prescribed by rule.

4. The Board shall have the power to:

a. Adopt, amend, or repeal all rules necessary for its government and all regulations necessary to carry into effect the provisions of this act, including the establishment and publication of standards of practice and professional conduct for the practice of veterinary medicine.

Box 4   AMERICAN VETERINARY MEDICAL ASSOCIATION MODEL VETERINARY PRACTICE ACT—*cont'd*

h. Adopt, promulgate, and enforce rules and regulations relating to specific duties and responsibilities; certification, registration, or licensure; and other matters pertaining to veterinary technicians, veterinary technologists, or nonlicensed persons consistent with the provisions of this act.

c. Initiate disciplinary procedures, hold hearings, reprimand, suspend, revoke, or refuse to issue or renew credentials, and perform any other acts that may be necessary to regulate veterinary technicians and technologists in a manner consistent with the provisions of this act applicable to veterinarians.

d. Examine by established protocol the qualifications and fitness of applicants for a license to practice veterinary medicine in the state.

e. Issue, renew, or deny the licenses and temporary permits to practice veterinary medicine in this state.

f. Limit, suspend, or revoke the licenses of disciplined veterinarians or otherwise discipline licensed veterinarians consistent with the provisions of the act and the rules and regulations adopted thereunder.

g. Establish and publish annually a schedule of fees for licensing, certification, and registration.

h. Conduct investigations of suspected violations of this act to determine whether there are sufficient grounds to initiate disciplinary proceedings. All investigations shall be conducted in accordance with the Administrative Procedures Act of this state or other applicable laws.

i. Inspect veterinary premises and equipment, including practice vehicles, at any time in accordance with protocols established by rule.

j. Hold hearings on all matters properly brought before the Board and in connection thereto to administer oaths, receive evidence, make necessary determinations, and enter orders consistent with the findings. The Board may require by subpoena the attendance and testimony of witnesses and the production of papers, records, or other documentary evidence and commission depositions. The Board may designate one or more of its members to serve as its hearing officer or may employ a hearing officer defined by state law. All hearings shall be conducted in accordance with the Administrative Procedures Act of this state or other applicable laws.

k. Employ full or part-time personnel necessary to effectuate the provisions of this act and purchase or rent necessary office space, equipment, and supplies.

l. Appoint from its own membership one or more members to act as representatives of the Board at any meeting within or outside the state where such representative is deemed desirable.

m. Bring proceedings in the courts against any person for the enforcement of this act or any regulations made pursuant thereto.

5. The powers enumerated above are granted for the purpose of enabling the Board to effectively supervise the practice of veterinary medicine and veterinary technology and are to be construed liberally to accomplish this objective.

SECTION 4. LICENSE REQUIREMENT

No person may practice veterinary medicine in the state who is not a licensed veterinarian or the holder of a valid temporary permit issued by the Board unless otherwise exempt pursuant to Section 6 of this act.

SECTION 5. VETERINARIAN-CLIENT-PATIENT RELATIONSHIP REQUIREMENT

1. No person may practice veterinary medicine in the state except within the context of a veterinarian-client-patient relationship.
2. A veterinarian-client-patient relationship cannot be established solely by telephonic or other electronic means.

SECTION 6. EXEMPTIONS

This act shall not be construed to prohibit:

1. Any employee of the federal, state, or local government performing his official duties.
2. Any person who is a student in an accredited college of veterinary medicine or an accredited program in veterinary technology performing duties or actions assigned by instructors or working under the direct supervision of a licensed veterinarian.
3. Any person advising with respect to or performing acts that the Board has designated by rule as accepted livestock management practices.
4. Any person providing consultation to a licensed veterinarian in this state on the care and management of a patient.
5. Any member in good standing of another licensed or regulated profession within any state, or any member of an organization or group approved by the Board within the rules and regulations, providing assistance requested by a veterinarian licensed in the state, acting with informed consent from the client, and acting under the direct or indirect supervision and control of the licensed veterinarian. Providing assistance involves hands-on active participation in the treatment and care of the patient. The licensed veterinarian shall maintain responsibility for the veterinarian-client-patient relationship.
6. Any veterinarian employed by an accredited college of veterinary medicine providing assistance requested by a veterinarian licensed in the state, acting with informed consent from the client, and acting under the direct or indirect supervision and control of the licensed veterinarian. Providing assistance involves hands-on active participation in the treatment and care of the patient. The licensed veterinarian shall maintain responsibility for the veterinarian-client-patient relationship.
7. Any pharmacist, merchant, or manufacturer selling at his regular place of business medicines, feed, appliances, or other products used in the prevention or treatment of animal diseases as permitted by law.
8. Any person lawfully engaged in the art or profession of horseshoeing.
9. Any person rendering advice without expectation of compensation.
10. Any owner of an animal and any of the owner's regular employees caring for and treating the animal belonging to

Continued

Box 4 AMERICAN VETERINARY MEDICAL ASSOCIATION MODEL VETERINARY PRACTICE ACT—*cont'd*

such owner, except where the ownership of the animal was transferred for purposes of circumventing this act. Notwithstanding the provisions of this subsection 10, a veterinarian-client-patient relationship must exist when prescription drugs or nonprescription drugs intended for extralabel use are administered, dispensed, or prescribed.

11. Any person who provides appropriate training for animals that does include diagnosing or the prescribing or dispensing of any therapeutic agent.

12. Any instructor at an accredited college of veterinary medicine or accredited program in veterinary technology performing his regular functions or any person lecturing or giving instructions or demonstrations at an accredited college of veterinary medicine or accredited program in veterinary technology or in connection with a veterinary or veterinary technology continuing education course or seminar.

13. Any person selling or applying pesticides, insecticides, or herbicides as permitted by law.

14. Any person engaging in bona fide scientific research that reasonably requires experimentation involving animals.

15. Any credentialed veterinary technician, veterinary technologist, or other employee of a licensed veterinarian performing duties other than diagnosis, prognosis, prescription, or surgery under the direction and supervision of such veterinarian who shall be responsible for the performance of the employee.

16. Any graduate of a non-accredited college of veterinary medicine who is in the process of obtaining an ECFVG® certificate and is performing duties or actions assigned by instructors in an accredited college of veterinary medicine.

17. Any person who, without expectation of compensation, provides emergency veterinary care in an emergency or disaster situation.

18. Any animal shelter employee acting under the supervision of a licensed veterinarian or authorized by the Board to perform euthanasia in the course and scope of employment.

SECTION 7. VETERINARY TECHNICIANS AND TECHNOLOGISTS

1. No person may practice veterinary technology in the state who is not a veterinary technician or technologist credentialed by the Board.

2. A veterinary technician or technologist who performs veterinary technology contrary to this act shall be subject to disciplinary actions in a manner consistent with the provisions of this act applicable to veterinarians.

3. Credentialed veterinary technicians and technologists shall be required to complete continuing education as prescribed by rule to renew their credentials.

SECTION 8. STATUS OF PERSONS PREVIOUSLY LICENSED

Any person who holds a valid license to practice veterinary medicine in this state on the date this act becomes effective shall be recognized as a licensed veterinarian and shall be entitled to retain this status so long as he complies with the provisions of this act, including periodic renewal of the license.

SECTION 9. APPLICATION FOR LICENSE: QUALIFICATIONS

1. Any person desiring a license to practice veterinary medicine in this state shall make written application to the Board. The application shall show that the applicant is a graduate of an accredited college of veterinary medicine or the holder of an ECFVG® certificate. The application shall also show that the applicant is a person of good moral character and such other information and proof as the Board may require by rule. The application shall be accompanied by a fee in the amount established and published by the Board.

2. If the Board determines that the applicant possesses the proper qualifications, it shall admit the applicant to the next examination, or if the applicant is eligible for license by endorsement under Section 11 of this act, the Board may forthwith grant him a license. If an applicant is found not qualified to take the examination or for a license by endorsement the Board shall notify the applicant in writing within 30 days of such finding and the grounds therefore. An applicant found unqualified may request a hearing on the questions of his qualifications under the procedure set forth in Section 16.

SECTION 10. EXAMINATIONS

1. The Board shall provide for at least one examination for licensing, certification, or registration during each calendar year and may provide for such additional examinations as are necessary. The Board shall give public notice of the time and place for each examination at least 120 days in advance of the date set for the examination or in compliance with state law. A person desiring to take an examination shall make application at least 60 days before the date of the examination.

2. The preparations, administration, and grading of examinations shall be governed by rules prescribed by the Board. Examinations for veterinary licensure shall be designed to test the examinee's knowledge of and proficiency in the subjects and techniques pertaining to the practice of veterinary medicine commonly taught in an accredited college of veterinary medicine. The passing score for the examination shall be established by the testing entity. The Board may adopt and use the results of the examinations prepared by the National Board of Veterinary Medical Examiners.

3. After examination, each examinee shall be notified of the result of the examination, and the Board shall issue a certificate of registration to the new licensees. Any person who fails an examination may be admitted to any subsequent examination on payment of the application fee.

SECTION 11. LICENSE BY ENDORSEMENT

1. The Board, in its sole discretion, may issue a license by endorsement to a qualified applicant who furnishes satisfactory proof that he is a graduate of an accredited college of veterinary medicine or holds an ECFVG® certificate. The applicant must also show that he is a person of good moral character, and:
   a. is currently licensed to practice veterinary medicine in at least one state, territory, or district of the United States and

has practiced veterinary medicine in one or more of those states without disciplinary action by any state or federal agency for at least the three years immediately prior to filing the application, or

b. has within the three years immediately prior to filing the application passed the licensing examination prepared by the National Board of Veterinary Medical Examiners.

2. The Board may, in its sole discretion, issue a limited license by endorsement to a qualified applicant who furnishes satisfactory proof that he currently holds a license to practice in at least one state, is an active diplomate in an AVMA-recognized veterinary specialty organization, and will limit his practice to his certified specialty.

3. At its sole discretion, the Board may examine any person qualifying for licensing under this Section.

SECTION 12. TEMPORARY PERMIT

The Board, in its sole discretion, may issue a temporary permit to practice veterinary medicine in this state:

1. To a qualified applicant for license pending examination, provided that such temporary permit shall expire the day after the notice of results of the first examination given after the permit is issued and provided that the grantee is under indirect supervision of a licensed veterinarian. No temporary permit may be issued to any applicant who has previously failed the examination in this state or in any other state, territory, or district of the United States or a foreign country.

2. To a nonresident veterinarian who is a graduate of an accredited college of veterinary medicine or an ECFVG® certificate holder validly licensed in another state, territory, or district of the United States or a foreign country who pays the fee established and published by the Board, provided that such temporary permit shall be issued for a period of no more than 60 consecutive days and that no more than one permit shall be issued to a person during a calendar year. A temporary permit may be summarily revoked or limited by the Board without a hearing.

SECTION 13. LICENSE RENEWAL

1. All licenses shall expire periodically but may be renewed by registration with the Board and payment of the registration renewal fee established and published by the Board. At least 30 days in advance, the Board shall mail a notice to each licensed veterinarian that his license will expire and provide him with a form for re-registration. The Board shall issue a new certificate of registration to all persons registering under this act.

2. The Board shall establish the continuing education requirements that must be met for license renewal. The Board shall also define the types of continuing education that will meet its requirements.

3. Any person who shall practice veterinary medicine after the expiration of his license and willfully or by neglect fail to renew such license shall be practicing in violation of this act. Any person may renew an expired license within five years of the date of its expiration by making written application for renewal, paying the current renewal fee plus all delinquent renewal fees, and complying with current continuing education requirements.

4. The Board may by rule waive the payment of the registration renewal fee of a licensed veterinarian during the period when he is on active duty with any branch of the armed services of the United States.

SECTION 14. DISCIPLINE OF LICENSEES

Upon written complaint sworn to by any person the Board, in its sole discretion, may, after a hearing, revoke, suspend, or limit for a certain time the license of, or otherwise discipline, any licensed veterinarian for any of the following reasons:

1. The employment of fraud, misrepresentation, or deception in obtaining a license.

2. The inability to practice veterinary medicine with reasonable skill and safety because of a physical or mental disability, including deterioration of mental capacity, loss of motor skills, or abuse of drugs or alcohol of sufficient degree to diminish the person's ability to deliver competent patient care.

3. The use of advertising or solicitation that is false or misleading.

4. Conviction of the following in any federal court or in the courts of this state or any other jurisdiction, regardless of whether the sentence is deferred.
   a. Any felony
   b. Any crime involving cruelty, abuse, or neglect of animals, including bestiality
   c. Any crime of moral turpitude
   d. Any crime involving unlawful sexual contact; child abuse; the use or threatened use of a weapon; the infliction of injury; indecent exposure; perjury, false reporting, criminal impersonation, forgery and any other crime involving a lack of truthfulness, veracity, or honesty; intimidation of a victim or witness; larceny; or alcohol or drugs.

5. For the purposes of subsection 4, a plea of guilty or a plea of nolo contendere accepted by the court shall be considered as a conviction.

6. Incompetence, gross negligence, or other malpractice in the practice of veterinary medicine.

7. Aiding the unlawful practice of veterinary medicine.

8. Fraud or dishonesty in the application or reporting of any test for disease in animals.

9. Failure to report, as required by law, or making false or misleading report of, any contagious or infectious disease.

10. Failure to keep accurate and comprehensive patient records as set by rules promulgated by the Board.

11. Dishonesty or gross negligence in the performance of food safety inspections or the issuance of any health or inspection certificates.

12. Failure to keep veterinary premises and equipment, including practice vehicles, in a clean and sanitary conditions as set by rules promulgated by the Board.

13. Failure to permit the Board or its agents to enter and inspect veterinary premises and equipment, including practice vehicles, as set by rules promulgated by the Board.

14. Revocation, suspension, or limitation of a license to practice veterinary medicine by another state, territory, or district of the United States on grounds other than nonpayment of registration fee.

Continued

15. Loss or suspension of accreditation by any federal or state agency on grounds other than nonpayment of registration fees or voluntary relinquishment of accreditation.
16. Unprofessional conduct as defined in regulations adopted by the Board.
17. The dispensing, distribution, prescription, or administration of any veterinary prescription drug, or the extralabel use of any drug in the absence of a veterinarian-client-patient relationship.
18. Violations of state or federal drug laws.
19. Violations of any order of the Board.
20. Violations of this act or of the rules promulgated under this act.

SECTION 15. IMPAIRED VETERINARIAN

1. The Board shall establish by rule a program of care, counseling, or treatment for impaired veterinarians.
2. The program of care, counseling, or treatment shall include a written schedule of organized treatment, care, counseling, activities, or education satisfactory to the Board, designed for the purposes of restoring an impaired person to a condition whereby the impaired person can practice veterinary medicine with reasonable skill and safety of a sufficient degree to deliver competent patient care.
3. All persons authorized to practice by the Board shall report in good faith any veterinarian they reasonably believe to be impaired as defined in Section 2, subsection 13.

SECTION 16. HEARING PROCEDURE

All hearings shall be in accordance with the Administrative Procedures Act of this state or other applicable state law.

SECTION 17. APPEAL

All appeals shall be in accordance with the Administrative Procedures Act of this state or other applicable state law.

SECTION 18. REINSTATEMENT

Any person whose license is suspended, revoked, or limited may be reinstated at any time, with or without an examination, by approval of the Board after written application is made to the Board showing cause justifying relicensing or reinstatement.

SECTION 19. VETERINARIAN-CLIENT CONFIDENTIALITY

1. No licensed veterinarian shall disclose any information concerning the licensed veterinarian's care of a patient except on written authorization or by waiver by the licensed veterinarian's client or on appropriate court order, by subpoena, or as otherwise provided in this Section.
2. Copies of or information from veterinary records shall be provided without the owner's consent to public, animal health, animal welfare, wildlife, or agriculture authorities, employed by federal, state, or local governmental agencies who have a legal or regulatory interest in the contents of said records for the protection of animal and public health.
3. Any licensed veterinarian releasing information under written authorization or other waiver by the client or under court order, by subpoena, or as otherwise provided by this Section shall not be liable to the client or any other person.

4. The privilege provided by this Section shall be waived to the extent that the licensed veterinarian's client or the owner of the patient places the licensed veterinarian's care and treatment of the patient or the nature and extent of injuries to the animal at issue in any civil criminal proceeding.

SECTION 20. IMMUNITY FROM LIABILITY

Any member of the Board, any witness testifying in a proceeding or hearing authorized under this act, any person who lodges a complaint pursuant to this act, and any person reporting an impaired veterinarian shall be immune from liability in any civil or criminal action brought against him for any action occurring while he was acting in his capacity as a Board member, witness, complainant, or reporting party, if such person was acting in good faith within the scope of his respective capacity.

SECTION 21. CRUELTY TO ANIMALS: IMMUNITY FOR REPORTING

Any veterinarian licensed in this state who reports, in good faith and in the normal course of business, a suspected incident of animal cruelty, as described by law, to the proper authorities shall be immune from liability in any civil or criminal action brought against such veterinarian for reporting such incident.

SECTION 22. ABANDONED ANIMAL

1. Any animal placed in the custody of a licensed veterinarian for treatment, boarding or other care, which is unclaimed by the client for more than ten days after written notice by certified mail, return receipt requested, or US priority mail, confirmation of receipt, is sent to the client at the client's last known address shall be deemed to be abandoned. Such abandoned animal may be turned over to the nearest humane society or animal shelter, or otherwise disposed of or destroyed by the licensed veterinarian in a humane manner.
2. If notice is sent pursuant to subsection 1 of this Section, the licensed veterinarian responsible for such abandoned animal is relieved of any further liability for disposal. If a licensed veterinarian follows the procedures of this Section, the veterinarian shall not be subject to disciplinary action under Section 14 of this Act, unless such licensed veterinarian fails to provide the proper notification to the client.
3. The disposal of an abandoned animal shall not relieve the client of any financial obligation incurred for treatment, boarding, or other care provided by the licensed veterinarian.

SECTION 23. ENFORCEMENT

1. Any person who practices veterinary medicine without a valid license or temporary permit issued by the Board shall be guilty of a criminal offense and upon conviction for each violation shall be fined [an appropriate amount of money according to the Board or the laws of the state] or imprisoned [an appropriate amount of time according to the Board or the laws of the state], provided that each act of such unlawful practice shall constitute a distinct and separate offense.
2. Any person not licensed under this act is considered to have violated this act and may be subject to all the penalties provided for such violations if he:
   a. Performs any of the functions described as the practice of veterinary medicine as defined in this act, or

Box 4 AMERICAN VETERINARY MEDICAL ASSOCIATION MODEL VETERINARY PRACTICE ACT—*cont'd*

b. Represents, directly or indirectly, publicly or privately, an ability and willingness to perform any of the functions described as the practice of veterinary medicine as defined in this act, or

c. Uses any title, words, abbreviation, or letters in a manner or under circumstances that induces the belief that the person using them is qualified to perform any of the functions described as the practice of veterinary medicine as defined in this act.

3. The Board may bring an action to enjoin any person from practicing veterinary medicine without a currently valid license or temporary permit issued by the Board. If the court finds that the person is violating or is threatening to violate this act, it shall enter an injunction restraining him from such unlawful acts.

4. Not withstanding other provisions of this act, the Board may take immediate action if there is an imminent threat to the health, safety, or welfare of the public. The Board shall find that this action is necessary for the protection of the public and necessary to effectively enforce this act. If the Board takes immediate action pursuant to this subsection 4, efforts shall be made as soon as possible to proceed in accordance with a hearing pursuant to Section 16 of this act.

5. In addition to any other penalty or remedy provided by law, the Board shall have the authority to implement a system of Cite and Fine procedures for licensed and nonlicensed persons who violate the state veterinary practice act. The Board may also impose a civil penalty, upon conviction, for each separate violation. This civil penalty shall be in an amount not to exceed [dollar amount] for each violation and shall be assessed by the Board in accordance with the provisions set forth in Section 16 of this act.

6. The success or failure of an action based on any one of the remedies set forth in this Section shall in no way prejudice the prosecution of an action based on any other of the remedies.

SECTION 24. SEVERABILITY

If any part of this act is held invalid by a court of competent jurisdiction, all valid parts that are severable from the invalid part remain in effect.

SECTION 25. EFFECTIVE DATE

This act shall become effective on _____ 1st, 20___. This act does not affect rights and duties that matured, penalties that were incurred, and proceedings that were begun before its effective date.

Box 5 NAVTA'S MODEL PRACTICE ACT FOR VETERINARY TECHNICIANS

SECTION I. TITLE

This act shall be known and may be cited as the "Model Practice Act."

SECTION II. LEGISLATIVE INTENT AND PURPOSE

The practice of veterinary technology is privilege granted by legislative authority to maintain public health, safety and welfare and to protect the public from being misled by unauthorized individuals.

SECTION III. DEFINITIONS

When used in the text that follows, except where otherwise indicated by context, the words and phrases below shall have the following meanings:

Animal—Any mammalian animal other than man, and any avian, amphibian, fish or reptile, wild or domestic.

Board—The _____ State Board of Veterinary Medical Examiners or Board of Governors.

Veterinary Technology—The science and art of providing all aspects of professional medical care and treatment for animals with the exception of diagnosis, prognosis, surgery and prescription.

Emergency—When an animal has been placed in a life-threatening condition and immediate treatment is necessary to sustain life; or where death is imminent and action is necessary to relieve pain or suffering.

Licensed Veterinarian—An individual who is validly and currently licensed by the Board to practice veterinary medicine in _____ .

Veterinary Technician (Licensed, Registered or Certified)—An individual who has graduated from a veterinary technology program that is accredited according to the standards adopted by the American Veterinary Medical Association's Committee on Veterinary Technician Education and Activities and who has passed the examination requirements as prescribed by the Board in _____ shall be known as a licensed, registered or certified veterinary technician.

SECTION IV. TASKS

Certain tasks may be performed ONLY by a licensed veterinarian OR licensed, registered or certified veterinary technician under the direction, supervision and control of a veterinarian licensed to practice in the state of _____ .

See the Rules and Regulations Document for a list of tasks.

SECTION V. EXAMINATION FOR LICENSURE, REGISTRATION OR CERTIFICATION

Veterinary technicians applying for licensure, registration or certification shall be required to pass the Veterinary Technician National Examination, with scores as set by the Board prior to licensure, registration or certification.

See the Rules and Regulations Document for a list of tasks.

Continued

Box 5 Navta Model Practice Act for Veterinary Technicians—*cont'd*

SECTION VI. CONTINUING EDUCATION

All licensed, registered or certified veterinary technicians shall be required to continue their professional education as a condition of maintenance of his/her status in the state of _____ .

See the Rules and Regulations Document for a list of tasks.

SECTION VII. DENIAL, SUSPENSION, OR REVOCATION OF VETERINARY TECHNICIAN LICENSES, REGISTRATIONS OR CERTIFICATIONS

The Board may suspend, revoke or deny the issuance or renewal of license, registration or certification of any veterinary technician if after a hearing by his/her peers, has been found guilty of any of the following:

1. Fraud or misrepresentation in applying for license, registration, or certification.

2. Criminal offense relating to veterinary medicine.

3. Any violation of the Uniform Controlled Substances Act or the Legend Drug Act.

4. Convicted of cruelty to animals.

5. Violation of any of the rules or regulations stated in the Rules and Regulations Document.

From the 2005 American Veterinary Medical Association (AVMA) membership directory.

---

the task force completes the proposed amendments, they are often circulated within the state veterinary medical association and within the state veterinary technician association to obtain feedback and to ensure that most members support the proposed changes. The task force may then hire a lobbyist who can help locate state senators and representatives who would be willing to support the bill. These senators and representatives are called sponsors. The House and the Senate will each have a head sponsor and a team of co-sponsors. It is helpful if the sponsors are well-respected members of the legislature and if they have influence among their colleagues. The lobbyist can help to advise the task force in selecting influential and supportive sponsors. He or she can also advise the task force about whether it is better to begin the legislative process in the House or in the Senate. It is important to start in the arena where there is the greatest likelihood for success.

Before the bill goes to the House or Senate "floors" for passage, it is put into "committee." If the task force decides to start the lobbying process in the House, for example, then the bill will be sent initially to the House Professional Licensure Committee where the language will be examined for legal consistency (i.e., that the language is in keeping with other professions' practice acts) and accuracy (i.e., that the language legally says what the people who wrote it think it says). If the bill is controversial, the committee may decide to hold a hearing in which the supporters and opponents of the bill have an opportunity to testify for and against it, respectively. If the committee is not aware of any opposition to the bill, the bill may be passed, given an official bill number, and sent to the House majority leader, who puts it on the House agenda. Controversial bills can be tied up indefinitely in committee and in the offices of the House or Senate majority leaders.

When the bill goes to the floor of the House or the Senate, it can be further amended before it is passed. Sometimes bills come out of the House and the Senate looking very different from the way they did when they were first presented. For this reason, it is important to stay abreast of amendments that are made during the legislative process. Additional guidelines for developing and introducing a legislative proposal can be found on the NAVTA website at http://www.navta.net/modelpracticeact.htm.

RULES AND REGULATIONS

Based on the laws outlined in the practice act, more specific laws, called rules and regulations, are written by the state veterinary board. Refer to Box 6 for NAVTA's model of rules and regulations. As previously mentioned, the board may be formally known as the board of veterinary medical examiners, the board of veterinary governors, or the licensing board of veterinary medicine, depending on the state. Typically, there is a state board for every profession that requires licensure. However, unlike the human nursing field, which has its own state boards, there are currently no state boards of veterinary technology. Veterinary technology falls under the governance of the state board of veterinary medicine or under a private governing body such as the state veterinary medical association or the state veterinary technician association.

In veterinary medicine, state boards are responsible for writing the rules and regulations, distributing licenses, collecting renewal fees, and evaluating complaints of malpractice or unethical conduct perpetrated by veterinarians and veterinary technicians (if they are licensed in the state). With adequate evidence of wrongdoing, a board can revoke the license of a veterinarian or veterinary technician. Members of a state board are typically recommended by members of the veterinary profession but are officially appointed by the governor. Although it is recommended that every state board include a least one veterinary technician, some state boards do not. In addition to representatives from the veterinary profession, the board may also include one government official and one or two members of the general public. In addition, each board is given legal counsel by the state to ensure that the laws (both in the practice act and the rules and regulations) are interpreted and upheld

Box 6 MODEL RULES AND REGULATIONS FOR VETERINARY TECHNICIANS

I. Licensed, Registered or Certified Veterinary Technician Activities
A. Tasks
1. Levels of supervision defined
a. Immediate supervision—A licensed veterinarian is within direct eyesight and hearing range
b. Direct supervision—A licensed veterinarian is on the premises, and is readily available
c. Indirect supervision—A licensed veterinarian is not on the premises, but is able to perform the duties of a licensed veterinarian by maintaining direct communication
2. The following tasks may be performed ONLY by a licensed, registered or certified veterinary technician (or licensed veterinarian) under the direction, supervision and control of a veterinarian licensed to practice in _____ provided said veterinarian makes a daily physical examination of the patient treated:
a. Immediate supervision
1. Induction of anesthesia
2. Dental extraction not requiring sectioning of the tooth or the resectioning of bone
3. Surgical assistant to a licensed veterinarian within the rules and regulations issued by the Board of Veterinary Medical Examiners and the laws of the state of _____
b. Direct supervision
1. Euthanasia
2. Blood or blood component collection, preparation and administration
3. Application of splints and slings
4. Dental procedures including, but not limited to the removal of calculus, soft deposits, plaque and stains; the smoothing, filing and polishing of teeth; or the flotation or dressing of equine teeth
c. Indirect supervision
1. Administration and application of treatments, drugs, medications and immunological agents by parenteral and injectable routes (subcutaneous, intramuscular, intraperitoneal and intravenous) except when in conflict with government regulations
2. Initiation of parenteral fluid administration
3. Intravenous catheterizations
4. Radiography including settings, positioning, processing and safety procedures
5. Collection of blood; collection of urine by expression, cystocentesis or catheterization; collection and preparation of tissue, cellular or microbiological samples by skin scrapings, impressions or other non-surgical methods except when in conflict with government regulations
6. Routine laboratory test procedures
7. Supervision of the handling of biohazardous waste materials
d. Other
1. Services which a licensed, registered or certified veterinary technician is competent to perform under the appropriate degree of supervision

3. Under conditions of emergency, a licensed, registered or certified veterinary technician may render the following life-saving aid and treatment:
a. Application of tourniquets and/or pressure bandages to control hemorrhage
b. Administration of pharmacological agents and parenteral fluids shall only be performed after direct communication with a veterinarian authorized to practice in _____ and such veterinarian is either present or en route to the location of the distressed animals
c. Resuscitative procedures
d. Application of temporary splints or bandages to prevent further injury to bones or soft tissue
e. Application of appropriate wound dressings and external supportive treatment in severe wound and burn cases
f. External supportive treatment in heat prostration cases
4. HOWEVER, nothing shall be construed to permit a licensed, registered or certified veterinary technician to do the following:
a. Make any diagnosis or prognosis
b. Prescribe any treatments, drugs, medications or appliances
c. Perform surgery
II. Examinations
A. Examinations of applicants for licensure, registration or certification as a veterinary technician in _____ shall be held at least annually at a time, place and date set by the Board no later than ninety (90) days prior to the scheduled examination.
B. An applicant shall be required to pass the Veterinary Technician National Examination (VTNE) with scores as set by the Board prior to licensure, registration or certification.
III. Continuing Education Requirements for Licensed, Registered or Certified Veterinary Technicians
A. All licensed, registered or certified veterinary technicians shall be required to continue their professional education as a condition of maintaining his/her license of veterinary technology in the state of _____ with _____ hours of continuing education required annually.
IV. Removal of Veterinary Technician Licenses, Registrations or Certifications
A. All licenses, registrations or certifications issued to veterinary technicians in the state of _____ shall expire on _____ of every year unless renewed.
B. All license, registration or certification holders shall submit renewal fees and a current mailing address by the dates determined by the Board on a renewal form that shall be provided by the Board and mailed to all license, registration or certification holders.
C. All license, registration or certification holders will be required to submit evidence of the necessary amount of continuing education in the fields of veterinary medicine to the Board as required by the Board for license, registration or certification renewal.

Continued

correctly. The state's legal counsel also assists the board in writing the rules and regulations. Although the rules and regulations do not need approval by the state House or Senate, as does the practice act, they must be reviewed and approved by the state's independent regulatory review commission and must be made available to the public before their implementation.

The rules and regulations must support the practice act and cannot overrule it. They tend to be more specific laws than those of the practice act. For example, the practice act might define the profession of veterinary technology in general, whereas the rules and regulations might list the specific application fees associated with certification, registration, or licensure. The rules and regulations might also list the specific tasks that veterinary technicians perform and separately list those that may be completed by a veterinary assistant. Finally, the rules and regulations might define the indirect, direct, and immediate levels of veterinary supervision that further delineate the scope of practice of the veterinary technician from that of the veterinary assistant. Because of the variability of laws among states, it is important for veterinary technicians to be aware of the particular laws in their state that govern what they can and cannot do in practice.

TECHNICIAN NOTE

Because of the variability of laws among states, it is important for veterinary technicians to be aware of the particular laws in their state that govern what they can and cannot do in practice.

MALPRACTICE AND COMMON LAW

The society in which we live today is litigious. The workplace for the veterinary technician is no different and includes legal risks. Because veterinary technicians are becoming increasingly skilled and are taking on greater levels of responsibility in clinical practice, they become increasingly more vulnerable to the possibility of litigation against them. Although veterinarians typically bear the brunt of legal action, veterinary technicians can be and *are* sued. Therefore veterinary technicians should understand what constitutes malpractice.

As already mentioned, much of the legal framework of our society is defined by federal and state laws that are

written, approved, and enforced by federal and state governmental bodies. These rules constitute what is called legislative law, because the laws are written down. The veterinary practice act, professional rules and regulations, and local ordinances are examples of legislative laws. They define the profession of veterinary medicine and provide clear guidelines for the management of veterinary practices. In contrast, however, *common law* is not written down. Rather, it is a series of laws that have evolved over time on the basis of established professional conduct, customs, and practices. Common law is also derived from and enforced by the decisions of judges made during civil suits when someone has been injured. Thus common law is not enforced by governmental bodies, but by judges in courts of law.

Common law dictates many things to veterinary practices. For example, it dictates that practice owners must provide a reasonably safe environment for their employees and clients. Failure to provide this constitutes *ordinary negligence* (refer to Chapter 36 for additional information about laws that protect employees). In addition, common law dictates that veterinary practitioners must provide a level of medical care to their patients that is in keeping with a reasonably prudent veterinary practitioner of similar training under similar circumstances. Failure to comply with common law under these circumstances constitutes *professional negligence* or *malpractice*.

Malpractice may be subject to litigation if the plaintiff can prove the following three things:

1. The veterinarian or veterinary technician agreed to treat and *did* treat that particular patient.
2. The veterinarian or veterinary technician failed to provide a reasonable level of medical care to the patient and in this way was professionally negligent.
3. The patient was injured as a result of the negligence.

Although veterinary technicians can be and are sued for malpractice, it is still relatively rare. Legal responsibility for the clinical actions of veterinary technicians generally falls on the supervising veterinarian. Under the common law doctrine of *respondeat superior,* veterinarians may be found negligent for the injurious actions of veterinary technicians. For example, if a veterinary technician gives a cat 6 ml of insulin instead of 0.06 ml, as directed by the veterinarian, and the cat dies as a result of the overdose, the veterinarian, and not the veterinary technician, may be found to be negligent. On the other hand, there have been circumstances in which the veterinary technician has been sued and found to be negligent for carrying out the injurious instructions of the supervising veterinarian.

Most, if not all, veterinarians purchase malpractice insurance. The AVMA offers professional liability insurance to its members (veterinarians), which is supported by the Professional Liability Insurance Trust (PLIT). AVMA liability insurance includes coverage of the veterinary technician as well as the veterinarian (or practice) who bought the insurance. The insurance, however, is only protective when the veterinary technician is engaged in employment activities for the veterinarian (or practice) who bought the professional liability insurance policy. It also covers veterinary assistants and kennel workers while they are engaged in their work for the insured veterinarian or practice. The following quote from section E(3) of the Common Certificate Definitions Form of the AVMA-PLIT information brochure verifies coverage of "any employee or volunteer" of the insured veterinarian or practice. Notice that other veterinarians are NOT covered and must purchase their own insurance policies.

> *Insured means . . . any employee or volunteer of the Insured described in 1., or 2., above but only for liability arising out of a Veterinary Incident with the scope of his, her or their duties of the Named Insured, or for an insured Veterinary Partnership, Veterinary corporation, or Veterinary Limited Liability company. However, regardless of his, her or their duties a person other than the Named Insured who is a licensed veterinarian shall not be considered an Insured under this definition.*

For additional information about professional liability insurance, go to http://www.avmaplit.com or contact avmaplit@mackparker.com, 1-800-754-8329.

✎ TECHNICIAN NOTE

Although veterinarians typically bear the brunt of legal action, veterinary technicians can be and are sued. Therefore veterinary technicians should understand what constitutes malpractice.

ETHICS

Working and living within their respective communities, people are faced with ethical issues, which may be divided into three classifications: societal, personal, and professional.

SOCIETAL ETHICS

The ethics that are established by society are generally written into law. The laws may include federal legislation against major offenses such as committing murder, rape, embezzlement, and arson; or they may be local ordinances that require people to walk their dogs on leashes or that prohibit loitering. Individuals may not be aware of all the ordinances, rules, and regulations that govern what they should and should not do, but most people are taught from an early age about the most important laws, such as those that prohibit stealing. Thus federal, state, and municipal laws establish the societal ethics of our country.

PERSONAL ETHICS

In addition to the laws of society, each person is guided by an array of personal principles that give him or her a sense of what is right and wrong and what is fair and unfair. For example, issues concerning sexuality, gender roles, dress, family structure, religious choice, and political beliefs are left to the individual to consider. For Americans, the right to make personal choices regarding family, religion, and politics is a fundamental freedom; but this is not the case in all cultures. In some countries, these issues are controlled by legislative laws and thus become societal rather than personal ethics. In addition, personal ethics vary from culture to culture. In some areas of the world, for example, the concept of honor requires that vengeance for a slight be carried out, whereas in other areas of the world, it is considered honorable to forgive those who may have slighted you.

PROFESSIONAL ETHICS

Most veterinary technicians are drawn to the profession of veterinary technology because of a love of animals and a desire to help them. We see countless examples of suffering among living creatures on earth as we watch news clips, read articles, donate funds, and sign petitions. In this worldly context the compassionate work of the veterinarian and veterinary technician emerges as a welcomed counterweight to cruelty. With such an indelible image, the public sets high standards for the ethical conduct of animal healers.

As with all citizens, the individuals that make up a profession are bound by societal laws and personal ethics. In addition, a code of ethics is established by members of the profession to help define and encourage conduct specific to that profession. This code is important and helps to provide additional guidelines by which people carry out their jobs. In veterinary technology, NAVTA has established a nine-point code of ethics (refer to Box 7).

Veterinary technicians, like other professionals, may occasionally find themselves in uncomfortable situations. Taking responsibility for giving a medication incorrectly, for example, is the ethical thing to do, but it may not be easy. The veterinary technician is challenged to sort out the daily ethical choices that are to be made in practice. In addition to the study of the profession's code of ethics listed in Box 7, veterinary technicians may find asking

Box 7 NAVTA's Code of Ethics for the Profession of Veterinary Technology

Veterinary technicians shall:

1. Aid society and animals through providing excellent care and services for animals.
2. Prevent and relieve the suffering of animals.
3. Promote public health by assisting with the control of zoonotic diseases and informing the public about these diseases.
4. Assume accountability for individual professional actions and judgments.
5. Protect confidential information provided by clients.
6. Safeguard the public and the profession against individuals deficient in professional competence or ethics.
7. Assist with efforts to ensure conditions of employment consistent with the excellent care for animals.
8. Remain competent in veterinary technology through commitment to lifelong learning.
9. Collaborate with members of the veterinary medical profession in efforts to ensure quality health care services for all animals.

From the North American Veterinary Technician Association: http://www.navta.net.

themselves the following three simple questions to be helpful:

1. Is it legal? Would I be breaking the law if I carried out my proposed action?
2. Is it fair and balanced? Am I being biased in some way? Does one group or individual benefit more from my proposed action than another?
3. How would I feel about myself? If my family knew about my action, and if it were published in a newspaper, how would I feel?

PROFESSIONAL IDEALS

In addition, to the profession's code of ethics, NAVTA has established a list of ideals and recommended behaviors. These encourage veterinary technicians to take pride in their work, dress, and overall presentation; to participate in professional organizations; and to promote veterinary technology by participating in career days and by giving talks to community groups. As already mentioned, it is important for veterinary technicians to continue their education by attending professional conferences and by being receptive to new ideas and suggestions at work. In addition, veterinary technicians should be respectful of confidential information, should avoid gossip, and should be honest when dealing with co-workers and clients. Finally,

veterinary technicians should strive to improve the standards of their profession by contributing to the profession's body of knowledge and by supporting legislation that defines and strengthens the role of the veterinary technician.

PROFESSIONAL ORGANIZATIONS

NATIONAL ASSOCIATION OF VETERINARY TECHNICIANS IN AMERICA

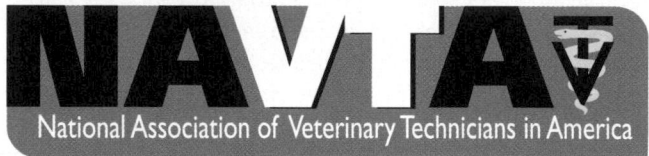

Many associations and professional societies support the education, professional interests, and activities of the veterinary technician. NAVTA, which represents the profession of veterinary technology in the United States, has been a particular leader in shaping and supporting the profession. NAVTA, for example, has written the code of ethics, the veterinary technician oath, and the veterinary technician portion of the model practice act and has brought about important changes in the profession's terminology. In addition, NAVTA is an important source of support and information for veterinary technicians. It publishes *The NAVTA Journal* and has established a website at http://www.navta.net. The website contains a plethora of information, ranging from important credentialing information for technicians relocating to another state to promotional materials for National Veterinary Technician Week. Therefore it is not surprising that NAVTA's mission statement is "to represent and promote the profession of veterinary technology. NAVTA provides direction, education, support and coordination for its members, and works with other allied professional organizations for the competent care and humane treatment of animals." In addition, the goals of NAVTA are to help its members do the following:

1. Influence the future of veterinary technology
2. Be part of the decision-making process that affects veterinary technology
3. Foster high standards of veterinary care
4. Promote the veterinary health care team

To be an active member of NAVTA, you must live in the United States; be a graduate of an AVMA-accredited program of veterinary technology; and/or be licensed, certified, or registered as a veterinary technician. In addition, there are associate members that might include veterinarians, veterinary technicians who live outside of the United States, and veterinary assistants. Associate members may serve on committees but may not vote or hold an elected office.

THE CANADIAN ASSOCIATION OF ANIMAL HEALTH TECHNOLOGISTS AND TECHNICIANS/ASSOCIATION CANADIENNE DES TECHNICIANS ET TECHNOLOGISTS EN SANTE ANIMALE

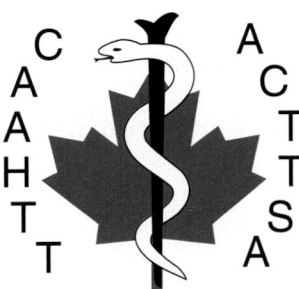

The CAAHTT was founded in 1989 and represents the joining together of seven provincial associations. This union makes CAAHTT a truly national body. CAAHTT is dedicated to promoting the profession of veterinary technology within the animal health care community and the public in general. It focuses on national issues and plays a role in international affairs. CAAHTT is a member of the International Veterinary Nurses and Technicians Association (IVNTA) and is allied with NAVTA. "The CAAHTT/ACTTSA is dedicated to fulfilling the goal of professional recognition nationally and internationally through communication, direction and support of the provincial AHT/VT associations."

Continued growth of veterinary technology depends heavily on the efforts of individuals within these and other professionally related organizations. Graduate veterinary technicians can assist in advancing their profession by joining and being active members of national, state or provincial, and regional veterinary technician associations, some of which are listed in the following sections.

INTERNATIONAL ASSOCIATIONS

International Veterinary Nurses and Technicians Association (IVNTA)
Website: http://www.vetweb.co.uk/sites/ivna/index.htm

NATIONAL ASSOCIATIONS

Academy of Veterinary Emergency and Critical Care Technicians (AVECCT)
Organizing Committee, c/o VECCS
15729 San Pedro, San Antonio, TX 78232
Phone: (210) 826-1488
Website: http://www.veccs.org/technicians

Academy of Veterinary Dental Technicians (AVDT)
Vickie Byard, CVT, VTS (Dentistry)
551 Creek Rd
Warminster, PA 18974
E-mail: Gr8vettek@aol.com

Academy of Veterinary Technician Anesthetists (AVTA)
Website: http://www.avta-vts.org

American Society of Veterinary Dental Technicians (ASVDT)
PO Box 1636
Venice, FL 34284-1636
Phone: (800) 613-3647 or (941) 488-6937

Association of Zoo Veterinary Technicians (AZVT)
Cheryl Purnell, LVT, Executive Director
North Carolina Zoological Park
4401 Zoo Pkwy
Asheboro, NC 27203
Phone: (336) 879-7636
Fax: (336) 879-7637
E-mail: Cheryl.purnell@ncmail.net
Website: http://www.azvt.org

Canadian Association of Animal Health Technologists and Technicians (CAAHTT)
Sandy Hass, RVT, Executive Director
Box 91
Grandora, SK S0K 1V0 Canada
Phone: (306) 329-4956; fax: (306) 329-4700
E-mail: s.vettech@sasktel.net
Website: http://www.caahtt-acttsa.ca

National Association of Veterinary Technicians in America (NAVTA)
A. Patrick Navarre, BS, RVT, Executive Director
Battleground, IN 47920
Phone or fax: (765) 742-2216
E-mail: navta@navta.net
Website: http://www.navta.net

Society of Veterinary Behavior Technicians (SVBT)
Amy Breton, CVT, VTS (ECC), Newsletter Editor
55 Littleton Rd, Unit 19E
Ayer, MA 01432
Phone: (978) 772-4695
E-mail: Newfieldamy@hotmail.com
Website: http://www.svbt.org

Veterinary Technician Anesthetist Society (VTAS)
Stephanie Plattner
Purdue University
1249 Lynn Hall
West Lafayette, IN 47907

STATE, PROVINCIAL, AND REGIONAL ASSOCIATIONS

State associations are listed on the NAVTA (http://www. navta.net) and AVMA (http://www.avma.org/care4pets/ vtassns.htm) websites. Provincial associations are listed on the CAAHTT website (http://www.caahtt-acttsa.ca) and on the VAVTA website. You can find additional regional associations by contacting your state veterinary technician association or provincial animal health technician association.

Provincial Association websites:

- British Columbia: http://www.ahta.bc.ca
- Alberta: http://www.aaaht.com
- Saskatchewan: http://www.savt.ca
- Manitoba: E-mail: ghunker@mb.sympatico.ca
- Ontario: http://www.oavt.org
- Quebec: http://www.spg.qc.ca/atsaq
- Atlantic Provinces: EVTA E-mail: b.sutherland@ns.sympatico.ca

RELATED ORGANIZATIONS

American Animal Hospital Association (AAHA)
PO Box 150899
Denver, CO 80215-0899
Phone: (303) 986-2800; fax: (303) 986-1700

American Association for Laboratory Animal Science (AALAS)
Michael Sonday, Executive Director
9190 Crestwyn Hills Drive
Memphis, TN 38125
Phone: (901) 754-8620
Website: http://www.aalas.org

American Association of Veterinary State Boards (AAVSB)
3100 Main Street, Suite 208
Kansas City, MO 64111
Phone: (816) 931-1504; fax: (816) 931-1604

American Veterinary Medical Association (AVMA)
Suite 100, 1931 North Meacham Road
Schaumburg, IL 60173
Phone: (847) 925-8070; fax: (847) 925-1329
Website: http://www.avma.org

Association of Veterinary Technician Educators (AVTE)
Terry Teeple, DVM
Pierce College
9401 Farwest Drive SW
Tacoma, WA 98498
Phone: (253) 964-6668; fax: (253) 964-6599
Website: http://www.avte.net

Committee on Veterinary Technician Education and Activities (CVTEA)
AVMA
Suite 100, 1931 North Meacham Road
Schaumburg, IL 60173
Phone: (847) 925-8070; fax: (847) 925-1329
Website: http://www.avma.org

Northeast Veterinary Technician Educators Association (NEVTEA)
Amy Shields, CVT
Director of Nursing and Critical Care Veterinary Referral Center
340 Lancaster Avenue
Fraser, PA 19355
Phone: (610) 674-2950

Professional Examination Service (PES)
475 Riverside Drive
New York, NY 10115-0089
(For information regarding the Veterinary Technician National Examination or the AALAS Animal Technician Certification Program)

Veterinary Emergency and Critical Care Society (VECCS)
8015 Broadway, Suite 201
San Antonio, TX 78209

Veterinary Hospital Managers Association, Inc. (VHMA)
48 Howard Street
Albany, NY 12207-1608
Phone: (518) 433-8911
E-mail: vhma@caphill.com
Web site: http://www.vhma.org

Recommended Reading

The Veterinary Technician
Professional Journal by Veterinary Learning Systems
Aggie Kiefer, Editor-in-Chief
780 Township Line Road, Yardley, PA 19067
Phone: (800) 426-9119, Ext. 2447
E-mail: akiefer.vls@medimedia.com

NAVTA Journal
Monthly publication by NAVTA
PO Box 224, Battleground, IN 47920
Phone or fax: (765) 742-2216
E-mail: navta@navta.net

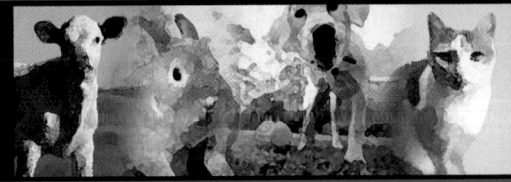

Restraint and Handling of Animals

DENNIS D. FRENCH • THOMAS N. TULLY, JR.

INTRODUCTION

Most people entering the field of veterinary medicine have had experience with some animals, but few have had the experience necessary to deal with all species that may be encountered. To assume all animals respond in the same manner is not correct and can be quite dangerous. Restraint techniques differ markedly among species, and the responses of different animals to restraint are also highly variable. The wise individual is able to ascertain what the body language of a particular animal means and respond to the actions of that animal appropriately. Animals that are herd oriented present unique problems for the uninitiated.

This chapter is intended to be a guide to the behavior, handling, and restraint of animals commonly encountered in veterinary practice. It is not intended to be an exhaustive text, but rather to provide a range of techniques to build confidence and competence.

Initial client reaction invariably results from how an animal is restrained and examined by veterinary personnel. The differences that exist in clients' perceptions of animal handling are as diverse as the animals on which veterinary technicians work. It is absolutely imperative that technicians and veterinarians appreciate the clientele by which they are employed and the differences in attitudes that these clients have with regard to restraint and examination of their animals. ■

INDICATIONS FOR RESTRAINT

The most obvious reason for restraint of an animal is to control it for an examination or a procedure. The reaction of the animal to unpleasant experiences, sometimes simply avoiding the people trying to restrain it, can be disastrous. Environmental factors must be considered when a plan for restraint is developed. Veterinary personnel should be aware from the time that they accept the animal from the owner that situations that are potentially dangerous for the animals may develop. Two dogs passing in the reception area may decide that they are mortal enemies, and a fight may ensue. Dogs and cats are generally examined on tables, and scrambling off the table may result in a damaging fall. Large animals are often held in extremely hazardous environments. Fences constructed of barbed wire can cause massive cuts to equine skin, an unacceptable outcome for all during attempts to catch a horse for a routine examination. Buildings with tin walls that do not extend completely underground will cause heel bulb lacerations when a horse wheels away from a would-be handler and catches its foot under the bottom of the tin. Protruding nails in a stall may cause skin lacerations or a puncture of the cornea as a horse spins away from a handler trying to halter it. Low sheds can result in severe damage to the head in both horses and cattle. Veterinary personnel must try to make the reception and examination areas as safe as possible. The unfortunate truth is that clients will blame the veterinary practice and the people involved if their animals are injured during an examination.

✎ TECHNICIAN NOTE

Assessing the situation before beginning any approach to an animal is necessary and extremely helpful to the practitioner.

Restraint for the purpose of physical examination or diagnostic or therapeutic procedures commonly performed on animals may be unpleasant for them, and most animals will attempt to escape or at least resist. To avoid excessive discomfort for the animal, the application of restraint should be to the minimum effective level. The procedure and the animal's response will determine the level of restraint. For example, the examination of a cat's mouth can usually be performed with a minimal hold on the animal, whereas the examination of a cow's mouth will require significant restraint to protect the cow and the examiner.

A major reason for proper restraint and handling is to prevent the animal from harming itself during the procedure. Venipuncture may result in torn vessels, hematomas, and free-flowing blood if the animal is not properly restrained for the procedure. In pigs, bleeding from the anterior vena cava without proper restraint may result in laceration of the vessel or the phrenic nerve and subsequent death. Rectal palpation of an inappropriately restrained horse may result in a rectal tear for the horse or serious musculoskeletal injury of the veterinary staff. Surgical procedures performed on inadequately restrained animals are doomed to failure. Restraining devices (Elizabethan collars, neck cradles) are used in many aspects of veterinary practice to protect the animal from self-mutilation following procedures.

Probably the most important reason for restraint is to protect the personnel involved in the procedure. All veterinary personnel rely on functioning body parts to perform their jobs and make a living. Slight injuries may result in significant loss of income or efficiency. Bruised and swollen hands from bites and scratches cannot assist in surgery. The use of crutches or wheelchairs severely limits mobility and restraint capabilities around large animals. Severe injuries, including disfigurement, or septicemia may result from bites. Kicks and body slams from large animals may also result in significant trauma to personnel, with subsequent loss of time and income. The veterinarian and associated personnel are legally responsible for any injuries to the client during performance of a veterinary procedure. This liability begins when the client enters the practice facility or the truck stops in the driveway. The liability includes injuries that occur during the initial capture of the animal.

> ✎ **TECHNICIAN NOTE**
>
> Protection of personnel involved in veterinary procedures may be the most important reason for the use of restraint.

Effective restraint is paramount to success of a veterinary practice. Quality practice begins with the physical examination, and this can only be accomplished with the animal properly restrained. Clients often base their impression of the care their animals receive on the manner in which their animals are restrained. The health and safety of the animals and people involved must be identified as the primary goal. Human perception of animal behavior can be used to better control and maneuver animals. This involves interspecies communication that is usually silent. The popularity of behavioral science and the "horse whisperers" is simply a study in animal-to-animal behavior into which humans have been interjected. The unspoken language of gestures, touches, and actions is a part of animal communication to which humans have become responsive.

> ✎ **TECHNICIAN NOTE**
>
> Clients often base their impression of the care their animals receive on the manner in which their animals are restrained.

We all possess innate abilities to control and manipulate animals; these abilities can be consciously developed according to interest or occupation. The perceptive student of animal communication may acquire these techniques quickly, and the use of these techniques will greatly facilitate handling of any animal. Caution and analysis of each situation are warranted, however, because animals that have disease do not react in the same manner as healthy animals. A healthy feedlot steer does not usually challenge pen riders, but a bad case of "foot rot" may make him charge the horse and rider in an effort to convince the threat to go away. Another consideration that will affect behavior, especially in herd situations, is the mixing of males and females. A normally docile stallion placed into a brood-mare band will protect his band of mares against intruders. The presence of young, unweaned animals still under the watchful eyes of their dams may totally change the expected reactions of a mare, cow, or sow.

Thoughtful assessment of the situation, careful application of the knowledge of species behavior, and the use of appropriate equipment will facilitate restraint of all animals.

ANIMAL PERCEPTION AND BEHAVIOR

All animals are aware of their environment and the changes occurring around them. They use their five senses just as we do, particularly sight, smell, and hearing. The question of how an animal senses your encroachment into its environment must be a primary consideration in approaching that animal.

SMELL

The sense of smell is well developed in all domestic mammals. The rabbit and cat have improved olfaction because of olfactory epithelium that is nearly 14 times more developed than that in humans.

Horses will snort when they encounter a smell with which they are unfamiliar. Bulls may react by pawing and blowing when they encounter a different smell. It is sometimes said that animals can smell fear. Behaviorists point out that body language is more likely to convey lack of confidence, and this may be misconstrued as the smell of fear. However, the language of smell undoubtedly has a more extensive vocabulary in animals than in humans.

HEARING

All domestic mammals have well-developed methods for collecting sound waves into the external ear. Domestic animals are able to move the pinnae, the skin-covered cartilaginous sound collectors of the ear, with muscles, which enables them to focus on the source of the sound. This is advantageous to the handler as an approach is made to a new animal. Slight sounds will elicit movement of the ears and allow the animal to become aware of the presence of someone new. Low, smooth, confidant tones will allow the animal to become comfortable with your presence. The response of the ear is important to assess the animal's attitude. The ears-back position in a horse or llama signals that the animal is upset or aggressive. A dog pricks its ears forward when dominant or actively aggressive, whereas a submissive dog wrinkles and flattens its ears. Cats with their ears pinned back should be considered dangerous.

> ✎ **TECHNICIAN NOTE**
> The position of an animal's ears provides an excellent clue to the attitude of the animal.

VISION

Domestic animals, with the exception of pigs, have a special layer behind the lens called the *tapetum* that permits them better vision in low light.

Herbivorous animals have wide fields of vision, enabling them to detect the encroachment of predators from various angles. This is particularly evident in the horse and rabbit, both of which enjoy nearly circumferential vision without moving the head.

> ✎ **TECHNICIAN NOTE**
> With the exception of pigs, domestic animals have a special layer behind the lens called the *tapetum,* which permits them better vision in low light.

The eyes of domestic animals focus by means of muscles controlling the shape of the lens. Most animals accommodate the eye on near objects much less readily than humans do. The horse has a particularly sluggish accommodation. What some handlers may perceive as fractious and spooky behavior may in fact be nothing more than the horse attempting to visually accommodate. This is particularly noticeable when an already nervous human makes fast movements near a horse. The horse moves about in a rapid manner, trying to ascertain what the human wants. Horses apparently have very acute vision at middle and far distances, which is not surprising for a prey species. Many of the behavioral displays of horses are visual in nature, and subtle movements by handlers at seemingly great distances will generate responses from horses.

The dog's ability to discriminate form and pattern is thought to be poor as compared with human abilities. This is particularly important when dealing with those dogs that are noted to be "fear biters."

Cats have excellent night vision, which is consistent with their nocturnal habits. They are also acutely aware of small movements, which facilitates the precision of their rush after stalking their prey. Unfortunately, this also enhances the ability of a fearful or vengeful feline patient to strike out against those humans who move too suddenly or come too close.

TOUCH

The sense of touch is becoming more important in the handling of animals. Behaviorists and trainers recommend that handlers touch horses on different parts of their bodies as a way of enhancing communication with them. Contact behaviors that appear to result from or resolve conflicts are the ones most described in handling. Dominant animals use biting, scratching, kicking, or striking to teach their young proper behavior. Dogs have been observed to bite or hold the scruffs of puppies' necks, hold their muzzles, or force them prone by the application of weight over the withers as a show of dominance if their behavior is unacceptable. This is why hanging dogs or shaking them by the scruff or collar is often a potent punishment. Horses kick or slam a shoulder into other horses to demonstrate dominance and make a point of their supremacy. Mares training foals and yearlings in a herd will actually keep a particularly hardheaded youngster out of the herd by biting and kicking at it. Some people will use blows to correct unacceptable equine behavior. However, when these techniques are used, the target must be carefully selected, and the individual must possess the physical strength to make the procedure effective. As a general rule, humans will end up hurting themselves much more than the horse they are trying to correct.

The actual method of how to touch animals is a matter of skill. A tentative, light touch or repeated patting makes many animals nervous and apprehensive. Steady, firm strokes are reassuring to most species. Watching behavior of animals in a natural setting provides the insight into how to most effectively touch them when they are nervous. You will never observe one animal slapping another to calm it down in a natural setting. Clever individuals learn to read the animals that they are asked to restrain and develop the touch necessary to keep them calm.

> ✎ **TECHNICIAN NOTE**
> The degree of restraint necessary for any animal is determined by the circumstances under which it is to be examined.

AGONISTIC BEHAVIORS

Agonistic behaviors are those associated with conflict. Many animals must be maneuvered into a position in which restraint is possible, or they must be restrained from the outset as a safety measure. These maneuvers are perceived by the animal as conflict, and the technician must understand the normal behavior of the particular species that he or she is asked to restrain to be effective in handling and restraint. Agonistic behaviors range from passive avoidance through the assertion of dominance to the extreme of aggression and fighting. In nature, overt aggressive attacks that lead to fights with animals of the same or different species are not common outside sexual or predatory behavior. Dominance and submissive behaviors represent the more common method of resolving disagreement over things such as territory and favors. Chapter 13 provides additional information on animal behavior.

Fight or Flight

When a stranger approaches an animal, the same basic principles apply, regardless of whether the animal is domestic or wild. Each species in a given environment has its own degree of response, but the factors or cues giving rise to the response are common to all animals in varying degrees. Each animal has a fight-or-flight distance. When that space is invaded, the animal goes into a state of alert. Herd animals demonstrate this by bunching together with a well-defined flight distance (Figure 1-1). In individual animals, reactions occur through activation of the sympathetic nervous system and the release of the hormone epinephrine from the adrenal glands. Epinephrine causes increased heart rate and subsequent increase in blood flow to the skeletal muscles, lungs, and brain. Further encroachment into the animal's space will lead to action that may take the form of avoidance (the cow or horse crashes through a fence, the dog runs off down the road) or aggression (the dog bites, the cow runs over the stranger). This action is aptly termed the *fight-or-flight response*. The response will vary from animal to animal of the same species and may vary from time to time for the same animal. When this happens, it is very difficult to come up with a good restraint plan.

AGGRESSIVE BEHAVIOR

Aggressive behavior is the form of agonistic or conflict behavior that leads to and includes fighting. Aggression is not the result of a single cause. The different forms of aggression are classified according to the stimuli or circumstances giving rise to the ferocity. The reader should refer to Chapter 14 for more information regarding animal behavior.

Irritability-Induced or Pain-Induced Aggression

Inevitably, pain-induced aggression is a common problem in the veterinary hospital and in field situations. Herd animals that have become incapacitated and are incapable of keeping up with the herd must resort to aggression to stay alive. Injections and certain manipulations, such as treatment of wounds, cause pain and discomfort that animals may resent. Even the initial injection of a local anesthetic can be most uncomfortable, no matter how skilled the anesthetist. The state of mind of the patient has a lot to do with the potential for aggressive behavior. If the animal is initially apprehensive and nervous, the probability for aggression is

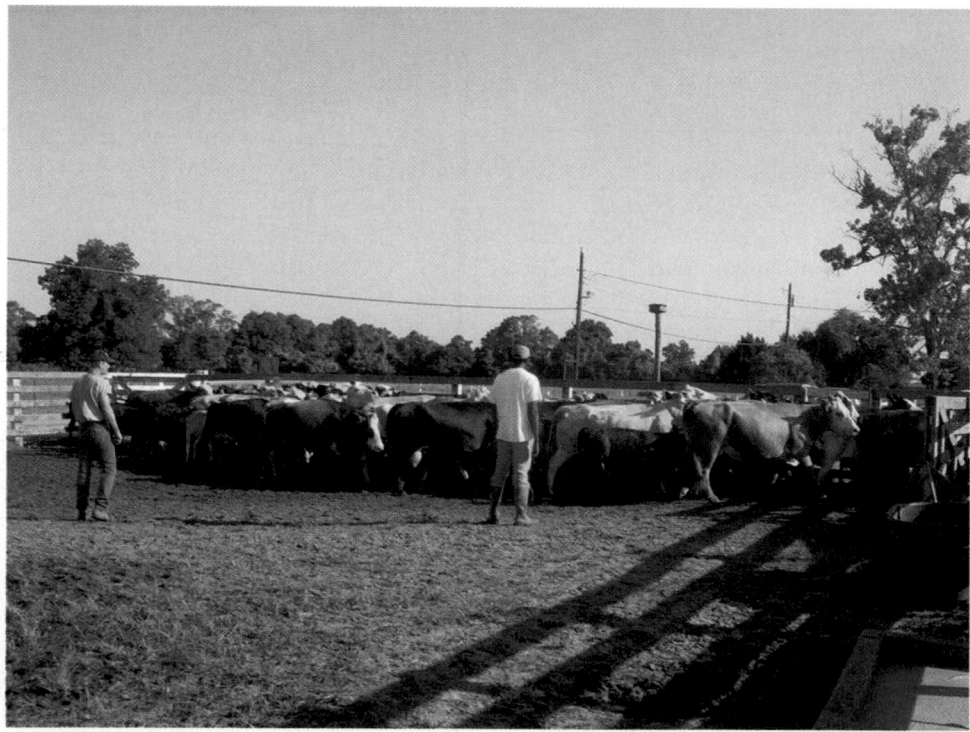

Figure 1-1 These cattle have established their flight zone, and the handlers are using that to their advantage as they move the cattle from one pen to the next. Note how the two handlers are alert yet not too demonstrative with their hands and arms. This keeps the cattle from becoming too agitated.

high. This is the reason that calming and familiarization of the patient are practiced whenever possible. Sedation may also be indicated for certain patients.

Maternal Aggression

All female domestic animals that are suckling their young are sensitized to interference with their offspring by strangers. The calmest, old brood mare in the herd may be extremely protective of her new foal. The bitch can be aggressive with strangers and even family members if she perceives a threat to her pups. A sow within earshot of her piglets when they are being restrained can become one of the most dangerous animals encountered. All parties working within a farrowing house must exercise caution, because the vocalization of any young piglet as it is manipulated can make all the sows in the house become sensitized.

> **✐ TECHNICIAN NOTE**
>
> All female domestic animals that are suckling their young are sensitized to interference with their offspring by strangers.

Predatory Aggression

Aggressive activity displayed by chasing and killing prey is observed in predatory domestic animals, such as the dog and cat, and is called *predatory aggression*. This form of aggression does not usually pose a threat to the animal handler, although large dogs may pull the handler down if they feel the urge to chase a cat while on leash.

Territorial Aggression

All domestic mammals have a degree of territorial domain. They will protect the area over which they range from intruders, and they may, in fact, exhibit territorial aggression. Separate groups of horses may share feeding sites and watering holes, but they remain apart from one another and retain control of their own separate home ranges. The domestic dog regards the yard as its territory or the territory of its pack (the dog's human family). Strangers are treated with suspicion, and this suspicion may lead to barking or attack. Dogs that harass the mail carrier or meter reader are acting within the norm of canine behavior. The female rabbit is strongly territorial in the captive situation. If a buck is taken to her cage, she will attack him aggressively, often causing serious injury. Thus the doe is always taken to the buck's cage for mating. This female territoriality may be associated with aggression that continues even when the nesting box is empty, and it can be directed at humans. While the concept of an "attack rabbit" may seem humorous, it becomes less so when one is reaching into the cage of an old doe and being growled at, struck, and bitten.

Fear-Induced Aggression

When an animal is terrified of an environment and the people in it and is not given an option to avoid the circumstances, it will resort to aggression. Fear is a common cause of aggression in dogs in such circumstances. Fear biting is the most commonly encountered type of attack in veterinary hospitals. The attack is not overtly dominant, and the dog is usually giving classic signs of being intimidated; avoiding direct eye contact with the head down, lips pulled back horizontally, ears flattened, and the tail between the legs (Figure 1-2). When the personal space of such a dog is encroached, a sudden attack may ensue. This is fear biting. The attack is usually confined to the proffered hand or forearm, and the purpose is simply to repel the invader.

Intermale Aggression

Aggression occurring between males can be a problem, particularly when stud animals are being kept together. Boars can be extremely vicious when confronting each other, and great care should be taken when handling them. A stallion can become extremely agitated when mixed with another stallion. Bulls and rams spend a great deal of time head butting and pushing one another around to establish the dominance order when they are turned out together.

Dominance Aggression

Certain dogs will establish their authority over a human family, other animals, and strangers because of their heritage as pack animals. Alternatively, a dog may accede to dominance from one family member but attempt to assert itself aggressively with other family members. Such animals are a menace in the clinic, since they will not only fear bite but also attack. Persuasion is of little value in handling these

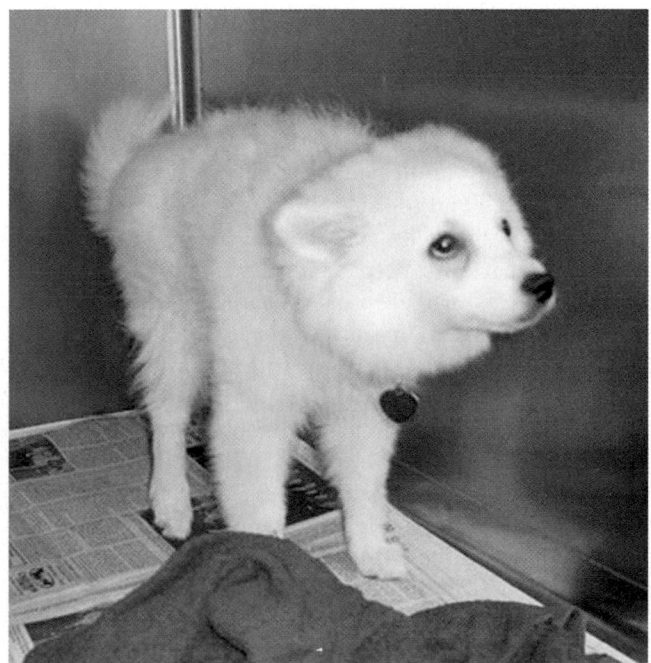

Figure 1-2 This dog demonstrates the posture of a classic "fear biter." Note the defensive stare with the ears laid back and the tail between the legs.

dogs. This type of animal is dangerous, and reliable restraint must be used at all times when handling them.

TYPICAL BEHAVIOR OF DOMESTIC ANIMALS IN AGGRESSION AND AVOIDANCE

Cattle

The individual that handlers should be most concerned about when dealing with cattle is the bull, regardless of size. Dairy breed bulls such as the Jersey and Holstein should be considered the most dangerous animals of all the species that veterinary personnel are asked to restrain or handle. They are powerful, unpredictable, and mean-spirited. Aggressive behavior is characterized by pawing the ground with the forefeet while holding the head with the frontal area nearly vertical with the ground and snorting. These bulls, after charging and knocking the person down, will make continued attempts to toss the victim, which will lead to goring if the bull still has horns. Bulls may also attempt to kneel on the victim or may continually smash the victim with their foreheads. Little can be done to dissuade or thwart a bull once this activity begins. Front-end loaders and pickup trucks have been used to try to push these animals away from their targets without success. Bulls, particularly the dairy breed types, should always be treated with the utmost respect and with the appropriate means of restraint and containment. Ironically, a hand-raised bull may prove more dangerous than an overtly aggressive and rarely handled one. The hand-raised bull may appear to be quite gentle, yet when approached, may react aggressively. Special handling considerations are made for those who work with semen donors at bull studs. These bulls are selected for their high-quality genetic potential, and their semen is worth considerable amounts of money. Insensitive handling before and during collection may give rise to reproductive behavior problems leading to decreased collection volumes and significant economic loss.

Aggressiveness in the heifer and cow seems to be directly related to breed and socialization. Dairy cows are generally very docile, probably because they are handled a great deal. Beef cows that have been handled frequently in a quiet, professional manner are very manageable. However, beef cattle that are raised on range with very little human interaction or those that are handled with lots of whipping and shouting tend to be apprehensive and may become quite aggressive. This aggressiveness is compounded when they are nursing calves.

The fight-or-flight distance for a herd of cattle will vary, depending on the previous degree and type of contact with humans. The handling of dairy cattle and beef cattle differs greatly. Flight distance for dairy cows is extremely short, with the animal veering off only when directly confronted by the handler. Most dairy cattle are used to a number of different people being around them during milking time and do not resent the introduction of someone new into the herd. This makes handling dairy cows easier for veterinary

personnel. Beef cattle have a much longer flight space, which is accentuated when they sense a new presence in a field or pen. It is common for ranchers to be able to walk or drive among their cattle at very close range. When a new pickup or person enters the pasture, the cattle's heads come up and they will gradually move further away. If the cattle are approached too quickly, they will break into a disorganized run, which makes them nearly impossible to maneuver. It is important to realize the impact that outsiders have on a herd of beef cattle before trying to handle and examine individuals.

The use of props as an extension of the body makes maneuvering cows easier. Cattle view canes, stock whips, or wiffle paddles used by a person on foot as an extension of the body. If the cattle can be kept calm, the visual barrier created by these devices allows the handler to maneuver them from pen to pen. If cattle are accustomed to being observed from horseback, maneuvering a herd can be quite easy for one or two riders. Mixing riders and walkers in a pasture is not a good idea and should only be done as a last resort when trying to maneuver a herd of cattle.

Calves

Calves are inquisitive and will become very attentive to the presence of someone new. The calf stretching its head or neck toward the new handler is the usual posture (Figure 1-3). Darting movements will cause the calf to panic, veer, and run away. The approach toward a calf should be slow and deliberate with the hands slightly away from the sides of the body. No loud noises are necessary, and movement of the hands and arms should be kept to a

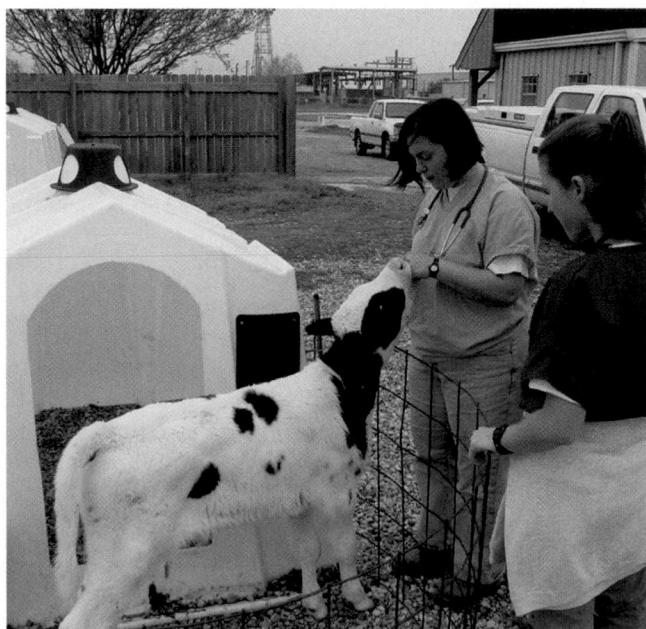

Figure 1-3 This Holstein calf demonstrates the curiosity that most bovids have at an early age. The heifer has come to the new handler without any reservations.

minimum. Using a fence line or wall, the handler should move to cut off escape routes and negotiate the calf into a corner and then grab it with one arm under the jaw; the other hand should reach and grab the tail.

Cats

Aggressive behavior in cats should never be underestimated. They can be formidable patients in situations of conflict because they will use the claws of all four feet, they have razor-sharp teeth, and when stressed they seem to have a spinal cord that is made much like a Slinky, which allows them to go in many different directions at once. It should be remembered that cats stalk their prey and run only short distances to pounce. They are stealth aggressors. The true speed of a cat never becomes apparent until it is actively avoiding conflict. When handling cats in any environment, all doors and windows must be closed to prevent escape.

> **TECHNICIAN NOTE**
> When handling cats in any environment, close all doors and windows to prevent escape.

Dogs

Overtly aggressive behavior in dogs is a significant social problem and one that will present difficulties for veterinary personnel. Dominance and submission are important in communication between two dogs in a conflict situation. Fixing the other animal in a direct stare signals dominance. The ears are raised and angled forward. The front end of the body is held high, and the hackles on the back of the neck are raised. The head is held up, and the lips curl to reveal the incisor and canine teeth. The tail will be raised. The clinical stare of veterinary personnel as they examine a dog can be interpreted as a dominance challenge by a dog.

Lowering the front end of the body and avoiding direct eye contact demonstrate the submissive role. Usually the tail will be held between the legs, and the dog may squat and urinate or defecate. The spine may adopt an S shape, and the animal may lie down on its side or back, raising the legs and exposing the undefended belly.

When confronted by a person, a dog may demonstrate potential aggression by adopting the dominantly aggressive posture, or it may adopt a submissive stance. The ears will flatten on the back of the head, and the lips may be pulled back at the corners of the mouth into a "grin." The tail is held between the legs. A dog in the active or dominant aggressive posture may attack if the threat is not removed from its fight-or-flight distance. A dog in this posture will bite only if you attempt to encroach on its space. Some dogs may show active aggression only when the owner is present. The protectiveness may actually be possessiveness as the dog defends its own favored object. Removing the owner from this situation may resolve the conflict. The opposite may occur when handling dogs that have developed a bond with their usual handlers. These dogs may be quite aggressive

without their human partner in the examination room. Retrievers, herding dogs, and guard dogs that tend to associate closely with only one individual may be quite difficult to handle without their owners present.

Certain dogs do not attempt to resolve conflict by dominance or aggression, preferring to avoid it if at all possible. Those that skillfully avoid conflict are described as having a passive defense reflex. Dogs that tend to face conflict are said to have an active defense reflex.

Horses

Blatant aggressiveness in the horse is not common. However, certain horses can be nasty with their aggression. This is most commonly seen in horses that are stalled most of the time. Racehorses and breeding stallions seem to be the worst offenders. Aggressive behavior may be observed on brood mare farms, with mares protecting new foals and stallions protecting their band of mares. Lunging forward and biting, kicking with the hind legs, and striking with the front legs characterize the aggressive acts of the horse. Although the field of vision of the horse is nearly 360 degrees, the binocular field of vision is only 60 to 70 degrees in front of the animal. Binocular vision is required for judging distance; therefore vision outside this range requires movement of the head and sometimes the entire body to allow the horse to further investigate what it perceives as a threat.

The approach to a horse should not be made from the blind spot directly behind the horse. The horse, as it detects new objects or people in its environment, will raise its head and observe. If no threat is perceived, the horse resumes its previous activity. If the threat is perceived as real, the head turns toward the object, the neck is raised, and the ears will turn toward the object. The nostrils will become dilated to further evaluate the threat. The tail will also become elevated, and the muscles of the torso and lower limbs will become more rigid, ready for fight or flight. Occasionally, the horse will snort, further alerting other horses to the presence of a potential threat. A mare with a foal will usually nicker, and a foal will move to the other side of its dam. Further encroachment results in rapid movement away from the intruder. If the horse is in a stall, it will circle rapidly away, always keeping its hind end toward the intruder.

> **TECHNICIAN NOTE**
> The approach to a horse should not be made from the blind spot directly behind the horse.

Pigs

Aggressive behavior in domestic pigs has serious economic and physical consequences. Adult boars that are mixed together will circle and threaten each other with grunts and jaw snapping. Fighting commences in the side-to-side position, with sideways pushing and slashing at one another with the tusks. Solid panels of plywood should be used to separate the combatants. Commercial pigs are reared in groups, which provide plenty of opportunity for fighting. When new pigs are introduced into a group, fighting will occur, especially if living space and trough space are limited. Introducing a sow into an established group may induce savage attacks and even deaths. Allowing more space and diversions for the group may reduce aggression.

Large numbers of unfamiliar pigs adapt better than smaller numbers. There is less fighting, probably because dominance is more difficult to establish in the larger social groups. Avoidance behavior in young pigs in confined areas involves running into corners and huddling, shoving, and climbing over one another. This does not present a problem if small groups are huddled, but larger groups that pile up may produce traumatic lesions and, in severe cases, death from suffocation.

Remember that the lactating sow can be extremely dangerous because of maternal aggression. When handling suckling pigs, always remove the sow to a secure area, out of earshot if possible.

> ✎ **TECHNICIAN NOTE**
>
> The lactating sow can be extremely dangerous because of maternal aggression.

Sheep

Avoidance behavior in sheep is the basis of maneuvering the flock. When sheep are approached, they will flock together and move as a single unit. This herding behavior is well understood by dogs. By carefully controlling their posture, speed of movement, and distance from the flock, dogs use the sheep's avoidance behavior to maneuver the flock into an enclosure. This is one of the most fascinating and complex interspecies relationships in domestic animal management.

Aggression between rams may lead to injuries between the combatants. Handling these rams may also be difficult because of the willingness of the ram to challenge the handler. Rams are most dangerous when they attempt to head butt and therefore should be treated with respect.

MANAGEMENT ETHOLOGY

Ethology is the study of animal behavior (see also Chapter 14). Capture, handling, and restraint might be called management ethology, which is the study of animal behavior as a means of determining how best to maneuver and control animals. The approach and handling techniques that are described for each species are in harmony with the typical behavior of the animals that we are asked to restrain, and the physical techniques described are compatible with their anatomy. Humans have great powers of observation, and it is important for students of the animal industries to enhance their powers of observation regarding animal behavior. Knowledge of body systems and anatomic structure is clearly important, but there is no substitute for alertness, observation, and perception of how the animal is reacting to its environment and to the presence of veterinary personnel. Mental preparation must begin well in advance of any potentially dangerous restraint situation. Confidence and knowledge that ensure the handler of a correct assessment in any situation will be acquired over time.

CAPTURE AND RESTRAINT OF HORSES

A cardinal rule when approaching any animal, *especially* a horse, is not to startle it. The handler should always make his or her presence known by talking or calling to the horse. Many horses have learned that being captured leads to work or some sort of unpleasantness, and these horses will practice avoidance. Horses also do not like to be closely confined or "squeezed." Close quarters will make many horses anxious, and some will attempt to escape, which may result in injury to the horses and people involved. By calling to a horse, the handler begins to have an appreciation of how that particular animal is going to respond. Refer to Chapter 28 for additional comments and information about restraint of horses.

> ✎ **TECHNICIAN NOTE**
>
> A cardinal rule when approaching any animal, especially a horse, is not to startle it.

The normal flight distance of most horses is between 3 and 10 meters (m). Events that occur outside this radius are of little concern to the horse. Within this area, sudden movements or sharp noises may easily startle it. Always be sure that the horse is observing you as you approach. A horse that is looking at you is less likely to be startled than one looking off at some other object. Be aware that if the horse decides to become nervous, the first evasive maneuver that it will perform is to wheel away, leaving you facing its hindquarters.

It should be obvious that approaching a horse from the rear should be avoided. Given the horse's zone of vision and its blind spot, the horse is not likely to see a person directly behind it. A horse's kicking zone extends 1.8 to 2.5 m behind it. The furthest extension of the heels is the most dangerous and is the area of potentially fatal kicks to the head or chest. Horses usually kick to the rear, rather than to the side, but many of them can "cow kick," or kick to the side very well. Therefore it is wise to allow a space of at least 3 m behind and to the side of a horse when dealing with the rear quarters of the horse. The other alternative is to stay in direct contact with the horse as you maneuver about the hind end (Figure 1-4). Staying close to the hindquarters will not allow the full force of a kick and will keep the force of the blow low on the recipient's body. This does not mean that the blow will not be painful or damaging. However, a fractured tibia is a less serious injury than a fractured skull. Grasping the tail may discourage some horses from kicking.

The prospective handler should also never stand directly in front of a horse. A horse that becomes agitated may strike out with a front foot and leg at any time. Agitated horses may also attempt to bite the handler.

The initial approach to the horse is best accomplished from the front and left side (Figure 1-5). The left side of the horse in equine terminology is known as the *near side.* This is the side from which the horse is accustomed to being handled because of tradition and the fact that most people lead their horses with their right hands. The first point of contact for the handler on the horse should be the withers. The handler should have a slightly outstretched arm that is no higher than his or her shoulder. The handler should make some low, confidence-building conversation as he or she moves toward the horse. This goes back to the natural behavior of the horse, from mares licking their foals to the social interaction between horses in which they will rub each other on the withers. If the horse moves away, the handler should stop and stay still until the horse has quieted again. Many times, if the handler will turn slightly away from the horse and not look directly at it, the horse will turn back to the handler (Figure 1-6). This movement mimics the communication found in herds of horses when an outsider is finally "welcomed" into the herd. It is always wise to move in slow increments without raising your hands or voice. Presenting the hands in an open and empty manner may help the horse to gain confidence. Sometimes it is beneficial to squat down. This works reasonably well with young foals and some horses. The shorter stature probably makes the figure less threatening and increases the horse's curiosity. Do not rush toward the horse at any time. Horses will assume you are giving chase and continue to move away, and some can become quite panicked. Once the would-be handler is behind the horse, the horse perceives even more of a threat, since it cannot see the presumed intruder.

The approach to halter the horse should also be unhurried and without sudden movements. Keeping the lead rope or halter hidden by your side may assist in the capture of the skittish horse. A small-diameter catch rope may aid in the capture of the horse's neck (Figure 1-7). The rope may be carried up along the neck after the horse's confidence has been gained by a moment of petting at the withers. If the horse moves away, attempt to stay with it by moving

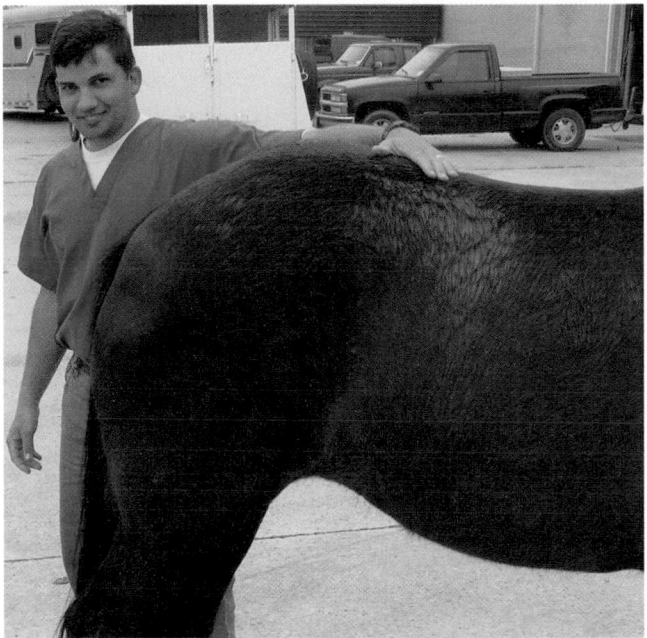

Figure1-4 Note how the handler maintains contact with the horse as he moves from the near to the far side of the horse. This is especially important because he is in the horse's blind spot.

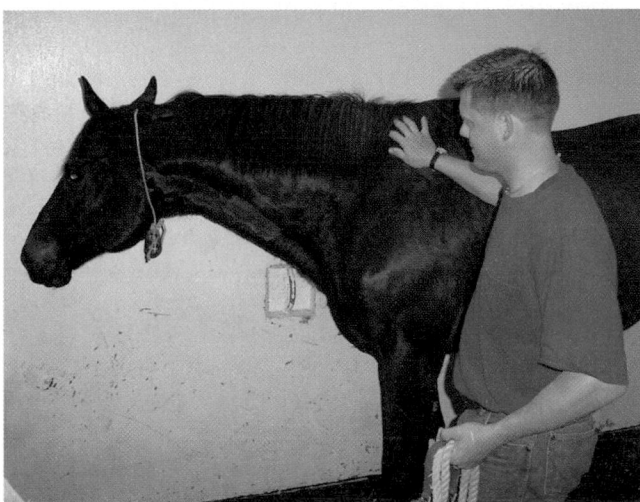

Figure 1-5 Initial approach to the horse should be from the left, or near, side. Note how the right hand leads to touch the horse at the withers. The left hand holds the halter and lead rope low and to the handler's side to avoid initiating an avoidance reaction.

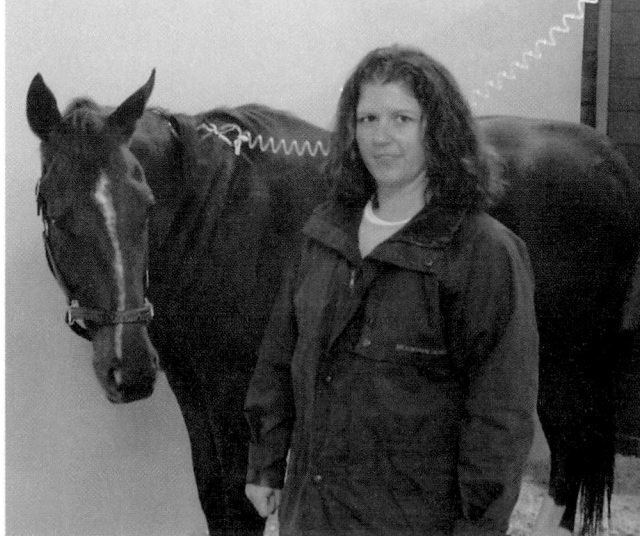

Figure 1-6 Note how the horse's ears and head are directed toward the would-be handler, almost as if the horse wants to know what is going to happen next.

along-side and holding onto the mane. Most horses will have sense enough to know that you mean business if you stay with them at this time.

When the horse is standing quietly, loop a rope around the neck by passing the rope over the horse's neck with the right hand and reaching under the neck to grab the free end with the left hand. When placing the rope over the neck, start as low on the back as possible. Remember that slow and steady movements are the key to success. Once the rope is around the neck, the horse may be held in the loop, and the rope can be maneuvered to the throat-latch area. The halter can then be placed by sliding the nose band over the nose and passing the crown strap to the right hand and then bringing the strap over the horse's head for fastening.

The horse that does not respond to any of the previously described techniques becomes the biggest problem encountered in a field service practice. The arrival of veterinary personnel may trigger memories of previous contact that the horse does not want to have repeated. The usual reaction is for the horse to move as far away from the handlers as possible. Of course, the simple solution is to have the horse caught before arrival of the veterinary team. However, this is not always possible. The usual solution to this problem is bribery with a handful or bucket of grain, which will entice the horse to approach or at least be approached. It is best to hold the bribe in the left hand and turn at right angles to the horse so that the neck is within easy reach for petting. As the horse's confidence is gained with some firm strokes along its shoulder, the right hand can then be eased around the neck to allow capture. Many horses will attempt to wheel

away when the arm is first placed over the neck, and this is where the small rope may be of assistance as a restraint aid. It is desirable to not allow horses to escape the first time, because if they do it once, they are likely to persist and become even harder to capture the second time. A horse that persists in whirling away becomes a candidate for trapping or, in extreme cases, roping.

Many horses that are impossible to catch in an open field will give up in an enclosed space. However, some become exceptionally nervous in a small area and will kick or try to jump out when approached. The use of another haltered, calm horse within the stall to trap the nervous one will work in most of these cases. Similar to catching an unbroken foal, one handler will use the calm horse to trap the other in a corner. Then with slow and steady movements, beginning at the withers, the second handler eases up the neck with a rope and makes the loop, which will allow temporary restraint of the nervous horse. A second technique that may be used is to have a solid panel that may be used to "squeeze" the horse into a corner. The panel needs to be sturdy enough to withstand the horse pushing against it and be movable enough to allow the handlers to back away in case the horse "blows up." This should be used as a last resort in attempting to capture a nervous horse. Remember that exciting a horse like this is self-defeating. Excited horses lose whatever sense they have and in fear will go over, under, or through whatever containment devices are present.

TECHNICIAN NOTE

Roping horses is the last thing any sane individual wants to do.

It is nearly impossible to rope a horse in a field, and holding on to the horse after it has been successfully roped is also very difficult. Dallying the rope off to the bumper of a truck is not an easy maneuver to accomplish, and then the roper must be able to stay out of the way of the rope as the horse swings back and forth on the other end. If you must rope a horse, only attempt to do so in a small, sturdy enclosure, such as a wooden round pen. Do not use a round pen made of pipes. This is an invitation to disaster! It is better to leave the horse uncaught than to have to destroy it because it became hung in pipes and fractured a leg. There are many trainers available who have the talents necessary to train both the horse and owner to get the horse comfortable enough with humans to be caught. The owner should contact these individuals before veterinary personnel make an attempt to rope a horse.

Horses that demonstrate signs of dangerous behavior or viciousness should not be given the opportunity to harm veterinary personnel by their physical proximity. Running the horse into a sturdy, small alleyway can be a very effective technique to capture the horse's head. Slow, calm movements must be maintained during this effort as well.

Other alternatives that may be used as a means of capture, such as tranquilization or anesthesia, do not require being close to the horse. The use of pole syringes, dart guns, and

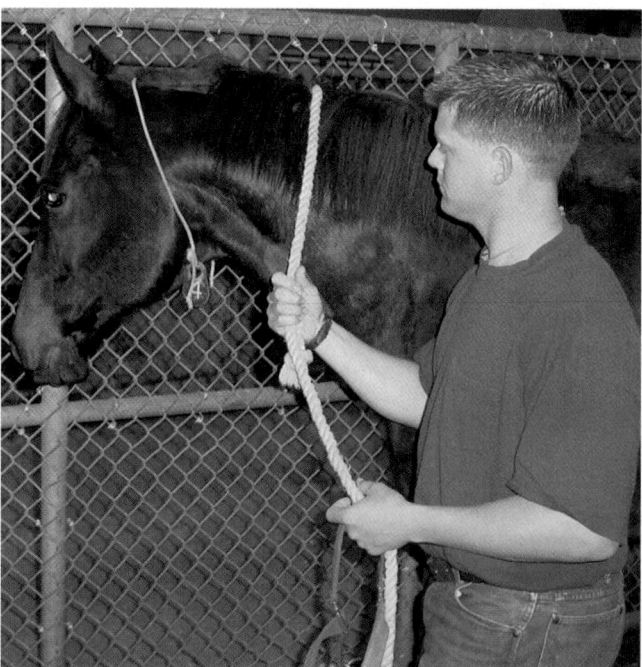

Figure 1-7 The use of a small rope looped over the horse's neck will aid in controlling the horse's head and allow the handler to place the halter over the nose.

capture guns, although not common in equine practice, can save handlers from serious injury.

CAPTURE AND RESTRAINT OF FOALS

Newborn foals act from instinct in avoiding strange creatures and will hide behind their dams for safety. Therefore capture of foals is somewhat more difficult and usually requires two people. Undoubtedly, these foals will not be halter-broken, and if they are sick or injured, they do not need the increased stress that accompanies training to halter. The easiest way to capture a suckling foal is to first catch the mare and back her in a corner of a stout wall or solid fence, allowing her foal to come into the corner between the wall and the mare. The barrier should not have any holes that the foal may try to climb through. Flimsy barriers or barbed wire fences should never be used in an attempt to capture foals. The handler of the mare should realize that when the foal starts to struggle against the restraint, it may vocalize in fear and the mare might try to attack those who appear to threaten her foal. The mare handler must be prepared to move the mare to a location away from the foal and its handlers immediately after capture of the foal.

The mare should be positioned about the length of the foal away from the corner of the barrier, forming an open box in the corner of the barrier. One person should then slowly go behind the foal; invariably, the foal will cower to

the hindquarters of the mare (Figure 1-8). The foal should be approached midway between the head and tail with the knowledge that once it senses hands or arms on it, it will try to escape by bolting, rearing, or kicking. Most commonly, the foal will bolt forward, into the mare's hindquarters, and the person should grab under the foal's neck and at the tail at this time. The tail should be held from underneath with the palm facing up. Grasping the tail is the most secure way to hold the hindquarters, even though the foal may be uncomfortable. It is possible for one person to restrain the foal after this by grabbing the tail and holding it straight up over the back, keeping the other arm under the foal's neck (Figure 1-9). With bigger foals, two people are necessary for restraint, although the technique is similar. The first person advances toward the hindquarters of the foal as previously described and makes the initial contact with the hindquarters of the foal. The mare is then moved forward slightly, and the second person passes behind the mare and grabs under the foal's neck. Handlers may have to push the foal against a fence until the foal stops struggling (Figure 1-10). There is a tendency to lift small foals off the ground when accomplishing this task, which is poor form. When the foal loses its footing, it may become more frightened and struggle more vigorously and batter the shins of the handler.

Attempts to capture foals only by the neck result in a rapid reverse by the foal and subsequent escape. Once a foal escapes, just like an adult horse, it becomes much harder to capture. Veterinary personnel should not contribute to the negative experiences of a foal. Extra care and gentle techniques should be used to get the foal to develop trust in people as much as possible.

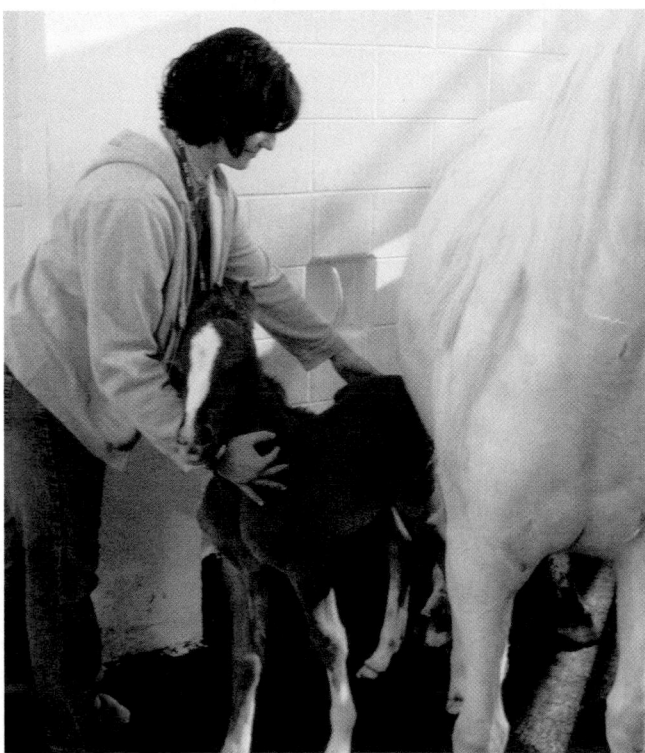

Figure 1-8 The mare is backed into a corner and the foal is driven in beside her to safely capture the foal. Note how the handler keeps the foal next to the mare. This is important in keeping the mare as quiet as possible.

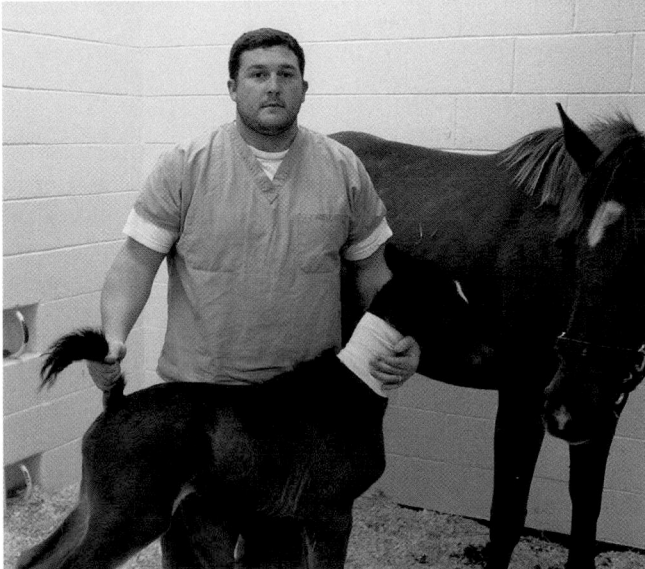

Figure 1-9 The handler must move in swiftly from the side of the foal and capture the tail first and then sweep the arm under the neck of the foal. The mare handler must move her to a safe location at the same time to protect the individual holding the foal.

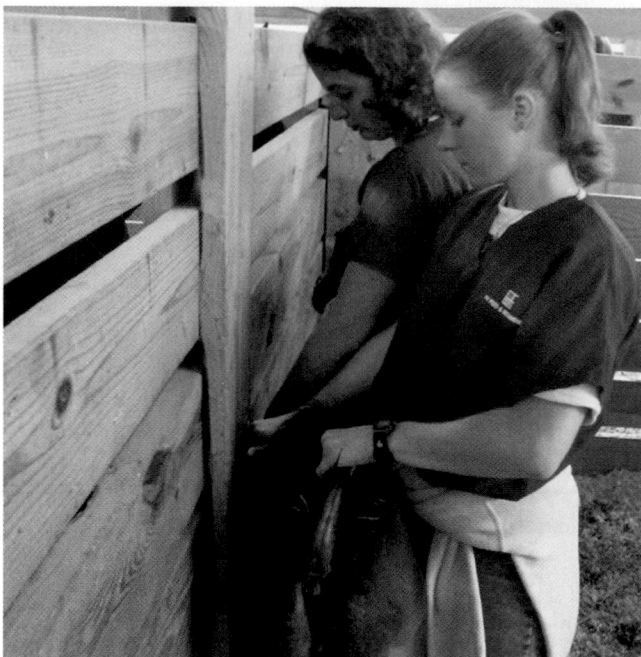

Figure 1-10 Two people may be needed to capture larger foals. The first approaches the foal from the rear, and the second comes around behind the mare and grabs the foal under the neck. The foal is then moved toward a solid wall for support.

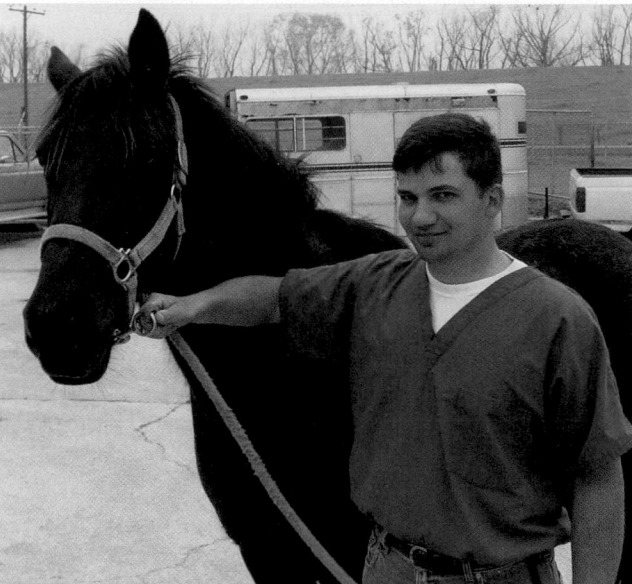

Figure 1-11 Halter and lead rope correctly placed on a horse. Note the position of the handler and the position of the arm. This allows the handler ample opportunity to sense impending movements.

After successful capture of the foal, it is usually in the best interest of all to position the mare and foal so that they face each other. They should be as close as possible without the mare becoming a nuisance for the procedure being performed. It is generally not recommended to separate the mare and foal because they both will fret until they are rejoined.

HALTER AND LEADS

The halter is the basic restraint tool for horses, and a lead shank should always be attached to the halter. Horses should never be led by the halter alone; a lead should always be attached (Figure 1-11). The halter and rope shank may be inadequate for some tasks. Halters that have rings at the side of the nosepiece may be made more effective if a chain lead is passed from one side to the other. The lead is snapped on the side of the halter that is away from the handler after being passed through the loop near the handler, usually on the near side. This arrangement allows finer control of the direction of the horse's nose and, when snapped against the bridge of the nose, reinforces the authority of the restraint because of the discomfort it causes. The chain lead should come in contact with the horse very lightly, if at all, when the horse is being led. Only when the horse misbehaves should the chain be used. Constant pressure is worrisome to the animal and does not leave the handler any reserve to use if necessary.

> **TECHNICIAN NOTE**
>
> Lead shanks should always be used when handling horses, and a chain shank should be used only when the horse misbehaves.

There are three possible positions for the chain lead on the halter. The least authoritative is under the jaw, which causes a squeeze around the nose. Horses with tender chins or those that are not accustomed to a chain lead may throw their heads or lunge backward when the lead is pulled. Horses that sense a squeezing of the nose as a signal to back up must be carefully restrained to respond correctly to this type of lead. It is often necessary to release pressure to allow the horse to stop its reverse. The chain over the nose is very effective in controlling many horses (Figure 1-12). The top of a horse's nose is sensitive, and a pull on the lead with the chain across the nose will make the horse drop the nose and stop forward progress. Very few stallions should be led without this technique. A variation of this technique is to carry the chain across the nose and then to the cheek-piece connection of the halter (Figure 1-13). This gives the handler far more control of the horse's head and nose. The most severe method of chain lead restraint is passing the chain over the upper lip and onto the gums of the upper jaw (Figure 1-14). This method works very well with horses that have a bad attitude and need to be reminded about the "chain" of command. When this technique is used, it is imperative that the chain be used only when the horse is

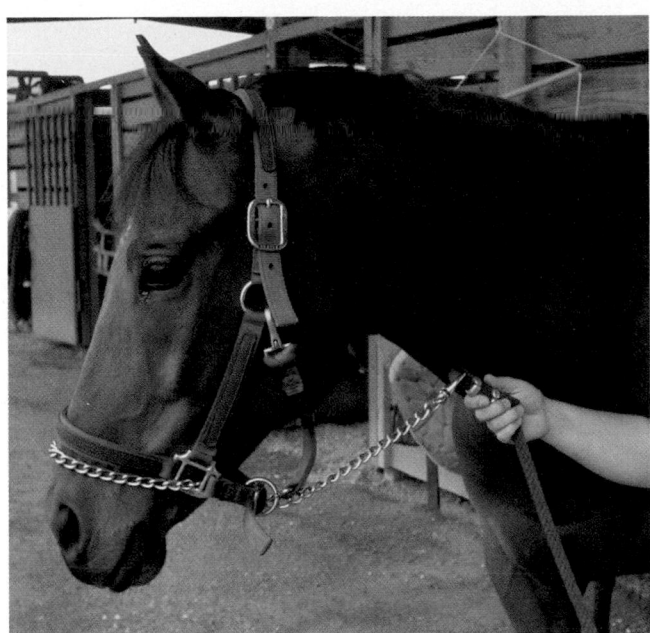

Figure 1-12 Lead shank with a chain positioned across the bridge of a stallion's nose to allow for more control.

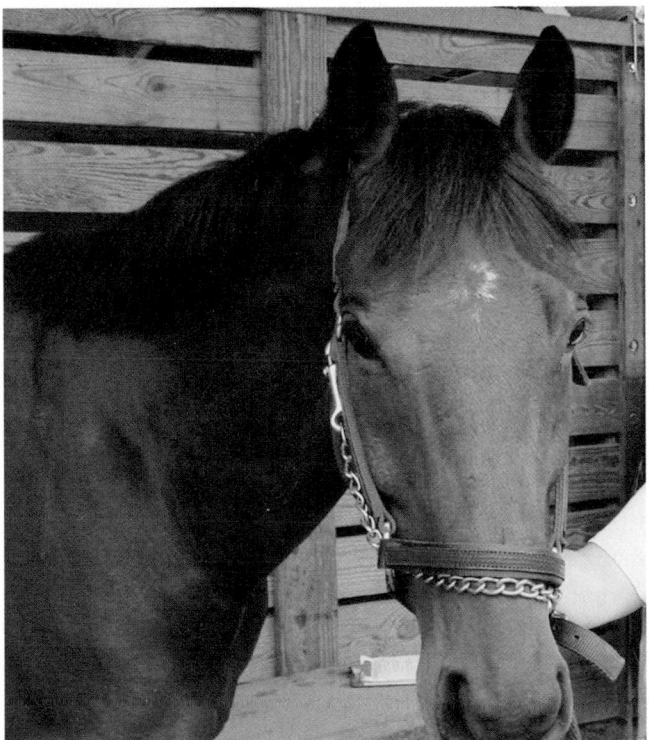

Figure 1-13 Lead shank across nose of this horse and then to the cheek piece of the halter. This allows the handler much more control of a feisty horse.

misbehaving, and it should only be used once or twice to get the horse's attention. Repeated attempts to restrain a horse with a chain may cause extreme resentment from the horse. When used correctly, this method of restraint replaces the use of a twitch and provides the handler with much

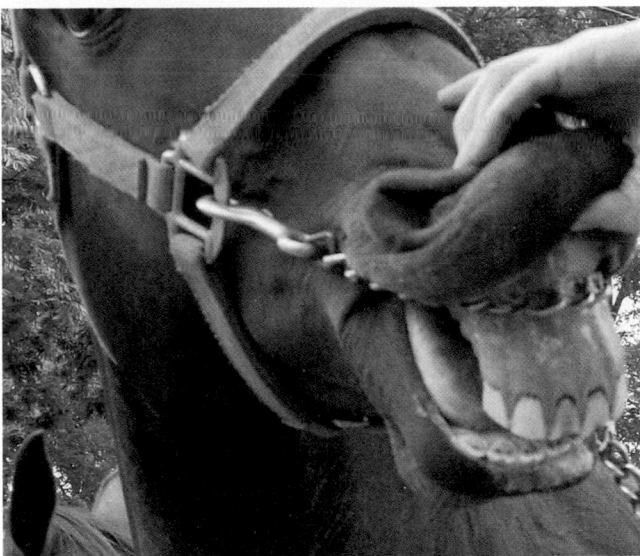

Figure 1-14 The chain of the lead shank has been placed under the top lip of this horse as an addition to the restraint. This technique maximizes the control for the handler and replaces the use of a twitch in many instances.

more stopping power over the horse. If the horse continues to resist, chemical restraint is warranted.

TYING THE HORSE

A horse should never be tied with a chain over or under its nose. This is an invitation for disaster. Seldom will it be desirable for a handler to tie a horse in order to perform a procedure. When a horse must be tied, the equipment must be strong and sound. The halter, rope, and whatever the rope is tied around must be in premier shape. Snaps on a rope, for example, often give way when a horse jerks back on them unless they are manufactured very well. If something breaks (the rope, halter, or post), the horse will be free and may have previously learned to pull back as an escape whenever it was tied. Another serious problem that can result from the horse pulling back occurs when it goes over backward and sustains head or neck trauma on landing. A horse should be tied to objects that are at the level of its shoulder or higher to prevent it from pawing and getting a foot over the rope. This also prevents the horse from trying to graze and becoming entangled in the tie rope. Horses should also be tied short; only 60 cm of rope should be present from the halter to the post to prevent the horse from having too much play in the rope and getting in trouble (Figure 1-15). Once a horse is tied, care should be taken to prevent the introduction of hazardous objects that might spook the horse into the area, and the horse should never be left unattended. The shorter the horse is tied, the less likely it is to get into trouble.

One technique that may be used to restrain (or train) a fitful horse is to place a cotton rope around the midsection of the horse just behind the rib cage and then pull it

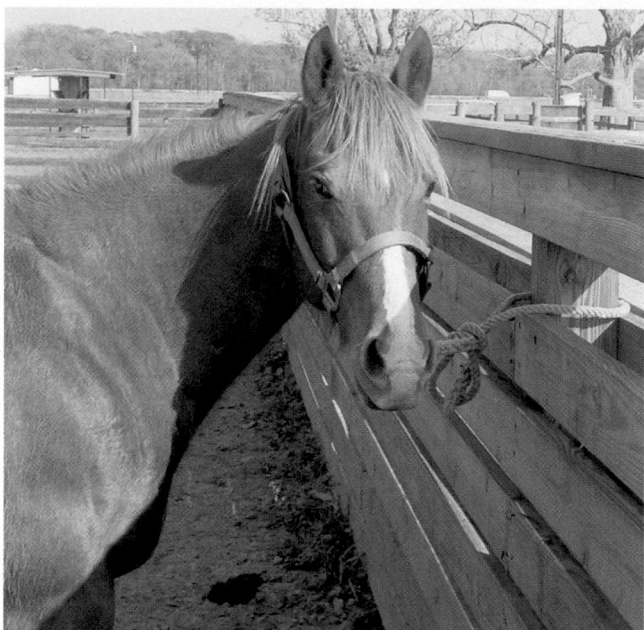

Figure 1-15 Properly tied horse at a rail. Note the level of the tie and the short amount of rope between the post and the halter.

through between the front legs and through the bottom of the halter. This rope is tied slightly shorter than the halter rope. The basis of this technique is that the horse will hit the cotton rope first and feel the pull against its abdomen, causing it to move forward and release pressure on the rope (Figure 1-16).

> **✎ TECHNICIAN NOTE**
>
> In general, horses should always be held, rather than tied, for veterinary procedures.

For veterinary purposes, it is generally preferable to hold a horse rather than tie it. Also, it is imperative for the holder to stand on the same side of the horse as the veterinarian, so that the horse's head, rather than its body or hindquarters, may be directed toward the practitioner (Figure 1-17). If the handler is on the opposite side and the handler bails out, the head of the horse follows the handler, leaving the back end of the horse swinging directly into the veterinarian. When the head is controlled and the horse acts up, the worst that will happen is that the body of the horse will swing away from both handler and veterinarian. No matter what the circumstances, this technique should be used, because in an emergency situation self-preservation of the holder will overcome protection of the practitioner.

THE TWITCH

The twitch is a nerve-stimulating device that may immobilize horses and can be helpful in equine restraint. Most twitches are applied to the upper lip of the horse. The most innocuous is the humane twitch, which is a hinged pair of

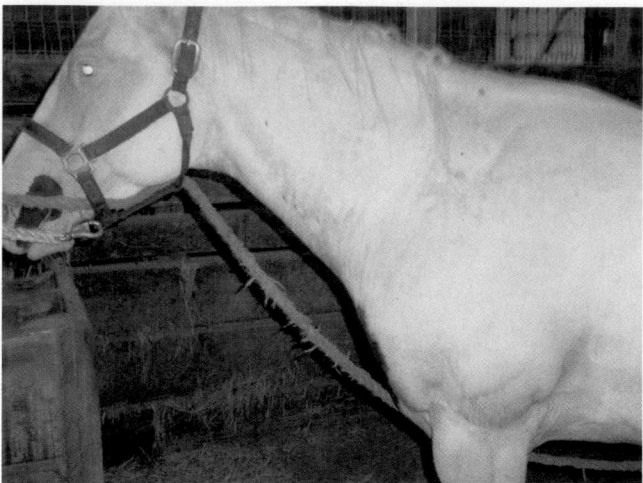

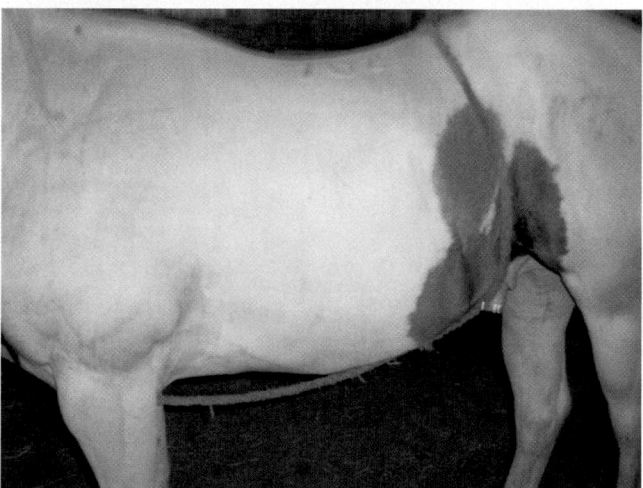

Figure 1-16 The technique necessary to place a belly rope on a horse that will not stand tied. **A,** A soft cotton rope is placed around the horse's abdomen and then run between the front legs. **B,** The rope is then run down the halter and tied, slightly shorter than the halter rope. Remember that most procedures performed by veterinary personnel will be done with the horse in hand.

long handles that squeeze down over the sides of the lip and may then be secured at the bottom by a thong and snapped back to the halter. The major advantage of this twitch is that once it is applied, it need not be held in place (Figure 1-18). Therefore one person may restrain a horse that is acting up. The disadvantage is that the pressure is fairly mild and most horses ignore it. More traditional twitches rely on a loop and a leverage device. The loop is either of chain or rope and is placed on the lip and tightened by twisting the leverage device. The leverage may be from a piece of wood or pipe that is about 50 cm long. The loop needs to be seated on the lip behind the heavy gristle pad at the tip and ahead of the nostrils. This area may be hard to find on thick-nosed horses. Horses that have been twitched become quite wise and will throw their heads into the air and tighten their lips when attempts are made to apply the twitch.

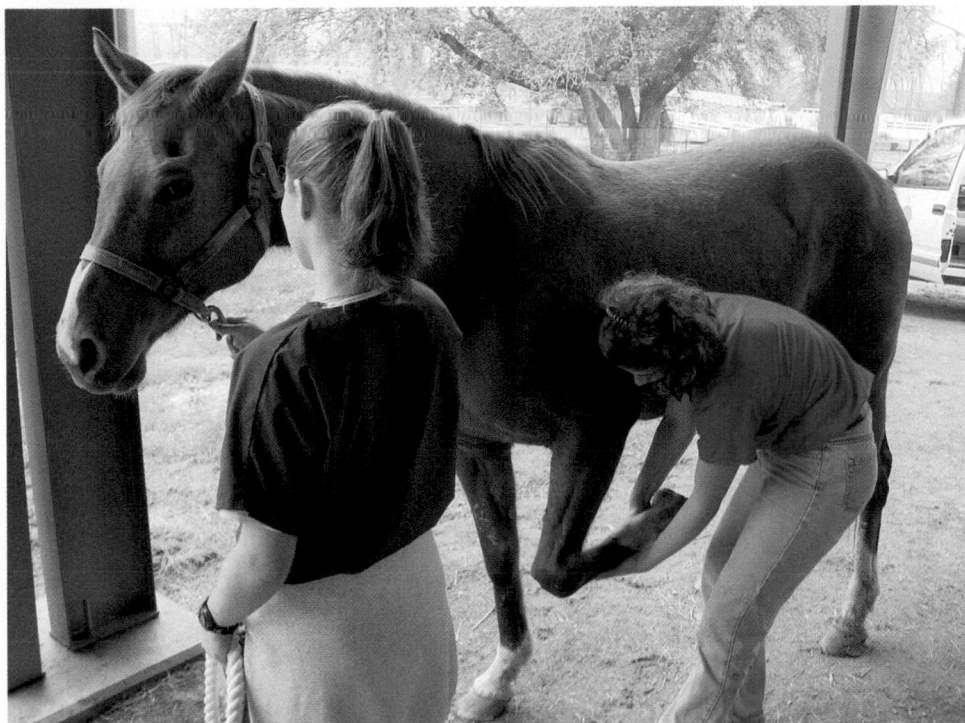

Figure 1-17 When horses are handled for any procedure, it is good technique for the holder and the individual working on the horse to be on the same side of the animal.

Application of the twitch should be done with the calmness and assuredness of the initial capture of the horse. It is best to have an assistant holding the horse by a lead rope when the twitch is applied. The loop should be placed over the thumb and three fingers, leaving the little finger out so that the twitch does not slide down the hand or arm (Figure 1-19). Grasp the end of the horse's lip, raise the hand with the twitch on it, and slide it onto the horse's nose. The end of the handle should be held in the opposite hand in case the horse throws its head. Twist the end of the handle until the twitch is snug and begins to elongate and distort the shape of the horse's upper lip (Figure 1-20). The twitch should be tightened until the horse responds by standing still. The average person cannot twist enough to damage the horse's nose. Once the twitch has been applied, the person holding it should also be holding the lead rope from the halter. He or she should be positioned on the side of the horse next to the shoulder and should be at the end of the handle of the leverage device (Figure 1-21). In the absence of a twitch, a person with a firm grip can hold the upper lip to accomplish a minor procedure. It should be remembered that horses are able to strike out with their front legs, and twitches may evoke this response. Never stand directly in front of the horse when applying or holding a twitch. As mentioned previously, the lip chain may be an alternative

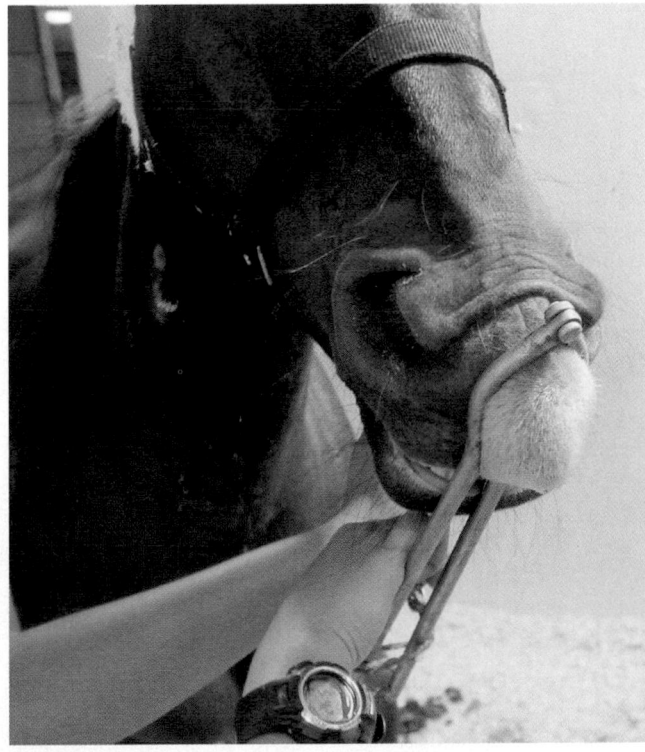

Figure 1-18 The humane twitch in place on a horse's lip.

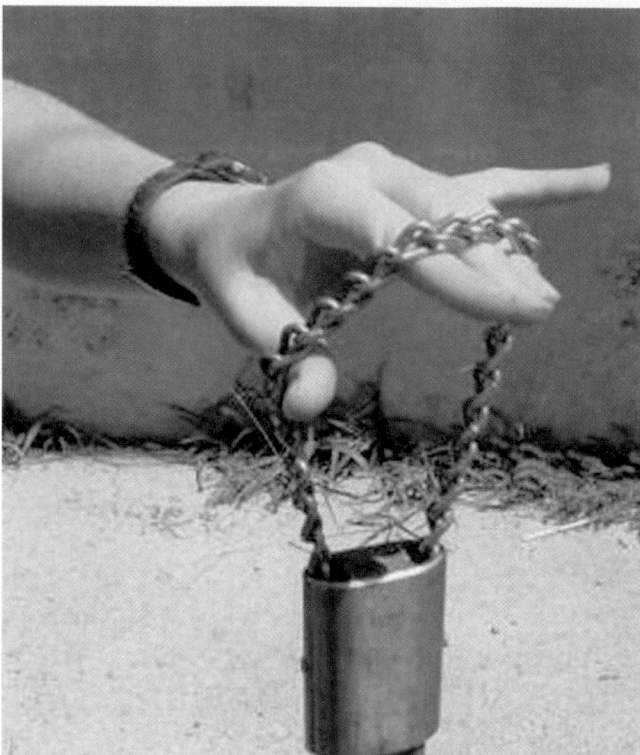

Figure 1-19 The proper placement of the fingers through the loop of chain before placement of the twitch on a horse's nose. This is important so that the twitch does not slide down the arm of the individual as it is secured onto the horse's nose.

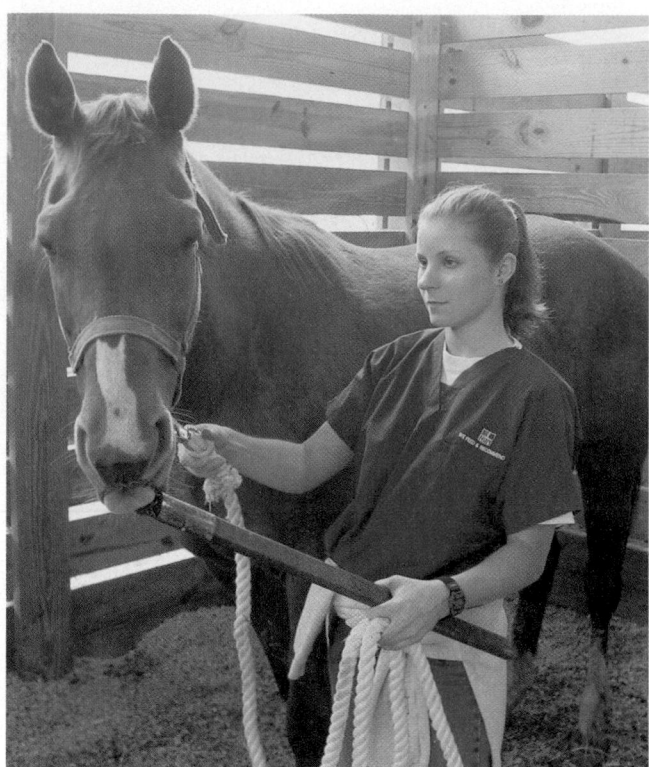

Figure 1-21 This individual demonstrates the proper position after placement of a twitch on the horse's lip in a stall. She has control of the lead rope in one hand and the twitch in the other and has positioned herself to the side of the horse.

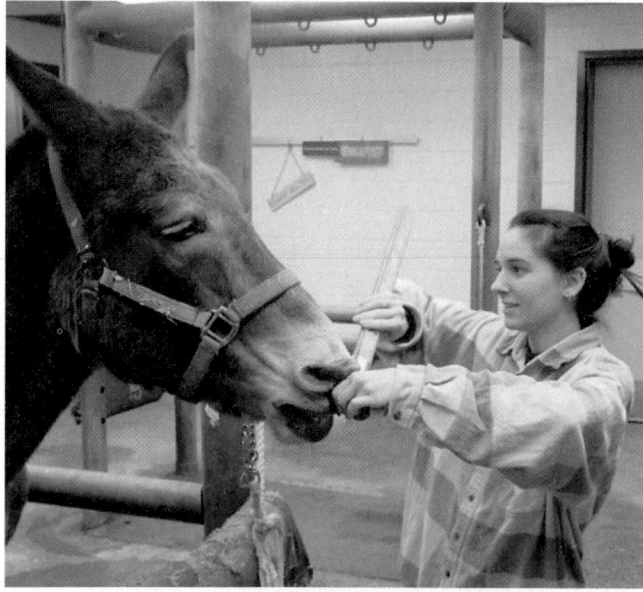

Figure 1-20 This individual demonstrates the proper positioning while placing the twitch on the lip of a horse in a stock. Note that the handler has both hands on the twitch and is off to the side, even though the horse is contained within a pipe stock.

that will produce similar results without having to dodge the flying wooden handle of a twitch or the helicopter feet of a horse that has been stimulated to strike.

✏ TECHNICIAN NOTE

Never stand directly in front of the horse when applying or holding a twitch.

A skin twitch may be a more acceptable form of restraint for many owners. This technique may also be helpful for those horses that seem to be very "light" on their front feet, attempting to strike when a regular twitch is applied to their noses. Grabbing the skin of the neck just in front of the shoulder and rolling it around a clenched fist will make many horses stand still (Figure 1-22).

The old cowboy notion of twisting the horse's ear and biting down on it as a means of restraint is poor practice. The supporting structures of the ear may be damaged, and it is extremely common for the horse to become head-shy after ear twisting. Owners are not keen on having this procedure done on their horses, and the handler risks a trip to the dentist after every attempt. Clearly, better forms of restraint are available.

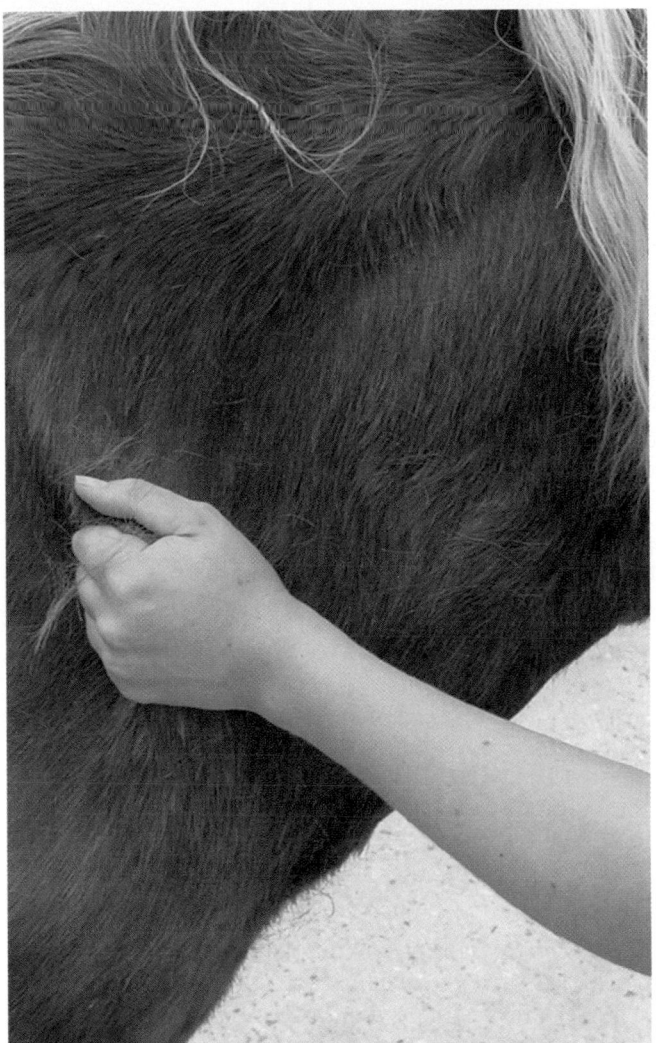

Figure 1-22 A skin twitch can be a powerful deterrent to an obnoxious horse. The skin just in front of the scapula is drawn into the clenched fist and rolled to accomplish this task.

LIFTING A FORELEG

Some horses will stand still if a foreleg is picked up and held. The theory is that with one leg in the air, the horse is less likely to leave the ground with the other three. To lift a horse's foreleg, face the rear and stand next to the horse slightly in front of the leg that is to be lifted (Figure 1-23). Bend from the waist and push your hips slightly into the horse as the hand closest to the horse palpates the suspensory ligament. The suspensory ligament is immediately palmar to the third metacarpal bone. Squeezing the suspensory ligament will cause the horse to flex its fetlock joint, and cradling the dorsal aspect of the fetlock as it flexes will allow the handler to pick up the foot. When holding the foot as a means of restraint, the handler should rotate and face forward with both hands supporting the foreleg (Figure 1-24). To handle the horse's hoof for procedures involving that area of the body, the handler should face

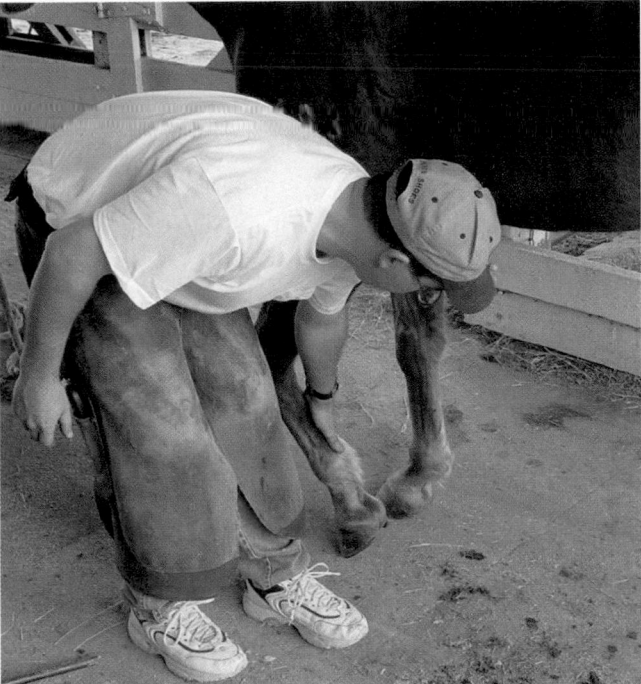

Figure 1-23 The proper foot positioning and bending at the waist to pick up a front foot of a horse. The inside hand is placed on the suspensory ligament of the horse's leg.

the rear of the horse. The foreleg should be placed between the handler's legs from the rear and held between the thighs just above the knees, freeing both hands to work on the foot (Figure 1-25).

LIFTING A HIND LEG

Lifting a hind leg will only be done as part of an examination procedure, not as a means of restraint. To lift a hind leg, the handler stands near the flank area of the horse and bends from the waist with a hand palpating down the horse's rear limb. A slight lean into the horse will aid in elevating the limb off the ground, and the leg should be pulled upward toward the handler. Then the handler should walk under the limb, staying close to the horse's body until the leg is outstretched behind the horse with the foot resting on the inside thigh of the handler. The horse's hock should be at the level of the handler's waist, and the tibial region should rest snugly against the side of the back (Figure 1-26). The leg should stay braced in this position without the use of hands. If the horse should resist, the handler's arm should clamp down over the horse's hock joint and attempt to quiet the horse.

There are descriptions of how to tie a horse's legs up for examination in the literature, but they have many disadvantages to both horse and handler. A horse with a leg tied up may fall and seriously injure itself. Too many chemical mediators are available in equine practice today to recommend rope restraints for lifting limbs.

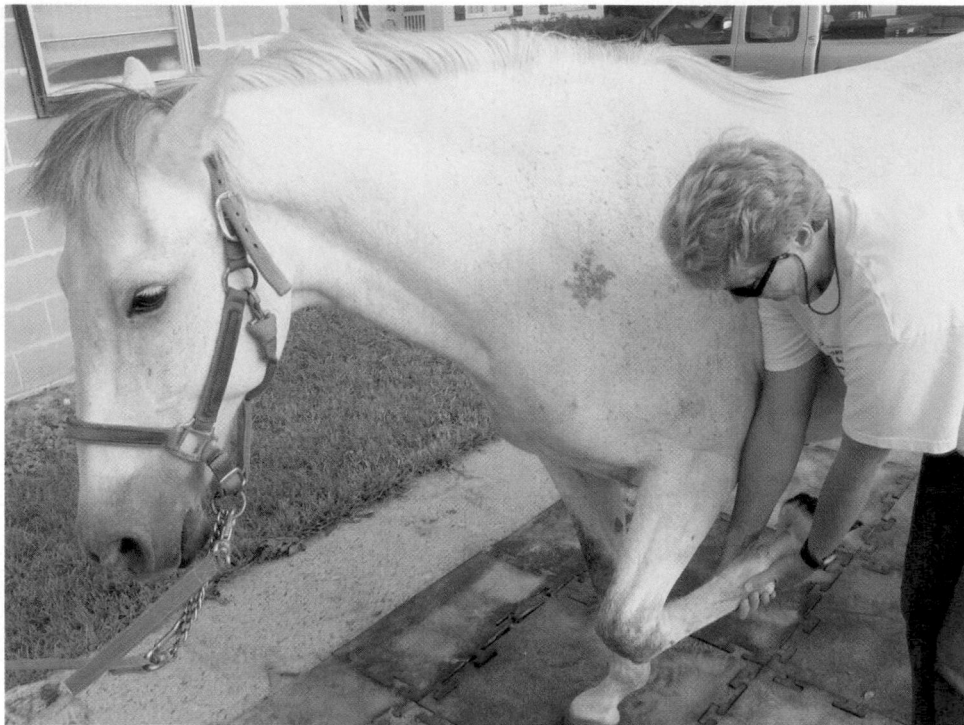

Figure 1-24 The handler is positioned properly to either examine or restrain the forelimb while a procedure is performed elsewhere.

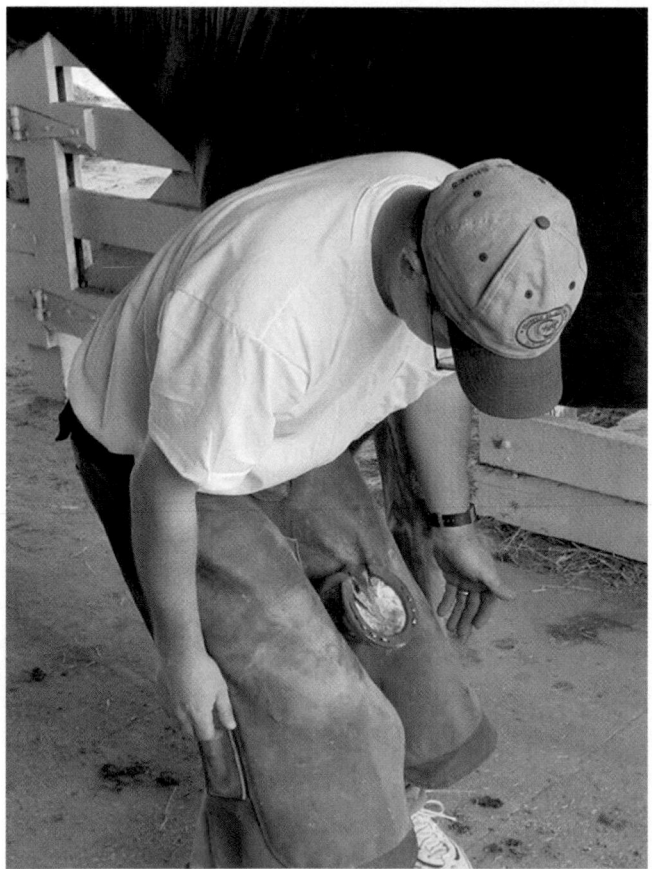

Figure 1-25 The hands-free stance while working on front feet. Note that the back is only slightly bent and the knees are directed together to hold the forelimb.

STOCKS

The use of stocks is clearly the safest way to manage fitful horses. The best stocks are made of heavy pipes or poles, anchored well to the ground surface, with the horizontal pieces set at the level of the horse's shoulder. Stocks are used for many procedures, such as administration of fluids, dental work, nasogastric intubation, rectal palpations, and injections of jittery horses. Many horses will require encouragement to get into the stocks. This can be done safely with voice commands, slight elevation of the arms of a second handler standing behind the horse, or a straw broom raised and lowered behind the horse (Figure 1-27). Again, every effort should be made to keep horses calm as they are loaded into the stocks. Some horses have an innate fear of being enclosed. These horses may do anything to get out of a set of stocks. Kicking, jumping, lunging, and striking are all ways in which a horse may try to escape. Therefore it is best to have a quick-release mechanism on the stocks, especially for the rear gate. The rear gate must be closed before the horse's head is tied after it has been loaded into the stocks. Once a horse is in the stocks, cross-ties can be placed on the horse's halter to keep its head centered in the stock (Figure 1-28). Do not assume that the horse cannot come over the front of the stocks, because many have done so in the middle of a tantrum. With this in mind, the principles discussed previously regarding where to stand apply to horses in stocks as well. Always remember that horses should never be left unattended in the stocks.

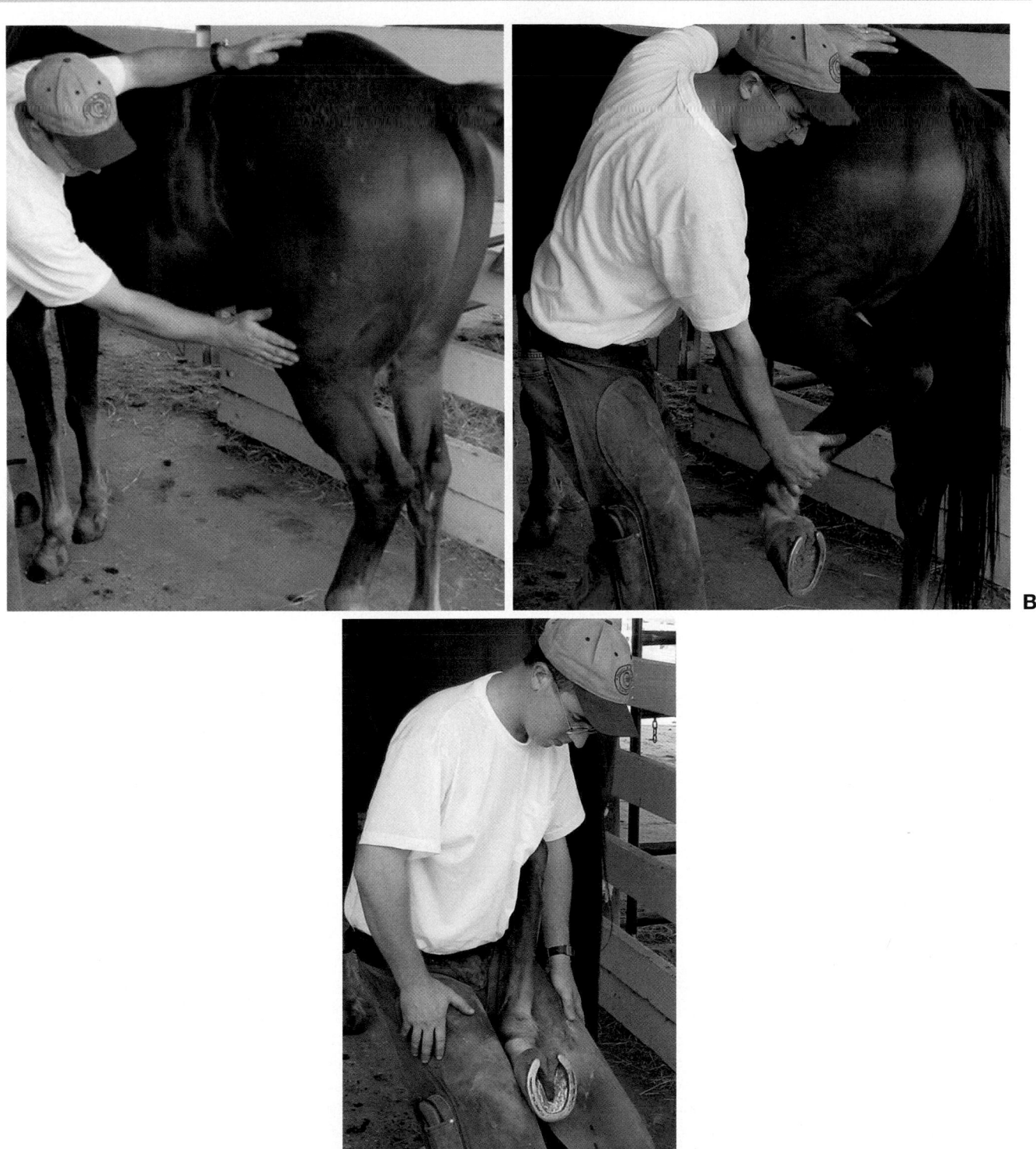

Figure 1-26 Lifting of the hind limb. **A,** The handler stands near the flank and palpates down the limb to give the horse knowledge of his presence. **B,** The leg is then brought forward toward the handler before he attempts to go out behind the horse. **C,** The handler then walks in underneath the horse's leg, supporting the tibia on his hip and placing the hoof over the inside thigh to support the lower leg.

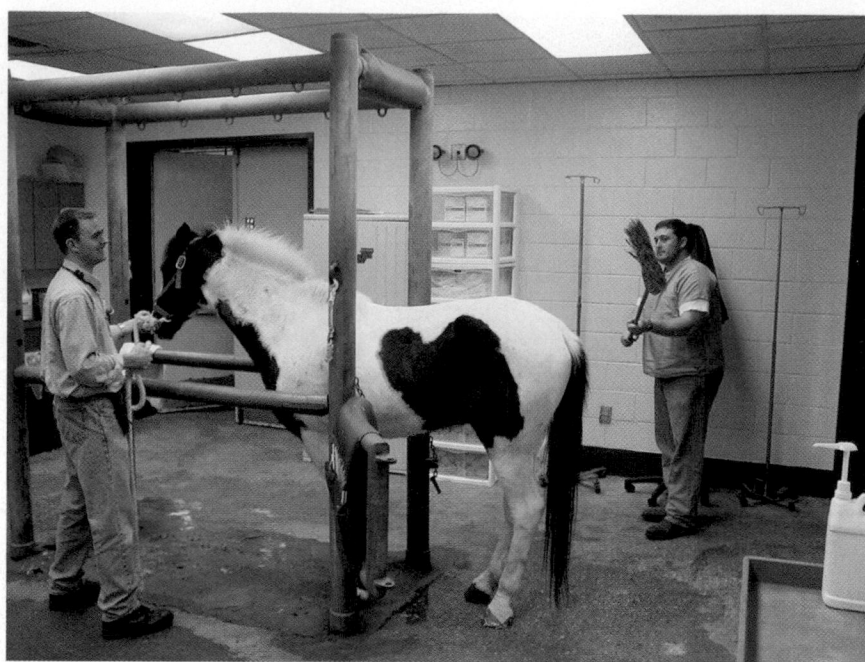

Figure 1-27 The rear end of the horse must always be respected and the back gate must be closed before the head of a horse is secured in the stock. The judicious use of the broom helps get many horses to make the final step into the stock.

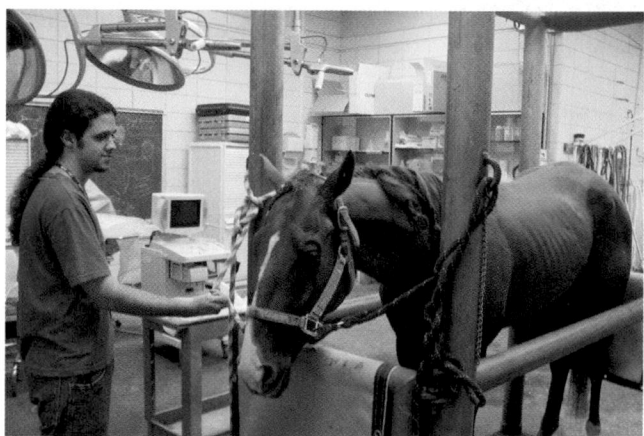

Figure 1-28 This horse is secured with cross-ties in a set of pipe stocks. Note the height of the side pipes, about the level of the horse's shoulder and stifle joints. This stock is well anchored in cement to avoid unsteadiness once the horse is in the stock. Note also the position of the cart and technician off to the side of the horse.

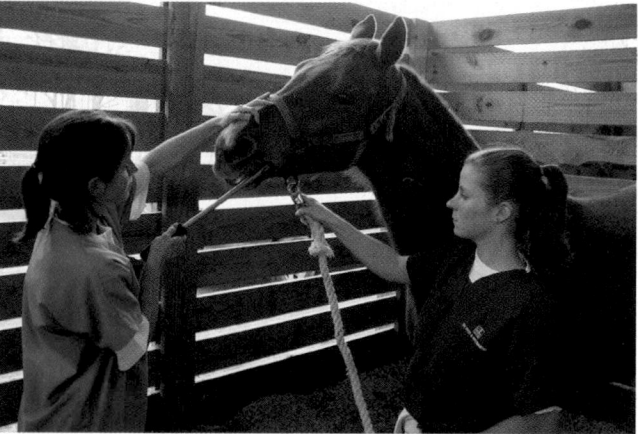

Figure 1-29 This horse is undergoing a dental procedure, and both the handler and the veterinarian are located on the same side of the horse for safety. Also note that the veterinarian's free hand is placed on the bridge of the nose, not on the halter. This is a critical point of safety because if the horse should rear, the hand in the halter can become hung.

✎ TECHNICIAN NOTE
The use of stocks is the safest way to manage fitful horses.

The lack of stocks presents a problem with restraint for more noxious veterinary procedures, such as dental work, nasogastric intubation, and rectal palpations. For dental work and nasogastric intubation without stocks, the horse should be backed into the corner of a secure and sturdy area and quieted. Make sure that the ceiling is not so low that if the horse rears it will hit its head. The handler and the veterinarian should be located on the same side of the horse when they are performing the procedure (Figure 1-29). For palpation without stocks, the horse should be placed along a

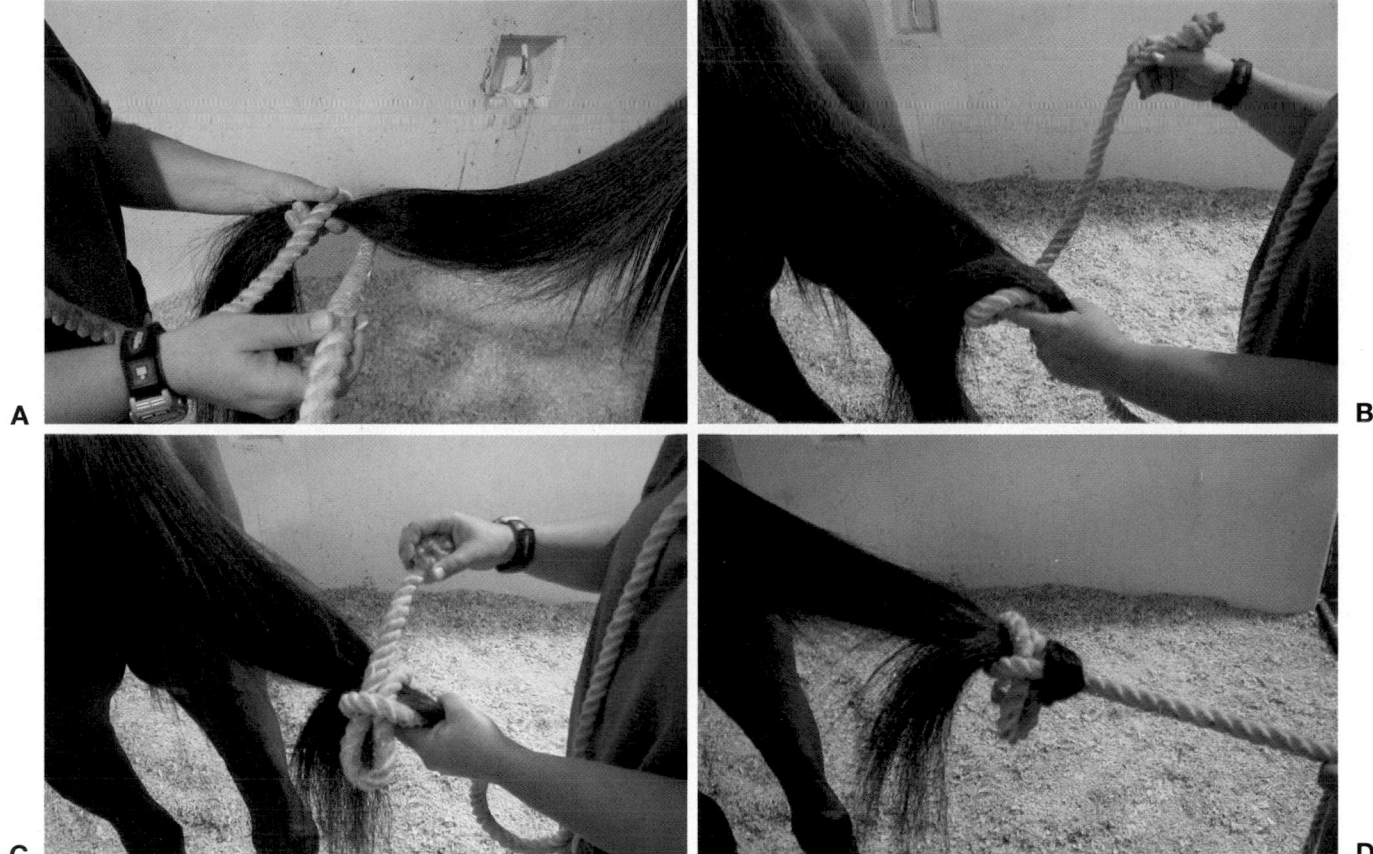

Figure 1-30   The steps in making a secure tail tie. **A,** The rope is placed around the tail. **B,** The tail is folded back on itself and on the rope. **C,** The short end of the rope passes over the folded tail, and a loop is pushed through the tail-encircling portion of the rope. **D,** Tension on the long end of the rope makes the knot snug. Pulling the short end of the rope will release the knot.

sturdy solid wall with the handler and veterinarian standing on the same side of the horse. The handler must "read" the horse, and everyone must have a clear idea of where the escape route is located when this procedure is performed.

TAIL TIE

The horse's tail may be tied during rectal palpations, vaginal examinations, and minor obstetric procedures. This is accomplished by using a small rope or a roll of gauze tied into the hair of the tail. The tail should never be tied to anything but the horse. Tying the free end around the neck of the horse is best. Should a horse get loose with the tail tied to a stationary object, serious injury could result. The tail tie is a simple quick-release knot in a rope or piece of gauze placed across the tail just below the fleshy portion (Figure 1-30), with the long end tied in a quick-release knot around the neck.

HOBBLES

Horses have been very seldom hobbled or cast (thrown to the ground with the aid of ropes) since the advent of

chemical restraint that is both powerful and short acting. Breeding hobbles are still commonly used on farms that have natural breeding operations. These hobbles prevent a mare from kicking effectively. They are fitted around the hocks with web or leather straps, which are tied to a neck strap or rope after being passed between the forelegs.

The scotch hobble is a means of drawing up a hind leg (Figure 1-31). This technique can be used as a form of restraint for examination of the opposite forelimb. It works by keeping the weight on the hind leg of the side that is being examined. Most often the scotch hobble will be used for holding the hind leg that is "up" out of the way during a castration. A heavy cotton rope should be used to avoid rope burn. A loop is placed around the horse's neck and tied with a bowline before initiation of anesthesia. Once the horse is down in a surgical plane of anesthesia, the rope is passed through the loop behind the pastern area and then brought back to the loop. Pulling the end of the rope by using the neck loop as a pulley then draws the leg forward. Care must be taken to avoid a rope burn in the pastern area. Some people actually have a leather sheath with two loops on it that is used behind the pastern to allow the rope to slide around the leg without the potential of producing a rope burn.

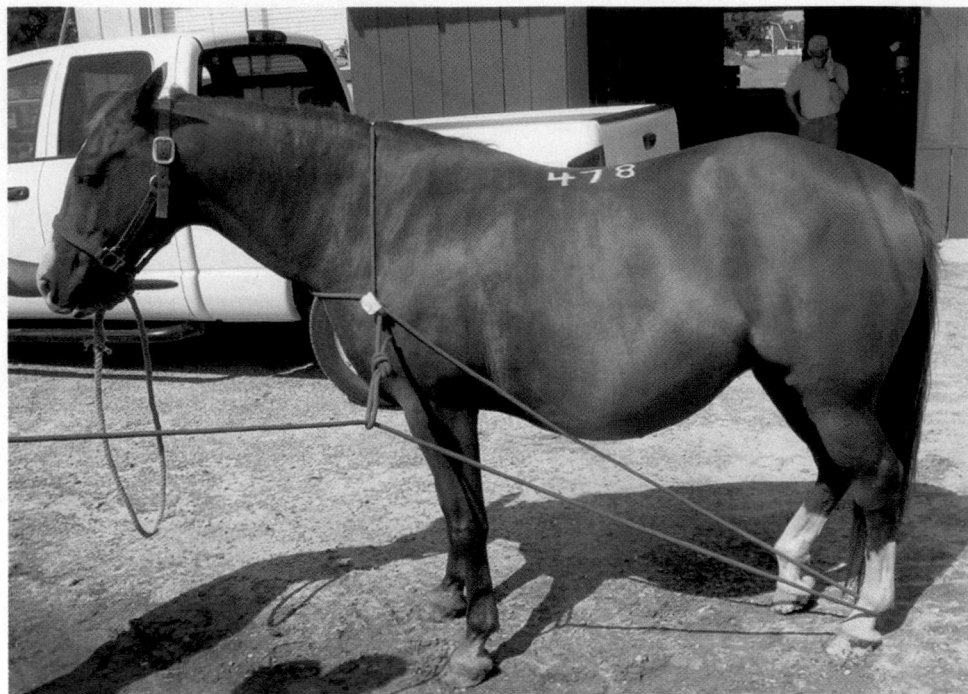

Figure 1-31 The scotch hobble on a standing horse.

RESTRAINT OF THE DOWN HORSE

Control of the head is the key to restraining a horse lying in lateral recumbency, because for the horse to get up, its head must be lifted. Kneeling on the neck near the head will keep most horses down. This should always be done from the back of the horse; in fact, any activities performed on a horse that is down must be done from the back. Approach from the belly side puts the handler in path of of thrashing legs and feet. To keep the horse from damaging the facial nerve and the down eye, the handler should cushion the lateral area of the face and orbital area. This may be done with a towel, inner tube, or foam mat placed under the horse's head. If such a protection is not available and the horse is thrashing its head, pulling up on the nosepiece of the halter will elevate the nose and prevent the horse from moving its head and producing traumatic wounds to the eye and face.

> **TECHNICIAN NOTE**
> Control of the head is the key to restraining a horse in lateral recumbency.

OTHER HEAD AND MOUTH RESTRAINTS

Horses will sometimes tear at bandages. Devices are available that may be used to prevent this by restricting the horse's ability to move the head laterally. One such device is the cradle. It is made of wooden slats and leather straps with a buckle that goes over the horse's neck to secure the

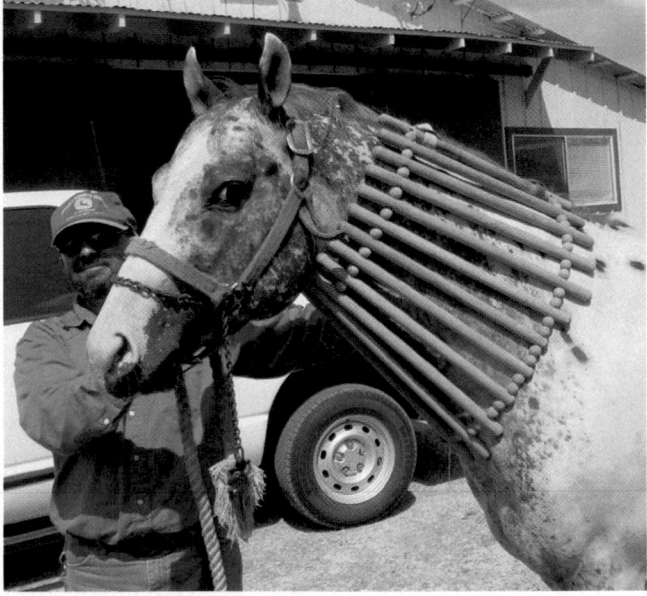

Figure 1-32 The horse wearing a neck cradle that will prevent excessive head and neck movement.

cradle and brace the neck in a straight line (Figure 1-32). This device prevents the lateral movement of the neck while allowing the horse to eat and drink. Another method of preventing the horse from chewing at bandages is to tether the horse to an overhead cable in the stall. Running the cable diagonally across the stall is the usual method. When this technique is used, the horse is able to move about the stall

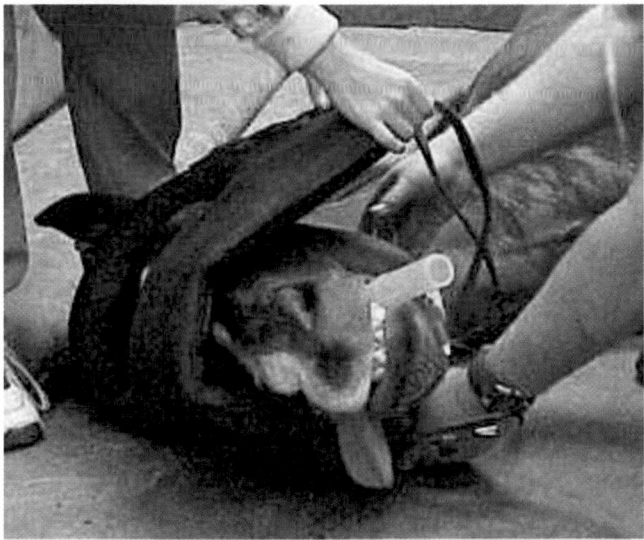

Figure 1-33 The handler is placing a protective foam and rubber helmet over the head of this anesthetized horse to protect the head during recovery from anesthesia.

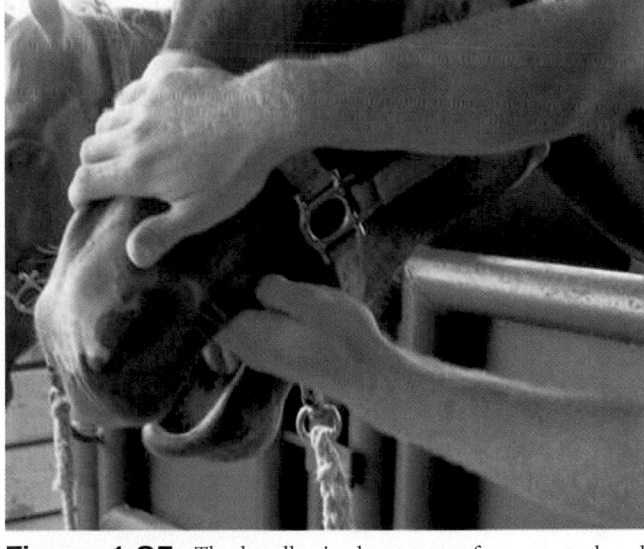

Figure 1-35 The handler is about to perform an oral and dental examination on this horse. It is critical that the examiner keep the hand in a vertical position while checking the teeth because the horse will bite down on a hand placed in a horizontal plane.

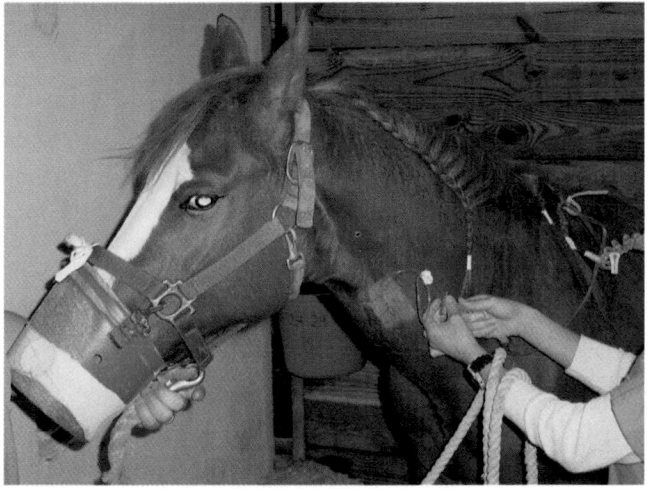

Figure 1-34 This horse is wearing a plastic muzzle to keep it from eating during the perioperative period. The muzzle does have holes to allow the horse access to water.

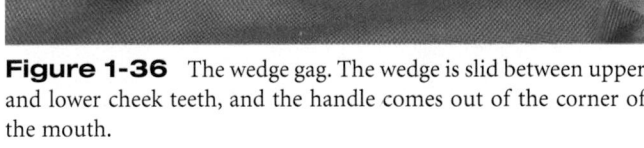

Figure 1-36 The wedge gag. The wedge is slid between upper and lower cheek teeth, and the handle comes out of the corner of the mouth.

freely but cannot reach far enough laterally to gain access to the bandage.

Horses with severe pain or neurologic disease or those undergoing anesthesia will frequently throw their heads, crashing into solid objects and mutilating themselves. Foam rubber and head protectors made to fit snugly over the head of the horse, much like a helmet, are available to prevent this (Figure 1-33). The use of these helmets and padded stalls help to prevent self-inflicted trauma.

Wire or plastic muzzles are used frequently on horses that are to be held off feed and to prevent them from eating bedding while still allowing them access to water (Figure 1-34).

Examination of a horse's mouth and dental arcades may be accomplished by standing to the side of the horse's head and placing the hand of the arm more caudal to the mouth over the bridge of the horse's nose. The hand nearest the horse's nose is then inserted into the interdental space (Figure 1-35). The hand must be kept in a vertical position. The fingers are then placed on the lingual surface of the dental arcade, and the thumb palpates the buccal surface. After dental examination has been completed, the tongue may be pulled out the side of the mouth through the interdental space. Mouth gags are available to allow for more complete visual examination of horses' mouths. A simple wedge (Figure 1-36), which is pushed up between the upper and lower cheek teeth with the handle hanging out, is commonly used. A variation on this is a round gag, used in a fashion similar to that used for the wedge. There is also a large hinged speculum that fits over the upper and lower incisors and hangs from the halter (Figure 1-37). The mouth can be cranked open by using this gag, allowing examinations and procedures to be performed on the caudal cheek teeth. Although this device is effective in getting the mouth open, it is heavy and cumbersome for both the handler and the horse. The use of this gag is usually coincidental with sedation of the animal.

MANUAL AND CHEMICAL RESTRAINT

Manual casting of horses has been replaced by chemical restraint and anesthesia. Casting always had inherent danger

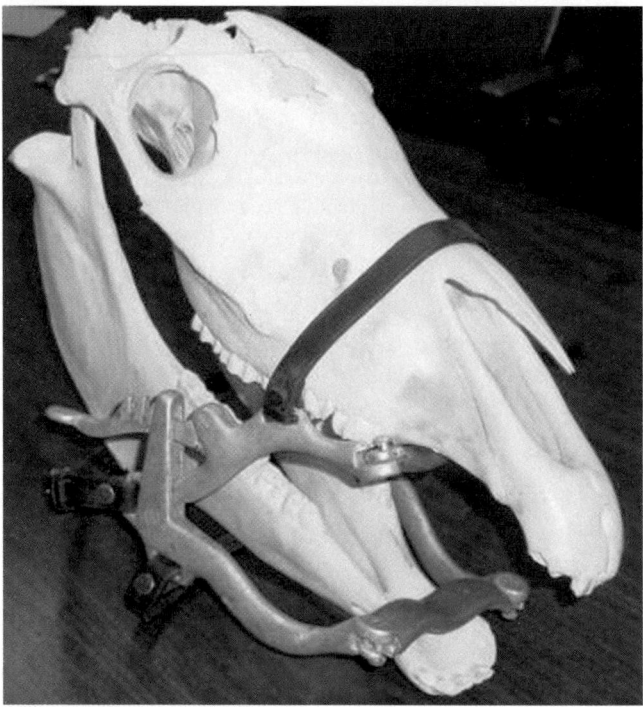

Figure 1-37 The position of the hinged speculum inside the horse's mouth to allow for visualization and work on the teeth.

for both horse and handler. Musculoskeletal damage was always possible when the forefeet of the horse were pulled from under it. Once the horse was cast, the thrashing about caused a variety of injuries.

Chemical restraint is now widely accepted and practiced. Many different agents and combinations of agents are used. These are discussed in Chapter 21. Whenever a horse has been sedated, tranquilized, or anesthetized, it is important for veterinary personnel to stay with that horse until it is steady on its feet. Also, when a horse is tranquilized, handlers must remember to maintain a safe distance from the horse. When a horse is under deep sedation, tranquilization, or proceeding through stage 2 of anesthesia, it may crash into an unwitting handler and cause significant injury. Once the horse is down, the handler should confirm the stage of anesthesia before placing restraint ropes or beginning surgical preparations. A slap to the flank of a horse awaiting castration may prevent damage from the kick of a partially anesthetized colt.

CAPTURE AND RESTRAINT OF CATTLE

Cattle are less difficult to capture than horses. They are also less discriminating than horses about what or whom they step on or run over. Generally, they are not directly approachable for haltering and leading. However, they are easier to drive into pens, alleyways, and chutes. Herds of cattle will vary in the amount of avoidance present. Some herds will allow a person to approach very closely before moving away. It is preferable to have the herd begin to move when the handlers come within about 12 m of the herd (Figure 1-38). Cattle are very herd oriented, so they will crowd and bunch together as they are driven, even climbing over other cows if they are driven too hard or fast. This should be avoided because bruising and other injuries are likely to occur.

It must be stressed that herding cattle into weak barriers is to be avoided. Most beef cattle will walk through

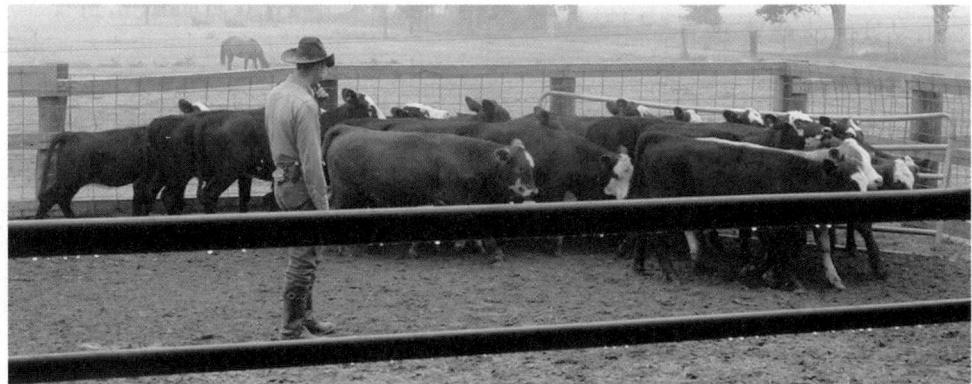

Figure 1-38 This individual is working a small herd of heifers from one pen to an alleyway. Note how the calves group together and that the corner of the pen is blocked by a gate to prevent them from crowding into the corner and turning around. This photo demonstrates the amount of "pressure" necessary to move this group without causing piling up or allowing them to turn back.

a barbed or smooth wire fence completely unconcerned and unscathed. Sometimes they even leave the wire in place, although much looser than it was. Calves become very adept at slipping through the lower strands of pasture fences.

Cattle are usually less spooky than horses about strange surroundings, but they may balk and then bolt suddenly. Generally, the balking occurs just as the cattle reach the open gate of a holding corral after being driven off a pasture. The clever cattle rancher avoids placement of strange things, such as dogs, new people, or strange trucks, at the entrance to a corral. Veterinary personnel should remain out of sight unless the owner requests assistance in driving cows. Nothing aggravates a rancher more than having all the cows bunched and ready to go into the pen and then having them spook at the last instant because something or somebody steps into their sight.

> ✏️ **TECHNICIAN NOTE**
> Do not stand in gates or alleyways where cattle are expected to go.

Once cattle are in the corral, they work best if they are funneled from larger areas into smaller pens and eventually into an alleyway leading to a chute. Usually there is a system of gates that will allow the handler to block the cattle into these progressively smaller areas. These gates may be used to "cut" calves from cows to facilitate handling. It is best to work larger stock separately from the nursing calves. The handler must be careful in closing gates on a large group of cattle. If they get turned back toward the opening and hit the gate before it is latched, there is a significant chance of injury to the handler.

The alleys leading to the chute should be built just wide enough for one animal to prevent attempts to turn around. People on foot may follow cattle in an alleyway to drive them toward the chute, but they should always be cautious and ready to climb out of the way. Never enter an alleyway that cannot be easily evacuated. The alleyway is usually arranged so that posts or boards may be slipped behind the cattle to prevent them from moving backward. "Tailing" may be used to push a cow ahead in the alley. Tailing is simply grasping the tail in the middle and twisting it forward onto the cow's back. This causes discomfort to the cow, and the usual and expected response is for the animal to move forward. Never underestimate the ability of a cow to get frightened or balk and begin moving backward. This may cause serious injury to the unwise handler. Cattle prods, wiffle paddles, and electric "hot shots" are available and may be used from outside the alley. When moving cattle through a chute, remember that less is better, and restrict the use of the battery-operated "hot shots." Producers and researchers do not want animals arriving in the head catch in a stressed and overexcited manner. Many alleyways will have an elevated walkway that allows handlers to move the length of the alley to assist in moving cattle forward to the chute. Pipes or boards may be inserted behind an alley full of cattle to prevent them from backing up (Figure 1-39). This is encouraged, but the handler must be sure to stand behind the board when placing it across the alley. If the handler is in front of the board and the cattle are backing up, the handler will become trapped between the walkway and the pipe, which may result in serious injury. If an alleyway and chute are not available, the next best solution is to run an individual cow into a gated corner. The handler must then move quickly to get behind the animal and tail it to keep it from backing up. It may be necessary to rope a cow if no other method of restraint is possible, but this is not a technique that is advantageous or desirable in modern veterinary practice.

> ✏️ **TECHNICIAN NOTE**
> The use of electronic "hot shots" or prods should be kept to the absolute minimum when driving cattle.

A single, calm cow restrained in a stall may be haltered without resorting to use of a chute. A bovine halter is all one piece and made from rope, as opposed to an equine halter. The halter is placed by loosening the nose loop first and then flipping the crown loop over the animal's ears. Once the crown loop is in place, the nose loop may be positioned and the slack in the free end of the rope may be taken up as the rope comes under the jaw (Figure 1-40). Always keep the cow's head at arm's length and bend forward from the waist, because an animal that becomes nervous will throw its head and may catch the handler in a compromised position. Animals with horns may be restrained by placing a loop of rope around the base of both horns and then dallying off to a solid post.

Calves are captured in much the same manner as foals. If a calf is small enough, it may be "flanked" and placed in lateral recumbency (Figure 1-41). The dam of the calf deserves respect and must be observed for aggression.

Bulls must always be respected for the aggression that they possess. Extreme caution should be used when driving bulls on foot. The use of feed to entice bulls into a capture area is often necessary. Once the animal is in the enclosed area, gates may be used to squeeze the animal into a position that will allow restraint. Capturing the nose ring by using a wire with a hook on the end and then snapping a long lead provides the necessary restraint for most bulls (Figure 1-42).

> ✏️ **TECHNICIAN NOTE**
> Extreme caution should be used when driving bulls on foot.

MOVEMENT OF CATTLE INTO PENS AND HEAD CATCH

Most modern cattle ranches will have a hydraulic chute at the front of their working alleys. These chutes are an efficient means of restraint for all sizes of cattle. Technicians should

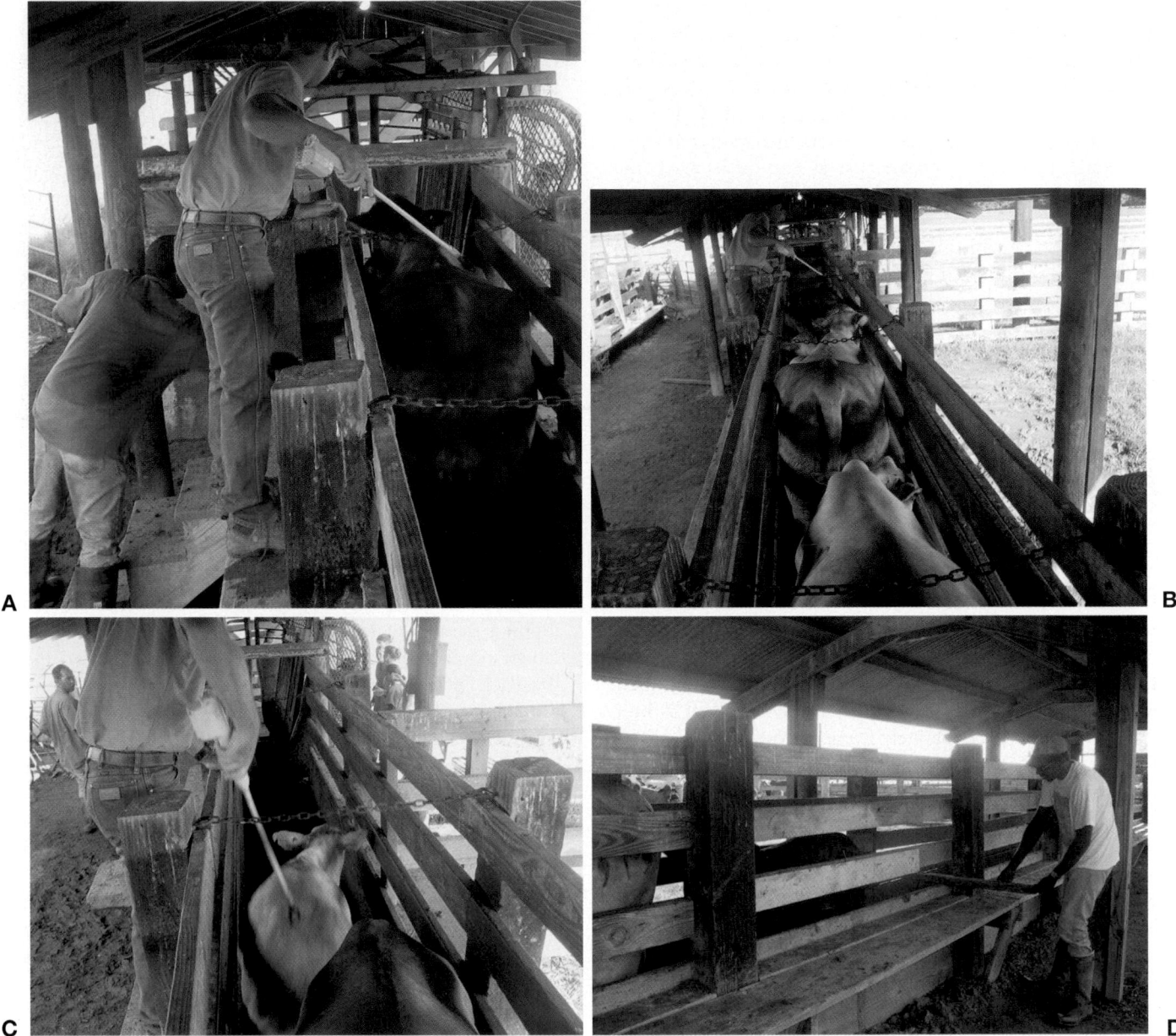

Figure 1-39 The alleyway that works best for moving cattle is only wide enough for one cow to pass through. **A,** Note that the alley is braced well with support posts and there are chains across the top of the alley to prevent it from spreading. **B,** The handler is positioned to encourage the cow to move when the gate is opened but is not in contact with her. **C,** Once the gate to the chute is opened, the handler encourages the cow to move forward by moving his hand and the hot shot toward the animal. **D,** Pipes or boards can be used to block backward movement of the cattle. The handler should always stand behind the pipe when placing it, because if the cow hits the pipe before it is set against the block on the other side of the alleyway, the pipe will come forward and pin the handler against the fence of the walkway.

become familiar with the operating handles of the chute before cattle are presented (Figure 1-43).

Cattle usually do not willingly put their heads through the head catch. It takes precise timing to close the head catch after the presentation of the head and ears and before presentation of the shoulders. Once a bovid gets its shoulders through the head catch, it will escape. Spring-loaded head catches are available, but their use is not as easy

as the manufacturers suggest. Most chutes can also squeeze the animal from side to side after the head is captured. This prevents the animal from moving about during examination. Many hydraulic chutes are equipped with a head sweep that will effectively restrain the animal's head for examination, blood collection, or ear tagging (Figure 1-44). Head catches on manual or hydraulic chutes can be dangerous. Rapidly swinging handles or closing panels provide opportunity for

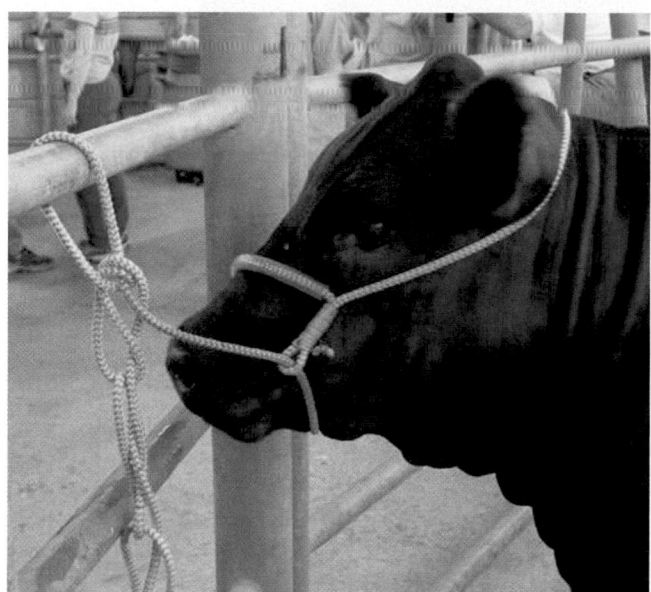

Figure 1-40 A rope halter placed correctly and tied to the pipe at an appropriate level to restrain this Angus heifer.

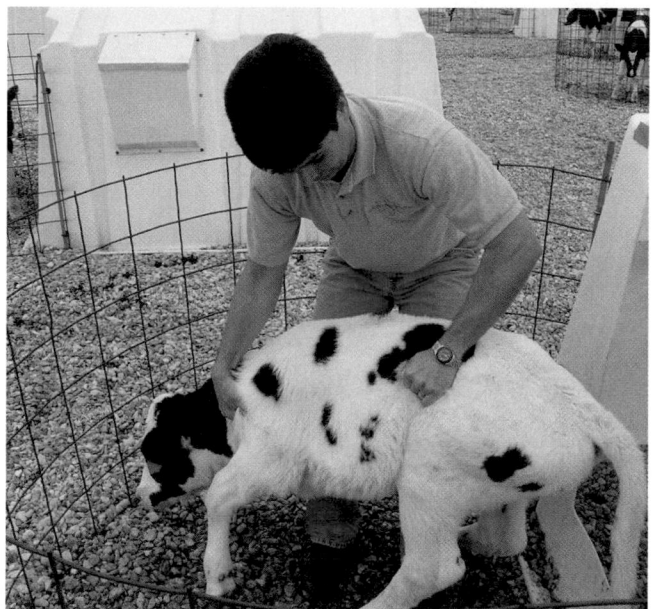

Figure 1-41 The proper positioning to "flank" a calf to the ground into lateral recumbency.

injury to the person who is unfamiliar with the equipment. Take time to become familiar with the operation of any chute and head catch before using it.

RESTRAINT OF THE HEAD

Many different techniques may be used as an adjunct to the head catch to restrain the animal for procedures more invasive than observation. Halters may be applied to pull

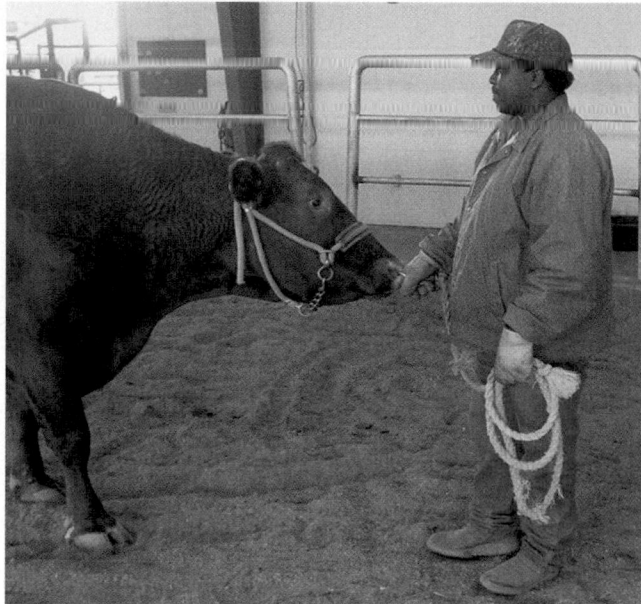

Figure 1-42 The handler has a long rope with a heavy snap in the nose ring of this bull and has also elected to hold the ring in his hand. Note that the handler has the rope coiled in his left hand so that in case of any sudden movement by the bull, he has an escape method without letting go of the animal.

the head to the side for exposure of the jugular veins. A strong person can grasp over the muzzle and place his or her hands into the mouth to allow for an oral examination. The nasal septum may be pinched between the thumb and forefingers or nose tongs may be placed in the nose to stabilize the head. The horn or ear should be used to provide leverage for the handler. Care must also be taken to perform these techniques at arm's length to prevent being hit in the head as the animal throws its head up (Figure 1-45). All dairy breed bulls and some beef bulls will have nose rings. They are easily led with the rings, but care must be taken because a ring may break or pull through the nasal cartilage. Likewise, a bull should not be tied by the nose ring. A combination of halter and nose ring may provide the most efficient means of leading a bull.

Grabbing the animal's tongue and moving it to one side of the mouth allow oral examinations to be performed in cattle. The handler can make this easier by grasping the tongue with a towel. Large, metal, hinged speculums may also be used in bovine oral examinations. These are placed and maintained as in the horse. Remember that cattle are not used to being restrained in the first place, and the use of additional hardware on the head may make them dangerous to the handlers, should they become panicked or aggravated.

TECHNICIAN NOTE

When working around the head of any bovine, be aware and stay an arm's length away from the head to avoid injury.

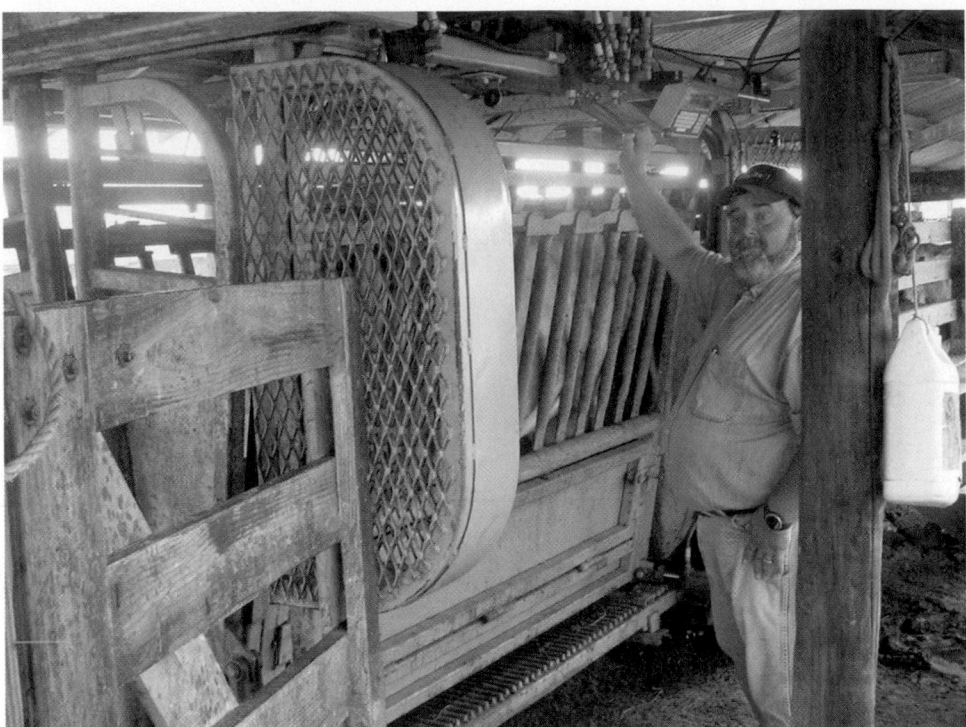

Figure 1-43 This photo demonstrates a hydraulic chute that has guards placed over most of the moving parts. The handler has his hands on the control levers that operate the gates at either end of the chute.

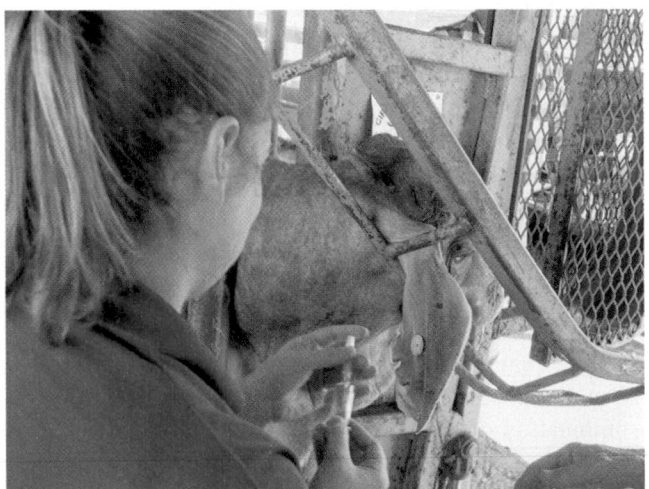

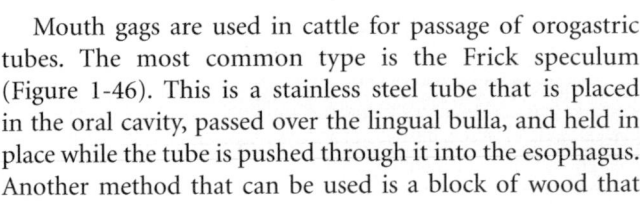

Figure 1-44 This individual is about to obtain a jugular blood sample from the cow restrained by the hydraulic head sweep of the chute. The use of the sweep allows for easy, safe access to any bovine head.

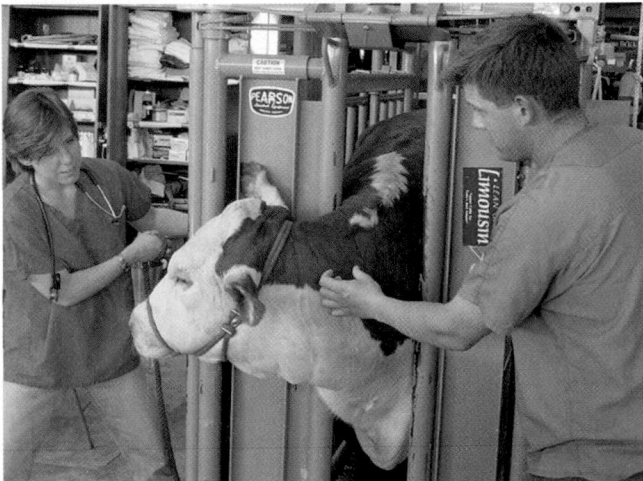

Figure 1-45 A chute with a Hereford cow captured inside of it. There are many varieties of chutes, and each has its own handling characteristics. They can be very dangerous if the handler is unfamiliar with the use of the different types of pulls and levers. Note how the individuals are working at arm's length as they proceed in restraining the head.

Mouth gags are used in cattle for passage of orogastric tubes. The most common type is the Frick speculum (Figure 1-46). This is a stainless steel tube that is placed in the oral cavity, passed over the lingual bulla, and held in place while the tube is pushed through it into the esophagus. Another method that can be used is a block of wood that extends across the animal's mouth and has a hole in the center to allow for passage of the tube. The gag is placed in the interdental space and held by a strap placed behind the head. During administration of any oral medications to cattle, care must be taken so that the speculum or dose syringe does not damage the pharyngeal mucosa.

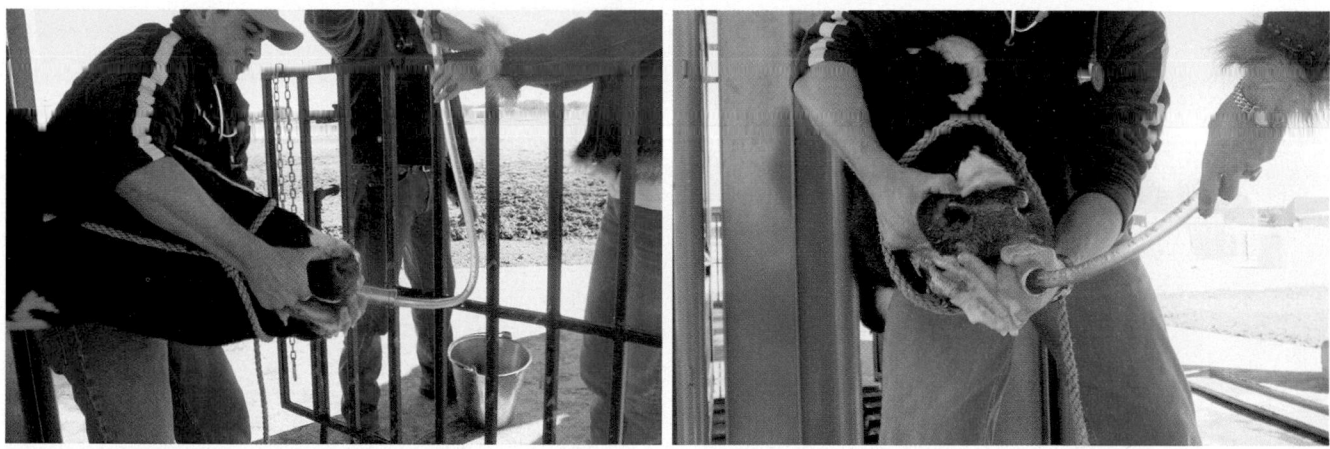

A   B

Figure 1-46 These photos demonstrate the use of a speculum as an aid in passing an orogastric tube in a bovine. **A,** The handler has placed a Frick speculum into the oral cavity of this cow. Note how the cow has been restrained in a chute before this procedure. Note the placement of the right hand and arm over the cow's head and in the interdental space to restrain the head. **B,** The left hand has firm control of the speculum to avoid advancing it too far into the pharyngeal region.

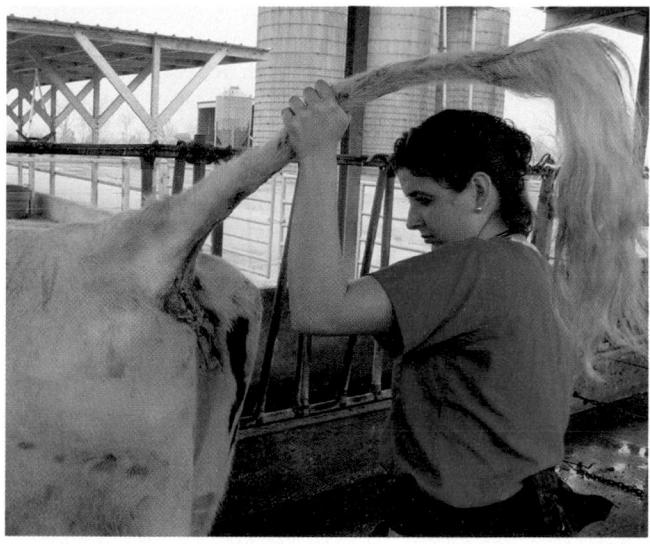

Figure 1-47 The tail "jack" technique. Handlers are reminded to keep the tail on the midline when pushing it forward and to keep their balance when pushing into the cow.

TAIL RESTRAINT

The tail of a cow can be tied just like that of a horse, with the same precautions necessary about tying the tail to anything other than the cow. The tail of a cow may also be used for driving it as mentioned previously. "Jacking" the tail of a cow will also provide a means of restraint for short procedures. This technique involves pushing straight up and forward on the tail, carrying it vertically in a plane directly over the cow's midline. The handler should remain balanced and have the tail about one third of the way down from the tail head (Figure 1-47). This technique works only when the tail is maintained vertically over the midline of the cow.

KICKING RESTRAINT

Cattle usually kick to the side and forward with a hooking action, rather than straight to the rear. Several commercial devices are available to prevent kicking and to restrain the hind legs. Milking hobbles are flat metal hooks with a chain in between that are placed over the tendons of the hind legs just above the hocks. The open end of the hooks is to the inside of the legs, and the chain passes around the front of the limbs. Once the hooks are in place, the chain can be drawn up until the hocks are close together.

Pressure on the flank seems to discourage cows from kicking. A device shaped like giant ice tongs may be squeezed over the flank (Figure 1-48), or a rope may be tied snugly around the abdomen just anterior to the udder or prepuce (Figure 1-49).

CASTING

The act of casting a bovid is quite simple. The animal must always be anchored to a sturdy post before one of the various rope harnesses is placed on it. Therefore a sturdy halter is the first requirement for casting. The simplest harness technique consists of a noose around the neck, a half-hitch around the girth, and a half-hitch around the flank. Care should be taken to avoid incorporating the udder of a cow or the testicles of a bull into the flank rope. The free end of the rope comes off the animal's back with all half-hitches positioned dorsally. Once the harness is secure, a strong pull toward the rear of the animal will make it lie down. One average-sized person can easily cast an adult cow in this manner.

The cow may be rolled onto her back if there are appropriate wedges available to keep her in dorsal recumbency. Square bales of hay may be used to wedge against the animal

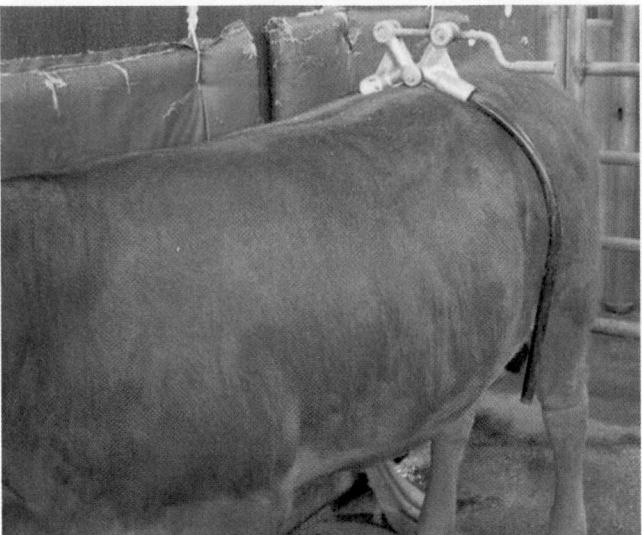

Figure 1-48 This commercially available restraint is known as the Can't Kick Device. The handle on the top turns to move the prongs of the device into the flanks of the cow for restraint and away from the flanks to remove restraint.

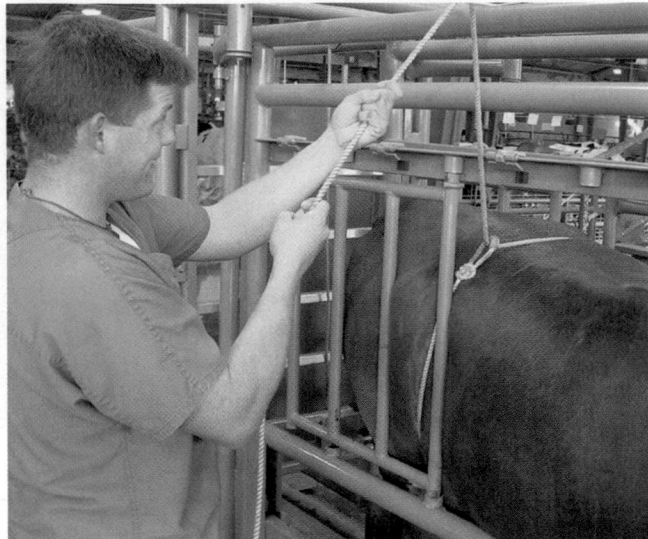

Figure 1-49 This technique involves the same concept as the Can't Kick Device but provides more control of the animal by encompassing the entire abdomen. The rope can be cinched down as tightly as necessary.

to keep it in position. The legs should be stretched to the front and rear with stout cotton rope. Cattle in sternal or dorsal recumbency are less likely to bloat than those in lateral recumbency when they are cast.

Many facilities now have restraint tables for cattle. These tables allow for access to the feet and ventrum of the bovid with minimal discomfort to the animal and veterinary personnel. The process of tabling a bovine is stepwise, and most cattle accept the ride without too much anxiety (Figure 1-50). Any bovid that must be placed in lateral recumbency should be restrained on its right side unless the procedure is of very short duration. This allows the veterinary personnel to observe the rumen for any signs of bloat that may occur. If the bloat becomes large, the procedure should be terminated. Kneeling on the animal's neck may provide additional restraint for a bovid in lateral recumbency. Standing cattle that are undergoing any procedure may go down at any time, for unspecified reasons. Therefore restraint of the head should always be with a halter because a rope around the neck may tighten and strangle the cow and the use of nose tongs may lead to ripping out the nasal septum.

TECHNICIAN NOTE

A bovid that must be placed in lateral recumbency should be restrained on its right side.

LIFTING FEET

Cattle are very reluctant to lift up their feet, which explains why many farms and facilities now have their own tilt tables.

However, in some situations it will be necessary to examine the feet in places where there is no table. To lift a bovine's front foot with the animal standing, tie a noose around the pastern and pass the free end of the rope over the back of the cow or around an overhead rail or pipe, which will then act as a pulley. The hind leg is more of a problem, because there is no portion of the cow's anatomy that will act as a pulley. The limb may be tied to an overhead beam or rail after placement of a clove hitch around the animal's hock joint (Figure 1-51). Realize that most of the time this will be done in a chute or narrow area, and maneuvering space will be limited. However, the use of this procedure will allow for visual and digital examination of the foot and interdigital space of all but the most recalcitrant cattle.

Chemical restraint is used for cattle; however, it must be remembered that ruminants are exquisitely sensitive to alpha$_2$ agonists, such as xylazine.

CAPTURE AND RESTRAINT OF SHEEP AND GOATS

Sheep and goats are more herd conscious than cattle and can be driven in bunches. Dogs are an excellent adjunct in working sheep and some goat herds, although goats will occasionally challenge the dogs.

Sheep can be worked in alleyways, and although they tend to climb on and over each other worse than cattle, they do less damage because of their smaller size. Sheep are much more athletic than cattle, yet they do not seem to want to climb out of enclosures or go over fences like cattle do when driven hard. Temporary fencing may adequately restrain sheep.

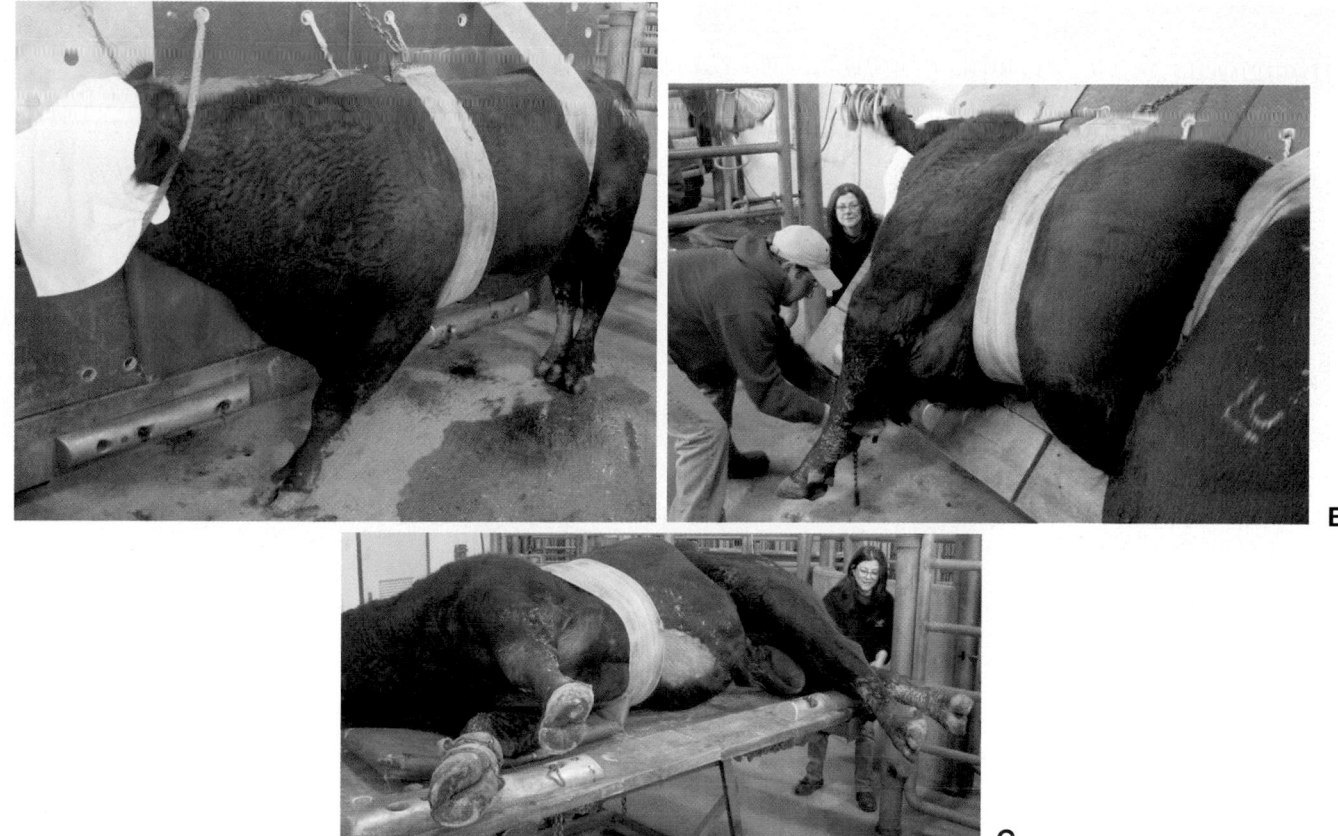

Figure 1-50 This series demonstrates the procedure for putting a bovine on the tilt table. **A,** The animal is maneuvered next to the table; the head is restrained and the eyes may be covered. The belly bands are then secured around the animal just behind the forelegs in front and in front of the rear legs and drawn tight to the table. Care must be taken to avoid incorporating the testicles or the udder under the rear belly band. **B,** The table is then tilted slightly to elevate the feet, and the inside foreleg is secured to the table at this time. One person secures the limb with the appropriate straps and the second tightens the leg to secure it to the table. **C,** The table is then tilted flat, and the other three limbs are secured to the table in succession.

The kids and lambs within a flock may be quite acrobatic, jumping into fences and climbing over structures to avoid being caught. These activities may result in traumatic injuries, and veterinary personnel should be alert to avoid dangerous situations.

Goats and sheep can be caught in small enclosures in the same way as foals or calves are caught, with a hand under the neck and one under the rump. It is important to remember that a sheep or mohair goat must not be restrained by grabbing the wool. The fleece may be damaged, or, in meat animals, a subcutaneous bruise may develop at the site, damaging at least the esthetics of the product.

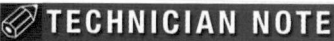

TECHNICIAN NOTE

Do not restrain sheep by grabbing their wool.

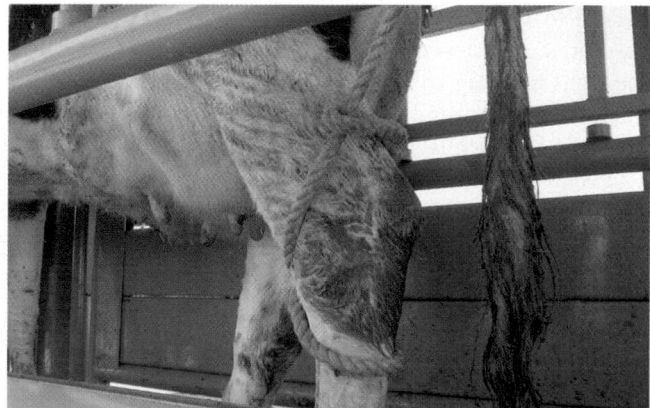

Figure 1-51 The hock of this cow is held by a clove hitch that has been placed in a sturdy rope. The rope restraint of the hock allows for the entire hind leg to be elevated by pulling the rope over a beam behind the cow.

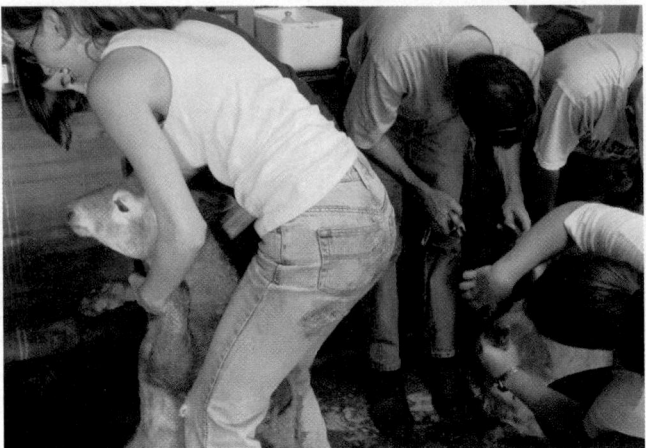

Figure 1-52 This photo shows how an individual handler can restrain and manipulate a sheep by setting it on its rump.

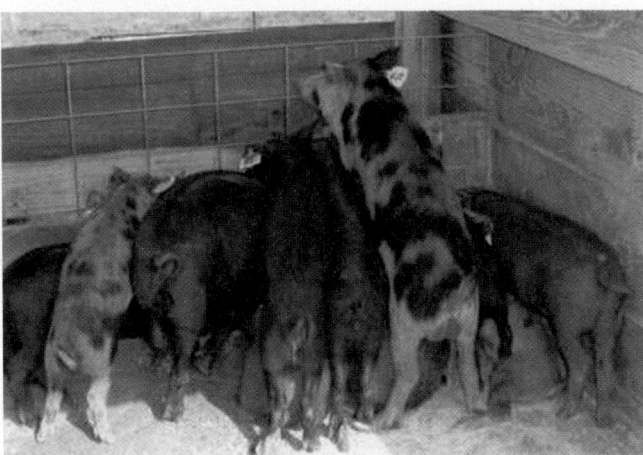

Figure 1-53 Piglets pile up in the corner when driven. It is now quite easy to capture one by grabbing onto the hind legs that are presented.

A helpful technique for capturing goats is the use of a shepherd's crook or cane. The goat can be hemmed in toward the fence, and then the crook can be placed in the throat-latch area to catch the head. Care must be taken to avoid trauma to the trachea when this technique is used.

> ### ✎ TECHNICIAN NOTE
> A helpful technique for capturing goats is the use of a shepherd's crook or cane.

Sheep are often set up on their rumps for the purpose of performing several different procedures. There are several different ways to end up with the sheep on its rump with its back leaning against the holder who retains a grip on the forelegs (Figure 1-52). The easiest method is for the person to begin on the sheep's left side. Reach under the base of the neck with the left hand and over the back to the right hind leg with the right hand. The sheep is gently lifted off the ground toward the right and upturned, as the right hind leg is lifted to get the animal's weight off it. The right hand moves to the right foreleg as the left hand moves to the left foreleg, and the sheep is held on its rump facing away from the handler. One person can shear a sheep or perform other procedures unassisted with the sheep on its rump by steadying its upper torso between his or her arms and the lower torso between his or her legs.

The method of holding the legs of lambs for docking and castration is the same, regardless of whether they are held by the handler, laid on a bench, or placed over a fence. The holder grasps the parallel hind and forelegs, bringing the hind leg forward while holding between the hock and fetlock. The foreleg is held just below the elbow.

CAPTURE AND RESTRAINT OF SWINE

Small piglets can be crowded into corners and then grasped by a hind leg (Figure 1-53). The leg hold should be rapidly changed to holding the pig in both hands around the torso for comfort of the pig. Obviously, this technique is not applicable to adult swine.

Veterinary personnel may be faced with castration of large boars based on an owner's perception of when the signs are right. One technique that can be used on a market-weight boar is to herd it to a corner and have two handlers grab the nearest hind leg. After capture, the hind end is then elevated so that the pig is standing on his head in the corner. This technique is not for the faint of heart; the coordination and strength of the two handlers are required to accomplish the task. Sedatives and anesthetic agents are available for use with pigs of this size and should be offered as the primary means of capture and restraint for larger swine.

Swine can be very aggressive, particularly boars and nursing sows. A fence or panel may be used to "haze" them, and this barrier also provides protection to the handler. When the panel is meant to be stationary, take care to push it all the way to the ground and plant it. Pigs will attempt to "root" underneath it. Always be aware of the escape route when entering a pen. Swine are intelligent and individualistic and may be difficult to direct in a large area. They tend to dart through small openings for escape. A cane is a valuable tool for a handler who is attempting to drive and direct swine. Tapping them on the side of the neck and face with the cane while following on foot gives the handler some degree of "steering" capability.

Once pigs are inside a small enclosure, a snare may be used to catch them. A hog snare is an adjustable metal cable loop at the end of a rigid handle. The usual procedure in

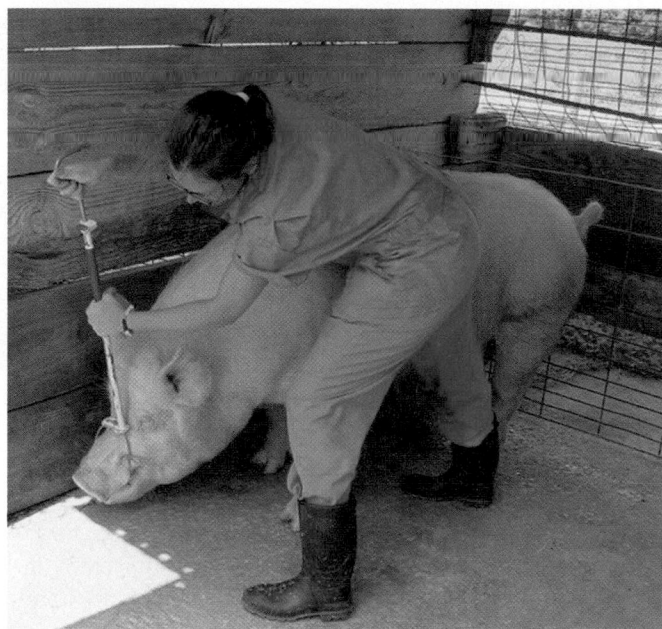

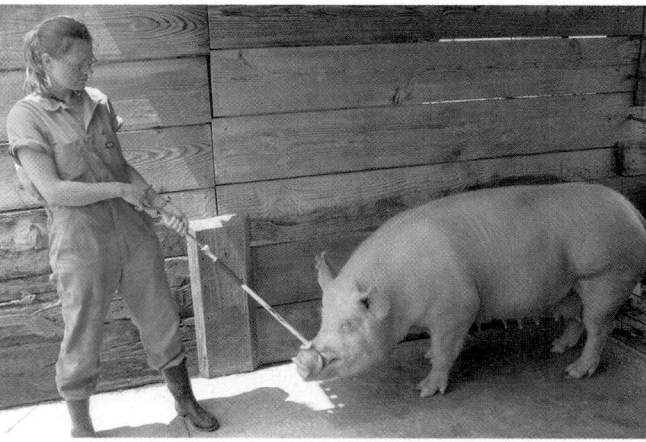

A   **B**

Figure 1-54 Demonstration of the capture of an adult pig with the hog snare. **A,** The handler approaches from the side of the pig and carefully loops the snare over the upper jaw just in front of the cheek teeth. **B,** After the snare is tightened, it is obvious that the pig resents this and will resist by pulling back against the snare. This allows the handler to brace against the pig and hold it steady for examination or sample collection.

capture of the pig is to push it into a corner and then step in, tight to the flank area, and slip the snare loop over the upper jaw from behind. The loop is tightened after it is placed behind the incisors. The snare has a rigid handle that allows the handler to direct the snout after the pig has been captured. Generally, swine will brace themselves by pulling backward when caught and are immobilized by use of a snare (Figure 1-54). However, the discomfort of the snare usually results in nonstop squealing until it is removed. Handlers are encouraged to wear ear protection when performing any restraint on pigs.

TECHNICIAN NOTE

Handlers should wear ear protection when performing any restraint on pigs.

Pigs can be restrained on their backs in a trough but find it unsettling and complain vocally (Figure 1-55). A sling of canvas with holes for the legs has been used with great success in laboratories and veterinary hospitals to cradle the pigs comfortably for certain procedures. The farrowing crate is the restraint device for sows, which keeps them from lying on their piglets.

Pigs can be restrained for castration or vaccination by holding them off the ground by the hind legs with their backs against the handler's legs. Large pigs will struggle less if their forefeet rest on the ground. Piglets can be given oral medications by holding them up by the forelegs and leaning their backs against the handler's legs while they stand on their hind legs.

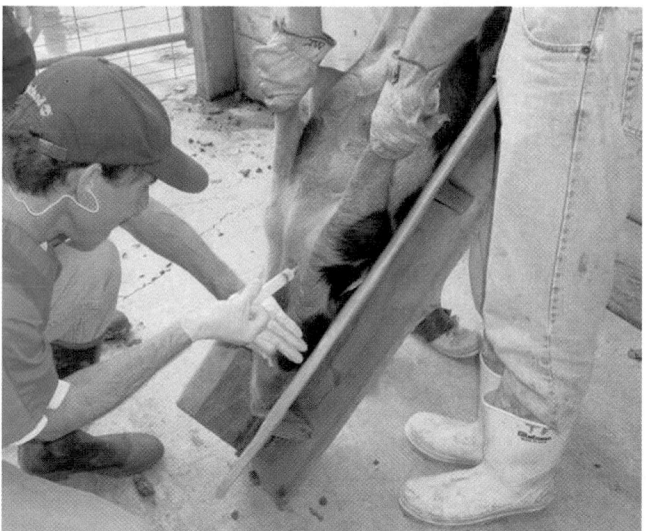

Figure 1-55 This feeder pig is being restrained on its back in a V trough. Both hind legs are held by an assistant and the forelegs are pulled back to allow access for blood collection. Procedures such as ear notching and bleeding can be done with the pig in this position. Note that pigs will squeal the entire time they are restrained in this fashion, and all handlers should wear ear protection as demonstrated by the individual performing the blood collection.

The pig is an intelligent animal that can be trained to tolerate minor discomforts; unfortunately, the time involved to train swine is often not profitable in agricultural animals. Miniature pigs, kept as pets, are most often seen these days in urban practices. Many of these are spoiled, willful creatures that dominate the household, and their owners are not impressed with rough handling. The support sling is the best method for restraint because it causes the animal no discomfort yet immobilizes the animal well. Many pet pigs are fond of having people scratch their backs and may stand or lie quietly for examination if this is done for them. Holding the pig cradled in the arms of a handler may seem to be a good idea until the pig struggles. Then the hind foot nearest the body will gouge the holder. Pigs also have powerful jaws, and some will bite, especially if in pain. Examination of the mouth can be accomplished by the use of a U-shaped gag, which is placed into the mouth from the front to behind the canines; the gag is then rotated to spread the jaws. Never put fingers into the side of a pig's mouth, since the cheek teeth are very sharp.

> ✎ **TECHNICIAN NOTE**
>
> Many pet pigs are fond of having people scratch their backs and may stand or lie quietly for examination if their backs are scratched.

Although a miniature pig may live in and control a house, it is still a pig. Pigs vocalize when they are uncomfortable or in pain. Do not be surprised when the cute little pig emits an ear-piercing shriek as it is picked up. This will continue until it is set free. Chemical agents for restraint are highly recommended for use on these animals.

CAPTURE AND RESTRAINT OF DOGS

CATCHING DOGS

The only time veterinary personnel should have to catch a dog that is not in a cage or run is if the animal has escaped. In a hospital, dogs are often motivated by fear, so personnel should learn to deal with the two types of behavior this produces. Avoidance with submissiveness when cornered is one, and the other is avoidance until cornered and then aggression, otherwise known as *fear biting*. Unfortunately, it may be difficult to discriminate between the two until the moment when hands are approaching the dog. It is the rare dog that will not snap at a handler who grabs it as it runs past, yet it is difficult to resist the temptation of doing so as a dog streaks past on its way to freedom.

Dogs that feel they are being chased will run, and a person is not going to outrun any but the smallest or most debilitated. It is best to try to keep the dog in sight until there is an opportunity to corner it. Sometimes it helps to have a canine companion to entice the dog to approach. In this situation it will never hurt to have a pocketful of bait to gain the dog's favor. Most dogs respond favorably to voice reassurance, and a higher-pitched voice usually gets better results. With many dogs, squatting in front of them to appear less large and overbearing will help. Moving slowly and deliberately, offer the back of your hand for the dog to sniff, at or below the level of its nose. The response to this action is the first indication of the tendency for the dog to try to bite. Never try to grab the dog's collar or pick it up until some reassurance is given to the animal. Do not confuse a wagging tail with friendliness in a dog with an unknown personality. Watch the ears, eyes, and face. It is not unusual for an aggressive dog to hold the tail erect with a tense, narrow, oscillating motion before biting.

> ✎ **TECHNICIAN NOTE**
>
> Chasing dogs is a frustrating and mostly futile exercise. Always make sure that runs and turn-out yards are closed and secure before turning any dog loose.

The back of the hand is offered to the dog for two reasons. The first is that it is probably less threatening than the open palm, which may appear to the dog as an attempt to slap. Second, the fingers are out of the way and the dog will be less likely to get the entire hand if it does bite. Caution should be exercised by all handlers in these situations, because dogs bite with lightning speed, and the position of the hand may have little to do with the ability to withdraw from danger.

Some dogs are naturally gregarious and trusting and require little in the way of preliminary introduction. The trusting dog will sniff the hand, begin wagging its tail, and approach for more petting. It is a good idea for the handler to run his or her hands over the entire dog in a friendly fashion before taking liberties with the body. Evaluating dogs requires knowledge of the relationship of the dog with the owner. Some dogs have trained their owners rather than the opposite, and the handler must forge his or her own relationship with the dog.

Many times, dogs act reasonably in an initial examination with the client present and then threaten to bite when approached after the client has gone. When faced with a dog that will bite if given the chance, the sensible approach is to keep your hands and body out of the way. Always remember to keep all outside gates and doors closed when working with difficult animals. The cage door should be held closed as much as possible when trying to catch these animals. They are trouble enough without trying to capture them after they have escaped. Small dogs may be managed by handling with heavy leather gloves. A dog will bite at the fingers of the glove of one hand while the clever handler grabs it by the scruff of the neck with the other. A large dog that wants to bite is more troublesome. The first step is to catch it by the neck. A lead rope with a slipknot can be tossed over a dog's head, but sometimes a rope or cable snare similar to a hog snare is required (Figure 1-56). Most dogs will give up when caught by the neck. The truly vicious or confirmed fear biters will continue to attempt to bite and even attack. These animals will require a muzzle or rope with a pole to keep the teeth away from veterinary personnel. When forced

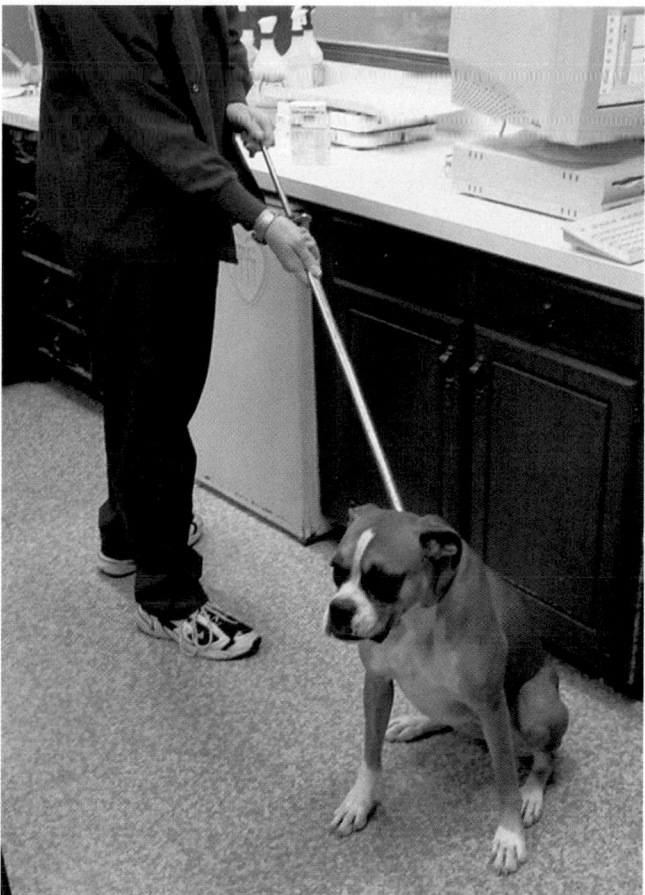

Figure 1-56 This dog has been captured with a cable snare. The steel handle allows the handler to keep the dog at a safe distance when maneuvering the animal.

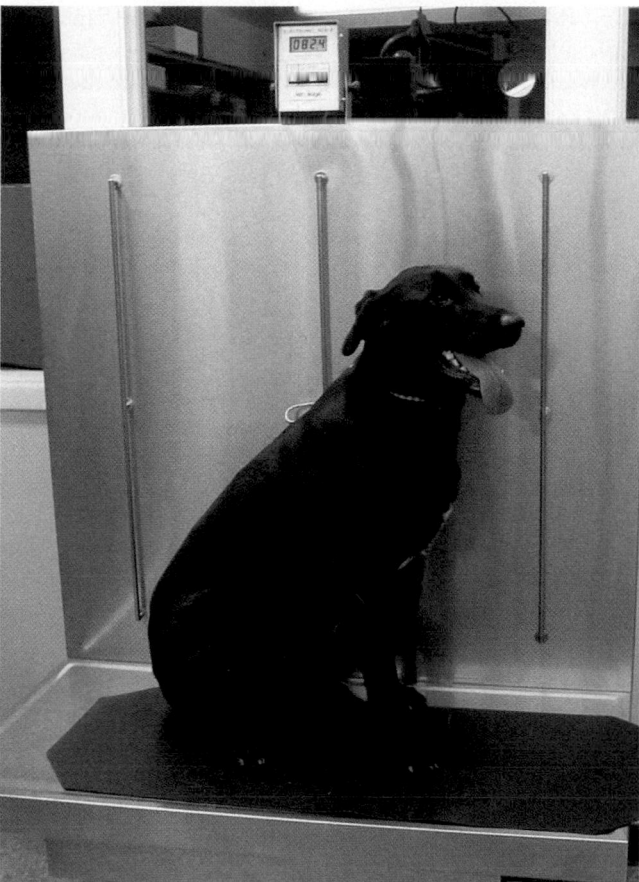

Figure 1-57 A stainless steel lift table that also has a self-contained scale. This allows large dogs or those that do not like to be picked up to step onto the table at floor level and then be raised to a comfortable height for examination. An attendant should always be present with the dog when the table is elevated.

to snare these dogs, remember that tracheal damage to the dog is possible and great care must be taken to avoid physical damage to the animal. However, some of these dogs are incorrigible and require force to gain respect.

TECHNICIAN NOTE

Often, dogs act reasonably in an initial examination with the client present and then threaten to bite when approached after the client has gone.

A truly vicious large dog is a major challenge. Such a dog must always be handled with at least one snare, possibly two, if the dog is strong. Once captured, the dog is stretched between the snares for leading. Many of these dogs are used as guard animals, and only one person can handle them. The owner may be able to place the muzzle on the dog before bringing it into the clinic. These dogs must always be treated with respect for their ability to harm the handler. A discussion of muzzles and how to place them occurs later in this chapter, and the reader is encouraged to become familiar with all types of muzzles that are available.

A dog at large may require the use of a capture gun or pole syringe. Animal control officers are experienced with the use of these devices and may be able to provide assistance.

LIFTING DOGS

Lifting a dog onto the examination table is usually the first step in any examination or procedure. Grasping on either side of the thorax behind the elbows allows the handler to lift small dogs. Putting the arms around the front of the chest and behind the rump will allow a handler to lift a medium-sized dog easily. This technique places the handler close to the animal's teeth, so care must be taken to avoid being bitten by a frightened dog. It may be appropriate to muzzle dogs that seem to have issues about being lifted before any attempt is made to do so. Large dogs are harder to lift. Their weight may be prohibitive, their bulk makes them awkward, and they are not accustomed to being lifted. One person can lift a large dog by using a forklift technique, placing his or her arms behind the dog's elbows and in front of its hind legs. If the animal struggles, there is danger that it will fall forward or backward. Two people can lift a dog together, if one lifts the forequarters and the other lifts the hindquarters. Both individuals should be on the same side, away from the table, to accomplish this technique.

Some dogs object to being lifted from under the flank area, especially males. Such dogs definitely need two people to lift them, and the person in back should make sure the placement of the hand or arm is well forward on the abdomen. Many practices now have lift tables that allow dogs to be walked onto the table at floor level and then elevated to a comfortable height for examination (Figure 1-57). Handlers are cautioned that lifting dogs may result in back injury. Lifting with the legs and keeping the back straight will help prevent muscle strains. Large dogs that are nervous about being lifted or react adversely to being on top of a table should be dealt with on the floor.

TECHNICIAN NOTE

Never let a dog jump down from a table.

Never let a dog jump down from a table. Tables and floors have slick surfaces that invite slips and possibly fractures. Lift the dog off the table in the same manner as it was placed on the table.

Injured or sick animals pose different problems in lifting. More support is required for patients with fractures or painful abdomens. A stretcher may be required for lifting a badly injured dog. Good judgment should be used in all instances when lifting is required.

TABLE RESTRAINT FOR EXAMINATION

The degree of restraint required for a dog on the examination table depends on the procedure. The forequarters and hindquarters must be controlled at all times to prevent the dog from jumping or falling off the table. The form of restraint most commonly used is to have the handler's arms either behind the rump or under the flank and in front of the chest, pulling the dog inward in much the same manner as lifting. The head may be pulled toward the handler's chest (Figure 1-58). This is adequate restraint on most dogs for examination and intramuscular or subcutaneous injections.

A rectal examination requires only slight adjustments for restraint. The handler's arm should not be behind the dog; rather, it can be placed over the dog's back to stabilize lateral movement by drawing the body toward the handler. Sometimes the hand must support the ventral abdomen to prevent the dog from sitting down.

Whenever procedures are done on puppies, it is wise to put the bitch into a crate, or better, remove her to a kennel outside the room. Care must be taken when removing newborn pups from the bitch for the reasons discussed previously.

RESTRAINT FOR VENIPUNCTURE

A dog must not be allowed to move during venipuncture because movement results in perivascular placement of the needle. The primary reason for struggling and movement

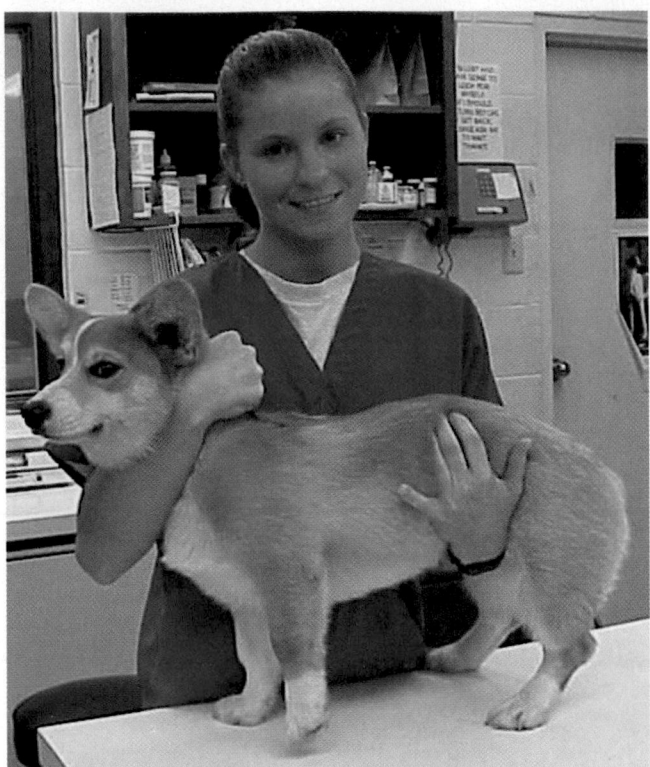

Figure 1-58 The handler is providing support for the dog and restraint for examination at the same time. Note the placement of the arms in a forklift position under the neck and in front of the flank. The handler is positioned to draw the animal closer if serious anxiety develops.

during venipuncture is anxiety. Calm, affectionate handling with petting and soothing words will help alleviate anxiety. The most painful portion of the venipuncture is the piercing of the skin and vessel, which is when the restraint must be most secure. Positioning is the most critical part of a venipuncture to allow for accurate location of the vessel. Diagnostic sampling is discussed in Chapter 3.

The holder must restrain the dog's body, present the forelimb, and occlude the vein to allow it to fill and be recognized under the skin for cephalic venipuncture. To accomplish this, the holder places the dog on the table near one end facing the edge. The holder stands beside the table facing in the same direction as the dog and nestles the animal on the table under his or her arm. The handler's forearm, elbow, and upper arm all exert pressure to bring the dog snugly to the handler's side. The hand of the same arm cradles the dog's elbow with the palm and fingers while the thumb clamps down on the cephalic vein (Figure 1-59). To ensure that the vein is under the thumb and on the dorsal surface of the dog's forearm, the holder grasps the limb just below the elbow with the thumb as far inside as possible and rotates the skin outward. The fingers should rest on the table, and the dog's elbow should be pushed slightly forward to stabilize the leg. The elbow should be near the edge of the table to allow good access to the vein.

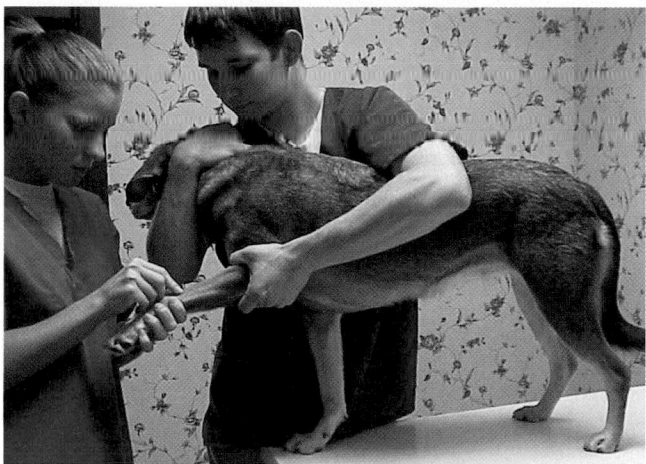

Figure 1-59 The correct positioning for obtaining blood samples from the cephalic vein. The handler has the dog well restrained, even though the dog remains standing, and has rolled the vein slightly outward to tighten the skin and provide easy access for venipuncture. If the dog becomes anxious, the handler will force the dog into sternal recumbency while maintaining the hold.

The handler's free hand is used to restrain the dog's head, and for most dogs, this is best accomplished by pressing the head into the chest of the handler by reaching under the neck and placing the hand behind the jaw. The hand may also go around the dog's muzzle to prevent biting when necessary. The handler must release the thumb when the veterinarian or veterinary assistant is ready to perform the injection. Failure to release the vessel will prevent the injected substance from reaching the general circulation and may result in rupture of the vessel.

Kneeling or squatting behind a large dog that is sitting on the floor allows cephalic venipuncture to be performed in the same manner. Most dogs submit to cephalic venipuncture quite readily. Dogs that are gentle may allow cephalic venipuncture while they are sitting up.

Jugular venipuncture may be necessary in some cases. This is accomplished by placing the dog close to the edge of the examination table and bracing against the dog so that it cannot retreat from this area. The forelegs are incorporated by one arm of the assistant with a finger between the legs for a secure grip. The hand of the other arm is then placed over the animal and is the one that restrains the head. The hand on the head grasps the muzzle with the fingers under the jaw, and the thumb is over the nose. Care must be taken when placing the hand to avoid cutting off the animal's ability to breathe. The fingers must not be placed too far caudally on the jaw, which may occlude the jugular vein and make it difficult to locate. The main advantage of this position is to provide a nearly straight plane from the angle of the jaw to the forefeet for easy access to the jugular vein. The dog should be "stretched" to a slight degree to achieve the correct position. Common errors in this position are pulling the forelegs too far forward, which interferes

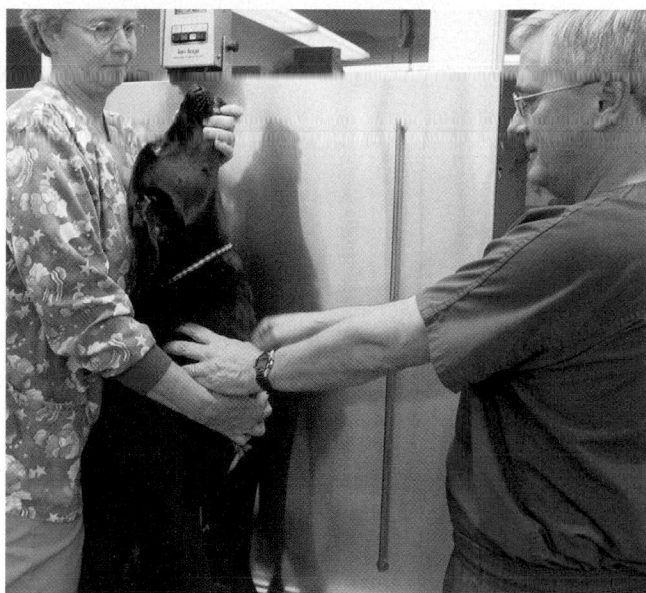

Figure 1-60 Method of holding the dog for jugular venipuncture. Note the straight line from the ramus of the mandible to the feet and the fact that the holder is positioned to help support the dog's back. Also note how the veterinarian is positioned at arm's length from the dog in case of a sudden pain response by the dog.

with the angle of entry for the syringe, and pulling the head too far backward, which stretches the skin and vessel and collapses the vein. The correct position of the head should be no more than slightly greater than 90 degrees from the neck. The head may be directed toward the holder's chest, allowing access to the vessel that is on the side opposite the holder. A large dog can be restrained on the floor with the holder steadying the chest with one hand and the muzzle with the other (Figure 1-60).

The saphenous vein, located on the lateral aspect of the hind leg, is an alternate venipuncture site; for this procedure, the dog must be restrained in lateral recumbency. (Refer to Chapter 3 for additional information about diagnostic sampling techniques.) To position a dog in lateral recumbency, the holder places the dog in sternal recumbency first and then reaches under the dog to grab the legs nearest to him or her. Then the dog is rolled from sternal to lateral recumbency, and the holder stands behind the dog with one forearm pressed across the animal's neck while that hand holds the forelegs with a finger between the legs. The other forearm presses across the dog's flank, and the hind legs are held in a similar manner (Figure 1-61). When venipuncture is being performed, only the down leg is held; the person making the puncture stabilizes the other leg.

🖎 TECHNICIAN NOTE

The saphenous vein, located on the lateral aspect of the hind leg, is an alternate venipuncture site for which the dog must be restrained in lateral recumbency.

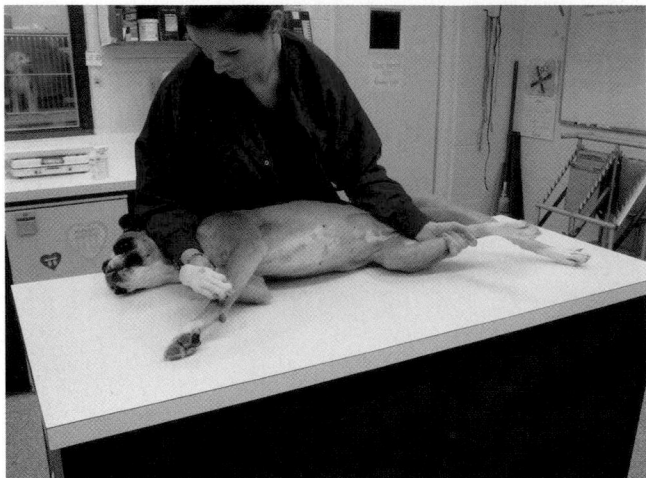

Figure 1-61 The correct positioning for holding a dog in lateral recumbency. Note how the handler has the downside limbs in her hands and the forearm that restrains the front limb rests across the dog's neck and the forearm restraining the hind limb rests across the dog's flank to aid in keeping the dog in lateral recumbency.

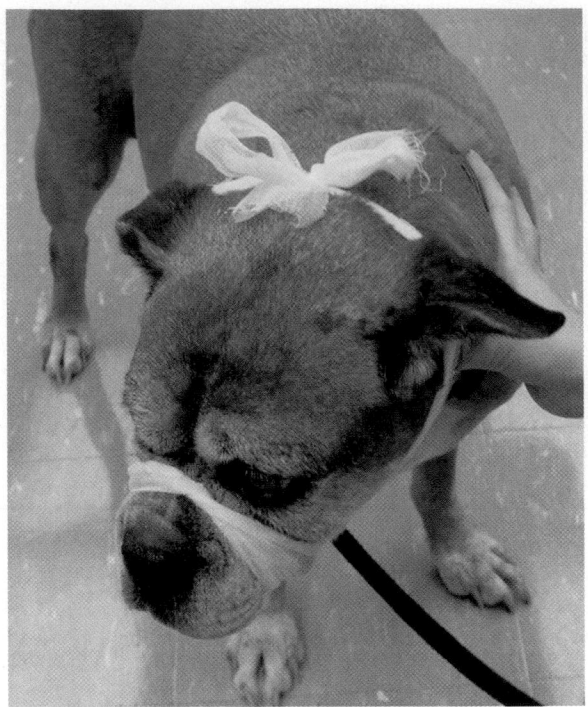

Figure 1-62 The gauze muzzle.

MUZZLES AND MOUTH GAGS

A dog's mouth can be restrained manually by bringing the hands forward from the rear on both sides of the face. The thumbs are placed on the forehead, and the fingers are looped under the mandibles. The palms of the hands should be below the ears.

Commercial muzzles are made of a variety of materials and come in various sizes. Several sizes should be available in any small animal clinic. Gauze or rope muzzles can be made if necessary. Nylon rope choke leads are sometimes handy as muzzling devices for snapping dogs. After capture of the dog, a loop of rope made with a single overhand knot is positioned from above the dog's nose until it is in place over the muzzle. This loop should be tightened quickly after it is positioned with the knot on top of the nose. Most dogs will try to push the rope loop off with their forepaws. The first knot must be held snugly while a second knot is made with the ends under the nose. The second knot may be a single overhand, or a square knot may be thrown. The two free ends are then passed behind the dog's head and tied again. This knot is extremely important because it holds the muzzle in place so it must be secure, yet it must be tied in such a manner to allow for quick release, should the animal have difficulty breathing.

Gauze roll bandage (7.5 to 15 cm) may be used as a muzzle in the same fashion as the rope (Figure 1-62). Gauze is preferable to rope because it is less slick. However, it also makes a less rigid loop to apply to a recalcitrant dog. The piece of gauze should be cut at least 90 cm long for most dogs. It is important to have sufficient length to begin with, because there may be only one opportunity to muzzle the dog without a significant battle.

Brachiocephalic breeds are difficult to muzzle and can be determined biters. For the purpose of muzzling them, a gauze bandage is first tied around the nose with the first knot tied underneath the jaw. The ends are then passed behind the head and tied with a square knot. Finally, one end is passed over the forehead and under the loop on top of the nose and then tied back to the other side. This keeps the loop from slipping off the top of the short nose.

The mouth of a dog can be examined in a variety of ways. The easiest, if the dog is a willing participant, is to open the mouth with the hands for visual examination. Placing one hand on the upper jaw and the other on the lower jaw and then forcing the lips over the teeth will allow the handler to separate the jaws of the mouth (Figure 1-63). A variety of mouth gags can also be used on dogs. A simple wooden dowel may be pressed toward the back of the mouth to rest between the carnassial teeth. The dowel can be tied in place behind the ears, or it can be held by hand. Stomach tubes may be inserted with the dowel in place. The commercial spring mouth gag has a hole on either end for the canine teeth, and it is inserted on one side of the mouth for a variety of procedures. The disadvantage to this type of gag is that it hangs outside the mouth, is heavy, and can fracture the teeth to which it is attached. A syringe case of appropriate size, placed over opposing canine teeth, makes a lighter and safer gag, especially for use in dental work.

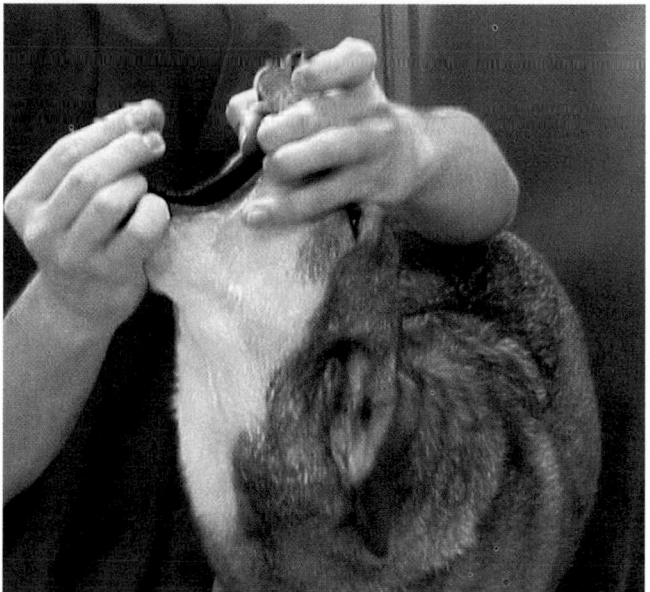

Figure 1-63 Technique for examination of the mouth. The lips of the upper jaw are pressed against the teeth by one hand while the lower lips are pressed into the teeth of the lower jaw. Forcing the lips apart then opens the jaw.

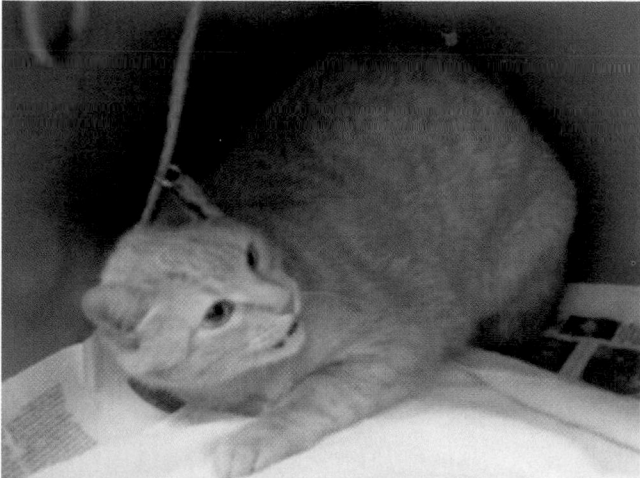

Figure 1-64 Trapped cats will display flattened ears and may hiss and growl before unleashing their claws.

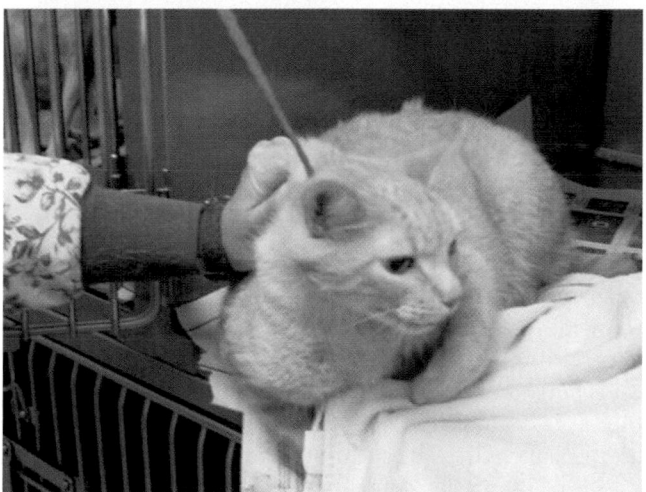

Figure 1-65 Capture of the head followed by grasping the scruff of the neck will restrain most cats.

MOBILITY-LIMITING DEVICES

Self-mutilation and tearing of bandages can be prevented with several devices. The most common is the Elizabethan collar. The concept is to place some type of stiff material extending from the collar area to the dog's nose so that it cannot chew or lick its body. Commercial plastic collars are available; or collars may be fabricated from buckets, large bottles, or heavy plastic sheets. It is most important to ensure that no sharp edges are present and that the collar is secured to the neck by gauze or the dog's collar. (It would be embarrassing for a veterinary practice if the dog traumatized itself with the collar, causing an injury more severe than the original lesion.) Attention must be given to the ability of the dog to eat and drink after the placement of these devices.

Fastening a pole along the body to a snug collar high on the neck makes another type of device that will limit movement of the head. This would mimic the cradle described for restraint of horses earlier in the chapter. Tape is usually used to keep the device from shifting.

CHEMICAL RESTRAINT

Many drugs are available for chemical restraint and sedation of dogs. The main reason for tranquilization is to alleviate anxiety, which is one of the major reasons that dogs bite. However, the handler is cautioned that tranquilizing effects vary among dogs and that dogs are still capable of biting even when heavily tranquilized. Chapter 21 provides more information on chemical anesthetic agents.

CAPTURE AND RESTRAINT OF CATS

CATCHING CATS

Cats are more apprehensive than dogs with strange people and surroundings. A cat that escapes will seek out a hiding place, whereas a dog that escapes will look for room to run away. This may be due to the lower endurance that a cat has for running and the security that cats feel in an enclosed space. A cat that is trapped may respond with flattened ears, hissing, scratching, and biting at hands and extended fingers (Figure 1-64). Heavy leather gloves or a large towel may be used to subdue these cats in the same manner as described for small dogs. Grasp the scruff of the neck to lift the cat (Figure 1-65). This may be followed by a rapid "stretch" restraint in which the hind legs are also grasped. Certain

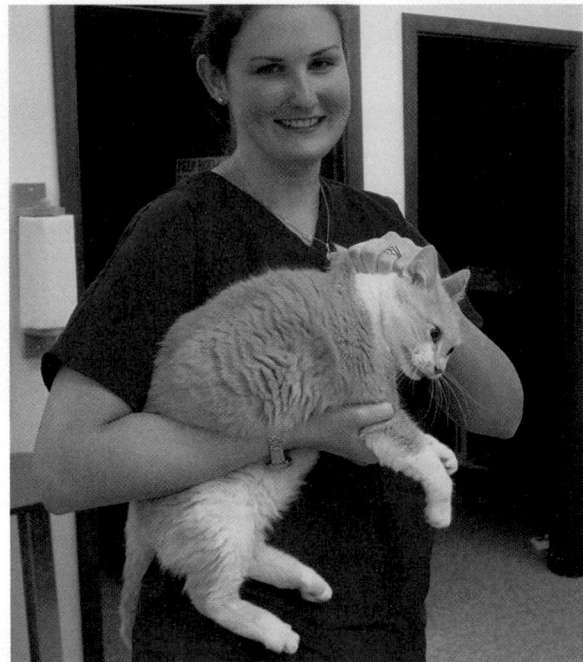

Figure 1-66 The proper carrying position for a cat. Note the support given to the abdomen, the grasp of the neck, and the restraint of both front feet.

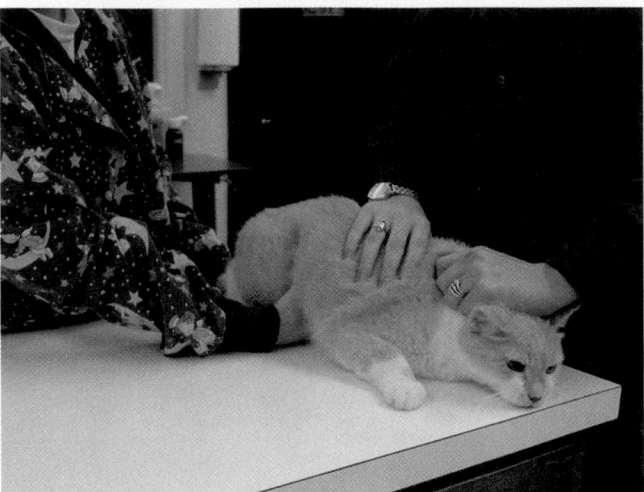

Figure 1-67 Restraint for examination of a cat. Note that both the handler and examiner have on long-sleeved lab coats.

cats are too fast and smart to succumb to either the glove or the towel technique. These cats may be caught by a neck rope or snare, but they react poorly to a choke compared with the scruff of the neck. One of the easiest ways to catch a cat is to force it into a box that is pushed into the cage where the cat is housed. Boxes that allow for anesthesia induction after the cat is captured, without additional handling of the cat, are available. All escapes from the box are blocked once the cage is placed in the kennel until the cat is safely inside and the top is closed.

A rope may be used to lasso a cat that is extremely un-cooperative. The rope is thrown over the cat and then quickly passed between the cage bars, and the front of the cage is closed. The cat is then brought to the front of the cage with the noose. Next, chemicals may be used to subdue the cat, either by oral spray or injection. If the tail can be hooked and pulled to the cage door while the cat's head is restrained in the noose, the hindquarters will be presented for intra-muscular injections. This provides the greatest amount of safety for handlers.

CARRYING CATS

Cats generally feel most secure in close quarters and seldom resist being put into a bag or rolled in a towel. They are best carried from place to place in a cat carrier or small cardboard box with a lid. They can also be carried with one arm if they are not particularly nervous. For the purpose of carrying a cat, its hindquarters are placed under the elbow area and pressed securely to the holder's body with the forearm

(Figure 1-66). The cat lies in a sternal position along the forearm while the hand, which has one finger between the legs, holds the forelegs. The cat may still use the hind claws to gouge the abdomen of the holder, who must be ready to grab the scruff of the neck and hold the cat at arm's length if it panics. Quickly grasping the hind legs and pulling away from the scruff of the neck will effectively immobilize almost any cat. This is not a position of comfort for the cat, and the cat will object, but it is clearly safer for the holder.

✎ TECHNICIAN NOTE

Cats usually feel most secure in close quarters, and they seldom resist being put into a bag or rolled in a towel.

RESTRAINT FOR EXAMINATION

Table restraint of cats is similar to that of dogs, except that cats tend to use their claws as their first line of defense (if they have them), rather than their teeth. Cats should be allowed supervised movement when it is not necessary for them to be still. Some cats are so terrified that they are best held or cuddled with the head buried under the holder's arm. Muzzles are available for cats that cover both the teeth and eyes and provide a sense of security for some. Cats are not necessarily malicious when they climb onto a person's chest or clamp nails into a forearm, but their actions will hurt if the holder is not prepared. It is a good idea to wear protective gowns or laboratory coats with long sleeves when dealing with cats (Figure 1-67). Cat scratches are potentially dangerous to veterinary personnel, and care should be taken to avoid movements and behavior that will agitate a cat.

RESTRAINT FOR VENIPUNCTURE

Cephalic venipuncture restraint can be applied to cats much as it is to dogs (Figure 1-68). However, cats will tend

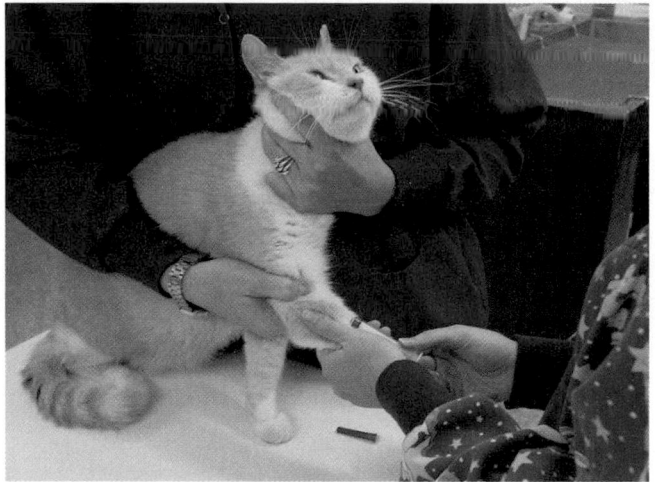

Figure 1-68 Proper restraint for cephalic venipuncture in the cat. The head, forearm, and back of the cat are all supported and well restrained by the handler.

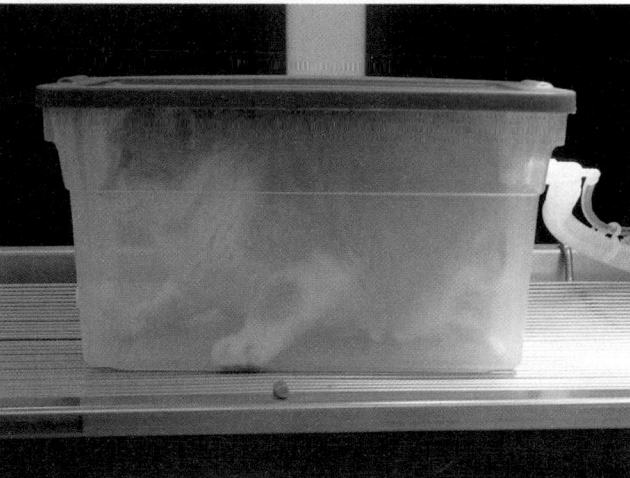

Figure 1-70 This cat is being restrained in a capture box that has inlet ports for inhalation anesthesia.

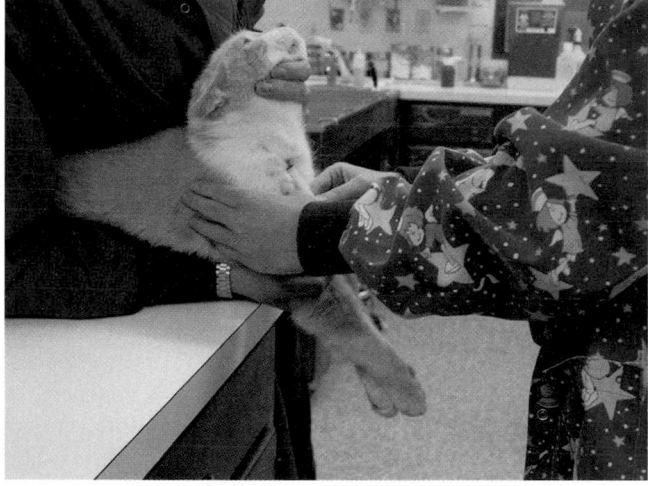

Figure 1-69 Restraint for jugular venipuncture in the cat. Note how the hind legs are tucked under the elbow of the handler and the forefeet are extended and held in one hand.

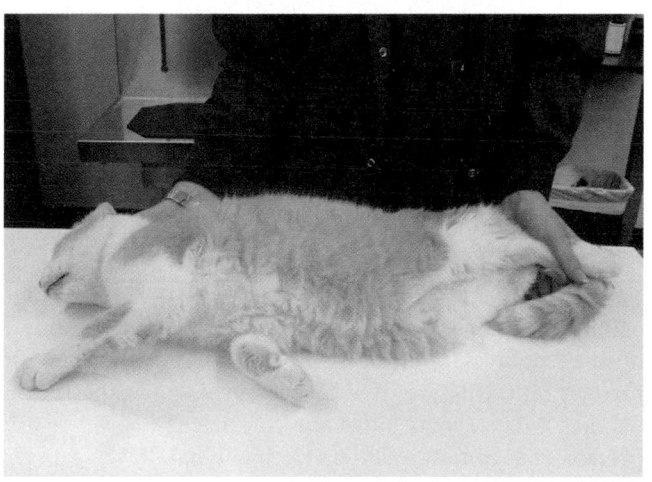

Figure 1-71 Stretching a cat on its side.

to engage their claws and teeth in an effort to get away from the handler. When a cat becomes agitated, it seems to lose its spine and develop legs that swirl about like a weed-eater. Once cats develop this attitude, they are impossible to hold like dogs, and other restraint techniques must be used. Jugular venipuncture may be more appropriate for some cats because the hold restrains the head and forefeet more securely than the cephalic technique (Figure 1-69). Wrapping the hindfeet with a towel disarms all but the most persistent cat. The head is held with the hand over the top of the head, and the jaw or zygomatic arch is grasped with the thumb on one side and two or three fingers on the other side. The other hand then restrains both forelimbs as is done for the dog.

There are other ways to hold a cat for jugular venipuncture. They involve the cat being placed on its back with the handler occluding the jugular vein and the person using the syringe pushing the chin down toward the table to make the head move backward to get a straight shot at the jugular. The holder can hold two legs in each hand with a finger between the legs while pushing the cat down on the table and using the little finger to press on the thoracic inlet to occlude the jugular vein. A cat can also be rolled in a towel or bag to engage the feet and legs. The handler need only steady the cat on its back and occlude the vessel in this case. Cat bags are made with zippers so a single limb may be withdrawn and used for cephalic venipuncture, and in a similar fashion, there are now restraint boxes made for cats that have different openings to allow for withdrawal of a limb (Figure 1-70).

Stretching a cat in lateral recumbency will provide access to the saphenous vein (Figure 1-71). Most cats do not seem to realize that they can use their forefeet to scratch the hand on the scruff of their neck when they are appropriately stretched. The medial saphenous vein can then be used for venipuncture by holding the hind leg that is up in a flexed position. The little finger can be used to hold off the vein on the down leg for the venipuncture. The person who is performing the venipuncture must restrain the down leg with one hand while handling the syringe with the other.

BATHING

Bathing a cat may be a trying experience for both the cat and the person. Most cats will try to climb up the person's arms to escape standing water or spray. Cats should be bathed on top of a screen suspended over a tub (a metal window screen will suffice) and washed with a light spray of warm water. Almost all cats will clamp their claws into the screen and stand still for the entire bath when this technique is used.

CHEMICAL RESTRAINT

The use of chemicals and anesthesia to restrain cats is common. The eyes should be treated with ophthalmic ointments to prevent corneal drying from the lack of blinking when these agents are used. See Chapter 19 for more information on anesthesia.

RESTRAINT OF EXOTIC ANIMALS

Minimal handling of all exotic animals is recommended and must be done efficiently, quietly, and confidently. The best method of learning restraint is by watching an experienced handler. Many clients judge the competency of veterinary professionals by how well they catch and handle the patient. Smooth handling and restraint of their animals reassure clients that the technician is well trained. It is often difficult to quantify the stress factor. The importance of fast, competent handling cannot be overemphasized. The sights, sounds, smells, and temperatures of the strange environment will stress the exotic animal in a veterinary hospital. As a general rule, the more tame the animal, the better it will tolerate handling. However, do not underestimate the added stress of disease and trauma. Always discuss the risk of stressing an ill or traumatized nondomestic pet with the owner before handling begins. All treatment and testing material (Culturettes, syringes) must be in place before the animal is restrained to minimize the stress. The patient work-up may have to be done incrementally because of the patient's poor physical condition or response to handling.

TECHNICIAN NOTE

Always discuss the risk of stressing an ill or traumatized nondomestic pet with the owner before handling begins.

RESTRAINT OF BIRDS

Psittacines

When holding and examining a psittacine patient, the medical team should avoid the strong beak, jaws, wings, and feet. The feet usually have sharp, pointed claws. The equipment needed to capture and handle these patients will include towels or drapes, perches, and nets. Gloves should never be used with psittacine birds in the clinical setting. Gloves are not supple enough for handlers to feel the patient within their grasp. Do not use gloves during stressful events with a pet bird because that bird will soon associate the shape of the human hand with negative experiences. The handler should first remove water bowls and perches from the cage or carrier. Room lights may be dimmed to take advantage of the bird's inability to rapidly accommodate to changes in lighting. The psittacine bird's primary weapon is the beak; therefore the head should be promptly secured.

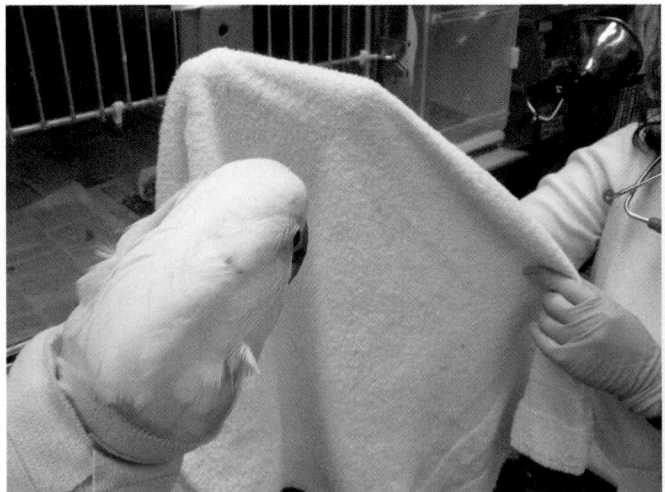
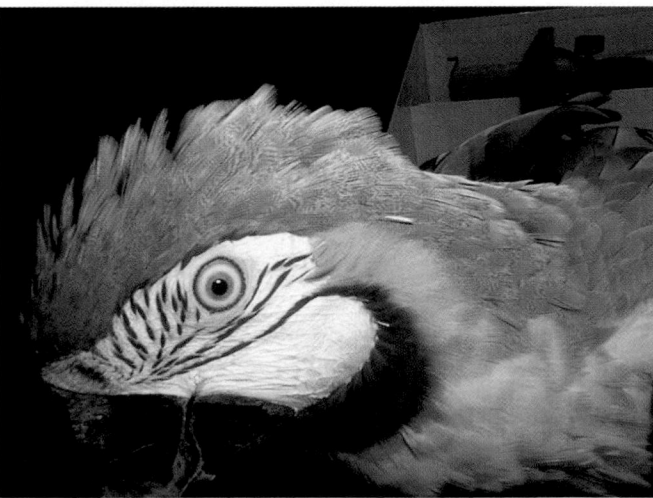

A   B

Figure 1-72 **A,** Allowing a bird to view the towel before capture often helps the bird to accept being held without the trauma associated with a blind grab from behind. **B,** Dilated pupils are often indicative of a stressed, angry parrot.

Placing a towel or drape over the bird's head and securing it with your hand is the best way to accomplish this. To prevent the bird from becoming afraid of the towel, you should come toward the bird with the towel, covering the grasping hand in a manner in which the bird can see (Figure 1-72). By approaching the bird in a nonthreatening manner, you can often often capture it with minimal stress. A wooden perch may be used to give the bird something to bite on other than fingers. The bird cannot bite the person attempting to catch it if it is chewing or biting the cage or carrier. Once the head is secured, the body is wrapped in the towel, the feet are held, and the bird is placed against the holder's body to control the wings. The towel or drape may then be slowly removed from the patient's head for examination, keeping the towel around the wings to secure them from flapping. Commercially available avian restraint boards allow for secure restraint with minimal risk to the patient or veterinary personnel (Figure 1-73). Care must be maintained to prevent restriction of the chest to allow the bird to breathe properly.

TECHNICIAN NOTE

Birds inhale and exhale air through mechanical chest movements. Any restriction of their ability to expand and contract their chests, such as improper restraint, may cause suffocation.

Passerines

Canaries and finches are the most common passerines seen in veterinary offices. These birds are easily stressed under normal conditions and are even more sensitive when they are ill. Catching the patient for an examination must be done quickly and efficiently. For an attempt to catch a passerine patient, all lights should be turned off after the cage door is slowly lifted and the hand has been inserted into the cage door opening. Grab the patient with one hand, and then turn on the lights. To hold the bird for examination, let the bird's head rest between the middle and index fingers while lying on its back. The fingers should not completely encircle the body but should stay on the sides of the bird. As with other avian species, do not put pressure on the breast or the patient may suffocate (Figure 1-74). Care should be taken to hold the head straight so the thumb does not slip to the anterior part of the neck and occlude the trachea.

Raptorial Species

Birds of prey use their anatomic weapons in a different way than psittacine species. With them, it is of utmost importance for the handler to secure the talons. Although many raptors will bite, their jaws are not tremendously strong, and they do little damage with their beaks. The mouth is soft except close to the very point of the beak, which the birds use for tearing flesh. The wings should also be considered a weapon and should be properly secured in a manner similar to that described for other avian species. Equipment needed for restraining raptors includes towels or drapes, gloves of appropriate size and thickness, and hoods.

TECHNICIAN NOTE

Most raptor species can be captured by using welding gloves or specialized raptor gloves of a similar design. Gloves for larger species, such as eagles, have special full cuff gauntlets to protect the arm from being injured by talons during the capture and handling of these birds.

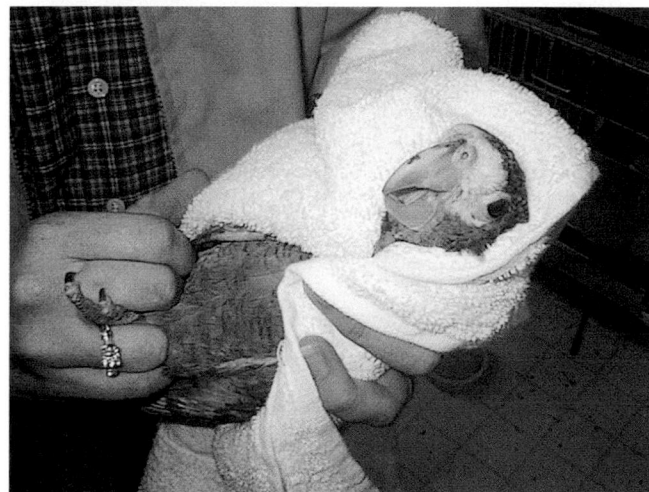

A

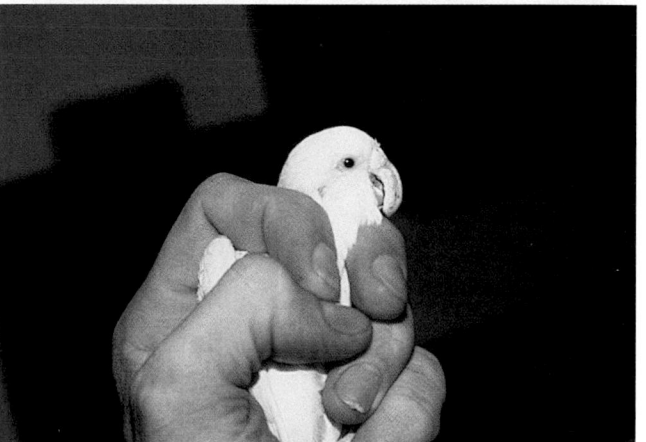

B

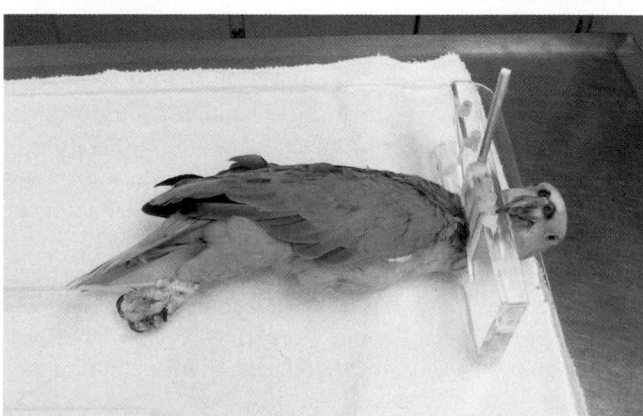

C

Figure 1-73 **A,** Restraint of a Hispaniolan Amazon parrot with the use of a towel and an Elizabethan hand grip. **B,** One-handed restraint techniques can be used for a budgerigar. No pressure is being placed on the pectoral area to allow for breathing. **C,** Restraint with a commercial avian restraint board.

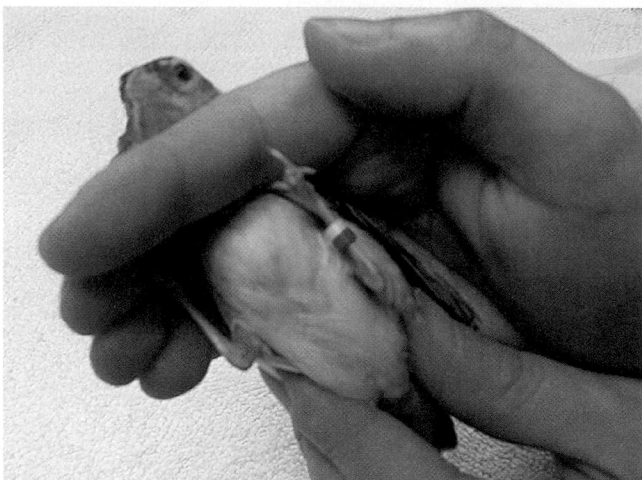

Figure 1-74 The proper technique for restraining a passerine for a physical examination.

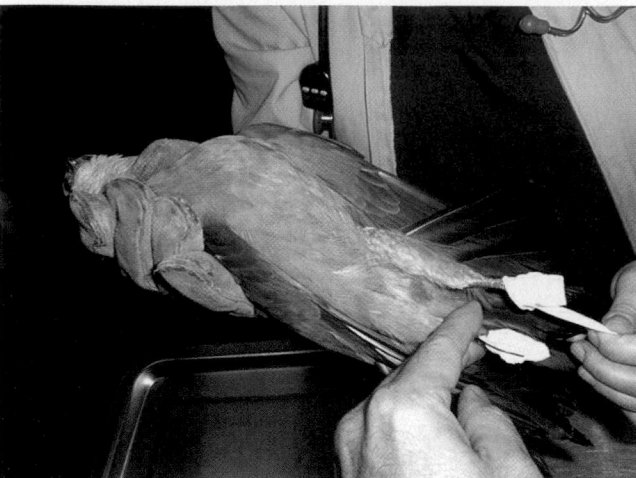

Figure 1-76 Taping the talons of a raptor with 1-inch white adhesive tape will help protect the technician. Leaving a tab on the end of the taped talon by folding over the tape will aid in tape removal at the end of the procedure.

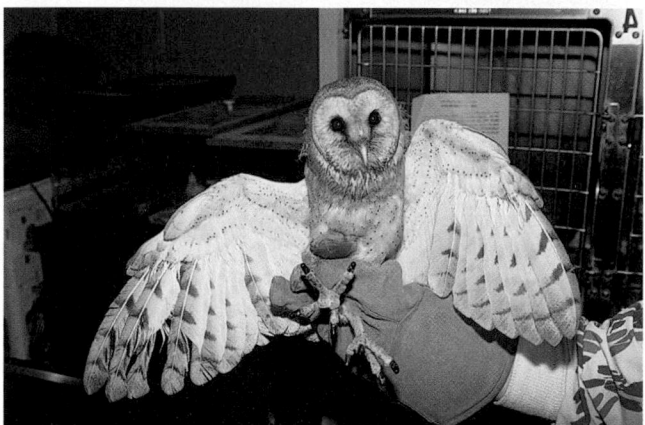

Figure 1-75 The restraint of a barn owl with the use of leather gloves. Note the restraint of the talons.

To approach a bird of prey using gloves, the handler should bend down low and quietly approach the patient. Dimming the lights may be a disadvantage for examining a species that hunts at night. The handler should present as little threat as possible to the raptor. As the handler places one hand in front of the raptor's face, the second hand should be brought in low toward the bird's feet. The upper hand should be held between the handler's face and the bird and may be used to distract the bird. The lower hand should quickly grasp the feet, in an attempt to place the index finger between the bird's feet (Figure 1-75). The bird is then smoothly and quickly pulled up out of the cage or off the floor so it does not beat its wings on any surfaces. It is important to hold the bird away from objects such as the examining table or cage. The bird can then be brought into a cradle position, with the wings secured between the handler's arm and body and the hood placed over the bird's head.

If hoods are not available, a towel may be draped over the bird's head, which will reduce visual and auditory stimuli and help to significantly calm the bird. An alternative approach to secure a bird of prey may be done with a towel or drape. The handler approaches the bird in the same manner, quietly and low, with the towel or drape spread in front with both hands. The handler moves in slowly until he or she is close enough to use the towel as a large glove, completely covering the bird. The handler's hands should contact the bird at the level of the bird's shoulders. It is important to avoid simply throwing the towel because the bird will be able to dodge it or move from under it. The bird is then pressed through the towel with enough pressure to make the bird push up, using its legs on the ground. The handler's hands are then worked downward, alongside the wings, toward the legs, and the legs are grasped at the tarsometatarsus (below the hock). Once the bird is covered by the towel and its feet are secured, the handler then lifts the bird up with the bird's back toward the handler's abdomen. A hood may replace the towel over the head. It is important never to release the feet of a bird of prey until someone else has secured them. A 10- to 15-cm long piece of 2.5-cm (1-inch) wide white cloth tape should be used to secure the talons to prevent accidents (Figure 1-76). If a bird has talons, the legs must be fully extended before the talons can be removed. Birds of prey under the control of a falconer are considered a different situation when being examined because the falconer is often adept at restraining the bird for a physical examination.

RESTRAINT OF REPTILES

Turtles and Tortoises

The veterinary technician should become as familiar as possible with anatomic and physiologic adaptations of reptiles

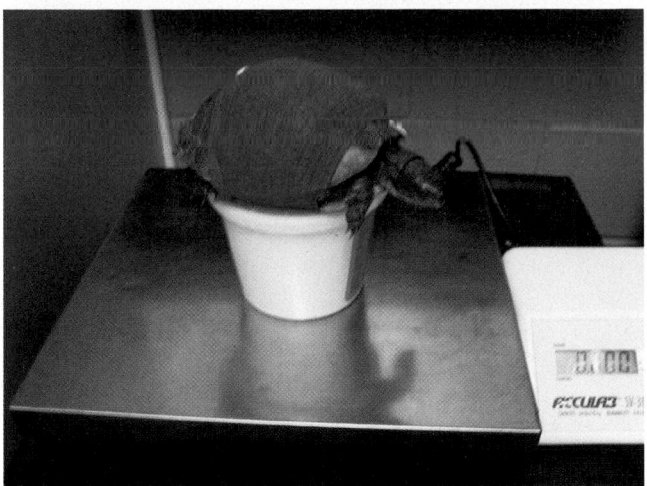

Figure 1-77 Placing a turtle or tortoise on a broad-based object will allow for easy handling and short-term restraint.

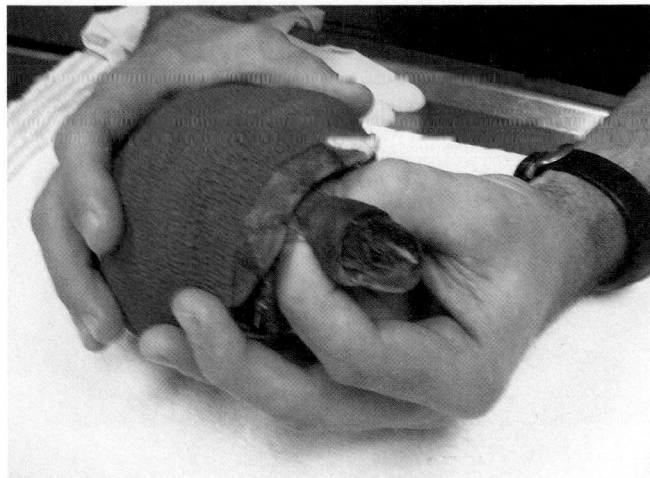

Figure 1-78 Gentle traction applied to the turtle's head with the thumb and forefinger is often effective in exposing the patient's head.

to handle them. Several sources of information are found in the recommended reading list at the end of this chapter. Restraint of turtles or tortoises should be done with caution. Some species of turtles have long necks and sharp powerful beaks (rhamphotheca) that can inflict a serious bite on the unwary handler. Some turtles may be able to extend their heads and necks nearly to the level of the hind limbs, two thirds of their body length. Many are quick and therefore should be approached from the rear, with the tail and legs securely held. Simply covering the head, neck, and forelimbs with a cloth towel is usually adequate to prevent injury to the turtle and handler. To prevent an animal from walking during an examination, the handler may place it on a broad-based object that will keep the chelonian limbs from touching the examination table surface (Figure 1-77). The legs may be kept in place by wrapping the shell, with the legs inside, with an elastic bandage. Straight ovoid delivery forceps or digital pressure may be used to remove a turtle's head from the shell for examination (Figure 1-78). Care must be taken; and steady, gentle traction must be used, without allowing the forceps to touch the eyes. The main force of the forceps' jaws should be applied away from the shell and not onto the head.

Snakes

Snakes are usually more difficult for the inexperienced handler. Equipment needed may include Plexiglas shields, Plexiglas tubes, tongs, canvas bags or drapes, snake hook, gas anesthetic machine, and plastic bags.

TECHNICIAN NOTE

Venomous reptiles are not recommended as pets and should be handled only by experienced snake handlers and veterinarians.

The general approach to restraint of any snake is to immobilize the head and grasp it firmly with the hands at the base of the skull. Several methods may be used to immobilize the animal's head initially; a drape, piece of paper, or Plexiglas shield may be used to block the snake's vision while the hands grasp the animal behind the head (Figure 1-79, *A*). The Plexiglas shield can be held in one hand, pressing the head of the snake to the floor, while the other hand grasps the snake at the base of the skull as the shield is slowly moved rostrally off the body. A snake hook may be used to pin the head to the floor.

When a snake hook is used, a suitable soft and resilient padded surface is useful to prevent trauma to the snake. A hand then replaces the hook. It is possible to injure a reptile by applying too much pressure with the hook; therefore only experienced technicians should use a snake hook on a client's animals. Most snakes can be easily maintained through hand control at the base of the skull. A few snake species can autotomize their tails as a defense mechanism. Snakes should not be picked up by their tails to prevent skin loss (degloving injury) and autotomization. Plexiglas tubes may be used in conjunction with a hook or pole. The hook is used to guide the snake into the Plexiglas tube, and the tube should be of sufficiently small diameter to prevent the snake from turning around and coming back out. The aim is to get the snake to crawl up the tube; when it reaches the halfway point, the technician grasps the junction of the snake and the tube, trapping the snake's head within the tube. The caudal half of the snake is accessible with this technique. A gas anesthetic unit may be attached to the open end of the tube for further restraint. Plastic tubes are not generally recommended for many elapine snake species (e.g., coral snakes, cobras) because of their ability to turn around and injure the handler.

Placing snakes in a plastic bag or box and filling it with anesthetic gases may also induce anesthesia. After induction of anesthesia, snakes are intubated and monitored on a gas anesthetic machine with intermittent ventilation

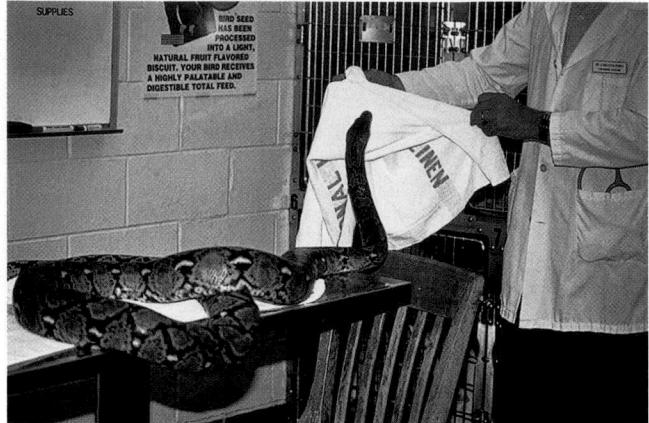

A

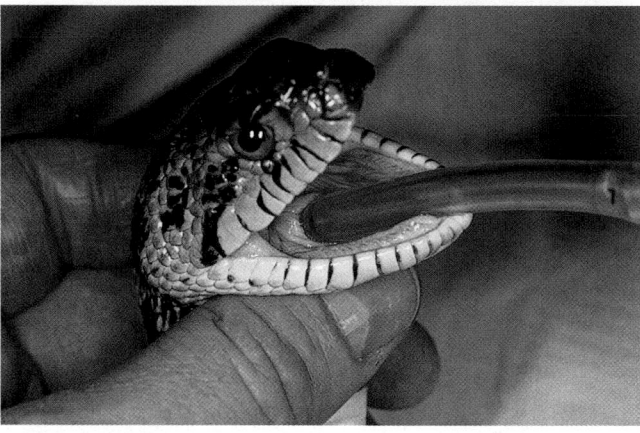

B

Figure 1-79   **A,** A towel may be used to block a snake's vision before grasping it from behind the head. **B,** Proper technique of holding a snake's head as an endotracheal tube is being placed.

(Figure 1-79, *B*). Snakes can be easily transported in canvas bags (Figure 1-80). When a snake is handled, its body should always be supported, and large species should always be handled by more than one person.

> ### TECHNICIAN NOTE
> It is always important to remember to wash your hands before handling reptiles, particularly if the previous patient was a rabbit or rodent (a snake's typical prey), because snakes attack primarily on the basis of smell.

Lizards and Crocodilians

Lizards and crocodilians may be restrained by using a combination of experienced hands and snare poles, towels, drapes, nooses, or Plexiglas shields. All lizards will bite, and some have strong jaws and sharp teeth. Most lizards will also use their claws and tails as weapons. The approach for small to medium lizards is to attempt to block their vision with a towel or sheet of paper, make a quick grab around the shoulder girdle at the base of the skull with one hand, and restrain the pelvic girdle with the other hand. The tail

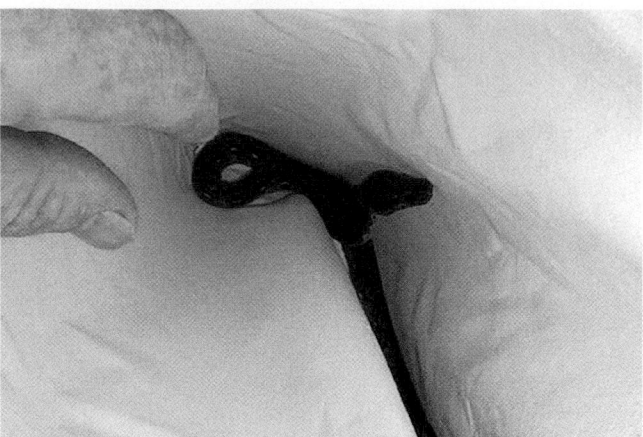

Figure 1-80   Snakes are often transported in canvas bags. An important point to remember is that the head should be identified before restraint is attempted.

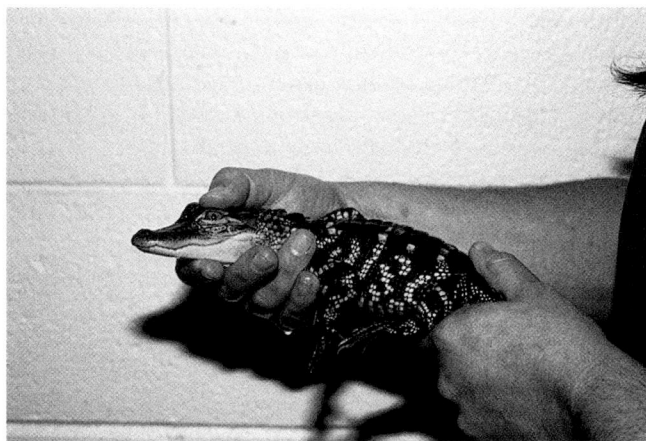

Figure 1-81   The proper restraint technique for a large lizard, in this case, an alligator. One hand is placed firmly about the pelvis, and the other is about the shoulders and neck. The tail may be tucked beneath the elbow.

may then be tucked in against the body, under the arm (Figure 1-81).

A noose made of fine fishing line at the end of a pole may be used for very small lizards. The noose is lowered over the animal's neck, the pole is quickly lifted with the noose tightened, and the animal is lifted by the neck. The animal should be restrained and removed from the noose as quickly as possible. For a large lizard or crocodilian, it is important to block the animal's vision and then quickly and safely immobilize the head and body simultaneously. This is best accomplished by grasping the animal at the base of the skull or neck with one or both hands, then sitting on it. Two or more people are needed to accomplish this task, and the animal's mouth should then be taped shut as soon as it is restrained. A noose or rabies pole may be used to help control the mouth before attempts to restrain the head, legs, and tail are made. Crocodilians, most large lizards,

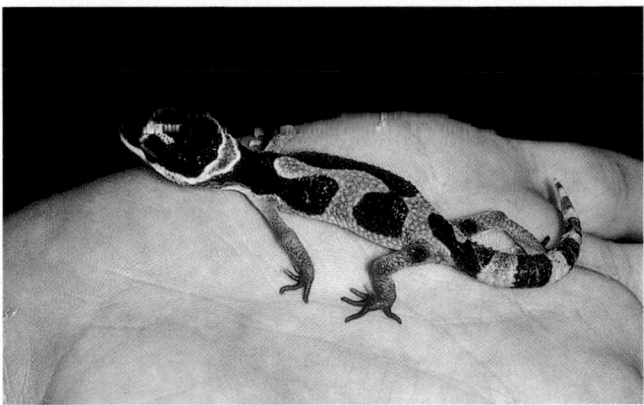

Figure 1-82 Great care must be used when restraining and treating patients that easily autotomize their tails, such as this gecko.

and some chelonians can be immobilized for short periods (up to 30 seconds) by application of gentle, inward pressure on their closed eyes for a few moments. The handler is cautioned that many lizards, particularly gecko species, have tails that autotomize when they are stressed or traumatized (Figure 1-82). Extreme caution should be used when lizard tails are handled.

RESTRAINT OF FERRETS

Ferrets that are not cooperative are a restraint challenge. Ferrets belong to the family group that includes weasels, and as such, they are quick, agile animals possessing sharp teeth. The ferret's primary weapons are its teeth, and when threatened, it will not hesitate to bite. Ferrets that are hand raised, which includes most pets, can make docile companion animals in the right circumstances. Proper precautions should be taken when restraining ferrets.

Primary restraint for a ferret is to secure the head and forelegs by gripping the animal by the skin in the dorsal cervical area (the scruff of the neck) (Figure 1-83). The other hand is used to support the bottom of the animal. For the highly aggressive ferret, a towel or drape may be placed over the animal to block its vision. The animal's head, neck, and shoulders can then be grasped through the drape or towel. The handler may want to use gloves. Remember, it is not good for any pet animal to associate negative experiences with gloved hands. Once the animal is restrained with this method, the handler may alter the grip on the head to perform a thorough physical examination and other necessary diagnostic procedures. Ferrets may be "stretched" in a manner similar to that used for cats, or they may be grasped with both hands around the forequarters, with one hand on the scruff of the neck and the other holding down the forelegs.

Ferrets are subject to hypnosis, although it is less likely to be effective when an animal is apprehensive in strange hands. For an attempt at hypnosis, a ferret is hung by the scruff with one hand and stroked around the entire length

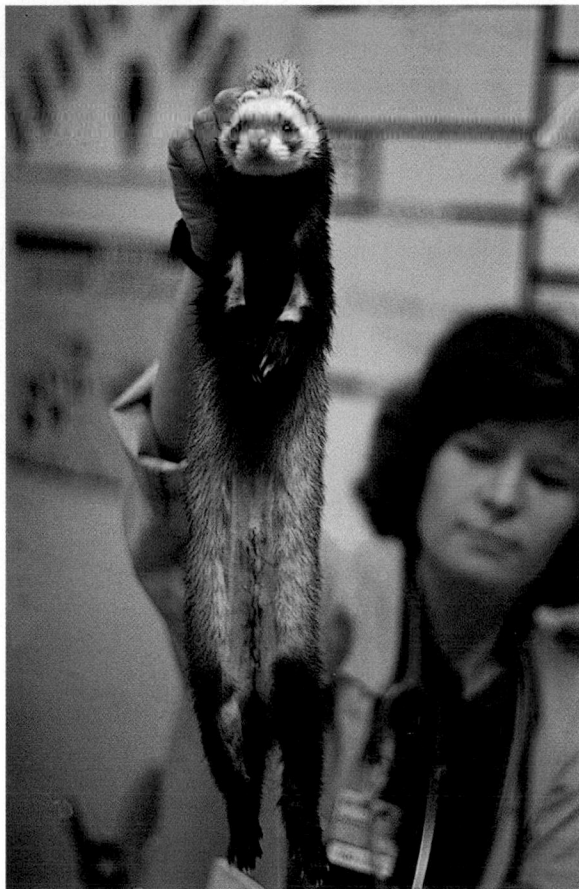

Figure 1-83 The proper technique for restraining a ferret. The scruff of the neck is held by one hand, and the other hand supports the body. Often this technique will elicit a "yawn," at which time the oral cavity may be examined.

of its torso with the other hand. The susceptible ferret will begin to yawn, and its eyelids will droop or close after repeated stroking. The effect is not long lasting, and many ferrets will be easily startled out of the trance.

RESTRAINT OF RABBITS

Proper rabbit restraint is important in reducing stress and injury to the patient (Figure 1-84, *A*). Rabbits have some peculiarities for restraint. Their muscle-to-skeleton ratio is very high, and their bones are small and light for animals of their size. Rabbits also have extremely powerful hind legs. Restraint of rabbits without controlling their hind legs may precipitate a kicking episode that could result in a "broken back." This terminology is not precise because the bones of the back may not be fractured, but there is definite loss of neural function in the hindquarters that results from trauma to the spinal cord. The hind legs become paralyzed, and bladder and anal tone are lost. The prognosis from recovery is poor in cases of total paralysis. Paralysis may be immediate or delayed, depending on the amount of hemorrhage and edema that surrounds the spinal cord.

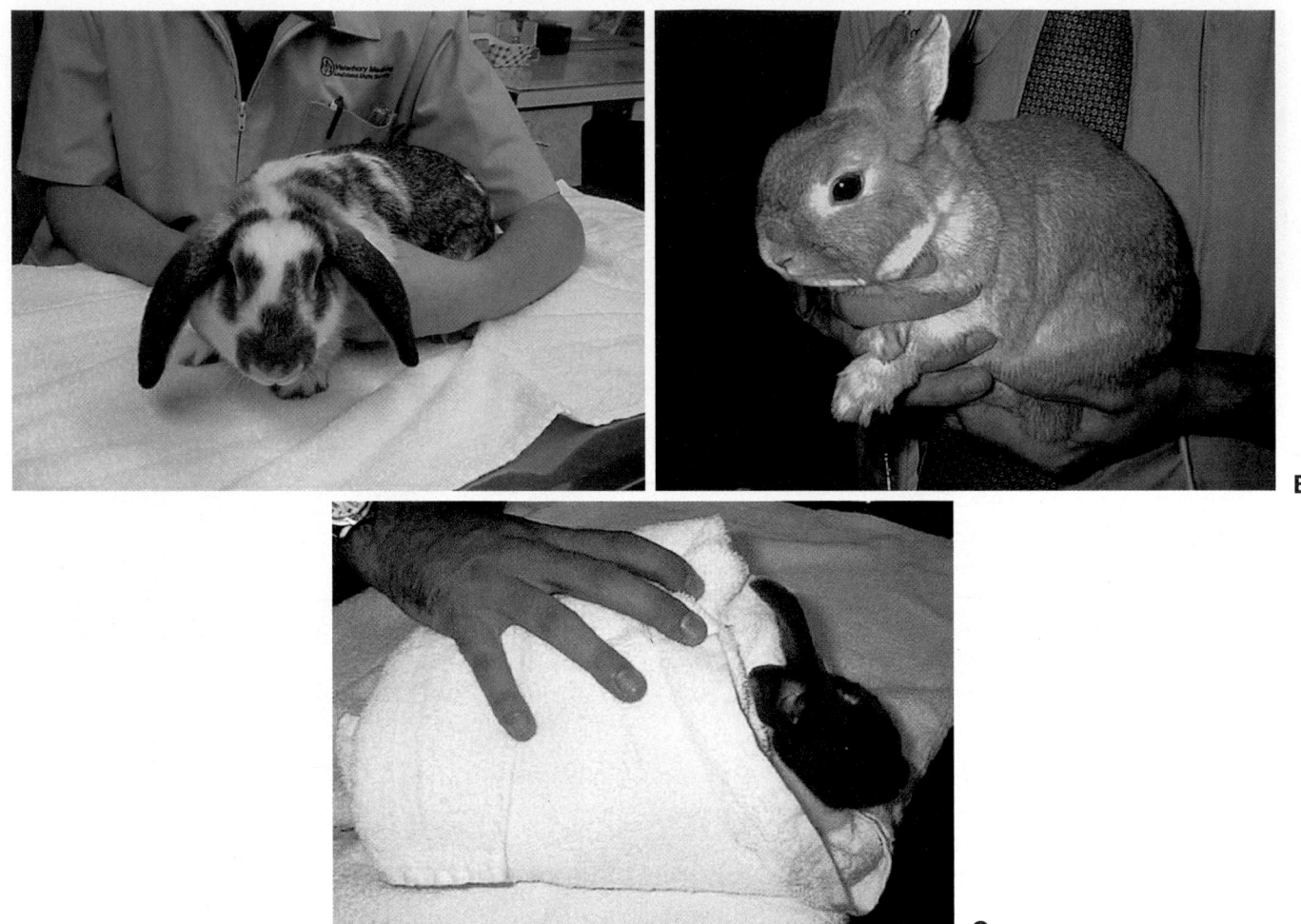

Figure 1-84 **A,** Proper holding technique for a rabbit undergoing a physical examination. **B,** The proper method of restraint for carrying a rabbit short distances. **C,** Wrapping a rabbit in a towel or "bunny burrito" is an effective way to restrain a fractious patient.

To avoid this situation, never pick up, carry, or restrain a rabbit by its ears. To carry a rabbit short distances, grasp the nape of the neck skin with one hand while supporting the rear legs with the other (Figure 1-84, *B*). The best way to replace a rabbit in a cage is by holding its skin fore and aft, placing it well inside the cage facing outward, and pressing its body down to the floor for a few moments before releasing it. Use of this technique forces the rabbit to turn in its cage before leaping to the safety of the rear of the cage. The ears should never be used to lift a rabbit of any age. Small plastic pet carriers should be used when rabbits are carried for long distances. A towel can be placed around the rabbit to help with restraint when the animal is carried or examined (Figure 1-84, *C*).

TECHNICIAN NOTE

Rabbits should never be picked up, carried, or restrained by their ears.

Rabbits do not like slick surfaces, and losing their footing agitates them. It is best to set them down on something on which they will have good traction, such as a rubber mat,

during an examination or treatment. Pressing the rabbit to the table and pulling the hindfeet to the rear allow for trimming of nails. The nails of the forefeet may be trimmed by lifting one foot at a time off the table while the rabbit is held to the surface.

Rabbits have sensitive whiskers and will flinch whenever these hairs are touched or the mouth is approached. For examination of the mouth, the head must be firmly held. To steady the head for an examination, the holder should place the rabbit facing away from his or her body with the forearms pressing down the entire length of the rabbit. The thumbs of the handler are placed behind the ears of the rabbit and the fingers are used to lift the head from below the mandible. The incisor teeth may be trimmed, aural examinations may be conducted, and ear venipuncture may be performed with the rabbit in this position.

TECHNICIAN NOTE

Rabbits may occasionally demonstrate signs of aggression by growling and scratching with the forelegs. Medium-weight gloves will prevent injury to the handler in these cases.

Rabbits will bite; therefore a conscious effort should be made to keep fingers away from the rabbit's mouth. Normally, the fight goes out of even the most aggressive rabbit once its forequarters are pressed to the floor and the body is restrained from free movement.

RESTRAINT OF RODENTS AND SMALL MAMMALS

Rodents and small mammals can be problematic to examine and treat because restraint without injuring such animals is difficult. These animals are generally very small and may bite when placed in a stressful situation. Commercial restraint devices are available for small rodents, but it is difficult to perform a good external examination because of their design. To catch these small animals, a technician can use bare hands or leather gloves. However, the teeth of rodents will penetrate leather gloves, so protection is minimal and may be more psychologic than physical for the handler.

Cornering or encircling the animal with both hands will allow the handler to capture a large rodent. Both hands should be used to pick the animal up, with the fingers underneath and the thumbs on top of the body. One hand should be behind the other to support the entire abdomen. Grasping the scruff of the neck and supporting the back legs provide restraint for larger rodents (e.g., guinea pigs, chinchillas, prairie dogs) (Figure 1-85). A large rodent that is standing on the examination table can also be restrained by wrapping a towel around its torso. Guinea pigs are different than most small mammals when restrained in that they can be quite vocal. Pregnant guinea pigs have pendulant bellies, and they may be lifted by grasping around the thorax with one hand and around the rump with the other to hold them up. Teeth of the guinea pig may be clipped by holding the head with one or two hands, with the forefinger under the jaw and the thumb behind the head. The guinea pig tolerates being placed upside down in a trough with the legs tied down in the same fashion as swine.

Smaller rodents and mammals are initially restrained by grabbing the tail (e.g. mouse, rat) or the scruff of the neck (hamsters, sugar gliders, gerbils) (Figure 1-87).

TECHNICIAN NOTE

Never grab a gerbil by the tail because the skin is easily removed (Figure 1-86). If the skin is removed, a tail amputation is required.

Hedgehogs are covered with sharp spines, and most will require anesthesia when examinations need to be performed or diagnostic samples need to be obtained (Figure 1-88). Once restrained, these small patients are held by the scruff or around the neck with one hand while the other hand supports the body. Hamsters have a large amount of redundant tissue associated with the cheek pouches, and this must be gathered up in the hand to hold them. Most small rodents may be restricted from movement on a surface by placing a hand over them to form a cage, with the head protruding between

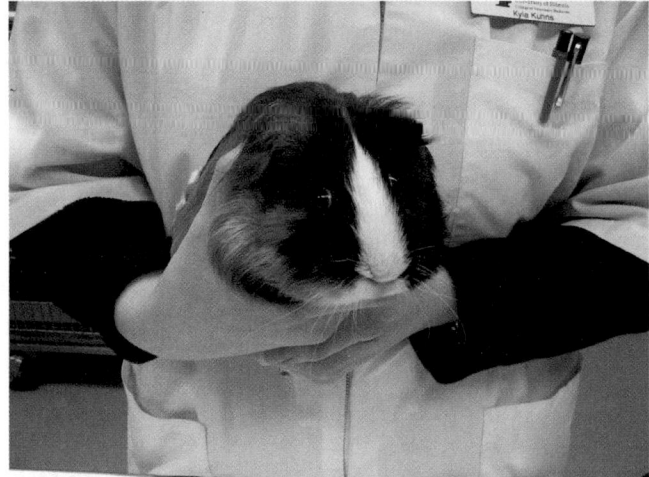

Figure 1-85 The proper restraint technique for a chinchilla or other large rodent.

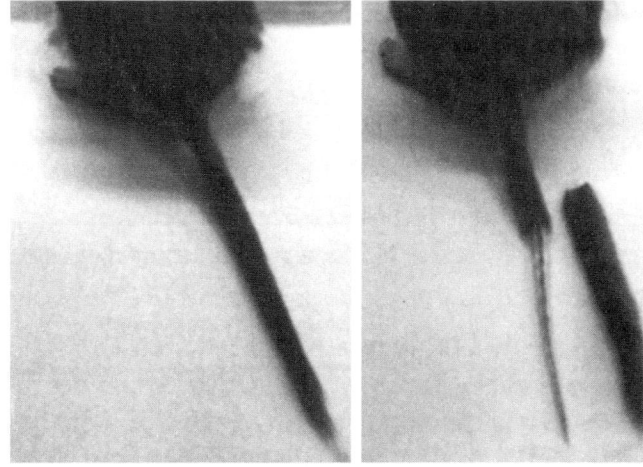

A   **B**

Figure 1-86 **A,** A normal gerbil tail, which should never be used to capture and restrain the patient. **B,** The skin has sloughed off the tail of this gerbil, which will require surgical amputation for correction.

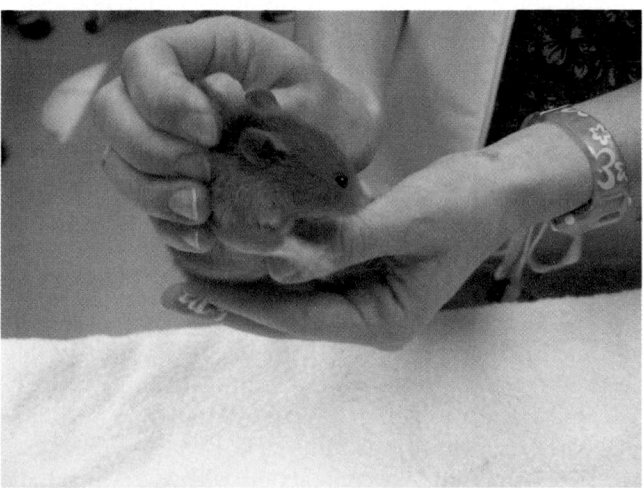

Figure 1-87 The proper restraint technique for a rat.

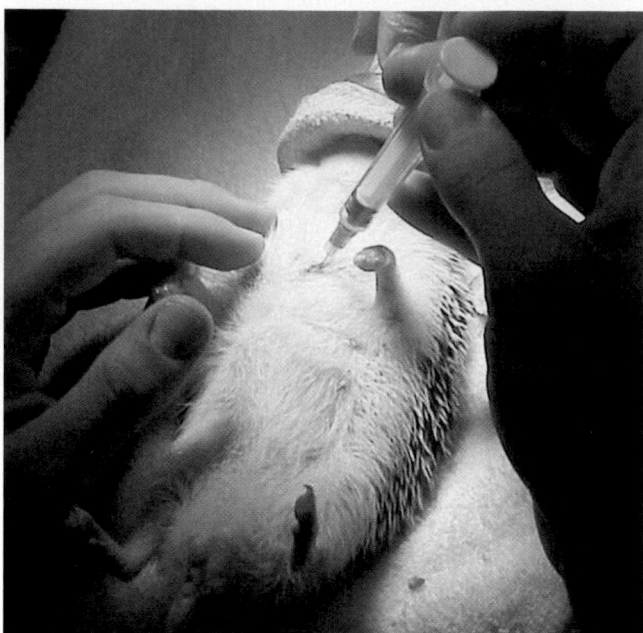

Figure 1-88 Hedgehogs are covered in sharp spines and often need to be anesthetized for examination or handled with thin leather gloves.

the first and second fingers. If a small rodent suddenly attempts to bite, it may be caught and restrained by driving it into a small tube. Rodent restraint tunnels are available in several sizes; usually they are made of Plexiglas and have several ports available for injection.

TRANSPORTATION AND SHIPPING OF ANIMALS

Control of animal health and surveillance of potential animal disease is part of the national duty of veterinarians and animal health technicians. The mobility of society today and the ability to transport animals quickly from one region to another makes this area of veterinary practice responsibility exceedingly important. As the average size of commercial livestock operations increases, more animals are at risk per outbreak. Increased agricultural trade increases exposure to diseases from foreign sources. Exotic animals are often found on modern hobby farms, hunting preserves, in aquaculture, and as pets; and the variety of backgrounds of these animals presents wide-ranging exposure to diseases for which immune systems are often unprepared. Although animal health control constitutes a "public service," it should be noted that it is necessarily implemented by both public institutions and private veterinary practices on whom the law imposes duties to report and act rapidly. The United States Department of Agriculture (USDA) has empowered veterinary personnel in conjunction with the Animal and Plant Health Inspection Service (APHIS) to be the central

component of this system. It is imperative that the veterinary profession follow the guidelines set forth by USDA/APHIS with regard to transport of animals both within and between states. Disease outbreaks are volatile, and as such, are continually changing. These guidelines are published on the APHIS website (http://www.aphis.usda.gov) and are listed for each state.

Most states have a minimum requirement of a negative result on a test for equine infectious anemia for entering horses or brucellosis for cattle more 20 months of age. Female cattle younger than 20 months must be vaccinated against brucellosis. Dogs and cats that are transported over state lines are legally required to have a certificate of veterinary inspection to cross state lines and are required to be vaccinated against rabies. This information is recorded on a certificate of veterinary inspection as well as the individual identification of all animals in the truck, trailer, or car.

Cats are often nervous when riding in cars and are usually best transported in carriers. They may be given a tranquilizer if they are excessively nervous, and most tranquilizers will also have an antiemetic effect. Cats and dogs may produce excess saliva when they become nervous, which can be controlled with atropine or a similar drug.

Most dogs and cats do not need tranquilization when shipped on airlines, because they feel secure in their shipping containers if they are accustomed to them before the trip. Even though the animals may be nervous in their crates, they are probably better off without tranquilization in this situation of minimal supervision. Air transportation requirements and regulations have been examined recently by the American Veterinary Medical Association, and their findings can be found at http://www.avma.org/grd/lac/Air_Transport. Commercial shipping crates of an acceptable size for the dog or cat are useful not only for shipping but also for containment at home. All animals traveling in air freight must be accompanied by a current certificate of veterinary inspection (within 10 days).

Recommended Reading

Fowler ME: Restraint *and handling of wild and domestic animals,* Ames, 1978, Iowa State University Press.

Fox MW: *Understanding your cat,* New York, 1974, Bantam Books.

Fox MW: *Understanding your dog,* New York, 1972, Coward, McCann and Geogheagan.

Fraser AF: *Farm animal behavior,* London, 1974, Balliere Tindall.

Grandon T: *Livestock handling and transport,* ed 2, Oxfordshire, England, 2000, CABI Publishing.

Hafez ESE: *The behavior of domestic animals,* ed 3, London, 1975, Balliere Tindall.

Hart BL: *Canine behavior,* Santa Barbara, Calif, 1980, Veterinary Practice Publishing.

Kiley-Worthington M: *The behavior of horses in relation to management and training,* London, 1987, JA Allen.

Roberts M: *The man who listens to horses,* New York, 1997, Random House.

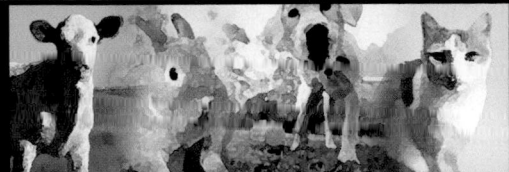

History and Physical Examination

ELLEN MILLER

Obtaining an Accurate History

Without an accurate history, even the best veterinarian may be unable to solve the problems of a particular patient. The history is the first step in reaching the ultimate diagnosis of the patient's illness. Although obtaining a history can be time-consuming, information elicited from the owner may save time and effort later in the diagnostic work-up of a particular problem. For example, a common mistake is the failure to differentiate true vomiting from regurgitation; the diagnostic plans for these two problems are costly and very different. An accurate history will help the veterinarian avoid errors of this kind. In a busy practice, the technician can begin the history-taking process for the veterinarian, freeing up time for the veterinarian to later discuss the primary problem in detail with the client.

The key to history taking is to obtain accurate information by asking the right questions. The specific questions asked will vary slightly, depending on the species of animal being evaluated. In this chapter the companion animal is the primary example. However, the principles discussed may be applied to other species. Specific species information concerning exotic animals, horses, and food animals may be found in Chapters 18, 29, and 30, respectively.

TECHNICIAN NOTE

The key to obtaining an accurate history is to ask the right questions.

Questions should be unbiased and not intended to lead the client toward a particular answer. For example, instead of asking, "Does Max drink more water than he used to?" it is preferable to ask, "Have you noticed a change in Max's water consumption?" Many people have such a desire to please that they will, without thinking, answer your questions affirmatively. Asking a question in an unbiased fashion

forces the client to think. He or she must decide whether there has been a change and, if so, whether the change is positive (more water than normal) or negative (less water than normal). Sometimes, questions need to be asked two or three times but be phrased differently to ensure the owner has understood the question and is consistent with answers. In asking questions, consider the owner's ability to observe the pet. An owner may tell you that the dog does not have diarrhea when he or she does not normally observe the dog defecating and does not know the answer to the question. It may be better to ask, "Do you observe your dog when it defecates?" and if so, "Does your dog have diarrhea?"

Because animal patients cannot talk, the owner must be relied on to provide accurate information. It is important to ask questions in terms that the client can understand. For instance, a client may know that his or her pet is drinking more than normal but may answer the question, "Does your pet exhibit polydipsia?" inappropriately because he or she doesn't know what polydipsia means. The intelligence of the client and any handicaps that might interfere with the client's ability to observe his or her pet or properly understand or hear the questions must be weighed in the interpretation of answers to these questions.

Active listening skills are important in the history-taking process. Often, paraphrasing what the client has said will help determine whether you understood him or her correctly.

Before entering the examination room with the client, it is important to know the client's name, the patient's name, and the type of animal that will be examined. Greet the client when you walk in the room and introduce yourself. Let the client know what you are doing each step of the way so that he or she feels informed.

SIGNALMENT OF THE ANIMAL

The signalment of the animal is the age, breed, and sex, including reproductive status, of that animal. This information is vital in developing a list of the most likely rule-outs for the patient's problem. For example, a young animal is more likely to be vomiting because of an infectious agent, toxin ingestion, foreign body obstruction, or intussusception; whereas an older animal with the same complaint may be more likely to have kidney, liver, or pancreatic disease as the cause of the vomiting. Certain diseases are heritable and occur in particular breeds of dogs and cats. Knowing the breed is the first step in identifying a possible genetic defect. Knowledge of the sex of the patient and whether it is spayed or neutered can obviously help rule out disorders that affect one sex or the other.

CHIEF COMPLAINT

> ✎ **TECHNICIAN NOTE**
>
> The chief complaint is the reason the client presented the patient for evaluation.

The chief complaint is the reason the client brought the animal to be evaluated. Discussing the chief complaint is the most important part of the history-taking process for the client. Although other problems may seem more important, failure to address the chief complaint can annoy the owner and imply that you are not listening. Be sure to spend time on the client's concerns before moving on to other questions. You may say something such as, "That is important information, and I am also interested in your observations regarding...."

HISTORY OF THE PRESENT ILLNESS

In the history of the present illness, detailed information about the chief complaint and any related problems is obtained. Duration, severity, progression, frequency, trigger situations, time of day, and character of the problem must be addressed if applicable. For instance, a miniature poodle that has a dry, hacking cough (character) in response to excitement (trigger) two or three times daily (frequency) for longer than 1 year (duration) without progression is likely to have a collapsing trachea at the root of the cough. All these clues will help narrow and prioritize the list of possible causes for the problem. In addition, the severity and progression will help determine the aggressiveness of the diagnostic work-up. The more severe the disease or rapid the progression, the quicker the diagnosis needs to be made.

MEDICAL AND SURGICAL HISTORY

> ✎ **TECHNICIAN NOTE**
>
> Medical and surgical history can provide valuable information related to the current problem.

The medical and surgical history can provide very important information related to the presenting problem in certain cases. Does the dog or cat have any medical problems or previous illnesses other than the chief complaint? Not only could the history have a bearing on the current problem, it may also affect the approach to the new problem, both diagnostically and therapeutically. For instance, knowing that a cat received megestrol acetate for a behavioral problem may provide a clue as to the reason for the increased thirst and urination the cat is experiencing. Increased thirst and urination are signs attributable to diabetes mellitus, which can be a sequela to progestogen therapy.

Has the animal ever had surgery, and if so, what type of surgery has it had? For example, a Yorkshire terrier presented with a draining tract from the medial aspect of the right stifle. The history revealed the dog had surgery to repair a ruptured anterior cruciate ligament in the right stifle 8 months earlier. Based on the knowledge that sutures were most likely used to repair the ligament, it was probable the suture was acting as a foreign body and providing a nidus, or point of origin, for infection. The current complaint was solved when the suture was removed. Had the history of the previous surgery not been known, an expensive work-up might have been undertaken.

ENVIRONMENTAL HISTORY

The type of environment in which the pet lives often helps narrow the list of possible causes of a particular problem. The environment may be primarily indoor, outdoor, or a combination. The animal may live in an outdoor kennel or roam free. All these situations imply potential hazards. An animal that spends the majority of its life indoors is less likely to be traumatized, ingest poisons, or be exposed to infectious diseases (unless in a kennel or cattery situation) compared with an animal that lives outdoors or is free to roam.

MEDICATION HISTORY

Information on any medication the animal is receiving is important for reasons that include prioritization of differential diagnoses, potential drug side effects, and possible drug interactions when additional drugs are prescribed. A dog receiving heartworm preventative is not likely to have heartworm disease as the cause of exercise intolerance if the correct dose is given at the appropriate time intervals. An animal that is presented with a history of increased thirst and urination while being treated with corticosteroids may not have a serious problem because these are common side effects of the drug. This knowledge can prevent an unnecessary work-up or help provide an explanation of abnormal laboratory results. An animal receiving corticosteroids for a skin disorder should not be given aspirin or other nonsteroidal antiinflammatory drugs (NSAIDs) at the same time for an acute lameness. If the history of corticosteroid therapy was not known and aspirin or an NSAID was prescribed at antiinflammatory dosages, life-threatening complications, including gastrointestinal ulceration and kidney failure, may result.

DIETARY HISTORY

It is important to know what type of food and how much food a patient is consuming, especially when dealing with problems of weight loss or obesity, vomiting, diarrhea, and anorexia. For instance, diet must be considered as a potential problem in a dog that has lost weight but has a good appetite. Knowledge of the diet will allow analysis of the digestibility and therefore the availability of nutrients to the animal. If the diet or amount of food the dog is fed is in question, this can be addressed before a costly diagnostic work-up is done by feeding the dog a high-quality diet in adequate amounts for a specific period and reassessing the body weight to evaluate a response. Another situation in which dietary history is imperative is in regard to the animal with unregulated diabetes. A semimoist type of diet with high quantities of simple carbohydrates will cause a post-prandial rise in the blood glucose level, resulting in polyuria and polydipsia.

Dietary history includes questions regarding the potential for toxin, garbage, or foreign body ingestion. Again, answers to these questions may provide crucial information as to the cause of the pet's problem.

✎ TECHNICIAN NOTE
A complete systems review requires that one or two questions be asked about each body system.

SYSTEMS REVIEW

The systems review is necessary to ensure that a complete history is taken. A systems review requires that one or two questions be asked regarding each body system to identify other problems that the owner may have overlooked or deemed unimportant. These problems, when put together with the chief complaint, may provide evidence to support a specific disease as the cause of the animal's illness. For example, when questioning the owner about water intake in a dog with bilaterally symmetric, nonpruritic alopecia, you find that polyuria and polydipsia are also problems. Because this combination of clinical signs is compatible with hyperadrenocorticism, the diagnostic work-up should include a screening test for this disease. Sample questions for each system can be found in Table 2-1. For ease of remembering, major systems can be listed on a standard history form (Figure 2-1). If a response to any of these

Table 2-1 SAMPLE HISTORY QUESTIONS FOR EACH BODY SYSTEM

System	Questions
General	How is your pet's attitude? Is it interested in the family? Is your pet playful?
Integument	Is your pet scratching, licking, or biting excessively? What do you think of your pet's hair coat?
Respiratory	Is your pet coughing or sneezing? Is there any nasal discharge?
Cardiovascular	Has there been a change in your pet's activity level? Do you exercise your pet regularly, and if so, have there been any changes in the amount of exercise your pet will tolerate? Does your pet cough?
Gastrointestinal	Has there been any vomiting? How is your pet's appetite? Have there been any changes in the stool character?
Genitourinary	Has your pet ever been bred? Has there been a change in the urinating habits of your pet? Do you think your pet drinks the same amount of water as before this problem started?
Musculoskeletal	Have you noticed any lameness?
Neurologic	Does your pet seem alert and aware of its surroundings? Is your pet weak or unable to support weight?
Special senses	Does your pet see sufficiently well? Does your pet hear normally?

questions is positive, then the problem should be pursued with further questions as to the duration, severity, character, and so on.

RECORDING THE INFORMATION

The information obtained from taking the history must be recorded in ink in the patient's medical record, usually on the history form (Figure 2-1). This is a legal document and should be signed by the person taking the information. The information should be written legibly and in terms that are professional and accurate. Abbreviations should be limited to medically accepted terminology.

Components of a Complete Physical Examination

A complete physical examination begins with a general impression of the dog or cat, including its attitude, awareness of its surroundings, gait, and general appearance (body

HOSPITAL NAME

ADDRESS

OWNER INFORMATION

HISTORY

HOSPITAL REGULATION: ALL POSITIVE AS WELL AS NEGATIVE FINDINGS SHALL BE RECORDED

DATE _____ HOUR _____ | A.M. | | P.M. |

ORDER
OF
RECORDING

1. (CC) CHIEF
   COMPLAINT

2. (HPI) HISTORY
   OF PRESENT ILLNESS

3. (PH) PAST
   HISTORY
   A. MEDICAL
   B. SURGICAL
   C. TRAUMA
   D. VACCINATIONS
   E. Coggins

4. (EH) ENVIRONMENTAL
   HISTORY

5. (SR) SYSTEM
   REVIEW
   A. GENERAL
   B. SKIN
   C. HEAD/NECK
   D. (EENT) EYES-EARS-
      NOSE-THROAT
   E. RESPIRATORY
   F. CARDIOVASCULAR
   G. (GI) GASTRO-
      INTESTINAL
   H. URINARY
   I. REPRODUCTIVE
   J. MUSCULOSKELETAL
   K. NERVOUS

6. SIGNATURE

ATTENDING CLINICIAN

HISTORY

14786

Figure 2-1 A sample standard history form.

weight, condition, appearance of the coat). This portion of the physical examination can begin as soon as you meet the pet and lead it to the examination room. Observe the animal in its new environment. Is it curious and exploring? Is it aware of noises outside the room? Is it totally uninterested in or unable to respond to the new stimuli? Is it favoring any legs when it walks into the room?

TEMPERATURE, PULSE, AND RESPIRATIONS

The temperature, pulse rate, and respiratory rate are often obtained and recorded by the technician. Rectal temperatures are the most accurate and are taken by inserting a thermometer into the rectum and holding it there until the temperature reading has stabilized. Mercury or digital thermometers can be used. Lubricant will ease insertion into the rectum. It is best to use a probe cover to minimize disease transmission from one patient to the next. Take care when obtaining the temperature because some animals may not appreciate the thermometer in the rectum. Go slowly and, if necessary, have an assistant hold the animal's head. The normal ranges are 99.5° to 102.5° F (dogs) and 100.5° to 102.5° F (cats).

The pulse rate should be taken from the femoral artery on the medial thigh. Count the number of pulses in 10 to 15 seconds and multiply by the appropriate factor to get the number of beats per minute. A normal heart rate for dogs is 60 to 180 beats per minute, while a normal heart rate for cats is 140 to 220 beats per minute. It is also helpful to auscultate the heart at the same time. The pulse and heart beat should be synchronous. If there are dropped pulses, that is, a heart beat without a pulse, it could signal the presence of an arrhythmia.

The respiratory rate can be taken by again counting the number of respirations in 10 to 15 seconds and multiplying by the appropriate factor to determine the number of respirations per minute. Dogs have a normal respiratory rate of 10 to 30 breaths per minute, while cats' normal respiratory rate is slightly faster at 24 to 42 breaths per minute. Note the quality of the respirations as well. Are the respirations shallow and rapid, slow and deep, or normal? Does the patient look distressed or uneasy? Is the patient breathing with an open mouth? Panting does not provide an accept respiratory rate. If the animal is panting, gently close the mouth and assess the rate again.

SYSTEMS ASSESSMENT

The systems assessment is comparable to the systems review section of the history. Each system is examined thoroughly for abnormalities. There is no particular order in which the systems are examined, but a routine pattern should be established by the individual performing the physical examination

so no system will be overlooked. Some clinicians prefer to examine the animal from nose to tail, intermingling the systems together, whereas other clinicians will examine each system separately. It does not matter how the examination is accomplished as long as it is complete and thorough. A standardized physical examination form (Figure 2-2) can provide prompting until a routine is developed. The systems can be listed and numbered at the top of the form, with boxes to check if normal or abnormal. Any abnormality can be listed in the space provided by the corresponding system number.

TECHNICIAN NOTE
Each of the 12 body systems must be thoroughly examined during the complete physical examination.

INTEGUMENT

The skin can be examined all at once or during the examination of other systems. Brush the coat with the hand in the opposite direction of the hair growth and observe the skin for redness (erythema) or lesions such as macules, papules, pustules, or crusts. Remember to examine the skin of the extremities and check the nail beds and nails and areas between the toes. Is there moistness between the toes or brown discoloration indicative of excessive licking in the area? Are the foot pads normal in appearance? Are there areas of hair loss, and if so, where are they located? Is the hair loss symmetric or patchy and random (see Figure 2-3)? Is the skin in areas of hair loss normal, or is it hyperpigmented, erythematous, or crusty? What is the general texture of the coat? Is it soft and fluffy like the undercoat hairs, or is it coarse like the guard hairs? Does your hand feel oily or dirty after touching the coat? If lumps are present, are they in the skin or under it? Are they hairless? Is their overall appearance smooth and round or irregular and cauliflower-like? Make a note of their size and location on the physical examination form. Are there areas of bruising in the skin? Is the skin excessively thin with tiny wrinkle lines and easily observed blood vessels? Are there blackheads (comedones)? All observations need to be recorded; the significance may be realized later.

RESPIRATORY SYSTEM

Examination of the respiratory system begins with the nose and throat, including the pharyngeal area. Is there a nasal discharge, and if so, is it unilateral or bilateral? What is the character of the nasal discharge? Does the animal sneeze or cough while being examined? Are the nares of normal size or stenotic as in some brachycephalic breeds? Palpate the bridge of the nose and the frontal sinus above the eyes. Are there any deformities or soft spots? In the oral cavity, examine the pharynx, tonsils, and, if possible, the edge of the soft palate and the epiglottis. Is the palate elongated? Are there any red or ulcerated areas? Are the tonsils normal and in their crypts? Use symmetry to assess for abnormalities.

Palpate the trachea and larynx. Does the animal cough easily? Are there any swellings or irregularities? Auscultate over the larynx and trachea for any wheezes.

Observe the animal breathe, and note the respiratory rate and pattern. Table 2-2 lists normal ranges for respiratory rates of four species. If the animal is having difficulty breathing, note when the problem is occurring (e.g., inspiration or expiration); this information may be important in the ultimate diagnosis of the problem. Auscultate the lungs in sections or quadrants (Figure 2-4). Normal respiratory sounds can usually be heard in a dog throughout inspiration and through the first third of expiration. The sounds are normally quiet, but with exercise they are louder because of the increased volume of air moving through the airways.

PHYSICAL EXAMINATION

(1) GENERAL APPEARANCE ☐ Normal ☐ Abnormal	(2) INTEGU-MENTARY ☐ Normal ☐ Abnormal ☐ Not examined	(3) MUSCULO-SKELETAL ☐ Normal ☐ Abnormal ☐ Not examined	(4) CIRCU-LATORY ☐ Normal ☐ Abnormal ☐ Not examined
(5) RESPIRA-TORY ☐ Normal ☐ Abnormal ☐ Not examined	(6) DIGESTIVE ☐ Normal ☐ Abnormal ☐ Not examined	(7) GENITO-URINARY ☐ Normal ☐ Abnormal ☐ Not examined	(8) EYES ☐ Normal ☐ Abnormal ☐ Not examined
(9) EARS ☐ Normal ☐ Abnormal ☐ Not examined	(10) NEURAL SYSTEM ☐ Normal ☐ Abnormal ☐ Not examined	(11) LYMPH NODES ☐ Normal ☐ Abnormal ☐ Not examined	(12) MUCOUS MEMBRANES ☐ Normal ☐ Abnormal ☐ Not examined

DESCRIBE ABNORMAL: (Use numbers above)   T _____   P _____   R _____   Wt. _____

_____

_____

_____

_____

_____

_____

_____

_____

_____

_____

_____

_____

_____

_____

_____

TEMPORARY PROBLEM LIST	Initial Plan	
(1)	Dx	Rx
(2)		
(3)		
(4)		

STUDENT SIGNATURE   CLINICIAN SIGNATURE

PHYSICAL EXAMINATION

Figure 2-2 A sample standard physical examination form.

The lung sounds of a normal cat often are heard only during inspiration. Feline lung sounds are more quiet than canine lung sounds, so loud lung sounds in a cat can be significant. If the animal is panting, all that can be heard is air moving through the large airways and the mouth noises. This is not a true representation of lung sounds, so be sure to close the animal's mouth to listen. Abnormal lung sounds are described as crackles (i.e., short, popping noises) or wheezes (i.e., longer, musical noises). Note the location and timing (expiration or inspiration) of any abnormal noises. The lack of normal respiratory sounds can also be significant and suggests a consolidated lung lobe or a lung lobe that has collapsed because of air or fluid accumulation.

CARDIOVASCULAR SYSTEM

Begin with an examination of mucous membrane color and capillary refill time; look for blanching, or loss of color, of the mucous membrane of the oral cavity over the canine tooth on the gingival mucosa or on the inner surface of the labial mucosa. It normally takes 1 or 2 seconds for the pink color to return to the area. The capillary refill time is often prolonged because of poor cardiac output as a result of dehydration or cardiac disease. Examine the jugular furrow in the neck. If the animal is standing, sitting, or lying in a sternal position, it is not normal to see a jugular pulse. Sometimes a jugular pulse can be seen in a normal animal in lateral recumbency. Palpate the femoral pulse, and describe the quality as strong or weak. Does the pulse vary in intensity from pulse to pulse?

Auscultate the heart over the areas shown in Figure 2-5. First, note the heart rate and rhythm. Table 2-2 lists the normal rates of four species. If the rhythm is irregular, decide whether the irregularity is related to the respiratory cycle. If the rhythm is irregularly irregular (e.g., no pattern at all), make a note of this. Palpate the femoral pulse while listening to the heart. Is there a pulse for every heartbeat? Next listen for any heart murmurs. Heart murmurs are described on the basis of five parameters: timing, location or

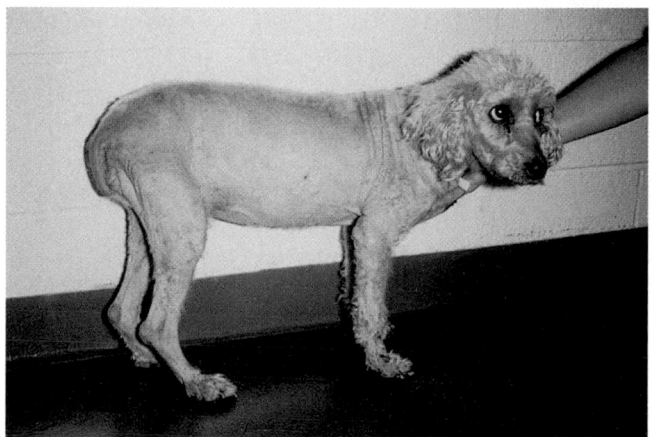

Figure 2-3 Symmetrical truncal alopecia.

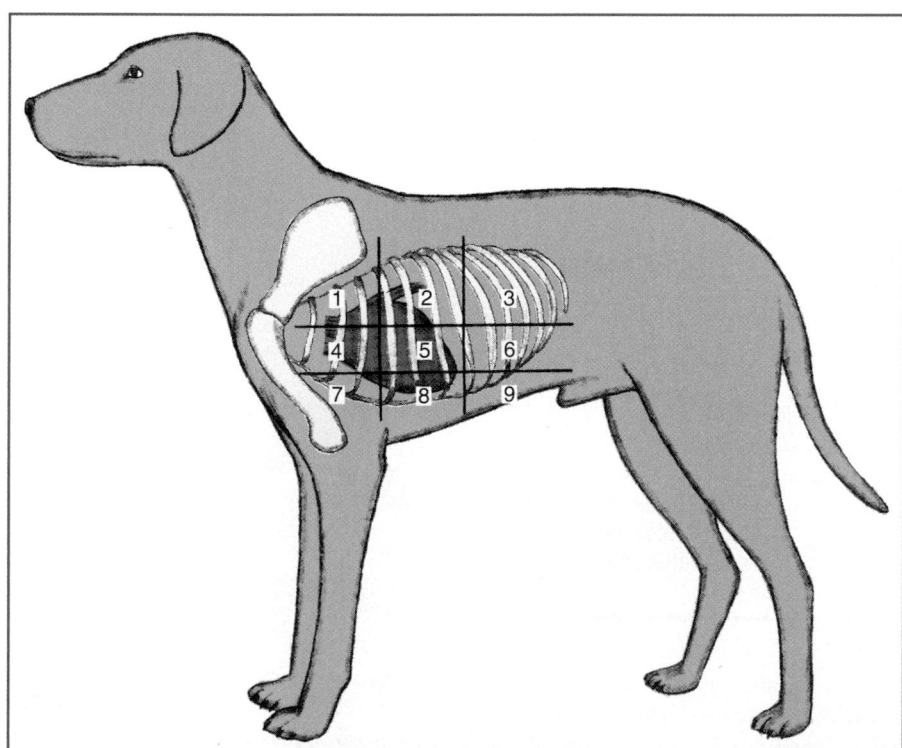

Figure 2-4 Division of the lungs into nine quadrants for auscultation and description of location of abnormal lung sounds. (From McCurnin DM, Poffenbarger EM: *Small animal physical diagnosis and clinical pro*cedures, Philadelphia, 1991, WB Saunders.)

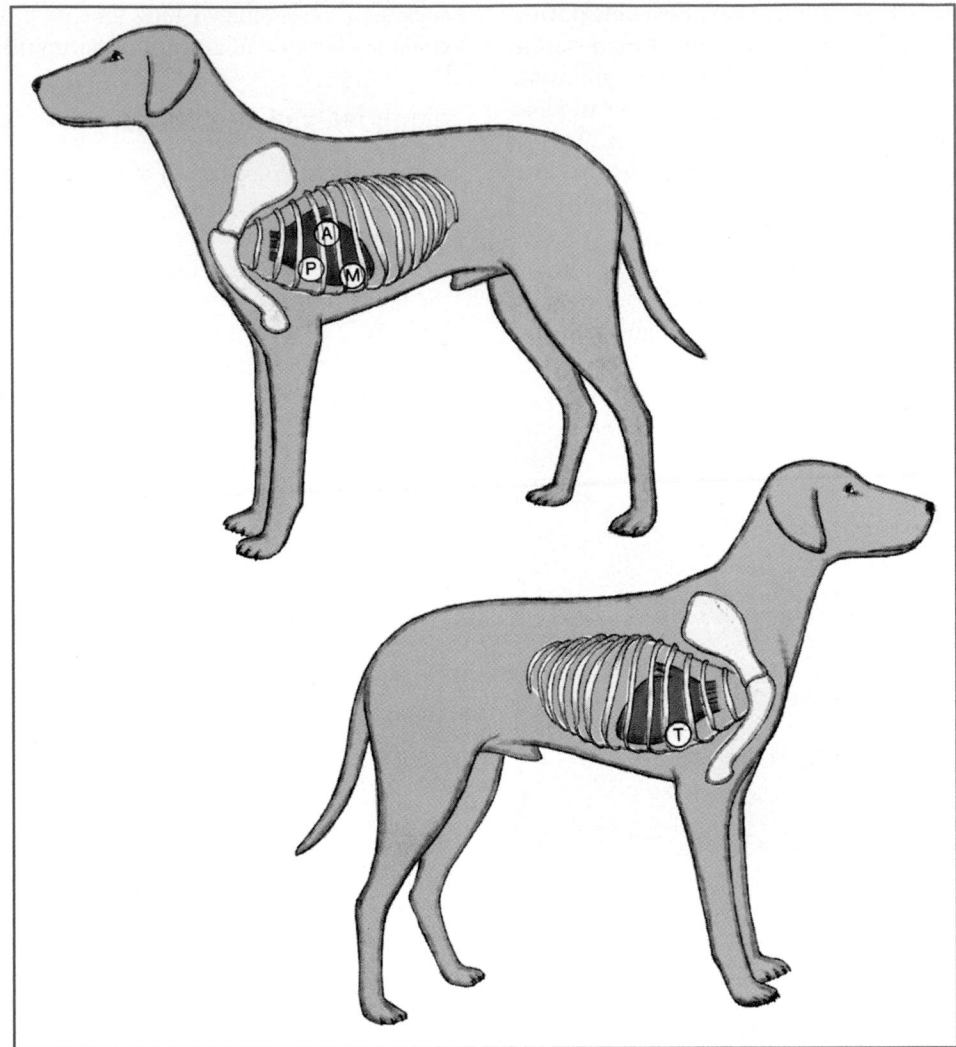

Figure 2-5 Location of heart valves as an aid in the determination of the origin of a heart murmur. *A,* Aortic; *M,* mitral; *P,* pulmonic; *T,* tricuspid. (From McCurnin DM, Poffenbarger EM: *Small animal physical diagnosis and clinical procedures,* Philadelphia, 1991, WB Saunders.)

Table 2-2	NORMAL RESTING RESPIRATORY AND HEART RATES	
Species	Respiratory Rate (breaths/min)	Heart Rate (beats/min)
Cat	16-30	160-240
Cow	20-30	50-70
Dog	16-24	70-180 (smaller breeds have higher rates; puppies can have rates up to 220)
Horse	8-12	36-50

point of maximal intensity, quality, grade, and radiation. Box 2-1 describes the various murmurs. These parameters will help the veterinarian generate a list of possible differential diagnoses for the cardiac disease and give the owner some information on prognosis for his or her animal.

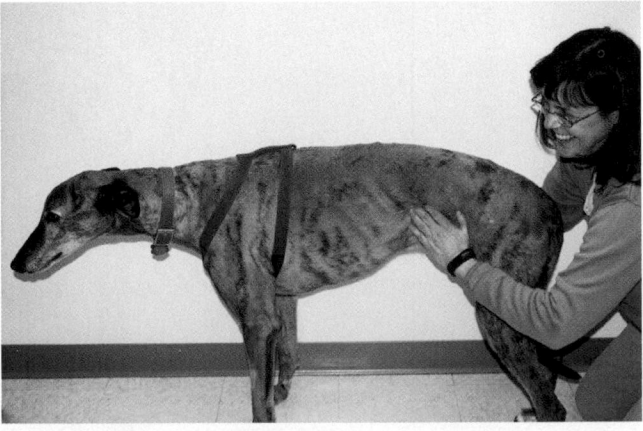

Figure 2-6 Two-handed abdominal palpation in the dog. (From McCurnin DM, Poffenbarger EM: *Small animal physical diagnosis and clinical procedures,* Philadelphia, 1991, WB Saunders.)

Box 2-1 Description of Heart Murmurs

LOCATION
This is usually the valve area over which the murmur is loudest.
Aortic
Mitral
Tricuspid
Pulmonic
The location may also be described in relation to chest structures, such as the sternal border.

TIMING
This refers to the part of the cardiac cycle during which the murmur is heard:
Systole
Diastole
Continuous

DURATION
This refers to the duration within systole or diastole in which the murmur is heard:
Early systole
Holosystolic (pansystolic)
Diastole

CHARACTER
This refers to the quality of the murmur:
Plateau or regurgitant type (same sound for the duration of the murmur)
Decrescendo, crescendo, crescendo-decrescendo, or ejection type (intensity changes throughout the duration of the murmur)
Machinery (heard throughout systole and diastole)
Decrescendo or blowing

GRADE
1/6—Can only be heard in a quiet room after several minutes of listening
2/6—Can be heard immediately but is very soft
3/6—Low to moderate intensity
4/6—Loud but without a palpable thrill
5/6—Loud with a palpable thrill
6/6—Can be heard with the stethoscope bell slightly off the thoracic wall

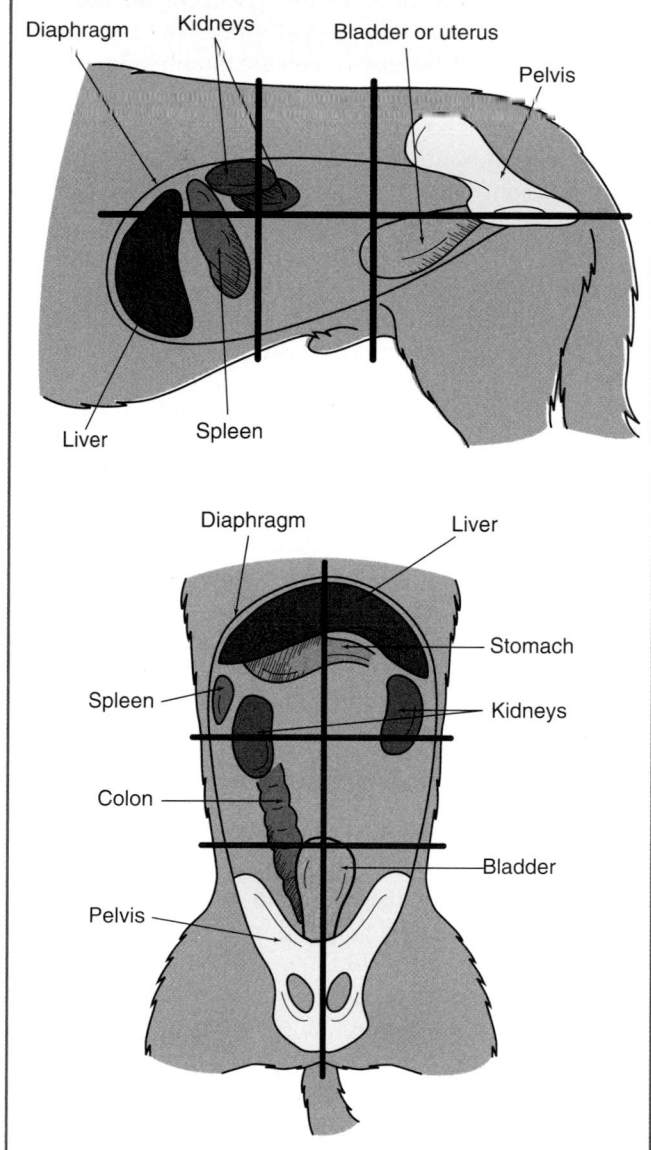

Figure 2-7 Location of internal organs within the abdominal quadrants. **A,** Lateral projection. **B,** Ventrodorsal projection. (From McCurnin DM, Poffenbarger EM: *Small animal physical diagnosis and clinical procedures,* Philadelphia, 1991, WB Saunders.)

GASTROINTESTINAL SYSTEM

Examination of the gastrointestinal system begins in the oral cavity and includes the teeth, tongue, oral mucosa, and pharyngeal area. Next, palpate the neck for any esophageal masses or foreign objects. Auscultate the abdomen, and note the presence or absence of gut sounds.

Abdominal palpation requires practice and patience to obtain any useful information. In most dogs, a two-handed technique is the best method (Figure 2-6). Stand on either side or to the rear of the dog. Put a hand on either side of the abdomen. The hands should be in a flat but relaxed position. Begin palpating the abdomen in the dorsal, cranial region. With gentle pressure, try to move your hands toward each

other. If you move slowly, the animal will usually relax. Do not use the fingertips or the animal will tense the abdominal muscles and palpation will become very difficult. Slowly move your hands toward the ventral, cranial abdomen and feel the structures as they slip past your fingers. When you have reached the ventrum, move to the dorsal, central region and repeat the same steps. Finally, examine the caudal abdomen in a similar manner. Figure 2-7 shows the organs found in the various abdominal quadrants. In a cat or small dog, the one-handed palpation technique is often easier to use (Figure 2-8). The thumb is placed on one side of the animal while the four fingers are placed on the other side of the abdomen. Again, using gentle pressure and a flat hand, begin palpating the dorsal, cranial region of the abdomen and move on to the other areas. Often, the four fingers can be used to trap a structure, and the thumb can be moved over its surface to get an idea of the texture, shape, and size of the structure.

With the gastrointestinal tract of a normal animal, you will not identify much except intestines slipping between your fingers. If the animal has recently consumed a meal, the stomach may be palpated behind the ribs as far caudal as the mid abdomen. Note any pain during palpation and where it is elicited. Are there any abnormal structures? If so, what are the shape, size, and consistency? Does the structure seem to have intestines coming from each end as with an intussusception, foreign body, or intestinal tumor? If the abdomen is distended and it is difficult to discern anything, make a note of that.

The perineal area should be examined for evidence of diarrhea caked on the hairs or inflammation of the surrounding skin. A rectal examination can be performed to determine whether any rectal masses, strictures, or enlargements are present. During a rectal examination, the anal glands can be palpated between the thumb and index finger on each side of the anus, ventrolateral to the anal opening.

UROGENITAL SYSTEM

The kidneys are readily palpated in the normal cat; however, because of anatomic differences, the right kidney of the normal dog is rarely palpated, and only the caudal pole of the left kidney can be palpated in a small percentage of cases. The kidneys should feel smooth on their surface. Note whether the shape is irregular or if the surface feels generally roughened. The size of the kidneys varies with the size of the animal. In the average 5-kg cat, the kidney is usually 2.5 to 3.5 cm in length and spherical.

The urinary bladder can usually be palpated in the caudal ventral abdomen, depending on its degree of fullness. It will be pear shaped with the small end directed caudally in a dog, whereas it is usually spherical in a cat. It should feel

fluctuant or fluid filled. Abnormalities might include a very firm bladder—as occurs with chronic infection, bladder stones, or neoplasia—or a gritty feel when multiple stones are present. The uterus can sometimes be palpated in the female dog if it is enlarged because of pregnancy, infection (pyometra), or neoplasia. The cervix is dorsal to the urinary bladder and can be palpated during certain stages of the estrus cycle and during pregnancy. It is a firm, tubular structure during these times. The uterine horns can be followed cranioventrally from the cervix.

The urethra can be palpated in the male or female dog rectally on the floor of the pelvis as a turgid tubular structure. In the male dog, the prostate gland can be felt as a widening in the pelvic urethra into a bi-lobed, firm, walnut-sized gland. Note any asymmetry, pain, or irregularities in the prostate gland and pelvic urethra. The urethra of the male dog can then be followed distally (caudally) through palpation of the perineal area on the midline. From here it becomes surrounded by penile tissue and is impossible to make out as a separate structure. The penis should be palpated to determine whether pain or abnormalities in shape are present. Extrude the penis from its sheath and note the color and surface texture.

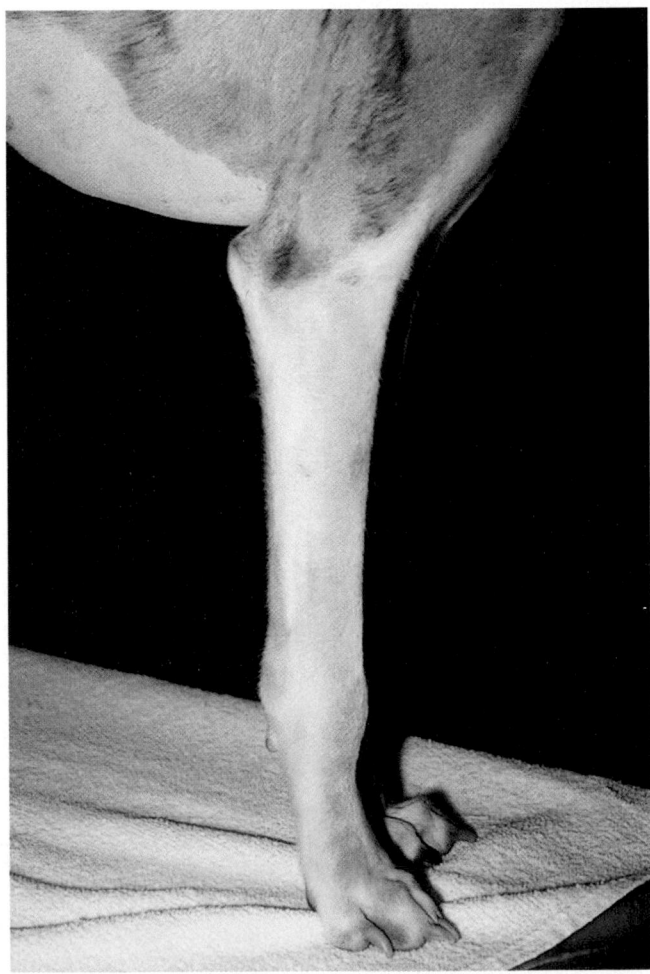

Figure 2-9 Swollen carpal joint.

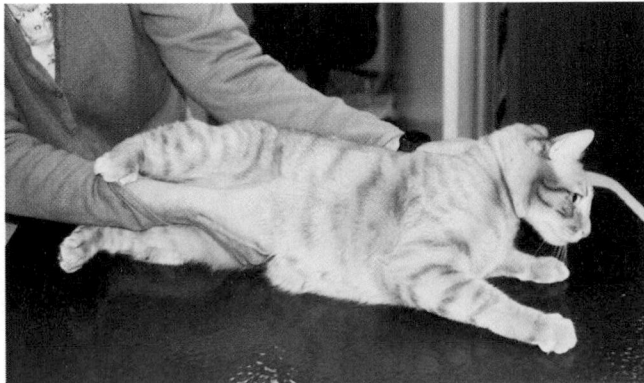

Figure 2-8 One-handed abdominal palpation in the cat. (From McCurnin DM, Poffenbarger EM: *Small animal physical diagnosis and clinical procedures*, Philadelphia, 1991, WB Saunders.)

The testicles of the intact male dog and cat are located in the scrotum in the caudal (cat) or ventral (dog) perineal area. They should be smooth on the surface and symmetric in shape and size. Note any pain on palpation or irregularity in size or shape.

Palpate the mammary chains of the female dog and cat for lumps. Note any pain or swelling. Milk can be expressed from the glands of lactating animals and during the last 1 or 2 weeks of gestation. Examine the milk for color changes; normal milk varies from white to a creamy yellow color.

MUSCULOSKELETAL SYSTEM

Palpate the muscles of the head and limbs, and note any pain or asymmetry. Are the underlying skeletal structures more easy to palpate than normal, indicating atrophy or degeneration of the muscles?

Beginning with the toes, palpate the bones and joints of each limb. Are the joints swollen (Figure 2-9)? Manipulate the joints through their full range of motion, and note any pain response or crepitus (crackling). Firmly palpate the long bones and note any pain response. With your thumb, put firm but gentle pressure on the dorsal spinous process of the thoracic vertebrae one at a time, moving caudally through the lumbar region to the sacrum. Note whether

the animal flinches or drops down to move away from the pressure.

NERVOUS SYSTEM

Complete examination of the nervous system is technically difficult and time-consuming. Some knowledge of neuroanatomy, structure, and function is necessary to accurately assess the location and cause of a neurologic problem. Therefore a complete neurologic examination is usually reserved for the patient with known or suspected neurologic disease. The general appearance of the animal, including mental attitude and ability to ambulate, can provide information regarding the need for a complete neurologic examination.

The central nervous system can be divided into the brain and the spinal cord for ease of examination and localization of lesions. In assessment of the brain, the mental status and cranial nerves are examined. Is the animal alert and aware of its surroundings? Does it respond appropriately to stimuli, such as noises or movement? Table 2-3 lists the specific cranial nerves, tests to assess them, and the expected normal and abnormal responses (Figure 2-10).

Localization and characterization of lesions within the spinal cord require assessment of spinal reflexes, postural

Table 2-3 EXAMINATION OF THE CRANIAL NERVES

Nerve	Test	TEST RESPONSE Normal	Abnormal
I. Olfactory	Volatile substance	Sniff, recoil, nose lick	No response
II. Optic	Menace	Blink	No blink
	Pupillary light reflex	Direct, consensual responses present	No direct or consensual responses
III. Oculomotor	Pupillary light reflex	Direct, consensual responses present	No direct response, consensual intact
	Observe eye follow an object	Normal eye movement	Impaired ocular movement in ventral, dorsal, and medial directions
IV. Trochlear	Observe	Normal eye position	Dorsomedial strabismus
	Palpate temporalis	Normal muscle tone	Muscle atrophy
	Corneal reflex	Eye blink	No blink
	Palpebral reflex	Eye blink	No blink
VI. Abducens	Observe	Normal eye position	Medial strabismus
VII. Facial	Observe	Facial symmetry	Lip droop
	Corneal reflex	Eye blink	No blink
	Palpebral reflex	Eye blink	No blink
	Menace	Eye blink	No blink
VIII. Acoustic	Hand clap	Startle response	No response
	Move head horizontally, vertically	Normal nystagmus	No response, resting or positional nystagmus
IX. Glossopharyngeal	Gag reflex	Swallow	No response
X. Vagus	Gag reflex	Swallow	No response
	Oculocardiac reflex	Bradycardia	No response
	Laryngeal reflex	Cough	No response
XI. Accessory	Palpate neck muscles	Normal muscle tone	Muscle atrophy
XII. Hypoglossal	Tongue stretch	Retraction of tongue	No response

From McCurnin DM, Poffenbarger EM: *Small animal and physical diagnosis and clinical procedures*, Philadelphia, 1991, WB Saunders, p 115.

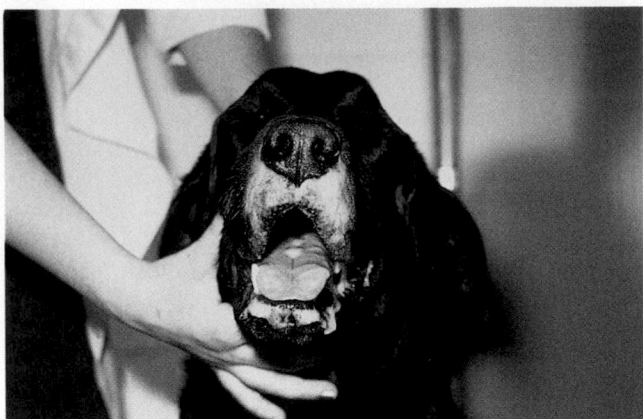

Figure 2-10 Examination of the head showing facial nerve paralysis (note the drooped lip on the left side of the face).

reactions, and response to painful stimuli. Spinal reflexes are assessed by gentle but firm tapping of a tendon to determine the degree of response (contraction) of the muscle. The most common reflexes assessed are the triceps in the front leg (Figure 2-11) and the quadriceps or patellar (Figure 2-12) and gastrocnemius reflexes (Figure 2-13) in the hind limb. The response is graded as shown in Table 2-4.

Postural reactions include conscious proprioception, wheel-barrowing, hemistanding and hemiwalking, and hopping. The most commonly performed test is the reaction of conscious proprioception, in which the foot is gently turned so that the animal is standing on the top of its foot. Each foot is tested individually. A normal animal will immediately right the foot. A slow or absent response usually indicates spinal cord disease. Wheel-barrowing is performed by holding the animal's rear legs in the air while slowly

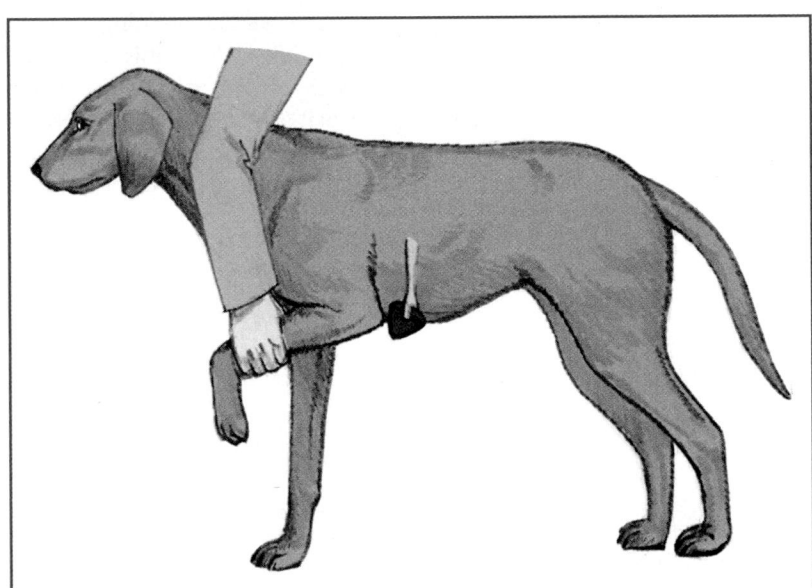

Figure 2-11 The triceps reflex can be elicited in lateral recumbency or standing, as shown. (From McCurnin DM, Poffenbarger EM: *Small animal physical diagnosis and clinical* procedures, Philadelphia, 1991, WB Saunders.)

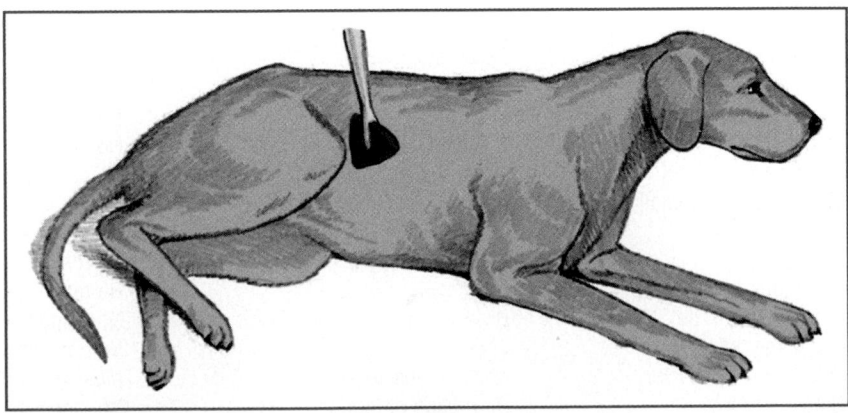

Figure 2-12 The femoral, or patellar, reflex. (From McCurnin DM, Poffenbarger EM: *Small animal physical diagnosis and clinical procedures,* Philadelphia, 1991, WB Saunders.)

moving forward; the normal animal will move the front legs forward and maintain an upright position. Hemistanding and hemiwalking require that the front and rear legs on the same side be supported while the animal is required to stand or walk, respectively. A normal animal can stand with ease and walk with minor difficulty. Hopping responses are assessed by holding three of four legs up with the fourth allowed to touch the floor or table. The animal is slowly moved toward the side with the leg down. A normal animal will move the leg laterally to attempt to support weight and maintain balance.

Superficial and deep pain perception is assessed by pinching the skin and bone of the toe area, respectively. The normal response is withdrawal of the leg with some acknowledgment of pain, such as turning to look at the toe, dilation of the pupils, or a growl or snap. If both responses are absent, the prognosis for recovery is poor.

The *panniculus reflex* is a simple test that aids in the localization of a spinal cord lesion. It is performed by gently pinching the skin of the back just lateral to the midline and watching for a reflex contraction of the skin. Start with the skin near the tail and slowly work forward. The lesion is approximately one vertebra caudal to the location where the first response is elicited.

Last, the anal tone and perineal reflex should be assessed. The anus should be closed and not gaping open. The perineal reflex is tested by gently stimulating the skin around the anus and watching for a "wink," or contraction, of the anal sphincter.

PERIPHERAL LYMPH NODES

The peripheral lymph nodes that can be palpated in the normal animal include the submandibular, prescapular, and popliteal. Usually, the axillary and inguinal lymph nodes will be palpated only if they are enlarged. Symmetry is often a clue to any abnormalities, so palpate both sides at the same time for comparison.

The submandibular lymph nodes are located at the ventral aspect of the neck near the angle of the jaw. There are usually two on each side, just cranial to the mandibular salivary gland. The trick to palpating them is to grab the extra skin of the ventral neck between the thumb and forefingers. Slowly move your hands rostrally, and the nodes should slip through your fingers. In the cat, these nodes are normally pea sized, whereas in the dog, they vary from pea sized (small dogs) to small grape sized (large dogs).

The prescapular lymph nodes lie in the connective tissue just cranial and dorsal to the shoulder joint. Again, it is easiest to grab the skin and muscles and then let the lymph nodes slip through your fingers as you pull your hands cranially. These lymph nodes may be similar in size to the submandibular nodes or slightly larger.

The popliteal lymph nodes can be palpated in the fat pad just caudal to the stifle joint.

EARS

Examination of the ears involves palpation and visual examination of the pinnae, or ear flaps, as well as visual inspection of the external ear canal. Common abnormalities of the ear flaps include hair loss, crusting margins as occur with mange or flea-bite dermatitis, hematomas (blood-filled pockets within the pinna), and skin tumors. The external ear canal should be free of exudate, debris, and hair. If exudate is present, the character of the discharge should be noted (dark brown and flaky as occurs with ear mites, dark brown and malodorous as occurs with yeast infections, or purulent as occurs with bacterial otitis).

If abnormalities are noted on visual inspection or ear disease is the chief complaint, an otoscopic examination should be performed. While the pinna is held up, the otoscope cone is gently inserted into the vertical ear canal (Figure 2-14). While the examiner looks through the otoscope, the otoscope is slowly advanced and rotated 90 degrees to examine the horizontal part of the ear canal. Note any redness, exudate, foreign objects, mites, polyps or tumors, or hemorrhage. The tympanic membrane or eardrum can be visualized at the end of the horizontal canal as a white translucent membrane. Note any color change or lack of translucency,

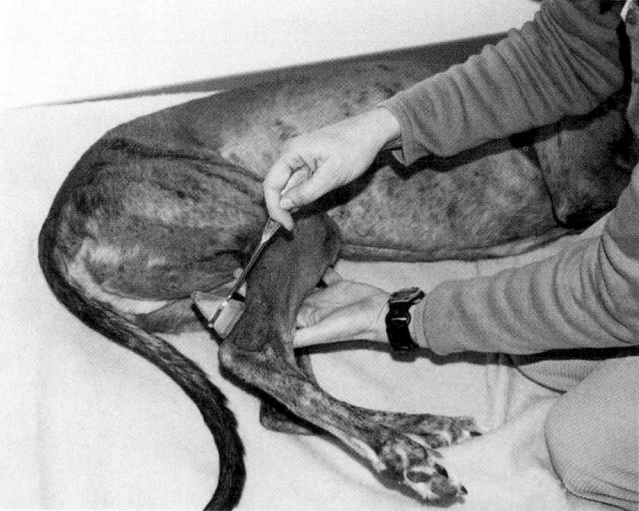

Figure 2-13 The gastrocnemius reflex. (From McCurnin DM, Poffenbarger EM: *Small animal physical diagnosis and clinical procedures*, Philadelphia, 1991, WB Saunders.)

Table 2-4 GRADING OR REFLEX RESPONSES

Grade	Description
0	No response
1	Hyporeflexia (less than normal response)
2	Normal response
3	Hyperreflexia (greater than normal response)
4	Clonus (repetitive response)

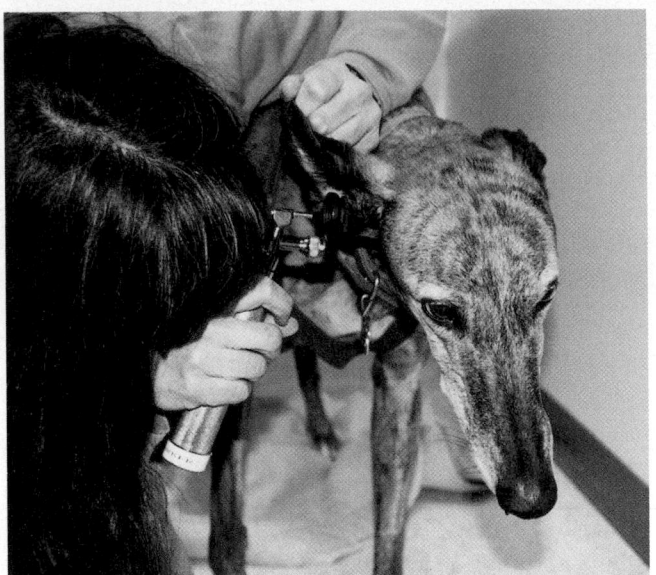

Figure 2-14 Examination of vertical canal.

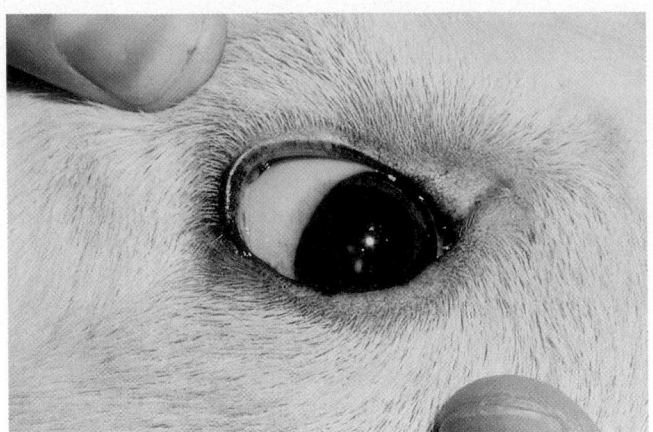

Figure 2-15 The yellow sclera indicates jaundice.

which indicates the presence of exudate or hemorrhage in the middle ear.

EYES

A good ocular examination includes an examination of the external ocular features (eyelids, sclera, cornea, third eyelid [nictitating membrane]) as well as internal ocular features (anterior chamber, iris, lens), all of which can be visualized without special equipment. First, note the character of any discharge present in or under the eyes. If present, is it watery, mucoid, purulent, or ropy? Examine the eyelid margins for small masses, aberrant eyelashes, and position. Do the eyelids seem to roll inward (entropion) so that the lashes rub on the cornea, or do the eyelids appear to be loose and not in contact with the eye (ectropion)? A normal sclera should be white. Is the sclera yellow (Figure 2-15), indicative of jaundice, or red, as in the inflamed eye? Is the third eyelid in its normal position, or does it appear to be bulging or protruding across the eye? Is the cornea clear or cloudy?

If it is cloudy, note the location of the cloudiness. Does the cornea appear wet? Are there small blood vessels present on the surface of the cornea?

The anterior chamber (portion of the eye in front of the lens and iris) should be clear, allowing easy visualization of the iris. Note any hemorrhage or purulent debris in the anterior chamber. Examine the iris, and compare with the opposite side for symmetry. Are the pupil sizes equal? Are there any brown spots on the iris? Does the iris appear to be tattered? Shine a light in one eye, and note the response in both eyes. Both pupils in a normal animal will constrict when a light is shined in either eye. Carefully record any deviations from normal.

Recommended Reading

McCurnin DM, Poffenbarger EM: *Small animal physical diagnosis and clinical procedures*, Philadelphia, 1991, WB Saunders.

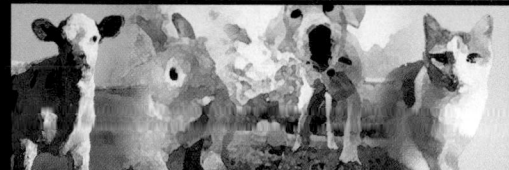

3

Diagnostic Sampling and Therapeutic Techniques

Tracy J. Jaffe

INTRODUCTION

A veterinary technician proficient in obtaining diagnostic samples and performing a variety of treatment techniques is an invaluable asset to any veterinary practice. Technicians should therefore have expertise in many basic procedures, such as blood and urine collection, intravenous catheter placement, and fluid and medication administration. As the practice of veterinary medicine becomes more specialized, technicians are increasingly being asked to perform more advanced diagnostic and therapeutic procedures. Many technicians, for example, are now employed by specialty practices in which performing certain advanced procedures has become routine. For this reason, a variety of advanced as well as basic procedures are addressed in this chapter. ■

BASIC GUIDELINES

Whenever possible, baseline blood or urine samples should be obtained before the initiation of fluid therapy. Administration of fluids and the recent ingestion of a high-fat or high-protein meal may alter blood or urine laboratory values.

All supplies needed for collection of samples and for therapeutic procedures should be gathered ahead of time. Samples should be collected and stored in appropriate containers with the patient's name and hospital identification number printed on each label.

Whenever a needle is inserted through the skin as part of a treatment (e.g., intramuscular injection) or a sampling procedure (e.g., blood collection), the skin should be clean, dry, and free from obvious inflammation and infection. Microbes and other contaminants present on the skin surface may be introduced into the underlying tissue when the needle is inserted. Needles and intravenous catheters from which the protective coverings have been removed should remain sterile and should only be handled at the hub; the shaft, for example, should not be touched or set down on a nonsterile surface.

SMALL ANIMAL SAMPLING AND THERAPEUTIC TECHNIQUES

BLOOD SAMPLE COLLECTION

VENOUS BLOOD SAMPLE

Most technicians perform venipuncture on a routine basis, either to collect blood samples for laboratory tests or to inject a drug or medication. Only through experience does one learn to collect a blood sample quickly with minimal trauma to the vessel and minimal stress and discomfort to the patient (Box 3-1). Proper animal restraint is as important as the venipuncture technique.

Venipuncture is performed with either a needle and syringe or a Vacutainer collection system. The method and needle gauge selected depend on the vessel size, amount of blood required, intended use of the sample, and technician preference.

The majority of venipunctures in cats and small dogs are performed with 22-gauge needles. Larger-gauge needles, such as 20- and 18-gauge, may be used in large-breed dogs and in most farm animals. For any venipuncture technique, the needle should always be inserted into the vein with the bevel facing upward.

Box 3-1 VENOUS BLOOD COLLECTION

- Attach a 20- to 25-gauge needle to a 1- to 6-ml syringe.
- Occlude the vein with a tourniquet or digital pressure.
- Wipe the skin and hair on top of the vein with an alcohol-soaked cotton ball to help identify the vein.
- Insert the needle with the bevel facing up through the skin and into the vein at a 25-degree angle.
- Slowly retract the syringe plunger, and collect a blood sample.
- Release the pressure on the vein, and release the syringe plunger when a sufficient volume of blood has been collected.
- Remove the needle from the vein.
- Apply digital pressure to the venipuncture site as soon as the needle is removed until hemostasis occurs.

TECHNICIAN NOTE

For venipuncture, the needle should be inserted with the bevel facing upward.

Blood collected for coagulation profiles (i.e., activated clotting time, prothrombin time, activated partial thromboplastin time) should be drawn rapidly through a 20-gauge needle. The needle should ideally penetrate the vessel on the first attempt to minimize the amount of tissue fluid that enters the sample; tissue fluid (thromboplastin) may hasten the clotting process.

Smaller, 25- to 28-gauge needles are used with smaller vessels, fragile vessels, or multiple venipunctures. Bihourly sampling to establish a blood glucose curve is a situation in which use of a small-gauge needle is appropriate. The amount of negative pressure applied to aspirate the blood into the syringe must not be excessive. Forceful retraction of the syringe plunger may result in hemolysis of the red blood cells as they pass through the needle, yielding erroneous laboratory values. Application of excessive negative pressure may also cause the vein to collapse.

Just before venipuncture, the hair and skin over the vessel are wiped with a cotton ball saturated with 70% isopropyl alcohol. This helps to remove some superficial skin contaminants, causes vasodilation, and improves visualization of the vein. In animals with dense hair coats, the vessel may be easier to identify if the hair over the vessel is parted with the use of an alcohol-soaked cotton ball or shaved with a clipper. When blood is drawn for bacterial culture, the region on top of the vein is shaved and aseptically prepared. Sterile gloves are worn when blood is collected for culture.

The most frequently used sites for canine blood collection are the cephalic, jugular, and lateral saphenous veins. The cephalic, jugular, femoral, and medial saphenous veins are used for feline venipuncture.

To collect blood from a peripheral vein, introduce the needle into the occluded vessel as far distally as possible. If the initial venipuncture attempt is unsuccessful, reinsert the needle more proximal to the previous entry site. For jugular venipuncture, the initial attempt is made in the caudal third of the jugular vein. Subsequent venipuncture attempts can be made in a more cranial region. If the vessel is damaged in the distal portion of the vein, a more proximal region is still patent and usable for blood collection.

TECHNICIAN NOTE

To perform venipuncture on a peripheral vein, introduce the needle into the most distal portion of the vein possible.

After blood is collected, the needle is detached from the syringe, and the stopper is removed from the collection tube before the blood is transferred into the tube. This reduces the amount of hemolysis that may occur if blood is forcefully ejected through the narrow lumen of a needle. If blood is transferred into a tube containing an anticoagulant, such as lavender-topped ethylenediamine tetraacetic acid (EDTA) tubes, the stopper is quickly replaced, and the tube is gently inverted a few times to mix the blood with the anticoagulant. Vigorous shaking can cause hemolysis. The tube containing the anticoagulant should be at least half filled with blood to achieve the appropriate blood/anticoagulant ratio.

Cephalic Venipuncture

When blood is collected from the cephalic vein, which is located on the cranial aspect of the foreleg, the animal is restrained in sternal recumbency or in a standing position. Small dogs may be picked up and held in the restrainer's arms with a foreleg extended. Some large-breed dogs prefer to remain standing or seated with a foreleg held in extension. Refer to Figure 3-1.

When venipuncture is performed on the right cephalic vein, the restrainer is positioned on the animal's left side. The left hand or arm is placed under the muzzle to pull the head toward the restrainer's body. The restrainer wraps the right arm over the animal's back, extends the right foreleg, and occludes the vein with the thumb at the elbow. Alternatively, a tourniquet may be secured just distal to the elbow joint to occlude the vein if an assistant is unavailable.

Once the patient has been restrained, the phlebotomist grasps the leg, places a thumb lateral to the vein, and pulls the skin distally to stabilize the vein. The cephalic vein is wiped with alcohol. A 22-gauge needle attached to a 3-ml syringe is slowly inserted at a 25-degree angle through the skin and into the vein. Approximately 0.5 to 0.75 cm of the needle is placed into the vein. Blood appears in the needle hub when the needle enters the vein. The syringe plunger is retracted, and blood flows into the syringe as shown in Figure 3-2. If too much suction is applied, the vein may collapse, and blood flow will cease. Blood flow may also be interrupted if the needle tip is lodged against the vessel wall. The needle is slightly rotated and repositioned to remedy this situation. If blood flows into the syringe too slowly,

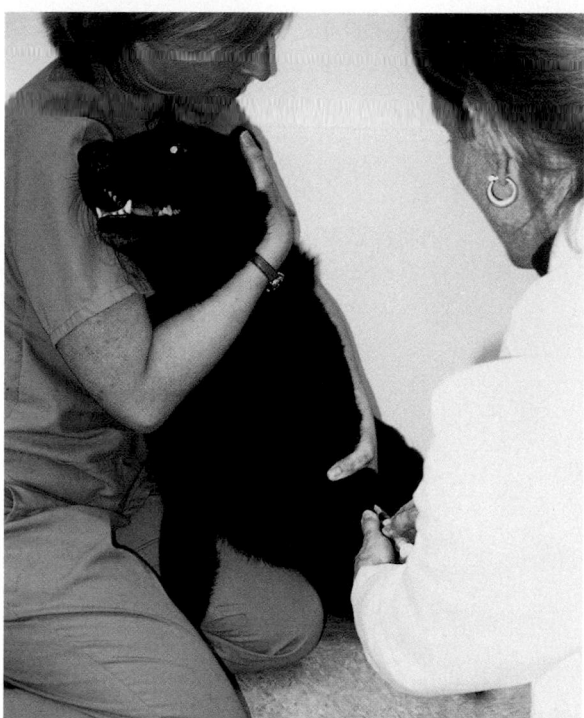

Figure 3-1 For venipuncture, some large-breed dogs prefer to remain seated on the floor with a foreleg extended.

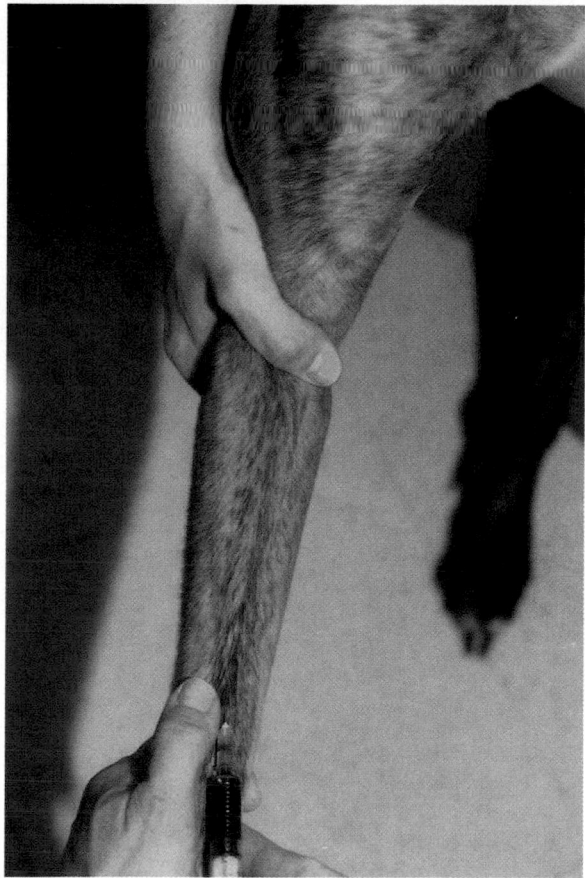

Figure 3-2 Restraint of a large-breed dog for venipuncture of the cephalic vein.

the animal's foot can be repeatedly pumped to augment blood flow.

After a sufficient volume of blood has been collected, the restrainer's thumb or the tourniquet is removed from the vein. The needle is withdrawn, and digital pressure is applied to the venipuncture site for 10 to 20 seconds. Insufficient application of pressure may result in blood leakage from the vessel into the surrounding tissue and the formation of a hematoma. If a hematoma occurs during venipuncture, the needle is promptly removed and a gauze sponge is held firmly over the site until the bleeding subsides. When venipuncture is reattempted, the needle is reinserted proximal to the initial needle entry site or in a different vein.

> ### ✎ TECHNICIAN NOTE
> The jugular vein is the preferred site for venipuncture if several milliliters of blood are needed.

Jugular Venipuncture

The jugular vein is the preferred venipuncture site if several milliliters of blood are needed. Cats and small to medium-sized dogs are held in sternal recumbency near the edge of a table. Large dogs are restrained in a seated position on the floor.

For left jugular venipuncture, the restrainer stands on the animal's right side. The left arm is draped around the patient's back and holds the patient's body. The holder grasps the front legs just proximal to the elbows. Front legs of a

cat or small dog may be stretched downward over the edge of the table. The assistant extends the neck and turns the head slightly away from the jugular vein to be sampled. Overextension of the neck may flatten the vein and should be avoided.

The jugular vein is occluded with the phlebotomist's thumb lateral to the trachea at the thoracic inlet. Once distended, the jugular vein is visualized or palpated as it courses from the thoracic inlet to the angle of the mandible. Wiping the neck with alcohol helps visualize the vein. In cats, water is sometimes used because the smell of alcohol is often repugnant to them. A 20- to 22-gauge needle on a syringe is inserted into the vein at a 25-degree angle with the bevel facing upward as shown in Figures 3-3 and 3-4. Prebending the needle to form a 150-degree angle with the syringe may make jugular venipuncture easier in cats and small dogs. After a sample is collected, digital pressure in the thoracic inlet is released from the vein, and the needle is removed. Pressure is applied to the puncture site for approximately 30 seconds or until the bleeding stops.

Use of a Vacutainer collection device may make jugular blood collection easier; however, some technicians prefer to use a needle and syringe. The Vacutainer collection system consists of three pieces: a two-way needle, a cylindrical

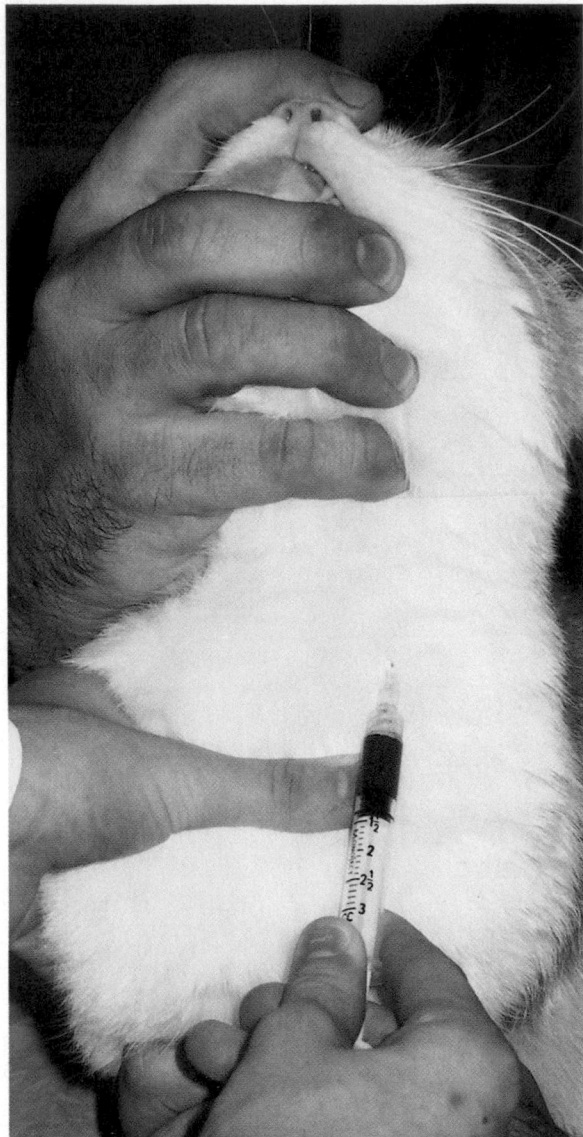

Figure 3-3 Venipuncture of the feline jugular vein.

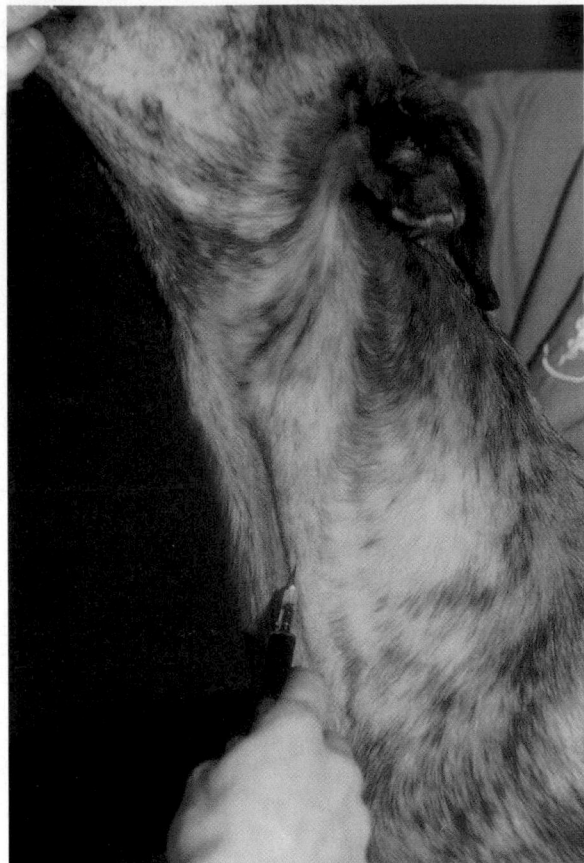

Figure 3-4 Venipuncture of the canine jugular vein.

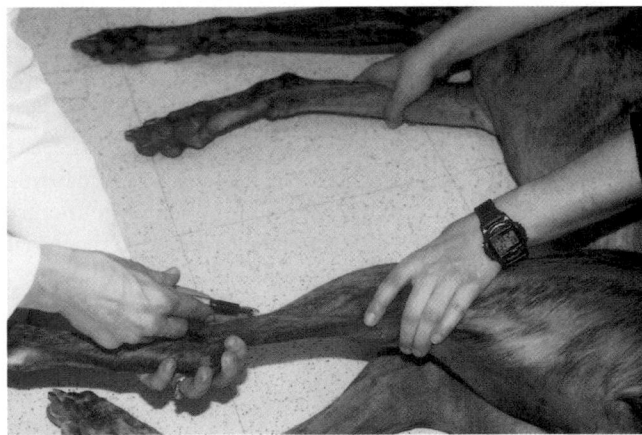

Figure 3-5 Restraint of a dog for venipuncture of the lateral saphenous vein.

plastic holder, and a glass tube. A needle is twisted into the top of the holder, and a Vacutainer tube sealed with a rubber stopper is held near the base of the holder. After the needle enters the vein, the tube is inserted into the base of the holder until the stopper is punctured. Blood is automatically suctioned into the tube until it is three fourths full. The tube is withdrawn from the holder to break the vacuum, and the needle is removed from the vein. If more than one tube of blood is required, the blood-filled tube is replaced with an empty one *without* removing the needle from the vein. The vacuum that draws the blood into the tube will be broken once the needle is withdrawn from the skin.

Lateral Saphenous Venipuncture

The lateral saphenous vein, which is located on the lateral aspect of the hind limb near the hock, is an ideal site for blood collection in the dog. This vein is often used in aggressive animals when the phlebotomist does not want to be positioned close to the dog's face.

When venipuncture of the left lateral saphenous vein is performed, the dog is placed in right lateral recumbency. The restrainer stands at the dog's back, places his or her right forearm across the thorax, and grasps the medial aspect

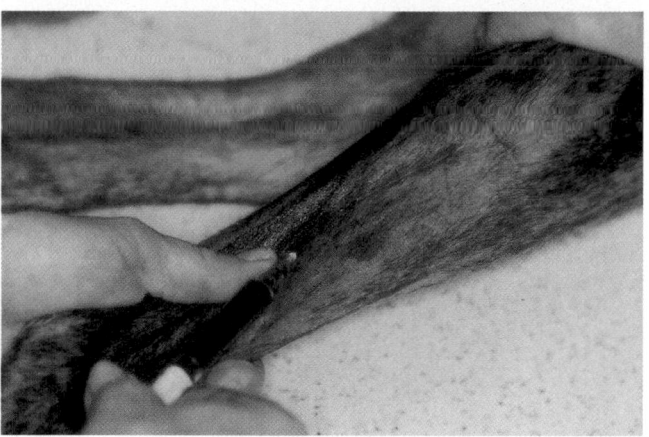

Figure 3-6 The thumb is placed alongside the lateral saphenous vein to stabilize the vessel.

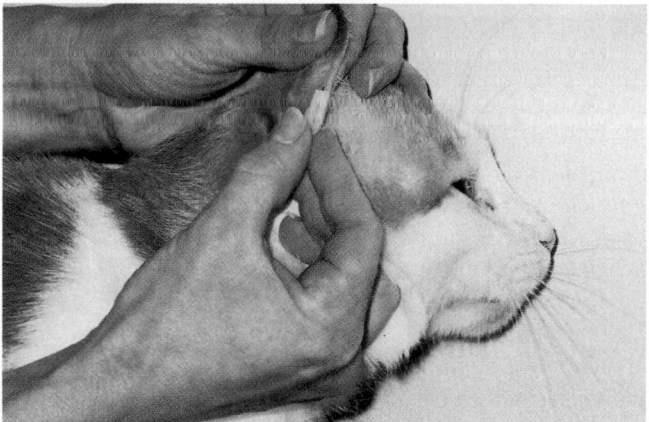

Figure 3-8 Collection of a peripheral capillary blood sample from the marginal ear vein of the cat with a lancet.

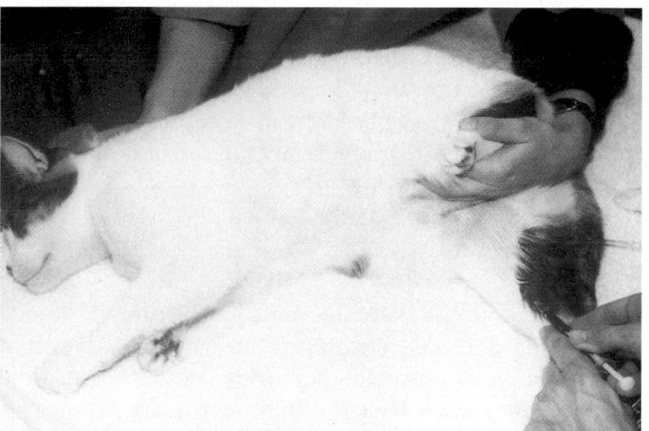

Figure 3-7 Venipuncture of the femoral vein in the cat.

of the right front leg. The left hand grasps and extends the left stifle; this occludes the vein and immobilizes the leg. As shown in Figure 3-5, the phlebotomist holds the left tarsus and pulls the skin taut to stabilize the vessel. Placement of the thumb parallel to the vein helps prevent the vein from rolling when the needle is introduced (Figure 3-6).

Medial Saphenous or Femoral Venipuncture

The medial saphenous or femoral vein, which is located on the medial aspect of the rear leg, is used to obtain small volumes of blood, primarily in feline patients. If the right vein is used, the cat is stretched in right lateral recumbency with the left rear leg abducted. The phlebotomist grasps the tarsus and extends the left leg. The vein is occluded with pressure applied by the restrainer's left hand in the right inguinal region. It is easy to identify the vein after the medial aspect of the leg is wiped with alcohol and the hair is parted over the vessel. Blood is collected with a 22- to 25-gauge needle attached to a 1- or 3-ml syringe (Figure 3-7). Firm pressure is applied to the puncture site for at least 60 seconds after venipuncture. This is particularly important at these

sites because the medial saphenous and femoral veins are prone to hematoma formation.

Marginal Ear Venipuncture

On occasion, the technician will collect blood from a peripheral capillary bed to check for erythroparasitic organisms, such as *Babesia* spp. or *Haemobartonella* spp. Collection of a small drop of capillary blood is also used by clients who monitor their diabetic pets' blood glucose levels at home. A peripheral capillary blood sample can be obtained by clipping the quick of a toenail or lacerating the buccal mucosa. A more desirable, less painful alternative is to collect a sample from the marginal ear vein, which is most easily visualized as it courses around the periphery of the dorsal aspect of the pinna.

When a capillary sample is collected, the pinna of the ear is first warmed with a heated cloth, light source, or the technician's hands to help vasodilate the marginal ear vein and then wiped with a small amount of alcohol. A 25-gauge needle or lancet is used to nick the vein, and then the pinna is massaged until a sufficient drop of blood is obtained (Figure 3-8). When a sample must be examined for erythroparasites, blood is collected into a heparinized capillary tube and is later smeared onto slides for microscopic examination. If blood is collected to measure blood glucose, a glucometer test strip is placed alongside the drop of blood on the pinna, and the blood is wicked directly onto the test strip. The test trip should be designed to measure a capillary, not venous, blood sample. The technician must make certain that the patient does not move its head or flick its ear, or the blood sample may be lost. After the blood sample has been obtained, firm pressure should be applied to the puncture site for approximately 15 seconds.

TECHNICIAN NOTE

An arterial blood sample is used to evaluate the acid-base and blood gas status of an animal.

ARTERIAL BLOOD SAMPLE

An arterial blood sample is used to evaluate the acid-base and blood gas status of an animal. Cost-effective, easy-to-use arterial blood gas analyzers are becoming increasingly available. It is not necessary to occlude an artery to obtain a blood sample. Femoral and dorsal metatarsal arteries are used to obtain samples in conscious companion animals. When arterial puncture is performed in anesthetized patients, the lingual, brachial, and radial arteries may also be used.

Arterial blood gas samples are collected in a heparinized 1-ml syringe fitted with a 25-gauge, 1.6-cm needle. Arterial blood is generally brighter red than venous blood.

Femoral Artery Sample

When a sample is collected from the right leg, the patient is placed in right lateral recumbency with the right rear leg extended and the left rear leg abducted. The mammary glands or the prepuce is retracted dorsally to access the femoral artery of the down leg. The inguinal region is wiped with 70% alcohol. Once the arterial pulse is palpated with the fingertips, the needle is introduced into the artery at a 60-degree angle. Gentle suction is applied to the syringe as it is advanced with a slight back-and-forth motion. When the artery is penetrated, blood should rapidly fill the syringe in a pulsatile manner. A sample of 0.25 to 0.5 ml of blood is collected (Figure 3-9). Air bubbles are expelled from the syringe, and the needle is promptly capped with a rubber stopper. Bending the needle in lieu of embedding it in a rubber stopper is not sufficient to maintain an anaerobic environment. Firm pressure is immediately applied to the arterial puncture site for several minutes to prevent hematoma formation.

Dorsal Metatarsal Artery Sample

Blood can be taken from the dorsal metatarsal artery, located on the dorsal aspect of the metatarsus, if the femoral artery is inaccessible or difficult to palpate. The skin is thicker over the metatarsal artery than over the femoral artery and is more difficult to penetrate. The dog is placed in lateral recumbency, with the hock extended. The dorsum of the metatarsus is shaved and wiped with alcohol. After the arterial pulse is palpated, the needle is introduced into the artery at a 30-degree angle, and a blood sample is obtained and handled in the same manner as described for a femoral artery puncture.

URINE SAMPLE COLLECTION

Because urine is often collected for gross and microscopic analysis and/or bacterial culture, the technician should be familiar with the many different methods of collection. For example, urine may be obtained as the patient voids, from manual bladder expression, from catheterization of the bladder, or by cystocentesis.

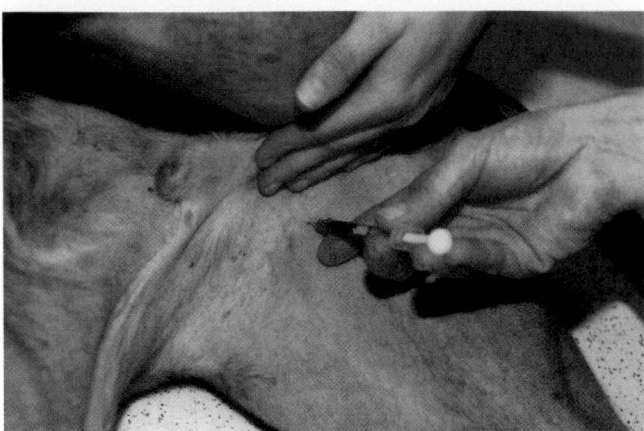

Figure 3-9 Femoral artery blood sample collection.

Routine samples are collected in clean, dry containers, but urine needed for bacterial culture is collected in sterile containers. Samples that cannot be analyzed within 30 minutes of collection should be refrigerated in airtight containers. Once they have been refrigerated, urine specimens should be returned to room temperature before urinalysis is performed.

VOIDED COLLECTION

It is easy to collect a naturally voided urine sample. Voided samples are adequate for routine urinalyses. However, a voided sample is unsuitable for urine culture because the sample may contain bacteria, cells, and debris from hair, skin, or the genitourinary tract. The initial portion of voided urine contains the greatest concentration of contaminants and is usually excluded from collection.

> **✐ TECHNICIAN NOTE**
> Urine is most easily obtained from a dog by walking it outdoors and catching a voided midstream sample.

Urine is most easily obtained from a dog by walking it outdoors and catching a voided midstream sample. A collection device is often helpful because many dogs stop urinating when a person gets close to them. These devices can be improvised by bending a loop in the end of an aluminum rod or straightened metal coat hanger. A paper cup placed in the loop serves as a urine receptacle.

Urine can be collected from a hospitalized animal by placing it on a raised grate in a clean cage. After the animal voids, the urine is collected from the cage floor with a syringe.

Confinement of the animal in a specialized metabolic cage is another means of collecting urine. These cages are made of stainless steel and include a grate raised above a slanted cage floor. The floor forms a funnel under which a container for urine collection is placed.

In addition, voided samples can be collected from empty clean litter pans or pans covered with plastic bags. Cats that prefer to urinate in a litter-type material may require use of specially designed plastic, nonabsorbent pellets, such as NoSorb (CATCO, Tifflin, Ohio). Shredded strips of wax paper can also serve as an inexpensive, convenient alternative to cat litter when a urine specimen needs to be collected at home. After the cat urinates in the litter pan, the urine is simply poured into a clean container or collected with a syringe.

MANUAL BLADDER EXPRESSION

Urine can be collected for routine urinalysis by manual compression of the bladder. Urine expressed from the bladder contains contaminants from the urogenital tract, skin, and hair. Therefore manual expression should not be used to obtain samples for bacterial culture.

Bladder expression may be difficult to perform in some patients, especially males, because transabdominal compression causes the pressure inside the bladder to increase, but the urethral sphincter may not relax simultaneously. Manual bladder expression can be done in patients that cannot initiate voluntary urination or completely empty the bladder, such as animals with neurologic impairments. In addition, unsuccessful attempts to manually express the bladder, especially in a male cat suspected of having a urethral obstruction, can serve a diagnostic purpose.

To express the bladder, support the animal in a standing or lateral position and place a hand on either side of the caudal abdomen. Isolate the bladder between the palmar surfaces of the fingers, and gently apply steady, firm pressure until a stream of urine is produced. It may be possible to express the bladder of cats and small dogs with only one hand.

If urine is not expelled with moderate compression, do not continue to exert pressure. An alternative method of emptying the bladder should be attempted. Care must be taken when attempting to express an overly distended bladder in the presence of urethral obstruction because urethral or vesicular rupture may occur.

CATHETERIZATION

Urinary catheterization is performed to collect urine, relieve a urethral obstruction, or empty the bladder (Box 3-2). Although catheterization is performed with aseptic technique, it may induce urethral inflammation and bacterial urinary tract infection. This is particularly problematic in cases in which the urinary catheter remains indwelling for prolonged periods. Trauma from catheterization may cause increases in the number of red blood cells, amount of protein, and number of transitional epithelial cells in the sample. Urine samples may contain contaminants from the genital region and urethra. Urine obtained by catheterization is acceptable for bacterial culture if a sample cannot be obtained by cystocentesis.

Urinary catheters are temporarily left indwelling in patients at risk for urethral obstruction, such as male cats

---

Box 3-2 MALE URINARY CATHETERIZATION TECHNIQUE*

- Retract the prepuce to expose the penis
- Wash the penis and prepuce with warm dilute antimicrobial solution, and rinse well with warm water.
- Lubricate the tip of the sterile urinary catheter with sterile, water-soluble gel.
- Wearing sterile gloves, insert the catheter into the urethra and advance it until the bladder is entered and urine flows through the catheter. If sterile gloves are not worn, keep the catheter in its wrapper and cut a freely moveable paper tab from the tip of the package.
- Use this tab to feed the catheter into the bladder to avoid directly touching the catheter. Do not allow the top edge of the tab to contact any surface.
- Do not force the catheter; if it does not advance easily, remove it and use a catheter with a smaller lumen. If it does not advance easily because of a urethral obstruction, flush a small volume of 0.9% saline solution into the end of the catheter as it is advanced to attempt to dislodge the obstructing material.
- Once the catheter enters the bladder, attach a syringe to the end and collect a urine sample if needed.
- Attach a closed collection system to the end of the urinary catheter.
- If the catheter is to remain indwelling, secure the catheter in place by inflating the balloon cuff (Foley catheter) or by suturing the tape tab wrapped around the catheter through suture loops placed in the skin of the prepuce. Use 4-0 to 3-0 nylon sutures.

*Male cats are sedated.

---

who have recently had urethral calculi removed. Indwelling urinary catheters are also placed in animals unable to stand to void and those with neurologic impairment that interferes with micturition. Catheterization is also an important part of quantitating urinary output.

The prepuce or vulva should be gently rinsed with warm antimicrobial solution and water and then dried twice daily. Gloves are worn to detach or connect the catheter to extension tubing or a collection system. A closed collection system is created by connecting the catheter, via intravenous tubing, to an empty sterile fluid bag. The bag serves as a urine reservoir. Its contents must be measured and emptied periodically.

Urinary catheters should be inspected for occlusion and adequate urine production every 4 to 6 hours. A normotensive, normovolemic patient with intact renal function should produce 1 to 2 ml of urine per kilogram of body weight per hour. If urine does not accumulate in the collection bag and the bladder is firm and distended, the catheter is probably obstructed. It should be slightly repositioned and inspected for kinks. The bladder can be gently compressed to determine whether urine will flow through the catheter. As a last resort, a small volume of sterile 0.9% saline solution can be flushed into the catheter in an attempt to relieve the obstruction.

The catheter should be removed as soon as possible to prevent or limit catheter-induced infection and inflammation of the urinary tract. If catheterization is required beyond 4 days, a new catheter should be placed.

Male Dog

It is usually not difficult to place a urinary catheter in a male dog unless a urethral obstruction exists. A wide range of sizes and types of urinary catheters is available. A 4 to 10 French (Fr) polypropylene urinary catheter is used. If the catheter is to remain indwelling, placement of a softer, flexible feeding tube or a self-retaining Foley catheter is a more comfortable alternative.

The dog is placed in lateral recumbency with the upper rear leg abducted. An assistant retracts the prepuce so the tip of the penis is exposed. The prepuce and glans penis are gently washed with warm, dilute antiseptic solution and rinsed with warm sterile saline solution or water. The package containing the catheter is cut open to expose the distal 3 cm of the catheter. Sterile, water-soluble lubricant or lidocaine ointment is placed on the catheter tip. If sterile gloves are worn, the catheter can be removed from its package. If sterile gloves are not worn, the catheter should be kept wrapped so it can be handled aseptically as it is advanced through the urethra.

When the catheter is placed, the lubricated tip is introduced into the urethra and slowly advanced. The catheter should never be forced. If the catheter cannot be passed, a catheter with a narrower lumen should be used. Resistance may be met when the catheter reaches the os penis or a portion of the urethra that curves around the ischial arch. Steady gentle pressure should overcome this resistance. The catheter can be guided around the flexure of the urethral canal by applying digital pressure on the perineum externally or pressing on the catheter with an index finger placed in the rectum.

Urine should flow into the catheter as it enters the neck of the bladder. The catheter is then advanced 1 cm further. A sterile 20- to 35-ml syringe is attached to the catheter, and urine is slowly aspirated from the bladder. The first several milliliters of urine suctioned from the catheter may contain contaminants and should not be submitted for urinalysis or culture.

If the urinary catheter is not self-retaining (i.e., not a Foley catheter) and it is to remain indwelling, it must be secured. Two 0.75-cm–diameter loops can be made through the skin on two sides of the distal prepuce with 3-0 or 4-0 nylon suture material to accomplish this. Adhesive tape is folded over on itself to make a "butterfly" around the catheter as it exits from the penis. A suture is passed through one side of the tape and then through the nylon loop in the prepuce. This "chain link" is repeated on the other side of the tape. This secures the catheter to the prepuce so it remains in place. If the catheter needs to be replaced, the suture ring

that courses through the tape is cut. Tape is wrapped around the replacement catheter and sutured through the existing loops in the prepuce. When a set of suture loops is left in the prepuce, the urinary catheter can be readjusted or replaced without having to pass another needle through the prepuce.

Female Dog

Catheterization is more challenging in the female dog than in the male. The dog is placed on a table in a standing position, in lateral recumbency, or in sternal recumbency with the hind legs dangling from the end of the table. The vulva is gently washed with a dilute, warm antiseptic solution and rinsed with sterile saline solution or water. The ventral vaginal floor is instilled with 1.0 ml of 2% lidocaine. A sterile flexible polypropylene urinary catheter is lubricated with sterile, water-soluble gel at the fenestrated end. Wearing sterile gloves, the technician places a lubricated finger into the vagina and slides it 3 to 5 cm along the ventral floor until the external urethral orifice is identified. The catheter is introduced into the vagina and guided into the urethral orifice by the finger in the vestibule. It is important to avoid inadvertently passing the catheter into the clitoral fossa. The catheter is advanced until it enters the bladder. If "blind catheterization" is not possible, a lighted vaginal speculum or an otoscope fitted with a large speculum can be inserted into the vagina and used to visualize the urethral orifice.

If the urinary catheter is to remain indwelling, a soft Foley self-retaining catheter with a removable stylet is used. Once the catheter is placed in the bladder, the cuff is inflated with a few milliliters of water to prevent the tip of the catheter from slipping out of the bladder. The catheter is then taped to the tail to prevent the dog from stepping on it. A urine collection device is placed on the free end of the Foley catheter.

🖉 TECHNICIAN NOTE

The most common reason for catheterizing a male cat is to relieve a urethral obstruction.

Male Cat

The most common reason for catheterizing a male cat is to relieve a urethral obstruction. Catheterization requires the use of a short-acting anesthetic, such as a ketamine-diazepam combination or propofol, either alone or in combination with a gas anesthetic.

The anesthetized or heavily sedated male cat is placed on his side or back with the hind legs drawn forward. As shown in Figure 3-10, the prepuce is retracted to expose the penis. The perineum is prepared aseptically, as described for male canine catheterization, and the penis is extended dorsally so the urethra is parallel to the vertebral column. Sterile gloves are worn and a sterile, lubricated, 3.5 Fr polyethylene or silicone tomcat catheter is passed into the urethra. If resistance is met, the catheter is retracted and then slightly rotated as it is readvanced. If the catheter

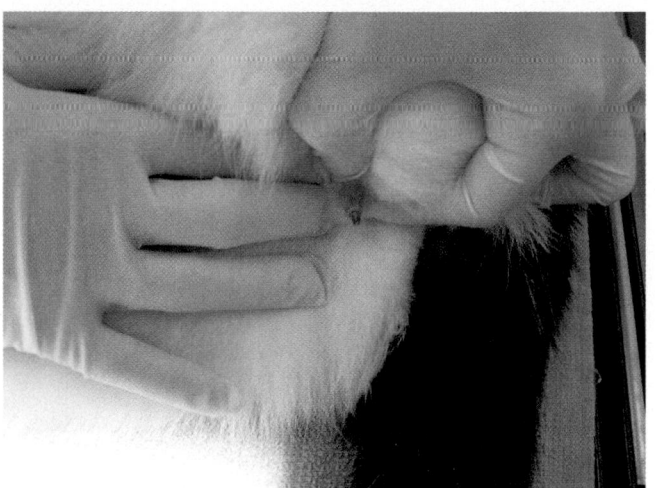

Figure 3-10 Retraction of the prepuce to expose the penis for feline urinary catheterization.

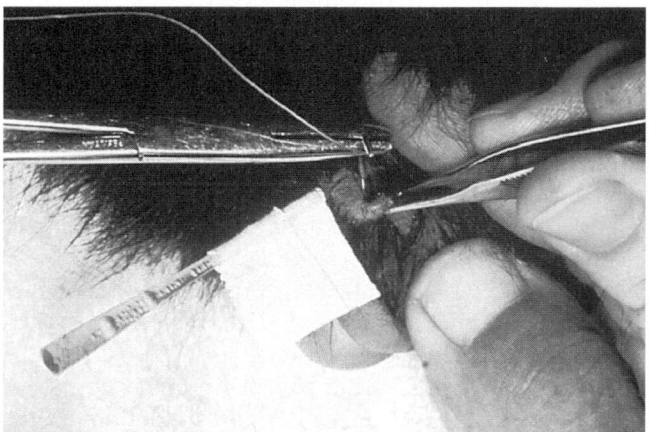

Figure 3-11 A urinary catheter is secured in place in a male cat. Tape wrapped around the catheter is sutured to the skin of the prepuce.

cannot be easily advanced, a small volume of sterile water or saline solution is instilled through the catheter. The pressure created often dislodges the obstructing material. Alternatively, saline solution can be flushed through a 24- or 22-gauge intravenous catheter placed in the urethra. After the obstruction is relieved, a 3.5 Fr catheter is placed to prevent reobstruction.

Once the catheter is in place, it is secured with 4-0 nylon in the same fashion as described for the male dog. Refer to Figure 3-11. The cat should be fitted with an Elizabethan collar to prevent removal of the catheter and urine collection system.

Female Cat

Catheterization of female cats is performed infrequently because of its difficulty, and, as with male cats, the requirement for sedation. The perineal region is aseptically prepared, and the vulva is pulled caudally. A sterile, lubricated,

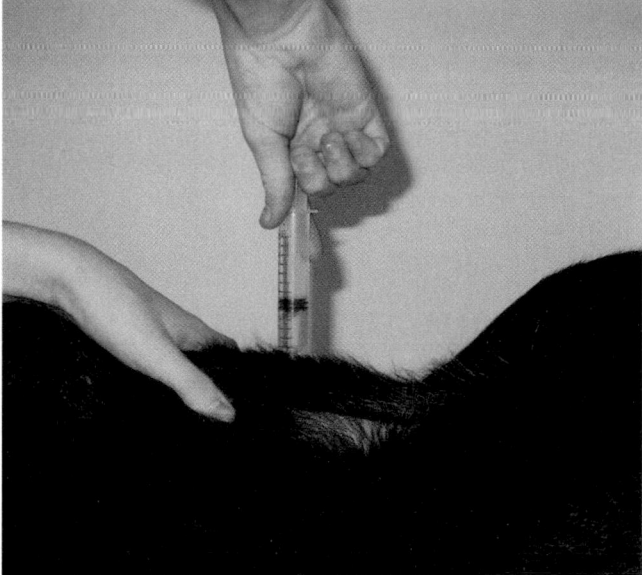

Figure 3-12 Collection of a urine sample through cystocentesis in a dog. The bladder is isolated, and urine is aspirated into a syringe.

open-ended 3.5 Fr tomcat catheter is inserted along the midline of the floor of the vagina and into the urethra.

> ✎ **TECHNICIAN NOTE**
> Cystocentesis is the percutaneous aspiration of urine from the bladder.

CYSTOCENTESIS

Cystocentesis is the percutaneous aspiration of urine from the bladder. It is performed to collect specimens for urinalysis or bacterial culture that will be free of contamination from the distal urethra and genital tract. Cystocentesis is used as a last resort to empty an overly distended bladder when a urethral obstruction prevents urinary catheterization. Recent abdominal surgery or trauma, suspected bleeding disorders, pyometra, or suspected caudal abdominal or bladder tumors are contraindications for cystocentesis.

When cystocentesis is performed, most but not all of the urine should be removed from the bladder. Excessive pressure from a full bladder might lead to extravasation of urine from the puncture site when the needle is withdrawn. On the other hand, removal of the entire volume of urine increases the risk of contact between the needle and the bladder wall, which may result in damage to the bladder.

When cystocentesis is performed, the animal is restrained in dorsal or lateral recumbency or in a standing position. The skin of the ventral or lateral abdomen is wiped with 70% alcohol. One hand is used to isolate the bladder. A 22-gauge, 2.5- to 3.75-cm needle attached to a 12- to 20-ml syringe is inserted through the abdominal wall and into the bladder at a 45- to 75-degree angle (Figure 3-12). In male dogs, the prepuce and penis are diverted laterally, and the needle is inserted on the ventral midline or slightly paramedian. The syringe plunger is slowly retracted, and urine is collected. If blood enters the needle, another cystocentesis attempt should be made with a different needle and syringe. The needle should not be redirected once it is within the abdominal cavity because accidental laceration of viscera may occur. Once a sufficient urine volume is collected, negative pressure is released and the needle is withdrawn.

OTHER COLLECTION PROCEDURES

FECES SAMPLE COLLECTION

Gross and microscopic examination of feces for intestinal parasites, ova, blood, and mucus is frequently performed in veterinary practice (see Chapter 7). Samples are most commonly obtained by collecting them from the ground or litter pan after defecation. Alternatively, a lubricated fecal loop or gloved finger can be inserted into the rectum to remove feces. Fresh samples are placed into a sealed container or bag or wrapped in aluminum foil. If feces are collected to check for parasites but samples are not examined for several hours, the samples should be refrigerated or placed in a formalin solution. Samples intended for parasitology examination can be refrigerated for up to 3 days.

THORACOCENTESIS

The thorax (chest cavity) contains the heart and lungs. Many medical conditions lead to the accumulation of air or fluid in the *pleural space.* This space is located between the lungs and the chest wall. When air or fluid accumulates in the pleural space, the lungs are unable to completely expand. This results in rapid and difficult breathing. *Thoracocentesis* is the process of removing accumulated air or fluid from within the pleural space.

When thoracocentesis is performed, the area between the fifth and twelfth ribs is clipped and surgically prepared with alternating chlorhexidine or povidone-iodine and alcohol scrubs. Thoracocentesis of pleural fluid is done at the seventh or eighth intercostal space, which is located by counting forward from the thirteenth rib. Needles used during the procedure are introduced at the cranial aspect of the rib to avoid penetration of the blood vessels that lie along the caudal aspect. For fluid removal, the needle is inserted in the ventral third of the thorax near the costochondral junction. For removal of air, the needle insertion site should be more dorsal.

When thoracocentesis is performed, the animal is placed in sternal recumbency or held in a standing position. A 21-gauge butterfly catheter or a 22-gauge needle attached to extension tubing is connected to a closed three-way stopcock. A 60-ml syringe is also attached to one of the stopcock ports. The needle is directed into the seventh or eighth intercostal space, perpendicular to the body wall, as

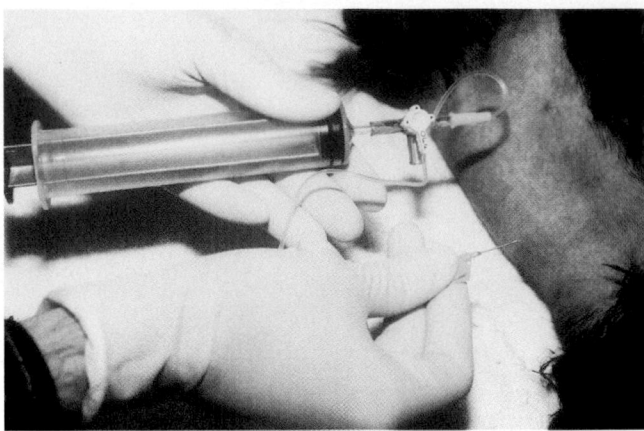

Figure 3-13 Materials used for thoracocentesis of a cat include a 21-gauge butterfly catheter attached to a three-way stopcock and 60-ml syringe.

shown in Figure 3-13. After the pleural space is penetrated, the needle is directed caudoventrally to avoid puncture of the lung, and the stopcock is then opened. Suction is applied with the syringe, and fluid or air is withdrawn from the pleural cavity. If only negative pressure is obtained, the needle is retracted 2 to 3 mm and carefully redirected. Caution should be used because redirection of the needle may lacerate a lung. If frank blood enters the needle, the needle should be removed. When the syringe is filled, the stopcock valve is closed, and the syringe contents are expelled into a container through the third stopcock port. This process is repeated until no additional fluid or air can be removed.

After thoracocentesis, the patient's respiratory pattern is monitored for approximately 2 hours. In addition, the technician must be observant of the stopcock apparatus. If the three-way stopcock is accidentally opened or any part of the apparatus is disconnected, air may enter the thoracic cavity and cause serious complications. In this situation, thoracocentesis should be repeated immediately.

> ✏️ **TECHNICIAN NOTE**
>
> Similar to thoracocentesis, *abdominocentesis* is the process of drawing fluid from the abdominal cavity.

ABDOMINOCENTESIS

Similar to thoracocentesis, *abdominocentesis* is the process of drawing fluid from the abdominal cavity. It is performed for both diagnostic and therapeutic purposes. Abdominocentesis is an important technique for use in some emergency and critical care cases, such as those in which abdominal trauma or peritonitis is suspected.

Patients should urinate before abdominocentesis to empty and avoid accidental puncture of the bladder. The patient is restrained in a standing position or lateral recumbency. A 5- to 10-cm area on the ventral abdomen between the umbilicus and bladder is clipped and aseptically prepared. A 20- to 22-gauge, 2.5- to 3.75 cm needle is inserted to the right of the ventral midline, 1 to 2 cm caudal to the umbilicus. This right paramedian approach is selected to avoid lacerating the spleen. Fluid is collected as it drips out of the needle hub, or it can be aspirated into a syringe attached to the needle. Sometimes rotation of the needle or insertion of a second needle into the abdomen 2 cm from the first will stimulate fluid flow. If the abdominal effusion is suspected to be compartmentalized, abdominocentesis can be performed in more than one quadrant, such as in the left and right craniolateral or caudolateral regions.

Abdominocentesis can also be performed with an 18- to 20-gauge, over-the-needle (OTN) intravenous catheter. After the catheter has been inserted into the abdominal cavity, the stylet is removed and a sample is collected.

Gastrocentesis, which is an emergency procedure, involves insertion of a large-gauge needle or metal trocar into the stomach to temporarily relieve pressure in animals with gastric dilation. The skin over the greatest point of abdominal distension is shaved and aseptically prepared. A 14- to 16-gauge needle or trocar is inserted through the abdominal and stomach walls. Gas and fluid will exit the needle once it enters the stomach lumen, but solid ingesta will not fit through the needle. Gentle compression applied with the hands helps evacuate the fluid and gas within the stomach. The needle is removed after the stomach is decompressed. Gastrocentesis may result in laceration of the stomach or other abdominal organs and the development of peritonitis.

DIAGNOSTIC PERITONEAL LAVAGE

Diagnostic peritoneal lavage is performed if abdominocentesis does not provide a sufficient abdominal fluid sample. Warm sterile water or 0.9% sterile saline solution is injected into the abdomen through an 18- to 20-gauge catheter at a volume of 20 ml/kg of body weight. With the catheter in place, the animal is gently rolled from side to side to disperse the fluid. A sample of abdominal fluid is aspirated through the catheter, and then the catheter is removed. Usually only a small percentage (less than 10%) of the volume of fluid infused into the abdominal cavity will be retrieved.

TRANSTRACHEAL WASH

A transtracheal wash is performed to obtain fluid samples from the lower respiratory tract for culture or cytology. Light sedation may be used in the dog, but the cough reflex should remain intact. In fractious or feline patients, general anesthesia is required.

Percutaneous Technique

The percutaneous technique requires one person to position the patient, one to place and secure the transtracheal catheter, and another to flush and aspirate the fluid. The patient is placed in sternal recumbency or a seated position with the

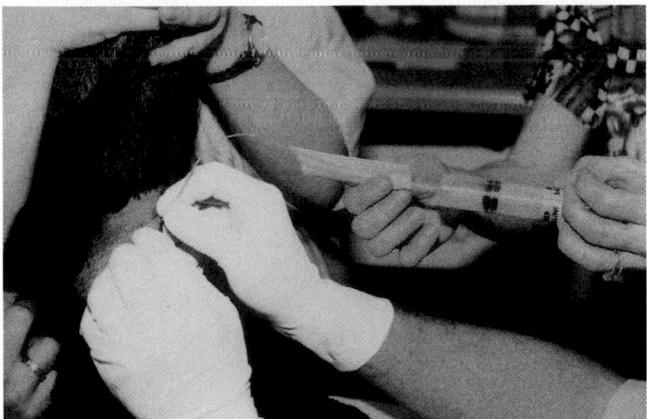

Figure 3-14 Transtracheal wash in a dog with a urinary catheter placed into the trachea.

head raised slightly. The laryngeal region is clipped and aseptically prepared. A sterile gloved finger is placed on the ventral aspect of the trachea and moved in a cranial direction until the protruding cricoid cartilage is palpated. Just above the cartilage is a flattened, triangular region called the cricothyroid membrane. From 0.5 to 1 ml of 2% lidocaine is injected into the skin, subcutaneous tissue, and cricothyroid membrane.

The needle from an 18-gauge, 20-cm, through-the-needle (TTN) catheter is disengaged from the catheter. The catheter is set aside but kept in its protective sleeve. One hand stabilizes the trachea. The needle is inserted at a 90-degree angle through the cricothyroid membrane with the bevel facing downward. Alternatively, the needle can be inserted between any tracheal rings in the cranial third of the trachea.

A burst of air accompanied by a cough occurs when the needle enters the trachea. The needle is repositioned at a caudal 120-degree angle. The catheter is advanced through the needle until it reaches the distal trachea. Placement of the needle with the bevel aimed downward decreases the likelihood of laceration of the catheter as it courses through the needle. The needle is withdrawn through the skin. The catheter, with the stylet removed, is left in place. In large dogs, a sterile 3.5 Fr polyvinyl urinary catheter can be passed through a 14-gauge needle and advanced into the distal third of the trachea in lieu of a TTN catheter (Figure 3-14).

A 3-ml syringe is attached to the catheter, and the plunger is retracted. Air is aspirated if the catheter is in the tracheal lumen. If only resistance is felt, the catheter should be repositioned because it may be kinked, occluded against the tracheal mucosa, or embedded in the tissue surrounding the trachea.

After the catheter is properly positioned in the trachea, the contents of a syringe containing warm, nonbacteriostatic sterile saline solution (0.5 to 1.0 ml/kg of body weight) is flushed through the catheter. When the animal coughs, the syringe plunger is immediately retracted several times to collect a sample. Only a small percentage of the volume of fluid infused down the trachea will be reaspirated; the remainder will be absorbed. Additional aliquots of saline solution are instilled into the catheter and reaspirated until a sufficient sample volume is collected. The catheter position may need to be adjusted during the procedure.

When transtracheal aspiration has been completed, the puncture site is covered with a povidone-iodine ointment-treated gauze sponge and bandaged. Respiration is monitored for 12 hours after the procedure. The needle insertion site is checked for air accumulation (subcutaneous emphysema) in the tissue surrounding the trachea, which would indicate laceration of the tracheal tissue from the needle.

Endotracheal Tube Technique

Tracheal aspirates in fractious or very small animals are obtained in a different manner. The animal is anesthetized and intubated with a sterile endotracheal tube. The plane of anesthesia is lightened. A sterile polypropylene urinary catheter longer than the endotracheal tube is threaded down the tube to just above the tracheal bifurcation. Warm sterile saline solution is injected through the catheter. When the animal coughs, the sample is aspirated into a sterile 12-ml syringe. The saline solution injection-aspiration procedure is repeated until a sufficient sample volume is obtained.

ARTHROCENTESIS

Aspiration of fluid from a swollen or painful joint, *arthrocentesis*, is performed by the veterinarian to help determine the cause of pain or swelling. Synovial fluid is collected for cytologic, bacterial, and biochemical analyses. The technique is reviewed so the technician will be familiar with the site preparation, materials needed, and sample handling.

The anatomy of the joint to be aspirated should be reviewed to determine the appropriate site of needle insertion. For the shoulder, the needle is inserted into the lateral aspect and is directed medially. Aspiration of the elbow is performed from the lateral or caudal aspect. The carpus is tapped from its dorsal surface. The coxofemoral joint is aspirated from its craniodorsal aspect. The stifle is approached from the craniolateral surface, just below the patella. A caudolateral approach is used for tarsal arthrocentesis.

When arthrocentesis is performed, the animal is sedated, and the skin over the joint is shaved and aseptically prepared. It is often helpful to flex the joint to facilitate needle insertion. The person who performs the aspiration should wear sterile gloves. A 22-gauge needle on a 3- to 6-ml syringe is inserted into the joint space with the needle directed into a bone-free location (Figure 3-15). If the needle comes in contact with bone, it is withdrawn slightly and redirected. After the joint is penetrated, the syringe plunger is retracted to collect the synovial fluid. Although some disease processes may cause a hemorrhagic effusion within the joint capsule, if frank blood enters the needle hub, the needle should be removed from the joint. Subsequent joint taps may be hemorrhagic.

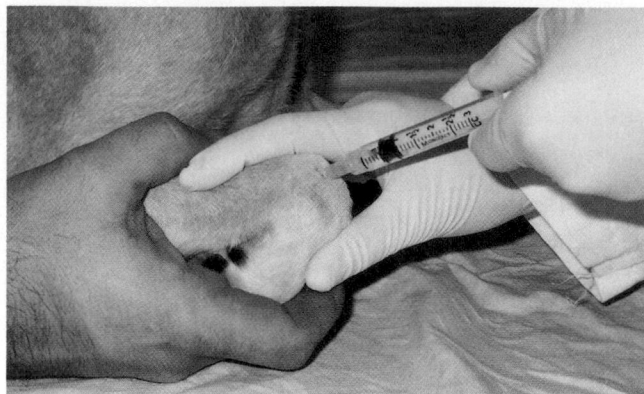

Figure 3-15 Arthrocentesis of the carpal joint through a dorsal approach.

The color, consistency, volume, and viscosity of the synovial fluid are noted. Normal joint fluid should be clear, pale yellow, and viscous. A fluid drop stretched between the thumb and forefinger should stretch out at least 10 cm long. Fluid is placed on a microscope slide to make a smear for cytologic analysis. A sample is saved for bacterial culture and further laboratory analysis.

BONE MARROW ASPIRATION

Bone marrow aspiration is performed to evaluate the cells in the bone marrow. It is most commonly performed in patients with nonregenerative anemia, persistent thrombocytopenia, or neoplasia. A complete blood count is done within 24 hours before or after the aspirate is obtained so the peripheral and marrow cell populations can be compared. *Because aspiration of bone marrow is a very uncomfortable procedure, heavy sedation or general anesthesia, in conjunction with local anesthesia, is advised.*

The most frequently aspirated sites include the iliac wing, humerus, and femur. Patient size and conformation generally determine which site is used.

Aspirations are performed with strict aseptic technique. Hair over the site is shaved, and the skin is surgically prepared. Sterile gloves are worn by the person performing the aspiration.

✎ TECHNICIAN NOTE

Common sites for bone marrow aspiration include the iliac wing, femur, and humerus.

Iliac Bone Marrow Aspiration

The animal is placed in lateral recumbency or in sternal recumbency with the rear legs drawn forward. The widest portion of the iliac crest region is clipped and aseptically prepared. From 0.5 to 1 ml of 2% lidocaine is infiltrated into the skin, subcutaneous tissue, and periosteum of the bone (Figure 3-16, *A*).

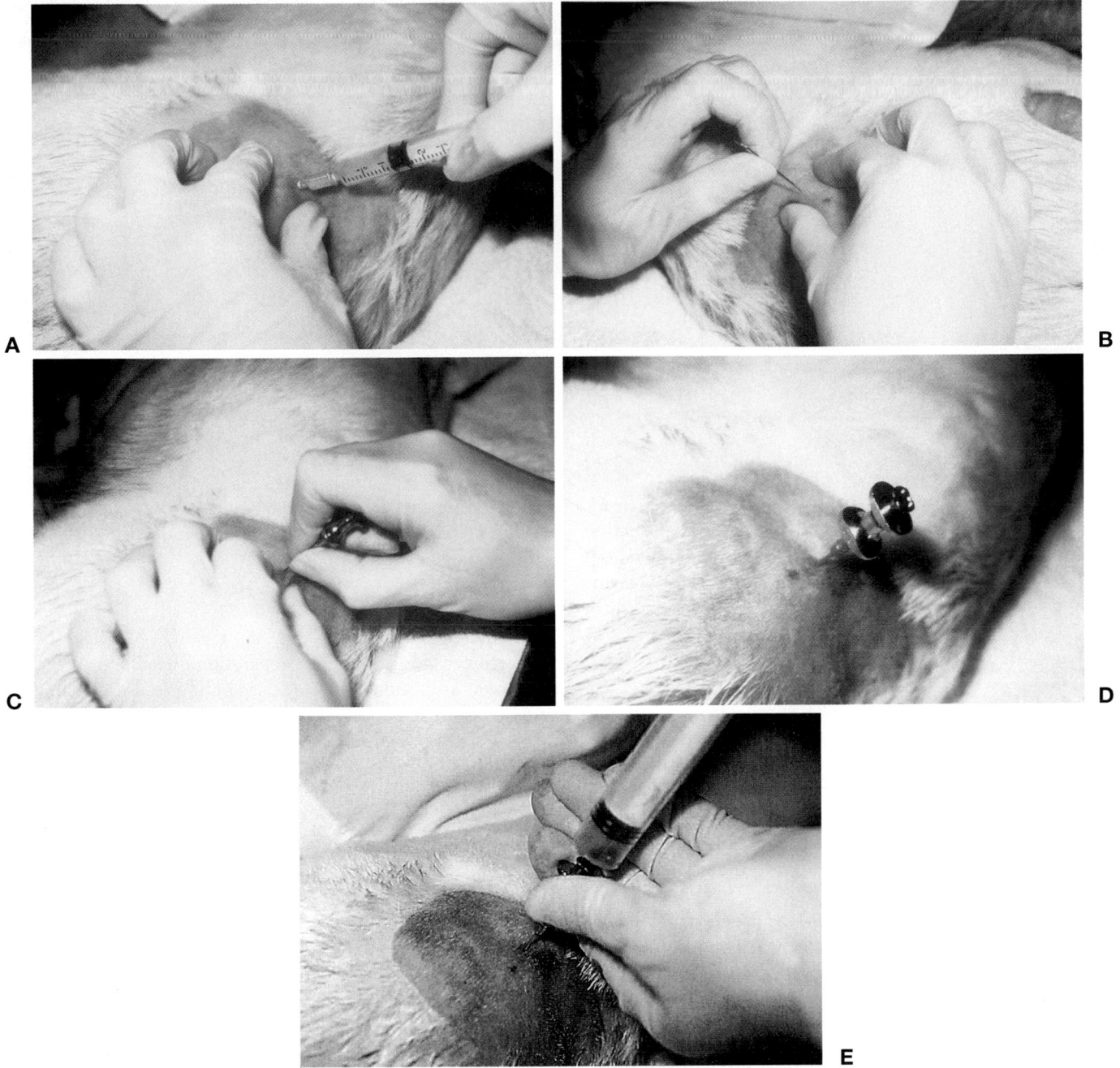

Figure 3-16 **A,** Injection of 2% lidocaine into the skin, subcutaneus tissue, and periosteum of the wing of the ilium of a dog. **B,** A No.11 scalpel blade is used to make a stab incision over the iliac crest. **C,** The bone marrow needle is inserted through the skin incision and into the marrow cavity. **D,** The bone marrow needle is seated in the dorsal aspect of the wing of the ilium. Note that the stylet has been removed after placement. **E,** One hand is used to stabilize the bone marrow needle as marrow is aspirated from the ilium.

A sterile 15- to 18-gauge bone marrow needle is flushed with an anticoagulant, such as a 2.5% to 3% EDTA solution. A No. 11 scalpel blade is used to make a stab incision through the skin over the iliac crest (Figure 3-16, *B*). One hand is placed on the ilium to stabilize it. The bone marrow needle, with the stylet in place, is introduced through the skin incision and advanced by application of firm pressure and rotation of the wrist in a clockwise-counterclockwise manner. The needle eventually penetrates the cortex of the

bone and enters the marrow cavity (Figure 3-16, *C*). If the needle slips off the bone during placement, which may occur if the iliac wings are narrow, the needle is repositioned and another attempt is made.

Once the needle is firmly seated in the bone and the tip is in the marrow cavity, the stylet is removed and placed on a sterile field (Figure 3-16, *D*). An anticoagulant-coated, 12-ml syringe is attached to the end of the needle, and negative pressure is rapidly and forcefully applied. One tenth of 1 ml

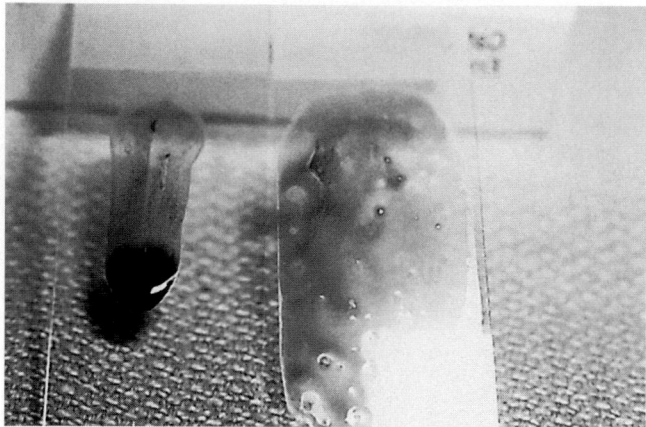

Figure 3-17 Drops of bone marrow are placed on the end of a microscope slide, which is tilted to allow blood to run to the other end. A pull smear is made with the bone marrow sample.

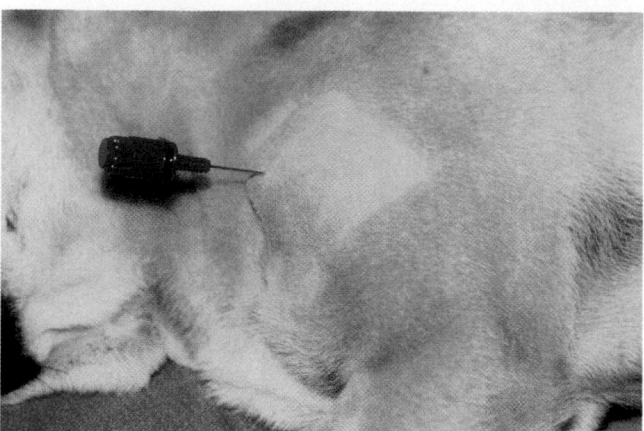

Figure 3-18 Jamshidi bone marrow needle placed into the craniolateral aspect of the proximal humerus to obtain a bone marrow aspirate.

of bone marrow is aspirated into the syringe (Figure 3-16, *E*). If a marrow sample does not enter the syringe when suction is applied, the stylet is replaced, and the needle is advanced or retracted a few millimeters until it enters the marrow cavity.

Once marrow enters the syringe, the syringe is detached, and a drop of the sample is placed onto a few tilted microscope slides. Marrow particles adhere to the tilted slides, and the excess blood trickles to the ends (Figure 3-17). Alternatively, the marrow sample can be emptied from the syringe onto a Petri dish. The dish is then tilted to separate the blood from the marrow. The marrow particles are transferred to a slide with the tip of a hypodermic needle. A pull slide is made with each sample. A pull slide is made by placing a clean glass slide on top of the slide containing the aspirate and pulling the slides apart to create two slides for cytologic analysis.

After marrow has been obtained, the needle is withdrawn, and firm pressure is held on the site until hemostasis occurs. An antibiotic ointment–treated gauze sponge is secured over the aspiration site for the next 24 hours.

Humeral Bone Marrow Aspiration
The craniolateral aspect of the greater tubercle of the proximal humerus is an excellent bone marrow aspiration site (Figure 3-18). The advantage of this site is that it has less tissue, fat, and muscle overlying the bone. Thus the humerus is preferred in heavily muscled or overweight dogs when the dorsal iliac crest is difficult to palpate. The humerus is also advantageous to use in animals with narrow iliac wings or in patients with thrombocytopenia when hemostasis is a concern.

The animal is placed in lateral recumbency with the humerus to be aspirated positioned on top. The proximal humerus is shaved, surgically prepared, and infiltrated with a local anesthetic. The needle is embedded perpendicular to the humeral shaft as the elbow is held flexed and the shoulder is rotated externally. The techniques for site preparation, needle placement, bone marrow aspiration, and slide preparation are the same as those described for iliac bone marrow aspiration.

Femoral Bone Marrow Aspiration
In small dogs and cats, the femur can be used for bone marrow aspiration. Site preparation, needle placement, marrow aspiration, and slide preparation techniques are the same as those described for bone marrow aspiration from the wing of the ilium. Needle placement within the femur is described in the discussion of placement of an intraosseous catheter.

Fine-Needle Aspiration
Fine-needle aspiration is a quick procedure frequently performed to collect a sample of fluid or tissue cells from a dermal or visceral mass or a lymph node. The skin overlying the tissue to be aspirated is wiped with alcohol to remove superficial contaminants. The mass is stabilized with one hand as a 22-gauge needle is inserted into the center. The needle is redirected once or twice within the tissue and then removed. A syringe containing 1 ml of air is attached to the needle. The syringe plunger is forcefully depressed, and the needle contents are expelled onto a microscope slide. Slides are then prepared with the pull technique described for iliac bone marrow aspiration.

An alternate technique for performing fine-needle aspiration is to use a needle attached to a 3- to 12-ml syringe. The needle is embedded in the mass, and suction is applied to aspirate cells into the needle. During this process, the needle may be redirected once or twice. Negative pressure is released before the needle is withdrawn from the mass. The needle is then detached to allow the syringe to be filled with 1 to 2 ml of air. Subsequently, the needle is reattached, and the syringe plunger is depressed so that the contents of the needle are sprayed onto a microscope slide. Slides are made by using the previously described pull technique.

Box 3-3 ROUTES OF FLUID OR MEDICATION ADMINISTRATION

- Intravenous
- Subcutaneous
- Intramuscular
- Intradermal
- Intranasal
- Intratracheal
- Intraosseous
- Intraperitoneal
- Topical ophthalmic
- Aural
- Transdermal
- Intrarectal
- Oral
- Per os
- Oroesophageal tube
- Orogastric tube
- Nasoesophageal tube
- Nasogastric tube
- Pharyngostomy tube
- Esophagostomy tube
- Gastrostomy tube
- Duodenostomy/jejunostomy tube
- Intramammary (primarily large animal)

Box 3-4 INTRAVENOUS INJECTION

- Occlude the vessel with digital pressure or a tourniquet.
- Grasp the extremity and pull the skin tautly in a distal direction.
- Wipe an alcohol-soaked cotton ball over the hair and skin covering a distal section of a peripheral vein.
- Insert a 22- to 25-gauge needle attached to a syringe, with the bevel facing up, through the skin and into the vein.
- Aspirate a small volume of blood into the syringe to ensure the needle is within the vein.
- Release the pressure from the vein.
- Inject the contents of the syringe into the vein.
- Remove the needle, and apply digital pressure to the needle insertion site for 30 to 60 seconds until hemostasis occurs.
- If a hematoma occurs when the needle is inserted, remove the needle and apply digital pressure over the hematoma until the bleeding subsides. Make another injection attempt either proximal to the initial site or in a different vein.

VAGINAL CYTOLOGIC SAMPLING

Vaginal cytologic sampling is performed to determine the patient's present stage in the estrous cycle for breeding purposes or to collect samples to help determine the cause of vaginal disease. When a vaginal smear must be obtained, the patient is placed in a standing position or lateral recumbency. The vulvar region is wiped with warm water. A gloved hand is used to separate the labia so that a cotton swab can be inserted and rolled against the vaginal wall. The swab is then removed from the vagina and is rolled onto a glass microscope slide for cytologic evaluation.

ADMINISTRATION OF MEDICATION IN THE SMALL ANIMAL

Multiple routes exist for the administration of fluids and medication (Box 3-3). The route used depends on many factors, including, but not limited to, patient condition and temperament, type of medication or fluid, urgency involved in administering the fluid or medication, cost, ease of administration, and whether a systemic or local effect is desired.

INTRAVENOUS ADMINISTRATION

Many medications are administered directly into a vein. Intravenous injection is used for drugs or fluids that must rapidly reach high blood levels or that would be irritating to tissue or insufficiently absorbed if given by another route (Box 3-4). Certain anesthetics, chemotherapeutic agents, anticonvulsant drugs, and drugs used in cardiopulmonary resuscitation are given intravenously. If an extremely rapid onset of action is required, the intravenous or intraosseous route is chosen.

The most frequently used sites for intravenous injection in the dog are the cephalic and lateral saphenous veins. Cats are most often given intravenous injections in the cephalic, medial saphenous, and femoral veins. The jugular vein is used to administer injections in both large and small animals if an intravenous jugular catheter is in place.

When an intravenous injection is administered, the vessel is occluded with a tourniquet or digital pressure. Air bubbles are expelled from the syringe before the needle is inserted into the vein. The skin and hair over the vein is swabbed with alcohol, and the needle is then inserted into the vein. Blood will appear in the needle hub when the needle penetrates the vein, but intravenous placement is confirmed by aspirating blood back into the syringe. Pressure is released from the vein, and the syringe contents are injected. The needle is withdrawn, and firm pressure is applied to the venipuncture site until hemostasis occurs.

Intravenous Catheter Placement

When intravenous fluids or drugs must be infused in large volumes, repeatedly, or continuously, a catheter is placed in the cephalic, jugular, or saphenous vein. The technician should be familiar with catheter selection, placement, and maintenance.

The four types of catheters used are the butterfly catheter, OTN catheter, TTN catheter, and single-lumen and multilumen guide-wire catheters. If the catheter is to remain indwelling, the OTN, TTN, or guide-wire type is used.

Box 3-5 INTRAVENOUS CATHETER PLACEMENT IN A PERIPHERAL VEIN

- Flush a 20- to 22-gauge, 2.5- to 3.75-cm over-the-needle catheter with a small volume of heparinized saline solution.
- Shave and aseptically prepare the skin over the distal portion of the vein.
- Occlude the vein with digital pressure or a tourniquet.
- Align the catheter, with the stylet in place, parallel to the vein.
- Insert the catheter into the skin and vein with the bevel facing upward.
- When blood enters the hub of the catheter, advance the catheter an additional few millimeters.
- Hold the stylet in place and slide the catheter into the vein. Remove the digital pressure or tourniquet as the catheter is advanced.
- Immediately place a catheter cap into the hub of the catheter.
- Inject 1 ml of heparinized saline solution into the catheter to check patency.
- If the fluid does not inject without resistance, the catheter may be kinked, occluded with a blood clot or tissue plug, or extravascular (i.e., outside the vein) and should be reflushed, repositioned, or replaced.
- If a hematoma occurs during catheter placement, remove the catheter and apply pressure to the hematoma site until hemostasis occurs. Reattempt catheter placement further proximal to the initial entry site or in a different vein.
- Secure the catheter in place with adhesive tape.

Single- or multi-lumen guide-wire catheters are most often placed in the jugular veins in critically ill patients. Detailed instructions for guide-wire catheter placement are available from the manufacturers. Butterfly catheters are used to administer small volumes of fluid and are generally not left indwelling for longer than a few minutes.

Indwelling catheters are placed by using aseptic technique to minimize subsequent thrombus formation, phlebitis, and infection. The hair is shaved from the skin on top of the vein, and the skin surface is cleansed a minimum of three times with an antimicrobial solution and alcohol. Ideally, the skin should be in contact with the antimicrobial solution for 2 minutes. If it is necessary to palpate the skin to identify the vein, the area should be rescrubbed or the individual placing the catheter should wear gloves.

✎ TECHNICIAN NOTE

Indwelling catheters are placed by using aseptic technique to minimize subsequent thrombus formation, phlebitis, and infection.

Catheters are inspected for irregular surfaces and are usually flushed with heparinized saline solution (1 unit of heparin per milliliter of 0.9% saline solution) before insertion. The heparinized saline solution may prevent development of blood clots within the catheter lumen.

Peripheral Vein Catheterization

When an OTN catheter is placed into a peripheral vein, the skin is aseptically prepared as previously described (Box 3-5). The vessel is occluded with digital pressure or a tourniquet. The extremity is held with the skin pulled tautly to stabilize the vein. A catheter (22-gauge, 2.5 cm long in cats and very young or small dogs; 20-gauge, 2.5 to 3.75 cm long in adult or medium to large dogs) with the stylet in place is aligned parallel with the vein. The tip is inserted through the skin and into the vein at a 20-degree angle in a distal a portion of the vein. When blood enters the hub of the stylet, the catheter and stylet are advanced an additional few millimeters to ensure that the catheter tip is well within the vessel lumen (Figure 3-19, A). The catheter is then slid off the stylet, which is held stationary, and into the vein. In a patient with sufficient blood pressure, blood will trickle out the end of the catheter if it is within the vein lumen. Digital pressure is removed once the catheter enters the vein. A cap is quickly and tightly placed on the end (Figure 3-19, B), and the catheter is flushed with 1 ml of heparinized saline solution. The saline solution should pass through the catheter without resistance.

Adhesive tape in 1.3- to 2.5-cm–wide strips is wrapped around the circumference of the catheter and leg to secure the catheter (Figure 3-19, C). An antibiotic ointment–treated gauze sponge is taped over the catheter entry site. Tape is placed underneath the catheter cap to isolate it from the skin. The tape should not be applied too tightly or the limb may swell. If this occurs, the catheter should be retaped or removed.

Jugular Vein Catheterization

A flexible, 16- to 22-gauge, 20- to 30-cm, TTN catheter is used to catheterize the jugular vein. The size required depends on the size of the animal. Gloves, preferably sterile ones, should be worn to place a TTN catheter in a central (jugular, medial saphenous/femoral) vein.

For jugular catheterization, the ventral surface of the neck is shaved and aseptically prepared. An assistant restrains the patient in lateral recumbency with the front legs pulled caudally and the neck extended. In feline patients, it may be helpful to slightly rotate the head externally. The vein that will be used faces away from the table and is occluded at the thoracic inlet.

The plastic needle guard is removed to expose the catheter needle. The needle is inserted through a fold of tented skin just lateral to the vein in the cranial third of the neck (Figure 3-20, A). After the needle penetrates the skin, the needle tip is inserted into the vein. Successful placement is usually denoted by a reflux flash of blood within the catheter lumen. Once the needle enters the vein, the catheter is fed into the vein through a protective sleeve (Figure 3-20, B).

If resistance is met as the catheter is advanced, the catheter is most likely extravascular (outside the vein). The catheter or the patient's head and neck are slightly repositioned, and

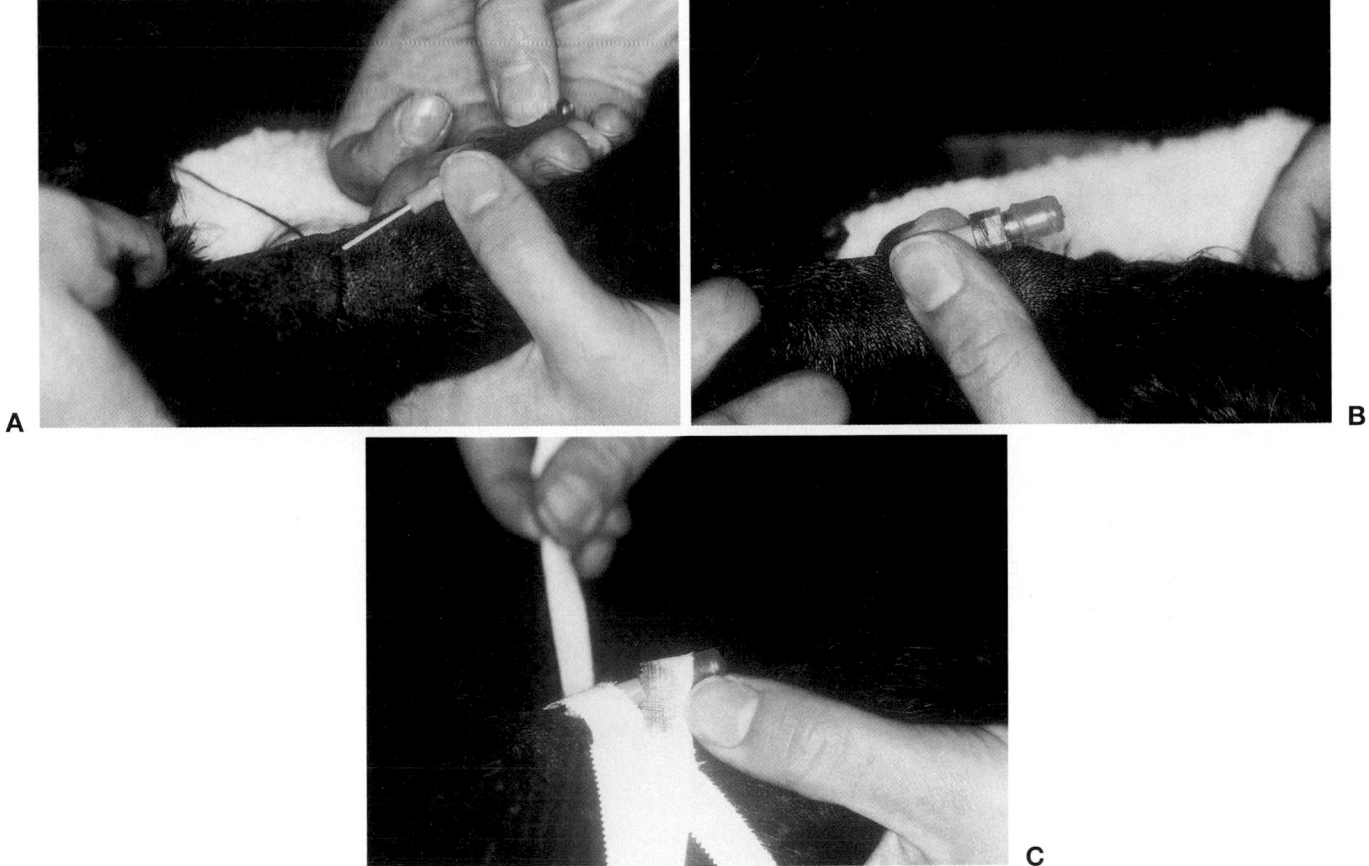

Figure 3-19 **A,** An over-the-needle type catheter is placed in the cephalic vein of a dog. Note the presence of blood in the stylet hub. The catheter is slid off the stylet into the vein. **B,** A cap is placed on the end of the catheter immediately after it is completely inserted into the vein. **C,** The catheter is kept in place by wrapping several strips of tape around the catheter and circumference of the front leg. The thumb presses against the catheter cap to prevent the catheter from backing out of the vein as it is taped.

catheter advancement is reattempted. If difficulty in threading the catheter persists, the catheter should be removed, and catheterization should be reattempted at a different site or with a new catheter. The catheter should never be backed out through the introducer needle because the bevel may sever the catheter and create an embolus.

Once the catheter is successfully placed within the vein, the needle is backed out of the skin and covered with the needle guard. Firm pressure is applied over the site of skin entry for 30 seconds to control bleeding. The plastic sleeve and stylet are removed, and extension tubing prefilled with heparinized saline solution is firmly placed on the end of the catheter. Approximately 3 ml of heparinized saline solution is flushed through the catheter to confirm placement within the vein. It should be possible to aspirate blood through a jugular catheter to check patency (Figure 3-20, *C*). In many instances, the animal's head position may need to be adjusted to aspirate blood from the catheter.

A 2.5-cm portion of the catheter is usually left exposed and looped at the skin entry site. If the entire length of a long catheter is inserted into a small patient's jugular vein, the end of the catheter may inadvertently enter the heart.

If this occurs, an additional length of catheter can be backed out of the skin.

After placement, the jugular catheter must be secured to the neck. A gauze sponge containing a small amount of antibiotic ointment is taped on top of the catheter entry site and covers any exposed catheter (Figure 3-20, *D*). A long strip of tape is placed longitudinally along the needle guard–hub interface to prevent the catheter from backing out of the needle hub. This strip of tape is also wrapped around the circumference of the neck. Stretch gauze is wrapped several times around the neck to cover the catheter and is taped to the skin at the cranial and caudal borders (Figure 3-20, *E* and *F*). If the patient has a history of vomiting, waterproof tape placed on top of the stretch gauze will help keep the bandage dry (Figure 3-20, *G*). Dogs with jugular catheters should be walked on a harness or leash looped behind one or both front legs to prevent the leash from rubbing against the catheter.

A long, TTN catheter can be placed in a saphenous vein by using the technique used for jugular catheter placement. It is advantageous to use the saphenous vein when the jugular vein is inaccessible or if the patient is vomiting or

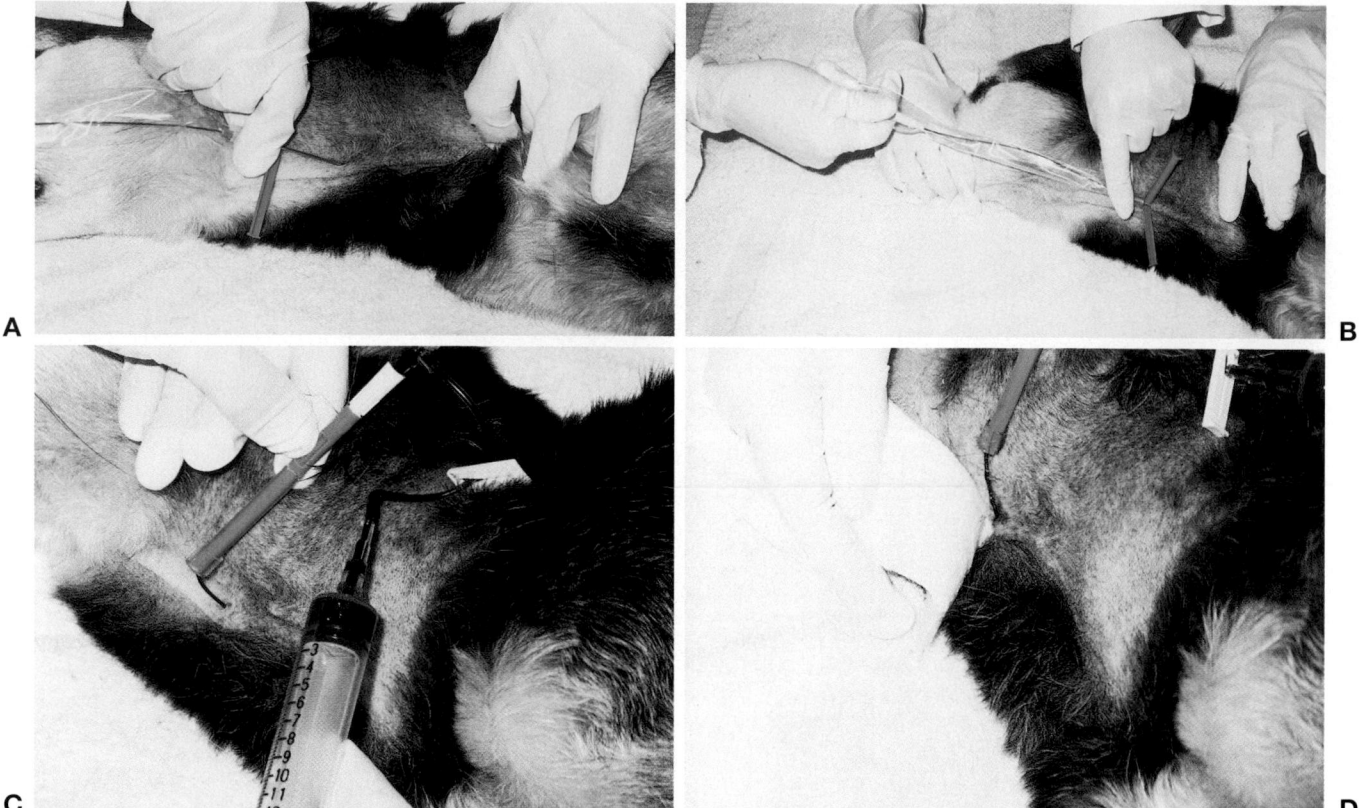

Figure 3-20 **A,** The needle (with blue plastic guard folded back) is inserted through skin just lateral to the left jugular vein. **B,** The catheter is fed into the vein through a protective plastic sleeve. **C,** Once the needle has been removed from the vein, the plastic guard is folded back over the needle. The catheter remains in the vein and exits the skin through the needle. The patency of the catheter is checked by aspirating blood through the syringe. **D,** Antibiotic ointment is placed on a gauze sponge and applied to the catheter entry site. *Continued*

has a disease affecting the neck (cervical disease). Saphenous catheter placement is not recommended in recumbent animals that cannot stand to void or have diarrhea or fecal incontinence. If a saphenous catheter is used for such patients, application of an outer layer of waterproof tape will help keep the bandage dry.

A long, TTN catheter placed in the jugular or saphenous vein is in direct communication with the vena cava. A major advantage of placement of a long catheter in a central vein is the ability to obtain blood samples directly from the catheter. For collection of blood from a long catheter, the "three-syringe technique" is used. The technician, wearing gloves, removes approximately 3 to 5 ml of blood from the catheter with a sterile, heparinized syringe and sets it aside. A second empty syringe is then attached to the catheter, and a blood sample is drawn. The blood from the first syringe is injected back into the catheter, and 2 ml of heparinized saline solution from a third syringe is flushed through the catheter.

Another advantage to the use of a TTN intravenous catheter is the ability to monitor central venous pressure. Central venous pressure can be monitored through a catheter placed into the anterior vena cava via the jugular vein or into the caudal vena cava via the saphenous vein.

However, TTN catheters are more expensive and require more expertise to place than short, OTN catheters.

Arterial Catheter Placement

Indwelling arterial catheters allow blood pressure monitoring and collection of multiple arterial blood samples. A 22-gauge, 2.5-cm OTN catheter is placed in the dorsal metatarsal artery. The method for arterial venipuncture is described in this chapter in the discussion of arterial blood samples. Arterial catheter placement technique is similar to venous catheter placement except that the artery is not occluded. Arterial catheter placement is more uncomfortable than venous catheter placement and is not well tolerated in awake animals. In addition, flushing the arterial catheter may cause the patient some discomfort. *Medications and fluids, with the exception of small boluses of heparinized saline solution, are never administered through an arterial catheter.* The catheter should be clearly labeled as "arterial" and "not for injection."

✐ TECHNICIAN NOTE

Indwelling arterial catheters are placed to allow blood pressure monitoring and collection of multiple arterial blood samples.

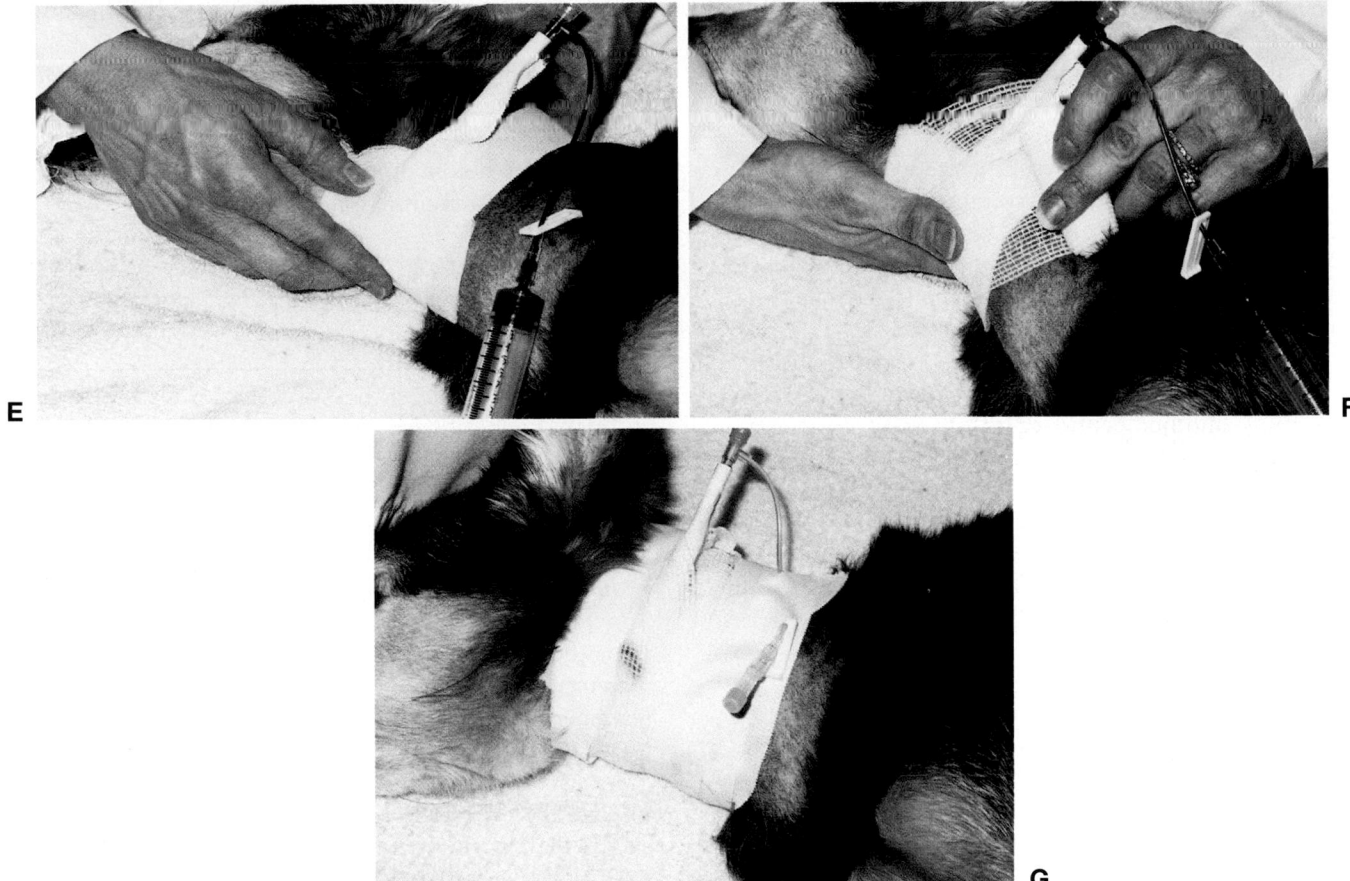

Figure 3-20 *cont'd* **E,** Tape is placed along the needle guard and is wrapped over the gauze sponge and the circumference of the neck. **F,** Roll gauze is used to secure the catheter to the neck. **G,** As a final step, the gauze wrap is covered with waterproof tape.

Intravenous and Intraarterial Catheter Maintenance

Several important points must be made with regard to maintenance of indwelling intravenous or intraarterial catheters. Catheters should be inspected every few hours and should not be left in place for longer than 72 hours. One exception to the 72-hour rule is catheters placed under strictly aseptic conditions in a central vein, such as those placed to administer total parenteral nutrition (TPN). Such catheters may remain indwelling for longer than 72 hours if catheter or catheter site complications are not noted. The type of material used for catheter construction (e.g., polypropylene, polyvinyl chloride, polyethylene, silicone rubber, polyurethane, or nylon) is also a factor in the determination of the length of time a catheter remains in place. Generally, catheters made of polypropylene and polyethylene are less likely to cause vessel irritation and thrombosis than those constructed of silicone rubber, nylon, polyurethane, or polyvinyl chloride.

The catheter site and the tissue proximal and distal to the catheter are checked frequently for pain, redness, swelling, and discharge; if any of these signs are noted, the catheter should be removed, and a new one should be placed in a different vein. If catheter-induced bacteremia or septicemia is suspected, the tip of the catheter is submitted for bacterial culture after removal. If a catheter becomes extravascular, subcutaneous swelling proximal to the catheter site may be noted, and the catheter should be removed and placed in a different site (Figure 3-21). When swelling is attributed to overly constrictive tape or bandage material and the catheter is still patent, the catheter can be rewrapped more loosely. If the bandage material feels damp, the bandage is removed and the catheter is inspected for leakage around the skin entry site and catheter cap. Sometimes blood or fluid leaks from a loosely applied catheter cap. It is not uncommon to find that bandage material has become wet from a spilled water bowl.

From 0.5 to 2 ml of heparinized saline solution is used to flush venous catheters every 4 to 6 hours and arterial catheters every 2 hours to maintain patency. If a patient is receiving a continuous infusion of fluids, the catheter is generally flushed every 8 to 12 hours. If the catheter cannot be flushed without resistance or if blood cannot be aspirated back into the syringe, the catheter may be bent, occluded with a blood clot, or extravascular or the catheter cap may be loose.

Catheters should be checked for patency before medication is injected and should be flushed with heparinized saline solution after drug administration. Nonheparinized saline solution is used to flush a catheter if the drug is known to precipitate with heparin. When multiple medications are given consecutively, it is important to flush the catheter after administration of each drug to prevent the precipitation that may occur if the drugs are mixed.

When a catheter is removed, a gauze sponge onto which a small amount of antibiotic ointment has been applied is taped over the puncture site. When an arterial catheter is removed, the puncture site is covered with a pressure bandage for 10 minutes, followed by application of a regular gauze bandage.

Intravenous Chemotherapy Administration

Use of chemotherapeutic agents to treat neoplasia is becoming more common in companion animal practices. The veterinary technician should be familiar with chemotherapy administration protocols and safety precautions (see Chapter 10). Because many chemotherapeutic agents are carcinogens, it is advisable to minimize exposure to the drugs during administration. Latex gloves, safety glasses, masks, and nonpermeable, long-sleeved, elastic-cuffed gowns should be worn. Materials used for chemotherapy administration should be discarded in leak-proof hazardous waste containers. Drug aerosolization is decreased if an alcohol-soaked gauze sponge is placed over the catheter cap when the needle on the chemotherapy drug syringe is inserted into or removed from the catheter.

> ### ✎ TECHNICIAN NOTE
> Materials used for chemotherapy administration should be discarded in leak-proof hazardous waste containers.

Intravenous catheters are used to administer cytotoxic solutions, especially those that cause tissue irritation when injected extravascularly. Examples of such drugs, which are termed *vesicants,* include doxorubicin, vincristine, vinblastine, and actinomycin D.

Intravenous chemotherapy catheters must be placed with extreme care. The catheter should be placed in a peripheral vein, and the vessel must be punctured only once during placement. If a "clean stick" is not achieved on the first placement attempt, a different vein should be used. This prevents tissue irritation caused by drug leakage from the previous puncture site. It is permissible, *but not advisable,* to place the catheter in the same vein, in a more proximal site, if the initial site has been given time to seal with a clot. Nonheparinized 0.9% sterile saline solution should be used to flush the catheter when specific chemotherapy drugs, such as doxorubicin, that precipitate when mixed with heparin are used.

Catheters used for drug administration should be frequently evaluated for patency. The area proximal to the catheter site should be freely visible so that extravasation may be observed. Signs that the chemotherapeutic agent has leaked out of the vein include loss of catheter patency, redness or swelling at or proximal to the injection site, and vocalization or signs of discomfort by the patient.

If extravasation occurs, as much of the drug should be removed from the site as possible by aspirating 5 ml of blood back through the catheter. The tissue surrounding the site should be infused with saline solution, corticosteroids, or 2% lidocaine; and either warm or cold compresses should be applied, depending on the chemotherapy drug used.

When chemotherapy administration is complete, the catheter is flushed with several milliliters of sterile, nonheparinized 0.9% saline solution. An alcohol-soaked gauze sponge covers the catheter as it is removed from the vein. The skin puncture site is covered with an antibiotic-treated gauze pad and securely bandaged.

When less than 2 ml of a chemotherapeutic drug, such as vincristine, is injected intravenously, a 23- or 25-gauge butterfly catheter is often used. After the drug has been administered, the catheter is flushed with several milliliters of saline solution. The tubing is crimped to prevent fluid from leaking back out of the catheter, and the needle is

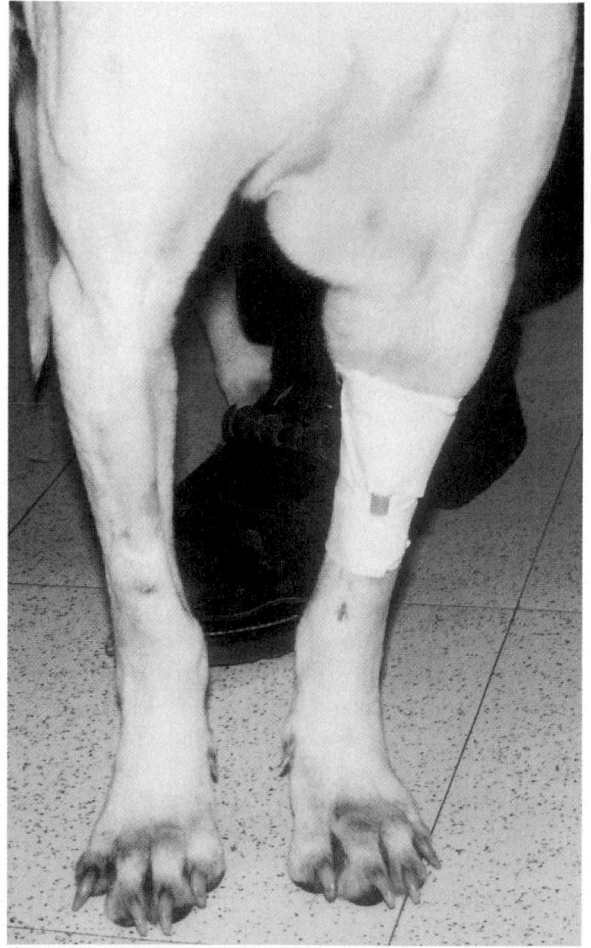

Figure 3-21 This patient's cephalic catheter was not properly positioned within the vein during intravenous fluid administration. Fluid accumulated in the subcutaneous tissue proximal to the catheter site and resulted in swelling of the left front leg and pectoral region.

removed from the vein. The needle is covered with an alcohol-soaked gauze pad as it is removed from the skin, and the venipuncture site is bandaged.

SUBCUTANEOUS ADMINISTRATION

The subcutaneous injection is easily and frequently performed and is the most common route for vaccine administration. Although absorption may be slow in obese animals because of the relatively poor vascular supply in fat, subcutaneous injections, in general, allow for relatively rapid absorption of the injected substance. However, the subcutaneous route is not recommended in severely dehydrated or critically ill patients when immediate absorption is required. In an emergency situation, the intravenous or intraosseous route provides much faster absorption. The intravenous route is preferred when large volumes of fluid must be administered.

Moderate volumes of isotonic fluids can be injected under the skin to rehydrate animals if intravenous or intraosseous access is unavailable. Approximately 50 to 100 ml of body temperature fluids can be injected per site, depending on patient size. Owners of patients that may require long-term fluid supplementation at home (e.g., those with chronic renal disease) can be instructed in how to administer subcutaneous fluids.

The preferred site for most subcutaneous injections is the dorsolateral region from the neck to the hips. The dorsal region of the neck and back should be avoided because of the difficulty in treating any abscesses or masses that may occur after injection. When vaccinations are administered, especially to feline patients, the intrascapular region should be avoided because of the incidence of vaccine-induced tumors. Feline vaccinations should be administered in as distal a portion of an extremity as possible (Figure 3-22). The following sites are recommended for feline vaccination: right front leg, rhinotracheitis-calici-panleukopenia; right rear leg, rabies: left rear leg, feline leukemia. The intra-scapular area should also be avoided for insulin injections because of the relatively poor absorption of insulin from that site and the fibrosis that may occur as a result of repeated injections. Insulin should be injected in alternating sites along the dorsolateral or ventrolateral aspect of the trunk.

When a subcutaneous injection is administered, a fold of skin is tented, and the needle is inserted at the base of and parallel to the long axis of the fold (Figure 3-22). If the needle is inserted perpendicular to the long axis, the needle may penetrate both sides of the skin, and the syringe contents may be accidentally deposited on the patient's hair. The syringe plunger is retracted slightly, and the needle hub is checked for blood before injection. If blood appears in the hub, a vessel has been penetrated, and the needle should be removed and reinserted in another location. After injection, the skin is briefly massaged to facilitate drug distribution. If multiple vaccinations or medications are to be administered, the injection sites should be a minimum of several centimeters apart.

⬥ TECHNICIAN NOTE
Vaccine injection into the intrascapular region should be avoided.

INTRAMUSCULAR ADMINISTRATION

The intramuscular route is appropriate for injection of small volumes of medication. Drugs are most often administered in the lumbosacral musculature lateral to the dorsal spinous processes or in the semimembranosus or semitendinosus muscles of the rear leg. Deep lumbar injections in the third to fifth lumbar region are used to administer heartworm treatment (Figure 3-23). Placement of the needle in the lumbosacral muscles is not recommended in very thin animals. When injections are made into the semimembranosus or semitendinosus muscles, the needle should

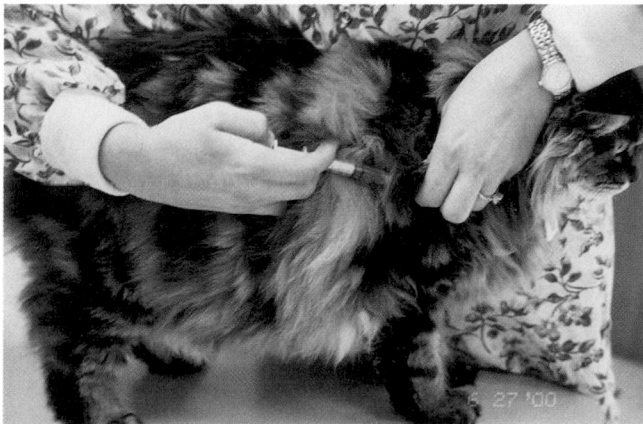

Figure 3-22 Subcutaneous injection made into tented skin on the lateral aspect of the front leg. Note that administration of feline vaccination in the intrascapular region is avoided.

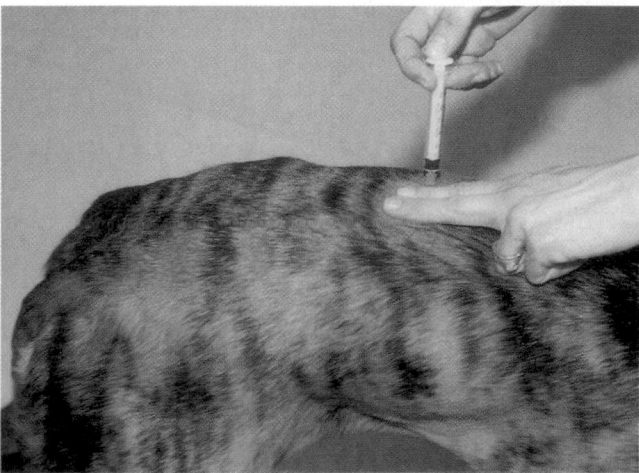

Figure 3-23 Deep intramuscular injection into the lumbar musculature of the dog.

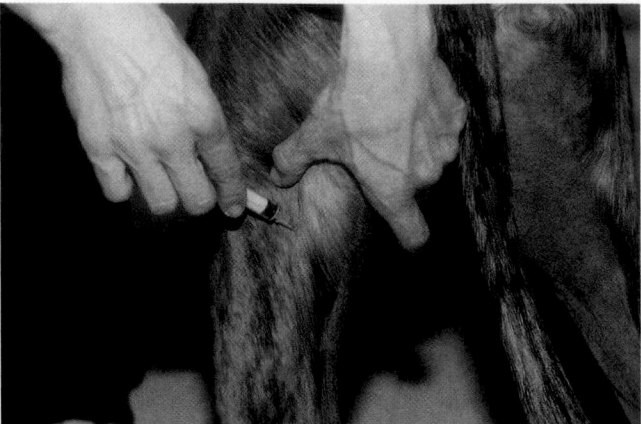

Figure 3-24 Intramuscular injection into the semimembranosus and semitendinosus muscles of the rear leg of the dog.

enter the lateral aspect of the muscle and be directed caudally to avoid penetration of the sciatic nerve (Figure 3-24). Contact of the needle with the sciatic nerve may cause pain and lameness. Occasionally, the triceps muscles on the caudal aspect of the front legs are used as injection sites. The neck is never used as a site for intramuscular injection.

When an intramuscular injection is performed, the muscle is isolated between the fingers and thumb, and a 22- to 25-gauge needle attached to a syringe is embedded in the muscle. As with subcutaneous injections, the needle hub is checked for blood before administration of medication to make certain a vessel is not inadvertently penetrated. If blood is observed, the needle is removed and inserted in another site. Once placement within the muscle has been verified, the drug is slowly injected. The site is massaged for a few seconds after injection to help distribute the substance.

INTRADERMAL ADMINISTRATION

Intradermal injections are performed to desensitize the skin with a local anesthetic or to perform allergy skin testing. Most animals will not tolerate skin testing unless they are sedated. Hair on the lateral aspect of the trunk is shaved with a No. 40 clipper blade. The skin is carefully wiped with a water-moistened gauze sponge. Vigorous scrubbing or use of an antimicrobial cleaning solution is contraindicated because skin irritation that may occur interferes with testing. For an intradermal injection, a fold of skin is lifted, and a 25- to 27-gauge needle attached to a 1-ml syringe is inserted, with the bevel up, into the dermis. A 0.1-ml volume of allergen is injected. The injection site will look like a translucent lump if the injection is performed correctly. The skin is then examined for tissue reaction.

INTRANASAL ADMINISTRATION

Certain vaccines—such as those for feline infectious peritonitis, feline viral rhinotracheitis-calici-panleukopenia,

and *Bordetella bronchiseptica*—are formulated for intranasal (and/or intraocular) administration. The patient's muzzle is held in one hand and elevated slightly. The tip of the vaccine dispenser is placed into the nostril, and the dispenser is compressed. Alternatively, the patient's head can be tilted back, and the pipette containing the vaccine can be squeezed to dispense the liquid onto the plane of the nose. The vaccine runs into each nostril as the animal inhales. This method frequently results in less sneezing after administration than when the dispenser tip is placed directly into the nostril.

Diazepam can be administered intranasally for the immediate treatment of status epilepticus if intravascular access cannot be obtained. Diazepam is absorbed more rapidly into the systemic circulation by the intranasal route than by the intrarectal route.

INTRATRACHEAL ADMINISTRATION

In an emergency situation, such as during cardiopulmonary resuscitation, drugs can be injected directly into the trachea of an unconscious animal. Absorption by this route is extremely rapid.

When an intratracheal injection is performed, a polypropylene urinary catheter or rubber feeding tube is inserted into the trachea, either directly or through an endotracheal tube. The drug (e.g., epinephrine, atropine, or lidocaine), contained in a syringe, is forcefully injected through the urinary catheter or feeding tube. Approximately 10 ml of air or 3 to 10 ml of sterile saline solution is injected through the catheter or tube immediately afterward to disperse the drug. If a urinary catheter or feeding tube is not available, the drug is sprayed down the endotracheal tube with a syringe and followed by a burst of air. The intratracheal dosage of drugs is usually greater than the intravenous dosage.

✎ TECHNICIAN NOTE

In an emergency situation, such as during cardiopulmonary resuscitation, medications can be injected directly into the trachea because absorption of the drug by this route is extremely rapid.

INTRAOSSEOUS ADMINISTRATION

Needles are placed directly into the bone marrow cavity to deliver fluids, drugs, and blood products when intravenous catheterization is not possible or cannot be performed rapidly. The intraosseous route is often overlooked and may be useful in emergency situations. Medications and fluids quickly enter the central circulation via the intramedullary vessels in the marrow cavity. Intraosseous placement of a needle or catheter allows rapid fluid delivery to neonates, small animals, and patients with circulatory collapse. Intraosseous needles are removed as soon as intravenous access can be established.

Placement of an intraosseous needle or catheter is contraindicated in patients with sepsis. Catheters are not placed in bones that are fractured or infected. Skin overlying the insertion site should be free of infection so that skin surface pathogens are not introduced into the underlying tissue during intraosseous needle placement. If the bone cortex is punctured multiple times during insertion attempts, a different bone should be used; fluid that is administered may leak from the bone into the subcutaneous tissue.

Sites for intraosseous administration include the tibia, femur, humerus, and occasionally the iliac wing or ischium. The intraosseous catheter or needle should have a stylet that helps prevent the needle from bending or becoming occluded with a core of bone as it is inserted. Needles used include 15- to 18-gauge bone marrow needles specially designed for intraosseous access. If intraosseous access is needed in a neonate, an 18- to 22-gauge hypodermic needle can be used. If the hypodermic needle plugs with a core of bone, it can sometimes be flushed out with saline solution. A 22-gauge, 3.75-cm needle can be nested inside an 18-gauge, 2.5-cm needle to serve as a stylet during placement.

Needle placement for the purpose of delivering medications or fluids into the intraosseous space follows the protocol described for needle placement for bone marrow aspiration. When an intraosseous catheter or needle must be placed in the femur, the hip region is shaved and aseptically prepared. The patient is placed in lateral recumbency, and the technician stands at the dorsum of the patient. The trochanteric fossa of the femur of the upside leg is identified on the medial aspect of the greater trochanter of the proximal femur.

Approximately 0.5 to 1.0 ml of 2% lidocaine is injected into the skin, subcutaneous tissue, and periosteum over the trochanteric fossa to provide local anesthesia. A stab incision is made through the skin. The femur is grasped, and the hip is held in a flexed position. The intraosseous needle is introduced medial to the greater trochanter and parallel to the femoral shaft. The needle is inserted through the skin incision and into the femur by using firm, steady pressure as the wrist is rotated back and forth. Insertion of the needle through a skin incision helps decrease the likelihood that skin contaminants will be carried into the bone. During needle insertion, care is taken to avoid piercing the sciatic nerve, which is posteromedial to the greater trochanter of the femur. When the needle enters the marrow cavity, the needle will feel firmly embedded. Placement can be ascertained through aspiration of bone marrow into a syringe attached to the needle hub.

Once placed, the needle is secured by wrapping a "butterfly" tab of tape around it as it exits the skin. The tape is sutured to the skin. A povidone-iodine ointment-treated gauze pad is applied to the skin entry site. A bulky, gauze bandage is placed around the needle for further stabilization. Patency of the intraosseous needle is maintained by flushing every 6 hours with 1 to 2 ml of heparinized 0.9%

saline solution. The needle may remain in place for up to 3 days but is difficult to maintain in an ambulatory patient.

INTRAPERITONEAL ADMINISTRATION

The intraperitoneal route involves placement of substances directly into the abdominal cavity. This route is occasionally used to administer noncaustic fluids, blood products, or medications. It may be used in neonates when intravascular or intraosseous access is difficult to obtain. Specific chemotherapy drugs, such as asparaginase, can be given intraperitoneally. Body temperature fluids may be infused into the abdominal cavity to lavage the abdomen in animals with peritonitis or pancreatitis. Warm or cool fluid intraperitoneal lavage may be used to help treat patients with severe hypothermia or hyperthermia.

Substances injected into the peritoneal cavity are absorbed more rapidly than those administered subcutaneously but more slowly than those given by the intravascular or intraosseous route. When a drug or fluids must be administered into the peritoneal cavity, the ventral abdomen between the umbilicus and the bladder is shaved and aseptically prepared. An 18- to 22-gauge needle or catheter is inserted into the abdominal cavity on the ventral midline, a few centimeters caudal to the umbilicus. A syringe is attached and aspirated. If the needle is in the proper location in the peritoneal cavity, no blood or fluid will be aspirated into the syringe. If blood or fluid enters the syringe tip, the needle may have punctured a vessel or abdominal organ. The needle is removed, and a new needle is inserted in a different site. If the syringe remains empty when negative pressure is applied, the medication or fluids have been injected.

TOPICAL OPHTHALMIC ADMINISTRATION

The topical ophthalmic route of administration is required for medications used to treat ocular diseases or for specific vaccines, such as feline rhinotracheitis-calici-panleukopenia (a formulation designed for intranasal/intraocular administration is available). For placement of medication onto the surface of the eye, good restraint is essential or the medications will be inadvertently placed on the eyelids or face. The tip of the medication dispenser should not come into contact with any surface, including the cornea, because it may become contaminated or scratch the cornea. Eye medication should be used exclusively by the patient for whom it is dispensed. Sharing ophthalmic medications may transmit ocular infections between patients. If the solution appears to be contaminated (e.g., a clear solution now looks cloudy), contains flecks of material, or has a color change, it should not be used.

When a substance must be administered by the ophthalmic route, the solution or ointment is slightly warmed by holding the container in the palm of the hand for 1 or 2 minutes. This makes administration more comfortable for the patient. The lids are held open with the thumb and index finger of one hand as one drop of medication is deposited onto the sclera (Figure 3-25). It is helpful to rest the hand holding the medication on the patient's head as the drops are dispensed. When ointment is administered, the lids are held open with the thumb and index finger of one hand, and a 5-mm strip of ointment is squeezed onto the upper sclera or lower palpebral border. The ointment is dispersed across the cornea when the patient blinks. Some technicians find it easier to administer medication if the patient's upper lid is held closed and the medication is placed inside the lower lid.

If multiple topical medications are to be administered into the same eye, they should be applied a minimum of 3 to 5 minutes apart to allow for sufficient absorption. If both a solution and an ointment are to be applied, the liquid should be placed in the eye at least 3 to 5 minutes before the ointment. If the ointment is given first, it may coat the cornea and interfere with absorption of the solution.

AURAL ADMINISTRATION

The ear should be cleared of debris before medication is placed in the ear canal. Precleaning increases the amount of contact between the drug and the epithelium and enhances medication absorption.

When medication is placed in the ear canal, the pinna is grasped and pulled upward and back toward the head. The tip of the medication dispenser is placed into the vertical ear canal, and the dispenser is squeezed. The base of the ear is then massaged to distribute the medication.

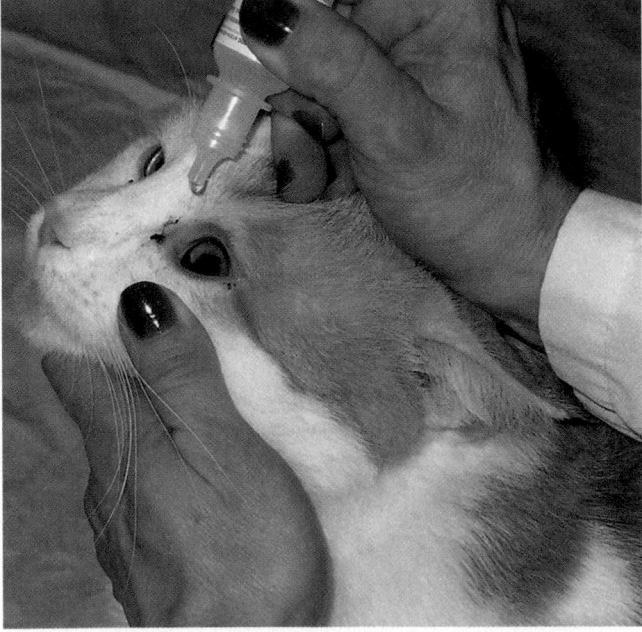

Figure 3-25 Ophthalmic drop is directed onto the cornea of a cat.

TRANSDERMAL ADMINISTRATION

Certain medications applied topically to the skin have systemic as well as local effects. Many drugs commonly administered by the oral route, such as prednisone or methimazole, can be formulated into an ointment for transdermal application. Other medications, such as nitroglycerin, are manufactured as a cream to be applied directly on the skin.

Medications such as nitroglycerin may be absorbed by the individual making the application; therefore disposable gloves should be worn to prevent absorption. A small quantity of ointment is applied to a sparsely haired region, such as the pinna of the ear, the groin, or a shaved area on the ventral thorax. If gloves are unavailable, the ointment can be applied to a small piece of wax paper and wiped onto the skin. The treated area is covered with a light bandage so it will not be accidentally touched. A note is placed on the front of the patient's cage specifying the medication used, the site to which the medication has been applied, and the duration of time that must pass before the application site can be safely touched.

Many topical medications are dispensed in a liquid or aerosol form to control fleas, ticks, mites, heartworms, and intestinal parasites. Depending on the product, the medication is either sprayed on the hair on the entire body or applied to the skin between the shoulder blades. Manufacturers directions regarding application should be followed closely. Gloves are worn during application, and the site of administration should not be touched for a specified period after application.

Transdermal application of analgesics is gaining popularity. One analgesic manufactured in a form specifically for transdermal application is fentanyl citrate. A fentanyl-impregnated self-adhesive patch is placed directly onto a shaved, dry region of skin. The technician should not touch the adhesive side of the patch containing the fentanyl because the medication is absorbed topically. Gentle pressure is applied with the palm of the hand over the patch application site for 1 minute to help the patch adhere to the skin. Each patch can only be applied once because it may not adhere to the skin and deliver the complete dose of fentanyl if it is removed and reapplied. The patch can be covered with tape on which the date and time of placement have been recorded.

It is important to place the fentanyl patch in a location from which the animal cannot remove it, such as on the intrascapular region. It should not be applied to skin that will be in contact with a heating pad, heat lamp, or other external heat source. The rate of drug delivery is increased when the skin beneath the patch warms and the cutaneous vessels vasodilate.

Topical application of creams (e.g., EMLA cream, lidocaine, and prilocaine) desensitizes the skin so that venipuncture is more comfortable for the patient. This topical anesthetic must be in contact with the skin for at least several minutes (ideally 30 to 60) for it to reach its maximum effectiveness.

INTRARECTAL ADMINISTRATION

The mucosa of the large intestine is capable of absorbing medications delivered intrarectally. Medications delivered by this route may have both local and systemic effects. Absorption is most effective when the intestine is free of fecal material. Antiemetic tablets or suppositories can be administered intrarectally to vomiting patients that cannot be medicated orally. A gloved, lubricated finger is used to insert the tablet into the rectum a distance of at least 5 cm. The medication is then gradually absorbed.

Antiseizure drugs, such as diazepam, can be given intrarectally if intravenous or intranasal administration is difficult to perform. A lubricated short rubber feeding tube or urinary catheter is inserted 8 to 10 cm into the rectum. The diazepam is placed into a syringe and injected through the catheter. Several milliliters of warm water are then flushed into the catheter to disperse the drug. Diazepam can also be injected directly into the rectum with a needleless syringe.

Enemas are also administered per rectum. A syringe containing the enema is lubricated and inserted into the rectum. After the enema is injected, the animal should be placed in an area where it can defecate, such as outdoors or near a litter box.

Warm water enemas are administered through lubricated plastic tubing inserted through the rectum and into the large intestine. Water is funneled or injected into the end of the tube held in a raised position. The tube is moved back and forth and is slowly advanced up the intestinal tract as fecal material is expelled.

When a medication, such as lactulose, is added to the enema solution, it must be retained within the large intestine for a specified length of time. The solution is injected into a urinary catheter or feeding tube placed into the descending colon. The rectum is held closed with a gloved hand to prevent the enema from exiting. After the allotted time has passed, the catheter is removed and the intestine is evacuated.

ORAL ADMINISTRATION

Administration of medication by direct placement into the oral cavity is frequently and easily performed. Technicians should be adept at administering oral medications to animals and capable of demonstrating techniques to pet owners.

✎ TECHNICIAN NOTE

Technicians should be adept at administering oral medications to animals and able to demonstrate techniques to pet owners.

Oral medications are usually administered in liquid, capsule, or tablet form. Liquids are easy to administer through a dropper or syringe. Pulverized tablets and the contents of capsules can be mixed with a small volume of food, water, or flavored liquid. When liquids must be administered with a syringe or dropper, the patient's lower lip is pulled out at the commissure. The tip of the syringe or dropper is placed between the cheek and the gums, and small volumes of liquid are injected. The muzzle should be held at a neutral angle and not elevated. Hyperextension of the neck or movement by the patient during administration may result in fluid aspiration into the trachea. If the patient struggles or coughs or if fluid spills out of the mouth, the patient should be allowed to rest before further administration attempts.

A tablet or capsule is most easily administered to a dog if it is hidden in meat, cheese, or a chunk of canned pet food. Cats rarely consume pills hidden in food. Cats will meticulously eat the food that surrounds the pill and leave the medication. If a patient has a diminished appetite, it may not consume the entire amount of medication-laced food and will not receive a sufficient dose of medication.

An animal that will not consume baited food is medicated by tilting the head back, prying open the jaws, and placing the pill far back on the base of the tongue (Figures 3-26 and 3-27). The tablet will be expelled if it is not placed far enough back in the pharynx. The technician holds the muzzle closed, rubs under the animal's chin, taps the tip of the nose, or blows air into the nostrils to stimulate the animal to swallow. When the animal licks its nose, it can be assumed that the tablet has been swallowed.

A specially designed device is available to administer tablets to fractious cats and dogs. The tablet is secured in the tip of a plastic rod that is inserted into the back of the mouth. The rod plunger is quickly depressed, and the pill

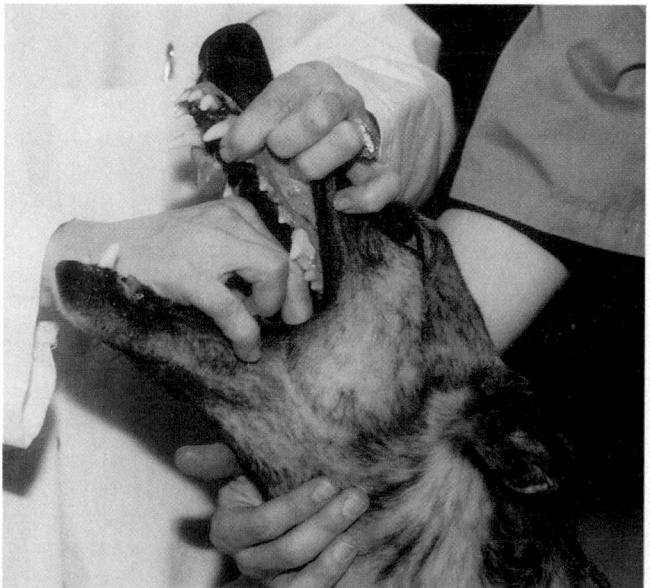

Figure 3-26 A dog's muzzle is held open as a tablet is placed into the back of its mouth.

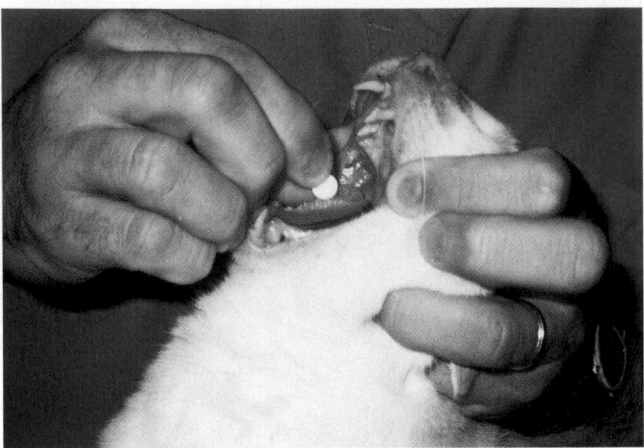

Figure 3-27 A cat's neck is hyperextended so its nose points toward the ceiling. The lower jaw is held open as a tablet is placed in the back of its mouth.

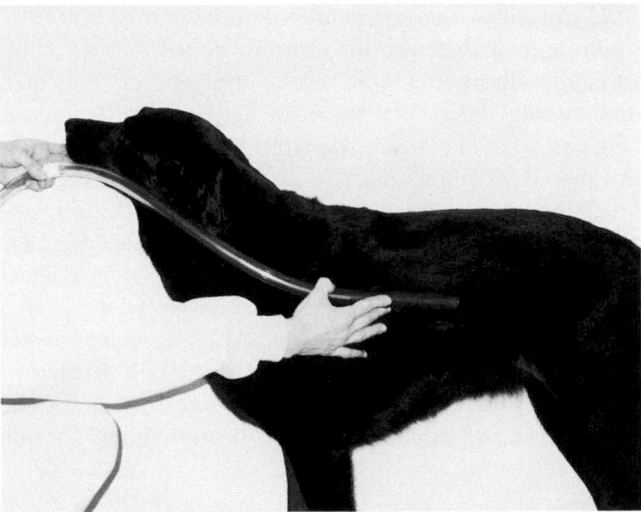

Figure 3-28 A length of stomach tube is measured from the nose to the thirteenth rib. It is then marked with tape.

is propelled down the esophagus. Technicians can demonstrate the use of the "pill gun" to owners for administration of medication at home.

Orogastric Intubation

Sometimes it is necessary to administer medication, food, or fluids through a tube passed through the mouth and directly into the stomach. This technique is used to administer activated charcoal solutions or lavage the stomach to treat animals that have ingested toxins. Orphan or weak neonates who cannot nurse can be fed milk replacer via a tube passed through the mouth and into the distal esophagus or stomach. An orogastric tube is also passed in an attempt to decompress a patient with gastric dilation (bloated stomach). Dogs usually permit orogastric tube placement with moderate resistance. Cats, with the exception of neonates, usually require sedation.

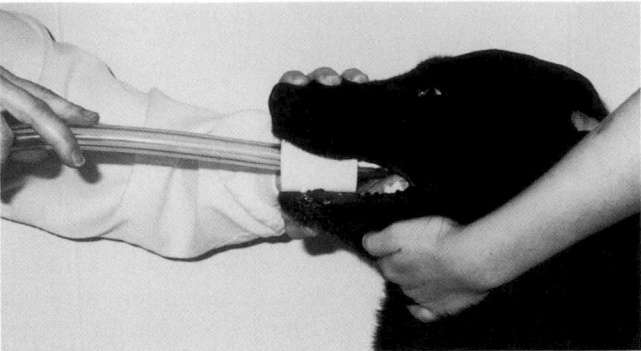

Figure 3-29 A roll of tape holds the mouth open as a stomach tube is placed into the oral cavity.

The length of 10 to 22 Fr plastic or rubber tube required to extend from the tip of the nose to the thirteenth rib is measured and marked on the tube with tape or ink (Figure 3-28). If the tube is to be placed in the distal esophagus to feed an animal, the distance between the tip of the nose and the eighth rib is marked. Water-soluble gel is used to lubricate the tip of the tube. The animal is restrained in sternal recumbency or in a standing or seated position. A roll of tape, a plastic or wooden speculum with a hole in the middle, or a plastic syringe case with smooth ends is placed behind the canine teeth to hold the mouth open. The muzzle is kept in a normal position and held so the mouth speculum does not become dislodged.

The tube is slowly passed through the speculum (Figure 3-29). Swallowing will be noted as the tube passes over the base of the tongue and into the esophagus. If the animal coughs, the tube may have entered the trachea and should be removed. Once the tube is in the esophagus, it is advanced the premeasured length until it enters the stomach.

Correct placement of the tube in the gastrointestinal tract should always be verified before the introduction of any medications or fluids. Refer to the discussion of nasoesophageal and nasogastric tubes for instruction on how to check tube placement.

Fluid is added to the tube with a 60-ml syringe, metal drench pump, or funnel. After the fluid has been administered, the tube is bent to occlude it and then withdrawn in a downward direction. This technique prevents a backflow of fluid from entering the trachea.

ENTERAL FEEDING TUBES

Critically ill animals may not be able to normally consume enough calories for proper nutrition and therefore require nutritional support. If the gastrointestinal tract is capable of digestion and absorption, then food slurries, fluid, or medication can be administered through tubes placed directly into the pharynx, esophagus, stomach, duodenum, or jejunum. The technician needs to be familiar with the technique that the veterinarian uses to place enteral feeding tubes and be knowledgeable about tube maintenance.

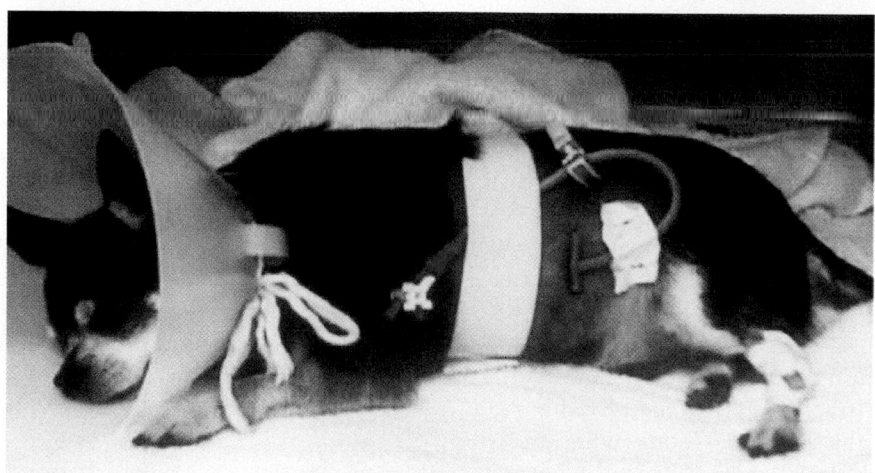

Figure 3-30 A gastrostomy tube is placed to feed a patient that has undergone esophageal surgery. The Elizabethan collar prevents chewing on the tube or intravenous lateral saphenous catheter.

Nasoesophageal tubes are occasionally used for short-term feeding and the administration of medications. If nutritional support is required beyond 10 days, placement of a gastrostomy tube is preferred (Figure 3-30). If the stomach must be bypassed completely, a duodenostomy or jejunostomy tube is surgically placed.

Enteral feeding tubes should be flushed before and after use with a small volume of warm water to help prevent lumen obstructions. Fluids should always be injected slowly. Before the injection of fluid into a gastrostomy tube, the tube is aspirated with a syringe to make certain the stomach contents have emptied from the previous feeding. If the stomach is still full, the veterinarian should be consulted; the full volume of the next meal should not be instilled into the gastrostomy tube until the previous meal has passed from the stomach. The tube insertion site and tube position are inspected daily to make certain that the tube has not shifted and the skin is free from inflammation, redness, tenderness, and discharge.

Nasoesophageal and Nasogastric Tubes

Nasoesophageal tubes are easy and inexpensive to place in an animal that requires short-term force-feeding, such as a severely anorexic cat. These tubes are inappropriate for use in patients that are vomiting or do not have a gag reflex. A 5 to 8 Fr pediatric feeding tube is held up to the animal to determine the appropriate length that is required. For nasoesophageal placement, the distance between the nares and distal esophagus is marked on the tube with ink or tape. Likewise, for nasogastric placement, the distance from the nares to the eighth rib is measured. The patient is held in sternal recumbency, in a seated or standing position. The head is held securely with the neck slightly extended. From 0.5 to 1 ml of 2% lidocaine is infused into one nostril of the dog, and 5 drops of 0.5% proparacaine are placed into one nostril of the cat. The tip of the tube is coated with Xylocaine ointment and placed in the nostril dorsomedial

to the alar fold. The tube is advanced into the nostril and directed ventrally. The tube then continues down the ventral meatus and into the nasopharynx. The animal will usually swallow when the tube enters the pharynx.

The tube is placed in the distal esophagus. Proper placement may be checked by injecting a few milliliters of air into the tube and simultaneously auscultating the cranial abdomen. If gurgling sounds are present, the tube has been placed in the gastrointestinal tract. Alternatively, 5 ml of sterile saline solution may be injected into the tube; if the animal coughs, the tube is in the trachea and should be removed. A radiograph can also be taken to evaluate tube placement.

Suture material or tissue adhesive is used to secure the tube to the patient. The tube should be sutured or glued close to its entrance to the nostril, onto the bridge of the nose, and onto the forehead. The remainder of the tube should be taped to the dorsum of the neck, and the animal should be fitted with an Elizabethan collar to prevent chewing of the tube. A cap is placed on the end of the tube to prevent reflux.

Pharyngostomy Tube Placement

A red rubber feeding tube or silicone pharyngostomy tube, ranging in size from 8 to 14 Fr for cats and small dogs and from 14 to 28 Fr for medium-sized to large dogs, is used for pharyngostomy tube placement. One end of the tube is flared, and the other is fenestrated. The length of tube needed to span the distance from the angle of the mandible to the distal esophagus is measured and marked on the tube with tape or ink.

Placement of a pharyngostomy tube is performed surgically and requires general anesthesia with endotracheal intubation. The patient is placed in lateral recumbency, and a speculum is placed between the canine teeth to hold the mouth open. The lateral neck area is clipped and aseptically prepared. A gloved index finger is inserted into the mouth and placed between the hyoid apparatus and esophagus. Skin directly over the fingertip is incised with a scalpel blade. A large, curved hemostat is placed through the skin incision and used to bluntly dissect the underlying tissue, muscle, and oral mucosa. The flared end of the premeasured tube is brought into the mouth, grasped with the hemostats, and pulled exteriorly through the pharyngostomy site. The fenestrated end of the tube is then directed into the esophagus. Tube placement is checked in the same manner as described for nasoesophageal tubes.

The tube is secured by placing a butterfly tape around the proximal end and suturing the tape to the skin. Alternatively, a Chinese finger-trap suture may be placed around the tube to secure it to the skin. A povidone-iodine–treated gauze sponge should be placed around the skin-tube interface. The tube tip should either be cut so it extends a few centimeters from the skin surface or left long and bandaged over the dorsum of the neck. The exposed tube end is capped with a catheter adapter and a catheter cap.

Esophagostomy Tube Placement

Placement of a feeding tube directly into the esophagus to provide nutritional support has proved to be an effective technique. Esophagostomy tubes are better tolerated by patients than are pharyngostomy tubes because they cause less laryngeal irritation and obstruction and are less likely to induce emesis and become dislodged. Therefore animals fed through esophagostomy tubes are less likely to aspirate their food than are those fed through pharyngostomy tubes. Placement requires the use of heavy sedation or short-acting anesthesia.

> **✎ TECHNICIAN NOTE**
>
> Patients tolerate esophagostomy tubes better than pharyngostomy tubes because they cause less laryngeal irritation and obstruction and are less likely to induce emesis and become dislodged.

A specially designed instrument is available to place esophagostomy tubes, the ELD Gastrostomy Tube Applicator (Jorgensen Laboratories, Inc.). Long hemostats are usually used in lieu of the ELD Applicator by most veterinarians to place esophagostomy tubes; therefore the placement technique in which hemostats are used is given. An instruction sheet detailing the procedure involved in using the ELD Applicator to place an esophagostomy tube is available from the manufacturer.

An esophagostomy tube is placed in the midcervical esophagus on the left side of the neck (Figure 3-31). The animal is placed in right lateral recumbency, and the left cervical region is shaved and surgically prepared. The scapulohumeral joint and the angle of the mandible are used as guides to measure the distal and proximal limits of the cervical esophagus. The length of a 20 Fr red rubber feeding tube needed to extend from the skin of the midcervical region to the seventh rib is measured and marked on the tube with ink or tape. A pair of extra long curved hemostats

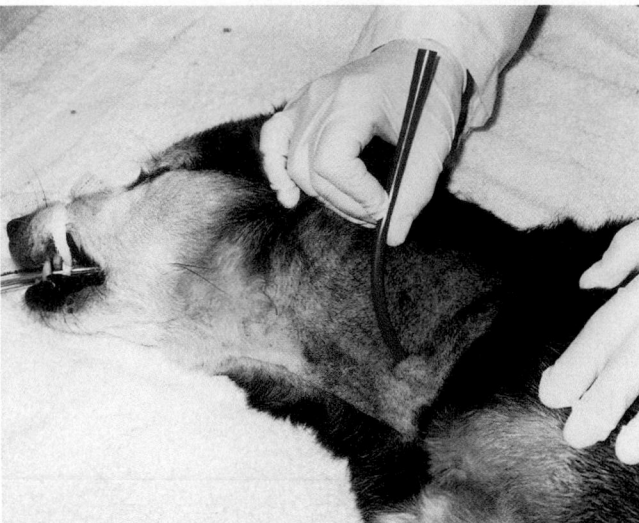

Figure 3-31 An esophagostomy tube for enteral feeding is placed into the midcervical esophagus on the left side of the neck.

is placed into the oral cavity and advanced to the left mid-cervical region of the esophagus. It is difficult to reach the midcervical region of the esophagus in large-breed dogs when hemostats are used instead of the longer ELD Tube Applicator. The hemostat tips should be palpable on the patient's neck. A stab incision is made with a scalpel blade through the skin and subcutaneous tissue over the tips. The scalpel blade is used to carefully dissect the subcutaneous tissue over the esophagus until the hemostats are able to bluntly penetrate the esophagus. The tips of the hemostats are then brought to the exterior and opened just enough to grasp the fenestrated end of the feeding tube. The hemostats with the attached feeding tube are then withdrawn back through the skin and into the esophagus toward the oral cavity. Once the fenestrated end of the tube reaches the mouth, the tube is bent and redirected back down the esophagus to the level of the seventh rib. Esophagostomy tubes are secured and maintained in the manner described for pharyngostomy tubes. Once esophagostomy tubes are removed, healing occurs by second intention. Stricture of the esophagus at the site of tube removal is minimal.

LARGE ANIMAL SAMPLING AND THERAPEUTIC TECHNIQUES

VENOUS BLOOD SAMPLE COLLECTION

As with small animals, blood is drawn from large animals to screen for disease and help diagnose the cause of illness.

The venipuncture site used depends on the volume of blood needed and the type of restraint available. Venipuncture should not be attempted unless the patient is firmly restrained. The individual who draws the blood or helps with restraint should stand at the side, and not in front of, the animal. Ideally, cattle and horses should be confined in a chute or stanchion.

BOVINE VENIPUNCTURE

Blood is collected from cattle from the jugular vein, the coccygeal vein, or—as a last resort—the subcutaneous abdominal (milk) vein. Either a Vacutainer collection device or a syringe topped with a 16- to 18-gauge, 4-cm needle is used. The skin and hair on top of the vein are wiped with an alcohol-soaked gauze pad before venipuncture to remove superficial contaminants. The vessel is occluded and blood is collected. Digital pressure is applied to the venipuncture site after sample collection until hemostasis occurs.

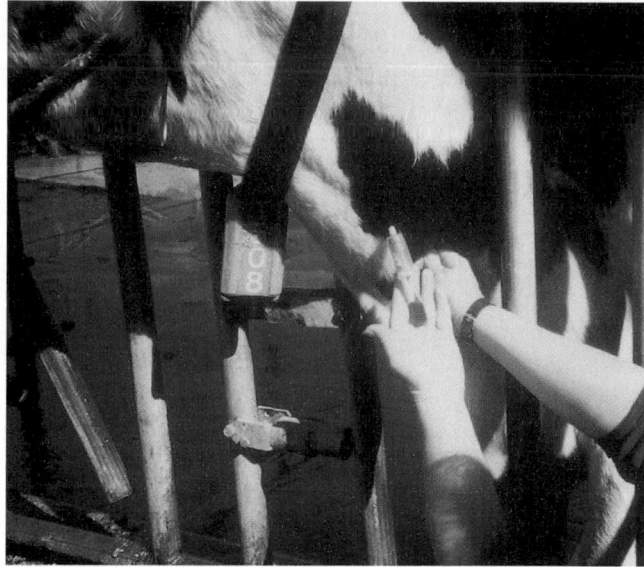

Figure 3-32 Bovine jugular venipuncture with a Vacutainer collection device.

> **✐ TECHNICIAN NOTE**
>
> Blood is collected from cattle from the jugular or coccygeal vein. The subcutaneous abdominal vein is used on rare occasions.

Jugular Venipuncture

When jugular venipuncture is to be performed, the head is placed in a halter with an attached lead. The head is elevated slightly and drawn to the side opposite the vein to be used. The restraint rope is tied to a stationary object.

The vein is occluded with digital pressure applied to the lower third of the jugular groove. Stroking the groove several times in a downward direction with an alcohol-soaked gauze sponge helps visualize the vein. A needle is placed into the jugular vein at a 45-degree angle. When blood flows out of the needle, the Vacutainer tube is inserted into the needle, and a blood sample is collected (Figure 3-32). When the desired volume has entered the tube, digital pressure is removed. The tube is withdrawn from the needle, and the needle is removed from the vein.

Coccygeal Venipuncture

Blood collection from the coccygeal vein, or "tail vein," is performed when the jugular vein is thrombosed or inaccessible. The coccygeal artery lies close to the vein and should be avoided.

The animal is restrained in a chute, and the tail is grasped and bent toward the back. The ventral surface of the tail is cleaned well with 70% isopropyl alcohol to remove dirt and fecal material. An 18- to 20-gauge, 2.5-cm–long needle with a syringe attached is inserted between the sixth and seventh coccygeal vertebrae, perpendicular to the midline. The needle is inserted until bone is felt and then slowly withdrawn as suction is applied with the syringe. When blood flows into the needle hub, the needle is held in place as a sample is collected (Figure 3-33).

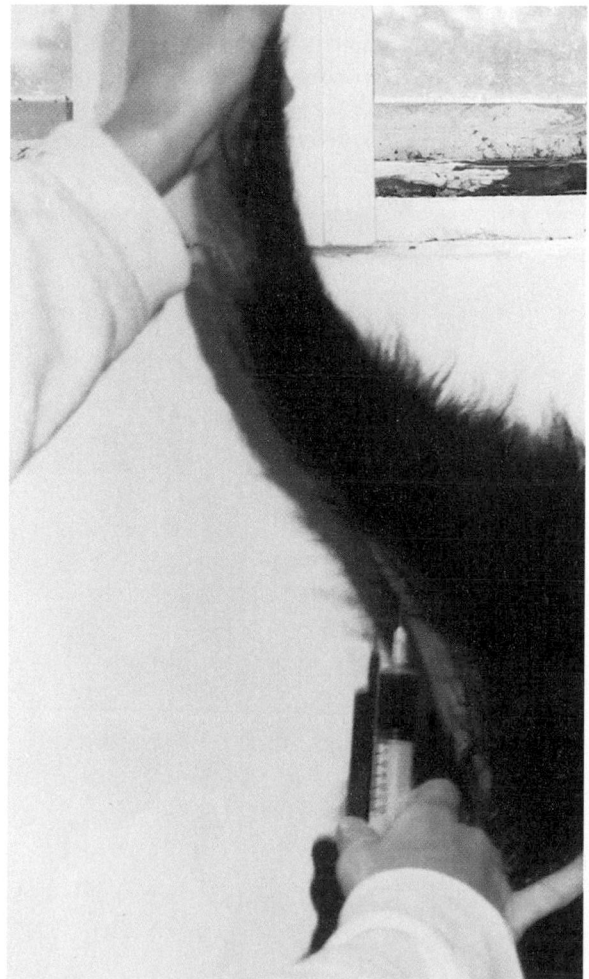

Figure 3-33 Venipuncture of the ventral coccygeal vein in the cow.

Subcutaneous Abdominal (Milk Vein) Venipuncture

The subcutaneous abdominal vein, located on the mammary gland, can be used as a venipuncture site if the jugular and coccygeal veins are unavailable and only a small volume of blood is needed. Because of the risk of being kicked, the milk vein is only used as a last resort. It is imperative to confine the cow in a stanchion. The technician should stand close to the cow's flank and face toward the cow's head. For collection of blood, the skin around the vein is held tautly to stabilize the vein. A 20-gauge, 2.2-cm–long needle attached to a 3-ml syringe is inserted into the vein, and a blood sample is drawn.

EQUINE VENIPUNCTURE

The jugular vein is used to collect most blood samples from the horse. Many horses can be restrained with a halter and lead rope, but fractious ones may need to be placed in a stock. The restrainer turns the head slightly away from the vein to be sampled. Pressure is placed on the jugular groove in the lower third of the neck to occlude and distend the vein. The vessel is stroked several times in a downward direction with an alcohol-soaked gauze sponge. A 20-gauge, 2.5- to 3.75-cm needle is placed in the jugular vein at a 45-degree angle, and a blood sample is collected (Figure 3-34). After the needle has been withdrawn, firm pressure is applied to the venipuncture site for several seconds. A Vacutainer collection device can be used in lieu of a needle and syringe.

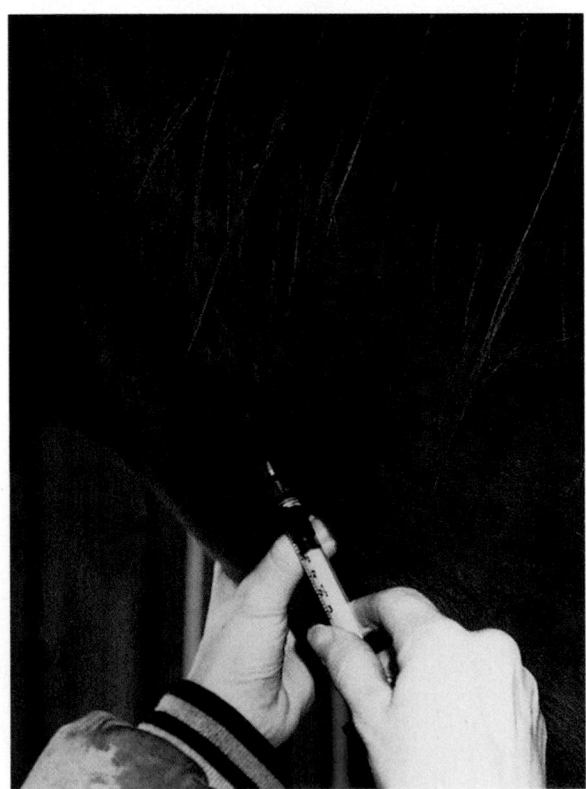

Figure 3-34 The thumb is used to occlude a horse's jugular vein during venipuncture.

TECHNICIAN NOTE

The jugular vein is used to collect most blood samples from the horse.

In a calm horse, the transverse facial vein of the head is occasionally used to obtain a small volume (less than 1 ml) of blood. The vein courses beneath the facial crest and above the transverse facial artery. A 22- to 25-gauge needle is inserted perpendicular to the skin and into the vein, and blood is collected into a syringe or hematocrit tube.

The external thoracic vein on the cranioventral thorax, the cephalic vein on the medial aspect of the front leg, and the medial saphenous vein on the medial aspect of the rear leg are alternative sites for blood collection. They are generally only used if the jugular and transverse facial veins are inaccessible.

PORCINE VENIPUNCTURE

Blood is collected from pigs via the cranial vena cava, external jugular vein, auricular vein, or occasionally the orbital sinus or tail vein. It is more challenging to draw blood from a pig than from most other animals.

Cranial Vena Cava

The right anterior vena cava is used for venipuncture. Because the phrenic nerve courses near the left exterior jugular vein, the left side of the neck should be avoided as a venipuncture site.

When a blood sample must be obtained from a small pig, the animal is positioned on its back on a 45-degree incline with the head lower than the hips. The head is extended, and the front legs are crossed and caudally displaced (Figure 3-35). A 20-gauge, 2.5- to 3.75-cm needle is used in pigs weighing less than 25 kg.

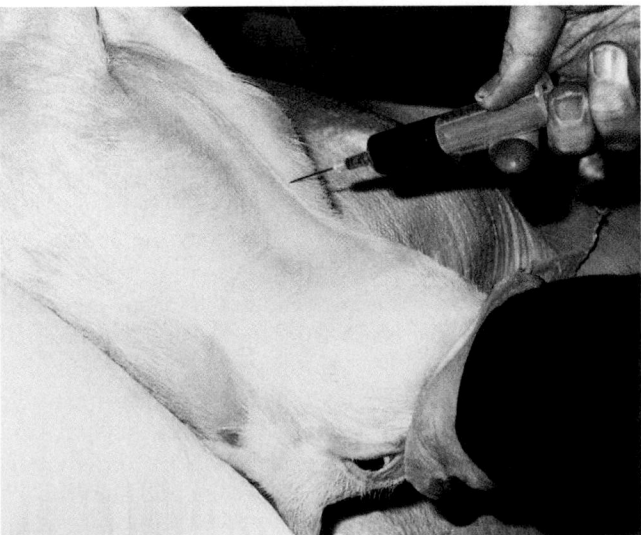

Figure 3-35 Venipuncture of the right anterior vena cava in a small pig in dorsal recumbency.

Pigs that weigh more than 25 kg are restrained in a standing position with the front legs parallel and symmetric to each other. An assistant places a hog snare around the maxilla and holds the head slightly elevated in a parallel plane with the body. The individual who takes the blood sample crouches in front of the right side of the pig. An 18- to 20-gauge, 3.75- to 9.0-cm–long needle with attached syringe is completely inserted into the right jugular fossa just lateral to the manubrium sterni (Figure 3-36). It is placed at a 90-degree angle to the skin of the neck and directed toward the left shoulder. The needle is slowly withdrawn as the syringe plunger is retracted. When blood enters the syringe, the needle is held in place until a sufficient volume is collected.

External Jugular Vein

Blood is frequently collected from the external jugular vein. The needle is inserted near where the internal and external

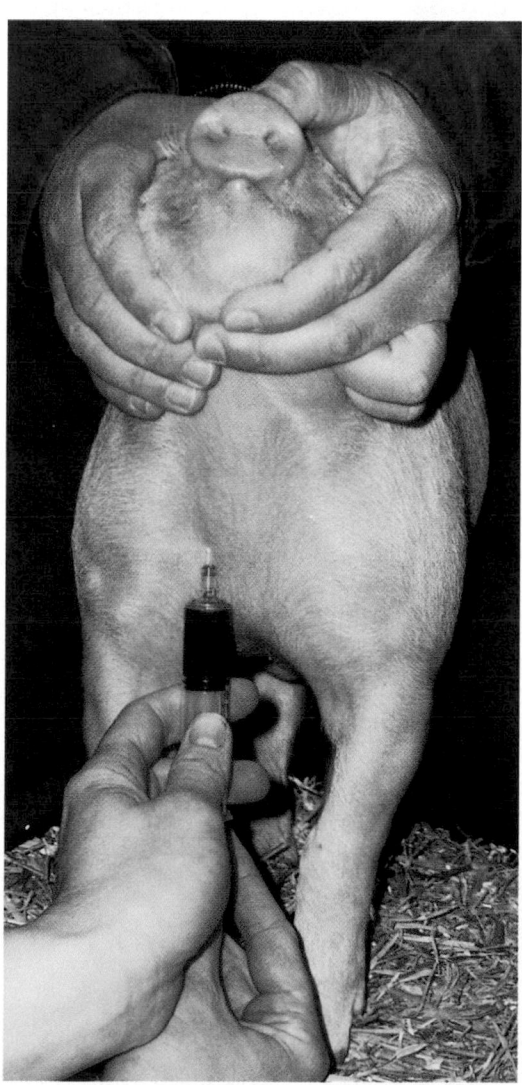

Figure 3-36 A blood sample from the right anterior vena cava is taken with the needle directed into the jugular fossa just lateral to the manubrium sterni.

jugular veins merge to become the brachiocephalic vein. A shorter (20-gauge, 3.75-cm–long) needle than the one used for cranial vena caval venipuncture is used, and therefore jugular venipuncture is considered safer for the animal. Because a shorter needle is used and the jugular vein is smaller than the vena cava, the jugular vein may be more difficult to penetrate in heavier pigs. Venipuncture is performed on the right side of the neck to avoid puncture of the phrenic nerve.

The pig is restrained in a standing position as previously described for vena cava venipuncture. An imaginary horizontal line that passes through the shoulders and manubrium sterni is visualized. A second line is visualized that extends from the manubrium sterni to the scapula at an angle of 45 degrees with the first line. The needle is inserted perpendicular to the skin at the intersection of the second line with the deepest part of the right jugular fossa. The needle is directed caudodorsally and should not be angled toward either scapula. Because the vein is superficial, the syringe plunger should be retracted slightly as soon the needle penetrates the skin. The needle is advanced until blood is aspirated into the syringe. Once a sufficient volume of blood has been collected, the needle is removed.

Auricular Vein

The auricular vein on the dorsal aspect of the pinna is used to collect up to 5 ml of blood. The pig is restrained with a hog snare. A rubber band is placed around the base of the ear to serve as a tourniquet. The ear is held in place, and a 20-gauge, 2.5-cm needle attached to a syringe is inserted into the vein. The sample is slowly aspirated into the syringe. When a sufficient volume of blood is collected, the tourniquet is removed and the needle is withdrawn from the vein.

Orbital Sinus

Small quantities of blood can be collected from the venous sinus near the medial canthus of the eye. A 22-gauge needle is inserted into the medial canthus until it comes in contact with bone. The needle is then rotated between the fingers until blood enters the hub. A microcapillary tube with the end broken to form a rough point can be used in lieu of a needle (Figure 3-37). When collection is complete, the needle or capillary tube is removed, and digital pressure is applied over the medial canthus with the head in an elevated position.

Tail Vein

A 20-gauge, 2.5-cm–long needle is occasionally used to collect small volumes (usually less than 5 ml) of blood from the tail vein in adult pigs with intact tails. The vein is located on the ventral midline of the tail.

OVINE AND CAPRINE VENIPUNCTURE

The jugular vein is the most accessible site for venipuncture in the sheep and goat. Blood collection is easiest to perform

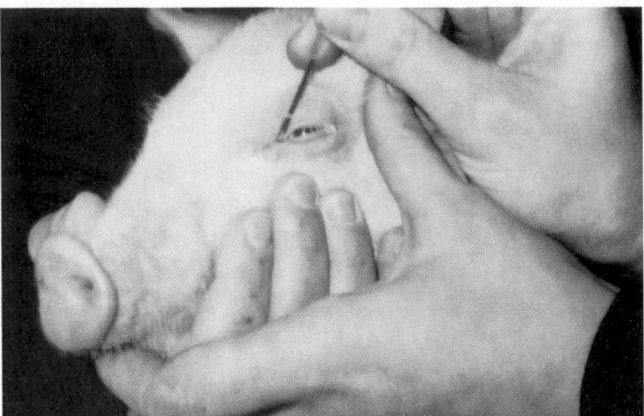

Figure 3-37 Small quantities of blood can be collected from the orbital sinus of the pig.

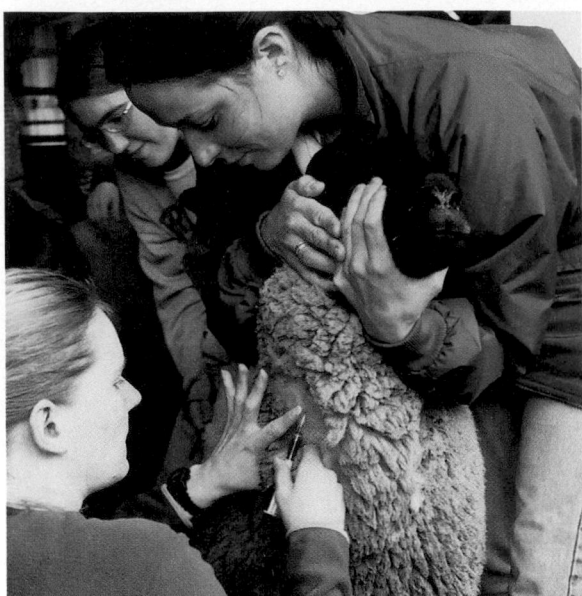

Figure 3-39 A technician crouches in front of a standing sheep to collect blood from the jugular vein. Note that the assistant at the rear of the sheep prevents the sheep from backing away from the technician.

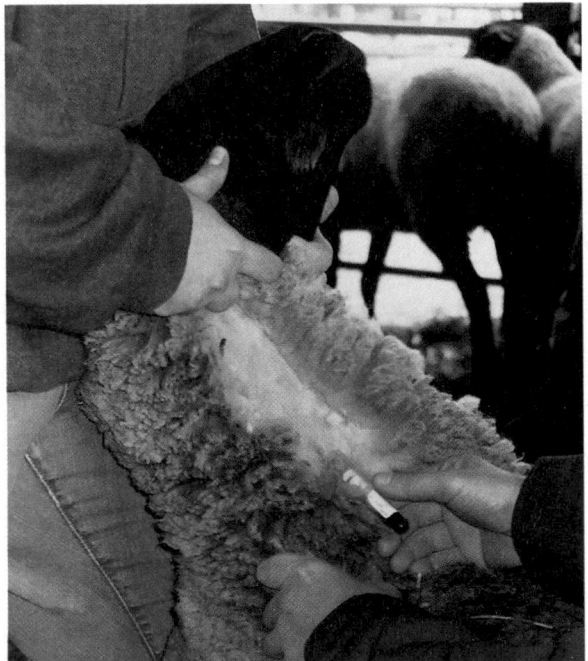

Figure 3-38 Sheep placed in a seated position to allow blood to be collected from the jugular vein.

with a Vacutainer collection system, but a 20- to 22-gauge, 2.5-cm needle and syringe can be used. If the jugular vein is difficult to identify in the sheep, wool is pulled over the jugular furrow until the vessel is visualized.

Sheep become passive when tipped up on their rumps. For a single-person venipuncture technique, the phlebotomist crouches or stands behind the tipped sheep and slightly moves the head in the direction opposite the vein to be used. One hand occludes the jugular vein, and the other hand holds the Vacutainer collection device. The needle is inserted at a 45-degree angle into the jugular vein, and a sample is collected. If additional helpers are available, the sheep is tipped up on its rump, and an assistant stands behind the sheep. The assistant uses his or her legs to

support the back of the sheep and holds the sheep's neck in slight extension and turned slightly away from the jugular vein. The phlebotomist crouches in front of the sheep, occludes the jugular vein, and draws the blood sample with a Vacutainer device or a needle and syringe (Figure 3-38).

Blood can be drawn from a standing sheep or goat by a single person facing forward and straddling the animal over the shoulders. It is helpful to back the animal into a corner to further limit its movement. The phlebotomist holds the sheep's head to the side with the arm that is used to occlude the vein. The other hand is used to collect the blood sample. If assistants are available, one assistant can hold the sheep or goat in a standing position with the neck slightly extended and rotated away from the side of the vein to be used, while another stands near the rear of the animal to prevent it from backing up. The technician, positioned at the front of the animal, occludes the jugular vein and obtains a blood sample (Figure 3-39).

Although the jugular vein is the easiest site from which to collect a blood sample, the cephalic vein can also be used. The procedure previously described for cephalic venipuncture in the dog can be applied to the sheep and goat.

ARTERIAL BLOOD SAMPLE COLLECTION

Arterial blood samples are obtained to evaluate the respiratory and acid-base status of an animal. Evaluation of blood gas values is most often performed intraoperatively in horses under general anesthesia. Information provided from serial intraoperative blood gas values allows the patient's medical status and plane of anesthesia to be monitored more closely.

The carotid and transverse facial arteries are the most frequently sampled arteries in conscious horses. The great metatarsal artery, located on the lateral aspect of the third metatarsal bone, is sometimes used in the foal. When a needle is placed in an artery, bright red blood is expelled from the needle hub in a pulsatile manner. In contrast, if a needle enters a vein, darker red blood will drip out at a slow, constant rate.

The carotid artery lies within in the dorsal aspect of the jugular groove deep to the jugular vein. The artery feels like a cord, and a pulse is not palpable. Skin superficial to the artery on the lower third of the right side of the neck is wiped with alcohol. An 18-gauge, 3.75-cm needle is directed into the artery at a 90-degree angle. As the needle in the carotid artery is stabilized with one hand, a heparin-coated syringe is attached and a sample is collected. Bubbles are expelled from the needle and syringe, and the needle tip is embedded in a rubber stopper. Firm pressure is applied over the needle insertion site for several minutes.

The transverse facial artery is palpated near the lateral canthus of the eye. When a blood sample must be collected from this site, the skin over the artery is numbed with an injection of 0.25 ml of 2% lidocaine. A 22-gauge, 2.5-cm needle is inserted into the artery. The sample is collected and handled as described previously.

A short, OTN catheter can be placed in the artery of an anesthetized patient to monitor intraoperative blood gas values and systemic blood pressure. The catheter can be placed in any of the arteries described previously; however, the transverse facial and dorsal metatarsal arteries are most frequently used. The technique for placing and maintaining arterial catheters is described in the discussion of intravenous administration of medication in the small animal.

URINE SAMPLE COLLECTION

Urine is collected from large animals to screen for either systemic or urinary tract disease. Urine is routinely collected from race horses for drug analysis. Certain drugs or their by-products can be detected as they are excreted in the urine.

BOVINE URINE COLLECTION

Several techniques are used to collect urine from cows. One method to stimulate urination is to stroke the perineum with a piece of straw or your fingers. The tail should not be held aside because it may distract the animal. If stroking the perineum fails to produce a sample, the lips of the vulva can be repeatedly opened and closed to stimulate urination.

Once micturition occurs, a midstream sample is collected in a dry, clean container. If urine is collected for bacterial culture, a sterile specimen cup is used. The initial portion of the stream contains the largest amount of contaminants and should not be included in the sample collected for urinalysis.

Urinary catheterization of the cow is accomplished through use of a sterile flexible or rigid urinary catheter. The perineal region is gently scrubbed with an antiseptic solution and rinsed with warm water. A sterile-gloved, lubricated hand is inserted into the vagina. Fingers are slid approximately 10 cm along the floor of the vagina until the urethral orifice is identified. The catheter is guided into the urethra and advanced until it enters the bladder. Urine will flow through the catheter when it has reached the bladder.

EQUINE URINE COLLECTION

Catheterization of the mare is performed in a manner similar to that described for the cow. The tail is wrapped to prevent hair from entering the vagina. After the vulvar region is aseptically prepared, a sterile-gloved, lubricated hand is placed into the vagina. The urethral opening is located approximately 10 to 12 cm from the ventral commissure of the vulvar lips. The catheter is slid into the urethral orifice and advanced 5 to 10 cm until it enters the bladder. Urine should flow into the catheter once it enters the bladder; however, it may be necessary to apply negative pressure with a syringe to stimulate urine flow. The transverse fold of the vagina overlies the opening of the urethral orifice. It is not uncommon to slide the catheter over the transverse fold and miss the urethral orifice beneath it.

Urinary catheterization of the male horse requires tranquilization. Administration of detomidine or a combination of xylazine, butorphanol, and acepromazine sedates the horse and helps extrude the penis from the prepuce. The prepuce and penis are cleansed with warm, dilute antibacterial solution and then rinsed with water. The tip of a sterile, flexible, 24- to 28 Fr, 137-cm–long urinary catheter is coated with sterile, water-based lubricant. Sterile gloves are worn to grasp the penis and place the catheter, with stylet, approximately 50 to 70 cm into the urethra. It is usually easily advanced through the penile urethra, but resistance may be felt as it passes around the ischial arch. At this point, the stylet is gradually withdrawn as the catheter is passed over the pelvis and into the bladder.

When the catheter enters the bladder, urine should flow through the catheter. If it does not, a 60-ml syringe is attached to the catheter and slowly aspirated. If urine still does not flow, a small volume of air can be injected into the catheter, or the catheter can be repositioned.

OVINE AND CAPRINE URINE COLLECTION

A 5- to 10 Fr lubricated, sterile canine urinary catheter can be used to blindly catheterize ewes and does. The technique used is the same as that described for canine catheterization. Urine can be collected from ewes by holding the nostrils and mouth closed for up to 45 seconds. A ewe will soon struggle to breathe and will urinate. This technique is not highly recommended. A more humane and less stressful way to obtain a urine sample from sheep or goats is to wait until they stand up from a lying down position. They will often urinate when they move from a lying down position to a standing position.

Rams and bucks have anatomic obstacles that make urinary catheterization extremely difficult. Urine samples are primarily collected by free catch of voided samples.

FECES SAMPLE COLLECTION

Feces are collected to check for intestinal parasites or to culture for organisms such as *Salmonella* spp. Samples can be obtained by simply picking them up from the ground. Alternatively, feces can be manually retrieved from the rectum with a gloved or sleeved hand. The glove or sleeve is turned inside out as it is removed and tied in a knot to store the sample.

RUMEN FLUID COLLECTION

Rumen fluid is collected for analysis from both large and small ruminants. Sometimes rumen fluid is transferred from healthy to sick or weak sheep to inoculate the weak animal's rumen with microorganisms that aid in food digestion.

A medium-sized stomach tube lubricated with water-based gel is used to obtain rumen fluid from cattle. Tubes with internal diameters less than 1.5 cm may become obstructed with ingesta and are not recommended for rumen fluid collection.

When orogastric intubation is performed, the cow is confined in a head catch. The restrainer wraps one arm around the muzzle and places either nose tongs or one finger into one of the cow's nostrils and a thumb into the other nostril and pulls the nose upward. The mouth will open. The technician stands to the animal's side and carefully places a Frick speculum (Figure 3-40) into the mouth and over the base of the tongue (Figure 3-41). One end of the tube is inserted into the speculum, and the other is held in the intubator's mouth. As the animal swallows, the tube is advanced down the esophagus. The intubator blows into the tube to dilate the esophagus, which helps the tube pass through the esophagus and into the rumen.

Placement of the tube within the rumen is confirmed by auscultation of the abdomen as air is simultaneously blown into the tube. Air should be heard bubbling through rumen contents. The distinctive odor of fermented gas will be detected coming from the end of the tube.

Rumen fluid samples are withdrawn from the tube with a dose syringe. The initial fluid portion should be discarded because it often contains an excessive amount of saliva. This erroneously elevates the pH of the fluid.

When rumen fluid collection is complete, the tube is kinked and removed with a downward motion. This prevents rumen contents from leaking out of the tube and entering the trachea as the tube is withdrawn.

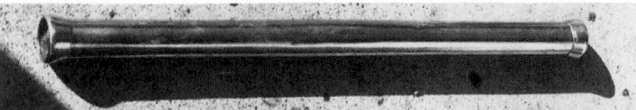

Figure 3-40   Frick speculum.

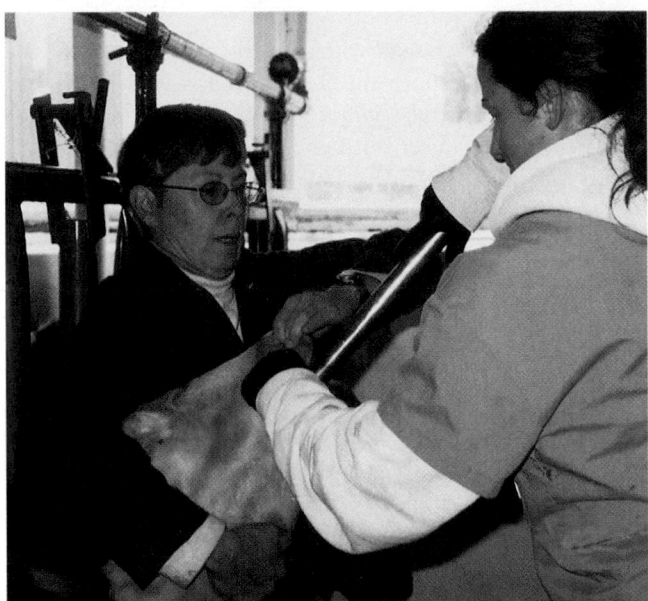

Figure 3-41   A Frick speculum is placed in the mouth of a cow.

ABDOMINOCENTESIS

Abdominocentesis is performed to obtain samples of abdominal fluid for laboratory evaluation. It is used as a diagnostic technique in horses with suspected peritonitis, colic, chronic diarrhea, weight loss, or fever of unknown origin.

> **✏ TECHNICIAN NOTE**
>
> Abdominocentesis is used as a diagnostic technique in horses with colic, chronic diarrhea, weight loss, or fever of unknown origin.

EQUINE ABDOMINOCENTESIS

When abdominocentesis is performed, the standing horse is restrained in a chute or stanchion. The individual who performs the centesis stands close to the front legs and faces the abdomen to avoid being kicked by the rear legs.

The most dependent site on the ventral midline of the abdomen is clipped and aseptically prepared. Approximately 2 ml of 2% lidocaine is infused into the skin and subcutaneous tissue at the abdominocentesis site. Sterile gloves are worn to make a stab incision through the skin with a No. 15 blade. Obvious cutaneous vessels should be avoided.

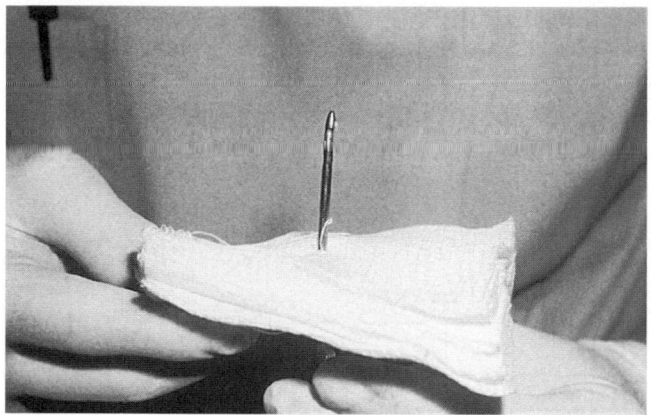

Figure 3-42 A teat cannula is pushed through sterile gauze sponges before being inserted into the abdominal cavity to prevent peripheral blood from contaminating the abdominocentesis sample.

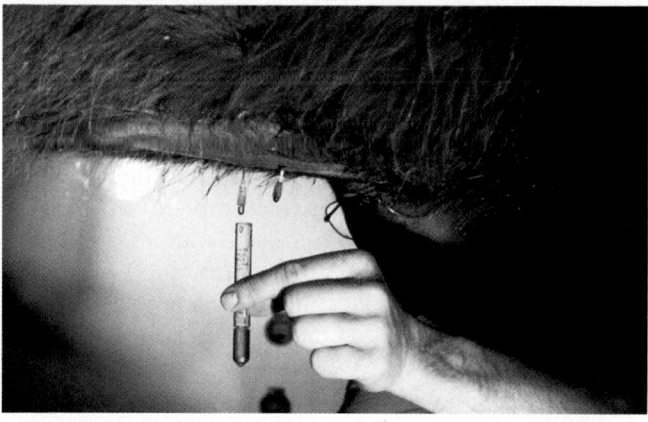

Figure 3-43 Abdominocentesis is performed in a horse by passing a teat cannula into the abdominal cavity.

The blade is rotated to form an entrance through which a sterile, 9-cm–long, blunt-ended teat cannula or stainless steel canine urinary catheter may pass. The cannula is pushed through the center of a 4-by-4 sterile gauze sponge and is then inserted through the incision and into the abdominal cavity (Figures 3-42 and 3-43). The gauze prevents blood that drips down the outside of the cannula from contaminating the sample.

The first few drops of fluid that drip from the cannula often contain blood or other contaminants. These first drops should not be included in the collected sample. The sample is collected in sterile tubes with and without anticoagulants. If fluid does not drain, the cannula is rotated or redirected, or a syringe is attached to the end and negative pressure is applied.

If a teat cannula is not available, an 18-gauge, 3.75-cm hypodermic needle can be used for abdominocentesis in horses and large ruminants; and a 20-gauge, 3.75-cm needle can be used in small ruminants. Centesis is performed as previously described, except that neither a local anesthetic is used nor a blade incision is made before needle insertion. If fluid does not flow through the needle, 1 to 2 ml of air is injected to dislodge any particles that might be plugging the needle. Rotation or redirection of the needle or insertion of an additional needle several centimeters away from the initial one may stimulate fluid flow.

RUMINANT ABDOMINOCENTESIS

The site selected for abdominocentesis in a ruminant is determined by which abdominal disorder is suspected. If traumatic reticuloperitonitis is suspected, the centesis site is the ruminoreticular recess. In large ruminants, this recess is in the left cranial quadrant of the abdomen approximately 5 cm caudal to the xiphoid process and 5 cm to the left of midline. If uterine or small bowel rupture is the concern,

centesis is performed 5 cm cranial to the udder and medial to the right flank fold. Care is taken to avoid penetration of the large subcutaneous mammary vessels on the surface of the ventral abdomen. Peritonitis in ruminants is often highly compartmentalized; therefore additional sites are tapped if the initial centesis does not yield fluid.

Abdominocentesis is usually performed in small ruminants to diagnose a urinary tract obstruction or a bladder rupture. The needle is inserted approximately 3 cm to the right of the midline in the most dependent part of the ventral abdomen. Insertion at this site helps to prevent accidental rumen puncture. The procedure is the same as that described for large ruminants.

Complications of abdominocentesis in horses and ruminants are (1) bowel laceration; (2) introduction of bacteria at the centesis site, resulting in peritonitis or cellulitis; and (3) damage to the xiphoid process if the centesis site is too cranial.

THORACOCENTESIS

Thoracocentesis is performed in large animals, primarily horses, to drain fluid or air from the pleural cavity. Fluid is submitted for cytologic analysis or bacterial or fungal culture. Light sedation with a combination of xylazine and butorphanol may be required. A 12- or 14-gauge, 6.0- to 7.5-cm teat cannula is used to remove small volumes of air or fluid. If the fluid is thick or large in volume, a wider-bore, 5- to 7.5-cm–long sterile metal bitch urinary catheter or human thoracic drainage cannula is used.

The ventral thoracic region from the fifth to the ninth ribs is clipped and surgically scrubbed. Centesis to remove fluid is performed in the ventral portion of the sixth or seventh intercostal space, 10 to 12 cm dorsal to the olecranon. If air is expected to be withdrawn, the needle is inserted further dorsal in the intercostal space. The needle is inserted along the cranial border of the rib to avoid the intercostal vessels and nerves that run along the caudal border of the ribs. The lateral thoracic vein, which courses subcutaneously over the ventral aspect of the thorax, should also be avoided. From 3 to 5 ml of 2% lidocaine is injected into the skin, subcutaneous tissue, and intercostal muscles down to the parietal pleura. A stab incision is made with a scalpel blade into the anesthetized skin on the cranial aspect of the rib. The cannula, connected to a three-way stopcock with the valve closed, is inserted through the skin incision until it penetrates the pleura. A 60-ml syringe is connected to the stopcock with extension tubing. The stopcock valve is opened, and air or fluid is aspirated into the syringe. After thoracocentesis is completed, the cannula is withdrawn. Skin sutures are usually only needed if the human cannula or bitch urinary catheter is used.

TRANSTRACHEAL WASH

A transtracheal wash is performed on occasion to help determine the cause of lower airway disease. It involves the collection of fluid from the lower respiratory tract for cytologic and microbiologic analysis. The following procedure is described for equine and bovine patients. The technique for transtracheal aspiration in small ruminants is similar to that previously described for small animals.

The middle tracheal region is clipped and aseptically prepared. Approximately 2 ml of 2% lidocaine is injected intradermally and subcutaneously over the center of the trachea. A stab incision is made with a scalpel blade through the skin between the tracheal rings. As the trachea is stabilized with one hand, a 12- to 14-gauge needle is inserted, with the bevel facing downward, through the incision and into the tracheal lumen. A burst of air will exit the needle when it penetrates the lumen.

A sterile, 5 or 6 Fr polyvinyl urinary catheter with the tip cut off is threaded through the needle until it reaches the tracheal bifurcation. A syringe is attached to the flared end of the catheter, and the plunger is retracted. Air is aspirated if the catheter is within the tracheal lumen. If air is not aspirated, the catheter may be outside the trachea, bent, or occluded against the tracheal mucosa and should be repositioned.

Once the catheter is within the tracheal lumen, the needle is withdrawn and the catheter is left in place. Extension tubing connected to a 60-ml syringe filled with sterile 0.9% saline solution is inserted into the flared end of the catheter. A 30- to 50-ml aliquot of saline solution is injected into the trachea. Saline solution is reaspirated, and a sample is collected. Approximately 10% of the infused volume will be reaspirated. The catheter may need to be adjusted and redirected during the procedure. Additional aliquots of saline solution are instilled through the catheter and reaspirated until a sufficient sample volume is obtained.

After the sample has been collected, the catheter is removed. The site is covered with an antibiotic-coated sterile gauze pad and wrapped with a bandage for 24 hours. Cellulitis at the tracheal puncture site is the most common complication. If swelling occurs, warm compresses are applied.

ADMINISTRATION OF MEDICATION IN LARGE ANIMALS

INTRAVENOUS ADMINISTRATION

Bovine Administration

The jugular vein is used for intravenous administration of medication or fluids. The haltered animal is restrained in a chute or stanchion with the head elevated and pulled to the side. Digital pressure is applied to the jugular groove to occlude the vein. The skin overlying the vein is wiped with an alcohol-soaked gauze sponge several times in a downward direction to remove superficial skin contaminants and to help identify the vein.

A 16- to 18-gauge, 3.75- to 5.0-cm needle is inserted through the skin and into the vein at a 45- to 90-degree angle with the skin. When blood flows from the end of the needle, it is inserted completely to the hub in either an upward or a downward direction. The syringe containing the medication is attached to the needle. Before injection of the syringe contents, the plunger is retracted slightly to ensure that blood enters the syringe. The digital pressure is removed from the jugular groove, and the medication is injected. As the needle is removed, pressure is placed on the venipuncture site until hemostasis occurs.

✎ TECHNICIAN NOTE

When an animal requires repeated intravenous injections or large volumes of fluids, a catheter is placed in the jugular vein.

When an animal requires repeated intravenous injections or large volumes of fluids, an intravenous catheter is placed in the jugular vein. The procedure for jugular catheterization in cattle is similar to that of equine jugular catheterization and is described in detail in the discussion of equine venipuncture.

The ventral coccygeal vein, on the ventral aspect of the tail, can be used as a site for injection of small volumes of medication. Because of the proximity of the coccygeal vein to the coccygeal artery and the fecal contamination around the tail, the vein is not recommended for injections.

Equine Administration

The jugular vein is used for intravenous injections in the horse. It is large and easily palpated in the jugular groove on the neck. Injection into the right jugular vein is preferred over injection into the left jugular vein because the esophagus lies in the left jugular groove.

When an injection is made into the jugular vein, the vessel is occluded with digital pressure on the jugular groove. The vein is more easily visualized in the proximal third of the neck if the jugular groove is wiped with an alcohol-soaked cotton ball several times in a downward direction.

An 18-gauge, 2.5-cm needle is embedded into the vein, up to the hub, at a 90-degree angle and then directed caudally (Figure 3-44). Blood will trickle constantly from the needle hub if it is in the vein. If the needle inadvertently enters the carotid artery, blood will forcefully spurt out of the hub in a pulsatile manner, even when the jugular vein is not occluded. If the needle enters the carotid artery, it should be removed immediately, and firm pressure should be applied for several minutes to ensure hemostasis. Use of a large-bore needle and insertion of the needle without the syringe attached decreases the likelihood that an injection of medication will accidentally be given intraarterially.

TECHNICIAN NOTE

If the needle inadvertently enters the carotid artery, blood will be ejected from the needle hub in forceful spurts, even when the jugular vein is not occluded.

Once it has been determined that the needle is placed intravenously and not intraarterially, the needle is stabilized and the syringe is attached. The plunger should be retracted slightly to ensure that venous blood flows back into the syringe. Digital pressure on the vein is removed, and the contents of the syringe are slowly injected.

If repeated administration of large volumes of fluid or intravenous medication is required, an intravenous catheter is placed in the jugular vein. Although intravenous catheters can also be placed in the cephalic and lateral thoracic veins, fluids can be administered at a more rapid rate in the larger jugular vein.

For placement of a jugular catheter, the hair over the cranial third of the vein is clipped, and the skin is aseptically

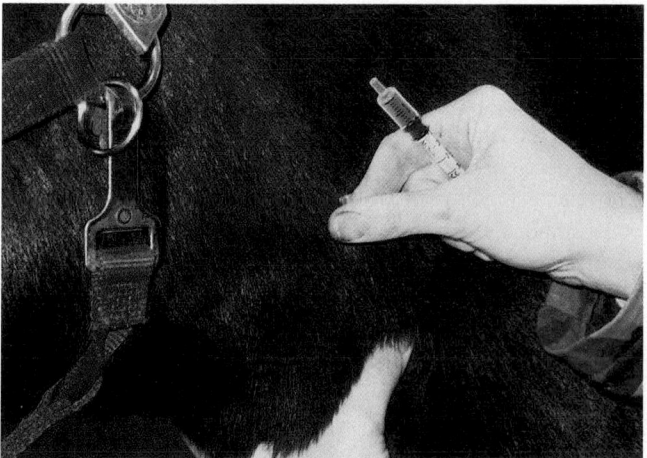

Figure 3-44 A needle is placed into the jugular vein to administer intravenous medication to a horse.

prepared. Approximately 1.0 ml of 2% lidocaine is instilled into the skin over the vessel. Latex gloves, ideally sterile ones, are worn to place the catheter. A small incision is made through the desensitized skin with a scalpel blade or 14-gauge needle. The vein is occluded by the application of digital pressure in the jugular furrow.

A 10- to 16-gauge, 13-cm OTN catheter, with a stylet, is inserted through the skin incision and into the vein. (Figure 3-45, *A*). The tip should be at a 45-degree angle, pointing downward and parallel with the vein. Blood will appear in the catheter hub when the tip enters the vein. The catheter is advanced an additional 5 mm. It is then laid parallel to the vein as it is slid over the stylet and threaded completely into the vein (Figure 3-45, *B* and *C*). Digital pressure on the vein is released. A cap or extension set is placed on the hub, and the catheter is flushed with heparinized 0.9% sterile saline solution.

Glue, tape, or suture is used to secure the catheter to the skin. A gauze sponge onto which a small amount of antibiotic ointment has been applied is placed over the venipuncture site. The catheter is secured with layers of bandage material and adhesive tape wrapped around the neck (Figure 3-45, *D*).

The catheter site should be checked several times daily for patency and monitored for signs of inflammation or infection. If excessive warmth, redness, firmness, swelling, pain, extravasation of fluid, or discharge is noted around the catheter site, the catheter should be removed and placed in a different vein.

TECHNICIAN NOTE

If excessive warmth, redness, firmness, swelling, pain, extravasation of fluid, or discharge is noted around the catheter site, the catheter should be removed and placed in a different vein.

Ovine and Caprine Administration

The injection technique used with goats and sheep is similar to that described for small animals. An 18- to 20-gauge, 2.5-cm hypodermic needle is used in adults, and a 20- to 22-gauge, 2.5-cm needle is used in lambs and kids.

The jugular vein is the most convenient site for intravenous injection in the sheep and goat. To obtain access to the vein, a handler restrains the goat, backs it into a corner, straddles it over the withers, and turns its head to one side. Restraint of a sheep for intravenous injection involves either sitting the sheep up on its rump or straddling the sheep over the withers and stretching the neck laterally. It may be necessary to part the wool or hair to visualize the vein.

Porcine Administration

The auricular vein, located on the dorsal aspect of the pinna, is the most commonly used vein for administration of drugs or fluids to pigs. A 19- to 21-gauge butterfly catheter or an 18-gauge OTN catheter can be placed in the ear vein

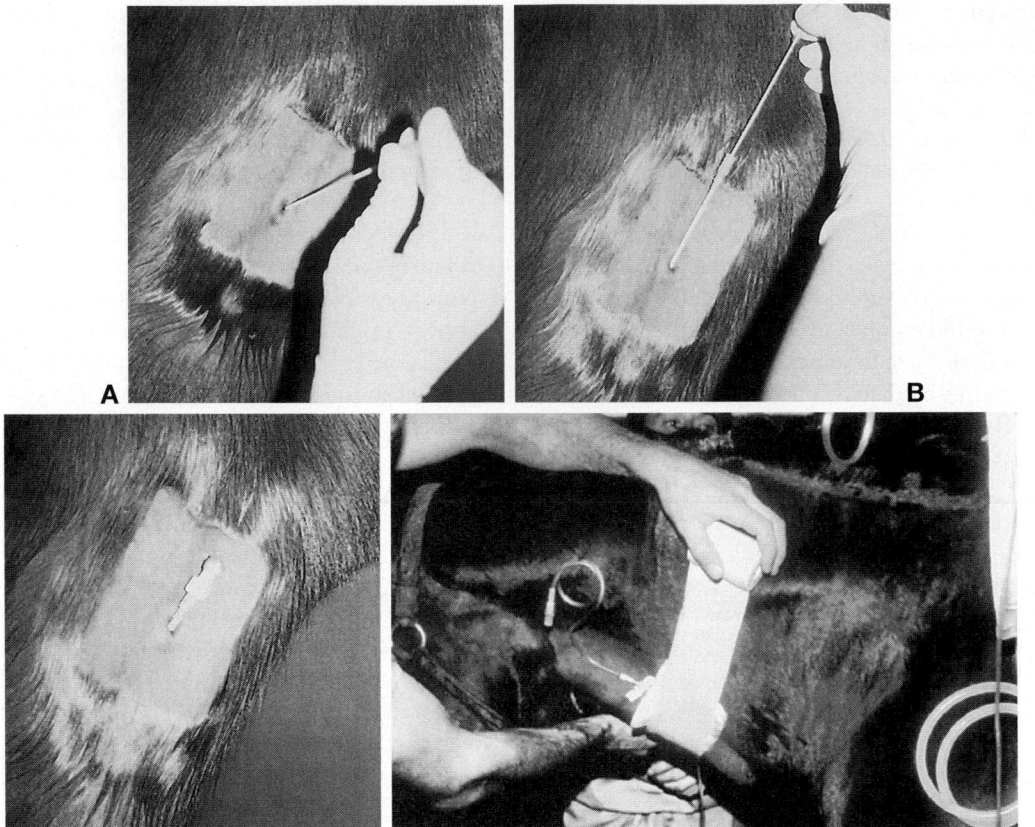

Figure 3-45 A jugular catheter is placed in a horse for intravenous fluid therapy. The catheter is secured in place by bandage material that is wrapped around the neck. (**A** through **C**, from Sirois M: *Principles and practice of veterinary technology*, St Louis, 2004, Mosby.)

if large volumes of fluid or multiple intravenous injections are needed.

When the auricular vein is catheterized, a rubber band tourniquet is wrapped around the ear base to distend the vein. The dorsal aspect of the pinna is aseptically prepared. The catheter is inserted into the vein. After the catheter is threaded into the vein, the tourniquet is released. The catheter is capped, and the hub is affixed to the pinna with quick-setting glue. A dry gauze sponge is placed flat against the underside of the pinna to serve as padding. A partially used roll of 5.0-cm–wide tape is placed next to the gauze sponge to support the underside of the pinna. The margins of the ear are bent around the roll of tape. Several strips of adhesive tape are wrapped around the ear to secure the catheter to the pinna.

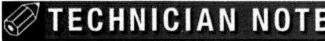

> **TECHNICIAN NOTE**
>
> The only muscles recommended for intramuscular injections in cattle are those in the neck.

INTRAMUSCULAR ADMINISTRATION

Bovine Administration

The only muscles recommended for intramuscular injections in cattle are those in the neck. Injection into the gluteal muscle should be avoided because this area is prone to abscessation. Intramuscular injections are performed when the animal is restrained in a stanchion or crowded into a confined area. In cattle and horses, a maximum of 5 to 10 ml, depending on the site and size of the animal, should be administered at each site. It is best to alternate sites if repeated injections are needed over a multiday period.

The injection site is wiped with 70% isopropyl alcohol to remove gross skin contaminants. A 16- or 18-gauge, 3.75- to 5.0-cm needle is grasped, and a fist is formed with the same hand. The injection site is struck several times with the flat of the fist. The hand is then rotated slightly, and the animal is struck again as the needle is embedded in the skin and muscle. Striking the animal in this manner distracts it and decreases its awareness of the needle insertion. Once the needle is inserted to the level of the hub, the syringe is attached. Before the medication is injected, the plunger is retracted, and the hub is checked for blood. If a vessel has been inadvertently penetrated, the needle should be removed, and the injection should be made in another location. After injection, the site is briefly massaged to help distribute the injected fluid.

Equine Administration

The neck and rear legs are used for intramuscular injection in the horse. As with cattle, the gluteal region should be

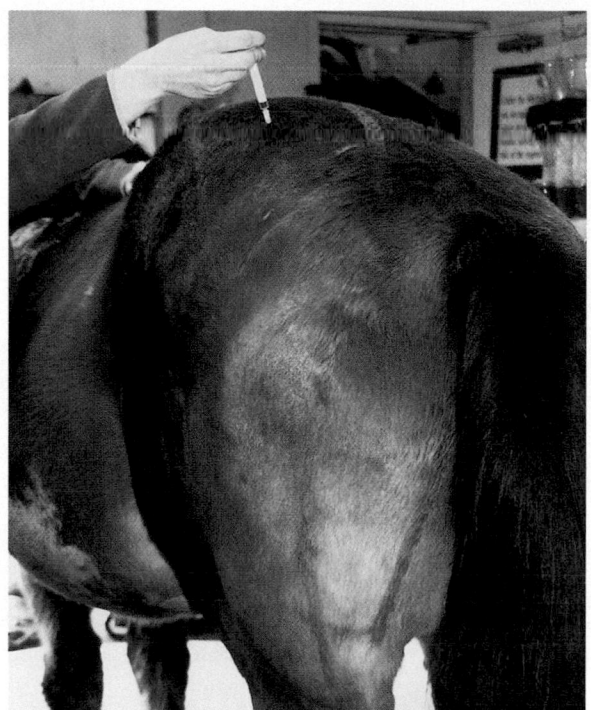

Figure 3-46 The gluteal region (dorsal blue outlined region) may be used for intramuscular injections, but the pectoral or semimembranosis/semitendinosis muscles (ventral blue outlined region) are preferred sites for intramuscular injections.

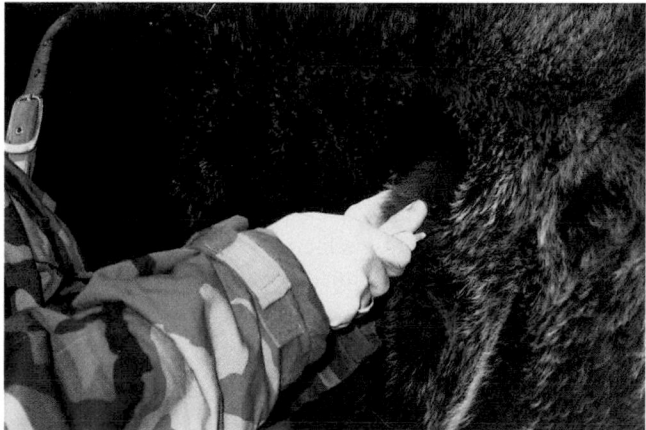

Figure 3-47 Intramuscular injection into the cervical muscles in a horse.

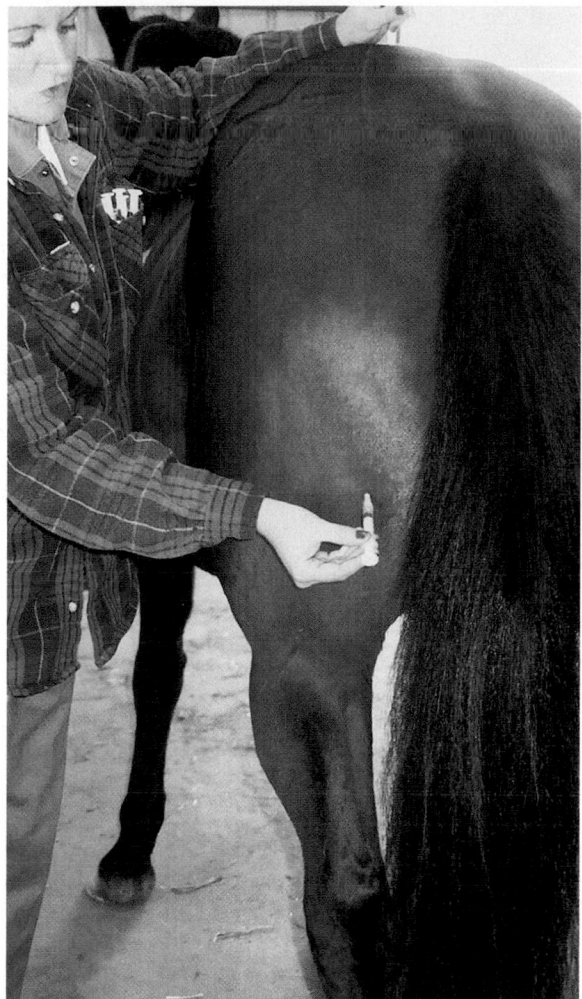

Figure 3-48 Intramuscular injection into the semimembranosus and semitendinosus muscles in a horse.

avoided because of the difficulty in treating any injection-induced abscesses (Figure 3-46). The pectoral muscles may be used as sites for injection, but there is an increased likelihood of inflammation. Abscesses that may develop subsequent to injection in the pectoral region are easier to drain than are those in the gluteal muscles.

Intramuscular injections in the neck are given in the indented triangular region bordered by the nuchal ligament, cervical spine, and shoulder blade (Figure 3-47). Medication administered into the nuchal ligament is poorly absorbed. Volumes of up to 10 ml can be injected intramuscularly

into the neck. Postinjection muscle tenderness is a relatively common sequela.

The lower half of the semimembranosus and semitendinosus muscles in the caudal aspect of the rear leg are excellent injection sites, but the injector is at risk of being kicked (Figures 3-46 and 3-48). The individual giving the injection stands on one side of the horse and reaches around the rear to inject the opposite leg. If the horse kicks, it usually kicks toward the side of the injection. It is best to stand as close to the horse's body as possible to avoid a kick. It is not always possible to stand on the side opposite the injection. In such a case, the restrainer should stand on the same side as the individual giving the injection and pull the horse's head toward them both. If the horse kicks, it will attempt to straighten itself and spin its rear end away from the side on which the injection is received and from the restrainer.

Equine intramuscular injections are administered in the same manner as described for cattle, except that an 18-gauge, 3.75-cm needle is used. The site is tapped with the back of the hand or fist once or twice, and then the needle, without the syringe attached, is inserted through the skin and deep into the muscle.

Ovine and Caprine Administration

Intramuscular injections in the sheep and goat are administered in the semimembranosus and semitendinosus muscles of the rear leg, triceps, neck muscles, or longissimus muscles over the lumbar region. Occasionally, the gluteal muscles are used. Goats and sheep do not have sufficient muscle mass for large-volume intramuscular injections. A maximum of 5 ml is injected in any single site.

Porcine Administration

In pigs, intramuscular injections are made into the cervical muscles or the semimembranosus or semitendinosus muscles of the rear leg. Lameness may occur after injection into the caudal muscles of the rear leg. Use of the muscles of the "ham" for intramuscular injections is avoided in animals intended for use as food because the injection may mark the muscle and downgrade the quality of the meat. Because of the tendency of pigs to store a thick layer of subcutaneous body fat, a needle that is at least 3.75 cm long is needed to penetrate to the muscle. Medications deposited in fat are absorbed much more slowly than are those deposited in muscle, so the onset of action of the injected substances is delayed.

> ✎ **TECHNICIAN NOTE**
>
> The use of the muscles of the "ham" for intramuscular injections is avoided in animals intended for use as food because the injection may mark the muscle and downgrade the quality of the meat.

SUBCUTANEOUS ADMINISTRATION

Bovine and Equine Administration

The neck is the site recommended for subcutaneous injections in the horse. Any region on the lateral aspect of the neck or trunk can be used for subcutaneous injections in cattle. For both horses and cattle, when a subcutaneous injection is given, the site is first wiped with a gauze sponge saturated with 70% isopropyl alcohol to remove superficial skin contaminants. A fold of skin is tented, and an 18- to 20-gauge, 2.5- to 3.75-cm needle with attached syringe is inserted at the base of the tented skin (Figure 3-49). Slight negative pressure is applied by retraction of the plunger to ensure that the needle has not entered a vessel. If placement is satisfactory, the medication is injected under the skin, and the needle is withdrawn. The area around the site is rubbed to promote distribution of the injected substance.

Ovine and Caprine Administration

The neck and shoulder region is frequently used for subcutaneous injections in the sheep and goat. Axillary or flank subcutaneous injections are made in show animals if the

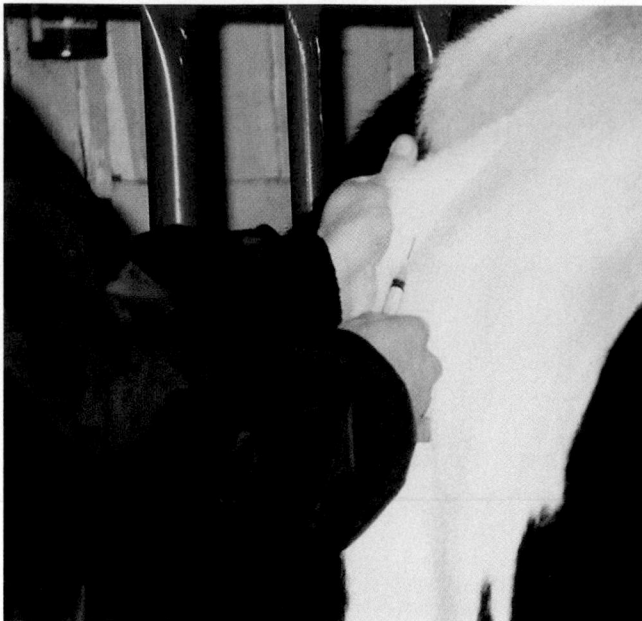

Figure 3-49 A needle is inserted into the base of a fold of skin to make a subcutaneous injection in a cow.

injections contain medications or vaccines, such as clostridial vaccines, that may cause nodular swellings or abscesses. Subcutaneous masses, if located in the prescapular region, may be mistaken by show judges as caseous lymphadenitis. The back or upper flank areas should be avoided as injection sites in goats if the skin will be marketed. Injection of sheep should be done when the wool is dry. Sheep have a greater tendency toward injection site reactions if the needle is introduced through wet wool.

Porcine Administration

The skin of pigs is tightly adhered to the body. This limits the volume that can be injected subcutaneously. Subcutaneous injections are made into the lateral side of the neck, immediately posterior to the base of the ear, with a 16- to 18-gauge, 2.5- to 3.75-cm needle.

INTRADERMAL ADMINISTRATION

In large animals, as in small animals, intradermal injections are made primarily for the purpose of skin testing or to provide local anesthesia. Cattle and sheep are tested for tuberculosis by means of an intradermal injection into the caudal tail fold (Figure 3-50). Intradermal injections are also used to treat nodular skin lesions and sarcoids. The technique for intradermal injection is as previously described for small animals and can be adapted for use in large animals.

INTRAPERITONEAL ADMINISTRATION

Intraperitoneal injections are usually reserved for treatment of neonatal kids or lambs with umbilical infections

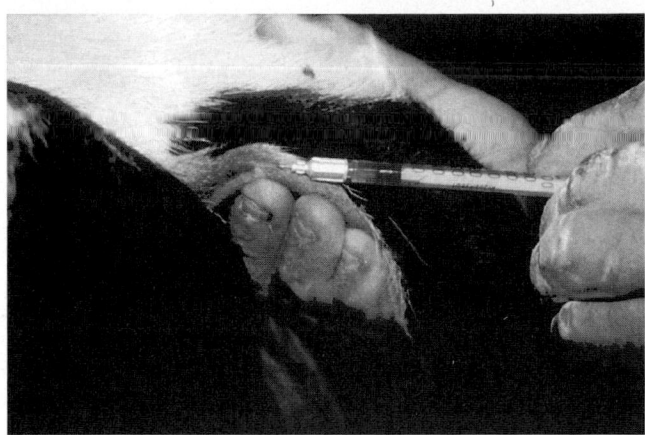

Figure 3-50 Intradermal injection is made into the caudal skinfold to test for tuberculosis in the cow.

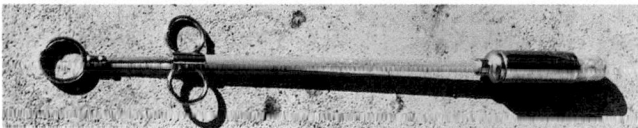

Figure 3-51 Metal balling gun for use in cattle. Smaller, plastic balling guns should be used with sheep and goats.

or hypoglycemia. The neonate is lifted by the front legs, and a 20-gauge needle with attached syringe is introduced to the left of the umbilicus to a depth of 1.0 cm. The plunger is retracted to ensure that the needle has not penetrated a vessel or an abdominal organ. Once intraperitoneal placement has been confirmed, the syringe contents are injected into the peritoneal cavity.

In baby pigs, fluids are usually administered intraperitoneally because of the impracticality of placing an intravenous catheter. Fluids should be body temperature, nonirritating, and isotonic. The site of needle introduction is aseptically prepared. When intraperitoneal fluids are administered to a baby pig, the pig is grasped by the rear legs, and an 18-gauge, 1.25- to 2.5-cm needle is inserted paramedially between the midline and flank. Intraperitoneal injection in a mature standing pig requires the insertion of a 16- to 18-gauge, 7.5-cm needle.

INTRANASAL ADMINISTRATION

Certain vaccines or local anesthetics are administered intranasally in large as well as small animals. The head is restrained with the nose tilted slightly upward. Excessive nasal exudate is removed from the nostril to be injected. This is best accomplished by cleaning the nares with damp gauze sponges or cotton balls. The needleless syringe containing the vaccine or local anesthetic is injected into the nostril. It is not uncommon for the animal to sneeze out some of the injected substance.

ORAL ADMINISTRATION

The easiest but least reliable method of administering oral medication to a large animal is to mix it with food or drinking water. If the animal detects a different taste or smell, it may refrain from ingesting the off-flavored food or water. If the animal is sick, it may have diminished appetite and will not consume the entire medication dose.

Ovine and Caprine Administration

Balling Gun
Administration of tablets to adult sheep and goats can be a challenge. A balling gun is used to help perform the task (Figure 3-51). The end of the gun should be smooth and, ideally, made of soft plastic. It should be inspected for sharp edges before each use. Care should be taken not to insert the balling gun too forcefully or too far back into the oral cavity. The tip of the gun should not scrape the roof of the mouth. Improper use can cause trauma to the mouth, pharynx, and esophagus.

When the balling gun is used, the animal is backed into a corner and straddled over the shoulders by the handler. The head and neck are held in normal position. A balling gun is placed in the interdental space of the mouth and positioned over the base of the tongue. The bolus is released, and the gun is withdrawn. Observation of the animal after administration is required to ensure that the pill has been swallowed.

Dosing Syringe
Small volumes of liquid are administered orally with the use of a 60-ml catheter-tipped syringe, dosing bottle, or dosing syringe. When a syringe is used, the tip is introduced into the side of the mouth and over the base of the tongue. The liquid is slowly injected with the head held in a normal position. If coughing occurs, administration should be ceased until the trachea is cleared of fluid. If the animal struggles and becomes upset, it should be allowed to rest before administration is reattempted.

Nasogastric Intubation
A nasogastric or orogastric tube can be used to administer larger fluid volumes, medication, electrolyte solutions, rumen fluid, or colostrum. Nasogastric intubation is generally better tolerated than orogastric intubation (Figure 3-52).

The sheep or goat is restrained in a standing position by a handler who straddles the withers. The nasal passageway is desensitized by the instillation of 0.5 ml of 2% lidocaine into one nostril. A length of flexible plastic or rubber tube needed to extend from the nostrils to the rumen is premeasured and marked. The tube should have a smooth, rounded end and have a sufficiently small diameter to pass through the ventral nasal meatus.

Water-soluble lubricant or water is placed around the tube tip. The tube is inserted into the nostril and slowly

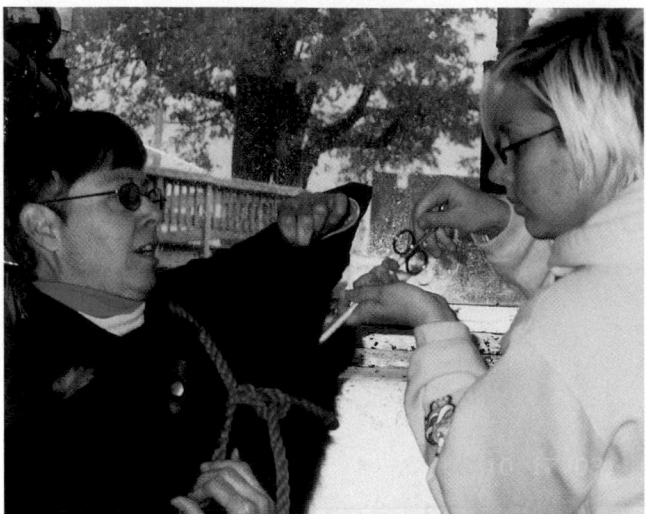

Figure 3-52 A cow opens its mouth when the handler pulls the nose dorsally, using a finger and thumb inserted into the nostrils. This allows the technician to place the balling gun over the base of the tongue.

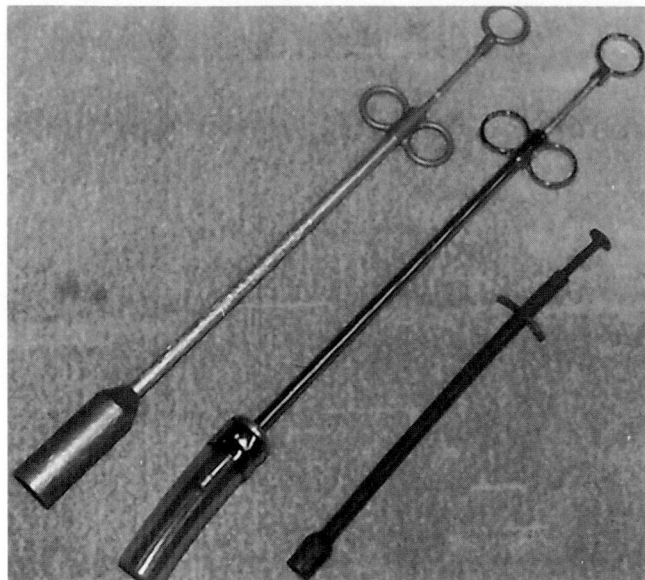

Figure 3-53 Nasogastric intubation of a sheep with a stallion urinary catheter.

advanced into the ventral nasal meatus and nasopharynx. The animal should be observed swallowing the tube as it is advanced. The tube is palpated on the neck as it passes down the esophagus. If the animal coughs, the tube has entered the trachea and should be promptly removed.

Once the nasogastric tube has been inserted to the pre-measured mark, the placement is checked to ensure that the tube is definitely within the rumen. If the tube is properly placed, when air is blown into the end of the tube, an assistant who auscultates the area over the rumen with a stethoscope can hear bubbling as air passes through rumen contents. The smell of rumen contents also emanates from the end of the tube.

Fluid or medication is flushed through the tube with a dose syringe or drench pump. A bolus of water is generally flushed through the tube after the medication has been introduced. After the medication and water bolus have been administered, the tube is kinked to occlude it. The tube is withdrawn in a downward direction. This technique prevents rumen contents from leaking from the tube and entering the trachea as the tube is removed.

Orogastric Intubation

Orogastric intubation is performed with the animal re-strained in a standing position. The diameter and length of tube needed depends on the size of the animal. A 9.5-mm–diameter foal tube is used with adult sheep and goats. A narrower, 37-cm–long soft rubber feeding tube or metal lamb probe is used to intubate lambs or kids. Because the diameter of the tube used for orogastric intubation is wider than that used for nasogastric intubation, fluids placed into an orogastric tube can be more viscous and can be delivered at a more rapid rate.

A partially used roll of tape is used as a speculum to hold the mouth open. The length of orogastric tube needed to span the distance from the tip of the chin to the last rib is marked on the tube. The distal third of the tube is lubricated with water or water-soluble gel. It is placed through the speculum, over the base of the tongue, and into the esophagus. The tube is advanced until it enters the rumen. Placement of the tube in the rumen is verified before any substances are administered.

Bovine Administration

Balling Gun

A balling gun is used to administer medication boluses to cattle (Figure 3-51). The tip of the gun should be inspected for sharp edges, and the animal's mouth should be emptied of food before the balling gun is inserted. The animal is confined in a head catch. The handler inserts a finger into one nostril and a thumb into the other and pulls the nose dorsally. This causes the animal to open its mouth so the balling gun can be placed over the base of the tongue (Figure 3-52). Care should be taken to avoid pressing the balling gun too deeply into the oral cavity and injuring the pharynx. Alternatively, a hand can be placed into the interdental space to open the mouth.

Orogastric Intubation

Fluids and medications can be administered to cattle through a stomach tube passed from the nose or mouth directly into the rumen (Figures 3-53 and 3-54). Refer to the discussion of rumen fluid collection for a description of the technique used for orogastric intubation of large ruminants with a Frick speculum as a guide (Figure 3-41). The previously

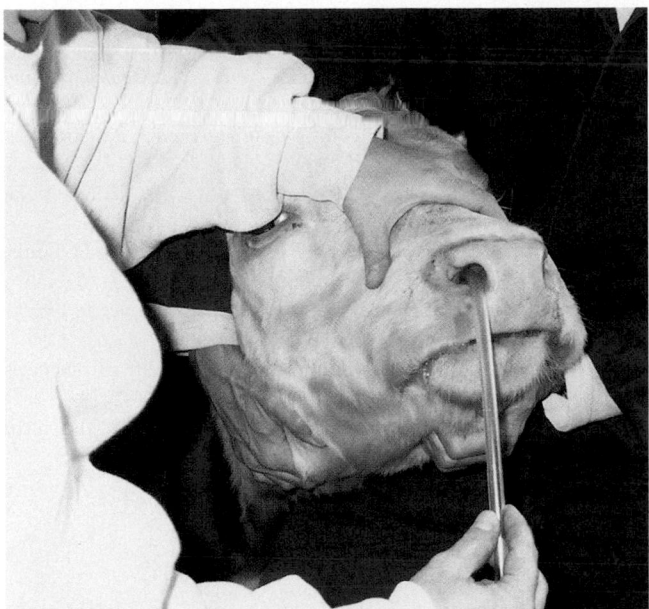

Figure 3-54 Nasogastric intubation of a bovine with a foal stomach tube.

described technique for nasogastric intubation of the sheep and goat can be adapted for cattle.

Equine Administration

Syringe Administration

Oral medications are frequently administered to horses. A variety of preparations are available in paste form, including anthelmintics, vitamin-mineral supplements, antibiotics, and antiinflammatory agents. Some pastes are available pre-packaged in syringes for oral administration. Other pastes must be poured or aspirated into syringes by the technician. Tablets can be pulverized and then combined with water and administered through a syringe or mixed with corn syrup, applesauce, or molasses and added to the feed.

Before oral suspensions are administered, the oral cavity is checked to ensure that it is free of food. The head is raised slightly, and the syringe is inserted into the interdental space on the side of the mouth. As the plunger is depressed, the syringe contents are slowly emptied onto the base of the tongue. The horse should be sufficiently restrained so that it does not move as the injection is made. If the horse moves, the medication may trickle out of the side of its mouth. The horse should not be permitted to drink water immediately after administration because some medication may be lost in the drinking water.

Nasogastric Intubation

Boluses of medication can also be delivered via nasogastric intubation. This procedure should only be performed by a technician while under the direct supervision of the veterinarian. A detailed description of the technique used to pass a nasogastric tube is given in Chapter 28.

> ### 🖉 TECHNICIAN NOTE
>
> Boluses of medication can also be delivered via nasogastric intubation, but a technician should only perform this procedure under the direct supervision of the veterinarian.

INTRAMAMMARY ADMINISTRATION

Intramammary infusion of antibiotics is used to treat or control mastitis. Because potential exists for the introduction of contaminants into the udder during the infusion process, the procedure must be performed aseptically. After the udder is milked out, the teat is cleaned with a dip and thoroughly dried. A separate cloth is used to dry each teat to prevent cross-contamination. The teat is then wiped with 70% isopropyl alcohol and air dried. The teats on the far side of the udder are cleaned before those on the near side.

Teats on the near side are infused before those on the far side. The infusion cannula on the antibiotic syringe is partially inserted into the teat canal. The teat end is grasped and occluded as the udder is massaged to distribute the infused medication. Partial insertion of the cannula into the teat canal delivers fewer contaminants into the udder than does full insertion. Because antibiotic is deposited directly into the streak canal, infection in the canal may be controlled better than when the entire volume of medication is placed in the cistern. Teat dip is reapplied after infusion.

ACKNOWLEDGMENTS

The author wishes to acknowledge the senior students and the faculty members K. Hrapkiewicz, DVM, M. McGonagle, LVT, and M. Robson, LVT, of the of the Wayne County Community College Veterinary Technology program at Wayne State University; M. Seeley, manager of The Charles L. Bowers Farm, Bloomfield Hills, Michigan; and K. Wolfsheimer, DVM, and D. M. McCurnin, DVM, of the Veterinary Teaching Hospital and Clinics, School of Veterinary Medicine, Louisiana State University, who assisted in obtaining photographs for the manuscript. The author also wishes to acknowledge the work of Dr. M. J. Lucas and Ms. S. E. Lucas in the second edition of this book.

Recommended Reading

Baldwin K: Placing an intraosseous catheter in the canine trochanteric fossa, *Vet Tech* 12:656-659, 1999.

Bistner SI, Ford RB, Raffe MR: *Kirk and Bistner's handbook of veterinary procedures and emergency treatment,* ed 7, Philadelphia, 2000, Harcourt Health Sciences.

Crowe DT: Nutritional support for the hospitalized patient: an introduction to tube feeding, *Compend Contin Educ Pract Vet* 12:1711-1720, 1990.

Devitt CM, Seim HB III: Clinical evaluation of tube esophagostomy in small animals, *J Am Anim Hosp Assoc* 33:55-60, 1997.

Ettinger SJ, Feldman, editors: *Textbook of veterinary internal medicine,* ed 5, Philadelphia, 2000, WB Saunders.

House JK, Smith BP, Van Metre DC, et al: Ancillary tests for assessment of the ruminant digestive system, *Vet Clin North Am Large Anim Pract* 8:203-232, 1992.

Kopcha M, Schultze AE: Peritoneal fluid. II. Abdominocentesis in cattle and interpretation of nonneoplastic samples, *Compend Contin Educ Pract Vet* 13:703-710, 1991.

Lawhorn B: A new approach for obtaining blood samples from pigs, *J Am Vet Med Assoc* 192:781-782, 1988.

Orsini JA, Divers TJ: *Manual of equine emergencies,* Philadelphia, 1998, WB Saunders.

Otto CM, Kaufman GM, Crowe DT: Intraosseous infusion of fluids and therapeutics, *Compend Contin Educ Pract Vet* 11:421-430, 1989.

Pratt PP, editor: *Principles and practice of veterinary technology,* St Louis, 1998, WB Saunders.

Raskin RE: Bone marrow. In Slatter D, editor: *Textbook of small animal surgery,* ed 2, Philadelphia, 1993, WB Saunders.

Rose RJ, Hodgson DR: *Manual of equine practice,* ed 2, Philadelphia, 2000, WB Saunders.

Smith MC, Sherman DM, editors: *Goat medicine,* Philadelphia, 1994, Lea & Febiger.

Smith BP, editor: *Large animal internal medicine,* ed 3, St Louis, 2002, Mosby.

Taylor FGR, Hillyer MH, editors: *Diagnostic techniques in equine medicine,* Philadelphia, 1997, WB Saunders.

Terry C, Rashmir-Raven A, RL Linford: Placing an intravenous catheter in horses, *Vet Tech* 4:207-212, 2000

Williams CSF: Routine sheep and goat procedures, *Vet Clin North Am Large Anim Pract* 6:737-758, 1990.

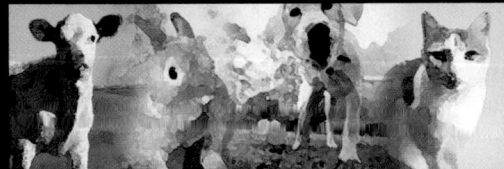

4

Wound Healing, Wound Management, and Bandaging

GISELLE HOSGOOD • DANIEL J. BURBA

INTRODUCTION

The veterinary technician can play an important role in assisting the veterinary surgeon in the management of wounds. The nature of the wound often dictates the method of wound management. Knowledge of the physiology of wound healing and the factors that alter wound healing is required to understand the methods of wound management. The methods of wound management, the role of bandaging in wound management, and the different types of bandages can then be more clearly understood. ■

WOUND HEALING

A wound is created when an insult, either purposeful, such as a surgical incision, or incidental, such as a traumatic injury, disrupts the normal integrity of the tissue. Wound healing is a complex biologic event that is well characterized at the microscopic level, but its regulation at the molecular level is only just beginning to be understood. The process of wound healing begins immediately after the insult and is described in four physical phases: the inflammatory, debridement, repair, and maturation phases (Figure 4-1 and Table 4-1). Wound healing is a dynamic process, and more than one phase of wound healing is usually occurring at any time.

Peptide growth factors appear to play a key role in initiating and sustaining the phases of wound healing (Table 4-2). The platelet appears to initiate the wound healing process through the release of growth factors; the process is then amplified or sustained by wound macrophages, endothelial cells, and fibroblasts. The *inflammatory phase* begins immediately after injury. Blood fills the wound and cleans the wound surface. The blood vessels constrict immediately to slow hemorrhage, but vasoconstriction lasts only 5 to 10 minutes. The blood vessels then dilate and leak fluid

containing clotting elements into the wound. This fluid, combined with blood, causes a blood clot to form. The blood clot stabilizes the wound edges, and fibrin within the clot provides the limited wound strength of this phase. In a sutured wound, the sutures will also provide wound strength at this time. The blood clot will dry and form a scab, which protects the wound, prevents further hemorrhage, and allows healing to progress under its surface. The scab does not provide any wound strength. The blood vessels also leak white blood cells into the wound. This marks the beginning of the debridement phase.

The *debridement phase* begins approximately 6 hours after injury, when white blood cells, namely neutrophils and monocytes, appear in the wound. These cells remove necrotic tissue, bacteria, and foreign material from the wound. The white blood cells, in combination with the fluid that has leaked into the wound, form the exudate commonly associated with wounds.

✎ TECHNICIAN NOTE

During the first 3 to 5 days of wound healing, known as the lag phase, wound strength is minimal.

The *repair phase* begins after the blood clot has formed and necrotic tissue and foreign material have been removed from the wound. The repair phase, which is usually active by 3 to 5 days after injury, is associated with invasion of fibroblasts into the wound. The fibroblasts produce collagen that will mature into fibrous or scar tissue. The repair phase is characterized by a significant increase in wound strength. In contrast, the first 3 to 5 days after injury are associated with a minimal increase in wound strength. Consequently, the first 3 to 5 days are also known as the "lag phase" of wound healing.

Capillaries appear in the wound at the same time fibroblasts appear. The combination of new capillaries, fibroblasts, and fibrous tissue forms the characteristic red, fleshy granulation tissue that fills the wound, often lying underneath the scab.

Granulation tissue characteristically appears in the wound after 3 to 5 days. Poor granulation tissue is white and has a high fibrous tissue content with fewer capillaries. Granulation

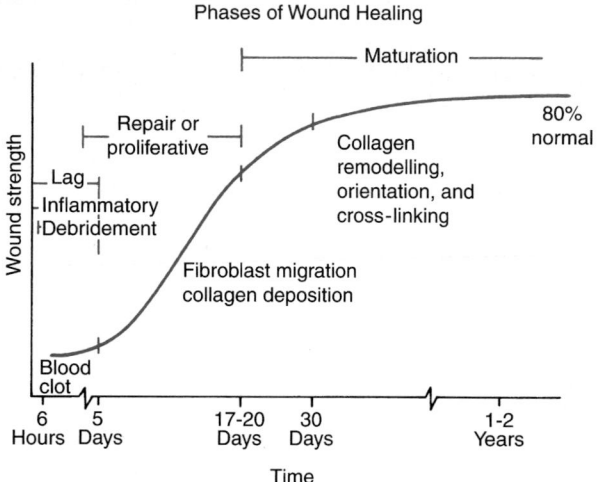

Figure 4-1 Schematic representation of the phases of wound healing and associated changes in wound strength.

Table 4-1 CHARACTERISTICS OF THE MICROSCOPIC PHASES OF WOUND HEALING

Phase	Characteristics
Inflammatory	Begins immediately after injury; characterized by formation of blood clot; platelets stimulate other stages by release of growth factors
Debridement	Part of inflammatory phase; characterized by influx of white blood cells (macrophages, monocytes) into wound; occurs approximately 6 hours after injury; wound healing is sustained by release of growth factors from multiple cell types
Repair (fibroblastic)	Begins 3 to 5 days after wounding; characterized by invasion of fibroblasts and development of granulation tissue; wound strength increases exponentially
Maturation	Characterized by remodeling of the collagen of the scar and slow gain in wound strength; begins approximately 3 weeks after injury and may take weeks to years to complete

Table 4-2 CHARACTERISTICS OF SELECTED GROWTH FACTORS AND EFFECTS ON WOUND HEALING

Growth factor or cytokines	Sources	Effect on Wound Healing and Target Cells
Platelet-derived growth factor (PDGF)	Platelets, macrophages, fibroblasts, endothelial cells	Stimulates replication of fibroblasts and vascular smooth muscle
Transforming growth factor β1 and β2 (TGF-β1, TGF-β2)	Macrophages, lymphocytes, fibroblasts, bone cells, epidermal cells, platelets	Affects wound fibrosis and tensile strength; inhibits replication of most cells (epidermal cells, endothelial cells, lymphocytes, and macrophages); may inhibit or stimulate fibroblasts; may have a modulating effect on wound healing
Transforming growth factor β3 (TGF-β3)	Macrophages	Antiscarring effects
Transforming growth factor α (TGF-α)	Macrophages, eosinophils, epidermal cells	Stimulates replication of epithelial cells, fibroblasts, and endothelial cells; has more potent effect on endothelial cells than EGF
Epidermal growth factor (EGF)	Almost all body fluid, platelets	Stimulates replication of epithelial cells, fibroblasts, and endothelial cells
Insulin-like growth factor (IGF)	Most tissues, fibroblasts, macrophages	Stimulates replication of fibroblasts, endothelial cells, bone cells, neural tissues, and hemopoietic cells; influences granulation tissue formation
Fibroblast growth factor (FGF)	Fibroblasts, bone cells, smooth muscle cells, endothelial cells, astrocytes	Stimulates replication of neural tissue, bone cells, muscle cells, and fibroblasts; influences angiogenesis
Keratinocyte growth factor (KGF)	Fibroblasts	Affects epidermal cell motility and proliferation
Vascular endothelial growth factor	Epidermal cells, macrophages	Enhances angiogenesis and increases vascular permeability
Colony stimulating factor 1	Many cells	Activates macrophages and influences granulation tissue formation

tissue is important in wound healing because it fills the tissue defect, protects the wound, provides a barrier to infection, provides a surface for new epithelial cells to form across, and provides a source of special fibroblasts called *myofibroblasts*, which are responsible for wound contraction.

The formation of new epithelium on the wound surface (epithelialization) occurs during the repair phase and begins once an adequate granulation tissue bed has formed. New epithelium is usually visible on a wound in 4 to 5 days. In an incised wound that is sutured, in which the skin edges are close together, epithelialization can occur almost immediately (as early as 24 to 48 hours after injury), because there is no defect that needs to be filled with granulation tissue. The normal epithelial cells at the edge of the wound divide and produce new cells that migrate across the granulation tissue. Some hair follicles and sweat glands may also regenerate, depending on the extent of damage. The new epithelium is only one cell layer thick initially and is fragile, but it gradually thickens over time as more cell layers form.

Wound contraction helps to reduce the size of the wound but occurs independently of epithelialization. No new skin is formed during contraction. Wound contraction is a result of contraction of the myofibroblasts in the granulation tissue, which pulls the full-thickness skin edges inward. If the skin around the wound is tight and under tension, wound contraction will be limited. Visible wound contraction usually occurs 5 to 9 days after injury.

The *maturation phase* is the final phase of wound healing, during which the wound strength increases to its maximum level because of changes in the scar. Remodeling of the collagen fibers in the fibrous tissue, with alteration of their orientation and increased cross-linking, improves wound strength. The number of capillaries in the fibrous tissue gradually decreases, causing the scar to become paler. The maturation phase begins once collagen has been adequately deposited in the wound and may continue for several years. The wound never regains the strength of normal tissue.

FACTORS AFFECTING WOUND HEALING

Many factors affect wound healing, including host factors such as the health of the animal and the characteristics of the wound and external factors such as the type of wound management and treatment.

HOST FACTORS

Old animals tend to heal slowly, probably because they are often debilitated and have other ongoing health problems. Animals that are malnourished or have a disease causing low serum protein concentrations below 2 g/dl (e.g., liver disease with poor protein production or kidney disease with excessive loss of protein) will have delayed wound healing and decreased wound strength. In addition, the lag phase of wound healing will be prolonged in these animals.

Wound healing is delayed by certain diseases, such as hyperadrenocorticism or Cushing's disease, in which there is an excess of circulating corticosteroids. Corticosteroids delay all phases of wound healing.

Animals with diabetes mellitus have delayed wound healing and a predisposition to wound infection. Animals with liver disease may have clotting factor deficits in addition to low serum protein concentrations.

> **TECHNICIAN NOTE**
> Corticosteroids delay all phases of wound healing.

WOUND CHARACTERISTICS

Foreign material in the wound, such as sutures, surgical implants, drains, or extraneous material, can cause an intense inflammatory reaction that interferes with normal wound healing. Soil particles can contain specific infection-enhancing factors.

Compared with a sharp surgical incision, the incision created with an electroscalpel or electrocoagulation during surgery causes more necrosis at the wound margin, increases the chance of wound infection, and results in a slower gain in early wound strength.

Contaminated tissue becomes infected if the bacteria multiply to a critical number of 10^5 organisms per gram of tissue and then invade the tissue. Whether this occurs depends on the degree of tissue trauma, the amount of foreign material present, the delay between injury and treatment, and the effectiveness of host defenses. Infection stops the repair phase.

Bacterial toxins and associated inflammation directly damage the cells. The wound exudate produced during inflammation can accumulate and separate the tissue, leading to wound infection and delayed wound healing.

> **TECHNICIAN NOTE**
> Infection stops wound repair.

The blood supply to the wound is obviously important for wound healing and is responsible for delivering oxygen and metabolic substrates to the cells. Damage to the blood supply during surgical treatment should be avoided. Tight bandages that compromise the wound's blood supply should not be used. Movement in a healing wound is also detrimental, because it disturbs the fine cellular structures of the healing tissue. Movement across a wound should be limited. It may be necessary to apply a bandage to the affected limb to reduce movement.

EXTERNAL FACTORS

Certain drugs and radiation therapy delay wound healing. Corticosteroids depress all phases of wound healing and increase the chance of infection. Antiinflammatory drugs (aspirin, phenylbutazone, ibuprofen) have little effect on wound strength but will suppress early inflammation. Prolonged aspirin therapy may delay blood clotting. Chemotherapeutic drugs can have an adverse effect on wound healing, depending on their mechanism of action and the time of administration in relation to the time of injury. Radiation can have a profound adverse effect on wound healing, depending on dose and time of exposure in relation to time of injury.

Wound Management

IMMEDIATE WOUND CARE

The wound should be covered with a clean, dry bandage as soon as possible after injury to prevent further contamination and reduce hemorrhage. The bandage should remain in place until definitive treatment is initiated. Water-soluble antibiotic ointments may be applied and may be useful in keeping the wound moist and reducing the microorganism load that is initially contaminating the wound. Antibiotic creams or powders act as foreign bodies and delay wound healing and thus should not be applied.

Once the animal is stabilized and other, life-threatening injuries have been treated, the wound can be prepared for treatment. The bandage is removed, and the wound is packed with sterile gauze or filled with a sterile water-soluble lubricant, such as K-Y Jelly (Johnson & Johnson, Arlington, Texas), or temporarily closed with sutures, towel clamps, or Michel clips (Figure 4-2). This allows skin around the wound to be clipped and prepared for aseptic surgery without the introduction of hair into the wound.

Hair from the edges of the wound can be removed with scissors dipped in mineral oil to prevent it from falling into the wound. Once the skin has been prepared, the lubricant

can be flushed out or the sponges can be removed from the wound.

WOUND LAVAGE

Wound lavage is necessary to remove debris and loose particles and tissue from the wound. It also reduces the number of bacteria in the wound. If infection is suspected, a piece of tissue should be sampled for bacterial culture before lavage. Large volumes of warm, sterile, balanced electrolyte solution are preferred for lavage.

🖉 TECHNICIAN NOTE

Wound lavage with warm, sterile, balanced electrolyte solution is preferred.

Antibiotics should not be added to the fluid. Soaps, detergents, and antiseptic solutions should not be used, because they damage the tissue. The mechanical action of the lavage is the most important factor for successful lavage. Moderate pressure (7 psi) can be generated with a 35-ml syringe and 19-gauge needle; this method is more effective than pouring fluid over a wound. The syringe can be connected to a bag of fluid with a three-way stopcock to facilitate refilling of the syringe (Figure 4-3). A pulsating, high-pressure (70 psi) stream can be generated by means of a Water Pik (Teledyne, Fort Collins, Colo), which is even more effective in reducing the bacterial population and removing necrotic tissue and foreign material from heavily contaminated wounds.

WOUND DEBRIDEMENT

Wound debridement is necessary to remove all contaminated, devitalized, or necrotic tissue and foreign material from the wound (Table 4-3). This can be performed surgically

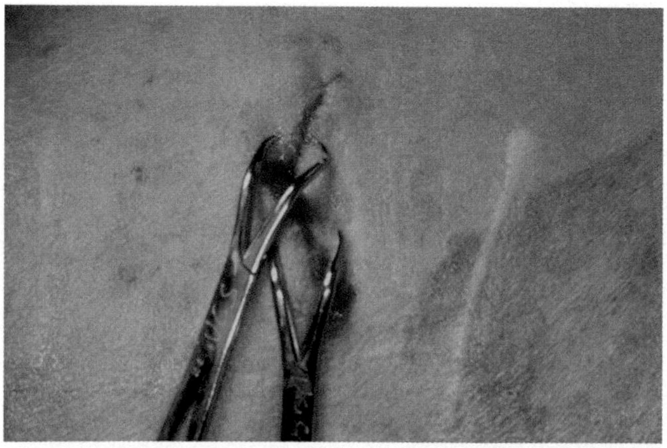

Figure 4-2 The wound is temporarily closed with towel clamps to allow aseptic preparation of the surrounding skin.

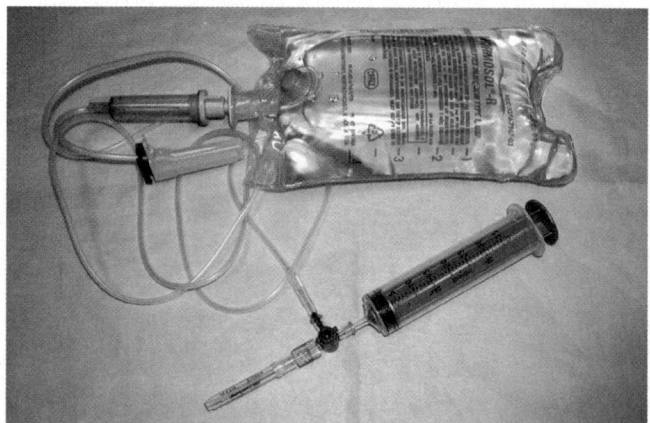

Figure 4-3 Connection of a 35-ml syringe and 19-gauge needle to a three-way stopcock and bag of sterile balanced electrolyte solution to facilitate copious lavage of a wound.

by excising the affected tissue in layers, beginning at the surface and progressing to the wound depths. Alternatively, the entire wound can be excised en bloc if there is sufficient healthy tissue surrounding the wound and vital structures can be preserved (Figure 4-4). Enzymatic debridement with a commercial solution containing trypsin (e.g., Granulex, SmithKline Beecham, Pittsburgh, Pa) can be used for wounds that are not suitable for surgical debridement. Enzymatic debridement is slower and may damage normal tissue.

WOUND CLOSURE

Selection of one of the four methods of wound closure depends on the nature of the wound (Table 4-4). *Primary*

Table 4-3 METHODS AND INDICATIONS FOR WOUND DEBRIDEMENT

Method	Indications
Layered debridement	Conservative debridement beginning at superficial layers of wound and progressing to depths; indicated for large wounds with substantial tissue trauma; may be repeated for heavily contaminated/traumatized wounds
En bloc	Complete excision of wound; indicated for small wounds in areas with loose skin that can be closed primarily
Enzymatic	Use of trypsin products that dissolve necrotic tissue; very slow method of debridement; indicated in minimally contaminated/traumatized wounds or as an adjunct to surgical debridement

wound closure results in healing by first intention. First-intention healing, also known as appositional healing, is achieved by suturing or grafting of a wound soon after injury (Figure 4-5). Primary wound closure is indicated in fresh, clean, sharply incised wounds with minimal trauma and minimal contamination that are seen within hours of injury. Wounds treated within 6 to 8 hours of injury are treated within the "golden period"; that is, bacteria

Table 4-4 METHODS OF WOUND CLOSURE

Method	Comments
Primary closure	Closure of a wound with sutures; indicated for fresh clean wounds with minimal contamination/trauma or surgically created wounds; results in *first-intention healing*
Delayed primary closure	Closure of a wound before 3-5 days after injury; that is, before development of granulation tissue; indicated for moderately contaminated/traumatized wounds
Contraction and epithelialization	Wound allowed to heal without surgical closure; wound closes as a result of contraction and epithelialization; may not be possible or desirable in all wounds; results in *second-intention healing*
Secondary closure	Closure of a wound after 3-5 days; that is, after granulation tissue has developed in the wound; indicated in severely contaminated/traumatized wounds that require considerable debridement and prolonged wound management; takes advantage of the positive effects of granulation tissue; results in *third-intention healing*

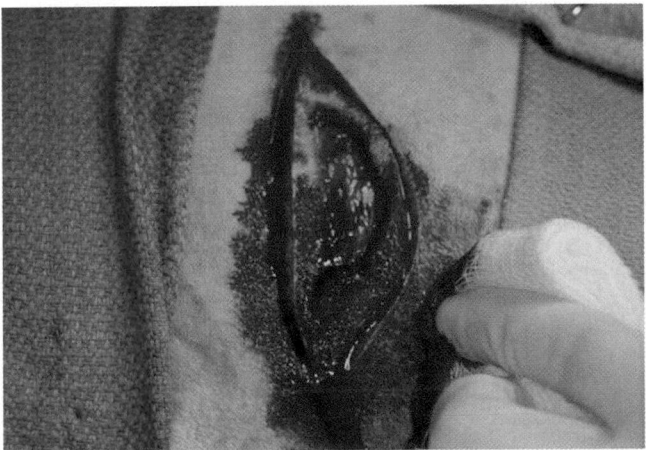

Figure 4-4 For small wounds in areas of loose skin, the entire wound is excised en bloc, and the clean surgical wound that is created is closed primarily.

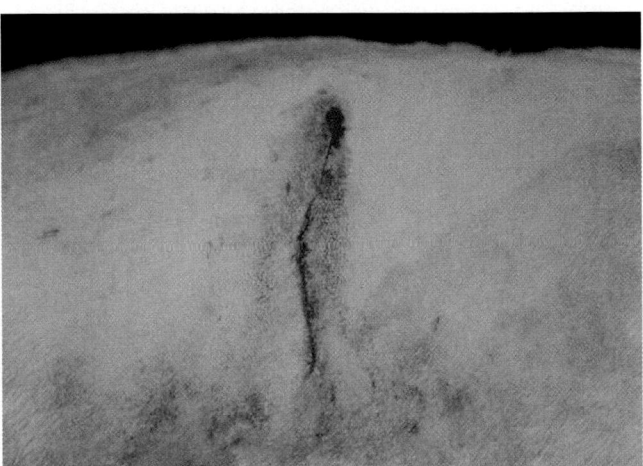

Figure 4-5 A fresh laceration or a surgical wound created after en bloc debridement is closed primarily to allow first-intention healing.

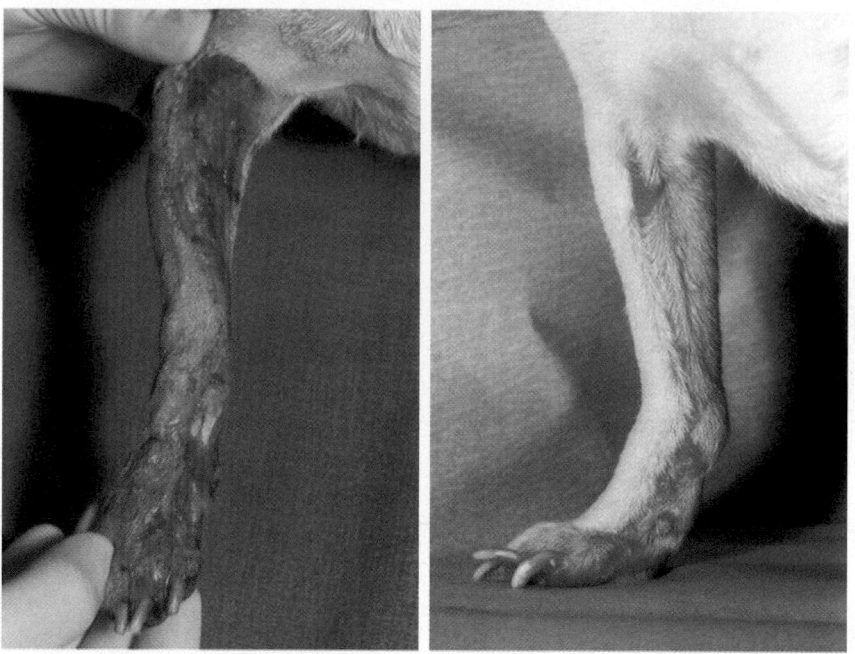

Figure 4-6 **A,** A degloving injury on the antebrachium of a dog. After surgical (layered) debridement and open wound management, the wound healed by second intention with contraction and epithelialization. **B,** After several weeks, the wound is completely closed. Note the hairless, shiny new epithelium and the reduced outline of the wound caused by contraction. The epithelium will thicken over time but will always remain fragile. The pink color will become reduced as the wound remodels underneath the epithelium and the vascular granulation tissue becomes organized fibrous tissue.

contaminating the wound have not multiplied to the critical number of 10^5 organisms per gram of tissue and the tissue has not become infected. Wounds treated after the golden period should not be closed, because infection is likely.

Delayed primary closure is primary closure of a wound 1 to 3 days after injury, before granulation tissue has appeared in the wound. It is indicated for mildly contaminated, minimally traumatized wounds that require some cleansing and debridement or for relatively clean wounds seen 6 to 8 hours after injury. This method allows any local contamination or infection to be controlled before closure.

Healing by contraction and epithelialization is also known as second-intention healing and is indicated for dirty, contaminated, traumatized wounds when cleansing and debridement are necessary and when closure may be difficult. Adequate, loose skin surrounding the wound is necessary to allow contraction. Closure by second intention may not always be desirable because the new epithelium is fragile and easily abraded. In addition, contraction may impede normal function, depending on the location of the wound (Figure 4-6).

Secondary closure results in third-intention healing (Figure 4-7). The wound is sutured at least 3 to 5 days after injury. Granulation tissue will be present in the wound by the time of closure. The granulation tissue helps to control infection in the wound and fills in the tissue defect. Secondary closure is indicated when (1) the wound is severely contaminated or traumatized, (2) epithelialization

and contraction will not completely close the wound, or (3) second-intention healing is undesirable.

The decision about whether to treat a wound primarily or to have it remain open initially and follow up with delayed closure, second-intention healing, or secondary closure depends on the (1) time lapse since injury; wounds greater than 6 to 8 hours old should be kept open initially; (2) degree of contamination; wounds obviously contaminated should be kept open initially and thoroughly cleansed; (3) amount of tissue damage; wounds with substantial tissue damage have reduced host defenses, are more likely to become infected, and consequently, should remain open initially; (4) thoroughness of debridement; if the initial debridement was conservative, the wound should remain open until definitive debridement is performed; (5) blood supply to the wound; a wound with questionable blood supply should remain open until the extent of nonviable tissue is determined; (6) animal's health; if the animal is unable to endure prolonged surgical debridement, the wound should be kept open and possibly undergo enzymatic debridement until the animal can withstand surgery; (7) closure without tension or dead space; if excessive tension or dead space is present, the wound should be allowed to remain open because dead space allows accumulation of fluid, separation of tissues, and formation of seromas, which may predispose to infection and delay wound healing; and (8) location of the wound; certain locations may not be amenable to closure (e.g., a large wound on a limb) (Box 4-1).

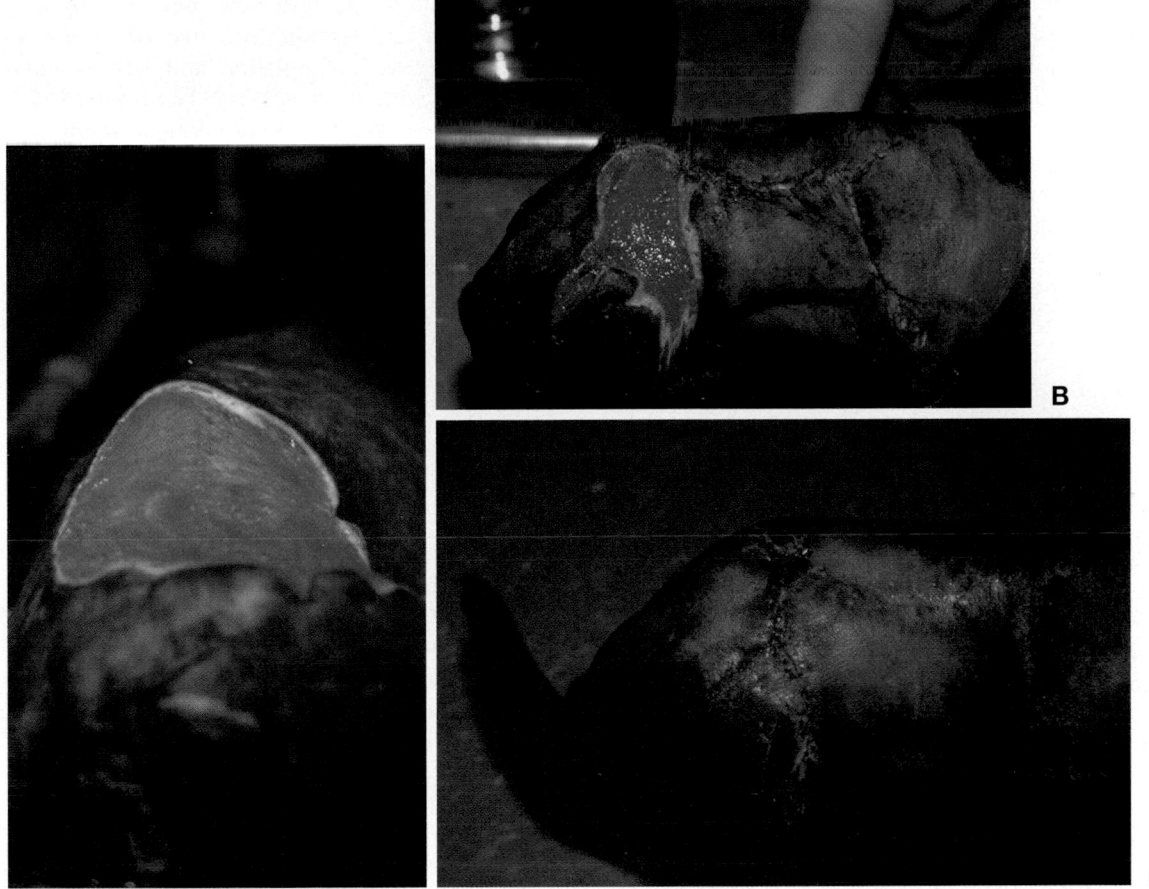

Figure 4-7 **A,** A healthy granulation tissue wound bed on the dorsum of a dog after open wound management of a thermal burn injury (the dog's head is toward the top). **B,** Staged, partial closure of the wound over the granulation tissue allows third-intention healing of the wound (the dog's head is to the right). **C,** Closure of the remaining portion of the wound.

Box 4-1 FACTORS IMPORTANT IN WOUND MANAGEMENT DECISION MAKING

- Time since injury
- Degree of wound contamination
- Degree of tissue trauma
- Thoroughness of initial debridement
- Blood supply of wound
- Animal's physical status
- Wound tension and possibility of closure
- Location of wound

TECHNICIAN NOTE

Nonadherent bandages are indicated for granulating wounds.

Wound Bandaging

Bandages promote wound healing by protecting the wound from additional trauma and contamination, by preventing wound desiccation, by preventing hematoma and seroma formation through compression to obliterate dead space, and by immobilizing the wound to prevent cellular and capillary disruption. Bandages minimize postoperative edema around incisions and minimize exuberant granulation tissue formation in open wounds on the lower limb region (below the carpus or tarsus) of horses. In addition, the bandage can absorb wound exudate and lift away foreign material and loose tissue that has adhered to the bandage as it is removed. Covering a wound with a bandage promotes an acid environment at the wound surface by preventing carbon dioxide loss and absorbing ammonia produced by bacteria. An acid environment increases oxygen dissociation from hemoglobin and subsequently increases oxygen availability in the wound. The bandage also keeps the wound warm. Higher temperatures improve wound healing and facilitate oxygen dissociation (Box 4-2). Leaving a wound open to dry and form a scab is never indicated.

A bandage usually consists of three layers: the primary or contact layer, the secondary or padded conforming layer, and the tertiary or holding and protective layer (Table 4-5). The primary bandage layer has direct contact with the wound surface (if present) and may be adherent or nonadherent.

Adherent primary bandage layers are no longer recommended. The recent consensus among wound care professionals is that moist wound care is the most important management principle. This involves the use of nonadherent primary bandage layers that act to keep the wound surface moist. Nonadherent primary layers that facilitate moist wound care usually include a hydrophilic layer. Moist wound care enhances epithelialization, particularly in partial-thickness skin wounds or abrasions. Moist wound care also enhances natural debridement within the wound by drawing the exudate from the wound and allowing the wound to "bathe" in this cytokine-rich material. Moist wound care results in less inflammation and less wound disruption compared with dry or adherent bandages. Allowing wounds to be exposed and the use of drying techniques such as dry-to-dry (applica-tion of dry gauze sponges) or wet-to-dry (application of wet sponges that later dry out) bandages are no longer acceptable as standard care practices.

The nonadherent primary bandage layer is either occlusive or semiocclusive. An occlusive primary bandage layer is impermeable to moisture but allows some air transfer, whereas a semiocclusive primary bandage layer allows air and moisture vapor to move through the dressing. A semiocclusive primary bandage layer is indicated for wounds with moderate to copious exudate and must be changed frequently (daily to every third day, depending on the volume of exudate production) to avoid maceration of the surrounding normal tissue and skin. An occlusive primary bandage layer is indicated for minimally exudative wounds and is particularly useful for wounds in which promoting epithelialization is the goal, for example, a partial-thickness abrasion or a wound with healthy granulation tissue. Occlusive bandages require changing less frequently (every 4 to 7 days, depending on exudate production) and will accelerate

---

Box 4-2 BENEFICIAL EFFECTS OF BANDAGING A WOUND

- Protects from further contamination
- Prevents wound desiccation
- Prevents hematoma and seroma formation
- Immobilizes the wound and prevents cellular disruption
- Minimizes surrounding edema
- Absorbs wound exudate and debris
- Promotes retention of carbon dioxide and creation of an acid environment, which facilitates oxygen dissociation
- Keeps wound warm, which facilitates healing

Table 4-5 CHARACTERISTICS OF PRIMARY, SECONDARY, AND TERTIARY BANDAGE LAYERS

Layer	Type	Indication and Purpose	Example
Primary	Adherent	No longer indicated in wound care	Dry gauze (dry-to-dry) Wet gauze (wet-to-dry)
	Nonadherent semiocclusive	Moderately or copious exudative wounds; keeps wound surface moist, draws tissue debris from wound. Note: Petrolatum may delay epithelialization.	Transparent polyurethane film (e.g., Polyskin II*) *Without hydrophilic material:* Petrolatum-impregnated gauze (e.g., Adaptic[†]; rayon or Teflon pads (e.g., Telfa pads[†]) *With hydrophilic material:* hydrogel (e.g., Curagel*); hydrocolloid (e.g., Ultec Hydrocolloid Dressing*)
	Nonadherent occlusive	Minimally exudative wounds; partial-thickness wounds (abrasions); keeps wound surface moist and promotes epithelialization; protects new epithelium	*Without hydrophilic material:* OpSite*, Tegaderm Transparent Dressing,* Bioclusive Transparent Dressing[†] *With hydrophilic material:* hydrogel (e.g., Nu-Gel); hydrocolloid (e.g., Hydrocol Dressing)
Secondary	Padding	Absorbs exudate; pads and supports the wound	Cast padding (e.g., Specialist Cast Padding[‡]) Roll cotton
Tertiary	Conforming gauze	Conforming and holding layer	Conforming gauze (e.g., Kling*)
	Nonocclusive elastic adhesive tape	Holding and protective layer, permeable to moisture	Elasticon*
	Nonocclusive elastic bandage	Holding and protective layer, permeable to moisture	3M Vetrap Bandage Tape[§]
	Occlusive tape	Contraindicated	Waterproof tape
	Occlusive wrap	Contraindicated	Plastic wrap

*Tyco Healthcare/Kendall, Mansfield, Mass.
[†]Johnson & Johnson Medical, Arlington, Tex.
[‡]Johnson & Johnson Orthopaedics, Rayham, Mass.
[§]3M Animal Products, St. Paul, Minn.

epithelialization considerably, up to 50% compared with an exposed wound. The occlusive primary bandage layer can also be used as a protective layer for new epithelium, preventing desiccation and abrasion of the fragile tissue. Although the occlusive bandage is nonadherent at the wound surface, some products will adhere to the surrounding local skin. Examples of nonadherent occlusive products that do not include a hydrophilic material include OpSite (Smith and Nephew, Largo, Fla), Tegaderm Transparent Dressing (3M Medical, St Paul, Minn), and Bioclusive Transparent Dressing (Johnson & Johnson Medical, Arlington, Tex). Examples of nonadherent occlusive products that include a hydrophilic material are Nu-Gel (hydrogel) Wound Dressing (Johnson & Johnson Medical) and Hydrocol (hydrocolloid) Dressing (Bertek Pharmaceuticals Inc, Morgantown, WV).

Examples of nonadherent, semiocclusive products (i.e., nonhydrophilic) include petrolatum-impregnated gauze (e.g., Adaptic, Johnson & Johnson Medical) and Teflon- or rayon-based bandages (e.g., Telfa Pads, Johnson & Johnson Medical). These products keep the wound moist yet draw exudate and debris from the wound. All these products are nonadherent, nonirritating, and nontoxic. Petroleum-based products have been shown to enhance wound contraction but may delay epithelialization.

Nonadherent, semiocclusive hydrophilic bandage layers include hydrogel and hydrocolloid bandages. Hydrogel bandages (Curagel, Tyco Healthcare/Kendall, Mansfield, Mass) have a thin layer of hydrogel adhered to a fine synthetic fiber mesh that is semiocclusive. Hydrogel also comes as a water-based paste. The hydrogel layer absorbs the wound exudate, which keeps the wound moist. As the wound exudate is absorbed, particulate matter and microorganisms are also removed, facilitating wound debridement. Hydrocolloid bandages (Ultec Hydrocolloid Dressing, Tyco Healthcare/Kendall, Mansfield, Mass) are starch polymers in an adhesive matrix with semiocclusive polyurethane backing. Hydrocolloid bandages are indicated for granulating wounds. The hydrocolloid becomes gel-like after contact with a moist surface and forms a protective layer at the wound surface. Hydrocolloid bandage layers are indicated for minimal to moderately exudative wounds. Hydrophilic gels and colloids are also available as powders, flakes, beads, and sponges. These materials can be placed in wounds with large defects and act to absorb exudate and remove debris. They are usually covered by a semiocclusive polyurethane film (Polyskin II Transparent Dressing, Tyco Healthcare/Kendall, Mansfield, Mass).

Polyurethane film is a semiocclusive, transparent bandage layer that can be used to cover hydrophilic dressings or used alone as a primary bandage layer on partial-thickness skin wounds if they incorporate a nonadhesive pad (e.g., Tegaderm Transparent Dressing). They are indicated for moderately exudative wounds in which the amount of wound exudate is declining. The polyurethane film is adhesive to the surrounding tissue, and if left on too long, can lead to maceration of the surrounding tissue and damage to the epithelium on removal.

The secondary bandage layer is an absorbent, padded, conforming layer of cast padding (e.g., Specialist Cast Padding, Johnson & Johnson Orthopaedics) or roll cotton that covers the primary contact layer and supports the wound. The tertiary layer is the holding and protective layer, which includes some form of gauze (e.g., Kling, Johnson & Johnson Medical) and elastic (3M Vetrap Bandage Tape, 3M Animal Care Products) or adhesive tape (Elasticon, Johnson & Johnson) to hold the bandage in place. The tertiary layer should be nonocclusive to allow air transfer. However, nonocclusive layers will allow moisture to enter or exit the wound through this layer. When the outer tertiary layer becomes wet, known as strike-through, the wound is at risk for contamination from the environment because bacteria can wick through the moist bandage material. Once the tertiary layer is wet, the bandage must be changed. Although use of an occlusive, water-resistant tertiary layer such as waterproof tape or plastic wrap would prevent this, such materials do not allow air transfer to the wound. Occlusive tertiary layers also trap excessive amounts of fluid at the wound surface, resulting in tissue maceration. For these reasons, occlusive tertiary bandages are contraindicated.

Specific bandages and their indications for use in small animal practice are described in the following sections. The standard procedure for application of any bandage to a limb requires (1) application of anchoring tape strips (stirrups) to the distal portion of the limb; (2) application of a primary bandage layer over the wound; (3) application of the padded secondary layer over the stirrups; (4) application of the gauze tertiary layer; (5) application of the splint; (6) reflection and twisting of the stirrups to adhere to the gauze layer; and (7) application of the protective tertiary layer of tape (Box 4-3). The middle two toes of the bandaged limb should always be exposed to allow for assessment of color, warmth, and swelling. A stockinette can be applied under the secondary layer to help keep the bandage from slipping. Other modifications are also acceptable.

🖉 TECHNICIAN NOTE

The middle two toes of a bandaged limb should always be exposed to allow for assessment of color, warmth, and swelling.

Box 4-3 Steps in Bandage Placement*

- Apply anchoring tapes (stirrups)
- Apply primary (contact) layer on wound
- Apply secondary (padded) layer
- Apply tertiary (conforming) gauze layer
- Apply splint
- Reflect, twist, and adhere tape stirrups to gauze
- Apply tertiary (protective) tape

*Some steps may not be indicated.

WOUND BANDAGING IN SMALL ANIMALS

CASTS

Fiberglass cast materials (DeltaLite "S," Johnson & Johnson Orthopaedics, Arlington, Tex) are currently used almost routinely because of their light weight, extreme rigidity, rapid setting time, and ventilation and waterproof proper-

ties. Casts are indicated for stabilization of certain fractures distal to the elbow or stifle and for immobilization of limbs to protect ligament or tendon repairs. The cast must extend one joint above and below any fracture or structure to be immobilized; hence, a cast is unsuitable for a humeral or femoral fracture. The cast material is applied instead of a tertiary layer; however, minimal padding is suggested to prevent cast loosening and movement and excessive compression (Figure 4-8). Animals with casts should be monitored at least weekly.

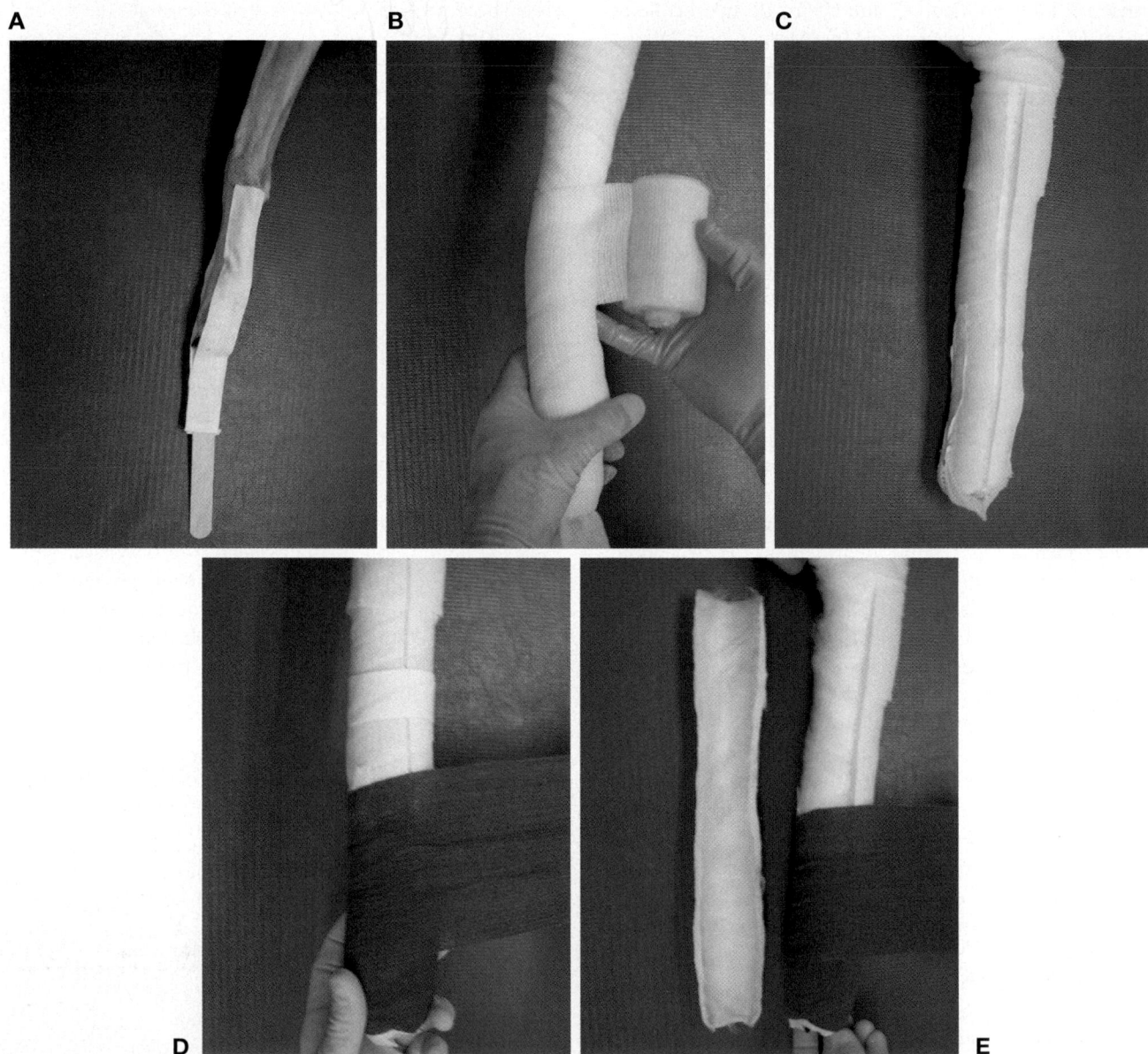

Figure 4-8   Cast. **A,** Tape stirrups are placed on the lateral aspects of the limb. A tongue depressor is placed between them to prevent adherence of the stirrups to each another. **B,** A stockinette is applied over the limb, and a lightly padded, secondary layer is then applied firmly around the leg. The fiberglass casting material is applied firmly but not tightly to the leg, with care taken to avoid compression of the cast material with the fingers. **C,** The cast can be bivalved by cutting it lengthwise. This reduces the risk of excessive compression of the leg. **D,** The two halves are taped together, the stockinette ends are reflected over the cast, and the tape stirrups are reflected onto the cast. Protective tape is applied over the cast. **E,** The caudal half of the cast can be used alone as a custom-fitted splint (see Figure 4-12).

BANDAGES AND SPLINTS

The *Robert Jones bandage* is most commonly used for temporary immobilization of fractures distal to the elbow or stifle before surgery. The bandage must extend one joint above and below any fracture or structure to be immobilized; hence, it is unsuitable for humeral or femoral fractures. It is a large bulky bandage that provides rigid stabilization because of the extreme compression of the thick cotton secondary layer (Figure 4-9).

The *modified Robert Jones bandage,* or simple padded bandage, is a less bulky bandage and is used to reduce postoperative swelling of limbs (Figure 4-10). It provides little or no splinting of the limbs. Less padding is used in the

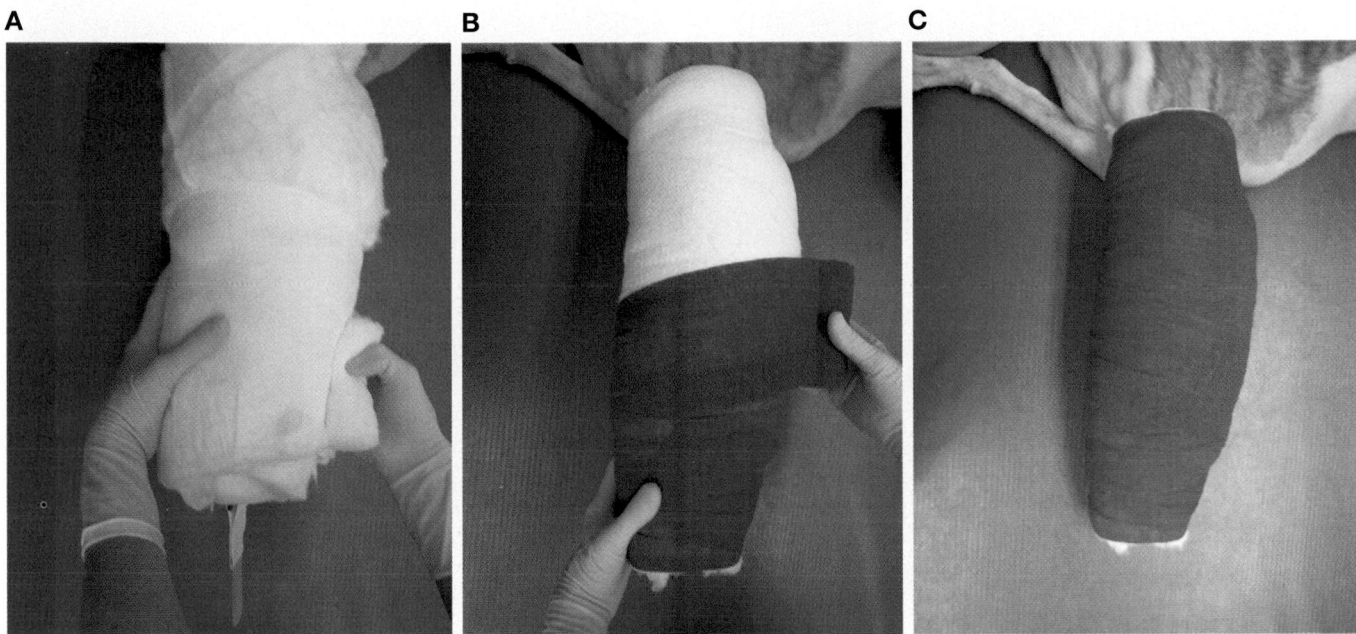

Figure 4-9 Robert Jones bandage. **A,** Tape stirrups are applied, and the limb is wrapped in a secondary layer of roll cotton that extends beyond the joints above and below the fracture or injury. The roll cotton is compressed tightly with a conforming gauze layer. Excessive twisting of the leg should be avoided as the gauze layer is tightened. **B,** The stirrups are reflected on top of the gauze. Protective tape (nonocclusive) is then firmly applied. **C,** The completed bandage should feel solid, and a "ping" should be heard on percussion.

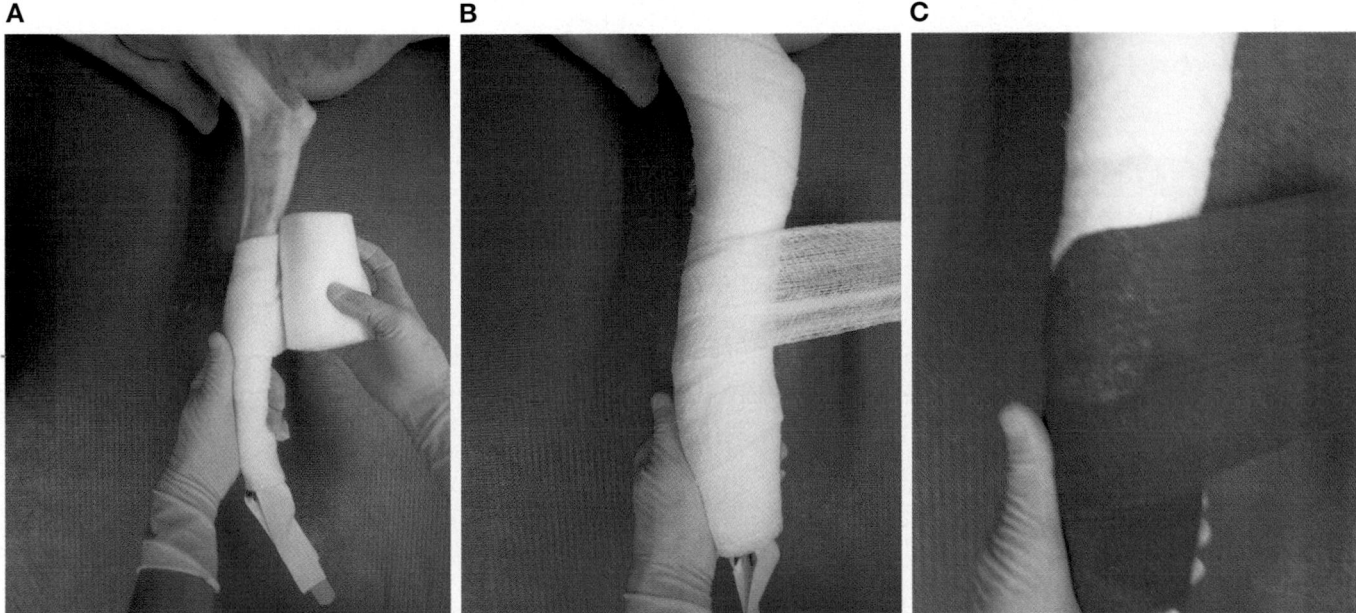

Figure 4-10 Modified Robert Jones or simple padded bandage. **A,** Tape stirrups and a padded secondary layer are applied to the limb. **B,** This is followed by application of a gauze tertiary layer. **C,** The stirrups are reflected to adhere to the gauze, and the bandage is covered by protective tape.

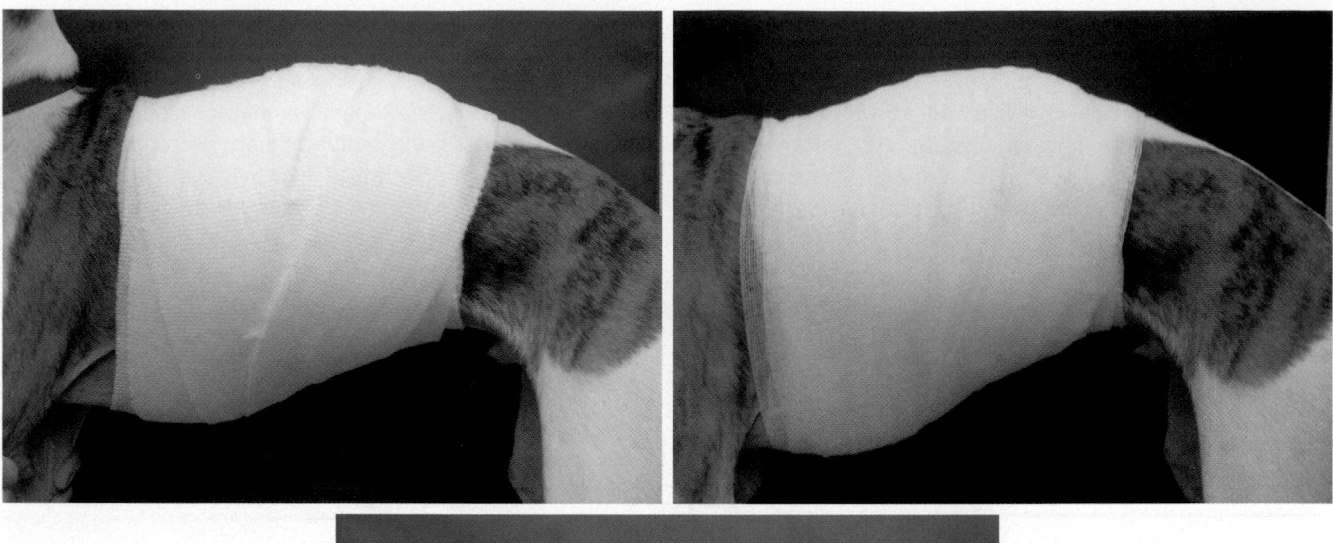

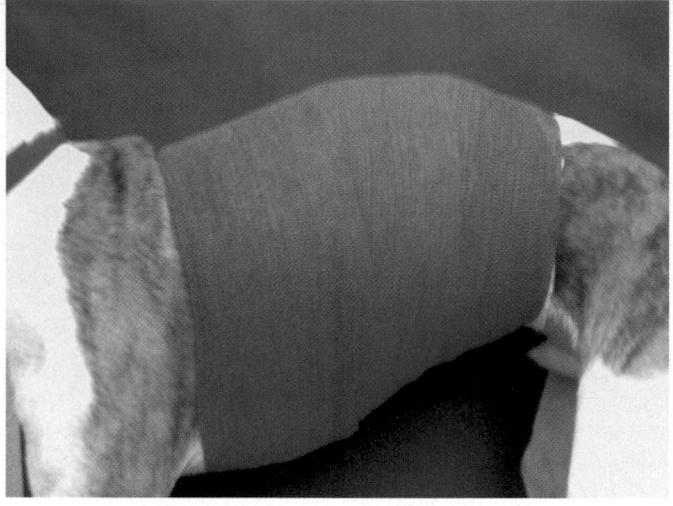

Figure 4-11 Abdominal or chest bandage. **A,** After a primary layer is placed on the wound, the padded secondary layer is applied. **B,** This is followed by application of a gauze tertiary layer. **C,** Protective tape is then applied.

secondary layer, and cast padding is used instead of roll cotton.

> ### ✎ TECHNICIAN NOTE
> The Robert Jones bandage is not appropriate for fractures of the femur or humerus.

A *chest* or *abdominal bandage* is applied in the standard three layers. These bandages should be applied firmly but without constricting the chest or abdomen (Figure 4-11). If an abdominal bandage is used to control abdominal bleeding, the layers are applied more firmly. A rolled towel can be used to reinforce the bandage along the midline, and it is applied before application of the protective tape. The effectiveness of a compression bandage lasts for only 1 to 2 hours, and it should not remain in place longer than 4 hours.

Distal limb splints can be made with tongue depressors for very small animals—or with aluminum splints, cast material, or thermoplastics (Figure 4-12). They are indicated for temporary immobilization or definitive stabilization

of certain fractures of the distal radius and ulna, carpus, tarsus, metacarpals and metatarsals, and phalanges. They can also be used to support a traumatized distal limb. The limb should be well padded to prevent the development of pressure points. The splint should always be placed on the caudal aspect of the limb.

SLINGS

The *Ehmer sling* is used specifically to immobilize a hind limb after reduction of craniodorsal coxofemoral luxation and to prevent weight-bearing after surgery on the pelvis. Correct application results in internal rotation and adduction of the coxofemoral joint (Figure 4-13). Minimal padding is suggested, and the sling is usually applied with adhesive tape alone to prevent slippage.

> ### ✎ TECHNICIAN NOTE
> The 90-90 flexion sling is critical in preventing quadriceps contracture after distal femoral fracture repair in young animals.

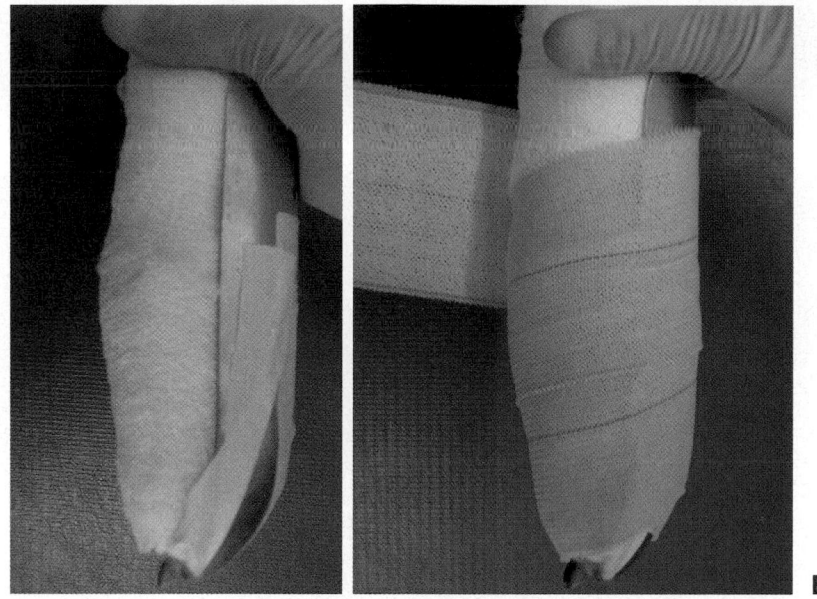

Figure 4-12 Splint. **A,** After application of a modified Robert Jones or simple padded bandage (see Figure 4-10), the splint is applied to the caudal aspect of the limb, and the stirrups are reflected onto the splint. **B,** Protective tape is then applied to hold the splint in place.

The *90-90 flexion sling* is applied with the stifle and hock placed in 90-degree flexion, and no attempt is made to adduct and internally rotate the coxofemoral joint (Figure 4-14). The 90-90 flexion sling is used to prevent stifle joint stiffness and hyperextension caused by quadriceps muscle contracture after distal femoral fracture repair in young animals. It can also be used as a non–weight-bearing sling to protect other surgical procedures on the hind limb.

The *Velpeau sling* holds the flexed forelimb against the chest and prevents movement in all joints (Figure 4-15). It is used as a non–weight-bearing sling for the forelimb. The Velpeau sling is indicated after reduction of scapulohumeral joint luxation or for immobilization of scapular fractures.

The *carpal flexion sling* is a non–weight-bearing forelimb sling (Figure 4-16). The degree of carpal flexion can be reduced by partially cutting the crisscross of tape formed at the caudal aspect of the carpus.

Hobbles can be applied to the hind limbs to prevent excessive abduction of the limbs. They are specifically indicated after reduction of ventral coxofemoral luxation and to prevent excessive tension in the inguinal region. They can be used to prevent excessive activity after pelvic fracture repair or for nonsurgical, conservative management of pelvic fractures (Figure 4-17).

AFTERCARE OF CASTS, BANDAGES, SPLINTS, AND SLINGS

Close monitoring of animals with casts, bandages, splints, or slings is extremely important and should be performed daily for inpatients and at least weekly for outpatients. Client education for outpatients is essential. The toes should be monitored daily for warmth, color, and swelling. Abnormal findings indicate a tight cast. Monitoring the bandage for a foul odor that would indicate tissue damage is necessary. Observation for areas of chafing from the cast is important. The animal should be restrained from chewing at the bandage (e.g., by means of an Elizabethan collar), and exercise should be restricted to brief leash walks. While the animal is outside, the bandage should be protected from dirt and moisture by application of a plastic bag or other waterproof material. The plastic covering should not remain on for more than 30 minutes, because it prevents the bandage from "breathing" and allows the underlying tissue to become moist and macerated.

Specific Wound Management

Characteristics of certain wounds may influence the type of wound management performed. The characteristics of certain wounds and management indications are listed in the following sections.

ABRASIONS

Abrasions are partial-thickness wounds of the epidermis with exposure of the deep dermis. Abrasions can be very painful. Abrasions are associated with minimal bleeding and develop minimal exudate. Abrasions heal by reepithelialization. Healing of abrasions will be enhanced by keeping the wound surface moist and protected rather than allowing

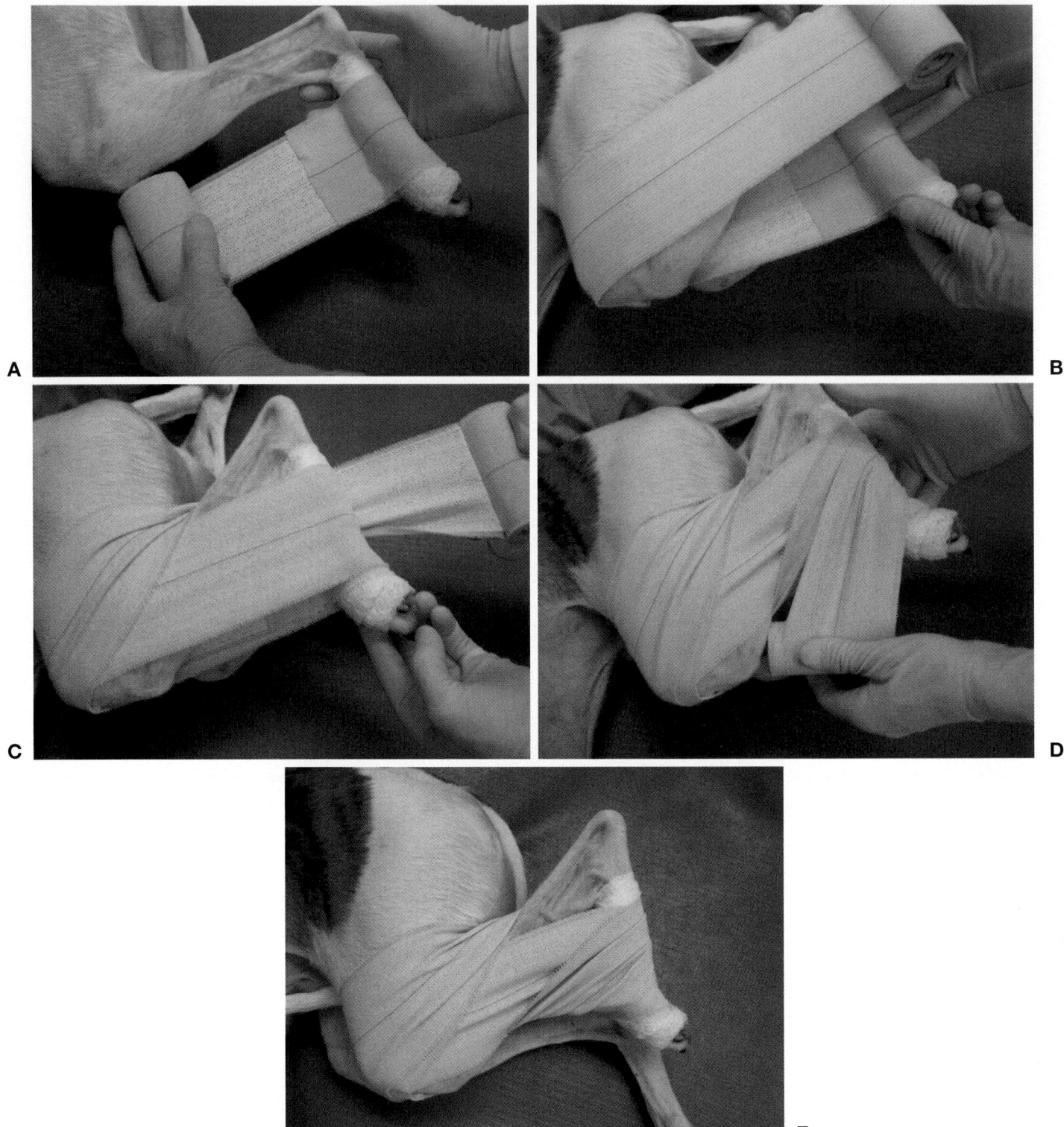

Figure 4-13 Ehmer sling. **A,** After minimal padding has been applied to the tarsus, a sling of adhesive tape is passed along the medial aspect of the limb. **B,** The tape is then wrapped around the hind limb with the stifle and hock held in maximum flexion for one or two passes. **C,** On the third pass, the tape is brought over the flank and twisted behind the hock. **D,** The tape is then passed over the front of the metatarsus. **E,** This wrapping is repeated for three or four passes.

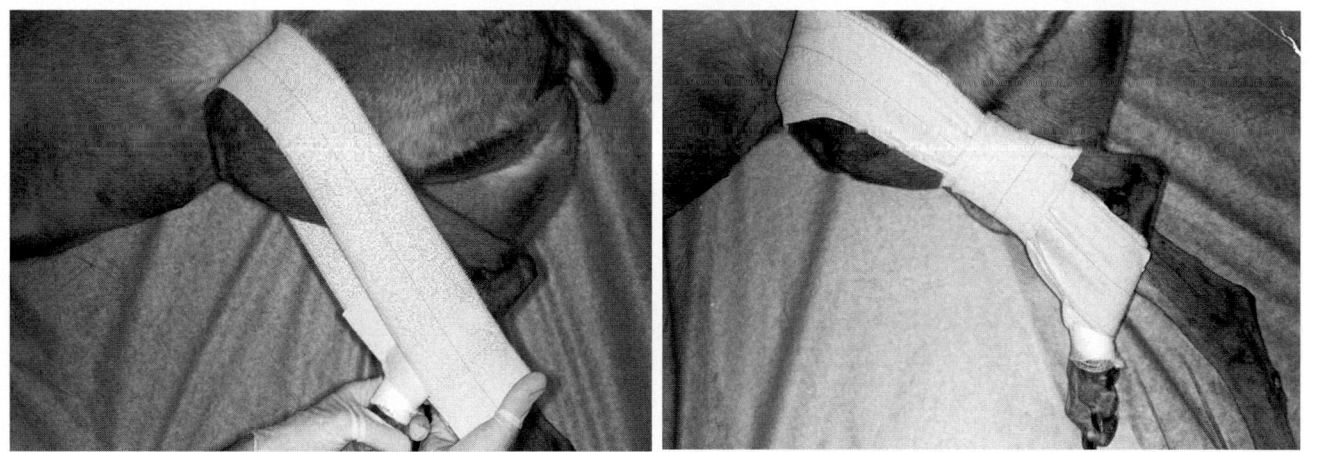

Figure 4-14 A 90-90-degree flexion sling. After minimal padding has been applied to the tarsus, a sling of adhesive tape is passed along the medial aspect of the limb (see Figure 4-13, *A*). **A,** The tape is then wrapped around the hind limb with the stifle and hock held in 90-degree flexion. **B,** A second layer of tape is passed horizontally around the tibia to hold the previous layer in place.

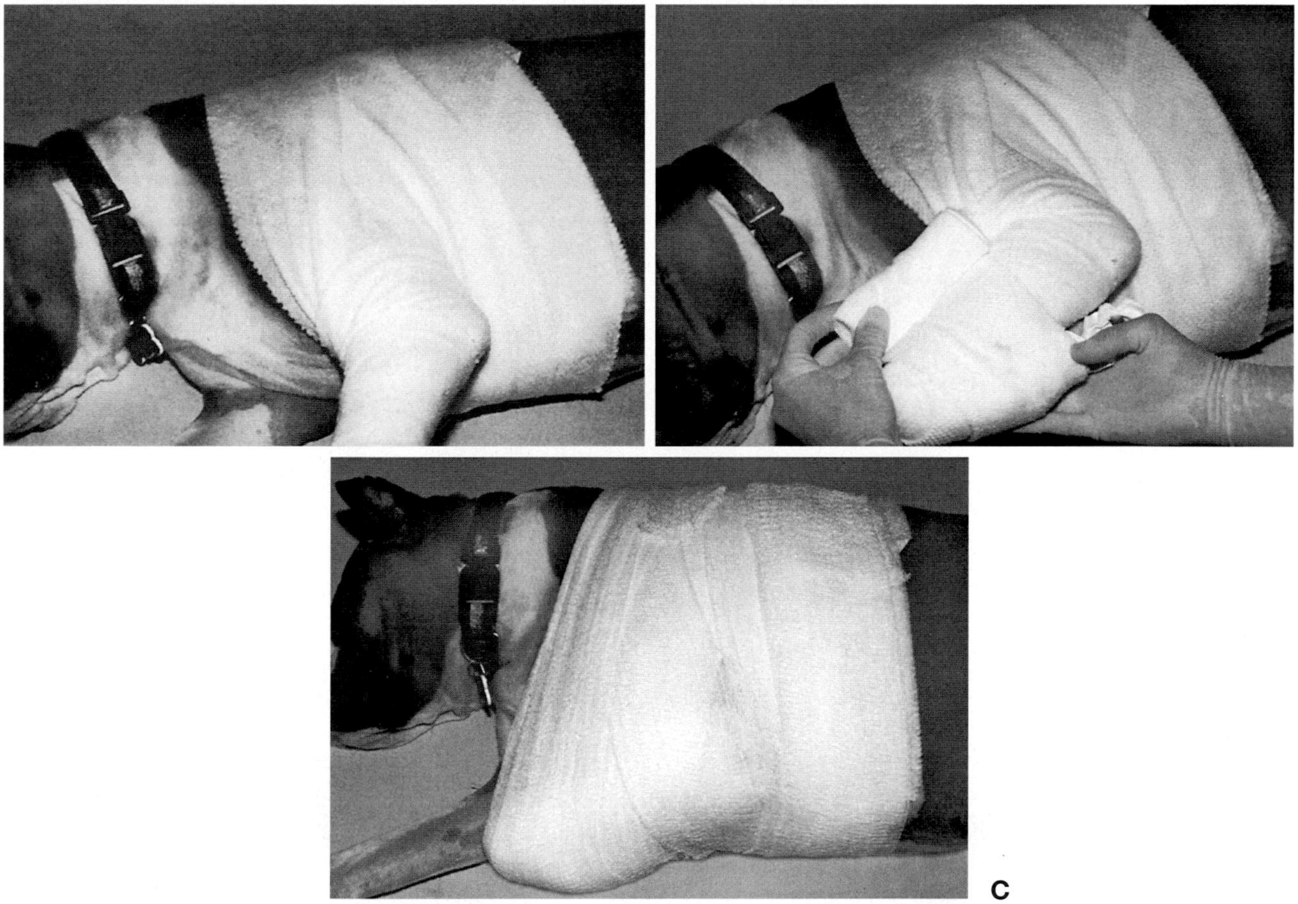

Figure 4-15 Velpeau sling. **A,** Stirrups are applied to the forelimb. The entire forelimb and chest are covered with a light padded bandage. **B,** The carpus is then flexed and covered with an additional layer of a light padded bandage. **C,** The flexed carpus and foreleg are then compressed against the chest and held in place with a conforming gauze layer.

Continued

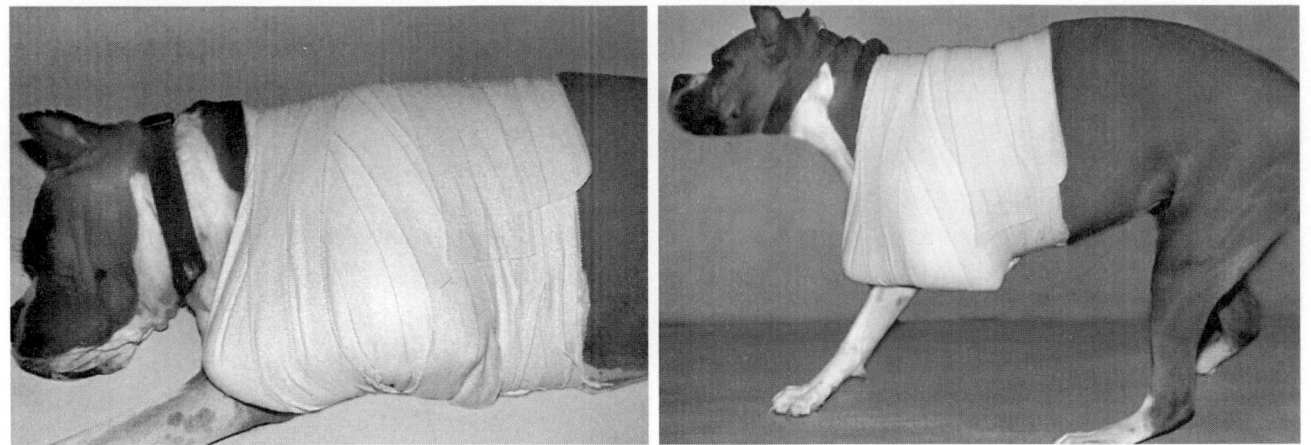

Figure 4-15 *cont'd* Velpeau sling. **D** and **E,** The entire leg and chest area are then covered by protective (nonocclusive tape).

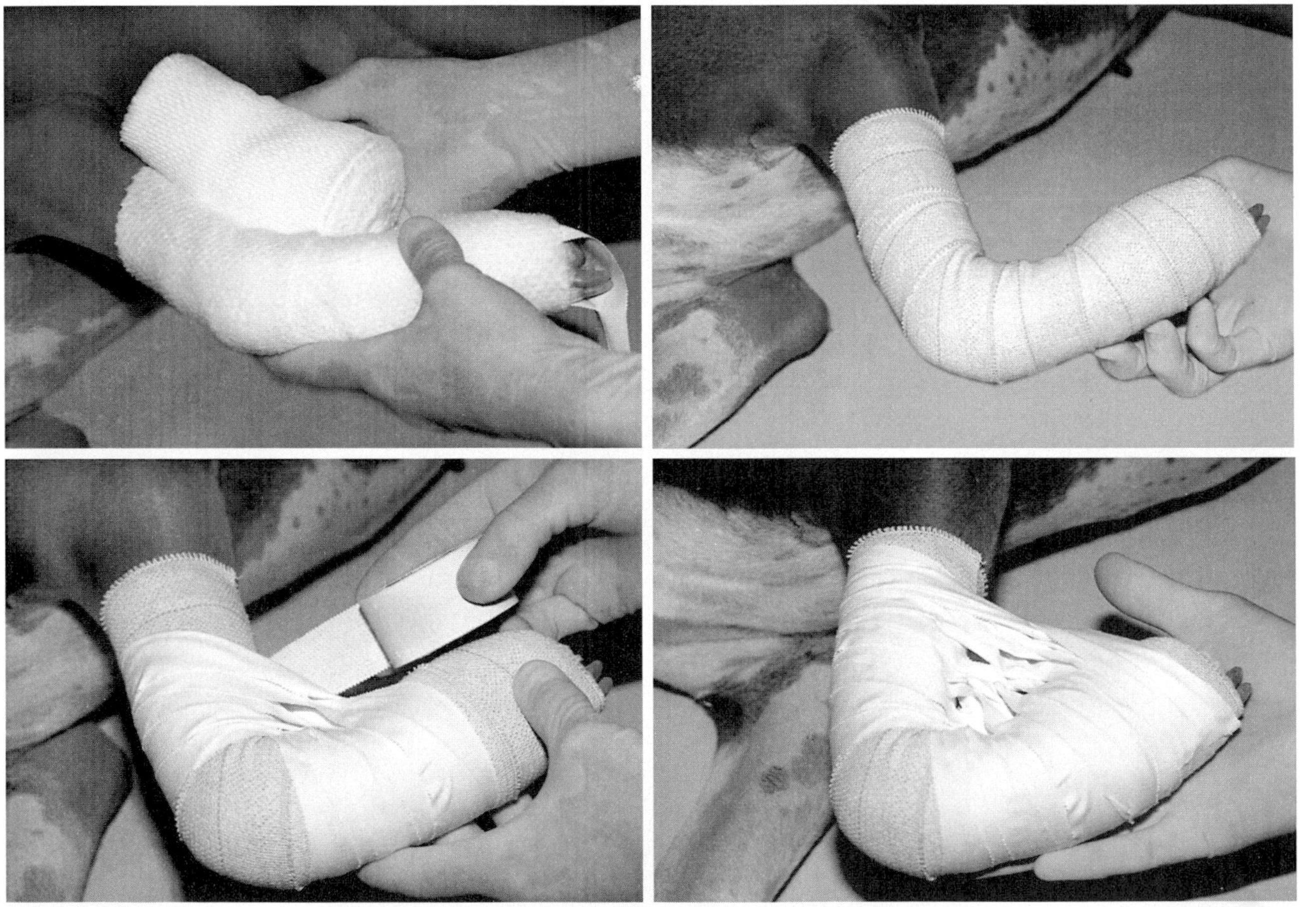

Figure 4-16 Carpal flexion sling. **A,** Stirrups are applied. With the limb in flexion, a lightly padded bandage is applied. **B,** The stirrups are reflected, and protective (nonocclusive) tape is applied. **C** and **D,** One-inch tape is then applied in a figure-of-eight fashion around the carpus to support it. The tape starts at the middle of the carpus and then extends proximally and distally, forming a web of tape behind the carpus.

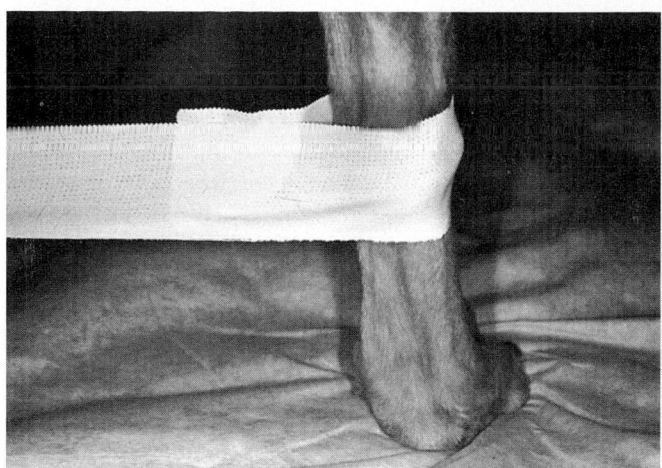
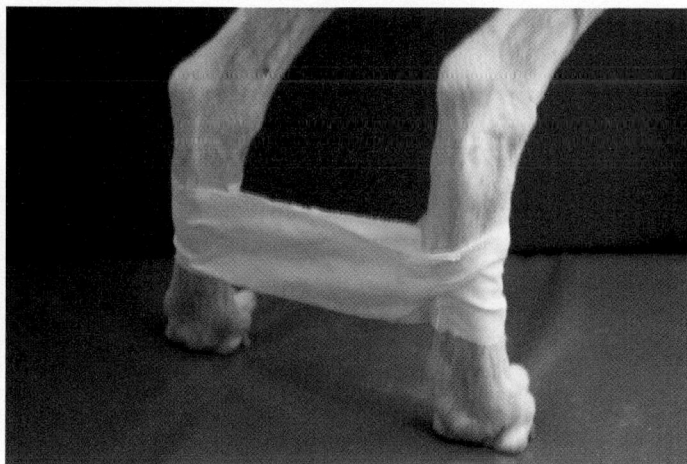

A   **B**

Figure 4-17 Hobbles. **A,** Adhesive tape wide enough to cover half of the metatarsal region is placed loosely around the metatarsal region. **B,** The tape is then adhered together between the legs and placed around the opposite metatarsus. The hind limbs are positioned apart at a distance equal to the width of the pelvis.

a scab to dry on the surface. Application of a nonadhesive, semiocclusive primary layer with a minimal amount of padding and a nonocclusive tertiary layer is indicated. Hydrophilic primary layers are ideal for these wounds because they promote epithelialization. Bandages can be changed every 3 to 4 days, and an abrasion should be kept bandaged until the surface has completely resurfaced with new epithelium.

LACERATIONS

Lacerations are characterized by sharply incised edges with minimal tissue trauma. They may be superficial (skin) or deep (tendons, muscle). If tissue is torn away, the wound is called an *avulsion.* Lacerations presented within 12 hours of injury are amenable to minimal debridement of the tissue edges, lavage of the wound, and primary closure. Lacerations seen later than 12 hours after injury may be best treated by en bloc debridement of the wound and primary closure. Although uncommon, heavily contaminated lacerations or old lacerations may be best treated by debridement, lavage, and delayed primary or tertiary closure.

BURNS

Burns are classified by degree of tissue injury (Table 4-6).

The most common causes of burns in companion animals are fire, cage dryers, prolonged contact with heating pads, heat lamps, spillage of hot liquid, and contact with electrical cords. Unfortunately, these causes often result in fourth-degree burns characterized by extensive tissue damage. Animals with more than 50% of the body surface burned rarely survive.

Table 4-6 CLASSIFICATION OF THERMAL BURNS

Classification	Description
First degree	Very superficial burn that involves only the epidermis. Does not blister but becomes erythematous because of dermal vasodilatation and is painful. Over 2 to 3 days, the pain subsides, and the damaged epidermis desquamates.
Second degree	Superficial burn that involves all layers of dermis. Characteristically forms blisters with fluid collection at the interface of the epidermis and dermis. Blistering may not occur for several hours after injury.
Third degree	Full-thickness burn that involves all layers of the dermis. The surface may appear white or black and leathery, firm, and depressed compared with surrounding skin.
Fourth degree	Full-thickness burn that involves not only the dermis, but also subcutaneous fat and deeper structures

Animals with fourth-degree burns require intensive management. The large surface area of tissue damage and the extent of the deep tissue damage result in large volumes of fluid, electrolyte, and protein loss through the wound surface. Burn wounds are prone to infection because of the extensive tissue damage, the large surface area exposed to the environment (contamination), and the compromised condition of the animal.

Treatment of an animal with severe burns requires intravenous crystalloid and colloid fluid administration, antibiotic administration, nutritional support, and intensive wound management. Nutritional support is extremely important because the metabolic requirements of the animal may increase up to 200%. The animal is unlikely to take in adequate nutrition voluntarily. Force feeding or enteral feeding through a pharyngostomy, esophagostomy, or gastrostomy tube is indicated.

The wounds must be debrided and managed as open wounds. Any dead skin (eschar) must be removed. Debridement may have to be repeated, particularly for fourth-degree wounds, because the extent of the tissue damage may not be evident initially. Burn wounds tend to produce copious, often viscous exudate. Use of hydrophilic primary bandage layers will keep the wound moist yet absorb the exudate and facilitate removal of any tissue debris. A padded bandage to absorb the exudate with a nonocclusive tertiary layer is required. Ideally, sterile bandage material should be used. Bandages should be changed as often as required to prevent strike-through of the bandage by exudate from the wound. Once healthy granulation tissue is apparent in the wound, application of a semiocclusive, nonadherent primary bandage layer is indicated. Coating the wound with salves or lotions is contraindicated because they can be occlusive and prevent oxygen transfer to the wound. In addition, they trap wound exudate over the normal margins of the wound, which may macerate the tissue. After a healthy granulation tissue wound bed has developed, the wounds are then amenable to tertiary closure or skin grafting.

PUNCTURE WOUNDS

Puncture wounds are characterized by small skin openings with often extensive deep tissue damage. Penetrating injuries caused by sharp objects (e.g., sticks), gunshots, bite wounds, and insect stings are all types of puncture wounds. Foreign material and bacteria are carried deep into the wound. Puncture wounds should be treated by exploration, debridement, lavage, and primary closure if all the damaged contaminated tissue and all foreign material can be removed from the wound. If the wound remains contaminated, or if there is a large amount of deep tissue damage with resultant dead space in the wound, a drain may be placed. Ideally, a closed suction wound drain that connects to a closed reservoir should be used to reduce contamination of the wound from the environment via the drain. A closed drain also allows the volume and nature of the drainage to be monitored.

DEGLOVING INJURIES

Degloving injuries are commonly seen in small animals and are typically the result of being hit by a car and dragged over the road surface. An anatomic degloving injury results in skin and varying amounts of deep tissue (muscle, tendon, ligament, bone) being torn off a limb. A physiologic degloving injury is characterized by an intact skin surface with disruption of the skin attachment and neurovascular supply at the deep fascial level. Necrosis of the detached skin becomes apparent 3 to 5 days after injury.

Degloving injuries require intensive management over a prolonged period. Initial debridement, lavage, and management of the open wound are required. It may take several weeks before the wound is covered by a healthy granulation tissue bed. At this time, skin grafting is indicated. Some degloving injuries will completely heal by second intention, although the tension on the skin of the distal extremities can be a limiting factor. In addition, the resultant skin contracture and friable new epithelium may not always be a desirable outcome.

DECUBITUS ULCERS

Decubitus ulcers are the result of compression of soft tissues and skin between a bony prominence and the surface on which an animal is lying. Thin, debilitated animals that are recumbent for long periods are at risk, as are the naturally thin breeds (e.g., Afghan hounds, Greyhounds, Whippets). The soft tissue and underlying bone of decubitus ulcers may become secondarily infected by environmental microorganisms.

Prevention is the key to management. Adequate soft bedding (water beds) is essential for an at-risk animal. The animal's position should be changed frequently throughout the day. Likely pressure points should be examined daily. Physical therapy and hydrotherapy three or four times per day help to keep the skin clean and promote peripheral circulation. The bedding should be kept clean, dry, and free of excreta. Vulnerable sites can be padded. Maintaining the animal on a high nutritional plane (high-protein, high-carbohydrate diet) is essential.

Closure of existing decubitus ulcers is desirable. Minimal debridement is usually required. Closures often fail because the line of wound closure also overlies a pressure point, and tension is often apparent on the wound edges. In some instances, skin flaps may be preferred.

Large Animal Wound Management

WOUND CARE OF HORSES

Basic wound management is no different in large animals than in small companion animals. However, the size and nature of the animal as well as the location of the injury may dictate the way a wound is approached. Thus some additional points are briefly discussed.

When a wound on a horse is prepared, a water-soluble lubricant or saline solution–soaked gauze can be used to fill the depths of the wound. Electric clippers are usually used to remove the hair from around the edges of the wound. However, if clippers are not available, the wound edges can be lathered with antiseptic scrub, and a straightedge razor or No. 22 scalpel blade can be used to shave the hair (Figure 4-18).

> **✎ TECHNICIAN NOTE**
>
> It is important to clip or shave the hair surrounding a wound.

Methods used to lavage a wound are similar to those described for small companion animals, earlier in this chapter. Local anesthesia with tranquilization or general anesthesia may be needed before a fresh wound can be properly treated. If tranquilization is used, local or regional anesthesia is necessary for debridement and closure of the wound. Local infiltration is performed by injecting a local anesthetic, mepivacaine or lidocaine, approximately 1 cm from the wound edge, subcutaneously around the entire wound. A 22-gauge hypodermic needle is used in most situations and is reinserted repeatedly through the skin, each time at the end of the bleb formed by the preceding injection of local anesthetic (Figure 4-19). In this way, the patient will not react to the successive injections. If the wound is located on the distal portion of a limb, a ring block or nerve block (e.g., a palmar nerve block) can be applied, and the portion of the limb distal to the block will be anesthetized.

If a wound is to be sutured, the same considerations for wound closure in small companion animals apply to large animals. It is important to remember that open wounds on the distal aspect of the limb (below the carpus or tarsus) of the horse are notorious for developing exuberant granulation tissue. Exuberant granulation tissue, commonly referred to as "proud flesh," can form rapidly in horses. Various measures must be undertaken to keep exuberant granulation tissue in check, or it can become excessive (Figure 4-20). Methods of controlling granulation tissue include immobilizing the limb (as with a cast), wound bandaging, surgical excision, caustic agents such as equal parts of copper sulfate and boric acid powder, cryotherapy, electrocautery, and topical corticosteroids. Regardless of the decision to allow a wound on the limb of a large animal to heal by first or second intention, a bandage should be placed on the limb.

BANDAGING AND CAST APPLICATION TECHNIQUES FOR HORSES

Bandages and casts serve many purposes and are named for the location and purpose they cover and serve, respectively. Various materials are available for use in a bandage or cast, but the important aspect is their proper application and function. Development of good bandaging and cast application skills is important to ensure proper function of the bandage or cast. The application and purpose of the different types used on horses are discussed.

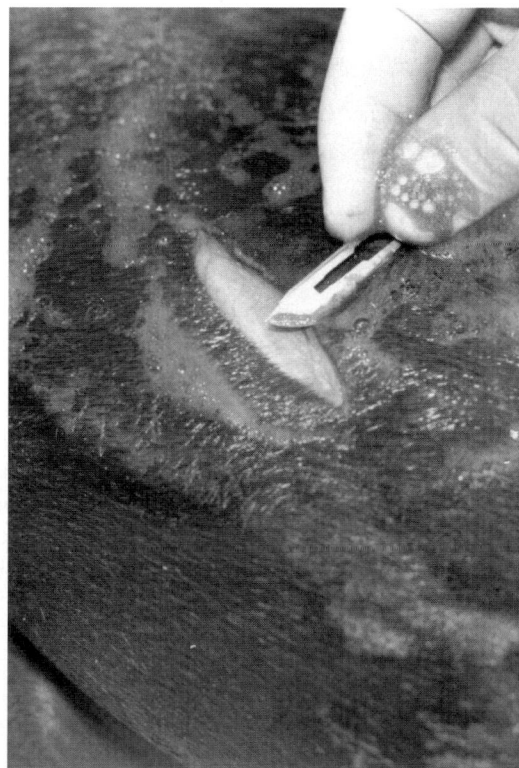

Figure 4-18 Once the hair has been lathered with antiseptic (Betadine) scrub, a No. 22 scalpel blade can be used to shave away the hair from the wound edges.

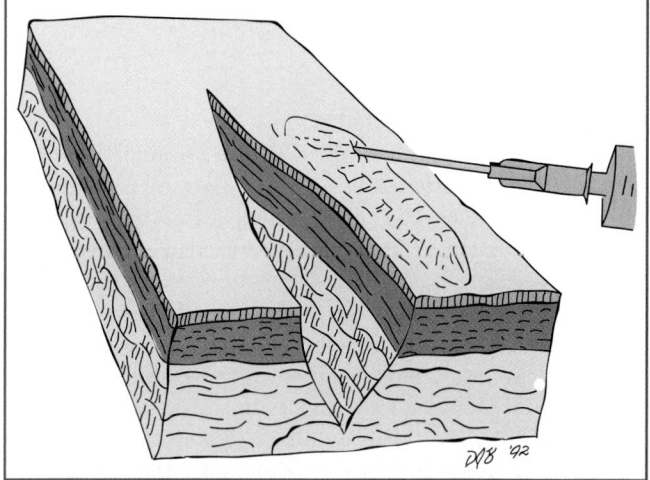

Figure 4-19 Proper technique for infiltration of a wound edge with a local anesthetic. The needle should enter through the skin at the point of the last injection.

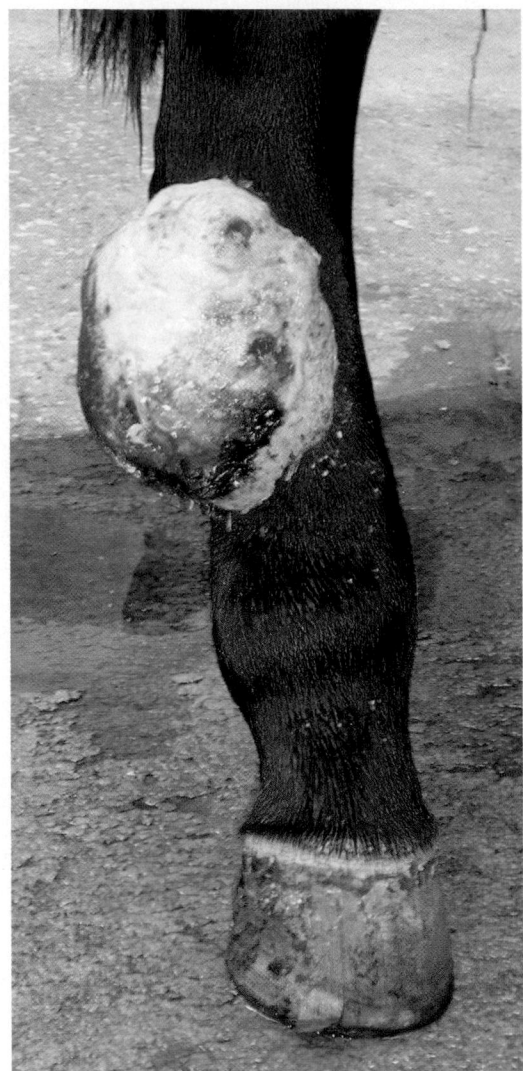

Figure 4-20 Exuberant granulation tissue on the metatarsus of a horse.

BANDAGES

Lower Limb Wound Bandage

A *lower limb wound bandage* covers a wound on a limb distal to the carpus or tarsus. When the wound is traumatic, after it has been cleaned and debrided, a topical medication is usually applied if it is left unsutured. A nonadherent dressing is then placed directly over the wound. The wound dressing is secured to the limb with rolled conforming gauze. The conforming gauze is wrapped around the limb with *light* pressure, overlapping, and without wrinkles to prevent formation of pressure lines, which may cause skin sloughing if applied too tightly. It is wrapped proximal and distal to the wound edges approximately 2 to 4 cm (Figure 4-21).

The padded layer is applied next. Combine cotton sheets cut from a roll, rolled cotton, layered cotton sheet, quilted leg wraps, or a military field bandage can be used (Figure 4-22).

If cotton sheets are available, five are used, folded in half and neatly rolled. The fifth sheet is folded in the opposite direction to the other sheets to conceal the edges. The padded layer is secured to the limb with a roll of conforming gauze. Pressure is applied during wrapping to compress and conform the padding to the limb. The outer shell of the bandage is finished with elastic wrap (3M Vetrap Bandage Tape or an Ace bandage), adhesive elastic tape (Elasticon, Johnson & Johnson), or a flannel track wrap. If an Ace bandage or track wrap is used, it is secured with white tape cut into strips or placed around the bandage in a "barber pole" fashion. Elasticon is placed around the top and bottom of the bandage, with half of the tape sticking to the wrap and half to the skin, to prevent slippage and to keep debris (e.g., bedding shavings) from getting inside the bandage (Figure 4-23).

Lower Limb Support Bandage

A lower limb support bandage is used to provide support for the soft tissues (e.g., ligaments, tendons) of the limb contralateral to the injured leg, which is bearing excessive weight because of decreased weight-bearing on the injured limb. The bandage also minimizes static limb edema in a confined, inactive horse. A support bandage is placed on the lower limb, just like the lower limb wound bandage described previously, except that the underlying wound dressing and inner conforming gauze layer are not used. It is also unnecessary to place wide adhesive elastic tape around the top and bottom.

SPLINT APPLICATION

A splint is an addition of a rigid material to a limb bandage to reinforce immobilization of a particular part of a limb. Various materials can be used as the reinforcement, including wooden slats, metal bars, low-temperature thermoplastic, and casting material. However, the most common material used is polyvinyl chloride (PVC) pipe, because of its light weight and strength. The pipe used is 10 cm in diameter and is split in thirds. It can be bent by heating with a cutting torch to conform to the fetlock angulation. The length and width of the splint vary with the size of the leg and the area being splinted. Depending on the amount of immobilization required, splints can be placed the full length of the forelimb or from just below the carpus or tarsus all the way to the ground surface. In most situations, they are placed on the flexor surface of the limb. Splints are used in situations such as cases of extensor or flexor tendon lacerations and flexure deformities in foals or as needed limb support (as in radial nerve paresis).

A thick bandage is first placed on the limb. It should be long enough to cover the limb above as well as below the ends of the splint. This will prevent the development of pressure sores. Once the bandage is in place, the splint is secured to the limb with adhesive tape (Figure 4-24). Splints should be reset frequently (at least once per day) in foals.

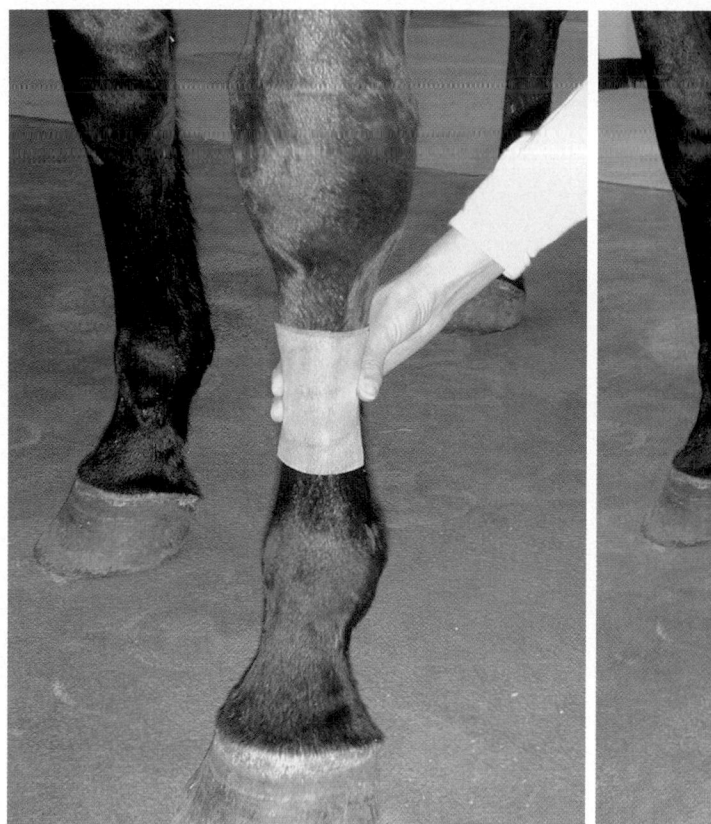
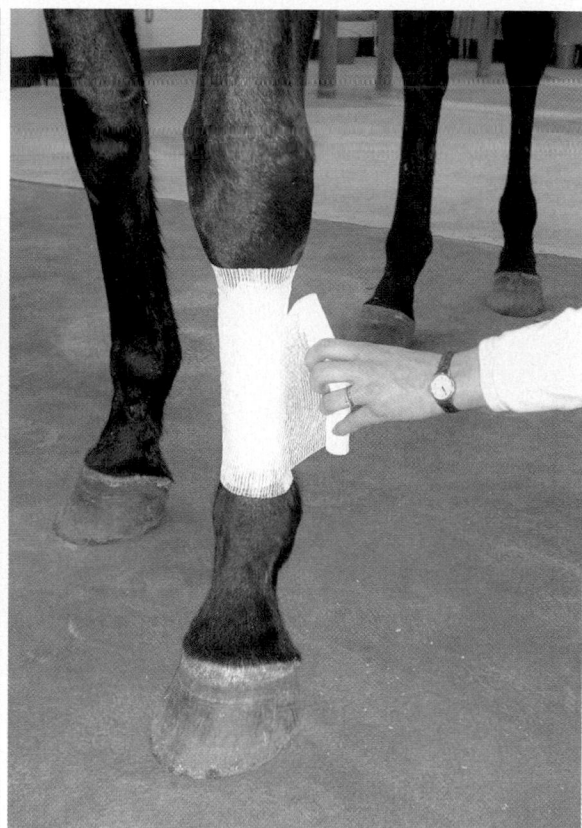

A   B

Figure 4-21 Application of wound dressing on the distal region of the limb of a horse. **A,** Nonadherent dressing is applied directly over the wound. **B,** Conforming gauze is applied to maintain a nonadherent dressing over the wound.

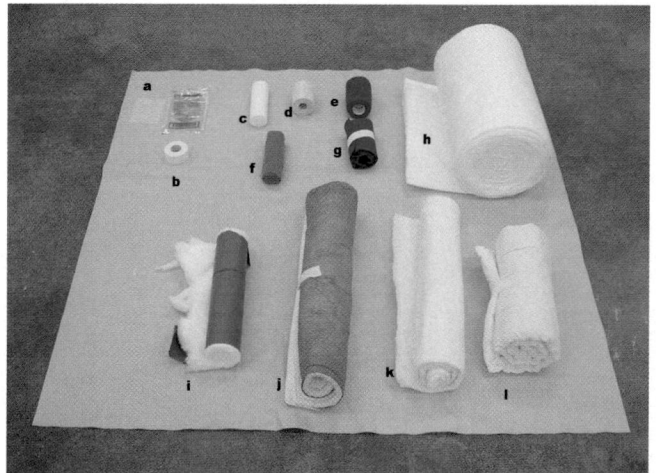

Figure 4-22 Various materials can be used in a leg bandage for large animals. Nonadherent wound dressing *(a)*, white tape *(b)*, white roll gauze *(c)*, Elasticon *(d)*, 3M Vetrap Bandage Tape *(e)*, brown gauze *(f)*, track wrap *(g)*, cotton combine *(h)*, rolled cotton *(i)*, military field bandage *(j)*, layered cotton sheets *(k)*, quilted leg wraps *(l)*.

✎ TECHNICIAN NOTE

A bandage should cover the limb well above and below the ends of a splint to prevent pressure sores.

CAST APPLICATION

A cast is the most frequently used external coaptation to manage various orthopedic injuries or problems when maximum support and immobilization are required. Casts are commonly used for lower limb problems; however, full-limb application is sometimes indicated in large animals. Indications for use of a cast include lower limb fractures; tendon lacerations; support of the lower limb during recovery from orthopedic surgery; heel bulb lacerations; and luxations of the tarsus, fetlock, or pastern. A cast may also be used as an adjunct to internal fixation.

For optimal effectiveness in immobilization, a cast must immobilize the joint proximal and distal to the injury. Full-limb casts must extend up to the elbow or stifle as far as possible. The most frequently used material today is fiberglass. Fiberglass (e.g., DeltaLite, Johnson & Johnson) is appealing because it is lightweight, strong, and relatively easy to apply. However, some veterinarians prefer to use an initial layer of the traditional plaster of Paris under the fiberglass. Plaster conforms well to the contour of the limb, reducing the risk of pressure sores.

Before cast application is begun, several things must be considered. A limb cast must be applied properly or serious problems such as pressure necrosis can occur. Because of its importance, application of a limb cast is described here in detail.

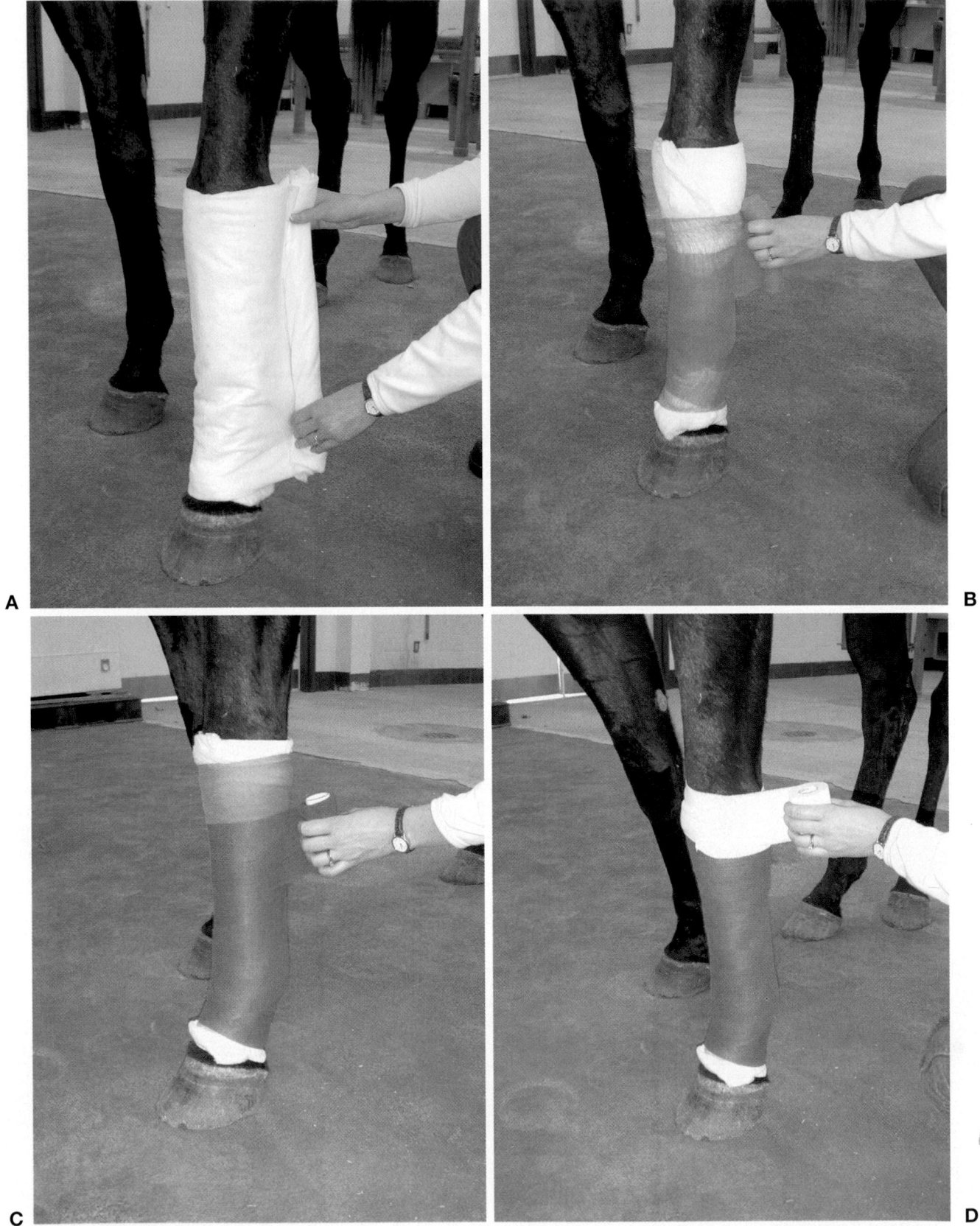

Figure 4-23 Application of padded layer of a wound bandage. **A,** Cotton wrap is applied snugly around the limb. **B,** Conforming gauze is used to secure the padded layer to the limb. **C,** 3M Vetrap Bandage Tape is applied as the outer shell of the bandage. **D,** Wide adhesive tape is used to provide a seal between the skin and bandage.

Before the procedure is begun, all the materials needed should be collected: orthopedic stockinette (3-inch), orthopedic felt, towel clamps, white tape (1-inch), wire (approximately 30 cm), 1/8-inch drill bit and hand drill, broom handle, hoof-trimming equipment, bandage scissors, and cast material (Figure 4-25). Proper application of a cast is essential, especially if it is to remain on the limb for a prolonged period (4 to 6 weeks).

In general, it is best to apply the cast with the horse under general anesthesia. The horse is positioned in lateral recumbency so that the limb to which the cast will be applied is uppermost. Debris are cleaned from the sole, the horseshoe is removed, and the hoof is trimmed. The limb is placed in an extended position perpendicular to the body. Effective support of the leg to maintain the limb in alignment is essential. Traction achieved by using wire looped through holes drilled in the hoof can be helpful. Two holes are drilled in the hoof wall, 5 cm apart near the toe, in the same direction as that in which a horseshoe nail is driven. The ends of the wire are twisted together to form a loop through which a broom handle is placed to apply traction (Figure 4-26).

The frog (the central soft tissue of the hoof) can be packed with povidone-iodine, especially if thrush is present. If a wound is present, a three-layer bandage consisting of a nonadherent dressing, conforming gauze, and adherent elastic tape is used to cover it. The skin must be clean and dry. It can be powdered with talcum or boric acid to help keep the area under the cast dry. The limb is then covered with a double layer of stockinette. The length of the region that the cast will cover is measured, and approximately 20 cm is added to this to determine the length of stockinette needed. One end is rolled outward and the other is rolled inward until they meet at the midpoint of the stockinette (Figure 4-27).

The traction wire is threaded through the opening in the stockinette. A broom handle is placed through the wire loop, and traction is applied. The outward roll is first unrolled up the leg. A twist is placed in the stockinette just beneath the toe, and the inward roll is unrolled up the leg (Figure 4-28). Any wrinkles are smoothed out, and towel clamps are used to secure the stockinette to the medial and lateral aspects of the limb, above the area to which the cast will be applied (Figure 4-29).

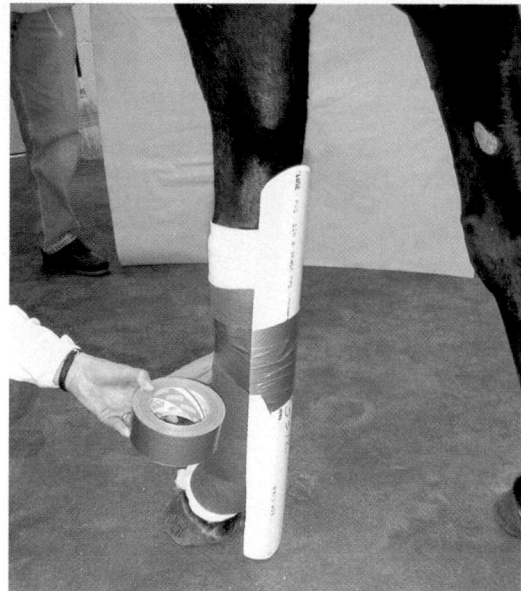

Figure 4-24 Application of a lower limb splint. A thick bandage is placed on the limb. The splint (polyvinyl chloride [PVC] pipe) is positioned along the flexor surface and secured to the bandage with duct tape.

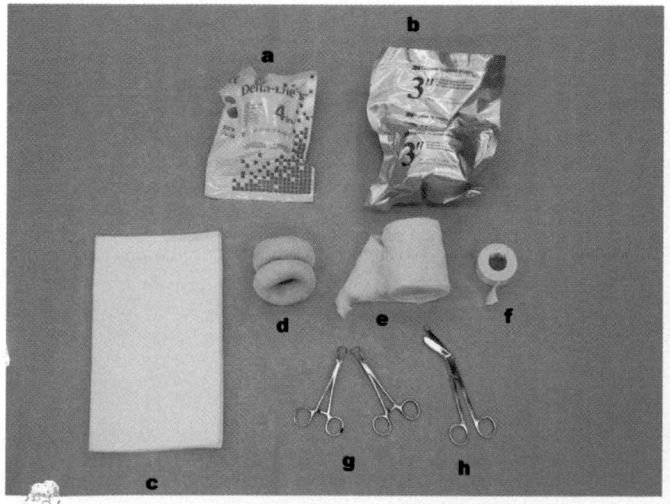
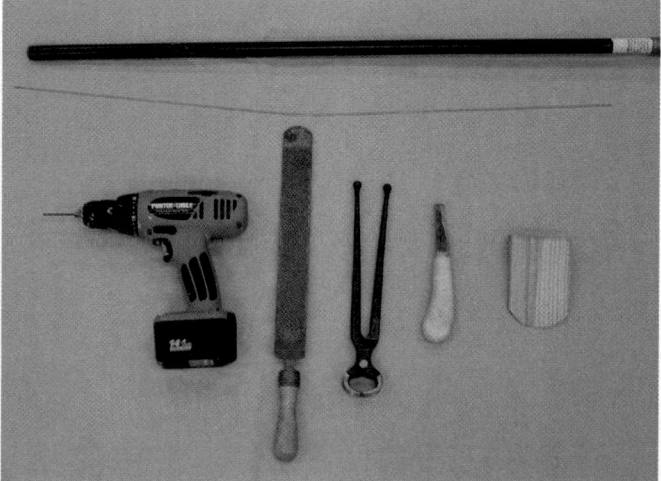

Figure 4-25 Materials needed to apply a limb cast on a large animal. **A,** Cast material *(a)*, support foam *(b)*, orthopedic felt *(c)*, orthopedic stockinette (3-inch) *(d)*, cast padding *(e)*, white tape (1-inch) *(f)*, towel clamps *(g)*, and bandage scissors *(h)*. **B,** Wire (approximately 30 cm), 1/8-inch drill bit and hand drill, hoof-trimming equipment, wooden wedge block, and broom handle.

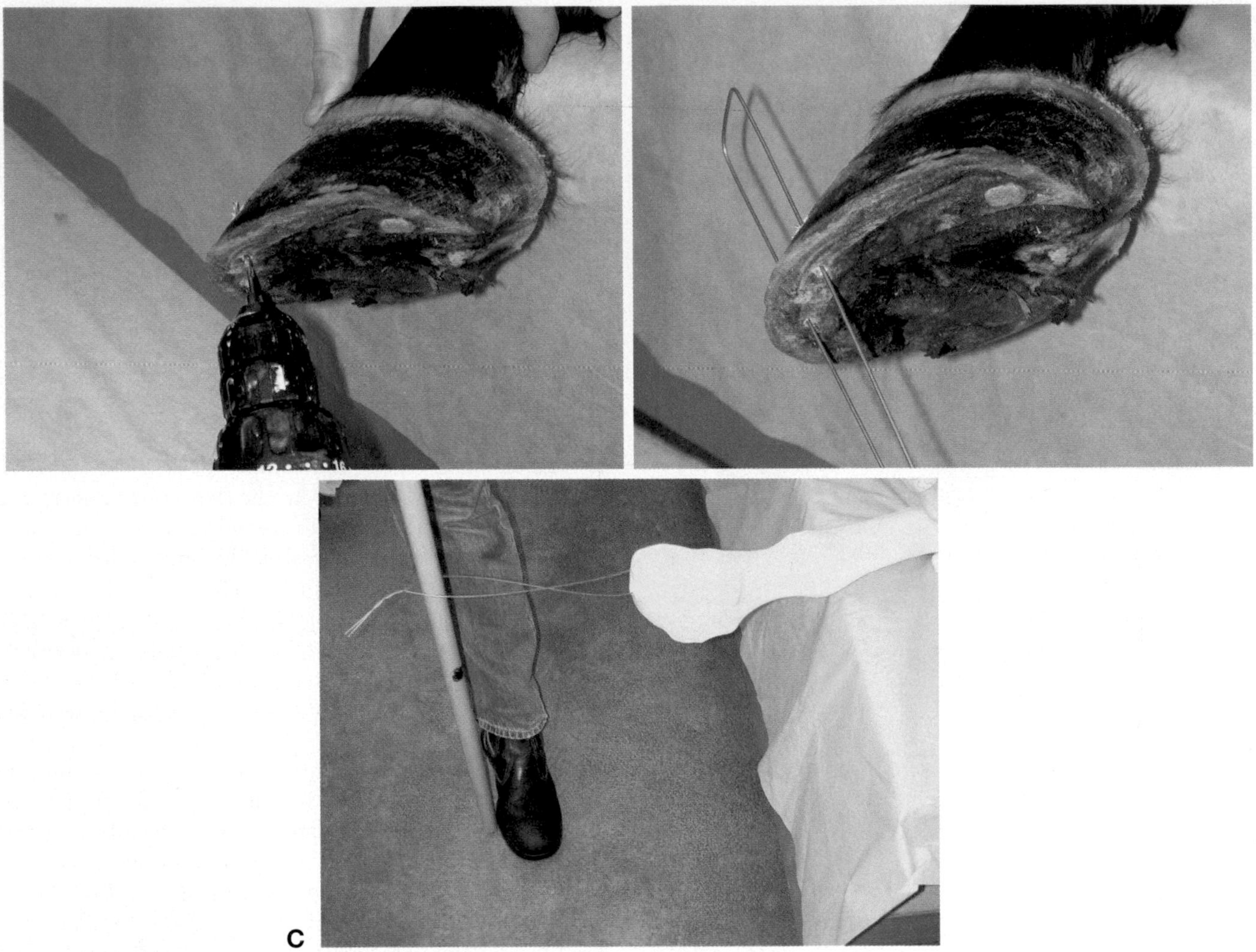

Figure 4-26 Traction can be applied to a limb before cast application by drilling two holes in the toe of the hoof (**A**) and threading a loop of wire through the holes (**B**) with a broomstick placed in the loop to apply traction (**C**).

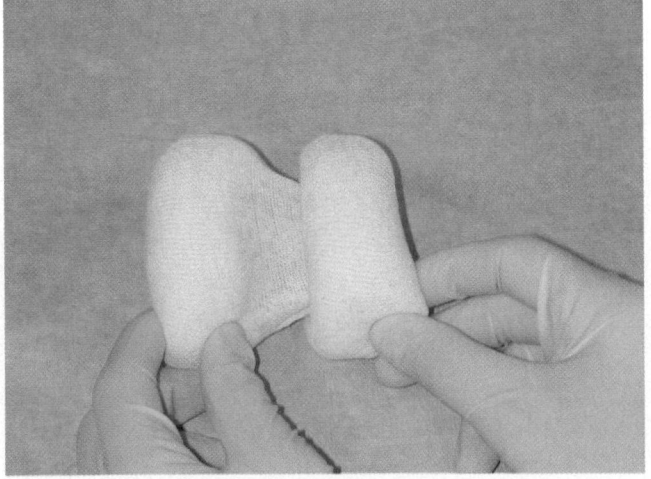

Figure 4-27 Orthopedic stockinette used under a cast is prerolled. One end is rolled outward and the other end is rolled inward until they meet at the midpoint of the stockinette.

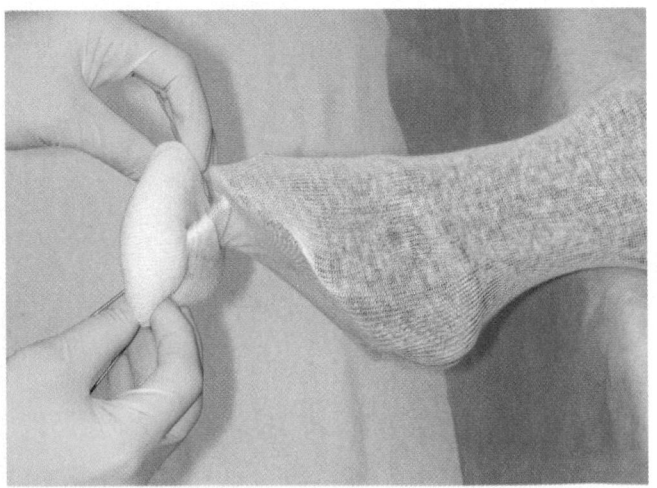

Figure 4-28 A twist is placed in the stockinette just beneath the toe, and the inward roll is unrolled up the leg.

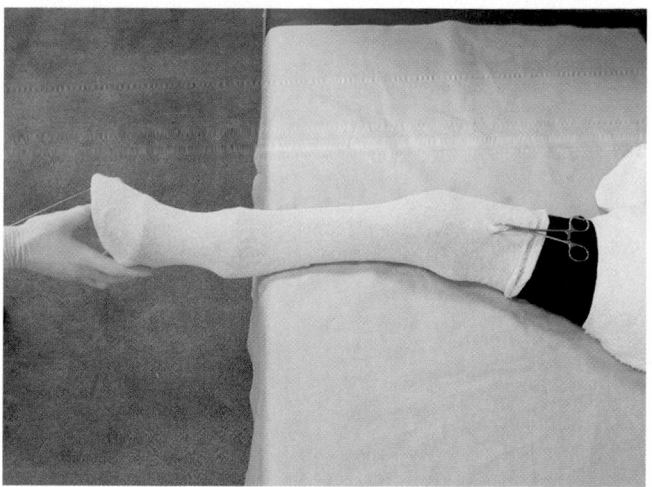

Figure 4-29 Before cast material is applied, the orthopedic stockinette is secured with towel clamps to the medial and lateral aspects of the limb, above the area to which the cast will be applied.

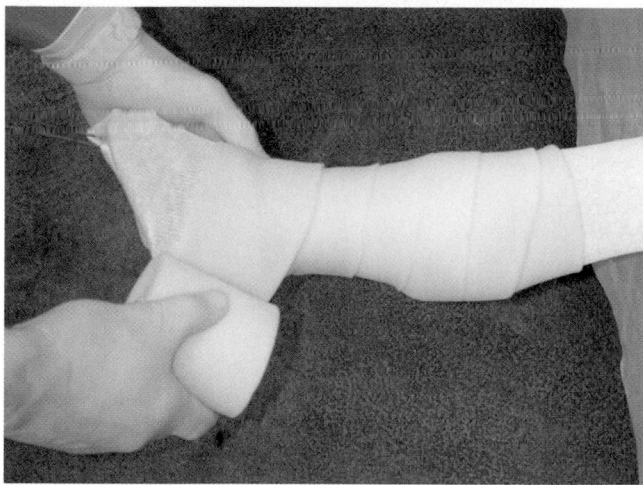

Figure 4-31 A roll of support foam can be applied over the stockinette to provide padding under the cast to prevent formation of pressure sores.

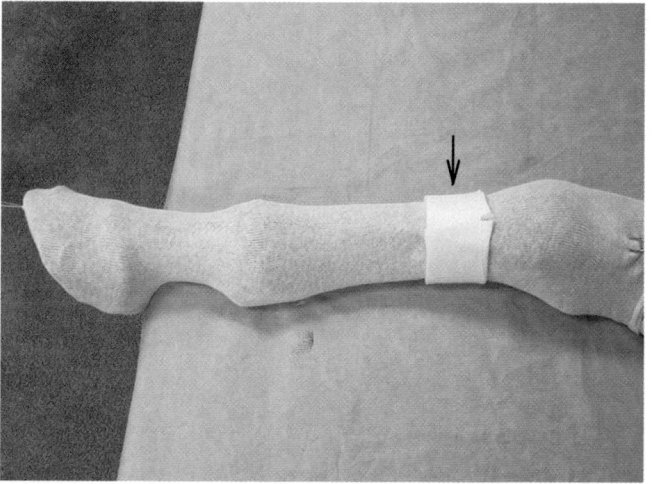

Figure 4-30 A strip of orthopedic felt (5 to 7 cm wide) *(arrow)* is placed around the leg at the most proximal limit of cast. The ends are held in place with 1-inch white tape.

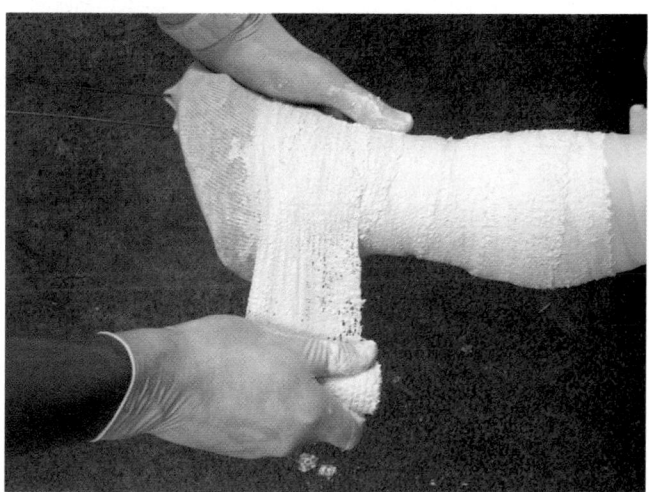

Figure 4-32 Application of plaster of Paris.

A strip of orthopedic felt (5 to 7 cm wide) is placed around the leg at the most proximal limit of the cast. This is held in place with 1-inch white tape (Figure 4-30). When a full-limb cast is used, a doughnut pad cut from orthopedic felt is placed over the accessory carpal bone of the forelimb. A thin strip of orthopedic felt is placed over the gastrocnemius tendon and the point of the hock of the hind limb to prevent the development of pressure sores. A roll of support foam can be applied next. It is applied over the stockinette and its purpose is to provide padding under a cast to reduce the development of pressure sores (Figure 4-31). Additional padding on the leg should be avoided because this can become compressed, thus allowing the leg to move within the cast and cause sores.

Two layers of 3-inch plaster material are first carefully and snugly applied to the limb. These layers should be applied without wrinkles to prevent development of pressure sores. Application of the cast material is usually started at either the proximal or distal aspect of the limb. (The authors) prefer to start distally (Figure 4-32). A roll of plaster is started at the level of the fetlock and worked distally and then proximally. Approximately 1 cm of the orthopedic felt is left exposed above the top of the cast to prevent formation of a sore.

Gloves should be worn when the casting material is applied. To save time in identifying the end on a wetted plaster roll, unroll 2 to 3 inches of the plaster material and hold onto it while wetting the roll in a bucket of warm water (Figure 4-33). The excess water is removed by shaking and squeezing the roll. Do not squeeze excessively or much of the plaster will be lost. Fiberglass material is held in a bucket of clean water until it is thoroughly wet, and the excess water is shaken out.

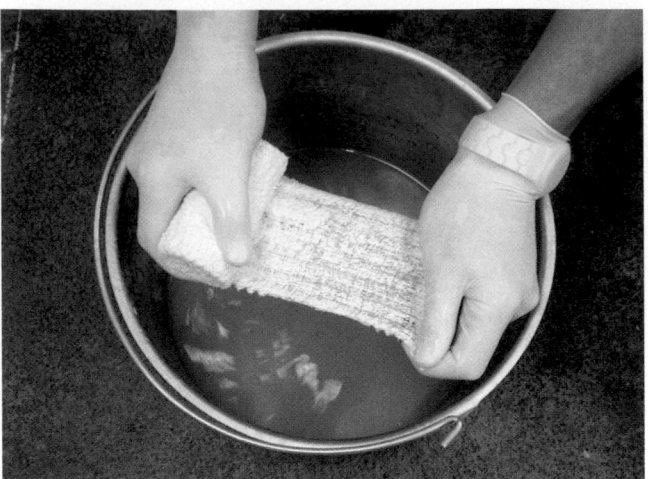

Figure 4-33 The end of plaster of Paris cast material is held away from the roll while it is being moistened.

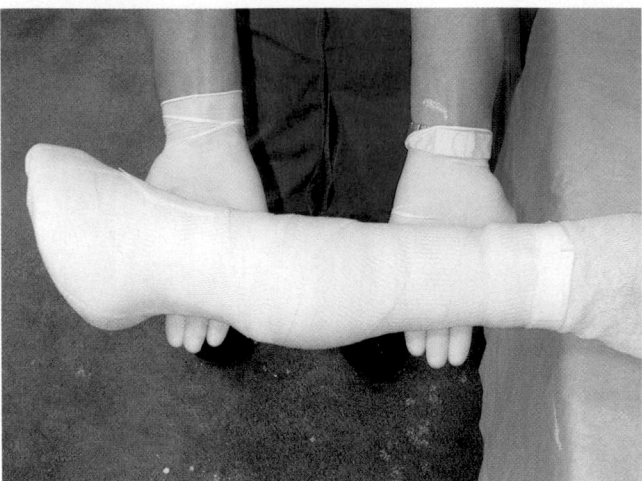

Figure 4-34 As the fiberglass cast material is being applied, an assistant holds the leg out by resting it on the palms of his or her hands under the metacarpus/metatarsus region. This method prevents finger impressions from being made in the uncured cast material.

Next, the fiberglass cast material is applied. Usually it is easier to begin with 3-inch material because it conforms to the limb better. The cast material is overlapped by one third to one half. As the fiberglass casting material is worked toward the foot, the traction wires are cut, and an assistant holds the leg out at the upper limb region or by resting it on the palms of his or her hands, which are placed under the metacarpus or metatarsus region. It is imperative to prevent formation of finger imprints in the cast because they could cause pressure sores to develop (Figure 4-34).

> ### ✎ TECHNICIAN NOTE
> It is very important that the initial layer of casting material be applied to the limb without wrinkles or finger imprints, which may create pressure sores.

More pressure is applied to the succeeding layers of fiberglass. This will allow them to laminate better. Generally, two layers of 3-inch fiberglass cast material are applied, followed by two or three layers of 4- or 5-inch fiberglass. At the time the last roll of cast material is applied, the stockinette is unclamped and the excess is cut off, leaving approximately 4 cm. This 4-cm excess is turned down over the top of the cast and incorporated in the last layer.

A wooden wedge block or a 3-inch roll of wet plaster cast material is placed underneath the heel and also incorporated with the last layer (Figure 4-35). A heel wedge allows the horse to walk more easily while wearing a cast because it decreases the breakover force, reduces pressure on the dorsal proximal limits of the cast at the metacarpus or metatarsus, and allows more even axial weight bearing down through the cast.

When application of the cast is completed, the outer layer is smoothed by running wetted, gloved hands up and down

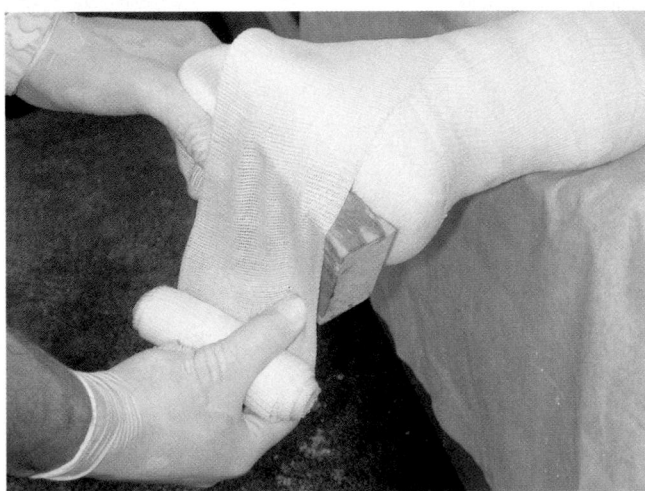

Figure 4-35 A wooden wedge block is placed underneath the heel and incorporated with the last layers of cast material.

the cast. The bottom of the cast is protected from wear by capping it with hard acrylic (e.g., Technovit, Jorgensen Laboratories, Loveland, Cólo) (Figure 4-36). Finally, elastic adhesive tape is placed around the top of the cast and attached to the skin (Figure 4-37), or a piece of stockinette is pulled over the top and taped to the cast and the limb above the cast to prevent debris (wood shavings) from getting inside the cast.

Stall confinement is mandatory after cast application. The patient must be monitored daily. Indications for cast change or removal include breakage, increased lameness, swelling, or exudates coming out of the top of the cast. Horses vary in their reaction and tolerance to a cast. If there is any doubt, a cast should be removed, and the limb should be evaluated.

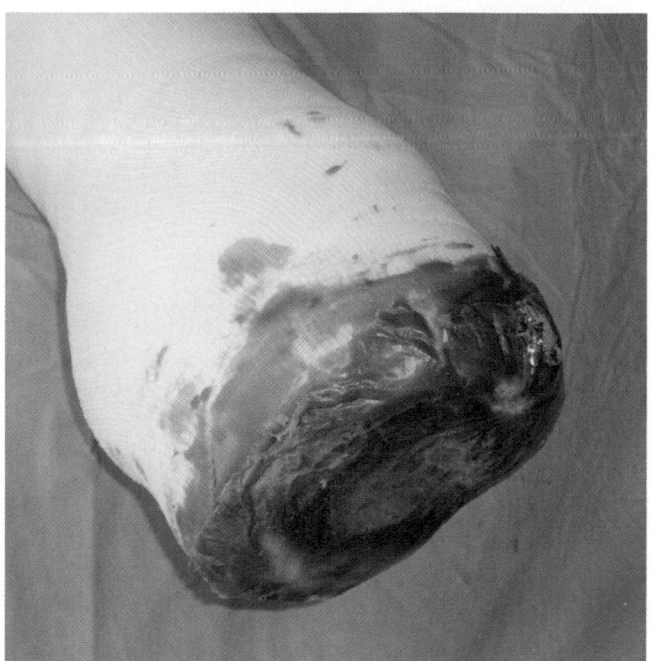

Figure 4-36 The bottom of the cast is protected from wear by capping it with hard acrylic (Technovit, Jorgensen Laboratories).

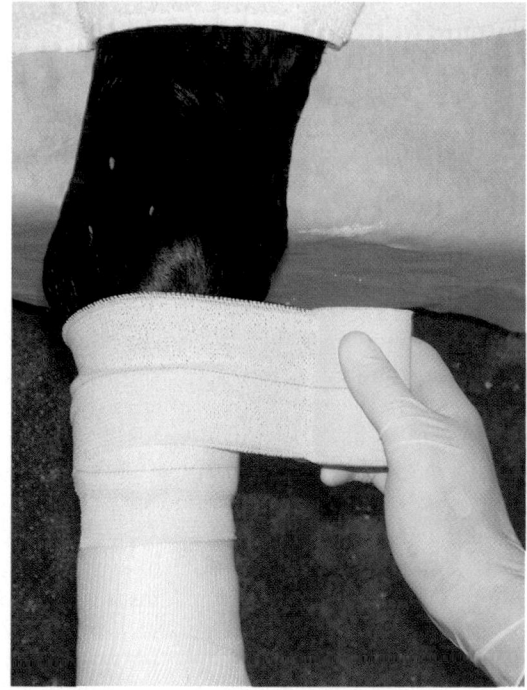

Figure 4-37 Elastic adhesive tape is placed on top of the cast to form a seal between the skin and cast that prevents debris from getting inside the cast.

CAST REMOVAL

Removal of a cast is best performed with the animal standing, unless another cast is to be reapplied. If cast removal is performed under general anesthesia, there is

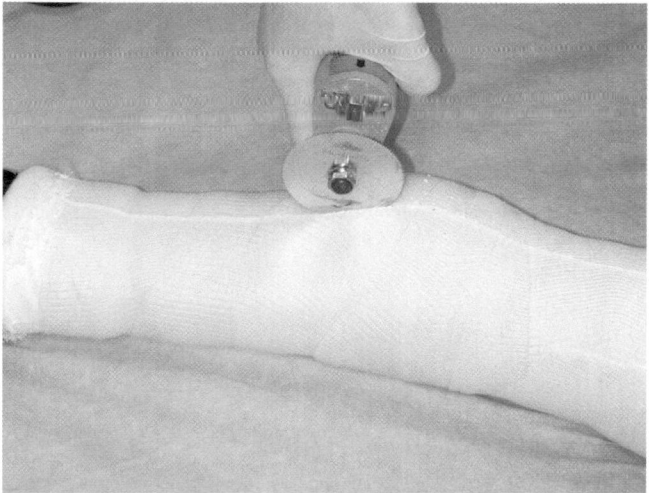

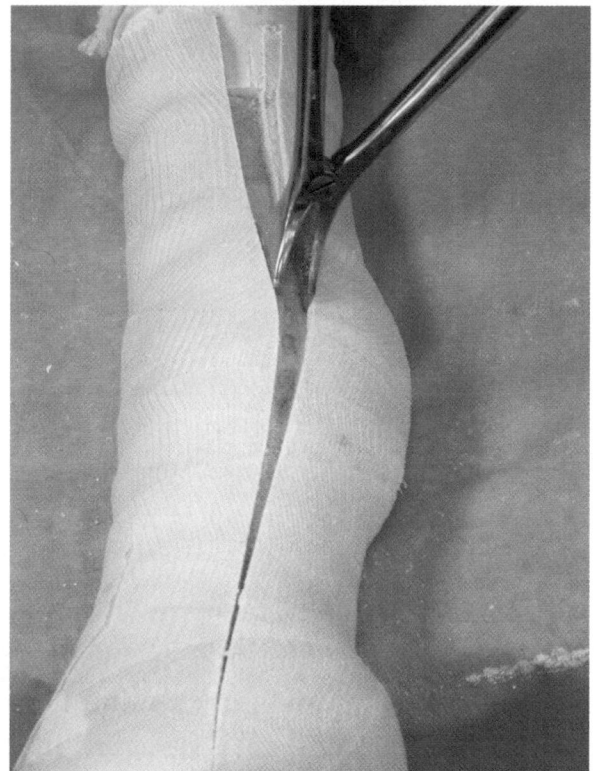

Figure 4-38 Removal of a limb cast from a horse. **A,** With a Stryker saw, the cast is split on the medial and lateral surface, and the cut is continued under the foot. **B,** Once the cast is completely cut, the two halves are separated with cast spreaders.

a risk of reinjury to the limb when the animal is trying to recover from anesthesia. However, general anesthesia is used if the cast is being changed. The cast is split on the medial and lateral surfaces, and the cut is continued under the foot with a Stryker saw (Figure 4-38, *A*). With this approach, injury to the flexor and extensor tendons with the cast saw can be avoided. When cutting over bony prominences, one should be careful to avoid lacerating the skin. Once the cast is completely cut, the two halves are separated with

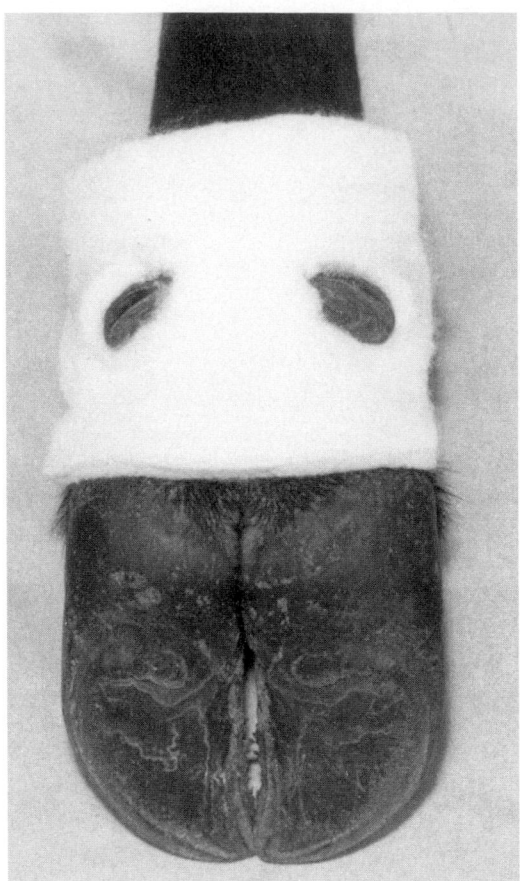

Figure 4-39 A piece of orthopedic felt, with holes cut out, can be placed between the dewclaws to reduce the motion under a cast and help prevent development of pressure sores.

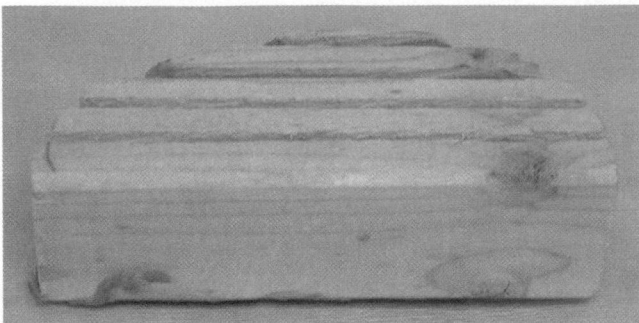

Figure 4-40 A claw block made from wood. Grooves are cut on both sides of the block to improve traction and bonding.

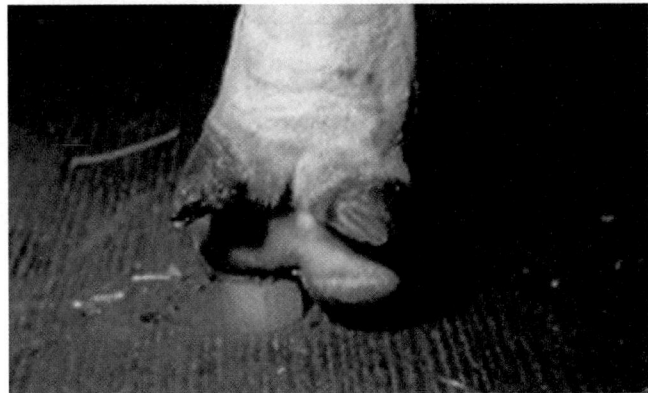

Figure 4-41 A wooden block is cemented to the unaffected claw with acrylic. (Photograph courtesy Dr. Marge Gill.)

cast spreaders (Figure 4-38, *B*). A support wrap is then placed on the limb.

> **✎ TECHNICIAN NOTE**
>
> A cast is split on the medial and lateral surfaces to avoid injury to the flexor and extensor tendons with the cast saw.

BANDAGING AND CAST APPLICATION TECHNIQUES FOR CATTLE

The principles applied to limb bandaging and cast application are the same in cattle as in horses, but there are specific techniques for cattle. Cattle are often not as cooperative as horses, and more restraint is required.

With cattle, a cast can be applied directly over the dewclaws without causing major problems. However, sores caused by motion of the cast can occur in this area because of the inability to closely fit the cast. This can be remedied by placing a pad of orthopedic felt, with holes cut out for the dewclaws, between the dewclaws (Figure 4-39).

APPLICATION OF A CLAW BLOCK

A wooden block is applied to an unaffected claw for various reasons: to alleviate weight-bearing on an adjacent claw if it is fractured or injured or to protect an operated area by raising it higher off the ground (e.g., after amputation of an adjacent claw). The block is usually made from a piece of wood 5 cm thick and cut to the shape of the sole surface of the claw. Grooves are cut in the ground surface for traction (Figure 4-40).

The claw is first trimmed, and debris is removed by means of an electric sander or rasp. This is an important step for effective bonding of the acrylic to the claw. The block is then bonded to the horny surface of the claw with acrylic cement, such as Technovit (Jorgensen Laboratories) (Figure 4-41).

MODIFIED THOMAS SPLINT

Despite advances in external and internal skeletal fixation, modified Thomas splints are still often used in cattle and small ruminants as a means of external skeletal fixation. The modified Thomas splint is often used in combination with internal fixation or a cast. The indications for its use

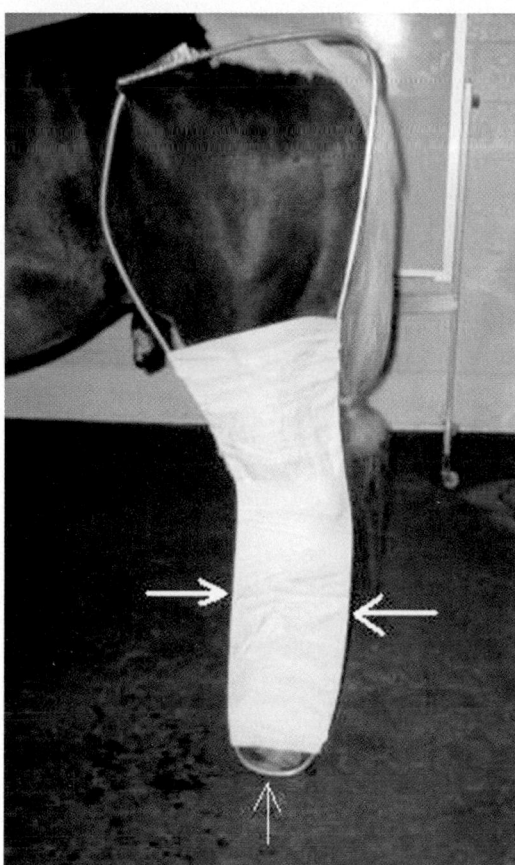

Figure 4-42 A modified Thomas splint. Extensions of the splint *(large arrows)* come off the edge of the ring and are positioned medial to the leg. The construct is made long enough to fit under the animal's foot *(small arrow)*. (Courtesy Dr. Marge Gill.)

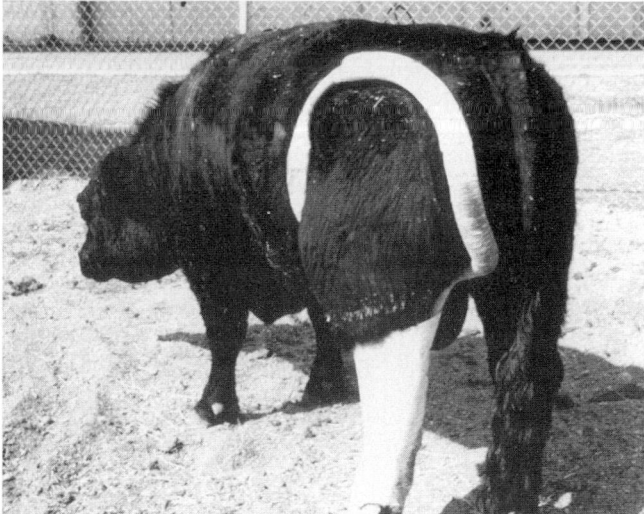

Figure 4-43 The limb and modified Thomas splint are covered with layers of cast material and thereby incorporated to stabilize the limb. (Photograph courtesy Dr. Dwight F. Wolfe.)

include fractures of the tibia or radius and ligamentous injuries of the stifle. Pressure sores in the inguinal or axillary region are a problem when a Thomas splint is used, despite padding of the metal ring part of the splint that fits in that area.

Application of a modified Thomas splint in large ruminants does require special equipment, such as a conduit bender, to bend the round rod iron used to construct the splint. The design of the splint varies somewhat among clinicians, but the purpose is the same.

The animal is first placed in lateral recumbency with the affected leg uppermost. A template to fit the individual animal, devised from a nasogastric tube or other similar flexible tubing, is used to construct the ring that will encircle the proximal part of the leg. The ring should be large enough so as not to impinge on any bony prominences. The rod iron is bent in a ring the same size as the template. The variation in design occurs with the extensions that come off the ring to support the animal's limb.

One design has the extensions coming off the ring cranially and caudally to the leg (Figure 4-42). The extensions of the splint must be shaped to conform to the angles of the hock and stifle. These extensions are also bent away

(lateral) from the flat plane of the ring to allow the ventral part of the ring to fit into the axillary or inguinal region. Another design has the extensions coming off the ventral aspect of the ring. The ring is then bent so that the extensions are positioned medial to the limb and so that the ring itself fits the contour of the upper limb (see Figure 4-43).

The next portion of the splint to be constructed is the distal part of the splint (foot plate). A foot plate can be constructed in various ways. In one method, two threaded rods are attached to the extensions of the splint. This splint is devised with these types of extensions so that the length of the splint can be adjusted. Another construct has a piece of rod iron instead and is bent in a U shape, positioned under the foot, and connected to the ends of the extensions of the splint. The ring is padded with cotton. Holes are drilled into the toes of the hoof walls and wired to the bottom of the splint. A slight amount of traction is placed on the limb as the splint is applied. Traction should be minimal within the splint, so as not to create excessive pressure in the axillary or inguinal regions, which could interfere with venous drainage or distract the fracture fragments.

Once the splint is in position, the limb and splint are then covered with layers of cast material and thereby incorporated (see Figure 4-43). Cast material should first be placed around the carpus or tarsus to give these areas initial support, which should keep them from bowing medially. The cast material should be applied as proximal as possible.

Recommended Reading

Small Animal

Hosgood G: Wound repair and specific tissue response to injury. In Slatter D, editor: *Textbook of small animal surgery,* ed 3, Philadelphia 2003, WB Saunders, pp 66-86.

Knecht CD et al: *Fundamental techniques in veterinary surgery,* ed 2, Philadelphia, 1981, Saunders.

Lozier SM: Topical wound management. In Harari J, editor: *Surgical complications and wound healing in the small animal practice,* Philadelphia, 1993, WB Saunders, pp 63-88.

Mason LK: Treatment of contaminated wounds. In Harari J, editor: *Surgical complications and wound healing in the small animal practice,* Philadelphia, 1993, WB Saunders, pp 33-62.

Swaim SF, Henderson RA: *Small animal wound management,* ed 2, Baltimore, 1997, Williams & Wilkins.

Waldron DR, Zimmerman-Pope N: *Superficial skin wounds.* In Slatter D, editor: *Textbook of small animal surgery,* ed 3, Philadelphia 2003, WB Saunders, pp 259-273.

Large Animal

Adams SB, Fessler JF: Treatment of radial-ulnar and tibial fractures in cattle, using a modified Thomas splint-cast combination, *J Am Vet Assoc* 183:430, 1983.

Stashak TS: Bandaging and casting techniques. In Stashak TS, editor: *Equine wound management,* Philadelphia, 1991, Lea & Febiger, pp 258-272.

Stone WC: Drainings, dressings, and external coaptation. In Auer JA, Stick JA, editors: *Equine surgery,* Philadelphia, 1999, WB Saunders, pp 104-113.

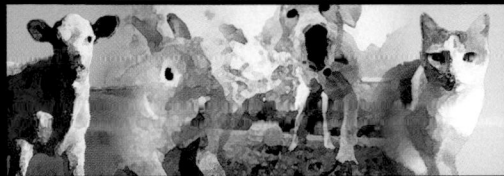

5

Basic Necropsy Procedures

Thomas J. Van Winkle • Perry L. Habecker

INTRODUCTION

A *necropsy* is the examination of an animal, after it has died, to determine the abnormal and disease-related changes that occurred during its life. The term *necropsy* originates from the Greek language and means "viewing the dead." Necropsy is also known as *autopsy*, which is Greek for "seeing with one's own eyes." ■

Before beginning our discussion of the necropsy, it is important to understand the meaning of terms that are used frequently in this chapter. *Pathology*, for example, is the science and study of disease, especially the causes and development of abnormal conditions. *Gross pathology* refers to pathologic changes in tissue that are visible with the unaided eye, whereas *histopathology* refers to pathologic changes in tissue that are microscopic and can be seen with the use of a microscope. *Lesions* are alterations or abnormalities in a tissue (pathologic changes), and the *pathogenesis* is the sequence of events that leads to or underlies a disease.

Necropsies are done for a variety of reasons. A necropsy is often done on an animal for the following reasons:

- To determine the disease process or processes that led to the animal's death
- To determine the accuracy of the clinical diagnosis
- To evaluate the positive and negative effects of therapeutic measures

In situations in which more than one animal is at risk, such as in multiple-animal households, farms, and laboratory animal facilities, the necropsy is also helpful in determining whether other animals are at risk for infection, inherited conditions, or injury caused by toxins or environmental hazards.

Successful performance of a necropsy requires a knowledge of anatomy and gross pathology and a systematic technique for examination of the animal's body. Well-trained technicians, working with appropriate supervision, perform necropsies in many diagnostic laboratories and in most laboratory animal facilities (Figures 5-1 and 5-2). In practice situations, technicians trained in necropsy techniques, and supervised by a veterinarian familiar with the case, can and should perform necropsies. Necropsies should be performed frequently enough so that the techniques are familiar to the technician and the supervising veterinarian. In the necropsy all abnormalities and disease processes should be exposed and described. If necessary, appropriate samples are collected for histopathology, cytology, bacteriology, virology, parasitology, and toxicology. Descriptions of the gross findings should be recorded and included in a report together with the animal's species, age, sex, and breed (signalment); the history; and the clinical findings. Samples that are submitted to the laboratory for further testing should be packaged with a copy of the report. In addition, the report should be added to the animal's record together with the histopathology and other reports. Digital photos of lesions are also helpful and can be sent to the lab along with the reports or as a separate electronic file by E-mail.

TECHNICIAN NOTE

The owner's permission for the necropsy must be obtained, and the animal for necropsy must be correctly identified.

Before we begin describing the necropsy procedure, several important things must be considered. First, be sure that the owner's permission is obtained before the necropsy is performed. Second, make sure that the animal for necropsy is correctly identified. The species, breed, sex, age, and identifying tags or tattoos should be carefully matched with the information on the owner's permission form and the medical record. This step is critical to avoid performing the necropsy on the wrong animal. In addition, the owner's preference for disposition of the body (e.g., cremation, private

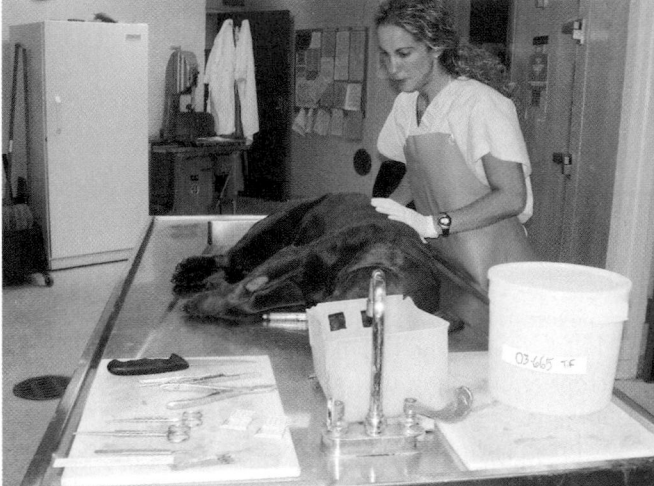

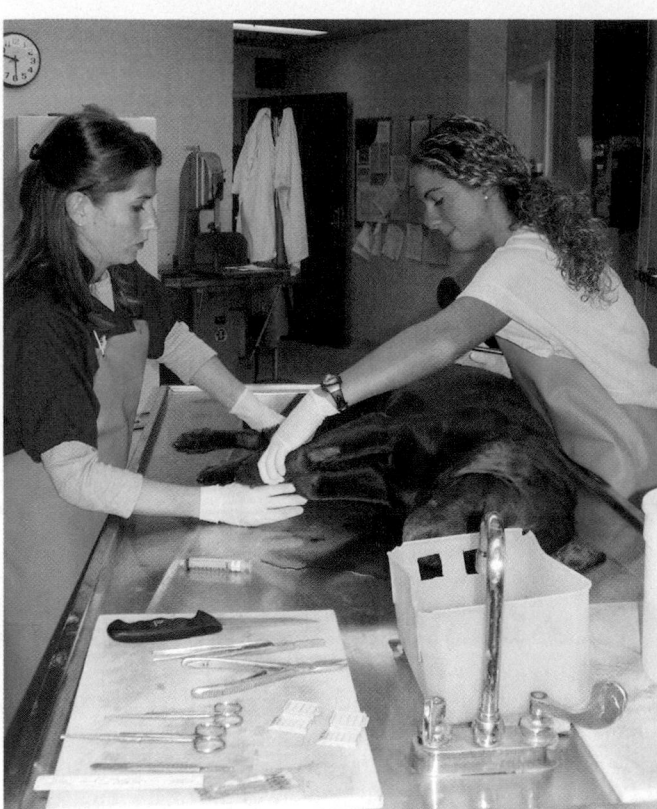

Figure 5-1   **A and B,** Prosectors ready to begin a small animal necropsy.

cremation, burial) should also be determined before the necropsy, if possible. It is also important to perform the necropsy as soon as possible after the animal's death to avoid decomposition (autolysis). If the necropsy must be delayed, the body should be refrigerated as soon as possible. Small animals should be placed in thin plastic bags with identification tags secured on both the body and the outside of the bag. Decomposition occurs most rapidly in large, obese animals at high temperatures. It is particularly troublesome in large animals that rely on gut fermentation for their nutrients, because the rumen continues to generate heat long after the animal's death. The body should not be frozen, because freezing and subsequent thawing cause many postmortem artifacts.

✎ TECHNICIAN NOTE

If the necropsy must be delayed, the body should be refrigerated as soon as possible. The body should not be frozen, because freezing and subsequent thawing cause many postmortem artifacts.

The signalment, history, and clinical findings should be reviewed before the necropsy is started. The record should include the owner's name, address, and phone numbers; names of other veterinarians involved with the case; the animal's species, breed, age, sex, name or identification; and the hospital record number. The history should include

vaccination history, owner's observations of the clinical signs, length of illness, and a list of other animals at risk. The clinical findings should include results of the physical examination and clinical tests (e.g., complete blood count [CBC], clinical chemistries, radiographs), surgical procedures, and the date and time of death or euthanasia.

NECROPSY REPORTS

While the necropsy is being performed, all abnormalities should be described and recorded. A report in which the findings are described should be written after the necropsy has been completed. Tentative conclusions (diagnoses) may be made at the end of the report (refer to Appendix I of this chapter).

All lesions are described and recorded by using the following criteria (examples are given in parentheses):

- Location (caudal dorsal left lung lobe, left ventricle, cornea)
- Number (one, two, hundreds)
- Color (red, green, yellow-tan)
- Size (either measurements such as $3 \times 5 \times 4$ cm or weights for liver and heart)
- Shape (round, flat, spherical, stellate)
- Distribution (focal, multifocal, diffuse)

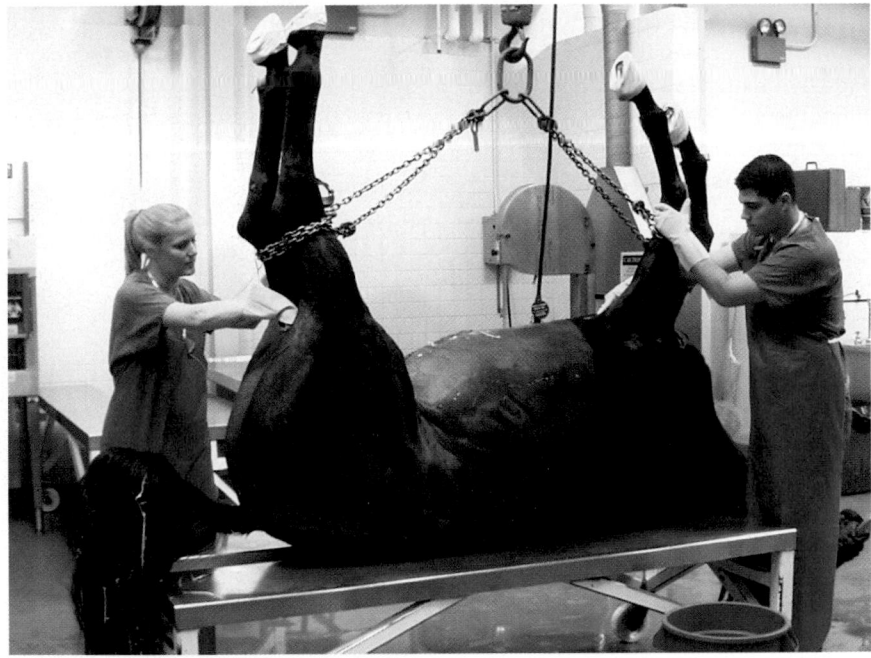

Figure 5-2 Prosectors ready to begin a large animal necropsy.

- Consistency (soft, firm, hard, rubbery)
- Odor (sweet, sour, ammonia)

The findings are usually recorded in the order in which they were encountered in the necropsy. Either the present or past tense should be used (not both), and the descriptions should be as specific as possible without drawing conclusions. For example, "There are multiple dark red 1- to 4-mm – diameter soft nodules in all lung lobes" rather than "hemangiosarcoma." On the basis of the descriptions, the veterinarian formulates a morphologic diagnosis, which includes severity, time, distribution, lesion, and anatomic site. An example of a diagnosis might be "severe acute multifocal interstitial pneumonia."

FIXATIVES

Ten percent buffered formalin is the most widely used fixative for the preservation of tissues. Slices of tissue (generally no thicker than 1 cm) should be placed in large volumes of formalin. Generally, there should be 10 times as much formalin solution as tissue (by volume). This solution may be purchased from a variety of sources and is also easily prepared. It is made by mixing nine parts of water with one part of commercially available formaldehyde solution (37% to 40% HCHO). The addition of 6.5 g of dibasic anhydrous sodium phosphate and 4 g of monobasic sodium phosphate per 1000 ml of solution creates neutral buffered 10% formalin. This is an excellent general purpose fixative, which is somewhat more desirable than plain (acidic) 10%

formalin. The addition of buffers is important because it eliminates the formation of undesirable hematin pigment in tissue sections. Formalin (and all fixatives) should be handled with care. Formalin is a contact irritant and a carcinogen. Protective plastic gloves, preferably of nitrile composition, should always be worn when fixatives or fixed tissues are handled. Containers with fixatives should be kept closed except when tissues are being placed in them, and fixatives should be handled and used in a well-ventilated space.

> **✎ TECHNICIAN NOTE**
>
> Ten percent buffered formalin is the most widely used fixative for the preservation of tissues. Tissues should be placed in large volumes of formalin (10:1, formalin to tissue ratio).

For the preservation of whole brains, intact spinal cords, and bones, 50% formalin, made by mixing one part 10% buffered formalin with one part of commercial formaldehyde (37% to 40% HCHO), is superior to the 10% solutions. The stronger 50% solution penctrates and fixes the large tissue mass more rapidly and more thoroughly than 10% formalin. Formalin fixation is usually complete within 24 hours (large brains may take 48 hours). Tissues fixed in 10% formalin are traditionally stored in 10% formalin, but storage in 70% alcohol is superior.

Bouin's fixative is less widely used than 10% formalin, but it is preferred in some instances because it produces less tissue shrinkage and better preservation of cellular detail. Fetal tissues, intestinal epithelium, eyes, testes, endocrine glands, and the inclusion bodies associated with several important diseases are particularly well preserved with this fixative. Bouin's fixative may be purchased from a variety of sources or can be made by mixing 750 ml of a saturated aqueous solution of picric acid, 250 ml of 37% to 40% formaldehyde, and 50 ml of glacial acetic acid. Picric should be handled with caution because it is explosive!

> ✐ **TECHNICIAN NOTE**
>
> All containers of fixed tissue samples should be clearly labeled. Appropriate caution should be used in handling, shipping, and disposal of all fixatives.

FACILITIES AND INSTRUMENTS

Necropsies should be performed in a well-lit, well-ventilated space, ideally outside the usual surgical and treatment areas. The area should be easy to clean and disinfect, have adequate drainage for fluids and water, and be large enough to comfortably move around in (Figure 5-3). When necropsies are performed in the field (outdoors), the appropriate disposal of tissues and the inadvertent spread of disease become particular concerns.

The person performing the necropsy (called the prosector) should wear protective clothing, such as a plastic apron, laboratory coat, or scrubs, which can be removed and either discarded or cleaned after the necropsy (Figure 5-4). Latex or other protective plastic gloves should be worn at all times. In addition, a surgical mask should be worn when dealing with animals that have died from infectious diseases that can be spread through aerosolization. Protective footwear (boots or booties) is appropriate when dealing with larger animals.

Necropsies do not require specialized equipment or instruments. Most instruments can be obtained from surgical suppliers and hardware stores (Figures 5-5 and 5-6). The following instruments are used in a typical necropsy:

- Necropsy knives (sturdy ones that can be sharpened) and honing steel
- Scalpel handle and blades
- Scissors (large and small operating, Mayo, or Metzenbaum scissors work well)
- Forceps (large- and small-toothed)
- Serrated, all-purpose, plastic-handled utility scissors
- Bone-cutting forceps
- Hacksaw, meat saw, or Stryker saw (for brain removal)
- Lopping (pruning) shears for cutting ribs and bones
- String or hemostats for closing off bowel ends
- Labeled plastic buckets or screw-top plastic containers containing formalin
- Tissue cassettes (for very small tissues) and clip-on laundry tags for identifying tissues
- Labeled, sealable, plastic bags and plastic vials or bottles for refrigerated and frozen samples
- Culturettes for aerobic and anaerobic cultures

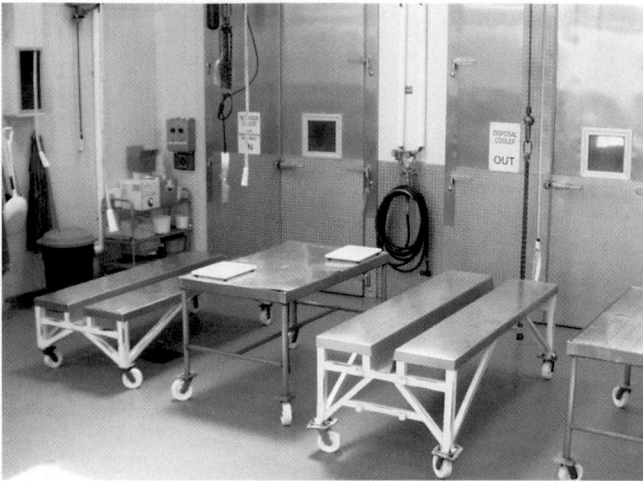

Figure 5-3 A view of a large animal necropsy room.

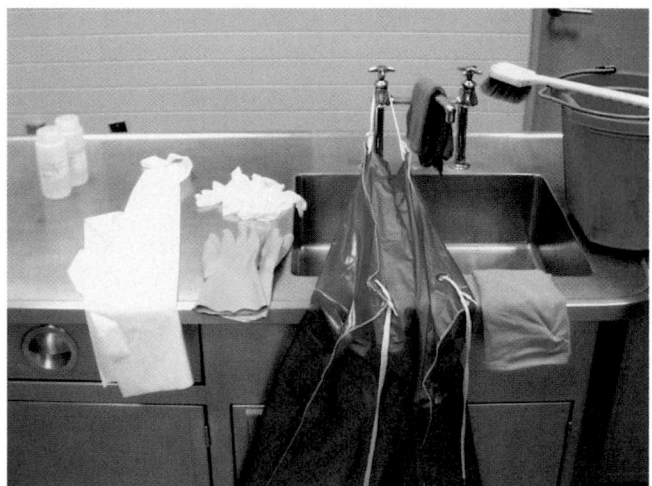

Figure 5-4 Personal protective clothing and equipment commonly used in a large animal necropsy.

> ✐ **TECHNICIAN NOTE**
>
> All equipment and instruments should be thoroughly cleaned and disinfected after the necropsy. Instruments should be dedicated for necropsy use only to prevent the spread of pathogens.

ANCILLARY PROCEDURES

Before samples are collected for examination in the microbiology, parasitology, and toxicology departments, the diagnostic laboratory should be contacted for specific advice on which samples should be collected, how they should be collected, and how they should be packaged and submitted. This minimizes potential errors and provides the laboratory with the best possible specimens.

Tissues and specimens for bacteriology, mycology, and mycoplasma cultivation are collected aseptically, placed in

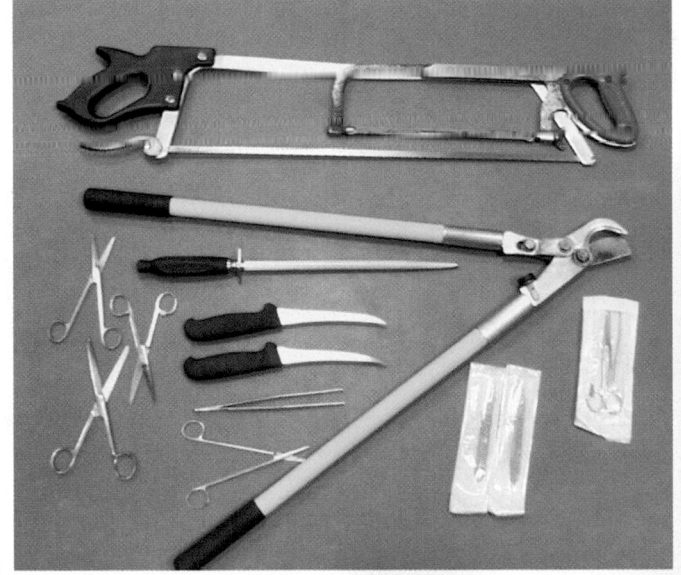

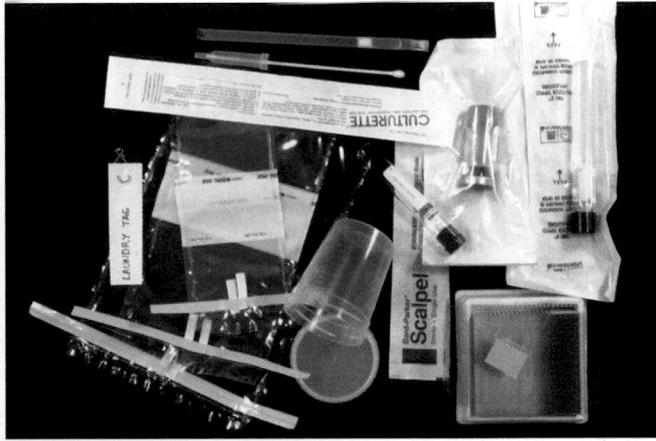

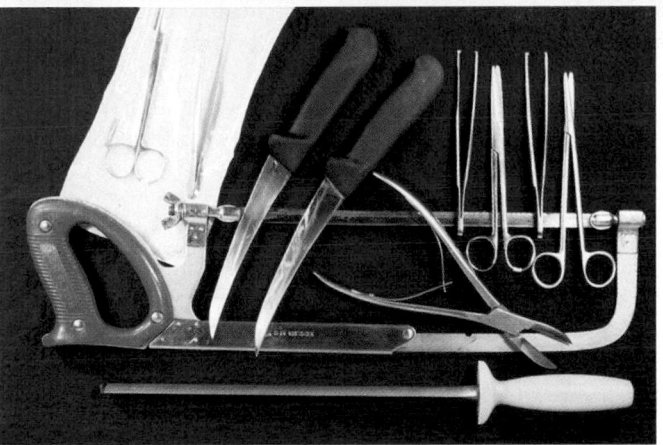

Figure 5-5 **A** and **B,** Instruments commonly used in a large animal necropsy. **C,** Equipment commonly used in a large animal necropsy.

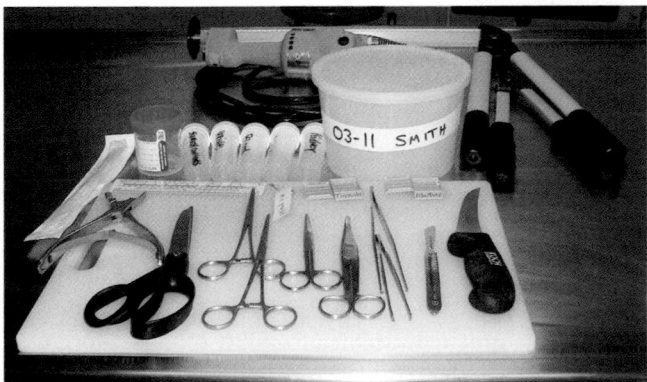

Figure 5-6 Instruments and equipment commonly used in a small animal necropsy.

either culturettes or sterile containers without preservatives, and submitted to the laboratory *without delay.* Frozen specimens should not be submitted. Sterilized instruments should be used to collect samples for microbiologic testing. If the surface of the tissue is contaminated, it can be seared with a flamed spatula, the surface can be cut with a sterile blade, and a culturette or needle attached to a sterile syringe can be inserted to swab/aspirate the tissue for testing.

Specimens collected for microbiology include the primary site of disease and its regional lymph nodes. Other samples may include heart, blood, lung, liver, spleen, stomach contents of aborted fetuses, placenta, exudates, synovia, bone marrow, cerebrospinal fluid, brain, and small intestine. When intestine is submitted, a 10-cm segment of intestine is tied off at each end to prevent excessive contamination by the internal contents. The instruments used to do this are heavily contaminated by the microbes exposed at the cut ends. For this reason, intestine should be collected last and placed in a separate container to prevent contamination of other tissue samples. Tissue sections of $2 \times 3 \times 1$ cm and fluid specimens of 3 to 5 ml are desirable.

> ### ✐ TECHNICIAN NOTE
> Contact the diagnostic laboratory for specific advice on which samples should be collected, how they should be collected, and how they should be packaged and submitted.

Tissues for virus isolation are collected aseptically and either refrigerated in a sterile container or immersed in sterile 50% buffered glycerol in sterile containers and preserved by freezing. Fresh, refrigerated tissue immersed in virus transport medium (available from the virology laboratory) is the preferred method of tissue submission. Lung, liver, spleen, kidney, and brain are prime specimens. Sections need to be $5 \times 5 \times 10$ mm. Contact the virology laboratory for the appropriate technique.

For toxicology, blood, liver, stomach contents, kidney, fat, brain, and urine may be saved. Blocks of tissues $10 \times 5 \times 4$ cm (approximately 200 g), 10 to 20 ml of blood, and 50 to 100 ml of fluids are desirable. They may be frozen.

If rabies is suspected, the animal's head should be sent to the appropriate laboratory for testing according to the guidelines and laws of the state. In cases in which rabies is suspected, decapitation or other necropsy procedures should not be attempted unless the technician has been specifically trained to perform this procedure. A necropsy should only be performed on the rest of the carcass if the brain is found to be negative for rabies.

For cytologic examination, smears are made (after gentle blotting on absorbent paper) by either scraping the cut surface of the specimen with a new scalpel blade and then spreading the scraped material onto a slide or lightly pressing small pieces of tissue against the surface of a clean slide. Several impressions are made across the slide. They are generally submitted unstained to the laboratory, or they can be stained and examined at the time of the necropsy.

NECROPSY PROCEDURE FOR A SMALL MAMMAL

The following procedure is appropriate for dogs, cats, ferrets, rodents, and rabbits. See also Appendix II of this chapter for the steps in the necropsy procedure.

TISSUE COLLECTION

Tissues being collected for histologic examination must be handled carefully before fixation and must be properly labeled for identification. Tissue sections should not be squeezed, stretched, or rinsed with water; and epithelial surfaces should not be rinsed or rubbed with fingers or instruments before samples are obtained for histopathologic examination. Tissues become rigid with fixation, so if there is a need to retain the flatness of the tissue, it can be placed on a piece of cardboard. The tissue will remain adhered to the cardboard after immersion in formalin.

Sections from paired organs may be trimmed differently from one another to distinguish them from one another. For example, the left kidney may be sectioned longitudinally, and the right kidney may be cut transversely. In addition, sections can be labeled with clip-on laundry tags to identify them. If there is any possibility that a section of tissue may lose its identity (i.e., be difficult to distinguish) when mixed with other specimens, the sections should be tagged with clip-on laundry tags. If tissue samples are small, they may also be placed in separate labeled containers, such as tissue cassettes. The pituitary gland of a small animal, for example, is well differentiated from other tissues when placed in a small tissue cassette.

In all cases it is desirable to save sections of critical tissues for histopathologic examination. These include lung, myocardium, liver, spleen, pancreas, stomach, small intestine, kidneys, lymph nodes, whole brain, endocrine organs, urinary bladder, colon, and muscle.

DISSECTION

The method of dissection described here is a standard technique that can be applied to all mammalian species and that is based on the following two precepts:

1. In stepwise fashion, each part of the carcass is examined in situ (as it first appears in the carcass); it is then isolated from the carcass and examined as a whole; finally it is dissected and examined.
2. Once a part has been taken from the body, it is dissected to completion (exceptions include tissues from the gastrointestinal tract, brain, spinal cord, and eyes). Sections for histologic or laboratory examination are collected before further dissection is undertaken.

This method is the opposite of those that call for evisceration now and dissection later, methods that disrupt the entire carcass all at once and that lead to tissues being forgotten or lost. The immediate complete dissection of one part at a time reduces the possibility of lost or forgotten parts and leaves the remainder of the carcass intact. In this way, if the findings in one organ suggest that another part or parts of the carcass should be explored in situ, this is still possible and has not been precluded by previous dissection.

PRELIMINARY OBSERVATIONS

Before the necropsy begins, the prosector should review the signalment (species, breed, color, sex, age, weight, animal identification), the clinical history, and the laboratory data available. It is important that the time of death and time of necropsy be recorded. The animal should then be weighed, and the weight should be recorded in grams or kilograms. All organs that are abnormal in size or shape should be measured and/or weighed.

> ### 📝 TECHNICIAN NOTE
>
> Before the necropsy begins, the prosector should review the signalment (species, breed, color, sex, age, weight, animal identification) of the animal, the clinical history, and any available laboratory data.

EXTERNAL EXAMINATION

The exterior of the animal is examined: body conformation, hair coat, skin, nose, mouth (lips, cheeks, gums, teeth, tongue), eyes (eyelids, conjunctiva, cornea, sclera, anterior chamber, iris, lens), ears, mammae, penis, prepuce, scrotum, vulva, anus, and feet. Because the retina undergoes rapid decomposition after death, dissection begins with the eyes. The upper and lower eyelids are examined and excised. The membrana nictitans is grasped with tissue forceps, the globe is lifted, and the soft tissue attachments to the bony orbit are incised with scissors or a scalpel in a 360-degree arc. As the globe is freed from the orbit, care must be taken to avoid application of excessive tension to the optic nerve. The optic nerve is carefully severed at the optic canal. The excised globe is examined; and then extraocular muscles, fascia, fat, conjunctiva, and membrana nictitans are dissected from the globe. The interior of the eye can be examined by immersing the globe in clear, cool water. The sclera is

examined, and the unopened globe is immersed in Bouin's fixative or formalin.

REFLECTION OF SKIN AND LIMBS AND EXAMINATION OF SUPERFICIAL ORGANS

The animal is placed in left lateral recumbency (on the left side). A midline incision is made beginning at the right axilla and extending cranially to the mandibular symphysis (Figure 5-7). The incision is continued in the opposite direction caudally as a median or paramedian incision, passing between the mammae and around the penis, prepuce, and scrotum to the perineum (Figure 5-8). The upper forelimbs are reflected by dissection between the scapula and the ribs. Fat, fascia, and superficial muscles are reflected back together with the skin. Skin of the ventral aspect of the neck and throat is reflected. Abdominal skin is reflected, and the hind limbs are reflected by extending the incision into the coxofemoral (hip) joints. The animal is now placed in dorsal recumbency (on its back) (Figure 5-9).

Skin incisions are extended down the cranial medial aspects of both rear legs, and the skin is reflected. As they are exposed in the dissection, superficial organs are examined and samples from these organs are collected: lymph nodes (mandibular, superficial cervical, prescapular, axillary, inguinal, popliteal), mammary glands, testes, and skin.

In all necropsy examinations, several joints are examined before the body cavities are opened. The coxofemoral joints are opened and examined during the initial incision. The scapulohumeral and stifle joints are also examined during all routine necropsies. The atlantooccipital joint will be examined when the head is removed.

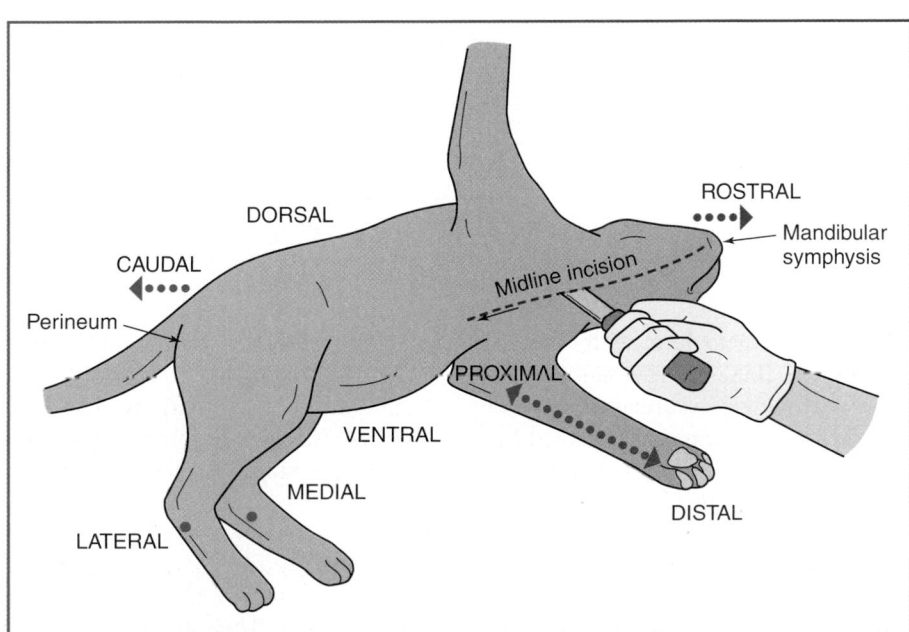

Figure 5-7 The necropsy begins with the animal placed on its left side. A midline incision is made from the mandibular symphysis caudally.

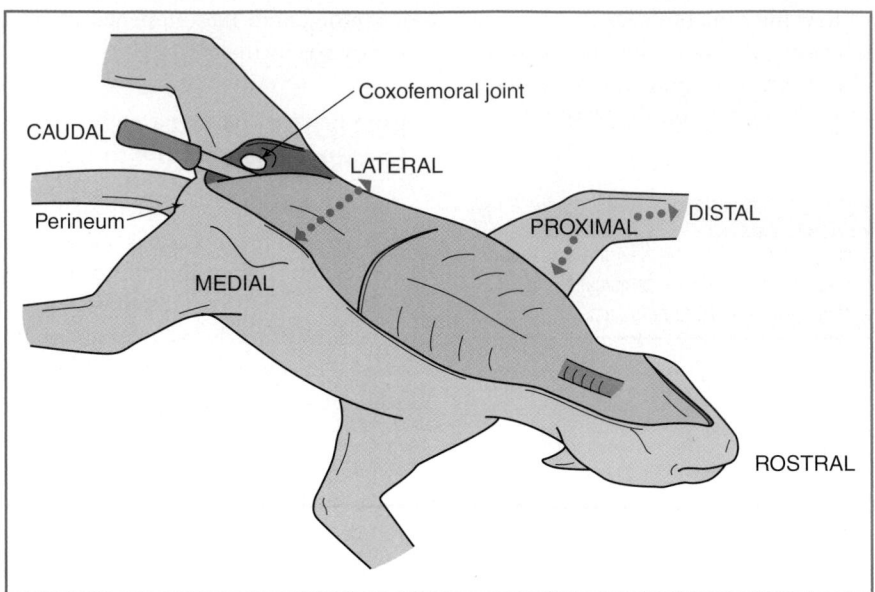

Figure 5-8   The front limbs are reflected by making incisions between the ribs and the scapulae. The hind legs are reflected by incising the coxofemoral (hip) joints.

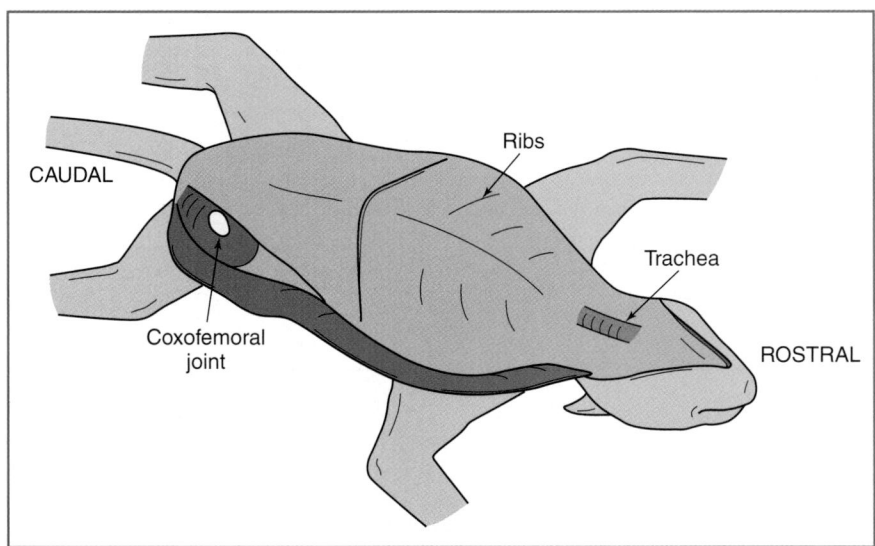

Figure 5-9   After all four limbs have been reflected, the animal is positioned in dorsal recumbency (on its back).

Samples of the sciatic nerve, synovium with patella, and skeletal muscle are collected. Bone marrow samples for impression smears or histopathologic examination should be collected at this time. Generally, marrow is obtained by cracking the upper midshaft femur with pruning shears.

You should, at this point, have already collected the following: eyes, lymph nodes, testes or mammary glands, skin, synovium, sciatic nerve, skeletal muscle, and bone marrow.

Next, the three major body cavities (peritoneal, pleural, pericardial) are opened. All organs are examined in situ, and any abnormalities are noted. The abdomen is opened by making a midline incision from the sternum to the symphysis pubis and making incisions laterally from the sternum along both caudal costal margins. The abdominal wall is then reflected laterally to expose the abdominal cavity (Figure 5-10).

The diaphragm is now punctured to check for negative pleural pressure, and the diaphragm is cut away from the ventral and lateral rib cage. The ventral rib cage is removed by cutting the ribs bilaterally (on both sides) midway between the costochondral junction and the vertebral column (Figure 5-11). This should be done with utility scissors or pruning shears. Examine the pleural surface of the rib cage. In young animals the costochondral growth plate may

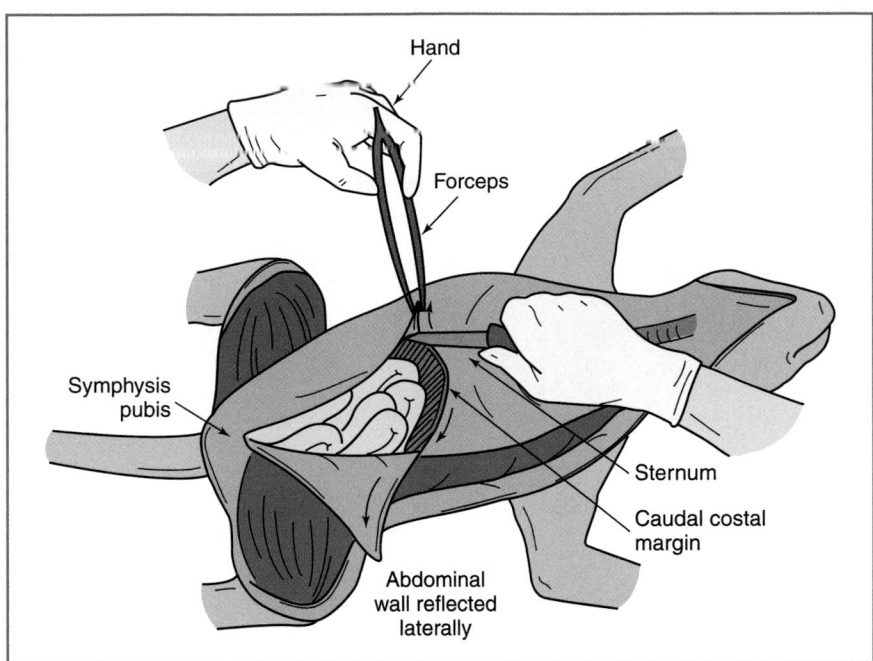

Figure 5-10 The abdominal wall is incised with a midline incision. The right and left halves of the abdominal wall are reflected laterally by making incisions from the sternum along both right and left caudal costal margins.

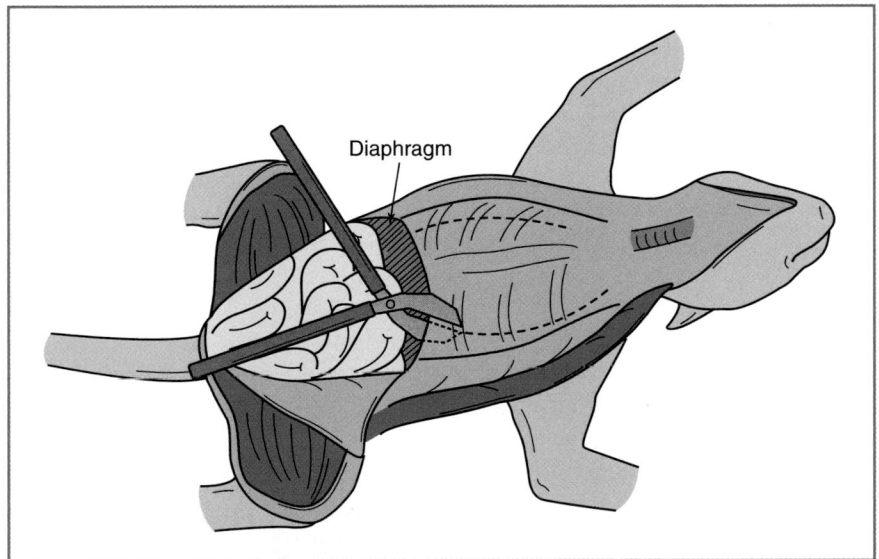

Figure 5-11 The ventral portion of the rib cage is removed by cutting the ribs bilaterally (on both sides) with heavy pruning shears.

be examined and saved for histopathologic examination. Next, the pericardial sac is opened, and the exterior of the heart is examined.

> **TECHNICIAN NOTE**
> The history and preliminary findings are reviewed with the clinician after all body cavities have been opened.

The thyroid, parathyroids, and thymus should be identified at this time and removed. The adrenal glands should then be identified and removed. The adrenal glands are sectioned, and the corticomedullary ratio is noted. The mandibular salivary glands, parotid salivary glands, parotid lymph nodes, jugular veins, and parapharyngeal and retropharyngeal lymph nodes are examined.

EXAMINATION OF SKULL AND BRAIN

Remove the tongue from the oral cavity; and reflect the tongue, tonsils, larynx, and esophagus caudally (Figure 5-12).

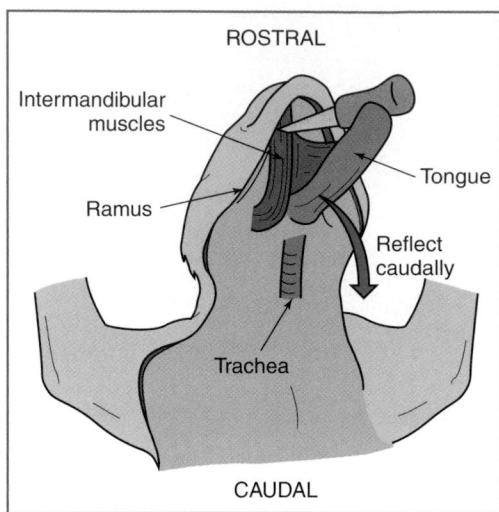

Figure 5-12 Examination of the tongue, tonsils, larynx, and esophagus. These are reflected caudally after the intermandibular muscles have been incised.

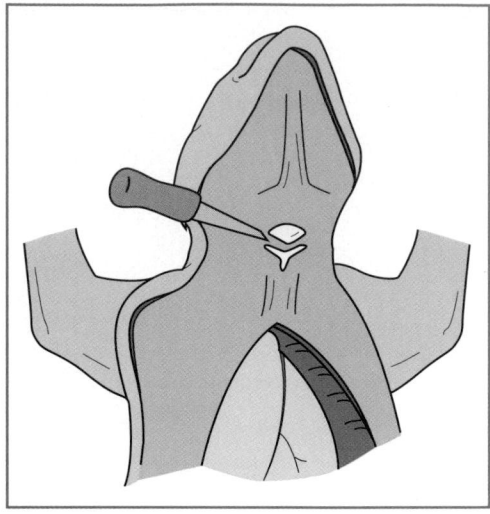

Figure 5-13 The spinal cord is transected ventrally by first making an incision into the atlantooccipital joint. The head is disarticulated from the vertebral column.

An incision is made through the intermandibular muscles, along the medial surface of the ramus of each mandible, from the angle to the symphysis. The frenulum of the tongue is incised, and the tongue is pulled (or pushed) ventrally between the rami. The tongue is used as a handle, and right and left paramedian incisions are extended from the larynx to the thoracic inlet, exposing the length of the trachea and esophagus. It is necessary to cut or disarticulate the hyoid bones dorsal to the pharynx to free the tongue, larynx, pharynx, trachea, and esophagus as a unit.

The spinal cord is transected by an incision into the ventral atlantooccipital joint. Atlantooccipital membranes, ligaments, and joint capsule are transected, disarticulating the head from the vertebral column (Figure 5-13). The skin is removed from the head by leaving it attached to the skin of the body and peeling the head forward out of the skin. The superficial muscles of the head are removed. External ears are opened and examined. Temporal muscles are removed, exposing the calvaria (skull cap) (Figure 5-14).

The calvaria and caudal wall of the cranial cavity are removed from the skull as a unit, exposing the dorsum of the brain. Three cuts are made with a Stryker saw, hacksaw, or meat saw to accomplish this. The first is a transverse cut through the frontal bones. This cut is usually made immediately caudal to the orbits. Care is taken to make the cut just deep enough to transect bone but not deep enough to engage the brain beneath.

The second and third cuts are made through the side walls and caudal wall of the cranial cavity. At 45-degree angles to the longitudinal axis of the skull, they extend from the lateral ends of the transverse cut to the medial faces of the occipital condyles (Figure 5-15). In very small animals the bone may be broken away piecemeal, progressing cranial from the foramen magnum with scissors, bone-cutting forceps, or postmortem shears. The calvaria and caudal wall, as a unit, are pried loose from surrounding bones and removed. The meninges (the three membranes that cover the brain) and the surface of the brain are examined in situ (Figure 5-16).

For removal of the brain, the dorsal meninges are removed and the cranial nerves are transected, progressing rostrally from the foramen magnum. The brain is examined, tagged, and then immersed in 50% formalin. Brain slicing is postponed until after the brain has been thoroughly fixed in formalin.

The pituitary gland is removed from its fossa with the brain and examined. The middle ears (tympanic bullae) are opened ventrally by using rongeurs. For examination of the nasal septum, turbinates, and frontal or maxillary sinuses, the skull is sectioned longitudinally with a saw. The oral cavity is examined.

DISSECTION AND EXAMINATION OF THE NECK AND THORACIC VISCERA

The cervical and thoracic viscera are removed from the body and examined. The trachea and esophagus are used as a handle, and the thoracic organs are removed from the body by cutting between the dorsal mediastinum and the vertebral column from the thoracic inlet back to the diaphragm. The dorsal incision is carried above the aorta. At the diaphragm, the aorta, postcava, and esophagus are transected; and the throat, neck, and thoracic viscera are removed as a unit. This unit is dissected and examined from tongue to aorta. The tongue is examined and sliced transversely. The pharynx is opened middorsally with scissors, and the pharynx and tonsils are examined. The esophagus is opened longitudinally by a middorsal incision. The larynx is opened middorsally

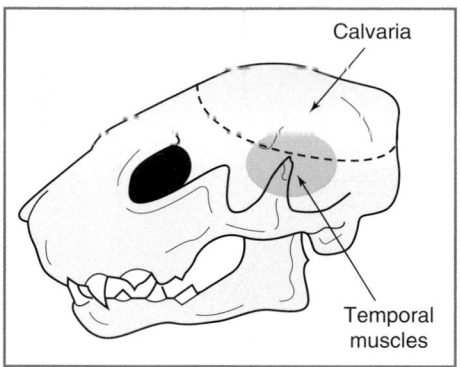

Figure 5-14 The temporal muscles are removed to reveal the skull cap, or calvaria.

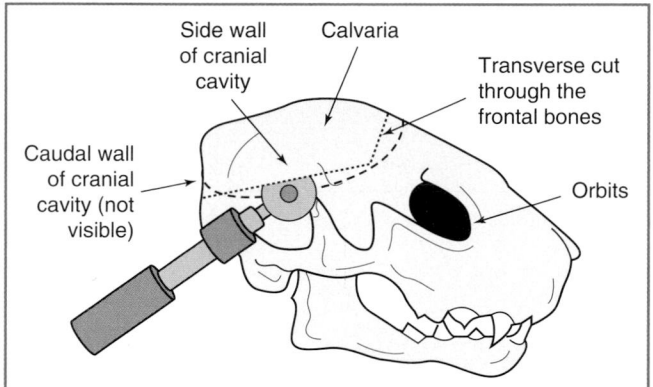

Figure 5-15 The cranial cavity is opened by removing the calvaria and caudal wall as a unit.

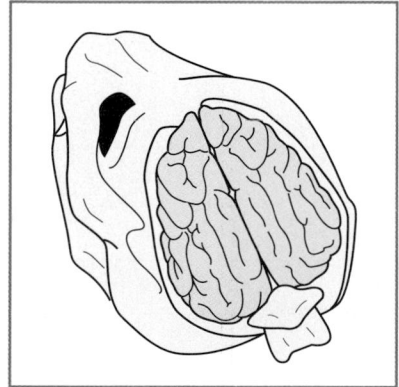

Figure 5-16 The meninges and surface of the brain are examined in situ.

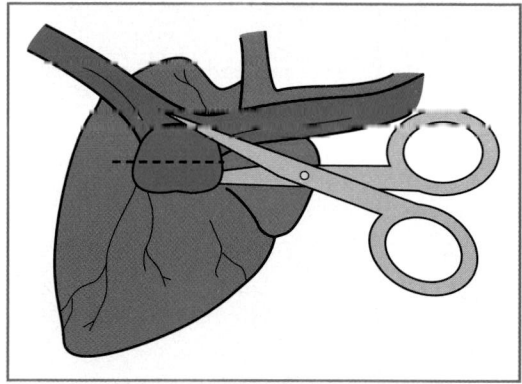

Figure 5-17 Dissection of the heart begins with an incision into the right auricle.

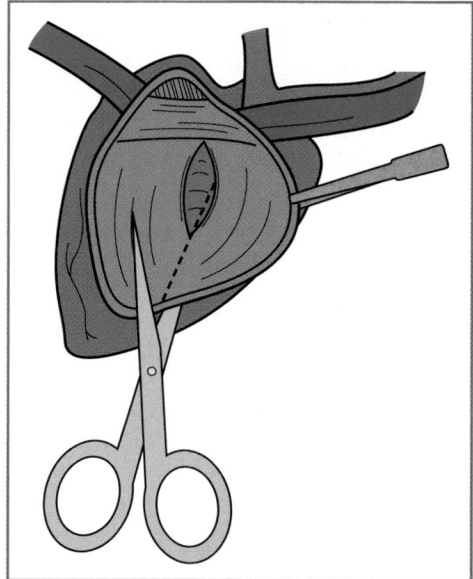

Figure 5-18 The heart is incised through the right atrium and ventricle following the interventricular septum. The incision is then continued into the pulmonary artery.

with utility scissors or a knife, and the incision is extended through the trachea to the lungs. The lungs are examined and palpated. (For fine fixation, the lung may be "inflated" with 10% formalin, gravity-fed into the trachea or bronchi.)

The right side of the heart and pulmonary arteries are examined before the lungs are cut. The heart is held so that the right side is on the prosector's left and the left side is

on the right. The right auricle is incised, and the incision is extended away from the prosector to the far end of the right atrium (Figure 5-17). The incision is then directed downward through the right atrioventricular (AV) valve and along the interventricular septum to the apex of the right ventricle. The incision is then continued up along the interventricular septum through the pulmonic valve into the pulmonary artery (Figure 5-18). The right free wall of the heart is reflected, and the valves and endocardial surfaces are examined. The pulmonary arteries are opened into each lung lobe (Figure 5-19). Air passages and transected lung tissue are examined. Sections of lung are squeezed gently to assess fluid content. Bronchial lymph nodes are examined and sliced longitudinally.

The heart and major vessels are then removed from the lungs. The heart is again held so that the right side is on

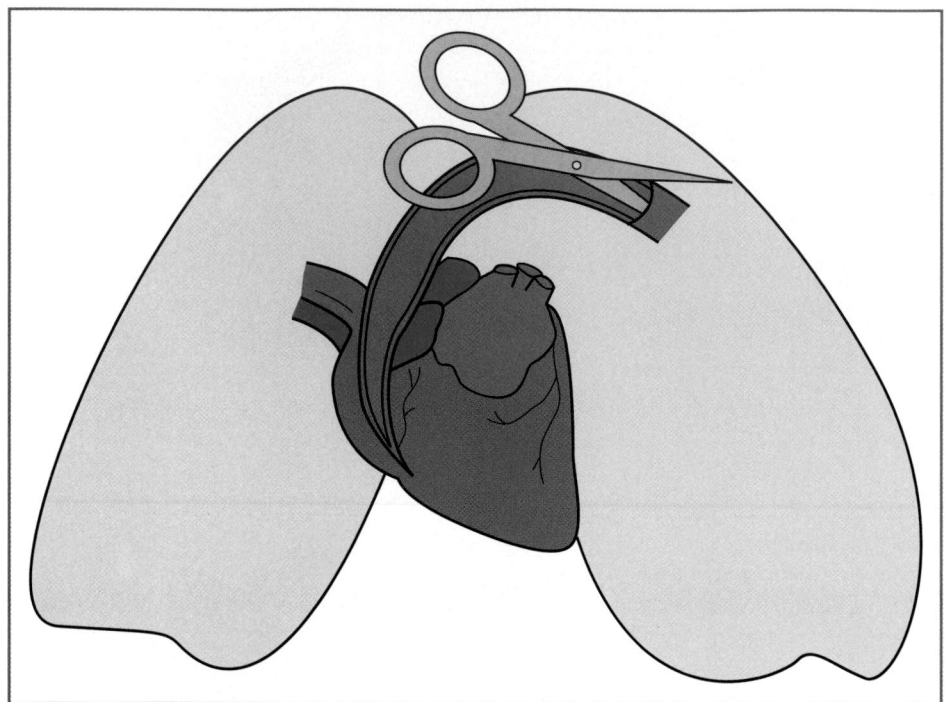

Figure 5-19   The pulmonary artery is incised, and the incision is continued into each lung lobe.

the prosector's left and the left side is to the right. The left auricle is incised, and the incision is extended away from the prosector to the far end of the left atrium (Figure 5-20). The incision is then directed downward through the left AV valve and along the center of the left ventricular free wall to the apex of the left ventricle (Figure 5-21). The aortic valve and aorta are examined by cutting up through the septal leaflet of the left AV valve and into the aorta (Figure 5-22). The valves, endocardium, and endothelial surfaces are then examined. The heart may then be weighed after all major vessels have been removed at the base of the heart. Next, the myocardium is sliced longitudinally for examination, and samples are collected. Small hearts should be fixed whole after they have been opened.

ABDOMINAL CAVITY

Examination of the abdominal cavity begins with examination of the portal vein as it enters the liver and removal of the intestinal tract. The intestine is removed by stripping the mesentery from the small intestine and colon. The duodenum is clamped or tied and transected distal to the tail of the pancreas. The colon is transected at the pelvic inlet, and the intestinal tract is removed and set aside for later examination. If the animal is thought to have intestinal disease, the intestines are examined at this time.

The stomach, liver, spleen, pancreas, and duodenum are removed by cutting the attachments between these organs and the diaphragm and ventral body wall. The spleen is

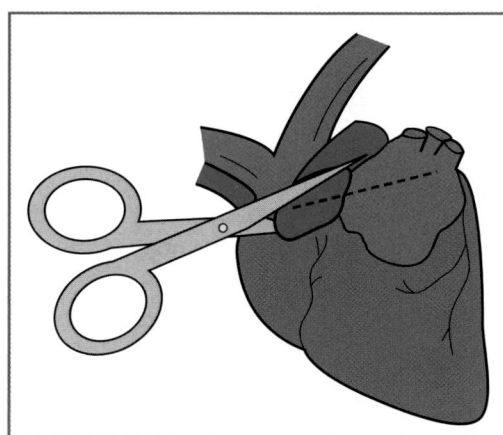

Figure 5-20   The second half of the heart is dissected by incising the left auricle and continuing the incision into the left atrium.

examined and sectioned. The stomach is opened along the greater curvature, and the duodenum is opened. The gallbladder is squeezed to determine patency of the bile duct; the gallbladder is opened; and the stomach, duodenum, and pancreas are dissected from the liver, examined, and sectioned. A section of the right side of the pancreas is collected with the duodenum, and a section of the left side is collected separately. The liver is then examined and sectioned. Multiple slices (approximately 1 cm apart) are made in the liver, and samples are collected from each lobe.

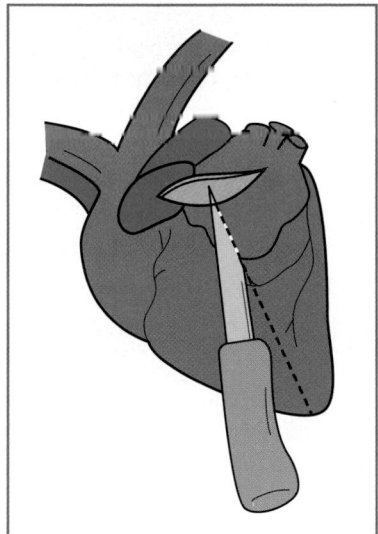

Figure 5-21 From the left atrium, the incision is continued through the left atrioventricular (AV) valve into the left ventricle to the apex.

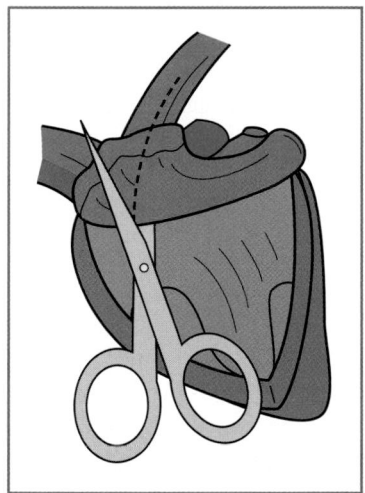

Figure 5-22 The incision is then continued into the aorta.

FEMALE REPRODUCTIVE TRACT, URINARY TRACT, AND ACCESSORY MALE REPRODUCTIVE ORGANS

The floor of the pelvis should be removed to facilitate examination and removal of the urogenital tract. This is accomplished by making paramedian cuts through the obturator foramina on the floor of the pelvis. The mesovarium, mesosalpinx, and mesometrium are examined. Ovaries, oviducts, and uterus are freed from mesentery and reflected toward the pelvis.

The left kidney is dissected free from the abdominal wall but remains attached to the ureter. It is sliced longitudinally, and the capsule is peeled from one half of the kidney (Figure 5-23). The surface, cortex, medulla, and pelvis are

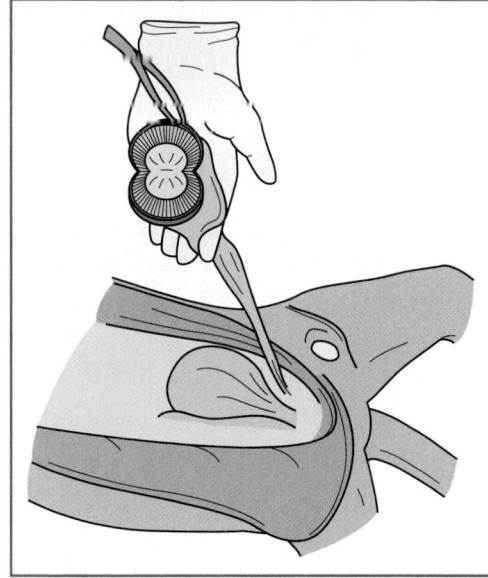

Figure 5-23 The kidney is dissected with a longitudinal incision. The renal capsule is then peeled away to reveal the renal surfaces.

examined. The ureters are examined and palpated. If the ureters or renal pelvis is dilated, the ureters are opened from kidney to bladder with scissors. The ureter is cut near the bladder, and the kidney is removed. Sections are taken from the middle of both halves, one with the capsule intact and one with the capsule removed. Samples are also collected from any other renal lesions. The right kidney is then examined in the same manner.

The urinary bladder is incised and opened. Serosa, mucosa, and cut surfaces are examined. Care should be taken not to rub mucosal surfaces. The urethra is opened and examined, and the prostate is examined and sectioned.

⬛ TECHNICIAN NOTE

Care should be taken not to rub the mucosal surfaces of the tissues being examined.

Ovaries, oviducts, uterus, cervix, vagina, and vulva are removed from the carcass as a unit. Large ovaries are sliced longitudinally; oviducts are examined and palpated; and uterus, cervix, vagina, and vulva are opened with scissors or a knife. Serosa, contents of the uterus, endometrium, cut surfaces, cervical folds, and luminal surface of vagina and vulva are examined.

INTESTINAL TRACT

The intestinal tract is examined by laying it out on the table and examining the serosal surface. The tract is then opened from the duodenum through the colon by using scissors. The mucosa is examined; and sections are taken from the jejunum, ileum, and colon, including lesions. The mucosa should be handled carefully to prevent creation of artifacts. Once sections have been taken, the mucosa can be gently rinsed with water to reveal mucosal details.

ABDOMINAL AORTA, RECTUM, AND ANAL GLANDS

The abdominal aorta is opened longitudinally and examined, and a section is taken for histologic examination. The rectum is opened, and the anal sacs are examined.

VERTEBRAL COLUMN AND SPINAL CORD

The manner and extent to which the vertebral column is dissected will depend on the history and size of the animal. For more extensive examination of the vertebral column and spinal cord, the remaining rib cage, the four limbs, and most of the dorsal spinal musculature are removed from the vertebral column and pelvis. A dorsal laminectomy is performed to demonstrate ventral or lateral impingements on the spinal cord of small animals. The spinal cord is covered dorsally by the vertebral arches; each arch consists of a right and left lamina, which unite to form the spine. Beginning at the atlas, the right and left laminae of each vertebra are cut with bone shears or, in larger specimens, with the Stryker saw. The laminae of atlas and axis are broad and difficult to cut, but the remainder of the vertebrae

present little difficulty. Once several dorsal arches have been freed, the connected arches are held as a handle and used to reflect succeeding arches dorsally and caudally. When the entire roof of the vertebral canal has been removed, meninges, spinal cord, and vertebrae are examined in situ. Spinal cord and meninges are removed by cutting spinal nerve roots, and then the floor of the vertebral canal and the intervertebral disks are examined.

NECROPSY VARIATIONS

The following sections describe variations on the basic small mammal necropsy procedure that are useful in dealing with ruminants, horses, pigs, fetal farm animals, birds, and laboratory animals.

RUMINANTS

Necropsy of a ruminant is done with the animal in left lateral recumbency. This positions the rumen on the down side, which facilitates removal of the abdominal organs (Figure 5-24). The right inguinal area is incised, and the coxofemoral joint is penetrated. Muscles near the pelvis are severed, and the right hind limb is reflected away from the body. Each mammary gland is undermined at its body wall attachment and retracted caudally. The mammary

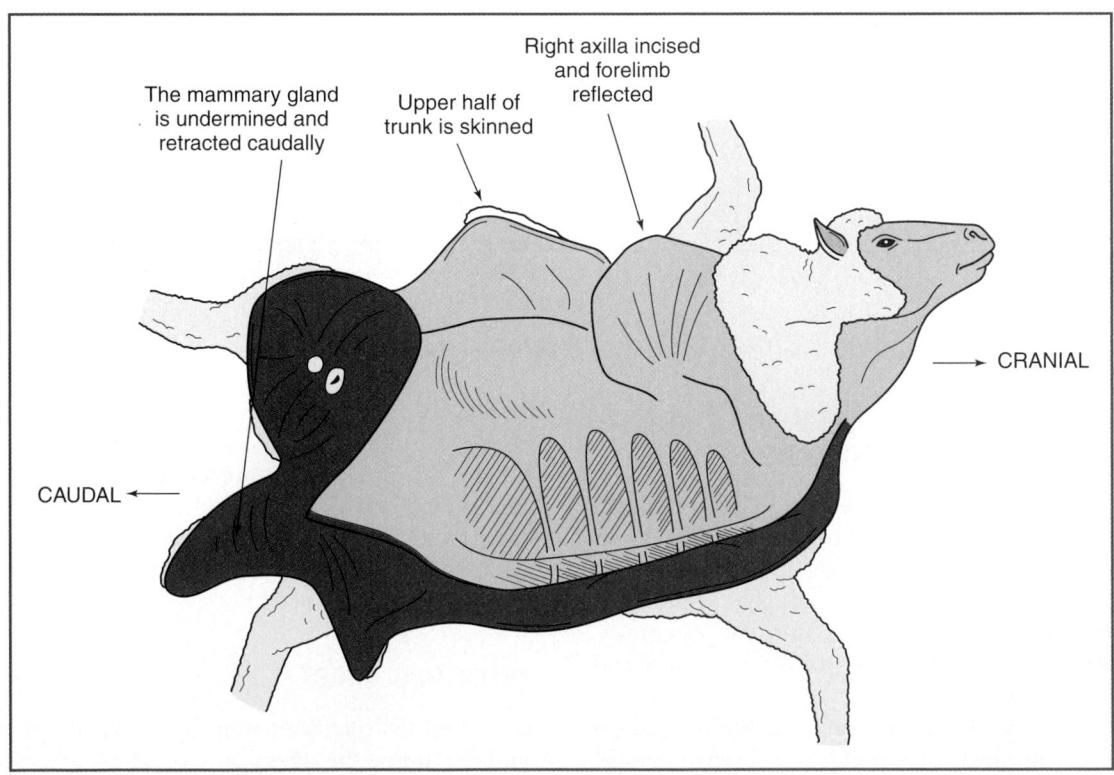

Figure 5-24 The ruminant is positioned in left lateral recumbency, which positions the rumen on the "down side." This facilitates access to the abdominal organs.

glands should remain attached to the body by the perineal skin so that gland position can be maintained when they are serially sectioned. The right axilla is incised so that the entire forelimb can be reflected away from the body. The upper half of the trunk is then skinned.

Entry into the abdomen is initiated by cutting the body wall behind the last rib. Cuts along the midline and upper flank permit exposure of the cavity (Figure 5-25). After an in situ inspection, the omentum is stripped from the forestomachs; double-string ligatures are placed on the duodenum (near the pylorus) and rectum, and a single ligature is placed around the esophagus near the reticulum. This prevents excessive leakage of contents. If the rumen is severely distended with gas, a tiny nick in the wall will release the gas without excessive contamination. The entire intestinal tract is removed by severing the mesenteric root; and the intestines are opened, examined, and sampled while still attached to the mesentery (Figure 5-26). The dorsal attachments to the rumen are cut, and the forestomachs and abomasum are rolled onto the floor. Ruminoreticular contents should be examined for foreign objects or undesirable plant material.

Because of the size of the chest cavity and difficulty in cutting the ribs in mature animals, the thoracic contents are usually removed via the abdominal cavity. The right side of the rib cage is easily removed with lopping shears in young animals. The diaphragm is incised along its costal attachment, and the ventral mediastinal attachments are severed. The tongue, larynx, and trachea are freed of their attachments and threaded into the thoracic inlet. The entire unit is pulled into the abdomen.

The remainder of the necropsy is similar to that described for the small mammal.

HORSE

Left lateral recumbency is the preferred body position for necropsy of a horse. Reflect the right forelimb and right hind limb as described for the ruminant. Skin the trunk, and enter the abdomen. The intestines are removed in the following multistep process:

1. Retract and drape the free portion of the large colon over the horse's body to ease access to the abdominal viscera.
2. Sever the ileum at the ileocecal junction, and remove the small intestine by cutting along the mesenteric insertion.
3. Cut the duodenum where it wraps around the mesenteric root; a string ligature here will reduce contamination by digesta.
4. Next, remove the small intestine mesentery.
5. Sever the small colon near the pelvic inlet, and detach along the mesocolon.
6. With careful blunt dissection, peel the soft connective tissue and pancreas adhering to the large colon near the mesenteric root. When your hand can encircle the mesenteric root, advance the knife to cut as close to the aorta as possible.
7. Obtain samples from the large colon and cecum and empty them of their contents. Rinse and examine the mucosal surfaces.

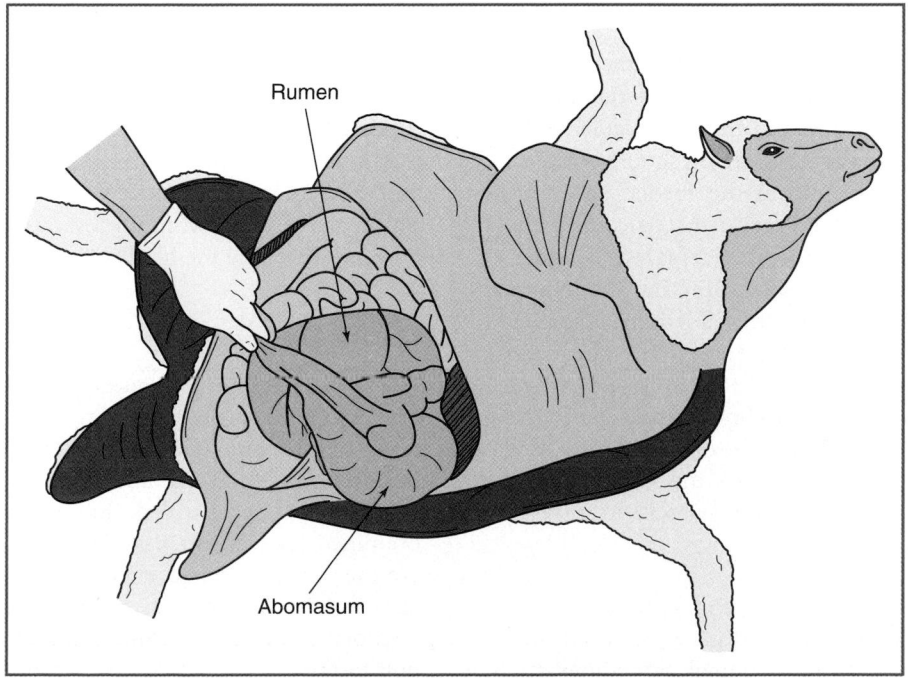

Figure 5-25 Access to the abdominal cavity is achieved by making an incision along the midline, followed by cuts along the last ribs.

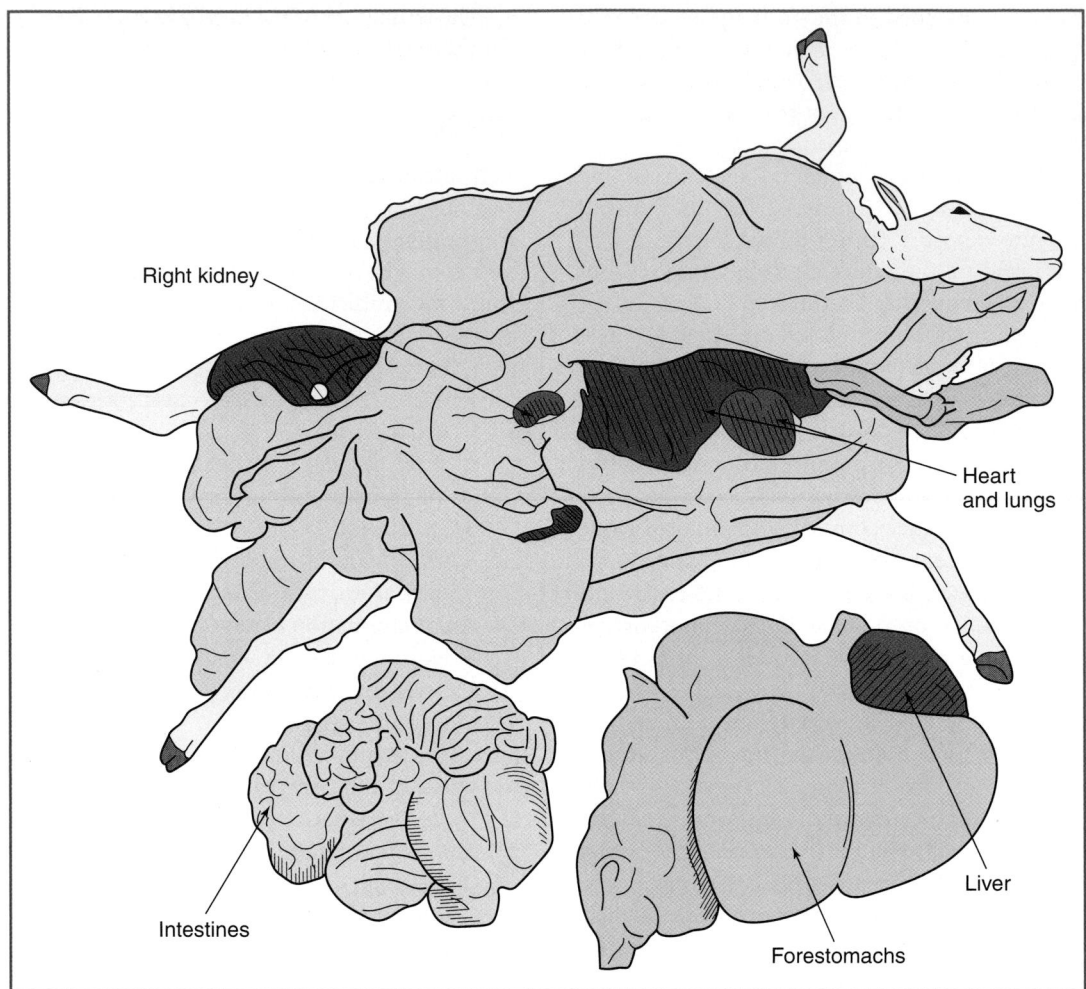

Figure 5-26   After the omentum is examined in situ, it is stripped from the forestomachs. The duodenum, rectum, and esophagus are ligated; and then the entire intestinal tract is removed by severing the mesenteric root.

The remainder of the necropsy is similar to the procedure done on ruminants and small mammals. Special attention should be given to the guttural pouches and jugular veins.

All joints of the appendicular skeleton should be opened. Joints are best approached from the medial and cranial aspects after the skin has been reflected. The coffin joint is the most difficult joint to access, but access is easier if the foot can be split (with a saw). Splitting the foot also facilitates examination of the hoof wall lamina. Spinal cord removal is extremely tedious without access to a meat-cutter's band saw. Alternatively, the cervical cord can be extracted by disarticulating the cervical vertebrae, one by one. Remove as much muscle as possible before disarticulating at the facets and annulus fibrosus. Sever the nerve roots by advancing a pair of thin, long-handled scissors along the wall of the spinal canal.

PIG

For necropsy of a pig, small mammal procedures apply. Because enteric disease is a frequent reason for necropsy,

attention should be focused on collecting the freshest possible gut tissues. It is customary to examine the nasal turbinates of market-weight pigs. This is accomplished with a transverse saw cut of the snout at the level of the second and third premolars. Mature swine have sinus bone covering much of the calvaria. Brain removal is best accomplished by hemisectioning the head.

FETUS

Fetuses are often severely autolyzed, sometimes mummified, because of in utero retention after death. Nevertheless, sample collection is justified. Fetal membranes (placenta) should be carefully examined, and all abnormal-appearing sites should be sampled. Equine fetal membranes are examined for completeness. Fetuses from cattle and horses are measured (weighed if possible) to estimate gestational age. Standardized charts are available in many veterinary textbooks. Crown-to-rump length (the distance from the poll to the tail base along the dorsum) is determined with a flexible tape measure.

The fetus is placed in right lateral recumbency because fetal abdominal organs are most easily sampled from the left side. The left limbs are removed, and the body wall is skinned. The abdominal wall is incised behind the rib, and the incision is extended along the ribs, sublumbar flank, and midline without touching the underlying viscera or allowing the body wall to drop onto the viscera. The left hemidiaphragm and costosternal cartilage are cut with the tip of the knife, and, similar to the abdominal approach, the rib cage is retracted without touching the underlying tissues. The ribs usually break along the vertebral column.

Organs are sampled in situ with sterile tools and aseptic technique. The organs of greatest interest for viral cultures are lungs, liver, kidneys, and lymphoid tissue (e.g., spleen and thymus). Samples for bacterial culture are usually taken from stomach fluid, lungs, and liver. The body can now be routinely examined for anatomic correctness, and samples can be obtained for histologic examination. The umbilical stump and brain should always be examined and collected.

BIRDS

Birds suspected of having infectious or zoonotic diseases (psittacosis) should be submitted to a diagnostic laboratory for necropsy. If avian necropsies are done, the prosector should wear protective clothing, gloves, and a mask. The carcass should be wetted by immersing it in warm soapy water or disinfectant to decrease the spread of infectious agents and reduce the amount of irritating aerosolized dander and feathers. After the external examination, the bird is placed in dorsal recumbency, and the feathers are parted along the ventral midline. For small birds, one wing may be pinned to a cork board or cardboard for easier dissection. A skin incision extending from the beak to the vent is made, and the skin is reflected. The legs are reflected laterally by cutting into and exposing the coxofemoral joint. The abdomen is opened as in the small mammal necropsy technique; and the sternum and lateral ribs are removed by cutting through the sternum, ribs, coracoid bones, and clavicles with scissors, utility scissors, poultry shears, or pruning shears, depending on the size of the bird. Air sacs and abdominal and thoracic contents are examined, and samples are taken for examination by a microbiologist if necessary.

✎ TECHNICIAN NOTE

Birds suspected of having infectious or zoonotic diseases (psittacosis) should be submitted to a diagnostic laboratory for necropsy.

For very small birds (e.g., hummingbirds or finches), the entire carcass can be fixed after the body cavities have been opened. For larger birds, the joints, nerves, muscles, eyes, brain, and spinal cord can be examined as in the small mammal necropsy technique. The spinal cord in small birds is difficult to remove without damaging it. The entire vertebral column with the spinal cord inside should be collected and fixed after the limbs, head, and muscles surrounding the vertebral column have been removed. The vertebral column and spinal cord can be submitted whole and decalcified and trimmed by the pathology laboratory.

In larger birds, the thyroid and parathyroid glands, located at the thoracic inlet adjacent to the carotid arteries, are removed. The heart is removed and examined. The entire gastrointestinal tract, liver, pancreas, and spleen are removed, beginning with the esophagus. The spleen, liver, and gastrointestinal tract are examined; and specimens are collected as in the small mammal necropsy. The tongue, trachea, and lungs are then removed and examined; and samples are collected. The gonads (only the left ovary is present in birds) and adrenal glands are removed and fixed whole in small birds; and then the kidneys are removed, examined, and sampled.

LABORATORY ANIMALS

The necropsy technique for small mammals can be used for most laboratory animals including rodents; however, for evaluation of the health status of laboratory animal colonies, more extensive testing is required. Complete health monitoring includes serology, bacteriology, parasitology, and genetic monitoring in addition to gross pathology and histopathology. It is beyond the scope of this chapter to include techniques for blood collection for serology, bacteriologic sampling techniques, techniques for ectoparasite and endoparasite examination, and genetic monitoring. Many laboratories provide complete diagnostic services and health monitoring for laboratory animals, and such laboratories should be contacted before specimens (either live animals or samples from necropsies) are submitted to them.

✎ TECHNICIAN NOTE

The necropsy technique for small mammals can be used for most laboratory animals. However, for evaluation of the health status of laboratory animal colonies, more extensive testing is required.

The technique for small mammals is followed except for the following variations for small rodents. An entire hind limb can be removed at the coxofemoral joint; the skin can be removed; and the limb can be fixed whole for bone, bone marrow, synovium, nerve, and skeletal muscle samples. For very small rodents (e.g., mice, hamsters, gerbils), the lungs should be inflated with formalin after the thorax has been opened but before the lungs and heart are removed from the thorax. A 5- to 10-ml syringe with a small- to medium-bore needle is filled with formalin. The needle is threaded caudally for a few millimeters from the middle of the trachea, and the trachea is clamped with a hemostat rostral to the needle insertion site. The lungs are gently inflated until they fill the thorax. The trachea is then clamped or tied below the needle insertion site, and the lungs and heart are removed from the chest as described on p. 175. The heart is often too small to open easily, and before fixation, it can be cut longitudinally through the middle of the right and left ventricles.

The intestinal tract can be opened in a few places and then infused with formalin by using a 5-ml syringe and a small-bore needle, or the entire tract can be opened up and pinned to cardboard before fixation. The kidney and adrenal gland on each side can be removed as a unit and left together for fixation after the kidney has been incised longitudinally to evaluate the pelvis for hydronephrosis. The uterus and ovaries or the testes and seminal vesicles/coagulating gland can be removed along with the urinary bladder and fixed whole without sectioning.

The spinal cord in very small animals is difficult to remove without damaging it. The entire vertebral column with the spinal cord inside should be collected and fixed after the limbs, head, and muscles surrounding the vertebral column have been removed. The vertebral column and spinal cord can be submitted whole and decalcified and trimmed by the pathology laboratory.

COSMETIC NECROPSIES

Cosmetic necropsies, although of more limited value than complete necropsies, can be performed when the disease processes are limited to the abdomen and chest. A midline incision is made in the ventral abdomen from the xiphoid to the pubis. The abdominal organs are examined in situ, and the diaphragm is cut away from the ventral rib cage. The colon and urethra are tied off at the pelvic inlet and transected caudal to the tie. By reaching up through the diaphragm, the prosector can grasp and transect the trachea and esophagus at the thoracic inlet. The thoracic and abdominal contents are removed as a unit and dissected and described as in a noncosmetic necropsy. The body cavities are examined. The cavities are filled with paper towels, and the ventral abdominal incision is sutured.

✎ TECHNICIAN NOTE

Cosmetic necropsies, although of more limited value than complete necropsies, can be performed when the disease processes are limited to the abdomen and chest.

Recommended Reading

King JM et al: *The necropsy book,* Gurnee, Ill, 2000, Charles Louis Davis, DVM Foundation.

Necropsy examination. In Richie BW, Harrison GJ, Harrison LR, editors: *Avian medicine: principles and application,* Lake Worth, Fla, 1994, Wingers Publishing, pp 355-379.

APPENDIX I

SAMPLE NECROPSY REPORT

Owner: Brown
Clinic #: 01-34567
Animal name: Ralph
Clinician: Smith
Date/time of death: 01/17/01 (9 am)
Date/time of necropsy: 01/17/01 (11 am)

This is a 3.0-kg, $7^1/_2$-year-old, spayed, female seal-point Siamese cross cat in adequate postmortem and emaciated nutritional condition. There is a clipped area on the distal aspect of the right front leg with an electrocardiogram (ECG) lead taped in place. The left antebrachium is clipped, and a catheter is in the left cephalic vein. The ventral cervical area and the ventral and lateral abdomen are clipped. There is very little body fat, and the muscle mass is reduced.

There is approximately 100 ml of yellow stringy fluid in the abdomen. There are multifocal, 2- to 10-mm, yellow-tan clots of fibrin throughout the abdomen and loosely adherent to abdominal organs. There are white-tan, multifocal to confluent, 1- to 5-cm diameter plaques on the surface of the liver, spleen, small intestine, omentum, mesentery, diaphragm, and body wall. The small intestine and colon are dilated (1 to 2 cm in diameter), and the wall of the small intestine is multifocally thickened. In the most severely affected area, at the jejunoileal junction, the serosa is corrugated and the wall is 3 to 5 mm thick. The abdominal and sternal lymph nodes are enlarged (0.5 to 2.0 cm in diameter) and white on the capsular surface. On section, they have a normal lymph node architecture with a thick white cortex.

The lungs are heavy, wet, and red-purple, and they sink in formalin. There is approximately 5 ml of serosanguineous fluid in the pericardium.

GROSS FINDINGS

Lungs: Moderate to severe acute pneumonia, presumptive
Abdomen: Severe fibrinous peritonitis
Small intestine and colon: Severe chronic enteritis and colitis, presumptive
Pericardium: Moderate serosanguineous effusion
Abdominal and sternal lymph nodes: Severe reactive hyperplasia, presumptive

GROSS DIAGNOSIS

- Euthanasia
- Feline infectious peritonitis (FIP)
- Severe enteritis and colitis, presumptive
- Severe pneumonia, presumptive

COMMENT

I am not sure if the changes in the small intestine and colon are due to FIP or some other process. The lung lesion is also not typical for FIP. Impression smears of the peritoneal surface lesions reveal a mixed population of inflammatory cells, including neutrophils, lymphocytes, plasma cells, and macrophages consistent with the diagnosis of FIP.

Samples of lung and small intestine are submitted for bacterial culture. Samples of lymph nodes, small intestine, colon, lungs, liver, and spleen are submitted for histologic examination.

APPENDIX II

NECROPSY PROCEDURE OUTLINE

1. Before you begin dissection, be sure you have the owner's permission, correct animal, disposition instructions, body weight, labeled formalin container, instruments, cassette for bone marrow, tag for brain, cardboard for nerve and skin, and an understanding of the clinical history.
2. All routine tissues and all lesions are collected; all lesions are described (measured and weighed if appropriate); and all necessary microbiologic, cytologic, and toxicologic samples are collected for every necropsy.
3. Do the external examination; remove eyes; then place body in left lateral recumbency; and make a midline skin incision extending into axillary and inguinal areas to reflect limbs and extend the incision rostrally to the mandibular symphysis and caudally to the perineum.
4. Dissect/examine, section, and collect (DESC) skin, lymph nodes, salivary glands, and testes or mammary glands. Open the coxofemoral, stifle, and scapulohumeral joints. DESC synovium, skeletal muscle, sciatic nerve, and bone marrow.
5. Open abdomen (midline); puncture diaphragm; open chest (bilateral, cutting ribs) and pericardium; collect microbiologic samples; and examine organs and vessels in situ. (NOTE: Discuss case with clinician at this time.) DESC thyroid, parathyroids, and adrenal glands.
6. Remove tongue from oral cavity; and reflect the tongue, tonsils, larynx, and esophagus caudally. Cut spinal cord and vertebral column at atlantooccipital joint; remove skin and muscle from calvaria; cut calvaria with Stryker saw in hood; and remove caudal-dorsal calvaria and dorsal meninges. Transect cranial nerves, and remove brain and pituitary. Open tympanic bullae. Section head longitudinally, and examine nasal and oral cavities.
7. Remove tongue, tonsils, esophagus, trachea, lungs, heart, and thoracic aorta together. DESC tongue, tonsils, esophagus, trachea, right atrium, right ventricle, pulmonary arteries, lungs, lymph nodes, left atrium, left ventricle, and thoracic aorta.
8. Remove distal duodenum, jejunum, ileum, colon, and mesenteric lymph nodes together (open later unless critical). Remove liver, duodenum, pancreas, stomach, and spleen en bloc. DESC spleen; open stomach and duodenum; express gallbladder; and DESC liver, stomach, duodenum, and pancreas.
9. Remove floor of pelvis; and DESC right kidney and ureter, left kidney and ureter, urinary bladder, urethra, prostate, ovaries and uterus, cervix/vagina, rectum, anal glands, and abdominal aorta. DESC small intestine, colon, and mesenteric lymph nodes.
10. Remove spinal cord if necessary.

The size of these items depends on the size of the animal being necroscopied.

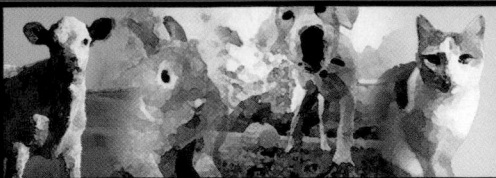

6

Clinical Pathology

JAN L. VANSTEENHOUSE

INTRODUCTION

Accurate clinical pathology data are an invaluable component of the minimum database used in the diagnosis of diseases in all species. Repetition of selected test results also provides a means of monitoring and evaluating the success of chosen treatment regimens. Erroneous data, however, may result in misdiagnoses and be a more serious disadvantage than a lack of data.

Each practice will be faced with the decision of whether laboratory data will be generated within the clinic or be obtained from a reference laboratory. The practice's caseload, availability and turnaround time of a qualified reference laboratory, and experience of the technician are important criteria used to make this determination. Having clinical laboratory data available within 1 hour can be a great advantage to the veterinarian in determining the diagnosis, especially during life-threatening emergencies.

Whether samples are submitted to a reference laboratory or analyzed in the practice, the appropriately trained veterinary technician can be an invaluable asset in ensuring that valid, reliable data are obtained. In either case, knowledge of proper sampling techniques and proper sample handling is essential. The veterinary technician should be familiar with the type and amount of sample to submit for various tests, whether an anticoagulant should be used, and how the sample should be prepared, transported, and stored if it is not immediately analyzed.

It is the veterinary technician's responsibility to have a thorough working knowledge of any in-house analyzer, its sample requirements, its routine maintenance procedures, and basic quality control procedures to ensure accurate laboratory results. The technician should also be familiar with the care and maintenance of all supportive laboratory equipment necessary to keep instruments functioning properly.

Should it be decided that a reference laboratory is more time or cost efficient for an individual practice, the veterinary technician must communicate with the personnel of that laboratory. The laboratory should be consulted regarding appropriate sample submission for specific tests to prevent unnecessary delays and invalid results. Precautions must be taken to ensure that the samples are not damaged or destroyed during transport. This chapter addresses the more commonly used clinical laboratory techniques and procedures in veterinary hematology, urinalysis, clinical chemistry, and cytology. Techniques and methods are emphasized rather than interpretation. The recommended reading list provides detailed reviews. Laboratory instrumentation and necessary quality control systems for clinical chemistry and hematology are reviewed and summarized. In addition, errors in sampling and sample handling and the consequence of misleading values, which complicate the interpretation of laboratory data, are discussed. ▪

Hematology

The basic equipment necessary for hematologic analyses includes a microscope, microhematocrit centrifuge, refractometer, hemacytometer, clean slides, and modified Wright's stain. The benefits of conscientious care and cleaning of these items cannot be overlooked. The complete blood count (CBC) provides the veterinarian with invaluable information regarding the patient's red blood cell (RBC [erythrocyte]) mass, white blood cell (WBC [leukocyte]) number and distribution, platelet number, and plasma protein. The CBC consists of a packed cell volume (PCV), WBC count, RBC count, hemoglobin determination, RBC indices, platelet count or estimate, total plasma protein determination, and evaluation of the blood smear for RBC morphology and a WBC differential count. Hematologic procedures are performed on anticoagulated whole blood. The preferred anticoagulant is ethylenediaminetetraacetic acid (EDTA) because it does not interfere with blood cell morphology and staining. EDTA is commercially available in purple-top Vacutainer tubes in a variety of sizes. Choosing the correct size is essential to obtaining accurate results because having a small amount of blood in a large tube will alter some of the values. The various types of sample tubes available and their appropriate uses are listed in Table 6-1.

The morphology of the normal and abnormal blood cells is briefly reviewed, but it is strongly recommended that the technician have on hand and consult the appropriate references listed at the end of this chapter. Table 6-2 contains sample reference ranges for normal hematology values in common domestic species.

EQUIPMENT

When a microscope is chosen, the laboratory's needs must first be assessed. The fewer "extras" that are included will reduce the requirements for maintenance, service, and

repairs. A good-quality binocular microscope with a mechanical stage, an adjustable substage condenser, and good-quality objective lenses will accommodate the needs of any hematology laboratory. The most important aspect, and often the cost determinant, of a good laboratory microscope is the objective lens. Planachromatic lenses are recommended because they provide a flat field of vision with superior optical properties. The entire field will be in focus, resulting in reduced eyestrain and improved microscopic images. The basic laboratory microscope should have 10×, 40× (high dry), and 100× (oil immersion) objective lenses in addition to standard 10× ocular objectives. Many microscopists find an additional 50× oil immersion objective lens useful for evaluation of both blood films and cytology specimens. The manufacturer's manual should provide directions for adjusting the light for optimal intensity (Kohler illumination), which enhances the clarity of the image.

Proper care of the microscope is essential to providing accurate results for an extended period. Great care should be taken to follow the manufacturer's directions for proper use, cleaning, and maintenance. The oil immersion lenses require a drop of special immersion oil on the blood film to achieve the appropriate optics. The immersion oil should be wiped from the objective after use to prevent damage to the lens. It is essential that all other objectives be kept free of oil. Lenses should be cleaned with lens paper only. A dust cover should be placed over the microscope when it is not in use to prevent collection of dust and hairs on the lenses and other surfaces.

Table 6-1 RECOMMENDED SAMPLE TUBES

Color of Top	Anticoagulant	Purpose
Purple	EDTA	CBC, platelet counts
Red	None	Chemistries
Tiger (red-black)	Separator gel	Chemistries
Green	Heparin	Electrolytes, stats
Turquoise	Citrate	Coagulation assay

CBC, Complete blood count; *EDTA*, ethylenediamine tetraacetic acid.

✎ TECHNICIAN NOTE

No laboratory equipment or instrument, regardless of cost, is any better than the care and maintenance it receives.

Table 6-2 HEMATOLOGY VALUES

	Canine	Feline	Equine	Bovine
PCV (%)	37-55	30-45	32-48	24-46
Hemoglobin (g/dl)	12-18	8-15	10-18	8-15
Reticulocytes (%)	0-1.5	0-1.0	0	0
WBCs (n/μl)	6,000-17,000	5,500-19,500	6,000-12,000	4,000-12,000
Segments	3,000-11,400	2,500-12,500	3,000-6,000	600-4,000
Bands (n/μl)	0-300	0-300	0-100	0-120
Lymphocytes (n/μl)	1,000-4,800	1,500-7,000	1,500-5,000	2,500-7,500
Monocytes (n/μl)	150-1,350	0-850	0-600	25-850
Eosinophils (n/μl)	100-750	0-750	0-800	0-2,400
Basophils (n/μl)	Rare	Rare	0-300	0-200
TP (g/dl)	6.0-7.5	6.0-7.5	6.0-8.5	6.0-8.0
Fibrinogen (mg/dl)	150-300	150-300	100-400	100-600
Platelets (n/μl)	200,000-500,000	300,000-700,000	100,000-600,000	100,000-800,000

n, Number; *PCV*, packed cell volume; *TP*, total protein; *WBCs*, white blood cells.

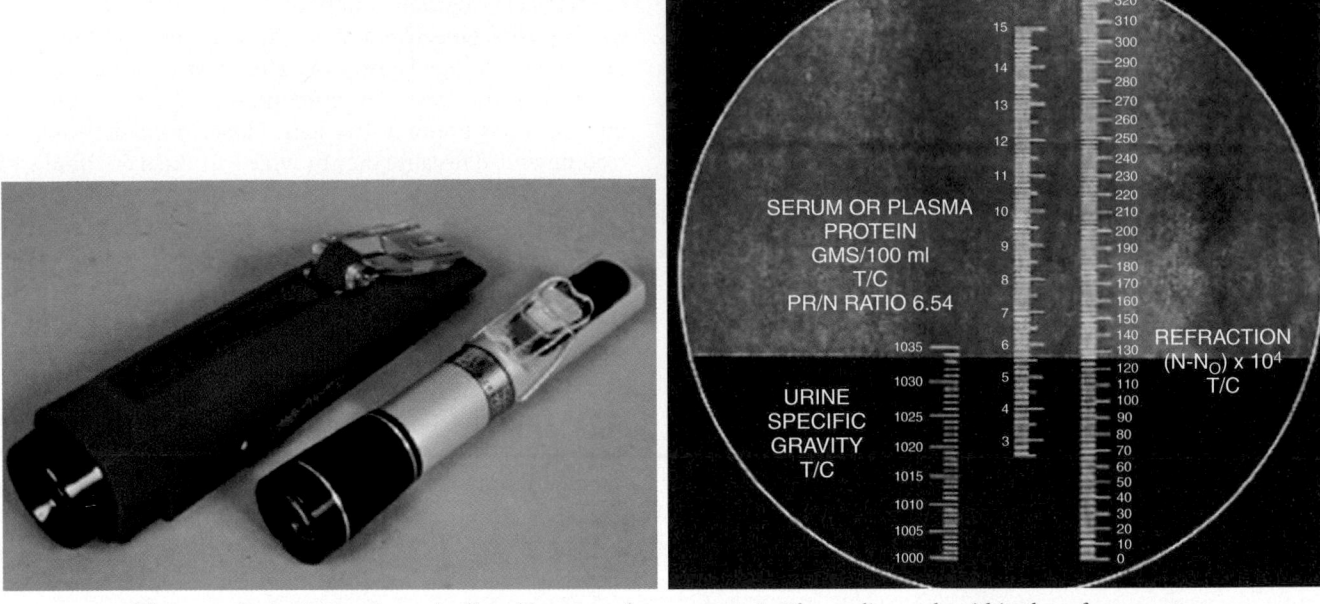

Figure 6-1 **A,** Veterinary (red) and human refractometers. **B,** The reading scale within the refractometer.

A microhematocrit centrifuge is required for determination of the PCV. The force generated by the centrifuge separates the cellular components of blood from the plasma. The manufacturer's manual should be consulted for recommended speed settings for the sample being spun. As with all laboratory equipment, the accuracy and functional longevity of the centrifuge are directly related to proper care and use. For the purpose of safety, the centrifuge should not be operated unless the lid is closed and properly secured. Samples should always be balanced to ensure accurate separation and reduce wear on the motor. Periodic maintenance, such as lubricating the bearings and checking the commutator, should be scheduled according to the manufacturer's recommendations to extend the life of the centrifuge and ensure accurate results.

The refractometer is used to determine the plasma protein concentration by measuring the refractive index of the plasma. Careful cleaning of the sample surface is imperative to prolonging the accuracy and functional life of the refractometer. Several models are available, including one designed specifically for veterinary use (Figure 6-1). The veterinary model is less expensive, has a more shock-resistant casing, and is appropriate for use in veterinary determination of urine specific gravity (SG). Calibration of the zero setting should be checked periodically with distilled water and adjusted according to the instructions in the manufacturer's manual if necessary.

The Neubauer (recommended) hemacytometer is a small but valuable specialized counting chamber used for determining WBC and platelet counts per microliter of blood (Figure 6-2). With the 1:100 dilution Unopette system (Becton Dickinson Inc, Franklin Lakes, NJ) for WBC and platelet counts, all nine of the large primary squares are

counted for WBCs at 10×, and platelets are counted in all 25 squares within the center primary square at 40×. Appropriate calculations are provided with the system used to determine cells per microliter. The hemacytometer has a special coverglass calibrated for accuracy; a regular coverglass cannot be substituted, should it be damaged. Both the hemacytometer and coverslip must be cleaned carefully to prevent scratching of the surfaces.

New, clean glass slides are essential for making usable blood films. Slides that are frosted on one end are preferred for labeling purposes.

SAMPLE HANDLING

In general, EDTA is the required anticoagulant for hematology. Be sure to use a tube of the appropriate size for the sample being drawn. It is often difficult to obtain large samples from small dogs and cats; the 2-ml pediatric collection tube is best for a patient of this size. There are collection tubes for smaller volumes (0.5-ml Microtainer tubes, Becton Dickinson Inc. Franklin Lakes, NJ). These tubes are excellent for samples from puppies, kittens, and small exotic animal species. Excess anticoagulant resulting from a small amount of blood in a too-large tube can erroneously decrease the PCV and increase total protein values determined with a refractometer.

Anticoagulated blood samples should be immediately mixed by gentle inversion of the tube. Blood films should be made from well-mixed blood within 15 minutes of obtaining the sample to decrease in vitro morphologic changes in the blood cells. If the practice uses a reference laboratory, unstained blood films should be sent with the EDTA sample.

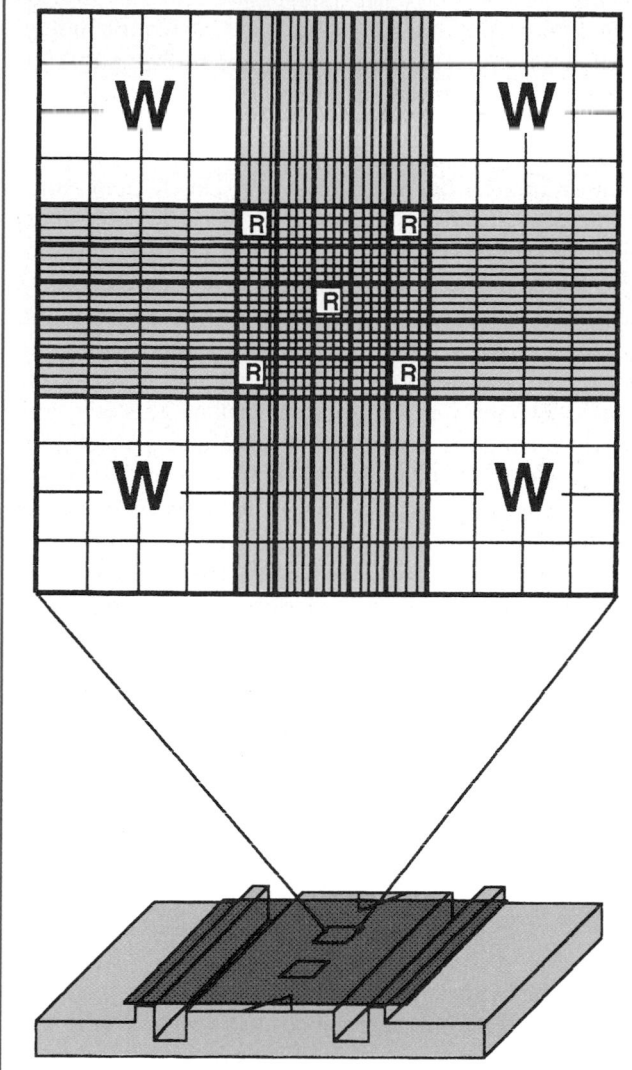

Figure 6-2 Neubauer hemacytometer. The large *W*s indicate the squares that are counted for a total white blood cell (WBC) count with the 1:20 dilution WBC Unopette system. The small *R*s indicate the squares that are counted for a red blood cell (RBC) count with the RBC Unopette system.

If samples must be held overnight, refrigerate the whole blood but do not refrigerate the blood film. Water will condense on the surface of the blood film if it is placed in the refrigerator and cause lysis of the RBCs. The blood film, as well as cytology slides, should be protected from formalin vapors because formalin will interfere with cell preservation and staining. If samples are being sent out, they should be packaged in separate bags.

🖉 TECHNICIAN NOTE

Blood films should always be made from fresh blood, before refrigeration, regardless of whether the CBC will be performed in the clinic or sent to a reference laboratory.

DETERMINATION OF ERYTHROCYTE NUMBERS

Determination of the PCV, the percentage of total blood volume accounted for by RBCs, is the easiest and most common means of evaluating the RBC mass. This is achieved by filling a plain microhematocrit capillary tube with anti-coagulated blood, sealing one end of the tube with a specific clay, and spinning the sample in a microhematocrit centrifuge. The spun sample is then applied to a chart to determine the PCV. This method provides a quick and accurate measurement if samples are spun for a standard length of time at a consistent speed. The specific time and speed depend on the particular centrifuge being used. Accuracy also depends on the care and operation of the centrifuge. Blood samples from cattle, sheep, and goats may require centrifugation for a longer time because their smaller RBCs do not pack as well as dog and cat RBCs. The plasma portion at the top of the tube should be evaluated for color and clarity and will also be used for determination of plasma protein values. The *hematocrit* provides basically the same information but is obtained by calculation when an auto-mated analyzer is used and thus may be slightly different from the measured PCV. This is most commonly seen in blood samples from collection tubes that have an inadequate volume of blood (less than 1 ml in a 5-ml tube or less than 0.5 ml in a 2-ml tube). The excess anticoagulant causes the RBCs to shrink, erroneously decreasing the PCV. When the blood is diluted by the electronic cell counter, the diluent reexpands the RBCs to their true size, providing the true value for the hematocrit.

The actual number of erythrocytes may be determined by using an automated cell counter, which is primarily available in reference laboratories. Erythrocyte counts may also be performed manually but are too tedious and inaccurate to be of diagnostic value. RBC counts vary proportionately with PCV and have little to no advantage over PCV. The major advantage of automated cell counters is that they also measure hemoglobin and measure or calculate the RBC indices. Hemoglobin is the protein in RBCs that is responsible for carrying oxygen from the lungs to the tissues.

RED BLOOD CELL INDICES

RBC indices are commonly provided when automated analyzers are used; these indices include mean corpuscular volume, mean corpuscular hemoglobin (MCH), and mean corpuscular hemoglobin concentration (MCHC). The MCH is of little value, but the mean corpuscular volume and MCHC are useful in evaluating and determining the cause of anemias (decreased RBC number). MCH and MCHC values calculated with an electronic cell counter will be artifactually affected by hemolysis, Heinz bodies, and lipemia. Samples with these properties therefore cannot be used to determine MCH and MCHC.

$$\text{Mean corpuscular volume (femtoliters)} = \frac{\text{PCV} \times 10}{\text{RBC} (10^6)}$$

$$\text{MCH (picograms)} = \frac{\text{Hemoglobin} \times 10}{\text{RBC} (10^6)}$$

$$\text{MCHC (g/dL)} = \frac{\text{Hemoglobin} \times 100}{\text{PCV}}$$

DETERMINATION OF LEUKOCYTE COUNTS

The total WBC count may be determined manually with the hemacytometer or an automated cell counter. Either way, it is important that the blood tube be well mixed before the sample is taken. Figure 6-2 shows the hemacytometer grid that will be seen microscopically and indicates the areas on the grid in which WBCs will be counted. The glass coverslip is one specifically designed for the hemacytometer, and regular coverslips cannot be substituted, so it must be handled and cleaned carefully to prevent damage and should never be used for other purposes. Use of the Unopette dilution system is the most accepted method for performing manual WBC counts. Several Unopette systems are available for counting various cell types (Table 6-3), but the system preferred for counting leukocytes is also used for counting platelets and determining cell counts on samples such as synovial fluid. This system consists of a disposable reservoir containing diluent and an agent to lyse RBCs to accommodate the counting of leukocytes. Each Unopette system comes with detailed instructions for obtaining reliable results and a capillary pipette with which to draw a specific volume of blood. The interchangeable use of pipettes from another cell counting system, such as one for RBCs, to obtain WBC counts will result in significant errors and inappropriately decreased WBC counts.

The accuracy of a manual WBC count depends on adherence to the directions and the proper performance of each step. Care must be taken to accurately fill the capillary tube and wipe off any excess blood on the outside of the tube without touching the tip of the pipette and drawing any of the sample out of the pipette. The blood sample must be carefully transferred to the reservoir with careful mixing to ensure complete delivery of the sample into the diluent. Blood left in the capillary tube or accidentally expelled from the top of the pipette during mixing will result in erroneous WBC counts. It will take practice and may require multiple attempts to completely and accurately fill the hemacytometer chamber. The chambers on both sides of the hemacytometer must be filled for accurate results. Counting both sides and comparing results also serve to check accuracy because the number of cells on one side should closely approximate the number of cells on the other side. Overfilling or underfilling the chamber will cause errors in the final cell count. After the hemacytometer chambers have been charged, the hemacytometer must be allowed to sit for several minutes to allow the cells to settle. WBCs will be counted with the use of the 10× objective; lowering the condenser on the microscope will increase the contrast, making the cells more prominent and easier to identify and count accurately.

Nucleated RBCs (NRBCs) will be counted along with WBCs by either manual or automated electronic counting methods, resulting in falsely elevated WBC counts. The number of NRBCs encountered on the blood film is counted while the differential count is performed on 100 leukocytes. The WBC count is then corrected by using the following formula if more than 10 NRBCs are counted:

$$\frac{100}{100 + \text{Number of NRBCs} \times \text{WBC}} = \textbf{Corrected WBC count}$$

For example, if 15 NRBCs are counted while the 100-cell differential count is performed and the initial WBC count is 30,000/µl, the corrected count is then calculated as follows:

$$\frac{100}{100 + 15 \times 30,000} = \textbf{26,087 WBCs}$$

Increased WBCs are referred to as *leukocytosis,* whereas decreased WBCs are referred to as *leukopenia.* The diagnostic significance of either leukocytosis or leukopenia cannot be appreciated without the WBC differential count. The differential count is performed by examining the blood film (see the discussion of blood film evaluation). At least 100 leukocytes are identified and counted according to cell type (as neutrophils, bands, lymphocytes, monocytes, eosinophils, or basophils). The more cells that are counted, the more accurate the differential count will be. The percentages of each cell type counted are then multiplied by the total WBC count to provide absolute numbers of the cell types present. These numbers are the values used for interpreting changes in the leukogram.

Table 6-3 UNOPETTE SYSTEMS FOR COUNTING DIFFERENT CELL TYPES

Test	Pipette Volume	Dilution	Diluent
Red cell count	<10 µl	<1:200	<0.85% Saline
White cell count	20 µl	1:100	3% Acetic acid
White cell count	25 µl	1:20	3% Acetic acid
Platelet count	20 µl	1:100	1% Ammonium oxalate
Eosinophil count	25 µl	1:32	Phloxin

Dramatic increases or decreases in WBC count may also be noted by looking at the *buffy coat.* The buffy coat is the white band of concentrated WBCs between the RBCs and plasma in the microhematocrit tube.

AVIAN AND REPTILIAN LEUKOCYTE COUNTS

Unlike mammals, birds and reptiles have NRBCs (Figure 6-3), and this prevents determination of their WBC counts by the methods described. However, the WBC counts of these nonmammalian species may be determined indirectly by using another Unopette system for eosinophil determination. This special Unopette is filled with anticoagulated blood, mixed well, and allowed to incubate for approximately 5 minutes to allow uptake of the stain by the cells. If the sample is allowed to stand for a prolonged time, all the cells will take up the stain and results will be erroneous. The hemacytometer is filled as for the manual WBC count described, and the red-staining cells are counted in all nine squares of the grid. With proper staining, only the eosinophils and heterophils (nonmammalian equivalent of neutrophils) will be stained. In contrast to performance of the mammalian manual count, it is important to keep the microscope condenser up to decrease contrast. If the condenser is down, it will be more difficult to count the heterophils and eosinophils because of RBC interference.

The number obtained does not represent the WBC count but is used in conjunction with the differential count to calculate the WBC count. When the differential count is completed and the percentages of the various cell types present are known, the WBC count is calculated with the following formula:

$$\frac{\text{Cells counted on hemacytometer} \times 32 \times 100}{\text{\% Heterophils} + \text{Eosinophils}} = \text{WBCs}/\mu l$$

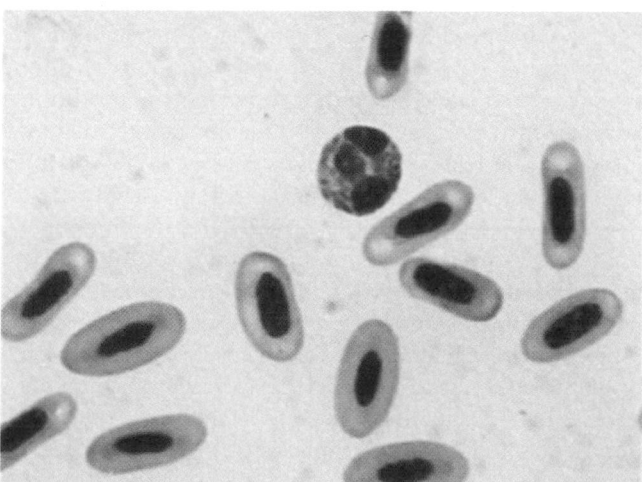

Figure 6-3 Nucleated red blood cells (RBCs) and a heterophil from a Cockatoo.

For example, if 282 cells are counted on one side of the hemacytometer and you have 70% heterophils and 5% eosinophils on the differential count, the total WBC count would be as follows:

$$\frac{282 \times 32 \times 100}{70 + 5} = 12,032 \text{ WBCs}/\mu l$$

PLATELET DETERMINATION

Determination of platelet numbers is important because platelets play an important role in *hemostasis,* or control of blood flow. Several diseases cause decreased numbers of platelets, and these can often be diagnosed and treated before a severe bleeding disorder develops. Like WBCs, platelets can be counted manually on a hemacytometer or with an automated cell counter. Feline platelets, in particular, have a tendency to clump, which interferes with obtaining accurate platelet counts; whether the count is done manually or by automation, an erroneously low platelet count can result. For this reason, it is important to always examine the blood film for platelet clumping. In addition, because cats often have relatively large platelets and cat RBCs are small, automated electronic counts are often inaccurate because of the inability to separate the cells by size.

Manual platelet counts can be performed by using the same Unopette system and sample used for the manual WBC count. This task can be very tedious, especially if the hemacytometer and coverglass are not properly cared for. Scratches and small dust particles are very difficult to differentiate from platelets. If platelet clumps are present, the resultant count will be inaccurate. It would be best to obtain another sample with special attention given to ensure a clean venipuncture and adequate mixing of the blood with the anticoagulant. Platelets are identified with the use of the 40× objective and will be easier to see if the condenser is lowered and the light intensity is moderate. The instructions that accompany the Unopette must be followed with regard to the squares of the grid that are counted and the method of determining the total count.

> ### ✎ TECHNICIAN NOTE
> The blood film should always be scanned for platelet clumps, especially for cats, to avoid reporting erroneously low platelet numbers.

When platelet counts are not available or when it is necessary to verify counts obtained manually or electronically, the number of platelets can be estimated from the blood film. During examination of the appropriate area of the blood film in which RBCs are spaced in a uniform monolayer, the average number of platelets per 100× oil immersion field in several fields (10 or more) is determined. This average number of platelets multiplied by 15,000 will provide an adequate estimation of the number of platelets per microliter.

Decreased platelet counts can have serious implications for the patient. Therefore before low platelet counts are reported, all technical problems must be considered. The feathered edge of the blood film must be checked for platelet clumping. The tube of blood from which the sample was taken should be checked for small clots, which could deplete platelets. Either or both of these problems may occur despite the use of an anticoagulant. If neither the blood film nor the tube reveals evidence of platelet aggregation, the low platelet count should be reported as determined. If platelet clumping or clots are found, another sample should be drawn, and the counts should be repeated.

BLOOD FILM EVALUATION

Examination of the stained blood smear is one of the most valuable parts of the CBC, and its importance cannot be overstressed. For the sake of time, many technicians are tempted to skip this portion of the CBC, but the numbers alone can be very misleading and result in incorrect diagnoses and inappropriate treatment. Anemias cannot be classified and changes in the WBC count cannot be accurately interpreted until the differential count is completed and the cells are examined for morphologic changes. Examination of the blood film is especially important as an internal quality control when automated electronic cell counters are used. If there appears to be a discrepancy between what the technician sees on the film and the numbers reported by the instrument, the counts should be repeated with special attention given to determining what could be causing the difference. A common cause is that the blood tube was not adequately mixed before sampling for either the count or the blood film. Another common problem is seen, particularly in cats with leukopenia, with considerable platelet clumping. The platelet clumps are large enough that they are counted as WBCs in the automated system, resulting in falsely higher WBC counts made by the instrument. With time and experience, the technician will be able to scan the blood film and recognize the discrepancies between the number of leukocytes apparent on the film and the number of WBCs reported by the instrument. As a general rule, there should be approximately 20 leukocytes per 10× field in a normal canine blood sample.

There are a variety of ways to make quality blood films. New slides should always be used, and they should be handled only by the edges because transfer of oils from fingers to the slide will result in poor-quality films. If the slides have inadvertently been exposed to dust and debris, it may be helpful to clean them with a nonabrasive tissue such as Kimwipes. (The reader is referred to Recommended Reading for examples of the different techniques.) What is most important is to try several methods, find the one that is most comfortable, and then practice repeatedly until quality films are consistently produced. Most commonly, a small drop of blood is placed at one end of a slide, and

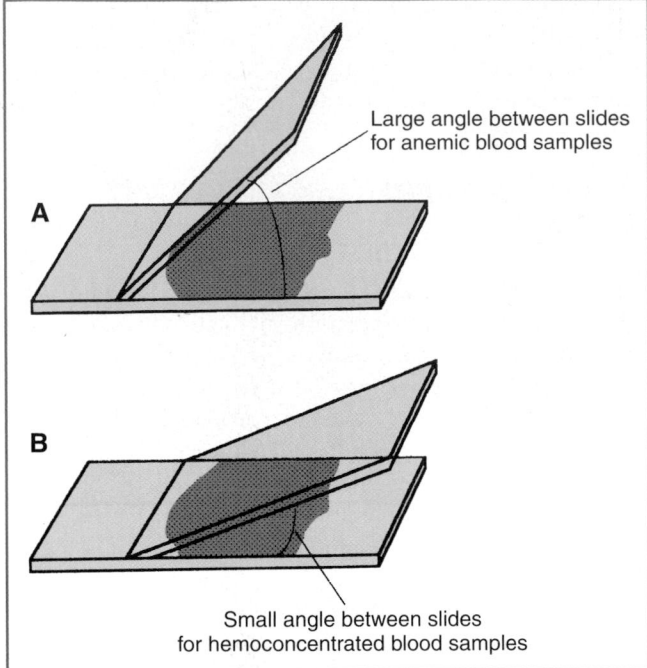

Figure 6-4 Difference in slide angle necessary for making blood films from anemic or hemoconcentrated blood. *A,* Large angle for anemic blood. *B,* Small angle for hemoconcentrated blood.

the edge of a second slide is used to spread the drop. It is important to make the film in one even stroke and not use excessive downward pressure. Increased downward pressure on the spreader slide can cause the leukocytes to be carried to the feathered edge and may even cause the cells to rupture or become distorted. In either case the accuracy of the differential count will be decreased. The thickness of the blood film can be altered to accommodate samples from severely anemic or dehydrated animals. Increasing the angle between the two slides will concentrate the cells when the PCV is very low. Conversely, decreasing the angle will allow greater spreading of the cells in a concentrated sample (Figure 6-4).

Manual counts with Wright-Giemsa stains are labor intensive and require frequent filtering of the stains. More equipment, a source of distilled water, and critical timing are necessary. Several modifications of the traditional Wright's stain are available for suitable staining of blood films for veterinary practices. Stat Stain (VWR Scientific, Philadelphia, Pa), Diff-Quik (Baxter S/P, McGaw Park, Ill), and CAMCO Quik Stain (Baxter S/P) are commonly used. They are relatively economical, less time consuming, and technically easy to use and maintain. The components may be kept in individual Coplin jars. The lids should always be securely replaced after use, and the stains should be freshened or refilled as necessary. Bacteria are rarely a problem in these stains, but care should be taken to avoid gross contamination of the jars. The disadvantages of these stains are few. Polychromatophilic RBCs do not stain as obviously as they do with Wright-Giemsa stain, and some mast cell and eosinophil granules may be washed out.

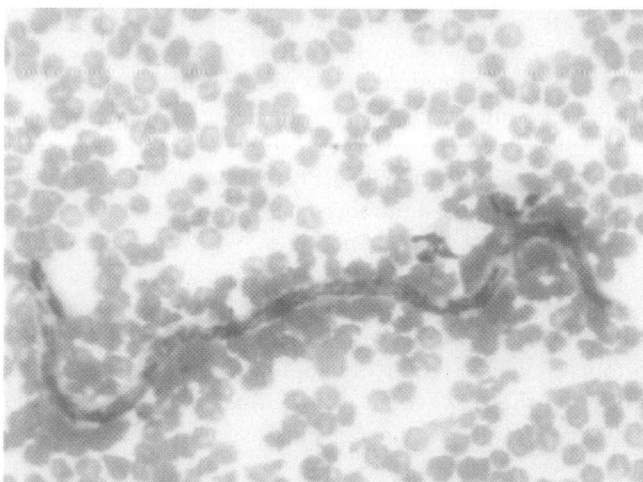

Figure 6-5 A microfilaria of *Dirofilaria immitis* in a canine blood smear. The parasite is about the same width as an erythrocyte.

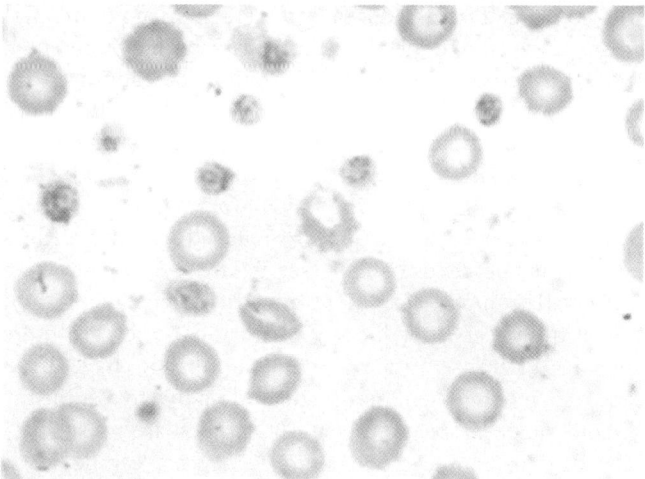

Figure 6-6 Canine blood smear showing hypochromic erythrocytes with increased central pallor as seen in iron-deficiency anemia. Several platelets are also present between the erythrocytes.

It is best to develop a routine for evaluating a blood film and follow the same approach each time to prevent oversights and mistakes. The blood film should first be examined under low power (10×). While scanning on 10×, one can get an impression of the general distribution of nucleated cells (clumped at the edges or spread evenly throughout), estimate the total WBC count (low vs. normal vs. high), and examine the feathered edge of the blood film for aggregates of platelets, the larger leukocytes, neoplastic cells, and microfilaria of *Dirofilaria immitis* or *Dipetalonema reconditum* (Figure 6-5). During the low-power examination, one may identify structures or areas that need a closer look. Last, on low power, one should identify the appropriate area in which RBCs are distributed in a uniform monolayer and the leukocytes are sufficiently spread so that morphologic identification on high power is possible. It is especially important to avoid being too far into the body of the blood film, where the WBCs are rounded and darkly stained. In this area, it is often difficult to differentiate the leukocytes.

The blood film is then studied under high power, generally under oil immersion (100×). The WBC differential count is performed at this power. Erythrocytes should be evaluated for morphologic changes and parasites, and platelets should be evaluated for morphology and counted to make the estimated count. These evaluations may be made before or after the differential count is performed, but they should be done consistently as part of the routine so they are not overlooked. Platelets are cytoplasmic fragments, so they have no nuclei. They are generally round to oval or spindle shaped with purplish granules and multiple pointed projections (Figure 6-6). They may vary greatly in size, but increased numbers of large platelets may indicate an increased output from the bone marrow. After the platelets have been evaluated, the erythrocytes should be studied.

ERYTHROCYTE EVALUATION

The erythrocytes of most mammals are disk shaped and anuclear. They appear flat with a varying degree of *central pallor* (pale area in center of cell with less hemoglobin), depending on the size. The RBCs of different domestic species differ markedly in size, with those of the dog having the largest diameter (7 μm), followed by those of the horse, cow, and cat (5.8 μm), the sheep (4.5 μm), and the goat (3.2 μm). Some species have RBCs that vary in size, which is termed *anisocytosis*. Cows normally have more anisocytosis than do other species. In other species, extreme anisocytosis implies either that many of the RBCs are smaller (microcytic), which may indicate iron deficiency, or that many are larger (macrocytic), which may indicate increased production and release of immature cells from the bone marrow in response to anemia. Some poodles normally have larger RBCs than do other dogs. Some Japanese Akita dogs normally have smaller RBCs. These are genetic traits and do not indicate a change in RBC dynamics.

Poikilocytosis is the general term used to indicate changes in RBC shape. *Leptocytes* are RBCs with an increased surface area that makes them highly deformable. Target cells and cells with a transverse fold are two common forms of leptocytes. Because leptocytes can occur for many reasons, they are rarely of any diagnostic significance. Immature polychromatophilic cells often appear as leptocytes.

Acanthocytes are RBCs with a membrane abnormality that causes them to develop multiple, irregularly spaced, club-shaped projections from the cell surface (Figure 6-7). These must be differentiated from crenated cells, which have numerous rounded, evenly spaced projections. *Crenation* is an artifact resulting from high temperatures or slow drying of the blood film. Acanthocytes may be encountered in normal cattle, but in other species, they are often associated with some neoplasms (especially visceral hemangiosarcoma) or disorders of lipid metabolism. *Schistocytes* are fragmented RBCs formed as a result of the trauma of colliding with intravascular fibrin strands; schistocytes are associated with disseminated intravascular coagulopathy, heartworm disease, and, occasionally, diseases of the spleen or liver that involve fibrin deposition within the vasculature of those organs. *Spherocytes* are RBCs that appear smaller than normal RBCs and exhibit no central pallor (see Figure 6-6). Spherocytes are most commonly seen in immune hemolytic anemia and can also be seen after blood transfusions. They are more spherical because bits of their membrane have been removed, making them more rigid and unable to assume the discoid shape more typical of RBCs. They are most easily identified in canine blood, because normal canine RBCs

are larger and have a distinct zone of central pallor. In the other species with smaller RBCs, which typically exhibit little or no central pallor, spherocytes are difficult to confirm (Figures 6-8 and 6-9).

NRBCs, or *metarubricytes,* may be seen in peripheral blood films. An occasional NRBC may be found in a normal animal, but increased numbers are a significant finding and should be reported as the number of NRBCs per 100 WBCs. Care must be taken to avoid confusing NRBCs with lymphocytes. NRBCs of a size similar to small lymphocytes will have more cytoplasm relative to nuclear size, and the cytoplasm will be faintly eosinophilic (reddish). Remember to correct the WBC count if more than 10 NRBCs per 100 WBCs are found (see previous discussion of determination of leukocyte counts).

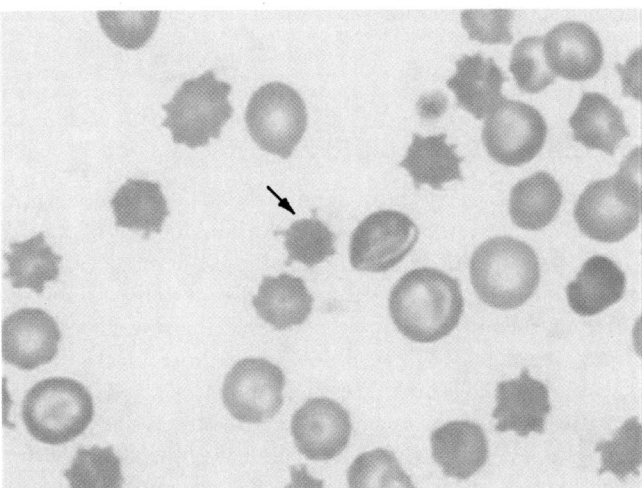

Figure 6-7   Canine blood film with acanthocyte.

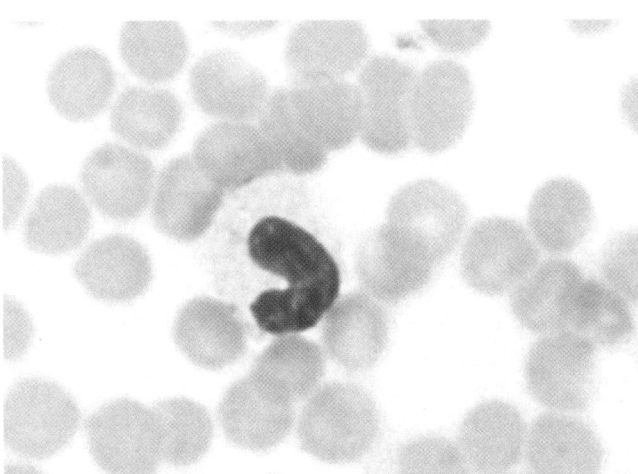

Figure 6-8   Feline erythrocytes. Note the lack of central pallor. There is also a toxic band neutrophil.

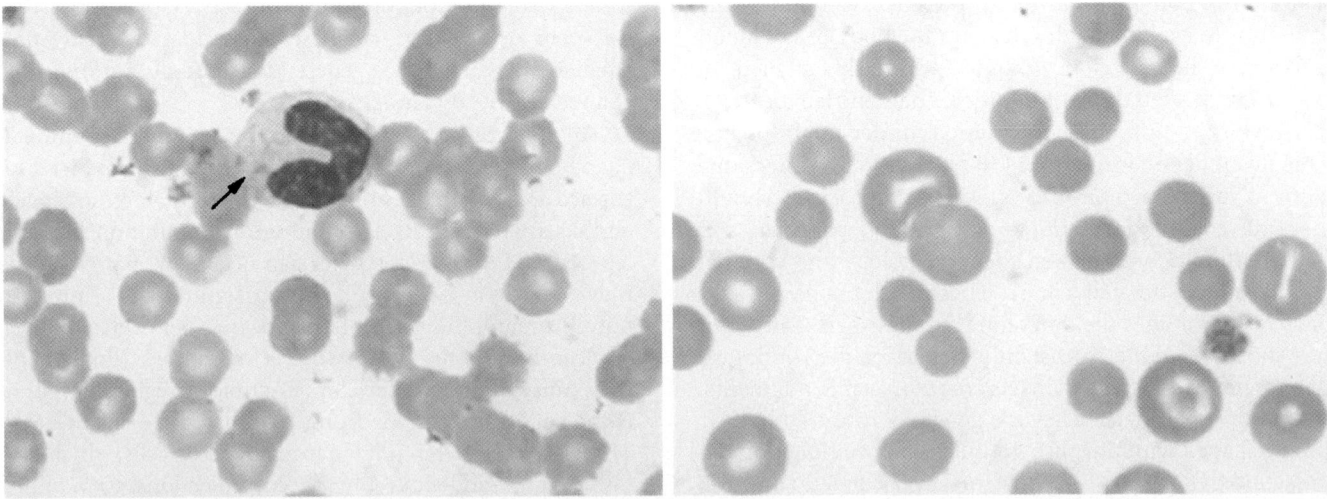

A

B

Figure 6-9   **A,** Normal canine red blood cells. Note the distinct central pallor. There is also a toxic band with Döhle bodies *(arrow)* in the cytoplasm. **B,** Blood from a dog with immune-mediated hemolytic anemia. Note the lack of central pallor in several smaller cells (spherocytes) and the large polychromatophilic cells.

The color of erythrocytes should be noted during examination of the blood film. *Polychromasia* is the term used to describe a variation in the color of RBCs. *Polychromatophilic RBCs* (Figure 6-10) are bluish, although this is not as consistently evident with Diff-Quik stain as it is with Wright's stain. Some polychromasia may be seen in normal, healthy animals, but increased polychromasia in animals with anemia suggests the anemia is regenerative; in other words, the bone marrow is responding to a need for RBCs and releasing immature RBCs. Little or no polychromasia detected on a blood film from an anemic animal suggests the anemia is nonregenerative; that is, the bone marrow is not responding appropriately. Although the presence of polychromasia may be suggestive of a bone marrow response to anemia, confirmation cannot be made without a reticulocyte count.

Polychromatophilic RBCs can be identified as *reticulocytes* (Figure 6-11) when the blood is stained with new methylene blue (NMB). Equal amounts of blood and stain (2 to 5 drops) are mixed in a small tube and left to stand for 5 to 10 minutes. Stain kits (ReticSet, Curtin Matheson Scientific, Houston,

Texas), in which liquid stain is not used, are available for reticulocyte counts. Instead, these kits include stain-coated plastic tubes into which 3 to 5 drops of whole blood are placed and then agitated. Whichever method is chosen, a blood film is then made from the mixed sample.

Normal RBCs appear yellowish green with NMB. The reticulocytes will be the same color but will contain deeply basophilic (bluish) dots or strands. Cats have two types of reticulocytes, punctate and aggregate (see Figure 6-11). Only the reticulocytes that have prominent clumps of reticulum (aggregate reticulocytes) are counted. The RBCs with small single dots (punctate reticulocytes) are generally not included in the count, but their presence should be noted. A reticulocyte count is the number of reticulocytes noted in a count of 1000 RBCs expressed as a percentage. In dogs and cats, reticulocyte counts expressed as percentages should then be corrected to account for the patient's PCV, or hematocrit. Or, absolute reticulocytes per microliter can be reported by multiplying the percentage of reticulocytes by the RBC count.

$$\% \text{ Reticulocytes} = 40 \text{ Reticulocytes counted in } 1000 \text{ RBCs} = \frac{40}{1000} \text{ or } 4\%$$

$$\text{Corrected reticulocyte per unit} = \frac{\% \text{ Reticulocytes} \times \text{Patient's PCV}}{45 \text{ (dog) or } 37 \text{ (cat)}}$$

Increased reticulocytes indicate regenerative anemia. Horses do not release immature RBCs from the bone marrow even when they are severely anemic, so polychromasia and reticulocytosis are not seen in equine peripheral blood.

Hypochromic RBCs have an increased area of central pallor with a narrow, peripheral rim of hemoglobin resulting from an abnormally low amount of hemoglobin within the cell. The most common cause of hypochromasia is iron deficiency. Hypochromasia can be confirmed by a low MCHC provided by automated instruments. True hypochromic RBCs (see Figure 6-6) must be differentiated from "punched out" RBCs, which are normochromic but have a more distinct central pallor with a thick dense rim of hemoglobinized cytoplasm. These cells are an artifact of blood film preparation, not a significant pathologic change. Hyperchromasia, or increased hemoglobin content, does not occur in RBCs.

Rouleaux are groupings of RBCs that resemble stacked coins (Figure 6-12). Marked rouleaux formation is normal in horses and, to a lesser extent, in cats. In dogs, rouleaux formation may occur in inflammatory or neoplastic diseases. It is important to differentiate rouleaux from true *agglutination* (clumping) of RBCs. Agglutinated RBCs tend to appear as clumps rather than as stacked coins (Figure 6-13). Often, agglutination of RBCs can be noted on the side of the blood tube as well as on the blood film. If there is some question about whether a blood sample is exhibiting rouleaux or true agglutination, a saline test can be performed. The blood cells are washed by adding 1 drop of blood to 5 ml of saline solution and centrifuging for 3 minutes. The supernatant

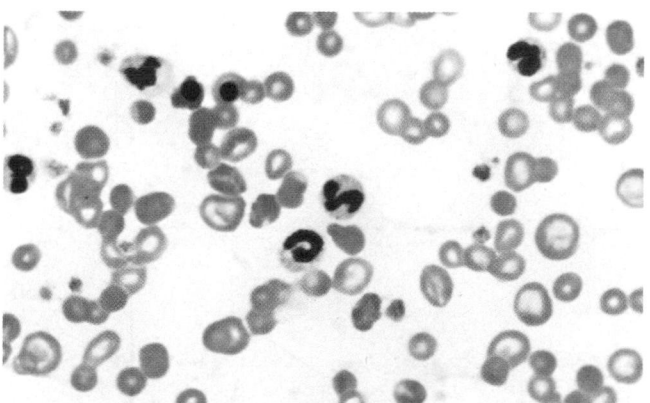

Figure 6-10 Canine blood film with several polychromatic erythrocytes, two nucleated erythrocytes, and neutrophils.

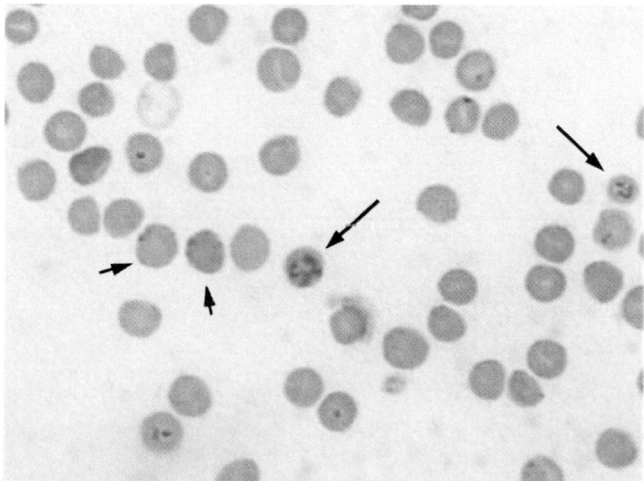

Figure 6-11 Feline blood smear with both punctate *(short arrows)* and aggregate reticulocytes *(long arrows)*.

is poured off, the RBCs are resuspended in saline solution, and a wet mount preparation is made. Rouleaux will disperse, but agglutinated RBCs will remain clumped.

The evaluation of erythrocytes under oil immersion should also include a search for RBC parasites, particularly in cases of anemia. *Haemobartonella felis,* the parasite responsible for feline infectious anemia, appears as small coccoid or rodlike structures on the surface of RBCs (Figure 6-14, *A*). A careful search for *H. felis* organisms should be performed on any anemic cat. These parasites may be very difficult to identify because they can be easily confused with protein and stain precipitates adhered to the cell surface. *Haemobartonella canis* is rarely seen but is more readily identified (Figure 6-14, *B*). *Eperythrozoon* spp., which are found in cattle, sheep, and swine, may appear similar to *H. felis* or may occur as ring forms on the RBCs. *Anaplasma marginale,* a parasite of bovine RBCs, appears as a small spherical body within the RBC, close to the cell margin. This parasite closely resembles Howell-Jolly bodies but is not as apt to be distributed throughout the cell. Another RBC parasite is *Babesia,* which has various species that can infect any domestic animal. *Babesia* spp. are larger and lighter

staining than the previously mentioned parasites, and they tend to occur as piriform structures (often paired) within the RBCs.

Other RBC morphologic abnormalities include *Howell-Jolly bodies, basophilic stippling, Heinz bodies,* and *viral inclusions.* Howell-Jolly bodies are small, often singular, deeply basophilic nuclear remnants that are occasionally seen on normal blood films. Increased numbers of Howell-Jolly bodies can be seen with regenerative anemias. Basophilic stippling is due to staining of small amounts of cytoplasmic RNA in RBCs. These inclusions are multiple tiny, lightly basophilic dots in the RBC cytoplasm. They can be found in cases of markedly regenerative anemia in dogs and cats but are found more commonly in cattle. Basophilic stippling may also be seen occasionally in cases of lead poisoning. The most consistent finding in lead poisoning is increased numbers of NRBCs with mild to no anemia. Heinz bodies are denatured hemoglobin that has fused to the RBC

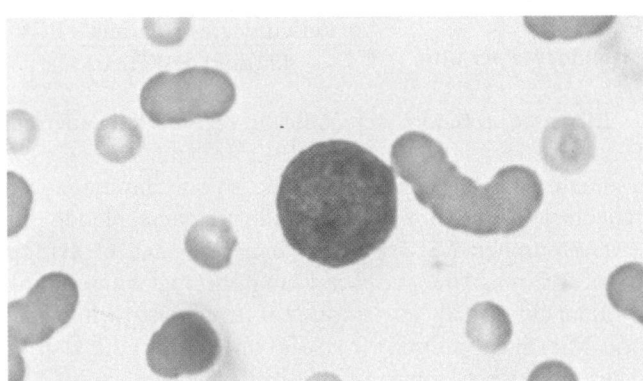

Figure 6-12 Feline blood film showing rouleaux formation.

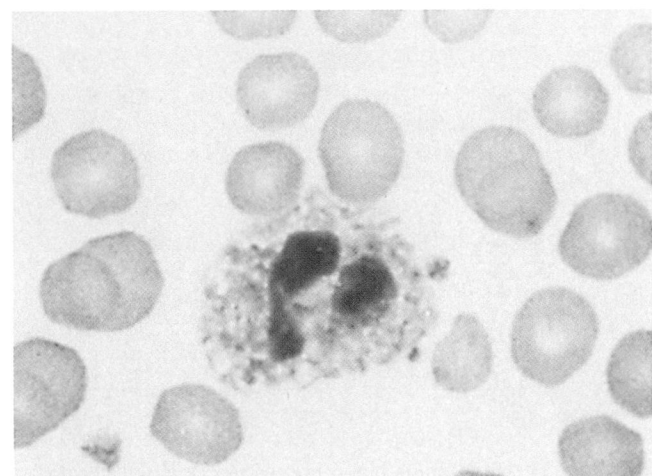

Figure 6-13 Feline blood film showing agglutination.

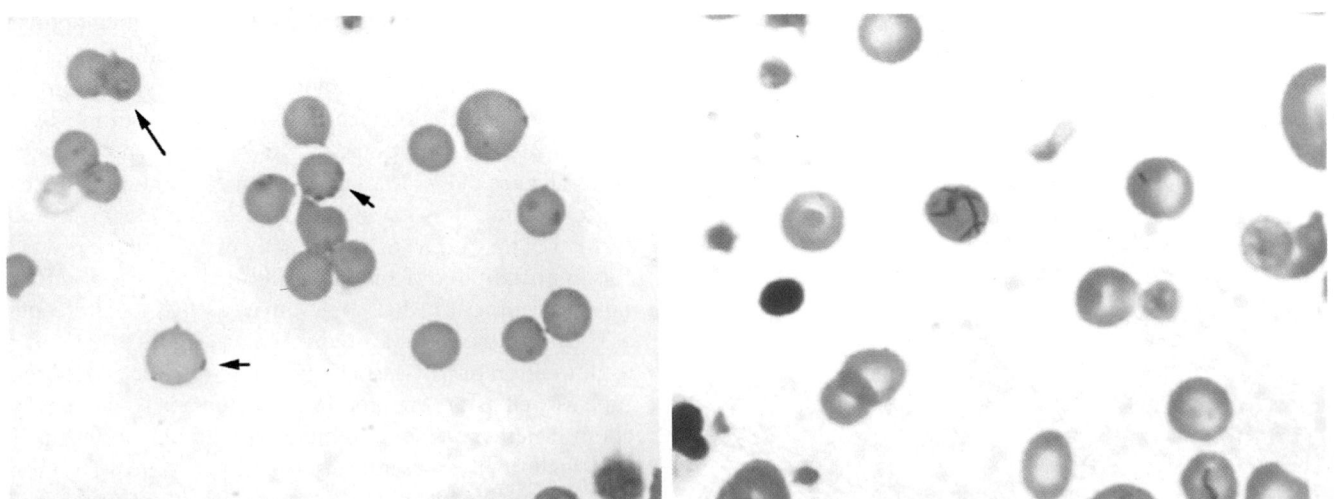

A   B

Figure 6-14 **A,** *Haemobartonella felis* on periphery of RBCs. **B,** *H. canis* with stands of organisms across the surface.

membrane and appear as refractile projections from the RBC membrane (Figure 6-15). These inclusions are most readily seen when the reticulocyte (NMB) stain is applied. They appear as distinct, darkly staining inclusions protruding from the cell surface (Figure 6-16). Distemper virus inclusions may be seen in either RBCs or WBCs. These appear as distinct, spherical eosinophilic inclusions (Figures 6-17 and 6-18).

LEUKOCYTE EVALUATION

The WBCs are categorized as granulocytes *(neutrophils, eosinophils, basophils)* and agranulocytes *(lymphocytes, monocytes)*. The granulocytic cells are characterized by *segmented,* or lobed, nuclei and, except for the neutrophil, are distinct cytoplasmic granules. The agranulocytes are also referred to as mononuclear cells and do not have segmented nuclei.

Neutrophils

In most species the predominant WBC is the neutrophil (Figure 6-19). Neutrophils have phagocytic and bactericidal capabilities, which means they have an important role in inflammatory conditions. The average time spent by the neutrophil in the blood is only about 10 hours, so it is clear that neutrophil numbers can rise or fall in a matter of hours, depending on the stimuli present. Normal neutrophils have deeply staining, clumped, segmented nuclei (three to five lobes) with relatively clear cytoplasm or, at most, a very faint, almost indiscernible dusting of tiny granules. Equine neutrophils tend to have more distinct nuclear segmentation than canine neutrophils.

> **✎ TECHNICIAN NOTE**
> Extra care must be taken in differentiating monocytes from toxic band neutrophils, particularly in horses.

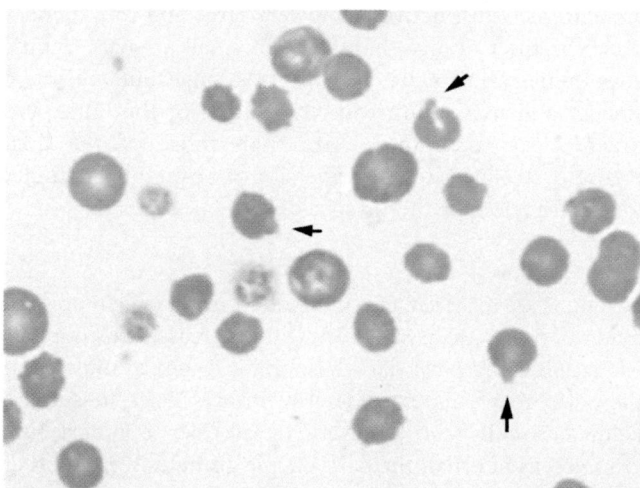

Figure 6-15 Feline blood film showing Heinz body formation. Note the red blood cells with variably distinct, pale, rounded projections from their surface (Wright's stain, 100×).

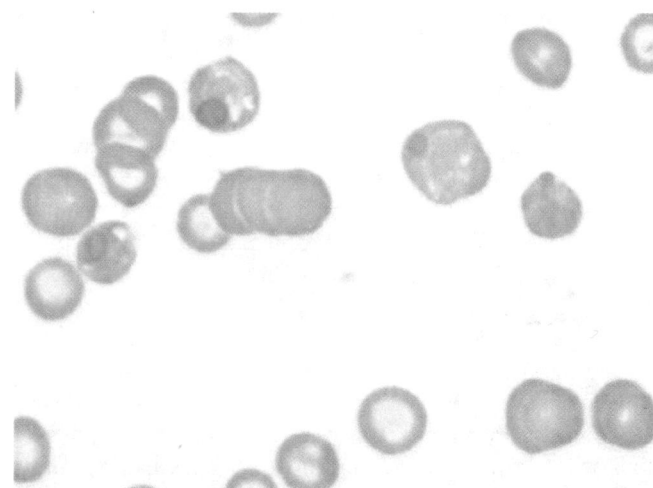

Figure 6-17 Canine blood film with viral (distemper) inclusions in red blood cells (Wright's stain, 1000×).

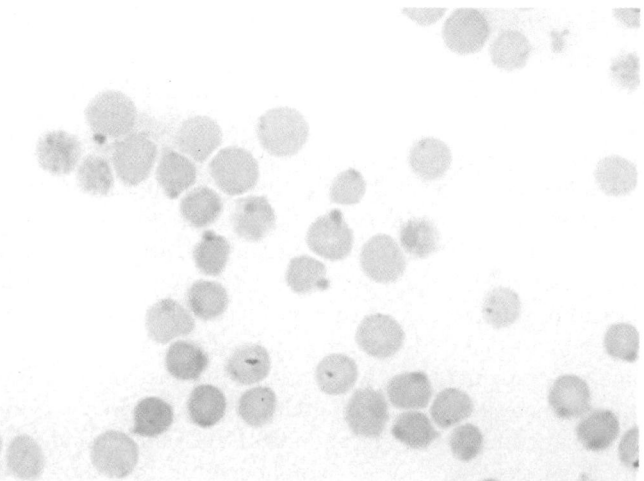

Figure 6-16 Distinctly basophilic, protruding Heinz bodies stained with new methylene blue (NMB).

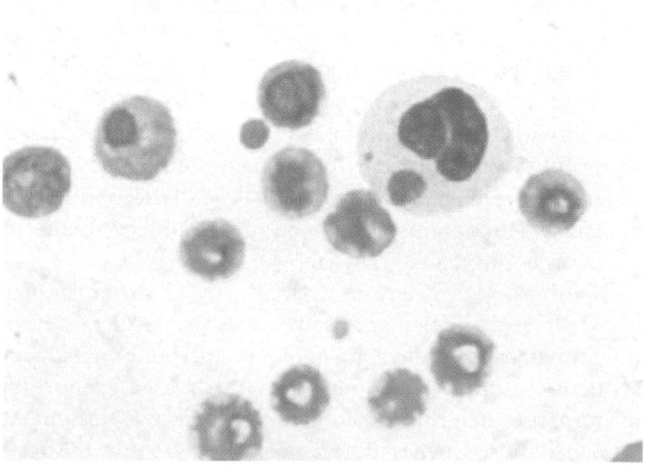

Figure 6-18 Canine blood smear with viral inclusions in red blood cells and neutrophil (Diff-Quik stain).

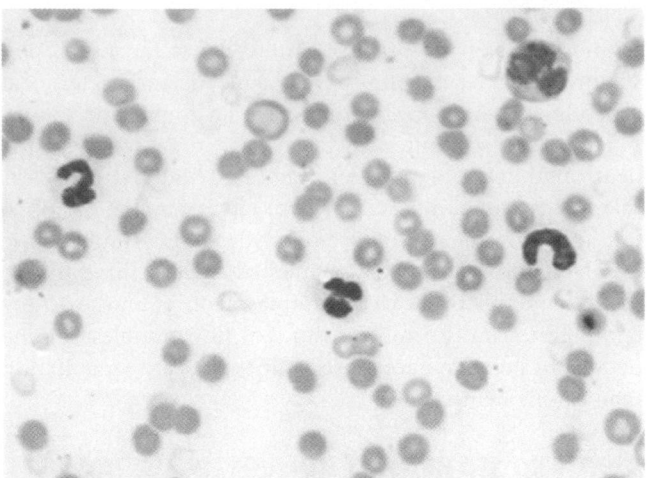

Figure 6-19 Canine blood film. Two segmented neutrophils, a band to the right, and a monocyte in upper right corner.

An important morphologic change in neutrophils is the appearance of band-shaped nuclei, which indicate the release of immature neutrophils, referred to as bands, from the bone marrow. A band nucleus lacks the segmentation seen in the mature segmented nucleus but instead has parallel borders (Figures 6-8, 6-9, and 6-19). Even more immature cells, with oval or bean-shaped nuclei, may be seen in cases of extreme tissue demand for neutrophils. Neutrophils, mature or immature, may also show evidence of inflammatory disease as demonstrated by certain cytoplasmic characteristics. *Toxic neutrophils* are characterized by any combination of *Döhle bodies, cytoplasmic vacuolation, basophilia,* and, rarely, cytoplasmic granulation. Cats apparently show toxic neutrophils during many kinds of illnesses, but in other species, toxic changes usually imply severe inflammatory disease. Döhle bodies are small, pale bluish-gray irregular inclusions in the cytoplasm that usually indicate mild toxemia. Generalized basophilia of the cytoplasm and cytoplasmic vacuolation are slightly more severe toxic changes. Toxic neutrophils are frequently seen with inflammatory leukograms, characterized by an increased total number of neutrophils *(neutrophilia)* and an increased number of band or other immature neutrophils. In contrast to these cytoplasmic changes, *nuclear hypersegmentation* (nuclei with five or more lobes) is a normal aging change that implies a nontoxic environment and prolonged circulation of neutrophils. They are most frequently seen in steroid or stress leukograms, in which neutrophils remain in circulation longer than normal.

Neutropenia, a decrease in circulating neutrophils, may occur when tissue demand is excessive as a result of severe inflammation exceeding the ability of the bone marrow to supply neutrophils. There may be an increased proportion of immature neutrophils along with the decreased number of neutrophils, which is indicative of the attempt by the bone marrow to meet tissue demands. This can be a very serious, sometimes life-threatening, situation if it is prolonged

because neutrophils are necessary for the body to fight serious inflammation or infection.

Eosinophils

Eosinophils help to control allergic or anaphylactic hypersensitivity reactions. They are attracted to the sites of these reactions by substances released from sensitized mast cells; therefore eosinophils tend to occur where mast cells congregate. The eosinophil is characterized by a segmented nucleus, colorless to pale blue cytoplasm, and distinct eosinophilic (reddish orange)–staining granules in the cytoplasm.

The morphologic appearance of eosinophil granules varies from species to species, so they can be used to identify the origin of a blood sample. The eosinophils of cats contain numerous tiny rod-shaped granules that may obscure the nucleus. The eosinophil granules of dogs are less numerous and are usually round but may vary considerably in size. Greyhounds often have eosinophils that have degranulated and appear vacuolated. The eosinophil granules of horses are extremely distinctive, being very large and round and a much brighter orange than those of small animals. Bovine eosinophil granules are also bright orange but are much smaller and more numerous than those of the horse and much more uniform in size than those of the dog. Figure 6-20 illustrates the diversity of eosinophil granules found in various domestic species.

Basophils

Basophils are relatively rare in blood films but, when present, tend to occur in association with increased eosinophils. Classically, they have dark basophilic (blue) granules, but they also may vary considerably from species to species. Feline basophils tend to have light lavender to almost pink granules, rather than the dark purple granules seen in other species. Canine basophils may have few to no granules and must be differentiated from neutrophils on the basis of an elongated nucleus and a more basophilic cytoplasm (Figure 6-21). Equine and bovine basophils tend to have variable numbers of the more typical dark basophilic granules. Basophils are frequently confused with mast cells because of similar granules, but the basophil nucleus is segmented, and the mast cell nucleus is round or oval.

Lymphocytes

Lymphocytes are usually small to medium-sized mononuclear cells with a thin rim of light to dark blue cytoplasm and a round, often eccentric, nucleus (Figure 6-22). Their cytoplasm may contain azurophilic (blue) granules. Cattle are notorious for their often large, bizarre-looking lymphocytes. In normal cattle, lymphocytes outnumber neutrophils and may be quite large, with indented (rather than round) nuclei, increased cytoplasm, and perhaps azurophilic cytoplasmic granules. During periods of antigenic stimulation in all species, some of the lymphocytes in the blood film may have extremely basophilic cytoplasm with a pale perinuclear zone (the site of the Golgi apparatus) and possibly

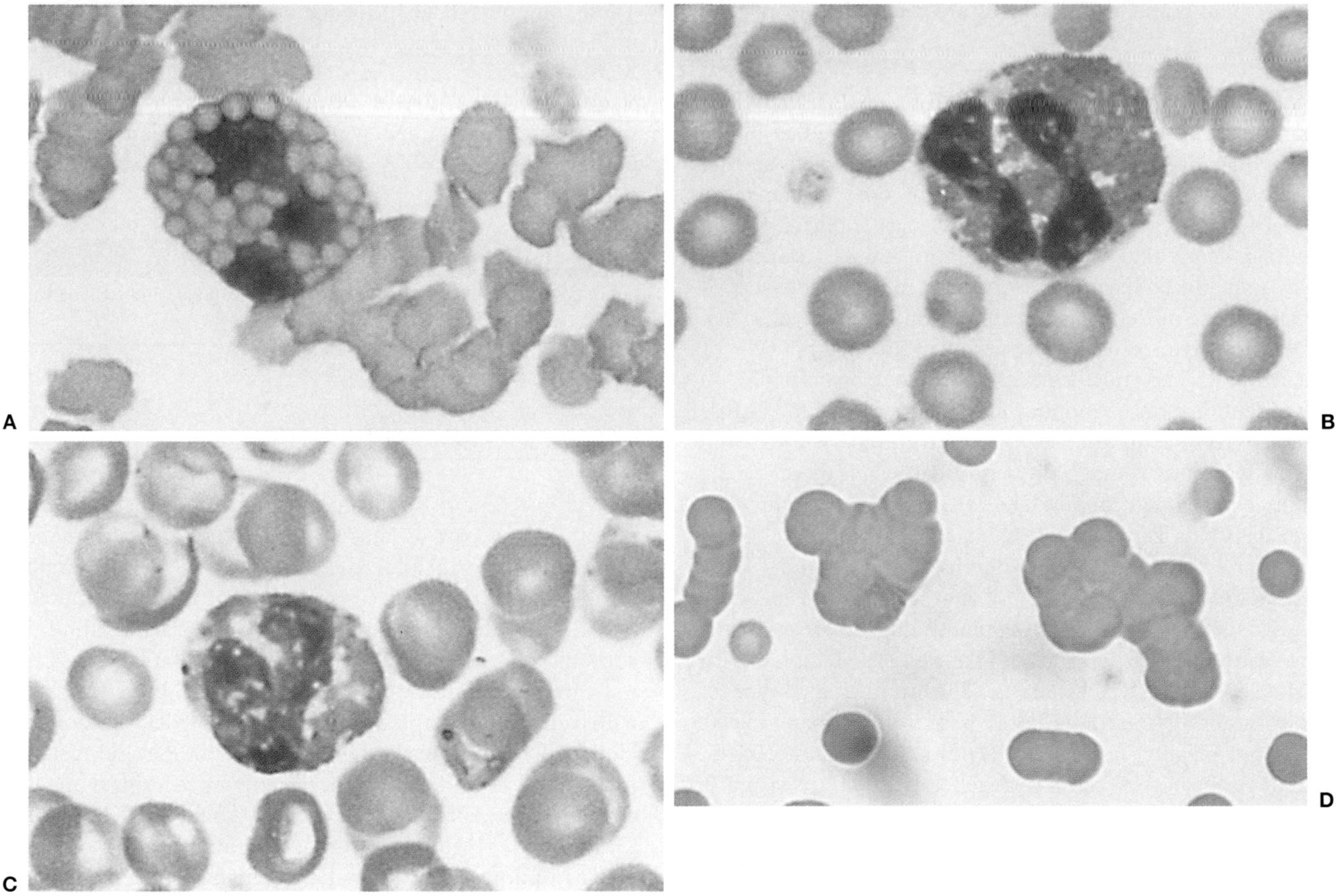

Figure 6-20 Species variation in eosinophil granules. **A,** Equine eosinophil. **B,** Bovine eosinophil. **C,** Canine eosinophil. **D,** Feline eosinophil.

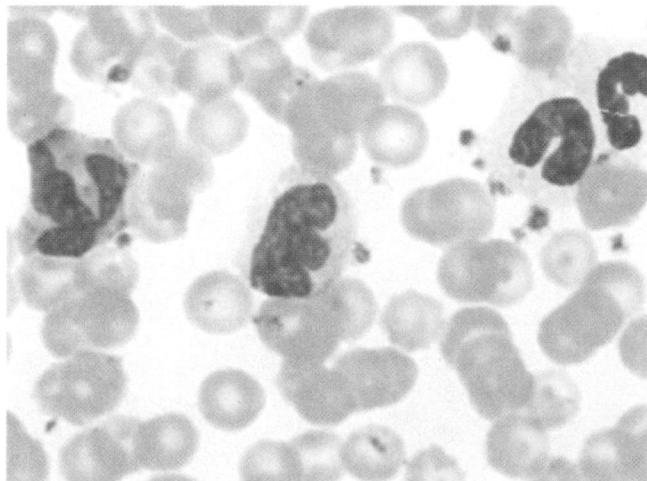

Figure 6-21 Canine blood film. *From left,* basophil, monocyte, band neutrophil, and segmented neutrophil. Note that the basophil has an elongated nucleus and darker cytoplasm but no distinct granules. There are several platelets between the red blood cells (RBCs) and few overlying RBCs.

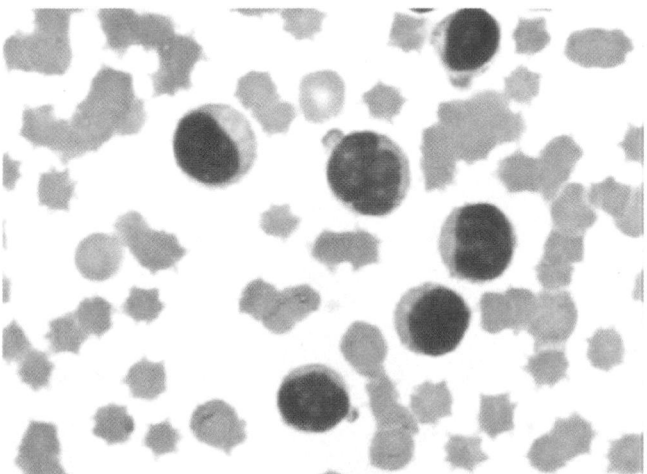

Figure 6-22 Canine blood smear with mature lymphocytes with scant, basophilic cytoplasm. The number of cells is compatible with lymphocytic leukemia.

azurophilic granules. These cells are referred to as *reactive lymphocytes.*

Monocytes

Monocytes (Figures 6-19 and 6-21) are derived from the bone marrow and circulate in the blood briefly before entering the tissues in which they become *macrophages.* Macrophages phagocytize (ingest) large particles and cellular debris that neutrophils cannot handle. Monocytes have gray-blue, often grainy, cytoplasm and a variable-shaped nucleus. The nucleus can be round, oval, ameboid, or lobed. The monocyte is usually larger than the lymphocyte or neutrophil. The most common problem associated with the identification of monocytes is the tendency to confuse monocytes that have a bean-shaped nucleus with a band neutrophil; this is especially a problem when there is toxic change in the neutrophils. The cytoplasm of the monocyte is usually a darker blue than the band neutrophil.

Other Cells

Occasionally, evaluation of the blood film reveals abnormal circulating cell types, such as mast cells, lymphoblasts, myeloblasts, and erythroblasts. The number and type of abnormal cells should be noted because they may indicate leukemia (Figures 6-23 and 6-24) or systemic mastocytosis. Smudge (or basket) cells are degenerated cells appearing as pale eosinophilic nuclear material lacking shape or form. These occur when excessive pressure is used in making the film or when old blood is used. A few of these are of little significance, but numerous smudge cells can affect the accuracy of the differential count. Blood films with unusual or abnormal cells can be sent to a reference laboratory for evaluation.

Absolute Versus Relative Numbers

The numbers obtained when doing the differential count are *relative*, or percentages of the whole cell population. These numbers have no diagnostic significance but are used to calculate the absolute numbers of the various WBCs. *Absolute numbers* are the only numbers with diagnostic significance and should always be calculated and reported as such. These are obtained by multiplying the relative percentages by the total WBC count and are expressed as cells per microliter.

⬥ TECHNICIAN NOTE

Only absolute numbers are significant for interpreting the differential count.

AUTOMATED CELL COUNTERS

Several instruments available for automated electronic cell counting may cost as much as $150,000. A basic understanding of the principles of electronic cell counting is useful for the veterinary technician, regardless of whether the practice has an in-clinic laboratory. Many practices find it convenient to use human reference or hospital laboratories, but these instruments must be specially calibrated for use with veterinary samples because of the wide variation in blood cell size among the different species. Several instruments have been designed specifically for veterinary medicine (e.g., Vet ABC-Diff Hematology Analyzer, Heska, Fort Collins, Colo [Figure 6-25]) that are computer driven with species options and automatically change the instrument settings for multiple species use. The major advantages of electronic cell counters are their speed, accuracy, and reproducibility. In addition to providing RBC and WBC counts, most cell counters will measure hemoglobin and calculate the RBC indices.

The disadvantage of electronic cell counters is their quality control and maintenance requirements. The veterinary technician must be able to recognize when the instruments

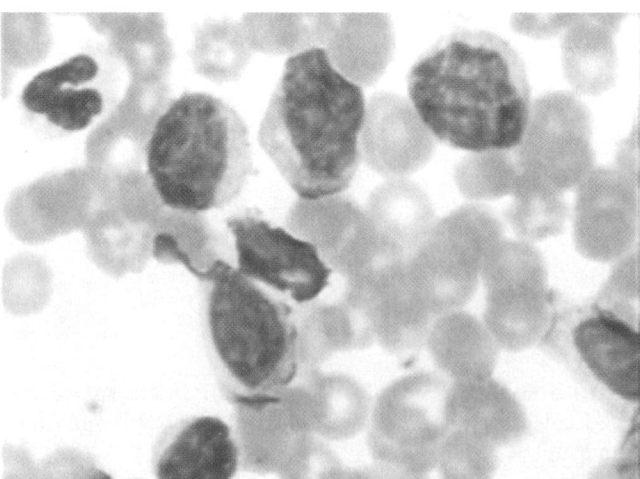

Figure 6-23 Canine blood film with large, atypical lymphs compatible with lymphoblastic leukemia.

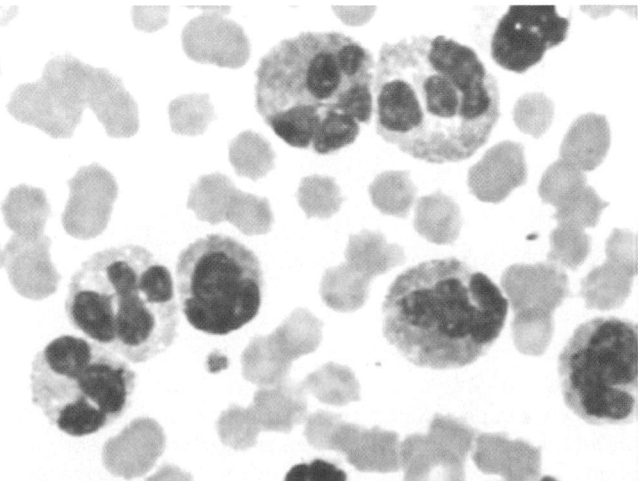

Figure 6-24 Feline blood smear. These are all eosinophils. The number of cells is indicative of eosinophilic leukemia.

are not functioning properly and determine the problem. The manufacturer should be willing to train the technician to perform quality control and calibration procedures, keep adequate quality control records, and handle minor adjustments. In addition, the manufacturer should be available for service calls if needed. In some practices, consideration should be given to the purchase of a service contract; this should be discussed before investing in a major instrument.

The operating principle involved in electronic cell counting is based on a type of flow cytometry (the counting of particles as they flow past a detection device). This technology allows the instrument to count blood cells and measure their size. Most instruments use a simple orifice through which an electrical current passes. As particles (e.g., blood cells) move through the orifice, they disrupt the current by increasing the resistance (impedance) proportional to the size of the particle. The instrument is set to detect and count only particles that produce a signal that exceeds a specific resistance or threshold. The threshold settings will determine what particles are counted, based on their size. This principle is important when an instrument is evaluated for use in veterinary medicine. Many instruments developed for human medicine do not accurately count RBCs with a volume of less than 55 femtoliters (fl). The RBCs of the cat, horse, cow, goat, and pig have mean cell volumes below this value.

WBCs from different species also have varying sizes after exposure to RBC lysing solutions. Total WBC counts on some instruments can be falsely decreased in the dog because of their small leukocytes. The reverse is true in the cat. The cat's platelets tend to form large clumps that are counted as leukocytes, thus falsely elevating the WBC count. Close inspection of the blood film will help the technician identify this problem.

Whole blood can be diluted for counting either before introduction of the sample into the machine (predilution) or by the instrument as part of the sampling cycle. In the newer instruments, whole blood is aspirated and diluted for the RBC count, and a portion of the sample is lysed to remove the RBCs and allow the WBCs to be counted. The lysed sample is often used for hemoglobin determination.

It is important to remember, however, that the limited differential counts obtained should not replace the blood film examination; nor should the automated reticulocyte or platelet count be taken at face value. Blood cell morphology is important in evaluating the numbers obtained in the blood cell counts. The automated instruments cannot tell the technician whether band neutrophils, toxic neutrophils, polychromatophilic RBCs, RBC parasites, or NRBCs are present.

TECHNICIAN NOTE

The differential count provided by automated analyzers is not an adequate substitute for microscopic evaluation of the blood film.

PLASMA PROTEIN DETERMINATION

Determination of the plasma protein concentration is another standard component of the routine CBC. After plasma color and turbidity have been noted, the capillary tube used for measuring the PCV is broken at a point slightly above the *buffy coat* (cream-colored layer of WBCs and platelets just above the RBCs), and the plasma is allowed to run through the unbroken end onto the prism of a refractometer by capillary action. Lifting the cover and tapping the hematocrit tube on the prism may scratch the surface of the prism. Plasma protein values obtained with a refractometer are accurate as long as the plasma is clear. If the plasma is lipemic, hemolyzed, or otherwise cloudy, the refractive index will be increased and provide an erroneously high protein measurement. Often, the lipemic samples have a very indistinct or unfocused line on the refractometer scale. In contrast to the dilution effect of a small blood sample in a large tube, excess anticoagulant will artifactually increase the plasma protein value obtained.

Semiquantitative determination of plasma *fibrinogen* levels may be useful in the detection of inflammatory processes, particularly in cattle and horses. Two capillary tubes of blood are centrifuged; one is used for the PCV and plasma protein determination, as described. The second tube is placed in a 56° C to 58° C water bath for 3 minutes to cause the precipitation of fibrinogen. The tube is then recentrifuged so the fibrinogen settles just above the buffy coat. The tube is broken above the fibrinogen, and the

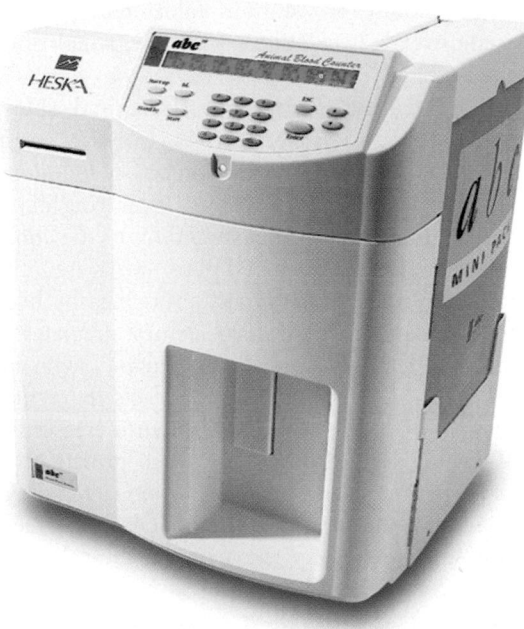

Figure 6-25 Heska Corporation's ABC-Diff impedance hematology analyzer for in-house use provides a complete blood count. (Image courtesy Heska Corp., Fort Collins Colo.)

remaining plasma is placed on the refractometer for protein determination. The difference between protein concentration of the first tube and protein concentration of the second tube is the fibrinogen concentration.

Fibrinogen is usually expressed in milligrams per deciliter; therefore if the first tube had a protein concentration of 7.3 g/dl and the second tube has a protein concentration of 6.9 g/dl, the plasma fibrinogen concentration is 0.4 g/dl, or 400 mg/dl. Plasma from cattle with markedly increased fibrinogen may completely coagulate during incubation; when the specimen is respun, the fibrinogen does not settle out, and a fibrinogen value cannot be determined.

COAGULATION TESTING

Animals will occasionally be presented with abnormal bleeding tendencies. *Hemostasis,* the maintenance of proper blood flow, depends on a complex interaction of vascular integrity, platelet number and function, and several coagulation factors counterbalanced by several thrombolytic factors to prevent excessive thrombosis. When vascular injury is present, the platelets are exposed to collagen fibers normally secluded within the vessel wall. They begin to adhere to the periphery of the lesion and then aggregate to form the initial plug to stem the flow of blood. The coagulation factors are a group of chemicals, enzymes, and cofactors that interact to stabilize the platelet plug. They, too, are activated by exposure to subendothelial tissue and factors released from the tissues and platelets. Once activated, they subsequently activate the next factor, thus forming a cascade of activated factors, resulting in a final formation of fibrin and stabilization of the plug and stemming the flow of blood. Without this stabilization, the platelet plug would gradually dissolve with subsequent rebleeding at the site of injury. Basic coagulation testing includes a platelet count and activated partial thromboplastin time and prothrombin time to evaluate factor activity. Each of these assays will evaluate a group of factors, and together, generally provide diagnostic or prognostic information. Identification of specific factor deficiencies requires special procedures at specific labs specializing in these disorders.

Most of these tests require special instrumentation and are submitted to a reference laboratory; however, sample collection and submission are critical for obtaining valid results. The venipuncture must be accurate to avoid tissue injury, which will invalidate the coagulation assays. In addition to collection in an EDTA tube for the platelet count, blood must be collected in tubes with citrate anticoagulant (turquoise top) for coagulation assays. The proper amount of blood must be drawn to maintain the 9:1 ratio of blood to anticoagulant for reliable results. Only plastic or siliconized glass should be used in handling these samples because contact with regular glass will invalidate the results. The samples should be centrifuged, and the plasma should be tested immediately or frozen. The reference laboratory should always

be contacted for additional directions before samples are obtained and submitted for coagulation testing.

TECHNICIAN NOTE
Proper filling of the citrate collection tube for coagulation testing is essential for reliable results.

Clinical Chemistry

Numerous chemistry parameters can be assayed. The basic chemistry panel consists of groups of analytes that reflect dysfunction or injury in various organ systems. Aspartate aminotransferase and alanine aminotransferase are intracellular enzymes that may be elevated as a result of damage to hepatocytes. Aspartate aminotransferase, in particular, may also be increased with muscle injury. Alkaline phosphatase and γ-glutamyltransferase are also indicative of liver damage but are membrane bound and more often associated with cholestatic disease. They may also be increased because of steroid use. Bilirubin and albumin may also be associated with liver disease but may also be altered as a result of injury to other systems.

Blood urea nitrogen and creatinine concentrations are used to indicate renal dysfunction or disease. The interpretation of concentrations of these two analytes requires a concomitant urinalysis, most specifically the urine SG.

Measurements of total protein, albumin, and globulins are generally included in the basic panel. Variations in these proteins may be indicative of a variety of disorders. Values may be increased with dehydration, inflammation, or autoimmune disease. Albumin values may be decreased in association with liver failure, gastrointestinal disorders, or renal glomerular disease.

Levels of serum sodium, potassium, and chloride—collectively referred to as electrolytes—can also be affected by various disorders. They may reflect changes in fluid balance, gastrointestinal disorders (vomiting/diarrhea), acid-base disturbances, renal dysfunction, or metabolic and endocrine disorders. Calcium and phosphorus are intimately associated with bone growth, and levels may be higher in younger animals than in adults. Calcium circulates bound to albumin; therefore calcium levels may be low in cases of decreased albumin levels. Phosphorus levels are regulated in the kidney, so the phosphorus level often increases in cases of renal dysfunction. Phosphorus is also present in RBCs, so if there is hemolysis or serum is allowed to remain on the cells, serum phosphorus results may be falsely elevated.

Several small, relatively inexpensive clinical chemistry instruments have been developed. As with all equipment, veterinary practices must have a demand for them and must be able to justify their expense. Two general types of chemistry analyzers are commonly used: liquid reagent chemistry and dry chemistry. Instruments that use liquid reagents require more technical expertise and time in preparing reagents and monitoring their performance. The dry chemistry instruments are simpler to use and provide consistent performance. The principles of operation differ significantly between the two types of instruments, as does the extent to which specimen quality affects the measurement.

EQUIPMENT

Regardless of whether an in-house chemistry analyzer is maintained and operated, veterinary practices will need a sample collection system consisting of either syringes and needles or Vacutainers plus clean plastic or glass tubes in which to store or transport samples. A centrifuge and pipettes will be necessary for separation of the serum or plasma from the cells.

CLINICAL CHEMISTRY INSTRUMENTATION

The liquid reagent–based instruments use the principle of photometry (the measurement of light transmittance by a solution). Beer's law states that the concentration of a substance in a liquid is indirectly proportional to the amount of light that passes through the liquid. Most instruments have a spectrophotometer to measure the amount of light transmitted. A spectrophotometer consists of a light source directed through a specific path and a photosensitive detector that converts light into electrical energy. Each substance will transmit light at a specific wavelength. For the purpose of increasing the specificity of the measurement, filters are placed between the light source and the sample to allow only a specific wavelength to pass through the sample. The magnitude of the electrical current produced by the detector corresponds to the concentration of the substance being measured. Solutions that contain a known concentration of specific substances are called standards and are used to calibrate the instrument. Each instrument has specific procedures for *calibration,* which should be carefully followed to ensure optimal performance.

The instruments that use dry reagents are becoming more popular for in-clinic use. The major advantage of these instruments is the elimination of liquid reagents, which must be reconstituted or diluted before use. Dry chemistry instruments use reagent slides or cartridges. A specific amount of the patient's sample is added as directed, and the intensity of the color that develops is measured by the principle of reflectance. Light is transmitted to the analyte slide, and the reflected light is conducted to a photodetector. The density of the color formed by the chemical reaction is determined and is proportional to the concentration of the substance being measured. Because this method does not depend on reading light transmitted through a liquid as with the spectrophotometer-based instruments, there is less interference from lipemia or hemolysis.

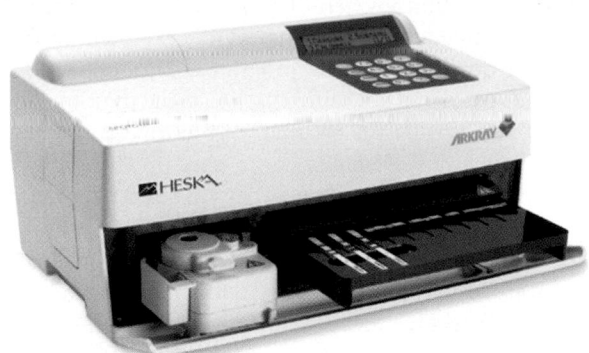

Figure 6-26 Heska Corporation's Spotchem dry chemistry and electrolyte analyzer offers a complete panel of analytes for routine and emergency needs. The i-STAT (not pictured) is a portable, hand-held analyzer with cartridges, which provides a variety of hematology, chemistry, and blood gas evaluations. (Image courtesy Heska Corporation, Fort Collins, Colo.)

Several dry chemistry instruments (e.g., Heska Spotchem and i-STAT, Abaxis VetScan, IDEXX VetTest) that are designed specifically for use with veterinary samples are available (Figure 6-26). Available tests may vary from analyzer to analyzer, and new tests are often added. The primary advantage of using an instrument intended for veterinary testing is the availability of predetermined reference ranges, which can be used until the laboratory can establish its own values. In most cases with these instruments, little variation occurs from instrument to instrument or operator to operator. Veterinary samples can vary significantly from human samples in the concentration of particular substances. If an analyzer not specifically designed for veterinary samples is used, the limits of the chemistry test (range of values that have a linear relationship within the method used) must be adhered to.

QUALITY CONTROL PROGRAMS

Any veterinary practice that decides to establish an in-house laboratory must make a commitment to quality control. Laboratory instruments will provide valid accurate results only if the samples are handled correctly, a well-maintained instrument is used, and the tests are performed correctly. The importance of routine maintenance and calibration procedures for all instruments cannot be overemphasized. However, even the most sophisticated, accurate, and well-maintained instrument cannot overcome errors in technique or poor sample quality. The technician should be familiar with the principles and limitations of all assays performed in the laboratory. Some of the more common causes for inaccurate results because of technical errors or sample quality are listed in Box 6-1. A quality control program consists of monitoring results of known *control samples* for identification of irregularities in reported values and following generally accepted laboratory procedures. Several textbooks on clinical chemistry and laboratory medicine (see Recommended Reading) provide excellent in-depth reviews of quality assurance programs. The following discussion deals primarily with the basics in monitoring an instrument to ensure the accuracy of reported data.

The three levels of quality control are preanalytic procedures, analytic procedures, and analytic quality monitoring procedures. The *preanalytic procedures* deal with how the patient is prepared (fasting vs. nonfasting samples), patient and specimen identification, specimen acquisition, and specimen processing. Establishment of standard procedures for each of these steps will decrease the likelihood of samples being misidentified or being of poor quality (hemolysed or lipemic). This aspect of quality control is important even in clinics that send their clinical pathology samples to a reference laboratory. *Analytic variables* include the analytic method, standardization and calibration procedures, documentation of analytic protocols and procedures, and monitoring of equipment during use. This aspect of quality control is usually well defined by the manufacturer of the

instrument and should be followed closely. The final level, *monitoring of analytic quality* by using statistical methods and control charts, is the aspect that involves the use of control products and record keeping. This aspect is the responsibility of the technician performing the tests.

> ### ✎ TECHNICIAN NOTE
> In spite of sales claims, valid results cannot be ensured without inclusion of appropriate control samples and proper calibration.

CONTROLS

Control products are biologic solutions, usually serum based, that have known concentrations of the various constituents or analytes that can be assayed by the instrument. These products should be stable, be available in aliquots to prevent alterations caused by refreezing, and have little vial-to-vial variation. Control products can be purchased from an independent source or from the company that makes the test kit or instrument. Most control products are available as normal, high abnormal, and low abnormal ranges. The control products are analyzed in a manner identical to that used for patients' samples, and the values reported by the instrument are compared with the known values provided with the product.

Many control products are provided in a lyophilized form that requires rehydration with distilled water or a diluent provided by the manufacturer. The solution must be diluted properly to ensure that the concentration of the analytes is correct. Imprecision in diluting the controls will be reflected by values that are not in concert with the

---

> **Box 6-1** COMMON CAUSES FOR INACCURATE RESULTS
>
> - Poor-quality or outdated reagents
> - Failure to calibrate or run controls
> - Improper pipetting techniques
> - Improper maintenance of instrument
> - Lipemic or hemolyzed samples
> - Allowing serum to sit on clot
> - Use of inappropriate cuvettes
> - Power surges or failure

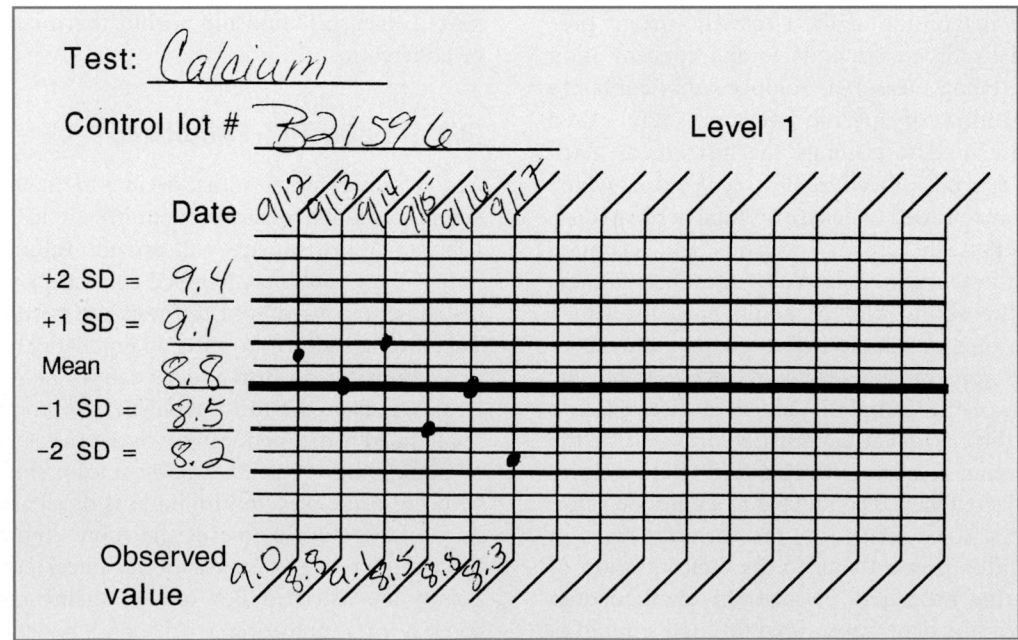

Figure 6-27 Levy-Jennings chart illustrating the common procedure used for following the performance of an individual test control serum.

known values of the product, even though the instrument is working properly. It is highly recommended that volumetric or other precise pipettes be used to dilute the control products (a graduated cylinder is not acceptable).

The control values must fall within a specific acceptable range, which usually encompasses the mean ±2 SD. This range is established by the manufacturer of the product by repeated assay of the solution. When the instrument reports a control value above or below the established range, there is a problem with the procedure, and test results for that particular sample should not be reported until the problem is identified.

A separate log of the control results should be kept and reviewed periodically. A useful visual display of the instrument's performance for quick inspection and review is the Levy-Jennings chart. Figure 6-27 shows the use of the Levy-Jennings chart to keep track of quality control data. By inspection of control data over 1 month, a technician can see the control values gently drift upward or downward, indicating possible deterioration of the control product or a change in the light source intensity. Wide scatter of values outside the range on both the low and high ends indicates imprecision on the part of the instrument or technician. It is best to keep the chart close to the instrument, not hidden in a file drawer. Everyone who uses the instrument must be willing to run controls and chart the results. Other useful laboratory records include calibration logs, sample logs, and maintenance logs.

SAMPLE HANDLING

Sample handling is a critical step in obtaining accurate laboratory data. Several factors can interfere with analysis of a sample. The most common problems in veterinary medicine are hemolysis and lipemia. Difficulty in performing the venipuncture or excess pressure applied to the syringe during collection can cause significant hemolysis. The most common cause of lipemia is collection of a postprandial sample. At times, both hemolysis and lipemia are unavoidable because they are the result of a disease process.

The effect hemolysis and lipemia will have on laboratory data is method dependent. There are no general rules to assist interpretation of changes caused by sample quality. A good reference laboratory will provide information on how each of its tests is affected by these two changes. Manufacturers of the instruments and reagents should provide information on how interfering factors such as hemolysis and lipemia affect the methods used in their instrument. Hemolysis will commonly affect inorganic phosphorus and potassium values in horses and some Akita dogs. Lipemia will interfere with any method that depends on optical density read on a spectrophotometer. Some chemistry instruments can compensate for this change. Again, the reference laboratory should be able to indicate which tests are affected. Errors in processing the sample can also cause artifactual changes in laboratory data. It is important to use the appropriate collection tube for the test being performed.

Samples collected for chemistry profiles can be collected in *clot tubes* (red tops), which contain no anticoagulant, or in lithium heparin tubes (green tops). Blood collected in clot tubes (tubes without anticoagulant) must be allowed to completely clot before the sample can be centrifuged and the serum removed; complete clot formation usually takes about 30 minutes. Clot tubes with activator gels (tiger tops) will promote clotting, thus decreasing the time required for complete clot formation and facilitating separation of the serum from the RBCs. The sample should not be refrigerated before complete clot formation because this inhibits good serum separation. In addition, a fibrin clot forms above the RBCs if the blood is centrifuged before complete clot formation or at too fast a speed.

✍ TECHNICIAN NOTE
Serum must be removed from the clot as soon as possible to avoid inaccurate results.

Blood collected in *lithium heparin tubes* (green tops) is excellent for emergency needs because it does not have to clot before it can be separated for analysis. Heparin may interfere with a few chemistry tests, so the reference laboratory should be consulted before submission of heparinized plasma for chemistry panels. Lithium heparin is also excellent for emergency electrolyte panels. EDTA tubes (purple tops) are unacceptable for most chemistry tests because EDTA binds calcium to prevent clot formation and thus interferes with many of the assays, particularly those that are enzyme based. In addition, potassium EDTA will markedly increase serum potassium levels.

The necessity of separating serum from the clot as soon as possible cannot be overstressed. Prolonged exposure of serum to the cells will erroneously decrease the glucose level; will increase the phosphorus level; may increase the potassium level, depending on species (especially in the horse); and may affect some enzyme activities. Do not depend on the reference laboratory courier service to get the sample to the laboratory in time to prevent these changes. It is best to take the time and responsibility to separate the serum and ensure the quality of the sample.

Urinalysis

Urinalysis is one clinical laboratory procedure that should be performed as a part of any minimum database in all veterinary practices but is frequently skipped for a variety of reasons. It is an important diagnostic test that should be done on fresh urine when possible. The techniques involved are simple and require no special instrumentation. Urine samples should be collected into clean glass or plastic containers. In general, no preservatives are necessary. The best time to collect urine for urinalysis is usually in the morning when the animal awakens. Urine that accumulates during the relative inactivity of the night is less likely to be influenced by feeding or exercise. It is generally concentrated, and therefore abnormal constituents, if present, are more easily detected.

EQUIPMENT

The equipment necessary for performing the urinalysis is minimal. A supply of clean glass or plastic collection containers, a centrifuge and conical centrifuge tubes, chemical reagent strips, clean glass slides and coverslips, a refractometer, plastic pipettes, and a microscope are all that are required.

URINE COLLECTION

Urine may be collected by several methods. The simplest (if the animal will cooperate) is to catch a free-flow nonsterile sample as the animal voids spontaneously or is assisted by gentle manual expression. If this method is used, the initial stream of urine should not be caught because the first portion may contain cells and debris from the urethra and lower genital tract, resulting in contamination of the sample that may interfere with interpretation. It is better to collect a midstream sample, avoiding collection of the very beginning or the very end of a voided urine sample.

A second method that may be used to collect urine is *cystocentesis*. This procedure involves placing a needle (with a syringe attached) through the ventral abdominal wall into the lumen of the bladder and aspirating urine. Aseptic technique must be used. By performing cystocentesis, secretions and debris of the lower urogenital tract are avoided, and interpretation of urinalysis findings is simplified. Iatrogenic hemorrhage can occur during cystocentesis; therefore it is not unusual to have a widely varying number of RBCs in the sediment of samples obtained by this method.

Another method for collecting urine is by catheterization of the bladder. This procedure must be done as aseptically as possible to prevent introduction of bacteria into the urinary tract. Extreme care should be taken to avoid traumatizing the lining of the urethra with the catheter, or the sample may contain increased numbers of erythrocytes and epithelial cells. Additional information on cystocentesis and catheterization can be found in Chapter 3.

Regardless of how the urine sample is collected, it should be analyzed as soon as possible. Many changes begin to occur immediately. Bacteria present in the urine will multiply, cells may degenerate, casts may dissolve (especially if the urine is alkaline), and bacteria that produce urease will convert urea to ammonia, causing the pH to increase. If there is to be any delay in performing the urinalysis, the sample should be refrigerated to slow these processes. However, refrigeration may cause a change in urine SG and interfere with some of the chemistry reactions on the chemistry reagent strip. Before a urinalysis is performed on refrigerated urine, the specimen should be allowed to come to room temperature.

EVALUATION OF PHYSICAL PROPERTIES

As with all laboratory procedures, it is wise to follow the same routine protocol with every urine sample analyzed. The physical properties evaluated in most routine urinalyses include color, appearance or turbidity, and SG. After making sure the sample is mixed well, the color (e.g., yellow, gold, red) and appearance (e.g., clear, hazy, flocculent) should be recorded.

COLOR

Normal urine is yellow to amber, depending on its concentration and constituents. Bright red urine indicates *hematuria* (RBCs in the urine) or *hemoglobinuria* (hemoglobin in the urine). Reddish brown urine usually suggests hemoglobinuria or *myoglobinuria* (myoglobin in the urine); note that these two pigments cannot be distinguished from one another solely on the basis of color. High concentrations of bilirubin or urobilin cause yellowish brown urine that, when shaken, may produce yellowish foam. Whenever an unusual discoloration of the urine occurs, the history of any drug therapy should be evaluated because many drugs can produce abnormally colored urine. Urine that is markedly discolored may make it difficult or impossible to interpret color changes when chemical reagent strips are evaluated.

TURBIDITY

Fresh urine is normally transparent, but as it cools, some salts may precipitate, causing the urine to become cloudy. Except for equine urine, fresh urine that is cloudy is often pathologic, and it must be examined microscopically to identify the cause: pus, blood, mucus, bacteria, casts, or crystals. Fresh equine urine is normally cloudy because it contains mucus and calcium carbonate crystals Even clear urine should be examined microscopically because some abnormal constituents may be present in small amounts that may not cause urine to be visually cloudy.

SPECIFIC GRAVITY

SG determination is one of the most important parts of a urinalysis. It may be determined before or after centrifugation because the material that settles during centrifugation has little to no effect on SG. The SG value depends on the number and size of particles in solution and is an indicator of the ability of the kidney to concentrate urine. The SG is most accurately determined with a refractometer, which is used for determining plasma protein and requires only 1 drop of urine. If the urine sample is turbid, the SG may be determined from the supernatant after centrifugation. Reagent strips are inaccurate for determination of SG.

The normal range for SG is extremely wide: 1.001 to 1.060 in dogs and 1.001 to 1.080 in cats. The major determinant of urine SG is salt concentration because of the large number of particles involved. Protein, in contrast, has little influence on SG, because although the particles are large, they are few in number. Glucose, likewise, has relatively little effect on SG. Both of these components, however, when found in large amounts in the urine, will increase the SG by about 0.001 to 0.002. SG provides a very good indication of how well the kidneys are able to function in maintaining the body's water and osmotic balance. In addition, SG is important in interpretation of other test results. Because of the usual inverse relationship between SG and volume, a 2^+ protein in dilute urine (SG <1.012) suggests a greater loss of protein than a 2^+ protein in concentrated urine (SG >1.030).

Isosthenuria is the continued excretion of urine at the SG of glomerular filtrate (1.008 to 1.012). Isosthenuria indicates that the tubules have not attempted to concentrate urine. A single, routine urine sample with an isosthenuric SG is not necessarily abnormal because this is within the normal range and could be a chance occurrence. However, if an animal is dehydrated, azotemic, or uremic, the renal tubules are under pressure to concentrate urine; and under those circumstances, an SG lower than 1.035 in cats, 1.030 in dogs, and 1.025 in large animals indicates that the kidneys are not functioning appropriately.

CHEMICAL EVALUATION

Reagent strip chemistries should be performed on unspun urine, unless the urine is very turbid (cloudy). If it is turbid, the chemistry tests may be done after the sample has been centrifuged. Levels of protein, glucose, ketones, blood, and bilirubin in the urine are routinely determined as well as urinary pH. The strips contain pads that are impregnated with reagents and result in a color change when the appropriate urine constituents are present. Although the strips are simple to use, proper technique and accurate timing for reading the results are critical. The strips must be properly stored, the urine must be at room temperature and well mixed, and excess urine must be shaken from the strips to obtain valid results. Significantly discolored urine may interfere with the ability to discern colors and color changes on the reagent pads.

Some commercially available strips contain reagent pads for other components, such as leukocytes. These are being evaluated for reliability but are not yet accepted as accurate.

✎ TECHNICIAN NOTE

Refrigerated urine samples must be brought to room temperature before chemical analysis is performed.

PH

Urine pH is detected by reagent strips with chemical indicators. The symbol *pH* is used to express the hydrogen ion concentration (acidity) of a fluid. pH 7 is the neutral point. Readings above 7 are said to be alkalotic, and those below 7 are acidotic. In general, dogs and cats tend to have more acidic urine than do cattle and horses. A fresh sample must be used because as urine stands, it loses carbon dioxide, and bacteria that are present may produce ammonia, both of which result in increased alkalinity (raising the pH). The body's acid-base status may affect urine pH, but it is a mistake to use urine pH to evaluate the systemic acid-base balance. Too many other factors influence urine pH; in fact, urine pH may be completely contrary to the body's pH. For example, some cows with metabolic alkalosis have a paradoxical aciduria because the kidneys attempt to maintain electrolyte balance at the expense of acid-base balance.

PROTEIN

Most commercial urine reagent strips include a test for *protein.* It is often stated that normal urine contains no protein, but almost all urine contains a small amount of protein, which is due to normal leakage and secretion from the urinary tract lining. However, this normal amount of protein is not detected by routine methods. The strips depend on color changes in tetrabromophenolphthalein blue to detect protein levels that are above a very small amount (>10 mg/dl) present in normal urine. The test reaction is usually graded *trace* or 1^+ through 4^+, which supposedly corresponds to various protein concentrations. As mentioned, a positive protein reaction in dilute urine implies a greater protein loss than the same level of reaction in a concentrated sample. As with most reagent strip chemistry tests, results are at best only semiquantitative and are subject to several types of error. False-positive results may occur when urine is very alkaline. Second, the strips are more sensitive to albumin than to globulins and therefore can produce false-negative readings when proteinuria is caused by globulins. Because interpretation of the change in color of the reagent strip pad is subjective, different technicians may make different readings on the same urine sample.

Protein loss into urine can be a significant drain on the body's protein stores. One can make a subjective evaluation of the amount being lost by comparing the results with the SG, as previously mentioned; however, a more exact method is to collect all urine produced in a 24-hour period and calculate its total protein content. The collection of 24 hours of urine output generally requires a metabolism cage and is not very practical. The ratio of urine protein to urine creatinine (P/C ratio) in any single sample is a good index of protein loss in the urine. A urine P/C ratio of less than 1.0 is considered normal; a ratio greater than 2.0 indicates abnormal urinary protein loss; and a ratio from 1.0 to 2.0 suggests protein loss. A urine sample with sediment that indicates inflammation (presence of WBCs) is not suitable for determination of the urine P/C ratio. The inflammation must first be successfully treated. If the patient still has proteinuria once all evidence of inflammation is gone, a urine P/C ratio can be requested. Urine P/C ratios are usually done at a reference laboratory because they require a sensitive protein determination.

In interpreting the cause for a positive urine protein test, one must also consider the results of the test for blood and the microscopic examination of sediment. These results may aid in identifying the source of urinary protein. Proteinuria without a positive blood reaction or significant cells indicates glomerular disease, in which defective glomeruli allow passage of albumin into the urine, often resulting in protein readings of 3^+ or 4^+. There are a few extrarenal factors that may temporarily alter glomerular permeability to protein and result in proteinuria; they include fever, strenuous exercise, shock, cardiac or central nervous system disease, and the postcolostral period in neonates.

When excessive hemorrhage into the urinary tract occurs, the result of the test for urine protein will be positive, and erythrocytes will be seen in the sediment. Possible causes of urinary tract hemorrhage include trauma, neoplasia, and inflammation. Hemoglobin or myoglobin in the urine will cause a positive protein test result as well as a positive blood test result. In either of these cases, intact RBCs are not a significant part of the sediment.

When proteinuria occurs in conjunction with increased leukocytes in the urine sediment, inflammation of the urinary tract should be suspected. Inflammation rarely causes a urine protein test result of more than 2^+, unless hemorrhage is associated with the inflammatory process. In some urinary tract infections, bacteria may be seen in the sediment. Determination of the location of the inflammation may depend on the method of collection. If testing is done on voided samples, the inflammation may be anywhere in the genitourinary tract, whereas if test samples were collected by cystocentesis, the inflammation may be localized to the bladder or kidney.

GLUCOSE

In addition to urine protein, a common reagent strip test for urine is the test for glucose. The reagent strips usually use glucose oxidase to detect glucose and for this reason are quite specific for glucose. However, as with all reagent strip tests, they are not quantitative. Tablets that detect glucose, which are somewhat more quantitative but not specific, are available. The tablets use a copper reduction method that detects many sugars and reducing agents other than glucose.

Normally, urine contains no detectable glucose. Glucose is filtered by the glomerulus, but the body preserves this energy source by reabsorbing it in the proximal renal tubules. This resorption ability is exceeded once the blood glucose level rises above 180 mg/dl in most species or above 100 mg/dl in the cow. This is the "renal threshold" for glucose, above which it will "spill" into the urine. The primary cause for *glucosuria* therefore is *hyperglycemia*. For confirmation of hyperglycemia as the cause, the blood glucose level should be determined at the same time as the urine glucose level. Diabetes mellitus is a common cause of hyperglycemia and glucosuria.

KETONES

A test for urine ketones is included on many reagent strips; tablets are also available. Both use a nitroprusside method that detects acetone and acetoacetic acid but not beta-hydroxybutyric acid, so false-negative results are possible. Ketones will appear in the urine before they build up to a detectable level in the bloodstream, so *ketonuria* may occur before a detectable *ketonemia* occurs. Ketonuria indicates excessive fat metabolism, a deficiency in carbohydrate metabolism, or both but is most commonly seen in conjunction with glucosuria as a complication of diabetes mellitus.

BILIRUBIN

There are reagent strips and tablets for detecting *bilirubinuria,* both of which use a similar reaction (diazotization), but the tablets are less subject to interference by urine color. The tablets are also highly sensitive, so a 1^+ reading, especially in concentrated urine, may not be significant. Both strips and tablets detect conjugated bilirubin and not unconjugated bilirubin. Bilirubin in urine can also be crudely detected by the *foam test.* If yellowish foam appears when the urine sample is shaken, bilirubin is likely present. Bilirubin may be oxidized on exposure to light, so if there is much delay between obtaining the urine sample and performing the urinalysis, the sample should be protected from light to avoid false-negative results. Many normal dogs, and sometimes cattle, will exhibit bilirubinuria because the kidneys, as well as the liver, have an enzyme that can conjugate bilirubin. However, this enzyme is lacking in cats, and any bilirubinuria is a significant abnormality in cats.

BLOOD

The designation "blood" is somewhat misleading because this test actually detects intact RBCs, hemoglobin, and myoglobin. Both reagent strips and tablets make use of the peroxidase property of free hemoglobin or myoglobin, which oxidizes orthotoluidine to a blue-colored derivative. If the urine is red and cloudy and erythrocytes are present in the sediment, *hematuria* is the reason for the positive blood reaction.

Hemoglobinuria (hemoglobin pigment in the urine) results in red to brown urine with a positive urine blood reaction and no erythrocytes in the sediment. A positive urine protein test result may also be apparent. In contrast to hematuria, hemoglobinuria will be accompanied by *hemoglobinemia*, imparting a pink to reddish discoloration to the serum or plasma.

Myoglobinuria (myoglobin pigment in the urine) will similarly result in red to brown urine with no erythrocytes in the sediment, a positive urine blood reaction, and a positive urine protein test result. However, during myoglobinuria, the blood serum or plasma generally remains clear. Myoglobin, which is derived from muscles, is a smaller molecule than hemoglobin and does not bind to serum proteins; thus it is rapidly excreted into the urine before reaching levels sufficiently high to produce discoloration of the serum. Animals with myoglobinuria generally do not show evidence of anemia but have some type of muscle disease, such as exertional myopathy in horses ("tying up" syndrome), trauma, electrical shock, or pressure necrosis from prolonged recumbency. If not apparent by clinical signs, hemoglobinuria and myoglobinuria may be differentiated by electrophoresis or a more cumbersome ammonium sulfate precipitation test.

MICROSCOPIC EXAMINATION

The sediment should be prepared for microscopic examination. Urine sediment examination may reveal extremely useful diagnostic information and be crucial for correct interpretation of the chemical analyses. A few cells and a few casts may be found in normal urine, but increased numbers of various elements indicate certain diseases. A reference is provided for assistance with sediment evaluation.

SAMPLE PREPARATION

Pour a standard volume (10 ml is recommended) of urine into a conical-tip centrifuge tube. If the sample available is less than 10 ml, use all that is left after the reagent strip chemistries and SG determinations have been completed. Centrifuge the urine at a slow speed (1500 rpm) for 5 minutes. Higher speeds for centrifugation may disrupt the cells and casts that are present. Decant the supernatant, leaving the sediment in the bottom. Gently tap the tube to resuspend the sediment in the small amount of urine remaining on the sides and in the bottom of the tube. With a small pipette, transfer a drop of suspended sediment to a glass slide and place a coverslip on it. Commercial stains (e.g., SediStain, Clay Adams, Parsippany, NJ) are available for evaluating urine sediments, but with practice and experience they are not necessary.

A phase-contrast microscope is ideal for examining unstained urine sediment. A more practical and highly satisfactory alternative is to lower the condenser of the light microscope and reduce the intensity of the light (as for the manual mammalian WBC count). The slide should first be examined at 10× magnification to obtain an overall impression of how much and what type of sediment is present. The 40× or 45× power (high dry) is then used to make the final identification and count of various components. At least 10 microscopic fields must be evaluated, and the average numbers of various cells and casts per high-power field are reported. The presence and relative amounts of other components are also noted.

EPITHELIAL CELLS

Three types of epithelial cells can be found in urine sediment: squamous, transitional, and renal tubular. *Squamous epithelial cells* (Figure 6-28) are very large, with angular

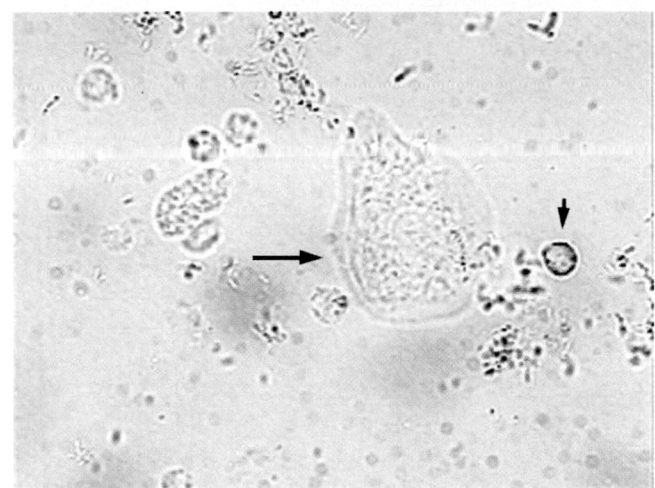

Figure 6-28 Urine sediment with a large squamous epithelial cell *(long arrow)*, crenated red blood cells *(short arrows)*, and bacteria in the background.

borders and small nuclei. They originate from the lining of the distal urethra and vagina or prepuce and are not generally indicative of disease. *Transitional epithelial cells* are medium-sized and oval, spindled, or caudate cells found lining the proximal urethra, bladder, ureters, and renal pelvis. They may occur in groups, especially if the urine was obtained by catheterization. If transitional epithelial cells are very large and variable, very basophilic, or found in large clusters, they should be further evaluated for possible neoplasia. *Renal tubular epithelial cells* are small, round cells and may indicate tubular degeneration.

BLOOD CELLS

Erythrocytes in unstained sediment appear colorless or yellowish and are round and slightly refractile, with no internal structure. They may be confused with fat droplets, but erythrocytes are fairly uniform in size and do not float in and out of planes of focus as do fat droplets. If there is doubt, a drop of diluted acetic acid will lyse erythrocytes, helping to differentiate them from fat droplets. In concentrated urine, erythrocytes may lose fluid and become *crenated* (shrunken and spiked). In dilute urine, they may imbibe water and swell or even lyse, becoming *ghost cells*. *Leukocytes* in urine sediment are round and granular and larger than erythrocytes but smaller than epithelial cells (Figure 6-29). The presence of more than five to eight WBCs per high-power field indicates inflammation of the urinary or urogenital tract, depending on the method of collection. When this occurs, a careful check for bacteria should be made.

CASTS

Casts are another prominent feature of urine sediment. They are elongated structures composed of protein from plasma and mucoprotein from the renal tubules. In general, they form in the distal tubules, in which the urine is more

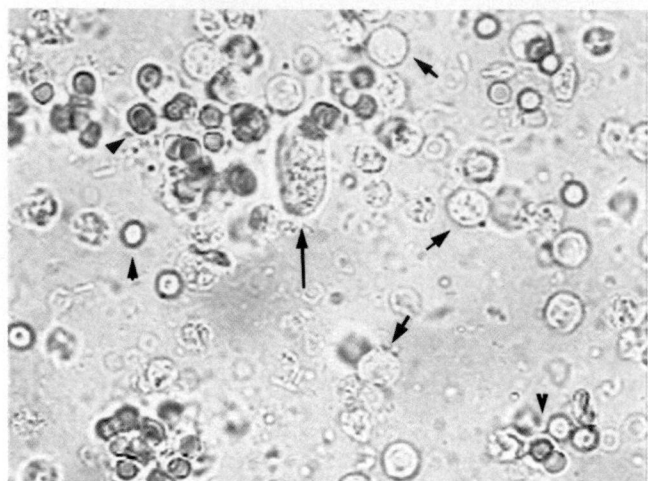

Figure 6-29 Urine sediment with a cast *(long arrow)* and several red blood cells *(arrowheads)* and white blood cells *(short arrows)*.

concentrated and acidic. Any structures that happen to be in the tubules at the time the casts form (erythrocytes, leukocytes, or epithelial cells) become embedded in the casts. The presence of increased numbers of casts helps to localize the renal disease to the tubules, but the numbers do not necessarily correlate with the severity of disease. For instance, severe chronic nephritis may be accompanied by just a few casts.

The five main types of casts are as follows:

1. *Hyaline casts* are colorless, homogeneous, and semitransparent. They may be difficult to see unless the light is reduced. They indicate mild glomerular leakage.
2. *Cellular casts* contain recognizable cells embedded in the protein matrix. They may be epithelial cell casts that contain sloughed tubular epithelial cells, erythrocyte casts that indicate renal hemorrhage, or leukocyte casts that indicate renal inflammation or pyelonephritis.
3. *Granular casts* are derived from degenerating cells or cellular casts. They are characterized by a nonspecific granular matrix and are designated as either coarsely or finely granular, depending on the degree of degeneration. They are probably the most common type of cast found in animals.
4. *Waxy casts* are wide and homogeneous, usually with distinct blunt or squared ends. They indicate a more chronic tubular lesion.
5. *Fatty casts* contain fat globules from degenerating tubular epithelial cells and are most common in cats because of the high lipid content of feline tubular epithelium.

CRYSTALS

Crystals are another major component of urine sediment. Their precipitation and presence depend on urine pH and the solubility and concentration of the substance forming them. Urine crystals that accompany pathologic conditions include *ammonium biurate, monohydrate calcium oxalate, bilirubin, triple phosphate* (struvite, ammonium, magnesium phosphate), and *cystine* crystals. Dihydrate calcium oxalate crystals can be found in normal urine but appear distinctly different from the monohydrate calcium oxalate crystals found with ethylene glycol (antifreeze) toxicity. Figure 6-30 shows these two types of calcium oxalate crystals. Bilirubin crystals generally occur in conjunction with bilirubinuria with little to no additional significance. Triple phosphate crystals (Figure 6-31) are often found in alkaline urine when urease-producing bacteria, associated with lower urinary tract disease, are present. Ammonium biurate crystals (Figure 6-32) are dark with very distinct, multiple, irregular protrusions and are often associated with portal caval shunts, a specific liver disorder. Cystine crystals (Figure 6-33), although sometimes seen in urine of healthy dogs, are also found in the urine of dogs with a congenital defect of cystine metabolism that leads to cystinuria. Drugs, such as sulfonamides, may precipitate in the urine of animals, resulting in the formation of crystals.

MICROORGANISMS

Bacteria in unstained urine sediment may be difficult to detect. Rods may appear singly or in chains, but cocci may be lost in Brownian movement. For this reason, whenever the presence of bacteria is suspected, the sediment should be stained to examine it more thoroughly. Usually, the regular examination of the unstained sediment is completed and recorded first, and then the coverslip is removed and the underlying sediment on the slide is allowed to dry. Once dry, the slide can be stained with Gram's stain or one of the modified Wright's stains, and any bacteria present can be identified. On Gram's stain, the gram-negative, rod-shaped bacteria may be difficult to see among all the pink-staining cellular debris. With Wright's stain, all bacteria stain dark purple and are relatively easy to find.

Bacteria in a voided sample are often not significant because they may be normal flora from the distal urogenital tract, especially from the prepuce or vagina. Bacteria are significant if they occur in catheterized or cystocentesis samples. Their presence should be correlated with leukocytes in urine because bacteria with no leukocyte response should raise suspicion of contamination of the sample. If bacteria are present in a urine sample, they can multiply as time passes, so this should be taken into consideration when the sample is being analyzed. Rarely, *fungal* organisms are found in urine sediment. The majority of these are insignificant contaminants, although some, such as *Blastomyces* organisms, may be significant.

MISCELLANEOUS FINDINGS

Usually insignificant components of urine sediment include mucus, fat, sperm, and parasites. Mucus appears as narrow,

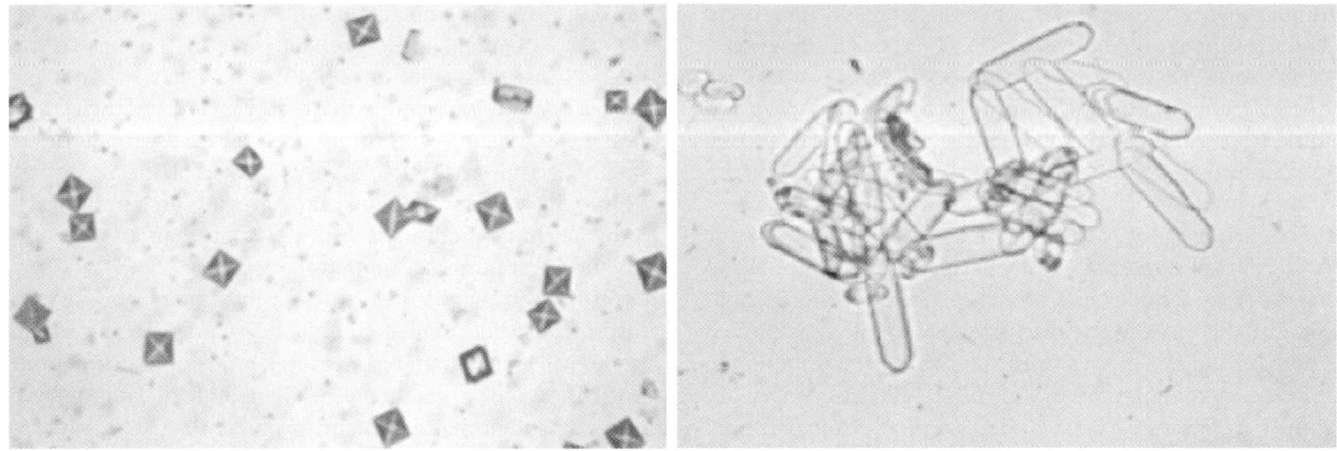

A   B

Figure 6-30   Canine urine sediment showing the two forms of calcium oxalate crystals. **A,** Dihydrate form. **B,** Monohydrate form.

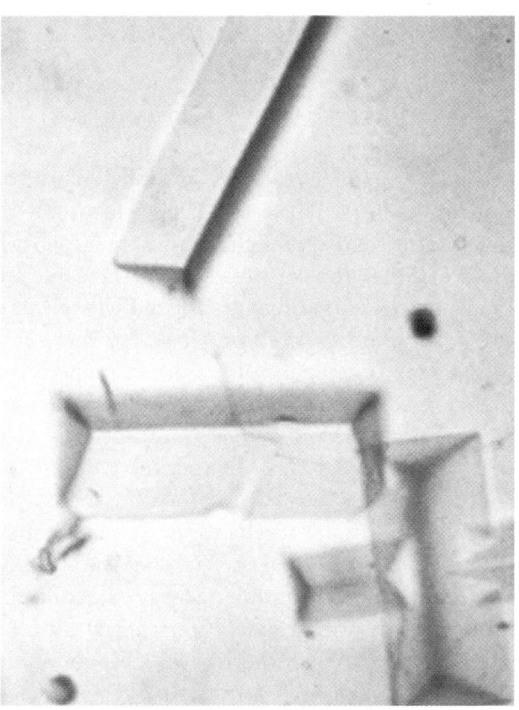

Figure 6-31   Urine sediment with triple phosphate crystals.

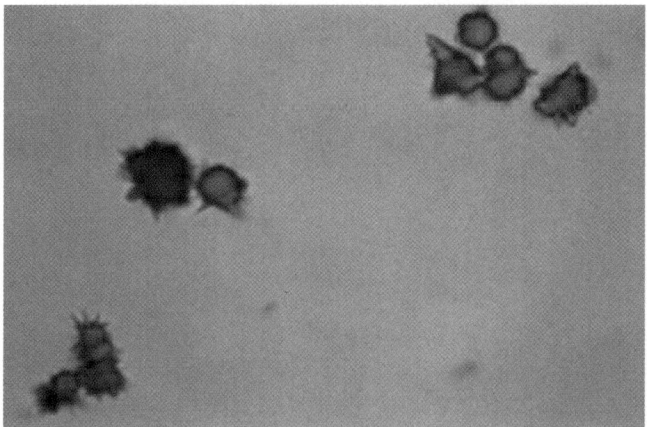

Figure 6-32   Urine sediment with ammonium biurate crystals.

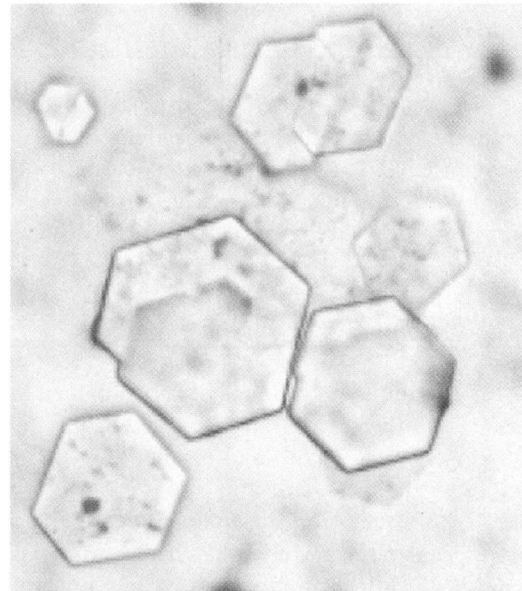

Figure 6-33   Urine sediment with cystine crystals.

twisted, ribbonlike strands. It is normal in equine urine and can be seen in other species as well because of genital secretions or irritation of the urethra. Fat, as previously noted, takes the form of refractile, variably sized spheres in many planes of focus. Fat is rarely significant. Sperm are commonly seen in male canine urine samples. Parasites that can occur in urine include the ova of *Stephanurus dentatus, Dioctophyma renale,* and *Capillaria plica* and microfilaria of *Dirofilaria* immitis.

Cytology

Cytology is the study of cells, specifically involving the microscopic examination of individual cells that have exfoliated from a tissue or structure. Unlike histopathology, cytology is not an evaluation of the architecture of a tissue. In most instances, cytology can be used to differentiate an inflammatory lesion from a neoplastic mass. Sometimes cytologic appearance reveals a very specific diagnosis, and for certain samples, such as bone marrow or mast cell tumors, it may be more helpful than histopathology. It should be emphasized that cytology is an adjunct diagnostic tool and not a replacement for histopathology.

Cytology requires a significant degree of expertise that can be acquired only through experience, especially for cytology of solid masses. Most veterinary practices prefer to send cytology samples to a reference laboratory for evaluation. For this reason, the discussion on cytology is limited to preparation of samples from solid tissues for submission to a reference laboratory and fluid analysis. Veterinary technicians interested in becoming adept at cytology should obtain specific training through continuing education workshops. Excellent reference material is available.

EQUIPMENT

One of the advantages of cytology is that it requires no special equipment or supplies other than those used in performing a CBC. A good microscope, clean glass slides, a modified Wright's stain, and a centrifuge for fluid samples will suffice for most cytologic examinations.

SAMPLE PREPARATION

Most cytology samples of solid masses are obtained through *fine-needle aspiration*. Cells are aspirated from the mass with a syringe (usually 6 ml) and needle (22- to 25-gauge) inserted into the mass and the application of negative pressure. It is not necessary to aspirate so strenuously that material appears in the barrel of the syringe or even the hub of the needle. Gentle aspiration will usually pull sufficient material into the needle. The sample can then be expelled onto a glass slide. Depending on the consistency of the sample, it can be spread in a manner similar to that used in making a blood smear or by what is referred to as the *squash prep* for more viscous samples. Placing a second slide on top of the slide containing the sample does this. The weight of the top slide should cause the sample to spread, and then the top slide is pulled off across the bottom slide, resulting in even spreading of the cells. This method works well for many types of samples, and it may result in fewer broken cells than the traditional technique. It is important not to exert excessive pressure on the top slide or pull the slides apart too rapidly because cells are often fragile, and this will distort or "squash" the cells and make identification difficult, if not impossible.

When handling excised pieces of tissue for cytologic study, keep them wrapped in gauze and slightly moistened with saline solution so they do not dry out. Do not allow any contact with formalin, or even with formalin fumes, until after the cytologic slides have been made and stained. Excised solid masses should be blotted with absorbent paper

to remove blood and tissue fluid and then gently touched to a slide to make an impression slide. If the mass is of a dense consistency that does not exfoliate cells easily, it may be necessary to scrape it with a scalpel blade and then spread the material gently and thinly onto the slide. An alternative method is to crosshatch cut the surface of the tissue with the scalpel blade and make an imprint preparation. The crosshatching method is often gentler than the scraping method and preserves the cells better.

If the slides are to be sent to a reference laboratory, the use of flat slide mailers should be avoided because many slides will arrive shattered. Most reference laboratories prefer unstained slides, which can be stained at the laboratory by means of their standard stain protocol. If a slide has been stained and there are questions pertaining to that slide, it is a good idea to include that slide for comparison purposes.

FLUID ANALYSIS

For fluid analysis, a refractometer and a cell-counting method (e.g., Unopettes and a hemacytometer) are also needed. Once a sample for cytology has been obtained, slides should be made as soon as possible, before the cells degenerate in the fluid. This is especially true of low-protein fluids, such as cerebrospinal fluid and tracheal washings. Many fluid samples can be prepared in the same manner as a blood film, leaving a feathered edge where the largest cells tend to migrate. If the fluid has very few cells, as is the case with cerebrospinal fluid, a direct preparation may not provide a sufficient number of cells for a thorough examination. Some *cytocentrifuges* are specially designed to make cytologic slides from hypocellular fluids; they are gentler to cells because they spin at a slow speed and have gradual acceleration and deceleration. They also may have a special apparatus that causes cells to be deposited directly onto a slide, with filter paper taking away excess fluid. However, cytocentrifuges are probably impractical for all except the largest practices. As an alternative, these low-cellularity samples can be concentrated in a manner similar to the preparation of urine sediment. The fluid is centrifuged at slow speed, and the slide is prepared from the sediment after the supernatant is decanted or removed with a pipette. It is always advisable to make one or two direct preparations in case the techniques used to concentrate the cells result in too many ruptured cells or other artifacts.

A routine fluid analysis of samples such as abdominal, thoracic, or synovial fluid usually includes a WBC count, which is more appropriately referred to as a total nucleated cell count, because some of the cells (mesothelial cells, synovial cells, etc.) may not be derived directly from blood. The total nucleated cell count can be performed in the same manner as a WBC count. If there are numerous cells present, these can be counted on an automated instrument, but lower cell counts will require use of the hemacytometer as for a manual WBC count but with no dilution.

Total protein is another helpful parameter in fluid analysis and can be done by refractometer, generally with

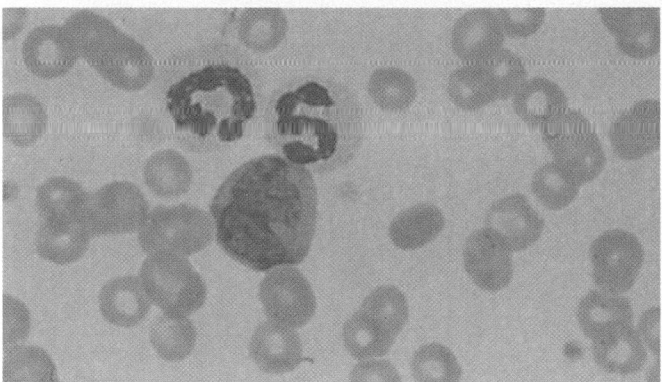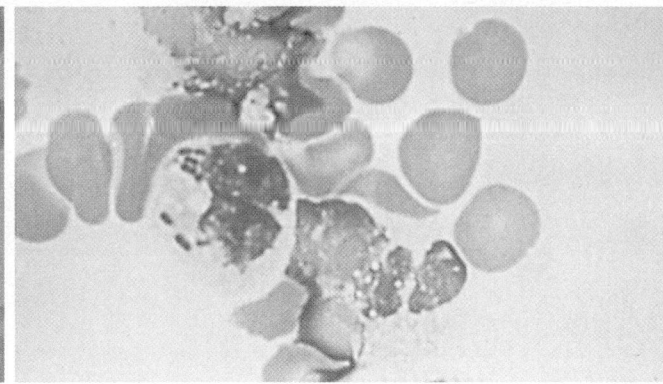

Figure 6-34 Equine abdominal fluid showing a degenerative neutrophil with intracellular rod-shaped bacteria. Two smudge cells are also present.

the supernatant portion of a centrifuged fluid sample. Total erythrocyte (RBC) count is often included in the fluid analysis if done on an automated instrument, but the RBC count alone is rarely helpful in evaluating fluid because of the frequency of peripheral blood contamination of samples. It is more important to check for *erythrophagocytosis* (phagocytosis of RBCs by macrophages) during the cytologic examination because erythrophagocytosis generally implies that the RBCs were present in the fluid before sampling rather than as contaminants.

Fluid samples that have neutrophils as the predominate cell type should be closely evaluated for the presence of bacteria. Bacteria should be present within cells (intracellular) to be considered significant (Figure 6-34). If they are only extracellular, the possibility of contamination of the sample should be considered. If no bacteria are found, it should not be assumed that they are absent. They may be present in very low numbers and difficult to find.

JOINT FLUID

The analysis of certain fluids includes specific tests that may add more information than routine tests. For instance, the *mucin clot test* is done on synovial fluid by mixing a diluted acetic acid solution (0.1 ml of 7N acetic acid in 4 ml of distilled water) and then adding 1 ml of synovial fluid. Normal synovial fluid contains mucin, which forms a tight white clot in the acetic acid; if the mucin has been digested by bacterial or cellular enzymes, the clot will be less distinct or may not form at all, leaving only hazy or cloudy fluid. Therefore good mucin clot formation usually accompanies normal or noninflamed joints, whereas a poor or absent mucin clot indicates inflammation, infection, or both. The precipitation of mucin in joint fluid by acetic acid precludes the use of the WBC Unopette system because this system contains acetic acid as the diluent in the reservoir. Total nucleated cell counts of joint fluid samples should be done with the Unopette system for both WBCs and platelets. The reservoir in this system contains ammonium oxalate, which will not precipitate mucin.

Recommended Reading

General
Duncan JR, Prasse KW: *Veterinary laboratory medicine/clinical pathology,* Ames, 1994, Iowa State University Press.

Laboratory Equipment
Tietz NW: *Fundamentals of clinical chemistry,* ed 4, Philadelphia, 1995, WB Saunders.

Hematology
Harvey JW: *Atlas of veterinary hematology: blood and bone marrow of domestic animals,* Philadelphia, 2001, WB Saunders.
Jain NC: *Essentials of veterinary hematology,* Philadelphia, 1993, Lea & Febiger.
Reagan WL et al: *Veterinary hematology: atlas of common domestic species,* Ames, 1998, Iowa State University Press.

Urinalysis
Graff L: *A handbook of routine urinalysis,* Philadelphia, 1983, JB Lippincott.
Osborne CA, Finco DR: *Canine and feline nephrology and urology,* Philadelphia, 1995, Lea & Febiger.

Chemistry
Coffman JR: *Equine clinical chemistry and pathophysiology,* Bonner Springs, Kan, 1981, Veterinary Medicine Publishing.
Kaneko JJ, editor: *Clinical biochemistry of domestic animals,* New York, 1989, Academic Press.

Quality Assurance Programs
Henry JB: *Clinical diagnosis and management by laboratory methods,* ed 19, Philadelphia, 1996, WB Saunders.

Avian and Reptilian Hematology
Campbell TW: *Avian hematology and cytology,* Ames, 1988, Iowa State University Press.
Frye FL: *Biomedical and surgical aspects of captive reptile husbandry,* Edwardsville, Kan, 1981, Veterinary Medicine Publishing.

Cytology
Cowell RL et al: *Diagnostic cytology and hematology of the dog and cat,* ed 2, St Louis, 1999, Mosby.
Menard M, Papageorges M: Fine-needle biopsies: how to increase diagnostic yield, *Compend Cont Educ Pract Vet* 19:738, 1997.

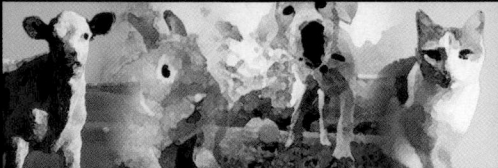

7

Parasitology

JOHNNY D. HOSKINS

INTRODUCTION

Most parasites are capable of causing significant damage to the host. This potential may be a function of the number of parasites present, location within the host, production of toxins, or interference with normal physiologic processes. Clinical signs associated with parasitism may include life-threatening anemia, hypoproteinemia, diarrhea, vomiting, and intestinal obstruction; however, the damage is often more insidious, such as interference with normal weight gain or milk production. Parasitism is most severe in animals younger than 1 year, but it may affect animals of any age.

Ectoparasites (external parasites)—including mites, ticks, lice, fleas, chiggers, and myiasis-inducing flies—and endoparasites (internal parasites)—including protozoa, trematodes, tapeworms, and nematodes—have representative parasites on or in all animals and in every organ or tissue. Some parasites are host specific, whereas other parasites are capable of infesting or infecting a broad range of animal hosts. Modes of transmission vary considerably from simple, direct transmission to an extremely complex life cycle involving the use of an intermediate host or transport host or specific environmental conditions. The nematode parasites have five stages in their development. Various nematodes, such as the strongyle nematodes of ruminants and horses, produce eggs that pass into the environment. A first-stage larva develops within each egg. This free-living larva grows and molts (sheds the skin or cuticle) to a second-stage larva, which then grows and molts into a third-stage larva—the infective larva. The infective larva is usually ingested and develops into a fourth-stage larva and finally into a fifth-stage larva within the host.

Some nematodes have developed modifications of this life cycle. For example, hookworm larvae generally penetrate the skin and circulate in the host's tissue before completing their development in the small intestine.

Others, such as roundworms and whipworms, develop into the infective stage within the eggs, which do not hatch until they are ingested by the host. Other important nematodes, such as *Strongyloides* spp., have first-stage larvae in the eggs when passed. Treatment, including selection of the proper medication and appropriate control in the environment, always necessitates a thorough knowledge of the biology of each parasite.

The following sections discuss specific parasites as they relate to animal host and parasite class within each host. The veterinary technician should become familiar with both the common and scientific names (e.g., roundworm = *Toxocara canis*) of the common parasites. Each section contains information on the life cycle, tissue location, and treatment and control of the specific parasite discussed. Sections on diagnostic procedures and public health are also included. ■

TECHNICIAN NOTE

The diagnosis of parasitism is not difficult; but timing, choice of technique, and interpretation of the results are often crucial for effective treatment and control.

Endoparasites

PARASITES OF DOGS AND CATS

ROUNDWORMS (*ASCARIDS*)

Toxocara canis, Toxocara cati, and *Toxascaris leonina* are ascarids that are thick, white to cream-colored nematodes. Mature specimens measure about 3.5 to 5 cm (males) and 10 to 15 cm (females). Eggs of the *Toxocara* spp. are large, oval, and dark colored with thick, rough shells. *Toxascaris leonina* eggs are lighter in color and more egg shaped and

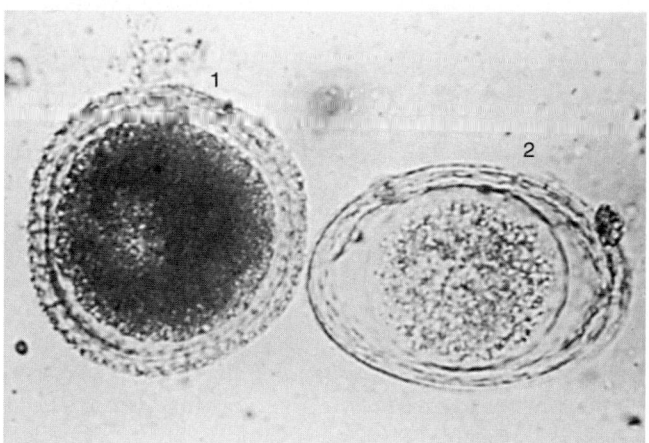

Figure 7-1 *1, Toxocara* egg measuring approximately 66 × 42 μm. *2, Toxascaris* egg measuring approximately 85 × 75 μm.

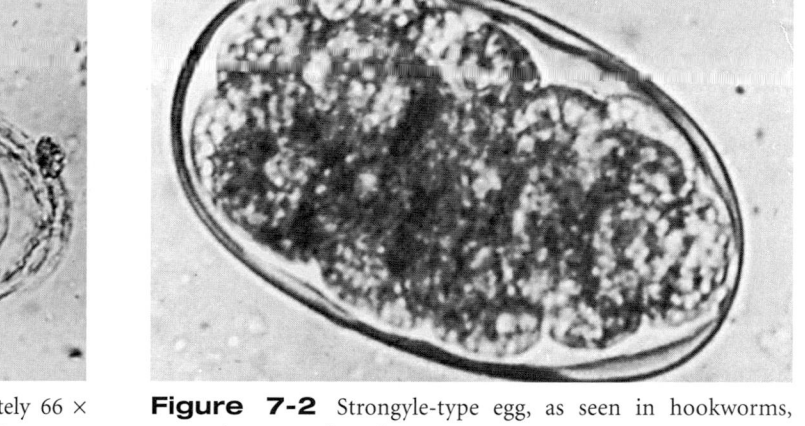

Figure 7-2 Strongyle-type egg, as seen in hookworms, measuring approximately 62 × 40 μm.

have thick, smooth shells (Figure 7-1). All three species are common in most geographic regions of the United States. The larval stage develops within the eggs, and the second stage consists of the infective larvae. Eggs are highly resistant to adverse conditions and, in ideal environmental conditions, become infective in about 2 weeks. Once ingested, *Toxocara* spp. hatch in the small intestine, penetrate the mucosa, migrate through the liver, pass through the heart, and go into the lungs, in which they develop within a short period. Larvae are coughed up and swallowed, and they mature in the small intestine within 4 to 6 weeks.

Toxascaris leonina eggs hatch in the small intestine, and the larvae penetrate the intestinal mucosa to develop for about 2 to 3 months and then return to the lumen as adults. In dogs older than 5 weeks, most of the larvae leave the circulation and are stored in the somatic organs until the dog becomes pregnant. Between the 42 and 56 days of gestation, these larvae leave the somatic tissues, cross the placenta, enter the fetal lungs, and remain there until birth. The larvae then complete the cycle already described. Consequently, a high percentage of dogs are infected via the prenatal or transplacental route. In pregnant dogs and cats, some of the activated *Toxocara* larvae migrate to the mammary glands. These larvae are ingested by puppies and kittens when they start to nurse. Transmammary infections are more common in cats than in dogs. The eggs of all three ascarids can be ingested by other animals (e.g., mice, chickens) and remain infective in their tissue until these animals are eaten by an appropriate host. All three species are readily identified by several techniques, and they are amenable to treatment with several anthelmintics. Control is difficult because the eggs are resistant, and control measures include thorough cleansing of kennels, runs, yards, and so forth.

HOOKWORMS

Ancylostoma caninum is found in dogs, foxes, coyotes, wolves, raccoons, and badgers; *Ancylostoma braziliense* is found in dogs and cats; *Uncinaria stenocephala* occurs in dogs, cats, foxes, coyotes and wolves; *Ancylostoma tubaeforme* is found in cats and wild Felidae. Hookworms are all short, thick parasites; adult males measure 6 to 12 mm, and females measure 6 to 20 mm. Hookworms produce strongyle-type eggs (Figure 7-2). *Ancylostoma* spp. are generally found in coastal areas of high rainfall, whereas *U. stenocephala* is found in the northeastern United States. All hookworm species have a similar life cycle. Undeveloped eggs pass into the environment, develop and hatch, releasing first-stage larvae that undergo a free-living existence until they develop to the third-stage infective larvae. Hookworms are capable of establishing themselves in the host after ingestion, but the normal mode of infection is skin penetration. After larvae penetrate, they enter the venous circulation, going ultimately to the lungs, in which they develop for a short period. They are then coughed up and swallowed, and they enter the small intestine and mature. This generally occurs within 4 to 6 weeks.

> ### ✎ TECHNICIAN NOTE
> Hookworms are capable of establishing themselves in the host after ingestion, but the normal mode of infection is skin penetration.

Ancylostoma caninum has developed the additional modes of *transplacental* and *transmammary infection*. Third-stage larvae penetrate the skin and circulate in the pregnant female host, ultimately crossing the placenta. The larvae are also stored in somatic tissues until the female host becomes pregnant. In dogs, most of the somatic larvae activated at the time of pregnancy migrate to the mammary glands of the bitch and are passed on to nursing puppies. Diagnosis can be made by identification of the eggs with a number of techniques, and these species are amenable to treatment with a number of anthelmintics. Control is difficult, especially in warm, humid geographic regions, necessitating regular thorough cleansing of yards, kennels, and other areas.

INTESTINAL THREADWORMS

Strongyloides stercoralis is a nematode that is a parasite of dogs, cats, foxes, humans, primates, and possibly other wild carnivores. Only the female nematode is parasitic, and she reproduces by parthenogenesis (without fertilization). Parasitic females live embedded in the mucosa of the small intestine. The eggs develop in utero, and nematodes give birth to first-stage larvae (Figure 7-3) whose chromosome number determines whether they will develop into a free-living generation before producing larvae destined to be parasitic or whether they will become a larval stage possessing a unique chromosome and be destined to develop into third-stage infective larvae. The infective larvae are capable of establishing infection by oral ingestion, after which they penetrate the small intestine and develop there. However, the primary mode of infection is skin penetration. If the larvae penetrate the skin, they then penetrate the venous circulation, going ultimately to the lungs to develop for a short period. Larvae are then coughed up and swallowed and penetrate the mucosa of the small intestine. In immunologically compromised animals, infections may be severe. *S. stercoralis* is widespread in tropical and subtropical regions, as well as in kennels and pet shops, in which environmental conditions are suitable. Diagnosis is not difficult. Frequently, a direct smear of fresh feces is suitable for identification. Treatment is not always satisfactory, and alternative anthelmintics should be considered. Control necessitates thorough cleaning of facilities and allowing the facilities to dry.

WHIPWORMS

Trichuris vulpis occurs in the cecum of the dog, fox, and coyote. Like all whipworms, *T. vulpis* has a slender anterior extremity and a thickened posterior extremity, resulting in a whip-like appearance. Males and females are about the same length, measuring 45 to 75 mm. The eggs are distinctive, possessing thick, brown-yellow shells with a clear polar plug at each end (Figure 7-4). *T. vulpis* is widespread in temperate zones, and the incidence of infection is frequently high. The life cycle is simple and direct. The infective larvae develop within the eggs. When the eggs are ingested, the larvae are released in the intestine, which they penetrate. Larvae develop within 8 to 10 days, return to the surface of the intestine, go to the cecum, and attach and mature in an additional 60 to 80 days. Diagnosis can be effectively accomplished by a number of procedures, but eggs are quite heavy, and interpretation of the severity of infection based on the number of eggs present is not possible. Several treatments are available. Control is difficult because eggs are highly resistant to environmental conditions. Sanitation, as applied for ascarids, is the best approach.

Whipworm infection is uncommon in cats and wild Felidae in the United States; however, *Trichuris campanula* has been reported to occur in the United States. Occasionally, *Capillaria* spp. have been found in feces of both dogs and cats. The eggs of *Capillaria* spp. are similar, but not as dark in color, and on average, the eggs are somewhat smaller than those of whipworms.

TAPEWORMS

✎ TECHNICIAN NOTE

Whipworm eggs are distinctive, possessing thick, brown-yellow shells with a clear polar plug at each end.

Dogs, cats, the wild Canidae, and some of the wild Felidae are susceptible to infection by a number of tapeworms. The most commonly found tapeworm species are *Dipylidium*

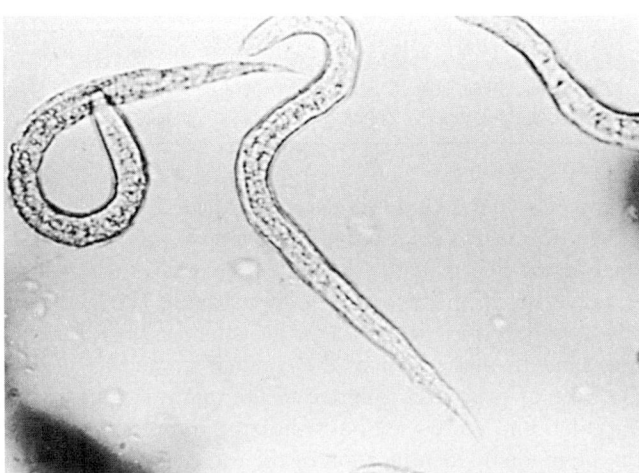

Figure 7-3 *Strongyloides* larvae from a dog. Note that the larvae are distorted in appearance because of the flotation solution.

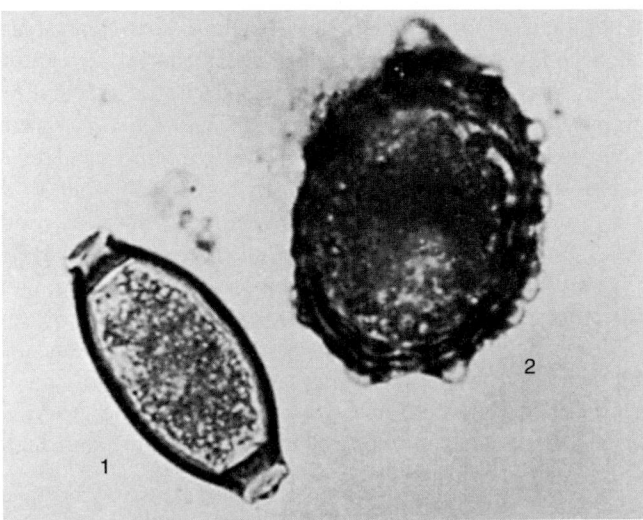

Figure 7-4 *1,* Trichurid egg, as seen in whipworms, measuring approximately 80 × 36 μm. *2,* Ascarid egg measuring approximately 60 × 50 μm.

caninum, *Taenia hydatigena*, *T. pisiformis*, *T. ovis*, *T. krabbei*, *Multiceps serialis*, and *Echinococcus granulosus*. Cats, and some of the wild Felidae, are generally infected with *T. taeniaeformis* and *D. caninum*. The species of tapeworms found in dogs and cats depends on their geographic location and the amount of free-ranging activity the animals are allowed.

All tapeworms have an intermediate host in which the larval stage (cysticercoid) develops; *D. caninum* uses a flea. *T. hydatigena*, *T. ovis*, and *T. krabbei* use ruminants—usually sheep, deer, elk, and moose—in which the larval stage (cysticercus) develops in the body cavity (*T. hydatigena*) or muscles (*T. ovis* and *T. krabbei*). *T. pisiformis* develops in the body cavities of rabbits, and *T. serialis* develops in subcutaneous areas or in the muscles (as a coenurus) of rabbits. The larval stage of *T. taeniaeformis* (strobilocercus) develops in the livers of mice, rats, and other small rodents. *E. granulosus* uses ruminants—such as sheep, deer and elk, and humans—as intermediate hosts. The larval stage is a rather large, fluid-filled bladder called a hydatid cyst that is easily recognized by its large size (25 to 100 mm in diameter), the presence of numerous small pieces of larval tapeworms (brood capsules) on the inner surface, and the presence of compartments within the body of the cyst in which daughter cysts have grown and fused together.

Diagnosis of *Taenia* spp. and *D. caninum* infections is normally made by finding the proglottids (body segments), or chain of proglottids, around the host's anal region or on its hocks. Although the eggs will float, they are usually not released to mix with the feces (Figure 7-5). *Taenia* spp. have one genital opening per proglottid, whereas *D. caninum* has two, one on either side. Further identification of *Taenia* spp. beyond the genus designation is extremely difficult, requiring morphologic study of the intact parasite.

> ✎ **TECHNICIAN NOTE**
>
> Diagnosis of *Taenia* spp. and *Dipylidium caninum* infections is normally made by finding the proglottids, or chain of proglottids, around the host's anal region or on its hocks.

E. granulosus eggs frequently mix with the feces (unlike *Taenia* spp.), but the eggs are typical *Taenia*-type eggs, possessing thick, striated shells. *D. caninum* eggs, if seen in feces, occur in packets contained within a thin-walled membrane. Several treatments are available. Control depends on the tapeworm species. The presence of *D. caninum* obviously necessitates vigorous control of fleas. When *Taenia* spp. are present, dogs and cats should not have access to the flesh or viscera of the infected intermediate host.

HEARTWORMS AND *DIPETALONEMAS RECONDITUM*

Dirofilaria immitis and *Dipetalonema reconditum* are the two filarial nematodes found commonly in dogs and the wild Canidae in the United States. *Dirofilaria immitis* infections may also occur in cats and the wild Felidae, but not as commonly as in dogs. The heartworm, *Dirofilaria immitis*, is found primarily in the right ventricle and pulmonary arteries of the host, whereas *Dipetalonema reconditum* is found in the subcutaneous tissue. Both nematodes produce a larval form called a microfilaria, which circulates in the blood (Figure 7-6). These filarial nematodes are found commonly in areas of the United States where the intermediate hosts occur; however, heartworm is becoming more widespread as infected dogs and cats are brought into areas where the parasite is not normally found.

Dirofilaria immitis males measure 12 to 20 cm, and the females are 25 to 31 cm long; whereas *Dipetalonema reconditum* males are 9 to 17 mm long, and the females are

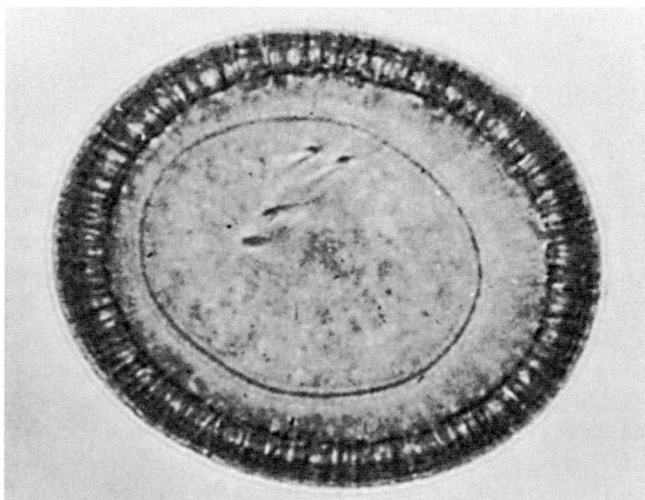

Figure 7-5 Typical *Taenia* egg measuring approximately 34 μm. *Dipylidium* eggs appear similar but are contained in packets of 1 to 20 eggs.

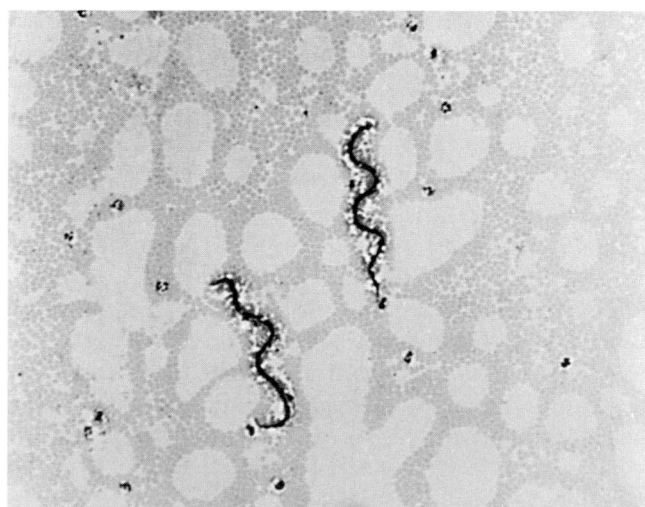

Figure 7-6 Stained microfilaria of *Dirofilaria immitis*.

20 to 32 mm long. Both nematodes need an intermediate host to complete their life cycle. *Dirofilaria immitis* uses several different species of mosquito, and *Dipetalonema reconditum* uses the common dog and cat flea. Microfilariae, when ingested by the intermediate host, undergo reorganization and development to the third-stage infective larvae. Once infective, they go into the mouthparts of the arthropod and remain there until the arthropod feeds on a susceptible host. *Dirofilaria immitis* infective larvae enter the tissue for 85 to 120 days and develop into young adults. They then go to the heart and reach sexual maturity in another 60 to 70 days, for a total of 145 to 190 days. *Dipetalonema reconditum* apparently goes directly into the subcutaneous tissues to develop to sexual maturity.

> ### ✒ TECHNICIAN NOTE
> Diagnosis of heartworm disease in the dog is based on identification of microfilariae in the peripheral blood or a positive serologic test result.

A microfilaria of *Dirofilaria immitis* is 295 to 325 μm long (average = 313 μm) and 6 to 7 μm in diameter (average = 6.9 μm), whereas a microfilaria of *Dipetalonema reconditum* is somewhat shorter and more slender, measuring 250 to 288 μm in length (average = 276 μm) and 4.5 to 5.5 μm in diameter (average = 4.6 μm).

Diagnosis of heartworm disease in the dog is usually based on identification of microfilariae in the peripheral circulation. Various techniques have been used to detect microfilariae, including the fresh blood/saline preparation; the capillary hematocrit tube test; and Knott's (or the filtration concentration) test. Fresh blood/saline preparations are helpful in differentiating *Dirofilaria immitis* and *Dipetalonema reconditum* microfilariae. *Dirofilaria immitis* microfilariae move in place without directional motion, whereas *Dipetalonema reconditum* microfilariae have a directional movement across the microscopic viewing field. Concentration tests are best used for the detection of *Dirofilaria immitis* microfilariae because they are much more accurate than fresh blood/saline preparations or capillary hematocrit tube tests. Occult heartworm infections (adult heartworms without circulating microfilariae) occur in approximately 25% of dogs and 90% of cats. Several serologic tests are available in commercial kits to test sera of dogs and cats for occult infection. Treatment of *Dipetalonema reconditum* infestation is unimportant, because these parasites are nonpathogenic. The treatment for *Dirofilaria immitis* infestation requires the use of an agent effective against adult heartworms, followed by a microfilaricide. Control of *Dirofilaria immitis* necessitates daily or monthly heartworm preventive therapy and mosquito control in enzootic areas.

GIARDIA SPECIES

Giardia spp. are common protozoan parasites of dogs and cats in the United States. A higher incidence of infection occurs in dogs, cats, humans, and beavers than in other

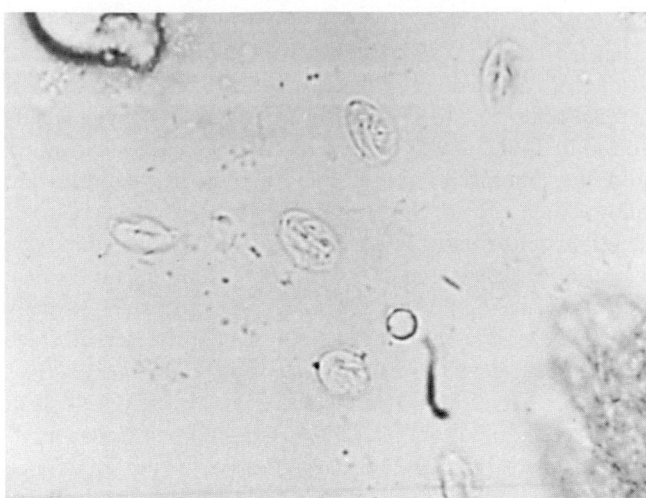

Figure 7-7 Cysts of *Giardia* sp. from a dog fecal flotation with zinc sulfate at a specific gravity of 1.18.

animals such as deer, sheep, moose, and antelope. There are two forms of *Giardia*. The motile trophozoite, which is approximately 12 to 17 μm long and 7 to 10 μm wide, is found in the small intestine. The cyst form (the infective stage) is approximately 9 to 13 μm long (Figure 7-7). When the cyst form is ingested, the cyst wall is digested away in the small intestine, releasing the trophozoite, which immediately divides into two organisms. These organisms attach to the epithelial cells lining the small intestine and continue to multiply by binary fusion over the next 6 to 10 days until a large population exists. At that time, diarrhea develops and *Giardia* spp. begin to produce cysts. Diagnosis can be accomplished by means of the direct fecal/saline smear or, more effectively, with the zinc sulfate centrifugal flotation technique. Treatment is available. *Giardia* infection is more commonly found among young dogs and cats crowded into kennels and animal shelters. The most effective control procedure is cleanliness and disinfection with quaternary ammonium compounds.

COCCIDIA

Dogs and cats are hosts for many species of *Isospora* (also called *Cystoisospora*), *Cryptosporidium*, and *Sarcocystis*; and the cat is the definitive host for *Toxoplasma gondii*. The incidence and severity of coccidial infection depend on the host's age and immune status, conditions in which the hosts are housed, and their diet and quality of drinking water.

The species of *Isospora* have a direct life cycle; however, some *Isospora* spp. (*I. canis* and *I. felis*) can use an intermediate host, such as a mouse. The life cycle starts with an oocyst in the feces (Figure 7-8). This oocyst must sporulate (develop into the infective form); it does so in less than a week, given optimum conditions of warmth and moisture. Once infective, the oocyst encloses two sporocysts, each of which encloses four small, spindle-shaped infective forms called sporozoites or a total of eight infective forms in each oocyst. When ingested, the oocyst and sporocyst walls are digested

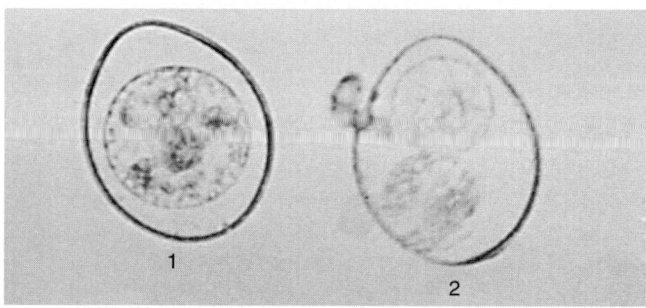

Figure 7-8 Unsporulated oocyst of *Isospora (1)* and sporulated oocyst of *Isospora (2)* measuring approximately 25 × 20 μm.

in the intestine, releasing sporozoites to penetrate the intestinal epithelium and enter a cell for subsequent development. Within the intestinal cell they become spherical and begin to grow to a large size. The nucleus replicates several times, and ultimately, thousands of small, spindle-shaped organisms called merozoites develop. This asexual process of reproduction is called schizogony, and the large structure filled with the merozoites is called a schizont.

Once mature, the schizont ruptures, releasing merozoites. The next step in the life cycle is species dependent, but usually the merozoites move further down the intestine, penetrate a cell, and repeat the asexual process, but with smaller schizonts containing fewer merozoites. When released, the merozoites then penetrate a cell, and some of them become macrogametes (ova) and some become microgametes (sperm). Once fertilization occurs, the oocyst is produced and passes in the feces to begin the life cycle again. Although the life cycle is finite (e.g., only a given number of oocysts can be produced from a single oocyst infection), the reproductive potential is great for some species.

Species of *Cryptosporidium* have essentially the same type of life cycle. *Cryptosporidium* organisms inhabit the respiratory and intestinal epithelia of many hosts including birds, mammals, reptiles, and fish. Dogs and cats develop intestinal tract infection almost exclusively. Enteroepithelial development is limited to the luminal enterocytes; extraintestinal tissue cysts do not develop. The enteroepithelial life cycle begins with ingestion of sporulated oocysts by a suitable host. After ingestion of oocysts, four sporozoites are released from each oocyst that penetrate intestinal epithelial cells. Asexual reproduction at the intestinal surface occurs with the production of merozoites that are released and penetrate other cells. Gametogony and sporogony occur, resulting in the production of thin-walled and thick-walled oocysts. Sporulated thick-walled oocysts are shed in the feces of an infected host and are immediately infective to a susceptible host. Thin-walled oocysts passed into the intestinal lumen rupture, releasing the sporozoites, which penetrate additional host cells and reinitiate the developmental cycle.

Species of *Sarcocystis* have essentially the same type of life cycle, except that carnivores act as hosts for the sexual stages (oocyst and sporocyst), and omnivores and herbivores act as hosts for the asexual (schizogony) stage. Infected carnivores pass a thin-walled oocyst, which will eventually rupture; the oocyst contains two small, thick-walled sporocysts in which four sporozoites have already developed and are immediately infective to the alternate host. Once ingested, the sporozoites are released and penetrate the epithelial tissue of the intestine. Generally, they enter the circulatory system and begin the first asexual (schizogony) phase in the kidneys. The first schizont releases its small, spindle-shaped organisms, which then enter cardiac or smooth muscle, in which they develop into rather large schizonts called sarcocysts. When sarcocysts are ingested by a specific carnivore, and most species are specific for each carnivore-herbivore, the small, spindle-shaped organisms penetrate superficial epithelial cells of the intestine and immediately begin the sexual phase, terminating as a thin-walled oocyst about 11 to 14 days after ingestion of the infected flesh.

The life cycle of *Toxoplasma gondii* is similar to that of *Sarcocystis* spp. except that most animals are suitable hosts for the development of the asexual (schizogony) stages, but only the cat is suitable as a host for the sexual stages. The typical life cycle occurs when a cat ingests the small sporulated oocyst. In the intestine, the parasite goes through two asexual stages and then into the sexual phase, producing oocysts. If, for example, a mouse should eat the oocyst, the first asexual phase occurs in this animal. When a cat eats these schizonts, the parasite goes into one asexual cycle, in the cat's intestine, followed by the sexual cycle. If the first mouse is eaten by another mouse, *Toxoplasma* goes into the second asexual cycle in this mouse. When the second mouse is eaten by a cat, the parasites go directly into the sexual phase. The asexual cycle can go on indefinitely as animals eat the flesh of infected animals.

Diagnosis of *Isospora, Cryptosporidium, Sarcocystis,* and *Toxoplasma* infection is based on recovery of the oocyst or sporocyst (for *Sarcocystis*) by a number of diagnostic procedures. Treatment is seldom administered for *Sarcocystis* or *Cryptosporidium* infection, but when clinical disease occurs, treatment is recommended for *Isospora* and *Toxoplasma* spp. infection. Control of *Isospora* and *Cryptosporidium* infections requires cleanliness, removal of the animal to clean premises, or both; however, the oocysts are extremely resistant to environmental conditions. Control of *Sarcocystis* infection is generally not practiced for the carnivore host because it is considered nonpathogenic. If control is exercised, the best approach is to prevent consumption of raw flesh from any source, including ground beef. The best control for *Toxoplasma* in cats is to prevent consumption of raw flesh and contact with feces of infected cats.

PARASITES OF HORSES

ROUNDWORMS

The ascarid of horses *(Parascaris equorum)* has a creamy white color. The males measure about 28 cm, whereas females are about 50 cm in length. They produce dark brown, thick-shelled oval to spherical eggs that are very resistant to environmental conditions. The horse ascarid is common throughout the United States, and the incidence of infection, especially among younger horses, is frequently high. The larval stage develops within the eggs, and the second stage is infective. Development to the infective stage requires about 2 weeks. When the eggs are ingested, the larvae are released in the intestine, penetrate the intestinal mucosa, enter the circulatory system, and pass through to the liver, heart and, ultimately, the lungs, in which they develop for a short period. Subsequently, larvae pass up the bronchial tree, enter the mouth, and are swallowed. They are passed into the small intestine and mature. This entire life cycle requires 10 to 12 weeks. Diagnosis is readily made by using a number of techniques, and these parasites are amenable to treatment by several anthelmintics. Control is difficult because eggs are extremely resistant to environmental conditions, and the coprophagous habits of foals tend to ensure infection.

> **⬛ TECHNICIAN NOTE**
> The horse ascarid is common throughout the United States, and the incidence of infection, especially among younger horses, is frequently high.

PINWORMS

The pinworm of horses, *Oxyuris equi*, is a white to slate gray–colored nematode with a slender, sharply pointed tail. Males are very small, measuring less than 12 mm, and females are 75 to 150 mm long. The eggs are slender and somewhat flattened along one side (Figure 7-9). Frequently, they contain first-stage larvae when deposited. Pinworms are common in horses in the United States. The life cycle is simple and direct. Female parasites living in the cecum pass out though the anal sphincter and deposit masses of eggs on the perineum. Eggs are cemented into masses with a gelatinous material. Eggs drop off, either singly or in masses, landing on ground or feed and become infective in 3 to 5 days. Once ingested, the larvae are released in the small intestine, penetrate the intestinal mucosa, and develop for several days. Larvae then return to the mucosal surface, move to the large intestine, and reach maturity about 50 days after the initial ingestion of the eggs. Diagnosis can be made effectively only by the adhesive tape technique. Pinworms are amenable to treatment with several anthelmintics. Control is difficult because of the coprophagous habits of foals.

SMALL AND LARGE STRONGYLES

Strongylus vulgaris, *Strongylus equinus*, and *Strongylus edentatus* are the three species of "large strongyles," along with 40 species of "small strongyles" of horses. The 40 or

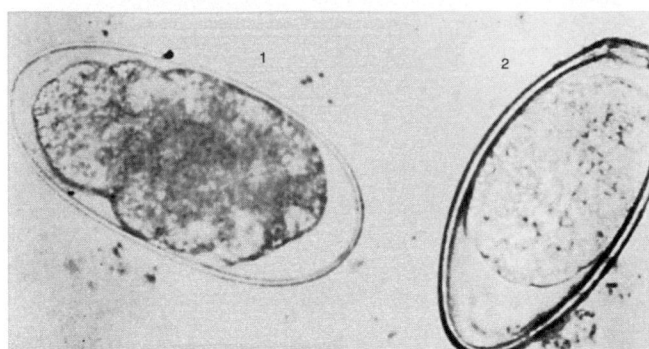

Figure 7-9   *1, Strongyle* egg measuring 95 × 50 µm. *2,* Egg of *Oxyuris equi* measuring 90 × 42 µm.

more species of small strongyles, of which there are several different genera, are bloodsucking nematodes. Strongyles vary in length from less than 12 mm (small strongyles) to 38 to 47 mm (large strongyles). However, some small strongyles, such as *Triodontophorus* spp., are nearly as large as *S. vulgaris*, the smallest of the large strongyles. All of the strongyles produce similar thin-walled eggs, each of which contains 4 to 16 brownish-colored cells when deposited, that are referred to collectively as "strongyle eggs," a term that refers to the order of nematodes to which this group belongs (order Strongyloidea, the bursate nematodes).

> **⬛ TECHNICIAN NOTE**
> All equine strongyles produce similar thin-walled eggs, each containing 4 to 16 brownish cells.

All of the strongyles are common in horses throughout the United States, and the incidence of infection is generally high. The small strongyles that have been studied have a simple, direct life cycle. The eggs pass in feces, and first-stage larvae develop within the eggs. Once developed, the larvae hatch and undergo a free-living existence, developing and molting to second-stage free-living larvae. They then develop to third-stage larvae that do not feed and await ingestion. In ideal environmental conditions, development from the egg stage to the infective larval stage will occur in less than 1 week. Once small strongyles have been ingested, the larvae go to the cecum, penetrate the cecal mucosa, and develop for 1 to 2 weeks. The larvae then return to the mucosal surface and mature in an additional 1 to 2 weeks. The species in the genus *Strongylus* all have very complex life cycles.

The development of the larval stages for large strongyles in the environment is the same as that for the small strongyles, and once ingested, large strongyles also penetrate the mucosa of the cecum and develop in a short period. *S. vulgaris*, the most important of the large strongyles, leaves the mucosa and by some means goes to the cranial mesenteric artery and its branches and develops in the lumen of the arteries over the next 6 months, becoming a young adult. It then returns to the cecum and matures;

the entire prepatent period (the period after ingestion and before eggs pass in feces) requires about 180 to 200 days. *S. equinus* leaves the cecal mucosa and enters the peritoneal cavity. It then goes to the liver and develops into a young adult. The route taken back to the cecum is incompletely understood, but it may enter the pancreas. The entire prepatent period may be as long as 265 days.

S. edentatus leaves the mucosa and enters the subperitoneal tissue, particularly in the right dorsal flank. Eventually, it enters the venous circulation and goes to the liver. Supposedly, it leaves the liver and about 2 months later migrates in the mesenteries to the perirenal fat for an additional 3 months. It again migrates in the mesenteries to the large intestine, which it penetrates, and develops to maturity in the lumen of the cecum. The entire prepatent period requires 300 to 322 days. Identification of the strongyles can be accomplished by a number of techniques, and strongyles are amenable to treatment by several anthelmintics. Control is difficult because the parasites are prolific egg producers and development of the larvae occurs rapidly. Control is best achieved by a treatment and management regimen based on environmental conditions and by limiting the number of horses on the pasture.

INTESTINAL THREADWORMS

Strongyloides westeri is a common parasite of horses, principally of foals 2 weeks to 6 months of age, and is widespread across the United States. The life cycle is essentially the same as that of *Strongyloides stercoralis* of the dog, except that the parthenogenetic female produces thin-walled eggs containing first-stage larvae when deposited (Figure 7-10). Diagnosis can be made by a number of techniques; however, fresh feces must be used because the eggs will hatch in older feces. Control requires good hygiene, together with treatment, because the parasite can be transmitted by the transmammary route.

> ### ✏ TECHNICIAN NOTE
> Identification of cattle and sheep lungworms is best achieved by use of the Baermann funnel technique.

TAPEWORMS

Anoplocephala perfoliata, Anoplocephala magna, and *Paranoplocephala mamillana* are the tapeworms of horses. They are broad, thick, and white and vary in length from about 2.5 cm *(A. perfoliata)* to 75 cm *(A. magna),* though most tapeworms are about 15 cm. The eggs of all species are similar and tend to have an amber color or almost no color. The eggs often have a peculiar shape, varying from almost round to somewhat square. The life cycles of all three tapeworms are similar in that the eggs are ingested by a free-living mite for further development. In the mite, a small larval form, the cysticercoid, develops to the infective

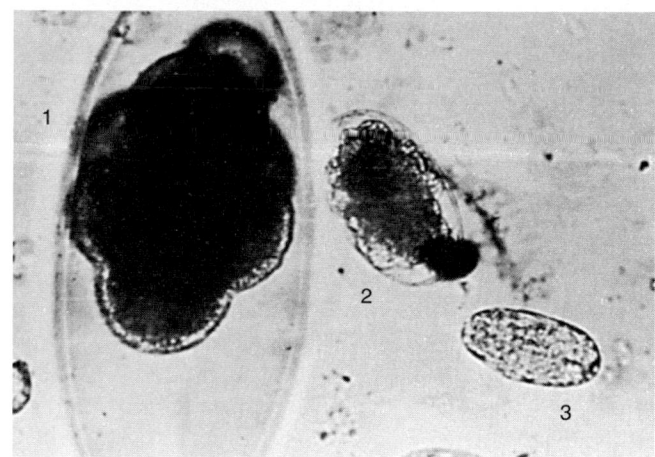

Figure 7-10 *1,* Egg of *Nematodirus* measuring approximately 200×95 μm. *2,* Strongyle-type eggs measuring approximately 86×40 μm. *3,* Egg of *Strongyloides* measuring approximately 52×25 μm.

stage within 2 to 4 months. Once ingested by the horse, the larval stage is released from the mite and develops into an adult tapeworm in 6 to 10 weeks. Diagnosis is readily made with a number of techniques because the eggs mix with the feces. Treatment or control is seldom practiced.

PARASITES OF RUMINANTS

STRONGYLES

Cattle and sheep in the United States are commonly infected by a number of species of strongyle nematodes (order Strongyloidea, the bursate nematodes). Species in the genera *Haemonchus, Ostertagia, Trichostrongylus, Cooperia,* and *Nematodirus* are the most common. These nematodes vary in size from about 6 mm (*Trichostrongylus* spp.) to about 25 to 30 mm (*Haemonchus* spp.). All except *Nematodirus* spp. produce similar "strongyle-type" eggs, which are thin walled and contain 4 to 16 brown-colored cells when deposited (Figure 7-10). *Nematodirus* spp. produce extremely large eggs (see Figure 7-10). These parasites are widely distributed throughout the United States, but their incidence depends on their ability to develop in the external environment. Some, such as *Haemonchus* spp., need considerable warmth and moisture; whereas others such as *Ostertagia, Trichostrongylus,* and *Nematodirus* spp. will withstand colder, drier climates.

The life cycles, though somewhat variable among species, are similar. The first-stage larvae develop within the eggs and hatch to undergo a free-living existence. The larvae develop within the eggs and grow and molt to the third-stage infective form in less than 2 weeks. Once ingested by the host, the larvae generally penetrate the mucosa in the site they normally inhabit (stomach, small intestine, large intestine) and develop in a short period, then return to the surface of the mucosa and mature. Diagnosis can be effectively made with most techniques. Several treatments are available. Control is best achieved by a combination of treatment and pasture management in areas where there is an abundance of warmth and moisture to promote survival of the larval stages.

LUNGWORMS

The lungworms of cattle and sheep are *Dictyocaulus viviparus* (cattle) and *Dictyocaulus filaria* (sheep). They are slender, white nematodes; males are 3 to 8 cm long, and females are 3 to 10 cm long. Females produce eggs containing first-stage larvae that hatch in the lungs. The first-stage larvae pass up the bronchial tree and are swallowed, passing with the feces. Lungworms occur in animals throughout the United States, but their distribution is discontinuous because the larval stages require a certain amount of warmth and moisture to survive. The life cycle is simple and direct. The first-stage larvae live on stored food granules, developing to the third-stage infective form within less than a week in optimum environmental conditions. Once ingested, the larvae enter the intestine, penetrate the intestinal mucosa, enter the lymphatic vessels, and develop for a short period in lymph nodes. They then go to the heart, enter the circulatory system, and then into the lungs to mature in a total of 25 to 30 days. Diagnosis is best made by use of the Baermann funnel technique. Only a few anthelmintics are considered acceptable. Control is best achieved by proper management, ensuring that cattle and sheep do not occupy wet, swampy pastures.

TAPEWORMS

Tapeworms in cattle and sheep are *Moniezia expansa* and *Moniezia benedini*. In addition, *Thysanosoma actinioides* occurs in sheep. The *Moniezia* spp. reach lengths of 4 m, whereas *T. actinioides* is generally 25 to 30 cm long. *Moniezia* spp. are widespread across the United States, but *T. actinioides* is found only in the western regions. The life cycle of *Moniezia* spp. is the same as that of the *Anoplocephala* spp. found in horses, and they use similar free-living mites. The cycle of *T. actinioides* is not known. Diagnosis of *Moniezia* spp. infections is readily accomplished by several acceptable techniques because the eggs mix with the feces; however, diagnosis of *T. actinioides* infection can be accomplished only by observation of the pearly white bell-shaped proglottid on the fecal mass. Treatment is seldom applied to *Moniezia* spp. or *T. actinioides*. Control would be difficult, necessitating control of the mites.

LIVER FLUKES

The common trematodes of cattle and sheep are *Fasciola hepatica* and *Fascioloides magna*. Both trematodes are greenish, flat, and leaf-like in shape. *Fasciola hepatica* is about 25 mm long, and *Fascioloides magna* is about 50 to 75 mm long. The eggs of both trematodes are very similar and are large and yellow-brown with an operculum or "lid" at one end (Figure 7-11). *Fasciola hepatica* and *Fascioloides magna* are widespread throughout the United States, but only in wet, swampy or subirrigated areas that will support substantial populations of the snail intermediate hosts. The natural hosts for *Fasciola hepatica* are cattle and sheep, but the natural hosts for *Fascioloides magna* are members of the deer family. *Fascioloides magna* cannot complete its life cycle (by passing eggs into the environment) in cattle and sheep.

The life cycles of both trematodes are similar and quite complex. Eggs passing in the feces must land in water to develop. Inside each egg, a small, ciliated miracidium develops, leaves the egg, and penetrates the tissue of a specific snail, in which it undergoes a sexual replication through larval stages called sporocysts and rediae, ultimately developing into a cercaria, which leaves the snail to encyst on vegetation and await ingestion. Once ingested, the cercaria goes into the intestine, penetrates through to the body cavity, and penetrates the surface of the liver in which it wanders for several weeks. *Fasciola hepatica* eventually enters the bile ducts, whereas *Fascioloides magna* will form a cyst wall around itself with an opening into a bile duct if it infects members of the deer family. In cattle, a calcified cyst is found, whereas in sheep, the parasite continues to wander throughout the liver. The eggs are very heavy and will not float; consequently, a sedimentation procedure is used for diagnosis. Effective treatment is available. Control necessitates draining and drying wet, swampy pastures to prevent an overabundance of snails.

COCCIDIA

Several species of *Coccidia* infect cattle and sheep, and all belong to the genus *Eimeria*. *Coccidia* spp. are common throughout the United States, and most animals are infected with at least one of the *Eimeria* species. The severity of the infection depends on environmental conditions (warmth, moisture), stocking intensity, age, and previous exposure. Oocysts of the *Eimeria* spp. sporulate in the environment and reach the infective stage in the same manner as do *Isospora* spp. *Eimeria* spp., however, develop four sporocysts, each of which contains two sporozoites, for a total of eight

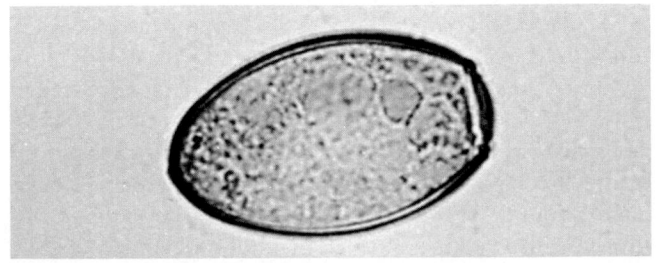

Figure 7-11 Egg of *Fasciola hepatica* measuring approximately 130 × 70 μm.

infective forms per oocyst. The life cycle of *Eimeria* spp. is identical to that of *Isospora* spp., except that an intermediate host is not required. Diagnosis may be accomplished effectively by a number of techniques. Several treatments are available for the clinical disease. Control is difficult because oocysts are highly resistant. Proper management for coccidiosis includes prevention of overcrowding, prevention of contamination of feed and water, and the use of dry bedding.

> ### ✐ TECHNICIAN NOTE
> *Coccidia* spp. are common throughout the United States, and most animals are infected with at least one of the *Eimeria* spp.

TRICHOMONIASIS

Trichomonas foetus is a common protozoan parasite of cattle. This small, flagellated protozoan is equipped with three anterior flagella, an undulating membrane, and a trailing flagellum. Generally, *T. foetus* is a slender, pear-shaped organism. The bull acts as a carrier, with the parasite living on the surface of the penis or in the prepuce. When transmitted by coitus to the cow, the organism develops in the vagina and uterus, causing abortion or fetal resorption. *T. foetus* multiples by binary fission; consequently, large populations can be generated in a short period. The cows, given a rest through two or three estrous cycles, will usually develop partial immunity. Diagnosis and treatment are performed on the bull. Diagnosis is difficult and complex. Control necessitates resting the cows and allowing immunity to develop, treatment or elimination of infected bulls, and purchase of virgin bulls for breeding.

PARASITES OF SWINE

STOMACH WORMS

Three stomach worms occur in swine: *Hyostrongylus rubidus*, *Ascarops strongylina*, and *Physocephalus sexalatus*. *H. rubidus* is the most common and the most pathogenic of the three, usually occurring in adult pigs. Its parasitic development is similar to that of *Ostertagia* spp. in ruminants. Diagnosis is based on finding strongyle eggs in the fecal sample, but the eggs can be confused with the eggs of *Oesophagostomum* spp., which also occur in pigs. *Ascarops* and *Physocephalus* spp. use beetles as their intermediate hosts and are rarely a problem in swine.

ASCARIS SPECIES

Ascaris suum is the large roundworm and is by far the most common parasite encountered in pigs. Its parasitic development is similar to that of *Parascaris* spp. in the horse. *A. suum* is usually more common in pigs younger than 1 year. Diagnosis is based on finding ascarid eggs in fecal samples.

> ### ✐ TECHNICIAN NOTE
> *Ascaris suum* is the large roundworm and is by far the most common parasite encountered in pigs.

STRONGYLOIDES RANSOMI

Strongyloides ransomi is found in the small intestines of young swine. Its parasitic development is similar to that of *Strongyloides* spp. in the horse. Diagnosis is based on finding embryonated eggs in fresh fecal samples.

OESOPHAGOSTOMUM SPECIES

Several species of *Oesophagostomum* occur in the large intestines of pigs. Their life cycle is similar to that of *Oesophagostomum* spp. in ruminants. Diagnosis is based on finding typical strongyle eggs in fecal samples. Again, these eggs can be confused with the eggs of *Hyostrongylus* and *Trichostrongylus* spp.

WHIPWORMS

The whipworm of swine is *Trichuris suis*. These worms usually occur in the cecum, and their parasitic development is similar to that of *Trichuris* spp. in dogs. Diagnosis is based on finding typical *Trichuris* eggs in the feces.

LUNGWORMS

Three species of *Metastrongylus* occur in the lungs of swine. Earthworms act as the intermediate hosts for the swine lungworm. Most commonly, the posteroventral part of the diaphragmatic lobe of the lung is involved. Diagnosis is made by finding rough-shelled, embryonated eggs in the feces.

Kidney Worms

Stephanurus dentatus is the kidney worm in swine. The adult worms live in the kidneys and perirenal tissue and pass eggs into the urinary bladder. Infection in pigs occurs by ingestion of third-stage larvae, ingestion of earthworms containing third-stage larvae, skin penetration, and in utero infection. Although eggs can be identified in urine, diagnosis is usually made at necropsy.

Ectoparasites

PARASITES OF DOMESTICATED ANIMALS

The ectoparasites of domesticated animals are generally members of the phylum Arthropoda. There are many different types of ectoparasites, including fleas, mites, lice, ticks, chiggers, bloodsucking flies, and myiasis-inducing flies.

Some are host specific, whereas others infect any number of animals. Diagnosis is generally based on the external morphologic appearance, with the use of taxonomic keys. Control is often very difficult, sometimes necessitating treatment of the premises and prevention by prohibiting interaction with infected animals (e.g., companion animals with fleas, ticks, or lice).

FLEAS

Ctenocephalides canis (Figure 7-12) and *Ctenocephalides felis* are the most common fleas of dogs and cats. Of these, *Ctenocephalides felis* is the most common. They are not host specific and will attack other animals and humans. They are widely distributed but are much more common in warm, humid environments. When environmental conditions are favorable, fleas have a great reproductive potential. Fleas thrive at low altitudes in temperature ranges of 65° F to 80° F (18.2° C to 26.6° C). Under these conditions, the flea life cycle can be completed, from hatching of an egg to the laying of the next generation of eggs, in as few as 16 days.

> ### ✐ TECHNICIAN NOTE
> The flea life cycle can be completed in as few as 16 days.

The female flea lays her eggs in the fur of dogs and cats. The eggs are not sticky and tend to fall out of the fur and survive in the protected places where a dog or cat sleeps or plays. The eggs will hatch into very small worm-like larvae. The larvae feed on organic debris, especially the dried blood droppings (flea dirt) left by adult fleas. Thus larvae depend on an animal to return time after time to the places where the eggs dropped off. The larvae molt and form pupae that spin cocoons and then emerge as young and hungry adults in about 3 weeks. An important source of fleas to a dog and cat is these newly "hatched out" young fleas.

Once fleas have had a chance to establish the life cycle in a house and yard environment, no program that does not emphasize environmental control will be successful. Mechanical cleaning of the house and yard environment should precede any application of insecticides. In general, the same environmental control methods may be used in households with young dogs and cats as in those with adult animals. Care should always be taken that animals and people are not directly exposed to insecticides used in household extermination. All effective in-house programs should take advantage of new technologies in flea control. There are new insecticides that have truly long residuals (synthetic pyrethroids or microencapsulated products), and there are insect growth regulators (methoprene and fenoxycarb) marketed for preadult flea control.

Advances in outdoor environmental flea control have been less remarkable. At present, the use of insecticides (compounds that contain chlorpyrifos, malathion, or diazinon as their active ingredient) labeled for outdoor flea control is still the best and most economical approach. Such programs must incorporate repeated applications at 2-week intervals throughout the flea season where temperature and humidity are favorable for flea reproduction.

All topical insecticides should be used exactly according to label directions, because it is not legally permissible to use or recommend the use of insecticide products beyond label restrictions. In general, the use of organophosphate preparations on puppies younger than 16 weeks or on kittens younger than 6 months should be avoided. Any product containing lufenuron, fipronil, or imidicloprid as its active ingredient should never be administered to or used on nursing animals. Pyrethrin-based products are generally safe for frequent application; the most effective products are synergized pyrethrin sprays or foams. Very small animals and nursing animals sprayed with alcohol-based or other volatile organic solvents may be severely chilled as the solvent evaporates. Water-based sprays are preferable, and small animals and nursing animals should never be thoroughly saturated with a spray. The safest effective products are sprays and foams with microencapsulated pyrethrins. Flea collars that are safe for use on puppies or kittens are not effective in most environments. Topical treatments should be coordinated with in-home environmental flea control.

> ### ✐ TECHNICIAN NOTE
> All topical insecticides should be used exactly according to label directions, because it is not legally permissible to use or recommend the use of insecticide products beyond label restrictions.

RABBIT BOTS AND FOX MAGGOTS

Cuterebra spp., the rabbit bot, and *Wohlfahrtia* spp., the fox maggot, occasionally infest dogs, cats, rodents, rabbits, and other wildlife. *Cuterebra* spp. flies usually deposit eggs around burrows or runs. Eggs hatch, and the larvae penetrate the skin of the host, developing to the third stage

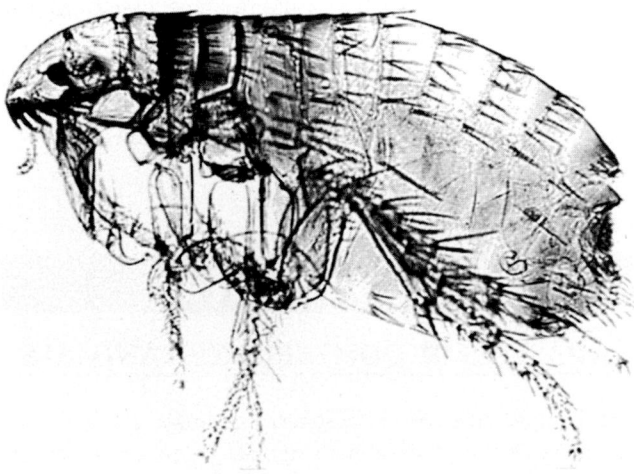

Figure 7-12 Ctenocephalides canis, the common dog flea.

in subcutaneous tissue without migrating in the host. The larvae then emerge from a hole in the host's skin and pupate in the soil. Females of the *Wohlfahrtia* spp. deposit larvae on the skin of the host, which is usually a young animal. The larvae penetrate and develop in the subcutaneous tissues with limited migration. When they become third-stage larvae, they drop out and pupate in the soil. Diagnosis of *Cuterebra* infection is based on the morphologic appearance of the larvae, whereas diagnosis of infection by *Wohlfahrtia* spp. requires use of the morphologic appearance of the stigmatal plates and, sometimes, the morphologic appearance of the cephalopharyngeal skeleton. Treatment consists of surgical removal of the larvae and supportive wound treatment.

BOT FLIES

Gasterophilus intestinalis, Gasterophilus nasalis, and *Gasterophilus hemorrhoidalis*—the bot flies of horses—are widespread and common wherever horses are found; but *Gasterophilus intestinalis* is the most common species. The adult fly cements eggs to the hair of the horse. The eggs either hatch by themselves and the larvae crawl into the horse's mouth or the eggs are stimulated to hatch by the horse licking them. Once in the mouth, the larvae penetrate the mucosa and burrow down the esophagus to the stomach, in which they emerge and develop into the third stage. They usually spend about 10 months as larvae. Ultimately, the larvae pass out with the feces, burrow into the soil, pupate, and later emerge as adult flies, usually in late summer. Diagnosis is based on the type of egg and means of attachment of the spines on each segment (single row, *Gasterophilus nasalis;* double row, *Gasterophilus intestinalis;* double row, smaller spines, *Gasterophilus hemorrhoidalis*). Treatment is generally applied in the fall with a combination of insecticides and anthelmintics or a broad-spectrum compound. Control is difficult.

HEEL FLIES

The heel flies of cattle, *Hypoderma lineatum* and *Hypoderma bovis,* whose larval stages are called *grubs* or *warbles,* are widely distributed wherever cattle are found. Emergence of these flies depends on environmental conditions. For example, they are active in early January in southern Texas and in early August in Montana. When both species are present, *Hypoderma bovis* emerges about 1 month later than *Hypoderma lineatum.* After emergence, *Hypoderma bovis* lays single eggs attached to hair, and *Hypoderma lineatum* lays a row of eggs just above the hooves. The larvae hatch from the eggs, penetrate the skin, and wander in the subcutaneous tissue for 4 to 5 months. *Hypoderma lineatum* then goes to the esophagus for 2 months, and *Hypoderma bovis* goes to the epidural fat of the spinal cord for 2 months. Both then go to the subcutaneous tissue along the back for about 2 months. They develop and drop out and burrow

in the soil, in which they pupate for 1 month to 3 months. Diagnosis is generally based on the presence of warbles on the backs of cattle; however, species can be identified on the basis of the morphologic appearance of the larvae. Several treatments are available, but they must be applied at a specific time of year.

> ✎ **TECHNICIAN NOTE**
>
> Identification of *Hypoderma* spp. of cattle is usually based on the presence of lumps (warbles) on the backs of cattle.

SHEEP NASAL FLIES

The sheep nasal fly (*Oestrus ovis,* often called the sheep nose bot) is common wherever sheep are found. Flies emerge from spring through fall and deposit first-stage larvae around the nasal opening. Larvae then enter the nasal cavity for 2 weeks to 9 months and migrate to the paranasal sinuses for a short period to complete their development. They leave through the nose and pupate in the soil for 15 to 60 days. The life cycle may be completed in 2 to 11 months, depending on environmental conditions. Diagnosis is based on the presence of these larvae in the nose or sinuses. There is no preferred treatment available.

LICE

Domesticated animals are commonly infested with lice of the orders Anoplura (sucking lice) (Figure 7-13) and Mallophaga (chewing lice). Lice live on the host continuously and infest other animals by direct contact. Lice may be a problem year-round on dogs and cats but are more commonly a problem in the winter months on cattle, sheep, and horses (Box 7-1). Lice deposit eggs, referred to as *nits,* cemented to the hair or wool of the host. The eggs hatch, and the small larvae are similar to the adults (incomplete metamorphosis). They develop into nymphs and then into adults; the entire life cycle requires 3 to 5 weeks.

Diagnosis is based on the morphologic appearance of the larvae, nymphs, or adults. Lice of the order Mallophaga have broad heads, and those of Anoplura have pointed heads. Treatment consists of dust, sprays, sponge-on dips, or shampoos, depending on the host and environmental conditions.

MITES

The mites commonly found on domesticated animals are listed in Box 7-2. Most mites are host specific, and even though they are morphologically similar, subspecies will not cross-infest other hosts. Mites live on the host continuously and infest other animals by contact. The life cycles of mites are all slightly different because some burrow, whereas others live on the surface of the skin. *Sarcoptes* spp. and *Notoedres cati* females burrow in the skin and deposit

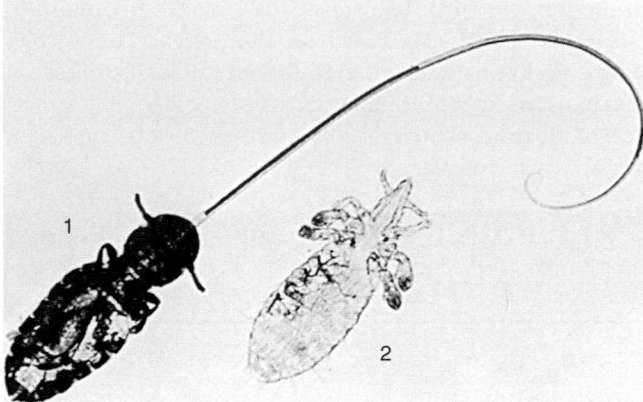

Figure 7-13 *1,* Chewing louse of the order Mallophaga attached to a hair shaft. *2,* Sucking louse of the order Anoplura.

Box 7-1 LICE ON DOMESTIC ANIMALS

CATTLE
Haematopinus eurysternus, sucking
Linognathus vituli, sucking
Solenopotes capillatus, sucking
Haematopinus quadripertusus, sucking
Damalinia bovis, chewing

SHEEP
Haematopinus tuberculatus, sucking
Linognathus pedalis, sucking
Linognathus ovillus, sucking
Linognathus africanus, sucking
Damalinia ovis, chewing

HORSES
Haematopinus asini, sucking
Damalinia equi, chewing

DOGS
Linognathus piliferus, sucking
Trichodectes canis, chewing

CATS
Felicola subrostratus, chewing

---

eggs. The eggs hatch into six-legged larvae, which develop and molt to eight-legged nymphs, which develop and molt into adults. The entire cycle requires 9 to 17 days.

Species of the genera *Chorioptes, Psoroptes, Psorergates, Otodectes,* and *Cheyletiella* have similar life cycles except that they do not burrow to deposit eggs. *Demodex* spp. generally live in the hair follicles. Their life cycles are probably direct, like those of the previously mentioned mites, but they can be found in tissues of the body other than hair follicles.

Identification of mites is based on the morphologic appearance of adults and generally requires a thorough skin scraping (Figures 7-14 and 7-15). Sometimes mites,

---

Box 7-2 MITES ON DOMESTIC ANIMALS

- *Sarcoptes scabiei*
  Varieties are found on the bodies of cattle, sheep, horses, goats, swine, and dogs.
- *Psoroptes communis*
  Varieties are found on the bodies of cattle, sheep, horses, goats, and rabbits.
- *Chorioptes* spp.
  Species occur on the bodies of cattle, sheep, goats, and rabbits.
- *Psorergates* spp.
  Species occur on the bodies of cattle and sheep.
- *Otodectes cynotis*
  Occurs in the ears of dogs, cats, and other related animals.
- *Notoedres cati*
  Occurs on the heads of cats.
- *Cheyletiella* spp.
  Occur on the bodies of dogs, cats, and rabbits.
- *Demodex* spp.
  Occur in hair follicles of dogs, cats, cattle, sheep, humans, and horses.

✎ TECHNICIAN NOTE

Mites are usually identified by appearance of the adults after a skin scraping.

---

especially *Cheyletiella* and *Demodex* spp., can be identified by fecal flotation in dog and cat feces because infected animals often ingest mites as a result of biting and licking their skin. Treatment consists of dusts, sprays, sponge-on dips, or shampoos.

TICKS

The ticks found on domesticated animals are not host specific, although they do have host preferences, and their distribution is subject to environmental conditions. The species, and their host ranges, are listed in Box 7-3. Ticks are identified as being soft or hard ticks. The most important soft tick is *Otobius megnini,* the spinose ear tick, which lives in the ear of its host. It attaches as a larva, enters the ear, and develops through the larval, nymphal, and adult stages. Adults mate and then drop off. The female deposits eggs and dies.

The hard ticks are generally classified as one-, two-, or three-host ticks. Some, such as *Dermacentor albipictus,* are one-host ticks, attaching as larvae and developing into adults on that host. Adults drop off, lay eggs, and then die. The three-host ticks attach as larvae, feed, drop off, and molt in the environment to nymphs; reattach to a host, feed, drop off, and molt to adults; then as adults attach, feed, mate, and drop off to lay eggs and die. *Rhipicephalus sanguineus,* a three-host tick, uses the same host (dog) for all three stages, whereas *Dermacentor venustus* uses small rodents for the larval stage; larger rodents and rabbits for

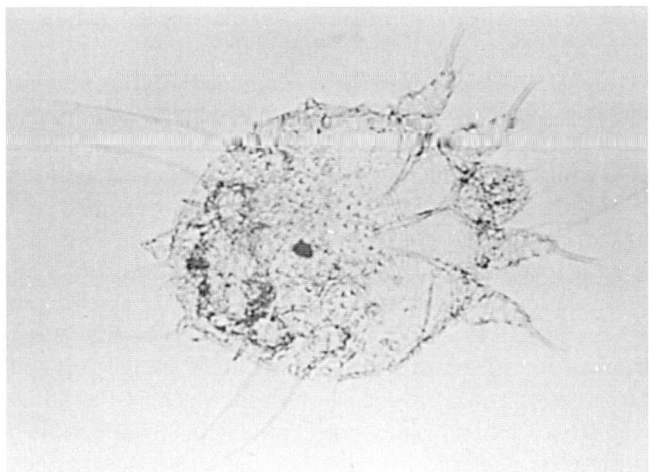

Figure 7-14 *Sarcoptes* sp. mite commonly found on dogs and swine.

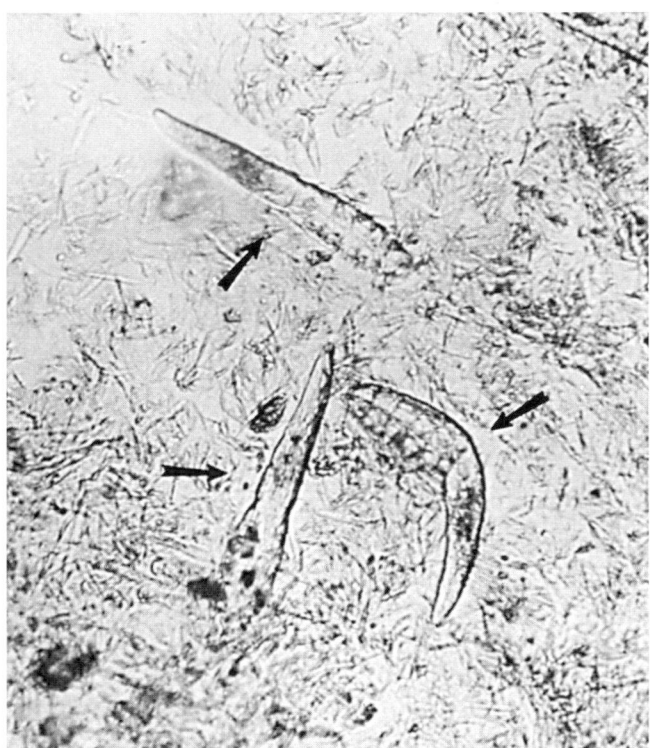

Figure 7-15 *Demodex* sp. mite commonly found on dogs.

the nymphal stage; and dogs, horses, cattle, and so on for the adult stage. Three-host ticks may complete the cycle in a short period (*Rhipicephalus* spp.), whereas other ticks (*Dermacentor* spp.) require 2 years, with 1 year between each stage before they reattach to a host.

Treatment necessitates the use of dusts, sprays, sponge-on dips, or shampoos, depending on the host. Control of *Rhipicephalus sanguineus* requires treatment of the premises and, often, the house or kennel. Control of the other ticks is difficult at best, and the precaution of keeping animals away from infested areas should be practiced.

Box 7-3   TICKS COMMONLY FOUND ON DOMESTIC ANIMALS

- *Otobius megnini:* the spinose ear tick
  Most warm-blooded animals
- *Dermacentor albipictus:* the winter tick
  One-host tick; cattle, sheep, horses, deer, elk, moose
- *Dermacentor venusutus* (no common name)
  Three-host tick; cattle, sheep, horses, wild ruminants, dogs, humans; immature stages on rodents
- *Dermacentor variabilis:* the American dog tick
  Three-host tick; dogs, primary host; immature stages on rodents
- *Dermacentor nitens:* the tropical horse tick
  One-host tick; horses, donkeys, and mules
- *Amblyomma americanum:* the lone star tick
  Three-host tick; cattle, sheep, goats, horses, dogs, cats, and wildlife; nymphs on rodents; larvae often found on birds
- *Amblyomma maculatum:* the Gulf Coast tick
  Three-host tick; cattle, sheep, goats, horses, dogs, cats, and wildlife; nymphs on rodents; larvae often found on birds
- *Amblyomma cajennense:* the Cayenne tick
  Three-host tick; mostly horses, but also cattle, sheep, goats, and wildlife
- *Ixodes pacificus:* the Western black-legged tick
  Three-host tick; adults feed on deer, dogs, horses, humans; immature stages found on small mammals, especially white-footed mice
- *xodes scapularis:* the black-legged tick
  Three-host tick; adults feed on deer, dogs, horses, humans; immature stages found on small mammals, especially white-footed mice
- *Rhipicephalus sanguineus:* the brown dog or kennel tick
  Three-host tick; usually found on dogs

MYIASIS-PRODUCING FLIES

Some of the myiasis-inducing flies (those developing in the tissue of animals), such as *Hypoderma, Oestrus,* and *Gasterophilus* species, are host specific and are discussed according to the appropriate host. Others, such as *Wohlfahrtia* spp. and *Cuterebra* spp., have a more limited host range and have been considered with the hosts generally infested. Blowflies in the genera *Lucilia, Calliphora,* and *Phormia;* the flesh flies; species of *Sarcophaga;* and the screw worm fly, *Cochliomyia hominivorax,* are not host specific and cause problems on several domesticated and wild animals. Blowflies and flesh flies generally deposit eggs (larvae for *Sarcophaga*) on the flesh of dead animals but can deposit eggs in wounds of living animals. The eggs hatch, and the larvae develop through three larval stages and then drop out of the wound to pupate in the soil. Development of the larvae (maggots) is a function of temperature and varies from 2 to 19 days. Pupation lasts 3 to 7 days. The screw worm fly has essentially the same life cycle but will deposit eggs only in fresh wounds.

Diagnosis is based on the morphologic appearance of the stigmatic plates of the third-stage larvae, except for *Cochliomyia hominivorax,* for which the presence of pigmentation of the tracheal trunks is used for diagnosis. Treatment is usually applied topically. Control measures usually require that procedures such as docking and castration be performed before fly season, dead carcasses be disposed of, and environmental spraying take place.

Diagnostic Procedures

FECAL FLOTATION

The nematodes that are parasitic in animals and humans may produce undeveloped eggs, eggs containing larvae, or free larvae. Consequently, special diagnostic procedures are often required to determine with which parasite an animal is infected. For nematodes producing undifferentiated eggs or eggs containing larvae, fresh feces is mixed with a chemical solution of higher specific gravity than water. The chemical solutions most frequently used are sodium chloride, magnesium sulfate, zinc sulfate, sodium nitrate, and sucrose. Eggs in feces mixed with any of the preceding chemical solutions will float to the top and can be removed for examination and identification.

DIRECT FECAL SMEAR

The direct smear is best used to aid in the detection of certain protozoan trophozoites found in fecal samples, such as *Trichomonas, Giardia,* and *Balantidium* species. The morphologic appearance and the motility of these organisms can be seen in a direct smear. A direct smear is not satisfactory for demonstrating eggs of tapeworms, nematodes, or coccidia, and, in fact, this method should not be used. The correct procedure is to mix a small quantity of fresh feces with a drop of tap water or physiologic saline solution on a clean microscopic slide. The sample is spread into a thin film, a coverslip is placed on the slide, and the resulting smear is examined.

TECHNICIAN NOTE

A direct smear is not satisfactory for demonstrating eggs of tapeworms, nematodes, or coccidia.

QUALITATIVE FECAL EXAMINATION

WILLIS TECHNIQUE

A qualitative fecal examination will reveal which parasites are present but not how many. Several procedures can be used for this type of examination, but the simplest technique is the Willis technique. The equipment needed is a sputum vial (or any 48-mm-deep cylinder about 24 mm in diameter), a glass microscope slide, a coverslip, and a tongue depressor. A small amount of feces, about the size of a large pea, is placed in the vial, and sufficient flotation solution is added to cover the feces. This is then macerated and mixed. Solution is added until the vial is about half full, and the material is mixed again. The vial is filled with flotation solution until the meniscus bulges slightly, and a clean microscope slide is applied over the vial. This slide is left in place for 10 minutes and is then lifted straight up and turned over, and a coverslip is affixed. Much of the liquid will drain from the slide, but eggs remain firmly attached if the glass is clean. To determine the best level at which to seek eggs, the examiner should focus on an air bubble. The chemical solutions most frequently used for this type of examination are sodium nitrate, magnesium sulfate, and sodium chloride.

DISPOSABLE FECAL FLOTATION KITS

Several commercial disposable kits that are modifications of the Willis technique are available. These kits require 1 g to 2 g of fecal material, depending on which kit is used. All of the kits have some method for preventing the large particles of fecal material from floating to the top of the vial. As in the Willis technique, a clean microscope slide is placed on top of the vial to collect the eggs that float to the top. It is recommended that the microscope slide be left on top of the flotation vial for 15 to 20 minutes.

PAPER CUP TECHNIQUE

One modification of the Willis technique occasionally used is mixture of the chemical solution with a large amount of feces in a paper cup. After thorough maceration, the fluid is strained through several (two or three) layers of cheesecloth (gauze) into a sputum vial. The remainder of the procedure is the same as with the Willis technique. The advantages are that the cup and feces can be discarded, eliminating the need to wash containers, and paper cups are handy for use in field situations. This technique often is used for horses and sheep because of the amount of fiber in the feces. The disadvantages are the same as those of the Willis technique.

The advantages of Willis-type techniques are that they are quick and simple and will provide the observer a qualitative examination for many nematode and tapeworm eggs and some protozoan cysts. These techniques are effective for the recovery of all strongyle-type eggs, as well as eggs of ascarids, *Trichuris, Capillaria,* and *Strongyloides* (egg-producing species only); the protozoan cysts of *Eimeria, Isospora, Cryptosporidium, Sarcocystis,* and *Toxoplasma;* and all of the tapeworm eggs that mix with feces. Thus these techniques can be used effectively in horses and ruminants when the presence of fragile cysts, larvae, or both is not suspected. However, the disadvantages inherent in these techniques are that they destroy or render unrecognizable fragile cysts and larvae. Therefore for dogs, cats, ruminants, and horses in which parasites such as lungworm (any species), *Giardia* spp., *Entamoeba* spp., and *Strongyloides stercoralis* are suspected, another technique, the zinc sulfate centrifugal flotation technique, is recommended.

None of these techniques are suitable for trematode eggs of *Fasciola* and *Fascioloides,* because these eggs are too dense to float, but eggs of *Paragonimus* and *Nanophyetus (Troglotrema)* species will float when these techniques are used.

ZINC SULFATE CENTRIFUGAL FLOTATION TECHNIQUE

The zinc sulfate centrifugal flotation technique is used almost exclusively for parasites of dogs, cats, and primates. It can also be used for other animals, such as exotic animals or native wild species. The reason it is used for these animals is that the technique is much more versatile, and when such animals are examined, a more complete technique is necessary. The technique does not destroy fragile cysts and larvae and is just as effective in recovering the other eggs and cysts as the Willis-type techniques.

> ### ✎ TECHNICIAN NOTE
> The zinc sulfate centrifugal flotation technique is used almost exclusively for parasites of dogs, cats, and primates.

Zinc sulfate, at a specific gravity of 1.18 or 1.20, is usually used. Both specific gravities are effective, but 1.20 is probably best. A small amount of feces (about the size of a large pea) is inserted into a round-bottomed, 10-ml or 15-ml, plastic centrifuge tube. (Conical 15-ml tubes can be used and are effective, but removal of fecal matter from the tube, especially cat feces, is almost impossible.) The feces should be pushed to the bottom of the tube. Five to ten drops of Lugol's iodine solution are then added, and the mixture is quickly but thoroughly stirred. Sufficient zinc sulfate is then added to fill the tube to approximately half full, and the mixture is thoroughly macerated. The Lugol's iodine solution should not remain in contact with feces for more than 1 minute before it is diluted with zinc sulfate; otherwise, fragile protozoan cysts (e.g., those of *Giardia* spp.) will distort and rupture.

Fill the tube with zinc sulfate until the meniscus bulges slightly, and then affix an 18 mm × 18 mm or a 22 mm × 22 mm glass coverslip to the top. Be certain to grasp the coverslip at the periphery, because human body oils will prevent eggs and cysts from attaching. Gently press the coverslip on the tube, being certain that it makes physical contact without any fecal debris disturbing the seal; otherwise, the centrifuge will "throw" the coverslip.

Place the tube into a swinging head centrifuge and centrifuge for 3 to 5 minutes at 1000 to 1500 revolutions per minute (rpm). When the centrifuge stops, remove the coverslip, place it on a clean glass slide, and examine the slide microscopically. The purpose of the Lugol's solution is to stain cysts of *Giardia* and *Entamoeba* species. It will also stain tapeworm eggs, larvae, and some strongyle eggs, and so on, but the purpose of the stain is to facilitate recognition of the aforementioned protozoan cysts.

The zinc sulfate technique is excellent for any of the strongyle-type eggs—*Strongyloides* (both eggs and larvae), ascarids, *Trichuris* spp., *Capillaria* spp., *Physaloptera* spp., coccidia, *Entamoeba* spp., *Giardia* spp., all tapeworm eggs that mix with feces, eggs of *Paragonimus* and *Nanophyetus* species, and mites such as *Demodex* and *Cheyletiella* species. Moreover, the lungworm larvae of dogs and cats, as well as those of ruminants and horses, will float without distortion. The technique cannot be used for *Fasciola* and *Fascioloides* species because their eggs are too dense to float in any chemical solution. The technique is also not effective for the trophozoites of rumen or cecal ciliates such as *Balantidium* spp. or the trophozoites of *Trichomonas hominis* (no cyst stage) because they are too fragile for demonstration by any technique other than direct fecal smear.

FORMALIN–ETHYL ACETATE SEDIMENTATION TECHNIQUE

The formalin–ethyl acetate technique has wide application in human parasitology and has the advantage that all eggs, cysts, and larvae form sediment and are preserved, regardless of whether they will float. This is also the inherent disadvantage: most other fecal debris will likewise form sediment.

For this technique, 2% formalin (vol/vol) and ethyl acetate are needed; the remainder of the equipment is the same as that used in the zinc sulfate technique.

In this technique, a small sample of feces (the size of a large pea) is placed into a small beaker, the beaker is half filled (or filled) with 2% formalin, and the feces sample is thoroughly macerated. A two- or three-thickness layer of cheesecloth (gauze) is placed over the beaker, and the material is strained into a centrifuge tube. The resulting tube of strained material is filled with 2% formalin and is centrifuged at 1000 to 1500 rpm for 1 to 2 minutes. This step is repeated until the supernatant is clear (two or three centrifugations). About half of the liquid is poured off, and the fecal matter is dislodged and stirred. Ethyl acetate is added to this half-filled tube. The tube is then stoppered and shaken vigorously. The stopper is removed, and the mixture is centrifuged for 1 to 2 minutes at 1000 to 1500 rpm. When the centrifuge stops, the tube is removed, and an applicator stick is used to gently "ring" the debris at the ethyl acetate–formalin interface (the two liquids are not miscible). The purpose of the ethyl acetate is to trap the lighter debris, removing it from the sediment. Once "ringed," the supernatant is poured off, leaving the bottom 1 to 2 ml of fecal material and formalin. A small amount of this sediment, or centrifugate, is pipetted onto a microscope slide; a coverslip is affixed; and the material is examined for eggs, cysts, larvae, trophozoites of protozoa, and so forth. A drop of Lugol's solution is added to the periphery of the coverslip and is allowed to spread beneath to stain cysts.

The advantage of this technique is that all eggs (including trematode eggs), fragile cysts, larvae, and trophozoites of non–cyst-forming (or even cyst-forming) protozoa are present.

The distinct, and often overwhelming, disadvantage of this technique is that most of the debris in the fecal sample (except the very low specific gravity material trapped in the ethyl acetate layer) is in the sediment, making examination extremely difficult. Moreover, the technique is time consuming.

QUANTITATIVE FECAL EXAMINATION

In many situations, especially in food-producing animals, it is not sufficient just to know whether the animal has parasites, because most food-producing animals will have parasites to some degree. The livestock producer wants to know how severe the infestation is and whether deworming will increase the animals' performance and the net return on their investment. Several procedures are used to perform a quantitative fecal examination for parasitic eggs and larvae. The most common method is described.

STOLL DILUTION TECHNIQUE

A special Stoll flask is available for use with this technique. The flask has two graduations, one at 56 ml and one at 60 ml. However, any 75-ml to 100-ml flask can be substituted for a Stoll flask. The method is as follows:

1. Fill the flask with decinormal caustic soda solution (0.1 N sodium hydroxide) or water to the first graduation.
2. Add feces until fluid goes to the top graduation (4-g displacement).
3. Add several glass beads, stopper the flask, and shake until the sample is mixed well. Samples can be stored and soaked overnight or longer in a refrigerator.
4. With a micropipette, transfer either 0.15 ml or 0.075 ml from the thoroughly mixed sample to a clean microscope slide. Cover the fluid with a coverslip and examine under the microscope, using low power (100×).
5. Examine the entire area under the coverslip, and count the eggs. Next, multiply by the proper dilution factor, either 100 (for 0.15 ml) or 200 (for 0.075 ml) for the eggs per gram of feces.

STOLL CENTRIFUGATION TECHNIQUE

The greatest advantage to the centrifugation modification of the Stoll technique is that it is more sensitive and will

allow detection of parasitic eggs when other techniques do not. The method follows.

A regular Stoll flask or a plastic vial is prepared with 56 ml of water and 4 g of feces. Fill the flask or vial with 56 ml of water to the lower mark. Add feces until the vial is filled to the upper mark (approximately 4 g of fecal material). Mix feces with the water, and when possible, allow feces to soak 3 to 8 hours. (Mixture should be refrigerated if it is allowed to stand for more than 2 hours.) Mix vial thoroughly, and immediately remove 1.5 ml of mixture with a 3-ml syringe. Place the 1.5-ml sample in a 10-ml to 15-ml test tube, and add flotation solution until a convex meniscus forms at the top of the tube. Place tube in a swinging head centrifuge, and place a coverslip on top. Centrifuge at 1500 to 2000 rpm for 2 to 5 minutes. Remove coverslip, and place on a clean microscope slide. Identify and count all the eggs under the coverslip. The count made multiplied by 10 gives the number of eggs per gram. (If more than 50 eggs are seen on the first coverslip and highly accurate results are desired, the test tube should be topped off with the chemical solution and a second coverslip should be added before centrifuging again.)

INTERPRETATION OF QUANTITATIVE FECAL EXAMINATION

There is no direct or positive correlation between the number of eggs or larvae found in the feces and the severity of parasitism in the animal. It must also be remembered that during the prepatent period, no eggs or cysts will be seen, although the animal may have severe parasitism.

Specialized Diagnostic Tests

LUNGWORMS

The Baermann funnel technique (Figure 7-16) is primarily used to recover larvae of lungworms, although it does have other uses. The funnel consists of a 12.5-cm to 22.5-cm diameter plastic or glass funnel to which a short piece of rubber tubing is affixed and a centrifuge tube is attached. The funnel is filled with lukewarm tap water, and a screen, piece of gauze, or single layer of facial tissue is lowered into the water. Feces, finely chopped tissues, or culture material is carefully added, and the system is allowed to stand for 24 hours. Larvae filter into the centrifuge tube at the bottom, and the coarse material is held back. The system should not be left for more than 24 hours, because eggs of some nematodes will hatch after this period and confuse the results. After 24 hours, the rubber hose is clamped, and the centrifuge tube is removed. The bottom 1 or 2 ml of fluid is examined microscopically for larvae.

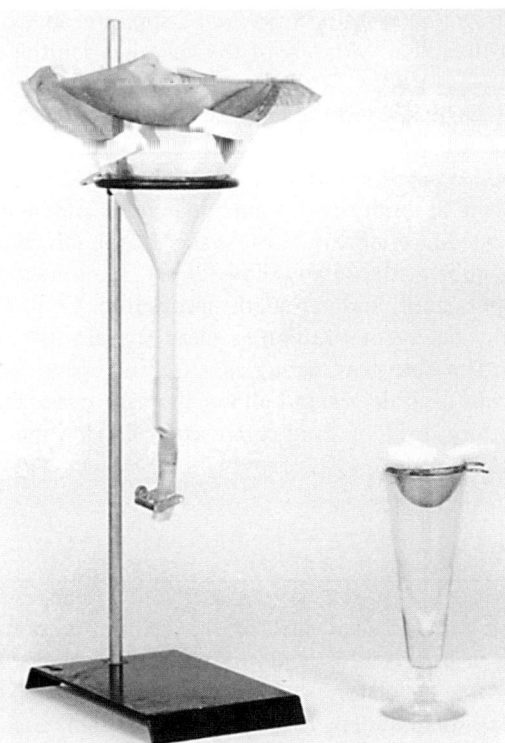

Figure 7-16 Baermann apparatus used for recovery of larvae from feces, soil, or minced tissues of an animal.

MICROFILARIA

Filarial nematodes infect many different tissues of the body and produce undifferentiated larvae called microfilaria. Depending on the species, microfilaria may be found in the blood or dermis of the host.

Species producing microfilaria that accumulate in the dermis are diagnosed by the skin maceration technique. A biopsy specimen of skin measuring at least 12 mm in diameter is finely macerated and allowed to soak for at least 6 hours in physiologic saline solution at approximately 37° C or about 8 to 10 hours at room temperature (21° C). At the end of this time, the tissue is strained off, the liquid is centrifuged, and the bottom 1 or 2 ml is examined for microfilaria. Another method is histologic sectioning of the skin, a procedure that is much more time consuming and not as sensitive as maceration.

For microfilaria of filarial nematodes that occur in the blood, several procedures can be done.

TESTS FOR BLOOD MICROFILARIA

Direct Smear
A thin film of blood is smeared on a slide and dried, and the film is stained with Wright's or Giemsa stain. This is a very poor technique and will work only if microfilaria are numerous.

Saline Preparation. A few drops of freshly drawn blood are mixed with physiologic saline solution, and the resultant preparation is examined microscopically for motile microfilaria. It has the same disadvantages as the direct smear, but when used by technicians experienced in working with microfilaria, it can be very effective.

Microhematocrit Technique. The microhematocrit tube is examined for microfilaria after centrifugation. Microfilaria will be found at the plasma-blood interface (buffy coat). It has the same disadvantages as the direct smear.

Knott's Technique. One milliliter of blood is added to 9 ml of 2% formalin (or 2 ml of blood to 18 ml of formalin). The mixture is then shaken until the blood is hemolyzed and is centrifuged at 1500 rpm for 5 minutes. The bottom 0.5 ml or 1 ml is then examined for microfilaria. Microfilaria are preserved, lay straight, and are easily measured. Measurements are often necessary to distinguish species and must be done to separate *Dirofilaria* and *Dipetalonema* species. This is the preferred technique for identification of microfilaria.

Filter Technique. Several filter techniques for the recovery of microfilaria from the blood are available commercially. These techniques require 1 ml of blood, which is then mixed with the lysing solution (usually 9 ml) to hemolyze the red blood cells. The mixture is then passed through a plastic chamber containing a filter membrane on which the microfilaria are collected. The membrane filter is then removed and placed on a clean microscope slide. A drop of stain is placed on top of the membrane, which is covered with a coverslip for examination under the microscope.

The two simplest and most effective techniques described here are the filter technique and Knott's technique. Both have advantages, depending on the host and parasite.

PINWORMS

Pinworms in horses and humans must be diagnosed by the adhesive tape technique. With this technique, adhesive tape is folded over a test tube or a smooth, round rod with the adhesive side out. The perianal folds are spread, and the tape is applied to the skin in several places, then the tape is placed on a clean microscope slide with the stickyside down. A few drops of xylene are allowed to seep under the tape to clear the fecal debris, and the slide is then examined microscopically for typical pinworm eggs (always flat on one side).

TAPEWORMS

Most tapeworms are found in the small intestine of their host as adults or, as with *Thysanosoma* spp., have access to the intestine. All tapeworms use an intermediate host; and because swine, domestic and wild ruminants, and rabbits frequently serve in this capacity, diagnostic procedures for both adult and larval stages must be performed.

ADULT TAPEWORMS

Some adult tapeworms such as *Moniezia* spp. in ruminants and the anoplocephalids in horses shed gravid proglottids that are destroyed in the intestine, releasing the eggs to mix with the feces. Any of the flotation procedures described for detection of nematodes are satisfactory for diagnosis. However, *Thysanosoma* spp. in ruminants and *Dipylidium caninum* and the *Taenia* spp. in carnivores produce proglottids that do not break up in the intestine. These proglottids usually pass intact when the animal defecates. Thus diagnosis requires visual observation of the proglottids (or chain) on the feces or around the anal region, which is frequently done by observant clients. *Echinococcus* spp. (taeniform tapeworm) in carnivores is an exception in that the eggs usually appear in the feces.

The fish tapeworms found in humans, bears, and wild carnivores shed eggs from the proglottids. Thus the eggs mix with the feces like those of *Moniezia* spp. and the anoplocephalids, but these eggs are very heavy and will not float; therefore the procedures used for diagnosis of trematodes (or the formalin–ethyl acetate technique) must be applied.

LARVAL TAPEWORMS

Most species of tapeworms use arthropods, fish, or mammals as intermediate hosts (an exception is *Hymenolepis diminuta*, which can use an intermediate host but does not need one). Some tapeworms that use mammals have larvae that occur as large bladderworms (cysticerci) on the mesenteries or the liver; others produce small bladderworms that occur in the muscles. The heavily exercised muscles are the preferred sites for these larvae. Diagnosis may be made by visual observation of the small bladderworms in the heart, diaphragm, or jaw muscles; by pressing thin slices of tissue between two slides for microscopic examination; by digestion with pepsin–hydrochloric acid; or examination of a histologic section. If the latter technique is used, remember that all tapeworms have small egg-shaped bodies called calcareous corpuscles that stain blue or purple with hematoxylin. This will identify a larva as a tapeworm, but it does not identify the species. For species identification, the specific host and the site within the host must be known.

TREMATODES

Trematodes (flukes) occur in the bile ducts of the liver, parenchyma of the liver, rumen, lungs, small intestine, and other sites, such as skin and oviducts.

Fluke eggs (except *Troglotrema* and *Paragonimus* spp. in the dog) are too heavy to float with the usual chemical solutions available for floating nematode and tapeworm eggs. *Troglotrema* and *Paragonimus* spp. are an exception in that they float with any of the chemical solutions listed earlier.

The diagnostic technique recommended for the recovery of fluke eggs, especially liver fluke and fish tapeworm eggs, is to add a small amount of material (one fecal pellet or equivalent amount) to a centrifuge tube and add 0.1% detergent. Macerate the feces, shake thoroughly, and then fill the tube with water. Allow to set 5 minutes, decant the supernatant, and repeat the procedure. Continue this until the detergent solution is clear (usually two to five times). The detergent, acting as a wetting agent, separates eggs from fecal debris and allows them to settle. Examine the bottom 1 ml of fluid microscopically for the typical operculated eggs.

PROTOZOA

Single-celled parasites, such as the helminths, occur in a variety of sites within the animal body. Various species occupy the circulatory system, especially the blood cells, gastrointestinal system (from mouth to anus), and reproductive system. A variety of techniques must be used for correct diagnosis.

BLOOD PARASITES

Parasites occurring in the blood of an animal, such as *Plasmodium, Haemobartonella, Cytauxzoon, Babesia, Theileria, Leucocytozoon,* or *Trypanosoma* spp., can be identified by the direct smear technique. The slide is air dried and then stained with Giemsa or Wright's stain. *Trypanosoma* spp. may not be demonstrable by the direct smear technique; therefore culture in blood agar slants overlaid with liver infusion tryptase medium is the best approach.

GASTROINTESTINAL PROTOZOA

TRICHOMONAS SPECIES

Trichomonas gallinae from the oral cavities of birds, *Trichomonas equi* from the gastrointestinal tracts of horses, and *Trichomonas hominis* from dogs and humans are best demonstrated by direct smear of fresh samples. Lesions suspected of being caused by *T. gallinae* can be scraped (or swabbed), and this material can be mixed with some physiologic saline solution on a clean microscope slide and examined for these typical flagellates. The presence of an undulating membrane is diagnostic. For *T. equi* of horses, a drop or two of fluid expressed from the feces can be examined. If the feces are dry, add saline solution, mix, and then examine a drop.

HEXAMITA MELEAGRIDIS

Hexamita meleagridis is the organism responsible for catarrhal enteritis of turkeys and is diagnosed by demonstration of the fast-moving flagellate in the upper part of the small intestine from freshly killed birds.

COCCIDIA

Eimeria, Isospora, and *Toxoplasma* spp. produce oocysts, whereas *Sarcocystis* and *Cryptosporidium* spp. generally produce sporulated sporocysts, all of which pass with the feces and may be easily demonstrated by either qualitative or quantitative concentration (flotation) techniques.

Sometimes, diagnosis of acute coccidiosis (in sheep or cattle) must be done at necropsy examination. In this situation, a scraping of the intestinal mucosa is mixed with physiologic saline solution on a clean microscope slide and is examined for schizonts, oocysts, and the small, motile, teardrop-shaped merozoites.

GIARDIA SPECIES

Giardia spp. found in domestic, wild, and laboratory animals ostensibly can be diagnosed by the direct smear technique, but a more effective procedure is the zinc sulfate centrifugal flotation technique. The cysts may be stained with Lugol's solution to make the internal structures easily identifiable.

ENTAMOEBA HISTOLYTICA

The dog is sometimes a transient host for *E. histolytica* and, on occasion, will show clinical signs of infection. As with *Giardia* spp., the cyst form is best demonstrated by the zinc sulfate centrifugal flotation technique. Iodine will tint the cyst, facilitating identification. This is an extremely small cyst with four to eight nuclei.

ENDAMOEBA SPECIES

This commensal ameba is often found in primates, rodents, humans, and other animals. The techniques used for identification of *Entamoeba histolytica* are effective. Each has eight nuclei.

BALANTIDIUM SPECIES

This large ciliate reportedly causes diarrhea in swine and humans, even though it is usually a commensal organism. Diagnosis is possible by direct smear, observing the large, motile trophozoite or by using zinc sulfate centrifugal flotation technique and recovering the large cyst. Iodine will stain the sausage-shaped macronucleus as an aid in identification.

HISTOMONAS MELEAGRIDIS

Histomonas meleagridis forms a cyst within the egg of the nematode parasite *Heterakis gallinae,* the cecal worm of poultry. In the event of an outbreak of "black head" in turkeys, recovery of the eggs of *Heterakis gallinae* from carrier birds and the presence of pathognomonic lesions in sick poults are sufficient to delineate the cause of the infection as well as the source.

TRICHOMONAS FOETUS

A positive diagnosis of trichomoniasis requires demonstration of the trichomonad in one or more infected animals. There is no serologic test or other test based on immunologic reactions that has yet proved practical or specific for trichomoniasis.

Diagnosis in the bull consists of checking the breeding records and determining which bulls are probably infected. After a few days of rest from mating, these bulls should be confined, the preputial hairs should be clipped, the preputial orifice should be washed with soap and water and dried, and each bull should be examined. For collection of the smegma sample, a dry plastic insemination pipette is attached to a 10-ml to 12-ml syringe. The pipette is introduced into the prepuce to its full length. A negative pressure is then created in the syringe, and the pipette is moved vigorously back and forth, scraping the glans penis and the preputial membrane. In most bulls, 0.5 to 1 ml of smegma can be collected in the pipette. This material is flushed into a vial containing 2 ml of lactated Ringer's solution or physiologic saline solution. The sample is then layered on Diamond's medium for culturing.

Trichomonas foetus may occur in small numbers; therefore proper handling after collection is necessary to avoid extremes of temperature, contact with harmful chemicals, and evaporation. It is highly desirable to examine samples within a few hours after collection. Samples should be refrigerated but not frozen if they cannot be cultured immediately. The liquid transport medium (lactated Ringer's solution) is layered on the surface of Diamond's medium and is incubated at 37° C for 48 to 72 hours.

Diamond's medium is very difficult to prepare and is not available commercially but is available from some diagnostic laboratories. Do not use other *Trichomonas* culture media, because the majority will not grow *T. foetus.*

ARTHROPODS

Infestation with ectoparasites means the presence of mites, lice, ticks, chiggers, fleas, or the larval stages of Diptera such as screw worm flies, blowflies, *Hypoderma, Gasterophilus, Oestrus, Cuterebra, Cephenemyia* (wild ruminants), or *Wohlfahrtia.* Fortunately, except for mites, the arthropod parasites are sufficiently large that identification is not as difficult as with the other parasites. In general, examination of the host and the site on each host will be sufficient.

MITES AND CHIGGERS

Some mites live on the surface of the skin (e.g., *Cheyletiella, Otodectes, Chorioptes,* and *Psoroptes* spp. and many bird mites), whereas others are burrowing types (such as *Demodex, Knemidokoptes,* and *Sarcoptes* spp.). Consequently, there is no uniform procedure for examination and recovery.

Mites and/or chiggers living under the skin, or even on the surface of the skin, are recovered by a deep scraping (deep enough to draw blood) at the periphery of the lesion. Sites of suspected *Demodex* lesions, or even any sites of suspected mite or chigger infestation, should be clipped of hair and "squeezed" at the time the skin is scraped to ensure adequate sample collections. This scraped material is then placed on a clean microscope slide, covered with a coverslip, and examined with a microscope.

TICKS, FLEAS, AND LICE

Ticks, fleas, and lice are all of a sufficient size to see with the unaided eye. Ticks and fleas are usually removed and identified. Sometimes lice are difficult to find; therefore a careful examination for nits (louse eggs) attached to the hair may reveal their presence. Accurate louse identification often requires the service of a specialist.

DIPTERA

The species of Diptera that infest domestic and wild animals are often easily identifiable because they are host or site specific, or both (e.g., *Hypoderma* spp., *Gasterophilus* spp., *Oestrus ovis,* and *Cuterebra* spp.). The larval stages of other dipterous insects are not as easily identified. Screw worm larvae can be identified by the presence of two black, pigmented tracheal trunks leading from the spiracle of the body. They can be clearly seen in the living third instar larva with the unaided eye. If a larva does not have pigmented tubules, it is one of myriad blowflies, which can be identified by the pattern of the spiracle at the caudal extremity of the body.

The larval stages of *Wohlfahrtia* spp. are parasitic in the very young, for skin must be tender for this parasite to penetrate. Identification of the larvae is based on the morphologic characteristics of the spiracular plates and cephalopharyngeal skeleton of the third instar larva.

PRESERVING PARASITIC SAMPLES

Ectoparasites and endoparasites may be adequately preserved in 10% formalin or 70% alcohol. Preservation of tapeworms and flukes for morphologic study is best accomplished by placing the specimen in a dish of water in the refrigerator until it relaxes (overnight) and then replacing this water with cold preservative (10% cold formalin). Preservation of feces can be done with 10% formalin, but this is only satisfactory for some eggs and larvae. Eggs of ascarids, as well as oocysts, will continue to develop. Refrigeration (or even freezing) of feces is often the best approach.

Parasitology and Public Health

Many infections and parasitic diseases are transmitted between animals and humans (zoonoses). These diseases are always of concern to occupational groups who come into daily contact with a variety of exotic, wild, and domesticated animals. Consequently, the zoonoses described in the following sections are the ones these groups might encounter. Control of most parasitic diseases requires strict attention to personal hygiene and avoidance of contaminated materials. Other zoonoses and public health issues are discussed in Chapter 35.

Cryptosporidiosis is caused by *Cryptosporidium* spp. The mode of infection is by direct contact with infected animals and consumption of feces-contaminated water or food. Dogs, cats, and birds are considered probable sources of infection.

Giardiasis is caused by *Giardia* spp. The mode of infection is by direct contact with infected animals and consumption of feces-contaminated water. Dogs and cats are considered probable sources of infection.

Toxoplasmosis is caused by *Toxoplasma gondii*. Infection can be acquired from sporulated oocysts in cat feces or ingestion of raw or insufficiently cooked meat.

Hydatidosis is caused by infection with the hydatid cyst of the eggs of *Echinococcus granulosis* or *Echinococcus multilocularis*.

Tapeworms are acquired by ingestion of raw or poorly cooked beef *(Taenia saginata)* or pork *(Taenia solium)*.

Creeping eruption is caused by penetration of the skin by larval stages of dog and cat hookworm of the genus *Ancylostoma*.

Visceral larva migrans is caused by ingestion of the infective larvae (within the eggs) of *Toxocara canis,* especially by very young children.

Strongyloidosis is caused by infection, generally by *Strongyloides stercoralis,* which infects humans, dogs, cats, and foxes.

Trichinosis is caused by infection with *Trichinella spiralis,* generally from consumption of raw or insufficiently cooked pork or bear.

Scabies include the mites that are not strictly host specific and can live for varying amounts of time on alternate hosts. Such mites include *Sarcoptes, Notoedres,* and *Cheyletiella* spp.

can establish the diagnosis. Serum can be tested for the presence of specific antibodies, or skin tests can be performed. Another diagnostic method is *direct examination* of exudates and tissue biopsy specimens. Some microorganisms present such unique morphologic characteristics, host inflammatory responses, and lesions that a preliminary diagnosis can be established without the need for further laboratory testing.

Recent developments in biotechnology are providing new methods for direct detection of infectious agents. Direct *nucleic acid hybridization probe* and *gene amplification* protocols have tremendous potential for detecting microbial pathogens. These procedures are highly specific and can be extremely sensitive. Because they detect the genes (or portions of genes) of organisms and can differentiate closely related organisms based on the presence of a unique genetic sequence, the identified strains are frequently described as genotypes. DNA probe assays are particularly well suited for in situ hybridization in tissue in which the location and distribution of the organisms must be determined, identification of slow-growing or difficult-to-isolate organisms, and identification of toxicogenic strains of bacteria that cannot be differentiated from nontoxicogenic strains through the use of conventional methods. Nucleic acid amplification assays use primers and polymerase chain reaction to provide specificity and sensitivity to detect as few as one organism or 1 to 10 copies of the specific gene sequence. Because of this exquisite sensitivity, specimen collection and handling procedures are critical. Cross-contamination of samples with as little as a single copy of a microbial gene carried on gloves, laboratory bench tops, or aerosolized droplets may result in false-positive test results.

✎ TECHNICIAN NOTE

Reference laboratories should be consulted for preferred methods of specimen collection and handling for nucleic acid detection methods to avoid false-positive results from minute contamination of samples.

Ultimately, the goal of these molecular techniques is the direct determination of identities and antimicrobial susceptibility patterns of microorganisms in clinical specimens.

As the technology for nucleic acid amplification currently stands, application of the procedure is limited to large referral laboratories and research laboratories. Partial or full automation and improved technology will begin to reduce costs and increase access to these assays. Despite their sensitivity, molecular detection procedures will not totally replace conventional culture and serologic procedures because the results of nucleic acid amplification procedures and the results of culture or serology mean different things. Nucleic acid amplification procedures are used to determine whether DNA or RNA from a particular organism is present in the specimen; they reveal nothing about the viability of the organism (because they can detect DNA from dead organisms) or whether the organism is involved in an infectious process. Culture, on the other hand, clearly demonstrates the viability of the organism, whereas a rise in titer of antibody to a specific organism strongly suggests infection.

COLLECTION OF SPECIMENS

There is tremendous diversity of microbial agents, specimen sources, and samples to be considered in the microbiology laboratory. Specimen selection, collection, and transport requirements may also vary significantly, depending on the agent to be detected and the assay to be performed. Therefore it is important that technicians be alert to the potential of receiving and implementing specific instructions about specimen collection and handling for each patient rather than anticipating generic procedures.

PROPER SPECIMEN COLLECTION

The goal of specimen collection is to obtain a sample from the patient that is representative of the disease process. Therefore the culture specimen must be from the actual *infection site* (Figure 8-1). It must be collected with a minimum of contamination from adjacent tissues or secretions. Material swabbed from superficial body surfaces (skin or mucous membranes) will usually yield a mixed growth

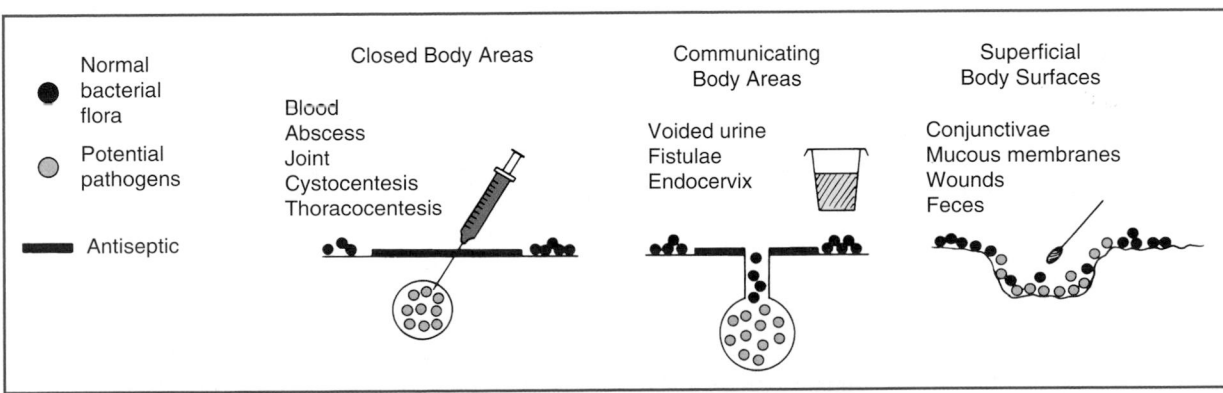

Figure 8-1 Methods used to collect bacterial culture specimens and probable sources of contamination.

of bacteria, often making it difficult to identify a significant pathogen. Culture specimens recovered from body orifices and draining tracts are frequently contaminated with normal flora. The most useful specimens are those aspirated from normally sterile, closed body compartments after the surface has been aseptically prepared.

Optimal times and *sites* for specimen collection must be observed. Infections by some viruses and mycoplasmas are acute processes that are followed by secondary invasion by opportunistic bacteria; therefore sampling must be performed early in the course of disease. When viruses and bacteria localize in specific tissues, collection should target such sites. Specimens obtained at necropsy for culture should be collected as soon as possible after the death of the animal (see Chapter 5).

Whenever possible, culture specimens should be obtained before the administration of antimicrobials, especially if the suspected pathogen may be susceptible to the antimicrobial or the antimicrobial may be concentrated at the site of infection. However, the administration of antimicrobials does not necessarily preclude the usefulness of cultures. The antimicrobial drug may be diluted to an ineffective level in culture medium, thereby allowing the pathogen to grow. Antimicrobial-resistant or superinfecting bacteria may still be recovered. In addition, the effectiveness of therapy can be evaluated by determining the relative numbers of bacteria present.

An *adequate quantity* of material should be obtained for complete examination. Aliquots of body fluids (>1 ml), exudates, or pieces of tissue (>3 cm^3) are always more useful than a swab. Smears can be prepared for direct examination, and multiple culture media can be inoculated when adequate material is submitted. Quantitative results can also be obtained if needed.

Appropriate collection devices and specimen handling must be used to ensure optimal survival and recovery of significant microorganisms (Figure 8-2). Sterile swabs are acceptable for transferring most samples from the patient to culture media. If the culture medium is not immediately inoculated, the swab must be placed in a swab transport system (CultureSwab, BD Diagnostic Systems; Copan Transport Swabs, Copan Diagnostics, Inc.) or into a transport medium. *Transport media* are designed to maintain optimal conditions for survival of the suspected pathogen without allowing overgrowth by contaminating saprophytes. Semi-solid transport media, such as Amies transport medium with charcoal for *aerobic bacteria* (growth in the presence of oxygen) or the Port-A-Cul Anaerobic Transport System (BD Diagnostic Systems) for *anaerobic bacteria* (requires absence of oxygen), can preserve specimens on swabs for several days. Swabs should not be placed in nutritive broths before inoculation of isolation media because an insignificant nonpathogen may overgrow and prevent recovery of the pathogen. Specimens can be collected in various sterile containers that do not contain preservatives or anticoagulants for transport. If tissues are collected for

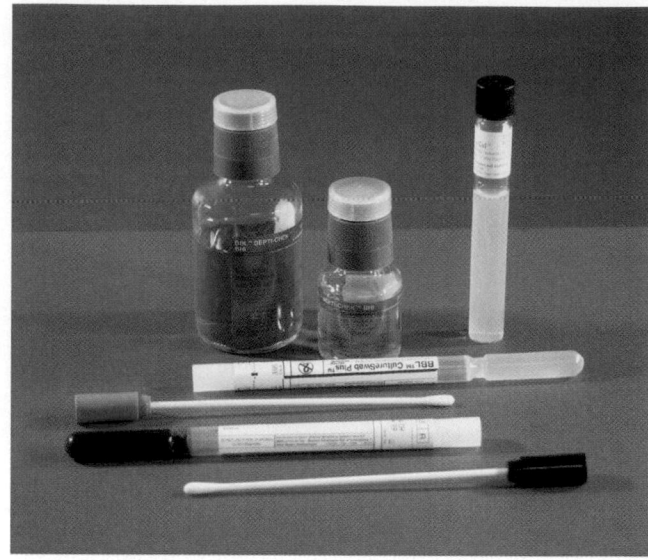

Figure 8-2 Culturette swab transport systems with transport media (black medium is Amies transport medium with charcoal), Port-A-Cul Anaerobic Transport Tube (BD Diagnostic Systems), and blood culture bottles. Swabs are used to collect culture inoculum and placed into transport systems or tube of medium for preservation of the viability of bacteria during transportation to the laboratory for culture. Blood culture bottles are inoculated with blood to prevent coagulation and contamination during transport to the laboratory for incubation.

culture, each piece must be packaged separately in a leak-proof, sterile container.

✎ TECHNICIAN NOTE

Transport media can serve as excellent vehicles for submitting a bacterial isolate to a reference laboratory for further characterization. A heavily inoculated swab of the pure culture should be placed in the appropriate medium for shipping rather than being submitted in an inoculated growth medium (plate or tube).

Each culture specimen container must be *properly labeled*. Identification of the patient by name, species, case number, or owner, as appropriate, should be legibly indicated. If more than one veterinarian works in the practice, the one in charge of the case should be identified so that questions about history and preliminary reports can be communicated efficiently. The source of the specimen should also be included on the label. As discussed later, the source of the specimen will be a significant factor in deciding how to set up the culture, which bacteria to identify, and how to interpret the results. If the culture specimen is to be sent to a referral laboratory, additional clinical history should be included. Results of previous culture attempts, other laboratory tests, and antimicrobial treatments should be reported, as well as the major clinical manifestations and duration of illness, so laboratory personnel will be able to recognize and identify significant findings.

SPECIAL COLLECTION AND HANDLING PROCEDURES

Some groups of microorganisms require special collection and handling for optimal isolation. Anaerobic bacteria must be protected from oxygen. Often, a sterile syringe with a fine-gauge needle (22- to 23 gauge) is the best collection device for aspirating exudates from an infected site. The specimen can be transported to the laboratory in the syringe if air is expressed, the needle is removed to prevent injuries, and the syringe is capped to prevent leakage. Otherwise, the specimen should be transferred to an appropriate anaerobic transport device. Survival and subsequent isolation of anaerobes are enhanced by keeping them in the reduced microenvironment in which they are found. Therefore, as stated previously, exudate and pieces of tissue are better specimens than swabs. If a swab is collected, it must be placed in an appropriate anaerobic transport device. Handling a specimen as if it contains anaerobes will not jeopardize the viability of aerobic bacteria. Exudates, biopsy material, and tissue should be submitted as quickly as possible to the microbiology laboratory.

In attempts to isolate fungi and mycobacteria, swabs are usually not the best specimens. These agents tend to cause chronic infections, often with small numbers of organisms present. Too few organisms may be present on a swab, or in the case of mycobacteria, they may adhere to the swab, and culture results will be negative.

The more fastidious groups of microorganisms (e.g., *Mycoplasma*, *Chlamydia*, and *Rickettsia* species and viruses) require special selective transport media. These media are usually formulated to contain antimicrobials that will inhibit the growth of other microorganisms while preserving the viability of the desired agent. Specific transport media and instructions for proper use should be obtained from a referral laboratory that is capable of providing the desired culture service.

> **TECHNICIAN NOTE**
>
> Selective transport media differ from anaerobic transport systems because they usually contain antimicrobial agents. Anaerobic systems only reduce the availability of oxygen to maintain viability of the anaerobes, but the lack of oxygen is not detrimental to other microorganisms during transport.

PROCESSING SPECIMENS

Each specimen received in the microbiology laboratory should be carefully and individually evaluated, with consideration given to anatomic source and condition of the specimen, animal family of the patient, clinical history, and special requests from the veterinarian. Each pathogen has a preferred habitat in which it will grow and specific mechanisms for causing disease. Therefore, for a particular manifestation of disease, there will be a limited number of agents that should be considered as likely pathogens. Table 8-1 lists the most common bacterial species associated with infections of various sites in animals. If the technician can focus the search for pathogens on these most likely agents, results will often be obtained much more rapidly and with less expense.

CONDITION OF THE SPECIMEN

If there is evidence that the specimen has become grossly contaminated or dried out, if it is of insufficient quantity, if there has been excessive delay in receipt, or if any other evidence of mishandling is present, an attempt should be made to obtain a second sample. Specimens should be processed the same day they are collected, or they should be kept refrigerated if a delay is anticipated.

DIRECT MICROSCOPIC EXAMINATION

Direct microscopic examination of exudates, impression smears from tissues, or infected body fluids is the most important laboratory procedure that can be used for microbiologic diagnosis. It provides immediate information on the types and numbers of microorganisms present as well as the type of host cellular inflammatory response. The likelihood of infection can be determined, as can the probable type of agent (i.e., virus, bacterium, or fungus), which in turn determines the nature of the diagnostic assays needed. The most likely pathogen (or predominant organism) may tentatively be identified. This information may be used to provide guidance in selection of optimal culture conditions and as the basis for the interpretation of the significance of subsequent culture results. In some cases it may be all the information the veterinarian needs.

In many situations, application of Gram's stain is the procedure of choice because it allows differentiation of gram-positive and gram-negative bacteria. However, some bacteria do not stain well with Gram's stain. Gram-negative bacteria may not be well differentiated from the background in exudates and tissue impression smears.

Other tissue stains (i.e., Giemsa and Wright's stains or methylene blue wet mounts) may be more useful for detecting all microorganisms present in the smear. Although these stains are more efficient in demonstrating the presence and morphology of bacteria, they do not provide differentiation of gram-positive and gram-negative bacteria. Careful direct examination may be sufficient for diagnosis without cultures, or it can narrow the diagnostic likelihood to a few bacterial species. This information helps in the selection of optimal culture conditions for identification of suspected pathogens.

> **TECHNICIAN NOTE**
>
> Microscopic examination of urine for bacteria should not be used as a substitute for urine culture. Caution must be exercised in the examination of unstained preparations of urine sediment to avoid interpreting artifacts as bacteria. Cocci are difficult to detect without staining, whereas rod-shaped bacteria may be more readily detected. Significant bacteriuria is rarely present in the absence of an inflammatory response, and the detection of bacteria within the cytoplasm of phagocytes suggests phagocytosis rather than contamination of the sample.

Table 8-1 COMMON BACTERIAL SPECIES ASSOCIATE WITH INFECTIONS

Type of Infection	Canine	Feline	Equine	Porcine	Ruminants
Conjunctivitis	Staphylococcus Streptococcus Pasteurella Pseudomonas	Staphylococcus Staphylococcus Chlamydia	Streptococcus Staphylococcus	Streptacoccus Branhamella	Moraxella bovis Streptococcus Staphylococcus Escherichia coli
Central nervous system	Rare	Rare	Streptococcus Actinobacillus Escherichia coli	Streptococcus Escherichia coli	Haemophilus somnus Listeria Escherichia coli Pasteurella haemolytica
Gastroenteritis	Salmonella Clostridium perfringens Campylobacter	Salmonella	Salmonella Escherichia coli Actinobacillus Rhodococcus equi	Salmonella Escherichia coli Brachyspira Clostridium perfringens	Salmonella Escherichia coli Clostridium perfringens Mycobacterium paratuberculosis
Genital tract	Brucella canis Escherichia coli Streptococcus Staphylococcus Mycoplasma	Streptococcus Pasteurella Escherichia coli	Streptococcus Escherichia coli Klebsiella Pseudomonas	Brucella suis Streptococcus Leptospira	Brucella Listeria Arcanobacterium pyogenes Campylobacter Mycoplasma
Mastitis	Staphylococcus	Staphylococcus	Streptococcus	Streptococcus Staphylococcus Escherichia coli Actinobacillus Arcanobacterium pyogenes	Streptococcus Staphylococcus Arcanobacterium pyogenes Nocardia Mycobacterium Escherichia coli Klebsiella
Musculoskeletal	Staphylococcus Escherichia coli Pseudomonas Brucella canis Anaerobes	Rare	Streptococcus Actinobacillus Escherichia coli Rhodococcus equi Staphylococcus	Streptococcus Mycoplasma Escherichia coli Erysipelothrix Arcanobacterium pyogenes	Clostridium Arcanobacterium pyogenes Escherichia coli Streptococcus Erysipelothrix Haemophilus somnus Mycoplasma Chlamydia
Otitis	Staphyloccus Pseudomonas Streptococcus Clostridium perfringens	Rare	Rare	Rare Streptococcus	Rare Streptococcus Pasteurella Arcanobacterium pyogenes
Upper respiratory tract	Bordetella bronchiseptica	Pasteurella multocida	Streptococcus equi	Bordetella bronchiseptica Pasteurella multocida	Arcanobacterium pyogenes Haemophilus somnus Arcanobacterium pyogenes Fusobacterium

Pneumonia	Bordetella bronchiseptica Pasteurella Kebsiella Escherichia coli Mycoplasma Streptococcus Staphylococcus	Rare Pasteurella Chlamydia Bordetella	Streptococcus Actinobacillus Rhodococcus equi Pasteurella Staphylococcus Klebsiella Pseudomonas Bordetella bronchiseptica	Bordetella bronchiseptica Pasteurella multocida Mycoplasma Haemophilus Pasteurella Streptococcus Actinobacillus	Haemophilus somnus Arcanobacterium pyogenes Fusobacterium Pasteurella, Mannheimia Arcanobacterium pyogenes Haemophilus somnus Mycoplasma
Pleuritis	Fusobacterium Prevotella Porphyromonas Actinomyces	Prevotella Porphyromonas Fusobacterium Pasteurella Nocardia	Streptococcus	Actinobacillus	Pasteurella, Mannheimia Arcanobacterium pyogenes
Skin wounds, abscesses	Staphylococcus Streptococcus Pseudomonas Nocardia Actinomyces Fusobacterium	Pasteurella multocida Streptococcus Staphylococcus Anaerobes	Streptococcus Corynebacterium pseudotuberculosis Pseudomonas Dermatophilus Staphylococcus	Streptococcus Staphylococcus Arcanobacterium pyogenes	Arcanobacterium pyogenes Dermatophilus Actinomyces Actinobacillus Staphylococcus
Urinary tract	Escherichia coli Proteus Staphylococcus Streptococcus Klebsiella Pseudomonas	Staphylococcus Escherichia coli	Streptococcus Eschericia coli	Actinobacterium suis Streptococcus	Corynebacterium renale Arcanobacterium pyogenes

Gram's Stain Procedure and Interpretation

The technique for preparing a gram-stained slide is as follows:

1. Prepare a thin smear from tissue exudates or bacterial suspension on a clean slide and allow smear to air dry.
2. Fix material to the slide so that it does not wash off during the staining procedure by passing the slide, right side up, through a flame three or four times.
3. Flood smear with crystal violet solution, and let stand for 1 minute.
4. Wash smear briefly with tap water.
5. Flood smear with Gram's iodine solution, and let stand for 1 minute.
6. Wash with tap water, and decolorize until solvent flows colorlessly from the slide. This usually requires 5 to 10 seconds.
7. Wash briefly with tap water, and flood the slide with safranin counterstain for 30 to 60 seconds.
8. Wash briefly with tap water, blot and air dry, and examine.

The stained smear is best examined by using the 100× (oil immersion) objective of the microscope. Gram-positive bacteria retain the crystal violet iodine complex and appear dark blue or purple. Gram-negative bacteria lose the primary complex, take up the secondary dye safranin, and appear red. Fungi (yeasts) appear gram-positive. Inflammatory cells appear gram-negative, and epithelial cells may appear gram-positive or gram-negative, depending on the thickness of the smear. Backgrounds usually appear gram-negative but may appear gram-positive if they are thick and inadequately washed. Fibrin, mucus, and erythrocytes often stain gram-negative and may mask detection of gram-negative bacteria.

BACTERIAL ISOLATION AND IDENTIFICATION PROCEDURES

EQUIPMENT

The equipment and supplies required for the performance of basic diagnostic bacteriology tests depend on the scope of services to be provided. Some of the more common items are as follows: binocular microscope, incubator, anaerobic culture system, staining reagents or kits, specimen collection devices, swabs, transport media, isolation and identification media (Table 8-2), packaged identification systems (Boxes 8-1 and 8-2), and miscellaneous instruments, supplies, and reagents as appropriate for the diagnostic procedures to be performed.

The most expensive item is a good-quality binocular light microscope with a 100× oil immersion objective. Dark-field and phase-contrast options are useful but not essential. Small countertop incubators are available. Important

---

> **Box 8-1** COMMERCIAL KIT SYSTEMS FOR IDENTIFICATION OF MICROORGANISMS
>
> **ENTEROBACTERIACEAE**
> API 20E (BioMérieux, Inc.)
> Enterotube II (BD Diagnostic Systems)
> MicroID (Remel)
>
> ***STAPHYLOCOCCUS***
> API Staph (BioMérieux, Inc.)
>
> ***STREPTOCOCCUS***
> API 20 Strep (BioMérieux, Inc.)
> Small Gram-Positive Bacilli
> API Coryne (BioMérieux, Inc.)
> Other Gram-Negative Bacteria
> API 20E (BioMérieux, Inc.)
> Oxi/Ferm Tube II (BD Diagnostic Systems)
>
> **YEAST**
> API 20C AUX (BioMérieux, Inc.)
>
> **ANAEROBIC BACTERIA**
> API 20A (BioMérieux, Inc.)

See Box 8-2 for addresses of product manufacturers and distributors.

characteristics of a quality incubator include (1) insulated walls to maintain a constant temperature; (2) an adequate seal to maintain a humid atmosphere; (3) a capacity for plates, tubes, and candle jars; (4) a thermometer to check the temperature, which should not fluctuate more than ±2° C; and (5) an adjustable, thermostatically controlled heating element.

CULTURE MEDIA

Several different media are needed in the bacteriology laboratory for isolation of various microbial agents and for identification of these microorganisms. Both dehydrated and prepared media are readily available today. It is usually much more convenient for small laboratories to purchase prepared media than to prepare their own. In addition, the quality of purchased media will be much more consistent, and these media will usually be quality tested before they are distributed. There are numerous distributors of prepared media throughout the United States. A few national and regional distributors are listed in Box 8-2. Names and addresses of other suppliers can be obtained from local hospitals and by searching the World Wide Web. Some microbiology supply distributors usually have a full line of prepared plates and tubes of media available, as well as the ancillary biochemical reagents, stains, and miscellaneous supplies.

Table 8-2 BACTERIOLOGIC PLATE AND TUBE MEDIA FOR THE PRACTITIONER'S LABORATORY

Media	Purpose and Inoculation	Reactions and Interpretations
Blood agar plate (trypticase soy agar with 5% sheep blood)	Primary isolation medium for all specimens in which pathogenic bacteria are suspected. Always streak for colony isolation.	Observe growth rates, colony morphologic characteristics, hemolysis. Test selected colonies for Gram's reaction, catalase, and oxidase. Inoculate differential tests and antimicrobial susceptibility tests from well-isolated colonies.
MacConkey agar	A primary isolation and differential plating medium for selection and recovery of Enterobacteriaceae and related gram-negative bacteria. Inoculate by streaking for isolated colonies.	Growth is usually gram negative. Pink to red colonies (with increased redness of the medium) are lactose fermenters (e.g., species of *Escherichia*, *Klebsiella*, and *Enterobacter*). Colorless colonies (often with a slight change of the medium to yellow) are non–lactose fermenters.
Hektoen enteric agar	A direct plating medium for fecal specimens that is highly selective for *Salmonella*. Inoculate by streaking for isolated colonies.	Disaccharide fermenters are moderately inhibited and produce bright orange to yellow to salmon to pink colonies. *Salmonella* colonies are blue-green, typically with back centers from hydrogen sulfide. *Proteus* colonies may resemble *Salmonella*.
Selenite broth or tetrathionate broth	Enrichment broth for the selective enhancement of growth by *Salmonella* from specimens containing heavy concentrations of mixed bacteria, such as feces. Inoculate relatively heavily, and incubate 18-24 hr.	Subculture to MacConkey agar and Hektoen enteric agar for isolation of *Salmonella*.
Triple sugar iron (TSI) agar slant	A differential medium for detection of carbohydrate (glucose, lactose, sucrose) fermentation and production of hydrogen sulfide. Inoculate by stabbing the butt once with an inoculating needle and by streaking the slant. Incubate with a loose cap.	Yellow color change indicates acidification caused by carbohydrate fermentation. In the butt, glucose fermentation is detected; in the slant, lactose and sucrose fermentation is detected (includes glucose fermentation as an intermediate product). Red color change indicates alkalinization caused by lack of carbohydrate fermentation. Black color indicates hydrogen sulfide production. Results are recorded as slant/butt; A = acid (yellow), K = alkaline (red), or NC = no change.
Christensen's urea agar slant	A differential medium for detection of urease production by an organism. Inoculate by streaking heavily over the slant.	Urease-positive bacteria produce a pink-red color change in the slant and sometimes throughout the butt. Urease-negative bacteria allow the medium to remain the original yellow color.
Motility media*	A test medium for determining if an organism is motile or nonmotile. Inoculate by stabbing the center of the tube with an inoculating needle. Incubate at 35° C for most organisms; incubate at room temperature if *Listeria* is suspected.	Motile organisms migrate from the stab line, flaring out to cause turbidity in the medium. Nonmotile organisms grow only along the stab line; the surrounding medium remains clear.
Indole test media*	A test medium for detecting the ability of bacteria to produce indole as one of the degradation products of tryptophan metabolism. Inoculate, incubate 24-48 hr, then add Kovac's reagent to detect indole.	Development of a red color at the interface of the reagent and the broth within seconds after adding the reagent indicates a positive test result.

*Combination media that provide for several tests in the same tube, such as SIM (sulfide-indole-motility), MIO (motility indole ornithine), or MIL (motility indole lysine), can be purchased.

Purpose of Specific Media

Solid media in plates are used for primary isolation of bacteria from clinical specimens. This type of medium allows distribution of the specimen in such a way that *isolated colonies* develop, each representing a single bacterial cell. Some primary isolation media contain inhibitory ingredients that allow them to be *selective* for specific groups of bacteria.

MacConkey agar is selective for bacteria that can grow in the presence of bile salts, which is similar to the environment found in the intestines. A *differential* medium contains an indicator system that can distinguish different bacteria, even though both types may grow. The lactose-fermenting ability of bacteria on MacConkey agar is a differential reaction. Table 8-2 lists some of the more commonly used

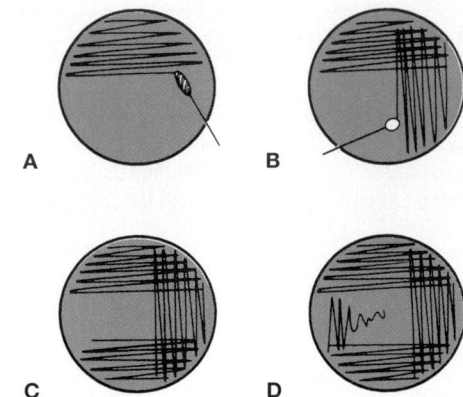

Figure 8-3 Plate inoculation and streaking method for
isolation of bacterial colonies. **A,** Inoculate with swab, covering one
fourth to one third of plate. **B,** Streak lightly, overlapping previous
area. **C,** Flame loop, allow it to cool, and streak next area. **D,** Repeat
as in **C.**

can be used to transfer inoculum material from liquid and
tissue specimens to isolation media. The same swab can be
used for inoculation of several media if the least inhibitory
medium is inoculated first and the most inhibitory medium
is inoculated last; for example, blood agar can be inoculated
first, and then MacConkey agar can be inoculated.

Between one fourth and one third of the surface of the
agar plates should be inoculated with the specimen. The
inoculum is then progressively diluted across the agar by
successive steps of streaking with a bacteriologic loop
(Figure 8-3). There are several different streaking technique
modifications, and any method that yields isolated colonies
is satisfactory. With the practice of a light touch to avoid
tearing the agar and experience in anticipating the amount
of bacterial growth that will occur, slight modifications
can be made in technique from one specimen to the next
to achieve the best isolation of colonies.

Media dispensed in tubes may be a broth or semisolid
agar, or media may be poured as a slant. Broth media can
be inoculated with a loop or an inoculating wire by touching
the side of the tube just below the surface of the medium.
Depending on the purpose of the slant medium, it may
require inoculation by stabbing the deep (or butt) portion
of the agar (e.g., triple sugar iron [TSI] slants); the slant
surface is then streaked from bottom to top (Figure 8-4).
When a semisolid medium for motility testing is inoculated,
it is important for the inoculating wire to be inserted and
removed along the same tract within the medium.

culture media, the indicated use of the media, and selective
and differential characteristics.

TECHNICIAN NOTE

Common laboratory media are optimized to support growth of many, but
not all pathogens. Occasionally, strains of common organisms such as
Staphylococcus, Streptococcus, and *Clostridium* spp. that grow very
poorly, if at all, in the laboratory are observed.

Inoculation of Media

Before media are inoculated, each tube or plate should be
labeled with a distinct identification and the date of
inoculation. Plates should be labeled on the bottom with a
waterproof marker. Most clinical specimens are collected for
culture on swabs. These swabs are used for direct inoculation
of primary isolation media. In the laboratory, a sterile swab

INCUBATION CONDITIONS

Inoculated plates are incubated in an inverted position to
prevent condensation of water on the lid. If water drops
to the agar surface, it can mix the bacterial growth rather
than allowing it to develop as isolated colonies. If tube media
have screw tops, they should be left loose during incubation.

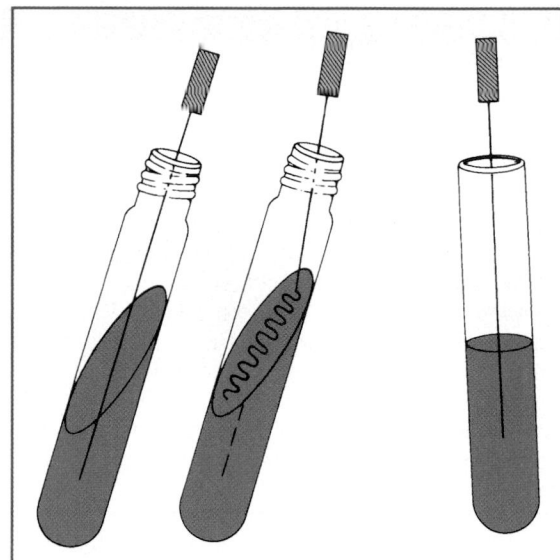

Figure 8-4 Inoculation procedure for tube media. **A,** Inoculation of agar slant and butt, such as triple sugar iron. The inoculation needle is first stabbed into the butt and then removed and streaked over the agar slant surface in a back-and-forth motion. **B,** Inoculation of motility test media. The inoculation needle is stabbed into the medium and withdrawn along the same tract.

Temperature

Cultures should be placed in incubation at an optimal temperature as quickly as possible. The majority of cultures for isolation of pathogenic bacteria are incubated at 35° C. Although optimal growth may occur at other temperatures, in most cases, alternate temperatures are more important for differentiation of bacteria than for primary isolation.

Atmosphere

Most common pathogenic bacteria are aerobes or facultative anaerobes and will grow well in an atmosphere of room air. However, oxygen is toxic to obligate anaerobic bacteria, requiring that a special culture container from which all oxygen has been removed be used for incubation. Two excellent anaerobic systems for the small laboratory are the BioBag Type A environmental chamber and the BBL GasPak anaerobic system (BD Diagnostic Systems). Each system consists of a hydrogen generator, a catalyst to facilitate the depletion of oxygen from the atmosphere by combining with the hydrogen, and a sealable container to hold these components and the culture plates. Certain bacteria—such as *Campylobacter, Brucella, Haemophilus,* and *Mycoplasma* spp.—have specialized atmospheric requirements and are best forwarded to reference laboratories.

Time

All inoculated plates should be examined after 15 to 24 hours of incubation (overnight). Most cultures will have sufficient growth for evaluation and identification at this time. Culture specimens that contained bacteria on direct microscopic examination but yield negative results after this time or specimens that may be expected to contain slow-growing bacteria should be incubated for up to 3 days before a final negative report is issued. Incubation of primary isolation plates beyond 3 days is rarely indicated unless there is reason to suspect the presence of an unusually slow-growing pathogen.

ROUTINE CULTURE SYSTEM

The majority of specimens for culture in the veterinary microbiology laboratory can be processed in a routine manner with a minimum of media. The approach presented in this section is not represented as a comprehensive culture system that will successfully isolate and identify all potentially pathogenic bacteria; rather, it is meant as a basic guideline for the veterinary technician who has the opportunity to provide a diagnostic bacteriology service within a private veterinary practice. The system is designed to be cost effective when used for routine aerobic cultures, which will usually account for 80% to 90% of culture requests. Often, the veterinarian's immediate objective is for the laboratory to characterize the isolate sufficiently to guide antimicrobial selection or to perform an antimicrobial susceptibility test rather than to pursue definitive identification. The challenge for the technician is to discern when it is better to refer a specimen to another laboratory for more sophisticated diagnostic evaluation.

Primary Isolation Media

Blood agar, containing 5% sheep blood, is the most widely used primary isolation medium because of its ability to support growth of most pathogenic bacteria. It is also a standard medium used extensively for describing colony morphologic characteristics and hemolytic patterns. MacConkey agar is also commonly used as a primary isolation medium. Although use of MacConkey agar is not always essential, it often provides significant information about bacteria and may provide presumptive identification, or at least group classification, of the isolate. If MacConkey agar is inoculated as a primary isolation medium, rather than used as a differential medium for subcultures, the identification process is often moved forward by 1 day.

In many laboratories, it is customary to include an enrichment broth as part of the primary isolation medium. One of the most common broth media used for this purpose is thioglycolate. This medium can support growth of many anaerobic or facultative anaerobic bacteria that might not be recovered on primary plates incubated aerobically.

Primary growth in a broth medium is frequently difficult to interpret. It must always be compared with a direct microscopic examination because contaminating bacteria from the environment or indigenous flora may overgrow a pathogen in the specimen. Specimens should never be cultured solely in a broth medium for primary isolation.

Further discussion of the interpretation of broth subcultures is presented later.

When specific pathogens are sought in specimens, modifications of the basic culture setup can be incorporated into the laboratory routines. Procedures that may enhance the likelihood of recovering specific pathogens are discussed later in this chapter.

Preliminary Evaluation of Cultures

Efficient evaluation of primary cultures requires considerable skill, which is acquired through experience in the microbiology laboratory. Decisions that must be made about isolated bacteria include their possible significance as pathogens, which bacteria require further identification, and what additional tests are needed. As the veterinary technician gains experience in the laboratory and becomes acquainted with common bacterial pathogens, these decisions will become less challenging. Clinically useful results usually only require that identification of bacteria is usually carried to the presumptive level by a few key characteristics rather than to a definitive identification. Only isolates considered to be clinically significant need to be identified. Identification of bacterial growth that results from environmental contamination or indigenous flora is wasted effort.

From the initial examination of primary cultures, considerable information can be obtained to help distinguish which bacteria should be characterized in further detail. The important characteristics of primary cultures to be noted include (1) the number of different types of bacteria isolated, (2) the relative number of each type, (3) the colonial morphologic characteristics of the various isolates, and (4) the changes in the media surrounding the colonies. While making the preliminary evaluation of primary cultures, the technician must keep in mind the source of the specimen. If it was obtained from a normally sterile body site (e.g., joint fluid) and was properly handled, any growth is likely to be significant. If the specimen is from a site normally colonized by microflora (e.g., intestinal tract), interpretation becomes much more difficult. In general, if there is scant aerobic growth of three or more bacteria, the result probably reflects normal flora. Most bacterial infections, other than mixed anaerobic infections, are usually caused by only one or two agents. When a specimen from an infectious process is carefully collected, growth of a single organism in nearly pure culture will often be observed. Therefore the most abundant colony type is usually the most important.

Some general guidelines for selection of significant isolates can be derived from colony morphologic characteristics, although exceptions will always occur. Usually circular, smooth, raised or convex, opaque to gray colonies with an entire edge are more likely to be significant. Large, rough, granular, irregular, spreading, or heavily pigmented colonies are likely to be insignificant unless large numbers are recovered in nearly pure culture.

Changes in the media should be carefully noted. Hemolysis in blood agar is often a good indication of a possible pathogen. Sometimes the hemolytic pattern provides adequate identification, such as the double zone of hemolysis produced by many coagulase-positive isolates of *Staphylococcus* spp. Pigment production can be an important characteristic to note on primary cultures. The differential features of MacConkey agar (i.e., ability to grow, lactose fermentation) are important bits of information that can aid in the identification of an isolate. Odors produced by bacteria are difficult to describe adequately but, after experience is gained, become another useful identifying characteristic.

The novice microbiologist may be required to rely on several differential tests for the identification of isolates. As experience is gained and confidence develops, more isolates will be recognized on the primary plates. Knowledge of the more common bacterial species to expect from a specimen (Table 8-1) will provide a differential list of bacteria to consider so that it is not necessary to face each culture as a complete unknown.

Recording, Interpreting, and Reporting Results

Although it is impossible to devise rigid rules that provide for adequate processing of all specimens, some routines are helpful for observing and recording results of cultures. A laboratory worksheet should be developed for recording all observations. These records should contain sufficient detail so that anyone who works in the laboratory can take over and complete the culture without a special briefing. A worksheet that provides adequate room for a flow chart type of illustration of culture processing and observation is easy to follow (Figure 8-5). These work records may become part of the medical record, so care should be taken to ensure that they are complete and accurate (see Chapter 33).

As an aid to interpreting culture results, the relative abundance of growth of each type of colony should be recorded. A convenient system of recording is a scale of

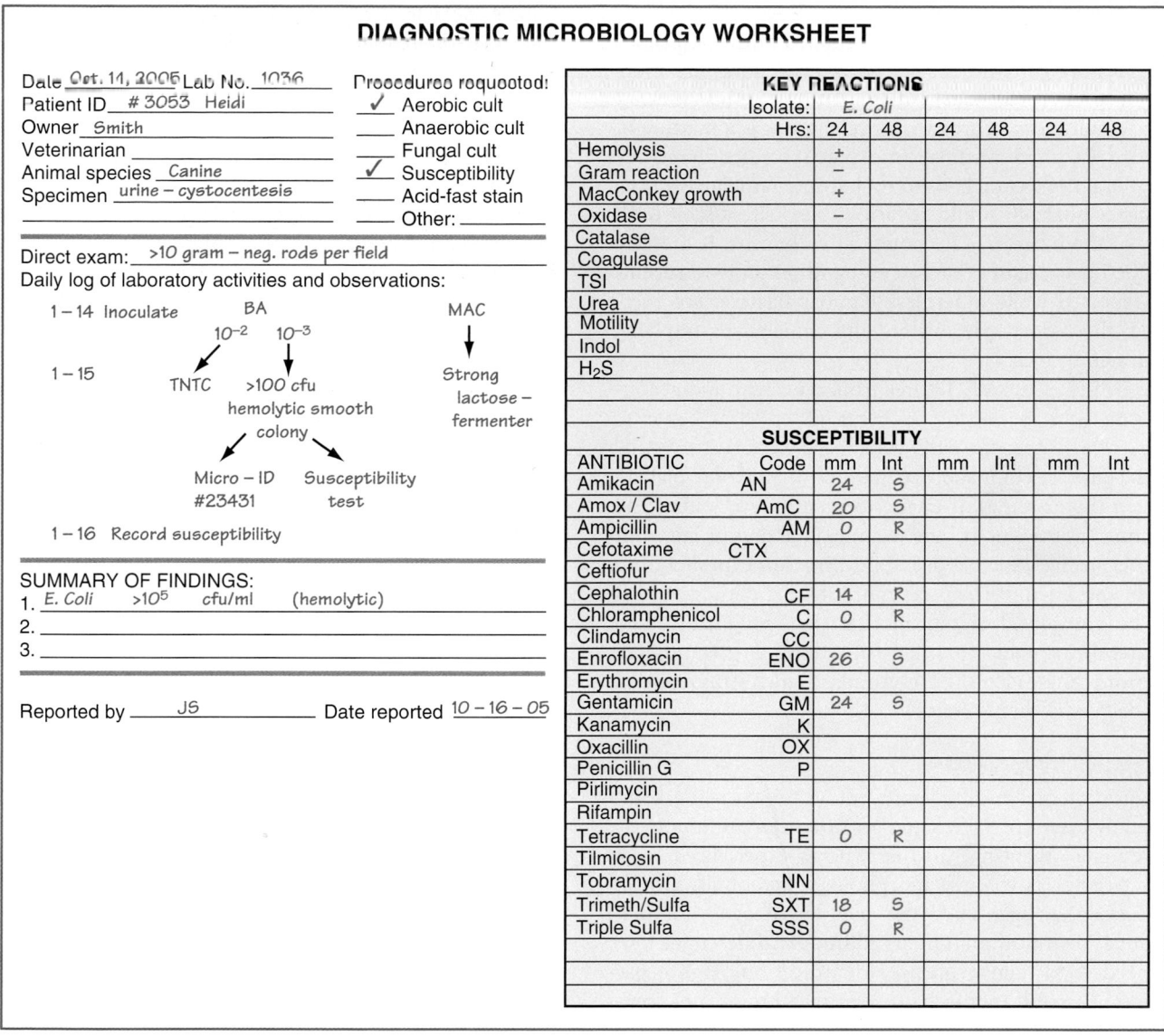

Figure 8-5 Example of a laboratory worksheet for recording results of various laboratory procedures, including microbial identification and susceptibility tests.

1+ to 4+, in which each step on the scale represents the number of quadrants of the primary culture plate in which the colony is growing. For example, if the only colonies are in the initial streak lines in which the specimen was inoculated on the plate, growth would be rated 1+. If growth is so abundant that colonies are found in the fourth quadrant (the final streak lines), growth is rated 4+. Any bacterium isolated from broth subculture, but not on primary inoculated plates, is rated 1+, regardless of the abundance of growth on the subculture plate. Bacterial cultures should not be evaluated empirically as positive or negative because this semiquantitative method helps the clinician to interpret the significance of the results. Specimens from most acute bacterial infections that have not been treated with antimicrobials will yield 3+ to 4+

growth. However, because of poor collection technique, mishandling the specimen, presampling antimicrobial therapy, or chronic infections, a smaller number of bacteria may be recovered. The clinician must decide whether these smaller numbers of bacteria are significant. If the culture is from a normally sterile body site, these culture results are often significant.

TECHNICIAN NOTE

With the advances in molecular taxonomy, many names of many bacterial species have recently been changed, and more changes are expected. A useful source of information for updates in nomenclature and cross-references to synonyms can be found on the Web at *http://www.dsmz.de/ bactnom/bactname.htm*

Indigenous Flora

Specimens cultured from sites populated with indigenous bacterial flora (often described as normal flora) are more difficult to interpret. Usually these cultures are insignificant if they result in scant growth, especially if it is a mixture of bacteria. To avoid wasting time precisely identifying the microflora, the technician should become familiar with the organisms normally found at various body sites (Table 8-3). Many of these bacteria are potential pathogens. If they are identified because of common recognition and are specifically reported while other, less familiar bacteria are overlooked, the report may mislead the clinician by implying undue significance.

Reporting results of cultures from sites with indigenous flora can be a perplexing problem. Often, it is better to specify which specific pathogens have been *excluded* by careful cultural examination, such as "no *Salmonella* isolated." Between the extremes of trying to identify everything and reporting "normal flora," the technician and clinician must agree regarding the most useful information expected from a given specimen. Perhaps certain potential pathogens that may be considered significant for the specimen should be carefully sought. In other situations a predominant bacterium can be identified or groups of organisms reported (e.g., coliforms, diphtheroids).

Identification Procedures

Identification of clinically significant bacteria is best accomplished by means of a few rapid tests that can presumptively differentiate organisms. To one who is experienced, such characteristics as colonial morphology, hemolysis, growth on MacConkey agar, and odor may be adequate for presumptive identification. Often, additional differential tests are needed for more precise identification. Figure 8-6 presents a useful approach to identification of unknown isolates when needed.

Gram's Reaction

The first differential characteristic to be considered is the reaction to *Gram's stain*. Staining with Gram's stain can be performed on thin smears of bacteria from a single colony (see Gram's Stain Procedure and Interpretation). Potassium hydroxide, 3%, may be used as an alternate and more rapid test for Gram's reaction of isolated colonies. A small drop of 3% potassium hydroxide (no larger than a colony) is dispensed on a slide, and a colony of bacteria is picked from the blood agar plate with a bacteriologic loop and mixed into the 3% potassium hydroxide. The loop is slowly and gently lifted at 5-second intervals to see whether a viscous gel is sticking to the loop. The formation of any sticky strand that can be lifted with the loop indicates a gram-negative bacterium. The reaction should appear within 20 to 30 seconds. Gram-positive organisms will diffusely mix in the 3% potassium hydroxide. Cellular morphologic

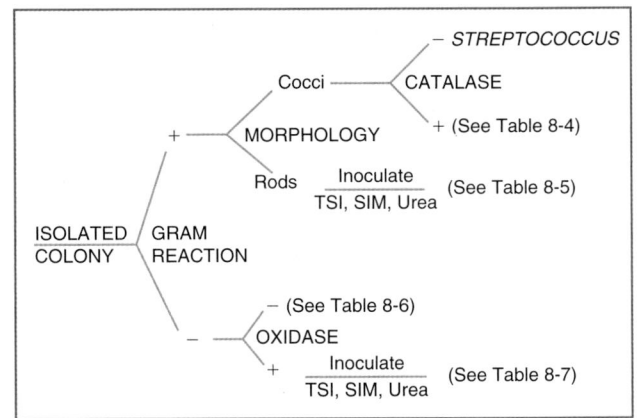

Figure 8-6 General flow chart for identification of common aerobic veterinary bacterial pathogens. *TSI*, Triple sugar iron; *SIM*, sulfide-indole-motility.

Table 8-3 INDIGENOUS FLORA

Site	Aerobes	Anaerobes
Skin, ear	*Staphylococcus, Micrococcus,* diphtheroids, and transient environmental and fecal contaminants	
Mouth, nasophyrynx	*Micrococcus, Staphylococcus, Streptococcus* (alpha and beta), *Bacillus,* coliforms, *Proteus, Pasteurella, Actinobacillus, Haemophilus,* and *Myocoplasma*	*Bacteroides, Prevotella, Porphyromonas, Fusobacterium, Actinomyces,* spirochetes, and others
Trachea, bronchi, lungs	No residents, only transient contaminants	
Stomach, small intestine	Small numbers of alpha-*Streptococcus*	*Lactobacillus*
Large intestine	*Streptococcus, Escherichia coli, Klebsiella, Enterobacter, Proteus, Enterococcus,* and others	*Clostridium, Fusobacterium, Bacteroides, Porphyromonas, Prevotella,* spirochetes, *Lactobacillus*
Vulva, prepuce	Diphtheroids, *Micrococcus, Staphylococcus,* and fecal organisms	
Conjunctiva, uterus, mammary glands	These areas may occasionally contain small numbers of insignificant bacteria.	

characteristics of the gram-positive bacteria are important differential characteristics that require careful examination of a stained smear.

TECHNICIAN NOTE

Luxuriant growth on a MacConkey agar plate is presumptive evidence of a gram-negative organism and usually does not need to be confirmed by Gram's stain.

Catalase Test

Catalase activity is an important and rapid test for differentiating *Staphylococcus* from *Streptococcus* spp. and *Erysipelothrix* spp. and *Arcanobacterium pyogenes* from other small gram-positive rods. Hydrogen peroxide (3%) is the only reagent needed and can be readily purchased from any drugstore. It should be stored in a dark bottle in the refrigerator. The *slide catalase test* is performed by picking bacteria from the center of a colony with a needle or loop and smearing the bacteria on a clean, dry slide. A drop of hydrogen peroxide is added over the bacteria and immediately observed for bubbling. Lack of bubbling is a negative test result. The order of the test procedure must not be reversed, or false-positive results may be obtained. If any blood agar is introduced into the test, it can also cause a false-positive result.

Oxidase Test

Cytochrome oxidase activity should be determined for all gram-negative bacteria except strong lactose fermenters, which will be negative. Commercial cytochrome oxidase test reagents are readily available. The reaction is supposed to be clearly visible within a few seconds, but with some reagents, the reaction may be delayed for up to 2 minutes for *Pasteurella* and *Actinobacillus* spp. A heavy inoculum must be used for accurate testing. A wooden stick or platinum loop should be used to pick colonies for testing, because trace amounts of iron from other loops can cause false-positive results.

Presumptive Identification

When Gram's reaction, cellular morphologic characteristics, and catalase and oxidase results have been determined,

the bacteria can be tentatively grouped, and differential tests can be selected as indicated in Figure 8-6 for identification.

Isolates of *Streptococcus* are usually characterized by the type of hemolysis they produce. Beta-hemolytic *Streptococcus* isolates are usually considered to be potential pathogens. Alpha-hemolytic and nonhemolytic *Streptococcus* isolates usually originate from normal flora of skin and mucous membranes and are not considered significant unless they are obtained from normally sterile sites.

Isolates of *Staphylococcus* should be differentiated from those of *Micrococcus* (Table 8-4), which are considered to be nonpathogenic. Glucose-fermenting ability, determined in TSI agar slants, can be used for differentiation of these genera. If a double zone of hemolysis is observed on the blood agar plate, the bacterium can be identified as a coagulase-positive *Staphylococcus* without need for further testing. All other *Staphylococcus* isolates should be tested for coagulase activity because coagulase activity correlates with pathogenicity. Speciation of coagulase-positive and coagulase-negative *Staphylococcus* spp. may be attempted in special cases, if desired, by using a range of tests or commercial identification kits.

The small gram-positive rods can be differentiated by inoculating TSI, urea, and sulfide-indole-motility (SIM) medium. The results of these tests, as well as colonial morphology and catalase activity, can identify the isolate (Table 8-5). Individual characteristics of the important pathogens in this group will be discussed later.

Most gram-negative, oxidase-negative bacteria are members of the Enterobacteriaceae family. These bacteria are reactive in biochemical tests and can be identified by one of several different systems. The most rapid and economical methods for differentiating the Enterobacteriaceae family members are the commercially available packaged multitest systems. These systems are discussed later. A few other organisms that are oxidase negative may be isolated infrequently. The most common reason for nonenteric oxidase-negative results is a false-negative oxidase test result. When such results are suspected, further differentiation of oxidase-negative bacteria, as shown in Table 8-6, is necessary.

The most frequently isolated oxidase-positive, gram-negative bacteria of veterinary importance can be differentiated by using three tubes of media (TSI, urea, SIM) as shown in Table 8-7.

Table 8-4 DIFFERENTIATION OF GRAM-POSITIVE, CATALASE-POSITIVE COCCI

Organism	Hemolysis	Hyaluronidase	Glucose Fermentation	Coagulase
Staphylococcus aureus	+*	+	+	+
Staphylococcus intermedius†	+*	−	+	+
Staphylococcus coagulase-negative sp.	±		+	−
Micrococcus	−		−	−

*Double zones of complete and incomplete hemolysis are frequently observed.
†*S. intermedius* is positive for pyrrolidonyl arylamidase activity when PYR disks are used; this quickly differentiates it from *S. aureus*.

Table 8-5 DIFFERENTIATION OF SMALL, NON–SPORE-FORMING GRAM-POSITIVE RODS

Organism	Motility (22° C)	Catalase	Hydrogen Sulfide in TSI	Urease	Hemolysis	Colony Morphologic Characteristics
Listeria monocytogenes	+	+	–	–	Complete	Very small
Erysipelothrix rhusiopathiae	–	–	+	–	Slow, greenish	Very small
Arcanobacterium pyogenes	–	–	–	–	Complete	Very small
Corynebacterium renale	–	+	–	+	V	Medium size, entire
Corynebacterium pseudotuberculosis	–	+	–	+ (w)	V	Dry, grainy white
Rhodococcus equi	–	+	–	+ (d)	–	Large, mucoid, pink
Other diphtheroids	–	+	–	V	V	V

d, Delayed, may require up to 2 weeks; *TSI*, triple sugar iron (agar); *V*, variable results; *w*, weak.

Table 8-6 DIFFERENTIATION OF GRAM-NEGATIVE, OXIDASE-NEGATIVE BACTERIA

	Growth on MacConkey	TSI	Motility	Identification Method
Enterobacteriaceae	+	A/A, K/A	+*	MicroID (Remel) or API 20E (Bio Mérieux, Inc.)
Pasteurella, Actinobacillus, Mannheimia	–	A/A, A/NC	–	See Table 8-4†
Pseudomonas	+	K/NC	+	
Acinetobacter	+ (w)	K/NC	–	

A, Acid; *K*, alkaline; *NC*, no change; *TSI*, total sugar iron (agar); *w*, weak.
Klebsiella is a nonmotile.
†Negative oxidase results are caused by very weak reactions.

Table 8-7 DIFFERENTIATION OF GRAM-NEGATIVE, OXIDASE-POSITIVE BACTERIA

Organism	Glucose Fermentation in TSI Agar	Growth on MacConkey Agar	Motility	Hemolysis	Urease	Indole
Aeromonas spp.	+	+	+	+	–	+
Actinobacillus spp.	+	±	–	+*	–	–
Mannheimia haemolytica	+	±	–	+*	–	–
Pasteurella multocida	+	–	–	–	–	+
Pasteurella spp.	+	–	–	–	±	–
Pseudomonas aeruginosa	–	+	+	+	±	–
Pseudomonas spp.	–	+	+	V	V	–
Bordetella bronchiseptica	–	+ (w)	+	–	+	–
Moraxella bovis	–	–	–	±	–	–
Moraxella spp.	–	–	–	–	–	–
Brucella canis	–	–	–	–	+	–

TSI, Total sugar iron; *V*, variable; *w*, weak.
*Hemolysis under the colony.

Definitive Identification

The identification procedures discussed in this chapter are presumptive methods. Definitive identification of some isolates may require extensive testing. The cost of such identification in time, media, and specialized techniques is usually not justifiable in a small practice laboratory.

Unusual isolates should be forwarded to a referral laboratory for further identification. The isolate should be subcultured to an agar slant medium that does not contain a fermentable carbohydrate, or it should be heavily inoculated onto a swab. The swab can be transported in a transport medium, such as Amies transport medium. Do not attempt to ship agar plates. Invariably, they become contaminated and overgrown, dehydrated, or broken.

Commercial Identification Kits

Commercial development of kit systems for identification of bacteria has been one of the most important advances in clinical bacteriology. These systems provide a cost-effective method for identification of bacteria in low-volume laboratories. Most kits consist of a number of test compartments arranged in a compact unit. The systems generally involve the use of microtechnique tests in various types of media systems. They may include compartments of solid agar, dehydrated broth, substrate or reagent disks, and supplementary conventional tests. All compartments are inoculated with organisms from an isolated colony or colonies. After the specified period of incubation and the addition of required reagents, the results are recorded as positive or negative for each test. For many of the systems, these reactions have variously weighted values so that the positive results will produce a unique profile number for each combination of positive and negative results. Most systems provide profile directories or registers for identification of the isolate most likely to produce the set of observed reactions.

It is advantageous for the low-volume laboratory to use these systems because they are usually more cost effective than attempting to maintain a large inventory of conventional media. They have a reasonable shelf life (6 to 18 months) and require minimum storage space because of the compact construction. Accuracy is better than that achieved with conventional media in most small laboratories, because most reactions are easy to interpret and results can be decoded more rapidly compared with sorting through conventional identification tables. Finally, depending on the specific system, most bacteria can be identified within 4 to 24 hours after isolation.

It is essential that the manufacturer's directions and precautions be carefully observed or misidentification will occur. If the system is limited to oxidase-negative enteric bacteria, only those organisms should be inoculated. Other organisms can still yield a profile number, which will result in an incorrect identification. Problems can also arise from inoculation with an older culture, improper concentration of inoculum, or mixed cultures. As experience is gained, accuracy will be increased.

> **✎ TECHNICIAN NOTE**
>
> Identification kits can only correctly identify organisms listed in their database. New or rare organisms are likely to be either incorrectly identified or not identified at all.

When one of these systems is selected, factors to consider include the ease of inoculation, manipulations required to add reagents, the availability of interpretive charts or numeric coding devices, and the database used in development of profile registers. Often, it is difficult to discover whether significant numbers of veterinary pathogens are included in the databases for there to be a reasonable probability of correct identification of unique veterinary pathogens. The most beneficial use of these systems is the identification of members of the Enterobacteriaceae family (Box 8-1). All enteric identification systems have essentially the same degree of accuracy and reliability of performance. The systems that seem to have gained widest acceptance in veterinary bacteriology include API 20E (BioMérieux, Inc.), MicroID (Remel), and Enterotube II (BD Diagnostic Systems). They provide excellent results.

Several packaged kit systems are marketed for identification of bacteria other than Enterobacteriaceae (Box 8-1). Although these systems may provide more definitive identifications of some organisms, they have limited usefulness in small veterinary laboratories. Presumptive identification methods outlined in this chapter are frequently adequate.

The identification kits for yeast and anaerobes are useful for large-volume laboratories, but usually, the need for them in the small laboratory is not adequate to be cost effective.

SPECIAL CULTURE PROCEDURES

Blood Cultures

The detection of viable bacteria in an animal's blood has considerable diagnostic and prognostic importance. Blood cultures are indicated for fever of unknown origin; suspected bacteremia associated with endocarditis, arthritis, or meningitis; and neonatal septicemias. Blood cultures should be obtained from dogs that have antibodies to *Brucella canis* to aid in confirmation of the diagnosis.

> **✎ TECHNICIAN NOTE**
>
> Special care must be taken to avoid contaminating blood cultures with skin microflora because some of these same organisms are frequently associated with significant bacteremia (usually <10 bacteria/ml of blood). Blood culture systems are not designed to differentiate small numbers of contaminants from bacteremia.

Special care must be taken to avoid contamination of blood cultures with skin microflora. The venipuncture site should be decontaminated by using surgical scrubbing procedures (see Chapter 22) and should not be palpated after preparation unless a sterile glove is used. Blood can be obtained by using a syringe and needle or a closed-vacuum bottle system. Often, the concentration of bacteria in blood is too low to detect by direct inoculation of plate media. Therefore inoculation of commercially available blood culture media bottles is recommended. Ideally, a sample of 5 to 10 ml of blood should be obtained for culture. Blood samples in anticoagulants, such as heparin and ethylenediaminetetraacetic acid (EDTA), are not acceptable for culture because of the poor survival of some bacteria in the presence of these anticoagulants.

Blood culture bottles should be incubated at 35° C to 37° C for at least 7 days and examined daily for macroscopic evidence of growth. Positive cultures can be recognized by one or more of the following characteristics: turbidity, gas bubbles, fluffy or compact colonies, and hemolysis of the blood. When growth is observed, smears and subcultures on plate media should be prepared with Gram's stain for examination and identification of the organism. Negative-appearing blood culture broths should be subcultured in blinded fashion before being discarded and reported as negative. Blood cultures in which attempts to isolate *Brucella* spp. have been made should be incubated for 2 to 4 weeks before being discarded as negative.

Urine Cultures

Urine is an excellent growth medium for many bacteria because it contains electrolytes, water-soluble vitamins, residual amounts of glucose, and various nitrogenous compounds. Therefore careful attention must be given to proper collection and handling of urine for culture, or a small and insignificant number of bacteria can rapidly multiply to significant numbers. Urine specimens for culturing can be collected in three ways: free catch, catheterization, or cystocentesis (see Chapter 3). The distal urethra and genitalia are colonized with microflora that contaminate free-catch and catheterization specimens. If the skin has been adequately prepared for cystocentesis and the needle does not come in contact with any abdominal organ other than the bladder, any bacteria isolated from the specimen should be significant. Cultures should be set up within 2 hours of collection to reduce overgrowth with insignificant bacteria that may contaminate urine specimens. If cultures cannot be established within 2 hours, the sample must be refrigerated to slow the bacterial growth. Refrigeration begins to fail after 18 to 24 hours. Therefore the best method for identifying urinary tract infections is to establish cultures as soon as possible.

The use of blood agar and MacConkey agar as selective and differential isolation media is recommended for the culture of all urine specimens. There is no need for broth medium for enrichment culturing. The bacteriologic examination of urine specimens collected by methods other than cystocentesis should provide an estimate of the number of microorganisms per milliliter of urine as an aid to interpreting the results. This can be accomplished by inoculating the blood agar plate with a standard dilution loop calibrated to deliver approximately 0.001 ml (Figure 8-7). Each colony that grows represents 10^3 organisms/ml in the specimen; therefore the number of colonies is multiplied by 1000 to obtain the concentration of organisms in the specimen. The number of bacteria can also be estimated through direct microscopic examination of a Gram-stained smear of uncentrifuged urine. If one or more bacteria per oil immersion field are observed, usually more than 10^5 organisms/ml should be present in cultures. If more than two types of bacteria are isolated, a second specimen should be collected

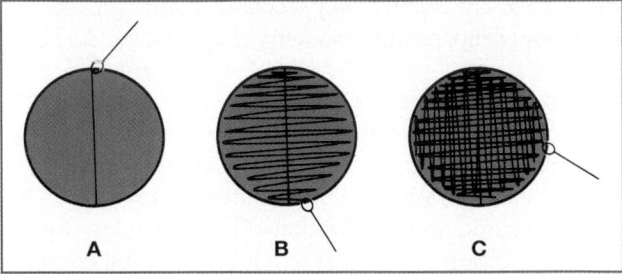

Figure 8-7 Procedure for inoculating media for semi-quantitative bacterial colony counts when culturing urine. **A,** Primary inoculation with calibrated loop. **B,** Streak at right angles to primary inoculation. **C,** Streak at right angles to previous streak.

and cultured to distinguish a mixed infection from contamination or mishandling of the specimen. Bacterial counts can be low because of improper handling of the specimen, dilution from forced fluid therapy, or cystocentesis samples from patients with urethritis that has not become established as a concomitant cystitis.

📋 TECHNICIAN NOTE

The following guidelines can be used for interpretation of urine cultures:

- For a single species, more than 10^5 bacteria/ml indicates significant bacteria.
- Between 10^3 and 10^5 bacteria/ml suggests infection if the urine has been properly collected and neutrophils are present.
- Fewer than 10^3 bacteria/ml suggests contamination or mishandling of the specimen. If there is doubt about interpretation of a colony count, the culture should be repeated with a second specimen.

COMMON BACTERIAL SPECIES

The bacterial pathogens frequently associated with many infectious processes are listed in Table 8-1. Some of the colony morphologic, growth, and identifying characteristics of these bacteria are listed in Table 8-8. Additional details are given in the following discussion of special isolation and identification techniques. Clinically important characteristics are noted.

GRAM-POSITIVE COCCI

Staphylococcus *Species*

Staphylococcus spp. are catalase-positive cocci that occur in grapelike clusters. They are frequently isolated from pyogenic lesions, such as wounds, dermatitis, otitis, mastitis, cystitis, and osteomyelitis. They are usually divided into coagulase-positive and coagulase-negative groups. The coagulase-positive species, *S. aureus* and *S. intermedius*, are more important pathogens, and the others are usually considered to be less pathogenic. One of the most important

Table 8-8 IDENTIFYING CHARACTERISTICS OF COMMON VETERINARY BACTERIAL PATHOGENS

	Blood Agar	MacConkey Agar	Other Characteristics
GRAM-POSITIVE			
Staphylococcus	Smooth, glistening, white to yellow pigmented colonies	No growth	Catalase-positive glucose fermenter; double-zone hemolysis usually indicates coagulase positive; coagulase activity is a useful differential test
Streptococcus	Small, glistening colonies; hemolysis	No growth except some enterococci	Catalase-negative, usually identified by type of hemolysis; beta-hemolytic strains more likely to be pathogens; others are often part of flora; streptococcus agalactiae CAMP-positive
Arcanobacterium pyogenes	Small, hemolytic, streplike colonies	No growth	Catalase negative; slow growth, often requiring 48 hr for distinct colonies; growth enhanced in candle jar
Corynebacterium pseudotuberculosis	Slow-growing, opaque, dry crumbly colonies; usually hemolytic	No growth	Catalase positive; weak urease positive
Corynebacterium renale	Small, smooth, glistening colonies (24 hr); become opaque and dry later	No growth	Catalase positive; urease positive
Rhodococcus equi	Small, moist, white (24 hr); become large, pink colonies; no hemolysis	No growth	Catalase positive; delayed urease positive
Listeria monocytogenes	Small, hemolytic, glistening colonies	No growth	Catalase positive; motile at room temperature
Erysipelothrix rhusiopathiae	Small colonies after 48 hr; greenish (alpha) hemolysis	No growth	Catalase negative; hydrogen sulfide positive
Nocardia	Slow-growing, small, dry, granular, white to orange colonies	No growth	Partially acid fast; colonies tenaciously adhere to media
Actinomyces	Slow growing, small, rough, nodular white colonies	No growth	Require increase carbon dioxide or anaerobic incubation; not acid fast
Clostridium	Variable, round, ill-defined, irregular colonies; usually hemolytic	No growth	Obligate anaerobes
Bacillus	Variable, large, rough, dry or mucoid colonies	No growth	Usually hemolytic; large rods with endospores
GRAM-NEGATIVE			
Escherichia coli	Large, gray, smooth, mucoid colonies; hemolysis variable	Hot pink to red colonies; red cloudiness in media	Hemolysis frequently associated with virulence
Klebsiella pneumoniae	Large, mucoid, sticky, whitish colonies; not hemolytic	Large, mucoid, pink colonies	Nonmotile; require biochemical tests to differentiate from Enterobacter
Proteus	Frequently swarming without distinct colonies	Colorless; limited swarming	
Other enterics	Gray to white, smooth, mucoid colonies	Colorless colonies	Biochemical tests for identification; serotyping indicated for Salmonella
Pseudomonas	Irregular, spreading, grayish colonies; variable hemolysis; may show a metallic sheen	Colorless, irregular colonies	Oxidase positive; fruity odor; may produce yellow greenish soluble pigment in clear media
Bordetella bronchiseptica	Very small, circular dew-drop colonies; variable hemolysis	Small, colorless colonies	May require 48 hr for distinct colonies; oxidase positive; rapid urease positive; citrate positive
Brucella canis	Very small, circular, pin-point colonies after 48-72 hr, not hemolytic	No growth	Oxidase positive; catalase positive; urease positive
Moraxella	Round, translucent, grayish white colonies; variable hemolysis	No growth	Oxidase and catalase positive; often nonreactive in routine biochemical tests; colonies may pit media
Actinobacillus	Round, translucent colonies; variable hemolysis	Variable growth; colorless colonies	Glucose fermenter, non-motile; urease positive; sticky colonies
Mannheimia haemolytica	Round, gray, smooth colonies; hemolysis under the colony	Variable growth; colorless colonies	Glucose fermenter in TSI; weak oxidase positive
Pasteurella multocida	Gray, mucoid, round to coalescing colonies; no hemolysis	No growth	Glucose fermenter in TSI; weak oxidase and indole positive

TSI, Triple sugar iron (agar).

identifying characteristics that should be noted is the development of a double zone of hemolysis (an inner zone of complete hemolysis and a second zone of incomplete hemolysis). This is a common identifying characteristic of most coagulase-positive isolates from animals. Mannitol fermentation is not a reliable correlate of coagulase activity in staphylococcal isolates from animals. Because of a high incidence of acquired antimicrobial resistance, these organisms should be tested for antimicrobial susceptibility.

Streptococcus *Species*

Streptococcus spp. are catalase-negative cocci that occur singly, in pairs, or in short chains. Chain formation is more easily demonstrated in broth cultures. *Streptococcus* is the most common bacterial pathogen of the horse and can be found to cause pyogenic infections and mastitis in all species of animals. However, each species tends to be rather host specific. Therefore the streptococcal pathogens of humans rarely cause infections in animals, and animals are usually not reservoirs of human pathogens. Some species cause specific diseases. *Streptococcus equi* ssp. *equi* is the cause of strangles in horses. *Streptococcus agalactiae* is an important cause of bovine mastitis. It can be identified by the CAMP test. Definitive biochemical and serologic (Lancefield typing) testing is usually not clinically important. For clinical interpretation, it is important to evaluate the hemolysis produced on blood agar. Beta-hemolysis (complete clearing) usually correlates well with potential pathogenicity; alpha-hemolysis (incomplete greenish discoloring) and gamma-hemolysis (nonhemolytic) are usually indications of normal flora of skin and mucous membranes. However, when isolated in nearly pure culture from normally sterile body sites, these organisms can be considered to be clinically significant. Susceptibility to antimicrobials is usually predictable, which means antimicrobial susceptibility testing may be an unnecessary expense.

The enteric group D streptococci have been renamed as *Enterococcus* spp. Urinary tract infections are the most common presentation of these organisms; and *Enterococcus* spp. occasionally infect wounds and cause bacteremia. They are emerging as significant nosocomial agents and are particularly troublesome because they are likely to be resistant to many antimicrobials.

ANAEROBIC COCCI

Anaerobic cocci belong to the genera *Peptococcus* and *Peptostreptococcus*. When isolated, these agents are usually associated with mixed anaerobic infections.

GRAM-POSITIVE RODS

Spore Formers

Bacillus spp. are common contaminants isolated in the laboratory. They are ubiquitous in soil, water, air, and dust. They are large spore-forming rods that usually grow as large, rough, granular, or spreading colonies. They are usually hemolytic. Occasionally, strains of *Bacillus* will be isolated that react as if they are gram-negative and oxidase-positive. However, they can be identified by the presence of spores in stained smears. *Bacillus anthracis* (the agent that causes anthrax) is the important pathogenic species. It is extremely virulent for humans. *Do not attempt to culture it.*

Clostridium spp. are large, spore-forming anaerobic rods. The pathogenic species are noted for their potent toxins and extensive destruction of tissue. Infections may be accompanied by an accumulation of gas (emphysema) in the tissues. Laboratory diagnosis of the toxic diseases (tetanus, botulism, enterotoxemia) and differentiation of the infectious diseases (blackleg, malignant edema, bacillary hemoglobinuria, etc.) require the assistance of reference diagnostic laboratories. Often a Gram-stained smear is useful for ruling out clostridial disease or indicating it as a possibility. *Clostridium perfringens* is occasionally isolated from deep wounds with extensive tissue necrosis, such as compound fractures. The bacterium requires an anaerobic atmosphere for growth and frequently produces a double zone of hemolysis.

C. perfringens is also associated with enteritis and diarrhea in dogs. In some cases, the presence of enterotoxigenic strains of *C. perfringens* can be presumptively identified in fecal smears by evaluating the smears for the presence of increased bacterial spores because sporulation is associated with the release of enterotoxin. Spores appear as unstained, small, oval structures and are usually surrounded by a halo of stained bacterial cells unless a specific spore stain is applied.

Small Rods

Corynebacterium spp. are small, club-shaped rods that tend to occur in palisades or in an angular arrangement because of their "snapping" division. Colonies are usually quite small at 24 hours but continue to enlarge and vary markedly by species. Most species are catalase positive. *Arcanobacterium pyogenes* (previously called *Actinomyces pyogenes*) produces a small pinpoint colony, hemolysis, and a negative catalase reaction. Cellular morphologic characteristics must be evaluated carefully to differentiate it from *Streptococcus* spp. It is the most common pyogenic agent in ruminants. *Rhodococcus equi* is a cause of pneumonia and abscesses in foals. Morphologically, individual cells are coccobacillary and larger than other those of *Corynebacterium* organisms. *Corynebacterium pseudotuberculosis* causes chronic abscesses in goats and sheep. The *Corynebacterium renale* group causes pyelonephritis and cystitis in cows. There are many other *Corynebacterium* spp. that are nonpathogenic commensals of the skin; they are frequently referred to collectively as diphtheroids.

Listeria monocytogenes is a small, non–spore-forming rod that is catalase positive. It is the only small gram-positive rod that is motile at room temperature. It is an infrequent cause of abortion in large animals and septicemia in young animals. In ruminants, it causes an encephalitis known as *circling disease*. The bacteria localize in the pons and medulla (brainstem). Cultures from other parts of the brain may be negative. Isolation may require specific selective and enrichment techniques. The brain is stored in a refrigerator and cultured weekly for up to 12 weeks before the results are considered negative.

Erysipelothrix rhusiopathiae is a pleomorphic rod that is usually slender and small. The colony is small, and an incomplete, greenish hemolysis (alpha like) is produced. The cellular morphologic characteristics must be carefully evaluated to differentiate it from *Streptococcus* spp. because both are catalase negative. A definitive characteristic that differentiates it from other gram-positive rods is the production of hydrogen sulfide. *E. rhusiopathiae* is most commonly encountered as a cause of septicemic or arthritic disease of pigs, but it is occasionally a cause of endocarditis in dogs.

Filamentous Rods

The Actinomycetaceae family contains several clinically important bacteria that are distinguished by forming branching, filamentous gram-positive rods. Most *Actinomyces* spp. are anaerobic bacteria that may tolerate low levels of oxygen. Therefore some species can be isolated in a candle jar, but the most efficient isolation can be achieved with an anaerobic system. *Actinomyces* spp. colonies are slow to develop, requiring up to 5 days, and are usually raised and irregular in shape. When isolated, they are usually recovered from pyogranulomatous lesions of soft tissue, pyothoraces, or osteomyelitis. *Nocardia* spp. are partially acid fast, which means a modified staining procedure must be used to differentiate them from *Actinomyces* spp. In place of the acid-alcohol decolorizer, only an acid decolorizer is used to demonstrate acid fastness. *Nocardia* spp. are aerobic bacteria with colonies usually appearing after 2 to 5 days of incubation. The colonies are rough and have a dry, granular texture. They adhere tenaciously to the media. *Nocardia* spp. are occasionally isolated from pyothoraces and wounds. They may be serious mastitis pathogens in some dairy herds. *Dermatophilus congolensis* is another branching, filamentous bacterium. It often has a beaded appearance with transverse and longitudinal divisions. It is an uncommon cause of skin infections of horses and ruminants. The organism can be demonstrated in smears of pus from under the elevated scabs containing tufts of hair. *Streptomyces* spp. are aerobic, filamentous bacteria that are not acid fast. They are abundant in soil and may be isolated as contaminants.

Anaerobes

Anaerobic, gram-positive, non–spore-forming rods belong to the genera *Bifidobacterium*, *Eubacterium*, and *Propionibacterium*. If definitive identification of these organisms is needed, culture specimens should be sent to a reference diagnostic laboratory. They are usually isolated in mixed cultures from pyogenic lesions.

ACID-FAST BACTERIA

Mycobacteria are mostly small, short rods but are occasionally pleomorphic. They stain poorly with Gram's stain but are acid fast. These bacteria are rarely isolated in veterinary practice laboratories because special procedures and media are usually required. However, preparation of an acid-fast stained impression smear can be a useful diagnostic procedure for making a presumptive diagnosis of mycobacterial infection. Positive findings are significant; however, negative findings have limited predictive value. *Mycobacterium avium* ssp. *paratuberculosis* may be demonstrated in acid-fast stained smears prepared from intestinal mucosa or mesenteric lymph nodes of ruminants. *Mycobacterium avium* infection of birds can frequently be confirmed by examination of acid-fast smears prepared from the liver or intestinal mucosa. Occasionally, abundant acid-fast organisms can be demonstrated in the feces.

Isolation of the zoonotic agents of tuberculosis, *Mycobacterium bovis* and *Mycobacterium tuberculosis*, should not be attempted in a clinic laboratory. Infrequently, a rapidgrowing *Mycobacterium* sp. may be isolated from a case of bovine mastitis. The colonies will usually appear at 3 to 5 days of incubation. These organisms should be forwarded to a reference laboratory for definitive identification.

GRAM-NEGATIVE BACTERIA

The Enterobacteriaceae family of bacteria is the largest group of potential pathogens and the most frequently isolated bacteria. The normal habitat of these organisms is the digestive tract and soil; therefore they will usually grow on MacConkey agar and are frequently insignificant contaminants of specimens. They are small gram-negative rods, with some pleomorphism. Some of the common identifying characteristics include oxidase negativity, glucose fermentation, and motility (except *Klebsiella* spp.). Genus and species identification requires numerous biochemical tests, and serotyping is frequently needed to identify pathogenic strains. Acquired antimicrobial resistance from R factors (plasmids) is common in this family of bacteria, making antimicrobial susceptibility testing a necessary clinical evaluation of isolates.

Most non-Enterobacteriaceae, gram-negative bacteria are oxidase positive, and growth on MacConkey agar is variable.

Coliforms

Escherichia coli can frequently be presumptively identified by the strong lactose fermentation reaction it produces on MacConkey agar. Strains causing tissue infections and cystitis are frequently hemolytic. *E. coli* is frequently associated with diarrhea in neonates (especially pigs, calves, and lambs). The pathogenic strains causing diarrhea are best identified by genotyping and other specialized laboratory testing, such as use of the *Escherichia coli* K99 test kit (Pilitest, VMRD, Inc.). However, presumptive evidence of *E. coli* involvement in diarrhea (scours) can be obtained by Gram staining a smear taken from small intestinal mucosa shortly after the death of the animal. If a large number (>25) of gram-negative rods are observed in each oil immersion field, it is a strong indication that *E. coli* is a cause of diarrhea. *Klebsiella* spp. and *Enterobacter* spp. are occasionally involved in infections of the respiratory and urinary tracts and in mastitis. They are becoming more important in veterinary medicine as superinfecting agents after antimicrobial therapy.

Salmonella *Species*

Salmonella spp. can cause diarrhea and septicemia in all animals and in humans. When feces are to be cultured, selective and enrichment media should be used to increase the probability of successful isolation of *Salmonella*. Hektoen enteric agar and selenite enrichment broth (Table 8-2) are recommended (brilliant green agar and XLD agar are also commonly used selective media). The enrichment broth should be subcultured to both MacConkey and Hektoen enteric agar. Non–lactose-fermenting colonies can rapidly be screened with *Salmonella* polyvalent O antiserum to identify them. For the purpose of defining the epidemiology of salmonellosis outbreaks, the isolates should be forwarded to a reference laboratory for serotyping.

Proteus *Species*

Proteus spp. are frequently isolated as specimen contaminants or secondary invaders. They are important pathogens of the urinary tract. Related genera of bacteria that do not swarm on blood agar are *Morganella* and *Providencia*, and they can be readily identified by using kits. The swarming *Proteus* spp. sometimes interfere with isolation of other organisms. This problem can be solved by using phenylethyl alcohol (PEA) blood agar plates. *Proteus* and other gram-negative organisms will be inhibited, providing easier isolation of gram-positive organisms.

Other Enteric Organisms

There are many other members of the Enterobacteriaceae family—including *Serratia, Citrobacter, Edwardsiella, Enterobacter, Pantoea,* and *Hafnia* spp.—which are infrequently isolated. Careful clinical evaluation is necessary to determine their significance. Often a repeated culture helps confirm the significance of isolation.

Aeromonas *Species*

Aeromonas spp. are oxidase-positive rods that grow on MacConkey agar. They are commonly found in soil, water, and sewage and frequently infect aquatic animals. They are infrequently a cause of septicemia in terrestrial animals.

Actinobacillus

Actinobacillus spp. are oxidase-positive, small rods that usually grow on MacConkey agar. The colony morphologic characteristics are similar to those of *Pasteurella* spp.

Actinobacillus equuli is the most frequently isolated species. It produces a very sticky colony. It is frequently the cause of septicemic infections in foals. It can be isolated from most horses as part of the mucosal flora but is generally only an opportunistic pathogen in older horses.

Pasteurella *Species*

Pasteurella spp. are usually associated with respiratory tract infections in most animals. In cats, they are frequently recovered from abscesses. They are small, oxidase-positive coccobacilli. *Pasteurella multocida* produces a characteristic musty odor. Identification can be aided by noting the typically weak glucose fermentation reaction in a TSI tube. *Pasteurella* spp. tend to be nonreactive in most commercial identification kit systems and may be misidentified. Hemolytic strains, previously known as *P. haemolytica*, have been renamed *Mannheimia haemolytica* for bovine respiratory isolates, and some ovine strains are now called *P. trehalosi*. Antimicrobial resistance is a growing problem in isolates from food animals, indicating a need to perform susceptibility tests.

Haemophilus *Species*

Haemophilus spp. are often part of the normal flora of mucous membranes. A few species are important pathogens, usually of the respiratory system. They are small coccobacilli that require specially enriched media for growth. They may grow as satellite colonies around *Staphylococcus* spp. on blood agar. In addition to the nutritional growth requirements, an increased concentration of carbon dioxide is necessary. These bacteria are very susceptible to antibiotics and environmental stress factors, such as drying; therefore specimens must be collected and handled carefully or isolation will be unsuccessful.

Pseudomonas *Species*

Pseudomonas spp. are common soil and water bacteria. They are usually considered to be opportunistic pathogens of wounds and otitis. Infrequently, they are isolated from the respiratory and urinary tracts. There are many species, but *Pseudomonas aeruginosa* is the most common pathogen. It produces water-soluble yellow-green pigments that diffuse into the medium, and it has a distinctive odor that aids in recognition. Most isolates are quite resistant to antimicrobials and should routinely be tested for susceptibility.

Bordetella *Bronchiseptica*

Bordetella bronchiseptica is a small coccobacillus that is frequently recovered from respiratory tract infections of dogs and is emerging as an important respiratory pathogen of cats. It is associated with atrophic rhinitis in pigs and is infrequently isolated from respiratory tract infections of other animals. Colonies are slow to develop and may only be pinpointed after 48 hours. Growth occurs on MacConkey agar. It is oxidase positive, urease positive (often within 4 hours), and citrate positive.

Brucella *Species*

Brucella spp. are very small coccobacilli that are usually associated with reproductive failure: abortion and infertility. Some species require increased carbon dioxide for growth, however, *Brucella canis* can be isolated in an aerobic atmosphere. Growth is slow, often requiring 3 to 7 days for colonies to be detectable. Suspected *Brucella* isolates should be sent to a reference laboratory for definitive identification because of the regulatory and zoonotic importance of these agents.

Other Gram-Negative Rods

Many gram-negative bacteria have limited or undetermined clinical importance. Included are bacteria such as *Moraxella, Acinetobacter, Neisseria,* and *Branhamella* spp. and related pleomorphic coccobacilli. These organisms are commonly found as part of the flora of mucous membranes and are usually secondary, opportunistic pathogens. They are relatively nonreactive in most conventional biochemical tests. Thus identification is usually difficult, even for reference diagnostic laboratories.

Anaerobes

The gram-negative anaerobes (*Bacteroides, Porphyromonas, Prevotella, Fusobacterium* spp.) are frequently involved in mixed infections in abscesses and necrotic tissue. They are normally found in the digestive tract, so infections resulting from contamination of tissues with mucous membrane flora or intestinal contents frequently contain these organisms. If obligate anaerobes are isolated, evaluation of the cellular morphologic characteristics provides adequate clinical information. Species identification is rarely important. Taxonomic advances have resulted in the reclassification of some former *Bacteroides* spp. into the genera *Dichelobacter, Porphyromonas,* and *Prevotella.*

> **✐ TECHNICIAN NOTE**
>
> Observation of bacteria that do not grow aerobically in Gram's stained exudate from a pyonecrotic lesion is often a significant indication that obligately anaerobic bacteria are present.

SPIROCHETES AND CURVED BACTERIA

Leptospira spp. cause febrile infections, often followed by abortion and infertility. These spirochetes are difficult to isolate and usually die within a few hours while being transported to a laboratory. Darkfield examination of urine may aid in establishing a diagnosis. Most diagnoses are made by serologic testing.

Borrelia burgdorferi is a tick-transmitted spirochete that causes Lyme disease in humans and arthritis and lameness in dogs. Canine borreliosis may be accompanied by high rectal temperature and lymphadenopathy. Detection of serum antibodies to *B. burgdorferi* is the diagnostic test of choice in dogs. Isolation of *Borrelia* by culture is difficult and often nonproductive. Borreliosis is of importance in the United States in dogs and other animals only within areas infested by ticks carrying this agent.

Brachyspira hyodysenteriae (formerly called *Serpulina hyodysenteriae*) is a spirochete that causes dysentery in pigs. Cultural isolation is beyond the capability of most laboratories. Diagnosis of this infection may be made by examining smears of colonic mucosa for numerous large spirochetes.

Campylobacter spp. cause two different types of disease conditions. One group contains important reproductive pathogens, causing abortion and infertility. Because of special needs for enrichment and selective media and a microaerophilic atmosphere, specimens for isolation of *Campylobacter* spp. should be sent to veterinary diagnostic laboratories specially equipped for *Campylobacter* culture. The second group includes important zoonotic enteric pathogens. Most public health and hospital laboratories are equipped to isolate this group. *Campylobacter* spp. are curved gram-negative rods. They can be recognized by darkfield or phase-contrast microscopy by their darting motility.

Helicobacter spp. are helical or curved gram-negative bacteria that colonize the gastric mucosa of humans, dogs, and cats and the intestinal tracts of some rodents, birds, and swine. Some species have been associated with gastritis and peptic ulceration, whereas other species are considered to be nonpathogenic flora of the gastric mucosa of animals. They can be detected and identified in histologic sections, by culture in reference laboratories, and by association with strong urease activity in gastric mucus.

MYCOPLASMA SPECIES

Mycoplasma spp. are small bacteria that lack cell walls and, as a result, are not easily stained and observed in exudates. Arthritis and pneumonia are the most common mycoplasmal diseases. The role of *Mycoplasma* spp. in urogenital infections is not well characterized. Occasionally, strains can be isolated on blood agar plates inoculated with urine from dogs with cystitis. Special media and techniques are required for isolation and identification of most *Mycoplasma* spp. Therefore arrangements should be made with a reference laboratory for *Mycoplasma* transport media and specimen shipping instructions.

The agent of feline infectious anemia (formerly *Haemobartonella felis*) has recently been renamed *Mycoplasma haemofelis*. Examination of a stained blood smear frequently results in identification of clinical cases. Molecular detection assays are also available.

OTHER FASTIDIOUS BACTERIA

Diagnosis of several fastidious bacterial infections is best accomplished by using molecular detection systems specific for gene sequences of nucleic acids or serology. Some of the agents most amenable to molecular detection include *Bartonella*, *Rickettsia*, *Neorickettsia*, *Chlamydophila*, *Chlamydia*, *Ehrlichia*, *Mycoplasma*, and *Mycobacterium* spp.

ANTIMICROBIAL SUSCEPTIBILITY TESTING

One of the most important functions of the clinical microbiology laboratory is to provide information that can assist in the selection of appropriate therapy for infectious diseases. All antimicrobial agents have limitations in their spectra of activity. Therefore a universal antimicrobial for all infections is not available. Some organisms are intrinsically resistant to an antimicrobial, whereas others acquire resistance. The most common mechanism for acquired resistance is the acquisition of extrachromosomal pieces of DNA, such as plasmids (R factors) and bacteriophages. As a result, the bacteria are able to produce enzymes that modify or inactivate the antimicrobial, enable the cell to resist accumulation of the drug, or alter target sites and reduce the activity of the drug. Because the acquired resistance traits are not static, the antimicrobial susceptibility pattern *(antibiogram)* is not predictable for many organisms. Therefore susceptibility tests are necessary.

TECHNICIAN NOTE
Antimicrobial susceptibility testing by means of standardized test systems is indicated for clinically significant bacterial isolates with unpredictable (changing) patterns of susceptibility.

INDICATIONS FOR SUSCEPTIBILITY TESTING

Susceptibility testing is indicated for most rapidly growing, aerobic and facultative anaerobic, clinically significant bacteria. Testing should be avoided for isolates representing normal flora and for those bacteria with predictable susceptibility to the antimicrobial of choice. Gram-positive bacteria other than *Staphylococcus* spp. have rather predictable antibiograms; therefore routine testing is not needed. However, susceptibility testing may be indicated if the antimicrobial of choice cannot be safely and economically administered to the patient. Unpredictable resistance patterns are frequently observed with the gram-negative bacteria, thus requiring testing. Most slow-growing and anaerobic bacteria have rather predictable antibiograms, so testing is not necessary. If acquired resistance is found to be a problem in these organisms, special methods will be necessary for testing them.

In most cases the veterinarian will have started antimicrobial therapy before the laboratory results are available. When the test results become available, therapy can be altered or modified to provide safe, effective, least-cost therapy. In some situations the culture specimen will be from a moribund or dead animal. Susceptibility testing may still be important because it can establish patterns of antimicrobial susceptibility for the organism when encountered in other animals in the herd or region.

SUSCEPTIBILITY TEST METHODS

The simplest type of susceptibility test is one that determines the presence of an enzyme that can inactivate an antimicrobial. Penicillin resistance in *Staphylococcus* spp. is acquired by gaining the ability to produce beta-lactamase, an enzyme that inactivates most penicillin derivatives. Sensitive and rapid tests, such as Cefinase (BD Diagnostic Systems), are available for detection of this enzyme. If the test result is negative, penicillin or a penicillin derivative is usually the drug of choice, and no further testing is needed. If the isolate is producing beta-lactamase, further antimicrobial susceptibility testing will be needed to select an alternative therapy. A beta-lactamase test can be a very useful part of a mastitis culture procedure to rapidly evaluate the appropriateness of penicillin therapy because penicillin is one of the most frequently administered antimicrobials.

In most cases, tests for antimicrobial-inactivating enzymes are not available. Therefore most routine susceptibility tests measure the degree of susceptibility of the isolate to each of several antimicrobials. The broth dilution susceptibility test system is the most precise method and is considered the reference method. This test is performed by introducing a standardized inoculum of an organism into a series of tubes (or wells in a microculture plate) containing serial dilutions of an antimicrobial in medium (Figure 8-8). The lowest concentration of antimicrobial that macroscopically inhibits growth of the organism is the *minimal inhibitory concentration (MIC)*. The MIC of an antimicrobial for a given isolate represents the degree of susceptibility to the drug. If the antimicrobial is going to be used in therapy, the MIC must be achieved at the site of infection to effectively inhibit bacterial growth.

The most commonly used method of antimicrobial susceptibility testing in small laboratories is the *agar diffusion test* in which antimicrobial-impregnated paper disks are applied to the surface of agar that has been streaked with a standardized inoculum. As the antimicrobial is absorbed from the disk into the agar, it begins diffusing in a radial pattern (Figure 8-9). As the antimicrobial diffuses, it becomes more dilute, thereby creating a gradient effect of decreasing concentrations. The bacterial inoculum on the agar begins to grow in all areas except the places in which the antimicrobial concentration exceeds the MIC of the isolate. Zones of inhibition of growth can be observed around the disks. In carefully controlled studies, the diameters of the zones of inhibition have been correlated with MIC values. The results of the diffusion test can then be semiquantitatively interpreted, usually as susceptible, intermediate, or resistant.

The diffusion test is easy to set up, but it requires careful attention to detail to ensure that the results are accurate. Mueller-Hinton agar has been selected as the standard

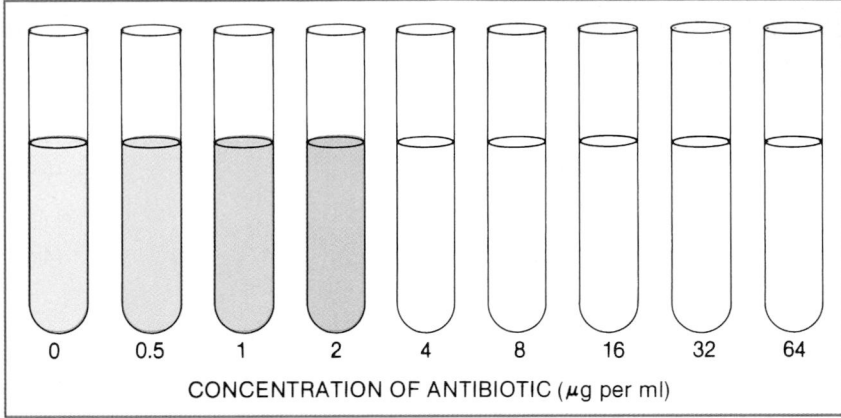

Figure 8-8 Broth dilution susceptibility test. The organism grew in broth containing antibiotic in the amounts of 0.5, 1, and 2 µg/ml, but growth was inhibited in the tube containing 4 µg/ml. Therefore the minimal inhibitory concentration is 4 µg/ml.

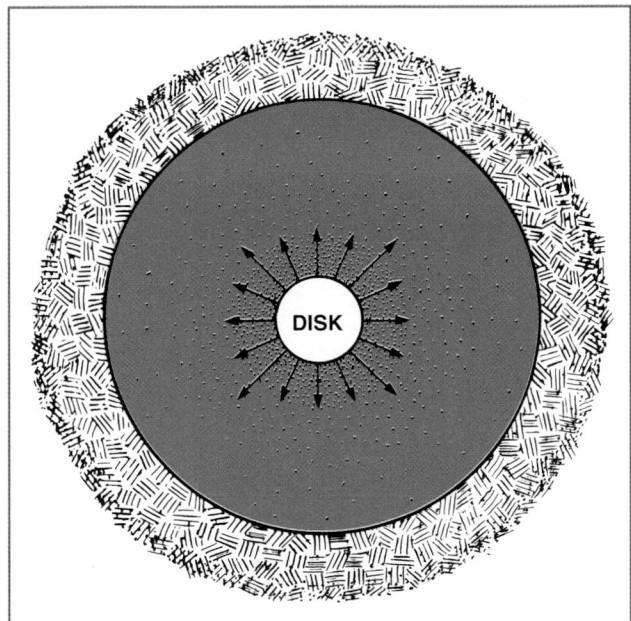

Figure 8-9 Principle of antibiotic diffusion in agar from a disk. The concentration of antibiotic is highest near the disk and logarithmically diluted as it diffuses radially into a larger area. At some point, the antibiotic is diluted below the minimal inhibitory concentration for the test organism, which allows the organism to grow. The resulting zone of inhibition is measured and interpreted with the use of Table 8-9.

culture medium so that the composition of the agar can be more uniformly controlled. However, this medium will not support growth of some fastidious pathogens, such as *Streptococcus, Listeria, Corynebacterium, Erysipelothrix,* and *Pasteurella* spp. and some other gram-negative bacteria. For these bacteria, serum or blood enrichment is necessary. Therefore it may be more practical to use blood agar plates for susceptibility tests in low-volume laboratories. Results

are usually comparable to those obtained with Mueller-Hinton agar; however, false-resistant results will often be obtained on the blood agar during testing of trimethoprim and sulfonamide activity. Fresh plates with the proper depth of agar must be used to avoid altering the kinetics of antimicrobial diffusion in a shallow or dehydrated plate.

Inoculum density should be standardized to avoid significant variations in zone sizes and misinterpretations. Susceptibility tests should always be performed with a *pure culture* of bacteria. Bacteria in mixed cultures can inhibit growth of slower-growing or fastidious organisms. Therefore if mixed cultures are tested, antimicrobial resistance of a pathogen may not be detected. Direct susceptibility testing of clinical specimens is discouraged, and, if performed, the results should always be verified by testing isolates in pure culture.

Standard antimicrobial disks should be purchased rather than attempting to prepare them from therapeutic drug solutions. It is important to make certain that the disks contain the same amount of antimicrobial as is listed in the interpretation chart (Table 8-9). Otherwise, the results will not correlate with the desired MIC values. All cartridges of disks not in current use should be stored in a −20° C freezer; those currently in use should be kept in the refrigerator to prevent deterioration of the antimicrobials.

DIFFUSION TEST PROCEDURE

Inoculum

Select four or five well-isolated colonies of the same morphologic type from an agar plate culture. Touch the top of each colony with a wire loop, and transfer the growth to a tube containing 0.5 to 1 ml of saline solution or broth. The turbidity of the bacterial suspension should be equivalent to a MacFarland No. 0.5 standard, which is just turbid enough that a slight change in optical density of the tube is macroscopically visible. Within 15 minutes after

Table 8-9 ZONE DIAMETER (MEASURED IN MILLIMETERS) INTERPRETIVE STANDARDS FOR SUSCEPTIBILITY TESTS

Antimicrobial Agent	Disk Content	Susceptibie	Intermediate	Resistant
Amikacin	30 µg	≥17	15-16	≤14
Amoxicillin/clavulanic acid (staphylococci)	20/10 µg	≥20		≤19
Amoxicillin/clavulanic acid (other organisms)	20/10 µg	≥18	14-17	≤13
Ampicillin* (gram-negative enteric organisms)	10 µg	≥17	14-16	≤13
Ampicillin* (staphylococci)	10 µg	≥29		≤28
Ampicillin* (enterococci)	10 µg	≥17		≤16
Ampicillin* (streptococci)	10 µg	≥26	19-25	≤18
Cefazolin	30 µg	≥18	15-17	≤14
Ceftiofur (respiratory pathogens only)	30 µg	≥21	18-20	≤17
Cephalothin†	30 µg	≥18	15-17	≤14
Chloramphenicol	30 µg	≥18	13-17	≤12
Clindamycin‡	2 µg	≥21	15-20	≤14
Enrofloxacin	5 µg	≥23	17-22	≤16
Erythromycin	15 µg	≥23	14-22	≤13
Florfenicol	30 µg	≥19	15-18	≤14
Gentamicin	10 µg	≥15	13-14	≤12
Kanamycin	30 µg	≥18	14-17	≤13
Oxacillin§ (staphylococci)	1 µg	≥13	11-12	≤10
Penicillin G (staphylococci)	10 units	≥29		≤28
Penicillin G (enterococci)	10 units	≥15		≤14
Penicillin G (streptococci)	10 units	≥28	20-27	≤19
Penicillin/novobiocin‖	10 units/30 µg	≥18	15-17	≤14
Pirlimycin‖	2 µg	≥13		≤12
Rifampin	5 µg	≥20	17-19	≤16
Sulfonamides	250 or 300 µg	≥17	13-16	≤12
Tetracycline¶	30 µg	≥19	15-18	≤14
Ticarcillin (Pseudomonas aeruginosa)	75 µg	≥15		≤14
Ticarcillin (gram-negative enteric organisms)	75 µg	≥20	15-19	≤14
Tilmicosin	15 µg	≥14	11-13	≤10
Trimethoprim/sulfamethoxazole**	1.25/23.75 µg	≥16	11-15	≤10

Modified from National Committee for Clinical Laboratory Standards document M31-A2, Table 2, pp. 55-59, 2002.

*Ampicillin is used to test for susceptibility to amoxicillin and hetacillin.

†Cephalothin is used to test all first-generation cephalosporins, such as cephapirin and cefadroxil. Cefazolin should be tested separately with the gram-negative enteric organisms.

‡Clindamycin is used to test for susceptibility to clindamycin and lincomycin.

§Oxacillin is used to test for susceptibility to methicillin, nafcillin, and cloxacillin.

‖Available as an infusion product for treatment of bovine mastitis during lactation.

¶Tetracycline is used to test for susceptibility to chlortetracycline, oxytetracycline, minocycline, and doxycycline.

**Trimethoprim/sulfamethoxazole is used to test for susceptibility to trimethoprim/sulfadiazine and ormetoprim/sulfadimethoxine.

preparing the inoculum suspension, dip a sterile nontoxic cotton swab into the suspension, and rotate the swab several times with firm pressure on the inside wall of the tube to remove excess inoculum from the swab. Then inoculate the agar plate by streaking the swab over the entire agar surface. Repeat the streaking procedure two or more times, rotating the plate approximately 60 degrees each time to ensure an even distribution of inoculum.

Test Procedure

Place the appropriate antimicrobial-impregnated disks, selected from the list in Table 8-9, on the surface of the agar.

Note that some disks serve as class disks for a group of related antimicrobials, thereby reducing the need for testing each drug individually. The disks should be distributed evenly on the surface of the agar so that they are no closer than 24 mm from center to center. This is best accomplished with a dispensing apparatus. Using a sterile forceps or needle tip, gently press each disk to the agar to ensure complete contact. Because some of the drug begins to diffuse immediately, a disk should not be moved once it has come in contact with the agar. Finally, invert the plates, and place them in the incubator. The inoculated test plate is incubated in an aerobic atmosphere at 35° C for 18 hours.

Measuring Zones of Inhibition

After 16 to 18 hours of incubation of a properly inoculated plate, zones of inhibition around the disks should be uniformly circular with a uniformly confluent or almost completely confluent lawn of growth between zones. If only isolated colonies grow, the inoculum was too light, and the test should be repeated. The zone diameters should be carefully measured, including the diameter of the disk, and recorded to the nearest millimeter. The end point should be taken as the area showing no obvious visible growth (not including faint growth of any colonies that can be detected only with difficulty at the edge of the zone of inhibited growth). Large colonies growing within a clear zone of inhibition should be subcultured, reidentified, and retested. Strains of *Proteus mirabilis* and *Proteus vulgaris* may swarm into areas of inhibited growth around certain antimicrobials. The zones of inhibition are usually clearly outlined, and the veil of swarming growth is ignored. With the sulfonamides, organisms may grow through several generations before they are inhibited. Slight growth (80% or more inhibition) with sulfonamides is therefore disregarded, and the margin of *heavy growth* is measured to determine the zone diameter.

Results

Interpret the sizes of the zones of inhibition by referring to Table 8-9, and report results for the organism as susceptible, intermediate, or resistant to each antimicrobial.

INTERPRETATION AND LIMITATIONS

It is important to understand that antimicrobial susceptibility is not an all-or-none phenomenon. Instead, bacteria have a *degree of susceptibility* as defined by the MIC value. Therefore interpretation of diffusion test results as "zone or no zone" is unacceptable. Small zones may represent organisms that can tolerate higher levels of the antimicrobial (high MIC) than can be achieved at the site of infection. The measured diameter of the inhibition zone must be compared with the standards in Table 8-9 to determine whether the degree of susceptibility is comparable to the therapeutic level of the antimicrobial. The classification of "susceptible versus resistant" is a practical simplification of the various susceptibilities of organisms in terms of expected clinical response to standard dose therapy.

Although the diffusion test has been accepted as a standard test and is used in most veterinary microbiology laboratories, some limitations should be kept in mind. This test system is not applicable to slow-growing isolates or for use in special atmospheres. In many cases the interpretative criteria (Table 8-9) are based on assumptions derived from knowledge of pharmacodynamics of antimicrobials in humans and efficacy in treating human pathogens. Dosages, absorption, and distribution of antimicrobials may be significantly different in the various species of animals. Levels of drug in tissues may significantly differ from levels in serum, such as low levels in cerebrospinal fluid. From the chart, a test result may be interpreted as susceptible, but the drug may not be able to penetrate to the site of infection. Conversely, ampicillin, for example, is concentrated several-fold in the urine and may exceed the MIC value for an organism that has a small zone of inhibition. Therefore susceptibility test results are not absolute rules for antimicrobial therapy. They should be used as guidelines in selecting therapy in addition to clinical judgment and knowledge of the pharmacokinetics and pharmacodynamics of the antimicrobials.

Some veterinary microbiology laboratories are using microdilution tests to determine the MIC of clinical isolates. The MIC value can be compared with the levels of drug that can be obtained in the animal for final interpretation.

> **✎ TECHNICIAN NOTE**
>
> *Susceptible* implies that infection caused by the strain may be appropriately treated with the standard dosage of antimicrobial recommended for that type of infection and infecting species, unless otherwise contraindicated.

Intermediate indicates infection caused by a strain with antimicrobial agent MICs that approach usually attainable blood and tissue levels for which response rates may be lower than for susceptible isolates. This category implies clinical applicability in body sites in which the drugs are physiologically concentrated (e.g., quinolones and lactams in urine) or when a high dose of drug can be used (e.g., lactams).

Resistant strains are not inhibited by the usually achievable systemic concentrations of the antimicrobial when normal dosage schedules are used, and/or they may have MICs that fall within the range in which specific microbial resistance mechanisms are likely and clinical efficacy has not been reliable in treatment studies.

MYCOLOGY

The fungal agents that technicians will most likely be expected to identify in a clinical laboratory are dermatophytes and some yeasts. Dermatophytes can be readily cultured and identified in local laboratories. The invasive *systemic mycoses* are usually encountered less frequently and require specialized laboratory facilities and procedures for identification.

DERMATOPHYTES

The dermatophytes are keratinophilic (keratin-seeking) fungi that invade hair, nails, and the superficial layers of the skin but not living tissue. They may cause chronic, mild inflammation rather than intense inflammation. Lesions are usually characterized by spreading areas of pruritus and accumulating crusty debris. Lesions can be single or multifocal, and hair loss is variable. Because of the peripherally expanding nature of the lesion, it is also referred to as ringworm. Lesions can be markedly different in various species of animals, from a dry, minimally inflamed lesion without hair loss on cats to a large, wartlike crusty lesion on ruminants.

Specimen Collection

Representative bits of hair, scale, or crust should be collected from the area of suspected dermatophyte lesions. Care must be exercised to prevent heavy contamination with saprophytic fungi or bacteria, which can overgrow the culture of the desired pathogen. If the lesion is likely to be contaminated, it should be cleansed gently with 70% alcohol before samples are collected. Various dermatophytes are best recovered from unique parts of the lesion, and so samples of scale, crust, and hair should be selected. Pluck broken, frayed, or distorted stubs of hair within the lesion area. Do not cut off hair to use as a specimen for culture. Brush sampling is the preferred method for obtaining a dermatophyte culture specimen from asymptomatic cats. Use a sterilized (or new) toothbrush to vigorously brush suspected lesions or brush the entire animal for 2 to 3 minutes as if grooming. Then lightly press the brush against the surface of the culture medium several times for inoculation. Avoid pressing too firmly because the agar may tear and subsurface inoculum will not grow well. Crush and separate large pieces of debris when inoculating media. To culture nails suspected of having dermatophytic invasion, make fine shavings with a scalpel. Scatter the specimen over the entire surface of the culture medium. Press the hair and scale onto the agar, but do not bury them in the medium. If samples are not placed directly on culture media, they should be placed in a clean, dry envelope. Do not seal them in a tube or place in transport media. When moisture is allowed to accumulate, bacteria and yeast may overgrow.

Direct Examination

All specimens for fungal culture should be evaluated by direct microscopic examination. Direct mounts can be prepared by mixing a small portion of the material in two or three drops of 10% potassium hydroxide on a microscope slide. Addition of black India ink to the potassium hydroxide solution will facilitate observation of fungal elements in the specimen. Add a coverslip over the wet mount, and examine for the presence of delicate hyphae in skin scales or for the accumulation of spores on the surface of an infected hair (ectothrix).

Culture Procedure

Sabouraud dextrose agar is the standard medium for isolation of fungi and can be used for the successful isolation of dermatophytes. Selective media, such as Mycobiotic (BD Diagnostic Systems), are modified with antibiotics to inhibit bacteria and saprophytic fungi. A selective and differential medium (DTM [dermatophyte test medium]) is the most convenient medium available (Synbiotics Corp.; BactiLab, Inc.). The medium contains a phenol red indicator, which turns red as a dermatophyte grows and produces alkaline metabolic products. Occasionally, dermatophytes do not sporulate as well on DTM as on Sabouraud medium, which can hinder identification. This problem can be overcome by using a supplemental medium, such as Rapid Sporulation Medium (BactiLab, Inc.), to enhance sporulation and identification of dermatophytes.

After the agar is inoculated, the cap should be replaced but left loose so that air exchange can occur. The culture is allowed to incubate at room temperature (22° C to 25° C). Placement on an open shelf or counter allows daily observation for up to 2 weeks for growth and color change in the medium. Dermatophytes are identified on the basis of both their gross colony characteristics and microscopic morphologic characteristics. Rate of growth, texture, pattern of growth, color of the colony, and pigmentation of the reverse of the colony should be noted. Most dermatophyte colonies are white or light shades of apricot, yellow, or cream to tan. Darkly colored brown or black fungi are likely to be contaminants. The dermatophytes rapidly change the color of the DTM agar to red, even before a colony is apparent. The red color may appear as early as 3 to 5 days after inoculation and rapidly spreads to most of the agar. Nonpathogenic fungi that grow on the medium do not produce an early color change, although the medium may become red after it is heavily overgrown.

Definitive identification of a dermatophyte and speciation require microscopic examination of wet tape mounts prepared in *lactophenol cotton blue stain*. The slide is examined for microconidia, macroconidia, hyphae structures, and other identifying characteristics. The distinguishing morphologic features of the common dermatophytes are illustrated in most clinical microbiology textbooks.

✏ TECHNICIAN NOTE

Morphologic features of fungi serve as the basis for identification, much like identification of plants. Although fungi can be identified by using dichotomous keys, most clinical microbiologists prefer to compare structures with photomicrographs published in atlases.

SYSTEMIC MYCOSES

The three most important systemic mycoses are coccidioidomycosis, histoplasmosis, and blastomycosis. They are serious zoonotic agents; therefore the small laboratory should not attempt to isolate them in culture systems. All culture work must be carried out in an approved biohazard safety hood. The small laboratory is limited to direct microscopic examination of clinical material. Stained smears and wet mounts are useful diagnostic tools. The size and structural characteristics of these agents in the tissue or yeast phase can serve as specific identifying criteria. If cultures are desired, the clinical material should be inoculated onto isolation media, and the inoculated tubes should be shipped to a reference laboratory. Delays in inoculation of isolation media will result in loss of viability and overgrowth of the sample by contaminating bacteria.

Sporotrichosis is a chronic infection characterized by nodular lesions of the skin or subcutaneous tissues. *Sporothrix schenckii* usually gains entrance by traumatic implantation into the tissue. Therefore there is little danger of contagion except from cats that frequently harbor very large numbers of yeast cells in lesions. The agent can be observed in direct examinations of tissue and exudates or isolated and identified by routine methods.

YEASTS

There are only a few clinical situations in which yeasts are significant veterinary pathogens. In general, animals seem to be much more resistant to yeast infections than humans. If yeasts are suspected, a direct smear of exudate should be stained for microscopic examination. The best approach to the isolation of yeast is to inoculate blood agar and Sabouraud dextrose agar. The blood agar is incubated at 35° C, and the Sabouraud agar, at room temperature. Media should be held at least 2 weeks before discarding them as negative. Therefore agar slants in tubes are preferable to plates because they do not dehydrate as rapidly. Culture and identifying methods for the most common pathogenic yeasts are described.

Malassezia pachydermatis

Malassezia pachydermatis is frequently found in cases of external otitis and is emerging as a cause of seborrheic and hypersensitivity reactions associated with dermatitis. It is readily observed in smears of exudate stained with Gram's stain as an oval, bottle-shaped, monopolar budding yeast. Isolation in cultures can be difficult but is best attempted by inoculating Sabouraud dextrose agar and incubating it at 35° C in a carbon dioxide incubator.

Cryptococcus neoformans

In direct smears, *Cryptococcus neoformans* may be presumptively identified by its abundant capsular material. Negative staining with India ink provides a black background that outlines the clear capsule for easier observation. It can be isolated on Sabouraud dextrose agar or blood agar. *Cryptococcus neoformans* can be differentiated from other nonpathogenic yeasts because it will grow at 35° C to 37° C and is urease positive. The urease test is performed by inoculating the same urea agar slant that is used for differentiating bacteria.

Candida albicans

Candida albicans is a frequently encountered opportunistic fungal pathogen. Infections usually involve mucous membranes. In direct microscopic examinations of wet mounts, unicellular budding yeasts without a capsule are observed. Limited hyphae development may also be observed. *Candida albicans* is readily isolated on Sabouraud dextrose agar or blood agar. Definitive identification can be made by demonstration of germ tube (pseudohyphae) development after 3 to 4 hours' incubation in rabbit serum.

Other Yeasts

Other yeasts are isolated much less frequently. It is usually not feasible for small laboratories to attempt to identify these rare isolates. They should be forwarded to a reference laboratory for definitive identification.

VIROLOGY

Laboratory diagnosis of viral diseases depends on the examination of appropriate specimens for evidence of viral infection and then attempting to correlate infection with disease. Because of the nature of viruses and the special laboratory procedures required, most clinical laboratories perform only limited viral diagnostic procedures. Viruses are obligate intracellular parasites. Therefore they are best recovered from living tissue. Isolation of viruses in dead tissues is reduced in direct proportion to the length of time since death and the extent of autolysis.

> **TECHNICIAN NOTE**
> Rapid detection of viral infection usually depends on some form of molecular diagnostics, such as antigen detection or nucleic acid detection.

VIRUS ISOLATION

Isolation and identification of viruses depend on the inoculation of susceptible living cells for cultivation of the virus. The major methods of providing these living cells include monolayer cell cultures, embryonated hen eggs, and laboratory animal inoculation. These techniques require special laboratory facilities and up to 2 weeks for recovery of a virus. Special care must be taken to ensure that viable virus is delivered to the laboratory for isolation attempts. Therefore specimens should be collected early in the course of infection when viruses are most numerous. At death, virus numbers in the tissues are usually reduced, and extensive secondary bacterial infection is often present. The presence of bacteria in the sample can be damaging to the cells that are being used as recovery hosts for the virus. Therefore specimens should be carefully collected, refrigerated, and promptly delivered to the diagnostic laboratory. Special arrangements should be made with the laboratory personnel so that they can be prepared to process the sample when it arrives. Transport media containing antibiotics and virus-stabilizing agents are often available from viral diagnostic laboratories.

MICROSCOPIC EVALUATION

In some cases, viral infection can be identified by microscopic examination of infected tissues for the presence of pathognomonic changes or of body fluids for the presence of viral particles. Some viral infections produce distinct changes in host cells, such as the intranuclear inclusions of infectious canine hepatitis, which can provide a definitive diagnosis. Electron microscopic examination of body fluids and washings allows the direct visualization of viral particles. This procedure is often used for diagnosis of respiratory and enteric viral infections because it is rapid and can detect mixed viral infections. The procedure does not require viable viruses, as long as they have retained their structural integrity. Direct electron microscopic examination is limited to cell-free viruses, such as those found in body fluids, rather than examination of infected tissue. Most diagnostic laboratories perform negative-contrast staining; therefore virus identification is limited to morphologic identification. If immunoelectron microscopy procedures are available, the type of virus within a group can be identified.

ANTIGEN DETECTION

Antigen detection methods are the most frequently used viral diagnostic procedures. Advantages of antigen detection compared with viral isolation include rapid results, less expense, less technically demanding procedures, and less dependence on the presence of viable virus in the sample because most viral antigens remain intact after death of the virus. The most common methods of antigen detection are immunohistochemical staining, hemagglutination, and solid-phase immunoassays. Hemagglutination assays are not easily standardized for use in clinical laboratories.

Immunohistochemical Staining

Examination of selected clinical specimens by using a specific antibody labeled with a marker as a probe to identify viral antigen is a rapid and highly reliable diagnostic method. Markers on the antibody can include fluorescent compounds, enzymes, or colloidal gold. The two most important limitations of these procedures are the need for specific antibodies to the viral antigens and a system for detecting the marker. For immunofluorescence, a microscope with an ultraviolet (UV) light source is required.

In the *immunoperoxidase method assay,* the specific antibody is labeled with an enzyme (usually horseradish peroxidase) instead of a fluorescent label. Attachment of the antibody to tissue sections or smears is detected by using a chromogenic substrate that is deposited at the site of enzyme-antibody attachment and produces a slide similar to other differential stains. The slide can then be examined by light microscopy. Several of these assays have been developed by using monoclonal antibodies to detect viral antigens in tissue, including examination of formalin-fixed specimens.

Solid-Phase Immunoassays

The use of enzyme immunoassays is based on the excellent ability of this method to be adapted to kits that meet practical needs, such as minimizing reagent cost, reducing technician time required to perform the assay, and simplifying the test protocol. These test systems are frequently referred to by the acronym ELISA (enzyme-linked immunosorbent assay). As a result, several kit systems are available for the detection of antigens from viruses and other infectious agents (Figure 8-10) and for detection of antibodies specific for infectious agents. Three typical configurations of ELISAs are illustrated in Figure 8-11. At present, there are several different solid phases commonly used in these assays. The most common solid phase for multiple tests is the microtiter well, but for individual clinical tests, dipstick, immunofiltration, immunomigration, and immunochromatographic formats are more efficient. Immunoassay diagnostic kit manufacturers usually offer technical assistance to kit users. If you have questions about a protocol or test result or are experiencing difficulty in conducting a test after carefully reading and following the manufacturer's instructions, call the company's technical services department and ask for assistance. Most companies provide a toll-free telephone number to facilitate this and will welcome an opportunity to assist you in using their products.

Assays that have been successfully developed for detection of viral antigen include feline leukemia virus (FeLV) in blood (Assure FeLV Leukemia Antigen Test and Witness FeLV Leukemia Antigen Test, Synbiotics Corp.; SNAP FeLV Antigen Test, IDEXX Laboratories, Inc.), FeLV in saliva (Assure FeLV Leukemia Antigen Test), canine parvovirus in

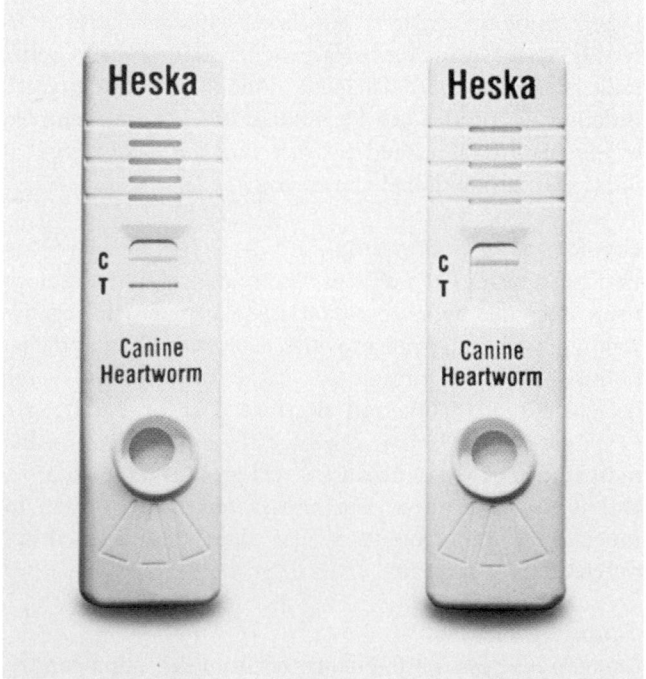

Figure 8-10 Solo Step CH (Heska Corp.) lateral flow immunoassay cassette for the detection of antigens produced by canine heartworms in serum. A positive test result has developed in the left cassette, and a negative test result is shown in the cassette on the right.

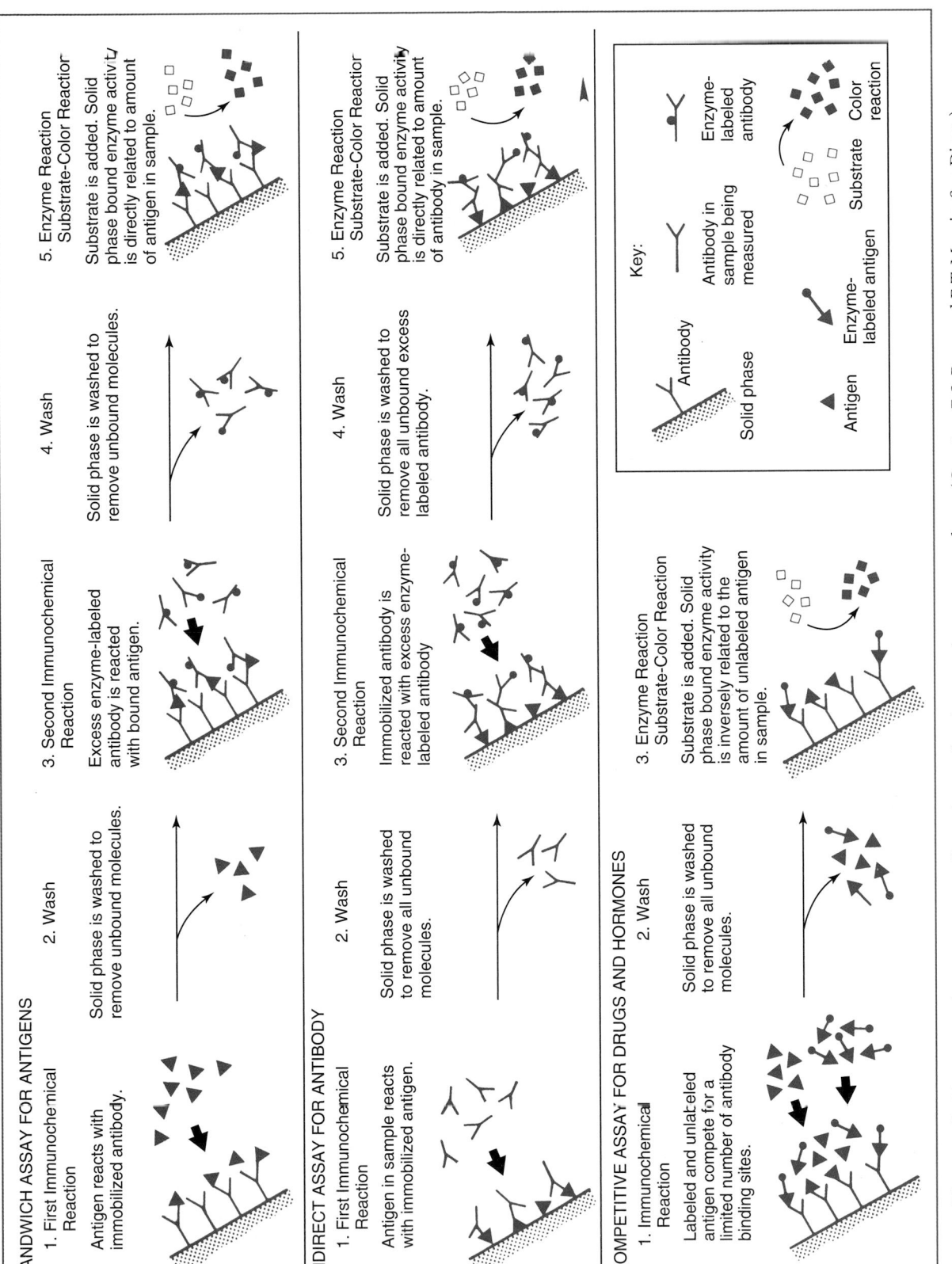

Figure 8-11 Enzyme immunoassay configurations and major steps in assay procedures. (Courtesy E.S. Bean and E.T. Maggio, San Diego.)

feces (Assure Canine Parvovirus Antigen Test, Synbiotics Corp.; SNAP Parvo Antigen Test, IDEXX Laboratories, Inc.), and influenza virus in respiratory tract specimens (Directigen Flu A, BD Diagnostic Systems). Kits are also available to detect bacterial antigens (*Escherichia coli* Antigen Test [K99 Pilitest], VMRD, Inc.) and heartworm antigens (Solo Step CH, Heska Corp.; SNAP Heartworm Antigen Test, IDEXX Laboratories, Inc.).

SEROLOGY

Serologic testing is an important tool in the diagnosis of infectious diseases. Serology is used extensively in the diagnosis of viral infections and in disease surveillance programs. Serologic tests for detecting a specific antibody have been developed for nearly every infectious agent. However, this indirect approach to diagnosing infection on the basis of a host immune response after exposure to an infectious agent has limitations. Serologic tests may vary in their sensitivity and specificity because of the type of test, immunogenicity and cross-reactivity of the antigen, and biologic variation of immune responses by individual animals. Nevertheless, serologic tests often remain the best diagnostic test available. In veterinary medicine, serologic tests are often required by regulatory agencies to prove an animal is not infected or a carrier of a particular infectious agent.

ANTIBODY RESPONSE TO INFECTION

The chronology of exposure to an infectious agent and subsequent development of an antibody response are illustrated in Figure 8-12. After exposure, there is a variable period of incubation, followed by clinical illness. During the time of clinical illness, the animal may be febrile, and this is when the greatest number of microorganisms are present. Therefore it is more likely to transmit the infectious agent, and the best samples can be obtained for recovery of the agent at this time. After a variable period from onset of clinical signs (usually after 5 to 10 days), the animal begins to produce antibodies to the agent. Continued production of antibodies after the animal is no longer ill, referred to as the convalescent phase, will cause the titer (serum antibody level) to rise for 1 month or longer.

INTERPRETATION OF SEROLOGIC TEST RESULTS

The presence of antibodies to a particular organism in an animal serum sample is not always a simple and absolute diagnosis of current or recent clinical illness caused by the organism. Sources of antibody in the serum of an animal include convalescent antibody after clinical disease or persistent infection, antibody response caused by exposure to an organism without clinical disease occurring, active immune response to vaccination, and passive transfer of maternal antibodies to the neonate. Therefore detection of antibodies in a single serum sample often has limited importance unless the finding can be correlated with other clinical indications of the disease. In most situations, it is necessary to collect two samples—the first one early in the course of the illness (*acute*) and the second one (*convalescent*) at a later time—to demonstrate a change in antibody titer that would indicate recent antigenic stimulation. The change must be at least two dilution increments (usually fourfold), such as an increase from 1:4 to 1:16 or greater, to be considered diagnostically significant. This change in titer is known as a *seroconversion*.

The presence of antibody in serum may be reported quantitatively as a titer or qualitatively as positive or negative. Qualitative tests have less diagnostic value than those tests that report titers, unless the result is negative, in which

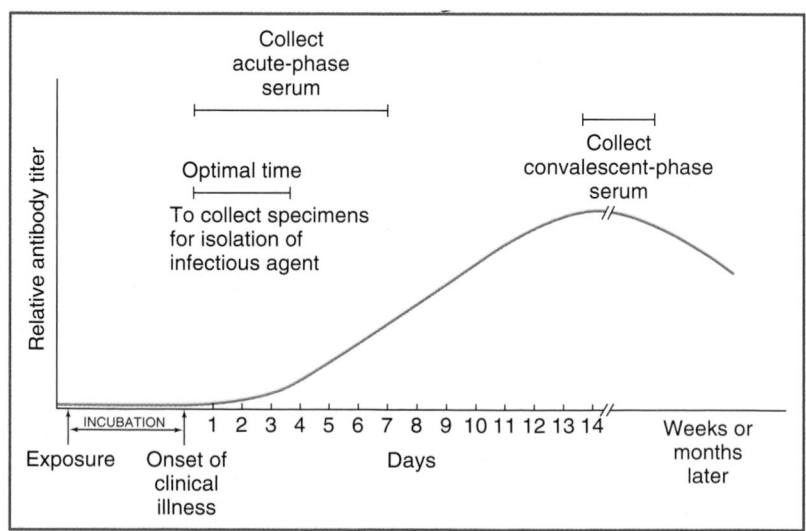

Figure 8-12 Antibody response to an infectious disease and optimal times for specimen collection.

case the test can exclude some agents from the differential diagnosis unless the serum was collected early in the course of disease. Most qualitative tests, such as immunodiffusion for equine infectious anemia (Coggins test) and bovine leukosis, are surveillance tests to identify animals that have been exposed and are possible carriers. Occasionally, a single, high-titered serum can aid in establishing a diagnosis, but it always leaves some question of whether the titer increased in association with clinical disease or is a stable, convalescent high titer.

When an animal is exposed to an infectious agent, the first antibodies produced are usually of the immunoglobulin (Ig) M class, with later antibody production being IgG. Some tests are designed to differentiate these antibody class responses, which can be helpful in confirming a diagnosis. If the antibody response to a virus is of the IgM type, the animal has recently been exposed. If the response is mostly IgG, it was probably exposed several weeks to months previously. Often IgM antibodies are less specific than IgG and may cross-react, resulting in false-positive test results. The test can be modified to exclude IgM reactions to prevent this from happening.

Serologic tests are frequently relied on as the only diagnostic procedures for abortion cases. Results are often difficult to interpret for two reasons. First, by the time abortion occurs because of infection of the fetus and its subsequent death, the dam is already in the convalescent phase of antibody production, so a seroconversion cannot be demonstrated. Second, the stress of abortion or other clinical illness may trigger reactivation of a latent viral infection. This provides an antigenic stimulus to the animal's immune system and increased antibody production. However, it is specific for the latent viral infection, not the current clinical illness.

COLLECTION OF SERUM

Technicians will frequently be responsible for collecting and handling serum samples. Improper methods can reduce the value of test results. The timing of serum collection is important (see Figure 8-12). The first sample should be collected as soon as possible after the animal begins to show signs of clinical illness. If the sample is not collected within the first 5 to 7 days, antibody titers might have already risen. The convalescent sample should be collected at least 10 days after the acute sample. Generally, 14 to 21 days between samples is recommended, but in young animals with a less efficient immune response, up to 4 to 6 weeks may be necessary to demonstrate a seroconversion. The technical procedures of serologic tests are difficult to duplicate exactly; therefore results of tests performed on different days or in different laboratories should not be compared to demonstrate a seroconversion.

Blood should be collected aseptically by venipuncture with a new needle and syringe or evacuated clot tube (Vacutainer tubes and SST Sterile Serum Separation Tubes,

BD Vacutainer Systems). Do not use recycled, washed needles, syringes, or tubes. Residual detergent may cause hemolysis or may be toxic to cell cultures used in the test systems. Blood should be allowed to stand at room temperature until a clot has formed; the serum should then be removed from the clot and placed in a new, sterile tube. It may be necessary to separate the serum from the clot by centrifugation to prevent transferring cellular components of the blood. Anticoagulants should not be used to collect plasma because they can be toxic in some test systems. Avoid freezing the whole blood because that will cause hemolysis. The transfer of serum from the original blood tube must be performed aseptically. Contaminating microorganisms can grow rapidly in serum and alter the immunoglobulin molecules. Therefore serum samples (separated from the clot and cells) should be refrigerated until testing is commenced, if within 72 hours. For longer periods of storage, serum may be preserved in a freezer ($-20°$ C). Frozen serum samples should be packaged and shipped with adequate insulation and ice to prevent thawing before arrival at the laboratory. If a second sample will be collected, the first sample should be held until both can be sent to the laboratory together for valid paired testing.

> ### ✎ TECHNICIAN NOTE
> The technical procedures of serologic tests are difficult to duplicate exactly; therefore results of tests performed on different days or in other laboratories should not be compared to demonstrate a seroconversion.

For shipment, the tubes of serum must be carefully labeled and packed so that they will not leak or break. When environmental temperatures are high, refrigerant and insulating materials should be used to preserve samples during transport.

SEROLOGIC TEST PROCEDURES

Only a few serologic tests have been standardized and packaged for efficient use in veterinary practice laboratories. When kits are used, it is important that the directions be followed carefully because modification of any part of the procedure can cause spurious results. A positive (or known titer) serum and a negative serum should be kept on hand (if not already included in the kit) and included in the test each time it is performed to verify accuracy of the results. Serology (antibody-detecting) kits are available for feline immunodeficiency virus (SNAP FIV Antibody/FeLV Antigen Combo Test, IDEXX Laboratories, Inc.), canine brucellosis (D-Tec Canine Brucellosis Antibody Test, Synbiotics Corp.), paratuberculosis (*Mycobacterium paratuberculosis* Antibody Test, ImmuCell Corp.), feline heartworm (Solo Step FH, Heska Corp.), and canine borreliosis and ehrlichiosis (Canine SNAP 3Dx Test: Heartworm Antigen, *Ehrlichia canis* Antibody and Lyme Antibody Test, IDEXX Laboratories, Inc.). The most frequent mistakes made in performance of serologic tests include the use of dirty or contaminated equipment, failure to adhere to instructions (especially incubation times), and unfamiliarity with reading results.

CLINICAL IMMUNOLOGY

PURPOSE OF EVALUATING IMMUNE SYSTEM FUNCTION

As the function and complexity of the immune system have been elucidated, an increasing need for laboratory diagnosis of dysfunction of the immune system has been recognized. Clinical immunologic laboratory support has become a well-established part of the diagnostic services and patient care procedures in human medicine. Similar assays are becoming available in veterinary medicine, but very few tests are readily available for use in practice laboratories.

Several types of diagnostic problems present the need for laboratory evaluation of possible immunologic disorders. These disorders can be classified into four types: allergies, autoimmune diseases, immunodeficiencies, and immunoproliferative diseases. In young animals, disorders of the immune system may be observed as developmental defects (sometimes inherited) or may be caused by a failure of passive transfer of maternal antibodies. However, immune function abnormalities can be observed in animals of all ages because of effects of aging, various drugs, or environmental exposure to immunomodulating toxins. A few simple procedures will be discussed in this section. The Recommended Reading list should be consulted for detailed and theoretic discussions of other immune system function assays.

LABORATORY TESTS FOR IMMUNOLOGIC DISORDERS

Allergies are usually diagnosed by physical examination, history, and response to intradermal inoculation of test antigens.

Autoimmune disorders can be diagnosed more efficiently by evaluating lesions obtained by biopsy. Morphologic evaluation, combined with various immunohistochemical staining procedures, provides the most definitive diagnosis. It is best to consult referral laboratories to learn which specimens they are able to analyze and how the sample should be submitted.

Immunoproliferative diseases may result in the production of abnormal amounts or unusual types of immunoglobulin proteins, referred to as *gammopathies*. The techniques of electrophoresis (usually on cellulose acetate) and immunoelectrophoresis are the laboratory tests most frequently used to diagnose these disorders. Abnormalities of routine laboratory tests, such as total protein in serum or urine and albumin/globulin (A/G) ratios, frequently indicate a need for these specialized tests. Because of the infrequent demand for these tests and the cost of electrophoresis equipment, most practices request these services from referral laboratories.

Immunodeficiency or immunosuppressive disorders are the most frequently encountered immune system dysfunctions. Most assays of immune cell function require specialized equipment and procedures that are usually available in only a few reference laboratories. Some cellular function assays require submission of viable cells for evaluation. Recently developed assays are used to detect and quantify receptors on the surface of cells, such as CD18 deficiency in Holstein calves. Assays are being developed in research laboratories for genetic analysis of lymphocytes to detect both immunodeficiency and immunoproliferative dysfunctions. Determination of immunoglobulin levels, as an indication of B-lymphocyte function or passive transfer status, is a readily available laboratory test that will be discussed.

FAILURE OF PASSIVE TRANSFER

The newborns of most domestic animals depend on absorption of maternal antibodies from colostrum for protection from infectious diseases. Failure of the neonatal animal to obtain and absorb adequate colostral immunoglobulins is frequently associated with increased morbidity and mortality from bacteremia and common neonatal diseases. Determination of the passive transfer status of foals and calves is an important evaluation that can modify patient care. Although total serum protein levels can indicate relative levels of immunoglobulins, this indirect measurement is subject to considerable variability. The reference method for quantitating serum immunoglobulins is the *radial immunodiffusion (RID) test*. The RID test consists of agar containing antisera specific for a particular antigen. In this case, the antigen is a particular immunoglobulin class, such as IgG. Each test requires that quantitated standards be tested at the same time for comparison. Therefore if single samples are being tested, the cost per sample will be more, and it might be more cost effective to send samples to a referral laboratory. (Commercially produced RID kits for canine, feline, bovine, llama, and equine immunoglobulins are available from Bethyl Laboratories, Inc. and VMRD, Inc.)

Passive transfer status of neonates can be evaluated rapidly and inexpensively in the practice laboratory. Field test kits that quickly assay plasma or blood concentrations of IgG are available for detecting failure of passive transfer in calves, foals, and llamas (VMRD, Inc. and Midland BioProducts Corp.).

> **✎ TECHNICIAN NOTE**
>
> Failure of passive transfer is the most common condition leading to infectious diseases and subsequent death in neonatal animals.

NOSOCOMIAL INFECTIONS

An infection that results from exposure to an infectious agent while the patient is in the hospital is considered to be *nosocomial* (hospital acquired). The nosocomial infection may become clinically apparent during hospitalization or after discharge from the hospital. Infections that are incubating at the time of admission are defined as *community acquired,* even though they become clinically apparent only during hospitalization. In veterinary practices, in addition to nosocomial infections of patients, zoonotic infections transmitted to the staff and clients can be considered part of the biosafety problem.

The incidence of nosocomial infections in veterinary hospitals is not well documented, but it is probably similar to the incidence in human hospitals, which ranges from 3% to 5% of hospitalized patients. The incidence is known to vary with the size and type of hospital and the sophistication of infection control programs. The highest incidence rates are observed in large referral or teaching institutions. The most important institutional risk factors appear to be an increased number of personnel having contact with the patient and an increased mean number of hospitalization days per patient. Therefore these infections are becoming an increasingly significant problem in teaching hospitals and large group practices in which intensive medical and surgical care is available through a large staff. These institutions also tend to care for patients with more critical and chronic diseases. Because these patients have increased susceptibility to opportunistic infection, the occurrence of a nosocomial infection does not necessarily indicate negligence by the hospital staff.

The stressed condition of hospitalized animals often makes them more susceptible to infections than the general population. Factors that predispose an individual animal to nosocomial infection may include extremes of age (old age or neonatal period); debilitating disease; diagnostic or medical procedures, such as urethral catheterization or immunosuppressive therapy (corticosteroids or cytotoxic drugs); long periods of hospitalization; antimicrobial therapy; presence of other infections; and presence of surgical hardware and drains. For some of the infectious diseases, such as canine distemper, the immunization status of the patient will determine its susceptibility.

Many nosocomial infections are caused by opportunistic microorganisms that infrequently cause infections in healthy animals. However, when the high-risk patient (increased susceptibility) is exposed, the agent can cause disease. Other highly virulent organisms, such as canine parvovirus and *Salmonella* spp., may cause disease in otherwise healthy patients. The greatest impact on the incidence of nosocomial infections can be made by understanding the sources of exposure and spread of these infectious agents. Microorganisms enter the hospital in or on people, animals, inanimate objects, air currents, and occasionally insects. Within the hospital, they are maintained in or on a variety of reservoirs, including patients with infections, healthy carriers, inanimate surfaces, solutions, food, staff, and insects. From these reservoirs, the potential pathogens may be disseminated by contact or by air to hospital personnel and patients.

The most important vehicles for the spread of nosocomial agents are the hands of hospital personnel. Therefore proper and frequent hand washing is the most important strategy for reducing the rate of nosocomial and zoonotic infections.

AGENTS OF NOSOCOMIAL INFECTIONS

Bacteria are the most frequent infectious agents involved in nosocomial infections, but viruses, fungi, and protozoa can also be involved. The commonly involved bacteria tend to be somewhat environmentally resistant, and the increasing use of antibiotic therapy has led to an increased level of antibiotic resistance by nosocomial agents. In the presence of limited antibiotic use, penicillin-susceptible, gram-positive cocci of the genera *Streptococcus* and *Staphylococcus* are the most common agents. With increased antibiotic use, penicillin-resistant *Staphylococcus* is frequently detected. Currently, the major problems are with multiple antibiotic-resistant, gram-negative bacilli, such as *Escherichia coli* and *Salmonella, Klebsiella, Enterobacter, Serratia,* and *Pseudomonas* spp. Methicillin-resistant staphylococci and vancomycin-resistant enterococci are beginning to emerge as the next wave of serious nosocomial agents. Colonization (growth and establishment) of the body surfaces of the patient by these nosocomial bacterial pathogens is usually a prerequisite to infection. Therefore the patient becomes its own major reservoir of these agents once the organisms are transferred to it during hospitalization. Common reservoir sites are the lower intestinal tract and the nasooropharyngeal area. Antimicrobial chemotherapy is the most important predisposing factor that allows the patient to become colonized because the antimicrobial suppresses normal flora and selects for resistant organisms. The most frequent locations of nosocomial bacterial infections are the urinary and respiratory systems and surgical wounds. Occasionally, infections become bacteremic. Clostridial enterocolitis in dogs has been identified as a nosocomial problem in several large teaching hospitals.

Viral infections are the second most frequent group of nosocomial infections in hospitalized patients but are probably the most important nosocomial infections of outpatients. This is because some of these agents are easily transmitted and are highly infectious to susceptible but otherwise healthy animals. Diseases in this group include canine distemper, canine parvovirus, feline panleukopenia, and respiratory viral diseases of all animals (feline viral rhinotracheitis, equine influenza, infectious bovine rhinotracheitis, canine tracheobronchitis, etc.).

Other viral diseases that are not as contagious can be transmitted to susceptible patients at a veterinary hospital if adequate preventive measures are not followed. The resulting disease would be classified as a nosocomial infection. Examples include transmission of viruses of feline leukemia and equine infectious anemia by blood transfusions.

Fungi have rarely been recognized as nosocomial agents in veterinary medicine. As the awareness level of this problem increases, no doubt more fungal infections will be identified, especially with improved intensive care of immunocompromised patients. Yeasts, such as *Candida albicans,* have occasionally been identified. The dermatophytes do not cause life-threatening infections and are usually overlooked, but they can also be transmitted as nosocomial agents to both patients and hospital staff.

Infection of animals by protozoan pathogens can be acquired in the veterinary hospital. *Cryptosporidium* spp. are relatively resistant to disinfectants and have been the cause of nosocomial enteritis. If litter pans are not properly cleaned, other animals and hospital staff could be exposed to toxoplasmosis. Hemotropic parasites (*Mycoplasma haemofelis* and *Anaplasma, Ehrlichia, Babesia* spp.) can be transmitted to other patients by blood transfusions or surgical instruments that have not been adequately washed and disinfected.

RECOGNITION AND CONTROL OF NOSOCOMIAL INFECTIONS

Technicians frequently have the opportunity to be the first persons to recognize a nosocomial infection problem by taking note of an unusual number of isolations of a single pathogen or the appearance of an unusual antibiogram. Excellent diagnostic microbiology laboratory support for accurate identification and antimicrobial susceptibility testing of infectious agents is an essential tool for defining the scope of the nosocomial infection problem.

Measures that can help reduce or control nosocomial infections include sterilization of equipment and supplies, aseptic treatment techniques, isolation practices, judicious use of antimicrobial drugs, diligent hand washing between examining patients, disposal of trash, and establishment of sound housekeeping protocols. These protocols should provide for adequate cleaning, disinfection, and maintenance of patient-care equipment and environmental surfaces, such as cages, tables, floors, and walls.

> ### 🖉 TECHNICIAN NOTE
>
> The hands of hospital personnel are consistently found to be the most important vectors of nosocomial bacterial infections. Diligent attention to hand washing after every contact with a patient or the use of exam gloves is essential to avoid contaminating the hospital environment and transmitting these agents.

The control measures that would be necessary to prevent all nosocomial infections are impractical and not economically feasible. Hospitals contain patients with increased susceptibility to infection, and short of total isolation in a controlled environment, few measures are biologically guaranteed. The risk for each patient of acquiring an infection must be individually evaluated. If the risk is sufficiently great, reverse isolation procedures may be indicated to prevent the patient from being exposed to potential pathogens.

If active or passive immunizing products are available, their use should be encouraged. Routine immunization programs can effectively prevent many of the viral infections that have been discussed.

ANTISEPTICS, DISINFECTANTS, AND STERILIZATION

The effective use of antiseptics, disinfectants, and sterilization procedures is an important factor in preventing nosocomial infections. Microorganisms vary widely in their susceptibility to germicidal treatments. Bacterial endospores are the most resistant type. In descending order of relative resistance after bacterial spores are mycobacteria, fungal spores, nonenveloped viruses, vegetative fungi, enveloped viruses, and vegetative bacterial cells. The differences in chemical resistance of various vegetative bacteria are relatively minor, except for the mycobacteria, which are relatively resistant to many disinfectants. Other factors that may have a significant effect on the results of disinfection are concentration of the chemical, length of exposure to the chemical, amount of organic matter (soil, blood, feces) present, type and condition (porosity, cracks, etc.) of the material to be disinfected, ambient temperature, and the nature and number of contaminating microorganisms. Good physical cleaning will allow better penetration of crevices and porous material. Generally, the higher the concentration of the chemical agent or the longer a process is continued, the greater its effectiveness. For temperature-based procedures, increasing temperatures will usually increase efficacy.

Veterinary clinics and hospitals should select disinfectants that are registered by the U.S. Environmental Protection Agency (EPA) and labeled as one-step cleaner-disinfectants for use in hospitals. The label should indicate that these products are effective in hard water up to 400 ppm hardness and in the presence of 5% serum. Most nonporous surfaces can be efficiently cleaned and disinfected with the newer combinations of twin-chain quaternary ammonium compounds (C_8/C_{10} dimethyl ammonium chloride) and alkyl dimethyl benzyl ammonium chloride. Product labels must always be consulted for proper mixing and diluting instructions and intended applications. Chemical incompatibilities may occur if products are mixed. Therefore do not attempt to combine germicides or alter treatment procedures from the manufacturer's specifications.

BIOLOGIC SAFETY

Potential hazards in the veterinary hospital may be associated with infectious or chemical materials, physical facilities, and animal handling. Management should develop a comprehensive safety program that includes consideration of these dangers as well as preparedness for fire, accidents, and other disasters. This discussion will deal primarily with biologic hazards related to infectious agents in the laboratory and hospital.

Each individual has responsibility for protecting himself or herself and others from accidental infection. Laboratory coats should be worn to prevent contamination of street clothes and dissemination of pathogens to homes and families. Disposable examination gloves should be worn when handling heavily contaminated materials. Good hand-washing procedures should become a habit in the laboratory—between procedures if there is a chance of contamination and always before leaving the laboratory. Mouth pipetting should be prohibited in laboratories handling infectious material. Automatic or bulb pipetting devices should be used. Syringes and needles are poor substitutes for pipettes because they tend to favor creation of aerosols that may be inhaled. There is also the inherent danger of self-inoculation when handling syringes and needles. Self-inoculation must be guarded against, both in the laboratory and when inoculating animals. Centrifuge accidents, which may produce infectious aerosols, should be avoided by selecting compatible tubes, performing proper balancing, and not exceeding recommended centrifugal forces.

Good housekeeping procedures that will maintain a neat, uncluttered work area should be adopted. Eating, drinking, and smoking should not be allowed in work areas, even during break periods when there is no laboratory activity.

Immunization of personnel is recommended when they are at increased risk of infection. A minimal prophylactic immunization for all personnel employed in veterinary hospitals and laboratories should include rabies vaccine and tetanus toxoid. Other immunization products may be recommended in areas in which there is an unusually high risk of exposure to a particular infectious agent.

Primary containment equipment and laboratory design features are important factors in biologic safety. Directional airflow should be from clean areas to areas of contamination and should then be exhausted from the building without recirculation. Small veterinary laboratories and hospitals usually cannot justify the cost of biologic safety cabinets for diagnostic procedures. However, some infectious agents are of sufficient hazard that they must be handled only in laboratories with special design features, including biohazard cabinets. Zoonotic pathogens that small laboratories should not attempt to isolate include the agents of anthrax, brucellosis, plague, tuberculosis, tularemia, and systemic mycoses.

The clinical laboratory has a responsibility to decontaminate potentially infectious materials and wastes before they are discarded. Many states have adopted statutes and regulations that stipulate how hazardous waste materials must be handled. Clinical veterinary laboratories are required to comply with these rules as well as EPA and U.S. Occupational Safety and Health Administration (OSHA) requirements (see Chapter 36). All diagnostic specimens (swabs), inoculated media, viable cultures, glassware, instruments, and equipment should be considered to be contaminated. Decontamination methods should be applied before waste materials are discarded or reusable products are cleansed. The most practical decontamination procedure for most infectious wastes is use of the steam autoclave. Other methods include physical procedures (incineration, boiling, irradiation) and chemical agents (phenolics, hypochlorites, formaldehyde).

Recommended Reading

Difco manual, ed 11, Sparks, Md, 1998, Difco Laboratories, Division of Becton Dickinson and Co.

Greene CE: *Infectious diseases of the dog and cat,* ed 2, Philadelphia, 1998, WB Saunders.

Hirsch DC, Zee YC: *Veterinary microbiology,* Malden, Mass, 1999, Blackwell Science Ltd.

Koneman EW et al: *Color atlas and textbook of diagnostic microbiology,* ed 5, Philadelphia, 1997, JB Lippincott.

Larone DH: *Medically important fungi: a guide to identification,* ed 4, Washington, DC, 2002, American Society for Microbiology.

Murray PR et al: *Manual of clinical microbiology,* ed 8, Washington, DC, 2003, American Society for Microbiology.

National Committee for Clinical Laboratory Standards: *Performance standards for antimicrobial disk and dilution susceptibility tests for bacteria isolated from animals; approved standard,* ed 2, NCCLS document M31-A2, Wayne, Pa, 2002, National Committee for Clinical Laboratory Standards.

Quinn PJ et al: *Clinical veterinary microbiology,* London, 1994, Mosby.

Quinn PJ et al: *Veterinary microbiology and microbial disease,* Osney Mead, Oxford, Great Britain, 2002, Blackwell Science Ltd.

Research Committee of the National Mastitis Council: *Laboratory handbook on bovine mastitis,* Madison, Wis, 1999, National Mastitis Council.

Rose NR, Hamilton RG, Detrick B: *Manual of clinical laboratory immunology,* ed 6, Washington, DC, 2002, American Society for Microbiology.

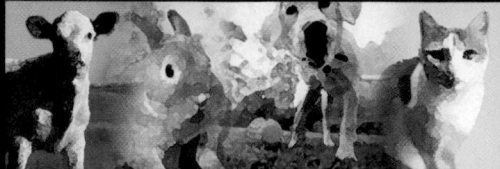

9

Diagnostic Imaging

BETH PAUGH PARTINGTON

INTRODUCTION

Radiology and ultrasonography are the primary diagnostic imaging techniques available to the veterinarian. However, for the veterinarian to arrive at the correct diagnosis on the basis of a radiographic or ultrasound examination, images of high quality must be available. The responsibility to provide useful diagnostic images usually falls to the veterinary technician.

This chapter deals with the basic but essential information needed to produce x-ray films and sonograms of diagnostic quality. It is not the intent of this chapter to offer a course in radiation physics, ultrasound physics, and proper positioning of animals for examination. Excellent textbooks on these subjects have been written and should provide the veterinary technician with the detailed information needed; see Curry et al. (1990), Douglas et al. (1987), Han et al. (2000), Lavin (2003), Morgan (1993), and Ticer (1984). These books should be consulted when the need arises.

This chapter discusses the basic information needed to support and assist the veterinary technician in the area of radiology and diagnostic ultrasonography. A short introduction to the use of nuclear imaging, computed tomography, digital radiography, computed radiography, and magnetic resonance imaging is included. Every effort is made to simplify the radiation and ultrasound physics. ■

RADIOLOGY

LEGAL RECORDS AND FILM IDENTIFICATION

Radiographs are part of the medical record and should be clearly labeled as to which animal has been examined. The identification should include the name of the patient and owner or patient identification number, date of the examination, and name of the hospital.

> ### 🖎 TECHNICIAN NOTE
> Radiographs are part of the legal medical record and must be correctly identified and carefully labeled.

Several methods of film labeling are available. In one method, leaded numbers and letters are placed on the cassette at the time of exposure (Figure 9-1, *A*). These show up as white markings on a finished radiograph. Also available is a special graphite-impregnated tape on which the desired information can be written or typed and placed on the cassette, or the information can be taped on a special filter at the time of exposure (Figure 9-1, *B*). One of the better film identification methods is a *light flasher system* (Figure 9-2). It is simple and inexpensive. The required information is typed on a card that is placed in the imprinter. This system requires placement of a small, leaded blocker in the upper left-hand corner of the film cassette, which will prevent exposure to that part of the film. The card is placed in the light flasher in the darkroom. The unexposed, left-hand corner of the exposed radiograph is placed underneath the card, and the light is flashed through the card. The information recorded on the card is transferred to the x-ray film and will be developed when the radiograph is processed (Figure 9-3).

One final identification method requires both a film identification camera and special windowed film cassettes. This method allows an individual to type the required information on a 3- × 5-inch card and place the card into the ID camera. The windowed corner of the cassette is then automatically opened and "flashed" by the camera, and the information is exposed on the x-ray film. The benefits of this system are that the camera will automatically identify the date and time of the examination, it can be done in

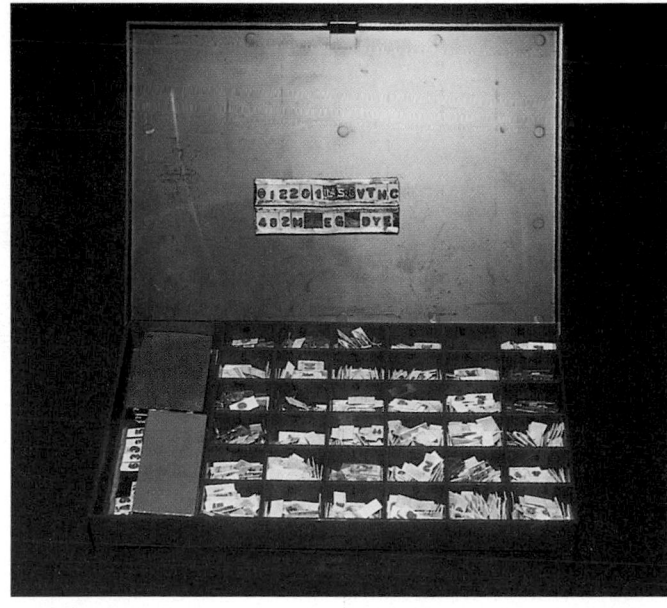
A

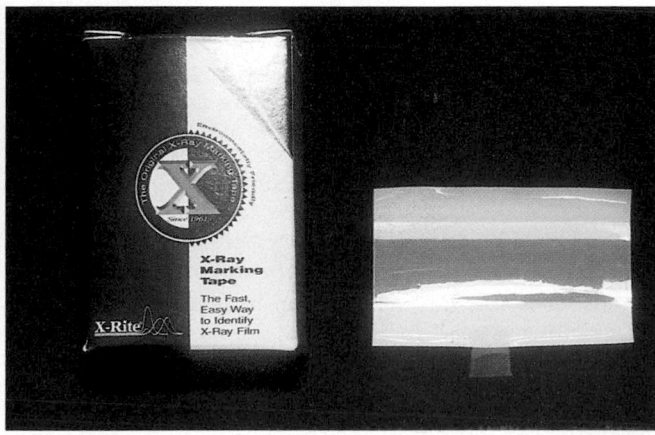
B

Figure 9-1 Film labeling. **A,** Leaded letters and numbers placed on the cassette at the time of exposure. **B,** Radiographic label tape.

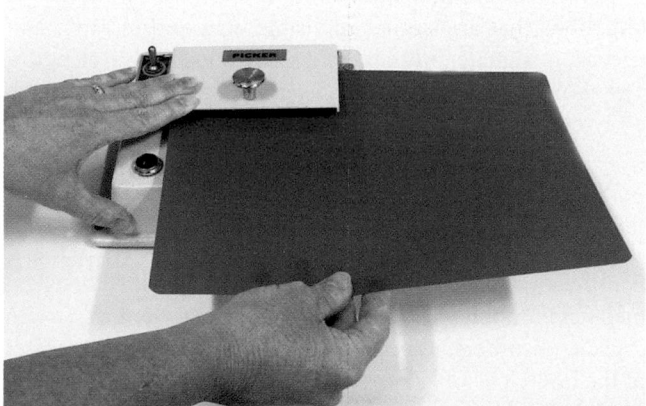

Figure 9-2 Light flasher. Patient information is printed onto a radiograph with an identification printer.

Louisiana State University
Veterinary Teaching Hospital & Clinics
No. 46478   Date 3/20/97
DOB 9/24/84 Owner Partington
Spec. Feline Sex F/S Breed Somali
Animal's Name Emmy
Baton Rouge, Louisiana

Figure 9-3 Film identification as it appears on a radiograph. The identification is flashed onto the film after x-ray exposure with a light flasher system or film identification camera.

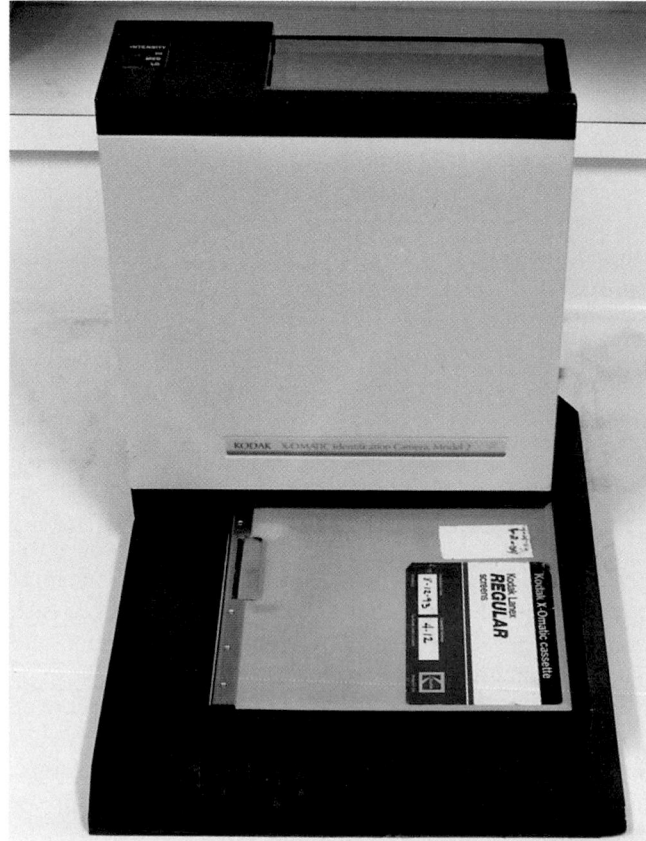

Figure 9-4 Film identification camera and special windowed x-ray cassette. Patient information is typed onto a 3- × 5-inch card and inserted into the top of the camera. The special cassette slides into the camera, which opens the window and flashes the identification onto the film.

daylight, and the area on the film in which the identification information is placed is constant (Figure 9-4).

In addition to the legal identification imprinted on the film, it is necessary to identify the part x-rayed at the time

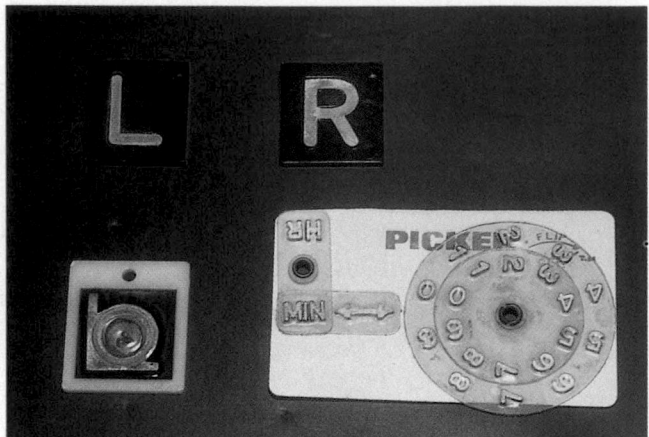

Figure 9-5 Leaded letters for film labeling. Left and right markers are used to label extremities and side of recumbency. The Mitchell marker *(lower left)* is used to identify gravitational direction, and the timer marker *(lower right)* is used with contrast studies to identify length of time since contrast medium administration.

of exposure. Leaded right and left markers should be placed on the cassette at the time of exposure to identify the extremity x-rayed or the side on which the animal is positioned for examination (i.e., right or left lateral recumbency). Additional specialty film markers include Mitchell markers, each of which consists of a plastic bubble containing two to four tiny lead balls that fall toward gravity. These are primarily used in standing radiography of the equine head to assist in identifying fluid levels in paranasal sinuses. Timing markers are used in contrast studies such as upper gastrointestinal studies and excretory urography to indicate when the film was obtained in relation to when the contrast medium was administered (Figure 9-5). Front leg versus hind leg and medial versus lateral side identification markers are critical for proper interpretation of equine lower-extremity radiographs.

FILING OF THE RADIOGRAPH

Because a radiograph is part of the medical record, one must be able to retrieve it when needed. The radiographs of each examination should be placed in an x-ray envelope and filed according to the filing system used for other hospital records (i.e., by last name or case number). The following information should be recorded on the envelope: owner's address, animal identification, date, and type of examination. In addition, the radiographic technique used for the examination can be recorded on the envelope to provide an easy reference for follow-up studies. Many of the veterinary clinic software programs have radiograph and film folder labels automatically available for printing when the patient information is entered. The film labels are convenient, but because they are printed and added to the radiograph after

it is exposed and developed, use of this system increases the risk for radiograph misidentification.

It would be most advantageous to the veterinarian if the envelope could be coded for use as a self-teaching file. Several color tape systems have been devised to code cases for specific purposes. The system could be refined to include a combination of color to identify species, breed, system examined, and so on. Morgan (1993) outlined an excellent color-coded system for x-ray retrieval purposes.

PRODUCTION OF X-RAYS

BASIC PRINCIPLES

A basic understanding of x-ray production, radiologic image formation, interactions of radiation with tissue, and radiation protection is essential. For those with little knowledge of physics or mathematics, the idea of having to learn basic radiation physics may be upsetting. However, the aim is not to teach radiation physics but rather to present basic concepts that are useful for those who use x-ray equipment.

X-rays can be defined as nonluminous electromagnetic radiations that are similar to visible light and to radio and television signals but are of much shorter wavelengths. The shorter the wavelengths, the greater is the energy of the x-ray beam. The greater the energy of the x-ray beam, the greater is its penetration.

X-rays are capable of penetrating opaque or solid substances, ionizing gases, and tissues through which they pass and affecting photographic plates and fluorescent screens. Because of these characteristics, x-rays are widely used in medicine for the study, diagnosis, and treatment of certain organic disorders, especially those of internal structures of the body.

Unfortunately, because of their short wavelengths, x-rays are not visible. As a consequence, many veterinarians, physicians, x-ray technologists, and veterinary technicians tend to become careless in the day-to-day use of x-rays by neglecting to use protective equipment or apply basic radiation safety rules.

THE X-RAY TUBE

Filament and Focusing Cup

The source of x-rays used in diagnostic radiology is the x-ray tube. The generators and transformers used in radiology exist only for the purpose of providing and controlling the amount of electricity reaching the x-ray tube. The x-ray tube is composed of an anode (+) and a cathode (−) enclosed in a vacuum within a glass envelope surrounded by a lead housing. The cathode contains one or two coiled wire filaments within hollowed-out wells or focusing cups. The filaments produce a source of electrons (e−) that are used to produce x-rays (Figure 9-6). The filament is heated to a critical temperature, and the electrons are boiled off

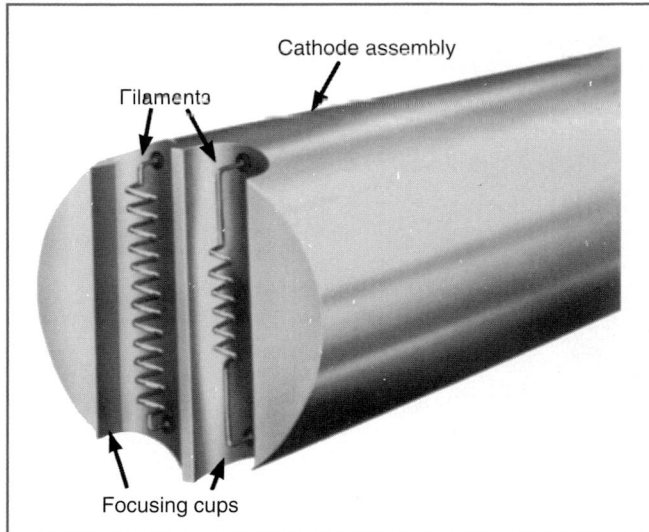

Figure 9-6 Cathode assembly showing focusing cups and filaments of two different sizes. Their arrangements produce electron beams that are focused onto narrow rectangles on the target. The smaller filament produces an electron stream of a smaller cross-sectional area and therefore a smaller focal spot. (From Eastman Kodak Company: *The fundamentals of radiography,* ed 12, Rochester, NY, 1980, Eastman Kodak Company, Radiographic Markets Division.)

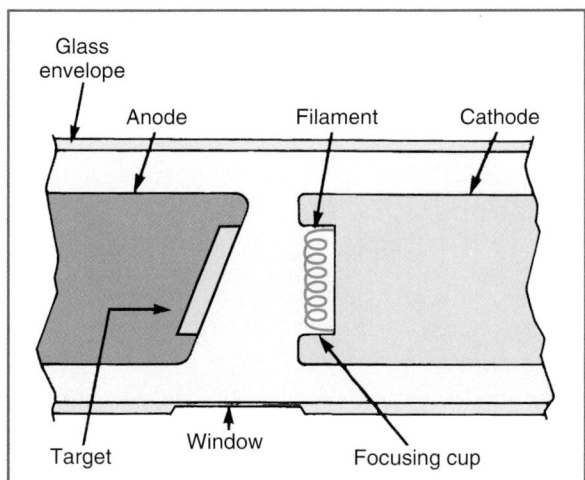

Figure 9-7 Stationary-anode x-ray tube. Diagram shows the relation of the anode and cathode. (From Eastman Kodak Company: *The fundamentals of radiography,* ed 12, Rochester, NY, 1980, Eastman Kodak Company, Radiographic Markets Division.)

and form an electron cloud within the focusing cup. The electrons are then accelerated very rapidly toward the positively charged anode. The collision of the speeding electrons into the anode results in the production of heat and x-rays. The x-rays are directed downward or vertically through the window of the tube by the angle of the anode and the lead shielding of the x-ray tube (Figure 9-7). Two electrical circuits are present in every x-ray tube: a high-voltage, or kilovoltage, circuit and a low-voltage,

or milliamperage, circuit. The kilovoltage circuit controls the electrical potential between the anode and cathode. This controls the speed of the electron acceleration and the energy level or penetrability of the resulting x-ray beam. The milliamperage circuit controls the electrical potential across the filament and affects the volume of electrons created and thus the number or volume of x-rays created.

The filament must produce electrons without melting. To this effect, an *alloy of tungsten* is used because it is less brittle and more efficient than pure tungsten for the production of electrons. This alloy has a high melting point and is used for the manufacture of most x-ray tube filaments.

The larger filament contains more tungsten than the small one and therefore can produce more electrons. As a result, the electron beam produced is larger and does not produce as sharp an x-ray picture as the smaller filament. Unfortunately, because of its size, the small filament may melt more rapidly than the larger one, if an excess load is placed on it. As a result, the veterinarian and veterinary technician must always be aware of the limits and capabilities of the equipment when selecting which filament (focal spot) to use for a given procedure.

Focal Spot

The smaller filament provides a small target region or focal spot for electrons at the anode. In general, the small filament is used to obtain images of higher quality. However, because of the limited number of electrons provided by a small filament, its use is generally restricted to lower mAs (milliamperage × time in seconds) settings used primarily in tabletop (nongrid) extremity radiography. When higher tube current and shorter exposure time are desired, the larger filament must be used, although there will be a loss of detail because the focal spot will be larger.

The size of the focal spot is determined by the size of the electron beam that is accelerated within the tube when high-voltage potentials are applied between the anode and cathode. Thus electrons traveling at an extremely high speed in the vacuum tube are suddenly stopped on the "target" area of the anode. As previously mentioned, the anode target is usually composed of an alloy of tungsten. Tungsten is used because it has the following special properties as a target material:

- High atomic number for the efficient production of x-rays
- High melting point to withstand the large amount of heat generated by the electron beam
- High capacity to transfer heat from the area in which electrons are absorbed
- High density to absorb the electron beam in a small surface area
- Low vapor pressure to maintain the vacuum inside the x-ray tube
- Relatively easy machinability into the appropriate shape at a reasonable cost

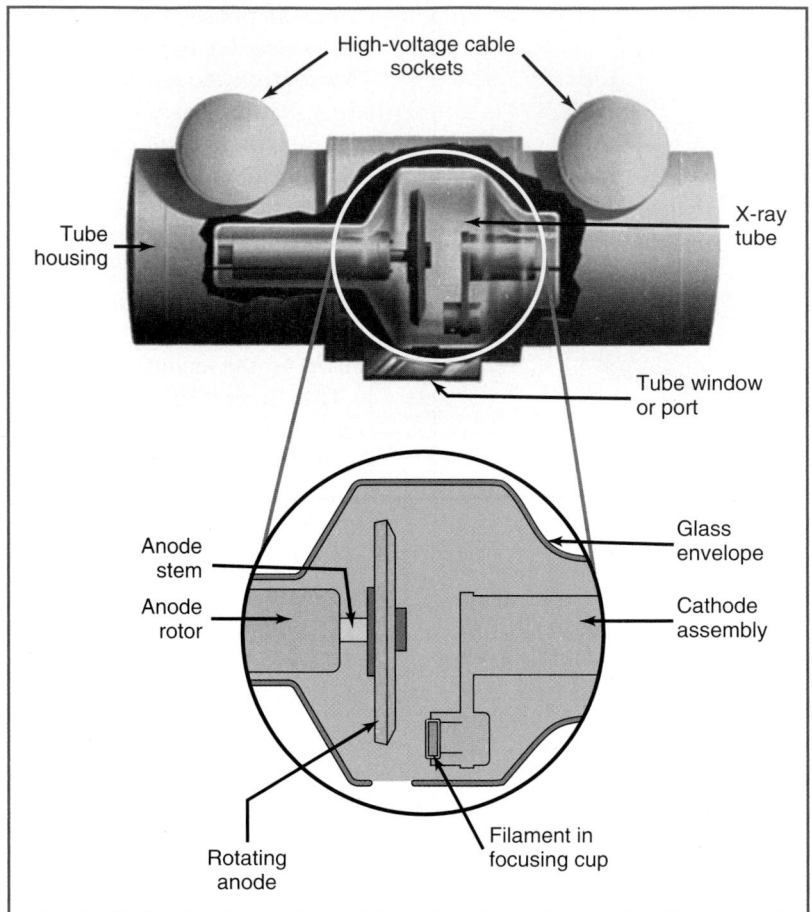

High-voltage cable sockets

Tube housing

X-ray tube

Tube window or port

Anode stem

Anode rotor

Glass envelope

Cathode assembly

Rotating anode

Filament in focusing cup

Figure 9-8 Modern rotating-anode radiographic tube. Exploded schematic view demonstrates the relationship of the filament to the rotating target. (From Eastman Kodak Company: *The fundamentals of radiography,* ed 12, Rochester, NY, 1980, Eastman Kodak Company, Radiographic Markets Division.)

Stationary Anode

In early x-ray equipment, stationary anodes were used in most x-ray tubes. This type of x-ray tube is still prevalent in some veterinary hospitals in which older equipment is used, in dental equipment, and in small portable units used extensively in large animal extremity radiology.

In x-ray tubes with stationary anodes, the target area is a small tungsten block about 3.18 mm thick embedded in a large block of copper. The copper is used to absorb and diffuse the tremendous amount of heat generated by the interaction of the electron beam with the target areas. This type of tube is popular and effective in radiography of the extremities of horses and dogs. However, it has limited application for the abdomen and thorax. The stationary anode x-ray tube cannot produce a sufficiently powerful x-ray beam to penetrate thicker body parts. It is also limited in its ability to produce a very rapid x-ray exposure of sufficient strength for chest radiography to eliminate respiratory motion artifact (Figure 9-7).

Rotating Anode

Rotating anodes became popular with the advent of more powerful x-ray machines and the requirement for radiologists to obtain x-ray pictures of higher quality. Rotating anode tubes can use much higher tube currents, shorter exposure times, and focal spots as small as 0.1 mm because the electrons deposit their energy over a larger target region as the anode rotates (Figure 9-8).

The target of a rotating anode is a tungsten alloy bonded to molybdenum or graphite to help diffuse the tremendous heat generated by a high-powered x-ray machine. Rotating anodes are 7.5 to 12.5 cm in diameter. These tubes must dissipate enormous amounts of heat. The apparatus used to rotate the anode and dissipate the heat must be of the highest quality and perfectly balanced to prevent the tube from wobbling. Any imbalance causes the anode to wobble, leading to loss of image quality and eventual tube destruction. Figure 9-9 is a diagram of a rotating anode tube. Some tubes may rotate at speeds varying from 3600 revolutions

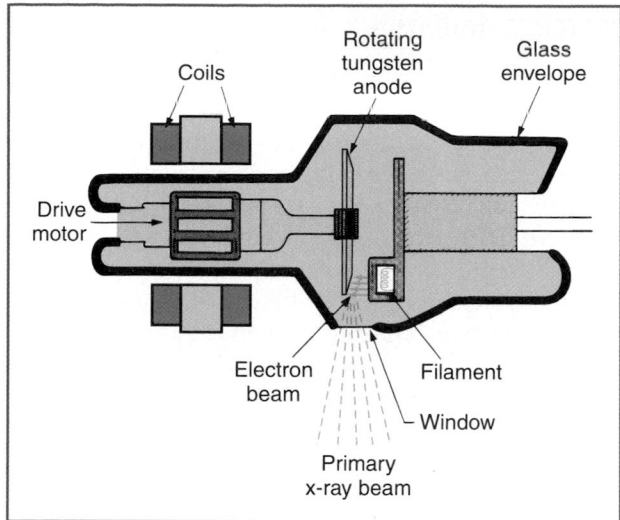

Figure 9-9 Rotating-anode tube. Heat is better dissipated by placing the target material at the circumference of a high-speed rotating disk.

per minute (rpm) to 10,000 rpm. Rotating anode x-ray machines generally have a two-step exposure switch. The first step of the switch starts the anode rotating, and the second step of the switch activates the high-voltage circuit, resulting in x-ray production. The anode is angled for two reasons. One, the angle directs the x-ray beam vertically to exit the tube window; and two, it creates a smaller, more compact effective focal spot to create better resolution and produce a higher-quality radiograph. The actual focal spot is the target on the anode. The effective focal spot is the tightly packed focused primary x-ray beam that exits the tube window. The actual focal spot is always larger than the effective focal spot (Figure 9-10).

Heel Effect

When an x-ray beam leaves the tube, it has an uneven x-ray photon distribution. This phenomenon is related to the angle of the target areas and the absorption by the anode and target material. As a result of this engineering feature, the x-ray beam is more intense at the side of the cathode than in the center of the beam or on the anode side. This phenomenon is called the *heel effect* (Figure 9-11).

This feature can be used to great advantage in veterinary radiology when x-raying parts of uneven thickness, a common problem in thoracic and abdominal radiography of deep-chested dogs. By placing the thickest part of the patient toward the cathode side of the x-ray tube, a more uniform density can be obtained on the radiograph.

✐ TECHNICIAN NOTE

Always place the thickest part of the area being x-rayed toward the cathode side of the x-ray tube.

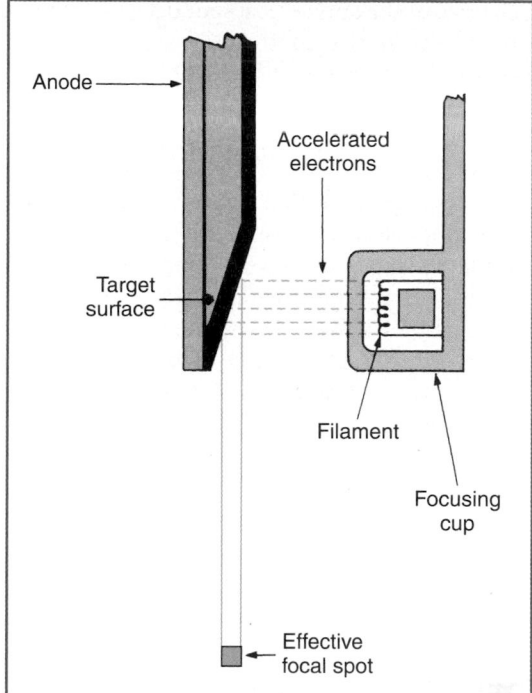

Figure 9-10 Effective focal spot. The surface area is decreased when the target area is constructed at a 20-degree angle to the electron beam.

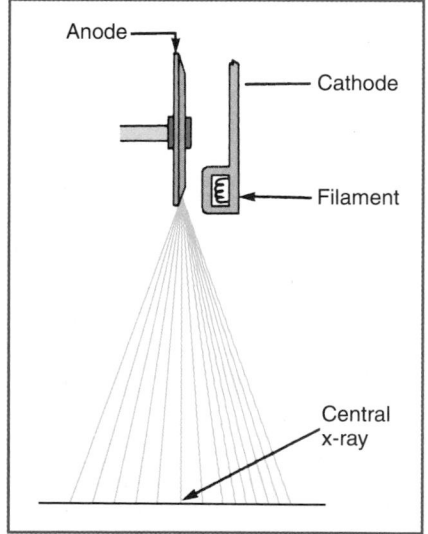

Figure 9-11 Heel effect, which is produced by the uneven intensity of the primary beam. The intensity decreases rapidly toward the anode.

Tube Rating Chart

A rating chart is provided by all manufacturers of x-ray tubes. The tube rating chart provides important information on the maximum safe exposure time that can be used with specific milliamperage and kilovoltage settings. If longer-than-designated exposure times are used, tube damage may occur. The size of the anode focal spot determines the rating of the tube because size controls the amount of energy it can absorb and convert into x-rays and heat.

THE PHYSICS OF X-RAY PRODUCTION

X-rays are produced when all the energy packed in extremely rapidly moving electrons comes to an abrupt stop on encountering the target in the x-ray tube. Most of the energy of the electrons is not converted into x-rays but is dissipated as heat. In fact, more than 99% of the energy dissipated in the target is lost as heat, and less than 1% is converted to x-ray energy. This explains the elaborate system of heat dissipation built into the x-ray tube described in the previous section.

Two events may occur when electrons approach the atoms of the target: (1) the electrons may miss the atom and its orbital electrons and go through the entire target and eventually be absorbed by the backing material of the target or the lead shielding of the x-ray tube, or (2) the incoming electrons may interact with the electron cloud of the atoms in the target material and produce x-rays by transferring their energy to these atoms. Both of these events produce x-ray photons, the majority produced by the slowing of the electrons as they are absorbed into the target. The faster the electrons travel, the greater is their energy and, therefore, the greater is the energy and penetrating power of the resulting x-ray beam.

SCATTERED RADIATIONS

In passing through a patient, an x-ray beam becomes attenuated; in other words, its energy decreases gradually. *Scattered radiations* are lower-energy x-ray photons that have undergone a change in direction after interacting with structures in the patient's body (Figure 9-12).

Scattered radiations are of concern because they decrease film quality and increase radiation exposure to the person taking the radiograph. Most scattered radiations contribute to the overall film blackness or radiographic density but do not contribute to the useful image. This results in reduced subject contrast. Scattered radiations are also the primary source of radiation exposure to technicians manually restraining patients. Scattered radiations are directly increased with increases in the following three factors: kilovoltage, thickness of the part being x-rayed, and size of the field (Figure 9-13).

Careful collimation with beam-limiting devices and close attention to technical factors to avoid the need for retakes are the best ways to decrease radiation exposure from scattered radiations. Several techniques are used to reduce scattered radiations and their effects on the radiograph. Beam-limiting devices, correct kilovolt peak (kVp) settings, compression radiography, and grids are a few devices that can be used to control scattered radiations. They are discussed later in this chapter.

> ### ✏ TECHNICIAN NOTE
> Scattered radiations coming from the area of the patient that is exposed during radiography are the main source of radiation exposure to the veterinary technician.

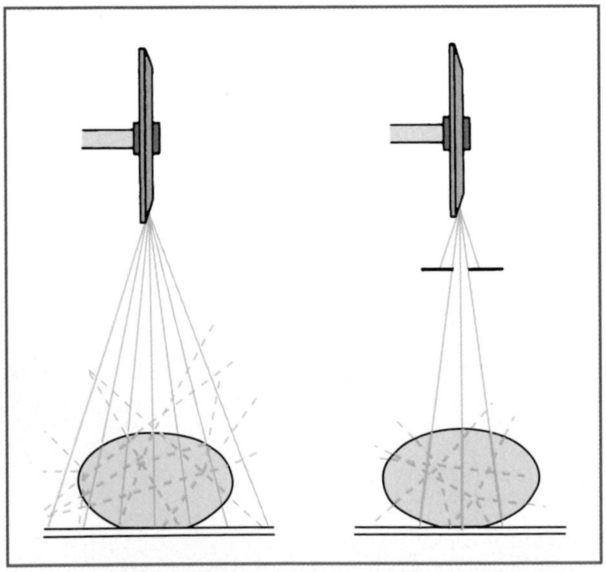

Figure 9-12 Scattered radiations. **A,** Scattered radiations are produced when the primary beam is redirected after interacting with structures in the patient's body. **B,** Reduction in the amount of radiation produced when the primary beam is restricted by a diaphragm or collimator.

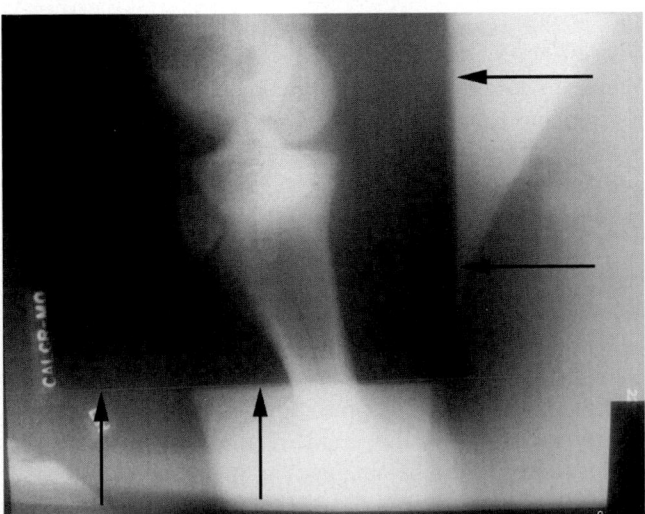

Figure 9-13 Lateral radiograph of an equine stifle. Note the close collimation on the joint *(arrows)* and that the scatter radiation from this area was of sufficient strength to penetrate the rest of the horse's leg and create an underexposed image of the leg on the rest of the radiograph.

X-RAY EQUIPMENT

The kind of x-ray unit encountered in a veterinary practice will vary according to the caseload and type of practice. Because one may be working with a large or small animal practitioner, in a large corporate practice, or in a veterinary teaching hospital, it is necessary to be familiar with the several types of x-ray units found in such practices.

Regardless of type and model, most x-ray machines share many features. For small animal radiology, an x-ray machine must have a table on which the animal can be positioned (Figure 9-14). For larger animals, hand-held or stationary cassette holders are most often used (Figure 9-15). All x-ray machines must have a control panel to select kilovoltage, milliamperage, and time of exposure. An x-ray machine may have numerous auxiliary meters, buttons, dials, or switches; but kilovoltage, milliamperage, and time of exposure are the three primary factors of x-ray production (Figures 9-16 and 9-17). Many x-ray machines have a common selector control for milliamperage and time of exposure. This mAs dial or setting automatically sets the highest milliamperage station and fastest time to provide the requested mAs. Milliamperage × time in seconds (mAs) controls the volume or number of x-ray photons produced. In older machines, milliamperage and time (in fractions of a second) must be set manually to produce a given mAs. The amperage (A) in mAs is always capitalized because it refers to Andre M. Ampere, the physicist credited with discovery of electric currents.

There are basically three types of x-ray machines used in veterinary practice: portable units, mobile units, and stationary units. Please refer to Chapter 28 for a discussion of dental radiographic units.

TECHNICIAN NOTE

Kilovoltage, milliamperage, and time of exposure are the three factors that must be set correctly to produce a properly exposed radiograph.

PORTABLE UNIT

As the name implies, portable units can be carried "easily" from one location to another. Weight varies from 6.75 to 20.25 kg or more. They are generally used on blocks or custom-made stands. From a safety perspective, these units should never be hand held. This recommendation applies especially to lighter models that have less shielding. Hand holding an x-ray machine not only places the operator close to the x-ray tube but also decreases film quality because of tube motion during exposure.

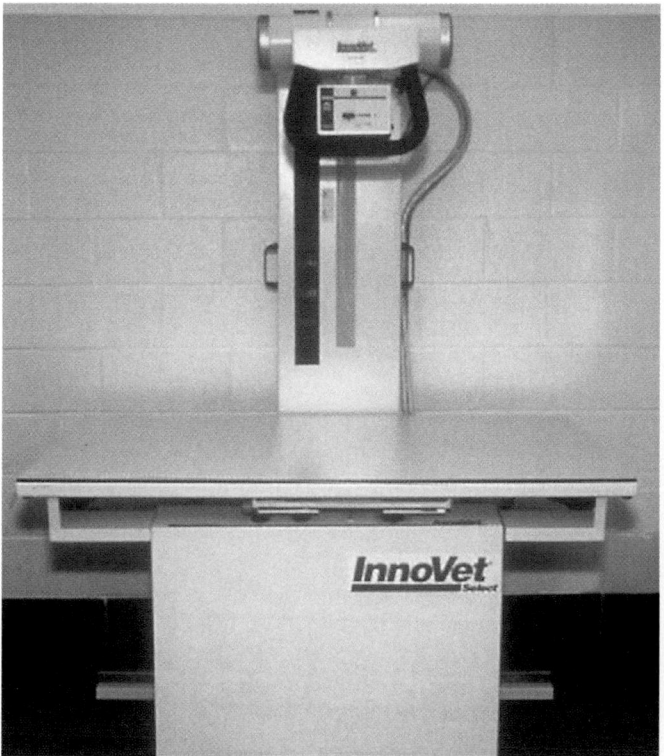

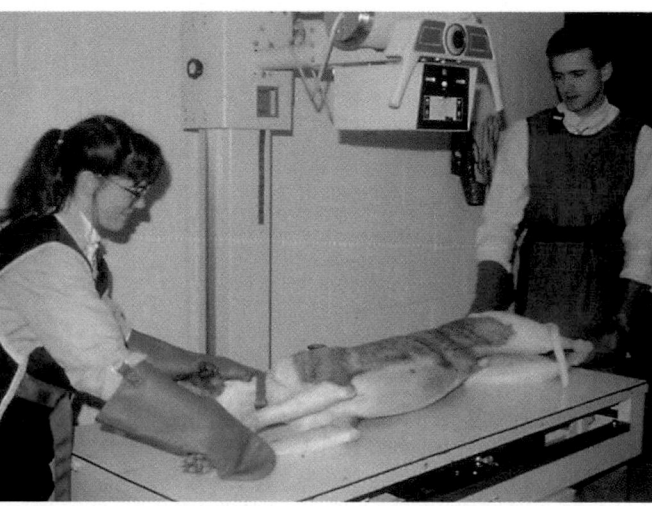

A   B

Figure 9-14 **A,** 300-mA x-ray machine commonly used in small animal practice. **B,** Canine patient correctly positioned on an x-ray table for a lateral thoracic radiograph.

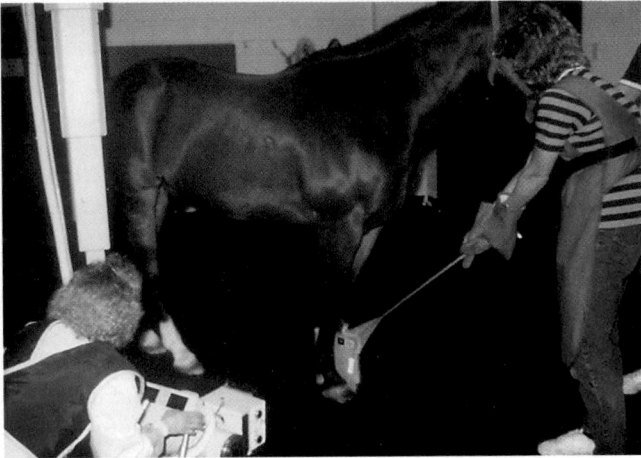

Figure 9-15 Large animal radiography unit with special film cassette holders for equine extremities.

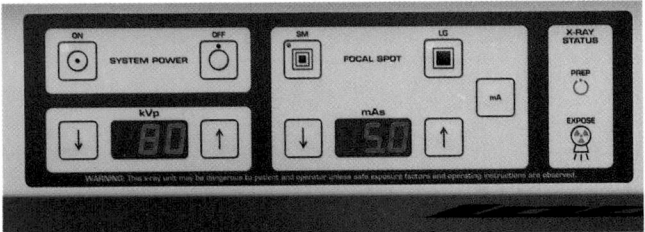

Figure 9-16 Typical instrument panel of an x-ray machine used by veterinarians showing digital panels with buttons for selection of milliamperage, time, and kilovolt peak (kVp).

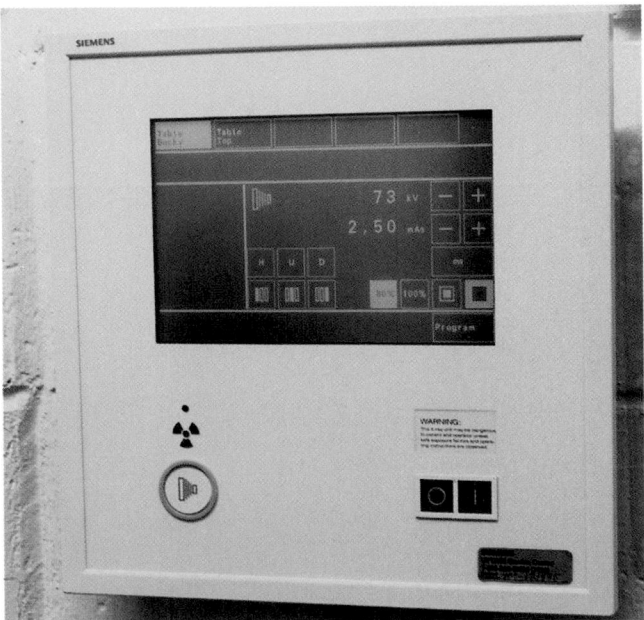

Figure 9-17 Wall-mounted operator control console used in some of the larger veterinary clinics and several veterinary teaching hospitals.

Common characteristics of portable units include the following:

- A single focal spot of about 1.2 mm, stationary anode tube, and single filament, although a few models have two filaments and focal spot sizes
- Collimation varying from lead adapter plate to adapt to film size to lighted collimator with adjustable field size
- Tube output varying up to 90 kVp at 10 mA, usually with settings at 10, 20, and 30 mA and at 70, 80, or 90 kVp
- Electronic timer ranging from 0.01 to 10 seconds
- Electrical input of 110 V with an adapter to 220 V

Some models may use 12 DC (direct current) or operate on an automobile battery with converter (Figure 9-18).

MOBILE UNIT

Mobile units are medium-powered, wheel-mounted units that can be moved around the hospital. In many small animal practices, these units are used as fixed units and remain in one room. They are also popular in a mixed practice, in which the same unit can be used for both large and small animals.

These units are powered by 220-V or 110-V outlets. The 220-V units require more extensive electrical wiring, especially if the same units must be used at several locations.

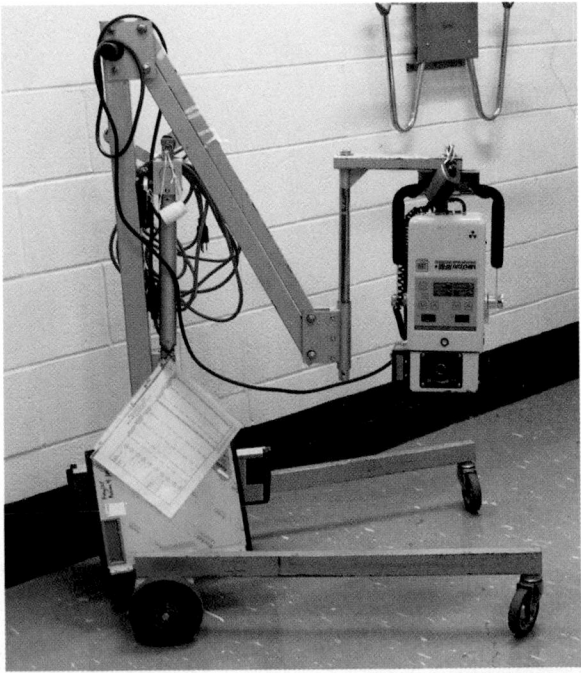

Figure 9-18 Portable x-ray unit. Such units are commonly used in large animal practices, mostly for the examination of extremities. This particular unit has a lighted collimator and a mobile operating stand.

These units are equipped with a long, heavy power cord that can be a problem when working with large animals. The 110-V units are usually lighter and therefore easier to move around, and the power cord is smaller, which can be an advantage when taking x-rays of equine extremities. However, these units are usually less powerful than the 220-V units.

STATIONARY UNIT

Stationary units are more powerful and are found in most small and large animal hospitals. A typical stationary small animal unit is shown in Figure 9-14. Custom large animal units and radiography/fluorography rooms are common in all veterinary teaching hospitals. Some of these units are among the most powerful diagnostic x-ray units installed in the United States.

They vary in size from 300 mA, 100 kVp up to 2000 mA, 150 kVp. They can be powered by single-phase or three-phase generators. The x-ray tube may be suspended from the ceiling or attached to a floor-stand support. The tube can rotate 90 degrees in all directions and usually has a heavy-duty collimator (Figure 9-19).

Stationary units commonly seen in small animal veterinary practices are of the 300 to 500 mA type with an exposure time of $1/60$ second to $1/120$ second. All these units can hold a cassette tray under the table with or without a Potter-Bucky grid. Some units have an image intensifier unit for fluoroscopic study or a fixed fluoroscopic screen.

FLUOROSCOPY

Fluoroscopic units are more suited to the study of moving structures and dynamic processes than are x-ray films. Although films exposed close together in time provide some information about these structures and processes, an image that is continuous in time is required for maximum information. The presentation of a continuous image is called *fluoroscopy*, and it involves directing the x-ray beam through the patient and onto an image intensifier. The image intensifier amplifies the x-ray coming through the patient, thus reducing the amount of radiation needed for the continuous exposure. The resulting images can be videotaped for analysis, and the tapes can be stored as part of the permanent medical record. The use of fluoroscopy is usually confined to gastrointestinal studies and myelography and is essential to heart and vascular studies. A fluoroscopic unit can be a very useful piece of equipment, but it is rarely used in veterinary medicine for economic reasons. For a more extensive discussion of fluoroscopy, review the chapters that cover this subject in Curry et al. (1990), Douglas et al. (1987), Eastman Kodak Co. (1980), Lavin (2003), and Morgan (1993).

DIGITAL RADIOGRAPHY

With the advent of high-performance computers and high-resolution high-luminance monitors digital radiography (DR) has been developed. In DR, an x-ray tube coupled to a specialized receiver that changes x-rays into electrical signals is used. The analogue image is digitalized and displayed on the integrated computer screen (Figure 9-20). The images can be printed on a dry laser camera and will closely resemble typical radiographs, or they can be printed on a variety of imaging printers that process digital data. In most practices, the images are read on the computer screen, and the data are downloaded onto digital videodiscs (DVDs), compact discs (CDs), or magnetic optical disks (MODs) for permanent storage. The advantages of these systems over traditional film/screen radiographs are numerous. They require

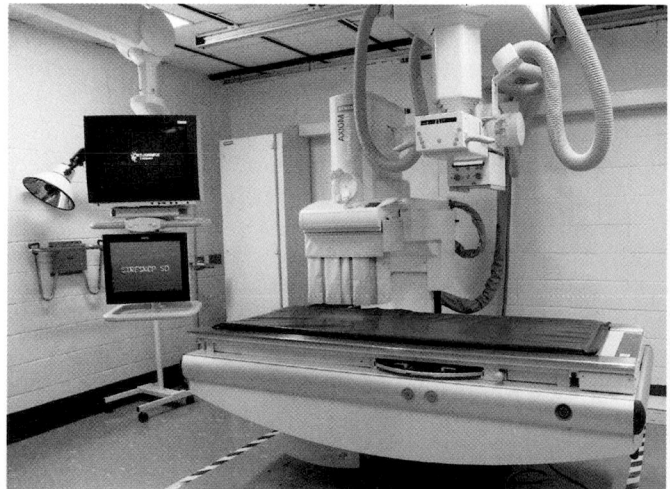
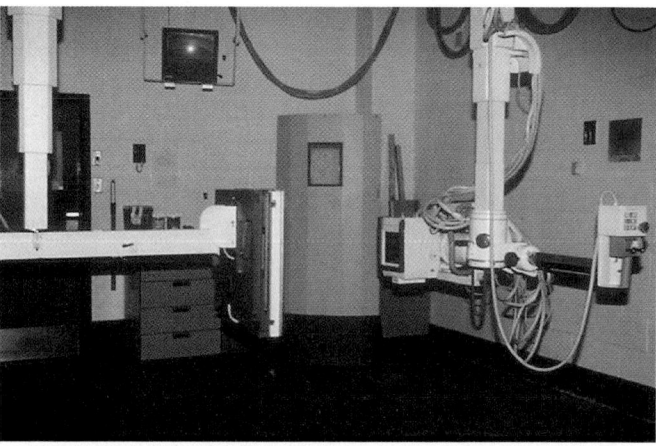

A   **B**

Figure 9-19 Stationary units. **A,** Radiography/fluorography used for special procedures, such as angiography, in a few large and small animal hospitals and all veterinary teaching hospitals. **B,** High-powered stationary large animal unit that includes a ceiling-suspended x-ray unit and a Potter-Bucky suspension system. The two units can be interlocked when needed for a fixed focal spot-film distance.

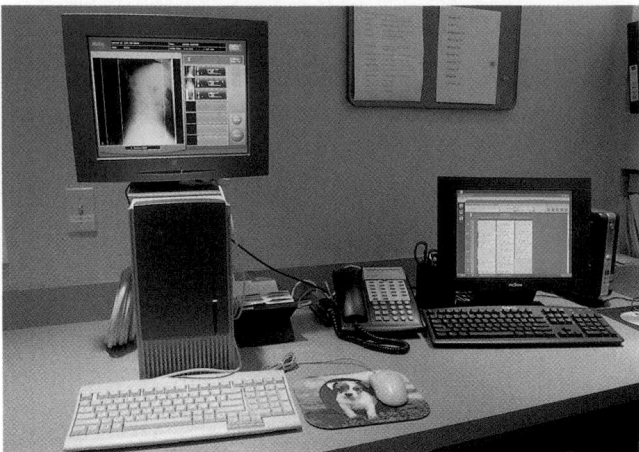

Figure 9-20 Digital radiology control system. The computer on the left is the digital radiography work station where the images are viewed, optimized. and then stored or printed. The computer on the right is an RIS, or radiology information system, used to couple patient data to the images.

no film, screens, or processing. The images can be manipulated after acquisition to adjust brightness and contrast so exposure parameters do not have to be as precise. Portions of an image can often be magnified, which improves visualization of small parts and enhances image interpretation in orthopedics and imaging of exotic animals. In equine practices, you can take as many images as you want without limitations because of cassette numbers, and because the image can be seen almost immediately, you know exactly which views need to be repeated or which additional views are needed without having to go back to the hospital and process your films. Because you can download 50 to 100 images on a single CD, DVD, or MOD film, much less storage space is required. Another big advantage is that because the data are digitalized, you can send these images via phone, T1, DSL, and cable lines to other specialists or referral centers almost instantly for a second opinion and not have to wait for the mail or courier services to transport the radiographs. Disadvantages include increased initial equipment cost, problems typical of any computer system such as power failures and lost data, and the possibility of increased radiation exposure as a result of overuse.

COMPUTED RADIOGRAPHY

Computed radiography (CR) is very similar to DR except that an x-ray receiver similar to a cassette is used and must be processed in a special machine (Figure 9-21). The special cassette contains a photostimulable phosphor that changes x-ray photons into a latent electronic image that is "read" by the processor and transferred to the computer. After that, the image data have all the advantages and disadvantages of DR. CR is primarily used in large human hospitals that have several x-ray machines in various departments and want a portable method to have digitized images from all of

them. CR will probably not be as popular as the DR system in veterinary medicine, except at large teaching hospitals or specialty clinics with several x-ray machines currently in use, because of the need for the special cassettes and latent image reader. There is some confusion about DR and CR in the veterinary marketplace, with some DR systems calling themselves "computed radiography." The question to ask is whether the x-ray receiver directly digitizes the image (true digital radiography) or whether a separate cassette and reader are needed to digitize the image (computed radiology).

EXPOSURE FACTORS

The veterinary technician is responsible for selecting an x-ray technique that will provide a diagnostic radiograph. The factors that must be selected are time of exposure, milliamperage, and kilovoltage. As previously mentioned, most recent x-ray machines have a common dial for time of exposure and milliamperage, called the mAs setting. The selection of each factor is based on an accurate technique chart. Preparation of a technique chart is discussed later in this chapter.

Other factors that enter into the production of a diagnostic radiograph are focal-film distance, type of intensifying screen, type of x-ray film, and tabletop versus grid technique. All of these variables are discussed in greater detail.

MILLIAMPERAGE

The milliamperage setting controls the quantity of electrons boiled off the filament in the x-ray tube. It is a *quantity factor*, because it controls the amount of x-rays that will be produced at the target area. Most diagnostic units used in small animal radiology are operated at settings from 50 to 300 mA. The smallest portable x-ray unit commonly used in large animal practices may use current flow as low as 10 or 20 mA, whereas the larger units used in small animal hospitals and veterinary teaching hospitals may have a current flow of 2000 mA.

Adjustments of the milliamperage setting control on an x-ray machine will control the amount of x-rays produced. When one increases the milliamperage setting, radiographic density, or film blackness, increases; conversely, when one decreases the milliamperage setting, a reduction in radiographic density, or a lighter film, results.

EXPOSURE TIME

The exposure time is the time in fractions of a second during which the anode is positively charged. The longer the exposure time, the greater is the number of electrons that flow from the cathode to the anode and the greater is the number of x-ray photons. Because both exposure time and milliamperage affect the number of photons created and because you want the shortest exposure time possible to

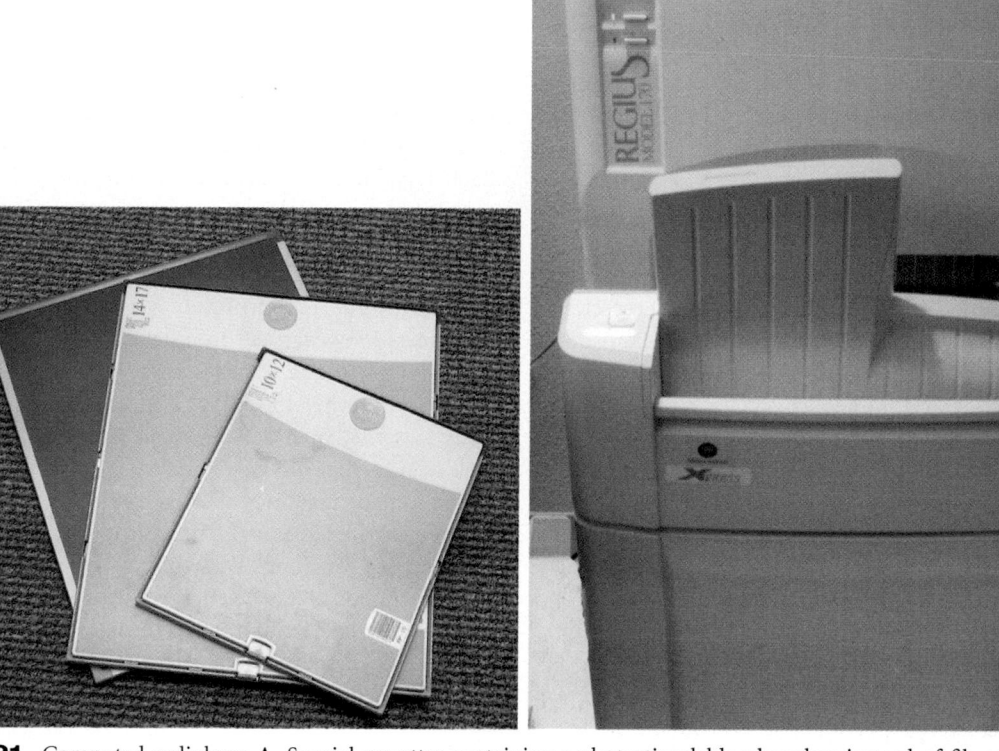

Figure 9-21 Computed radiology. **A,** Special cassettes containing a photostimulable phosphor instead of film to capture the latent x-ray image. **B,** The computed radiology reader that takes the specialized cassette and downloads the latent image into a computer.

decrease patient motion blur, you should always use the highest milliamperage setting and the lowest time setting to arrive at the desired mAs. By using the highest milliamperage setting, you are maximizing the number of electrons in the focusing cup so you only have to charge the anode for a very short period (exposure time) to get the number of electrons needed to the anode to create the desired number of x-ray photons.

> **✎ TECHNICIAN NOTE**
>
> Always use the highest milliamperage setting and the lowest time setting to arrive at a particular mAs. This will decrease motion blur on the radiograph.

As an example to illustrate this concept, an exposure made at 100 mA and $^1/_{10}$ second should produce a film of equivalent density to an exposure made at 200 mA and $^1/_{20}$ second. In both cases the mAs factor (milliamperage × time) is the same and is equal to 10 mAs. Shorter exposure times reduce the problem of motion, which may result in loss of detail. For this reason, a thoracic radiograph on a dog or cat should be taken at $^1/_{20}$ to $^1/_{60}$ second to prevent blurring of the radiograph as a result of respiratory motion.

KILOVOLTAGE

Kilovoltage is a *quality factor* that regulates the energy of the x-ray beam. This setting regulates the voltage differential applied between the anode and cathode in the x-ray tube. The higher the voltage, the faster the electrons are accelerated and the greater is the energy of the x-ray beam. The greater the energy, the greater is the amount of patient tissue that can be penetrated. Increasing the kilovoltage will also increase radiographic density, or film blackness, because of increased x-ray photons passing through the patient. The kilovoltage setting most often used in diagnostic radiology varies from 40,000 to 150,000 V (40 to 150 kV).

The kilovoltage setting affects the scale of contrast on a radiograph. The scale of contrast refers to the number of shades of gray that can be seen. In general, the higher the kVp, the greater is the scale of contrast, and the quality of the x-ray film is improved because small differences in soft tissue density are more visible. Higher kilovoltage lower mAs settings are used for soft tissue examination, such as thoracic examinations with low inherent contrast. Lower kilovoltage higher mAs settings are used for bone structures with high inherent contrast.

You must have a kVp setting high enough to penetrate your patient. If your radiographs are too light from exposure problems and you have increased your mAs with no increase in film density or blackness, you may have insufficient x-ray photon energy (too low a kVp) to penetrate your patient.

> ✎ **TECHNICIAN NOTE**
>
> You can increase radiographic density or film blackness by either increasing the energy level of the x-ray photons (kVp) or the total number of x-ray photons (mAs).

FOCAL-FILM DISTANCE

The focal-film distance refers to the distance between the target in the x-ray tube and the surface of the x-ray cassette. This factor is normally kept constant from one exposure to another. It is usually kept at a distance of 70 to 85 cm for large animal radiology and 90 to 105 cm for small animal radiology.

It is important to keep the focal-film distance constant from one exposure to the next because it has a significant influence on exposure factors. An increase in distance decreases the number of x-rays reaching the film. This is not a linear relationship. If you double the focal-film distance, the number of x-rays reaching the film will be reduced by a factor of four. This is often referred to as the *inverse square law,* which states that the intensity of the x-ray beam at a given point is inversely proportional to the square of the distance from the x-ray source.

> ✎ **TECHNICIAN NOTE**
>
> If you double the film distance from the x-ray source, you will decrease the x-ray beam intensity to one fourth of the original strength. Small changes in focal-film distance can result in big changes in radiographic density.

It is sometimes necessary to change the focal-film distance to obtain proper positioning. The following simple calculation will help you choose the new mAs setting when the distance is changed:

$$\frac{\text{Old mAs} \times \text{New distance F2}}{\text{Old distance F2}} = \text{New mAs setting}$$

For example, if an x-ray taken at 10 mAs at 100 cm must be taken at 50 cm, by using the formula given, the new mAs setting can be calculated as follows:

$$\frac{10 \text{ mAs} \times 50 \text{ F2}}{100 \text{ F2}} = 2.5 \text{ mAs}$$

This new mAs setting should produce an x-ray of similar radiographic density to the original setting of 10 mAs.

TECHNIQUE CHART

A technique chart is an essential component for obtaining diagnostic x-ray examinations in a consistent way. A technique chart must be formulated for each x-ray machine because there are differences in output with each machine (even those made by the same manufacturer). Therefore you should never use an x-ray chart formulated for another x-ray machine without making appropriate changes. If you select exposure factors from a good technique chart, consistent radiographic examinations of diagnostic quality will be obtained. In addition, there will be a saving on x-ray film because waste from repeated exposures will be avoided.

Several types of technique charts can be formulated. Each type must be formulated with the goal of using the maximum potential of a particular x-ray machine. Perhaps the most popular type of technique chart used by veterinarians is a variable kilovoltage chart. A variable mAs chart is probably more appropriate for the most powerful x-ray machines. However, a combination of variable kilovoltage and mAs technique charts is best. Such charts take into consideration the need to adapt a technique chart for different body systems, such as a thoracic and abdominal study, as well as examinations involving the musculoskeletal system.

This chapter cannot discuss appropriately every type of technique chart. The principle of how to prepare a variable kilovoltage technique chart, along with an example of such a chart (Table 9-1), is given. For a more extensive discussion of how to prepare different technique charts with examples of each, please refer to the discussions of this topic by Han et al. (2000), Lavin (2003), Morgan (1993), and Ticer (1984).

Formulation of a Technique Chart

A technique chart is formulated by a series of trial-and-error exposures. It is necessary, however, to standardize as many variable factors as possible before starting trial exposures. Factors such as the type of cassette and intensifying screen, type of x-ray film, and the focal-film distance must be constant, and a grid should be used if available. The darkroom procedures must be standardized to include fresh solution and developing time recommended by the manufacturer based on the temperature of the solution. All of these factors should be constant because the technique chart will be valid only under the conditions of formulation. If, for example, cassettes and intensifying screens in a veterinary practice are of different age or speed, the film density for a given technique will be different from one study to the next, even though the same factors are used.

For trial exposure, a normal dog with a lateral abdominal measurement of 8 to 10 cm should be selected. A trial exposure at a setting of 65 kV at 2.5 mAs is suggested. Two exposures are made at this setting. In selecting the mAs setting, the shortest possible time of exposure for a given mAs setting is selected. The two films are then developed according to standard technique and are examined for proper "diagnostic" density. If the films are either overexposed or underexposed, a second series of exposures is made by halving or doubling the mAs setting. The films are again processed and examined for diagnostic quality. All films should be examined and compared with each other for

Table 9-1 Variable kV Technique Chart for an X-Ray Machine of 300 mA, 125 kV, 1/120-Second Timer with FFD of 40 Inches

Thickness (cm)	kV	mA	Seconds	mAs	Grid 8:1
4	48	300	1/120	2.5	No
5	50	300	1/120	2.5	No
6	52	300	1/120	2.5	No
7	54	300	1/120	2.5	No
8	56	300	1/120	2.5	No
9	58	300	1/120	2.5	No
10	63	300	1/60	5	Yes
11	65	300	1/60	5	Yes
12	67	300	1/60	5	Yes
13	69	300	1/60	5	Yes
14	71	300	1/60	5	Yes
15	73	300	1/60	5	Yes
16	75	300	1/60	5	Yes
17	77	300	1/60	5	Yes
18	79	300	1/60	5	Yes
19	81	300	1/60	5	Yes
20	84	300	1/60	5	Yes
21	87	300	1/60	5	Yes
22	90	300	1/60	5	Yes
23	93	300	1/60	5	Yes
24	96	300	1/60	5	Yes
25	99	300	1/60	5	Yes
26	102	300	1/60	5	Yes
27	105	300	1/60	5	Yes
28	99	300	1/30	10	Yes
29	102	300	1/30	10	Yes
30	105	300	1/30	10	Yes

FFD, Focal-film distance; *kV*, kilovolts; *mA*, milliamperes; *mAs*, milliamperes per second.
Radiographs were taken with Kodak Lanex Regular screens and Kodak TML x-ray film.

consistent density between exposures. The best film is selected. If one of the techniques selected is completely satisfactory, a technique can be formulated starting with the factors that produced the "diagnostic" film. If, however, none of the films are totally satisfactory, a fourth series of exposures is started in which the kilovoltage setting is decreased or increased until an excellent film is obtained.

Because there is an increase in scattered radiation with an increase in thickness of a part to be x-rayed, it is recommended that a grid be used for thicknesses greater than 10 cm. If a grid of 8:1 ratio is used, it will necessitate a doubling of the mAs setting technique over the formulated technique. At this point, however, it is recommended that the accuracy of the technique chart be checked by making a few trial exposures of larger dogs by using a grid.

The technique chart is formulated by subtracting 2 kV for each decrease in centimeter of thickness and adding 2 kV for each increase in centimeter of thickness. You should keep in mind that a doubling of the mAs setting is necessary at thicknesses greater than 10 cm if a grid is used. At 80 kV and higher, the increase in kilovoltage should be in steps of 3 kV for each increase in centimeter thickness until the limit of the machine is reached.

Table 9-1 shows a variable kilovoltage technique chart formulated for an x-ray machine of 300 mA, 125 kV, and 1/120 second minimum time of exposure. Remember, however, that this is only an illustration of how to formulate a technique chart and should not be used with any one x-ray machine without adaptation to that particular machine.

✎ TECHNICIAN NOTE

Technique charts are developed for a specific focal-film distance, film, cassette screen, and development process. If you change any one of these factors, the technique chart will not be correct.

IMAGE FORMATION

When an x-ray beam penetrates a body system and reaches an x-ray film, a latent image is produced that will be revealed when the film is processed chemically. Several factors are

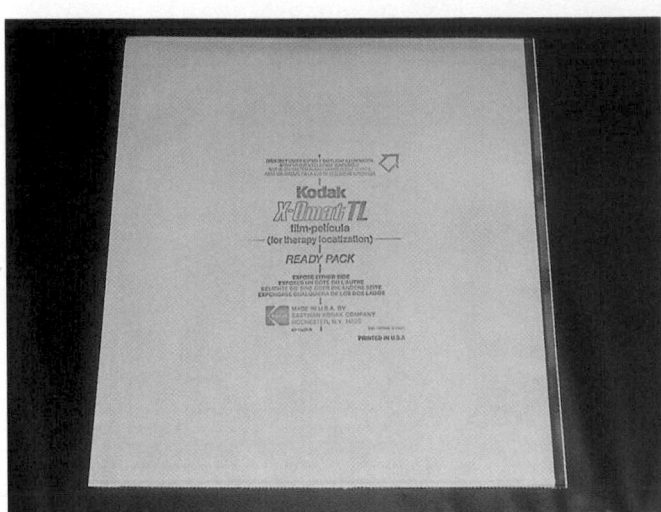
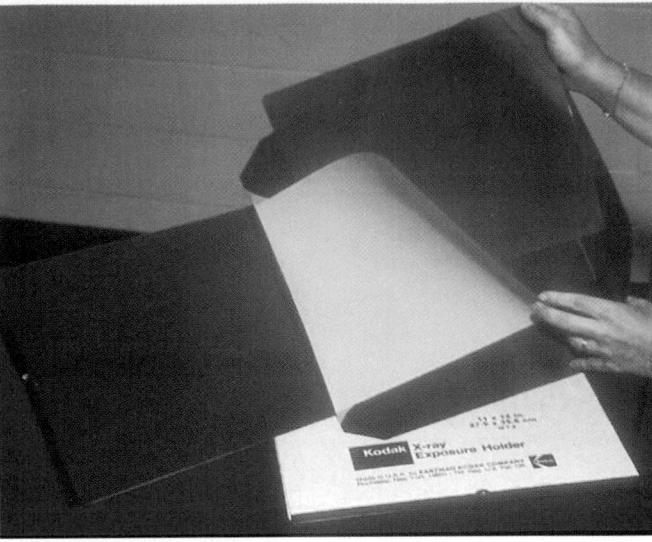

A **B**

Figure 9-22 Nonscreen film. **A,** Ready pack film with a special emulsion for direct exposure. **B,** X-ray exposure holder for regular screen film. Such a soft cassette necessitates exposure time in excess of 26 times the normal exposure time of a regular par screen cassette system. (From Eastman Kodak Company: *The fundamentals of radiography,* ed 12, Rochester, NY, 1980, Eastman Kodak Company, Radiographic Markets Division.)

involved in the formation of a high-quality latent image. This section discusses the factors that enter into the formation of an x-ray image.

X-RAY CASSETTE

Cassettes (film holders) used in veterinary medicine are of two types. The *nonscreen* type is a direct-exposure *cassette* in which the film is placed in a cardboard cassette or a plastic film holder (Figure 9-22). This nonrigid system must be light-proof and is used when great detail is needed for an examination. The disadvantage of this type of cassette is that it will require an exposure time in excess of 26 times the normal exposure time of a regular par screen cassette system. Nonscreen exposures should be used only when the animal is under general anesthesia or heavy sedation to stop motion and when no personnel are required for restraint in the radiology room. Nonscreen exposures are used primarily for intraoral occlusal studies of the nasal cavity and dental arches.

The second type is the more conventional *image intensifying screen,* which is placed in a *rigid cassette* (Figure 9-23). It is important that the hinges of the cassette be of the highest quality to ensure excellent and uniform contact between the x-ray film and the intensifying screen and to prevent light leakage that could fog or darken the film. Various materials are used in the manufacture of x-ray cassettes. Most cassettes have a solid front made of either plastic or light metal. Recently, carbon fiber (mostly graphite) has also been used. Such cassettes are excellent and may reduce the amount of x-rays needed to make an exposure by as much as 20%. The cassette back may be made of steel and can sustain moderate

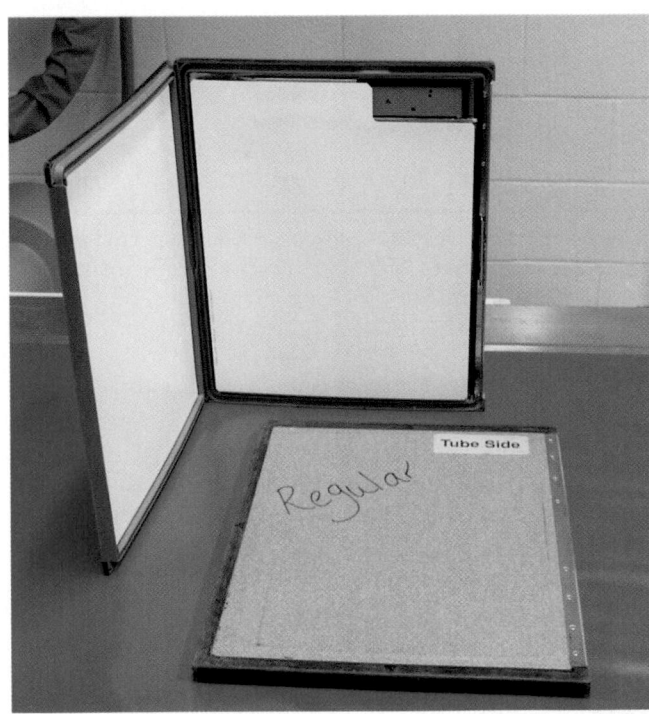

Figure 9-23 Open and closed rigid film cassette with image intensifying screens.

patient weight without being damaged. Sometimes a small area of about 7 × 3 cm is shielded from the primary beam for the purpose of film identification (Figure 9-4).

Cassettes are expensive and should be handled with care. When dropped, they may warp, or if the cover is forced, the hinges may be damaged, resulting in a cassette that does

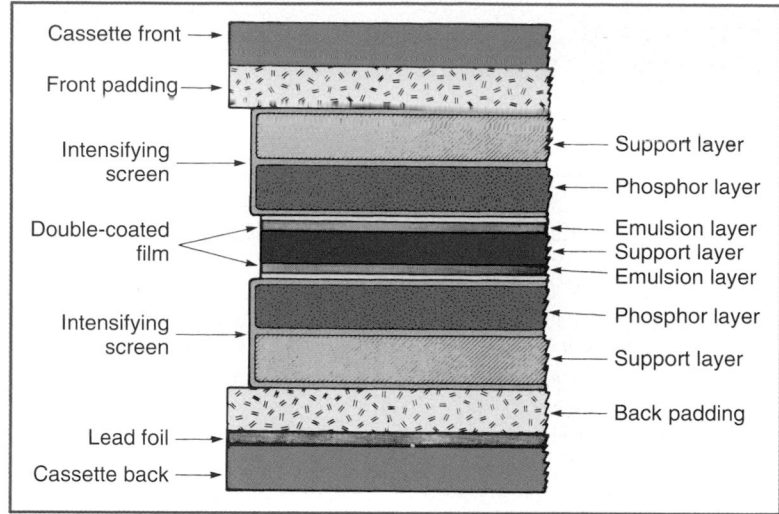

Figure 9-24 Cross section of a cassette intensifying screen system.

not close properly. If the film contact is not perfect along the surface of the cassette, distortion of the x-ray image will occur. The surface of the cassette should be kept clean at all times to prevent the creation of film artifacts.

INTENSIFYING SCREENS

Intensifying screens are the smooth shiny white inner surfaces of the film cassette. They are made of layers of tiny crystals bonded together on a plastic support and covered with a protective coating. These crystals fluoresce, or emit light, after exposure to x-rays. The screens are placed in the inner surfaces of the cassette, and the x-ray film is sandwiched between. Because film is more sensitive to light exposure than to radiation exposure, the use of fluorescent intensifying screens dramatically decreases the amount of radiation needed to produce a film of diagnostic radiographic density. Screens allow much lower mAs settings, which decrease loss of detail as a result of motion, decrease patient radiation exposure, and help to prolong the life of the x-ray tube. In addition, intensifying screens increase radiographic contrast and therefore improve radiographic detail.

Intensifying screens are mounted in pairs in an x-ray cassette (Figure 9-24). They are made of the following four components:

1. A backing of cardboard or plastic, most commonly a Mylar material
2. Reflecting layers, such as titanium dioxide, that reflect light from the active layer back toward the x-ray film
3. An active layer of light-emitting phosphor, such as calcium tungstate or rare earth material, that produces the fluorescence that exposes the film after absorption of x-rays
4. A plastic coating that reduces static electricity and provides a protective covering that can be cleaned

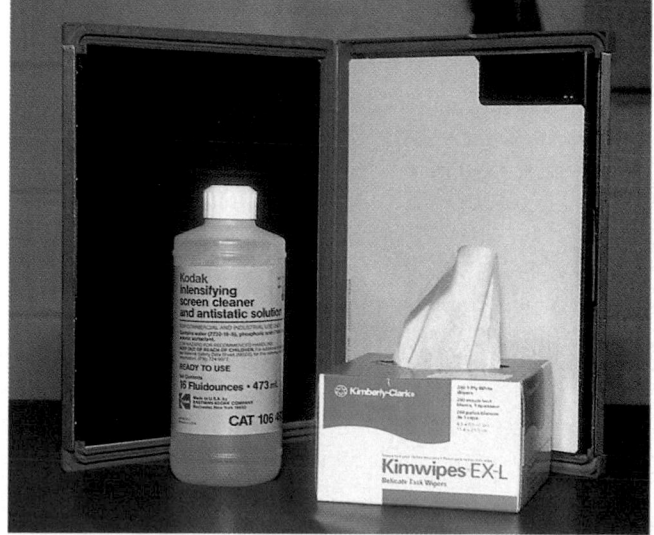

Figure 9-25 Open film cassette with a single intensifying screen (shiny white surface), used for detail extremity radiography. Screens should be handled carefully and cleaned regularly with approved solutions.

The screens must be cleaned on a regular basis—at least monthly or whenever screen artifacts are noted on a radiograph. It is best to use a cleaning product recommended by the manufacturer for this purpose. If such a product is not available, a 70% alcohol solution will work (Figure 9-25). The surface of the screen must be thoroughly dry before an x-ray film is inserted or the cassette is closed; otherwise, the film will stick to the screens and permanently ruin them. Any stain on the surface of the screen will interfere with transmission of light from the screen to the film and cause an artifact. The technician must be very careful not to spill or splash darkroom chemicals onto the surface of the

Table 9-2 RELATIVE SPEED OF CALCIUM TUNGSTATE* AND RARE EARTH† SCREENS

Screen Type	ASA Film Speed
Fine-detail calcium tungstate	30
Par calcium tungstate	100
Fine-detail rare earth	150
Regular calcium tungstate	200
Fast calcium tungstate	250
Medium rare earth	300
Regular rare earth	400
Fast rare earth	600

*Kodak X-O$_{MAT}$ with X-O$_{MAT}$ RP film.
†Kodak Lanex with T MAT L film.

screens, or they may be ruined. For this reason, emphasis is placed on the maintenance and cleanliness of screens.

SCREEN SPEED

The speed of a screen pertains to its ability to convert absorbed x-ray energy into visible light. Screen speed is a relative term that refers to the amount of radiation required by that screen to produce a film of diagnostic radiographic density. A fast screen requires less radiation than a regular, medium, or par screen to produce the same degree of blackness on the radiograph. The faster the screen, the poorer is the radiographic detail or resolution. Fast screens have a thicker phosphor layer and larger crystals to increase x-ray absorption and light production. Slower or detail screens have smaller crystals and are less efficient at light conversion but produce a radiograph of greater detail and resolution. Detail screens are also called *fine screens* and generally require four times the amount of radiation as a medium or par screen. These are best for obtaining radiographs of birds and small exotic animals. Regular screens are intermediate in speed between par or medium and fast screens.

The original phosphor used in intensifying screens was calcium tungstate. This phosphor produces light in the blue spectrum and is commonly found in veterinary hospitals that have acquired used cassettes and screens from local human hospitals. Improved rare earth phosphors introduced in 1975 emit light in the green spectrum and are able to produce the same degree of radiographic detail as calcium tungstate screens with less radiation exposure. Table 9-2 shows the relative speed of various calcium tungstate and rare earth screens. Rare earth screens are more efficient because they absorb more x-ray photons per crystal and produce more light per absorbed photon. These properties of rare earth screens have definite advantages in veterinary medicine and include the following:

- Reduced exposure time
- Reduced motion artifacts
- Decreased tube voltage, resulting in improved contrast
- Decreased tube current, which prolongs the life of the tube
- Reduced production of heat in the x-ray tube
- Reduced patient radiation dose

✎ TECHNICIAN NOTE

Rare earth screens are advantageous for veterinary radiography because they require fewer x-rays to produce a diagnostic radiograph. Lower exposures mean lower radiation doses to the patient and technician, fewer retakes because of patient motion, and longer x-ray tube life.

The main disadvantage of rare earth screens at this time is their cost, which is much greater than that of regular calcium tungstate screens. They have a definite place in large animal radiology because of their speed. This is an important factor when they are used with the smaller, low-capacity portable x-ray units. Table 9-3 presents an example of a technique chart that can be used with a small, portable x-ray unit in combination with the rare earth screen.

There is a misconception in veterinary medicine that intensifying screens last forever. This is not true. Screens have a predictable lifetime and gradually wear out with repeated use. Most rare earth screens are worn out after 10 to 12 years of regular use. The radiograph produced with a very old screen will have a white speckled pattern, most notable in the black areas on the film. This artifact is called *screen craze*. Most screens have a company name and screen number printed on the edge. By calling the manufacturer, the technician can find out the age of the screen and the best type of film to use with that particular screen.

X-RAY FILM

Because the recording medium for most x-ray examinations is photographic film, some basic principles of photography must be understood.

An x-ray film is prepared from a suspension of light and x-ray–sensitive granules embedded in a gelatin emulsion coated over a polyester base. The sensitive granules are usually silver bromide crystals of different sizes. The gelatin matrix is protected by a thin covering called the *T coat*. Just like the image-intensifying screens, the sensitive crystals come in various sizes. Images of exceptional detail can be recorded on films containing very fine crystals. In faster films the crystals are larger, which results in a loss of detail, which is compensated for, however, by possible shorter time of exposure. Because of the shorter time of exposure, faster films may sometimes provide better image detail because the images contain fewer motion artifacts.

X-ray film can be separated into two categories: *screen film* (Figure 9-26) and *nonscreen film*. Screen film is sensitive primarily to the wavelengths of light emitted from intensifying screens. Nonscreen films are designed for direct exposures to x-rays and are relatively insensitive to visible

Table 9-3 TECHNIQUE CHART FOR PORTABLE X-RAY UNIT OF 10 mA AT 90-kV, 15 mA AT 80-kV, AND 20 mA AT 70-kV CAPACITY KODAK CASSETTE WHEN RARE EARTH SCREEN OF REGULAR SPEED* IS USED

Examination	Size	View	kVp	Time (sec)	Distance (cm)
Fetlock	Foal	DP or obliques	80	0.02	60
	Large adult		80	0.04	70
Carpus	Foal	DP or obliques	80	0.02	70
	Large adult		80	0.04	70
Tarsus	Foal	Lat	80	0.02	70
		DP	80	0.04	70
	Adult	Lat	80	0.04	70
		DP	80	0.08	70
Stifle	Adult	Lat	80	0.1	70
		CdCa	90	0.25	70

DP, Dorsoplantar or dorsopalmar; *kV*, kilovolts; *mA*, milliamperes; *kVp*, kilovolt peak; *Lat*, lateral; *CdCa*, caudocranial.

*For a more complete treatment of cassette and image-intensifying screens, refer to Douglas et al. (1987) and Morgan (1993). Both have excellent discussion of all types of screen available on the market today.

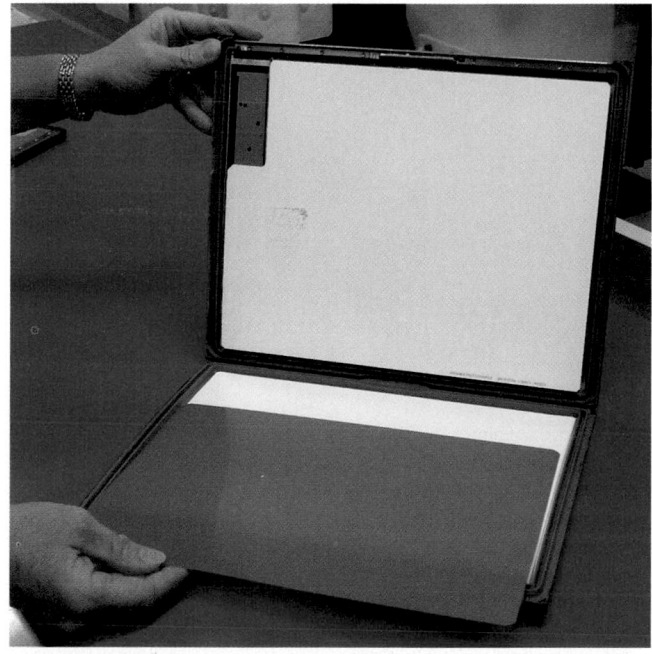

Figure 9-26 Screen film manufactured for the special purpose of being used with image-intensifying screens. Such film, when used with the proper combination of screen, will drastically reduce x-ray exposure time.

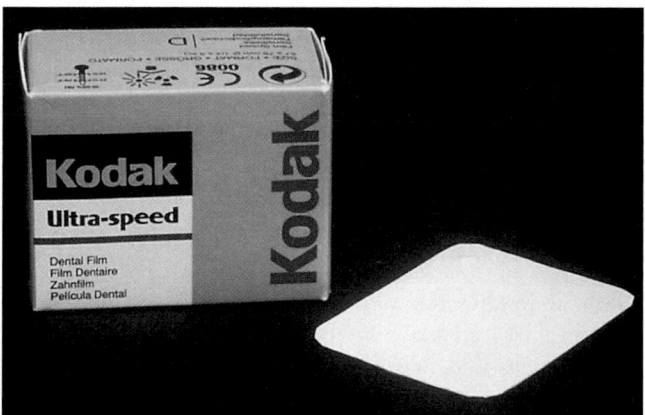

Figure 9-27 Prepackaged nonscreen film that can be used for dental and occlusal intraoral radiographic examinations. This type of film requires long exposure times because of the lack of intensifying screens. Patients should be under general anesthesia, and the technician should make the exposure from outside the room or behind a radiation safety barrier.

light from screens. Nonscreen films provide superb detail and are especially good for intraoral examination of the nasal cavity, dental studies, and bony extremities. Because this type of x-ray film is exposed by x-rays only, it has the disadvantage of needing very long exposure times to obtain necessary film density (Figure 9-27). Patients should be under general anesthesia and no personnel should be in the room during nonscreen film exposures.

Screen-type films are less sensitive to direct ionizing radiation but are very sensitive to visible light. This type of film requires less exposure to produce a radiograph because of its sensitivity to the fluorescence emitted by the intensifying screens. Remember that screens produce a specific color or spectrum of light. The film used should be matched in sensitivity to the light spectrum of the screen.

Rare earth screens do need special x-ray films to produce an optimal radiograph. Every x-ray film manufacturer produces a rare earth type of x-ray film. There is great confusion because of the endless names and types of combinations of x-ray film and image-intensifying screens available on the market. Again, please refer to Douglas et al. (1987) and

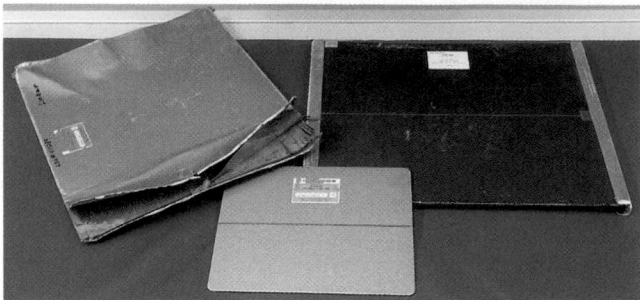

Figure 9-28 Three grids commonly used in veterinary radiology of large and small animals. The upper left grid has been damaged and opened, allowing you to see the hundreds of thin layers of metallic strips used to stop scattered radiation.

Morgan (1993) for a more elaborate discussion of this important topic.

> ✎ **TECHNICIAN NOTE**
>
> Be sure the x-ray film you are using is maximally sensitive to the spectrum of light your screens are emitting.

GRIDS

When x-rays enter a patient, some pass straight through to the film cassette, but a great many are scattered or redirected along a different path before exiting the patient. The purpose of a grid is to control the scatter radiation before it reaches the x-ray cassette. A grid is constructed of a sheet of lead strips interfaced with radiolucent spacers made of plastic or aluminum. These strips are encased in an aluminum protective cover for durability. Grids come in various sizes, similar to x-ray cassettes, and are placed directly over the cassette between the animal and the cassette, or more commonly, in a special tray just under the x-ray table above the cassette tray (Figure 9-28).

The purpose of a grid is to allow only the primary x-ray beam to pass through and prevent scattered radiations from reaching the film. The grid is constructed in such a way as to absorb all radiations that do not pass between the lead strips. This arrangement may absorb most scattered radiations if grids of high ratios are used. However, it has the disadvantage of absorbing part of the primary x-ray beam and therefore requires greater exposure time to obtain a given film density. Figure 9-29 shows how a grid absorbs scattered and secondary radiation and prevents it from reaching the film.

Grids are made of different ratios and number of strips per 2.5 cm. The ratio varies from 5:1 to 16:1 and from 60 lines (strips) per 2.5 cm to 120 lines per 2.5 cm. The higher the ratio and the number of lines per 2.5 cm, the more radiation is absorbed by the grid. The ratio of a grid refers to the relation between the height of the lead strips and the width of the radiolucent spaces. For example, if

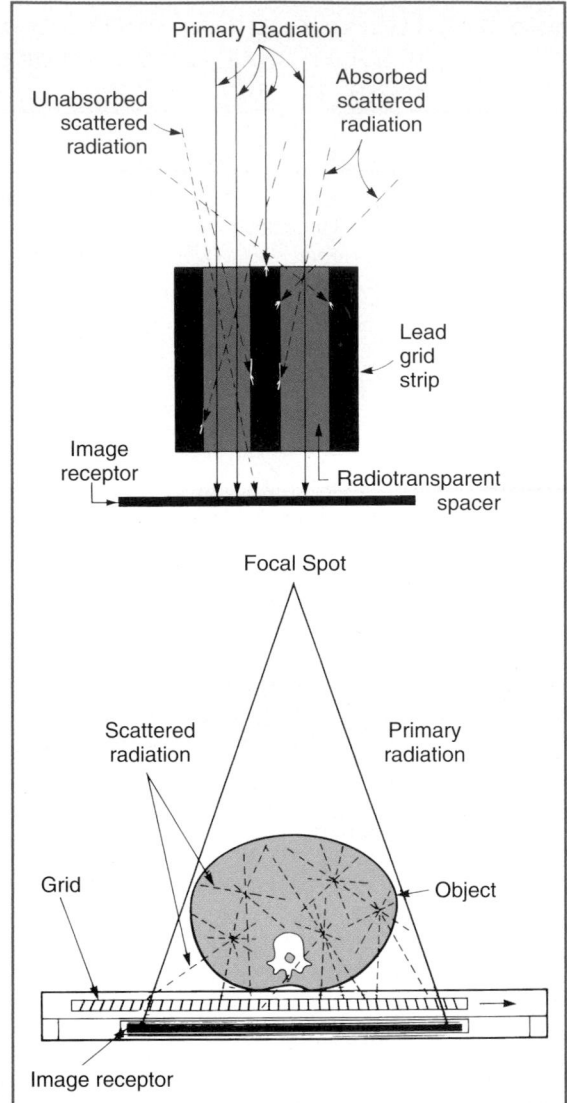

Figure 9-29 Cross section of a grid. **A,** Diagram of a small section of a grid showing how a large proportion of the scattered radiation is absorbed and image-forming primary radiation passes through to the image detector. **B,** Diagram of focused Potter-Bucky diaphragm being moved toward the right. (Modified from Eastman Kodak Company: *The fundamentals of radiography,* ed 12, Rochester, NY, 1980, Eastman Kodak Company, Radiographic Markets Division.)

the height of the lead strip is 12 times greater than the thickness of the space, the grid ratio will be 12:1, and if it is 10 times greater, the ratio will be 10:1. The greater the ratio, the more efficiently the grid absorbs scattered radiations. Figure 9-27, *A,* shows the ratio of a 5:1 grid. For veterinary work, a grid with a ratio of 8:1 at 103 lines per 2.5 cm is recommended.

The grid is most useful when x-raying parts of the body in which scattering is considerable, which in practice includes all thick parts of the body (e.g., thorax, abdomen, skull) and those joints and bones in excess of 10-cm thickness. The grid lines are visible on the resulting film, but this is made up for by the increased resolution of the image on the radiograph.

Grids may be *parallel* or *focused.* A parallel grid is one constructed with strips parallel to each other. A focused grid is one in which the lead strips and spacers are gradually angulated from the center to the periphery of the grid. The distance from the point of convergence, or focal point, is referred to as its focal distance, or radius. The advantage of a focused grid is that it allows unobstructed amounts of radiation to pass through it at the center and at the edge of the grid as long as the radiations are parallel to the axis of the lead strips. Such grids can be used only at a specific focal-film distance specified by the manufacturer. If distances above or below the focal-film distance are used, grid cutoff will occur, which means that part of the primary beam will be absorbed by the grid. With grid cutoff, large areas that are incompletely exposed will be found on the resulting radiograph.

Potter-Bucky Diaphragm

One other type of grid encountered in veterinary hospitals is the *Potter-Bucky diaphragm.* This is simply a movable grid. The movement of the diaphragm is timed to suit a particular exposure, and the grid moves across the film during the exposure so that the grid lines are not shown on the resulting film. When a movable grid is used, the exposure time must be increased by a factor of four, or the kilovoltage must be increased by about 20%. Usually, Potter-Bucky diaphragms are positioned under the table and electronically linked to the timer of the x-ray machine (Figure 9-29, *B*).

Another method of reducing scattered radiation is the *air gap technique.* It is a simple technique that consists of increasing the distance between the patient and the surface of the cassette. With this technique, the amount of scattered radiations produced is not reduced, but fewer scattered radiations reach the film because of the increased distance between patient and film. With the air gap technique, it is not necessary to increase the exposure factors, as must be done with a grid. However, this technique will decrease the sharpness of the image because of increased subject-to-film distance. It is also less effective at high kilovoltage settings, because the higher-energy scatter occurs in a forward direction. This technique is used most commonly in veterinary radiology for magnification purposes.

> ✐ **TECHNICIAN NOTE**
> Always use a grid between the patient and the film cassette when the body part being x-rayed is greater than 10 cm thick.

THE DARKROOM

The importance of the darkroom in radiography cannot be overemphasized. Radiography unquestionably begins and ends in the darkroom, in which films are loaded into cassettes ready for exposure and returned for processing into a finished radiograph. Most mistakes made in veterinary radiography are related to the processing of radiographs. It is necessary to keep the darkroom very clean and light proof. It is also essential for the technician to have a thorough knowledge of x-ray darkroom technique and of conventional or automatic processing. The chemicals should be changed, replenished, maintained, and mixed according to the strict directions of the manufacturer.

EQUIPMENT

A darkroom need not be spacious. For most veterinary practices, a small room of about 240×240 cm is adequate. However, it is essential that this room be made totally dark. If there is a window in the room, there is no reason not to open it for ventilation when the darkroom is not in use; however, the window should be light proof when closed. One can easily determine whether a darkroom is light proof by turning off all lights, including the safelight, closing the door tightly, and slowly turning around in the center of the darkroom, looking for any light leaking into the room. It is also important that a lock or light-proof cylindrical entrance be placed on the door to prevent its being opened while films are being processed. A darkroom need not be completely dark, because a safelight can be used during film processing. A safelight is a light bulb shielded by a plastic filter that stops any light to which the film is sensitive from penetrating the filter and entering the room. It is important, however, that the safelight bulb not exceed the wattage recommended for the type of filter used; otherwise, the exposed films will be "fogged," or partially exposed, and the quality of the radiographs will be compromised. The proper type of light filter must be used in the darkroom. Orange, red, or yellow filters may be used with most x-ray films; but with the rare earth type of x-ray film, a special red filter must be used (Figure 9-30). No films should be exposed to the safelight any longer than necessary. It is important to work rapidly but carefully when processing x-ray films and loading and unloading films in the cassettes.

There should be a worktable in the darkroom for loading and unloading cassettes, located as far away from the processing tanks as possible so that liquid or dry chemicals will not be spilled on it. Above or below the bench, there should be shelves to store film hangers and unexposed films and cassettes. X-ray film must be kept in a cool, dry place protected from extraneous x-rays.

> ✐ **TECHNICIAN NOTE**
> Remember that all film and safelights are not created equal. Make sure the wavelength or color of light to which your film is sensitive is completely blocked by your safelight filter.

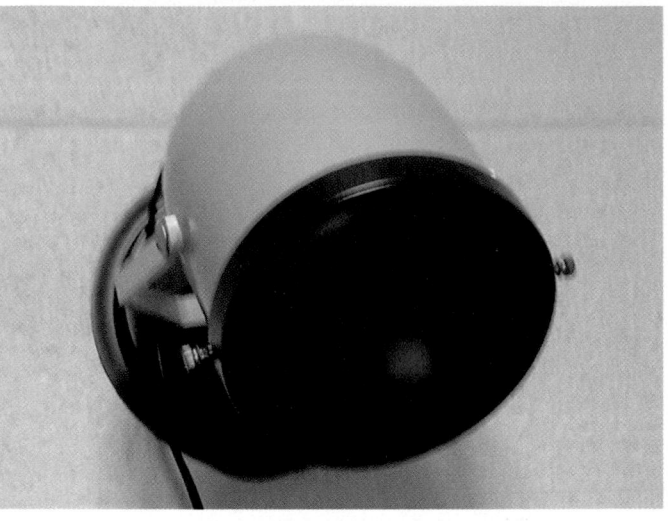

A   **B**

Figure 9-30   **A and B,** Two examples of darkroom safelights. The filters must be matched to the light sensitivity of the film being used in the darkroom and must not be cracked or incompletely sealed by the filter holder.

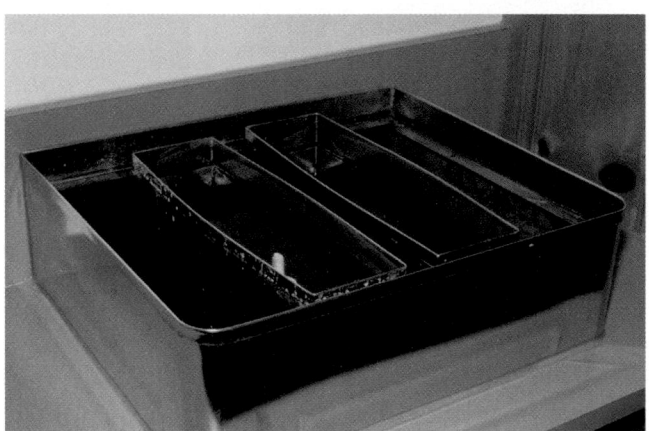

Figure 9-31   Processing tanks holding the developer *(left),* two central fresh water tanks to wash the films *(middle),* and fixer *(right).*

HAND PROCESSING EQUIPMENT

The processing equipment should include a developing tank, rinsing tank, and fixer tank. The tanks should be big enough to accommodate several 35-cm × 42.5-cm films at the same time. Running water in the rinsing tank is ideal. If it is not available, the water should be changed frequently. Development and fixer solutions should be changed every 90 days, regardless of use, and more frequently if radiograph volume is high. The tanks should ideally be made of stainless steel for ease of cleaning (Figure 9-31).

In certain areas of the United States, it will be necessary to heat up or cool down the solutions during certain times of the year. This may be accomplished with an electric heater or a cooling device. During the heat of the summer, it may be necessary to add ice to the washing water to keep the solutions at the proper temperature. An inexpensive way to keep the solution temperature constant in processing tanks is by installing a good-quality shower-bath mixer valve. This type of valve is sufficient and economical enough to maintain the solution at a constant temperature in a low-volume practice. It is also important to have separate stirring rods made of stainless steel, plastic, or rubber and to mix the solutions thoroughly every day before starting the processing of films. Good ventilation is necessary to keep the room dry and prevent accumulation of volatile chemicals.

AUTOMATIC FILM PROCESSORS

There are several makes and sizes of automatic processors on the market. In recent years, many veterinary hospitals have invested in automatic processing systems. There are small-capacity, 90-second processor units that can be installed in most darkrooms without remodeling. The larger processor units necessitate some remodeling because the input tray must be in the darkroom and the output side must be out of the darkroom. This usually requires some structural and plumbing modifications (Figure 9-32).

As with manual processing tanks, it is necessary to maintain fresh solution and ensure that the solutions are flowing properly within the processor. Automatic processors may speed up and standardize film processing but require similar, if not more, maintenance compared with manual processing tanks. It is important to provide ventilation in the darkroom when automatic processors are used. Usually, a good-quality, light-tight exhaust fan installed in the ceiling is adequate.

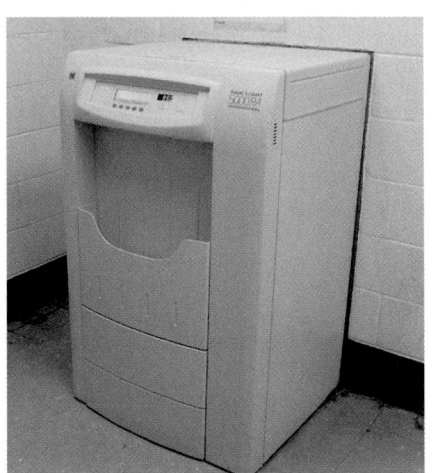

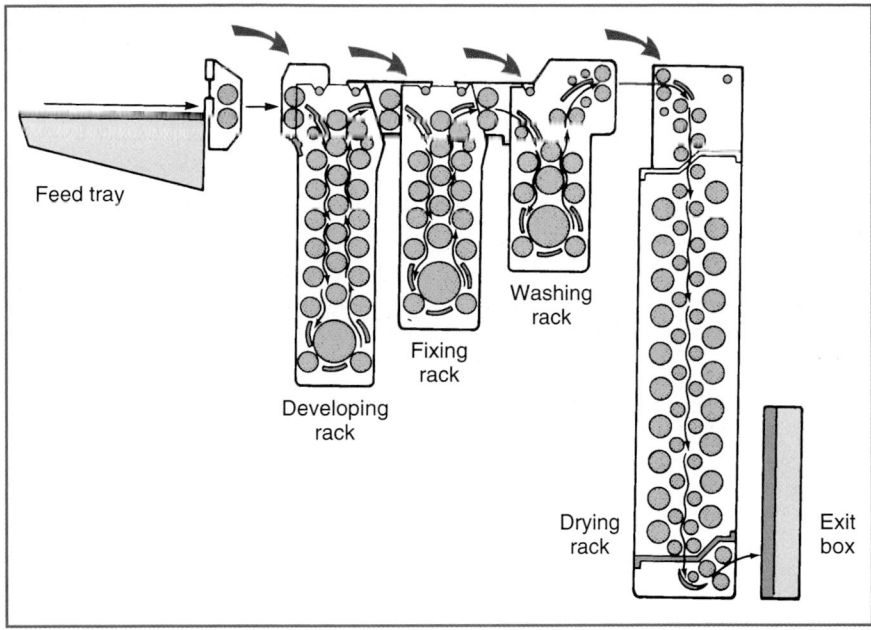

A

B

Figure 9-32 Automatic processor. **A,** Kodak X-OMAT processor (a 90-second processor). **B,** Diagram of a typical automatic x-ray processor.

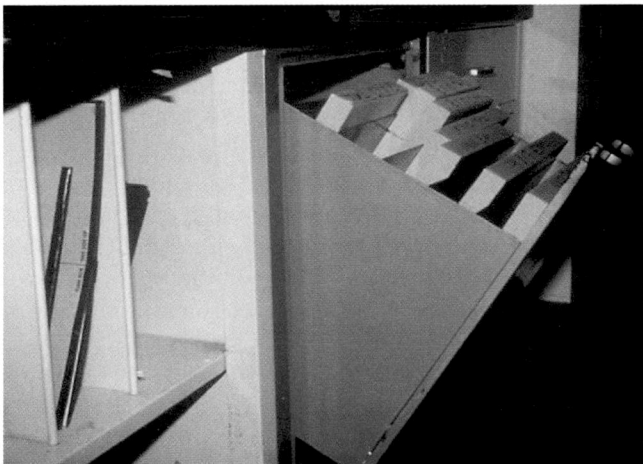

Figure 9-33 Film storage bin commonly used in darkrooms; it is designed to store open x-ray box films to load x-ray cassettes. This bin is wired to a switch that will automatically turn off the darkroom lights when opened.

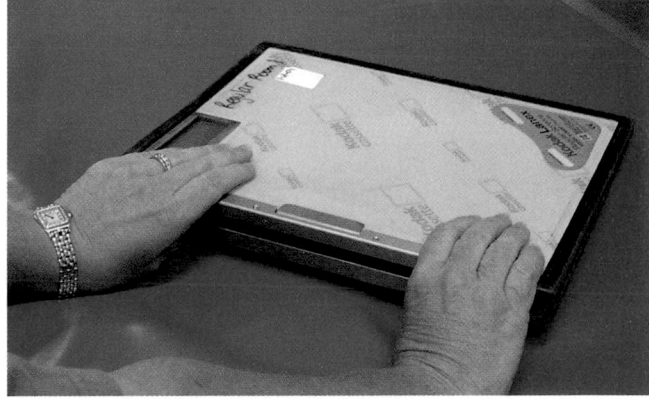

Figure 9-34 When loading a cassette, use both hands to avoid kink marks, and carefully place the film into the cassette. The cassette must be closed and latched gently.

FILM STORAGE

X-ray films must be handled and stored properly for maximum usefulness. The film must be protected from light, x-radiations, gamma radiations, heat, moisture, and pressure. All these hazards may result in film fogging and decrease radiograph quality. As previously mentioned, the darkroom can fulfill this function if the room is kept clean and free of moisture. It may be helpful if the x-ray films are kept in their original boxes and placed in a cabinet. Special bins to store x-ray films can be purchased, but they

are an unnecessary expense if proper care is used in storage (Figure 9-33).

CASSETTE LOADING AND UNLOADING

Care must be taken when transferring x-ray film from its box to the x-ray cassette to avoid static electricity, bending, creasing, or scratching. The film should be handled carefully, held only by the corners, and pulled from the box in a continuous and slow motion (Figure 9-34). The film should be carefully placed in the cassette, and the edges should not extend over the edge of the film cassette. Great care should also be taken in removing x-ray film from the cassette to prevent damage or soiling of the intensifying screen.

HANGING X-RAY FILM

When exposed films are placed on a film hanger or automatic processor tray, they must be handled carefully. X-ray film is more sensitive after exposure and before development than at any other time. The films should be handled *only* by the corners and attached to the stationary bottom clip first and then to the flexible top clip. It is most important to have dry hands when handling exposed, nonprocessed films. Any developer or fixer solution touching the film will create an artifact on the processed film.

DEVELOPING X-RAY FILM

As previously mentioned, processing solutions (developer and fixer) should be stirred before the film is inserted. When the film is placed in the developer, it should be agitated up and down a few times to remove air bubbles from its surface. The film should be developed for 5 minutes at 20° C (68° F). If the temperature is above or below 20° C, the developing time should be adjusted according to the directions of the manufacturer. Rapid (3-minute), high-temperature film development or sight processing is not recommended because of decreased radiograph quality.

In the developing solution, the chemicals reduce the exposed silver halides in the x-ray film to metallic silver, which is black. Gradually, through the developing process, the latent image is revealed. The film is then removed from the developer tank and quickly rinsed in the central water bath. It is then placed in the fixer solution, which stops the development process and preserves the film. The film should remain in the fixer for approximately twice the development time. The film is then placed in the central rinse tank for about 15 to 20 minutes. Films can be dried in a special air-circulated film dryer box or allowed to hang until dry in a well-ventilated, dust-free area. For a more complete discussion of the chemistry of x-ray processing, please refer to the Eastman Kodak publication *The Fundamentals of Radiography* (1980).

SILVER RECOVERY

In larger veterinary practices, the silver contained within the x-ray film emulsion may be removed and recovered. Most of the silver that is not exposed to x-rays is not converted to metallic silver and accumulates within the fixer solution. Silver recovery units can be attached to the fixer solution to remove the silver by an electrolytic process. This, however, is only economical for the larger-volume veterinary hospital. The silver can also be recovered from exposed and nonexposed x-ray film. A few companies specialize in recycling x-ray film for silver recovery. This could be the source of a small bonus at the time an x-ray file is purged from the old cases on file.

RADIOGRAPHIC FILM QUALITY

It is of utmost importance to produce radiographs of excellent quality to arrive at a radiographic diagnosis. A film of good diagnostic quality should have excellent detail, correct scale of contrast, and optimal density. Each of these film characteristics is briefly discussed.

DETAIL

Radiographic detail refers to the degree of sharpness that defines the edge of an anatomic structure. It is the best possible reproduction of an organ. Detail is influenced by every possible factor, but some factors are more influential than others.

The focal-film distance is one important factor in the loss of detail. If the focal spot is too close to the part x-rayed, there will be magnification and lack of distinction at the margins of the structures. Therefore it is important to keep the focal-film distance as long as possible without significantly reducing x-ray beam intensity. Most veterinary hospitals have radiographic technique charts that use a focal-film distance of 36 to 48 inches (80 to 110 cm).

Movement in veterinary radiology is a constant problem, especially with older units that have a minimum exposure time of $^1/_{10}$ second. It is difficult to produce diagnostic films of the thorax with a unit that does not have a minimum time of exposure of at least $^1/_{30}$ second and ideally $^1/_{120}$ second. With large animals, movement is a constant problem with a small, portable unit. This is why rare earth screens are becoming so popular in veterinary medicine; they have the advantage of requiring a much shorter exposure time.

The size of the focal spot is another important factor that regulates detail. The larger the focal spot, the poorer is the detail. Because most equipment in veterinary medicine has a rather large focal spot of 0.8 mm or more, loss of detail may be significant, especially with older units that have focal spots of 1.2 to 2 mm. Therefore it is important to place the part to be x-rayed as close as possible to the x-ray film. If the part is too far from the film, there will be magnification and distortion, resulting in a loss of detail. This is especially important in large animal radiology.

Other exposure factors that affect detail are poor film-screen contact and overexposed or underexposed radiographs that often result from an improper technique chart or carelessness. Poor radiographic processing causes more ruined radiographs than all other factors combined. All processing errors affect detail. It is therefore important to standardize the developing process by following exactly the instructions of the manufacturer.

RADIOGRAPHIC CONTRAST

Radiographic contrast refers to the density or opacity difference between two areas on a radiograph. High contrast means the opacity differences are large and there are fewer shades of gray. High-contrast radiographs are very black and white. Latitude refers to the range of different opacities on the radiograph. Long-latitude radiographs have a much larger number of shades of gray, but the difference or contrast between each shade is small. High-contrast radiographs are preferred for spine and extremity films. Long-latitude, low-contrast radiographs are preferred for thoracic films.

Kilovoltage is the exposure factor that has the greatest influence on radiographic contrast. The higher the kilovoltage, the greater the latitude and therefore the greater the number of shades of black, gray, and white. The absorption of the x-ray beam at high kilovoltage is more uniform among the various tissues in the body, resulting in less contrast. Therefore for thoracic examinations, a high-kilovoltage technique is recommended. For skeletal studies, a lower-kilovoltage technique is recommended.

Other factors reducing contrast are scattered radiations (which can be markedly improved by the use of a grid), light leakage, and rapid, high-temperature processing techniques.

RADIOGRAPHIC DENSITY

Radiographic density refers to the degree of blackness of the film. It is the result of the amount of light that was transmitted to the x-ray film after interaction of the crystals in the intensifying screens with the x-ray beam. When a film is properly exposed, the anatomic part x-rayed will have good contrast with good differential absorption of the x-ray beam by the various tissue densities. Therefore the part should be clearly seen but should not be so dark as to overexpose the anatomic structures to the degree that they are difficult to differentiate from the background film density. The thickness and density of the anatomic part x-rayed do affect density. The thickest part will absorb more radiation, sometimes as much as denser tissues of lesser thickness.

The primary factor affecting density is the mAs setting. As discussed previously, the mAs factor is a quantity factor that regulates the amount of x-rays produced. If more x-rays reach the film, more light will be emitted by the screens, and the film will be darker. Therefore it can be stated that high mAs settings will increase film density and low mAs settings will reduce film density.

Another factor that affects film density is the kilovoltage setting. At a higher kilovoltage, the x-ray tube is more efficient in producing x-rays and therefore increases the energy level of x-rays produced. If all other exposure and development factors are kept constant, increasing the kilovoltage will increase the radiographic density. This effect is more apparent at lower-kilovoltage settings for a given part than at higher-kilovoltage settings.

The distance from the focal spot to the surface of the film is another important factor in film density. If everything remains constant but the distance, a given examination could be markedly overexposed if the distance is reduced, or it could be underexposed if the distance is increased. This effect can be dramatic because the intensity of the radiation is reduced or increased as the square of the distance is changed. This effect is discussed in the section regarding inverse square law. It does emphasize the need for consistency and accurate measurement of the focal-film distance.

MAGNIFICATION

Magnification is a technique rarely used in veterinary practices, but it is popular in veterinary teaching hospitals. Magnification is based on the principle that a larger image of an anatomic structure can be obtained if the distance between the object and the film is increased. Generally, the object to be magnified is placed halfway between the film cassette and the focal spot of the x-ray tube. This results in an x-ray image twice as large as the actual anatomic structure. However, to obtain diagnostic films, it is necessary to have a very small focal spot. A focal spot of 0.3 mm or smaller is needed for radiographic magnification. If larger focal spots are used, the advantage of direct magnification is lost because of the blurring at the margin of an organ produced by the larger focal spot. This technique would be useful to veterinarians, especially for studies of extremities in small dogs and cats and for studies of the skull.

TECHNICAL ERRORS AND ARTIFACTS

Several errors can be made in handling x-ray films or in setting up a technique for an examination. In general, these errors will reduce the quality of the radiograph and in certain cases may nullify its diagnostic value. Boxes 9-1, 9-2, and 9-3 are intended to help the technician identify the cause of errors and take corrective measures. Box 9-1 deals with technical errors other than those occurring as a result of film processing. Boxes 9-2 and 9-3 deal with errors caused by poor film processing.

The advent of automatic processing equipment has helped tremendously in eliminating many errors made in hand tank processing techniques. It has standardized film processing and made it easier to trace the cause of processing mistakes, which are usually mechanically related. Even with automatic processors, many mistakes can be made and must be recognized and corrected to obtain the best possible radiographs.

Several other mechanical failures may occur with automatic processors. It is important to keep the processor clean at all times. It is especially important to wash the roller assembly thoroughly at least once each week. Processors are sophisticated machines that must be serviced regularly

Box 9-1 TECHNICAL ERRORS

INCREASED FILM DENSITY
Too high mAs or kV settings
Too short focal-film distance
Wrong measurement of anatomic part
Equipment malfunction
Speed of intensifying screen too fast

DECREASED FILM DENSITY
Too low mAs or kV settings
Too long focal-film distance
Wrong measurement of anatomic part
Speed of intensifying screen too slow

BLACK MARKS OR ARTIFACTS
Film scratches
Crescent mark from rough handling
Static electricity (linear dots or tree pattern)
Top of film black, resulting from exposure to light while still in box
Defective cassette that does not close properly, exposing margins of film to light

WHITE MARKS (ARTIFACTS)
Dirt or debris between the film and screen
Defect or crack in screen
Contrast medium on tabletop, skin, or cassette

GRAY FILM
Film accidentally exposed to radiation (scattered, secondary, or direct)
Lack of grid for examination of a thick part
Outdated film
Film stored in too hot or too humid place

DISTORTED OR BLURRED RADIOGRAPH
Motion: patient, cassette, or machine
Too great focal-film distance, causing magnification and distortion
Poor film-screen contact
Poor centering of primary x-ray beam

LINEAR ARTIFACTS
Gridlines
Grid out of focal range
Primary beam not centered
Grid upside down
Grid damage, causing distorted gridlines

MISCELLANEOUS ARTIFACTS
Cone cut, causing underexposed margins
Target damage, resulting in inconsistent film density: requires tube replacement
Double exposure
Blank film: faulty equipment, nonexposed film processed

kV, Kilovolts; *mAs,* milliamperes times seconds.

by professionals. It is unreasonable and cost ineffective for a veterinarian to expect the technician to service the processor. However, it is the responsibility of the technician to be able to recognize processor problems and correct them when possible. It is also the technician's responsibility to keep the processor clean at all times and to ensure that fresh developer and fixer solutions are provided as needed.

RADIATION SAFETY

Since 1970 there has been a tremendous growth in the use of x-ray equipment by veterinarians. There are few diagnoses in medicine or surgery that cannot be aided by the use of diagnostic radiology. It therefore behooves technicians to be aware of the hazard of using x-rays or any other type of ionizing radiation.

It is the responsibility of the veterinarian to ensure that proper radiation safety measures are observed in the hospital. It is also the veterinarian's responsibility to instruct the technician in the proper use of the equipment and to ensure that the design of the x-ray room meets state regulations.

All animal tissues are sensitive to radiation; that is, absorption of radiation doses above a certain minimum

roentgen value will change or alter the tissue. The following tissues (not in order of sensitivity) are most readily affected by ionizing radiation: skin, lymphatics, hemopoietic and leukopoietic (blood-forming) tissues, breast, thyroid, bone (especially the epiphysis or growing centers), and the germinal epithelium or gonads. These tissues are sensitive to all forms of ionizing radiation. All animal species are affected, including humans, even though there are different degrees of sensitivity among species. The more rapidly dividing tissues are affected most by radiation.

Technicians should remember that one of the best means of protection at their disposal is the ability to avoid retakes. Careful attention to patient positioning, thickness measurements, setting techniques, and film processing will decrease the need for radiograph retakes and reduce technician and patient radiation exposure. See Chapter 36 for additional radiation safety information.

RADIATION FILTRATION

The x-ray beam is a composite or spectrum of x-ray photons of various energy levels. The kVp setting is the highest energy level within the beam, but there are photons of all levels from the kVp on down. The useful portion of the x-ray beam (the portion that passes through the patient to interact

Box 9-2 FILM PROCESSING MISTAKES IN WET TANKS

INCREASED FILM DENSITY
Film overdeveloped
Temperature of solution too high
Wrong concentration of developer
Defective thermometer

DECREASED FILM DENSITY
Film underdeveloped
Temperature of solution too low
Exhausted developer
Contamination of developer
Developer too diluted or improperly mixed
Failure to add replenisher solution as needed
Defective thermometer

FOGGED FILMS
Light leakage in darkroom from defective safelight, door, windows; light leakage around processor pipes; or turning lights on in darkroom before film is cleared
Film exposed to radiation from any source: through wall if storage room adjacent to x-ray room, cassette left in x-ray room while exposure made
Overdeveloped film
Contaminated developer

YELLOW RADIOGRAPH
Fixation time too short
Exhausted fixer solution

WHITE SPOTS
Defective screens, pitted, scratched
Dust or grit on surface of film
Fixer on film before processing

BLACK SPOTS
Drops of developer solution on film before processing
Films stacked together in fixer

AIR BUBBLES
Film not agitated when placed in developer; air bubbles form on surface of film

RETICULATION
Solutions have uneven temperature from bottom to top of tanks
Need to stir up solution to even up temperature in tanks
Weak fixer or lack of hardening solution

BRITTLE RADIOGRAPHS
Drying temperature too high
Drying time too long

MISCELLANEOUS MISTAKES
Film wet: too short drying time
Grit on films: dirty tanks and solutions
Corner marks: wet or dirty fingers on hangers
Sticky film: film washed or dried improperly
Static electricity: low humidity and rough or too fast handling of films
Scratches: careless handling

Box 9-3 COMMON TECHNICAL ERRORS WITH AUTOMATIC PROCESSORS

INCREASED DENSITY
Temperature of developer too high
Overreplenishment
Light leak from cover or in darkroom
Speed too slow
Faulty thermostat

DECREASED DENSITY
Temperature of developer too low
Underreplenishment
Exhausted developer, necessitating thorough cleaning of tanks every 6 months
Faulty thermostat

PROCESSING STREAKS
Crossover rollers dirty

Dirty wash water
Air tubes need cleaning

SCRATCHES ON FILM
Guide shoes misaligned or dirty
Dryer air tubes mispositioned

WET OR DAMP FILM
Thermostat malfunction
Dryer temperatures too low
Insufficient air venting
Film not hardened sufficiently

FILM OVERLAP
Film fed too rapidly into processor
Tension on rollers too high

with the film and screens) is the upper two thirds of the energy levels. The lower third of the x-ray beam energies is too weak to pass through the patient. This radiation is called *soft radiation*. It is of no use for image formation and only causes increased radiation exposure of the patient. Aluminum has a marked effect on filtration of softer (lower energy level) x-rays. Insertion of 1 or 2 mm of an aluminum filter into the path of the primary beam at the portal of the x-ray tube is essential to filter out or absorb the soft x-rays that are a component of all x-ray beams in the diagnostic range. By absorbing these soft radiations, the filter reduces the amount of radiation absorbed by the patient. Increased aluminum filtration also generally improves latitude and detail by improving the quality of the x-ray beam.

RADIATION MEASUREMENT

To understand radiation safety and radiation dose units of measurement, it is necessary to define a few terms commonly used in the measurement of radiation exposure.

Roentgen

The roentgen (R) is defined as a unit of radiation exposure that will liberate a charge of 2.58×10^{-4} coulombs per kilogram of air. Roentgens are a measure of radiation exposure or x-ray machine output and are generally evaluated with an ionization chamber placed below the primary x-ray beam. As an example, 1 R is the approximate exposure to the body surface for an anteroposterior radiograph of the abdomen for an average adult human.

Rad

The unit of absorbed dose of ionizing radiations is called a *rad*. It is the energy imparted by ionizing radiations to a unit mass of irradiated material and is equal to 100 ergs/g of tissue. The number of rads deposited in tissue per roentgen of radiation exposure varies with the energy of the x-ray beam and with the composition of the absorber.

Rem

Rem is an abbreviation for rad equivalent man; it is the product of the dose in rads and the relative biologic effectiveness of the radiation used. This unit of measurement makes allowance for the fact that the effect of radiation on different tissue varies with the type of radiation or relative biologic effectiveness. A rem is equal to the absorbed radiation dose in rads multiplied by a quality factor:

$$\text{Rem} = \text{Rads} \times \text{Quality factor}$$

Because the quality factor for diagnostic radiation is 1, for all practical purposes in veterinary practice, 1 rem = 1 rad. For larger particles of radiation, such as neutrons, protons, and alpha particles, the quality factor increases from 3 to 20. These larger, more dangerous particles of radiation are not emitted from diagnostic x-ray machines.

Maximum Permissible Dose

The maximum permissible dose (MPD) should be of great interest to the veterinary technician because it is the maximum dose of radiation a person is allowed to receive during occupational exposure over a certain time. This dose is 0.1 rem for an average weekly dose or 3 rem over 13 weeks, 5 rem per year, and a maximum accumulated dose of $1(N-18)$ rem, where N is age in years. The N − 18 indicates that an individual should not have occupational exposure to radiation before the age of 18 years. The technician should remember that the MPD is the dose that the U.S. Nuclear Regulatory Commission has determined should not harm the person receiving it during her or his lifetime. The MPD is maximum occupational exposure allowed by law; technicians should try to keep radiation exposure as low as possible by carefully following radiation safety practices.

Personal Monitoring

To protect the staff from overexposure, the radiation that each person receives can be measured on a *film badge*. A film badge is a container that holds a special film designed to record a wide range of exposures. The film holder incorporates several different types of metal filters that permit differentiation of the type of ionizing radiation exposures. This badge should be worn outside the apron on the collar at the level of the thyroid gland (Figure 9-35). Film badges can be exposed by heat, pressure, and chemical fumes. The film badge should be taken care of and stored outside the radiology area so that the amount of radiation it detects is actually the amount to which the person is occupationally exposed.

Radiation monitoring badges come in several forms: rings, clips, and wrist badges. Several companies offer a badge service. These badges are mailed back to the company and analyzed on a monthly or quarterly basis.

Film badge readings are reported in millirem (mrem), or 1/1000 rem. The annual MPD equals 5000 mrem. Technicians using x-ray machines should insist that the veterinarian for whom they work provide them with a radiation monitoring device.

PROTECTION PRACTICES

- Always use a collimator and always use the smallest possible aperture that will cover the anatomic area of interest (Figure 9-36).
- Make sure there is an aluminum filter at the portal of the x-ray tube. This is to protect the patient, not the technician.
- Make sure the proper exposure factors are used to prevent the need for retakes.
- Make sure the animal is positioned properly the first time—again, to prevent the need for retakes.
- Never permit any part of your body to be in the path of the primary x-ray beam.

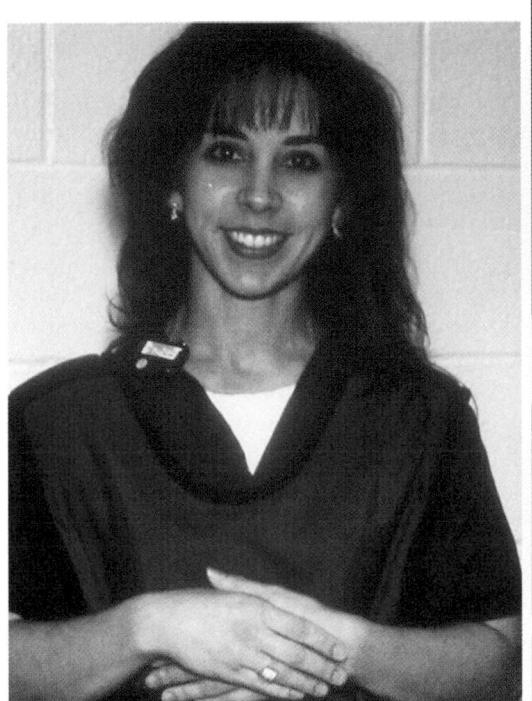
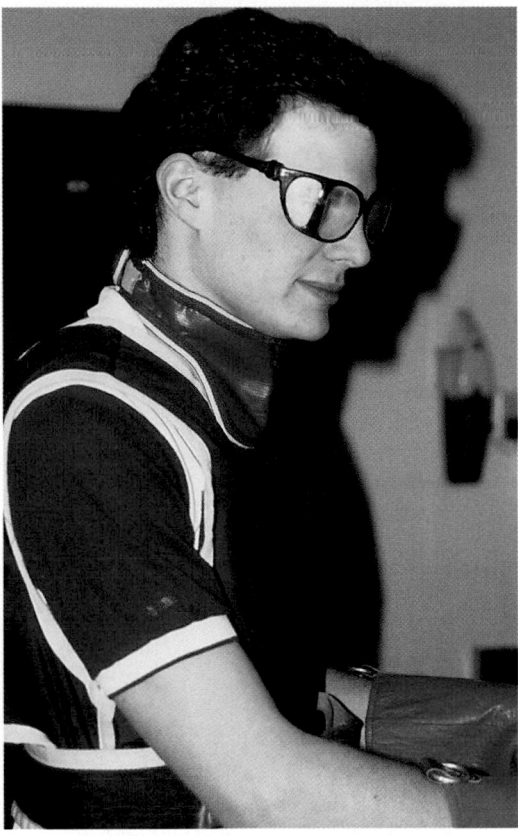

A   B

Figure 9-35 Each technician working in radiology should have a film badge to measure occupational radiation exposure. **A,** The film badge should be worn outside the lead apron at the level of the upper neck. This technician also wears a ring badge inside her lead gloves to measure dose to the hands. **B,** This technician who works in a very busy radiology department wears leaded glasses and a thyroid shield in addition to gloves and an apron.

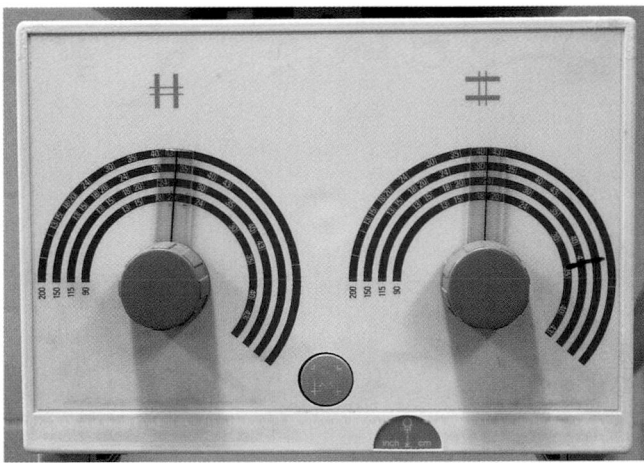

Figure 9-36 A collimator is used to limit the size of the x-ray beam to the part to be examined. By coning down on the area of interest, the amount of scattered and secondary radiation can be drastically reduced, improving image quality and decreasing technician exposure.

- Always wear an apron and gloves when holding an animal or an apron alone if you must be in the room when an exposure is made. The apron should have 0.5-mm lead equivalent minimum to ensure good protection from secondary and scattered radiations (Figures 9-37 and 9-38).
- Use accessory equipment designed to reduce radiation exposure, such as cassette holders, restraining devices, and positioning devices (Figures 9-39 and 9-40).
- Anesthesia or tranquilization of the patient should be used every time an animal cannot be controlled easily and adequately for a given examination.
- Only required personnel should be in the examining room at the time of exposure. A pregnant woman should not be in the room, nor should anyone younger than 18 years.
- Use good, fast screens to reduce the milliamperage (mAs) settings as much as possible.

TECHNICIAN NOTE

When working in radiology, always remember the "big three" of radiation safety: time, distance, and shielding.

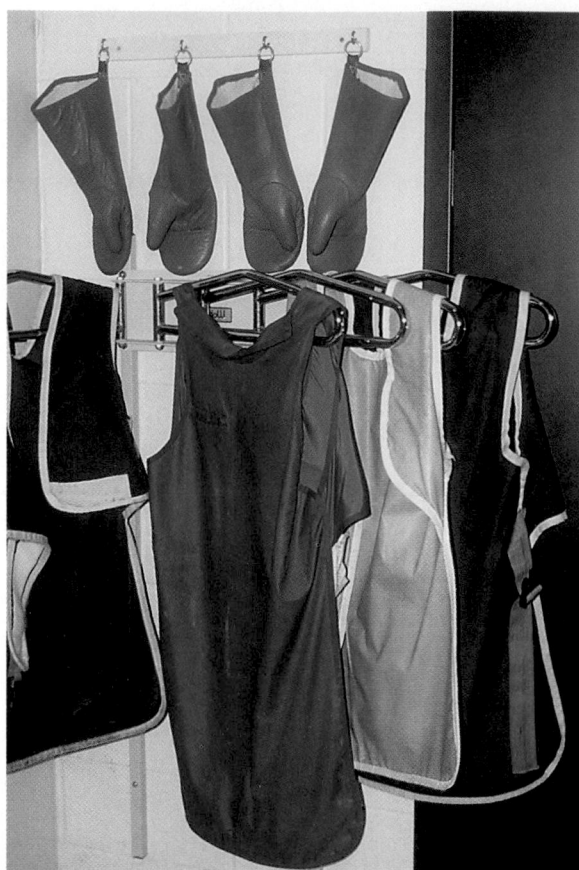

Figure 9-37 Aprons and gloves on a stand. It is important to keep the apron on a stand and the gloves well aerated when not in use to increase the useful life of the apron and gloves. The apron should have a minimum of 0.5 mm of lead equivalent.

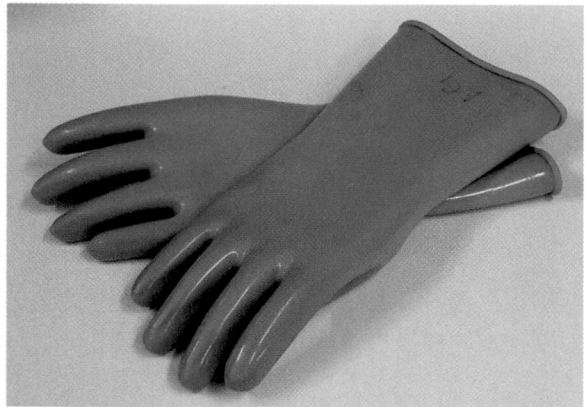

Figure 9-38 Lead gloves should have a minimum of 0.5 mm of lead equivalent; 1 mm of lead equivalent is ideal. They should always be worn when restraint is needed for examination.

Radiation safety is a frame of mind. It is a habit, and it requires awareness of the danger of radiation. It is easy to become careless with radiation because it is invisible, tasteless, and odorless and produces no external stimulation at diagnostic levels. Technicians should always remember that although invisible, radiations are dangerous to one's health. X-ray effects are cumulative. The ionization that results from continued exposure to x-rays and other high-energy rays constitutes the cumulative effect. These rays can destroy all living tissue if the absorbed doses are high enough. Secondary radiations are less harmful than primary radiations but are still extremely harmful. Therefore carelessness has no place in radiology. Remember the big three methods of radiation protection: *time, distance,* and *shielding.* Time means avoiding retakes; do it right the first time. Lower the time of exposures; keep the mAs as low as possible to still produce diagnostic radiographs. Distance means staying as far away as possible from the patient and x-ray beam. Shielding means always wearing an apron and gloves. It is important to take care of your apron and gloves. Hang them carefully after use, and do not allow the apron to be folded. Careless use causes creases and cracks to develop in the gloves and aprons and reduces their effectiveness.

RADIOGRAPHIC CONTRAST AGENTS

In radiology, *contrast* means density difference. In many radiographic examinations, there is insufficient natural or inherent contrast of the anatomy to make a diagnosis; this is especially true in gastrointestinal, urogenital, and spinal cord disease. The addition of positive or negative contrast medium can increase the radiographic density difference between anatomic structures and increase the likelihood of correct image interpretation. In veterinary medicine, the following four types of contrast media are used (Figure 9-41):

1. Radiolucent gases: air, nitrous oxide, carbon dioxide
2. Insoluble inert radiopaque medium: barium sulfate
3. Soluble ionic radiopaque medium: iothalamate, diatrizoate
4. Soluble nonionic radiopaque medium: iohexol, iopamidol

Radiolucent gases absorb very small amounts of radiation, resulting in images of greatly reduced radiographic opacity. These agents are used primarily in double-contrast gastrograms, double-contrast cystograms, and rarely, pneumoperitoneography. Contraindications for their use are primarily in patients with severe hemorrhagic cystitis, in which there is an increased likelihood for gas absorption into the circulation. Nitrous oxide and carbon dioxide are considered safer than room air because their increased solubility is less likely to cause serious air embolization.

Barium sulfate has a high atomic number and absorbs a large amount of radiation, resulting in greatly increased radiographic opacity. It is used almost exclusively for upper and lower gastrointestinal examinations. Barium sulfate is inert, nonabsorbed, and fairly soothing to the gastrointestinal tract. It coats the gastrointestinal mucosa better than organic iodides, improving visualization of the

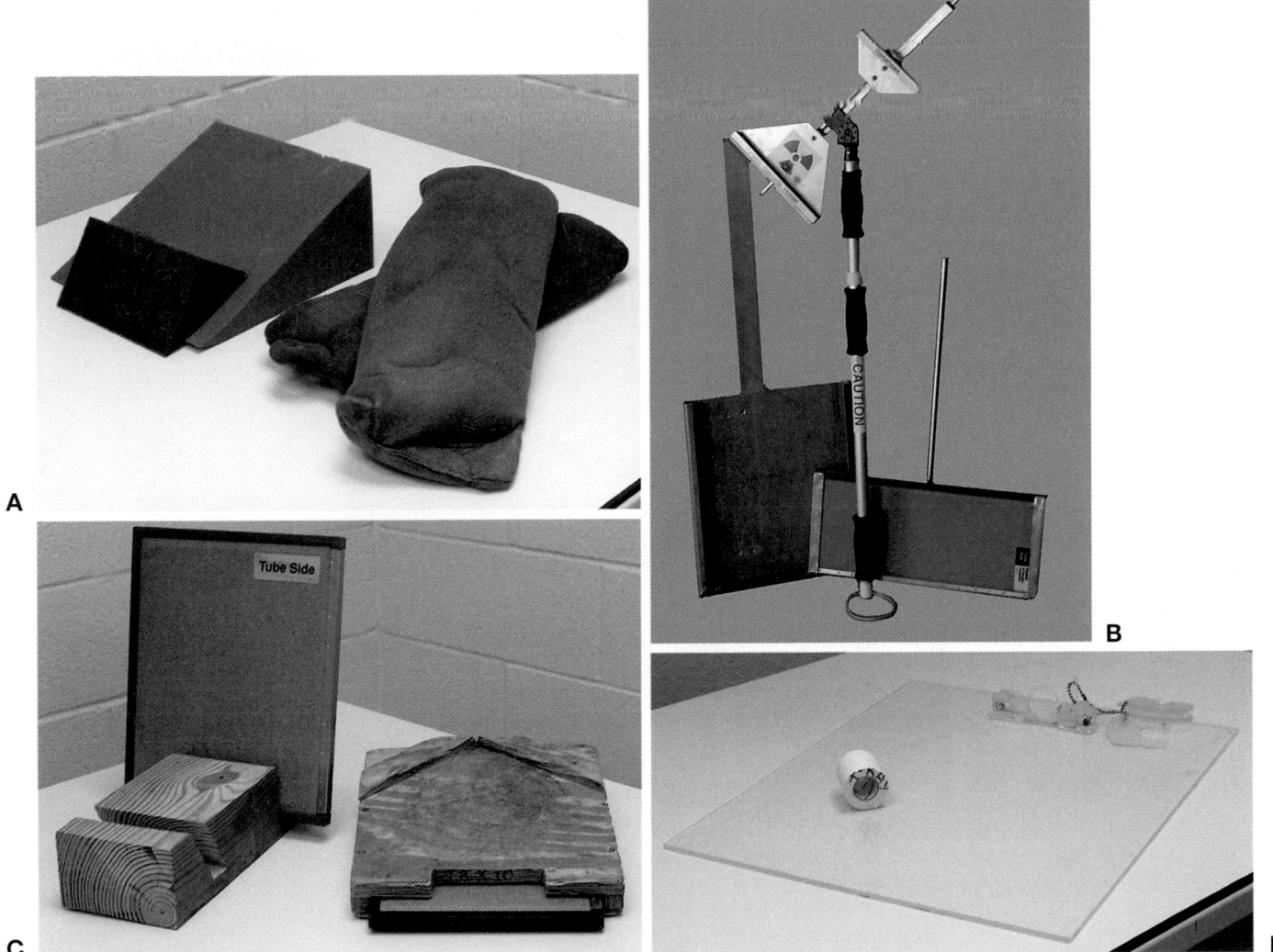

Figure 9-39 A number of commercially available positioning devices can be used to help position animals and reduce the time needed to perform the examination. **A,** Various foam wedges and sand bags used to position small animals. **B,** Cassette holder for large animal examinations. **C,** Wood blocks for examination of large animal feet. **D,** Lucite tray with neck restraint holder for avian radiology. Porous tape is used to position wings on anesthetized birds.

luminal surface. Barium sulfate is available in powder, paste, or liquid form. Micropulverized, solubilized barium sulfate solutions are vastly superior to powdered barium sulfate products because of the increased uniformity in mucosal coating. Contraindications for use include patients with severe constipation or upper or lower bowel perforations. As with all oral contrast media, care should be used in patients with known aspiration pneumonia or a high likelihood of aspiration.

Soluble radiopaque ionic contrast media include iothalamate and diatrizoate. The negatively charged iothalamate and diatrizoate are benzoic acid derivatives with three iodine molecules. They are coupled with positively charged sodium or meglumine to form a soluble salt. The high atomic number of iodine increases radiation absorption and increases radiographic opacity. These products can be used orally for gastrointestinal examinations; intravascularly for venous or arterial studies and excretory urography and in the peritoneal tract, bladder, and urethra; and intraarticularly and in draining wounds for fistulography and in salivary ducts for sialography. Ionic organic iodides should not be used in the respiratory tract or intrathecally for myelography. Because ionic iodides are essentially a hyperosmolar salt solution, they can result in an increase in intravascular fluid volume when used intravascularly followed by an osmotic diuresis. The hyperosmolarity can cause diarrhea when ionic iodides are administered orally. Because of these properties, these agents are contraindicated in dehydrated patients and patients with a known iodine sensitivity.

The newest class of positive contrast agents includes the nonionic organic iodides, represented by iohexol, iopamidol,

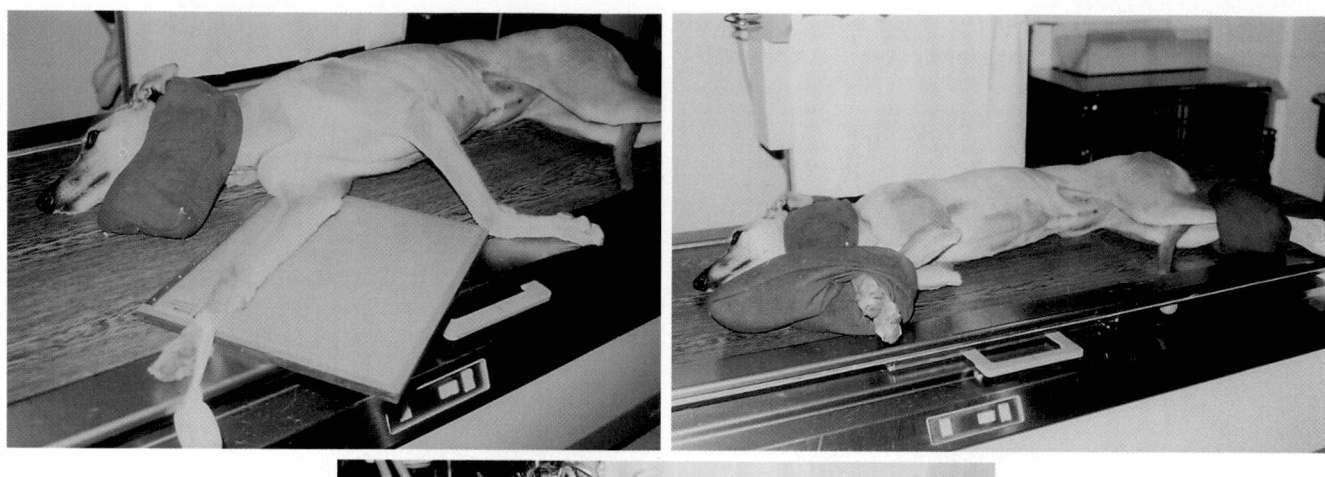

Figure 9-40 **A,** Sand bags and porous tape can help position tranquilized patients for some extremity radiographs. **B,** Sand bags can take the place of manual restraint for thoracic and abdominal lateral radiographs. **C,** Lucite positioning trays and sand bags can often take the place of technical restraint in postoperative radiography.

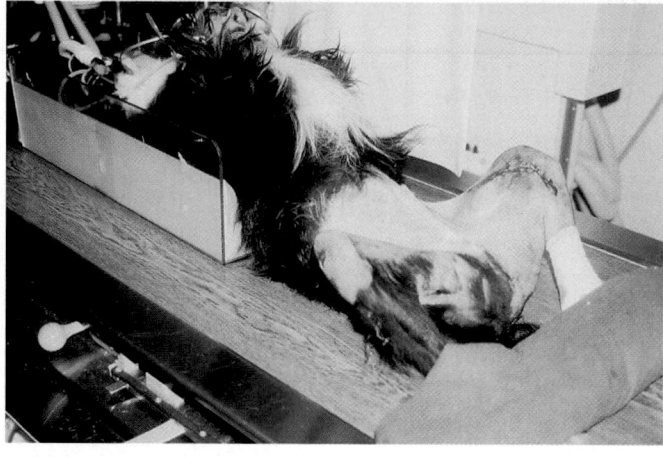

Figure 9-41 Positive contrast medium used in veterinary radiology. The first two containers are barium to be used orally or rectally only. The next four are ionic iodinated contrast, and the last two on the right are nonionic iodinated contrast.

iotolan, and, historically, metrizamide. These agents can be used like ionic organic iodides but have the advantage of not dissociating into positively and negatively charged ions in solution. This allows the agents to be used intrathecally (in the cerebrospinal fluid space around the spinal cord) for myelography as well as everywhere ionic iodides can be used. These contrast agents are still hyperosmolar but much less so than the ionic organic iodides. They appear to have a lower incidence of adverse effects and contrast reactions but have the disadvantage of increased cost.

Organic iodides (both ionic and nonionic) may cause serious contrast reactions, or adverse effects, when given intravenously, intraarterially, or intrathecally. These reactions are much less likely when the agents are used orally. Contrast reactions include nausea and vomiting, hypotension, cardiac arrest, and anaphylaxis. These reactions occur very infrequently, but it is advised to have a catheter in place when these agents are used and rapid access to fluids, oxygen, endotracheal tubes, and cardiovascular arrest resuscitation drugs during organic iodide contrast procedures. Do not leave these patients unattended after contrast administration. For a thorough discussion of contrast media and contrast procedures, see Douglas et al. (1987), Han et al. (2000), Lavin (2003), Morgan (1993), and Thrall (2002).

COMMON CONTRAST MEDIA AND APPLICATIONS

Esophagus
Contrast Agents
Barium sulfate, weight/volume (wt/vol) suspension 100%, is used alone and diluted to evaluate an enlarged esophagus or as a thick paste if the esophagus is not enlarged. Barium mixed with food may be more appropriate for diagnosis of esophageal strictures. Oral organic iodides (ionic or nonionic) are used when perforation of the esophagus is suspected.

Procedure
No special preparation is needed. Ideally, the study is done by using fluoroscopy. If this is not available, the exposure must be made when the animal swallows. The barium is administered with a syringe into the buccal pouch.

Stomach and Small Bowel (Upper Gastrointestinal Studies)
Contrast Agents
Three kinds of contrast agents are used for upper gastrointestinal studies: barium sulfate 25% to 30% wt/vol, oral iodides, and negative contrast, including air, carbon dioxide, and nitrous oxide. Barium sulfate is the most commonly used agent for upper gastrointestinal studies when perforation is not suspected. Negative contrast media are used in combination with barium sulfate for double-contrast studies. Oral iodinated products are given when perforation is suspected because barium sulfate will not be resorbed once it leaks into a body cavity.

Procedure
Food should be withheld for 24 hours, and warm water enemas should be administered about 2 to 3 hours before the gastrointestinal study. Acepromazine can be used without adverse effects on gastrointestinal motility.

Dosage
The dosage for barium sulfate is 10 ml/kg and for oral Hypaque or Gastrografin, 3 ml/kg.

Film Sequence
The survey film consists of a ventrodorsal and a lateral view. Immediately after administration of contrast medium, four films should be taken to completely evaluate the stomach: a ventrodorsal view, a dorsoventral view, and both a right and left lateral view. At 15, 30, and 60 minutes, the film sequence consists of ventrodorsal and right lateral views. These same views are taken at various intervals until contrast

reaches the large bowel. The timing sequence will vary with the patient and the suspected disease process.

Large Bowel (Lower Gastrointestinal Study, Barium Enema)
Contrast Agents
Barium sulfate 10% to 15% (wt/vol) or iodinated preparations, such as Gastrografin or oral Hypaque, are used for the lower gastrointestinal studies.

Precautions
Barium sulfate should not be used when a perforation is suspected. A barium enema should not be performed for 48 hours after a biopsy specimen of the colon or rectum has been obtained.

Preparation
The patient is fasted for 24 to 48 hours and may be given a gastrointestinal cleansing agent such as Golytely (Braintree Labs). Warm water enemas must be given before the examination because it is essential that the entire large bowel be cleansed before a barium enema is performed. A Bardex (French; Bard Hospital Division, C.R. Bard) catheter and barium container are needed for the study.

Procedure
The animal should be anesthetized. The balloon-tipped catheter is inserted into the rectum, and the cuff is inflated to form a firm seal against the colonic wall. The barium or iodine is placed in the colon by gravitational flow. A 15% wt/vol barium sulfate solution is used for barium enemas. The dose is 5 to 10 ml/0.45 kg of body weight. Ideally, the study is done by using fluoroscopy. Radiographic views needed are lateral, ventrodorsal, and right and left ventrodorsal oblique views. After completion, the barium is evacuated, and air is injected to obtain a double-contrast study of the large bowel.

Urinary Tract
Contrast Agents
Several kinds of contrast studies are available for evaluation of the kidneys. However, because the *intravenous pyelogram* (IVP) is the one most used in practice, this discussion is limited to it.

An IVP, or excretory urogram, is performed by injecting contrast medium intravenously. Ionic organic iodide products are most commonly used. A meglumine diatrizoate and sodium diatrizoate preparation is probably the most popular contrast product used for IVP examinations. The standard dose of contrast is 800 mg of iodine per kilogram, which may be increased by 50% in patients with poor renal function.

Complications
The most common complications encountered with an IVP are vomiting, anaphylactoid reactions, and hypotension.

Vomiting is a transient reaction of short duration and is not serious in nature. Care should be taken that the animal does not aspirate during the procedure. Anaphylactoid reactions are rare but must be attended to immediately. It is necessary to have epinephrine available for immediate administration whenever an IVP is done. Hypotension is rare, but when it occurs, it can be life threatening and may lead to renal failure.

Contraindications

The only serious contraindication is dehydration or iodine sensitivity.

Procedure

The animal should be fasted for 24 hours, but water should be available to prevent dehydration. Enemas should be given when needed, at least 2 to 3 hours before the IVP. Ventrodorsal and lateral films should be taken before the examinations. Films should be taken in the ventrodorsal and lateral positions immediately after injection of the contrast medium and at 5 and 15 minutes after injection. When needed, follow-up studies at 20 or 25 minutes after injection may be performed.

✍ TECHNICIAN NOTE

The intravenous pyelogram (IVP) is the most commonly used contrast study of the kidneys.

Urinary Bladder
Contrast Agents

Ionic organic iodide contrast materials are most desirable for retrograde cystography. Nonopaque contrast materials, such as air, carbon dioxide, and nitrous oxide, are used in addition to organic iodides for double-contrast cystography. Do not use barium sulfate.

Procedure

The colon should be cleansed. Depending on the breed and size of the animal, different catheters may be used. A Foley catheter, tomcat catheter, or soft flexible male catheter may be needed. In addition, a syringe and three-way valve are needed. Two types of cystography are commonly performed in veterinary practice: positive-contrast cystography and double-contrast cystography. Positive-contrast cystography is used to detect leaks or rupture of the lower urinary tract after trauma. Ionic organic iodide contrast at concentrations of 10% to 15% is injected retrograde into the urinary bladder at 5 to 15 ml/kg of body weight. Double-contrast cystography is used to detect all other forms of urinary bladder disease. A catheter is placed into the urinary bladder, and all urine is removed. Next, 3 to 10 ml of organic iodide contrast is injected, followed by carbon dioxide or room air at 5 to 15 ml/kg of body weight. Because of the variability of urinary bladder volume, it is best to fill the bladder to palpable turgidity. Lateral and oblique ventrodorsal radiographic views are most helpful.

Urethrography
Contrast Agents

Ionic organic iodide compounds at 20% concentration are best for urethrography.

Procedure

A balloon-tipped catheter (Foley type) is placed into the distal urethra. The cuff is inflated for a snug fit to prevent contrast from leaking around the catheter. Contrast, 10 to 20 ml, is hand-injected rapidly. The x-ray is taken during injections of the last few milliliters. A lateral view and two oblique views should be taken during the separate injections of the contrast material.

Spinal Cord

Myelography is the contrast examination most frequently performed to localize and characterize spinal cord lesions. Myelograms are always performed with the animal under general anesthesia. Nonionic iodinated contrast medium is injected into the subarachnoid space (cerebrospinal fluid space) at the cisterna magna (skull-C1 space) or in the caudal lumbar spine area (L4-L6). Myelography is most commonly performed before surgical intervention.

Contrast Agents

Two nonionic contrast agents are currently in wide use in veterinary medicine: iopamidol (Isovue, Bracco Diagnostics) and iohexol (Omnipaque, Sanofi Winthrop). The dose of contrast medium ranges from 0.25 ml/kg for cervical evaluation with a cisternal injection to 0.45 ml/kg for cervical evaluation from a lumbar injection. The concentration of iodine should be between 240 and 300 mg/ml, and injection volume should not exceed 15 ml.

Contraindications

Infection of the spinal cord and meninges and when the disease is to be treated medically only are contraindications.

Procedure

Survey films should be taken first. The site of injection should be aseptically prepared. Spinal needles of 20 to 22 gauge and 3.75 to 8.75 cm should be available because the size of the animal may vary considerably and some dogs may be so obese that even an 8.75-cm needle is short! Carefully collimated films are taken in the ventrodorsal and lateral positions immediately after administration of the contrast medium.

POSITIONING

Proper positioning is essential to obtain diagnostic radiographs. It is again the responsibility of the veterinary technician to properly position the animal. It is not the intent of this chapter to discuss positioning at length. Please refer to the excellent treatment of this topic by Butler et al. (2000), Douglas et al. (1987), Han et al. (2000), Lavin (2003), Morgan (1993), and Ticer (1984).

> **✎ TECHNICIAN NOTE**
> Proper positioning is essential to obtain diagnostic radiographs.

PRINCIPLES OF POSITIONING

To achieve proper positioning, the technician should remember that two views at right angles are necessary to obtain a diagnostic study. This principle applies to all examinations in small animals and to extremities in large animals. The exceptions to this rule are thoracic examinations and spinal examinations in the horse and examinations in cases of trauma or in debilitated animals when only lateral views can be taken without causing undue stress to the animals.

Another principle to remember is the importance of centering the primary beam on the lesion itself, when known. This is especially important in orthopedic cases in both small and large animals. For example, fracture healing may look very different when the x-ray beam is centered over the fracture line as opposed to a short distance away from it. Costly errors have been made by veterinarians who removed supporting devices before the correct time. These errors occurred because fractures may have appeared healed when the primary beam was centered away from the fracture line itself.

It is also important, when performing a radiographic examination, to use an x-ray film that is sufficiently large to completely cover the system to be examined. When x-raying very large dogs, it may be necessary to use two films for the abdomen: one for the cranial abdomen and one for the caudal abdomen, which is generally taken at a lower kilovoltage peak. For extremities, the primary beam should be directed at the lesion. It is good to have a radiograph large enough to include the proximal and distal portions of the joint to obtain a good spatial anatomic relationship of the lesion.

These principles are basic but essential. Proper positioning is achieved through practice. These topics are well illustrated and discussed in the references mentioned. A positioning reference textbook should be available in the radiology room of every veterinary practice.

RESTRAINT

The importance of restraint to achieve proper positioning cannot be overemphasized. It is part of radiation safety. Without proper restraint, many examinations should not be undertaken. In some cases, attempting to make examinations without restraint would be life threatening with large animals and dangerous with certain small animals.

There are many types of restraint; some are mechanical or manual, and some are chemical. For the purpose of radiation safety, manual restraint should be avoided as a routine procedure. When it is essential to be in the room with the animal, a protective lead apron and gloves should be worn, and the x-ray beam should be limited to the system to be examined by coning devices or by adjustment of the collimator.

Mechanical restraint comes in various forms. A number of commercial devices designed for animal positioning are available, varying in price from a few dollars to several hundred dollars. One of the most useful and inexpensive devices for use with dogs is a simple muzzle, which often has a calming effect on an animal (see Chapter 1). Sandbags and sponges can also be used to obtain excellent positioning. When the animal is positioned properly, it is most important to take the radiograph rapidly, because one can hope for only a few seconds of restraint before the animal moves.

Chemical restraint can be achieved with tranquilizers, analgesics, or anesthesia (see Chapters 19 and 20). Chemical restraint has contributed greatly to the progress made in radiology by allowing positioning that would otherwise be impossible to achieve. For example, complete examination of the skull should not be attempted without anesthesia. Every time total immobility or relaxation is required for proper positioning, general anesthesia should be used. Most spinal examinations will prove nondiagnostic unless the examination is done with the animal under anesthesia. In several circumstances, tranquilization is adequate to control most animals. Tranquilizers are excellent for control of frightened or aggressive dogs and cats. They are also most useful for controlling large animals.

> **✎ TECHNICIAN NOTE**
> Chemical restraint has contributed greatly to the progress made in radiology by allowing positioning that would otherwise be impossible to achieve.

Again, good positioning is essential in producing diagnostic x-ray films. It takes time to learn and become proficient in achieving every position needed for a variety of examinations in large and small animals. However, most organs can be x-rayed with proper techniques, equipment, and accessory devices and the use of mechanical or chemical restraint or both.

DIAGNOSTIC ULTRASONOGRAPHY

Ultrasound imaging is becoming an essential diagnostic tool in veterinary practice. It is portable; does not require the use of ionizing radiation; and is noninvasive, well tolerated by patients, and accepted by clients. As ultrasound equipment becomes affordable, the only problem with its introduction into practice is the long learning curve associated with its use. Recent veterinary graduates are more familiar with the uses and indications for ultrasonography, because veterinary schools have integrated ultrasonography into the curriculum. All new veterinary technicians are encouraged to familiarize themselves with the basics of diagnostic ultrasonography, but remember that ultrasonography is user dependent. The image and interpretation are only as good as the person doing the examination.

ULTRASONOGRAPHY BASICS

Sound is a mechanical pressure wave made up of a series of compressions and rarefactions transmitted through a medium. Sound waves are characterized by their wavelength or distance between compressions, their frequency in cycles per second, and their velocity or speed of transmission (Figure 9-42). These characteristics are integrated by the following formula:

$$\textbf{Velocity} = \textbf{Wavelength} \times \textbf{Frequency}$$

For simplicity, assume that the speed of sound in the body is 1540 m/sec. Therefore as the frequency of sound increases, the wavelength decreases. Shorter sound waves produce increased image resolution but decreased patient penetration. The frequencies used in veterinary diagnostic ultrasound examination generally range from 2.5 to 12 megahertz (MHz). A hertz (Hz) is 1 cycle per second. Therefore typical ultrasound frequencies will range from 2 to 12 million cycles/sec, or 2.5 to 12 MHz. Audible sound will range from 20 to 20,000 Hz.

Real-time, gray-scale ultrasonography is based on the *pulse-echo principle*. A short pulse of sound, usually 2 or 3 cycles long, is produced from the transducer and transmitted into the patient. The sound wave strikes an echogenic surface in the patient and returns some of the sound to the transducer. The strength of the returning sound wave

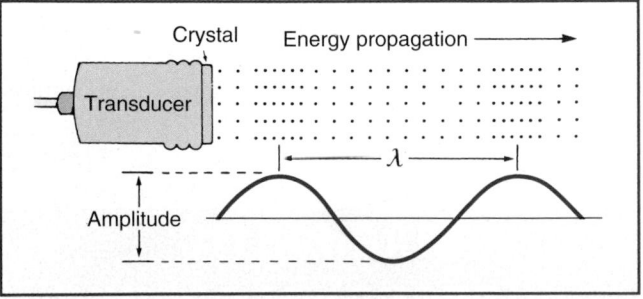

Figure 9-42 Sound wave with a wavelength = λ. *Closely spaced dots,* Compressions; *widely spaced dots,* rarefactions. The amplitude is proportional to the loudness.

determines the brightness of the image, and the time it takes for the sound to travel into the patient and back to the transducer determines where the echo will be seen on the screen. Remember that the time it takes for a sound wave to traverse a distance and be reflected back is a function of the distance between the sender and reflector and the speed of the sound wave in that medium. For all practical purposes, the speed of sound in small animal tissues is constant at 1540 m/sec.

Ultrasound production and reception are based on the *piezoelectric effect*. A piezoelectric crystal will change shape or thickness when subjected to a voltage pulse. Rapid pulses of electrical energy are transformed into mechanical energy or sound waves by the vibrating crystal. Returning sound waves cause the crystal to vibrate, and that mechanical energy is transmitted into electrical energy by the transducer. This electrical signal is transformed into the gray-scale image on the screen. The transducer acts as both the sound transmitter and the receiver. The operating frequency of the transducer is partially determined by the thickness of the piezoelectric crystal. The thinner the crystal, the higher the transducer frequency. The transducer transmits sound 0.01% of the time. It receives returning sound waves 99.9% of the time.

◢ TECHNICIAN NOTE

Ultrasound production and reception are based on the *piezoelectric effect*. A piezoelectric crystal will change shape or thickness when subjected to a voltage pulse.

ULTRASOUND-TISSUE INTERACTION

To better understand the ultrasound image, it is important to understand the interaction of ultrasound within tissue. As the sound wave proceeds through the body, it is progressively attenuated or weakened. This *attenuation* limits the depth of penetration of the sound wave and therefore limits the depth of structures that can be effectively imaged. The ultrasound beam is attenuated or weakened by absorption, reflection, scattering, refraction, and diffraction. Reflection is a redirection of the sound beam back to the transducer and is the basis of the diagnostic image. Absorption is sound energy converted to heat within the tissues. Scattering is the intertissue microreflection of sound, which is responsible for much of the echo texture of various organs. Refraction and diffraction are the bending of the sound beam as it crosses areas of differing tissue densities. Refraction attenuation is important in the generation of several ultrasound artifacts.

Sound reflection or echo production forms the basis of the ultrasound image. An echo is produced whenever the ultrasound beam crosses an acoustic interface. An acoustic interface is the boundary between two tissues of differing acoustic impedances, or Z. See the following equation:

$$\text{Acoustic impedance (Z)} = \frac{\text{Density (P)} \times \text{Speed of sound transmission (C)}}{}$$

$$\text{or Z} = \text{P} \times \text{C}$$

If we assume the speed of sound in soft tissue to be constant at 1540 m/sec, then the main factor that influences acoustic impedance is the density or composition of tissue. Thus the more different two adjacent tissues are, the greater will be the echo reflection between them. This is why very homogeneous populations of cells (lymphoma, lymph nodes, regenerative liver nodules) produce few echoes and are generally hypoechoic (darker). If the acoustic interface difference is small, only a small percentage of sound will be reflected. If the difference is large, a large portion of sound will be reflected. Most soft tissues have a Z, or acoustic impedance, within 1% to 2% of liver.

Interface	% Reflection
Fat-muscle	0.94
Fat-bone	49.00
Tissue-air	100.00

By looking at this list, one can see the acoustic impedance (Z) between fat and muscle is very low, whereas the acoustic impedance between fat and bone and between soft tissue and air is very high. This property is why ultrasound cannot be used to image through bone or gas. Too much of the sound beam is reflected back from bone and gas interfaces because of the large change in tissue density.

PATIENT PREPARATION

Patient preparation is important because 100% of the sound is reflected when the ultrasound beam intersects air. Hair traps air, which is how it insulates the animal, but if one tries to pass an ultrasound beam through hair, the majority of the beam is reflected before it ever enters the animal. A careful close clip of the area to be examined, as well as removal of dirt and scales, will improve the ultrasound image. A generous volume of ultrasound gel is also beneficial to displace air and couple the transducer to the skin (Figure 9-43). Small animals are placed in a padded V-trough table on their backs for abdominal examination and in lateral or sternal recumbency for cardiac examination. Most small animals tolerate abdominal and cardiac examinations well and rarely require tranquilization. A special cardiac table with large and small holes in it is very helpful for echocardiography. The animal is placed in lateral recumbency with the chest area over the appropriate-size hole, which allows for better ultrasound transducer access (Figure 9-44). Large animal examinations are done in the standing tranquilized animal. Again, close clipping, especially for tendon examinations, is critical for an optimal examination.

TECHNICIAN NOTE

Hair traps air, which is how it insulates the animal, but if one tries to pass an ultrasound beam through hair, the majority of the beam is reflected before it ever enters the animal. This is why good patient preparation is so critical.

ULTRASOUND DISPLAY MODES

The returning echo can be displayed in several ways. *A-mode*, or *amplitude mode*, displays the returning echoes as spikes from a baseline. The echo depth is determined by its location along the baseline. The echo intensity is displayed by the height of the spike. A-mode ultrasound machines are used predominantly in ophthalmology and have little value in veterinary practice.

B-mode, or *brightness mode*, forms the basis for two-dimensional imaging. The returning echoes are displayed as dots on the image screen. The brightness of the dot is a function of the strength of the returning echo. The placement of the dot is a function of the time it took for the echo to return to the transducer. The cross-sectional image is formed through data storage. The sound beam is automatically swept across the patient while the transducer is held steady and moved slowly over the area of interest. The rapid collection of images is called *real time*. This permits direct observation of moving structures, such as a beating heart or puppy motion. With B-mode real-time equipment, images are displayed in gray scale. Gray scale is a technique in which the various echo strengths are displayed in numerous shades of gray from black to white, similar to a black and white television picture.

M-mode, or *time-motion (TM) mode*, is produced by passing a narrow sound beam across a body part. Each echo interface is presented as a dot. The motion of the body part is displayed by sweeping the image across the screen or image recorder. M-mode can be thought of as a very thin sector of B-mode displayed as a function of time. M-mode is primarily used for echocardiography. Ideal ultrasound equipment for veterinary practice would be a real-time B-mode scanner with M-mode capabilities (Figure 9-45).

The selection of appropriate transducers is critical when ultrasound equipment is purchased. Transducers vary in type, size, style, shape, and frequency. Linear array transducers are made with several piezoelectric crystals stacked side by side. The crystals are fired in rapid sequence to produce a rectangular cross-sectional image. The major drawback for older linear array transducers is their large footprint or contact area. It is difficult to use these transducers for intercostal cardiac studies and for subcostal studies in the cranioabdominal area in small animals. Linear array transducers are primarily used for transrectal reproductive examinations in cattle and horses. Newer microcase,

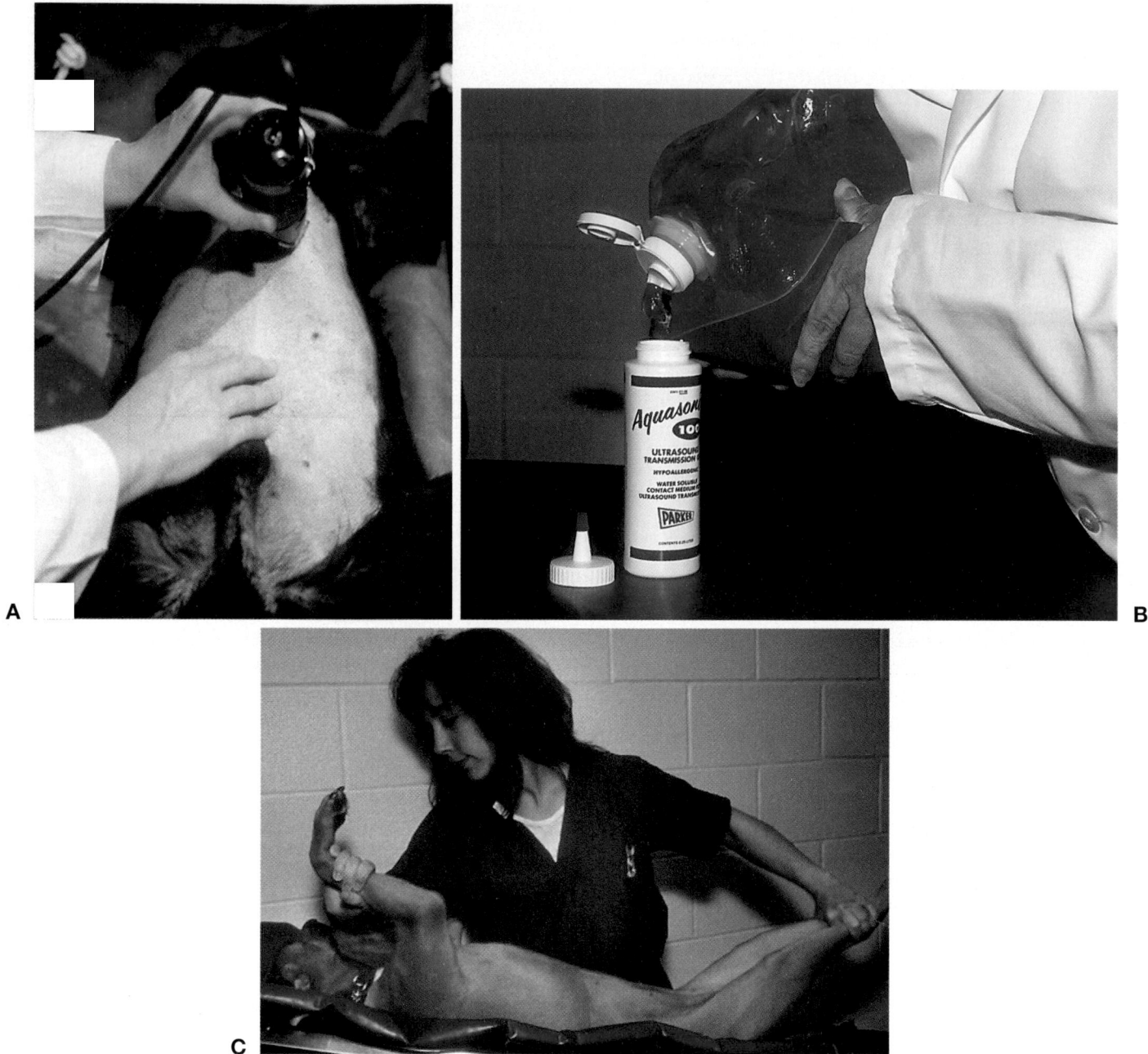

Figure 9-43 Patient preparation for abdominal ultrasound examination. **A,** Careful close clip of entire abdomen. **B,** Clean the skin surface, and use a generous volume of coupling gel. **C,** Place the animal in dorsal recumbency on a padded V-trough, and gently restrain during the examination.

small-footprint linear array transducers are used very effectively for small animal imaging.

Sector scanners produce a triangular field. The crystal is swept across the area by mechanical or electronic means, and the transducer generally has a small contact area. Newer, more expensive transducers may incorporate annular array and dynamic focusing technology. These transducers form the ultrasound beam by adding together many small beams from an array of small crystals. Dynamic focusing allows the operator to place any portion within the beam into maximum resolution without having to change transducers.

Deciding what frequency of transducer to use is easy. Use as high a frequency transducer as possible to maximize resolution while still allowing penetration to the needed depth. Remember that the higher the frequency of the transducer, the shorter will be the sound wavelength and the better will be the resolution. However, as the frequency increases, the depth of sound beam penetration decreases.

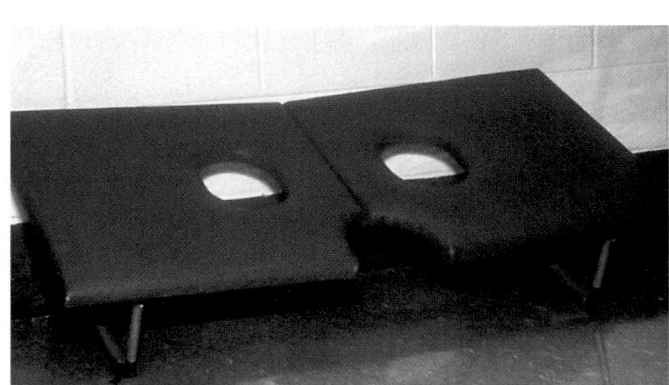
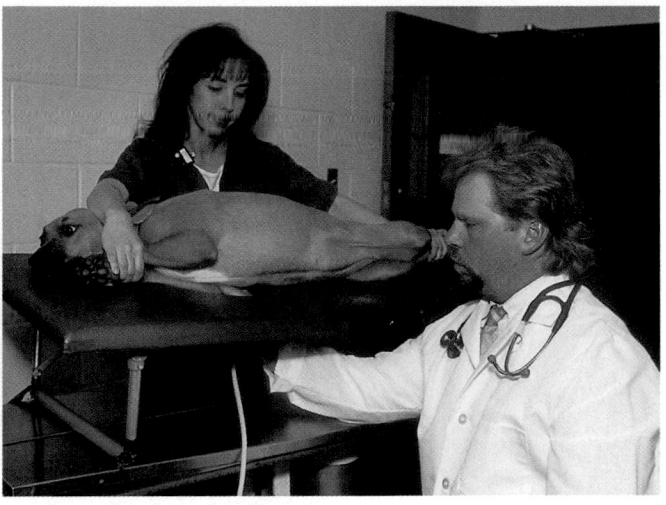

A **B**

Figure 9-44 **A,** Small animal cardiac ultrasound table. **B,** Patient properly positioned and restrained for echocardiography. The dog's cardiac notch is placed over the table hole so the sonographer can access the chest from beneath the table.

For abdominal ultrasonography in small dogs (15 kg or less) and cats, a 7.5-MHz transducer is ideal. For middle-size to large-breed dogs, a 5-MHz transducer works well. A guide for selecting a transducer is as follows:

High frequency:	Increases resolution
	Increases attenuation
	Decreases penetration
Low frequency:	Decreases resolution
	Decreases attenuation
	Increases penetration

TECHNICIAN NOTE

Use as high a frequency transducer as possible to maximize resolution while allowing penetration to the necessary depth.

The ultrasound equipment controls vary from machine to machine, but the concept of *time-gain compensation* (TGC) is fairly universal. The echoes coming from acoustic interfaces close to the transducer are stronger than the echoes returning from farther away from the transducer. Time-gain amplification compensates for the progressive attenuation with depth in the ultrasound beam. TGC is operator dependent and is set for the best-looking uniform image. TGC controls are most often a series of slide pods on the front of the machine. The top pod is the near field of the image, and the lowest pod is the far field, or bottom, of the image.

THE ULTRASOUND IMAGE

As one begins using ultrasound, the need to restudy anatomy increases. The ultrasound image is a thin cross-sectional slice through the body in a new or different orientation. It will help to use a standard image orientation, which places the head or front of the animal on the left in the sagittal or longitudinal view and the animal's right on the left of the screen on the transverse or axial view.

Ultrasound terminology is easy to remember. *Echogenicity* refers to the strength or amplitude of the returning echoes. A structure that is *sonodense* or *echogenic* (bright) produces echoes. A structure that is *anechoic* or *sonolucent* (dark) produces few or no echoes. A structure is *hyperechoic* (brighter than) if it produces more echoes than adjacent structures. A structure is *hypoechoic* (darker than) if it produces fewer echoes than surrounding structures. An *isoechoic* (same as) structure has a level of echogenicity similar to that of adjacent structures. Remember that echogenicity is a relative term. Any structure can be made bright by adjusting machine control settings. Compare organs at the same depth and control settings to avoid misinterpretation of relative echogenicities.

ULTRASOUND ARTIFACTS

Most people fail to take the time to fully understand ultrasound artifacts. They ignore artifacts because, by definition, an artifact does not contribute useful image information. This is not true of ultrasound artifacts. Ultrasound artifacts provide accurate clues to what makes up the ultrasound image.

REVERBERATION ARTIFACT

A reverberation artifact occurs when the ultrasound beam hits gas or air. Because of the large drop in acoustic impedance (soft tissue/air interface), all of the ultrasound

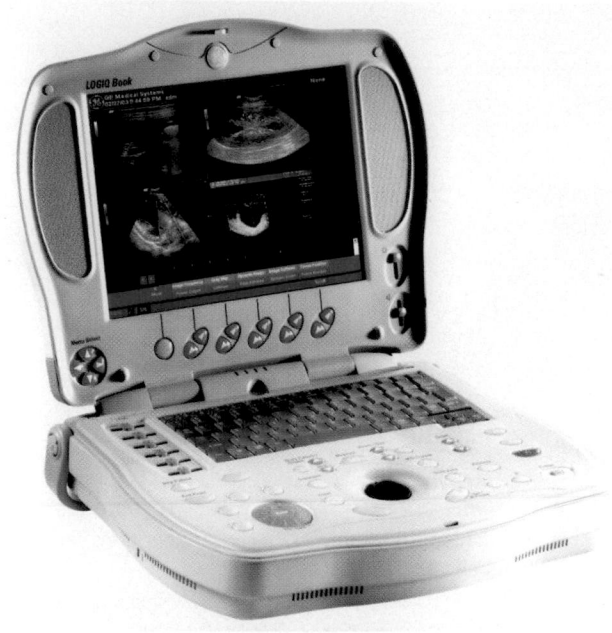

A

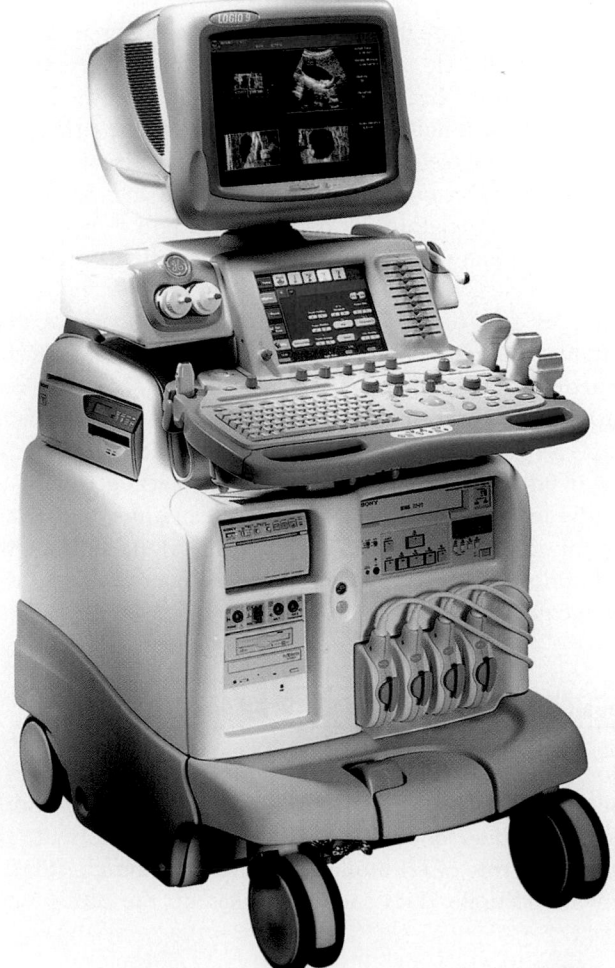

B

Figure 9-45 **A,** Portable notebook-style, real-time B-mode, M-mode, and color Doppler dedicated veterinary ultrasound unit that can be used on both large and small animals. **B,** Larger mobile veterinary ultrasound unit most commonly used in small animal practices. (Courtesy Sound Technologies, Inc, Carlsbad. Calif.)

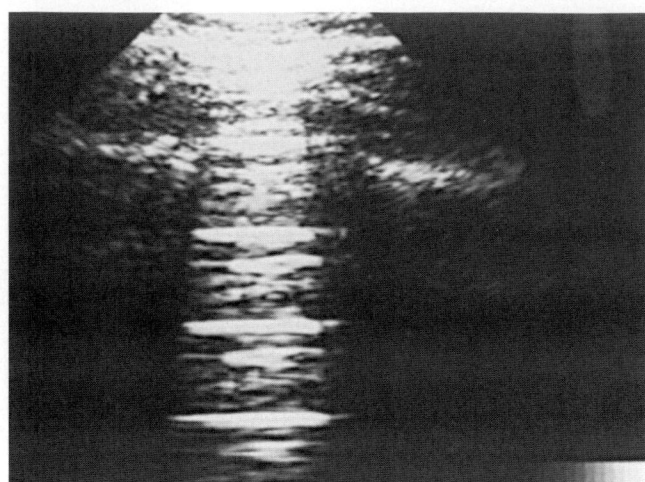

Figure 9-46 Reverberation artifact from the air-filled lung of a normal horse. The parallel, evenly spaced echogenic bands represent reverberation between the transducer and pleural surface.

beam is reflected back to the transducer. A portion of the reflected beam bounces off the transducer surface and reenters the patient. It hits the air interface a second time, and the same thing happens again. This occurs repeatedly and appears on the screen as a set of bright parallel lines that are the same distance from each other. Each parallel line represents the distance between the transducer and the gas interface. Reverberation artifacts can also be referred to as *dirty shadowing* or *comet tails* (Figure 9-46).

SHADOWING

A shadowing artifact occurs because of inadequate sound beam penetration through a highly reflective or sound-absorptive substance. Acoustic shadowing is an area of darkness or hypoechogenicity that occurs deep to very dense material, such as bone, calcium, or calculi. Very small objects cast an acoustic shadow only if they are within the focal zone or narrow portion of the ultrasound beam.

ACOUSTIC ENHANCEMENT

If the ultrasound beam passes through an area with few tissue interfaces (low attenuation region), the emerging ultrasound beam will have more intensity than would be expected and will be brighter or more echogenic distal to the nonattenuating structure. The best example of this is the normal gallbladder surrounded by the hepatic parenchyma. The liver tissue distal or deep to the gallbladder appears brighter than adjacent hepatic tissue (Figure 9-47). This artifact is seen deep to fluid-filled structures and is also referred to as *through transmission*.

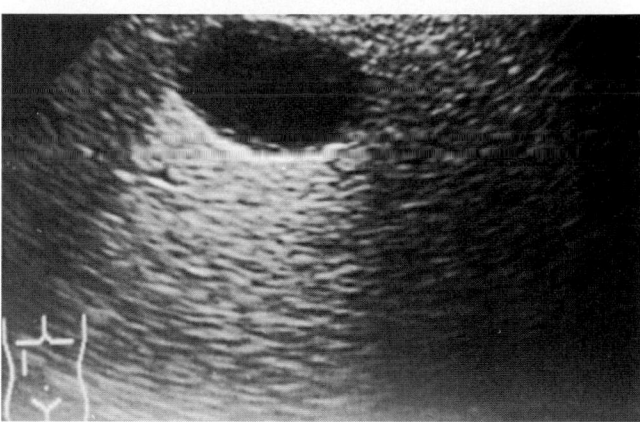

Figure 9-47 Bright echogenic band beneath the gallbladder represents acoustic enhancement. The ultrasound beam is not attenuated as much as it traverses the fluid-filled gallbladder as it is in the surrounding liver.

REFRACTION, OR EDGE ARTIFACT

Refraction is a hypoechoic band or stripe at the margin of a curved structure caused by the refraction or bending of the sound beam. The sound beam is deflected from its true path and never returns, with an effect similar to shadowing. An edge artifact is helpful in identifying very smooth round structures, such as early pregnancy vesicles.

MIRROR-IMAGE ARTIFACT

The ultrasound machine places the returning echo on the viewing screen as a function of the time it took the echo to return. If the sound wave reverberates within a highly echogenic structure before returning to the transducer, the image will be duplicated on the screen distal to the original image. This is most commonly seen as a duplication of the gallbladder in mirror image on the other side of the diaphragm.

SLICE-THICKNESS ARTIFACT

If the width of the ultrasound beam cuts through both the edge of a cystic structure and solid tissue, the solid tissue may look as if it is layered within the cyst. This artifact is responsible for the erroneous appearance of debris within the urinary bladder and gallbladder, although no debris are present. The erroneous appearance is the result of volume averaging of tissue by the ultrasound machine.

THE ULTRASOUND EXAMINATION

A complete ultrasound examination requires at least 20 to 30 minutes to perform. When ultrasound is used for a quick answer to a question such as pregnancy versus pyometra, the examination will be shorter. When ultrasound is used for abdominal disease diagnosis, a complete examination should be performed every time.

It is important to have a thorough understanding of the normal appearance of the various abdominal organs before trying to identify the abnormalities associated with disease. The ranking of small animal abdominal organs from least echogenic (darkest) to most echogenic (brightest) is as follows:

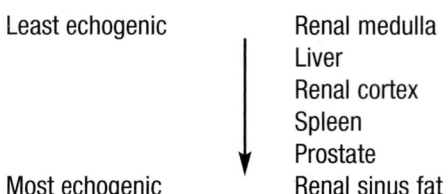

Least echogenic	Renal medulla
	Liver
	Renal cortex
	Spleen
	Prostate
Most echogenic	Renal sinus fat

Remember that echogenicity is a relative term, and one must compare organs at similar control settings and similar depths to avoid misinterpretation.

> **✎ TECHNICIAN NOTE**
>
> It is important to have a thorough understanding of the normal appearance of the various abdominal organs before trying to identify the abnormalities associated with disease.

CLINICAL USE

The clinical application of ultrasound in veterinary medicine has exploded during the past 10 years. Equipment designed for use in humans is readily adaptable for use in veterinary medicine, and several companies are producing dedicated veterinary ultrasound machines. Both 5- and 7.5-MHz transducers are popular for small animal and nonreproductive large animal imaging. The 3- and 5-MHz linear array transducers are extensively used for transrectal large animal reproductive ultrasonography. Traditional cardiac and solid abdominal organ examinations remain the mainstay, but ultrasound is used to answer hundreds of clinical questions in a wide variety of species. The following section lists common ultrasound applications in both large and small animals.

USES OF ULTRASOUND IN LARGE AND SMALL ANIMALS

- Tendon injury evaluation and response to surgery or therapy
- Diagnosis of tendon sheath infections, adhesions, and foreign bodies
- Evaluation of joint effusions, intraarticular injury, osteomyelitis, and neoplasms
- Congenital and acquired cardiac disease and response to therapy
- Pleural effusion, pleuritis, and pleuropneumonia
- Soft tissue, neck, thyroid, parathyroid, tongue, and mediastinal disease

- Hepatic, renal, splenic, adrenal, urinary bladder, gallbladder, and biliary disease
- Abdominal and peripheral vascular malformations
- Peritoneal and pleural fluid assessment and sampling
- Abdominal masses of unknown origin
- Intestinal foreign bodies, intussusceptions, infiltrative disease, and neoplasia
- Testicular and prostate evaluation and location of retained testicles
- Pregnancy diagnosis, fetal evaluation, twin removal, and complete fertility evaluations
- Soft tissue neoplasia, granulomas, abscesses, and foreign bodies
- Umbilical infections and persistent and patent urachus
- Ocular and orbital evaluation
- Vascular thrombosis and catheter foreign body evaluation
- Guidance for fine-needle aspiration, drain placement, biopsy, and culture

NUCLEAR MEDICINE

Many veterinary schools and several progressive specialized veterinary practices have nuclear medicine capabilities. Nuclear medicine can be divided into therapeutic and diagnostic procedures. Currently, veterinary therapeutic nuclear medicine involves the administration of radioactive iodine (^{131}I) for the treatment of hyperthyroidism and thyroid tumors. Diagnostic nuclear medicine involves the administration of radionuclides to the animal and detection of the electromagnetic radiation emitted from the animal with a gamma scintillation camera. Radionuclides are atoms with unstable nuclei that undergo radioactive decay. Radioactive decay is the transformation or disintegration of an unstable nucleus by spontaneous emission of electromagnetic radiation. Electromagnetic radiations that are of nuclear origin are termed *gamma rays,* in contrast to diagnostic radiations (x-rays), which originate from the electron cloud that surrounds the nucleus.

TECHNICIAN NOTE

Currently, veterinary therapeutic nuclear medicine involves the administration of radioactive iodine (^{131}I) for the treatment of hyperthyroidism and thyroid tumors.

Diagnostic nuclear medicine does not generate visual images equivalent to those of diagnostic radiology but detects functional or physiologic, pharmacologic, and kinetic data from the patient in image or numeric data form. Figure 9-48 shows a standard gamma scintillation camera, control panel, and nuclear medicine computer. Common clinical uses of veterinary nuclear medicine include bone scanning for detection of tumor metastasis to bone and radiographically undetectable bone injury or infection, lung scanning for detection of pulmonary embolism and as a pulmonary function test, renal scans for assessment of kidney perfusion

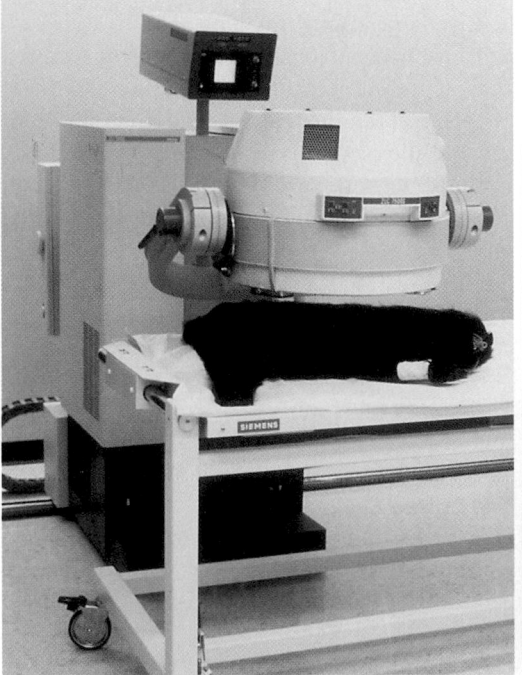

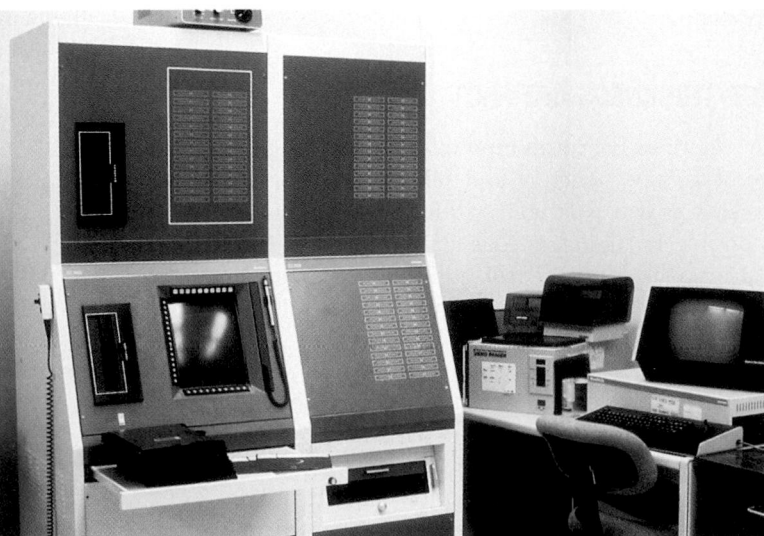

A **B**

Figure 9-48 **A,** Gamma scintillation camera in position over a dog during a whole-body bone scan to check for metastatic neoplasia. **B,** Control panel monitor, nuclear medicine computer, and matrix camera.

and function, and thyroid scans for the characterization of hyperthyroidism and the detection of metastasis. Other, less common nuclear medicine studies include hepatobiliary scanning, brain scans, labeled white blood cell scans for the detection of occult infection, lymphoscintigraphy, nuclear angiography, and scans for detection of an unknown focus of blood loss.

The most commonly used radionuclide is technetium 99m (^{99m}Tc). This agent is commercially available from a disposable technetium generator. Technetium is administered in an ionic form as ^{99m}TcO$_4$ (pertechnetate) or bound to a specific organ-localizing pharmaceutical agent before administration. Technetium is the radiopharmaceutical of choice because it has a 6-hour physical half-life and emits a 140-keV gamma ray, which is appropriate for most imaging studies. The radioactive or physical half-life of a radionuclide is the time required for the number of radioactive atoms to decrease by 50%.

Radiation safety practices are important with nuclear medicine. When working in a practice that uses nuclear medicine, one should insist on receiving comprehensive instruction in radiation principles and safety. This chapter is meant only as an introduction.

The primary route of radionuclide administration to veterinary patients is intravenous. Latex examination gloves should be worn, and careful injection techniques should be used to ensure that the entire dose is delivered intravenously and not perivascularly. This is especially important in equine bone scans for which a large dose of radionuclide is administered. Please refer to Chapter 29 for additional information on nuclear scintigraphy in horses. The routes of excretion of the radioactive imaging agents vary with the agent used. Technetium is primarily excreted in urine, with a lesser amount in the feces. Animals should be housed in a separate restricted area of the hospital, and their stool and urine should be carefully collected and held for decay until the levels are below exempt quantities. Always wear latex examination gloves, and limit contact with patients to only that necessary for their care. Never eat or bring eating utensils (coffee cups, spoons, etc.) into a nuclear medicine area. The dose of radiation to the patient is small, but repeated physical contact or accidental ingestion of radionuclides may be harmful to the nuclear medicine technologist. Animals should be held in the restricted area until they pose no radiation threat to their owners or the population at large. This is generally 3 to 10 physical half-lives of the radiopharmaceutical, depending on specific state regulations.

> ### ✐ TECHNICIAN NOTE
> The primary route of radionuclide administration to veterinary patients is intravenous. Latex examination gloves should be worn, and careful injection techniques should be used to ensure that the entire dose is delivered intravenously and not perivascularly.

COMPUTED TOMOGRAPHY

In the past 15 years, there has been an expansion of the diagnostic imaging techniques available to veterinary patients. Most veterinary schools and several specialty practices have access to computed tomography (CT) scanning. A CT scan is obtained by passing a very thin x-ray beam transaxially through the patient and measuring the x-ray attenuation at multiple sites in a thin slice of the patient's anatomy. The computer then reconstructs the transmitted x-ray data into a cross-sectional image on a video monitor. The image can then be captured on film or videotape or stored on magnetic tape for later use. The advantage of CT over standard radiography is the greatly improved radiographic contrast, spatial resolution, and cross-sectional anatomic presentation. The most common use of CT in veterinary medicine is head and spinal examinations for neurologic disease. CT allows the veterinarian a noninvasive look inside the patient's skull (Figure 9-49).

When a CT scan is performed, the patient is placed in the ventrodorsal or dorsoventral position on the long, narrow, movable CT table. The table then moves the patient through the circular gantry that houses the x-ray tube and detectors (Figure 9-50). The table moves in a measured stepwise fashion. During each table step, the CT scanner obtains a single cross-sectional slice of data. The patient must be heavily sedated or under general anesthesia to prevent any motion and must be positioned perfectly straight. Most studies are performed twice on the same animal. The first study is performed without contrast, and the second is performed after intravenous administration of iodinated contrast. Urographic contrast agents are commonly administered at a dose of 800 mg of iodine per kilogram of body

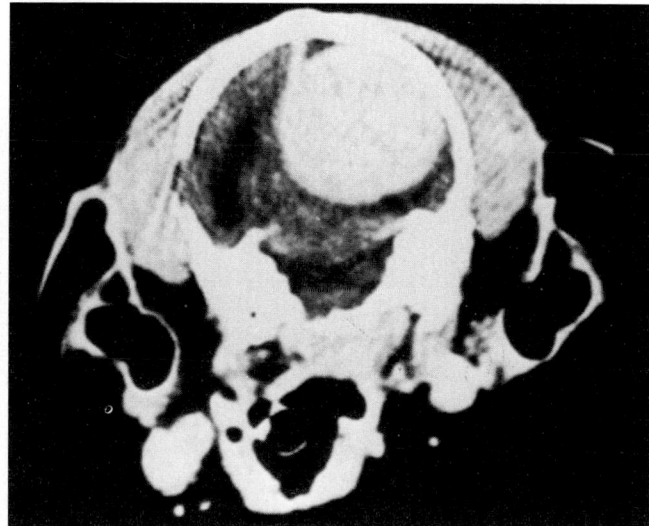

Figure 9-49 Computed tomogram of a dog brain showing a large contrast-enhancing brain tumor (meningioma) in the central cerebrum.

weight. Contrast will highlight vascular structures, and some neoplasms will have a characteristic contrast enhancement pattern. In addition to examination of the brain, CT can be used to identify and characterize musculoskeletal, thoracic, and abdominal disorders.

TECHNICIAN NOTE

When performing CT studies, you use the same contrast agents you use for radiographic contrast procedures; you just use much less concentrated contrast medium because CT is much more contrast sensitive.

MAGNETIC RESONANCE IMAGING

The newest imaging modality to be used in veterinary medicine is magnetic resonance imaging (MRI). MRI is similar to CT in that the image is a thin slice of cross-sectional anatomy made up of a matrix of volume elements. MRI differs from CT in that it uses no ionizing radiation to create the image. Instead, the MRI represents the intensity of a radio wave signal from tissue in which hydrogen nuclei have been disturbed by a characteristic radiofrequency pulse. MRI is superior to CT in image resolution, anatomic definition, and sensitivity to tissue composition differences. Because of this, MRI is vastly superior to CT for imaging of the brain and spinal cord and is currently used primarily for head and spine evaluation. Figure 9-51 is a sagittal canine brain magnetic resonance image of a patient with a large contrast-enhancing pituitary tumor.

TECHNICIAN NOTE

MRI differs from CT in that it uses no ionizing radiation to create the image. MRI is superior to CT in image resolution, anatomic definition, and sensitivity to tissue composition differences. Because of this, MRI is vastly superior to CT for imaging of the brain and spinal cord and is currently used primarily for head and spine evaluation.

Two general types of MRI units (also called *magnets*) are used in veterinary imaging: low field strength open magnets (Figure 9-52, *A*) and high field strength, or superconductive, magnets (Figure 9-52, *B*). Magnetic field strength is measured in tesla (T). Low field strength magnets are 0.4 T or less, and high field strength magnets are 0.6 T and above. The most typical superconducting magnet has a field strength of 1 or 1.5 T. Regardless of the type of magnet used, the technician needs to be aware of several safety measures and patient management concerns peculiar to MRI.

About half of the veterinary teaching hospitals have in-house MRI units. In most private veterinary practices, CT and MRI are often done off the clinic premises in an imaging center; a mobile, truck-based MRI unit; or a human hospital. Therefore everything needed to anesthetize, resuscitate, and recover a patient needs to be taken to the

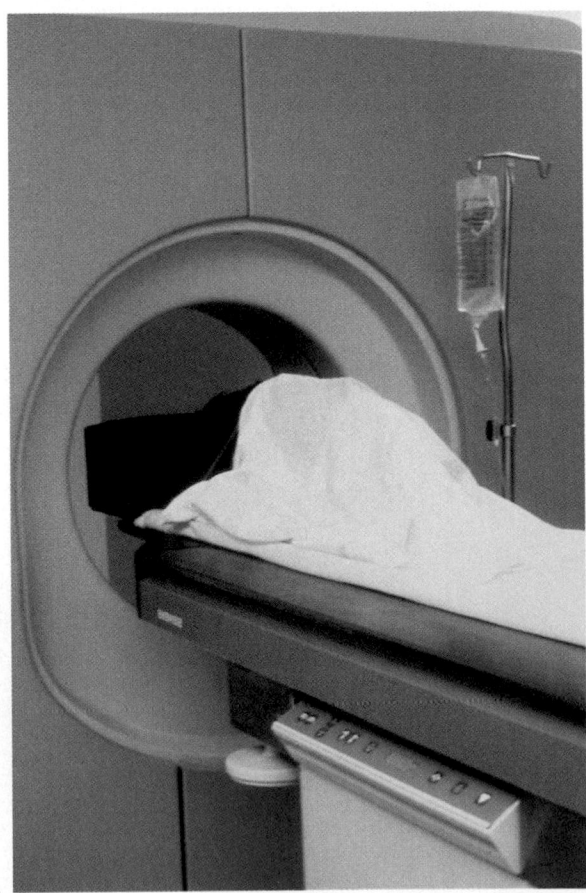

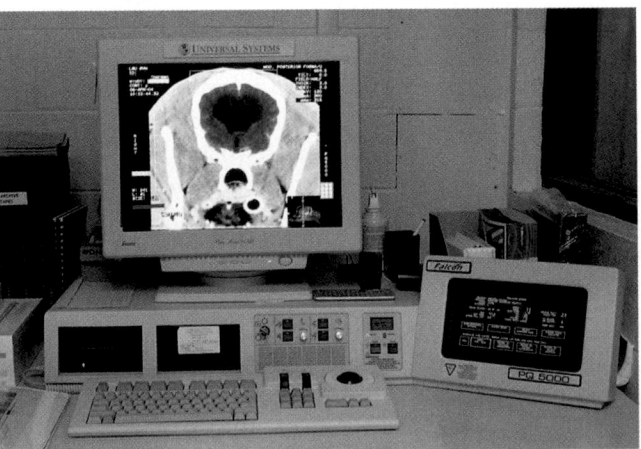

Figure 9-50 **A,** Dog in position for a brain computed tomogram. The large circular gantry houses the x-ray tube and detectors. The table moves the patient through the gantry in precise, measured, incremental steps. **B,** Computed tomography (CT) control panel located outside the shielded CT room.

imaging site. Most practices that perform off-site imaging have a large tackle box or physician's bag filled with all necessary drugs, fluids, catheters, intravenous access lines, syringes, needles, tape, gauze, and endotracheal tubes. It often helps to do a mock run or pretend case before a clinical case to ensure that everything is correctly packed. Imaging centers and hospitals appreciate clean, odor-free, and flea- and tick-free veterinary patients. It is a good idea to bathe the patient within 24 hours before the examination if possible and to ensure that the patient's bowel and bladder have been evacuated before the patient enters the hospital or imaging center.

A serious problem with MRI is the strong magnetic field (Figure 9-53). One cannot use anything made of ferromagnetic metal in or around the magnet. The magnetic field will rapidly and forcefully pull these objects into the magnet, potentially injuring anyone in its path. Such objects include the gas anesthesia machine, oxygen tank, intravenous poles, clipboards, ink pens, leashes, collars, and beepers. There are nonmagnetic products available for use during MRI, but they are generally prohibitively expensive for most veterinary hospitals. The exception is an aluminum oxygen tank. Because of this limitation, anesthesia is generally performed with injectable drugs and heavy tranquilization. Patients must be absolutely still for MRI; any motion will severely degrade the image, so they must be under fairly deep injectable anesthesia. This is sometimes complicated because it is often difficult to carefully monitor the animals during the examination because of the narrow tubular shape of some magnets and the inability to use mechanized monitoring devices. Patients that cannot tolerate deep injectable general anesthesia with minimal monitoring are not good candidates for out-of-clinic MRI. MRI examinations generally take 45 to 60 minutes to perform and are done with and without intravenous contrast, similar to CT examinations, but with a paramagnetic contrast agent (usually gadolinium pentetic acid). Organic iodide contrast will not work for MRI examinations.

In addition to the anesthesia and monitoring difficulties created by the high magnetic field, personal safety is a concern, and precautions must be taken. It is important to remember that even though no images are being produced and the MRI technician is not at the controls, the magnet is still on at full power at all times. Credit cards and watches may be permanently damaged if carried too close to the high

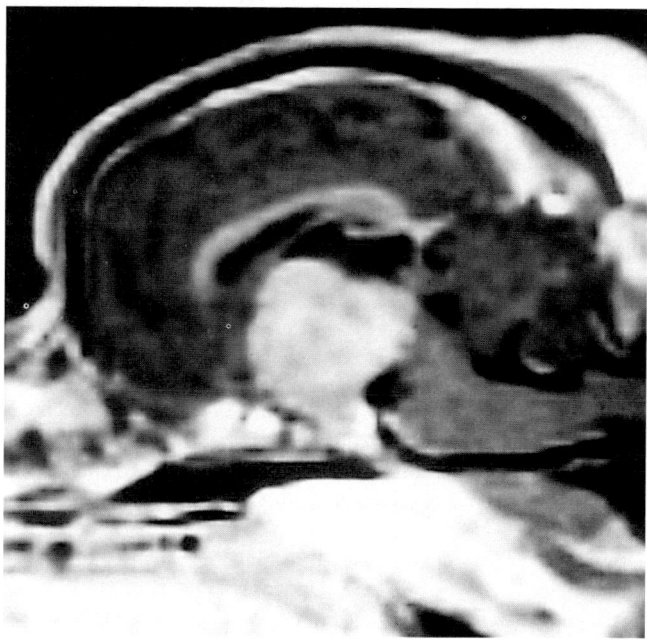

Figure 9-51 Sagittal T1 postgadolinium contrast magnetic resonance image of a dog with a large enhancing pituitary macroadenoma.

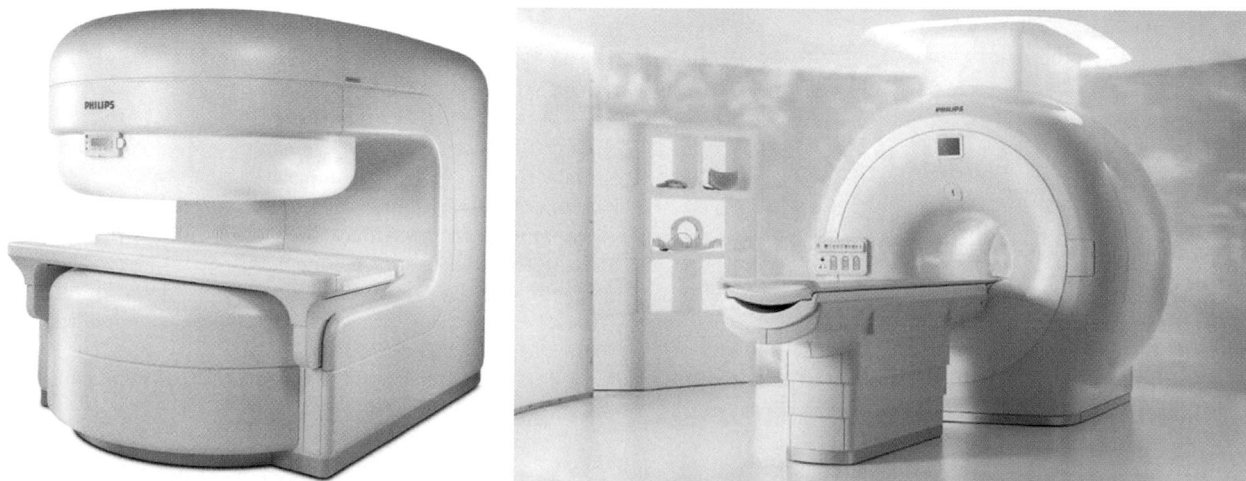

A   B

Figure 9-52 **A,** An open or low field strength magnetic resonance imaging (MRI) scanner. These machines make it easier to position and monitor the patient but may require longer scan times. **B,** Superconductive or high field strength MRI scanner. The circular closed MRI gantry can make patient positioning difficult.

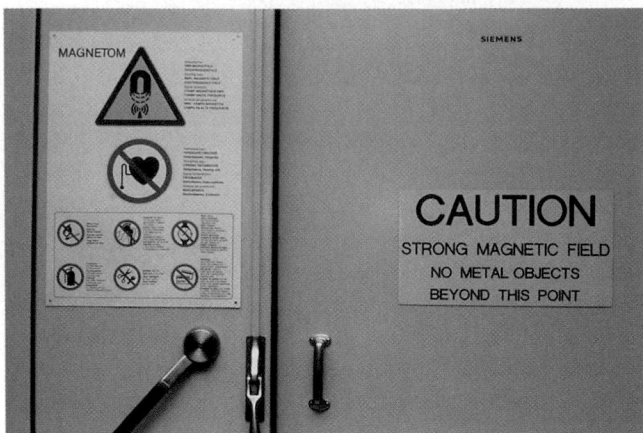

Figure 9-53 Warning signs positioned at the entrance to a magnetic resonance imaging (MRI) scanner. The technician must realize that the MRI magnet is always turned on and the high magnetic field may extend beyond the scanner room door. Never bring anything metallic into the MRI suite.

magnetic field. Any device that delivers a radiofrequency signal cannot be close to an MRI unit; these include but are not limited to televisions, radios, and pager transmitters. In addition, technicians with cardiac pacemakers, aneurysm or intracranial hemoclips, neural stimulators, metallic fragments within the orbits, or hearing aids should not be in charge of patient care during an MRI. If you ever have any questions regarding what can and cannot be brought into the MRI room, ask the MRI technician in charge before entering.

> **✎ TECHNICIAN NOTE**
>
> The high magnetic field in an MRI unit is always on. It is never safe to bring anything made of a ferromagnetic metal close to the machine.

TELERADIOLOGY, PICTURE ARCHIVAL COMPUTING SYSTEMS AND RADIOLOGY INFORMATION SYSTEM

As a consequence of the explosion in information technology, several new systems are becoming available for veterinary imaging. Teleradiology allows the transmission of digital data across phone, cable, T1, and ISDN lines from your clinic to referral centers around the world. Specialists can receive your images almost instantly, interpret them, and send back a written report very quickly. Now you do not have to package up all your films and send them via a mail carrier and wait several days for the answer. This has improved patient care and continuing education for the practitioner dramatically. Any digital data (MRI, CT, ultrasound, digital and computed radiology) can be sent directly, and analog data (regular radiographs and lab data) can be digitized or scanned into a computer and sent as well.

PACS units are "picture archival computing systems" and are used to move images around to several computer work stations within a single hospital or between hospitals and as a method of storing imaging data permanently. RIS systems are "radiology information systems" and are computer software programs that allow all the patient data to be available and coupled to the digital imaging data. These systems are fairly new and are just now being integrated into the veterinary marketplace.

Recommended Reading

Butler JA et al: *Clinical radiology of the horse*, ed 2, Oxford, England, 2000, Blackwell Scientific Publications.

Curry TS, Dowdey JE, Murry RC: *Christensen's introduction to the physics of diagnostic radiology*, ed 4, Philadelphia, 1990, Lea & Febiger.

Douglas SW, Herrtage ME, Williamson HD: *Principles of veterinary radiology*, ed 4, East Sussex, England, 1987, Bailliere Tindall.

Eastman Kodak Company: *The fundamentals of radiography*, ed 12, Rochester, NY, 1980, The Company.

Green RW: *Small animal ultrasound*, Philadelphia, 1996, Lippincott-Raven, ch 1-3.

Hall EJ: *Radiobiology for the radiologist*, ed 4, Philadelphia, 1993, Lippincott-Raven.

Han CM, Hurd CD, Kurklis L: *Practical guide to diagnostic imaging: radiology and ultrasonography*, ed 2, St Louis, 2000, Mosby.

Lavin LM: *Radiography in veterinary technology*, ed 3, Philadelphia, 2003, WB Saunders.

Morgan JR: *Techniques of veterinary radiography*, ed 5, Ames, 1993, Iowa State University Press.

Nyland TG, Mattoon JS: *Veterinary diagnostic ultrasound*, ed 2, Philadelphia, 2002, WB Saunders.

Rantanen NW, McKinnon AD: *Equine diagnostic ultrasonography*, Baltimore, 1998, Williams & Wilkins.

Stashak TS: *Adam's lameness in horses*, ed 5, Plymouth, United Kingdom, 2002, Plymbridge Distributors Ltd.

Thrall DE: *Textbook of veterinary diagnostic radiology*, ed 4, Philadelphia, 2002, WB Saunders.

Ticer JA: *Radiographic technique in veterinary practice*, ed 2, Philadelphia, 1984, WB Saunders.

10

Veterinary Oncology

Glenna E. Mauldin • G. Neal Mauldin

INTRODUCTION

Cancer is very common in both dogs and cats: it is estimated that 40% to 50% of animals older than 10 years will have potentially life-threatening malignant disease. The proportion of owners willing to pursue advanced diagnostics and treatment for these pets has grown significantly in recent years, so it is increasingly important that veterinarians and veterinary technicians have expertise in the practice of oncology. Some forms of cancer therapy, such as surgery or chemotherapy, can be performed easily in private practice with a minimum of specialized equipment. Other treatments, such as radiotherapy, necessitate referral to an institution that has the appropriate facilities. Regardless of the specific tumor and treatment being offered, however, oncology nurses and technicians play a central role in the treatment of companion animals diagnosed with cancer.

There are several reasons that the treatment of dogs and cats with cancer is worthwhile and should be encouraged. Important medical advances have been achieved by studying and treating tumors in pet animals, and participation in such clinical research programs can be extremely rewarding to both veterinarians and technicians. In addition, the strength and importance of the human-animal bond has gained wider recognition and acceptance, and providing effective cancer therapies helps to preserve this special relationship. Finally, many clients have had experience with cancer in their own lives and understandably feel fear and anxiety when their pet is diagnosed with a malignant disease. Veterinarians and technicians caring for dogs and cats with cancer must maintain a positive but realistic attitude toward the disease in general, recognizing and supporting the emotional needs of the client as well as providing quality medical care. Owners should never be made to feel that treating a pet with cancer is unreasonable or hopeless.

Box 10-1 gives the names and addresses of organizations for cancer information and treatment.

As part of the veterinary health care team, the veterinary technician plays a vital role in appropriate case management, quality patient care, and client support. The purpose of this chapter is to enhance the technician's knowledge of the basic principles of oncology. By understanding the unique diagnostic and therapeutic approach to neoplastic disease, the technician will become a more active and effective participant in the management of cancer in dogs and cats. ∎

TUMOR BIOLOGY

Oncology is the study of cancer. In general, cancer is defined as an uncontrolled growth of cells on or within the body. Virtually any type of normal cell may undergo the changes that eventually result in the development of cancer. Other terms that are commonly used to describe cancer include *tumor, mass, neoplasm,* and *growth.* Tumor growth can cause clinical signs in several ways: by destroying tissue and impairing normal organ function, by causing pain or inflammation, by predisposing the animal to infection, or by causing systemic symptoms that are indirectly associated with the cancer (called *paraneoplastic syndromes*). Paraneoplastic syndromes are characterized by symptoms that occur at systemic sites distant from the site of the primary tumor. These clinical signs are often caused by hormones or other substances synthesized by the tumor, which circulate systemically and affect multiple organ systems or tissues (Box 10-2).

Tumors can be either *benign* or *malignant.* The cells that make up benign tumors exhibit unchecked growth but do not destroy surrounding normal tissues. However, they can

---

Box 10-1 ORGANIZATIONS FOR CANCER
INFORMATION AND TREATMENT

VETERINARY
Veterinary Cancer Society
Barbara J. McGehee, Executive Director
P.O. Box 1763
Spring Valley, CA 91979-1763
Phone: 619-474-8929
Fax: 619-474-8947
http://www.vetcancersociety.org

HUMAN
American Cancer Society
National Home Office
1599 Clifton Road, NE
Atlanta, GA 30329
1-800-ACS-2345
http://www.cancer.org

National Cancer Institute
NCI Public Inquiries Office
Suite 3036A
6116 Executive Boulevard, MSC8322
Bethesda, MD 20892-8322
http://www3.cancer.gov/aboutnci/

Box 10-2 EXAMPLES OF PARANEOPLASTIC
SYNDROMES AND ASSOCIATED TUMORS

HYPOGLYCEMIA
Hepatocellular carcinoma
Insulinoma
Leiomyosarcoma

HYPERCALCEMIA
Lymphoma
Apocrine gland adenocarcinoma of the anal sac
Parathyroid tumors
Multiple myeloma

POLYCYTHEMIA
Renal carcinoma

DISSEMINATED INTRAVASCULAR COAGULATION
Hemangiosarcoma
Lymphoma
Thyroid carcinoma

ANEMIA
Multiple tumors

HYPERPROTEINEMIA
Multiple myeloma
Lymphoma

FEVER
Multiple tumors

Modified from Bergman PJ. In Withrow SJ, MacEwen EG, editors: *Small animal clinical oncology,* ed 3, Philadelphia, 2001, WB Saunders, p 36.

---

still impair tissue function and cause significant problems through their physical presence. For instance, even though most meningiomas (tumors of the meninges that surround the brain and spinal cord) are histologically benign, they can cause severe neurologic dysfunction and death if not identified and treated in a timely manner.

The cells in malignant tumors also exhibit uncontrolled growth, but unlike the cells of benign tumors, they are capable of local tissue destruction as well. They also have the potential for metastasis. *Metastasis* is the process by which cancer cells spread from a primary tumor to secondary locations, such as lungs, lymph nodes, and visceral sites (e.g., liver). The mechanisms of metastasis are not fully understood, but the metastatic process involves a series of basic steps that are similar regardless of the tumor type. First, cancer cells at the primary site proliferate and develop a blood supply. These cells then invade the blood vascular system and are transported to distant tissues. When they eventually reach the metastatic site, the cells arrest and leave the circulation (extravasation). A metastatic tumor is established when these cells are able to survive and grow in the new site.

In addition to being classified as benign or malignant, tumors are categorized according to their tissue of origin and their histologic features (Table 10-1). Carcinomas, for example, arise from epithelial tissues including skin, mucous membranes, glandular structures, and organs such as the liver or kidneys. Carcinomas generally spread through both the lymphatic system and the bloodstream, so regional

lymph node and lung metastases are commonly seen. Sarcomas, on the other hand, arise from mesenchymal tissues such as cartilage, connective tissue, or bone. These tumors spread through the bloodstream, and less frequently, through lymphatics. Because of this, pulmonary metastases are relatively more common with sarcomas, and local lymph node involvement is rarer.

The prefix of a tumor's name indicates the specific tissue of origin. For example, an osteosarcoma is a sarcoma originating from bone. The suffix of the name generally indicates whether the tumor is benign or malignant, with "-oma" designating a benign tumor (e.g., fibroma) and "-sarcoma" designating a malignant tumor (e.g., fibrosarcoma). Exceptions to this rule include *melanoma, insulinoma,* and *thymoma,* all of which are malignant tumors. More than 100 histologic types of cancer exist, and each requires individualized treatment and carries a different prognosis. It is also important to realize that the incidence and behavior of cancer in dogs is often quite different from its incidence and behavior in cats, even though the tumor names and histologic types may be the same.

Table 10-1 CLASSIFICATION OF TUMORS IN ANIMALS

Tissue Type	Benign	Malignant
CONNECTIVE TISSUE		
Bone	Osteoma	Osteosarcoma
Cartilage	Chondroma	Chondrosarcoma
Fibrous tissue	Fibroma	Fibrosarcoma
Fat	Lipoma	Liposarcoma
Smooth muscle	Leiomyoma	Leiomyosarcoma
Skeletal muscle	Rhabdomyoma	Rhabdomyosarcoma
Blood vessels	Hemangioma	Hemangiosarcoma
HEMOLYMPHATIC TISSUE		
		Lymphomas
		Multiple myeloma
EPITHELIAL TISSUE		
Skin	Papillomas	Squamous cell carcinoma
Sebaceous glands	Adenomas	Adenocarcinomas/carcinomas
Sweat glands	Adenomas	Adenocarcinomas/carcinomas
Ceruminal glands	Adenomas	Adenocarcinomas/carcinomas
Mammary glands	Adenomas	Adenocarcinomas/carcinomas
Nasal mucosa	Adenomas	Adenocarcinomas/carcinomas
Gastrointestinal mucosa	Adenomas	Adenocarcinomas/carcinomas
Biliary tract	Adenomas	Adenocarcinomas/carcinomas
Urinary tract	Adenomas	Adenocarcinomas/carcinomas

Modified from Powers BE. In Withrow SJ, MacEwen EG, editors: *Small animal clinical oncology,* ed 3, Philadelphia, 2001, WB Saunders.

> **TECHNICIAN NOTE**
>
> More than 100 histologic types of cancer exist, and each requires individualized treatment and carries a different prognosis.

Other methods used to classify tumors and help predict behavior and prognosis include the tumor's *grade* and *stage.* Tumors of the same histologic type are graded by the histopathologist according to defined microscopic features. For example, the cells in a low-grade soft tissue sarcoma have close to normal cellular architecture (well differentiated) and few mitotic figures (slow cell division) and exhibit minimal invasion of surrounding normal tissue. In contrast, the cells in a high-grade soft tissue sarcoma have very abnormal cellular architecture (undifferentiated) and numerous mitotic figures (rapid cell division) and exhibit aggressive invasion of surrounding normal structures. Well-established and reliable grading systems exist for some tumor types, such as canine mast cell tumors and soft tissue sarcomas.

Tumor staging is performed by the veterinarian according to physical characteristics of the tumor and results of diagnostic tests that assess the extent of malignant disease. The World Health Organization's staging system is known as the TNM system, and it categorizes tumors according to features of the tumor at the primary site (T), whether there is involvement of regional lymph nodes (N), and whether the tumor has metastasized to distant sites (M). Defined subclassifications, represented by numbers following the T, N, and M (e.g., $T_3N_1M_0$), describe the size and extent of the tumor in each of these locations. In addition, an animal's TNM system classification often includes assignment of a substage. Here, evidence of clinical signs of illness is usually designated "a" (denoting healthy) or "b" (denoting sick).

The exact cause of most cancers is not fully understood. Carcinogenesis is the process by which normal cells are transformed into cancer cells. In general, two events must take place before malignant transformation can occur: *initiation* and *promotion.* During the first event (initiation), the cell is exposed to a factor or factors that rapidly and irreversibly alter its DNA. Promotion, which follows initiation, is a prolonged process during which initiated cells are stimulated by an agent or agents to evolve into tumor cells. Under favorable conditions, a single transformed cell can proliferate and eventually develop into an invasive cancer. Factors with carcinogenic potential include inherited genetic defects, hormones, viruses, diet, immune system dysfunction, trauma, chronic inflammation, radiation, and a wide variety of chemicals. However, establishing a simple cause-and-effect relationship between a specific carcinogenic factor and subsequent tumor development in an exposed or affected individual is extremely difficult. Research must continue to focus on the underlying causes of cancer, with cancer prevention the being ultimate goal.

DIAGNOSTIC APPROACH IN THE DOG OR CAT WITH CANCER

The chances of long-term control of any cancer are much greater if the tumor is diagnosed early and treated appropriately. The most dangerous approach in any dog or cat with suspected cancer is to advise the owner to "just watch it." The American Veterinary Medical Association has published the following list of the early warning signs of cancer:

- Abnormal swellings that persist or continue to grow
- Sores that do not heal
- Weight loss
- Loss of appetite
- Bleeding or discharge from any body opening
- Offensive odor
- Difficulty eating or swallowing
- Hesitation to exercise or loss of stamina
- Persistent lameness or stiffness
- Difficulty breathing, urinating, or defecating

Although not every animal exhibiting these clinical signs has cancer, a geriatric animal with one or more of these symptoms should be carefully evaluated for the underlying presence of neoplasia. A systematic and logical approach, such as the one described in the following section, is necessary to accurately diagnose neoplastic disease.

HISTORY, PHYSICAL EXAMINATION, AND MINIMUM BASELINE DATA

The first steps in evaluating a dog or cat with suspected cancer are to obtain an accurate history from the client and to perform a thorough physical examination. Great care must be taken in gathering this information: there is no diagnostic test that can match the valuable data gained from these two sources. The history should include the owner's perception of the primary problem, the observed clinical signs, the duration of those signs, any treatments administered, and the response to those treatments. Concurrent or past medical problems should be characterized in detail. Owners should also be questioned regarding routine health maintenance, including vaccinations, parasite control, and diet.

Knowledge of the signalment (age, breed, and sex) of an animal may assist in the diagnosis of some cancers, because certain tumors occur more frequently in a particular species, breed, sex, or age-group. Most companion animals that have cancer are middle aged to geriatric; the average age at the time of diagnosis is 6 to 15 years. However, the age of the animal should never be used as an excuse not to pursue aggressive treatment. The animal's physiologic age, as determined by careful evaluation of cardiovascular, renal, and hepatic function, is more important for predicting treatment-associated risk than the chronologic age.

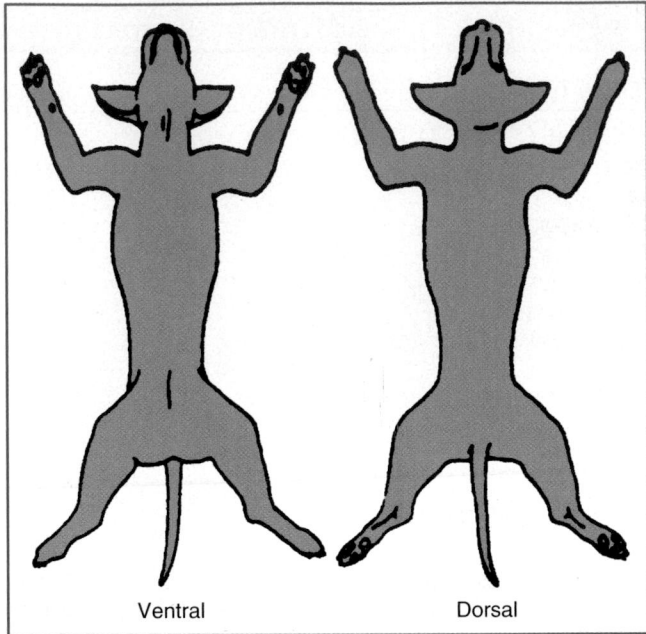

Ventral   Dorsal

Figure 10-1 Diagram for mapping the location of masses found during the physical examination. Masses of the skin and subcutaneous tissues are drawn on the diagram to scale, and it is placed in the animal's medical record for future reference.

After a complete history is taken, a detailed physical examination is performed (see Chapter 2). Each organ system should be carefully assessed, so that the primary problem as well as any concurrent conditions are identified and evaluated. Evidence of local tumor invasion, spread to draining lymph nodes, or distant metastases are all important in defining the stage or extent of the animal's cancer. Lymph nodes, especially those close to the tumor, must be carefully palpated for enlargement. Any skin or subcutaneous masses detected on the animal's body should be measured, and their location should be recorded in the medical record. Diagrams of the animal on which the location of any masses can actually be drawn are particularly useful in this regard (Figure 10-1).

Minimum baseline data are gathered next. These data generally consist of a complete blood count, serum chemistry diagnostic profile, urinalysis, and thoracic radiographs. The complete blood count is used to assess abnormalities in the red blood cells, white blood cells, and platelets. The biochemical profile should be evaluated for problems involving electrolytes, liver enzymes, creatinine, blood urea nitrogen, and serum protein concentrations. The urinalysis permits further assessment of renal function. Urine for urinalysis should be obtained by cystocentesis whenever possible: voided samples are often contaminated by debris washed out of the urethra, making microscopic evaluation of the urine sediment unreliable. However, cystocentesis is contraindicated in animals with bleeding disorders, as well as those suspected of having bladder cancer. Transitional cell carcinoma is by far the most common form of bladder cancer in the dog, and cells exfoliating from this tumor during cystocentesis will readily transplant into normal abdominal tissues. Finally, it is important to collect urine samples before any treatments are administered; urine specific gravity may be falsely lowered by fluid therapy.

All blood samples from dogs and cats with cancer should be obtained through venipuncture of the jugular vein if possible. Peripheral veins should be spared in the event that repeated catheterization for anesthesia or chemotherapy administration is indicated. Lack of venous access can be a frustrating problem in a dog or cat requiring multiple intravenous chemotherapy treatments. Some chemotherapy agents, such as the drug doxorubicin, can cause severe tissue damage if even a small amount is administered outside the vein. For this reason, an intravenous catheter must be placed whenever chemotherapy is administered.

RADIOGRAPHY

Radiography plays an important role in the diagnosis and staging of cancer (see Chapter 9). Radiographs of the chest, abdomen, and other anatomic structures are ordered on the basis of the tumor type and physical examination findings. The lungs are a common site for the development of metastases from certain malignant tumors. Chest radiographs should be obtained when the animal is in right lateral *and* left lateral recumbency, as well as in a ventrodorsal or dorsoventral position, to accurately evaluate all lung fields for metastatic nodules. Views in two planes are obviously necessary for all radiographic examinations, so that any lesions present can be localized. The additional lateral view of the chest in this case improves the ability to visualize both lung fields by allowing the "up" lung to be expanded and filled with air, thereby enhancing the radiographic appearance of nodules that may be present (Figure 10-2).

Imaging techniques other than radiography are now commonly used to assist in the clinical evaluation of dogs and cats with cancer. Ultrasonography, for example, is a noninvasive method that may be used to examine the architecture of specific organs or masses found in the thoracic cavity or abdomen. Computed tomography scans, magnetic resonance imaging, and nuclear medicine scans are noninvasive imaging techniques that are now available at many universities and some private referral hospitals. Each technique provides a different method for assessing virtually any area of the body. Computed tomography scans and magnetic resonance imaging, in particular, play an increasingly important role in cancer staging and also in the formulation of treatment plans, especially when radiotherapy is indicated (Figure 10-3).

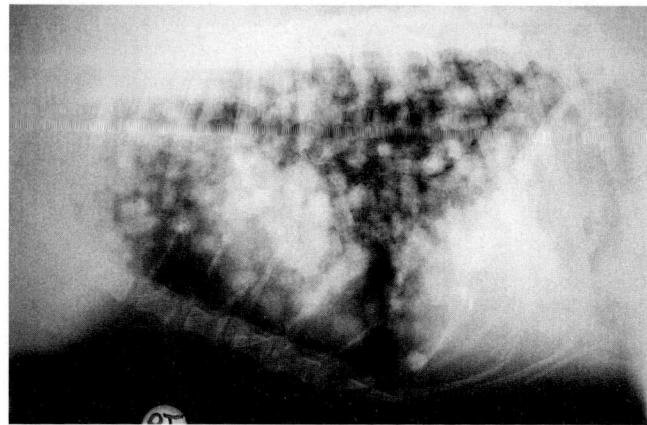

Figure 10-2   Chest radiograph showing numerous metastatic pulmonary nodules from a malignant mammary gland tumor in a dog.

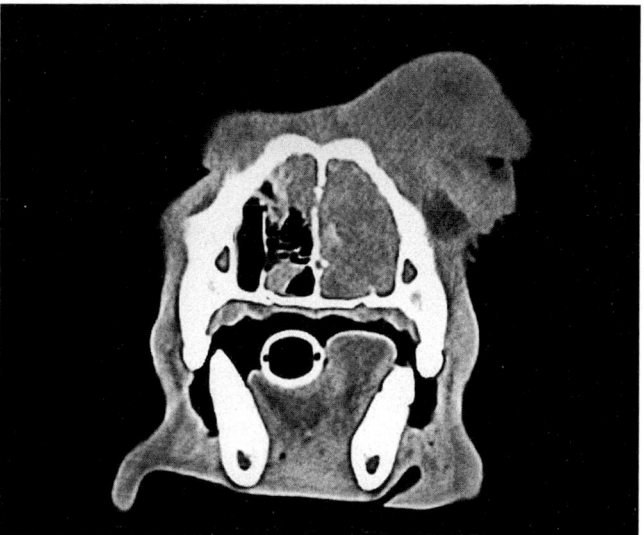

Figure 10-3   A cross-sectional computed tomographic image of a large nasal tumor in a dog. The tumor can be seen filling the nasal cavity and forming a large mass effect on the dorsolateral aspect of the animal's muzzle.

CYTOLOGY

Cytology is used to evaluate microscopic cell structure for the purpose of obtaining a clinical diagnosis (see Chapter 6). Although it is a practical and effective screening tool that is very valuable in differentiating neoplasia from inflammation or infection, it is not as reliable for establishing a definitive diagnosis of cancer as histopathology (see discussion of histopathology). Every skin or subcutaneous mass that is identified during the physical examination should be evaluated by either cytology or histopathology, and never simply by gross appearance.

Adherence to the proper techniques for collecting and preparing cytology samples is essential to obtain accurate results. Failure to collect sufficient cells or distortion of cellular architecture through poor handling techniques will make a reliable cytologic diagnosis impossible. Tumors that are easily diagnosed by cytologic examination are generally composed of cells that exfoliate or shed easily (e.g., mast cell tumors, many carcinomas). These loose cells can be placed onto glass slides with minimal distortion to their architecture and examined under a microscope. A positive cytologic report is highly suggestive of neoplasia and warrants further investigation (biopsy or surgical removal). A negative cytologic report must be interpreted with caution, because a false-negative finding is possible when sample acquisition or preparation was improperly performed. Samples for cytologic examination are easily gathered in many different ways: by fine-needle aspiration of the mass itself or accessible lymph nodes, by thoracocentesis or abdominocentesis, by impression smears of small biopsy samples or ulcerated lesions, or by needle biopsy of bone marrow. These procedures can be performed quickly with minimal discomfort to the animal. Except in the case of bone marrow aspiration, anesthesia or sedation is generally not necessary.

Fine-Needle Aspiration

Fine-needle aspiration is used to obtain samples for cytologic evaluation from cutaneous tissue masses and lymph nodes. Improvements in ultrasound and fluoroscopic instrumentation have also allowed fine-needle aspiration to be used safely for the collection of samples from structures within body cavities.

> **✎ TECHNICIAN NOTE**
>
> Fine-needle aspiration is used to obtain samples for cytologic evaluation from cutaneous tissue masses and lymph nodes.

A 6- or 12-ml syringe, a 22-gauge needle, and clean glass slides (preferably with frosted edges for labeling) are needed to perform a fine-needle aspiration of an external lesion. The lesion is stabilized between the clinician's fingers, and the needle is inserted into a representative area. The needle may be inserted with or without the syringe attached, and several core samples can be obtained by redirecting the needle several times without exiting the skin (Figure 10-4). Some clinicians use the attached syringe to aspirate while the needle is in place; others do not. Regardless, small portions of the needle contents are squirted onto a series of clean glass slides, and a second clean slide is used to smear the preparation.

Each slide should be labeled on the frosted edge with a graphite pencil before staining. The solvents used during the staining process will wash off most types of ink, including indelible ink. Identification of the slides should include the animal's name and identification number, as well as the specific location of the mass that was aspirated. The slides are air dried and sent to a qualified veterinary cytologist for evaluation, along with a complete and detailed description of pertinent clinical and historical information.

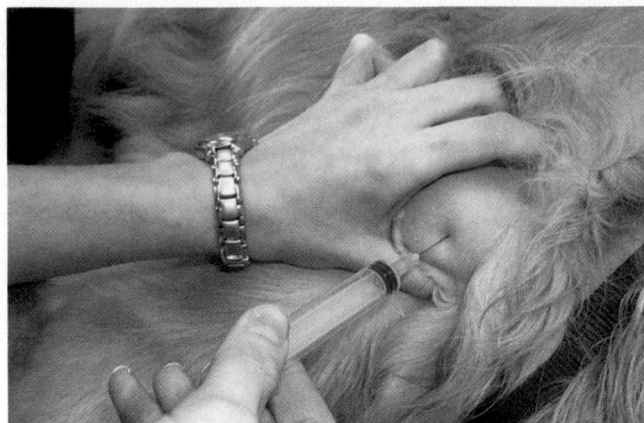

Figure 10-4 Fine-needle aspiration of an enlarged lymph node. A 22-gauge needle with a 6-ml syringe attached is inserted into the lymph node. The needle is redirected several times; concurrent suction on the syringe ensures a good sample of cells. Once aspiration is complete, suction is released, and the needle and syringe are withdrawn. The syringe is then detached from the needle, filled with air, and reattached to the hub of the needle. The needle contents are expelled onto clean glass slides and smeared for staining and microscopic examination.

> **✎ TECHNICIAN NOTE**
>
> Stain some of the prepared cytology slides for preliminary in-house review, saving the best and most representative slides for outside laboratory examination.

Stain some of the prepared cytology slides for preliminary in-house review, saving the best and most representative slides for outside laboratory examination. Slides that are evaluated in house must be fixed with an appropriate stain. The most common stains available include Wright's stain, new methylene blue, and Romanovsky stains such as Diff-Quik (American Scientific Products). It is important to realize that not all stains perform equally well under all circumstances. For instance, the characteristic granules diagnostic of mast cells may stain poorly or not at all when Diff-Quik stains are used.

Bone Marrow Aspiration

Evaluation of the cellular elements in bone marrow is sometimes indicated when abnormalities exist in the red cells, white cells, or platelets in the peripheral blood. Examination of bone marrow may also be performed to more accurately define the stage of certain tumors, such as lymphoma, multiple myeloma, and mast cell tumor. The most common technique used to collect a sample from the bone marrow is aspiration biopsy with a 16- or 18-gauge bone marrow needle (see Chapter 6). If this method fails to retrieve adequate cells, a core sample can be obtained with a Jamshidi bone marrow biopsy needle (American Pharmaseal Co.).

The preferred sites for biopsy of the bone marrow are the iliac crest, proximal humerus, and trochanteric fossa of

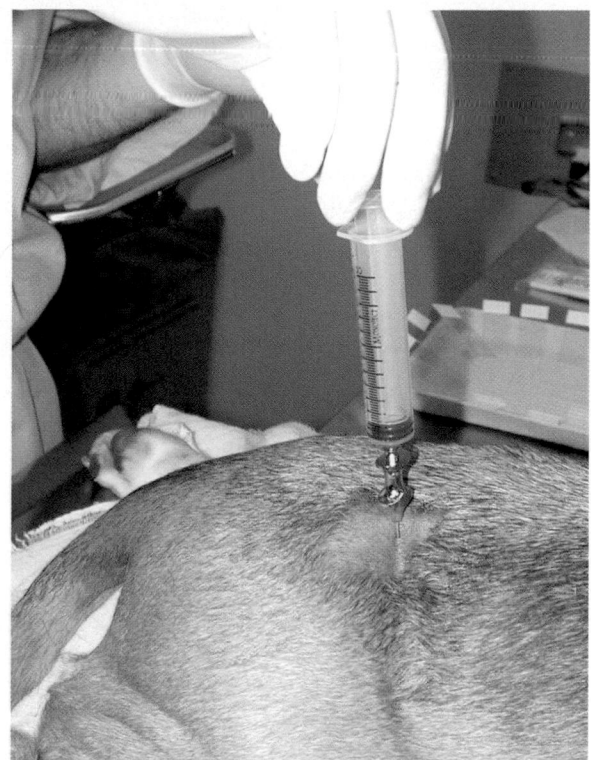
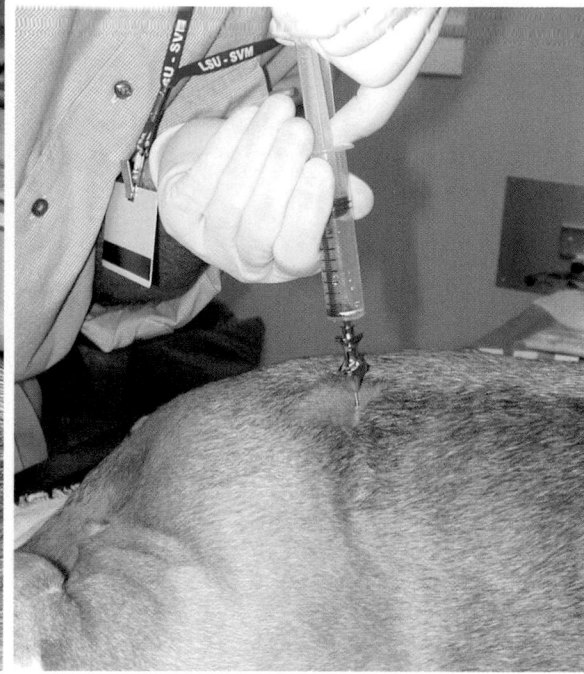

A   **B**

Figure 10-5 Bone marrow aspirate being obtained from the iliac crest of a Bassett hound. **A,** Bone marrow needle seated in the iliac crest. **B,** Suction being applied with a 6-ml syringe for retrieval of a sample of bone marrow.

the proximal femur (Figure 10-5). The most representative sample in a geriatric dog or cat will usually be obtained from a flat bone (iliac crest), because marrow in the long bones is replaced by fatty tissue as an animal ages. Some dogs will tolerate bone marrow aspiration after infiltration of the overlying skin with a small amount of local anesthetic alone; most cats require sedation.

HISTOPATHOLOGY

Obtaining a definitive histopathologic diagnosis is perhaps the single most important step in the overall diagnostic plan for the dog or cat with cancer. Histopathology determines what treatments should be considered and dictates the animal's prognosis, and these factors in turn influence the owner's decision about whether to treat. Every mass that is removed must be submitted for histopathologic examination, regardless of its location or gross appearance.

An advantage of histopathology over cytology is that the pathologist receives a larger sample that is less likely to be distorted by procurement and processing techniques. Individual tumors can exhibit significant cellular heterogeneity and may contain areas of necrosis, fibrosis, and inflammation, as well as neoplastic cells. Because of this variation in cellularity, entire masses or multiple sections of large tumors should be submitted for evaluation. All submitted tissue samples are then examined to determine

the cell type and tumor diagnosis, histologic grade, and surgical margins.

BIOPSY TECHNIQUES

Common methods used to obtain biopsy tissue include needle core biopsy, incisional biopsy, and excisional biopsy.

Needle Core Biopsy

Specialized needle biopsy instruments can be used to quickly and easily collect core samples of tissue through small (1- to 2-mm) skin incisions. The TruCut needle (Travenol Laboratories) is most commonly used for biopsy of cutaneous or subcutaneous masses; adaptations of this type of needle can be used for ultrasound- or fluoroscope-guided needle core biopsy of masses and organs within body cavities. These needles obtain a 1- to 1.5-cm sliver of tissue approximately the same diameter as a pencil lead.

When a needle core biopsy specimen must be obtained, the site is clipped and prepared for minor surgery. The mass is stabilized between the clinician's fingers, and a small incision (1 to 2 mm) is made in the skin with a scalpel. Infiltration of a local anesthetic into the incision site precludes the need for sedation or anesthesia in most cases. The needle is introduced, and a sample is obtained (Figure 10-6). The tissue sample is gently removed from the needle blade and placed in 10% buffered neutral formalin.

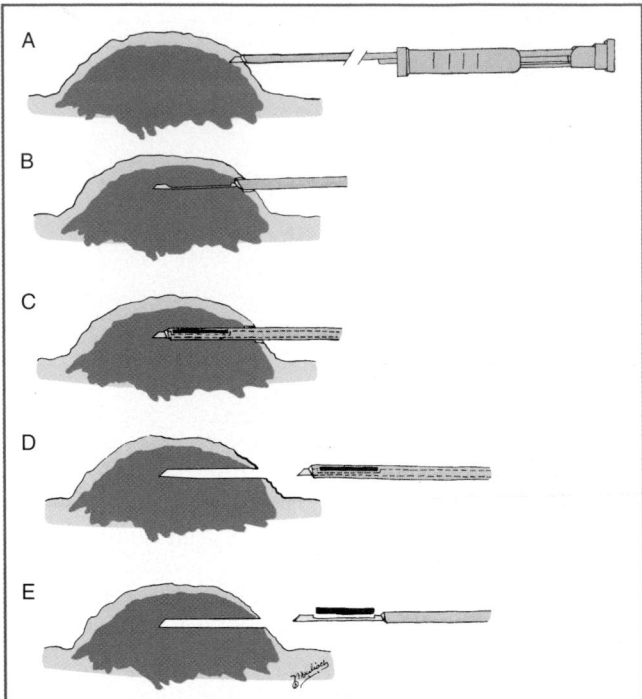

Figure 10-6 *Mechanism of action of TruCut biopsy needle used for typical nodular biopsy. A, With the instrument closed, the outer capsule is penetrated. A small skin incision is made with a No. 11 blade to allow insertion of the instrument. B, The outer cannula is fixed in place, and the inner cannula with specimen notch is thrust into the tumor. The tissue to be excised then protrudes into the notch. C, The inner cannula is now fixed, and the outer cannula is moved forward to cut off the biopsy specimen. D, The entire instrument is removed, with the tissue sample contained within. E, The inner cannula is pushed forward to expose the tissue in the specimen notch.*

Impression smears of this tissue can also be made by rolling the sample across a clean glass slide before placing it in formalin.

Incisional Biopsy

When an incisional biopsy specimen must be obtained, a small skin incision is made over the area to be evaluated and a wedge of the underlying tumor is removed. This technique is useful for obtaining more tissue than can reasonably be collected by needle core biopsy. Adequate biopsy size is especially important when cancer cells are intermixed with many necrotic or inflammatory elements, because these can complicate histopathologic evaluation.

Contamination of the biopsy tract with tumor cells is a potential complication when either the needle core or the incisional biopsy technique is used. For this reason, biopsy specimens should be obtained through small incisions and with minimal disruption of the surrounding tissue. In addition, the biopsy incision should be made with consideration of the eventual definitive surgery so that the biopsy tract can be removed with the tumor.

Excisional Biopsy

Excisional biopsy involves the complete removal of a mass for biopsy. Margins of normal tissue surrounding the tumor are included in the excision. Depending on the results of the histopathologic examination, this method of biopsy may be all that is required for both diagnosis and treatment. However, a second surgery or adjuvant therapy is indicated if the tissue margins are not free of cancer cells or if there is evidence that the tumor may have spread.

✎ TECHNICIAN NOTE
Excisional biopsy involves the complete removal of a mass for biopsy.

Biopsy Preparation

Once a biopsy specimen has been obtained, it should be handled gently so as not to distort the cellular architecture. In cases in which an excisional biopsy has been performed, evaluation of the surgical margins is extremely important for determining the success of surgical resection and assessing whether further treatment is indicated. The edges or surfaces of the resected tissue that need to be most carefully evaluated for presence of tumor should be marked so that the pathologist can easily identify them. While this is often accomplished with suture "tags," commercially available tissue "paints" are also extremely helpful in marking surgical margins. Paint will not distort the tissue and can be used to mark the entire margin. The paint will be present as a peripheral colored line when the tissue is examined under the microscope. If tumor cells are in contact with the paint-labeled margin, tumor cells probably remain within the animal and further surgery or other additional treatment is indicated.

After the margins have been marked, biopsy specimens should be placed in 10% buffered neutral formalin solution for fixation. The volume ratio of formalin to tissue for initial fixation is approximately 10:1. The tissue should be no thicker than 1 cm to allow effective penetration of the formalin. If it is thicker, it can be cut in the same manner as a loaf of bread to allow the formalin to penetrate. However, one edge should be left intact so that the pathologist understands the original orientation of the mass (Figure 10-7). Once the sample is fixed, it can be transferred to doubled or tripled plastic bags, or commercial mailers, with less formalin (1:1 ratio) for transportation to the laboratory.

A detailed information sheet should accompany the sample to the laboratory. Information that must be provided includes the clinic and veterinarian's name, the owner's name, the animal's name and signalment, the site of the biopsy, and a succinct clinical history including pertinent treatments and the suspected diagnosis. Any margins needing specific evaluation should be noted as well. For some tumors, such as mast cell tumors, a histologic grade may also be requested to help predict tumor behavior and prognosis.

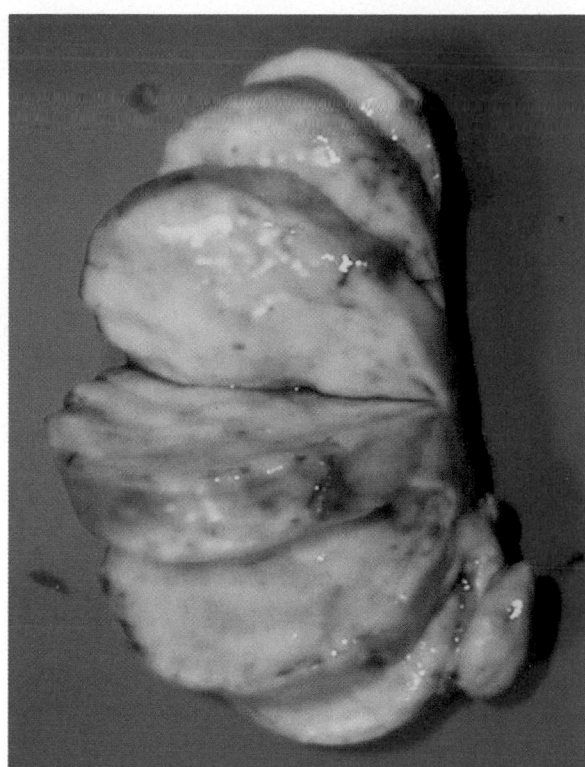

Figure 10-7 A large mass is sliced (loafed) into 1-cm sections. A 1-cm-thick base connecting all the slices is left to help orient the pathologist.

> ### 🖉 TECHNICIAN NOTE
> For proper fixation, allow a 10:1 fixative/tissue ratio and ensure that section samples are no thicker than 1 cm.

The pathologist is responsible for identifying the tumor type and providing information regarding completeness of surgical margins and histologic grade. However, the pathologist is limited by the quality of the sample submitted and the amount of information provided. It is ultimately the responsibility of the attending clinician to assess the compatibility of the pathologist's diagnosis with the animal's clinical presentation.

THERAPEUTIC OPTIONS

Once a definitive diagnosis has been made, the available therapeutic options can be identified. The clinician, technician, and client should discuss together the various choices with respect to the prognosis, benefits, potential complications, and cost. When speaking to the client, it is important to use simple terms that are easily understood. Information handouts are helpful to explain commonly performed procedures such as amputation, mastectomy, and the care and monitoring of incisions and bandages. Handouts can also be used to explain the nature, method of action, and expected side effects of common chemotherapy drugs as well as radiotherapy.

There are three primary treatment options for dogs and cats with cancer: surgery, chemotherapy, and radiotherapy. A single modality is recommended for some animals, whereas multimodality protocols combining more than one type of treatment are preferred for others.

SURGERY

Surgery is the treatment of choice for localized cancer in dogs and cats: it is practical and cost effective and will be curative in many cases. The primary limitations of surgery are its potential for damage to surrounding normal structures and its inability to address systemic spread of tumor. Animals whose tumors have metastasized generally undergo surgery as a diagnostic or palliative procedure only. Aggressive and complex resection and reconstruction surgeries should not be performed if long-term disease control is not possible; in such instances, surgery should be combined with other modalities (adjuvant therapy) if it is done at all. The oncologic surgeon must be familiar with all the potential therapy options to provide the best care for an individual animal.

Successful surgical resection of malignant cancer requires an aggressive approach. The tumor must be removed completely with a minimum of cosmetic and functional loss to the animal (Figure 10-8). A concerted attempt is made during resection to avoid incising the tumor and contaminating the surgical field with neoplastic cells: cells released in this manner may implant in the wound and result in local recurrence. Surgical resection should be performed in the normal tissues surrounding the mass so that a generous margin of normal tissue is removed together with the tumor.

Extensive surgical resections and prolonged surgery times may be necessary in animals that are severely debilitated from cancer or other concurrent diseases. These cases require careful perioperative planning and monitoring to avoid complications. It is the mutual responsibility of the clinician and technician to make sure that the animal has had a complete presurgical evaluation and that the surgical team is aware of any preexisting conditions. The anesthetic protocol must be tailored to the needs of the individual animal. It is best to perform major surgeries early in the day, so that the animal receives optimal monitoring from a full staff during the recovery period. Preparation for surgery should include clipping wide areas around surgical sites to accommodate extensive resections, should they be necessary. A thorough surgical scrub follows clipping. Perioperative antibiotics may be indicated if a prolonged operative period or potential contamination during surgery is anticipated. Intravenous fluids plus regional (epidural anesthesia or local anesthesia in regional nerves) or parenteral analgesic agents also provide for an improved recovery in most animals (see Chapters 19 and 20).

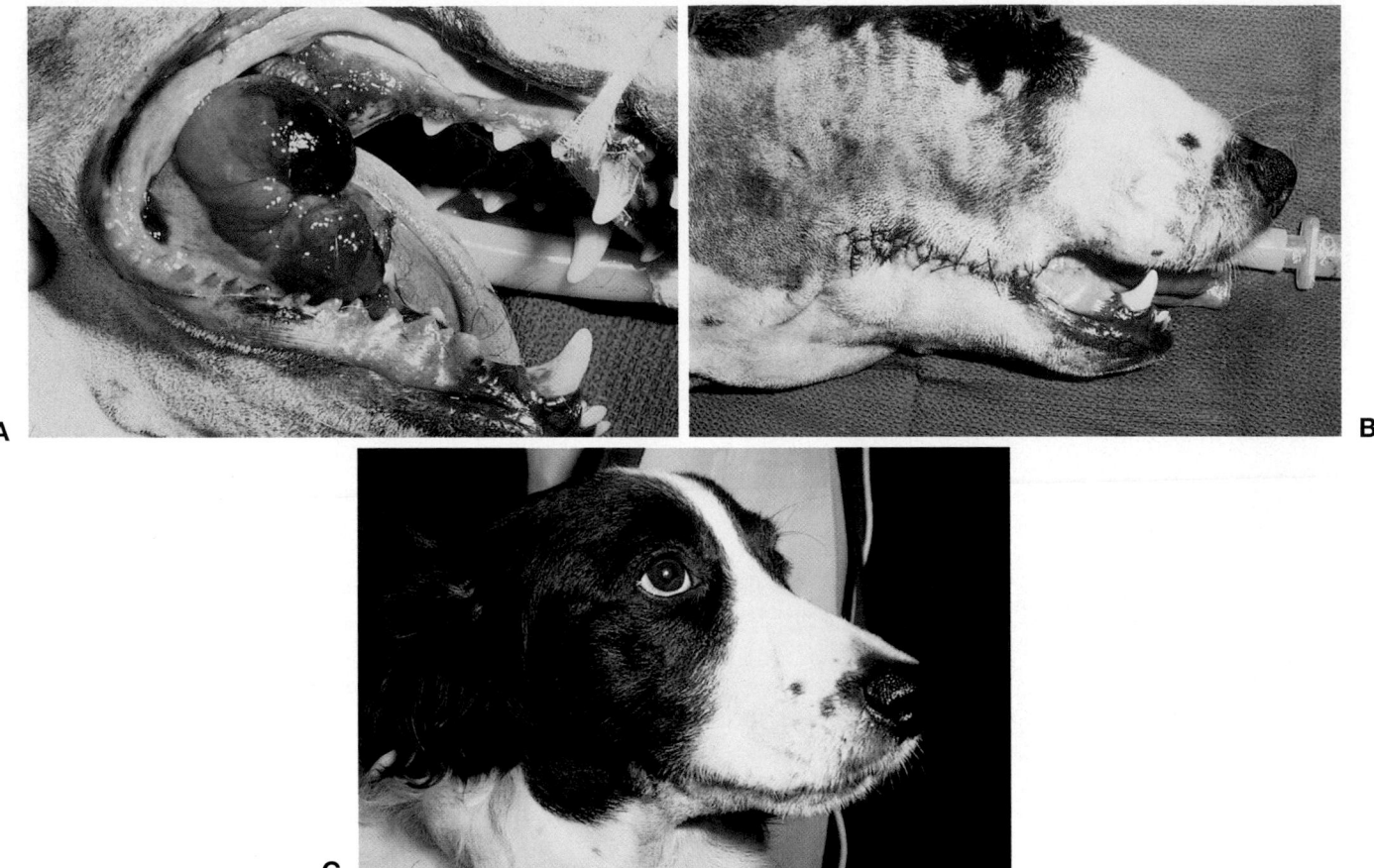

Figure 10-8 Surgical resection of an oral tumor in a dog. **A,** A large mandibular mass. **B,** Appearance of the surgical site immediately after tumor resection and reconstruction. **C,** The same animal after complete recovery and hair regrowth at the surgical site.

Another type of surgery used to treat cancer is cryosurgery. A cold source (usually liquid nitrogen) is used to freeze superficial cancers that are less than 2 cm in diameter. After freezing, the treated tissue dies and sloughs away, leaving a wound that later heals. There may be permanent discoloration or loss of hair associated with this process. Cryosurgery is useful for small, superficial lesions, such as eyelid, skin, and anal masses. A disadvantage of cryosurgery is that the completeness of tumor removal cannot be determined because there is no tissue to submit for margin evaluation. Cryosurgery should not be used to treat large, invasive masses or in cases in which a definitive histologic diagnosis has not yet been made.

The goal of surgery may be curative or palliative. The intent of curative surgery is complete and permanent removal of the animal's cancer. In the case of palliative surgery, the tumor is resected to improve the animal's short-term quality of life despite known tumor spread or an otherwise poor long-term prognosis. An example of this type of situation would be a dog with a painful primary bone tumor that has already metastasized. In this case, surgical resection of the mass (amputation) may improve the animal's quality of life but will not prolong survival, because the metastatic disease will continue to progress regardless of the surgical procedure.

> **TECHNICIAN NOTE**
>
> The intent of curative surgery is complete and permanent removal of the animal's cancer.

CHEMOTHERAPY

Chemotherapy is the treatment of cancer with chemical agents. Chemotherapy provides a means of delivering antitumor therapy to the whole body and is therefore most appropriate for animals who have systemic, as opposed to local, neoplastic disease. There are four primary indications for chemotherapy in dogs and cats. It is the most effective single treatment for some types of cancer, such as lymphoma (Figure 10-9) and transmissible venereal tumors. Chemotherapy is often recommended after surgical removal of malignant tumors to prevent the development of metastases and to inhibit local regrowth of tumor at the primary site. Canine osteosarcoma is routinely treated in this way (Figure 10-10). Certain chemotherapeutic agents, known as radiation sensitizers, are sometimes administered in

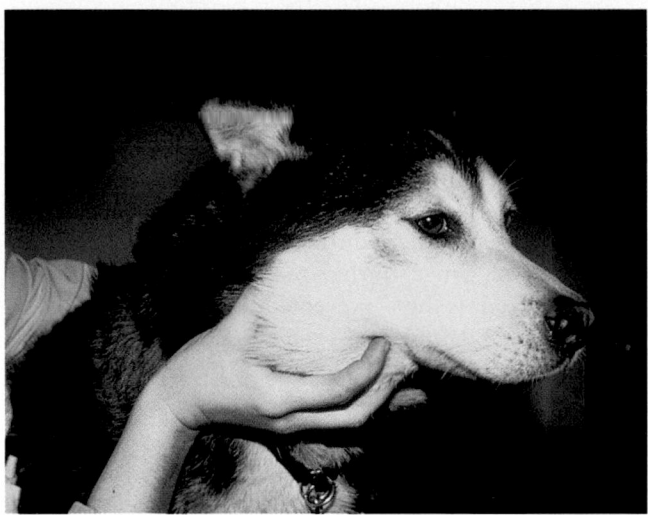

Figure 10-9 A dog with markedly enlarged lymph nodes caused by lymphoma.

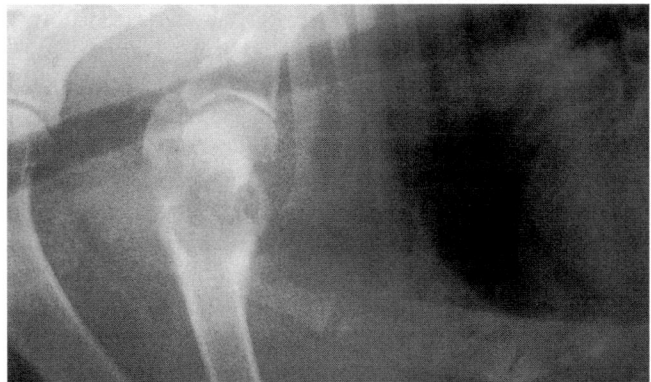

Figure 10-10 A lytic lesion caused by osteosarcoma in the proximal humerus of a dog.

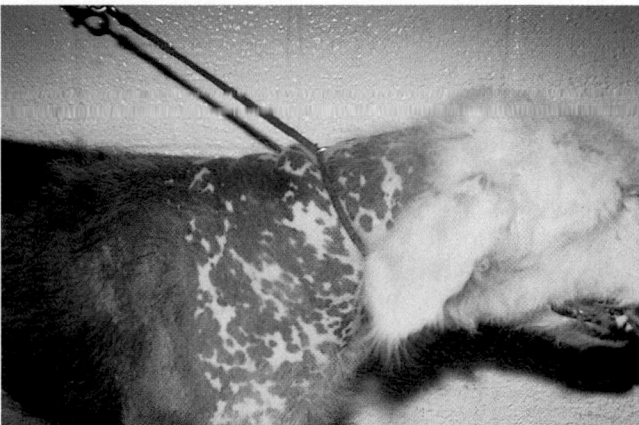

Figure 10-11 Hair loss caused by chemotherapy in an Old English Sheepdog.

conjunction with radiotherapy. These drugs increase the efficacy of radiotherapy. Cisplatin and doxorubicin are examples of radiation sensitizers. Finally, chemotherapy is occasionally used as a single modality for the treatment of cancers that are not amenable to surgical resection or radiotherapy or for tumors that have already metastasized. In most cases of this type, the goal of treatment is not to induce remission but rather to temporarily improve the animal's quality of life (palliate) by reducing pressure, bleeding, or pain.

Chemotherapeutic agents are categorized into groups based on their mechanism of action. However, regardless of category, most chemotherapeutic agents are cytotoxic and result in tumor cell death by injuring either the cell's DNA or its protective cellular membrane. Drugs that disrupt DNA typically target cells that proliferate rapidly, a characteristic of many neoplastic cells. Chemotherapeutic agents may also injure normal cells within the body that have high proliferation rates, such as the cells of the gastrointestinal tract, the bone marrow, and hair follicles. This is one of the basic mechanisms responsible for many of the toxicities classically

associated with chemotherapy: nausea, vomiting, diarrhea, bone marrow suppression, and hair loss (Figure 10-11).

The dose and timing of chemotherapy administration are predetermined to achieve maximum cancer cell destruction while minimizing the damage to normal cells and the resulting toxicities. Protocols that include a number of different drugs are preferred over single drug protocols, because they combine drugs that have complementary mechanisms of action and balanced toxicities. Chemotherapy drug dosages are generally based on the surface area of the body (meters squared) in the dog and on body weight in the cat. A meter-squared dosing chart that can be used in dogs and cats is included in Chapter 21.

In most cases, suppression of the bone marrow causing a decrease in the circulating neutrophil count is the toxicity that determines the highest dose of chemotherapeutic agent that will be tolerated by the animal. The interval between doses is determined in part by the time necessary for the bone marrow to recover from the previous treatment. The time at which the neutrophil count is at its lowest after the administration of a chemotherapy drug is known as the *nadir of leukopenia*. It is important to be familiar with the nadir of leukopenia for the different chemotherapeutic agents used in veterinary oncology and to understand that the greatest effect on an animal's bone marrow is likely to occur several days after the chemotherapy is administered. The nadir of leukopenia occurs approximately 7 to 14 days after drug administration for most chemotherapeutic agents, but for some drugs it is longer. Two critical questions to ask the owner of a systemically ill pet that is receiving chemotherapy are what drug was last administered and when that treatment was given.

TECHNICIAN NOTE

Suppression of the bone marrow causing a decrease in the circulating neutrophil count is the toxicity that determines the highest dose of chemotherapeutic agent that will be tolerated by the animal.

Chemotherapeutic agents have the potential to be teratogens (they may cause defects in a developing fetus), mutagens (they may cause injury to chromosomes), and carcinogens (they may cause DNA damage that ultimately leads to the development of a second cancer). The risks from long-term low-dose exposure are unknown, but no safe level of exposure has been identified. Since 1994, the U.S. Occupational Safety and Health Administration (OSHA) has required employers to protect their employees from occupational health hazards, such as handling chemotherapeutic agents. The veterinary community must recognize, promote, and institute policies and procedures that facilitate the safe mixing, handling, and administration of these drugs. In particular, women who are pregnant, may be pregnant, or are trying to become pregnant should not handle chemotherapy drugs, potentially contaminated materials (e.g., gloves, gowns, needles and syringes), or body wastes from treated animals under any circumstances (see Chapter 36).

All chemotherapy drugs should be clearly labeled and stored on shelves or in bins with front barriers that will prevent vials from accidentally rolling out. Chemotherapy drugs requiring refrigeration should be stored in a designated refrigerator in individually labeled Ziploc bags. All chemotherapeutics should be reconstituted in an isolated, draft-free section of the hospital where eating, drinking, and application of cosmetics are strictly forbidden. The work surface in this area should be covered with a plastic-backed absorbent liner that is replaced daily.

All hospital staff working with chemotherapeutics must be carefully protected from drug exposure. Inhalation of aerosolized drugs during reconstitution is especially dangerous and is best prevented by use of a biologic safety cabinet (Figure 10-12). This equipment is expensive and may be impractical in some practice situations, so commercially available venting devices (Figure 10-13) or high-efficiency respirator masks can also be used. Ordinary surgical masks do not prevent inhalation of aerosolized chemotherapy drugs. Cutaneous exposure during chemotherapy drug reconstitution and administration can be prevented by use of talc-free latex gloves, disposable low-permeability gowns, and protective eyewear or a face shield (Figure 10-14).

Reconstituted chemotherapy drugs should be transported to the treatment area in sealed and labeled Ziploc bags. The individual administering the drugs and the person restraining the animal being treated should always wear gloves, gowns, and face shields. Intravenous chemotherapy drugs are given through an aseptically placed butterfly or over-the-needle indwelling intravenous catheter (Figure 10-15). Routine use of Luer-Lok syringes further decreases the chance of inadvertent cutaneous or aerosol drug exposure during drug infusion. After the treatment has been administered, all potentially contaminated materials including Ziploc bags, syringes, catheters, gloves, gowns, and absorbent liners should be bagged separately and labeled for biohazard disposal according to appropriate local regulations. Contaminated sharps (i.e., needles) should also be placed in a specially designated container.

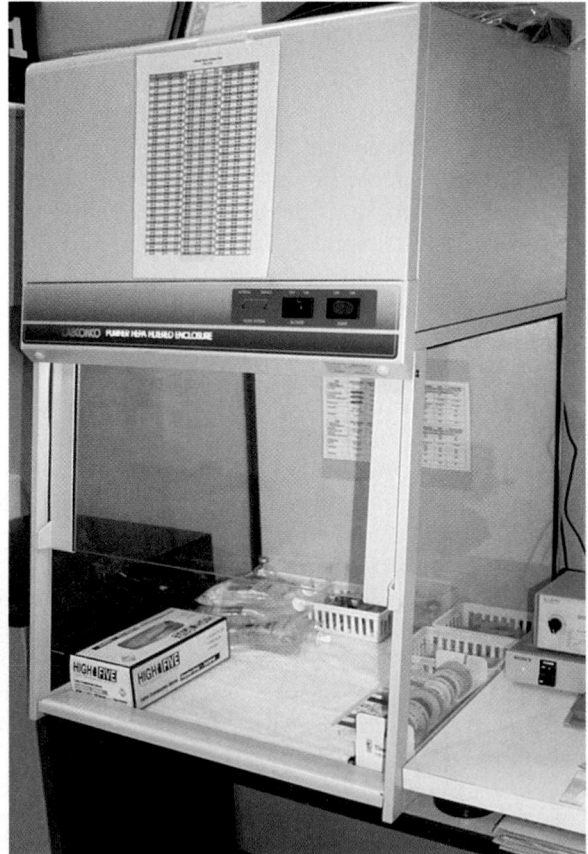

Figure 10-12 Biologic safety cabinet used to reconstitute chemotherapy drugs and prevent aerosol drug exposure.

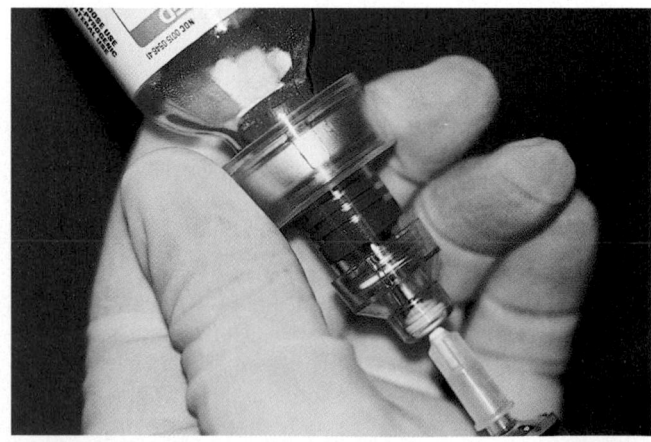

Figure 10-13 Venting device that prevents aerosolization of chemotherapy drug from the vial during reconstitution.

✐ TECHNICIAN NOTE

Protective gloves, mask, clothing, and eye shields, as well as appropriate and standardized drug-handling procedures, must be routine whenever chemotherapeutic agents are used.

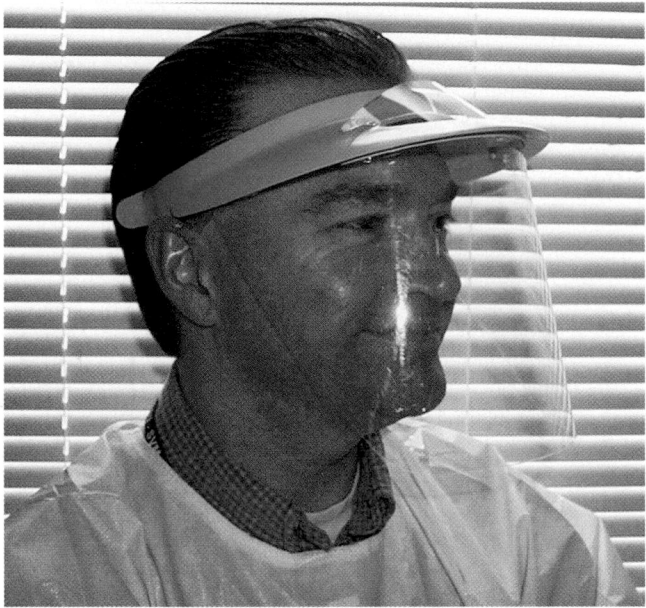

Figure 10-14 Face shield used during chemotherapy drug administration.

Chemotherapy drugs are excreted from the body in the urine or feces, and levels are usually highest in the first 72 hours after treatment. Hospital personnel and pet owners should take care to avoid exposure to excreted chemotherapeutics by wearing gloves when handling body wastes and soiled objects during this period. Dirty cages should be mopped with disposable sponges and never hosed, because water spray can aerosolize excreted drugs. Owners should be instructed to pick up and safely dispose of contaminated fecal material for the first 72 hours after treatment. In addition, during this time, dogs receiving chemotherapy should not be permitted to urinate in outdoor areas where children are likely to play.

There are many important nursing considerations with respect to the administration of chemotherapeutic drugs (Box 10-3). Toxicities such as myelosuppression (Box 10-4), extravasation (Table 10-2, Figure 10-16), and anaphylaxis (Box 10-5) are well documented. Additional potential toxicities include alopecia, gastrointestinal upset, sterile hemorrhagic cystitis, renal failure, cardiac toxicity, and neurotoxicity. Taking all necessary precautions to minimize risks to both the animal and the veterinary health care team is essential. There are many references that are useful in the development of appropriate hospital policies for the safe dosing, mixing, handling, and administration of chemotherapeutic agents (see Recommended Reading).

After each treatment, the animal should be monitored for signs of toxicity. Clients should be given detailed handouts describing known toxicities for each agent and the associated clinical signs. If the hospital staff or the client detects any

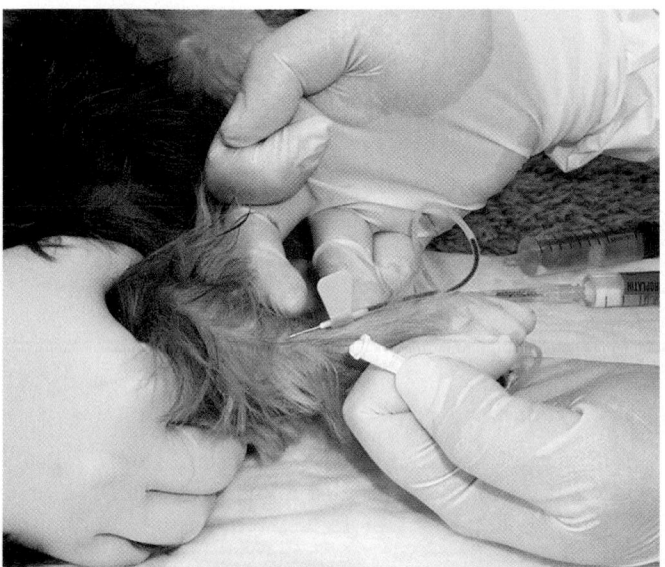
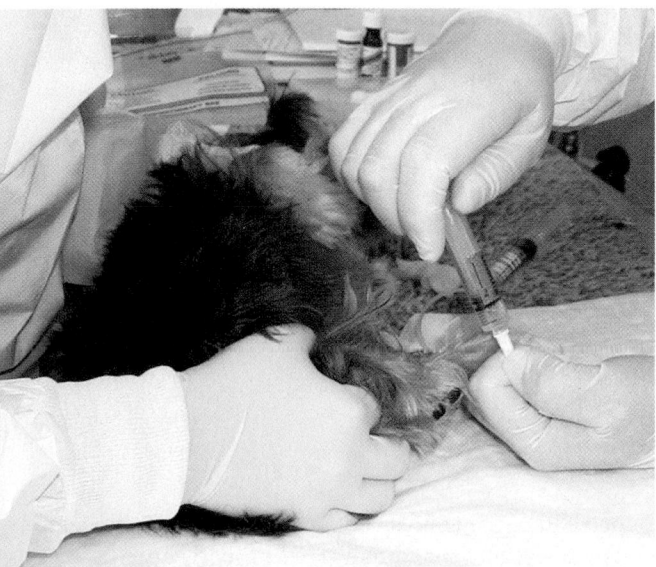

A   **B**

Figure 10-15 Administration of chemotherapy through a butterfly catheter. **A,** The catheter is placed in the lateral saphenous vein and checked for patency by using nonheparinized saline solution. **B,** The chemotherapy drug is given as a slow intravenous bolus through the catheter. The catheter is flushed thoroughly with nonheparinized saline solution after drug administration, before it is removed.

Box 10-3 Nursing Considerations for the Administration of Chemotherapy Drugs

CONCERNS BEFORE DRUG ADMINISTRATION

Admitting
1. Patient status
    a. History since last chemotherapy
    b. Physical examination
2. Appropriate diagnostics submitted
    a. Blood work
    b. Radiographs

Treatment Plan
1. Verification
    a. Drug and dosage
    b. Blood work
2. Appropriate catheterization
    a. Necessary equipment assembled
    b. Vein selection
    c. Aseptic technique
    d. Completely clean stick
    e. Intravenous challenge with saline bolus before and after drug administration
3. Appropriate protective equipment for person mixing and administering drugs
4. Appropriate protective equipment for person restraining animal
5. Knowledge of drug toxicities

6. Emergency protocols established
    a. Treatment of extravasation
    b. Treatment of anaphylaxis
    c. Treatment of chemical spill
7. Client informed of potential toxicities

CONCERNS DURING DRUG ADMINISTRATION
1. Extravasation of drug
2. Anaphylactic reaction
3. Patient comfort

CONCERNS AFTER DRUG ADMINISTRATION
1. Hematologic toxicity
2. Nonhematologic toxicity
3. Appropriate medications prescribed
    a. Chemotherapy drugs
    b. Antibiotics
    c. Other medications
4. Treatment documentation
    a. Patient medical record
    b. Future treatment plan
    c. Client information handouts

From Dickinson K: Unpublished data. Comparative Oncology Unit, Colorado State University Veterinary Teaching Hospital, May 1996.

Box 10-4 Myelosuppressive Chemotherapy Drugs Commonly Used in Veterinary Medicine

HIGHLY MYELOSUPPRESSIVE
Doxorubicin
Cyclophosphamide
Carboplatin

MODERATELY MYELOSUPPRESSIVE
Melphalan
Chlorambucil
Cisplatin

MILDLY MYELOSUPPRESSIVE
L-Asparaginase
Vincristine
Corticosteroids

Box 10-5 Chemotherapy Drugs With Potential to Cause Hypersensitivity or Anaphylaxis in Dogs and Cats

L-Asparaginase
Paclitaxel (Taxol)
Cisplatin
Anthracycline antibiotics (doxorubicin, daunorubicin, mitoxantrone)
Etoposide (VP16)
Bleomycin
Dacarbazine (DTIC)
Vinca alkaloids (vincristine, vinblastine)

---

abnormalities, the animal should be reevaluated. If chemotherapeutic agents are administered properly and the client is carefully educated regarding the potential risks, toxicity can be minimized and the animal should maintain an excellent quality of life during therapy.

RADIOTHERAPY

Ionizing radiation can also be used to treat cancer. Radiation causes cell death by disrupting the cell's DNA or by destroying important molecules required for normal cell function. Death occurs when the cell is so injured that it can no longer repair itself or divide. Radiotherapy is most appropriately prescribed for the treatment of localized cancers and will not address systemic disease. It can be used

Table 10-2	CHEMOTHERAPY DRUGS CLASSIFIED AS VESICANT OR IRRITANT AGENTS
Generic Name	**Brand or Other Name**
VESICANT*	
Dactinomycin	Actinomycin D
Doxorubicin	Adriamycin
Vinblastine	Valban
Vincristine	Oncovin
IRRITANT†	
Carmustine	BCNU
Cisplatin	Platinol
Dacarbazine	DTIC
Mitoxantrone	Novantrone

Modified from Brown KA, Esper P, Kelleher LO, et al: *Chemotherapy and biotherapy guidelines and recommendations for practice,* Pittsburgh, 2001, Oncology Nursing Society.
BCNU, 1,3-bis-(2-chloroethyl)-1-nitrosourea; *DTIC,* dimethyl triazenyl imidazole carboxamide.
*An agent causing tissue destruction or necrosis on extravasation.
†An agent causing pain and inflammation at injection site.

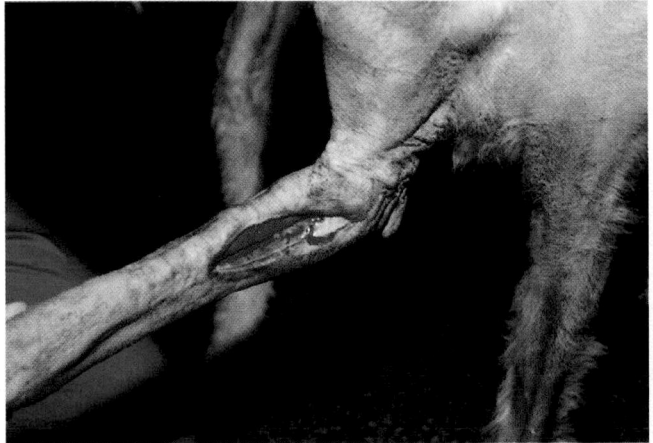

Figure 10-16 Tissue necrosis and sloughing caused by extravasation of a vesicant chemotherapy drug in a dog.

alone or in combination with surgery, chemotherapy, or hyperthermia. Most radiotherapy protocols involve the administration of multiple small doses (fractions) on a Monday, Wednesday, and Friday or a Monday through Friday schedule, usually for 15 to 21 fractions (Figure 10-17). Because radiation targets DNA, like chemotherapy, it is most effective against tumor cells with rapid rates of proliferation. Similarly, radiotherapy adverse effects are seen in normal tissues within the irradiated field that also have a high rate of cell turnover.

> ### ✏ TECHNICIAN NOTE
> Radiation causes cell death by disrupting the cell's DNA or by destroying important molecules required for normal cell function.

The potential adverse effects of radiation are divided into delayed and acute effects. Delayed side effects of radiotherapy develop months to years after treatment and usually involve permanent changes, such as necrosis or fibrosis of normal tissues. Acute effects are seen during the latter stages of a course of radiotherapy and, although they may require additional nursing care, are temporary. The most common acute effects of radiation occur because rapidly dividing normal cells in tissues such as the skin and mucosal linings have growth characteristics that are similar to those of cancer cells and are extremely sensitive to radiation (Figure 10-18). Therefore the damage to acutely responding normal tissues in the radiation field actually mimics damage to neoplastic tissue. For this reason, the acute toxicities of radiotherapy should never be permitted to limit the dose delivered: if radiotherapy is temporarily discontinued to provide time for the repair of acutely injured normal tissue, then tumor tissue will also be allowed to repair.

A frequent acute adverse effect of irradiation of oral or nasal tumors is mucositis of the oral cavity. Flushing the animal's oral cavity with prescription veterinary mouth washes can decrease the discomfort associated with this condition. Irradiation of skin may also induce a desquamative dermatitis or loss of the superficial layers of the epidermis. With regular cleaning and use of analgesics as needed, these conditions will resolve within 2 to 3 weeks. Oil-based or occlusive topical creams should be avoided, and self-trauma such as licking must be prevented. Elizabethan collars are especially useful, because they prevent self-trauma while still allowing access to the radiation field for topical treatments. Hair loss or change in color with the radiation field may be permanent, and the owner should be made aware of this possibility before the initiation of radiotherapy.

> ### ✏ TECHNICIAN NOTE
> The use of oil-based topical creams for the treatment of radiation-induced desquamative dermatitis should be avoided. Self-trauma must also be prevented when dealing with acute radiation dermatitis.

EUTHANASIA

Unfortunately, veterinary cancer therapy does not always result in a cure. In many cases, the most reasonable goal for both client and clinician is a long disease-free interval and improvement or preservation of quality of life. Euthanasia is an important component of pet cancer management. Euthanasia is the best option for some clients at the time of diagnosis; for others, this choice is made after therapy has

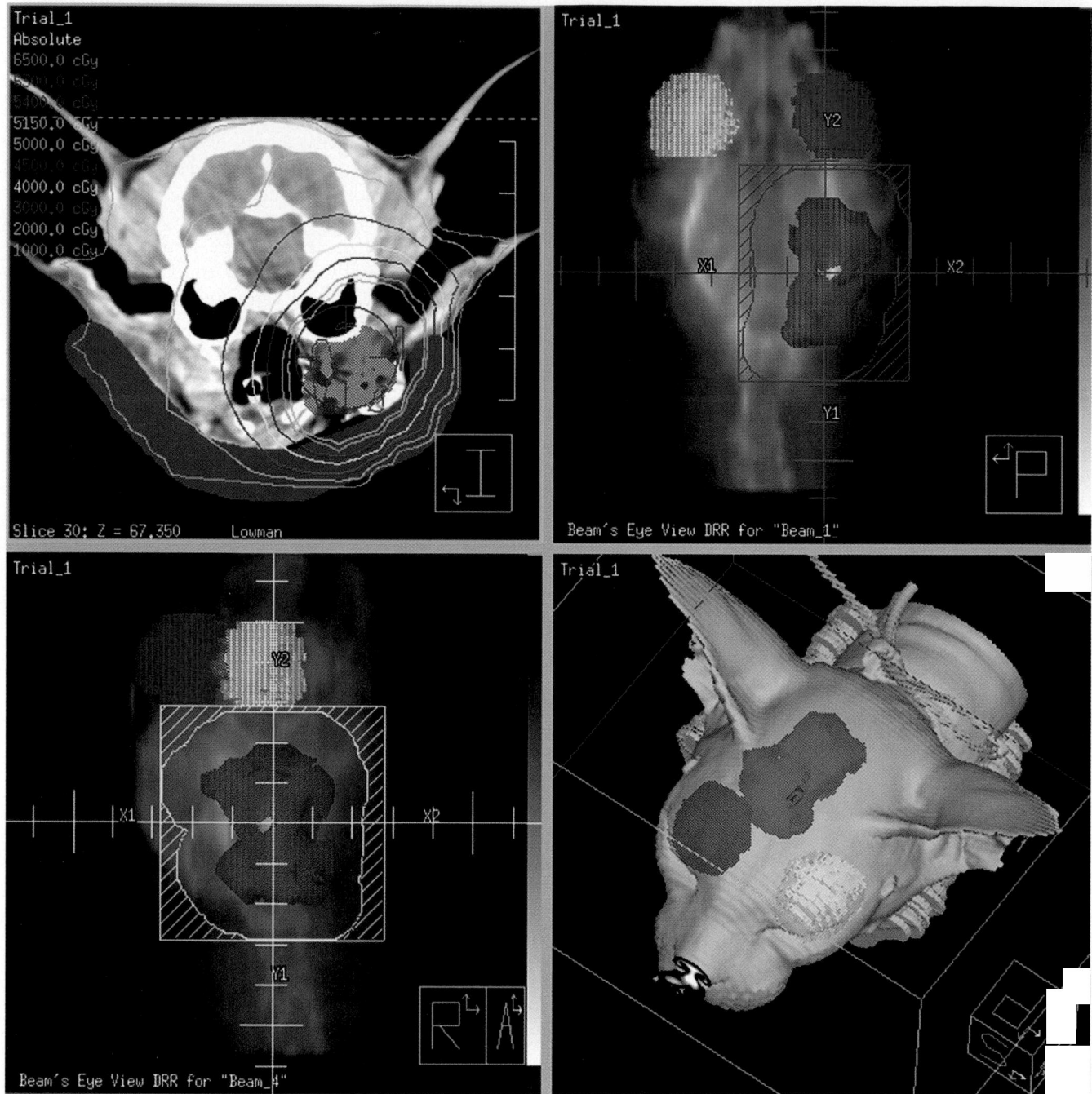

Figure 10-17 Example of a radiotherapy plan based on reconstruction of computed tomographic scan data. This treatment plan is for a salivary gland adenocarcinoma in a cat.

been instituted and has failed. In either situation, electing to euthanize a pet is an extremely difficult decision and one with which the client must be completely comfortable. Euthanasia should only be performed after careful consideration of all available options (see Chapter 37).

The veterinarian and technician must be prepared to provide medical information and expertise, as well as nonjudgmental emotional support and compassion to both the client and animal throughout the course of therapy. Much

of the emotional support comes from the technical staff. Clients may feel inhibited when talking to the veterinarian but can sometimes talk more freely with a nurse or receptionist. Technicians need to be aware of the important role they play in veterinary oncology, not only in providing treatment for the animal, but also in supporting the needs of the client. Good communication skills and compassion will be as important as the specific medical treatment provided to many dogs and cats with cancer (see Chapters 32 and 38).

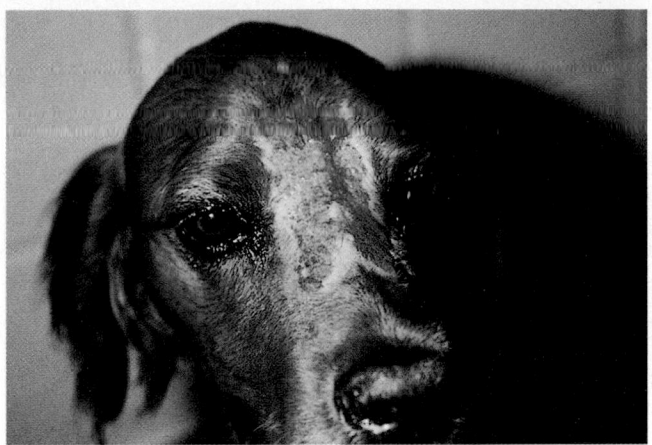

Figure 10-18 Moist desquamative dermatitis in a dog receiving radiotherapy for treatment of a nasal tumor.

Recommended Reading

Brown KA, Esper P, Kelleher LO, et al: *Chemotherapy and biotherapy guidelines and recommendations for practice,* Pittsburgh, 2001, Oncology Nursing Society.

Henry C: Chemotherapeutic agents. In Rosenthal RC, editor: *Veterinary oncology secrets,* Philadelphia, 2001, Hanley and Belfus.

Higginbotham ML: Safe handling of cytotoxic agents. In Rosenthal RC, editor: *Veterinary oncology secrets,* Philadelphia, 2001, Hanley and Belfus.

Kisseberth WC, MacEwen EG: Complications of cancer and its treatment: adverse effects. In Withrow SJ, MacEwen EG, editors: *Small animal clinical oncology,* ed 3, Philadelphia, 2001, WB Saunders.

Mauldin GN: Radiation oncology. In Rosenthal RC, editor: *Veterinary oncology secrets,* Philadelphia, 2001, Hanley and Belfus.

Morrison WB: *Cancer in dogs and cats: medical and surgical management,* Jackson, Wyo, 2002, Teton NewMedia.

Polovich M: *Safe handling of hazardous drugs,* Pittsburgh, 2003, Oncology Nursing Society.

Withrow SJ, MacEwen EG: *Small animal clinical oncology,* ed 3, Philadelphia, 2001, WB Saunders.

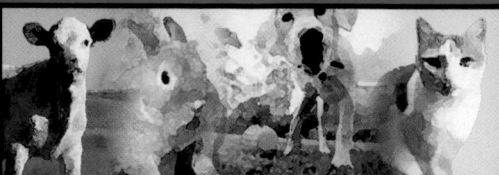

Preventive Health Programs

JOHNNY D. HOSKINS • SUSAN C. EADES • MARJORIE S. GILL

INTRODUCTION

In veterinary practice, preventive health programs are an integral part of providing for the general health needs of dogs, cats, horses, cattle, small ruminants, and swine. Regularly scheduled vaccinations alone do not represent a comprehensive preventive health program. Vaccinations are only one component of a preventive health program that attempts to meet the general health needs of an animal.

The time and effort invested in a preventive health program are rewarding not only to the animal but also to its owner or owners and those persons attending to the health needs of the animal. The veterinary technician can provide direct assistance to the consulting veterinarian by ensuring that the general goals of the preventive health program are met. ■

PREVENTIVE HEALTH PROGRAM FOR DOGS

For most dogs, a preventive health program usually begins when they are first presented to the veterinary hospital or clinic at 6 weeks of age. A general outline of one preventive health program and its implementation for dogs is presented in Box 11-1.

PHYSICAL EXAMINATION

Clinical evaluation of a dog initially focuses on taking a complete case history and performing the physical examination. Basic information about the animal, such as breed, age, and sex, as well as owner concerns or complaints, is essential to the case history (see Chapter 2). After the case history has been obtained, the physical examination should be conducted in a systematic manner. Body weight as part of the physical examination is recorded for several reasons. First, the weight provides information needed for dispensing medication; and second, it is an immediate indicator of the nutritional status of the animal. The body weight of a growing puppy steadily increasing at each office revisit is an indication that the puppy is receiving adequate nutrition (see Chapter 15).

VACCINATIONS

In the general, vaccinations for the prevention of canine distemper, canine parvovirus type 2 (CPV-2) disease, and rabies are the most important (Box 11-1). In addition to regularly scheduled canine distemper, CPV-2, and rabies vaccinations, other vaccinations can be incorporated into the preventive health program, as detailed in the following sections.

> ### ✎ TECHNICIAN NOTE
> In the general, vaccinations for the prevention of canine distemper, canine parvovirus type 2 disease, and rabies are the most important.

CANINE DISTEMPER VACCINE

Canine distemper (CD) is a viral disease of dogs and other carnivores; it has worldwide distribution. Since effective vaccines have become available, CD has been well controlled in domestic and zoo carnivores. Unvaccinated dogs and many feral species are susceptible to CD virus and can carry and spread the disease. The natural hosts include all animals in the Canidae family (e.g., dingo, fox, coyote, wolf, jackal), the Mustelidae family (e.g., ferret, mink, skunk, badger,

Box 11-1 OUTLINE OF A PEDIATRIC HEALTH CARE PROGRAM FOR A PUPPY

I. First office visit for health program is usually at 6 weeks of age
  A. Conduct a general physical examination and record the body weight
  B. Check for external parasites and dermatophytes and initiate appropriate therapy
    1. Fleas, ticks, and ear mites *(Otodectes cynotis)*
    2. Mange mites, especially *Demodex canis* and *Sarcoptes scabiei*
    3. Dermatophytes, particularly *Microsporum* species and *Trichophyton mentagrophytes*
  C. Conduct fecal examination, including both direct smear and flotation
  D. Initiate heartworm preventive management program
  E. Administer an anthelmintic such as pyrantel pamoate for hookworms and roundworms; if tapeworms are present, administer praziquantel or epsiprantel
  F. Vaccinate with DA$_2$PL-PC* and, possibly, with kennel cough vaccine,[†] *Giardia* vaccine, and canine Lyme borreliosis vaccine[‡]
  G. Advise owner on nutrition and routine grooming
  H. Provide the owner with client education pamphlets on topics such as the following:
    1. Identification, treatment, and control of fleas, ticks, and ear mites
    2. Benefits of preventive management for canine heartworm disease
    3. Management of normal and abnormal canine behaviors
    4. Skin, nail, and ear care
    5. "How to" on grooming and nutrition
  I. Fill in the puppy's health record for the owner
II. Second office visit for health program is usually at 9 weeks of age
  A. Conduct a general physical examination and record the body weight
  B. Check for external parasites and dermatophytes and initiate appropriate therapy
    1. Fleas, ticks, and ear mites *(O. cynotis)*
    2. Mange mites, especially *D. canis* and *S. scabiei*
    3. Dermatophytes, particularly *Microsporum* species and *T. mentagrophytes*
  C. Conduct fecal examination, including both direct smear and flotation
  D. Adjust dosage of heartworm preventive according to body weight
  E. Administer an anthelmintic such as pyrantel pamoate for hookworms and roundworms; if tapeworms are present, administer praziquantel or epsiprantel
  F. Vaccinate with DA$_2$PL-PC* and, possibly, with kennel cough vaccine,[†] *Giardia* vaccine, and canine Lyme borreliosis vaccine[‡]
  G. Adjust nutrition according to health needs, and if needed, change grooming procedures
  H. Provide owner with client education pamphlets on topics such as the following:
    1. Identification, treatment, and control of fleas, ticks, and ear mites
    2. Benefits of preventive management for canine heartworm disease

    3. Dental, skin, nail, and ear care
    4. "How to" on grooming and nutrition
    5. Management of normal and abnormal canine behaviors
    6. Exercise and its importance
  I. Fill in the puppy's health record for the owner
III. Third office visit for health program is usually at 12 weeks of age
  A. Conduct a general physical examination and record the body weight
  B. Check for external parasites and dermatophytes and initiate appropriate therapy
    1. Fleas, ticks, and ear mites *(O. cynotis)*
    2. Mange mites, especially *D. canis* and *S. scabiei*
    3. Dermatophytes, particularly *Microsporum* species and *T. mentagrophytes*
  C. Conduct fecal examination, including both direct smear and flotation
  D. Adjust dosage of heartworm preventive according to body weight
  E. Administer an anthelmintic such as pyrantel pamoate for hookworms and roundworms; if tapeworms are present, administer praziquantel or epsiprantel
  F. Vaccinate with DA$_2$PL-PC* and rabies vaccines and, possibly, with kennel cough vaccine,[†] *Giardia* vaccine, and canine Lyme borreliosis vaccine[‡]
  G. Adjust nutrition according to health needs, and if needed, change grooming procedures
  H. Provide owner with client education pamphlets on topics such as the following:
    1. Identification, treatment, and control of fleas, ticks, and ear mites
    2. Dental, skin, nail, and ear care
    3. "How to" on grooming and nutrition
    4. Management of normal and abnormal canine behaviors
    5. Recommendations for spaying and neutering
    6. Exercise and its importance
  I. Fill in the puppy's health record for the owner
IV. Subsequent visits for health program—usually annual visits
  A. Conduct a general physical examination and record the body weight
  B. Check for external parasites and dermatophytes and initiate appropriate therapy
    1. Fleas, ticks, and ear mites *(O. cynotis)*
    2. Mange mites, especially *D. canis* and *S. scabiei*
    3. Dermatophytes, particularly *Microsporum* species and *T. mentagrophytes*
  C. Conduct fecal flotation and occult heartworm examination, or all tests, for intestinal and heartworm infection screen
  D. Adjust dosage of heartworm preventive according to body weight
  E. Administer an anthelmintic according to fecal examination findings
  F. Vaccinate with DA$_2$PL-PC* and rabies and, possibly, with kennel cough vaccine,[†] *Giardia* vaccine, and canine Lyme borreliosis vaccine[‡]
  G. Adjust nutrition according to health needs and, if needed, change grooming procedures

---

Box 11-1 OUTLINE OF A PEDIATRIC HEALTH CARE PROGRAM FOR A PUPPY—CONT'D

H. Provide owner with client education pamphlets on topics such as the following:
   1. Identification, treatment, and control of fleas, ticks, and ear mites
   2. Dental, skin, nail, and ear care

   3. "How to" on grooming and nutrition
   4. Management of normal and abnormal canine behaviors
   5. Recommendations for spaying and neutering
   6. Exercise and its importance
I. Fill in the dog's health record for the owner

---

*This refers to the use of a vaccine to protect against the following: D—canine distemper; A₂ (canine adenovirus type 2)—infectious canine hepatitis; P—canine parainfluenza; L—leptospirosis; P—canine parvovirus type 2 disease; and C—canine coronavirus disease.

†This refers to the use of vaccine to protect against canine *Bordetella bronchiseptica*–induced disease. Puppies may be vaccinated with an intranasal vaccine as early as 2 to 4 weeks of age.

‡Lyme disease vaccine provides protection against canine Lyme disease. According to the manufacturer currently marketing canine *Borrelia burgdorferi* vaccine, puppies 12 weeks of age or older should receive two doses administered intramuscularly at 2- to 3-week intervals, and annual revaccination with a single dose is recommended.

marten, weasel, otter), and the Procyonidae family (e.g., raccoon, panda, kinkajou, coati).

CD virus spreads rapidly to epithelial cells and the central nervous system. Animals with CD have fever, depression, anorexia, ocular and nasal discharges, and signs related to disease of the respiratory and gastrointestinal tracts. The ocular and nasal discharges are initially serous and later become mucopurulent. Coughing is a frequent manifestation of the respiratory disease, and on physical examination, a mild breathing problem and increased lung sounds may be detected. Diarrhea and occasional vomiting reflect gastrointestinal tract involvement. The animal's condition almost invariably deteriorates from this point, and weight loss and dehydration develop. Eventually, animals become moribund and die with or without convulsions or other evidence of neurologic disease.

Vaccination is the preferred method of preventing CD. Active immunity can be induced in dogs with live-virus vaccines and heterotypic virus vaccines. Tissue culture–adapted live CD virus vaccines are highly effective if the recommended full doses are administered. The splitting of vaccine doses is never recommended. A heterotypic vaccine has been introduced to overcome the problem related to maternal CD antibody. Measles virus stimulates production of measles virus antibodies but not CD virus antibodies in dogs with low levels or without maternal CD antibodies. When dogs are vaccinated with measles virus and later challenged with virulent CD virus, the CD virus replicates. However, because of an anamnestic response, the CD virus does not spread to epithelial or neural tissues, and dogs recover rapidly. Because of the uncertain immune status of puppies between 6 and 12 weeks of age, a combined CD and measles virus vaccination can be used. If puppies have lost their maternal CD antibody, CD virus vaccine is preferred. If maternal CD antibody is still present, however, the measles virus vaccine will have some effect when CD virus vaccine would not.

CANINE PARVOVIRUS VACCINE

Canine parvovirus diseases are relatively new diseases in the general dog population. CPV-2 was initially described in the United States in 1978 and is the contagious enteric disease that most dog owners fear. Retrospective analyses of sera showed that CPV-2 did not exist in the general dog population before 1978. In 1967, a related parvovirus called canine parvovirus type 1 (CPV-1) (also referred to as minute virus of canines) was first isolated from the feces of military dogs. CPV-1 is not the same canine parvovirus as CPV-2. CPV-1 infection results in clinical disease only in puppies from birth to 42 days old. Affected puppies are usually presented with diarrhea, vomiting, dyspnea, and constant crying. Sudden death has also been observed. Lesions are restricted to the villi of the small intestine, lungs, and myocardium. The canine parvovirus vaccine used to protect dogs against CPV-2 does not protect puppies from CPV-1 infections.

Animals susceptible to CPV-2 enteritis may be of any breed, age, and sex, although young dogs are significantly more severely affected. Vomiting is often severe and is followed by diarrhea, anorexia, and rapid onset of dehydration. The feces appear yellow-gray and are streaked or darkened by blood. Elevated body temperature and leukopenia may be present, especially in severe cases. CPV-2 enteritis may progress rapidly, with shocklike death occurring as early as 2 days after the onset of illness. In severe cases, shock and disseminated intravascular coagulation are often responsible for the death of the animal. The recovery may be prolonged by secondary complicating factors such as the presence of bacteria, parasites, or other viruses.

Attenuated and killed CPV-2 vaccines are available, and they produce high, long-lasting levels of immunity while being safe when used alone or in combination with other canine vaccine components. All attenuated CPV-2 vaccines produce vaccine-virus shedding in the feces, but at a lower level compared with that in feces of dogs infected with and shedding virulent virus. Despite the shedding potential, the attenuated CPV-2 vaccines are safe for puppies and do not cause fetal infection; however, use in pregnant animals has not been recommended. Bitches should be vaccinated at least 1 month before conception to avoid any adverse effects that might occur. By vaccination of the bitch before conception, a high level of maternal immunity may be induced to help protect puppies from CPV-2 disease in utero or during the first weeks of life.

RABIES VACCINE

Rabies is acute infectious encephalitis characterized by altered behavior, aggressiveness, progressive paralysis, and in most species, by death. The rabies virus is usually present in the saliva of infected mammals, and in nature it is usually transmitted by a bite. Rabies most commonly affects the dog, cat, fox, skunk, raccoon, bobcat, coyote, bat, mongoose, and other small carnivorous mammals that are mainly responsible for the transmission of the disease.

Three phases of clinical signs are recognized in dog rabies: the prodromal, the excitative, and the paralytic. The term *furious rabies* refers to the syndrome in which the excitative phase is predominant; *dumb rabies* refers to those cases in which the excitative phase is extremely short or absent and the disease progresses quickly to the paralytic phase. The prodromal phase is often difficult to recognize. Changes in behavior and temperament may be seen. The animal may become restless, snap at imaginary objects, and vocalize at the slightest provocation. During this phase, there may be a slight rise in body temperature. Mydriasis, a sluggish corneal reflex, and some loss of appetite may be noticed. The prodromal stage usually lasts 2 or 3 days and sometimes only a few hours.

The excitative phase is usually not difficult to recognize when affected dogs become aggressive. It may last from 1 to 7 days, but it can be so short that it passes unrecognized and the typical aggression is never noticed. In the excitative phase, animals become increasingly restless and nervous. At the onset they may hide in dark places. Photophobia and hyperesthesia may become apparent. Chewing, biting, and swallowing unusual things such as sticks, straw, and stones are typical signs. Subsequently, the animal becomes more irritable and aggressive. During the excitative period, a dog may run as far as 20 miles per day and may attack any animal it encounters. Self-mutilation is very common. In most cases there is a characteristic change in the voice, caused by paralysis of the laryngeal musculature. Swallowing may become difficult, resulting in drooling. Convulsions and incoordination occur toward the end of this phase. If the animal does not die during a convulsion, it goes into the paralytic stage, becomes comatose, and dies. The total course may last as long as 10 days.

Paralytic rabies may be difficult to recognize. Paralysis of the pharynx and masseter muscles makes it impossible for the animal to eat or drink. After paralysis of the head and neck, the animal's entire body becomes paralyzed. Coma and death follow within 2 to 4 days of generalized paralysis. The animal with dumb rabies appears thin and dehydrated. The initial signs include drooling and slight protrusion of the tongue. The body temperature is usually normal or subnormal. After the animal has been unable to close its mouth for a while, its tongue and buccal mucosa may become red-brown and leathery. The animal's pupils may be dilated, or one or both pupils may be constricted. Strabismus may be unilateral or bilateral and either divergent or convergent. The congested third eyelid may protrude over much of the cornea. Poisoning is often suspected in rabid dogs, especially when they are found several days after their disappearance.

Inactivated rabies virus vaccines are currently licensed and available for preexposure vaccination of dogs against rabies. All rabies vaccines are administered in 1-ml doses intramuscularly at one site in the thigh or subcutaneously. The vaccines are licensed for immunization of dogs 3 months of age and older. Dogs vaccinated between 3 and 12 months of age should receive a second dose 1 year later. The vaccines are licensed for 1- to 3-year effective immune periods. Accidental exposure to licensed rabies vaccines for animals is not considered a hazard for humans.

✐ TECHNICIAN NOTE

Accidental exposure to licensed rabies vaccines for animals is not considered a hazard for humans.

CANINE ADENOVIRUSES VACCINE

Infectious canine hepatitis (ICH) is caused by one of the two recognized canine adenoviruses. The virus that causes systemic ICH is known as canine adenovirus type 1 (CAV-1). ICH is an uncommon disease in today's dog population. Certain strains of canine adenovirus have a strict affinity for the epithelial cells lining the respiratory tract and fail to produce infectious hepatitis in dogs. This strain of canine adenovirus infection is now known as canine adenovirus type 2 (CAV-2). Signs of CAV-2 infection include a fever that usually develops first and persists for 1 to 3 days after an incubation period of 5 to 6 days for susceptible dogs and a harsh, dry hacking cough of 6 to 7 days' duration, which may progress to a fatal pneumonia. Other signs include depression, anorexia, some difficulty in breathing, muscular trembling, and serous nasal discharge. In some dogs the nasal discharge becomes mucopurulent.

Products currently available for vaccination are attenuated virus strains of CAV-1 or CAV-2. Such vaccines have proved to be excellent immunizing agents, either alone or combined with attenuated canine distemper virus. The amount of virus required to immunize a puppy is the same as that required for an adult, regardless of breed, and all current vaccines are standardized for assured efficacy. Attenuated live virus (CAV-1) vaccines will occasionally cause immune-mediated corneal and iridal reactions 1 to 3 weeks after vaccination. The corneal edema disappears spontaneously and without sequelae if managed conservatively. Attenuated CAV-2 is now approved to replace CAV-1 in vaccines so postvaccination corneal opacity should no longer constitute a major problem. CAV-1 protects dogs against itself and against CAV-2, and CAV-2 protects dogs against itself and against CAV-1. Consequently, the currently available vaccines for ICH protect dogs against both types of canine adenoviruses.

INFECTIOUS TRACHEOBRONCHITIS VACCINE

Infectious tracheobronchitis (kennel cough) is a bacterial (*Bordetella bronchiseptica*) or viral (parainfluenza virus) respiratory disease in dogs that is characterized by spontaneously induced coughing, which usually appears suddenly after a dog has been recently boarded or exposed to another coughing dog. Kennel cough is extremely contagious. Vaccination can be an effective means of preventing or at least reducing the incidence of infectious tracheobronchitis in dogs of all ages. Intranasal vaccination, in particular, provides rapid, long-term immunity against *B. bronchiseptica* and parainfluenza virus infection and disease. Puppies can be vaccinated intranasally as early as 2 to 4 weeks of age without interference from maternal antibody, and the vaccine is safe for use in pregnant bitches during all trimesters. One dose is effective for a full year. Adult dogs can receive a one-dose intranasal vaccination at the same time as their puppies or at the time they receive their annual vaccinations. Puppies being prepared for shipment or entering a boarding kennel or veterinary hospital should be vaccinated at least 1 to 2 weeks before admission or shipping. Other infectious tracheobronchitis vaccines available include inactivated *B. bronchiseptica* parenteral vaccine. Parenteral vaccines are administered as two doses 2 to 4 weeks apart. When dogs have been vaccinated before the age of 4 months, they should be revaccinated after reaching the age of 4 months. Initial vaccination of puppies with parenteral vaccines is recommended at or about 6 to 8 weeks of age.

CANINE *LEPTOSPIROSIS* VACCINE

Canine leptospirosis had previously been characterized in natural infections into hepatonephric syndromes caused by two organisms: *Leptospira interrogans* serovars *canicola* and *icterohaemorrhagiae*. These serovars typically produced acute hemorrhagic diathesis, subacute icterus, and/or subacute uremia. Widespread use of a bivalent vaccine against *L. canicola* and *L. icterohaemorrhagiae* has led to a significant decreased incidence of leptospirosis in the general dog population. However, environmental and reservoir changes in canine leptospirosis have resulted in the introduction of other *Leptospira* organisms into the general dog population, such as *L. grippotyphosa*, *L. pomona*, *L. hardjo*, and *L. bratislava,* which have emerged as the most commonly identified serovars recognized in infected dogs. Currently, only one manufacturer has canine leptospirosis vaccine that contains the serovars *icterohaemorrhagiae*, *canicola*, *grippotyphosa*, and *pomona* in its product.

CANINE CORONAVIRUS VACCINE

Canine coronavirus (CCV) causes highly contagious viral enteritis and spreads rapidly through kennels of susceptible dogs. The primary source of infection is infectious fecal material. The incubation period is short, about 1 to 4 days. Dogs can have CCV and CPV-2 infections simultaneously. Other enteric microflora such as *Clostridium perfringens*, *Campylobacter* spp., and *Salmonella* spp. may increase the severity of the enteric illness. Animals are usually presented with a sudden onset of diarrhea and sometimes vomiting. The fecal material is characteristically orange in color, very malodorous, and infrequently contains blood. Loss of appetite and lethargy are also common signs. Fever is not constant, and leukopenia is not a recognized feature. CCV vaccines are available for protection against CCV infection.

CANINE *GIARDIA* VACCINE

Enteric infections with *Giardia* spp. are extremely common in dogs younger than 6 months and in immunocompromised dogs. Recurrent diarrhea is usually the primary presenting complaint. The *Giardia* vaccine acts at the intestinal level against both the trophozoite and cyst forms of the *Giardia* spp. When given twice, the *Giardia* vaccine lowers the number of organisms shed and decreases symptoms of clinical disease. The *Giardia* vaccine is most effective when dogs are frequently exposed to contaminated *Giardia*-laden water.

CANINE LYME BORRELIOSIS VACCINE

Canine Lyme borreliosis is caused by the pathogenic strains of *Borrelia burgdorferi*. The organism has been recovered from many different tissues of infected ticks, and simply crushing an infected tick between unprotected fingers has been reported to lead to human infection. *B. burgdorferi* infections in dogs cause fever, depression, anorexia, stiffness, and most important, joint pain and swelling. Joints frequently involved include the carpus, digits, shoulder, elbow, tarsus, and stifle joints. Many affected dogs will have multiple episodes of lameness with intervals between episodes of 1 to 23 months. Lymphadenopathy and renal disease have also been seen in dogs with Lyme borreliosis. Canine *B. burgdorferi* vaccine, available as killed bacteria and recombinant products, provides protection against canine Lyme borreliosis. According to the manufacturers currently marketing canine *B. burgdorferi* vaccines, puppies 9 to 12 weeks of age or older should receive two doses administered at 2- to 3-week intervals; with annual revaccination, a single dose is recommended.

Table 11-1 HEARTWORM PREVENTIVES

Trade Name	Drug(s)/Dosage	Application
Filarbits	Diethylcarbamazine 6.6 mg/kg	Oral/daily
Filarbits Plus	Diethylcarbamazine + oxibendazole 6.6 mg + 5 mg resp/kg	Oral/daily
Heartgard Tablets for dogs	Ivermectin 0.006 mg/kg	Oral/monthly
Heartgard Chewables for dogs	Ivermectin 0.006 mg/kg	Oral/monthly
Heartgard Plus Chewables for dogs	Ivermectin + pyrantel 0.006 mg + 5 mg resp/kg	Oral/monthly
Interceptor Flavor Tabs	Milbemycin 0.5 mg/kg	Oral/monthly
Iverhart Plus Flavored Chewables	Generic form of Heartgard Plus Chewables for dogs	Oral/monthly
ProHeart Tablets	Moxidectin 0.003 mg/kg	Oral/monthly
ProHeart 6	Moxidectin 0.17 mg/kg	Injectable/every 6 months
Revolution	Sclamectin 6 mg/kg	Topical/monthly
Sentinel Flavor Tabs	Milbemycin/lufenuron 0.5 mg + 10 mg resp/kg	Oral/monthly

Table 11-2 LABELED TIME OF EARLIEST ADMINISTRATION OF HEARTWORM PREVENTIVE TO PUPPY

Trade Name	Recommendation by Age
Interceptor Flavor Tabs	4 weeks or >2 lb
Sentinel Flavor Tabs	4 weeks or >2 lb
Heartgard Tablets for dogs	6 weeks
Heartgard Chewables for dogs	6 weeks
Heartgard Plus Chewables for dogs	6 weeks
Iverhart Plus Flavored Chewables	6 weeks
Revolution	6 weeks
ProHeart Tablets	8 weeks
Filarbits	8 weeks
Filarbits Plus	8 weeks
ProHeart 6	6 months

HEARTWORM PREVENTIVE THERAPY

Puppies can be started on a heartworm preventive program at 4 weeks of age and older (Tables 11-1 and 11-2).

OWNER EDUCATION

Owner education pamphlets on a variety of dog-related topics can be sent home with the owner each time the dog is seen for the preventive health program. Generally, only one or two well-written owner education pamphlets are given to the owner at the end of each office visit.

Veterinarians and veterinary technicians are in an excellent position to provide meaningful owner educational services and thus make owners more aware of their dogs and the associated responsibilities of dog ownership. By offering consultative advice and providing owners with educational pamphlets, the veterinary technician not only assists owners

who are seeking medical treatment for their dogs but serves a vital role in educating people in the community.

PREVENTIVE HEALTH PROGRAM FOR CATS

For most cats, a preventive health program usually begins when they are first presented to the veterinary hospital or clinic at 8 to 10 weeks of age. A general outline of one preventive health program and its implementation for cats is presented in Box 11-2.

PHYSICAL EXAMINATION

Clinical evaluation of a cat initially focuses on taking a complete case history and performing the physical examination (see Chapter 2). Basic information about the animal, such as breed, age, and sex, as well as owner concerns or complaints, is essential to the case history. After the case history has been obtained, the physical examination should be conducted in a systematic manner. Body weight as part of the physical examination is recorded for several reasons. First, the weight provides information needed for dispensing medication; and second, it is an immediate indicator of the nutritional status of the animal. The body weight of a growing kitten steadily increasing at each office revisit is an indication that the kitten is receiving adequate nutrition.

VACCINATIONS

In the general, vaccinations for the prevention of feline panleukopenia (FPL), feline viral rhinotracheitis (FVR), feline calicivirus (FCV) infection, and rabies are the most important (Box 11-2). In addition to regularly scheduled

Box 11-2 OUTLINE OF A PEDIATRIC HEALTH CARE PROGRAM FOR A KITTEN

I. First office visit for health program is usually at 8 to 10 weeks of age
   A. Perform a general physical examination and record the body weight
   B. Check for external parasites and dermatophytes and initiate appropriate therapy
      1. Fleas and ear mites (Otodectes cynotis)
      2. Mange mites, especially Notoedres cati, Demodex species, and Cheyletiella species
      3. Dermatophytes, particularly Microsporum species and Trichophyton mentagrophytes
   C. Perform fecal examination, including both direct smear and flotation
   D. Administer an anthelmintic such as pyrantel pamoate for roundworms and hookworms; if tapeworms are present, administer praziquantel or epsiprantel
   E. Vaccinate with FVRC-P,*† Chlamydophila,‡ feline leukemia virus,§ feline immunodeficiency virus, feline infectious peritonitis¶ Giardia, and Bordetella bronchiseptica vaccines
   F. Advise owner on nutrition and routine grooming
   G. Provide the owner with client education pamphlets on topics such as the following:
      1. Identification, treatment, and control of fleas, ticks, and ear mites
      2. Benefits of vaccination for feline leukemia virus infection
      3. Management of normal and abnormal feline behaviors
      4. Grooming "how to" and nutrition
   H. Fill in the kitten's health record for the owner
II. Second office visit for health program is usually at 12 to 14 weeks of age
   A. Perform a general physical examination and record the body weight
   B. Check for external parasites and dermatophytes and initiate appropriate therapy
      1. Fleas and ear mites (O. cynotis)
      2. Mange mites, especially N. cati, Demodex species, and Cheyletiella species
      3. Dermatophytes, particularly Microsporum species and T. mentagrophytes
   C. Perform fecal examination, including both direct smear and flotation
   D. Administer an anthelmintic such as pyrantel pamoate for roundworms and hookworms; if tapeworms are present, administer praziquantel or epsiprantel

   E. Vaccinate with FVRC-P,* Chlamydophila,‡ feline leukemia virus,§ feline immunodeficiency virus, rabies, and feline infectious peritonitis,¶ Giardia, and Bordetella bronchiseptica** vaccines
   F. Adjust nutrition and grooming procedures
   G. Provide owner with client education pamphlets on topics such as the following:
      1. Identification, treatment, and control of fleas, ticks, and ear mites
      2. Benefits of vaccination for feline leukemia virus infection
      3. Dental, skin, nail, and ear care
      4. Management of normal and abnormal feline behaviors
      5. Exercise and its importance
      6. Recommendations for spaying, neutering, and declawing
   H. Fill in the kitten's health record for the owner
III. Subsequent visits for health program—usually annual visits
   A. Perform a general physical examination and record the body weight
   B. Check for external parasites and dermatophytes and initiate appropriate therapy
      1. Fleas and ear mites (O. cynotis)
      2. Mange mites, especially N. cati, Demodex species, and Cheyletiella species
      3. Dermatophytes, particularly Microsporum species and T. mentagrophytes
   C. Perform fecal examination (fecal flotation)
   D. Administer an anthelmintic according to fecal examination findings
   E. Vaccinate with FVRC-P,* Chlamydophila,‡ feline leukemia virus,§ feline immunodeficiency virus, rabies, and feline infectious peritonitis,¶ Giardia, and Bordetella bronchiseptica** vaccines
   F. Adjust nutrition and grooming procedures
   G. Provide owner with client education pamphlets on topics such as the following:
      1. Identification, treatment, and control of fleas, ticks, and ear mites
      2. Benefits of vaccination for feline leukemia virus and feline immunodeficiency virus infections
      3. Dental, skin, nail, and ear care
      4. Management of normal and abnormal feline behaviors
      5. Exercise and its importance
      6. Recommendations for spaying, neutering, and declawing
   H. Fill in the cat's health record for the owner

*This refers to the use of a vaccine to protect against the following: FVR—feline viral rhinotracheitis; C—feline calicivirus infection; and P—feline panleukopenia.

†Cats being prepared for shipment or entering a boarding kennel or veterinary hospital or clinic should be vaccinated at least 1 to 2 weeks before admission or shipment.

‡The vaccine currently available apparently produces effective protection only against Chlamydophila infections. As is the case with other vaccines for respiratory ailments, complete protection is not afforded; however, clinically proven conjunctivitis or upper respiratory tract disease, if present, can be restricted to a short course and will be mild.

§This refers to the use of a vaccine to protect against feline leukemia virus infection. These vaccines are administered subcutaneously in healthy kittens or older cats as two doses, with the second dose given 3 or 4 weeks after the first. Annual revaccination with a single dose is recommended.

¶The feline infectious peritonitis vaccine is administered intranasally to healthy cats. Primary vaccination with two doses should be given, with the second dose administered 3 to 4 weeks after the first, and single-dose annual revaccination is recommended.

**This refers to the use of vaccine to protect against feline Bordetella bronchiseptica–induced disease. Kittens may be vaccinated with an intranasal vaccine as early as 4 weeks of age.

FPL, FVR, FCV infection, and rabies vaccinations, other vaccinations can be incorporated into the preventive health program, as detailed in the following sections.

⬥ TECHNICIAN NOTE

In the general, vaccinations for the prevention of FPL, FVR, FCV infection, and rabies are the most important.

FELINE PANLEUKOPENIA VACCINE

FPL is a highly contagious parvoviral disease that is characterized by an explosive, short course and a moderate to high mortality rate. The FPL virus causes fever, anorexia, diarrhea, weight loss, and leukopenia. This feline virus is similar to the canine parvovirus. There are many excellent vaccines available for immunization of cats against FPL. If these are used correctly and at the proper age, cats should be completely protected against FPL. Several slightly different programs for the immunization of cats against FPL have been presented during the past few years. The safest recommendation is to start the vaccination program at an early age and to vaccinate kittens at frequent intervals until they are at least 16 weeks of age. This might prove beneficial in certain circumstances, such as in catteries or colonies, in which kittens could be vaccinated at 6 weeks of age, followed by repeated vaccinations at 3-week intervals until the kittens are 16 weeks old. However, most kittens presented to the veterinarian are vaccinated with a minimum of two or possibly three vaccinations; revaccination with a single dose every year or every 3 years is recommended.

FELINE VIRAL RHINOTRACHEITIS VACCINE

FVR is a highly contagious viral disease of cats characterized by sudden onset of conjunctivitis, lacrimation, and nasal discharge accompanied by sneezing. The FVR vaccines may be obtained as a single vaccine or in combination with FCV vaccine. The FVR vaccines produce significant protection against FVR disease after vaccination and, as such, should be part of the routine vaccination program. The FVR vaccines are administered intranasally, subcutaneously, or intramuscularly to kittens at 9 weeks and again at 12 weeks of age; revaccination with a single dose every year or every 3 years is recommended.

FELINE CALICIVIRUS VACCINE

FCV-induced respiratory tract infections occur among cats at about the same frequency as FVR. Fever, lacrimation, and serous nasal discharges that soon become purulent are first manifestations of the disease. The fever tends to fluctuate after its initial appearance. Sneezing, anorexia, and depression are common. Ulceration of the glossal epithelium or the palatine mucosa occurs with FCV infection and may be the only sign of infection. The FCV vaccines may be obtained as a single vaccine or in combination with FVR vaccine. The FCV vaccines produce significant protection against FCV disease after vaccination and, as such, should be part of the routine vaccination program. The FCV vaccines are administered intranasally, subcutaneously, or intramuscularly to kittens at 9 weeks and again at 12 weeks of age; revaccination with a single dose every year or every 3 years is recommended.

RABIES VACCINE

Rabies is acute infectious encephalitis characterized by altered behavior, aggressiveness, progressive paralysis, and in most species, by death. The rabies virus is usually present in the saliva of infected mammals, and in nature it is usually transmitted by a bite. Rabies most commonly affects the dog, cat, fox, skunk, raccoon, bobcat, coyote, bat, mongoose, and other small carnivorous mammals that are mainly responsible for the transmission of the disease. As in dog rabies, three phases of clinical signs are recognized in cat rabies: the prodromal, the excitative, and the paralytic. For more details concerning rabies, refer to the discussion of rabies vaccine earlier in the chapter.

Inactivated rabies virus vaccines are currently licensed and available for preexposure vaccination of cats against rabies. All rabies vaccines are administered in 1-ml doses intramuscularly at one site in the thigh or subcutaneously. The vaccines are licensed for immunization of cats 3 months of age and older. Cats vaccinated between 3 and 12 months of age should receive a second dose 1 year later. The vaccines are licensed for 1- to 3-year effective immune periods.

FELINE *CHLAMYDOPHILA* VACCINE

Although feline *Chlamydophila* infection is not as prevalent as FVR or FCV infections, it is evident that in some cat populations *Chlamydophila* infection is contributing to persistent conjunctivitis and upper respiratory tract disease. The vaccines currently available produce effective protection only against *Chlamydophila felis* infections. As with other vaccines for respiratory ailments, complete protection is not afforded; however, clinical signs of conjunctivitis or upper respiratory tract disease, if they do occur, can be restricted to short courses and will be mild. Vaccines for feline *Chlamydophila* infection can be obtained from several manufacturers in various combinations with the more traditional feline vaccine components.

FELINE LEUKEMIA VIRUS AND FELINE IMMUNODEFICIENCY VIRUS VACCINES

Domestic cats may become infected with several retroviruses, including feline leukemia virus (FeLV) and feline immunodeficiency virus (FIV). FeLV and FIV cause a large number of diverse disease syndromes including lymphoreticular and myeloid neoplasms, anemias, immune-mediated disorders, and an immunodeficiency syndrome somewhat similar to human acquired immunodeficiency syndrome (AIDS). Excretion of FeLV occurs primarily by way of salivary secretions, although virus is also present is respiratory secretions, blood, milk, feces, and urine.

Several FeLV vaccines are currently available to protect cats of all ages against FeLV infection. The vaccines are administered subcutaneously in healthy kittens or older cats as two doses, with the second dose given 3 or 4 weeks after the first. Annual revaccination with a single dose is recommended. According to the manufacturers, the vaccines cause no interference with simultaneous vaccinations against rabies, panleukopenia, and respiratory viruses. The vaccines also do not affect red blood cell or white blood cell counts, weight gain, reproductive capability, or FeLV testing in kittens vaccinated as young as 6 weeks of age. In viremic cats, vaccines may produce minimal antibody responses and cats remain viremic, but they are not harmed by the vaccination.

A killed vaccine containing immunogens from two FIV isolates is licensed for use in cats. Efficacy was demonstrated in cats that received three doses of vaccine and were challenged 1 year after vaccination with a heterologous, or different, strain. The vaccine protected 67% of vaccinated cats against infection as shown by a lack of integration of the FIV provirus, whereas 74% of the control cats became persistently infected. The primary concern with FIV vaccination is that the FIV vaccine induces antibodies detectable by the currently available antibody test. After FIV vaccination, the veterinarian will be unable to determine whether the cat is infected with FIV.

FELINE INFECTIOUS PERITONITIS VACCINE

Coronavirus infection is of significant importance in the world's cat population. As many as 80% to 90% of cats are affected within individual catteries and multiple-cat households. Cats are susceptible to infection with several different strains of feline coronavirus. Depending on which strain of feline coronavirus is involved, clinical signs may range from asymptomatic infection to gastrointestinal disease of varying severity to widespread fibrinous serositis and disseminated vasculitis commonly referred to as feline infectious peritonitis (FIP). In FIP disease, young cats may be presented with nonspecific signs, such as nonresponsive fever, anorexia, lethargy, chronic weight loss, and pale mucous membranes. Icterus may be seen cases with severe liver involvement. Recurring episodes of diarrhea and constipation may be observed. Progressive abdominal distention occurs as a result of an accumulation of ascitic fluid in the peritoneal cavity.

A first-generation temperature-sensitive FIP virus (TS-FIPV) vaccine that affords protection against FIP virus challenge is available (Primucell-FIP Vaccine, Pfizer Animal Health). This TS-FIPV vaccine contains attenuated whole coronavirus and is recommended by the manufacturer to be administered intranasally to healthy cats. Primary vaccination should be given in two doses, with the second dose administered 3 to 4 weeks after the first; annual revaccination with a single dose is recommended. Cats vaccinated twice intranasally with the TS-FIPV vaccine have not developed a febrile response, nor have they had any blood dyscrasia indicative of FIP disease. Likewise, vaccinated pregnant cats, dexamethasone-suppressed cats, FeLV-infected cats, and feline enteric coronavirus–infected cats have not shown a febrile response or any blood dyscrasia.

FELINE *BORDETELLA* VACCINE

Feline *Bordetella bronchiseptica* (FeBb) is a primary respiratory pathogen in cats of all ages and breeds. FeBb should be considered in instances of feline upper respiratory tract infection and pneumonia. Even cats not showing signs of respiratory disease can be significant carriers of FeBb organisms. FeBb is readily transmitted from cat to cat, especially those living in multiple-cat environments. Proper husbandry, good nutrition, parasite control, and control of other respiratory tract infections can help reduce the risk of a cat contracting FeBb. An FeBb-specific vaccination can also help prevent acute infections. This vaccine is the only licensed product available for protection of cats against FeBb infection. The FeBb vaccine is safe in kittens as young as 4 weeks old and will not cause any serious disease or pneumonia. The vaccine is also safe in pregnant queens.

FELINE FUNGAL VACCINE

Common flaky skin lesions, referred to as ringworm, are usually caused by *Microsporum canis*. An *M. canis* killed fungal vaccine that affords protection against ringworm-induced skin lesions is available. The vaccine is used in cats 4 months of age and older as an aid in the prevention and treatment of clinical signs of disease caused by *M. canis*. Vaccination has not been demonstrated to eliminate *M. canis* organisms from infected cats. Primary vaccination should be given in two doses, with the second dose administered 3 to 4 weeks after the first; revaccination with a single dose every 6 months is recommended.

FELINE *GIARDIA* VACCINE

Enteric infections with *Giardia* spp. are common in cats younger than 6 months and in immunocompromised cats. Recurrent diarrhea is usually the primary presenting complaint. The *Giardia* vaccine acts at the intestinal level against both the trophozoite and cyst forms of *Giardia* spp. When given twice, the *Giardia* vaccine lowers the number of organisms shed and decreases the symptoms of clinical disease. The *Giardia* vaccine is most effective when cats are frequently exposed to contaminated *Giardia*-laden water.

VACCINE-ASSOCIATED SARCOMAS

Epidemiologic evidence has shown a strong association between administration of inactivated feline vaccines, specifically FeLV and rabies, and subsequent soft tissue sarcoma development at vaccine sites. The prevalence of sarcoma development after vaccination has been reported as 1 case per 10,000 vaccines administered. Sarcomas are believed to develop in areas of prolonged inflammation produced by the vaccine products. Although epidemiologic studies have failed to identify specific brands of FeLV or rabies vaccines involved, this may be due to the relatively low incidence of sarcomas found, large numbers of brands of FeLV and rabies vaccines administered to cats, or other factors. The vaccine component most commonly thought to be associated with local postvaccinal inflammation is the vaccine's adjuvant. Adjuvants of different types are used in many but not all inactivated feline vaccines.

Recommendations include a change in vaccination site location, decreased use of polyvalent vaccines, use of non-adjuvanted vaccines, and avoidance of overvaccination. The most important recommendation for prevention of vaccine-associated tumors would appear to be not to over-vaccinate. The National Vaccine-Associated Sarcoma Task Force studying vaccine site tumors recommends that no vaccine be given in the interscapular space, that rabies vaccine be administered in the distal right rear leg, that FeLV vaccine be administered in the distal left rear leg, and that all other vaccines be administered in the right shoulder. It appears that intramuscular and subcutaneous administration both result in local inflammation and sarcoma production. Subcutaneous sites are recommended for all vaccines because use of these sites will result in earlier detection of these sarcomas. The reasoning behind the use of these sites for vaccine administration is not based on prevention but rather on the likelihood of earlier diagnosis and a potentially higher cure rate with surgical treatment.

TECHNICIAN NOTE

The most important recommendation for prevention of vaccine-associated tumors would appear to be not to overvaccinate.

It is also recommended that any vaccine site lumps present after 3 months from the time of vaccination be removed, but only after a biopsy has been done. A biopsy will determine the magnitude of the surgery required (e.g., lumpectomy vs. extensive tissue removal). The mass should not be excised before a biopsy is done. Attempts at simple excision of these tumors are seldom curative and ultimately lead to local recurrence with a more difficult second attempt. Rear leg amputation has a higher rate of cure than surgery in the interscapular space for vaccine-associated sarcomas. Most chemotherapeutic attempts result in partial responses, but some complete responses have been observed with these

drugs. Although the vast majority of vaccine-associated tumors are only locally invasive, approximately 1 of 20 will metastasize to the lungs or other sites.

HEARTWORM PREVENTIVE THERAPY

Kittens can be started on a heartworm preventive program with ivermectin at 6 to 8 weeks of age. A heartworm preventive product that contains ivermectin should be administered orally at the recommended minimum dose level of 24.0 μg/kg of body weight at monthly intervals.

OWNER EDUCATION

Owner education pamphlets on a variety of cat-related topics can be sent home with the owner each time the cat is seen for the preventive health program. Generally, only one or two well-written owner education pamphlets are given to the owner at the end of each office visit.

Veterinarians and veterinary technicians are in an excellent position to provide meaningful owner educational services and thus make owners more aware of their cats and the associated responsibilities of cat ownership. By offering consultative advice and providing owners with educational pamphlets, the veterinary technician not only assists owners who are seeking medical treatment for their cats but also serves a vital role in educating people in the community.

EARLY SPAY-NEUTER PROCEDURES

Early spay-neuter involves the surgical removal of the gonads in sexually immature animals. Early spay-neuter of puppies and kittens as young as 8 weeks of age is now an accepted alternative to allowing sexually intact animals to leave most animal shelters or adoption agencies. Early spay-neuter allows for decreased operative time, improved visibility of intraabdominal structures, and rapid recovery from anesthesia. Puppies or kittens that undergo early spay-neuter are believed to be more people-oriented pets and are calmer, gentler, less likely to wander, and less likely to retain persistent juvenile behavior (seemingly desirable). Early spay-neuter in puppies and kittens is a safe and effective means of controlling the canine and feline population in animal control and private veterinary practice environments. The advantages of early spay-neuter far outweigh the risks.

HEREDITY DNA TESTS

DNA testing for inherited diseases in pedigree dogs intended for breeding purposes or for specific disease recognition became a reality in the late 1990s. DNA testing technology is now available for the clinical practice and for dog breeders.

Web sites that can provide this type of genetic service can be found on the Internet.

The principles of the DNA testing technology are as follows. The gene is the basic unit of heredity. All of the genes that constitute the hereditary makeup of an organism are called the genome. A dog is composed of a large number of cells that are genetically identical. The canine genome is made up of 39 pairs of chromosomes (one set from each parent) that contain approximately 3 billion base pairs of DNA, or around 100,000 or so genes. Each gene generally occupies a particular position within a particular chromosome. Scattered throughout the chromosome are short repeated groups of these base pairs known as microsatellites, or markers, that can be used to track defective genes. Hundreds of these distinctive sequences have been isolated along the canine genome for use in mapping genes.

To find a marker that is linked to a disease, researchers often examine hundreds of markers from dogs with and without the disease before they find one that is located so close to a disease gene that it is almost always inherited along with the disease caused by that gene. The closer the marker is to the disease gene itself, the more accurate is the test. Finding such a marker also narrows down where to look for the disease-causing gene, which could ultimately lead to a more specific DNA test for the gene itself.

A mutation is a genetic mistake that scrambles the instructions given by a gene. Mutations may be good, bad, or indifferent. In the case of inherited renal dysplasia in the Shih tzu, Lhasa apso, and Soft-coated wheaten terrier, it is believed that the presence of mutations in one or perhaps two different genes causes the glomeruli of the kidney to stop developing.

What are dominant and recessive genes? A dominant gene will express itself when the puppy inherits only one copy of the gene (from sire or dam). A recessive gene will express itself only when a puppy inherits two copies of the gene (one from the sire and one from the dam). If a disease-causing gene is recessive, a dog with the gene can be bred to a dog without it and will not produce the disease, although it will produce a carrier of the gene. If the gene is dominant, both parents must be free of it to avoid producing affected puppies. Again, more than one defective gene may be needed to produce a disease.

DNA testing can be done reliably at any age, and the results are accurate; that is, the DNA test results should never change with age and should be the same whenever the test is repeated. Dog breeders and veterinarians alike can separate the problem of some inherited disease into two distinct issues: getting rid of the disease and getting rid of the defective gene. There are three possible DNA testing results obtained: clear, carrier, and affected. A clear finding indicates that the gene is not present in the tested dog. Therefore when used for breeding purposes, dogs with clear status will not pass on the disease gene. A carrier finding indicates that one copy of the disease gene is present in the tested dog and that it will not likely exhibit signs of the disease. Carrier dogs will probably not have medical problems as a result. Dogs with the carrier status will not develop the medical problem but will pass on the disease gene 50% of the time. An affected finding indicates that two copies of the disease gene are present in the tested dog, and the disease will medically affect the dog. It is always best to breed "clear dog to clear dog." If followed by pedigree dog breeders, this strategy should ensure a significant reduction in the frequency of the targeted disease gene in future generations of dogs. However, to maintain a large enough pool of good breeding animals, some breeders may need to breed clear dogs to carrier dogs.

DNA testing procedures are available that identify coat color predilection for the Labrador retriever, Doberman Pinscher, American Cocker spaniel, Flat-coated retriever, Poodle, and Scottish terrier. DNA tests are available to assist in the elimination of copper toxicosis in the Bedlington terrier and inherited renal dysplasia in the Shih tzu, Lhasa apso, and Soft-coated wheaten terrier. Other available DNA tests for inherited diseases include the test for phosphofructokinase deficiency in the English springer spaniel and American Cocker spaniel, the test for progressive retinal atrophy in the Irish setter, and the test for pyruvic kinase deficiency in the Basenji. In addition, DNA tests are available to detect von Willebrand's disease in the Doberman pinscher, Scottish terrier, Shetland sheepdog, Manchester terrier, Poodle, and Pembroke Welsh corgi. DNA testing procedures are available to assist in the elimination of progressive retinal atrophy from the dog breeds *Chesapeake Bay retriever, English Cocker spaniel, Labrador retriever,* and *Portuguese water dog.* DNA tests to assist in the elimination of rod-cone dysplasia and canine leukocyte adhesion deficiency from the Irish setter and congenital stationary night blindness from the Briard are also available.

PREVENTIVE HEALTH PROGRAM FOR HORSES

A preventive health program for horses should be designed to meet the specific needs of the individual animal or herd. Such programs generally vary from one stable to another and from one veterinary practice to another, depending on expected exposures, management styles, and personal preferences of attending veterinarians and horse owners. An example of one preventive health program for horses is outlined in Box 11-3.

PHYSICAL EXAMINATION

New additions to a stable or an established herd should be Coggins' test–negative for equine infectious anemia and quarantined for 1 month before they enter the general

BOX 11-3 GENERAL OUTLINE OF A PREVENTIVE HEALTH PROGRAM FOR HORSES

FIRST QUARTER: JANUARY–MARCH
All Horses
Deworm at least every 8 wk. Exercise care in choice of anthelmintics for mares in the third trimester. Begin deworming foals at 2 mo of age.

Trim feet every 6 wk, more frequently in foals requiring limb correction.

Dentistry: Check twice yearly and float teeth as needed. Remove wolf teeth in 2-yr-olds and retained caps in 2-, 3-, and 4-yr-olds.

Immunize for respiratory disease: influenza, strangles, and rhinopneumonitis.

In southeastern United States, immunize for equine encephalitis.

Stallions
Perform complete breeding examination. Maintain stallions under lights if being used for early breeding.

Pregnant Mares
Immunize with tetanus toxoid, and open sutured mares 30 days prepartum. Develop a colostrum bank. Ninth-day breeding only for mares with normal foaling history and normal reproductive tract. Wash udders of foaling mares.

Open Mares
Maintain under lights if being used for early breeding. Perform daily teasing. Perform reproductive tract examination during estrus. Mares should not be too fat but should be in gaining condition during breeding season.

Newborn Foals
Dip navel in disinfectant.
Carefully, give a cleansing enema at birth.
Administer tetanus prophylaxis if indicated by history.
Perform immunoglobulin test at 12-24 hr.

SECOND QUARTER: APRIL–JUNE
All Horses
Deworm at least every 8 wk.
Trim feet every wk. Do not forget foals and yearlings.
Dentistry: Check teeth and remove or float teeth as needed.

Immunize for equine encephalomyelitis. Administer appropriate vaccine boosters.

Stallions
Maintain an exercise program.
Monitor semen quality.

Broodmares
Palpate at 21, 42, and 60 days after successful breeding.

Foals
Creep-feed the foals, and provide free-choice minerals.
Immunize at 3 mo of age.
Group foals by sex and size when weaned.

THIRD-QUARTER: JULY–SEPTEMBER
All Horses
Deworm at least every 8 wk. Clip and sweep the pastures.
Trim feet every 6 wk. Continue corrective trimming on foals.
Dentistry: Check teeth and remove or float teeth as needed.

Stallions
Maintain an exercise program.

Broodmares
Administer rhinopneumonitis boosters to pregnant mares according to manufacturer's labeled direction. Administer appropriate vaccine boosters to foals and yearlings.

Check condition of mare's udder at weaning, and reduce amount of feed given until milk flow is reduced.

Foals
Administer all appropriate immunization. Provide free-choice minerals. Maintain a protein supplement in creep feeders.

FOURTH QUARTER: OCTOBER–DECEMBER

All Horses
Deworm at least every 8 wk. Select anthelmintics appropriate for season.
Trim feet every 6 wk. Continue corrective trimming on foals.
Dentistry: Check teeth and remove or float teeth as needed.

Stallions
Continue exercise program.
Check immunizations.
Perform breeding examination.

Broodmares
Confirm pregnancy.
Begin treating open mares.
Check immunizations.

---

population. During this time, the first physical examination for the preventive health program can be performed. The physical examination should be completed in a manner that will gain the confidence of the new horse and allow the veterinarian to establish the current health status and soundness of the animal. These observations are then recorded in a permanent medical record at the stable.

The rectal temperature, respiratory rate, and heart rate before and after light exercise should be recorded, and the thorax should be thoroughly auscultated. The horse should be weighed or the body weight should be estimated with a thoracic tape, both to establish a weight baseline and for future reference in calculating doses. Both eyes should be completely examined for soundness. A dental examination should reveal incisor malocclusion and abnormal wear of the cheek teeth. Similarly, the musculoskeletal system and skin should be examined. Physical examination should be repeated at 2- to 3-month intervals as part of the preventive health program for horses of all ages. Obtaining a history and performing a physical examination are discussed in Chapter 2.

VACCINATIONS

A variety of vaccines approved for use in healthy horses can be obtained from manufacturers as individual components or in various combinations. Table 11-3 lists some vaccines currently available.

Horses that are immunologically naive or that have an unknown immunization history should receive an initial immunization, which is then followed in 4 weeks by a second immunization.

TECHNICIAN NOTE

Horses that are immunologically naive or have an unknown immunization history should receive an initial immunization, followed in 4 weeks by a second immunization.

Further booster vaccinations can be administered as indicated according to the risk of exposure and the veterinarian's experience with the vaccine. In rare instances, anaphylactoid reactions can occur with the use of any vaccine. These life-threatening crises must be handled quickly. Accordingly, it is essential that epinephrine be available for the treatment of anaphylactoid reactions. Other complications, such as fever, lameness, and swelling or abscess formation at the injection site, may also occur with the routine use of these vaccines. The horse owner should always be apprised of these possibilities before any vaccine is administered. Common diseases and vaccines used as an aid in disease prevention are discussed in the following sections.

TETANUS VACCINES

Tetanus, or lockjaw, is a disease characterized by muscular rigidity that may culminate in death from respiratory arrest or convulsions. Tetanus is caused by the toxins produced by the anaerobic bacterium *Clostridium tetani*. Active immunity to tetanus is produced by administration of a tetanus toxoid, which is a purified, inactivated toxin of *C. tetani*.

Tetanus antitoxin is produced by hyperimmunization of donor horses with tetanus toxoid. Administration of antitoxin to unvaccinated horses induces immediate protection, which lasts approximately 2 weeks. Acute hepatitis may be associated with use of tetanus antitoxin; therefore prophylaxis with tetanus toxoid should be emphasized.

EQUINE ENCEPHALOMYELITIS VACCINE

Equine encephalomyelitis is a viral neurologic disease of horses caused by eastern, western, and Venezuelan viruses. These viruses are maintained in nature by bird and animal reservoirs and are transmitted to horses by biting insects. Venezuelan equine encephalomyelitis occurs in South and Central America but has not been diagnosed in the United States for several years. The trivalent vaccine is commonly used for horses in states bordering Mexico to create a buffer zone, which may prevent the spread of Venezuelan equine encephalomyelitis into the United States. The clinical signs of equine encephalomyelitis may be as subtle as fever and partial anorexia or as severe as marked depression, convulsions, and death. The death rate varies with the type of virus infection, but it may range from 19% to 90%.

The equine encephalomyelitis vaccines currently used for active immunization are inactivated virus vaccines. They should be administered annually before the biting insect season. In areas where winter freezes are not common, semiannual vaccinations may be advisable. In endemic areas, frequent boosters (every 2 to 4 months) are recommended.

EQUINE RHINOPNEUMONITIS VACCINE

Equine herpesvirus (EHV) has caused sporadic infections and death in horses throughout the world. Four distinct equine herpesviruses have been identified: EHV-1, EHV-2, EHV-3, and EHV-4. EHV-1 and EHV-4 cause rhinopneumonitis. EHV-1 has been exclusively associated with the neurologic form of rhinopneumonitis, and it is also responsible for late-gestation abortions, stillbirths, and weak neonatal foals that fail to survive. EHV-4 is most frequently associated with upper respiratory tract disease in young horses and is rarely a cause of abortion.

Until recently all herpesvirus vaccines were prepared from EHV-1 virus. Vaccination of foals and young horses to prevent EHV-4 infections depended on the induction of cross-reactive antibody to EHV-1. The resulting immunity was short-lived and required revaccination at 2- to 3-month intervals. New vaccines that contain both EHV-4 and EHV-1 have been introduced and are approved for use in the prevention of respiratory tract infection.

Pregnant mares should be vaccinated during the fifth, seventh, and ninth months of gestation with an inactivated EHV-1 vaccine. Total protection from abortion cannot be achieved.

EQUINE INFLUENZA VACCINE

Equine influenza has a worldwide distribution and is frequently seen in mobile populations of horses. Disease outbreaks usually occur in horses 1 to 3 years of age after mixing with infected horses at the racetrack or show ground. Equine influenza may also occur in older horses, but the

Table 11-3 Equine Vaccines

Vaccine	Manufacturer	Type	Vaccine Components															
			EEE	WEE	VEE	EVA	A/1	A/2	EHV-1	EHV-4	TT	TAT	Rb	St	Anx	PHF	Bot	Rota
Anthrax vaccine	Colorado Serum	—													X			
Arvac	Fort Dodge Animal Health	MLV				X												
Calvenia EJV	Boehringer Ingelheim	I					X	X										
Calvenza EJV/EHV	Boehringer Ingelheim	I					X	X	X	X								
Calvenza EHV	Boehringer Ingelheim	I							X	X								
Bot Vax B	Neogen	I															X	
Encephaloid I.M.	Fort Dodge Animal Health	I	X	X														
Encephalomyelitis vaccine	Colorado Serum	I	X	X														
Encevac with Havlogen	Intervet	I	X	X														
Encevac-T with Havlogen	Intervet	I	X	X							X							
Encevac-T E with Havlogen	Intervet	I	X	X							X							
Encevac TC-4 with Havlogen	Intervet	I	X	X							X							
Encevac TC-4 with Havlogen	Intervet	I	X	X							X							
Equicine II with Havlogen	Intervet	I	X	X														
Equiflu EWT	Boehringer Ingelheim	I	X	X														
Equiflu VEWT	Boehringer Ingelheim	I	X	X														
Equiloid Innovator	Fort Dodge Animal Health	I	X	X							X							
Equine Rotavirus Vaccine	Fort Dodge Animal Health	I																X
Equivac EHV 1/4	Fort Dodge Animal Health	I							X	X								
Flu Avert I.N.	Heska	I						X										
Flumune	Pfizer Animal Health	I					X	X										
Fluvac Innovator Double EFT + EHV	Fort Dodge Animal Helath	I	X	X			X	X	X	X	X							
Fluvac EHV 4/1	Fort Dodge	I					X	X	X	X								
Fluvac Innovator Triple-EFT	Fort Dodge Animal Health	I	X	X	X		X	X			X							
Fluvac Innovator Double-EFT	Fort Dodge	I	X	X			X	X			X							
Fluvac Innovator	Fort Dodge Animal Health	I					X	X										
Fluvac Innovator Triple-EFT + EHV	Fort Dodge Animal Health	I	X	X	X		X	X	X	X	X							
Mystique	Intervet	I														X		
Mystique II	Bayer Intervet	I											X			X		
PHF-Vax	Schering-Plough	I														X		
Pinnacle I.N.	Fort Dodge Animal Health	LC												X				
Pneumabort-K + lb	Fort Dodge Animal Health	I							X									
Potomacguard	Fort Dodge Animal Health	I														X		
Potomac Shield	Novartis	I														X		
Potomacguard EWT	Fort Dodge Animal Health	I	X	X							X					X		
Prestige + Havlogen	Intervet	I						X		X								
Prestige II + Havlogen	Intervet	I					X	X	X	X								
Prodigy + Havlogen	Bayer	I							X									
Rabvac 3	Fort Dodge Animal Health	I											X					
Prestige V + Havlogen	Intervet	I	X	X			X	X	X	X	X							
Prestige V + VEE + Havloen	Intervet	I	X	X	X		X	X	X	X	X							

Continued

Table 11-3 EQUINE VACCINES—CONT'D

Vaccine	Manufacturer	Type	Vaccine Components														
			EEE	WEE	VEE	EVA	A/1	A/2	EHV-1	EHV-4	TT	TAT	Rb	St	Anx	PHF	BoT	Rota
Rhinomune	Pfizer Animal Health	MLV							X									
Equine Potomavac + Imrab	Merial	I											X			X		
Equine EWTF	Merial	I	X	X			X	X			X							
Imrab 3	Merial	I											X					
Strepguard with Havlogen	Intervet	I												X				
Super-Tet with Havlogen	Intervet	I									X							
Tetanus Antitoxin Equine Origin	Durvet	Antitoxin										X						
Tetanus toxoid	Fort Dodge Animal Health	I									X							
Tetanus toxoid	Colorado Serum	I									X							
Tetanus toxoid—concentrated	Colorado Serum	I									X							
Tetanus toxoid—concentrated	Professional Biological	I									X							
Tetnogen	Fort Dodge Animal Health	I									X							
Tetnogen-AT	Fort Dodge Animal Health	Antitoxin										X						
Tetanus antitoxin	Fort Dodge Animal Health	Antitoxin										X						
Tetanus antitoxin	Professional Biological	Antitoxin										X						
Tetanus antitoxin	Colorado Serum	Antitoxin										X						
Triple E	Fort Dodge Animal Health	I	X	X								X						
Triple ET Innovator	Fort Dodge Animal Health	I	X	X	X						X							
Surcocystis neurova	Fort Didge	I																
Equine Potomavac	Merial	I														X		
West Nile Virus	Fort Dodge Animal Health	I																
Tetguard	Boehringer Ingelheim	I									X					X		

Anx, Anthrax; *A/1*, equine influenza myxovirus A-equi; *A/2*, equine influenza myxovirus A-equi 2; *Bot*, botulism; *EEE*, eastern equine encephalomyelitis; *EHV-1*, equine herpesvirus 1; *EHV-4*, equine herpesvirus 4; *EVA*, equine viral arteritis; *I*, inactivated; *MLV*, modified live virus; *LC*, Live, Culture; *PHF*, Potomac horse fever; *Rb*, rabies; *Rota*, rotavirus; *St*, strangles; *TAT*, tetanus antitoxin; *TT*, tetanus toxoid; *VEE*, Venezuelan equine encephalomyelitis; *WEE*, western equine encephalomyelitis.

clinical signs are mild. Infection is characterized by fever, depression, anorexia, muscle soreness, and coughing.

The equine influenza viruses of importance in the United States are A/1 and A/2. Currently available vaccines contain inactivated virus that includes both A/1 and A/2 strains. Intranasal vaccines may increase protection via local immunity to A/2 strains. The duration of protective immunity from vaccination is short-lived, requiring revaccination every 2 to 3 months during periods of exposure (showing and racing).

STRANGLES VACCINE

Strangles is a respiratory disease caused by infection with the bacterium *Streptococcus equi*. Strangles is easily transmitted through direct contact with mucopurulent discharge from infected horses or from contaminated fomites, such as feeding utensils, buckets, or other equipment. Strangles is characterized by sudden onset of fever and upper respiratory catarrh, followed by acute swelling and abscess formation in submaxillary, submandibular, and retropharyngeal lymph nodes.

✎ TECHNICIAN NOTE

Strangles is easily transmitted through direct contact with mucopurulent discharge from infected horses or from contaminated fomites.

Several inactivated subunit M protein vaccines and one inactivated whole-cell bacterium are available for intramuscular injection as an adjunct to the prevention of strangles. All of these vaccines may cause postinjection reactions or abscesses at the site of administration. Because of these adverse effects, vaccination for strangles is performed only in immunologically naive horses with a high likelihood of exposure. Vaccination is not 100% effective for preventing disease but does often reduce the severity and incidence of disease. Most recently, live strangles vaccine for intranasal administration has become available. Purpura hemorrhagica (immune-mediated vasculitis) is a possible adverse effect of all strangles vaccines.

EQUINE VIRAL ARTERITIS VACCINE

Equine viral arteritis infection may cause subclinical to severe disease and death. The disease is characterized by fever, depression, nasal discharge, lacrimation, coughing, and limb swelling. Several attenuated live-virus vaccines have been developed. Only one serotype of virus appears to be relevant to the protection of horses. The vaccine induces partial to complete protection against the clinical signs of disease, but virus replication will still occur after virus challenge.

POTOMAC HORSE FEVER VACCINE

Potomac horse fever (equine monocytic ehrlichiosis) is caused by *Ehrlichia risticii*. It is most prevalent in eastern states, particularly near large waterways, but has been identified in many regions of the United States and in other countries. Although not proven, aquatic insect vectors, snails, and ticks are believed to be involved in disease transmission. Many approved vaccines are available for use in the prevention of Potomac horse fever, and their use should be considered in areas where the disease is known to occur. The efficacy of Potomac horse fever vaccine is unknown.

BOTULISM VACCINE

The currently available equine botulism vaccine is a *Clostridium botulinum* type B toxoid. The most common application for this vaccine is vaccination of mares 30 days before foaling for prevention of shaker foal syndrome in areas of high incidence. However, *C. botulinum* type C is an important pathogen in some regions of North America.

ANTHRAX VACCINE

Anthrax vaccines for use in horses are currently available but are not widely used except where a genuine risk is identified.

RABIES VACCINE

Horses with rabies initially display spinal cord or brainstem signs. Behavioral changes can occur as the disease progresses; however, aggressive behavior is rare. The disease is always fatal. Approved rabies vaccines are available for use in horses. Routine preexposure immunization should be considered in areas where wildlife rabies is epizootic.

SARCOCYSTIS NEURONA VACCINE

Sarcocystis neurona is a protozoa organism that parasitizes opossums without causing disease. Horses are an accidental dead end host; however, the exposure rate for horses appears to be relatively high (greater than 50% of horses in most parts of United States). The incidence of disease in exposed horses is quite low (<1%), and risk factors include stress (e.g., pregnancy, transport). The organism causes disease when it crosses the blood-brain barrier and gains access to the central nervous system, thereby causing clinical signs of multifocal, diffuse, asymmetric or symmetric, upper motor or lower motor neuron disease of the spinal cord and brain stem. Clinical signs often improve with treatment; however, residual deficits are likely, and only about one fourth of treated horses return to their previous function. A vaccine has been approved for use in horses based on safety but without studies of efficacy.

WEST NILE VIRUS VACCINE

West Nile virus was a foreign animal disease before 1999 when the disease was detected in humans and horses on the East Coast of the United States; however, West Nile virus is currently prevalent throughout the United States, with more than 14,000 equine cases reported in 2002. The disease is caused by a flavivirus that infects numerous species of birds and mosquitoes (and *Culicoides* spp.), causing death in some birds. Humans and horses are dead-end hosts. The mortality rate in horses is 30% to 40%. Nervous system signs in horses are highly variable, but weakness and muscle tremors are common. Protection in previously unvaccinated horses requires two doses of the vaccine given approximately 4 weeks apart.

DENTAL AND HOOF CARE

Many directional instructions from rider or driver reach the horse through the mouth. If the bit causes pain, the instructions given to the horse may be compromised. Wolf teeth cause extreme pain in some horses, especially with broken snaffle, overdraw checks, and gag bits. The mouth of the young horse should be examined, and if wolf teeth are present, they should be removed before training begins. Deciduous premolars that are retained and enamel points on cheek teeth may also cause pain in the mouth that interferes with normal feeding and willing response to the bit. In addition, the cheek teeth should be checked visually or by palpation for evidence of abnormal wear, such as wave mouth, step mouth, or shear mouth. Of course, all dental examinations should include inspection for malocclusion.

The role of the veterinarian and veterinary technician in hoof care is largely advisory, and advice can be provided through owner education pamphlets.

✐ TECHNICIAN NOTE

The role of the veterinarian and veterinary technician in hoof care is largely advisory, and advice can be provided through owner education pamphlets.

Frequent hoof cleaning helps in the prevention of thrush. This condition is caused by anaerobic bacteria that grow well in moist and dark conditions in the sulci of the frog or under dirt packed into the sole. Thrush appears as a moist malodorous accumulation in the sulci of the frog and sometimes over the sole. Frequent cleaning removes dirt and exposes these bacteria to drying, aerobic conditions. Copper- or iodine-based solutions can be applied to the sulci and frog to treat thrush.

Keeping the hooves trimmed short and maintaining the correct hoof-pastern axis helps to prevent excess stress on tendons and ligaments of the limb. In foals that are born splay-footed or pigeon-toed, frequent hoof trimming can often correct these conformation problems.

PARASITES

It is well accepted that the athletic horse cannot perform at its genetic peak potential if handicapped with a heavy parasite load. Likewise, the pet horse may not maintain its well-kept appearance if burdened with external or internal parasites. In addition, parasites can cause serious disease with weight loss, diarrhea, and/or colic. Therefore close attention to parasite control is extremely important in a preventive health program. Complete records are essential to ensure that each horse is being adequately treated. If all horses pastured together are not dewormed at the same time, the parasite control program will be ineffective. Pastured horses should be dewormed every 60 days or more often. Fecal flotations should be evaluated on 10% of the herd immediately before and 7 days after dewormer administration. Egg counts greater than 200 eggs/g before deworming indicate that the interval between treatments is too long. The presence of ova after treatment indicates resistance to the anthelmintic used. Horses that are never turned out in pasture may not require deworming as often. Feed additives are available that are lethal to developing housefly and stable fly larvae in treated horse feces (but not effective against existing adult flies). These types of feed additives are to be used with caution, because they are organophosphate larvicides with possible adverse effects if used concomitantly with other pharmaceutical products. Chapter 7 contains additional information on parasitology.

NUTRITION

Horses have evolved as forage eaters, and their digestive systems are able to handle most forage, such as grass and hay, efficiently. Further, metabolic diseases (e.g., laminitis, azoturia) are less likely to occur in horses fed diets composed primarily of roughage rather than grain. Therefore the horse's diet should contain mostly high-quality roughage with just enough grain supplements to maintain body weight. The amount of grain in the diet should increase as the amount of work performed increases. A complete vitamin and mineral supplement is usually added to the diet to ensure that the proper balance of vitamins and minerals is received. All guesswork can be removed from ration planning if there is a feed analysis laboratory in proximity. Equine nutrition is discussed in Chapter 16.

SANITATION

Advice on sanitation may be communicated orally to the horse owner or provided in owner education pamphlets. The fact that diseases are effectively spread from sick horses to susceptible horses via shared feed and water buckets, bits, twitches, chain shanks, trailers, and clothing is sometimes overlooked. Water and feed buckets should be cleaned and sanitized on a regular basis. Proper manure disposal is also important in preventing the spread of infectious diseases and in controlling flies and internal parasites. Fungal infections of the skin can be spread via brushes and blankets.

Box 11-4 GENERAL OUTLINE OF A PREVENTIVE HEALTH PROGRAM FOR BEEF CATTLE

COW CALF HERD RECOMMENDATION
At Birth
Ingestion of colostrum within the first few hours after birth is an important factor in baby calf survival. Immunize with oral bovine rotavirus and coronavirus enteric disease vaccine if a calf diarrhea problem exists in the herd.

Birth to 2 Weeks
Castrate, implant, and dehorn calves.

1- to 3-Month-Old Calves
Immunize with a 7- or 8-way *Clostridium* bacterin (depending on presence of liver flukes in the area) and vaccinate for *Haemophilus somnus*. Calves may also be vaccinated at this time with IBR-PI$_3$ (inactivated IM or MLV intranasal product), BVD (inactivated), and BRSV (inactivated). Deworm with commercial product effective against inhibited stages of *Ostertagia*.

At Weaning (around 6 mo)
Vaccinate calves for IBR-PI$_3$-BVD-BRSV (modified live vaccine) and 5-way leptospirosis, 7- or 8-way *Clostridium* (depending on presence of flukes), *Haemophilus somnus*, *Mannheimia haemolytica*, and *Pasteurella multocida*.

Vaccinate heifers with *Brucella abortus,* strain RB-51 ("calfhood" vaccination) between 4 and 12 mo of age.

Deworm with broad-spectrum commercial dewormer.

4-8 Weeks After Weaning Calves
Booster vaccination for IBR-PI$_3$-BVD-BRSV (modified live vaccine) and 5-way leptospirosis, *Mannheimia haemolytica*, and *Pasteurella multocida*.

Replacement Heifers (30-60 days prebreeding)
Deworm as needed with broad-spectrum commercial dewormer.

Immunize with IBR-PI$_3$-BVD-BRSV (inactivated) and 5-way leptospirosis and *Campylobacter*.

Adult Cows (30-60 days prebreeding)
Usually do not need to be dewormed with the exception of treatment for flukes in the fall.

Immunize with IBR-PI$_3$-BVD-BRSV (inactivated) and 5-way leptospirosis and *Campylobacter*.

Precalving Cows and Heifers (30-60 days precalving)
Vaccinate for 7- or 8-way *Clostridium* and bovine rotavirus, coronavirus, and/or *Escherichia coli* enteric diseases if needed.

Bulls (30-60 days prebreeding)
Deworm as needed (usually only for flukes in the fall).

Immunize with IBR-PI$_3$-BVD-BRSV (inactivated) and 5-way leptospirosis, *Campylobacter,* and anaplasmosis products.

FEEDLOT RECOMMENDATIONS
On Arrival Into the Feedlot
Deworm with a broad-spectrum dewormer, implant, and immunize for IBR, PI$_3$, BVD, BRSV (modified live vaccine), and clostridial diseases.

Castrate and dehorn if not already done.

Two Weeks After Arrival Into the Feedlot
Administer booster immunizations if necessary. Abort the heifers if necessary.

BRSV, Bovine respiratory syncytial virus; *BVD,* bovine virus diarrhea; *IBR,* infectious bovine rhinotracheitis; *IM,* intramuscular; *MLV,* modified live virus; *PI$_3$,* parainfluenza-3.

PREVENTIVE HEALTH PROGRAM FOR CATTLE

Preventive health programs for beef and dairy cattle are generally based on recommendations of the consulting veterinarian and the specific needs of the herd and the herdsman. Accordingly, the development of a vaccination program should be based on several factors. First, it is important to have an understanding of disease conditions present within a given herd and of the disease conditions present in the surrounding area. This should be based on accurate diagnosis or previous diagnoses of diseases in the specific herd and surrounding herds. Second, it is necessary to be familiar with the management procedures present on a farm that allow for a vaccination program designed around the working patterns of the herd; this is especially true for a cow-calf operation. Third, the population variances within a herd should be known. Vaccine choices and the frequency

of their use can vary depending on such factors as open versus closed herds, source of new replacement cattle, and feeding practices. General approaches to preventive health programs for beef and dairy cattle are presented in Box 11-4 and Table 11-4, respectively.

VACCINATIONS

Vaccines that may be included in preventive health programs for beef and dairy cattle can be obtained from manufacturers as individual components or in various combinations. Table 11-5 lists some vaccines currently available. Diseases for which vaccines are more frequently used in these preventive health programs are detailed in the following sections. In general, most cattle should be vaccinated for infectious bovine rhinotracheitis (IBR), parainfluenza-3, bovine respiratory syncytial virus, and bovine virus diarrhea (BVD) (to help prevent *shipping fever* or pneumonia and reproductive problems), as well as a 7- or 8-way clostridial

Table 11-4 GENERAL OUTLINE OF A PREVENTIVE HEALTH PROGRAM FOR DAIRY CATTLE*

CALVES
At Birth
Immunize with bovine rotavirus and coronavirus enteric disease vaccine, and administer *Escherichia coli* enteric disease vaccine orally.[†]

Weaning Age (about 2 mo) to Breeding Age (about 15 mo)

Immunizing Vaccine	Age for Vaccine Administration
Brucella abortus, strain RB-51 (calfhood vaccination—replacement heifers only)	4-12 mo
Clostridial diseases: *Clostridium perfringens* types C and D, *C. chauvoei, C. novyi,*	
C. septicum, C. sordellii, C. haemolyticum (if flukes are a problem)	2 mo, booster in 2 wk
IBR, PI₃, BVD, BRSV, leptospirosis, and campylobacteriosis	4-6 mo, booster in 2 wk, booster at 12-13 mo

DRY COWS AND BRED HEIFERS
The goal of dry cow immunization is to provide optimal protection for the newborn calf.

Immunizing Vaccine	Time of Vaccine Administration
IBR, PI₃, BVD, BRSV, leptospirosis, and campylobacteriosis	At time of dry-off
Bovine rotavirus and coronavirus enteric diseases[†]	At time of dry-off, booster in 2-3 wk
Escherichia coli enteric disease[†]	At time of dry-off, booster in 2-3 wk
Clostridial diseases: *C. perfringens* types C and D, *C. chauvoei, C. novyi, C. septicum,*	At time of dry-off, booster in 2-3 wk
C. sordellii, C. haemolyticum	

BRSV, Bovine respiratory syncytial virus; *BVD*, bovine virus diarrhea; *IBR*, infectious bovine rhinotracheitis; *PI-3*, parainfluenza-3.
*Other vaccines that may be incorporated into the vaccination program, depending on individual herd needs and diseases endemic to the area, include *Haemophilus somnus, Pasteurella* spp., *Salmonella* spp., *Clostridium haemolyticum*, anthrax, and anaplasmosis.
[†]Use if problem of neonatal calf diarrhea exists on the farm.

bacterin. In addition, breeding animals should routinely receive vaccination with a multivalent *Leptospira* bacterin in combination with a *Campylobacter* bacterin. It is strongly recommended that replacement heifers be vaccinated for brucellosis between 4 and 12 months of age.

> ✎ **TECHNICIAN NOTE**
>
> Most cattle are routinely vaccinated for the common respiratory viruses and clostridial diseases. In addition, breeding animals should receive protection against leptospirosis and campylobacteriosis, and heifers should be vaccinated for brucellosis.

Ideally, vaccination of the dam 4 to 6 weeks before calving against respiratory viruses and clostridial organisms allows provision of good colostral antibodies for the neonate. Reproductive bacterins such as those for leptospirosis and campylobacteriosis are most efficacious if given at least 4 weeks before breeding. Vaccine labels should be read carefully because some are not safe to use in pregnant cows or calves nursing pregnant cows. With the advent of the Meat Quality Assurance Program, proper administration of injections, including vaccines, is critical in all food animal species. All intramuscular and subcutaneous injections in cattle should be given in the neck if at all possible. An alternate site for subcutaneous injections is behind the

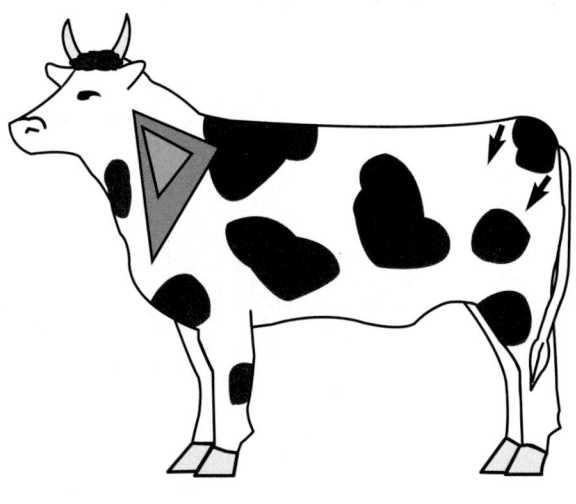

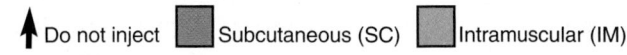
↑ Do not inject   ■ Subcutaneous (SC)   ■ Intramuscular (IM)

Figure 11-1 All injections in food animals should be given intramuscularly or subcutaneously in the neck region as outlined in this figure.

shoulder blade. Figure 11-1 shows the proper locations for injections in cattle (these sites are applicable to all food animal species). In general, no more than 10 ml of any product should be given per injection site, and multiple injections should be spaced several inches apart. A ¹/₂- to

Text continued on p. 362

Table 11-5 CATTLE VACCINES

Vaccine	Manufacturer	Type	Anthrax	BRSV	Brucella spp.	BVD Type I	BVD Type II	Campylobacter	Clostridium chauvoei	Clostridium haemolyticum	Clostridium novyi	Clostridium perfringens C &/or D	Clostridium septicum	Clostridium sordellii	Coronavirus	E. coli	Fusobacterium	Haemophilus somnus	IBR	Leptospira spp.	Moraxella bovis	Mycoplasma bovis	Neospora caninum	Papillomavirus	Pasteurella haemolytica*	Pasteurella multocida	Pl-3	Rabies	Rotavirus	Salmonella	Serpens spp	Serpulina (Treponema)	Staphylococcus spp.	Tetanus toxoid	Tritrichomonas
7-Gauge™	AgriPharm	K							X		X	X	X	X																					
7-Way	Aspen	K							X		X	X	X	X																					
7-Way/Somnus	Aspen	K							X		X	X	X	X				X																	
8-Way	Aspen	K							X	X	X	X	X	X																					
20/20 Vision® 7 with Spur®	Intervet	K							X		X	X	X	X																					
Alpha 7™	Boehringer Ingelheim	K							X		X	X	X	X																					
Alpha-7/MB™	Boehringer Ingelheim	K							X		X	X	X	X							X														
Alpha-CD™	Boehringer Ingelheim	K							X		X	X																							
Anthrax Spore Vaccine	Colorado Serum	LIVE	X																																
Antidote® PHM	AgriPharm	K																X			X				X										
Bar Somnus™	Boehringer Ingelheim	K																X																	
Bar Somnus 2P™	Boehringer Ingelheim	K																X							X	X									
Bar-Vac® 7	Boehringer Ingelheim	K							X		X	X	X	X																					
Bar-Vac® 7/Somnus	Boehringer Ingelheim	K							X		X	X	X	X				X																	
Bar-Vac® 8	Boehringer Ingelheim	K							X	X	X	X	X	X																					
Bar Vac® CD	Boehringer Ingelheim	K										X																							
Bar Vac® CD/T	Boehringer Ingelheim	K										X																						X	
Bovi-K® 4	Pfizer Animal Health	MLV/K		X		X	X												X								X								
Bovine 3	Durvet	MLV				X													X								X								
Bovine 8	Durvet	MLV/K				X	X												X	X							X								
Bovine 9	Durvet	MLV/K				X	X	X											X	X							X								
Bovine Pili Shield™	Novartis	K														X																			
Bovine Pili Shield™+C	Novartis	K										X				X																			
Bovine Rhinotracheitis-Parainfluenza-3 Vaccine	Colorado Serum	MLV																	X								X								
Bovine Rhinotracheitis Vaccine	Colorado Serum	MLV																	X																
Bovine Rhinotracheitis-Virus Diarrhea-Parainfluenza-3 Vaccine	Colorado Serum	MLV				X													X								X								
Bovine Virus Diarrhea Vaccine	Colorado Serum	MLV				X																													
Bovi-Shield™ 3	Pfizer Animal Health	MLV				X	X												X								X								
Bovi-Shield™ 4	Pfizer Animal Health	MLV		X		X	X												X								X								
BoviShield™ BRSV	Pfizer Animal Health	MLV		X																															
Bovi-Shield® FP 4+L5	Pfizer Animal Health	MLV/K		X		X	X												X	X							X								
Bovi-Shield™ IBR	Pfizer Animal Health	MLV																	X																

Continued

Table 11-5 Cattle Vaccines—cont'd

Vaccine	Manufacturer	Type	Anthrax	BRSV	Brucella spp.	BVD Type I	BVD Type II	Campylobacter	Clostridium chauvoei	Clostridium haemolyticum	Clostridium novyi	Clostridium perfringens C &/or D	Clostridium septicum	Clostridium sordellii	Coronavirus	E. coli	Fusobacterium	Haemophilus somnus	IBR	Leptospira spp.	Moraxella bovis	Mycoplasma bovis	Neospora caninum	Papillomavirus	Pasteurella haemolytica*	Pasteurella multocida	PI-3	Rabies	Rotavirus	Salmonella	Serpens spp.	Serpulina (Treponema)	Staphylococcus spp.	Tetanus toxoid	Tritrichomonas
BoviShield™ IBR-BRSV-LP	Pfizer Animal Health	MLV/K		X															X	X																
BoviShield™ IBR-BVD	Pfizer Animal Health	MLV				X	X												X																	
BoviShield™ IBR-BVD-BRSV-LP	Pfizer Animal Health	MLV/K		X		X	X												X	X																
BoviShield™ IBR-P13-BRSV	Pfizer Animal Health	MLV		X															X									X								
Breed-Back-10™	Boehringer Ingelheim	MLV/K		X		X	X	X											X	X								X								
Brucella Abortus Vaccine (Strain RB-51)	Professional Biological	LIVE			X																															
Calf-Guard®	Pfizer Animal Health	MLV													X															X						
Caliber® 3	Boehringer Ingelheim	K							X		X		X																							
Caliber® 7	Boehringer Ingelheim	K							X	X	X	X	X	X																						
Campylobacter Fetus Bacterin-Bovine	Colorado Serum	K						X																												
CattleMaster® 4	Pfizer Animal Health	MLV/K		X		X	X												X									X								
CattleMaster® 4+L5	Pfizer Animal Health	MLV/K		X		X	X												X	X								X								
CattleMaster® 4+VL5	Pfizer Animal Health	MLV/K		X		X	X	X											X	X								X								
CattleMaster® BVD-K	Pfizer Animal Health	K				X	X																													
Cattle-Vac™ 9-Somnus	Durvet	K		X		X	X											X	X	X								X								
Cattle-Vac™ EC	Durvet	K														X																				
Cattle Vac™ EC+C	Durvet	K										X				X																				
Cattle-Vac™ HS	Durvet	K																X																		
Cattle-Vac™ Pinkeye 4	Durvet	K																			X															
Cattle-Vac™ Salmo	Durvet	K																													X					
Cattle-Vac™ Vibrio-Plus	Durvet	K						X																												
C&D Toxoid	Aspen	K										X																								
Closti Bos™ BCD	Novartis	K										X																								
Clostridial 7-Way	AgriLabs	K							X	X	X	X	X	X																						
Clostridial 7-Way plus Somnumune®	AgriLabs	K							X	X	X	X	X	X				X																		
Clostridial 8-Way	AgriLabs	K							X	X	X	X	X	X																						
Clostridial BCD	Durvet	K										X																								
Clostridium Chauvoei-Septicum Bacterin	Colorado Serum	K							X				X																							
Clostridium Chauvoei-Septicum-Novyi-Sordellii Bacterin	Colorado Serum	K							X		X		X	X																						
Clostridium Chauvoei-Septicum-Pasteurella haemolytica-multocida	Colorado Serum	K							X				X													X	X									

Table 11-5 Cattle Vaccines—cont'd

Vaccine	Manufacturer	Type	Anthrax	BRSV	Brucella spp.	BVD Type I	BVD Type II	Campylobacter	Clostridium chauvoei	Clostridium haemolyticum	Clostridium novyi	Clostridium perfringens C &/or D	Clostridium septicum	Clostridium sordellii	Coronavirus	E. coli	Fusobacterium	Haemophilus somnus	IBR	Leptospira spp.	Moraxella bovis	Mycoplasma bovis	Neospora caninum	Papillomavirus	Pasteurella haemolytica*	Pasteurella multocida	PI-3	Rabies	Rotavirus	Salmonella	Serpens spp.	Serpulina (Treponema)	Staphylococcus spp.	Tetanus toxoid	Tritrichomonas
Clostridium Haemolyticum Bacterin (red water)	Colorado Serum	K								X																										
Clostridium Perfringens Types C&D – Tetanus Toxoid	Colorado Serum	K										X																							X	
Clostridium Perfringens Types C&D – Tetanus Toxoid	Prof. Biological	K										X																							X	
Clostridium Perfringens Types C&D Toxoid	Colorado Serum	K										X																								
Clostridium Perfringens Types C&D Toxoid	Prof. Biological	K										X																								
Clostri Shield® BCD	Novartis	K										X																								
Conquest™-4K	Aspen	K		X		X													X								X								
Conquest™-4K+H.S.	Aspen	K		X		X												X	X								X								
Conquest™-4KW	Aspen	K		X		X													X								X								
Conquest™-4KW+H.S.	Aspen	K		X		X												X	X								X								
Conquest™ 5K (oil base)	Aspen	K		X		X	X												X								X								
Conquest™5K+VL5 (oil base)	Aspen	K		X		X	X	X											X	X							X								
Conquest™-8K	Aspen	K		X		X	X												X	X							X								
Conquest™-9K	Aspen	K		X		X	X												X	X							X								
Conquest™-9K+H.S.	Aspen	K		X		X	X											X	X	X							X								
Conquest™ 10K	Aspen	K		X		X	X												X	X							X								
Covert™ 5	AgriPharm	MLV		X		X	X												X								X								
Covert™ 5-HS	AgriPharm	MLV/K		X		X	X											X	X								X								
Covert™ 10	AgriPharm	MLV/K		X		X	X												X	X							X								
Covert™ 10-HS	AgriPharm	MLV/K		X		X	X											X	X	X							X								
Covexin® 8 Vaccine	Schering-Plough	K							X	X	X	X	X	X																					X	
Cow-Vac® 9	Aspen	MLV/K		X		X	X	X											X	X							X								
Defensor® 3	Pfizer Animal Health	K																										X							
Durguard™ 4	Durvet	K		X		X													X								X								
Durguard™ 5	Durvet	K		X		X	X												X								X								
Durguard™ 5HS	Durvet	K		X		X	X											X	X								X								
Durguard™ 5HS+VL5	Durvet	K		X		X	X	X										X	X	X							X								
Durguard™ 5+VL5	Durvet	K		X		X	X	X											X	X							X								
Durguard™ 10	Durvet	K		X		X	X												X	X							X								

Continued

Table 11-5 CATTLE VACCINES—CONT'D

Vaccine	Manufacturer	Type	Anthrax	BRSV	Brucella spp.	BVD Type I	BVD Type II	Campylobacter	Clostridium chauvoei	Clostridium haemolyticum	Clostridium novyi	Clostridium perfringens C &/or D	Clostridium septicum	Clostridium sordellii	Coronavirus	E. coli	Fusobacterium	Haemophilus somnus	IBR	Leptospira spp.	Moraxella bovis	Mycoplasma bovis	Neospora caninum	Papillomavirus	Pasteurella haemolytica*	Pasteurella multocida	PI-3	Rabies	Rotavirus	Salmonella	Serpens spp.	Serpulina (Treponema)	Staphylococcus spp.	Tetanus toxoid	Tritrichomonas
Durguard™ 10HS	Durvet	K		X		X	X											X	X	X							X								
Electroid® 7 Vaccine	Schering-Plough	K							X		X	X	X	X						X															
Electroid® D	Schering-Plough	K										X																							
Elite 4™	Boehringer Ingelheim	K		X		X													X								X								
Elite 4-HS™	Boehringer Ingelheim	K		X		X												X	X								X								
Elite 9™	Boehringer Ingelheim	K		X		X													X	X							X								
Elite 9-HS™	Boehringer Ingelheim	K		X		X												X	X	X							X								
ENDOVAC-Bovi® with ImmunePlus®	Immvac	K														X														X					
EnterVene™-D	Fort Dodge	LIVE																												X					
Exalt™ 4	AgriPharm	K				X	X												X								X								
Exalt™ 4 + L5	AgriPharm	K				X	X												X	X							X								
Exalt™ 5	AgriPharm	K		X		X	X												X								X								
Exalt™ 5 + L5	AgriPharm	K		X		X	X												X	X							X								
Exalt™ 5 + Somnus	AgriPharm	K		X		X	X											X	X								X								
Exalt™ 5 + VL5	AgriPharm	K		X		X	X												X	X							X								
Express™ 3	Boehringer Ingelheim	MLV				X	X												X																
Express™ 3/Lp	Boehringer Ingelheim	MLV/K				X	X												X	X															
Express™ 4®	Boehringer Ingelheim	MLV/K		X		X	X												X								X								
Express™ 5	Boehringer Ingelheim	MLV		X		X	X												X								X								
Express™ 5-HS	Boehringer Ingelheim	MLV/K		X		X	X											X	X								X								
Express™ 5-PMH	Boehringer Ingelheim	MLV/K		X		X	X											X	X						X	X	X								
Express™ 10™	Boehringer Ingelheim	MLV/K		X		X	X												X	X							X								
Express™ 10-HS	Boehringer Ingelheim	MLV/K		X		X	X											X	X	X							X								
Express™ I	Boehringer Ingelheim	MLV				X	X												X																
Express™ IBP	Boehringer Ingelheim	MLV				X													X								X								
Express™ IBP/HS-2P	Boehringer Ingelheim	MLV/K				X												X	X						X	X	X								
Express™ I/Lp	Boehringer Ingelheim	MLV/L																	X	X															
Express™ IP/HS-2P	Boehringer Ingelheim	MLV/K																X	X						X	X	X								
Fortress® 7	Pfizer Animal Health	K							X	X	X	X	X	X																					
Fortress® 8	Pfizer Animal Health	K							X	X	X	X	X	X																					
Fortress® CD	Pfizer Animal Health	K										X																							
Fusion™ 4	Merial	MLV/K		X		X													X								X								
Fusoguard™	Novartis	K															X																		
Gauge™ C&D	AgriPharm	K										X																							

Table 11-5 Cattle Vaccines—cont'd

Vaccine	Manufacturer	Type	Anthrax	BRSV	Brucella spp.	BVD Type I	BVD Type II	Campylobacter	Clostridium chauvoei	Clostridium haemolyticum	Clostridium novyi	Clostridium perfringens C &/or D	Clostridium septicum	Clostridium sordellii	Coronavirus	E. coli	Fusobacterium	Haemophilus somnus	IBR	Leptospira spp.	Moraxella bovis	Mycoplasma bovis	Neospora caninum	Papillomavirus	Pasteurella haemolytica*	Pasteurella multocida	PI-3	Rabies	Rotavirus	Salmonella	Serpens spp.	Serpulina (T hyodysenteriae)	Staphylococcus spp.	Tetanus toxoid	Tritrichomonas
Herd-Vac™ 3	Biocor	MLV				X													X								X									
Herd-Vac™ 3 S	Biocor	MLV/K				X												X	X	X							X									
Herd-Vac™ 8	Biocor	MLV/K				X													X	X							X									
Herd-Vac™ 9	Biocor	MLV/K				X													X	X							X									
H. somnus Becterin	Aspen	K																X																		
IBL Vaccine	Aspen	MLV/K				X													X	X							X									
IBP-L5 Vaccine	Aspen	MLV/K				X													X	X							X									
IBP-SommuMune® Vaccine	Aspen	MLV/K				X												X	X	X							X									
IBP Vaccine	Aspen	MLV				X													X								X									
IL Vaccine	Aspen	MLV/K																	X	X																
Immrab® 3	Merial	K																										X								
Immrab® Large Animal	Merial	K																										X								
I-Site™	AgriLabs	K																			X															
J-5 Escherichia coli Bacterin	Hygieia	K														X																				
Jencine® 4	Schering-Plough	MLV		X		X	X												X								X									
J Vac®	Merial	K		X		X	X									X																				
Lepto 5	AgriLabs	K																		X																
Lepto-5	Boehringer Ingelheim	K																		X																
Lepto-5	Colorado Serum	K																		X																
Lepto 5	Durvet	K																		X																
Lepto 5	Premier Farmtech	K																		X																
Lepto 5 Vaccine	Aspen	K																		X																
Leptoferm-5®	Pfizer Animal Health	K																		X																
Lepto Shield™ 5	Novartis	K																		X																
Lepto Shield™ 5 Hardjo Bovis	Novartis	K																		X																
Lysigin®	Boehringer Ingelheim	K																																X		
Master Guard™ 10	AgriLabs	MLV/K		X		X	X												X	X							X									
Master Guard® 10	Intervet	MLV/K		X		X	X												X	X							X									
Master Guard® 10 + Vibrio	AgriLabs	MLV/K		X		X	X	X											X	X							X									
Master Guard® J5	AgriLabs	K														X																				
Master Guard™ Preg 5	AgriLabs	MLV/K		X		X	X												X	X							X									
Master Guard® Preg 5	Intervet	MLV/K		X		X	X												X	X							X									
Maxi/Guard® Pinkeye Bacterin	Addison	K																			X															
Mycoplasma bovis Bacterin	Biomune	K																				X														

Continued

Table 11-5 CATTLE VACCINES—CONT'D

Vaccine	Manufacturer	Type	Anthrax	BRSV	Brucella spp.	BVD Type I	BVD Type II	Campylobacter	Clostridium chauvoei	Clostridium haemolyticum	Clostridium novyi	Clostridium perfringens C &/or D	Clostridium septicum	Clostridium sordellii	Coronavirus	E. coli	Fusobacterium	Haemophilus somnus	IBR	Leptospira spp.	Moraxella bovis	Mycoplasma bovis	Neospora caninum	Papillomavirus	Pasteurella haemolytica*	Pasteurella multocida	PI-3	Rabies	Rotavirus	Salmonella	Serpens spp.	Serpulina (Treponema)	Staphylococcus spp.	Tetanus toxoid	Tritrichomonas
Nasalgen® IP Vaccine	Schering-Plough	MLV																	X								X								
Nasal-Vax™	AgriPharm	MLV																	X								X								
Neoguard™	Intervet	K																					X												
Ocu-guard® MB	Boehringer Ingelheim	K																			X														
Once PMH®	Intervet	MLV																							X	X									
OneShot®	Pfizer Animal Health	K																							X										
OneShot Ultra™ 7	Pfizer Animal Health	K							X		X	X	X	X											X										
One Shot Ultra™ 8	Pfizer Animal Health	K							X		X	X	X	X											X										
Papillomune™	Biomune	K																						X											
Pasteurella Haemolytica Multocida Bacterin	Colorado Serum	K																							X	X									
P.H.M. Bac® 1	AgriLabs	MLV																							X	X									
Piliguard® E. Coli-1	Schering-Plough	K														X																			
Piliguard® Pinkeye-1	Durvet	K																			X														
Piliguard® Pinkeye-1	Schering-Plough	K																			X														
Piliguard® Pinkeye + 7	Schering-Plough	K							X		X	X	X	X							X														
Pinkeye-3	Aspen	K																			X														
Pinkeye Shield™ XT4	Novartis	K																			X														
Poly-Bac B® 3	Texas Vet Lab	K																							X	X									
Poly-Bac B® 7	Texas Vet Lab	K																X							X	X				X					
Poly-Bac B® Somnus	Texas Vet Lab	K																X							X	X				X					
Presponse® HM	Fort Dodge	K																							X	X									
Presponse® SQ	Fort Dodge	K																							X										
Pre-Vent 6™	Agrilabs	K						X												X															
Prism™ 4	Fort Dodge	MLV/K		X		X	X												X								X								
Prism™ 9	Fort Dodge	MLV/K		X		X	X												X	X							X								
ProSystem® Pilimune	Intervet	K														X																			
Pulmo-guard™ PH-M	Boehringer Ingelheim	K																							X	X									
Pulmo-guard™ PHM-1	Boehringer Ingelheim	K																							X	X									
Pyramid® 4+Presponse® SQ	Fort Dodge	MLV/K		X		X													X						X		X								
Pyramid® 8	Fort Dodge	MLV/K				X	X												X								X								
Pyramid® 9	Fort Dodge	MLV/K		X		X	X												X	X							X								
Pyramid® IBR	Fort Dodge	MLV																	X																
Pyramid® IBR+Lepto	Fort Dodge	MLV/K																	X	X															

Continued

Table 11-5 CATTLE VACCINES—CONT'D

Vaccine	Manufacturer	Type	Anthrax	BRSV	Brucella spp.	BVD Type I	BVD Type II	Campylobacter	Clostridium chauvoei	Clostridium haemolyticum	Clostridium novyi	Clostridium perfringens C &/or D	Clostridium septicum	Clostridium sordellii	Coronavirus	E. coli	Fusobacterium	Haemophilus somnus	IBR	Leptospira spp.	Moraxella bovis	Mycoplasma bovis	Neospora caninum	Papillomavirus	Pasteurella haemolytica*	Pasteurella multocida	PI-3	Rabies	Rotavirus	Salmonella	Serpens spp.	Serpulina (Treponema)	Staphylococcus spp.	Tetanus toxoid	Tritrichomonas
Pyramid® MLV 3	Fort Dodge	MLV		X															X								X								
Pyramid® MLV 4	Fort Dodge	MLV		X		X													X								X								
Quick Shield™ Intranasal IBR+PI3	Novartis	MLV																	X								X								
Rabdomun® Vaccine	Schering-Plough	K																										X							
Reliant® 3	Merial	MLV		X		X													X								X								
Reliant® 4	Merial	MLV/K		X		X													X								X								
Reliant® 8	Merial	MLV/K				X													X	X							X								
Reliant® IBR	Merial	MLV																	X																
Reliant® IBR/BVD	Merial	MLV				X													X																
Reliant® IBR/Lepto	Merial	MLV/K																	X	X							X								
Reliant® Plus BVD-K (Dual IBR™)	Merial	MLV/K		X		X													X								X								
Reliant® Plus Plus (Dual IBR™)	Merial	MLV/K		X		X													X								X								
Resist™ 7	AgriPharm	K							X		X	X	X	X																					
Resist™ 7HS	AgriPharm	K							X		X	X	X	X				X																	
Resist™ 8	AgriPharm	K							X	X	X	X	X	X																					
Repishield™ 4	Merial	K		X		X													X								X								
Respishield™ 4 L5	Merial	K		X		X													X	X							X								
Respromune® 4	AgriLabs	K		X		X	X												X								X								
ResProMune® 4 I-B-P+BRSV	AgriLabs	K		X		X	X												X								X								
ResProMune® 4+SomnuMune® (I.M.)	AgriLabs	K		X		X												X	X								X								
ResProMune® 4+SomnuMune® (I.M., S.C.)	AgriLabs	K				X												X	X								X								
ResProMune® 5+VL5	AgriLabs	K		X		X		X											X	X							X								
ResProMune® 8	AgriLabs	K		X		X												X	X	X							X								
ResProMune® 9	AgriLabs	K		X		X												X	X	X							X								
ResProMune® 10	AgriLabs	K		X		X												X	X	X							X								
Resvac® 4/Somnumbac®	Pfizer Animal Health	MLV/K		X		X												X	X								X								
Resvac® BRSV/Somubac®	Pfizer Animal Health	MLV/K		X																															
Salmonella Dublin-Typhimurium Bacterin	Colorado Serum	K																												X					
Salmo Shield® T	Novartis	K																												X					
Salmo Shield® TD	Novartis	K																												X					
Salmo Vac	AgriPharm	K																												X					

Table 11-5 CATTLE VACCINES—CONT'D

Vaccine	Manufacturer	Type	Anthrax	BRSV	Brucella spp.	BVD Type I	BVD Type II	Campylobacter	Clostridium chauvoei	Clostridium haemolyticum	Clostridium novyi	Clostridium perfringens C &/or D	Clostridium septicum	Clostridium sordellii	Coronavirus	E. coli	Fusobacterium	Haemophilus somnus	IBR	Leptospira spp.	Moraxella bovis	Mycoplasma bovis	Neospora caninum	Papillomavirus	Pasteurella haemolytica*	Pasteurella multocida	PI-3	Rabies	Rotavirus	Salmonella	Serpens spp.	Serpulina (Treponema)	Staphylococcus spp.	Tetanus toxoid	Tritrichomonas
Scour Bos™ 4	Novartis	K										X			X														X						
Scour Bos™ 6	Novartis	K													X	X																			
Scour Bos™ 9	Novartis	K										X			X	X													X						
ScourGuard 3® (K)	Pfizer Animal Health	K													X	X													X						
ScourGuard 3® (K)/C	Pfizer Animal Health	K										X			X	X													X						
Scour Vac™ 2K	Durvet	K													X	X													X						
Scour Vac™ 3K+C	Durvet	K										X			X	X													X						
Scour Vac™ 4	AgriLabs	K										X			X	X													X						
Scour Vac™ 9	AgriLabs	K										X			X	X													X						
Scour Vac™ E coli + C	AgriLabs	K										X				X																			
SDT-Guard™	Boehringer Ingelheim	K																												X					
Serpens Species Bacterin	Hygieia	K																													X				
Siteguard® G	Schering-Plough	K										X		X																					
Siteguard® MLG Vaccine	Schering-Plough	K							X	X	X	X	X	X																					
SomnuMune®	AgriLabs	K																X																	
Somnu Shield™	Novartis	K																X																	
Somnu Shield™ XT	Novartis	K																X																	
Somubac®	Pfizer Animal Health	K																X																	
Staphylococcus aureus Bacterin-Toxoid	Hygieia	K																															X		
StayBred VL5™	Pfizer Animal Health	K						X												X															
Super Poly-Bac B® Somnus	Texas Vet Lab	K																X								X	X				X				
Super-Tet® with Havlogen®	Intervet	K																																X	
Surround™ 4	Biocor	K		X		X													X								X								
Surround™ 4+HS	Biocor	K		X		X												X	X								X								
Surround™ 8	Biocor	K		X		X													X	X							X								
Surround™ 9	Biocor	K		X		X													X	X							X								
Surround™ 9+HS	Biocor	K		X		X												X	X	X							X								
Surround™ HS	Biocor	K																X																	
Surround™ L5	Biocor	K																		X															
Surround™ V-L5	Biocor	K					X													X															
Syn Shield™	Novartis	K		X																															
Tetanus Toxoid-Concentrated	Colorado Serum	K																																X	
Tetanus Toxoid-Concentrated	Prof. Biological	K																																X	

Continued

Table 11-5 Cattle Vaccines—cont'd

Vaccine	Manufacturer	Type	Anthrax	BRSV	Brucella spp.	BVD Type I	BVD Type II	Campylobacter	Clostridium chauvoei	Clostridium haemolyticum	Clostridium novyi	Clostridium perfringens C &/or D	Clostridium septicum	Clostridium sordellii	Coronavirus	E. coli	Fusobacterium	Haemophilus somnus	IBR	Leptospira spp.	Moraxella bovis	Mycoplasma bovis	Neospora caninum	Papillomavirus	Pasteurella haemolytica*	Pasteurella multocida	PI-3	Rabies	Rotavirus	Salmonella	Serpens spp.	Serpulina (Treponema)	Staphylococcus spp.	Tetanus toxoid	Tritrichomonas
Tetanus Toxoid-UnConcentrated	Colorado Serum	K																																X	
Tetguard™	Boehringer Ingelheim	K							X	X	X	X	X																					X	
Tetni-Vax®	AgriPharm	K								X	X	X	X																					X	
Tetnogen®	Fort Dodge	K								X	X	X																						X	
Titanium™ 3	Agrilabs	MLV				X	X												X																
Titanium® 3	Intervet	MLV				X	X												X																
Titanium® 3+BRSV	Intervet	MLV		X		X	X												X																
Titanium™ 3+BRSV LP	Agrilabs	MLV/K		X		X	X												X	X															
Titanium® 3+BRSV LP	Intervet	MLV/K		X		X	X												X	X															
Titanium™ 4	Agrilabs	MLV				X	X												X									X							
Titanium™ 4 L5	Agrilabs	MLV/K				X	X												X	X							X							
Titanium™ 5	Agrilabs	MLV		X		X	X												X									X							
Titanium® 5	Intervet	MLV		X		X	X												X									X							
Titanium™ 5 L5	Agrilabs	MLV/K		X		X	X												X	X							X							
Titanium® 5 L5	Intervet	MLV/K		X		X	X												X	X							X							
Titanium™ 5+P.H.M. Bac®-1	Agrilabs	MLV		X		X	X												X						X	X	X								
Titanium® 5+P.H.M. Bac®-1	Intervet	MLV		X		X	X												X						X	X	X								
Titanium™ BRSV	Agrilabs	MLV		X														X	X							X								
Titanium® BRSV	Intervet	MLV		X														X	X															
Titanium™ BRSV 3	Agrilabs	MLV		X															X								X							
Titanium® BRSV 3	Intervet	MLV		X															X								X							
Titanium™ IBR	AgriLabs	MLV																	X															
Titanium® IBR	Intervet	MLV																	X															
Titanium™ IBR-LP	AgriLabs	MLV/K																	X	X														
Titervac™ 5	Aspen	MLV		X		X	X												X								X							
Titervac™ 5-HS	Aspen	MLV/K		X		X	X											X	X								X							
Titervac™ 10	Aspen	MLV/K		X		X	X												X	X							X							
Titervac™ 10-HS	Aspen	MLV/K		X		X	X											X	X	X							X							
Treponema Bacterin	Novartis	K																														X			
Triangle® 1 + Type II BVD	Fort Dodge	K				X	X																											
Triangle® 3 + Type II BVD	Fort Dodge	K				X	X												X								X							
Triangle® 3 V5L	Fort Dodge	K				X		X											X	X							X							
Triangle® 4+HS	Fort Dodge	K		X		X												X	X								X							

Table 11-5 CATTLE VACCINES—cont'd

Vaccine	Manufacturer	Type	Anthrax	BRSV	Brucella spp.	BVD Type I	BVD Type II	Campylobacter	Clostridium chauvoei	Clostridium haemolyticum	Clostridium novyi	Clostridium perfringens C &/or D	Clostridium septicum	Clostridium sordellii	Coronavirus	E. coli	Fusobacterium	Haemophilus somnus	IBR	Leptospira spp.	Moraxella bovis	Mycoplasma bovis	Neospora caninum	Papillomavirus	Pasteurella haemolytica*	Pasteurella multocida	PI-3	Rabies	Rotavirus	Salmonella	Serpens spp.	Serpulina (Treponema)	Staphylococcus spp.	Tetanus toxoid	Tritrichomonas
Triangle® 4+PH/HS	Fort Dodge	K		X		X												X	X						X		X								
Triangle® 4+PH-K	Fort Dodge	K		X		X													X						X		X								
Triangle® 4 + Type II BVD	Fort Dodge	K		X		X	X												X								X								
Triangle® 8 + Type II BVD	Fort Dodge	K		X		X	X												X								X								
Triangle® 9+HS	Fort Dodge	K		X		X												X	X								X								
Triangle® 9+PH-K	Fort Dodge	K		X		X													X						X		X								
Triangle® 9 + Type II BVD	Fort Dodge	K		X		X	X												X								X								
TrichGuard®	Fort Dodge	K																																	X
TrichGuard®V5L	Fort Dodge	K						X												X															X
TriVib 5L®	Fort Dodge	K						X												X															
Trustgard™ 5L	Vedco	K																		X															
Trustgard™ 7	Vedco	K							X	X	X	X	X	X																					
Trustgard™ 7/HS	Vedco	K							X	X	X	X	X	X				X																	
Trustgard™ 8	Vedco	K							X	X	X	X	X	X																					
Trustgard™ CD	Vedco	K										X																							
Trustgard™ CD/T	Vedco	K										X																						X	
Trustgard™ HS	Vedco	K																X																	
Trustgard™ MB	Vedco	K																			X														
Trustgard™ Vibrio/5L	Vedco	K						X												X															
TSV-2®	Pfizer Animal Health	MLV																	X								X								
Ultrabac® 7	Pfizer Animal Health	K							X	X	X	X	X	X																					
Ultrabac® 7/Somnubac®	Pfizer Animal Health	K							X	X	X	X	X	X				X																	
Ultrabac® 8	Pfizer Animal Health	K							X	X	X	X	X	X																					
Ultrabac® CD	Pfizer Animal Health	K										X																							
Ultrachoice™ 7	Pfizer Animal Health	K							X	X	X	X	X	X																					
Ultrachoice™ 8	Pfizer Animal Health	K							X	X	X	X	X	X																					
Ultrachoice™ CD	Pfizer Animal Health	K										X																							
Upjohn J-5 Bacterin™	Pharmacia & Upjohn	K														X																			
Vibralone™-L5	Intervet	K						X												X															
Vibrin®	Pfizer Animal Health	K						X																											
Vibrio-Lepto 5	Agriabs	K						X												X															
Vibrio-Lepto-5™	Boehringer Ingelheim	K						X												X															
Vibrio-Lepto 5	Durvet	K						X												X															
Vibrio-Lepto 5	Premier Farmtech	K						X												X															

Table 11-5 Cattle Vaccines—cont'd

Vaccine	Manufacturer	Type	Anthrax	BRSV	Brucella spp.	BVD Type I	BVD Type II	Campylobacter	Clostridium chauvoei	Clostridium haemolyticum	Clostridium novyi	Clostridium perfringens C &/or D	Clostridium septicum	Clostridium sordelii	Coronavirus	E. coli	Fusobacterium	Haemophilus somnus	IBR	Leptospira spp.	Moraxella bovis	Mycoplasma bovis	Neospora caninum	Papillomavirus	Pasteurella haemolytica*	Pasteurella multocida	PI-3	Rabies	Rotavirus	Salmonella	Serpens spp.	Serpulina (Treponema)	Staphylococcus spp.	Tetanus toxoid	Tritrichomonas
Vibrio–Lepto 5 (oil base)	Aspen	K						X												X															
Vibrio–Lepto 5 Vaccine	Aspen	K						X												X															
Vibrio/Leptoferm-5™	Pfizer Animal Health	K						X												X															
Vib Shield®	Novartis	K						X																											
Vib Shield® L5	Novartis	K						X												X															
Vib Shield® L5 Hardjo bovis	Novartis	K						X												X															
Vib Shield® Plus	Novartis	K						X																											
Vib Shield® Plus L5	Novartis	K						X												X															
Vira Shield® 2	Novartis	K				X	X																												
Vira Shield® 2+BRSV	Novartis	K		X		X	X																												
Vira Shield® 3	Novartis	K				X	X												X																
Vira Shield® 3+VL5	Novartis	K				X	X	X											X	X															
Vira Shield® 4	Novartis	K				X	X												X								X								
Vira Shield® 4+L5	Novartis	K				X	X												X	X							X								
Vira Shield® 5	Novartis	K		X		X	X												X								X								
Vira Shield® 5+L5	Novartis	K		X		X	X												X	X							X								
Vira Shield® 5+L5 Somnus	Novartis	K		X		X	X											X	X	X							X								
Vira Shield® 5+Somnus	Novartis	K		X		X	X											X	X								X								
Vira Shield® 5+VL5	Novartis	K		X		X	X	X											X	X							X								
Vira Shield®+VL5 Somnus	Novartis	K		X		X	X	X										X	X	X							X								
Vision® 7 Somnus with Spur®	Intervet	K							X	X	X	X	X	X				X																	
Vision® 7 with Spur®	Intervet	K							X	X	X	X	X	X																					
Vision® 8 Somnus with Spur®	Intervet	K							X	X	X	X	X	X				X																	
Vision® 8 with Spur®	Intervet	K							X	X	X	X	X	X																					
Vision® CD-T with Spur®	Intervet	K										X																						X	
Vision® CD with Spur®	Intervet	K										X																							
VL5-1X	Durvet	K						X												X															
VL5-1X Plus™	Durvet	K						X												X															
Volar®	Intervet	K															X																		
Wart Shield™	Novartis	K																						X											
Wart-Vac	Durvet	K																						X											
Wart Vaccine	AgriLabs	K																						X											
Wart Vaccine	Colorado Serum	K																						X											

BRSV, Bovine respiratory syncytial virus; *BVD*, bovine virus diarrhea; *IBR*, infectious bovine rhinotracheitis; *K*, killed; *MLV*, modified live virus; *PI-3*, parainfluenza-3.

Pasteurella haemolytica was renamed *Mannheimia haemolytica* in 1999.

³/₄-inch, 18- or 16-gauge needle is recommended for subcutaneous injections and a 1- to 1¹/₂-inch, 18- to 16-gauge needle is suggested for intramuscular injections.

> ✏ **TECHNICIAN NOTE**
>
> For compliance with meat quality assurance standards, vaccines should be administered as labeled (intramuscular or subcutaneous) only in the neck region of all food animal species, regardless of the use or age of the animal.

Administration of most vaccines requires observation of a slaughter withdrawal, some as long as 60 days. The veterinary technician can be instrumental in educating owners concerning proper vaccination administration and appropriate vaccine slaughter withdrawals.

> ✏ **TECHNICIAN NOTE**
>
> Use of most vaccines administered to cattle requires observation of a slaughter withdrawal and accompanying client education.

BOVINE RESPIRATORY DISEASE COMPLEX VACCINES

There are several viruses and bacteria that are widespread in the cattle population and are considered to be the major contributors to the bovine respiratory disease complex. Multiple infections may occur with these viruses, and secondary infections with these bacteria often exacerbate the primary diseases produced.

Parainfluenza-3 virus causes a mild respiratory disease that is often associated with shipment of cattle to the feedlot (and thus commonly referred to as *shipping fever*). Clinical signs may include fever, serous to mucopurulent nasal discharge, coughing, increased respiratory rate, weakness, depression, and weight loss.

IBR virus causes high fever, nasal discharge, conjunctivitis, increased respiratory rate, coughing, dyspnea, and severe hyperemia of the muzzle (commonly referred to as red nose). IBR can also be responsible for abortions in pregnant cattle.

BVD virus can cause respiratory disease and is often confused with or obscured by the other viruses of this complex. In addition to the respiratory disease, the virus may also cause a mild transient diarrhea and may be associated with abortions or birth of malformed or weak calves if the primary infection occurs during pregnancy. The chronic form of BVD, known as *mucosal disease*, often results in ulcerative lesions throughout the alimentary tract, causing persistent diarrhea and usually death. In general, attenuated (modified live virus) vaccines containing IBR or BVD should *not* be administered intramuscularly to pregnant cows or to calves being nursed by pregnant cows because abortion may result. Intranasal attenuated IBR vaccines *are* safe, however, for pregnant cows or calves being nursed by pregnant cows.

Bovine respiratory syncytial virus has been recognized in recent years as a major viral component of the bovine respiratory disease complex. Infection typically causes anorexia, coughing, increased respiratory rate, serous ocular and nasal discharge, fever, pulmonary edema and emphysema, as well as subcutaneous emphysema and intermandibular edema. Death may occur rapidly, as early as 48 hours after onset of infection.

The bacteria *Mannheimia haemolytica* (formerly *Pasteurella haemolytica*) and *Pasteurella multocida* are normal inhabitants of the bovine respiratory tract and therefore are common secondary bacterial invaders in cases of primary viral pneumonia in cattle. In addition, these bacteria contribute to a primary fibrinous pneumonia and pleuritis that are readily apparent at necropsy. Clinical signs associated with these *Mannheimia/Pasteurella* organisms may include fever, coughing, dyspnea, mucopurulent nasal discharge, depression, anorexia, and, in severe cases, death.

The bacterium *Haemophilus somnus* is another bacterial pathogen that can be a part of the bovine respiratory disease complex. It ranks second to *M. haemolytica* as the most frequent isolate from acute cases of fibrinopurulent pneumonia. *H. somnus* infection often develops as a septicemia, which can progress to fibrinous pleuritis, pericarditis, polyarthritis, or thromboembolic meningoencephalitis (also known as TEME or sleeper's syndrome).

> ✏ **TECHNICIAN NOTE**
>
> Respiratory virus infection in cattle marks the beginning of "shipping fever" and often leads to severe secondary bacterial pneumonia.

Many vaccines are currently available for these virus- and bacterium-induced bovine respiratory diseases. The vaccines contain these agents in various combinations and in the attenuated (modified live virus) or inactivated forms.

CLOSTRIDIAL VACCINES

Clostridial infections are caused by bacteria that live as spores in the soil. These spores may be ingested by cattle as they graze or may enter the body via wound contamination. The more common clostridial infections encountered in cattle are described briefly in the following paragraphs.

Infections with *Clostridium chauvoei* (the causative agent of blackleg), *Clostridium septicum* (the causative agent of malignant edema), and *Clostridium sordellii* primarily affect striated muscles. The spores of these organisms are deposited in muscles by the circulation after ingestion or via wound contamination. When conditions of reduced oxygen tension within these muscles exist (e.g., trauma during handling, transporting, butting, or riding), the spores vegetate and the resulting organisms multiply. Toxins released by the multiplying organisms rapidly destroy the muscles and cause death through destructive effects on vital organs. Death may occur suddenly, as early as 12 hours after onset of infection.

Infections with *Clostridium novyi* type B and *Clostridium haemolyticum* (also known as *Clostridium novyi* type D) primarily affect the liver. These spores are usually ingested and travel by the circulation to the liver, where they remain latent until some form of liver damage occurs, which allows the spores to vegetate and the resulting organisms to multiply. Predisposing factors that may activate the spores in the liver include the presence of liver flukes, migrating parasites, abscesses, bacterial hepatitis, fatty infiltration, and various hepatotoxins. Potent toxins produced by the multiplying bacteria are absorbed systematically and cause death through destructive effects on vital organs and blood vessels. Death may occur suddenly, as early as 24 hours after onset of infection. It is highly recommended that clostridial bacterins containing *C. haemolyticum* be used in cattle vaccination programs in regions of the country where liver flukes exist.

Infections with *Clostridium perfringens* types B, C, and D primarily affect the gastrointestinal tract. These organisms are normal inhabitants of the gastrointestinal tract of cattle and tend to proliferate under conditions of reduced oxygen tension created by consumption of large quantities of concentrate feed or sudden changes in feed. With favorable conditions, the organisms multiply rapidly and produce toxins that can cause several intestinal lesions leading to a hemorrhagic, necrotic enteritis and sudden death, particularly in young, rapidly growing animals.

Because these clostridial infections commonly occur in cattle, routine vaccination for clostridial infections is highly recommended.

> **✎ TECHNICIAN NOTE**
>
> Clostridial infections causing sudden death commonly occur in cattle; therefore routine vaccination is highly recommended.

LEPTOSPIROSIS VACCINE

Leptospirosis is a common bacterial disease of cattle that may cause hemolytic anemia, nephritis, decreased milk production, and late-term abortion. Abortion is probably the most economically significant effect of the disease. Regular vaccination of breeding animals for leptospirosis is strongly encouraged. Heifers should be vaccinated two or three times at monthly intervals before breeding and again at midgestation of the first pregnancy. Because leptospirosis bacterins produce immunity of fairly short duration, annual (prebreeding) or twice-annual (prebreeding and midgestation) boosters should be given.

CAMPYLOBACTERIOSIS (VIBRIOSIS) VACCINE

Campylobacteriosis is a venereal disease of cattle caused by the bacterium *Campylobacter fetus*. Infection of a cow's genital tract often causes early embryonic death, resulting in temporary infertility, repeat breeding, delayed conception, and a prolonged calving interval. The *Campylobacter* organism may be transmitted during coitus or by artificial insemination with contaminated semen. Systemic vaccination can cure and prevent *Campylobacter* infection. Vaccination of breeding stock is highly recommended.

BRUCELLOSIS VACCINE

Brucellosis is caused by the organism *Brucella abortus*. Infection in the cow can result in late-term abortion, usually around 5 months or more into gestation, and shedding of the *Brucella* organisms in the milk. In bulls, infection results in orchitis, impaired fertility, and shedding of *Brucella* organisms in the semen. Brucellosis is a serious human health hazard (zoonotic disease), so known *Brucella*-positive reactors must be culled from the herd, and vaccination of replacement heifers must be performed. *B. abortus* strain RB-51 vaccine is a live bacterial product that confers long-term, cell-mediated protection. Only female cattle are vaccinated for brucellosis with strain RB-51 live culture vaccine. Age at vaccination of heifers is critical and usually determined by federal and state regulations. Under current regulations, only heifers between the ages of 4 and 12 months can be vaccinated for brucellosis. Vaccination is only undertaken by accredited veterinarians or state or federal animal health representatives. Care must always be exercised when *B. abortus* vaccine is used, because accidental injection, ingestion, or exposure through broken skin or mucous membranes can result in human brucellosis (undulant fever). An alternative to vaccination of beef heifers destined for the feedlot is ovariectomy or spaying.

> **✎ TECHNICIAN NOTE**
>
> All heifers (dairy or beef) should be vaccinated for brucellosis between 4 and 12 months of age.

TRICHOMONIASIS VACCINE

Trichomoniasis, caused by *Tritrichomonas foetus*, is a venereal protozoal disease of cattle that manifests as infertility, relatively early abortion, or pyometra. It causes virtually no systemic illness, so its presence within a herd may go undetected for long periods, resulting in substantial economic losses. The bull serves as an asymptomatic carrier, and the organism may be spread by natural breeding or artificial insemination with contaminated semen. Inactivated protozoal vaccines are now commercially available to aid in prevention of the disease in known problem herds.

ANTHRAX VACCINE

Anthrax is caused by the bacterium *Bacillus anthracis* and is characterized by septicemia and sudden death. Often, affected animals are simply found dead without any prior signs of illness. Typically, the dead animal exhibits blood oozing from body orifices, failure of blood to clot, and absence of rigor mortis. Differential diagnosis of sudden death in cattle may include anthrax, lightning strike, clostridial diseases, and anaplasmosis. Vaccination for anthrax is recommended 4 weeks before anticipated exposure in those areas where the disease has historically been a problem.

ANAPLASMOSIS VACCINE

Anaplasmosis in the United States is a common rickettsial disease of cattle and is caused by the intraerythrocytic parasite *Anaplasma marginale*. Affected red blood cells are destroyed by the liver and spleen, resulting in a severe anemia. Clinical signs caused by an acute anemia may include pale mucous membranes, weakness, depression or aggressive behavior, and increased heart and respiratory rates. Anaplasmosis often causes sudden death and must be differentiated from anthrax and the clostridial diseases.

Currently, there is no vaccine commercially available for prevention of anaplasmosis. It is anticipated that a vaccine will be available again within the next several years.

ENTERIC DISEASE VACCINE

Bovine rotavirus and coronavirus, as well as enterotoxigenic bacterial strains of *Escherichia coli*, are often isolated from calves with diarrhea. These organisms may occur in combination or with other bacterial, viral, or protozoal pathogens. The combination of enterotoxins produced by *E. coli* and the cytopathogenic effects of rotavirus and coronavirus induces secretion of large amounts of fluid and electrolytes into the lumen of the gut, resulting in diarrhea, dehydration, and, in severe cases, death. Vaccines are currently available for immunization of pregnant heifers or cows before calving. Some of these vaccines are also designed for oral administration to newborn calves.

✎ TECHNICIAN NOTE

Cows and heifers can be vaccinated for rotavirus, coronavirus and/or *E. coli* 6 weeks before calving if neonatal calf diarrhea caused by any of these pathogens is a herd problem.

MORAXELLA VACCINE

Moraxella bovis is the principal cause of infectious bovine keratoconjunctivitis, commonly referred to as *pinkeye*. Infection may result in characteristic clinical signs, including epiphora, blepharospasm, photophobia, corneal ulcers, corneal edema, and chemosis. Healing may occur at any stage; but occasionally, with or without appropriate treatment, an affected cornea may perforate, resulting in loss

of vision. Several inactivated vaccines are now available for protection against infection by *M. bovis*.

EXTERNAL AND INTERNAL PARASITES

Control of external parasites, especially lice and grubs, may be achieved with repeated applications of approved insecticidal sprays or pour-on products or with the use of ivermectin. Many commercial products are currently available for effective treatment of lice and grubs. Always follow the manufacturer's labeled instructions carefully, and closely observe the slaughter and milk withdrawal times when using these products. Some products are not recommended for use in Brahmans, Brahman crosses, or exotic cattle breeds.

The most common internal parasites of beef and dairy cattle are the barber's pole worm (*Haemonchus* spp.), the brown stomach worm (*Ostertagia* spp.), the bankrupt worm (*Trichostrongylus* spp.), the hookworm (*Bunostomum* spp.), Cooper's worm (*Cooperia* spp.), the intestinal worm (*Nematodirus* spp.), the nodular worm (*Oesophagostomum* spp.), the lungworm (*Dictyocaulus* spp.), and the liver fluke (*Fasciola* spp.). In general, it is a good idea to deworm calves at least once before weaning and again at weaning. Cows, heifers, and bulls should be dewormed as needed. Many commercial dewormers are currently available. Product choice depends on the parasite or parasites identified by fecal examination within a herd and the resistance patterns of those parasites. Cattle raised in locales where liver flukes exist should be treated in the spring and/or fall. Chapter 7 contains additional information on parasitology and specific drug therapy.

Several commercial growth stimulant implants that are designed to improve feed efficiency and increase feed savings are currently available for beef cattle. Most implants contain anabolic agents, such as estradiol, progesterone, testosterone, zeranol, or combinations of these agents. The type of implant and its scheduled use depend on the sex and age of calves implanted, as well as the needs of the herdsman. Ruminant nutrition is discussed in Chapter 16.

MANAGEMENT RECOMMENDATIONS FOR DAIRY CALVES

The ultimate goal in raising replacement heifers is to produce healthy heifers that will calve and enter the milking herd by 24 months of age (Table 11-4). Probably the single most important factor in successful rearing of calves is to ensure that the calves ingest colostrum soon after birth. If a calf does not nurse on its own shortly after birth, the herdsman should administer at least 2 L of warm colostrum to the calf within the first hour. During the first 3 days of life, the herdsman should continue to administer the colostrum at 10% of the calf's body weight daily in two feedings (e.g., a 40 kg calf should receive 2 L of colostrum twice daily).

After this time, the calf can be switched to whole milk or a good quality commercial milk replacer administered at 10% of its body weight daily divided into two feedings. For the neonatal calf, it is important to use a milk replacer that contains 20% to 22% crude protein, all of which is milk derived, and 18% to 20% crude fat. Fresh water should be provided at all times, and grain (18% to 20% protein) and hay should be offered free choice beginning at 7 to 14 days of age.

Calves should be housed in individual huts until weaned. Separating calves helps to control direct transmission of disease, prevents postfeeding sucking among calves, reduces stress of competition, and allows for assessment of individual feed intake and fecal consistency. Most dairy calves should be weaned by 50 to 60 days of age.

> ✎ **TECHNICIAN NOTE**
>
> Ensuring ingestion of colostrum by the calf shortly after birth is essential to successful dairy calf rearing.

PREVENTIVE HEALTH PROGRAM FOR SWINE

An effective and economical preventive health program is an essential part of successful swine production.

> ✎ **TECHNICIAN NOTE**
>
> An effective and economical preventive health program is an essential part of successful swine production.

Preventive health programs should be individually designed by the consulting veterinarian and based on the specific needs of the swine herd and the producer. The preventive health programs should include immunization programs for disease prevention, well-proven methods of external and internal parasite control, recommendations for appropriate nutrition, and improvements in general management and sanitation procedures. Box 11-5 presents a general approach to a preventive health program for swine herds and its implementation.

Box 11-5 GENERAL OUTLINE OF A PREVENTIVE HEALTH PROGRAM FOR SWINE

PREBREEDING RECOMMENDATIONS FOR BOARS

Purchase boars 60 days before intended use. Quarantine new boars for 30 days, then allow fence line contact with gilts and sows for 30 days before breeding. Immunize boars for leptospirosis and erysipelas. Treat for external and internal parasites before breeding.

PREBREEDING RECOMMENDATIONS FOR SOWS AND GILTS

Immunize for leptospirosis, porcine parvovirus infection,* and pseudorabies* 2-4 wk before breeding. Flush gilts by increasing feed (energy) intake before breeding to increase ovulations. Treat for external and internal parasites before breeding.

PREFARROWING RECOMMENDATIONS FOR SOWS AND GILTS

Limit feed intake to about 4 lb per head per day or feed according to condition to avoid overweight sows or gilts at farrowing. Immunize for colibacillosis,* atrophic rhinitis, erysipelas, TGE, porcine rotavirus infection,* and *Clostridium perfringens* type C* according to manufacturer's labeled instructions. Treat for external and internal parasites before farrowing with approved products.

FARROWING RECOMMENDATIONS

Gradually increase feed intake so lactating swine are receiving full feed at peak milk production. (Rule of thumb: Feed daily 1 lb of feed for every pig being nursed [e.g., a lactating sow with a litter of 12 pigs should receive at least 12 lb of feed daily].)

GENERAL RECOMMENDATIONS FOR PIGS
At Birth

Perform newborn pig procedures (e.g., clip needle teeth, dock tails, castrate, ear-notch, and inject iron dextran).

One Week of Age

Immunize for TGE,* rotavirus,* and atrophic rhinitis.

Four to Five Weeks of Age

Weaning occurs at this time. Immunize for atrophic rhinitis, erysipelas, and *Actinobacillus* infection.*

Six to Eight Weeks of Age

Treat for external and internal parasites with approved products.

Older Than Eight Weeks of Age

Repeated treatments for external and internal parasites with approved products may need to be done during the growing-finishing period.

TGE, Transmissible gastroenteritis.
*Dependent on problems in the individual swine herd.

VACCINATIONS

Vaccines that may be incorporated in preventive health programs for swine herds can be obtained from manufacturers as individual components or in various combinations. The same injection recommendations made previously for cattle apply to swine as well. Table 11-6 lists some vaccines currently available. Most swine should be routinely vaccinated for erysipelas and leptospirosis. Additional vaccines may be added to the health maintenance program based on the needs of the individual herd. Diseases for which vaccines are commonly used in preventive health programs are described in the following sections.

> ### ✎ TECHNICIAN NOTE
> A minimum vaccination program for swine should include vaccination for erysipelas and leptospirosis.

ERYSIPELAS VACCINE

Erysipelas is caused by the bacterium *Erysipelothrix rhusiopathiae* and can occur as acute septicemia, skin discoloration (commonly known as *diamond skin disease*), chronic arthritis, and vegetative endocarditis. Erysipelas is extremely common among swine herds, and therefore routine vaccination of gilts and sows before farrowing and of pigs at weaning is highly recommended. Both killed bacterins and modified live vaccines are available for protection against erysipelas.

LEPTOSPIROSIS VACCINE

Leptospirosis is an important bacterial disease that affects domestic animals, as well as humans and wildlife. Leptospirosis (in particular, *L. pomona* and *L. bratislava*) in swine is characterized by poor production, anemia, kidney disease, and abortions. Abortions are especially common after infection during late pregnancy. Routine vaccination of breeding swine (gilts, sows, boars) 2 to 4 weeks before breeding has proved to be effective in prevention of this disease. Because immunity is short-lived, semiannual revaccination is generally recommended.

TRANSMISSIBLE GASTROENTERITIS VACCINE

Transmissible gastroenteritis (TGE) is a common viral disease of swine. TGE occurs in both epizootic and enzootic (endemic) forms. The disease affects swine of all ages but is most devastating to pigs younger than 2 weeks (especially the epizootic form). Clinical signs in very young pigs may include anorexia, vomiting, profuse watery diarrhea, and dehydration, which often progress to death. Older swine can exhibit similar but milder symptoms, and death is rare.

Vaccination of prefarrowing sows and gilts may be necessary for herds in which TGE has been diagnosed as a cause of neonatal diarrhea. In addition, vaccination of pigs within the first week of life may assist in the prevention of postweaning scours.

PORCINE ROTAVIRUS VACCINE

Porcine rotavirus infection causes a gastroenteritis that may be characterized by vomiting, watery diarrhea, dehydration, and death in young pigs. It is generally difficult to differentiate porcine rotavirus infection from TGE. Porcine rotavirus infection commonly occurs in both nursing and weaned pigs, and many swine herds have serologic evidence of its presence. Vaccination of prefarrowing sows and gilts, nursing pigs, and pigs 7 to 10 days before weaning is recommended for the prevention of postweaning scours in herds in which porcine rotavirus infection has been diagnosed as a cause of enteric disease in young pigs.

CLOSTRIDIUM PERFRINGENS TYPE C VACCINE

The bacterium *C. perfringens* types C and A can cause enteric disease in young pigs. In peracute infection, there is a rapid onset of bloody diarrhea and death within the first 2 days of life. Acutely infected young pigs usually have bloody diarrhea with shreds of necrotic mucosa and die within 2 days after onset of enteric disease. The subacute infection may result in persistent diarrhea, emaciation, and death after a 5- to 7-day course. In chronic infections, a gray mucoid diarrhea occurs and lasts for about 7 days. Some of these patients will die, whereas others survive and typically become chronic poor doers.

Vaccination of prefarrowing sows and gilts effectively assists in the control of *C. perfringens* type C infections in nursing pigs, although this vaccine does not protect against type A.

NEONATAL PORCINE COLIBACILLOSIS VACCINE

Neonatal porcine colibacillosis is caused by enterotoxigenic *E. coli* (ETEC). This disease is the most important cause of primary diarrhea in piglets less than 5 days of age. The results are diarrhea, dehydration, and, in severe cases, death. Vaccination of healthy, pregnant sows and gilts provides good protection against neonatal colibacillosis in their nursing pigs. Commercial bacterins and subunit vaccines containing specialized fimbrial antigens and inactivated enterotoxins are available.

PORCINE PROLIFERATIVE ENTERITIS VACCINE

Porcine proliferative enteritis is also known as porcine intestinal adenomatosis, regional ileitis and "garden hose gut." The causative agent, *Lawsonia intracellulare*, can cause disease in any age-group but primarily affects grower-

Text continued on p. 373

Table 11-6 SWINE VACCINES

Vaccine	Manufacturer	Type	A. pleuropneumoniae	Bordetella	Clostridium perfringens C &/or D	E. coli	Erysipelothrix	Haemophilus parasusis	Influenza	L. bratislava	Lawsonia sp.	Leptospira spp.	Mycoplasma	Parvovirus	Pasteurella haemolytica*	Pasteurella multocida	PRRS	Pseudorabies	Rotavirus	Salmone	Streptococcus spp.	TGE	Tetanus toxoid
Argus® SC/ST	Intervet	MLV																		X			
AR-Pac®-P+ER	Schering-Plough	K		X			X									X							
AR-Pac®-PD+ER	Schering-Plough	K		X			X									X							
AR-Parapac® +ER	Schering-Plough	K		X			X	X								X							
Atrobac® 3	Pfizer Animal Health	K		X			X									X							
Borde-Cell™	AgriLabs	MLV		X																			
Borde Shield® 4	Novartis	K		X			X									X							
Bordetella Bronchiseptica Intranasal Vaccine	MVP	MLV		X																			
BratiVac®	Pfizer Animal Health	K								X													
BratiVac®-6	Pfizer Animal Health	K								X		X											
Breed Sow™ 6	AgriLabs	K										X		X									
Breed Sow® 7	AgriLabs	K					X					X		X									
C&D Toxoid	Aspen	K			X																		
Clostridium Perfringens Types C&D-Tetanus Toxoid	Colorado Serum	K			X																	X	
Clostridium Perfringens Types C&D-Tetanus Toxoid	Professional Biological	K			X																		X
Clostridium Perfringens Types C&D Toxoid	Colorado Serum	K			X																		
Clostridium Perfringens Types C&D Toxoid	Professional Biological	K			X																		
DurVac™ Appear-HP	Durvet	K	X	X			X	X								X							
DurVac™ AR	Durvet	MLV		X																			
DurVac™ AR-4	Durvet	K		X			X									X							
DurVac™ E-AR	Durvet	MLV		X			X																
DurVac™ EC	Durvet	K			X	X																	
DurVac™ EC-C	Durvet	K			X	X																	
DurVac™ ERY	Durvet	K					X																
DurVac™ MYCO	Durvet	K											X										
Durvac™ P-E-L	Durvet	K					X					X		X									
Durvac™ Strep	Durvet	K																			X		
E-Bac™	Intervet	K					X																
Emulsibac® APP	MVP	K	X																				
Emulsibac® SS	MVP	K																			X		
End-FLUence® with Immugen® II	Intervet	K							X														
End-FLUence® 2	Intervet	K							X														
ENDOVAC-Porci® with ImmunePlus®	Immvac	K																		X			
Enterisol® Ileitis	Boehringer Ingelheim	MLV									X												

Continued

Table 11-6 Swine Vaccines—cont'd

Vaccine	Manufacturer	Type	A. pleuropneumoniae	Bordetella	Clostridium perfringens C &/or D	E. coli	Erysipelothrix	Haemophilus parasuis	Influenza	L. bratislava	Lawsonia sp.	Leptospira spp.	Mycoplasma	Parvovirus	Pasteurella haemolytica*	Pasteurella multocida	PRRS	Pseudorabies	Rotavirus	Salmone	Streptococcus spp.	TGE	Tetanus toxoid
Enterisol® 5C-54	Boehringer Ingelheim	MLV																		X			
Enterisol® SC-54 FF	Boehringer Ingelheim	MLV																		X			
Equisimillis Shield™	Novartis	K																			X		
ER Bac®	Pfizer Animal Health	K					X																
ER Bac®/Leptoferm-5®	Pfizer Animal Health	K					X					X											
ER Bac® Plus	Pfizer Animal Health	K					X																
ER Bac® Plus/Leptoferm-5®	Pfizer Animal Health	K					X					X											
Erycell™	Novartis	MLV					X																
Ery Shield™	Novartis	K					X																
Ery Shield™+L5	Novartis	K					X					X											
Erysipelas Bacterin	AgriLabs	K					X																
Ery Vac 100	Arko	MLV					X																
Ery Vac 500	Arko	MLV					X																
FarrowSure®	Pfizer Animal Health	K					X					X		X									
FarrowSure® B	Pfizer Animal Health	K					X			X		X		X									
FarrowSure® B-PRV	Pfizer Animal Health	MLV/K					X			X		X		X				X					
FarrowSure® Plus	Pfizer Animal Health	K					X					X		X									
FarrowSure® Plus B	Pfizer Animal Health	K					X			X		X		X									
FarrowSure® PRV	Pfizer Animal Health	MLV/K					X			X		X		X				X					
FluSure™	Pfizer Animal Health	K							X														
FluSure™/ER Bac Plus®	Pfizer Animal Health	K					X		X														
FluSure™/RespiSure®	Pfizer Animal Health	K							X				X										
FluSure™/RespiSure 1 One®	Pfizer Animal Health	K							X				X										
FluSure™/RespiSure 1 One®/ER Bac Plus®	Pfizer Animal Health	K					X		X														
FluSure™/RespiSure® RTU	Pfizer Animal Health	K							X				X										
FluSure™ RTU	Pfizer Animal Health	K							X														
Haemo Shield® P	Novartis	K	X																				
Ingelvac® APP-ALC	Boehringer Ingelheim	LIVE	X													X							
Ingelvac® AR4	Boehringer Ingelheim	K		X												X							
Ingelvac® ERY-ALC	Boehringer Ingelheim	MLV					X																
Ingelvac® HP-1	Boehringer Ingelheim	K						X															
Ingelvac® M. HYO	Boehringer Ingelheim	K											X										
Ingelvac® PRRS ATP	Boehringer Ingelheim	MLV															X						

Table 11-6 Swine Vaccines—cont'd

Vaccine	Manufacturer	Type	A. pleuropneumoniae	Bordetella	Clostridium perfringens C &/or D	E. coli	Erysipelothrix	Haemophilus parasuis	Influenza	L. bratislava	Lawsonia sp.	Leptospira spp.	Mycoplasma	Parvovirus	Pasteurella haemolytica*	Pasteurella multocida	PRRS	Pseudorabies	Rotavirus	Salmone	Streptococcus spp.	TGE	Tetanus toxoid
Ingelvac® PRRS-HP	Boehringer Ingelheim	MLV/K						X									X						
Ingelvac® PRRS-HPE	Boehringer Ingelheim	MLV/K					X	X									X						
Ingelvac® PRRS MLV	Boehringer Ingelheim	MLV															X						
Ingelvac® PRV-G1	Boehringer Ingelheim	MLV																X					
J-5 Escherichia coli Bacterin	Hygiela	K				X																	
Lepto 5	AgriLabs	K										X											
Lepto-5	Boehringer Ingelheim	K										X											
Lepto-5	Colorado Serum	K									X												
Lepto 5	Durvet	K										X											
Lepto 5 Vaccine	Aspen	K										X											
Leptoferm-5®	Pfizer Animal Health	K										X											
Lepto Shield™ 5	Novartis	K										X											
Litter Guard®	Pfizer Animal Health	K				X																	
Litter Guard® LT	Pfizer Animal Health	K			X	X																	
Litter Guard® LT-C	Pfizer Animal Health	K			X	X																	
Magestic™ 7 with Spur®	Intervet	K					X					X		X									
Maxi/Guard® Nasal Vac	Addison	MLV		X																			
MaxiVac® Excell™	SyntroVet	K							X														
MaxiVac®-FLU	SyntroVet	K							X														
MaxiVac®-M+	SyntroVet	K							X				X										
M+Pac®	Schering-Plough	K											X										
M+Parapac™	Schering-Plough	K						X					X										
Myco Shield™	Novartis	K											X										
Myco Silencer® BPM	Intervet	K		X									X			X							
Myco Silencer® BPME*	Intervet	K		X			X						X			X							
Myco Silencer® M	Intervet	K											X										
Myco Silencer® MEH	Intervet	K					X	X					X										
Myco Silencer® Once	Intervet	K											X										
Nitro-Sal	Arko	MLV																		X			
Nitro-Sal F.D.	Arko	MLV																		X			
Parapac™	Schering-Plough	K						X															
Parapleuro Shield® P	Novartis	K	X				X	X								X							
Parapleuro Shield® P+BE	Novartis	K	X	X			X	X								X							

Continued

Table 11-6 SWINE VACCINES—CONT'D

Vaccine	Manufacturer	Type	A. pleuropneumoniae	Bordetella	Clostridium pertringens C &/or D	E. coli	Erysipelothrix	Haemophilus parasuis	Influenza	L. bratislava	Lawsonia sp.	Leptospira spp.	Mycoplasma	Parvovirus	Pasteurella haemolytica*	Pasteurella multocida	PRRS	Pseudorabies	Rotavirus	Salmone	Streptococcus spp.	TGE	Tetanus toxoid
Para Shield®	Novartis	K						X															
Parvo Shield®	Novartis	K												X									
Parvo Shield® L5	Novartis	K										X		X									
Parvo Shield® L5E	Novartis	K					X					X		X									
Parvo-Vac®/Leptoferm-5®	Pfizer Animal Health	K										X		X									
PleuroGuard® 4	Pfizer Animal Health	K	X	X			X									X							
Pneumosuis® III	Pfizer Animal Health	K	X	X																			
Pneu Pac®	Schering-Plough	K	X																				
Pneu Pac® – ER	Schering-Plough	K	X				X																
Pneu Parapac® +ER	Schering-Plough	K	X				X	X															
Porcine Pili Shield™	Novartis	K				X																	
Porcine Pili Shield™ +C	Novartis	K		X	X	X																	
Prefarrow Shield™ 9	Novartis	K		X	X	X	X	X								X							
Prefarrow Strep Shield®	Novartis	K																			X		
Prevail™ MycoPlex™	Aspen	K											X										
Prevail™ Para Pleuro Bac+3DT	Aspen	K	X	X			X	X								X							
Prevail™ Parvoplex 6-Way++E	Aspen	K					X					X		X									
ProSystem® CE	Intervet	K			X	X																	
ProSystem® Pilimune	Intervet	K				X																	
ProSystem® RCE	Intervet	MLV/K			X	X													X				
ProSystem® Rota	Intervet	MLV																	X				
ProSystem® TGE	Intervet	MLV																				X	
ProSystem® TG-Emune® Rota with Imugen® II	Intervet	K																	X			X	
ProSystem® TG-Emune® with Imugen® II	Intervet	K																				X	
ProSystem® TGE/Rota	Intervet	MLV																	X			X	
ProSystem® TREC	Intervet	MLV/K			X	X													X			X	
PRRomiSE®	Intervet	K															X						
PR-Vac®	Pfizer Animal Health	MLV																X					
PR-Vac®-Killed	Pfizer Animal Health	K																X					
PR-Vac Plus®	Pfizer Animal Health	MLV																X					
PRV-Begonia with Diluvac Forte®	Intervet	MLV																X					
PRV/Marker Gold®	SyntroVet	MLV																X					
PRV/Marker Gold®-MaxiVac® FLU	SyntroVet	MLV/K							X									X					

Table 11-6 Swine Vaccines—cont'd

Vaccine	Manufacturer	Type	A. pleuropneumoniae	Bordetella	Clostridium perfringens C &/or D	E. coli	Erysipelothrix	Haemophilus parasuis	Influenza	L. bratislava	Lawsonia sp.	Leptospira spp.	Mycoplasma	Parvovirus	Pasteurella haemolytica*	Pasteurella multocida	PRRS	Pseudorabies	Rotavirus	Salmone	Streptococcus spp.	TGE	Tetanus toxoid
ReproCyc® PRRS-PLE	Boehringer Ingelheim	MLV/K					X					X		X			X						
RespiSure®	Pfizer Animal Health	K											X										
RespiSure 1 One®	Pfizer Animal Health	K											X										
RespiSure 1 One®/ER Bac Plus®	Pfizer Animal Health	K					X						X										
Rhinicell®	Novartis	MLV		X																			
Rhinicell® +E	Novartis	MLV		X			X																
Rhini Shield™ TX4	Novartis	K		X			X									X							
Rhinogen® BPE	Intervet	K		X			X									X							
Rhinogen® CTE 5000	Intervet	K		X			X									X							
Rhinogen® CTSE	Intervet	K		X			X									X					X		
Rotamune® with Immungen® II	Intervet	K																	X				
Salmo Shield® 2	Novartis	K																		X			
Salmo Shield® Live	Novartis	MLV																		X			
Score®	Intervet	K		X			X									X							
Scourmune®	Schering-Plough	K				X																	
Scourmune®-C	Schering-Plough	K			X	X																	
Scourmune®-CR	Schering-Plough	K			X	X													X				
Sow Bac® CE II	Intervet	K		X	X	X	X																
Sow Bac® E II	Intervet	K		X		X	X									X							
Sow Bac® TREC	Intervet	MLV/K		X	X	X	X									X			X			X	
SS Pac®	Schering-Plough	K																			X		
Strep Bac® with Imugen® II	Intervet	K																			X	X	
Super-Tet® with Havlogen®	Intervet	K														X							X
Surround™ L5	Biocor	K										X											
Suvaxyn® AR/E/EC-4	Fort Dodge	K		X		X	X									X							
Suvaxyn® AR/T	Fort Dodge	K		X												X							
Suvaxyn® AR/T/E	Fort Dodge	K		X			X									X							
Suvaxyn® E	Fort Dodge	K					X																
Suvaxyn® EC-4	Fort Dodge	K				X																	
Suvaxyn® E Oral	Fort Dodge	MLV					X																
Suvaxyn®-E	Fort Dodge	K					X																
Suvaxyn® LE+B	Fort Dodge	K					X			X		X											
Suvaxyn® PLE	Fort Dodge	K					X			X		X		X									

Continued

Table 11-6 SWINE VACCINES—CONT'D

Vaccine	Manufacturer	Type	A. pleuropneumoniae	Bordetella	Clostridium perfringens C &/or D	E. coli	Erysipelothrix	Haemophilus parasuis	Influenza	L. bratislava	Lawsonia sp.	Leptospira spp.	Mycoplasma	Parvovirus	Pasteurella haemolytica*	Pasteurella multocida	PRRS	Pseudorabies	Rotavirus	Salmone	Streptococcus spp.	TGE	Tetanus toxoid
Suvaxyn® PLE+B	Fort Dodge	K					X			X		X		X									
Suvaxyn® PLE+B/PRVgpI	Fort Dodge	MLV/K					X					X		X				X					
Suvaxyn® PLE/PRV gpl	Fort Dodge	MLV/K					X					X		X				X					
Suvaxyn® PRV gpl	Fort Dodge	MLV																X					
Suvaxyn® Respifend® APP	Fort Dodge	K	X																				
Suvaxyn® Respifend® HPS	Fort Dodge	K						X															
Suvaxyn® RespiFend® MH	Fort Dodge	K											X										
Suvaxyn® RespiFend® MH/HPS	Fort Dodge	K						X					X										
Swine Influenza Vaccine (H3N2 Subtype)	SyntroVet	K							X														
Swine Master M Plus™	AgriLabs	K						X					X										
Tetanus Toxoid	Fort Dodge	K																					X
Tetanus Toxoid-Concentrated	Colorado Serum	K																					X
Tetanus Toxoid-Concentrated	Professional Biological	K																					X
Tetanus Toxoid-Unconcentrated	Colorado Serum	K																					X
Tetguard™	Boehringer Ingelheim	K																					X
Tetnogen®	Fort Dodge	K																					X
TGE Cell™	Novartis	MLV																				X	
TGE Shield™	Novartis	K																				X	
Toxivac® AD+E	Boehringer Ingelheim	K		X			X									X							
Toxivac® Plus Parasuis	Boehringer Ingelheim	K		X			X	X								X							
TrustGard™ 5L	Vedco	K										X											

K, Killed virus; *MLV*, modified live virus; *TGE*, transmissable gastroenteritis.
Pasteurella haemolytica was renamed *Mannheimia haemolytica* in 1999.

finisher pigs. Clinical signs may be inapparent or mild with reduced feed intake and decreased growth rate. Pigs may exhibit intermittent diarrhea with anorexia and weight loss. Overall morbidity is variable, and the mortality rate is usually low. Melena and hemorrhagic diarrhea are more common in older pigs, and although occasional acute deaths occur, most affected pigs recover. Stress seems to precipitate the disease, so treatment is aimed at prevention. Recently, an avirulent live vaccine, which may help reduce the severity of this disease, has become available commercially.

BORDETELLA, PASTEURELLA, ACTINOBACILLUS, AND MYCOPLASMA VACCINES

Bordetella bronchiseptica and *Pasteurella multocida* are considered to be the major pathogens associated with development of atrophic rhinitis in swine. In combined infections, *P. multocida* and *B. bronchiseptica* can cause a more severe form of atrophic rhinitis than in cases in which either agent occurs alone. In young pigs, atrophic rhinitis is characterized by acute rhinitis that results in destruction of the nasal turbinates. Destruction of the turbinates leads to impaired filtering of air in the nasal passages, decreased rate of weight gain, and increased incidence of respiratory tract infections, including pneumonia. Vaccination of pregnant swine and nursing pigs can often reduce the incidence of clinical atrophic rhinitis. Several bacterin/toxoid combinations containing *B. bronchiseptica* and *P. multocida* are commercially available.

> **✎ TECHNICIAN NOTE**
>
> Combined infections of *Pasteurella multocida* and *Bordetella bronchiseptica* can cause a more severe form of atrophic rhinitis than when either agent occurs alone.

Actinobacillus pleuropneumoniae, the most common causative agent of respiratory disease in swine, causes a severe and often fatal disease affecting swine of all ages but, in particular, pigs 12 to 16 weeks of age. Manifestations of the disease are fibrinopurulent bronchopneumonia and fibrinous pleuritis. Acute *Actinobacillus* infections can cause death within 24 to 36 hours after the onset of clinical signs (e.g., coughing, cyanosis, blood-tinged nasal discharge). However, some animals may die suddenly without development of clinical signs. Chronic infections are usually subclinical and are characterized by decreased performance and an extended finishing period. In herds in which this disease is a problem, pigs should be vaccinated twice, 2 to 4 weeks apart, after weaning.

Mycoplasma hyopneumoniae or enzootic pneumonia is the most common cause of chronic pneumonia in swine. The disease is not usually evident until pigs are 3 to 6 months old. It is characterized by a chronic, nonproductive cough, often induced by exercise. The greatest economic loss from the disease is decreased growth rate; for every 10% of lung affected by pneumonia, average daily gain is reduced by 5.3%. Morbidity is variable, and the mortality rate is low in uncomplicated cases. Secondary bacterial infections may exacerbate clinical signs. Vaccination may reduce lesions and improve weight gains in herds in which *M. hyopneumoniae* is a problem.

> **✎ TECHNICIAN NOTE**
>
> The greatest economic loss from *Mycoplasma* pneumonia in swine is decreased growth rate and decreased feed efficiency.

PORCINE REPRODUCTIVE AND RESPIRATORY SYNDROME VACCINE

Porcine reproductive and respiratory syndrome (PRRS) is also known as swine infertility and respiratory syndrome, mystery pig disease, and blue ear disease. It is recognized as a viral disease of swine that causes respiratory problems in all ages of pigs, as well as reproductive problems in breeding swine. Clinical signs include transient, mild anorexia; lethargy; and fever in grower-finisher pigs and breeding animals. Cyanosis of the ears (blue ear disease), vulva, tail, abdomen, or snout is occasionally reported. Viral infection of breeding gilts or sows may result in premature farrowings with small, weak, or stillborn piglets and an increased incidence of fetal mummies. Respiratory distress ("thumping") and open-mouth breathing in suckling and weanling pigs may occur. The virus tends to increase the incidence of secondary respiratory tract infections in young pigs. Chronic infection in nursery and grower-finisher pigs may result in decreased growth rate and feed efficiency and increased morbidity and mortality rates as a result of secondary infections. Modified live virus vaccines for PRRS are available but should not be used in pregnant gilts or sows, in boars, or in seronegative herds.

PORCINE PARVOVIRUS VACCINE

Porcine parvovirus is believed to be the most common cause of infectious reproductive failure in swine. Infection of pregnant sows and gilts can result in stillbirths, birth of weak piglets, mummified fetuses, embryonic death, and infertility (formerly referred to as SMEDI [stillbirths, mummified fetus, embryonic death, and infertility]). Prebreeding vaccination is recommended in swine herds experiencing porcine parvovirus infections.

PSEUDORABIES VACCINE

Pseudorabies is a viral disease of swine that is characterized by fever, tremors, incoordination, convulsions, death, and, less frequently vomiting and diarrhea in baby pigs. Signs seen in older pigs include pneumonia and a "flu-like" syndrome. PRV infection can also be responsible for abortion, stillbirths, or mummies in pregnant swine. Available vaccines include killed virus modified live virus, and genetically engineered vaccines that allow differentiation between vaccine titers and titers resulting from natural infection. Vaccination of swine for PRV is controlled by state officials. There is currently a pseudorabies eradication program in place, so if PRV is diagnosed in a herd, it should be reported to the state veterinarian.

> **TECHNICIAN NOTE**
> Vaccination for pseudorabies in swine is controlled by state regulations. Pseudorabies in swine is a reportable disease.

STREPTOCOCCUS VACCINE

Streptococcus suis causes meningitis, polyserositis, polyarthritis, endocarditis, and pneumonia in recently weaned pigs. Clinical signs include fever, anorexia, depression, tremors, blindness, ataxia, convulsions, lameness, dyspnea, and death. *S. suis* can pose a significant human health hazard. Available vaccines may help to reduce the losses caused by *S. suis.*

> **TECHNICIAN NOTE**
> *Streptococcus suis* is a zoonotic disease and a significant human health hazard.

EXTERNAL AND INTERNAL PARASITES

Control of external parasites, especially lice *(Haematopinus suis)* and mange mites *(Sarcoptes scabiei* var. *suis),* may be done with repeated applications of approved insecticidal sprays or pour-on products or with the use of ivermectin. Treatment of external parasites should be done at the same time as treatment for internal parasites; however, always read the manufacturer's labeled instructions, because some types of sprays and pour-on products cannot be used concomitantly with dewormers or may not be used safely in pregnant or young nursing swine.

The most common internal parasites of swine are the roundworm *(Ascaris suum),* the whipworm *(Trichuris suis),* the threadworm *(Strongyloides* spp.), the nodular worm *(Oesophagostomum* spp.), the lungworm *(Metastrongylus* spp.), the red stomach worm *(Hyostrongylus rubidus),* and the kidney worm *(Stephanurus dentatus).* Many commercial dewormers are currently available. Product choice should depend on the parasites identified by fecal examinations within a herd, convenience of administration, and cost effec-tiveness. In general, it is a good idea to deworm adults before breeding, sows and gilts before farrowing, and pigs once or twice after weaning and once during the growing-finishing period. Chapter 7 contains additional information on parasitology and specific drug therapy.

PREVENTIVE HEALTH PROGRAM FOR PET PIGS

Although pot-bellied pigs as companion animals may never be as popular as dogs and cats, it is estimated that there are about 150,000 pot-bellied pigs in the United States. At one time, pot-bellied pigs were expensive, but as the fad passed, the prices fell, resulting in many owners acquiring these pigs with little to no planning before they purchased this unique pet. Many pot-bellied pig owners have difficulty finding veterinarians willing to treat their pets. Many first-time pot-bellied pig owners do not have the information necessary to properly care for their pet, nor do they know where to turn for answers to their questions. A knowledgeable veterinarian and veterinary technician can be invaluable resources for the new pet pig owner.

> **TECHNICIAN NOTE**
> A knowledgeable veterinary technician can be a valuable source of information to a new pet pig owner.

VACCINATIONS

Pet pigs should receive the same vaccinations as commercial swine. Most pigs visit the veterinarian for their first health maintenance check at around 6 weeks. At that time we recommend vaccination for erysipelas and leptospirosis (a combination product with a 2-ml dose is available and is recommended for these small pigs). The vaccination injection is given intramuscularly behind the ear. A booster dose should be given in 2 to 3 weeks. The erysipelas and leptospirosis vaccines should be repeated semiannually because neither vaccine provides long-term protection. We do not routinely recommend rabies vaccination of this species because there is no product approved for use in swine; however, in high risk areas it may be necessary to consider adding this to the vaccination program (contact your state veterinarian for more information). If a veterinarian is dealing with a breeding herd, it may be necessary to consider vaccination for other diseases, depending on existing disease problems in that herd (Box 11-5).

> **TECHNICIAN NOTE**
> Pet pigs should be vaccinated for erysipelas and leptospirosis twice a year.

EXTERNAL AND INTERNAL PARASITES

Most pet pigs have sarcoptic mange, so it is recommended that they be treated with ivermectin (1 ml per 75 lb) orally at weekly intervals for 4 consecutive weeks (dosage should be increased as the pig grows during this time). This protocol will simultaneously treat any internal parasites the pig may have. Owners should be educated that sarcoptic mange can be transmitted to them while they are holding their pets. It is a transient infestation that causes a skin rash and itching. Though it is self-limiting, owners should be advised to consult their physicians if necessary. After initial deworming, pet pigs probably do not need to be treated for parasites again unless they are exposed to other pigs. If in doubt, routine fecal exams may be performed at the semiannual health maintenance appointments.

> **✐ TECHNICIAN NOTE**
>
> Most pot-bellied pigs have mange, which can be transmitted to their owners.

NUTRITION

Without proper knowledge of the pot-bellied pig's husbandry and nutritional needs, health and behavior problems are inevitable. According to one report, approximately 50% of pot-bellied pigs are abandoned or re-homed before they are 1 year of age. This occurs because of unrealistic expectations of the owners and their unwillingness or inability to provide for the pig's environmental needs. The most common misconception held by pet pig owners is that their pot-bellied pig will only weigh 40 to 50 lb when fully grown. Although a few pigs remain small, most of them will weigh closer to 120 lb when mature, and they do not reach full size until they are 2 to 3 years old. Breed standards set by the North American Potbellied Pig Association describe a pig weighing no more than 95 lb and having a maximum height of 18 inches at the shoulder, at 1 year of age. The most common nutritional disease of pot-bellied pigs is obesity; however, many stunted and malnourished pigs are also seen, owing to their owner's misguided attempts to keep them small.

> **✐ TECHNICIAN NOTE**
>
> The most common nutritional disease of pot-bellied pigs is obesity.

Several companies have developed diets specifically for miniature pigs. Miniature pigs should never be fed commercial swine feeds; feeds for miniature swine are lower in protein and fat and have a higher fiber content than commercial swine rations. Miniature pig feeds are generally classified as starter, grower, breeder, or maintenance. Starter rations are intended for newly weaned pigs. The most appropriate ration for the average pot-bellied pig is the maintenance ration, which contains 12% protein, 2% fat, and 12% to 15% fiber. Most pot-bellied pigs are adopted by owners at 6 to 8 weeks of age and are spayed or neutered in the first few months. They begin to lead sedentary lifestyles early, so maintenance rations are probably the best choice for these pigs. If the pig is not spayed or neutered and/or it leads a very active life, grower rations may be a better choice.

Some commercially available pot-bellied pig feeds have urinary acidifiers to help prevent cystitis, so if this seems to be a problem, this specialty ration may be considered. Recommendations concerning amount to feed pot-bellied pigs vary; some references suggest 2% to 2.5% of their body weight; others suggest 1 cup of feed per 50 to 80 lb. These are general guidelines, and owners must be advised to feed their pets according to body composition. Although pot-bellied pigs should have rotund bellies, they should never have turgid, fat-filled jowls or rolls of fat hanging over their hocks. They should have ribs that can be felt but not seen.

Appropriate treats for the pig include low-fat, low-salt snack foods such as popcorn (air popped without salt or butter) and small amounts of dried or fresh fruit. Requiring that the pig earn its treats is one way of continually reinforcing the pig's position as a subordinate member of the family. Obesity is likely to be the leading cause of health problems and decreased life span in pet pigs. Arthritis, heart disease, and kidney failure are just a few possible geriatric diseases that may be hastened by obesity. Sometimes entropion and corneal damage occur in morbidly obese pigs. Water intake in pigs is important for prevention of cystitis, urolithiasis, and salt poisoning.

> **✐ TECHNICIAN NOTE**
>
> Salt toxicity (water deprivation) is a serious neurologic condition that may occur in pet pigs receiving excess dietary salt and/or inadequate water.

Pigs have a habit of alternating between eating and drinking and may make a mess at feeding time. Owners should be advised not to restrict water for this reason. Food and water should be provided in an easy-to-clean environment such as a shower stall; or the food and water can be placed in a large shallow tray to make cleanup easier. Pigs are also particular about the temperature of their drinking water, so the water should not be allowed to get too cold in the winter or too hot in the summer because this may restrict intake and cause problems. Pigs are foraging animals that normally spend much of their day either in search of food or at rest. When kept as pets, pigs are fed two to three small meals a day and spend little time looking for food or eating. There are a variety of ways to extend mealtime, which increases the pig's exercise and makes them more active participants in the acquisition of their food. In good weather the pig's ration may be broadcast over the grass in the yard. A rooting box can also be constructed out of wood or by utilizing a plastic wading pool. The box is filled with large smooth stones, and the pig's food can be spread among the stones. This not only extends feeding time but also allows the pig to fulfill its rooting needs in an acceptable place. Other useful techniques include the use of a food treat–dispensing toy (Manna Ball, Be Sure Training, Carnation, Wash), which allows the pig to slowly acquire its food while exercising at the same time.

PREVENTIVE HEALTH PROGRAM FOR SMALL RUMINANTS

In North America, sheep and goats are managed under a wide variety of conditions, including extensive range operations, semiconfinement, total confinement, and hobby farm systems; they are also kept as backyard pets. Meat-producing goats have gained popularity in recent years. One primary task of the small ruminant veterinarian and veterinary technician is to educate the producer about the value of careful observation, animal identification, and record keeping for improvement of herd and flock health and productivity. With adequate information, the veterinarian and veterinary technician can then make sound recommendations concerning nutrition, vaccination, parasite control, and management geared to the needs of a particular herd or flock.

VACCINATIONS

The number of vaccines licensed for use in small ruminants is limited. The veterinarian's first choice should be a licensed vaccine used in accordance with label instructions; however, products licensed for use in other species (particularly in cattle) are frequently considered to be effective in sheep and goats. Use of vaccines depends on the disease incidence within a given herd or flock, but vaccination for enterotoxemia and tetanus should be included in every herd and flock health program (Table 11-7).

> **TECHNICIAN NOTE**
> Vaccination for enterotoxemia (*Clostridium perfringens* types C and D) and tetanus should be included in every small ruminant health program.

ENTEROTOXEMIA VACCINE

Toxins produced by *Clostridium perfringens* types C and D may cause enterotoxemia in young sheep and goats. The organism is present in the gastrointestinal tract of healthy animals but may overgrow and produce potent toxins in the presence of rich ingesta and bowel stasis. Enterotoxemia is most likely to occur in young animals nursing from dams that are heavy milk producers or in animals receiving heavy grain rations, as in feedlot situations. For this reason,

the disease is called *overeating disease* (not to be confused with grain overload). Enterotoxemia is easily prevented by vaccination of the dams before lambing and kidding and vaccination of lambs and kids several times at 2- to 4-week intervals, beginning at 6 to 8 weeks of age. Protection provided by vaccination for enterotoxemia is effective but short-lived; therefore vaccination is recommended every 4 to 6 months in high-risk herds. Routine vaccination for enterotoxemia should be a part of all small ruminant herd health programs.

TETANUS VACCINE

Tetanus is caused by a toxin produced by the anaerobic organism *Clostridium tetani,* a bacterium that may be carried into wounds or surgery sites. Clinical signs may include muscular stiffness (sawhorse stance), difficulty in swallowing (lockjaw), prolapse of the third eyelids, labored breathing, and exaggerated response to external stimuli. Because small ruminants are particularly susceptible to infection, vaccination for tetanus at the time of vaccination for enterotoxemia is vital (combination products are available). In addition, booster vaccination is recommended any time an animal is wounded or has undergone any surgical procedure (e.g., dehorning, castration, tail docking).

CAMPYLOBACTERIOSIS (VIBRIOSIS) VACCINE

Campylobacteriosis is caused by *Campylobacter fetus* subsp. *fetus* and *Campylobacter jejuni.* The principal clinical sign with this disease is abortion, which usually occurs in the last 6 weeks of pregnancy. Losses from abortion may be substantial in individual flocks. Vaccines for *Campylobacter* alone or in combination with *Chlamydia* are now available for prevention of abortion in sheep.

> **TECHNICIAN NOTE**
> If a herd or flock is experiencing abortion problems, the producer may consider vaccinating for *Chlamydia* and *Campylobacter.*

CHLAMYDIA VACCINE

Chlamydia psittaci, the cause of enzootic abortion of ewes (EAE), is a major cause of abortion in sheep and goats. Abortions or stillbirths with placentitis usually occur in the fourth or fifth month of gestation; other animals in the flock or herd may concurrently show signs of arthritis or pneumonia. Vaccines for *Chlamydia* alone or in combination with *Campylobacter* are now available for prevention of abortion in sheep.

CONTAGIOUS ECTHYMA VACCINE

Contagious ecthyma (sore mouth, orf) is a viral infection of goats. Kids are primarily affected but may spread the

Table 11-7 Ovine Vaccines

Vaccine	Manufacturer	Type	Bacteroides	Bluetongue	Brucella ovis	Campylobacter	Chlamydia	Clostridium chauvoei	Clostridium haemolyticum	Clostridium novyi	Clostridium perfringens C &/or D	Clostridium septicum	Clostridium sordelli	Corynebacterium	Fusobacterium	Parapoxvirus (Orf)	Pasteurella haemolytica*	Pasteurella multocida	Rabies	Tetanus toxoid
7-Gauge™	AgriPharm	K						X		X	X	X	X							
7-Way	Aspen	K						X		X	X	X	X							
8-Way	Aspen	K						X	X	X	X	X	X							
Bar-Vac® 7	Boehringer Ingelheim	K						X		X	X	X	X							
Bar-Vac® 8	Boehringer Ingelheim	K						X	X	X	X	X	X							
Bar-Vac® CD	Boehringer Ingelheim	K									X									
Bar-Vac®-CD/T	Boehringer Ingelheim	K									X									X
Bluetongue Vaccine	Colorado Serum	MLV		X																
Caliber® 3	Boehringer Ingelheim	K																		
Caliber® 7	Boehringer Ingelheim	K						X		X		X	X							
Campylobacter Fetus Bacterin-Ovine	Colorado Serum	K				X														
Campylobacter Fetus-Jejuni Bacterin	Hygieia	K				X														
Case-Bac™	Colorado Serum	K												X						
Caseous D-T™	Colorado Serum	K									X			X						X
C & D Toxoid	Aspen	K									X									
Chlamydia Psittaci Bacterin	Colorado Serum	K					X													
Clostridial BCD	Durvet	K									X									
Clostridium Chauvoei-Septicum Bacterin	Colorado Serum	K						X				X								
Clostridium Chauvoei-Septicum-Novyi-Sordellii Bacterin-Toxoid	Colorado Serum	K						X		X		X	X							
Clostridium Chauvoei-Septicum-Pasteurella Haemolytica-Multocida Bacterin	Colorado Serum	K						X				X					X	X		
Clostridium Haemolyticum Bacterin (red water)	Colorado Serum	K							X											
Clostridium Perfringens Types C & D – Tetanus Toxoid	Colorado Serum	K									X									X
Clostridium Perfringens Types C & D – Tetanus Toxoid	Professional Biological	K									X									X
Clostridium Perfringens Types C & D Toxoid	Colorado Serum	K									X									
Clostridium Perfringens Types C & D Toxoid	Professional Biological	K									X									
Clostri Shield® BCD	Novartis Animal Vaccines	K									X									
Covexin® 8 Vaccine	Schering-Plough	K						X		X	X	X	X							X
Defensor® 3	Pfizer Animal Health	K																	X	
Electroid® 7 Vaccine	Schering-Plough	K						X		X	X	X	X							X
Electroid® D	Schering-Plough	K								X	X	X	X							

Continued

Table 11-7 OVINE VACCINES—CONT'D

Vaccine	Manufacturer	Type	Bacteroides	Bluetongue	Brucella ovis	Campylobacter	Chlamydia	Clostridium chauvoei	Clostridium haemolyticum	Clostridium novyi	Clostridium perfringens C &/or D	Clostridium septicum	Clostridium sordelli	Corynebacterium	Fusobacterium	Parapoxvirus (Orf)	Pasteurella haemolytica*	Pasteurella multocida	Rabies	Tetanus toxoid
Footvax® 10 Strain	Schering-Plough	K	X																	
Gauge™ C&D	AgriPharm	K									X									
Imrab® 3	Merial	K																	X	
Imrab® Large Animal	Merial	K																	X	X
Ovine Ecthyma Vaccine	Colorado Serum	LIVE														X				
Ovine Tetanus Shield™	Novartis Animal Vaccines	K																		X
Pasteurella Haemolytica Multocida Bacterin	Colorado Serum	K															X	X		
Prorab®-1	Intervet	K																	X	
Rabdomun® Vaccine	Schering-Plough	K																	X	
Ram Epididymitis Bacterin	Colorado Serum	K			X															
Resist™ 7	AgriPharm	K						X		X	X	X	X							
Resist™ 8	AgriPharm	K						X	X	X	X	X	X							
Siteguard® G	Schering-Plough	K									X									
Siteguard® MLG Vaccine	Schering-Plough	K						X	X	X	X	X	X							
Super-Tet® with Havlogen®	Intervet	K																		X
Tetanus Toxoid	Fort Dodge	K																		X
Tetanus Toxoid-Concentrated	Colorado Serum	K																		X
Tetanus Toxoid-Concentrated	Professional Biological	K																		X
Tetanus Toxoid-UnConcentrated	Colorado Serum	K																		X
Telguard™	Boehringer Ingelheim	K																		X
Tetni-Vax®	AgriPharm	K																		X
Tetnogen®	Fort Dodge	K																		X
TrustGard™ 7	Vedco	K						X		X	X	X	X							
TrustGard™ 8	Vedco	K						X	X	X	X	X	X							
TrustGard™ CD	Vedco	K									X									
TrustGard™ CD/T	Vedco	K									X									X
Ultrabac® 7	Pfizer Animal Health	K						X		X	X	X	X							
Ultrabac® 8	Pfizer Animal Health	K						X	X	X	X	X	X							
Ultrabac® CD	Pfizer Animal Health	K									X									

Table 11-7 OVINE VACCINES—CONT'D

Vaccine	Manufacturer	Type	Bacteroides	Bluetongue	Brucella ovis	Campylobacter	Chlamydia	Clostridium chauvoei	Clostridium haemolyticum	Clostridium novyi	Clostridium perfringens C &/or D	Clostridium septicum	Clostridium sordellii	Corynebacterium	Fusobacterium	Parapoxvirus (Orf)	Pasteurella haemolytica*	Pasteurella multocida	Rabies	Tetanus toxoid
UltraChoice™ 7	Pfizer Animal Health	K						X		X	X	X	X							
UltraChoice™ 8	Pfizer Animal Health	K						X	X	X	X	X	X							
UltraChoice™ CD	Pfizer Animal Health	K									X									
Vision® 7 with Spur®	Intervet	K						X		X	X	X	X							
Vision® 8 with Spur®	Intervet	K						X	X	X	X	X	X							
Vision® CD-T with Spur®	Intervet	K									X									X
Vision® CD with Spur®	Intervet	K									X									
Volar®	Intervet	K													X					

K, Killed; MLV, modified live virus.
*Pasteurella haemolytica was renamed Mannheimia haemolytica in 1999.

disease to the udders of does. Clinical signs include papules, vesicles, pustules, and scabs on the lips, muzzle, eyelids, oral cavity, udder, teats, and feet. Affected kids usually exhibit a decrease in feed consumption, and some kids become depressed, anorectic, and febrile. Contagious ecthyma is transmissible to humans, and so it is advisable to wear gloves when infected animals are handled. Effective live-virus vaccines are available but are not recommended for closed herds that are not experiencing contagious ecthyma. Proper precautions, such as wearing gloves during vaccine administration and disposal of contagious ecthyma vaccine containers, are necessary to prevent risks to human health.

> ### ✎ TECHNICIAN NOTE
> Contagious ecthyma is a highly contagious zoonotic disease. Care should be taken when infected animals are handled and when the live vaccine is administered to sheep and goats.

FOOT ROT VACCINE

Dichelobacter nodosus is the primary causative agent of foot rot in sheep. It is a highly contagious disease and is probably the most common disease of sheep in the United States, causing more economic loss than any other disease. Lameness in one or more feet is the most obvious clinical sign. The development of foot rot is facilitated by wet environmental conditions. A vaccine is available that, when combined with regular foot trimming and foot baths, significantly reduces the incidence of disease within a flock.

BLUETONGUE VACCINE

Bluetongue is a viral disease of ruminants; however, clinical disease is largely restricted to sheep. Clinical signs may include oral ulcers; edema of the face, lips, muzzle, and ears; excessive salivation; cyanosis of the tongue (thus the name); and lameness caused by coronitis. Teratogenic effects include abortions, stillbirths, and weak, live "dummy lambs." An attenuated live-virus vaccine is available for prebreeding vaccination of healthy sheep and goats; vaccination of pregnant females may produce teratogenic effects.

FOOT CARE

Foot rot is one of the most common diseases of sheep and goats.

> ### ✎ TECHNICIAN NOTE
> Foot rot is one of the most common and economically significant diseases of sheep and goats.

It is highly contagious, and infection can result in lameness in a significant number of animals within a herd or flock. Frequent foot trimming—combined with foot baths, foot soaks, or vaccination (or any combination of these)—is important in the control of the disease. Repeated foot soaking alone is an economic, practical, and effective treatment for foot rot in large commercial operations where hoof trimming is impractical. Products typically used for foot baths or foot soaks include zinc sulfate, copper sulfate, and formalin (care must be taken to prevent sheep from drinking solutions with a high copper content). There is some evidence of genetic susceptibility to development of foot rot in sheep; therefore culling animals with recurring infections may be helpful.

NUTRITION

Sheep and goats should be fed a good-quality commercial feed labeled for their particular species. Feeding horse or cattle feeds to small ruminants may result in copper toxicity because the copper levels in such feeds are much higher than those normally tolerated by sheep and goats. Feed commercial feeds according to the manufacturer's recommendations and based on the needs and use of the animal. Good-quality roughage may be fed ad libitum. Because castrated lambs and kids (wethers) are predisposed to the development of urinary calculi, it is advisable to feed a diet of good-quality roughage or pasture and no grain. If grain must be fed, it is advisable to supplement it with salt and a urinary acidifier, such as ammonium chloride (see Chapter 16).

> ### ✎ TECHNICIAN NOTE
> Care should be taken when feeding male small ruminants because obstructive urolithiasis is a common sequelae to improper feeding.

EXTERNAL AND INTERNAL PARASITES

There are few effective anthelmintics labeled for use in small ruminants. Most small ruminant veterinarians use cattle dewormers for the treatment of external and internal parasites in sheep and goats. Products commonly used include avermectins, fenbendazole, albendazole, and levamisole. Caution should be exercised when these products are used in lactating does and animals intended for slaughter. Recommendations for extra-label use of these products and suggested milk and slaughter withdrawal times may be obtained from the Food Animal Residue Avoidance Data Bank.

Frequency of deworming varies according to several factors, including concentration of animals in a given area and environmental conditions. Severe gastrointestinal parasitism can be life threatening, especially in subtropical climates, where it may be necessary to deworm small ruminants as often as every 3 to 4 weeks during the hot, humid summer months. Pasture management and careful rotation coupled with strategic deworming are critical to effective parasite control. Routine fecal examinations, either individual or composite samples, may be useful to determine the frequency of deworming and the effectiveness of various anthelmintics. See Chapter 7 for more information.

TECHNICIAN NOTE

Internal parasites are a serious, life-threatening problem in small ruminants. Control is accomplished with proper management, routine fecal egg counts, strategic deworming programs, and use of appropriate anthelmintics.

Recommended Reading

Dogs and Cats

Hoskins JD, editor: *Veterinary pediatrics: dogs and cats from birth to six months*, ed 3, Philadelphia, 2001, WB Saunders.

Hoskins JD et al: Isolation and characterization of *Bordetella bronchiseptica* from cats in southern Louisiana, *Vet Immunol Immunopathol* 65:173, 1998.

Lappin MR: Protozoal infections. In Morgan RV, editor: *Handbook of small animal practice*, ed 3, Philadelphia, 1997, WB Saunders, p 1169.

Cattle

Aldridge B et al: Role of colostral transfer in neonatal calf management: failure of acquisition of passive immunity, *Compend Contin Educ Pract Vet* 14:265, 1992.

Baker JC, Velicer LF: Bovine respiratory syncytial virus vaccination: current status and future vaccine development, *Compend Contin Educ Pract Vet* 13:1323, 1991.

Heinrichs AJ: Milk replacers for dairy calves. I, *Compend Contin Educ Pract Vet* 16:1605, 1994.

Larson BL: Immunization to decrease pregnancy wastage in beef cattle. II, Available vaccines, *Compend Contin Educ Pract Vet* 18:571, 1996.

Smith BP: *Large animal internal medicine*, ed 3, St Louis, 2002, Mosby.

Spire MF: Immunization of the beef breeding herd, *Compend Contin Educ Pract Vet* 10:1111, 1988.

Swine

Amass SF: *Streptococcus suis*: what's new? *Proc AASP*, 315-317, 2000.

Christianson WT, Joo HS: Porcine reproductive and respiratory syndrome: a review, *Swine Health Prod* 2:10, 1994.

Cooper VL: Diagnosis of neonatal pig diarrhea, *Vet Clin North Am Food Anim Pract* 16:117-133, 2000.

Cowart RP, Casteel SW: *An outline of swine diseases*, ed 2, Ames, 2001, Iowa State University Press.

Fedorka-Cray PJ et al: *Actinobacillus (Haemophilus) pleuropneumoniae*. I, History, epidemiology, serotyping, and treatment, *Compend Contin Educ Pract Vet* 15:1447, 1993.

Maes D et al: Enzootic pneumonia in pigs, *Vet Q* 18:104-109, 1996.

Marstella TA, Fenwick B: *Actinobacillus pleuropneumoniae* disease and serology, *Swine Health Prod* 7:161-165, 1999.

Primm ND et al: Deworming strategies for swine. II, Anthelmintics and their use in the control of endoparasites, *Compend Contin Educ Pract Vet* 12:889, 1990.

Tynes V: Potbellied pig husbandry and nutrition, *Vet Clin North Am Exotic Anim Pract* 2:193-207, 1999.

Wills RW: Diarrhea in growing-finishing swine, *Vet Clin North Am Food Anim Pract* 16:135-161, 2000.

Zimmerman JJ et al: General overview of PRRSV: a perspective from the United States, *Vet Microbiol* 55:187-196, 1997.

Small Ruminants

Council report: vaccination guidelines for small ruminants (sheep, goats, llamas, domestic deer, and wapiti), *J Am Vet Med Assoc* 205:1539, 1994.

Pugh DG: *Sheep and goat medicine*, ed 1, Philadelphia, 2002, WB Saunders.

Robinson A, Wolf C: American Association of Small Ruminant Practitioners survey of biologic usage, *Symposium on Health and Disease of Small Ruminants*, pp 197-214, 1991.

Zajac AM, Moore GA: Treatment and control of gastrointestinal nematodes in sheep, *Compend Cont Educ Pract Vet* 15:999, 1993.

12

Neonatal Care of Puppy, Kitten, and Foal

JOHNNY D. HOSKINS • DAVID M. BOLT • ANN M. CHAPMAN

INTRODUCTION

Caring for the ill puppy, kitten or foal from birth to young adulthood is often complicated by age-related changes in the body systems. These age-related changes occur because the normal development of specific body systems continues well after birth. Thorough clinical evaluation of the ill puppy, kitten, or foal may include the case history, physical examination, routine laboratory tests, electrocardiography (ECG) (lead II rhythm strip), and possibly radiography. ■

PUPPY AND KITTEN

PHYSICAL AND LABORATORY EXAMINATION

The physical examination of a sick puppy or kitten should be conducted in a systematic manner. Additional information on the physical examination can be found in Chapter 2. The first skill used in the examination is careful observation of the animal's responses, specifically noting the puppy's or kitten's general condition, mentation, posture, locomotion, and breathing pattern. Next, the body temperature, respiratory and heart rates, capillary refill time, and body weight should be recorded. After completing the observation and vital signs collection phase, the clinician should assess the function of specific body systems (Box 12-1).

Veterinarians often use a commercial laboratory facility for routine tests, such as hemograms, serum chemistry profiles, and urinalysis. However, collections from puppies and kittens younger than 6 weeks of age often result in inadequate samples for testing by these laboratories. As an alternative, the veterinarian can use in-house laboratory tests, including microhematocrit for the packed cell volume, blood film examination of erythrocyte and leukocyte structure, blood glucose and blood urea nitrogen by reagent strip for whole blood, urine evaluation by reagent strip for urinalysis and a urine sediment examination, and total plasma solids and urine specific gravity by refractometer. The results of these few tests may be sufficient to confirm illness or assist in case management of an illness.

An ECG can be used to diagnose life-threatening arrhythmias and conduction disturbances in puppies and kittens; however, ECG identification of right- or left-sided chamber enlargement or hypertrophy and alterations in mean electrical axis is usually not attempted. The ECGs of young kittens normally have smaller amplitude P waves and QRS complexes in all leads than those of puppies. Any ECG lead with easily recognizable P waves and QRS complexes can be used to identify arrhythmias.

Real-time, gray-scale ultrasonography is an invaluable diagnostic tool for the identification of selected abdominal and cardiac diseases in puppies and kittens. Ultrasonography is usually better tolerated by puppies and kittens and is safer for personnel than routine radiology. For ultrasonography in most puppies and kittens, a 5-MHz ultrasound transducer or, preferably, a 7.5-MHz transducer is required. The higher the transducer frequency, the better is the image resolution, but the greater is the ultrasound beam attenuation in soft tissue. Linear array transducers used transrectally for reproductive examination are inadequate for imaging in most puppies and kittens.

TECHNICIAN NOTE

Real-time, gray-scale ultrasonography is an invaluable diagnostic tool for the identification of selected abdominal and cardiac diseases in puppies and kittens.

Box 12-1 PHYSICAL EXAMINATION OF KITTEN OR PUPPY

- **Head and Oral Cavity:** Check for malformations of the skull, cleft lip, stenotic nares, or cleft palate. The mucous membranes should be light pink and moist. The teeth, if present, should be examined for early occlusion.
- **Ears:** External ear canals open between 6 and 14 days after birth and should be completely open by 17 days. When ear canals first open, cytologic examination shows an abundance of desquamative cells and some oil droplets. A thorough otoscopic examination can be performed on kittens older than 4 weeks of age.
- **Eyes and Eyelids:** The eyelids separate into upper and lower eyelids at 5 to 14 days after birth. Menace reflex may not appear until 3 to 4 weeks of life. Reflex lacrimation begins when the eyelids separate; therefore evaluation of tear production by the Schirmer tear test can be done thereafter. Pupillary light responses are present after the eyelids open but may not be evident until 21 days of age.
- **Nose:** Check appearance and patency of the nostrils and the presence of fluids (mucus, pus, blood, milk, clear discharges).
- **Thorax:** Check the thoracic wall, whether symmetric or deformed, and auscultate the thorax using a stethoscope with a pediatric chest piece (2-cm bell; 3-cm diaphragm). The heart rate approximates 220 beats/min, and the respiratory rate is from 15 to 35 breaths/min during the first 4 weeks of life and becomes similar to that of adults thereafter. The normal heart rhythm of puppies and kittens is a regular sinus rhythm. Heart sounds are localized to the left cardiac apex (left fifth to sixth intercostal space, ventral third of thorax), the left cardiac base (left third to fourth intercostal space above the costochondral junction), or the right cardiac apex (right fourth to fifth intercostal space opposite the mitral valve area). Heart murmurs are the most common type of abnormal sound heard, frequently being a functional murmur and not a murmur associated with congenital heart disease. Absence of lung sounds or audible asymmetry may indicate abnormalities within the thorax and/or lungs.
- **Abdomen:** Unless the liver margins extend beyond the ribs, the liver is not enlarged. The spleen is not normally palpable unless it is enlarged. Both kidneys are palpable in all kittens. The stomach may feel like a large, fluid-filled sac if it is full. The intestines palpate as soft, slightly fluid or gas-filled structures that are freely movable and nonpainful. The urinary bladder can be gently squeezed to determine resistance to urine outflow.
- **Skin and Umbilicus:** The skin should be inspected for wounds, state of hydration, and condition of foot pads. The skin and coat should also be examined for evidence of bacterial infection, external parasites, and dermatophytosis. The umbilicus should be carefully inspected for evidence of inflammation and/or infection or abnormalities of the abdominal wall. The umbilical cord normally drops off by 2 to 3 days of age.
- **Limbs, Tail, Anus, and Genitalia:** Check the limbs for deformities or absence of long bones, number and position of toes and pads, position of limbs at rest and during movement, presence of soft tissue (bruises, swelling, wounds), and condition of joints (deformities, range of mobility). The tail is inspected for length, mobility, and deformities. The anus should be evaluated for patency, redness, and signs of diarrhea; and the genitalia should be checked for position and appearance.
- **Nervous System:** Sucking reflex is present at birth and disappears by 3 weeks of life. Eliminative behaviors are controlled for first 3 to 4 weeks of life by anogenital reflex.

Most echocardiography is performed in puppies and kittens that are 6 weeks of age or older. Echocardiograms, whether obtained with the use of M-mode, two-dimensional, contrast, or Doppler echocardiographic technology, have facilitated evaluation of puppies and kittens with congenital heart disease or cardiomyopathy by improving the diagnostic accuracy and lessening the stress and risk to animals. For echocardiography in puppies and kittens, a 7.5-MHz transducer is preferred. Heart conditions readily identified with M-mode or two-dimensional echocardiography include pericardial effusion, valvular vegetations, abnormal chamber size, myocardial hypertrophy, and abnormal cardiac motion.

Contrast echocardiography may be helpful in confirming a right-to-left shunting lesion. Doppler ultrasonography is becoming increasingly available. Doppler imaging of high-velocity, retrograde, or turbulent flow through valves or intracardiac communications provides useful diagnostic and prognostic information in puppies and kittens with congenital heart defects. Interpretation of echocardiograms from puppies and kittens requires an awareness of the growth pattern and developmental anatomy of the heart during the first year of life. After birth, there is a decrease in right ventricular mass relative to the left ventricle and to body weight, a decrease that occurs by the third week of life in puppies.

Additional information on ultrasonography and radiology can be found in Chapter 9.

A finely tuned technique chart is necessary if good-quality radiographs are to be produced for all body parts of young puppies and kittens. Kilovoltage must be greatly reduced for radiography of a young puppy or kitten because of minimal absorption of x-rays by partially mineralized bones and because of the thinness of soft tissue body parts. A general guideline for reducing kilovoltage is to reduce the radiographic exposure to about one half of that used for adult dogs and cats of the same thickness. Extrapolations to thinner dogs and cats can be made based on the fact that each centimeter of soft tissue is the equivalent of 2 kVp at values equal to or less than 80 kVp. Most radiography of young puppies and kittens will be performed in the 40- to 60-kVp range; therefore a change of 4 to 6 kVp doubles or halves the film exposure.

An additional step that can be helpful in producing maximum-quality radiographs in young puppies and kittens is use of a single high-detail intensifying screen within the cassette. The single screen should be adhered to the back inner surface of the cassette. The screen should be a rare-earth, high-detail type. The emulsion side of the x-ray film must be positioned toward the screen.

The development of computer equipment that can average electrical signals by extracting low-amplitude, time-locked potentials from random background electrical activity has provided procedures for noninvasive evaluation of the auditory and visual systems. Recording of the brainstem auditory-evoked response is the best objective procedure for assessment of hearing in puppies and kittens. The electrical potential from the cochlea, cochlear nerve, and brainstem in response to an auditory stimulus is recorded. The brainstem auditory-evoked response approximates functional maturity by 4 to 6 weeks of age. If there is no response at all in puppies or kittens older than 6 weeks of age, the cochlea is not functioning, as may occur with congenital deafness.

The electroretinogram is the electrical recording of retinal response to light. The electroretinogram approximates functional maturity by 5 to 10 weeks of age. If there is no response at all after 10 weeks of age, the retina is not functioning, as may occur in retinal blindness from congenital or acquired causes. The visual-evoked response (VER) provides an objective evaluation of the central visual pathways. The VER is the cortical electrical activity that occurs in response to a light stimulus administered to the eye. The VER approximates functional maturity by 6 weeks of age. If there is an altered VER after 10 weeks of age, central visual pathways may not be functioning, as may occur in central blindness from congenital or acquired causes.

NEWBORN PUPPIES AND KITTENS

Newborn puppies and kittens are, for all practical purposes, completely helpless. They rely on their mother for warmth, food, elimination, cleanliness, and protection. They are incapable of thermal regulation for the first 6 days of life and require an external heat source to stay warm for the first 3 weeks of life. They nurse from the mother every 1 to 2 hours for the first week, and the mother licks their external genitalia both to stimulate urination and defecation and clean them after every feeding. Five to 14 days after delivery, the puppies' and kittens' eyes open but have limited vision; a day or so later, their external ear canals open. By 18 days of age, they begin to move around and explore their environment.

TECHNICIAN NOTE

Newborn puppies and kittens are, for all practical purposes, completely helpless.

Keep puppies and kittens in a small box with sides high enough both to keep them inside and to prevent drafts.

Raise the bottom of the box off the floor and cover it with a padded, disposable, or washable flooring such as indoor-outdoor carpeting and disposable diapers or cotton towels to keep the box as warm and dry as possible. Materials that become slippery when wet, such as newspapers, should not be used as bedding. Covered hot water bottles or heating pads set on the lowest setting may help keep the environmental temperature stable. Never set heating pads on higher settings, because severe burns can result. A puppy's or kitten's rectal temperature should be maintained at 96° F to 97° F for the first week of life and at 97° F to 100° F for the second, third, and fourth weeks. Do not cover the entire floor of the box with a heating pad; the puppy or kitten must be able to get away from the heat source if it gets too warm. A ticking clock placed in the box may help to keep puppies and kittens quiet.

PRINCIPLES OF ORPHAN ANIMAL CARE

Hand-raising orphan puppies and kittens requires a great deal of time and effort. The ideal solution to the problem of caring for a motherless puppy or kitten is to locate a lactating mother that will accept the puppy or kitten and raise it with its own. When a foster mother is not available, it is necessary to hand feed the puppy or kitten until about 4 to 6 weeks of age, but if possible, the puppy or kitten should be left with littermates between feedings during this time so it can interact with others and thereby learn appropriate social behavior. If neither of these options is possible, total care of the puppy or kitten must be undertaken. Puppies and kittens are usually mature enough to be sold between 6 and 8 weeks of age.

Successful rearing of orphaned puppies and kittens requires providing them with a suitable environment; the correct quantities and quality of nutrients for different stages of growth; a regular schedule of feeding, sleeping, grooming, and exercise; and the stimulus that provokes urination and defecation.

Newborn puppies and kittens are unable to effectively control their body temperature. They gradually change, during their first 4 weeks of life, from being largely poikilothermic to being homeothermic. That is, for the first week of life, their body temperature is directly related to the environmental temperature, and a steady ambient temperature of 86° F to 90° F is needed. Over the next 3 weeks, the ambient temperature can be gradually lowered to 75° F. Humidity should be maintained at 55% to 60%. It is equally important that sudden changes in environmental conditions be avoided and that disturbances outside of socialization, exercise, and hygiene activities be minimized.

TECHNICIAN NOTE

Newborn puppies and kittens are unable to effectively control their body temperature.

Feeding orphaned puppies and kittens that still require mother's milk can be rewarding. The most obvious alternative to a mother rearing her own young is for another nursing mother to act as a foster mother. If a foster mother is not available, it is necessary to hand feed the puppies or kittens a replacement food that is a prototype of nutritive substance formulated to meet the optimum requirements of the puppy or kitten. Mother's milk is the ideal food. Various modifications of homemade and commercially prepared formulas simulating mother's milk have been used with good success. Several homemade or commercial prepared formulas for puppies and kittens may be used (Box 12-2).

Commercially prepared milk formulas are preferred, because they more closely compare to mother's milk. These formulas generally provide 1 to 1.24 kcal of metabolizable energy per milliliter of formula. The caloric needs for most nursing-age puppies and kittens is 22 to 26 kcal per 100 g of body weight. Therefore the average puppy or kitten should daily receive approximately 13 ml of formula per 100 g of body weight during the first week of life, 17 ml of formula per 100 g of body weight during the second week, 20 ml of formula per 100 g of body weight during the third week, and 22 ml of formula per 100 g of body weight during the fourth week. These amounts of formula should be given in equal portions three or four times daily. For the first 3 weeks of life, the formula should be warmed before each feeding to about 100° F or to a temperature near the animal's body temperature.

After each feeding, the abdomen should be enlarged but not overdistended. When a milk formula is used, less than the prescribed amount should be given per feeding for the first feedings. The amount is then gradually increased to the recommended feeding amount by the second or third day. The amount of milk formula is increased accordingly as the puppy or kitten gains weight and a favorable response to feeding occurs. Puppies should gain 1 to 2 g/day/lb (2 to 4 g/day/kg) of anticipated adult weight for the first 5 months of their lives. At birth, kittens should weigh 80 to 140 g (most weigh around 100 to 120 g) and gain 50 to 100 g weekly.

When preparing the formula, always follow the manufacturer's directions for proper preparation, and keep all feeding equipment scrupulously clean. A good way of handling prepared formula is to prepare only a 48-hour supply at a time and divide this into portions required for each feeding. Once formula is prepared, it is best stored in the refrigerator at 4° C.

The easiest and safest way of feeding prepared formula to nursing-age puppies and kittens is by nipple bottle, dosing syringe, or tube. Nipple bottles made especially for feeding orphan puppies or kittens or bottles equipped with preemie infant nipples are preferred. When feeding with a nipple bottle, hold the bottle so that the puppy or kitten does not ingest air. The hole in the nipple should be such that when the bottle is inverted, milk slowly oozes from the nipple. It may be necessary to enlarge the nipple hole with a hot needle to get milk to ooze from the bottle when it is inverted. When feeding, squeeze a drop of milk onto the

---

Box 12-2 MILK REPLACER FOR NURSING PUPPIES AND KITTENS

COMMERCIAL PREPARED FORMULA FOR PUPPIES OR KITTENS
Begin Milk Replacer For Puppies (Performer Brand, St Joseph, Missouri)
Begin Milk Replacer For Kittens (Performer Brand, St Joseph, Missouri)
Esbilac Powder For Puppies (Pet-Ag Inc, Elgin, Illinois)
Esbilac Liquid For Puppies (Pet-Ag Inc, Elgin, Illinois)
GME Powder For Puppies (a Goat Milk Formula; Pet-Ag Inc, Elgin, Illinois)
Kitten Milk Replacer Formula (Eukanuba, The Iams Co, Dayton Ohio)
Kittylac Powder For Kittens (Landco Corp, Post Falls, Idaho)
KMR Liquid For Kittens (Pet-Ag Inc, Elgin, Illinois)
KMR Powder For Kittens (Pet-Ag Inc, Elgin, Illinois)
Multi-Milk For Multi-animals (milk replacer for animals with lactose intolerance; Pet-Ag Inc, Elgin, Illinois)
Nurturall Liquid For Puppies (Veterinary Products Laboratories, Phoenix, Arizona)
Nurturall Powder For Puppies (Veterinary Products Laboratories, Phoenix, Arizona)
Nurturall Liquid For Kittens (Veterinary Products Laboratories, Phoenix, Arizona)

Nurturall Powder For Kittens (Veterinary Products Laboratories, Phoenix, Arizona)
Puppylac Powder For Kittens (Landco Corp, Post Falls, Idaho)
Puppy Milk Replacer Formula (Eukanuba, The Iams Co, Dayton, Ohio)
Veta-Lac Powder For Puppies (Vet-A-Mix, Shenandoah, Iowa)
Veta-Lac Powder For Kittens (Vet-A-Mix, Shenandoah, Iowa)

HOMEMADE PREPARED FORMULA FOR PUPPIES
120 ml of cow's or goat's milk
120 ml of water
2 to 4 egg yolks
1 to 2 teaspoonfuls of vegetable oil
1000 mg of calcium carbonate

HOMEMADE PREPARED FORMULA FOR KITTENS
90 ml of condensed milk
90 ml of water
120 ml of plain yogurt (not low-fat)
3 large or 4 small egg yolks

tip of the nipple and then insert the nipple into the puppy's or kitten's mouth. Never squeeze milk out of the bottle while the nipple is in the animal's mouth; doing so may result in laryngotracheal aspiration of the milk into the lungs. In addition, prepared formula should never be fed to a puppy or kitten that is chilled or that does not have a strong sucking reflex. Only when the sucking reflex is present should nipple-bottle feeding be attempted.

Tube feeding is the fastest way to feed orphaned puppies or kittens. Most owners can do it easily with a little training. The following may be used: a No. 5 Fr infant feeding tube for puppies or kittens weighing less than 300 g; a No. 8 to 10 Fr infant feeding tube for puppies or kittens weighing more than 300 g; or an appropriately sized, soft, male urethral catheter. Once weekly, mark the feeding tube clearly to indicate the depth of insertion to ensure gastric delivery; that is, the distance from the last rib to the tip of the nose can be measured and marked off on the feeding tube as a guide. Never feed into the distal esophagus. When feeding, fill a syringe with warm prepared formula and fit it to the feeding tube, being sure to expel any air in the tube or syringe. Open the animal's mouth slightly, and with the animal's head held in the normal nursing position, gently pass the feeding tube to the marked area. If an obstruction is felt or if coughing occurs before the mark is reached, the tube is in the trachea. If this does not happen, slowly administer the prepared formula over a 2-minute period to allow sufficient time for slow filling of the stomach. Regurgitation of formula rarely occurs; but if it does, withdraw the feeding tube and interrupt feeding until the next scheduled meal.

A vital aspect of tending orphaned puppies and kittens is to simulate, after feeding, the mother's tongue action on the anogenital area, which provokes reflex micturition and defecation. Application of this stimulus must be taken over by the person tending the puppies or kittens. The necessary result can be achieved by swabbing the anogenital area with moistened cotton or dry, soft tissue paper to manually stimulate reflex elimination. It is sometimes possible to effect the same response simply by running a forefinger along the abdominal wall. This stimulation should be regularly provided after each nipple-bottle feeding or tube feeding. After they reach about 3 weeks of age, puppies and kittens are usually able to relieve themselves without stimulation.

Most puppies and kittens benefit from gentle handling before feeding to allow for some exercise and to promote muscular and circulatory development. In addition, at least once a week you should gently wash the orphaned puppy or kitten with a soft moistened cloth for general cleansing of the skin, simulating the cleansing licks of the mother's tongue.

As mentioned before, orphaned puppies and kittens should be encouraged to begin eating solid food at 3 and 4 weeks of age, respectively. Once they are eating satisfactorily from a bowl, gradually reduce the amount of prepared formula being given until only the puppy or kitten food designed for growth is being fed, at least three times a day.

Puppies and kittens should be checked for gastrointestinal parasites at 3 weeks of age, and they require fecal rechecks when they return for their vaccinations. Heartworm preventive medication should be started at 6 to 8 weeks of age in areas where heartworms are endemic. The initial vaccination series consists of one injection of a multivalent vaccine given at 6 weeks of age and two boosters given at 9 weeks of age and 12 weeks of age. Puppies and kittens whose immune status is uncertain may receive an additional injection of multivalent vaccine as early as 2 weeks of age. The rabies injection is given at 3 months of age in most states.

✐ TECHNICIAN NOTE

Heartworm preventive medication should be started at 6 to 8 weeks of age in areas where heartworms are endemic.

REASONS FOR NEONATE CARE

Puppies and kittens are commonly presented because of severe illnesses or to be reared as orphans during the period between birth and 12 weeks of age. Illnesses may have been acquired in utero, during the birth process, during the neonatal period (0 to 2 weeks of age), or in the postweaning period of 6 to 12 weeks of age. Illness during the postweaning period is primarily caused by infectious (bacterial, viral, protozoal, and parasitic) diseases and/or malnutrition potentiated by weaning stress, exposure to pathogenic organisms in the immediate environment, and diminished local or systemic immunity. In general, most puppy and kitten illnesses will occur because of congenital anomalies, nutritional diseases resulting from improper diets fed to the mother or her young, abnormally low birth weights, traumatic insults during or after the birth process (dystocia, cannibalism, maternal neglect), neonatal isoerythrolysis, infectious diseases, and other miscellaneous factors.

MALNUTRITION

Malnutrition occurs when basic nutritional requirements for puppies or kittens are not being met. Malnutrition is especially common during the time when they depend entirely on the mother. Several factors can contribute to malnutrition in the nursing puppy or kitten. The puppy or kitten may ingest insufficient or inadequate milk because the mother has died; the mother may disown her young; the litter may be larger than can be cared for properly; and partial or complete lactation failure may occur in the mother because of mastitis, metritis, or underdeveloped mammae. In addition, puppies and kittens may be born underdeveloped, be so weak and sick that they cannot suckle, or have a congenital anomaly that precludes adequate milk intake. Failure to provide an adequate growth diet at 3 to 4 weeks of age can also result in malnutrition.

Immediate recognition of a malnourished puppy or kitten is usually based on its smaller, lighter appearance; feeble attempts to feed; or inability to attain adequate weight gain for its age. High-pitched, constant crying and inactivity with an accompanying weak sucking reflex are advanced indications that the nursing puppy or kitten is receiving insufficient or inadequate milk. Reduced body tone and muscle strength may be evident on handling. A coexisting congenital anomaly that is not immediately life threatening may be detected on physical examination as well.

The management of malnutrition in the nursing puppy or kitten generally requires that proper nourishment be provided. Complications that are frequently encountered during the management of malnutrition are diarrhea, dehydration, hypoglycemia, and hypothermia. If diarrhea occurs during feeding of adequate amounts of commercial milk replacement formula, immediately reduce the amount of solids intake to one half of that offered. This can be done by diluting the milk replacement formula 1:1 with water, or preferably, with a mixture of equal parts of Ringer's solution and 5% dextrose/water solution. As the condition of feces improves, gradually increase the amount of solids to the recommended level. Hypoglycemia and dehydration occur quickly when the malnourished puppy or kitten is not adequately fed. Milk replacement formula should not be fed to a weak and severely chilled puppy or kitten that has a diminished sucking reflex or body temperature below 35° C (95° F). Giving an equal mixture of warm Ringer's solution and 5% dextrose/water solution parenterally or administering a warm nutrient-electrolyte solution orally every 15 to 30 minutes until the puppy or kitten responds can help to alleviate or prevent dehydration and mild hypoglycemia.

SIGNS OF NEONATAL ILLNESS

The clinical manifestations of neonatal illness do not always allow specific identification of the causative condition. Furthermore, many puppies and kittens have unusual or a wide variety of clinical presentations, which may not be immediately recognized as being associated with a specific illness. Death can occur so suddenly that noticeable signs are virtually absent. More typically, however, puppies and kittens will cry a lot, show signs of restlessness, weakness, hypothermia, diarrhea, altered respiration, hematuria, failure to thrive, and cyanosis; and in advanced stages, they may slough parts of their extremities.

The diagnosis of a neonatal illness is usually based on the case history and physical examination findings. Ideally, a complete blood count, plasma chemistry profile, urinalysis, urine and/or blood culture, and culture of suspected sources of infection are performed. When dealing with neonatal sepsis, it is imperative to conduct a thorough search for the primary source of infection and collect appropriate bacterial culture samples before initiating antimicrobial therapy.

The hemograms of septicemic puppies and kittens are usually characterized by a normochromic normocytic anemia. Thrombocytopenia and mild to moderate neutrophilia with a left shift may be present. Another laboratory finding that is consistent with, but by no means specific for, neonatal sepsis is hypoglycemia. The remaining laboratory values from the plasma chemistry profile and urinalysis may reflect specific organ failure.

MANAGEMENT OF NEONATAL ILLNESS

Early, prompt care for the ill puppy or kitten is required for satisfactory results. Because many neonatal diseases may cause sudden death, puppies and kittens suspected of having a severe illness should be treated immediately. In most instances, rewarming, fluid replacement, and antimicrobial therapy are started empirically. Severely ill puppies and kittens may also require glucose therapy if hypoglycemia is present (Box 12-3).

TECHNICIAN NOTE
Early, prompt care for the ill puppy or kitten is required for satisfactory results.

Meaningful advances in treating bacterial infections have been made in recent years, particularly in the development of antimicrobial agents. Many of these antimicrobial agents have either an increased spectrum of activity or fewer toxic effects compared with previously available antimicrobial agents. However, specific pharmacokinetic data for many of the antimicrobial agents have not been obtained in either adults or in puppies and kittens, and therefore the veterinary use of these antimicrobial agents remains somewhat empiric.

Unfortunately, clinical information necessary for appropriate dosing of antimicrobial agents in septicemic puppies and kittens is not always available. Drug distribution, especially in puppies and kittens younger than 5 weeks, differs from that of adults because of differences in body composition, such as lower total body fat, higher percentage of total body water, lower concentrations of albumin, and a poorly developed blood-brain barrier. Because of these differences, modifications of dosing amounts for adults, as much as 30% to 50% reduction of the adult dose, or changes in dosing frequency may be necessary when antimicrobial agents are administered to septicemic puppies and kittens.

Furthermore, fluid replacement therapy and antimicrobial agents should be administered intravenously or intraosseously in severely ill puppies and kittens, because systemic absorption after oral, subcutaneous, or intramuscular administration may not be reliable. Most drugs ingested by the lactating bitch or queen appear in her milk; the amount is generally 1% to 2% of the mother's dose. Therefore severely ill puppies or kittens should never be

---

Box 12-3 MEDICAL MANAGEMENT OF THE SEVERELY ILL PUPPY OR KITTEN

I. External warming procedure
  A. Use circulating hot water blanket, rice bags, or hot water bottle
  B. Take at least 20 to 30 minutes for gradual warming of the animal
  C. Turn the animal every hour
  D. Record rectal temperature every hour
II. Parenteral fluid therapy
  A. Use balanced multiple electrolyte solution supplemented with 5% dextrose solution
  B. Supplement the fluids with potassium chloride solution if plasma potassium concentration is less than 2.5 mEq/L
  C. Administer warm fluids slowly by intravenous or intra-osseous route
III. Glucose replacement therapy
  A. Administer 5% dextrose solution intravenously or intra-osseously to effect
  B. Administer 1 to 2 ml of a 10% to 20% dextrose solution per kilogram of body weight to the animal that is profoundly depressed or having seizures
  C. Maintain plasma glucose concentration at 80 to 200 mg/dl for euglycemia
IV. Antimicrobial therapy
  A. Collect bacterial culture samples (whole blood, urine, exu-date, and feces) before initiation of antimicrobial therapy
    1. For blood culture, collect 1 ml of whole blood aseptically and inoculate blood directly into enriched tryptic or trypticase soy broth, dilute the whole blood 1:5 to 1:10

in enriched broth, and examine broth for bacterial growth 6 to 18 hours later
    2. For urine culture, collect urine by cystocentesis, and culture it by standard methods
    3. For exudate and fecal cultures, collect and culture by standard methods
  B. Empirical treatment with antimicrobial agent(s) begins immediately after collection of appropriate bacterial culture samples
  C. Adjust the dosage and dosing interval of antimicrobial agent(s) selected
  D. Administer antimicrobial agent(s) by the intravenous or intraosseous route
V. Provide oxygen and nutritional therapy
  A. Administer oxygen by mask or intranasal catheter to counteract tissue hypoxemia
  B. Encourage food intake once animal is normothermic and adequately hydrated
VI. Monitor the effectiveness of medical management
  A. Observe for improvement in the animal's general demeanor
  B. Regularly assess the cardiopulmonary status (it is ex-tremely easy to overhydrate the ill puppy and kitten; thus attentive monitoring of breathing pattern is helpful for early recognition of overhydration.)
  C. Weigh the animal three to four times a day to record weight gain
  D. Observe for moistness and color of mucous membranes in assessing for adequate hydration

---

treated by only treating the lactating mother. The beta-lactam antimicrobial agents are considered to be the first choice in the treatment of septicemic puppies and kittens. The beta-lactam antimicrobial agents include the penicillins, cephalosporins, and the combination of beta-lactam antimicrobials and beta-lactamase inhibitors.

FOAL

The critically ill foal is one of the most challenging veteri-nary patients, and its survival is undoubtedly influenced by diligent nursing care. The overall survival rate of foals that require intensive care is constantly improving, and more immature foals of younger gestational ages are surviving. Specialized centers in equine neonatal care and an improved understanding of physiologic and disease states in foals appear to be responsible for these recent advances.

Management of ill foals requires a team approach, and competent veterinary technical support is a contributing factor of major importance for success. The skills required of an equine neonatal technician are extensive, and they are acquired and improved over years with growing expe-rience. This text merely provides an overview of these skills.

Veterinary technicians with aspirations in this area are advised to refer to more detailed information in textbooks that focus on equine and human neonatology and to obtain additional clinical training in facilities that have a specialized neonatal unit for foals.

THE HIGH-RISK MARE

Maternal factors play an important role in the development and health status of the neonatal foal, and early recognition of high-risk mares often allows identification of foals that are at increased risk of becoming critically ill. The most common conditions that place mares in the high-risk cate-gory are advanced age, poor general state of health, poor perineal conformation or vaginal discharge, and a history of difficulties during previous pregnancies or prolonged transport during late gestation. A variety of concurrent diseases in the mare can potentially compromise the health and ultimate survival of the fetus.

Mares must be routinely evaluated for risk factors before and during pregnancy. Although some risks can be avoided by changing management factors, some mares require intensive monitoring to prevent potential problems. Placement of a mare in the high-risk category necessitates monitoring of fetal viability and health for the whole period or the remainder of pregnancy.

Evaluation of fetal viability should include a rectal examination by a veterinarian. Gentle transrectal stimulation of the late-term fetus by ballottement often results in movement as a response. Although a rectal exam provides valuable information, the risk and potential complications associated with this diagnostic technique should be kept in mind. Transabdominal ultrasonography allows assessment of several important parameters including fetal activity, fetal heart rate, and the aortic diameter of the fetus. Additionally, the uteroplacental contact surface can be monitored for integrity, and its thickness can be evaluated. A low-frequency probe (e.g., 2.5-MHz linear probe) should be used for transabdominal ultrasonography. Image quality can be substantially improved by clipping the mare's hair and use of an ultrasound contact gel, or, alternatively, by wetting the hair on the flank with isopropyl alcohol.

The fetal heart rate is ultrasonographically detectable at approximately 160 days of gestation. The average fetal heart rate is 120 beats/min, although values are highly variable during late gestation and can range from 80 to 160 beats/min. Over the course of gestation, the fetal heart rate should decrease and become less variable during repeat measurements.

The uteroplacental unit should be between 8 and 16 mm thick, and no fluid should be detectable between the placenta and the uterine wall. Fluid between these two layers may be indicative of premature placental separation caused by placentitis or hemorrhage. Based on such findings, close monitoring of the uteroplacental unit for further separation by means of follow-up ultrasonographic exams is indicated. During late gestation, induction of labor may also be an option.

There are few reliable methods to predict the exact time of parturition. Enlargement of the mammae and the presence of "wax" on the tips of the teats have historically been used as predictors of imminent parturition. Although these signs are still considered valid today, as many as 15% of mares actually fail to demonstrate them before foaling. The rapid rise in colostral calcium represents one of the most consistent and significant changes before parturition. Calcium levels in colostrum samples can be rapidly measured in nearly every diagnostic laboratory or even just by the use of simple hard water test kits. Colostral calcium levels above 10 to 12 mmol/dl are considered significant enough to predict parturition within the ensuing 24 hours. Although colostral calcium levels appear to be the most reliable method for predicting the time of parturition, false-positive or false-negative results may still be obtained.

THE HIGH-RISK FOAL

The term *high-risk foal* refers to the equine neonate that is not necessarily exhibiting signs of disease but is at a high risk of becoming ill. These foals generally appear normal for the first 24 hours of life, but their condition may quickly deteriorate. Survival of these foals clearly depends on early recognition of the disease status. If foals exhibit the slightest signs of disease in the early postparturition period, they must be assumed to be abnormal, and there is an immediate need for accurate diagnosis and treatment of their condition. Physical exam findings, as well as laboratory results and historical factors, assist in the identification of high-risk foals.

The classic early signs of disease in foals are lethargy, depression, decreased suckle reflex, decreased appetite, increased periods of recumbency and sleeping, and decreased affinity for nursing. Historical factors increasing the probability of a high-risk foal are twin births, abnormal birth behavior (see Physical Examination), shortened gestational length, and failure of passive transfer (i.e., "leaking" of colostrum from the mare's teats for an extended period before parturition).

The equine gestational length may range from 315 to 365 days, with an average of 341 days. Premature foals are born before they reach 320 days of gestational age. Signs of prematurity include low birth weight, weakness, a delay in standing after parturition, soft pliant lips and ears, prominent domed forehead, soft silky hair coat, flexor tendon laxity, and angular limb deformities associated with incomplete ossification of the cuboidal carpal and tarsal bones on radiographs. Any physical sign of prematurity will categorize the foal as high risk. The term *dysmaturity* is used for foals that are of a gestational age of more than 320 days exhibit signs of prematurity. *Immaturity* is a collective term used to refer to foals of any gestational age that exhibit signs of prematurity. The veterinary technician familiar with neonatal foals should keep in mind that external signs of prematurity are correlated with immaturity of other organ systems. This results in an increased susceptibility to disease and injury. For example, premature foals with angular limb deformity are likely to have incomplete skeletal ossification, which can result in crushing injuries to the cuboidal carpal and tarsal bones from simple weight-bearing.

PHYSICAL EXAMINATION

To recognize high-risk foals, the veterinary technician needs to be familiar with the normal history, physical exam findings, and behavior of an equine neonate. The newborn foal should exhibit a suckle reflex at 20 minutes after birth, stand within 1 to 2 hours, and nurse within 2 to 3 hours. The first urination normally occurs within 10 hours, and the meconium should be passed by 24 hours after parturition.

A thorough observation from a distance should initiate a complete physical exam. When awake, the foal should be alert and easily aroused by environmental stimuli. Foals should develop a strong bond with the dam within the first 1.5 hours after parturition and normally nurse an average

Table 12-1 Diseases of Foals

Body System	Diseases
Infectious	Septicemia/bacteremia, pneumonia, meningitis, omphalophlebitis, nephritis, septic arthritis, osteomyelitis, septic peritonitis
Gastrointestinal	Meconium impaction, gastric and duodenal ulceration, enteritis, peritonitis, intussusception, intraluminal obstruction, volvulus, cleft palate, prognathism, brachygnathia, atresia coli, atresia recti, atresia ani
Respiratory	Respiratory distress complex, pneumonia, meconium aspiration, persistent pulmonary hypertension
Cardiovascular	Ventricular septal defect
Musculoskeletal	Flexural deformities, angular limb deformities, incomplete skeletal ossification, osteochondrosis, physitis, rib fracture
Urogenital	Patent urachus; rupture of the ureter, bladder, urethra, or urachus; umbilical hernia; scrotal hernia
Immunologic	Failure of passive transfer, combined immunodeficiency
Hematologic	Neonatal isoerythrolysis, anemia
Neurologic	Neonatal maladjustment syndrome, brain and spinal hemorrhage, epilepsy
Ocular	Corneal ulcer, entropion, ectropion
Miscellaneous	Hypoxemia, hypoglycemia, hypothermia

of seven times per hour. Head bobbing while searching for the udder of the mare is normal. Dried milk may be present on the foreheads and muzzles of foals that have not been nursing adequately. Severe mammary engorgement may indicate decreased nursing activity of the neonate. Within 24 hours of birth, the foal should be strong, alert, and capable of running. The foal's respiration undergoes an important change in the immediate postnatal phase and should be monitored closely. The respiratory rate increases from 20 to 40 breaths/min at birth to 60 to 80 breaths/min within the first hour. Respiration should be strong and regular when the foal is standing but may be irregular when it is sleeping. The extent of chest excursion during inspiration and expiration should be monitored to evaluate the foal for signs of respiratory distress.

The remaining body systems also need to be thoroughly examined. Special attention must be directed toward the identification of specific diseases that can affect the equine neonate (Table 12-1). The normal rectal temperature in the neonatal foal ranges from 37.2° C to 38.9° C (99° F to 102° F). The integument should be closely examined for decubital ulcers, urine and fecal scalding, as well as the presence of petechiae on the surface of mucous membranes and the inner ear (Figure 12-1).

Evaluation of cardiovascular stability is initiated by palpatation of the peripheral arterial pulses. At the facial artery, which courses beneath the ramus of the mandible, the arterial pulse should be easily identified. Arterial pulses should also be palpated at the brachial artery, located at the medial aspect of the elbow, and the great metatarsal artery, which is found on the lateral aspect of the third metatarsal bone. This latter vessel is also best suited for the collection of blood for arterial blood gas analysis (Figure 12-2). The distal limbs should feel warm to the touch. Cold limbs can indicate poor peripheral perfusion caused by septic shock as blood is directed away from the extremities to other

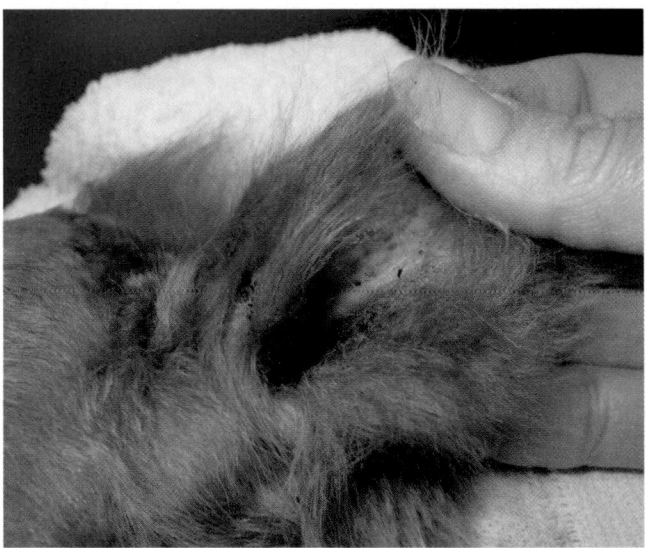

Figure 12-1 Examination of the inner ear reveals petechiation.

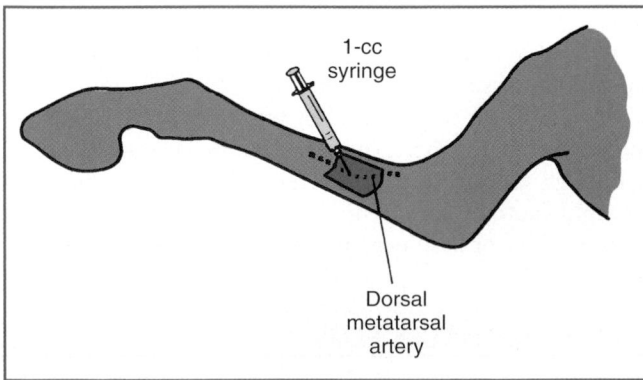

Figure 12-2 Location of dorsal metatarsal artery for collection of arterial blood samples in the foal.

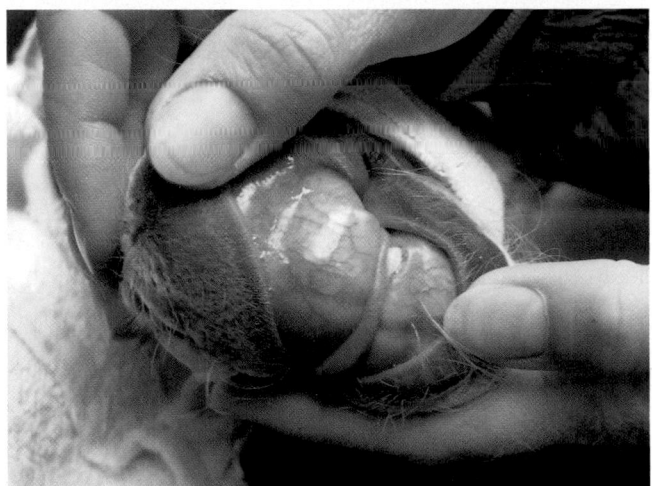

Figure 12-3 Abnormal reddening of the mucous membranes and tongue is termed injection.

important tissues. Cardiac auscultation of the newborn foal usually reveals a loud machinery or holosystolic murmur at the left heart base, which should abate within the first 72 hours of life. This murmur is believed to originate from a patent ductus arteriosus and can, on rare occasion, persist for up to 30 days after parturition. Bilaterally audible murmurs are most often pathologic and require closer examination. Rate and rhythm of the heart beat should be assessed and evaluated together with peripheral arterial pulses. The heart rate is 40 to 80 beats/min within 5 minutes after birth, increasing to 130 beats/min within the first hour, and should then be stabilized at 90 to 100 beats/min. A heart rate of up to 130 beats/min or higher can be observed on exertion (e.g., when the foal is standing). There should be no pulse deficits or jugular pulses present. Peripheral perfusion should be assessed by examining the mucous membranes of mouth, eyes, nares, vulva, and urethra. They should be pink with a capillary refill time of less than 2 seconds. All mucous membranes should be closely evaluated for ulceration or the presence of petechiae. Cyanotic, jaundiced, or injected mucous membranes are abnormal (Figure 12-3). It is important to know that membrane color does not provide an adequate assessment for peripheral oxygenation in the foal. Adequate oxygenation can only be assessed by means of an arterial blood gas analysis.

The respiratory tract provides a major route of infection for organisms that can cause septicemia. The boundaries of the equine lung begin at the seventeenth intercostal space at the level of the tuber coxae and slope in an arc to an area just above the olecranon. A thorough complete auscultation of the lung fields should always be performed. The lung sounds of a foal are normally harsh, making identification of lung disease subjective, rather insensitive, and difficult. An increased respiratory rate associated with exacerbated harsh lung sounds may be present with many other systemic diseases that do not specifically affect the lungs. Particular attention needs to be paid to abnormal sounds including crackles and wheezes, which always indicate lung disease. The chest should be grossly examined for possible rib fractures originating from parturition. Radiography represents the most sensitive diagnostic tool for the detection of pneumonia and other lung diseases in the foal. All high-risk foals that are referred to an adequately equipped facility should therefore have thoracic radiographs performed on admission. Thoracic ultrasonography may provide additional information in some cases, although it must be noted that this technique merely allows examination of the pleural surfaces of the thoracic cavity and the lungs.

The gastrointestinal system of the equine neonate also requires particular attention. Meconium impaction represents the primary cause of colic in the equine neonate. When the foal's temperature is taken, fecal matter should be detectable on the thermometer. If this is not the case and if the foal exhibits straining and signs of abdominal discomfort, the possibility of a nonpatent gastrointestinal system caused by an anatomic abnormality (atresia ani, atresia coli) should be considered. The gastrointestinal tract also represents the second major route of exposure for organisms causing neonatal septicemia. Diarrhea therefore represents a significant finding in the physical exam and requires appropriate treatment. Abdominal auscultation should reveal borborygmi in all four quadrants of the abdomen. Abdominal distention or "pings" (high-pitched tympanic sounds) detected during auscultation must always be considered abnormal findings. A thorough examination of the gastrointestinal tract should also include examination of the oral cavity for the presence of abnormal dentition or a cleft palate. However, the latter can often only be detected by means of an endoscopic exam.

The urogenital system also requires intense examination. The significance of the umbilicus as a major route of infection for septicemia is well known. The umbilical stump that is palpable outside the abdomen contains remnants of the urachus (which is connected to the urinary bladder), two umbilical arteries that travel caudally on the abaxial sides of the urachus to insert in the wall of the bladder, and one umbilical vein that courses forward to the liver. The umbilicus needs to be closely inspected for signs of infection, increase in size, and moistness, which is suggestive of patency. Because the predominant part of the umbilical structures lies within the abdomen, ultrasonography is required for a thorough examination. Examination of the urogenital system also includes palpation of the umbilical, inguinal, and scrotal areas for hernias and distention. Progressive distention and depression of the abdomen in the equine neonate may indicate patency of the urinary tract within the abdomen (e.g., rupture of the urinary bladder or a rent in the urachus). Because of the mainly liquid diet of foals, frequent urination should be observed.

The neurologic system of a newborn foal reveals distinct differences when compared with that of an adult horse. When the foal is standing for the first time, a base-wide stance and exaggerated steps when ambulating are considered normal. An increased response to visual, auditory, and tactile stimuli and jerky movements are also normal. In the recumbent foal, exaggerated responses to tests evaluating spinal reflexes are normally observed, including a myoclonus (rhythmic muscle contractions) in response to elicitation of the patellar reflex. The normal foal also exhibits a crossed extensor reflex (extension of a limb in response to squeezing of the opposite limb). This response can normally be observed as late as 4 weeks of age. When the normal standing foal is restrained, it will initially struggle and then fall limp, as if sleeping, into the arms of the handler. Loosening of the restraint will cause the foal to support its weight again. This specific behavior must be kept in mind by people who are restraining standing foals for procedures (e.g., placement of an intravenous catheter).

The ophthalmologic exam represents an integral part of the neurologic evaluation. Foals normally do not have a menace reflex during the first 2 weeks of life. The pupillary light reflex may be considerably slower if the foal is excited. The presence of entropion or ectropion should be noted during the exam because these conditions may provide information about the patient's hydration status and maturity. The eyes must also be thoroughly examined for corneal abrasions and ulcers. Other conditions that occur in foals include uveitis, hyphema (blood in the anterior chamber), hypopyon (purulent exudate in the anterior chamber), and congenital cataracts.

LABORATORY EXAMINATION

The laboratory parameters (hematology and serum chemistry values) of foals are distinctly different from those of adult horses (Table 12-2). The references provided in this text originate from the University of Florida, College of Veterinary Medicine, but because of variations in technique and equipment between different laboratories, reference ranges for values need to be established individually at each facility that is examining samples from veterinary patients. The packed cell volume of the normal foal during the first 24 hours of life is greater than that of an adult horse. Subsequently, a fall into the low normal range of an adult can be observed over the ensuing 2 weeks to 1 year. The total red blood cell count of a normal foal remains above that of an adult up to 1 year of age. Band neutrophils are uncommon in the normal foal, and values of more than 100 to 150 cells/μl are considered abnormal because they may be indicative of an ongoing infection or septicemia. If infection is suspected, the band neutrophil count should be evaluated in association with the plasma fibrinogen level, which should not exceed 420 mg/dl in foals up to 1 week

Table 12-2 SELECTED LABORATORY VALUES OF THE EQUINE NEONATE

Age	PCV (%)	RBC ($\times10^6$/Fl)	Plasma protein (g/dl)	
Presuckle	40-52	9.3-12.9	4.4-5.9	
≤12 hr	37-49	9.0-12.0	5.1-7.6	
1 day	32-46	8.2-11.0	5.2-8.0	
1 day-1 mo	28-46	7.2-11.6	5.1-7.9	
Adult	31-47	5.9-9.9	6.2-8.0	

Age	Serum Protein (g/dl)	ALP (IU/L)	GGT (IU/L)	SDH (IU/L)
Presuckle				
<12 hr	4.0-7.9	152-2835	13-39	0.2-4.8
1 day	4.3-8.1	861-2671	18-43	0.6-4.6
1 day-1 mo	4.4-7.76	137-1462	8-169	0.6-8.4
Adult	5.5-7.9	64-214	5-28	0.5-3.0

Age	Glucose (mg/dl)	Creatinine (mg/dl)	BUN (mg/dl)
Presuckle			
<12 hr	108-190	1.7-4.2	12-27
1 day	121-233	0.4-4.3	9-40
1 day-1 mo	101-221	0.4-2.1	2-29
Adult	57-96	0.9-2.0	12-24

Data from Koterba AM, Drummond WH, Kosch PC: *Equine clinical neonatology,* Philadelphia, 1990, Lea and Febiger; University of Florida, College of Veterinary Medicine.

ALP, Alkaline phosphatase; *BUN,* blood urea nitrogen; *GGT,* gamma glutamyl transferase; *PCV,* packed cell volume; *RBC,* red blood cell (count); *SDH,* sorbitol dehydrogenase.

of age. Before enteral absorption of colostral immunoglobulins, the plasma protein concentration of an equine neonate is considerably lower than that of an adult horse. Even after a successful passive transfer, the normal range for plasma protein remains below that of an adult. Serum concentrations (evaluated without the presence of fibrinogen) follow a similar trend.

The activities of various serum enzymes are distinctly different in foals than in adult horses. Alkaline phosphatase, gamma glutamyl transferase, sorbitol dehydrogenase, alanine transaminase, and glucose levels should be consistently higher in foals than in adults. An increase in alkaline phosphatase has been attributed to increased metabolic activities in bone, intestine, and liver. Increased gamma glutamyl transferase and sorbitol dehydrogenase activities are attributed to a greater activity in the liver in foals and may be associated with the greater mass of the liver in relation to the total body mass. Changes in alanine transaminase levels are of questionable clinical significance because this enzyme has not been shown to be specific for a particular organ system in the horse. The higher serum glucose concentration in normal foals compared with that in adults has been attributed to frequent nursing. A decrease in the serum glucose concentration below the normal reference range is a concern and is indicative of an insufficient caloric uptake of the foal by nursing, tube feeding, or intravenous supplementation. Consumption of glucose by circulating bacteria in cases of septicemia may also result in hypoglycemia. In normal foals, the serum levels of creatinine can be above the reference values for adults for the first 36 to 72 hours of life. The blood urea nitrogen concentration, however, should be within the normal adult range immediately after parturition. A decrease in blood urea nitrogen concentration between 3 days and 2 months of age can sometimes be observed and has been associated with an increased demand for amino acids required for the synthesis of structural and functional proteins. The urine specific gravity in normal neonates is low and ranges from 1.001 to 1.012.

ADMITTING THE CRITICALLY ILL FOAL

The labor involved in admitting, evaluating, monitoring, and treating the critically ill foal is intensive. A team approach to the diagnostic evaluation and management of the foal is vital to the success. For this reason, management of the severely compromised neonate has been most successful in specialized neonatal intensive care units.

Three conditions are immediately life threatening in the compromised foal: asphyxia, hypoglycemia, and hypothermia. Initial treatment of the foal should address these problems before proceeding to less life-threatening problems. Ambulatory foals should be gently restrained during examination to minimize stress. Recumbent foals should be examined on a well-padded, warm (25° C [77° F]) surface (Figure 12-4). Careful attention should be paid to protecting

the eye on the down side from excess rubbing and trauma (Figure 12-5). If respiratory distress is noted, immediate nasal insufflation of oxygen is warranted. Although it is ideal to collect blood samples for blood gas analysis before oxygen insufflation and to begin intravenous fluid administration after samples have been collected for blood culture and laboratory profiles, the stability of the patient should be the first priority and dictate the order of the admission protocol.

Once initial parameters are recorded (rectal temperature, heart rate, respiratory rate, etc.), heat lamps, circulating water blankets, or forced-air warming units (Bair Hugger, Augustine Medical, Eden Prairie, Minn) are applied if the foal's rectal temperature is less than 37.8° C (100° F). Foals should be warmed slowly to prevent cardiovascular collapse

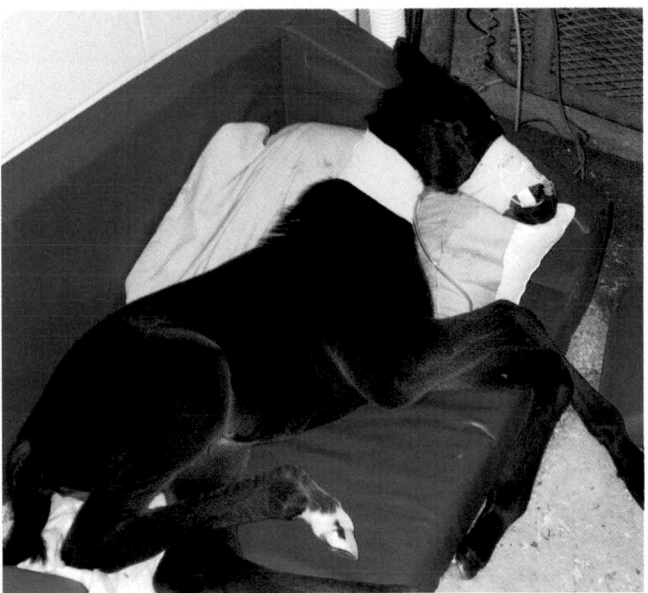

Figure 12-4 The critically ill neonatal foal should be placed on a warm, well-padded surface in semisternal recumbency.

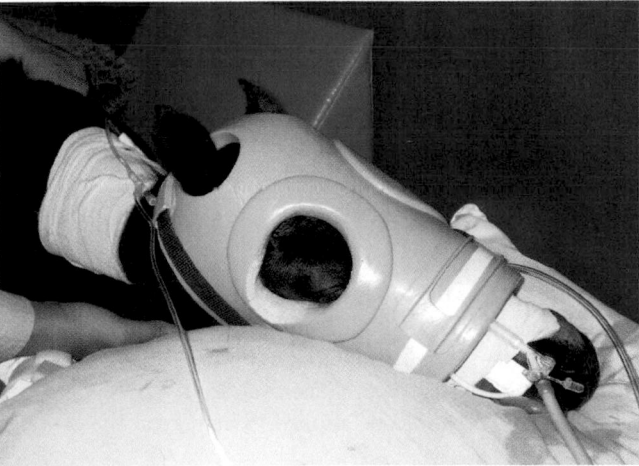

Figure 12-5 Padding of the head provides protection of the eyes in the recumbent foal.

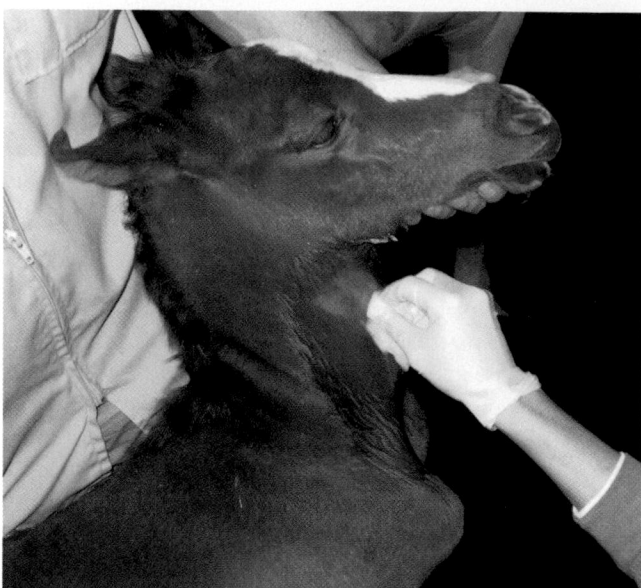

Figure 12-6 The jugular groove is widely clipped and prepared with sterile solutions before intravenous catheter placement.

and thermal burns. Heating blankets and heat lamps should not exceed 39.4° C (103° F). Foals have very sensitive skin and are extremely susceptible to burns, and therefore electric dry heating pads are not recommended. Next, a peripheral vein is prepared for venipuncture under sterile conditions. The cephalic vein is ideal because the jugular vein should be used only for venous catheterization. Blood is collected for aerobic and anaerobic blood culture, complete blood count, determination of fibrinogen level, serum chemistry, electrolyte analysis, and assessment of passive transfer. Once initial blood samples for culture have been collected, an intravenous catheter can be placed if warranted. An arterial blood gas sample is collected. A second set (and possibly a third) of blood samples for culture is collected in 15 minutes and 1 hour. Appropriate fluid therapy and oxygen therapy are administered if warranted.

Venous catheters are primary iatrogenic portals of infection and *must* be placed and maintained under condition of *rigid asepsis*. Always clip the hair and use sterile solutions to scrub the skin liberally before catheter placement (Figure 12-6). Wear sterile gloves when placing the catheter and use strict sterile techniques. An extension set and injection plug can be placed on the catheter to prolong the life of the catheter and assist in administration of intravenous solutions. The catheter should be secured by use of suture or cyanoacrylate glue. Finally, antibacterial ointment is applied to the insertion site and a sterile dressing of gauze sponges and elastic tape (Elasticon, Johnson & Johnson, Somerville, NJ) should be applied to help keep the catheter in place.

In the critically ill foal, fluid therapy may be required immediately after catheter placement. The fluid of choice

and rate of administration for initial therapy depends on the blood glucose, electrolytes, and hydration status. As a general rule, balanced polyionic fluids such as Ringer's lactate, Normosol-R, or Plasmalyte will remain in the intravascular space for longer periods than dextrose and water solutions and are the treatment of choice in shock therapy and maintenance fluid therapy. In the absence of laboratory values, these fluids are generally safe for replacement of fluid deficits. The normal maintenance fluid requirement in the equine neonate is 80 to 120 ml/kg/24 hr or 150 to 225 ml/hr for the average 45-kg foal. Shock therapy fluids can be administered at 20 ml/kg/hr for short periods. In foals with severe hypoglycemia, 5% to 10% dextrose solutions can be administered as a slow infusion. Careful monitoring of blood glucose levels is important because hyperglycemia can be detrimental to the neonate foal. Bolus doses of 25% to 50% dextrose solutions should never be administered because these solutions can exacerbate neurologic signs and result in a rebound hypoglycemia.

Once the foal's condition has been stabilized, the foal is weighed, thoracic radiographs are obtained, and a therapeutic plan is determined. Additional diagnostic measures that may be warranted include abdominal ultrasonography and radiography, transtracheal aspiration, arthrocentesis, cerebrospinal fluid collection, urinary catheterization, collection of feces, abdominocentesis, nasogastric intubation, and gastroduodenal endoscopy.

ROUTINE PERINATAL THERAPY

Certain aspects of neonatal care are common to all foals, regardless of risk category. At birth, the umbilicus should be allowed to tear without assistance. A 0.5% chlorhexidine or 0.5% iodine or Betadine solution should be applied to the umbilical stump. The use of stronger iodine solutions should be avoided because they may cause irritation and burns of the ventral abdominal skin. This treatment should be continued four times per day for 2 to 3 days. Foals from mares that were not vaccinated with tetanus toxoid in the last 4 to 6 weeks of gestation should receive 1500 international units (IU) of tetanus antitoxin intramuscularly. On some farms, an enema is routinely administered after birth. If the foal has not defecated within 24 hours or is straining to defecate, a pediatric sodium phosphate (Fleet) enema or warm, soapy water enema can be administered. This should be done with great care and generous lubrication, because the rectal mucosa of the foal is fragile. It is important to avoid repeated use of sodium phosphate enemas because rectal mucosa irritation can result.

FAILURE OF PASSIVE TRANSFER

Foals are born without appreciable quantities of circulating protective immunoglobulin. The mare's first milk is called colostrum, and it is rich in immunoglobulins. A foal must ingest and absorb colostrum to achieve adequate immunologic protection. Because the gastrointestinal cells that allow absorption of these immunoglobulins are lost soon after birth, the foal must ingest the colostrum by 6 hours of age. Inadequate absorption of colostrum is termed *failure of passive transfer* and is associated with increased susceptibility to infection or sepsis. Studies indicate that failure of passive transfer of maternal antibody occurs in approximately 25% of foals.

Assessing adequate passive transfer is an integral portion of the initial work-up because early detection is the key to intervention. Although there is some debate over what constitutes adequate passive transfer, most neonatal clinicians agree that high-risk foals should have serum immunoglobulin G (IgG) concentrations greater than 800 mg/dl. IgG levels are generally measured 18 to 24 hours after birth to allow time for absorption of ingested colostrum. Several tests that quantify IgG are available, each with advantages and disadvantages. At this time the gold standard is the radial immunodiffusion test. Although this appears to be the most accurate test, the expense, limited availability, and length of time required to run the assay preclude its use in routine screening. The commercial IgG screening kit with an enzyme-linked immunosorbent assay (ELISA) (SNAP ELISA, Idexx Inc., Portland, Maine) is the most commonly used test because it is quick, accurate, easily performed, and readily available. Of the rapid test methods (zinc sulfate turbidity, latex agglutination, glutaraldehyde coagulation test, SNAP ELISA), the SNAP ELISA is the only test that has sensitivity (and specificity) in the 800 mg/dl range.

Ensuring adequate passive transfer is an integral part of treatment for all equine neonates, regardless of disease process. When an immunoglobulin deficit is detected, the immunoglobulin can be replaced by one of two methods. The first is oral administration of good-quality colostrum or colostrum products. Good-quality colostrum is defined as having a value of >1.060 on a Colostrometer. Foals should receive 1 to 2 L of good-quality colostrum by 12 to 16 hours of age and have IgG levels measured 16 to 20 hours later. Oral therapy is not generally used because foals are often diagnosed with low IgG levels after the opportunity for maximum absorption has passed. Failure of passive transfer after 24 hours is treated with intravenous administration of plasma products from an appropriate donor. Commercial plasma is available, and although it is expensive, it is the safest and most reliable product. This plasma is harvested from hyperimmunized donors and has been shown to have IgG levels that far exceed normal plasma and is tested for anti-equine antibodies. If fresh plasma is given, a crossmatch should be performed to lessen the risk of a significant transfusion reaction. Plasma is administered via a sterile intravenous catheter. As a general rule, 1 L of commercial plasma raises the IgG level of a 45-kg foal by 200 mg/dl.

Antimicrobial therapy should always be based on isolation of infecting organisms and antimicrobial sensitivity testing. Special considerations need to be made regarding the physiologic features of the neonate, such as reduced hepatic activity and renal immaturity. Nevertheless, antibiotic therapy should be instituted as soon as sepsis is suspected, without waiting for culture results. In general, a combination of penicillin or ceftiofur sodium and an aminoglycoside (such as amikacin) provides appropriate coverage.

NUTRITION

The currently accepted minimum energy requirement of the compromised equine neonate is 130 to 150 Kcal/kg/day. To meet this requirement, a foal will consume approximately 20% of its body weight per day. Achieving this level via the enteral route (using the gastrointestinal tract) is practically impossible, and accordingly, many compromised foals require supplemental parenteral nutrition to achieve sufficient energy intake. Adequate nutrition is assessed on the basis of daily weight gain. The healthy 45-kg foal should gain 1 to 2 kg per day.

Every effort should be made to feed foals from their mares to promote maternal-neonate bonding. Some foals require assistance or encouragement to nurse. Foals that are unable or unwilling to nurse from their mares can be offered milk from a bucket or bottle (least desirable), provided that they can maintain a strong suckle reflex. Foals typically will not nurse well from commercial calf nipples and appear more receptive to a lamb's nipple. Orphan foals should be trained to bucket feed as soon as possible to limit human imprinting, which can become dangerous as the foal matures. Foals with weak or uncoordinated suckling behavior will require an indwelling nasogastric tube for feeding. The primary complication associated with enteral feeding is aspiration pneumonia. Before each use of the nasogastric tube, its position within the stomach or distal esophagus must be verified. Recumbent foals must be placed in sternal recumbency during feeding and for 30 minutes afterward to prevent regurgitation and aspiration of milk (Figure 12-7).

Mare's milk is the best source of enteral nutrition for the foal because of its digestibility and unique nutrient composition. When available, mare's milk should be used. The mare's udder and the caretaker's hands should always be cleaned before milking to prevent mastitis. Proper restraint of the mare is important during milking. Lubricating the hand or udder with sterile lubricating jelly helps to decrease chafing. Gentle massage or application of warm compresses before milking helps to soften the udder and assist in milk expression. Milk can be collected by hand-milking or by use of an inverted 60-ml dosing syringe (Figure 12-8). Several alternatives to mare's milk are available, but all have their drawbacks. Milk replacers are readily available and inexpensive but unpalatable and notorious for causing gastrointestinal upsets. Preparations formulated for enteral nutrition of other species are generally not

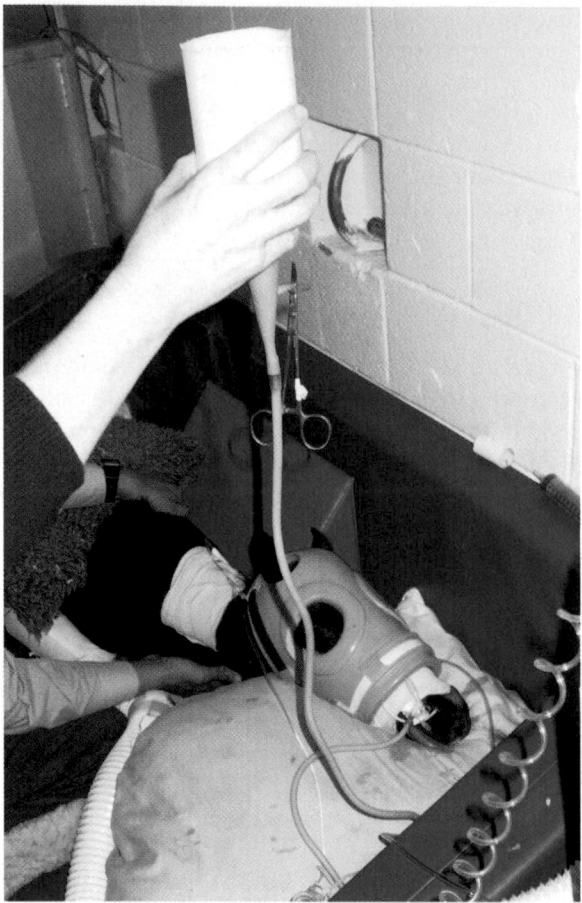

Figure 12-7 The recumbent foal is placed in sternal recumbency and fed by gravity flow with use of an indwelling nasogastric tube and simplex tubing.

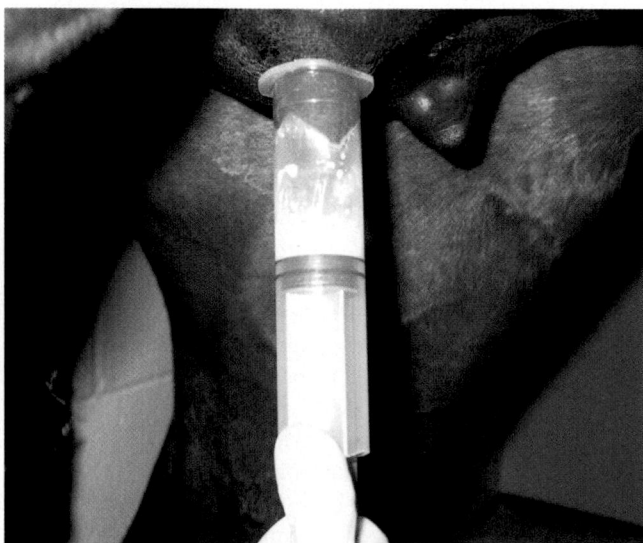

Figure 12-8 Milk can be expressed from the mammary gland by use of an inverted 60-ml dosing syringe to apply suction.

Box 12-4 CALORIC DENSITIES OF SELECTED MILK REPLACERS FOR FOALS

- Foal Lac (Pet Ag Inc, Hampshire, Ill): 260 kcal/pint
- Mare's Match (Land-o-Lakes, Fort Dodge, Iowa): 211 kcal/pint
- Nutri-Foal (Ross Laboratories, Columbus, Ohio) 345 kcal/pint

---

suitable for the foal. Goat's milk is palatable but causes some metabolic abnormalities and should not be used alone for extended periods. Goat's milk can be added to milk replacers to improve palatability. Milk replacers, when fed according to directions on the label, underestimate the caloric requirements of foals by 50% to 70%. Quantities to be fed should be calculated daily based on caloric requirement and the foal's body weight. Box 12-4 lists the caloric densities of several milk replacers.

All utensils used for feeding foals should be thoroughly cleaned and disinfected before and after use because the gastrointestinal tract is a potential portal for infection. Once reconstituted, milk replacers should be kept refrigerated. The preparations should be discarded after 2 hours at room temperature. Enteral nutrition should be started gradually. Begin at 50 to 100 ml every 30 to 60 minutes. If the foal tolerates these feedings, the volume of milk may be gradually increased to 5% to 10% of its body weight, divided into 12 feedings spaced every 2 hours. If well tolerated, milk feeding can be increased daily by 1% of body weight until total daily intake of 20% is achieved. Many high-risk foals will not tolerate enteral nutrition, and feeding should be discontinued if regurgitation, abdominal distension, colic, or severe diarrhea occurs. Foals receiving less than 100 Kcal/kg/day should be considered candidates for parenteral nutrition.

MONITORING AND NURSING CARE

Once the foal has been admitted to the veterinary hospital and initially examined, diligent monitoring is critical. The objective of frequent monitoring is to detect subtle changes in body parameters that signify a worsening or improvement in the foal's status. The primary complications that occur in foals are the development of resistant nosocomial infections, alternate sites of infection (arthritis, osteomyelitis, omphalitis, and pneumonia), corneal ulcers, decubital ulcers, and malnutrition. The severity of the patient's illness will dictate the required frequency of monitoring. Parameters should always be recorded on a flow sheet. Table 12-3 lists parameters that should be monitored and is basically an outline of a thorough, foal-oriented physical examination with the addition of blood pressure, blood gas, and ventilatory monitoring as needed. Particular attention should be paid to the catheter site for evidence of heat, pain, or swelling. Box 12-5 suggests physical exam parameters

Table 12-3 Monitoring the Critical Ill Foal

Body System	Parameters Monitored During Physical Examination
Cardiovascular	Pulse: rate, rhythm, strength
	Heart rate, rhythm, and murmurs
	Mucous membranes: color, CRT, petechiae, injection, hyperemia
Respiratory	Breathing: rate, effort, pattern
	Chest excursion
	Lungs: auscultation, percussion
Thermoregulatory	Body temperature: warmth of extremities
Gastrointestinal	Feces: volume, consistency; straining
	Borborygmi: frequency, character
	Abdominal distention, signs of colic and gastric reflux
Urinary	Urination: frequency, volume; straining
	Umbilicus: monitor for patency and signs of infection
Musculoskeletal	Joints: lameness, warmth, distention
	Tendon and ligament laxity
	Angular limb deformity
Integument	Decubital ulcers; urine and fecal scalding; linear dermal necrosis; coronitis
Ocular	Cornea: abrasions, ulcers, edema
	Anterior chamber: hypopyon, uveitis
	Lids: entropion
	Sclera: injection, petechiae
Nervous	Mental status, attitude, behavior
	Posture and muscle tone
	Gait: limb proprioception
	Cranial nerve and spinal reflexes

Modified from Koterba AM, Drummond WH, Kosch PC: *Equine clinical neonatology,* Philadelphia, 1990, Lea & Febiger.
CRT, Capillary refill time.

Box 12-5 Trends or Changes in Condition That Often Warrant Intervention

1. Trends
   A. Increasing or decreasing body temperature
   B. Increasing or increasingly irregular respiratory rate
   C. Increasingly rapid (>120 beats/min), slow (<60 beats/min), or irregular heart rate
   D. Weakening peripheral pulses and cool extremities
   E. Blood gases
      (1) Decreasing Pao_2: If foal is receiving oxygen therapy, check the flow rate and the pressure gauge for any disconnections or plugs in the tubing. Consider the amount of struggling and the length of time in lateral recumbency. If there are no equipment problems, consider the possibility that pulmonary function is worsening.
      (2) Increasing $Paco_2$, particularly with increased effort of breathing, suggests that the foal's respiratory system may be failing.
      (3) More negative base excess implies worsening metabolic acidosis. The cause should be determined.
2. Seizure activity
3. Colic
4. Decrease in amount nursed can be an early sign of deterioration in condition.
5. Gastric reflux
6. Diarrhea or constipation, excessive straining to defecate
7. Abdominal distention
8. Lack of or reduced urination
9. Eye abnormalities, most commonly corneal ulcers
10. Pitting edema, most commonly observed in the subcutaneous tissues of the ventral abdomen and legs, may indicate fluid overload, impaired renal function, infection, or capillary injury.

Modified from Koterba AM, Drummond WH, Kosch PC: *Equine clinical neonatology,* Philadelphia, 1990, Lea & Febiger.

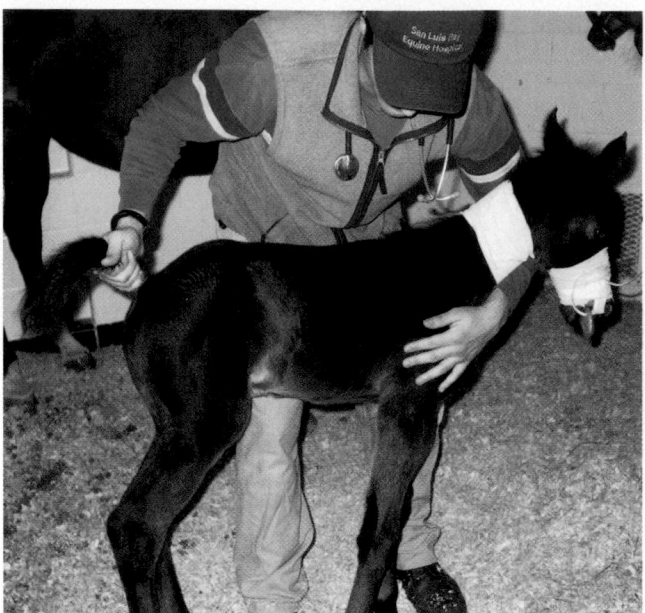

Figure 12-9 Proper restraint of the foal is achieved by gently cradling one hand under the neck and grasping the base of the tail with the other hand.

that may warrant intervention and should be brought to the attention of the attending clinician.

The hallmarks of nursing care for the foal are strict attention to asepsis and close observation of minor details. Providing care for critically ill foals is as much an art as a science. Ambulatory foals are generally restrained with one hand under the neck and the other grasping the base of the tail or surrounding the rump (Figure 12-9). Bracing the foal against a wall provides more security and better control during struggle. The recumbent foal can be a challenge to restrain. Use of two to three individuals in the restraint is vital. Briefly, while the foal is lying in lateral recumbency, its forelimbs are placed between the handler's legs and held in place without applying weight or pressure. The same is done by a second handler with the hind limbs. A third handler could restrain the head and neck carefully. A clean towel or blanket should be placed under the down eye to prevent trauma to the cornea. It is also very important to avoid compression of the chest or abdomen because severe injury can occur. Restraint should be safe for the foal, mare, and handlers; and the supportive intravenous lines and associated equipment should be protected.

If more than one foal is being treated by the technician, care should be exercised to avoid cross contamination. All skin injections should be made only after the area has been cleaned with alcohol and dried. Intramuscular injections are limited to the semimembranosus region and should not be given in the neck, pectorals, or gluteal region. Fluid lines should be changed daily to avoid contamination. Once a fluid line becomes disconnected, it should be considered contaminated and must be replaced. All intravenous ports should be capped with injection caps. Multidose vials of injectable drugs and injection caps or ports must be disinfected before needle insertion. Needles and syringes are *not* reused. Catheters should be flushed with heparinized saline solution every 4 hours. The interval for catheter changes depends on the type of catheter material used and the status of the vein. The commonly used Teflon catheter should be removed and replaced at least every 72 hours. Silastic or polyurethane catheters are less thrombogenic and may remain in place for several weeks, provided that they receive the proper care and monitoring. These catheters are expensive but quickly become cost effective when compared with Teflon because of the extended time they can remain in place and the decreased likelihood of developing thrombophlebitis associated with their use.

The foal should be kept clean, dry, and warm. Milk should be warmed to a tepid (not hot) temperature before it is fed to the foal. Physical therapy is a helpful modality for recumbent nonambulatory foals. All limbs should be put through a complete passive range of motion several times per day to maintain joint mobility. Because of the adverse effects of lateral recumbency on lung pathologic conditions and ventilation, foals should be kept in a semisternal position with the thorax and forelimbs in sternal recumbency and the hips and rear limbs in lateral recumbency. This position can be attained by use of wedge-shaped pads or sandbags positioned at the level of the elbow and thorax (see Figure 12-4).

The recumbent foal will require frequent turning from side to side every 2 hours to encourage complete ventilation of the lungs. Foals should be encouraged to stand and ambulate when possible. This effort may range form the handler suspending the foal and encouraging it to bear weight to taking short assisted walks with the mare.

SUMMARY

Working with compromised foals is an exhaustive endeavor. Despite intensive labor, many high-risk foals will die, usually taking with them a piece of each team member who has worked so hard to save them. Attention to detail must be unrelenting, and with the help of diligent, highly skilled technicians, more foals will survive.

Recommended Reading

Puppy and Kitten

Boothe DM, Tannert K: Special considerations for drug and fluid therapy in the pediatric patient, *Compend Contin Educ Pract Vet* 14:313-329, 1992.

Dow SW, Papich MG: Keeping current on developments in antimicrobial therapy, *Vet Med* 86:600-609, 1991.

Hoskins JD: Clinical evaluation of the kitten: from birth to eight weeks of age, *Compend Contin Educ Pract Vet* 12(9):1215-1225, 1990,

Hoskins JD: Nutrition and nutritional disorders. In Hoskins JD, editor. *Veterinary pediatrics: dogs and cats from birth to six months*, ed 3, Philadelphia, WB Saunders, 2001, pp 476-490.

Hoskins JD, Partington BP: Physical examination and diagnostic imaging procedures. In Hoskins JD, editor: *Veterinary pediatrics: dogs and cats from birth to six months*, Philadelphia, WB Saunders, 2001, pp 1-21.

Foal

Beech J: Symposium on neonatal equine disease, *Vet Clin North Am Equine Pract* 1(1):1-263, 1985.

Clabough DL: Disease of the equine neonate, *J Equine Vet Sci* 8(1): 5-10, 1988.

Drummond WH: Bridging the gap between the human and equine neonate. In Rossdale PD, editor: *The application of intensive care therapies and parenteral nutrition in large animal medicine*, Deerfield, Ill, 1986, Travenol Labs.

Koterba AM: IV fluid therapy and nutritional support in the sick neonate, *Equine Vet Educ* 3(1):33-39, 1991.

Koterba AM, Drummond WH, Kosch PC, editors: *Equine clinical neonatology*, Philadelphia, 1990, Lea and Febiger.

Madigan JE, editor: *Manual of equine neonatal medicine*, ed 3, Woodlawn, Calif, 1997, Live Oak Publishing.

McClure JT, Miller J, Deluca JL: Comparison of two ELISA screening tests and a non-commercial glutaraldehyde coagulation screening test for the detection of failure of passive transfer in neonatal foals. In *Proceedings of the Annual American Association of Equine Practitioners Convention, vol 49*, Lexington, KY, 2003, pp 301-305.

Paradis MR: Update on neonatal sepsis, *Vet Clin North Am Equine Pract* 10(1):109-135, 1994.

Pierce SW: Foal care from birth to 30 days: a practitioner's perspective. In *Proceedings of the Annual American Association of Equine Practitioners Convention, vol 49*, Lexington, KY, 2003, pp 13-21.

Vaala WE, House JK, Madigan JE: Initial management and physical examination of the neonate. In Smith BP, editor: *Large animal internal medicine: diseases of horses, cattle, sheep, and goats*, ed 3, St. Louis, 2002, Mosby.

Wilkins PA: Hypoxic ischemic encephalopathy: neonatal encephalopathy. 2003. In *Recent Advances in Equine Neonatal Care*. Available from http://www.ivis.org/advances/ Neonatology_Wilkins/wilkins_hie/chapter_frm.asp?LA=1

13

Geriatric Care of Companion Animals

JOHNNY D. HOSKINS

INTRODUCTION

Geriatrics is that branch of medicine and surgery that treats problems specific to old age. Aging is the accumulation of progressive body changes associated with or responsible for disease, decreased physiologic function, and death. Life span and life expectancy differ among species and among individual members of a species, and this variability suggests that a genetic component is responsible for the normal aging process. In addition to genetic factors, the variations in life expectancy are related to acquired diseases and environmental stressors.

Aging in a dog or cat is associated with gradual deterioration in the delicate interrelationships of the body systems. Box 13-1 outlines the common effects of aging. This then predisposes the dog or cat to acquired disease. Some diseases cause a dog's or cat's death indirectly through their effects on cells, tissues, and organs (e.g., ischemic heart disease or diabetes mellitus). However, death is frequently assumed to be from the normal aging process. If a dog or cat dies of natural causes at a young age, it is usually directly due to an underlying disease. If a dog or cat dies at an advanced age, it is attributed to disease or age or both. The dichotomy between age and disease in this circumstance is ambiguous. Death is a well-defined event with a strong correlation with age. ∎

LIFE STAGES GUIDELINES

A lifetime incorporates the sum of the various life stages of dogs and cats. Age by itself is not a disease. The following life stages apply to most dogs and cats:

- The pediatric life stage is the life stage between birth and 6 months old for both dogs and cats.

- The young adult life stage is the life stage from 6 months to 2 years through 5 years old for dogs. The age ranges of being a young adult vary according to the specific dog breed, because the large- and giant-dog breeds spend less time as a young adult. Young adult life stage is the life stage from 6 months to 4 years old for cats.

- Mature adult life stage is the life stage from 2 years through 5 years to 9 years through 12 years old for dogs. The age ranges of being a mature adult vary according to the specific dog breed, because the large- and giant-dog breeds spend less time as a mature adult. Mature adult life stage is the life stage from 4 years to 12 years old for cats.

- Senior life stage is the life stage after mature adulthood. The latter times in the senior dog's lifetime may be defined as the geriatric years, but dogs, just like humans, like being referred to as senior citizens. The oldest dog on record was 29 years old. The oldest cat on record was 34 years old.

✎ TECHNICIAN NOTE

The care of aging dogs and cats is a *proactive* comprehensive health care program that addresses the older animal's special needs.

INTEGRATING GERIATRIC CARE

The care for aging dogs and cats is a proactive comprehensive health care program that addresses the older animal's special needs. This specialized medical service is based on two premises: first, there are fundamental differences in specific diseases, behavior traits, and nutritional needs of the older animal; second, prevention, early detection, and timely intervention of medical problems can have a significant impact on the life span and quality of life of an older dog or cat.

Care for such older dogs and cats should focus on owner education, disease prevention strategies, and detection of medical and behavioral problems at the earliest possible stage when the prognosis is better and numerous treatment options still exist (Figure 13-1). The term "senior" or "geriatric" describes that life stage of progressive decline in physical condition, organ function, sensory function, mental function, and immunity. Although it is generally accepted that the senior life stage begins around 7 years of age for the average dog or cat, several interrelated factors, including size and individual genetics, will affect the onset and rate of the progressive decline.

Although care for the older animal begins at the first new puppy/kitten examination when the animal's entire life-stage health care program is outlined for the owner, the program is actually implemented when the animal reaches

---

Box 13-1 EFFECTS OF AGING

METABOLIC EFFECTS

Decreased metabolic rate plus lack of activity decrease caloric needs by 30% to 40%.

Immune competence decreases, despite normal numbers of lymphocytes.

Phagocytosis and chemotaxis decrease, and older animals are less able to ward off infections.

Autoantibodies and immune-mediated diseases develop.

PHYSICAL EFFECTS

Percentage of body weight represented by fat increases.

Skin becomes thickened, hyperpigmented, and inelastic.

Footpads become hyperkeratinized, and claws become brittle.

Muscle, bone, and cartilage mass are lost, with subsequent development of osteoarthritis.

Dental calculus results in tooth loss and gingival hyperplasia (Figure 13-1).

Periodontitis results in gingival retraction and atrophy.

Gastric mucosa becomes atrophic and fibrotic.

Hepatocyte numbers decrease, and hepatic fibrosis occurs.

Pancreatic enzyme secretion diminishes.

Lungs lose elasticity, fibrosis occurs, and pulmonary secretions become more viscous. Vital capacity decreases.

Cough reflex and expiratory capacity decrease.

Kidney weight decreases, glomerular filtration rate decreases, and tubules atrophy.

Urinary incontinence frequently develops.

Prostate gland enlarges, testes atrophy, and prepuce becomes pendulous.

Ovaries enlarge, and mammary glands become fibrocystic or neoplastic.

Cardiac output decreases, and valvular fibrosis and intramural coronary arteriosclerosis develop.

Bone marrow becomes fatty and hypoplastic, and nonregenerative anemia develops.

The number of cells in the nervous system decreases. Senility causes loss of house training.

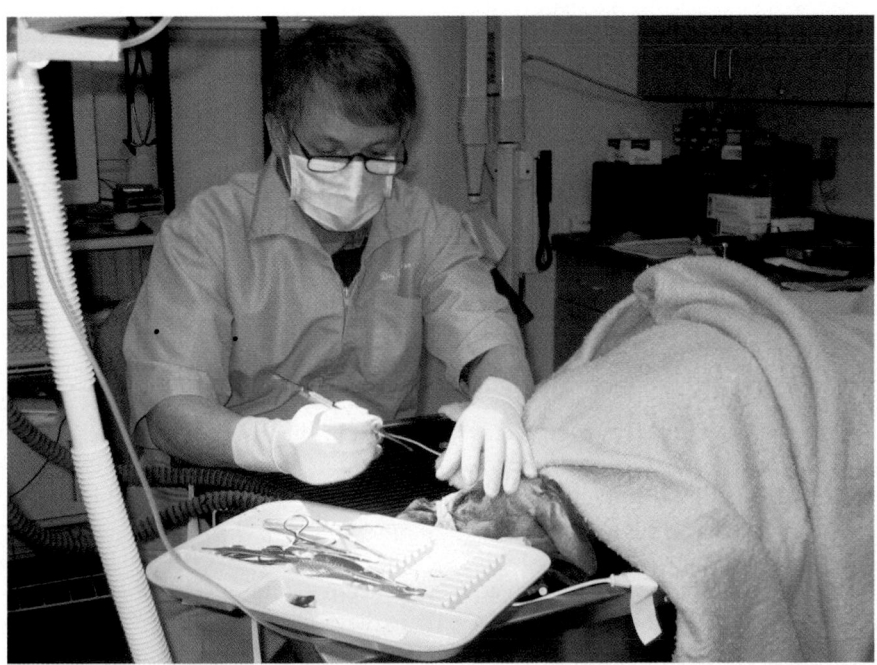

Figure 13-1 Halitosis is often related to orodental disease. Oral examinations and dental prophylaxis are therefore particularly important for the geriatric patient. This dog has had a canine tooth extracted.

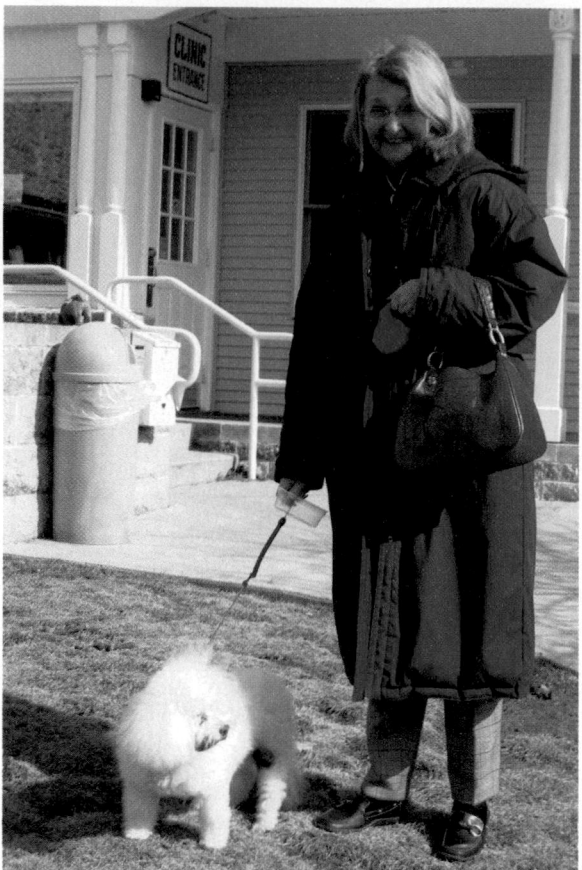

Figure 13-2 It is important to educate the owners of senior animals about the warning signs of age-related diseases. Early detection is important in providing effective treatment.

7 years of age. Starting at 7 years, senior care promotes routine examinations of healthy animals on a twice-a-year basis and advocates routine diagnostic screening for developing diseases. The healthy animal is just one component of the group that should be targeted for senior care. Another component is the older dog or cat that is asymptomatic or is exhibiting early signs of a problem, but the owner either does not recognize the signs or just attributes the signs to "old age" and fails to seek veterinary care.

Historically, veterinarians have reacted to existing problems in older animals waiting until the owner elects to seek professional help for the animal once the disease signs are blatantly obvious and/or no longer tolerable. When owners are not adequately educated on the early warning signs of disease or healthy animals are not regularly screened for age-related diseases, veterinarians are presented with animals that have moderate to advanced disease (Figure 13-2). As a result, considerable time and resources are transferred into effectively managing these diseases, and the available treatment options are often limited. Veterinarians should take a more proactive approach to common age-related problems.

Senior care is a proactive health care program that changes the way veterinarians traditionally approach older animals.

Senior health care has some distinct advantages over geriatric health care programs. Marketing surveys have indicated that the term "senior" is more owner-friendly than "geriatric." Senior care is also a more inclusive health care program, starting at 7 years of age and advocating twice-yearly examinations and regular health screening. However, most senior care programs are initiated by various commercial companies that provide all the marketing and implementation tools necessary to make senior care successful in the veterinary practice. Tools for owner education, health data gathering and reporting tools, and program implementation tips are currently provided. These companies also help raise owner awareness of age-related health issues by sponsoring a special Senior Health Month.

GERIATRIC HEALTH CARE PROGRAM

The basic services included in a geriatric health care program are as follows:

1. Complete patient evaluation (physical examination, blood/urine evaluation, other tests as needed)
2. Specific disease detection and treatment (e.g., nephritis, colitis, liver disease, skin disease, cardiovascular disease, musculoskeletal disease, and so on)
3. Preventive medicine, basic oncology information and normal aging counseling (including immunizations, dentistry, and nutritional counseling)
4. Bereavement counseling
5. Respite care

PHYSICAL EVALUATION

Clinical evaluation of the older dog or cat always begins with a complete medical, behavioral, and surgical history and a thorough physical examination. The signalment (breed, age, and sex), current or past medications, and owner concerns are obtained from the animal's history. Questions about a variety of behaviors should be asked, including specific questions about house soiling, incontinence, altered ability to recognize commands or people, muscle weakness or disorientation, disruption of the sleep-wake cycle, repetitive and compulsive disorders, persistent vocalization, intolerance to being left alone, and tremors or shaking.

After the history is obtained, a thorough physical examination is performed in a systematic manner. The body systems examination should be complete and address specific physical concerns about the animal that the owner may indicate (Box 13-2). Because cancer is an important concern of the owner of an older dog or cat, generalized or irregular enlargement of any organ should be considered serious, and ancillary diagnostic procedures should be recommended. Organ enlargement often indicates an infiltrative disease, inflammation, or cancer. Thorough

Box 13-2 PROBLEMS SPECIFIC TO GERIATRIC DOG
AND CAT

- Weight stasis—obesity
- Cancer—present or not
- Halitosis—orodental disease (Figure 13-1)
- Lusterless hair coat and skin changes
- Changes in behavior
- Altered ability to rise and/or walk
- Anesthesia risk
- Altered vision and hearing
- Heart murmur—heart failure
- Urine production—kidney failure
- Coughing—chronic bronchial disease
- Urinary or fecal incontinence

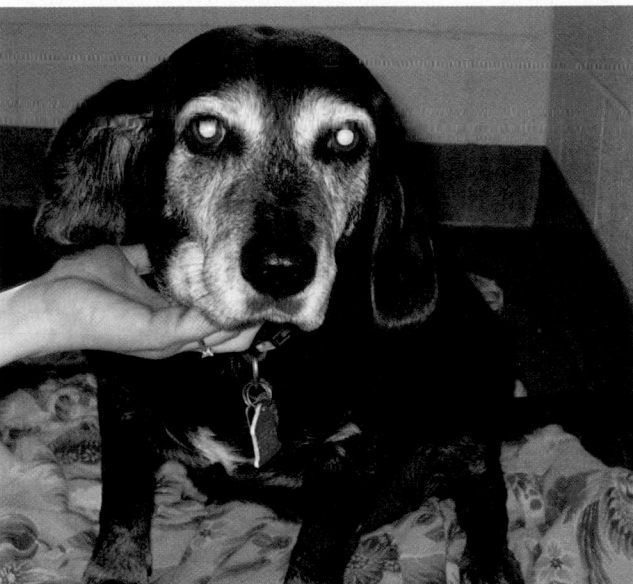

Figure 13-3 Detailed inspection of the skin, coat, nails, ear canals, and eyes may identify ongoing problems of infection, immune-mediated disease, degenerative disease, or cancer.

inspection of the mouth and teeth is especially important because of the increased incidence of orodental disease and oral tumors in older dogs and cats.

TECHNICIAN NOTE

Because cancer is an important concern of the owner of an older dog or cat, generalized or irregular enlargement of any organ should be considered serious, and ancillary diagnostic procedures should be recommended.

Because many older dogs or cats are presented with heart murmurs and breathing problems, thoracic auscultation should be done in a quiet room to determine the severity of the heart murmur and the presence of arrhythmias or conduction disturbances. Detection of abnormal heart or lung sounds may prompt thoracic radiography and electro-cardiography, and possibly echocardiography and indirect blood pressure measurements.

Detailed inspection of the skin, coat, nails, ear canals, and eyes may identify ongoing problems of infection, immune-mediated disease, degenerative disease, or cancer (Figure 13-3). Owners of older dogs and cats often complain of abnormal odors or discharges, so the body openings should be inspected and palpated.

The examination of the musculoskeletal system begins by observing the dog or cat standing (Figure 13-4). The animal is observed at rest for unequal weight-bearing and abnormal conformation of the bones, joints, and muscles. Next, the animal is observed while walking and trotting to detect lameness and, if lameness is present, which limb is affected. Hypermetria, shortened stride, and any other gait abnormality are noted. In cases of subtle musculoskeletal problems, it may be necessary to walk the animal in tight circles or up and down stairs to detect the abnormality.

Some neurologic disorders may cause signs suggestive of musculoskeletal problems. While watching the movement of an animal, it is necessary to distinguish between ataxia

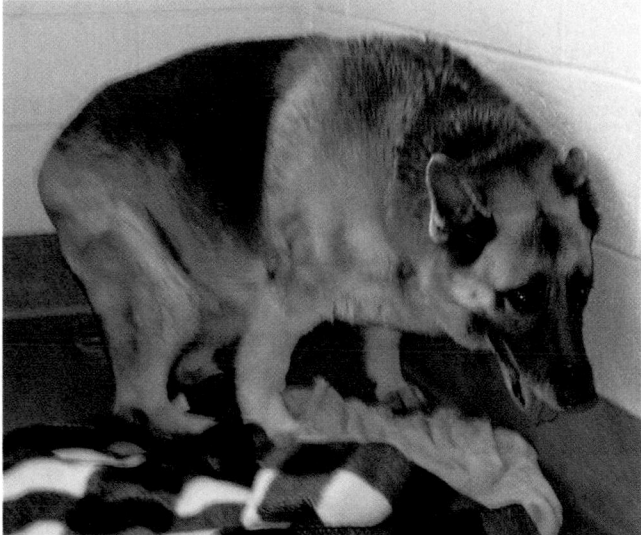

Figure 13-4 Examination of the musculoskeletal system begins by observing the patient standing. This dog has severe degenerative joint disease and shows evidence of muscle atrophy in the hind legs and hips.

(neurologic) and lameness caused by musculoskeletal problems. Conscious proprioception should be tested in both the front and rear legs. A complete neurologic examination should be performed in those cases in which neurologic disease is suspected.

While the animal is standing, animal's limbs and joints should be individually examined for any asymmetry in size, shape, heat, and sensitivity. The hind limbs are evaluated with the examiner behind the animal, and the forelimbs are evaluated with the examiner in front of the animal. A thorough examination of each leg is performed. Individual leg examination is started proximally and slowly progresses in the distal direction. Joint effusion and periarticular changes resulting in increased joint size should be recorded. While the animal is standing, attention is directed to the neck and back after the limbs have been examined.

Manipulation of each joint is performed with the animal in lateral recumbency. Joint manipulation includes assessment of the normal range of motion, response to hyperextension or hyperflexion, and stability of the ligaments supporting the joint. Crepitus, "clicks," and any pain response should be noted. Examination of each stifle joint includes evaluation for cranial and caudal cruciate ligament rupture and for patellar luxation. The hip joints are evaluated for laxity in the joint capsule and for pain response. Comparison with the opposite unaffected limb is helpful.

LABORATORY EVALUATION

Geriatric health care incorporates the use of blood and urine screening tests. Regularly performed laboratory tests of seemingly healthy or unhealthy animals allow for recognition of a spectrum of diseases previously thought to be uncommon, which are actually common (Box 13-3). Abnormal laboratory values should be pursued fully, and ancillary diagnostic procedures should be added as needed.

Educating owners about the benefits of obtaining baseline and regularly scheduled laboratory information sets the stage for continual monitoring during the animal's life. Thorough owner education allows a higher quality of services to be provided with a higher level of success and satisfaction for the older animal. When a veterinarian waits until disease is suspected to recommend blood and urine tests, it is difficult for the owner to understand the value of preventive medicine. The owner of an older dog or cat should be encouraged to have his or her animal examined at least annually. Regularly scheduled vaccinations and internal and external parasite control should be recommended and enforced. Specific vaccinations and frequency of administration should be recommended on the basis of an assessment of the individual animal's risk of exposure to infectious agents and risk of developing an immune-mediated disease.

TECHNICIAN NOTE

Educating owners about the benefits of obtaining baseline and regularly scheduled laboratory information sets the stage for continual monitoring during the animal's life.

Even in the older animal, examinations of feces should be done. If the animal has suggestive clinical signs, skin scrapings should be done as well. The most common parasites seen in older dogs and cats are fleas, ticks, ear mites, and tapeworms. Other parasites, such as hookworms, whipworms, *Giardia* species, and *Demodex* species, can also be found in older animals because of diminishing function of the immune system. Most animals should receive heartworm, flea, and/or tick preventive medication. These preventive products are safe to use even in older animals and breeding-age animals, as long as the label instructions

---

Box 13-3 COMMONLY ENCOUNTERED GERIATRIC DISEASES

GERIATRIC DOG	GERIATRIC CAT
Chronic pain	Chronic pain
Diabetes mellitus	Inflammatory bowel disease
Hyperadrenocorticism	Diabetes mellitus
Hypothyroidism	Secondary hepatic lipidosis
Prostatic disease	Chronic renal disease
Obesity	Pancreatic disease
Cardiovascular disease	Feline triad disease complex
Chronic airway disease/pneumonia	Obesity
Degenerative joint disease	Cancer
Cataract(s) and glaucoma	Orodental disease
Keratoconjunctivitis sicca	Cataract(s) and glaucoma
Cancer	Keratoconjunctivitis sicca
Orodental disease	Degenerative joint disease
Urolithiasis	Hyperthyroidism
Anemia	Urolithiasis
Urinary and fecal incontinence	Anemia
Hepatopathies	Hepatopathies
Chronic renal disease	Cardiovascular disease
Hypertension	Hypertension
Lumbosacral instability	Water imbalance problems

are followed. Annual retesting for canine and possibly feline heartworm disease is recommended.

Another important facet of preventive medicine is education of owners, especially in the areas of nutrition, proper exercise, natural aging process, cancer and its effects, and bereavement and hospice counseling services. This consultative advice provides owners with quality educational information. The veterinarian and hospital staff play a vital role in educating people of all ages in the local community about proper humane health care.

HEALTH CARE PROGRAMS

A comprehensive geriatric health care program can provide a means of targeting key age-related health problems and detecting disorders early enough for medical and surgical management to be effective (Box 13-4). The acceptance of an older dog or cat into the health care program depends on its general health status, which may be determined from the case history and findings from physical examination

---

Box 13-4 ANNUAL HEALTH EVALUATION FOR GERIATRIC DOGS AND CATS

GERIATRIC DOG

Perform complete physical examination and record accurate body weight. During the mature adult years, dogs have a tendency to steadily gain excessive body weight. Dietary management for the prevention of obesity and regularly performed exercise are extremely important points to emphasize to the owner to effectively control body weight. On the other hand, weight loss when there should not be weight loss is a definitive indication that a complete clinical and laboratory evaluation should be recommended.

Check for external parasites, such as fleas, ticks, mange mites, and ear mites, and institute treatment for specific parasites identified.

Perform examination of feces for intestinal parasites, specifically *Giardia* species, and deworm with broad-spectrum product.

Screen for canine heartworm infection, canine ehrlichiosis, and Lyme borreliosis.

Prescribe medications and canine heartworm/flea preventive products.

Perform blood and urine screening tests for detection of organ dysfunction.

Check the heart for rhythm disturbances using an electrocardiographic unit.

Examine the eyes for evidence of cataracts, glaucoma, and "dry eyes."

Administer vaccinations according to assessment of risk of exposure to infectious agent(s).

Adjust nutrition according to health needs, and institute regular grooming procedures.

Encourage trimming of nails and cleaning of ear canals monthly.

Discuss with owner natural age-related changes that are occurring and tendency of dogs to show clinical signs of preexisting medical conditions, such as heart, liver, kidney, and gastrointestinal tract dysfunction; diabetes mellitus; systemic hypertension; and recurrent eye, ear, and skin disease. Most geriatric dogs will be receiving daily medications for existing medical conditions; therefore discuss the administration and follow-up procedures for the medications being administered and possible drug interactions.

Fill in the dog's medical health record for each visit, and provide a readable copy to the owner.

GERIATRIC CAT

Perform complete physical examination and record accurate body weight. During the mature adult years, cats have a tendency to steadily gain excessive body weight. Dietary management for the prevention of obesity is an extremely important point to emphasize to the pet owner to effectively control body weight. On the other hand, weight loss when there should not be weight loss is a definitive indication that a complete clinical and laboratory evaluation should be recommended.

Check for external parasites, such as fleas, ticks, mange mites, and ear mites, and institute treatment for specific parasites identified.

Perform examination of feces for intestinal parasites, specifically *Giardia* species, and deworm with broad-spectrum product.

Prescribe medications and feline heartworm/flea preventive products.

Perform blood and urine screening tests for detection of organ dysfunction.

Check for heart rhythm disturbances using an electrocardiographic unit.

Examine the eyes for evidence of cataracts, glaucoma,* and "dry eyes."

Administer vaccinations according to assessment of risk of exposure to infectious agent(s).

Adjust nutrition according to health needs, and institute regular grooming procedures.

Encourage trimming of nails and cleaning of ear canals monthly.

Discuss with owner age-related changes that are occurring and tendency of cats to show clinical signs of preexisting medical conditions, such as heart, liver, kidney, and gastrointestinal tract dysfunction; diabetes mellitus; hyperthyroidism; systemic hypertension; and recurrent eye, ear, and skin disease. Most geriatric cats will be receiving daily medications for existing medical conditions; therefore discuss the administration and follow-up procedures for the medications being administered and possible drug interactions.

Fill in the cat's medical health record for each visit, and provide a readable copy to the owner.

---

*Kroll MM, Miller PE, Rodan I: Intraocular pressure measurements obtained as part of a comprehensive geriatric health examination from cats seven years of age and older, *J Am Vet Med Assoc* 219:1406, 2001.

Box 13-5 HEALTH SCREENING LEVELS FOR A GERIATRIC DOG AND CAT

PROGRAM ONE

Medical, behavioral, and surgical history

Physical examination, including ocular and thyroid gland examination

Complete blood cell count and comprehensive serum chemistry profile

Complete urinalysis, including urine sediment examination

Consultation regarding nutrition, teeth, ears, nails, and skin care

Weight control program

PROGRAM TWO

All components of Program One

Electrocardiography

Thoracic radiography

PROGRAM THREE

All components of Programs One and Two

Abdominal radiography

Ancillary diagnostic procedures

Echocardiography for cardiac failure or thoracic disease

Abdominal ultrasonography for any organ enlargement or organ dysfunction

Thyroid gland function tests for hypothyroidism and hyperthyroidism

Indirect blood pressure determination for heart, kidney, or endocrine disease

Liver (serum bile acids), pancreas (serum trypsin-like immuno-reactivity test), and small intestinal (serum folate/cobalamin) function assays for hepatic, gastrointestinal, or pancreatic disease

Schirmer tear test for keratoconjunctivitis sicca

Ocular tonometry for secondary glaucoma and uveitis

Urine early renal detection test or urine protein-to-creatinine ratio for proteinuria

Endoscopic examination and biopsy for chronic vomiting or diarrhea

Urine cortisol-to-creatinine ratio screening for hyperadrenocorticism

and other diagnostic procedures, and not on actual age. The health care program may include different levels of health evaluation (i.e., Program One for the apparently healthy animal, Program Two for the animal with minor health concerns, and Program Three for the animal with major health concerns) (Box 13-5).

IMPLEMENTATION OF HEALTH CARE PROGRAM

The first step in the initiation of a geriatric health care program is for the veterinarian to understand the full scope and need for geriatric health care services in the daily routine of the veterinary hospital. Next, the program should then be explained completely to the hospital staff, including how it fits into their daily activities. Ideas and changes should be solicited from the hospital staff, because these may improve the implementation of the program. Because the receptionist is the first person with whom the owner has contact, it is important for the receptionist to fully understand the health care program so that he or she can explain it in common terms to the owner. The technician also has an important and very visible role in this program; the technician can perform many in-hospital procedures on the geriatric animal, in addition to performing laboratory tests and obtaining radiographs and electrocardiograms.

The daily activities of the health care program should be worked out to include appointment schedules; office and examination room procedures; maintenance of health records; provision of laboratory support; and owner consultation periods in which to review all findings, recommendations, and subsequent examinations. When geriatric animals are scheduled, appointments should be made during the slower periods, if possible. Scheduling these

animals during less busy periods during the day, week, or year and encouraging owners to use these times allows for the provision of additional services with minimal additional overhead.

Adequate time is set aside for owner consultation so that a complete case review is possible. The consultation should start with a private discussion between the hospital staff and the owner, without the animal, regarding various test results or other important issues such as revisits or recommendations. The veterinarian should always participate in a portion of the consultation period. Specific recommendations to the owner should be provided in writing. Next, the owner makes payment for the services and schedules another appointment, if necessary. Finally, the animal is reunited with the owner, and any final issues are discussed or demonstrations with the animal are performed.

UTILIZING TECHNICAL SUPPORT STAFF

Most of the in-hospital evaluation procedures performed on geriatric dogs and cats can be carried out by a well-trained technician. All laboratory tests, radiographs, ultrasound examinations or electrocardiograms can be performed by the technician, and the results can be made available to the veterinarian before owner consultation. Veterinarians and hospital staff should have all necessary clinical materials, results, and recommendations organized and ready well in advance of owner consultation. The discharge and consultation process should begin with a private discussion between the owner, technician, and veterinarian without the dog or cat. The various tests and clinical findings should be discussed, and important items and information should be shared with the owner (e.g., radiographs, sonograms, electrocardiograms, and blood profiles). Specific recommendations should be provided to the owner in written form, and visual aids should be used as often as possible. The veterinary technician can be invaluable in providing additional owner education on specific conditions and home care needs. The older owner should always have an opportunity to ask questions about the findings, recommendations, follow-up care, and fees. After the consultation, the owner should be allowed to pay his or her account and make another appointment if necessary. Finally, the animal should be reunited with the owner, and any final items discussed and treatment recommendations demonstrated by the technician educator with the dog or cat.

RELIEF OF SUFFERING

For untreatable disease, comfort remains the primary goal, because the veterinarian can no longer use the elimination or treatment of the disease as the foremost means of restoring comfort. Instead, the veterinarian aims to achieve comfort using every means other than elimination of disease. Use of the terminology "transition from 'cure' to 'care'" implies a different approach to medical care (i.e., palliative care). Although the veterinarian and technician will experience grief over the death of each animal they treat, they must acknowledge that an animal's condition is terminal and avoid recommending treatments that decrease, rather than increase, the animal's comfort.

TECHNICIAN NOTE

Use of the home care concept maximizes the quality of life for terminal animals.

HOME CARE

When their pet is the hospital environment, the family is less available to stop procedures and practices that are not desired. Life of the animal may be prolonged, but so is suffering, and therefore such care may actually diminish rather than improve quality of life. Use of the home care concept maximizes the quality of life for terminal animals by supporting them with psychosocial services, providing respite care to relieve primary caregivers, and maintaining most animals in their homes (Figure 13-5). More than 62% of animals under home care die at home, allowing them and their owners to avoid the traumatic experience of the hospital.

The primary goal of owner services at the end of an animal's life should be to maximize the enjoyable interaction between the owner and the animal. Achieving this goal has the benefit of improving the quality of life for both. The animal should not suffer for the sake of the owner's

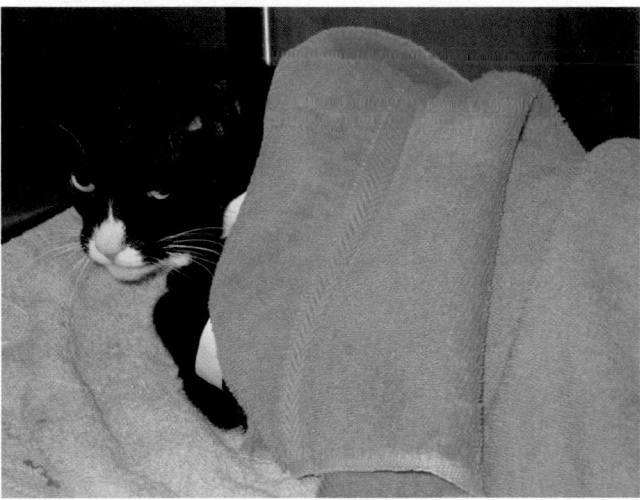

Figure 13-5 In the hospital environment, life may be prolonged, but so can suffering. Supporting terminally ill animals with the psychosocial benefit of home care, rather than hospital care, may maximize their quality of life.

quality of life, nor should the owner suffer needlessly in preserving the animal's quality of life. In most instances, the gains are mutual rather than competitive. Veterinarians and technicians are pledged to serve the animal, but this must usually be done through the owner. There are three realms that should be addressed in providing comprehensive care to geriatric animals, especially those coming to the end of their lives. The realms are physical, psychosocial, and spiritual care.

PHYSICAL CARE

High-quality nursing is the foundation of care for animals when there is no longer an expectation of achieving a cure. The major goals are maintaining maximum physical comfort, including assistance with the animal's bodily functions and activities of daily living, minimizing any complications and adverse effects, and preventing or relieving pain and all other physical discomforts (e.g., nausea, hunger, pruritus, constipation).

PSYCHOSOCIAL CARE

The responsibilities in psychosocial care involve both the animal and the family or household. The animal's attitude, responsiveness, and enthusiasm for interactions with the family must be assessed regularly. When the animal's psychosocial condition declines, it is important to re-assess the nursing interventions, pain relief, and owner activities to make adjustments that may restore the quality of life. A technician can be invaluable in helping people cope with behavioral changes and understanding an animal's behavior. Psychosocial care includes professional evaluation and assistance for the family members in dealing with conflicts exacerbated by the animal's condition, anticipatory grief, burden of caring for the animal, exhaustion, and other difficulties. Because veterinarians are not qualified to provide psychosocial services to people, a suitably credentialed counselor must be on retainer or available to take referrals.

✎ TECHNICIAN NOTE

Owners may need or appreciate help in talking through the questions and conflicts they are experiencing as a result of an animal's serious illness or death.

SPIRITUAL CARE

For many animal owners, spiritual support may be an important service. Spiritual care needs affect only the owners and family members, but just as with psychosocial services, veterinarians need to have spiritual counselors available through retainer or referral. It is very important that the spiritual counselors accept their roles as nondenominational caregivers and not try to promote their own religious beliefs. The death of an animal may prompt a spiritual crisis, especially if owners are experiencing internal conflicts over belief systems or if there are conflicting beliefs within the family or household. Owners may need or appreciate help in talking through the questions and conflicts they are experiencing as a result of an animal's serious illness or death.

Recommended Reading

Goldston RT: Geriatrics and gerontology, *Vet Clin North Am Small Anim Pract* 19:ix-x, 1, 1989.

Hoskins JD: Annual evaluation of senior and geriatric dogs, *Vet Forum* 17:42, 2000.

Kroll MM, Miller PE, Rodan I: Intraocular pressure measurements obtained as part of a comprehensive geriatric health examination from cats seven years of age and older, *J Am Vet Med Assoc* 219:1406, 2001.

Morse DR, Rabinowitz H: A unified theory of aging, *Int J Psychosom* 37: 5, 1990.

Mosier J: How aging affects body systems in the dog. In: *Geriatric medicine: contemporary clinical medicine and practice management approaches,* Lenexa, Kan, Veterinary Medicine Publishing, 1987, p 2.

Mosier JE: Effect of aging on body systems of the dog, *Vet Clin North Am* 19:1, 1989.

Turnwald GH, Baskett JJ: Effective communication with older owners, *J Am Vet Med Assoc* 209:725,1996.

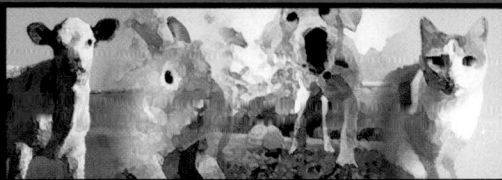

14

Animal Behavior

Suzanne Hetts

INTRODUCTION

Most veterinary technicians do not need to be convinced how important applied animal behavior is to veterinary medicine. Recent studies have shown that behavior problems are one of the most common reasons that dogs and cats are surrendered to shelters. Most dogs in shelters have not had basic training, and dogs who have been to basic training classes are less likely to be surrendered (Patronek et al., 1996a, 1996b; Salman et al., 1998). In addition, when owners have received advice about behavior problems that was either not helpful or not tried, their pets are at greater risk for surrender. ■

WHY BEHAVIOR WELLNESS?

Many owners who relinquish their pets have tolerated problems for months or years, often unable to find effective help (DiGiacomo et al., 1998). Owners often ignore or tolerate problems such as inappropriate elimination, phobias, or family pets not getting along until either the problem worsens or there is a lifestyle change that makes resolution of the problem a priority. Problems are usually much more difficult to resolve at these stages than if intervention had been obtained earlier.

In many cases, a window of opportunity for prevention and detection of problems and for providing timely intervention exists, but owners and veterinary care providers are not taking full advantage of it. For both general practice veterinary professionals, including technicians, and pet owners, making behavior wellness care an integral part of the delivery of pet health care services is more beneficial than a narrow focus on problem resolution, which is often sought at a crisis moment.

WHAT IS BEHAVIOR WELLNESS?

Behavior wellness has been defined as the condition or state of normal and acceptable pet conduct that enhances the human-animal bond and the pet's quality of life (Hetts, Heinke, Estep, et al., 2004).

Behavior wellness care is the planned attention to a pet's conduct and the active integration of behavior wellness programs into the delivery of pet-related services, including routine veterinary medical supervision.

Behavior wellness programs are protocols, procedures, services, and systems that educate pet owners and professionals about what constitutes the behaviorally healthy/well pet; promote behavioral wellness through positive proaction, behavior assessments, early intervention, and timely referrals; and decrease unrealistic human expectations and interpretations of pet behavior.

TECHNICIANS CAN PLAY A STRATEGIC ROLE IN BEHAVIOR WELLNESS CARE

When given sufficient education in behavior and behavior wellness care, including direction and support from the veterinarian, veterinary technicians can be the most strategically positioned individuals on the veterinary health care team to deliver many behavior wellness services.

TECHNICIAN NOTE
The technician is often the first person owners ask about why their pets behave the way they do.

The technician is often the first person owners ask about why their pets behave the way they do, how to prevent problems, and what to do once their pets' behavior has become a problem. Technicians are usually best positioned to have the first contact with clients during scheduled appointments.

409

With the support of the veterinarian, technicians can use these opportunities to deliver the appropriate elements of behavior wellness care. Elements of a complete behavior wellness program are listed in Box 14-1.

Practice management consultants are emphasizing the importance of veterinarians delegating health care tasks to their support staff when such tasks do not require the veterinarian (Wood, 1997). Increased use of technicians in history taking, nutrition, prophylactic dental services, and general client education has set precedents that provide the veterinary technician with an opportunity to play a leading role in behavior wellness programs as well. Doing so is beneficial to the technician, the clinic, and to pets and their owners (Box 14-2).

Box 14-1 COMPONENTS OF A BEHAVIOR WELLNESS PROGRAM

1. Promoting criteria for behaviorally healthy animals
2. Promoting helpful attitudes and realistic expectations
3. Promoting understanding of the behavioral needs of animals
4. Providing pet selection information
5. Promoting socialization of young animals
6. Promoting a positive plan for proaction to create good behavior
7. Conducting regular assessments of behavioral health
8. Making the veterinary hospital a behaviorally friendly place
9. Providing timely referrals when needed

Box 14-2 BENEFITS OF A BEHAVIOR WELLNESS PROGRAM

- The technician's job can be more rewarding and interesting.
- The technician and the clinic will better understand and meet both the clients' and the patients' needs. It is clear from the studies of animal shelters that the need for behavioral services is not being met.
- A behavior wellness program can help to make a visit to the clinic less stressful and more enjoyable for patients. This in turn can result in better health care for the pet. Many owners put off visiting the veterinarian if they know from past experience that this will be stressful and unpleasant for the animal.
- Pets become safer and easier to handle, and fewer staff members are bitten.
- A behavior wellness program increases the number of client visits per year.
- A program adds a significant dollar amount to the bottom line each year.
- A program attracts and retains top-of-the-line staff: the most motivated and best educated.
- A program decreases frustration in dealing with problem owners and problem pets because the technician can now provide them with services that can *prevent* pets from becoming difficult patients.

BEHAVIOR EDUCATION FOR TECHNICIANS

Technicians who deliver behavior wellness care must give up-to-date, scientifically accurate information. Scientific knowledge must replace nonscientific interpretations of behavior and information based solely on personal experience and beliefs.

Historically, most of the emphasis on continuing veterinary education in animal behavior has been on problem resolution. Lectures on resolving separation anxiety, aggression problems in both dogs and cats, and fears and phobias are common in veterinary technician continuing education programs. Time spent on these topics has often come at the expense of basic education in behavior.

As in other aspects of veterinary technician education, foundational skills must be acquired first. Whether within the veterinary technician curriculum or through continuing education, technicians must become familiar with basic concepts in applied ethology and animal learning. The former should include knowledge of species-specific communication signals and body postures, and the latter must include principles of operant and classical conditioning.

Continuing education opportunities focused on implementation of behavior wellness services, including implementing puppy classes in the veterinary clinic are now available[*][†][‡][§] (Hetts and Estep, 1999). Technicians can also consider continuing education opportunities other than, or in addition to, those traditionally provided within the field. National humane organizations, animal control associations, and dog training associations conduct training conferences that would be beneficial to technicians delivering behavior wellness services.

Problem resolution skills are the most advanced and complex and require the most education and experience. Technicians should first build a solid education in behavior basics and have experience with other aspects of behavior wellness care before participating in problem resolution activities.

A CHANGE IN PERSPECTIVE

A behavior wellness program requires that the technician not only *react* to questions when they are asked but also take a *proactive* approach and make behavior a part of every nonemergency appointment. This means initiating

---

[*]Hetts S, Estep DQ: *Implementing puppy classes in the veterinary practice: a two-day workshop,* Littleton, Colo, 2002, Animal Behavior Associates, Inc.
[†]Hetts S, Heinke ML: Implementing Behavioral Wellness Services Workshop, Lakewood, Colo, American Animal Hospital Association, 2000.
[‡]*Applied animal behavior for veterinary technicians,* Denver, Colo, 2004, Bel-Rae Institute of Technology.
[§]*Dogs! course,* West Lafayette, Ind, 2004, Animal Behavior Clinic, School of Veterinary Medicine, Purdue University.

discussions about the pet's behavior, whether the owner does or not.

Veterinary technicians who do not take the lead in asking questions about behavior are missing the point of behavior wellness. Owners are unlikely to initiate discussions about behavior unless a problem exists, which means missed opportunities for promotion of good behavior and early detection of problems that are at the core of behavior wellness.

BEFORE IMPLEMENTING BEHAVIOR WELLNESS CARE

Before offering any kind of behavioral information, technicians should clarify their role with the practice owner or their designated supervisor. Veterinarians usually determine what medical information or advice they wish technicians to impart to clients, and the same procedure should be followed when it comes to behavior.

When technicians' roles are not clearly defined, they may feel pressured and resentful of the time spent answering behavioral questions because this prevents them from completing other assigned tasks. On the other hand, if technicians spend significant time on behavior issues that is not charged to the client, this sets a dangerous precedent for the practice. It is one of the reasons that veterinarians believe, often erroneously, that providing behavior services is not financially feasible.

Behavior services should be professionally delivered, so that their value is fully recognized and they benefit not only clients and their pets, but the practice as well. The Society of Veterinary Behavior Technicians promotes and encourages the training of technicians in behavior and their appropriate involvement in the delivery of behavior services, making this organization an invaluable resource (Price, 2001). Information about the society can be found at the website listed in Box 14-3.

Box 14-3 Websites of Certifying Organizations and of Society of Veterinary Behavior Technicians and of the Delta Society

- http://www.veterinarybehaviorists.org—Website of the American College of Veterinary Behavior
- http://www.animalbehavior.org—Website of the Animal Behavior Society
- http://www.ccpdt.org—Website of the Certification Council for Pet Dog Trainers (CCPDT)
- http:// www.apdt.com—Website of the Association of Pet Dog Trainers (will also take you to the CCPDT site)
- http://www.svbt.org—Website of the Society of Veterinary Behavior Technicians
- http://www.deltasociety.org—Website of the Delta Society from which the document *Professional Standards for Dog Trainers: Effective, Humane Principles* can be obtained

---

> ### TECHNICIAN NOTE
> The first component of a behavior wellness program is defining characteristics of behaviorally healthy pets.

COMPONENTS OF A BEHAVIOR WELLNESS PROGRAM

DEFINING THE BEHAVIORALLY HEALTHY PET

Technicians are taught how to recognize healthy animals according to certain criteria. These commonly include good condition of the skin and coat, clear eyes, lack of external and internal parasites, proper weight, clean teeth and healthy gums, etc.

Criteria for behavioral health are often not considered. Behavioral health is more than the absence of behavior problems. As defined previously, it is the presence of normal and acceptable pet conduct that enhances the human-animal bond and the pet's quality of life (Hetts, Heinke, Estep, 2004).

Specifying the criteria for normal and acceptable pet conduct allows technicians to help pet owners set goals for promoting desirable behaviors, rather than just reacting when problems arise. Suggested criteria for behaviorally healthy cats and dogs are listed in Box 14-4. Technicians can use these as a basis for discussion with veterinarians and other co-workers to establish criteria within their hospitals. Criteria for other species can and should be established

---

Box 14-4 Criteria for Behaviorally Healthy Cats and Dogs

- Are affectionate, without being "needy."
- Are friendly toward or at least tolerant of people, including children, and other members of their own species.
- Enjoy or at least tolerate normal, everyday handling and interactions.
- Eliminate only in acceptable areas.
- Are not overly fearful of normal, everyday events or new things.
- Adapt to change with minimal problems.
- Play well with others by not becoming uncontrollable or rough.
- Are not nuisances or dangerous to the community.
- Can be left alone for reasonable time periods without becoming anxious or panicked.
- Readily relinquish control of space, food, toys, and other objects.
- Vocalize (bark, meow) when appropriate, but not to excess.

In addition, behaviorally healthy dogs:
- Reliably respond when told to sit, down, come, or stay.

In addition, behaviorally healthy cats:
- Scratch only items provided for this purpose.

as well. Assessment of behavioral health by using these and other criteria is another component of behavior wellness care that will be subsequently discussed.

ESTABLISHING REALISTIC EXPECTATIONS AND HELPFUL ATTITUDES

Anthropomorphic explanations for and unrealistic expectations about pets' behavior contribute to relationship problems between owners and pets. Technicians can play a vital role in educating clients in these areas.

Realistic Expectations

Technicians can routinely tell new pet owners to expect to lose something of value to their pet's house soiling or destructive behavior or to illness-related damage (e.g., diarrhea stains on the couch cushions). Most people expect some problem behaviors from puppies and kittens, but surprisingly many owners do not expect their 8- or 9-month-old cat or dog to still be prone to chewing and destructive play behaviors.

Clients who have recently acquired adult animals often make the erroneous assumption that their new pets are already "trained" and they will not have to worry about house training or chewing and other destructive behaviors. Adult animals new to the home, however, should be treated just like puppies or kittens would for the first few weeks to prevent problems as a result of owner expectations that are too high; adult pets often need training and supervision while they are making the adjustment to their new homes.

Reinterpreting Anthropomorphic Interpretations

Technicians can also help clients understand that their pets' behavior is not motivated by spite, revenge, rebelliousness, jealousy, or guilt. When owners realize that their pets are not being vindictive or mean-spirited or misbehaving even though they "know better," they are usually more willing to work with their pets' behavior and to listen to possible solutions.

Technicians can tell people that animals do what works for them—to meet a need, cope with stress, or control their environment. Destructive behavior that occurs when a pet is left alone, for example, is not motivated by revenge. Alternative explanations are separation anxiety, playful behavior, or the pet's realization that unpleasant consequences do not occur in the owner's absence.

PROVIDING PET SELECTION INFORMATION

The most proactive behavior wellness service is education of clients about pet selection. Unfortunately, few clients seek this service from the veterinary practice. Technicians can play a helpful role by regularly asking clients whether they are considering adding a new pet to the family and reminding them that the veterinary practice can assist them in selecting a pet that will best meet their expectations.

A closely related subject is helping owners introduce pets to one another. Better relationships between family pets could be created if introductions were also better managed. Pet owners don't usually ask for help until relationship problems exist, so creating opportunities for early intervention will be up to the veterinary professional. Introduction information that follows the Five-Step Plan for Positive Proaction (Hetts, Heinke, Estep, 2004), which will be subsequently discussed, should be provided when the new pet is first brought to the clinic for a medical examination and vaccinations.

IMPORTANCE OF SOCIALIZATION

Most species of social animals have a sensitive period during which socialization to their own species, to humans, and to other animals occurs most easily. Socialization refers to the process by which an animal develops appropriate social behaviors toward members of its own and other species (Bateson, 1979). In dogs, this period is from 4 to 12 weeks of age (Scott and Fuller, 1965); in cats, it is from 3 to 7 weeks of age (Karsh and Turner, 1988); and in horses, it begins at birth (Waring 2003). There may also be sensitive periods for the acclimatization of animals to new places, situations, and things, which occur around the same ages; but the precise time of these is unknown.

The process of socialization requires providing the young animal pleasant experiences with people, situations, inanimate elements of the environment, and other animals. Adequate socialization helps the animal to adapt to change and not react with fear or aggression to common, everyday events.

Technicians should educate pet owners about how early socialization can prevent the development of many behavior problems, especially those caused by fearful behavior. Cats are typically undersocialized, as evidenced by the tendency of many to hide when visitors come, be afraid in unfamiliar environments, and not enjoy human handling.

A practical approach to socialization advice is that during its sensitive period, a young animal should be exposed to elements of its world that are relevant to its adult role. A foal should have positive experiences with the horse trailer, kittens should be introduced to friendly dogs, and puppies should interact with friendly, well-behaved children.

Veterinarians have historically been reluctant to recommend early socialization programs for kittens and puppies because of concern about disease transmission. If recent outbreaks of contagious disease have been rare in the local area and the percentage of vaccinated animals is high, early socialization may present little hazard.

Although the veterinarian will set practice policy regarding early socialization programs, as one prominent veterinary behaviorist wrote ". . . the risk of a dog dying because of infection with distemper or parvo disease is far less than the much higher risk of a dog dying (euthanasia) because of a behavior problem" (Anderson, 1999).

With proper training and the support of the veterinary practice, technicians can offer puppy and kitten socialization classes. This limits concern over disease transmission if all attendees are immunized patients of the veterinary practice.

FIVE-STEP PLAN FOR POSITIVE PROACTION

The topic of preventing behavior problems is not a new one for technicians. However, a behavior wellness view focuses on promoting desirable behaviors, rather than preventing problems. The best time to share this plan is the first veterinary visit after a new animal has been acquired. Information may need to be repeated during future appointments, based on concerns discovered during behavior assessments.

This Five-Step Plan (Hetts, Heinke, Estep, 2004) organizes information and provides a framework technicians can use when they talk with pet owners about how they can create behavior patterns that define a behaviorally healthy pet. Having a means to organize information makes it easier to develop educational handouts on a variety of behaviors and may also ensure better coverage of the pertinent content. The five steps in the plan are as follows:

1. Elicit and reinforce appropriate behavior (Catch your pet doing the right thing).
2. Prevent or minimize inappropriate behavior (Don't let bad habits develop).
3. Meet your pet's behavioral and developmental needs.
4. Use negative punishment (the "take-away" method) to discourage inappropriate behavior.
5. Minimize positive punishment ("discipline") and use it correctly when necessary.

Each of these steps will be discussed in some detail.

TECHNICIAN NOTE
Animals need to be taught and encouraged to perform desirable behaviors.

Elicit and Reinforce Appropriate Behavior
Clients need specific instructions about how to proactively get their pet to do what they want rather than reacting to unwanted behavior. For example, technicians can tell owners to have treats at the door for occasions when people are greeted and to encourage the dog to sit, rather than yelling and pushing the dog off when he jumps up (Figure 14-1).

In some situations eliciting good behavior is integrally connected to meeting the pet's behavioral needs, another step in the Proactive Plan. For example, establishing reliable litterbox behavior is primarily dependent on creating a litterbox that meets the cat's behavioral preferences.

Technicians should also instruct owners to reward their pets when they catch them doing something right. It's easy to forget that behaviors that result in pleasant consequences are likely to be repeated. This is a very powerful

behavior modification method to which owners seldom devote enough effort.

Whenever the dog eliminates outside, the cat plays with its own toys, the foal nuzzles rather than nips at your hand, the puppy is lying down quietly, or the kitten is resting on a chair, the owner should reinforce these behaviors. Reinforcement may consist of a tidbit, presentation of a new or favorite toy, petting, or any other event the pet finds rewarding.

Praise alone, especially when an owner is first establishing a relationship with a new pet, is often not adequate reinforcement. Praise usually first needs to be paired with petting, play, or food for a time to become sufficiently reinforcing.

Technicians may need to educate owners about the value of using food in training. Both food and toys are very powerful ways to elicit and reinforce behavior when used correctly. The owner controls access to both, so the old adage that "a dog should work for me, not for food" is a useless argument. To prevent the "he'll only do it when he knows I've got a treat" objection, suggest the following:

- The food must be changed from being a lure to elicit the behavior to only being available as a reinforcer after the behavior has been performed.
- The food should be used as a reinforcer first on a continuous schedule to establish the behavior, and subsequently, on an intermittent, unpredictable schedule to maintain the behavior (petting or praise should always be used).
- All cues that the pet can use to predict whether or not food is available must be phased out.

TECHNICIAN NOTE
The fewer opportunities animals are given to engage in undesirable behaviors, the less likely such behaviors are to become habits.

Prevent or Minimize Inappropriate Behavior
When pets don't have the chance to make "mistakes," it's much easier to create good behaviors. The fewer opportunities an animal has to "practice" undesirable behaviors, the less likely such behaviors will become habits.

A cat that begins to eliminate on the carpet because the litterbox does not meet its behavioral needs may quickly develop a surface preference for carpet. If a puppy gets used to pulling on the leash while walking, this can quickly become a habit, making loose leash walking more difficult to teach. Playing with a kitten with hands and feet rather than its toys can result in a cat that bites hands and considers human body parts to be playthings.

The technician should instruct owners that they must manage the pet's environment to prevent bad habits from developing. Constant supervision of young animals and those new to the household is an absolutely critical

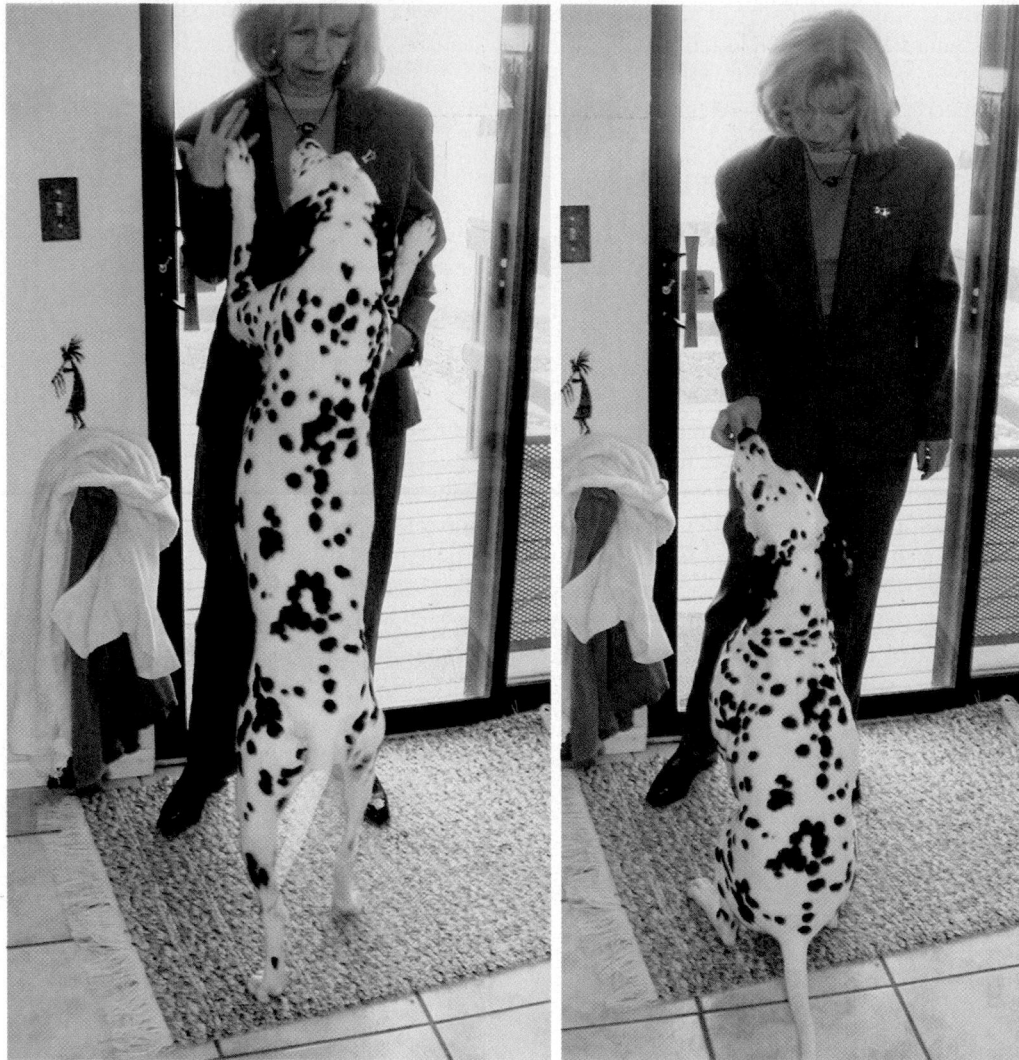

Figure 14-1 The lure-reward method of encouraging a dog to sit rather than jump on people.

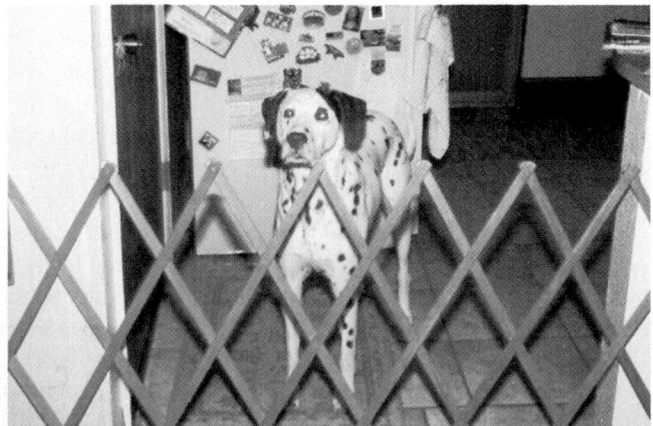

Figure 14-2 Environmental management with a baby gate to prevent opportunities for unwanted behavior.

Box 14-5 A Comparison of Dens and Crates

1. Wild canids become familiar with dens starting at birth. Dogs are not introduced to crates until much later, sometimes not until adulthood.
2. Wild canids are seldom, if ever, left alone in dens. If the dam is gone, the pups are usually together as a litter. For dogs, being confined in the crate is usually synonymous with being left alone.
3. Wild canids can choose when to come and go from the den. Dogs confined to crates when home alone cannot.
4. Once mobile, older pups and adult wild canids spend little time in the den. Dogs can spend as much as 50 hours a week or more confined in crates.

Box 14-6 Basic Steps in Crate Training

Goal 1: The dog enters and exits the crate willingly, without reluctance, with the door open.

Goal 2: The dog can stay in the crate for brief times while relaxing with a chew toy with the owner in view, with the crate door closed for about 15 to 20 minutes.

Goal 3: The dog can stay in the crate for brief times while relaxing with a chew toy with the owner not in view, with the crate door closed for about 30 minutes and/or overnight.

Goal 4: The dog can stay in the crate with the owner gone for 1 hour.

Box 14-7 Signs a Dog Is Not Tolerating the Crate

Even though a dog willingly enters a crate, this does not necessarily mean he is relaxed there when left alone. The only way to determine this is to audiotape or videotape the dog.

- Reluctance to enter the crate
- Excessive whining, barking, or vocalizing
- Attempts to get out of the crate
- Soiling in the crate, even if crated for brief time periods
- Finding your dog's fur wet from saliva when you return home
- Evidence that your dog has been so frantic that she has moved the crate
- Any damage to the crate, or injuries to your dog, from escape attempts

---

component of house training and also of teaching puppies and kittens to chew and scratch their own toys rather than household items.

Supervision can be accomplished in a number of ways, including crate training, use of baby gates to keep the pup in either a puppy-proof area or in the same room with the owner (Figure 14-2), or tethering the dog with a leash and collar to the owner or an object near the owner. Supervision of cats and kittens may mean closing doors to certain parts of the house.

A Word About Crate Training

A crate can be an extremely useful method of supervision, especially for puppies. Dog owners too often use crates incorrectly because they are not given good information about their use.

In the popular literature, crates are portrayed as analogous to dens. As the comparison points in Box 14-5 show, they are not. If technicians recommend crate training to pet owners they should also cover the following topics:

1. Correct Size of Crate. Dogs need to be comfortable in their crates. This means sufficient room to stand up to full height, easily turn completely around, and lay down on a side, fully relaxed. If the dog soils in the crate, it is *NOT* appropriate to recommend a smaller crate. Soiling the crate doesn't mean it is too large; it means something is wrong. The dog may be confined in the crate for longer than he can control himself, he may be anxious and frightened, or he may even have a medical problem. The technician should help the owner decipher why the dog is soiling, whether this means referral for a medical work-up or a behavior consultation.

2. How to Acclimate the Dog to the Crate. Dogs do not automatically like being confined in crates. They must be introduced to them gradually, by following steps similar to those listed in Box 14-6. This acclimation process may require just a day or two, or as long as several weeks with dogs who have previously been anxious when crated.

3. How to Acclimate the Dog to Being Left Alone in the Crate. This step is frequently overlooked. Just because the dog is comfortable in the crate when someone is home does not mean he will be when left alone. Technicians need to inform owners how to gradually acclimate the dog to being crated when alone; for example, technicians can tell owners to put the dog in the crate for periods of about 15 minutes.

4. How and When to Make the Transition to Leaving the Dog Alone, Free in the House. Crates should be a short-term management tool, not a way of life. The goal is for the dog to be unconfined in the home (perhaps with access to a backyard) when left alone. One study (Patronek et al 1996) revealed that dogs who spent most of their day crated were at increased risk of relinquishment.

5. Warning Signs That a Dog Is Not Adjusting Well to the Crate. An important related subject that should be discussed is guidelines for when a crate should not be used, such as when separation anxiety problems exist or when the dog becomes panicked when it is confined (Box 14-7).

Box 14-8 BEHAVIORAL NEEDS OF COMPANION ANIMALS

- Provision of a safe, comfortable place to rest and sleep.
- Freedom from, or the ability to escape from, unnecessary pain, fear, and threats or discomfort.
- Ability to control some aspects of the environment.
- Opportunities to express species-typical behaviors such as chewing, scratching, elimination, etc.
- Opportunities for exercise and play that are appropriate for that individual.
- Opportunities for mental stimulation.
- Opportunities for pleasant social contact with co-species and/or people to which the animals have been socialized and which are appropriate for that individual.

Meet the Pet's Behavioral and Developmental Needs

Animals do things in order to get their needs met. Technicians can teach owners how to meet their pets' needs in ways that encourage and provide for desirable behaviors. This is much more effective than owners vainly trying to suppress normal behaviors such as chewing, playing, or elimination. Instead, these behaviors should be directed onto appropriate targets, or steps should be taken to help the behaviors occur at appropriate times or locations.

Defining a list of widely accepted behavioral needs for pets, although difficult and controversial, has been proposed (Hetts, Heinke, Estep, 2004) and can be found in Box 14-8. This list presupposes that an animal's basic survival needs for food, water, and shelter have been addressed.

An Example of Meeting the Pet's Behavioral Needs: Elimination

Technicians can educate cat owners about cats' behavioral needs regarding a litterbox based on the list in Box 14-9. Many litterbox problems develop because the areas the cat is soiling meet the cat's behavioral preferences for elimination better than the litterbox area.

Figure 14-3, for example, shows a litterbox that is unacceptable in several ways, as follows:

- Dirty
- In an area where the cat is unlikely to spend much time
- Next to noisy appliances
- On a cold cement floor
- Not easily accessible

Compare it with a clean litterbox (Figure 14-4) located in a quiet, accessible, but private area. It's clear which box better meets the cat's behavioral needs and is therefore more likely to be used.

An Example of Meeting the Pet's Behavioral Needs: Play

Owners who do not realize they must be prepared to devote time to playing with their pets may become frustrated with

---

Box 14-9 LITTERBOX CHARACTERISTICS ASSOCIATED WITH MEETING CATS' BEHAVIORAL NEEDS

- Type and number of boxes
  - Size—average, smaller, larger
  - Cover or not—start without unless a good reason to cover
  - As many boxes as cats
- Litter
  - Type—the finer the better
  - Depth—1½ to 2 inches generally
  - Unscented preferred
- Liners or not
  - Some cats may dislike
  - Ease of cleaning may result in cleaner litterbox
- Location
  - Where in house
    Balance privacy with accessibility
    Avoid startling noises or other stimuli
  - Where in room
    Ability to see and be protected
    Escape routes—more than one
    Access routes—easy to access, no obstacle courses
    Comfortable surface—soft and warm generally
  - Multiple boxes not adjacent to one another
  - Away from food, water, and resting places
  - Cleaning
    Scoop at least daily
    Litter always appears dry and clean
    Wash with mild, odor-free cleaners—no dried urine or feces on box
    Self-cleaning litterboxes can be an option for some owners

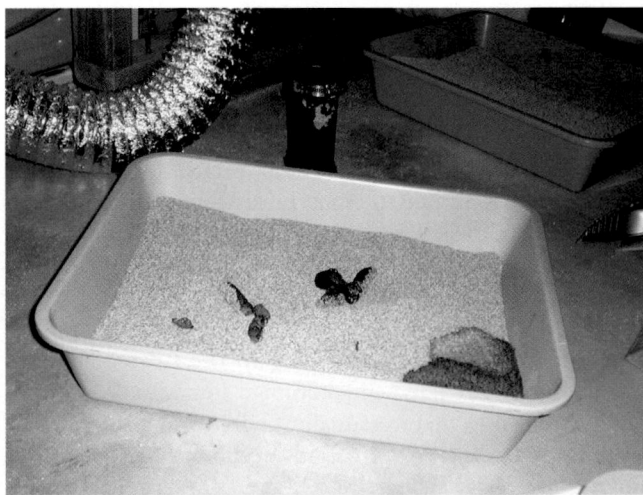

Figure 14-3 A litterbox that will not meet the behavioral needs of most cats. See text for reasons.

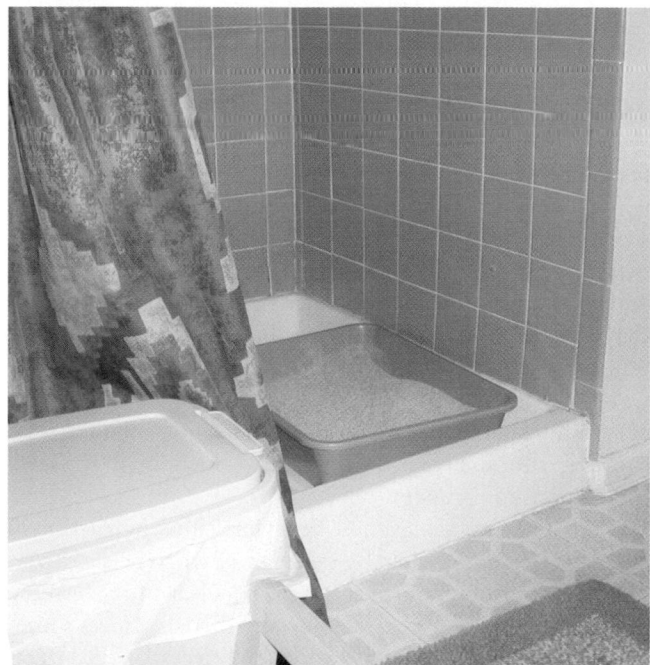

Figure 14-4 A cat-friendly litterbox. See text for important characteristics.

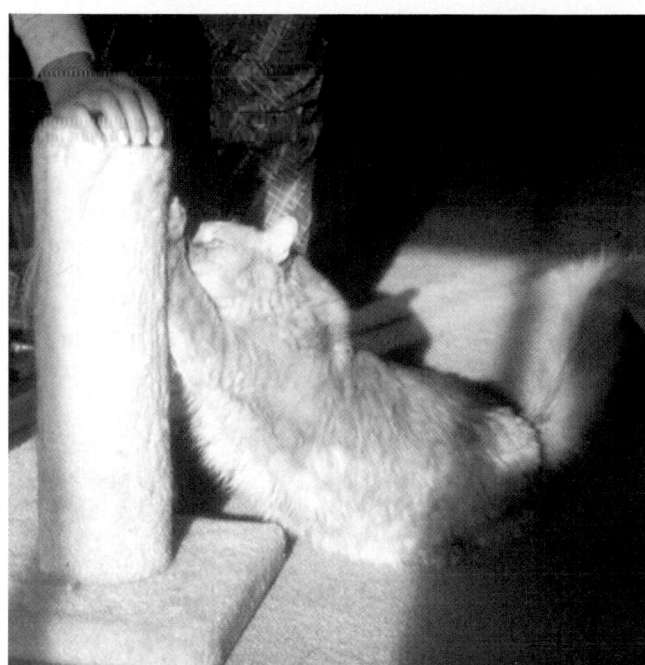

Figure 14-5 Cat with a preference for scratching vertical surfaces.

their pet's "hyperactivity" or pestering behavior that results when this need isn't met.

Pets need time for social play with their owners or other animals and for object play with toys. A variety of toys that allow for chewing, chasing, stalking (cats), and retrieving (dogs) should be provided.

Determine Individual Preferences

Technicians can explain to owners that sometimes it may be necessary to create choice situations so they can determine their pet's preferences, relative to various behavioral needs.

For example, cats need objects to scratch but individual differences exist for what they prefer. Most cats tend to prefer a scratching post that is oriented vertically (Figure 14-5), although some prefer a horizontal scratching area (Figure 14-6). An owner can discover the specific preferences of a cat by giving the cat choices among vertical and horizontal scratching posts presented at the same time in the same location and then noting which one is most used. Similar choice "tests" can be used to determine what individual animals prefer in the way of toys, bedding, litterboxes, and surfaces for elimination.

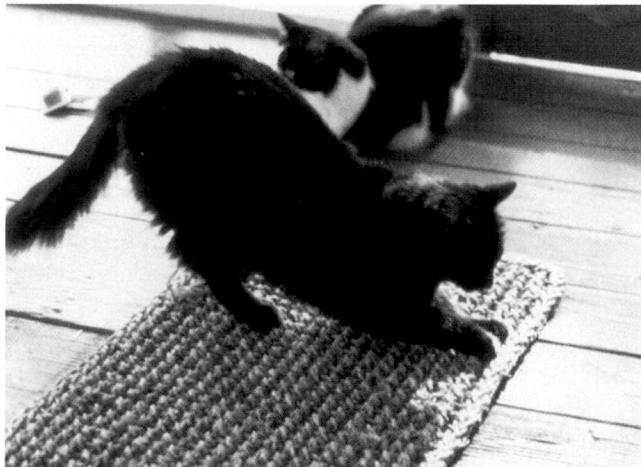

Figure 14-6 Cat with a preference for scratching horizontal surfaces.

Use Negative Punishment (The "Take Away" Method) to Discourage Inappropriate Behavior

Pet owners seldom make use of this technique. Because negative punishment does not involve the application of aversive stimuli, it is very often preferred over positive punishment.

Parents may be more familiar with the concept but rarely think to use it with animals. The "take away" method refers to a learning outcome called negative punishment. To stop an unwanted behavior, technicians can tell owners how to take away something the animal wants. This is similar to

---

✎ **TECHNICIAN NOTE**

Pet owners may need to set up choice situations to determine their pets' behavioral needs.

taking away a child's television privileges as a consequence of bad grades.

If a puppy is playing too rough, rather than yelling, pushing, or slapping the pup, the owner can walk away and ignore the puppy. The puppy learns that rough play loses him his chance to play at all.

If a horse becomes "pushy" when the handler enters the stall with grain, the handler doesn't feed the grain to the horse and leaves the stall.

There are many situations in which negative punishment can be applied instead of positive punishment, including the following examples:

- Cat meows at the owner to get attention—owner leaves the room.
- Dog paws at person who is petting her—person stops petting and walks away.
- Dog attempts to dash through door before being given permission—owner shuts door and walks away.
- Dog will not release toy for owner to throw—owner walks away and refuses to play with dog.
- When told to sit, dog lies down instead—owner withholds tidbit.
- Cat A stalks family cat B—cat A is put in a small bathroom for 3 minutes.

The last example is a time-out, a "take away" technique. Technically, the term is "time out from reinforcement." Practically, a time-out means that as a consequence of unwanted behavior, the animal is immediately taken to a place where he doesn't want to be. A kitten who bites during play can be immediately placed in a small, dark room for a few minutes. The difficulties in implementing a time-out are finding an appropriate location, getting the animal there in a timely fashion without adding inadvertent reinforcement, and remembering to keep the time-out brief.

Minimize Positive Punishment ("Discipline") and Use It Correctly When Necessary

When the other four steps are followed, discipline becomes less necessary. There are two kinds of punishment—positive and negative. In learning theory terminology, positive and negative do not refer to good or bad, but instead to adding something or taking something away.

Thus positive punishment is the addition, or presentation, of something unpleasant immediately after an undesirable behavior is observed. In contrast, negative punishment is taking away, or removing, something the animal wants as a consequence of undesirable behavior.

For example, a positive punishment (and not one recommended!) is kneeing a dog in the chest when it jumps on someone. A negative punishment is turning one's back, walking away, and ignoring the dog. This is negative punishment because the dog wants attention (something pleasant) and by jumping up it loses any opportunity to obtain that attention.

For punishment to be used effectively and humanely, several criteria must be met. These criteria are particularly important when the use of positive punishment is considered. Criteria for effective punishment are as follows.

Immediacy

Any punishment must be delivered within a very few seconds after the undesirable behavior occurs. Any longer delay prevents the animal from associating the punishment with the unwanted behavior and increases the likelihood that the pet has performed another behavior before the punishment is delivered. "Guilty looks" that dogs display when owners attempt to deliver punishment after the fact are nothing more than submissive behaviors. Rather than showing submissive behaviors, cats generally hide when they expect punishment.

Dogs and cats display these behaviors either in reaction to owners' threatening scolding behavior or when pets can predict that punishment is likely. Some pets learn to determine that when the owner comes home and there is a mess somewhere in the house (trash overturned, feces on the floor, a torn-up couch cushion), bad things will happen to them. If the owner comes home and there is no mess, nothing bad happens and the pet displays normal greeting behaviors.

Consistency

All occurrences of the undesirable behavior must be punished in order for punishment to be most effective. If an owner catches the pet misbehaving some of the time but not all of the time, it is likely the behavior will continue because the pet continues to play the odds that it will not be punished. With most behaviors, it is unrealistic to expect owners to be available to immediately and consistently deliver a positive punishment. This is one reason that owner-delivered positive punishment has limited value in changing behavior.

Appropriate Intensity

Animals will learn to tolerate higher levels of aversive stimuli if they are presented with such stimuli in gradually increasing intensity rather than a moderately intense stimulus initially. For example, an owner might gently tell his or her dog "no," which is not sufficient to stop the misbehavior. The owner may then say "no" in gradually increasingly threatening tones until it is necessary to scream at the dog to get him to stop the behavior. In contrast, an owner who says "no" in a more firm, authoritative tone of voice initially is more likely to successfully stop the misbehavior and not have to scream. Unfortunately, many aversive stimuli that are intense enough to inhibit behaviors can also elicit fearful and aggressive responses.

Remote Punishment Is Usually Preferable to Interactive Punishment

Positive punishment that comes from the owner has several potentially undesirable outcomes. First, the pet often learns that a behavior will be punished *only* in the owner's presence. The cat thus scratches the stereo speaker or the dog lifts his leg on the couch only when the owner is at work. This leads owners to incorrectly and anthropomorphically conclude the pet "knows better" because the behavior only occurs when the owner is not present. Second, owner-delivered punishment, especially if it is severe (scruff shakes, rollovers, hitting) or does not meet the other criteria, can result in the pet being afraid of or aggressive toward the owner and has a negative impact on the human-animal bond. Remote punishments or booby traps are more likely to be immediate and consistent. Examples of remote punishers are as follows:

- Citronella Anti-Bark Collar (Premier Pet Products) (Figure 14-7)
- Snappy Trainer (Interplanetary Pet Products, Inc.) (Figure 14-8)
- Motion detector (SSSCat, Premier Pet Products) (Figure 14-9)
- Scat Mat (Contech, Inc.) (Figure 14-10)
- Hand-held noisemaker, such as an air horn (Safety Sport) (Figure 14-11) or ultrasonic device (These require activation by the owner, who must be able to covertly, immediately, and consistently activate them.)

By definition, punishment decreases the frequency of the behavior it follows. If an owner has repeatedly attempted to punish a behavior, but the pet is still showing the behavior at the same frequency, then the behavior has not really been punished.

A general guideline technicians can give owners is that if positive punishment has not been successful after three to five applications, it probably will not be. Even more importantly, technicians should encourage owners to shift their perspective from "how can I get my pet to stop a certain behavior," which implies the need for some sort of aversive consequence, to "how can I get my pet to do what I want so I can reward it." With this perspective, the first three steps of the Five-Step Plan are usually the most important.

An example of how the Five-Step Plan can be applied to canine house training can be found in Box 14-10, and a list of behaviors and situations for which technicians should provide owners a Five-Step Plan is provided in Box 14-11.

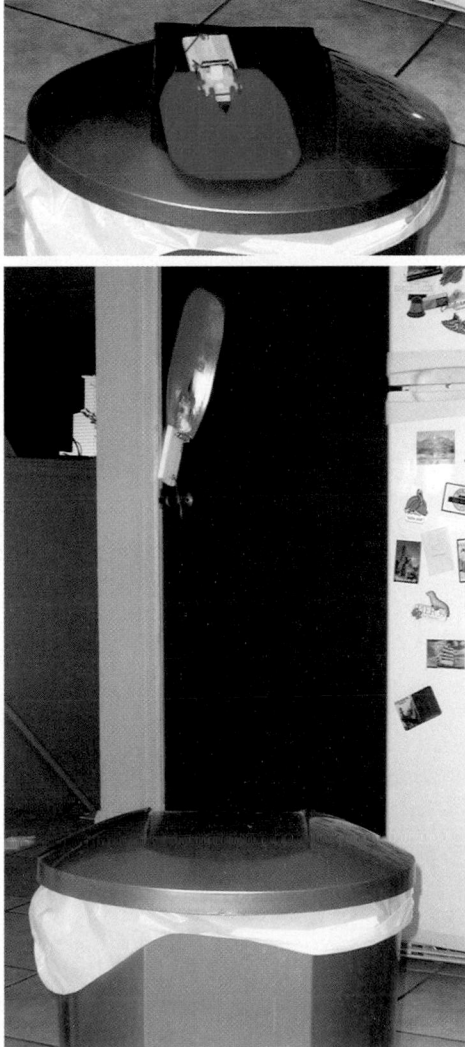

Figure 14-8 Snappy Trainer (Interplanetary Pet Products, Inc). A Snappy Trainer is a modified mousetrap that safely startles the pet. When triggered by the pet's touch, it snaps into the air but is unable to snap closed on the pet's body.

The most effective and humane solution to nuisance barking!

PREMIER

Gentle Spray™

Citronella Anti-Bark Collar

NO SHOCK NO PAIN

Figure 14-7 Citronella Anti-Bark Collar (Premier Pet Products).

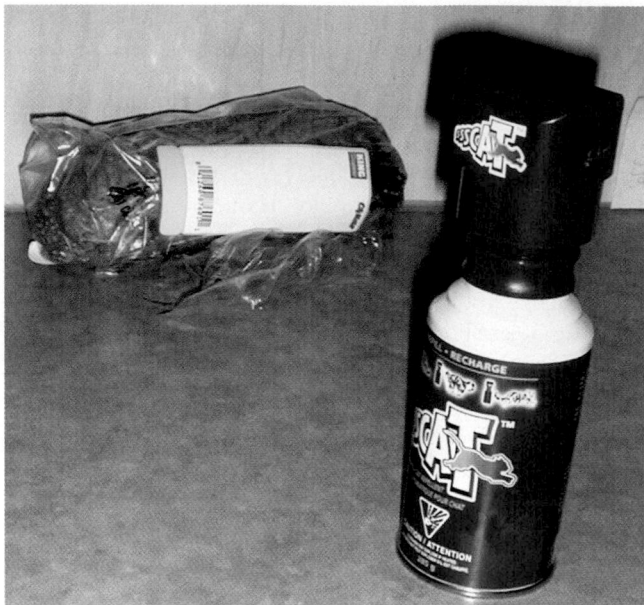

Figure 14-9 Motion detector (SSSCat, Premier Pet Products Inc).

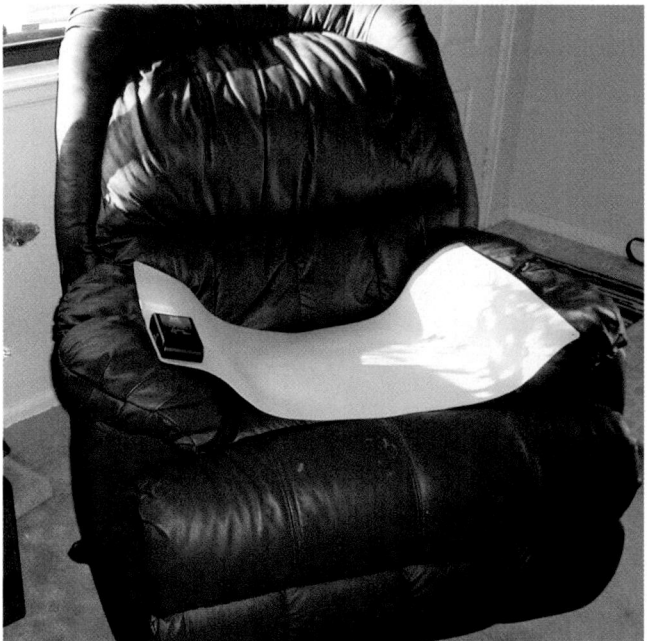

Figure 14-10 Scat Mat (Contech, Inc).

BEHAVIOR ASSESSMENTS

A recent study showed that as few as 25% of veterinarians routinely discuss behavior issues with clients, 17% never do, and only 11% of veterinarians thought it was their responsibility to initiate discussions about behavior problems with clients (Patronek and Dodman, 1999).

A behavior wellness approach *requires* that technicians and other veterinary professionals take the initiative during

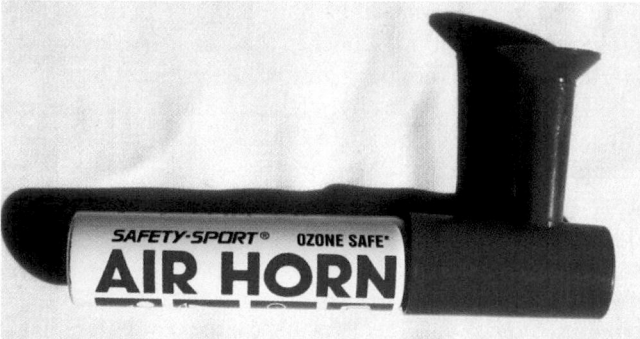

Figure 14-11 Hand-held noisemaker, such as an air horn (Safety Sport).

Box 14-10 USING THE FIVE-STEP PLAN TO FACILITATE CANINE HOUSETRAINING

1. Catch the dog doing something right. Reward the dog with a treat, praise, and/or petting for eliminating outside. Go to the dog rather than waiting for the dog to return to the door. If the treat is given after the dog has returned to the door, that's the behavior that is rewarded. If the dog enjoys leash walks, and eliminating terminates the walk, then eliminating is being negatively punished (it ends opportunity to continue walking).

2. Don't let bad habits develop. The dog should be constantly supervised (or crated when left alone during housetraining) so that he doesn't have an opportunity to house soil.

3. Meet the pet's behavioral needs. Provide the dog with sufficient opportunities for elimination, and locations that meet its behavioral preferences. Many dogs prefer soft surfaces, such as grass, so a gravel-covered pen may not be acceptable. Provide an outside area that is protected from weather extremes (wet and cold for small, short-coated dogs or hot and humid for heavy-coated dogs). Accustom puppies to those surfaces they will be expected to use for elimination as adults. For urban dogs, these may be city streets and curbs.

4. Use the "take-away" method to discourage unwanted behavior. This step is not directly applicable to housetraining. If the owner catches the dog soiling, the dog should merely be taken outside immediately. The owner should evaluate where the breakdown occurred that allowed the house soiling. Was the dog allowed too much freedom? Had too much time elapsed since his last chance to relieve himself?

5. Minimize "discipline" and use it correctly when necessary. Because the process of housetraining is creating the correct preferences for where and on what the dog likes to eliminate, and helping the dog learn that the entire house is his living area (or den) and shouldn't be soiled, discipline is not important in housetraining.

---

every nonemergency appointment to perform regular behavior assessments. If they do not, opportunities for helping owners create desirable behavior and for early detection and intervention when problems do arise will be lost.

Box 14-11 Behaviors and Situations for Which the Five Step Plan Should Be Given to Clients

- Elimination behavior
- Play behaviors
- Normal destructive behaviors (play, investigation, chewing, or teething)
- Barking
- Introducing new pets to family, especially children and resident pets
- Introducing new pets to resident family pets
- Acclimating dogs to being left alone
- Acclimating pets to being handled and examined

Box 14-12 Behavior Assessment: Questions About Family Lifestyle Changes That Put Pets at Risk for Problems

- Are you planning a move to a different house?
- Will the composition of your family change in the near future (new baby, marriage, divorce, children moving home, etc.)?
- Will any young children reach the crawling or walking stage in the near future?
- Will any family member's schedule undergo a significant change in the near future (e.g., resuming/leaving work, school, hours/shift change at work)?
- Will you be going on vacation?
- Will you be doing any home improvement or construction?
- Will you be acquiring another pet or have you recently lost a pet?

Owners will resort to inquiring about behavior only at the crisis stage in which the pet's continued presence in the home is at risk. With the support of the veterinarian, trained technicians are best positioned to conduct behavior assessments before the start of the medical appointment.

Behavior assessments involve the following five major areas:

1. How well the animal meets the criteria for a behaviorally healthy pet
2. Family conditions or changes that put pets at risk for surrender
3. The pet's daily routine, lifestyle, and whether its behavioral needs are being met
4. Identification of early warning signs and problems
5. The pet's behavior observed at the veterinary hospital

How Well the Animal Meets the Criteria for a Behaviorally Healthy Pet

For each behavior listed in Box 14-4, owners can be asked to rate their pet's behaviors on a 5-point Likert scale (always, usually, sometimes, rarely, or never). Technicians can discuss in depth those behaviors owners rank as "rarely" or "never." Certain behaviors may be sufficiently important to discuss even if an owner rated them as "sometimes." A pet who is only "sometimes" friendly with people may have an aggression problem that requires immediate assistance.

Family Conditions or Changes That Put Pets at Risk for Surrender

A move, addition of a new baby, a change in a family member's schedule, vacation, remodeling, and the addition or loss of another family pet are all examples of situations that frequently trigger behavior problems. If impending changes are identified, technicians can help owners be proactive and minimize potential negative effects on the pet's behavior. Examples of questions to ask are provided in Box 14-12.

The Pet's Daily Routine, Lifestyle, and Whether Its Behavioral Needs Are Being Met

Recent research shows that where a pet spends its time during the day may be a risk factor for relinquishment. One study revealed that dogs who were confined in crates, left outside, or confined to a small part of the house on a routine basis were at greater risk of surrender to a shelter than those who had free run of the house (Patronek et al., 1996a). Similarly, cats that were allowed outside were also at greater risk (Patronek et al., 1996b). Thus it may be very important to find out where the pet spends most of its time.

Problem behaviors can occur when an animal's behavioral needs are not being met or when the animal is getting its needs met by using inappropriate behaviors. Technicians can inquire about the pet's behavioral needs, based on the categories in Box 14-8. Box 14-13 gives examples of questions regarding the pet's routines and whether the pet's behavioral needs are being met.

Identification of Early Warning Signs of Problems

Owners often do not interpret behaviors as early warning signs of potential problems, such as the following:

- The dog leaves the room and avoids an infant whenever the infant is placed on a blanket on the floor. The owner may not understand that this is an indication that the dog is fearful, a behavior that could escalate to growling and snapping when the infant reaches the crawling or toddler stage.
- The cat often urinates right next to the litterbox. The owner tolerates and never mentions this behavior because it occurs on cement in the unfinished basement. The owner may not have the foresight to see that when he or she decides to finish the basement, this will likely result in the cat urinating on the new carpet.

> **Box 14-13** BEHAVIOR ASSESSMENT QUESTIONS REGARDING PET'S MANAGEMENT, LIFESTYLE, AND PROVISION FOR BEHAVIOR NEEDS
>
> - Does your pet have free run of the house when you are gone, or is she kept crated; left outside, in the basement, or in the garage; or confined to a small part of the house on a regular basis? If the pet is confined, why?
> - Where does your pet sleep at night?
> - Is your cat allowed outside? When and for how long? Supervised/leashed/confined or not?
> - Is your pet recently spending more time outside because its behavior inside the house has become more of a problem?
> - How do you discipline your pet? What does your pet need to be disciplined for? What's the strongest discipline procedure you've ever used?
> - How many hours does your pet spend alone?
> - How much exercise and play time does your pet receive each day?
> - What toys does your pet have? How does your pet like to play?

> **Box 14-14** BEHAVIOR ASSESSMENT: QUESTIONS TO ASK TO IDENTIFY EARLY WARNING SIGNS
>
> - Is there anything you (or any other family member) are afraid or reluctant to do with or to your pet?
> - What does your pet not like done?
> - What things is your pet afraid of? How does she behave when afraid?
> - What does your pet do when you do the following:
>   - Clip nails
>   - Brush her
>   - Take food or toys away
>   - Roll her over on her back
>   - Touch her body in certain places
>   - Discipline her
>   - Pick her up
>   - Pet her for a while
>   - Reach for her collar
>   - Walk by or disturb her when she's resting
>   - Tell her to move from the bed or furniture
>   - Disturb her while she's asleep

- A dog owner who is a teacher has been home all summer with a new puppy. She or he thinks it is cute that the puppy cries, paws, and becomes very distressed at the door when the owner steps outside for a short time to get the mail or mow the yard. The owner does not view this behavior as an indication of a potential separation anxiety problem when she or he goes back to work in the fall.

> **Box 14-15** POINTS FOR DISCUSSION WITH THE OWNER WHEN BEHAVIORS OF CONCERN ARE OBSERVED IN THE VETERINARY HOSPITAL
>
> - We are concerned about the pet not receiving top-quality care.
> - We are concerned about safety of staff.
> - Pet should be able to tolerate basic handling.
> - Discuss the pet's *behavior,* rather than labeling the pet as a problem.
> - We did everything we could to minimize his stress, yet he still became upset.
> - Behavior was out of proportion to the situation.

The important point in these examples is that the owners would never think to discuss these behaviors with the technician because they do not see them as problems or potential problems. People surrendering their pets to a shelter had often experienced some lifestyle change that either prevented them from continuing to tolerate the problem or, as in these examples, resulted in the same behavior becoming less tolerable (DiGiacomo et al., 1998; Scarlett et al., 1999). Behavior assessment can be used to detect these situations and identify problems or potential problems earlier.

Box 14-14 gives examples of questions technicians can ask owners for the purpose of identifying these warning signs. Things owners mention as the animal not liking and activities that elicit fearful, threatening, aggressive, or avoidance behaviors may later be associated with full-blown behavior problems.

The Pet's Behavior Observed at the Veterinary Hospital

Technicians should make note of the pet's demeanor at the veterinary hospital. This is important not only in assessing the pet's behavioral health, but in keeping staff safe when during handling of the pet. Occurrences of fearful, threatening, or aggressive behavior should be put in the patient's record, shared with staff, and discussed with the owner. It is a good idea to mark the front of a fractious or dangerous patient's file with a hard-to-miss symbol, so technicians are aware of the patient's behavioral history before attempting any interactions.

When technicians observe dangerous or threatening behavior from a patient, they must discuss this with the veterinarian. The veterinarian must in turn share this information with the owner. Under the veterinarian's direction, technicians may be asked to discuss these problems with the owner. Veterinarians and technicians can prepare a script for the conversation with the owner. Examples of discussion points are listed in Box 14-15. To gain a sense of the breadth of the problem, technicians should also ask the owner whether the pet has displayed similar behavior in other contexts.

Behavior Assessment Skills

Interviewing Skills: Asking Good Questions

Initiating discussions requires excellent interviewing skills. Such skills are important not only in behavioral wellness programs but also during the process of taking a medical history. The first important interviewing skill is asking nonleading, open-ended questions. Good questions do not lead the client into a particular answer and require more than a yes or no answer. Questions such as "Is your pet showing any problem behavior?" or "Do you have any questions about setting up a litterbox?" do not meet these criteria. A client could answer both questions "no" and yet have a 6-month-old dog who growls when people come too close to the food dish (the owner thinks this is normal and therefore not a problem), or the owner may have located a new kitten's litterbox in the basement on a cement floor next to the furnace (the owner sees nothing wrong with this placement and thus has no questions). More productive questions might be, "What does your pet not like you to do with him?" and "Would you describe in detail the characteristics of your cat's litterbox?" The technician may need to ask the same question in several ways to obtain concrete, detailed information.

The technician should try to not only obtain concrete descriptions about the animal's behavior but also discover how owners are raising and training the pet. Technicians need to evaluate these procedures and provide more appropriate alternatives when necessary. This topic is covered more thoroughly in the discussion of behavior assessments.

Interviewing Skills: Interpersonal Communication

For owners to provide good information about their pets, they need to feel comfortable talking to the veterinary technician. Clients need to know that technicians are not just "going through the motions" but are genuinely interested in them, their pets, and what they have to say. Even on a busy day, a harried technician can make a good impression and encourage clients to open up, while at the same time keeping the conversation on track, by using a few simple communication skills.

Put Clients at Ease by Sitting Down. Conducting the behavioral interview sitting down puts the technician and client at the same level and also helps relieve any tension or nervousness. The technician who remains standing gives the impression of being in a hurry or less approachable. Having clients sit down helps to relax them and put them more at ease.

Use Active Listening Skills. A technician should face a client when talking to him or her in order to communicate that the client is the focus of attention. If the technician's body is directed elsewhere, the message is that his or her attention is as well. The technician can keep an open body posture by trying not to cross legs or arms, hold a clipboard or folder at chest or face level, or stand behind a barrier such as an examination table. Doing so sends the message that the technician is not completely open to hearing the client. Maintaining casual eye contact by looking at the client from time to time, rather than burying one's face in papers, enhances communication. Looking up while still being able to take notes takes practice, but it is a skill worth developing. The technician can acknowledge what the client is saying by giving frequent feedback without interrupting, by nodding his or her head, and by saying "OK," "Hmmm," or "I see" or making other neutral, quick statements to let the client know the technician is engaged in the conversation. A warm or neutral tone of voice, rather than an abrupt or abrasive one, should be used.

Obtain Behavioral Descriptions, Not Interpretations. Owners often describe their pets' behavior in relatively vague terms, such as "He goes crazy at the door!" Consider the following three examples of what this statement might actually mean. When the doorbell rings the dog does the following:

- Barks, growls, runs to the door, and lunges at it
- Wildly jumps up, grabs his ball, races to the door, tail wagging, with a "happy face," and thrusts his wet, slimy ball into the visitor's hand
- Barks continuously, shies away from the door, hides behind the owner, and will not allow visitors to get near him

These are just three of many possible things that "He goes crazy at the door!" might mean. This illustrates the importance of obtaining behavioral *descriptions,* rather than *interpretations.* The technician can ask "What does your pet *do* at the door? Describe the behaviors you see." The technician should continue to probe for additional information until he or she is certain what a client is attempting to describe. Repeated questioning may be necessary to obtain a description that provides a mental picture of the behavior in question. While probing for more information, the technician should use good communication skills so that clients understand that he or she is genuinely attempting to clarify information rather than harassing them with repeated questions. The technician can paraphrase a client's description of the pet's behavior by asking, "So when the doorbell rings your dog barks and jumps on people—is that correct?" This question gives the client an opportunity to agree with the technician or provide additional information.

Using the Results of Behavior Assessments

The behavior assessment should be made part of the pet's permanent record, and the technician should discuss the results with the veterinarian. An action plan could include a medical examination, an in-house behavior consultation, referral to a behavior consultant, referral to a dog trainer for obedience classes, dissemination of educational materials, or a recommendation for particular behavior management products.

Follow-Up for Behavior Assessments

Once the veterinarian has created an action plan, technicians can be responsible for conducting behavioral follow-up telephone calls, just as many currently do for medical cases. After routine surgeries, suturing, or dental procedures, technicians are often given the responsibility of calling clients to inquire about the pet's status and progress. Behavior issues deserve the same type of follow-up. Technicians can call the client to determine whether the pet owner followed through with the suggested referral, implemented any training or behavior modification techniques that were suggested, or purchased behavior management products that were recommended. Technicians can also help owners implement a behavior modification plan created by the veterinarian or outside behavior consultant. Very few veterinary practices have routine procedures in place to follow up on behavioral problems in the same way they follow up on medical problems.

> 🖉 **TECHNICIAN NOTE**
>
> When behavioral concerns or issues are identified, a behavior wellness approach demands that these be addressed and not ignored. The practice should give pet owners specific recommendations or action plans.

MAKING THE VETERINARY CLINIC A BEHAVIORALLY FRIENDLY PLACE

Visiting the veterinary clinic is very stressful for some pets, and consequently, for their owners. An animal that is stressed or fearful is more likely to bite or scratch. This not only makes the animal more difficult to handle but also puts technicians and other veterinary professionals at risk of being injured and may prevent the pet from receiving the best medical care. Once pets have a bad experience and begin to associate the clinic with unpleasantness, future visits become more difficult.

One of the ways pet owners judge veterinary services is by how their animals are treated. Using behaviorally friendly methods with patients is "walking the talk" of behavior wellness care. Clients will better understand the idea of behavior wellness care when they see technicians use positive and proactive techniques when handling their pets. It is therefore to everyone's benefit to take a behavior wellness approach and help patients be more relaxed at the veterinary clinic. Rather than having to calm down animals who arrive at the clinic already stressed, a proactive behavior wellness approach seeks to create patients that have positive expectations when they arrive at the veterinary clinic.

The first step in lowering patient stress is to understand species typical behaviors when an animal feels threatened or challenged.

Understanding Aggressive Behavior

When animals feel threatened or challenged in a social interaction, they have a variety of choices as to how to respond. These choices are called agonistic behaviors. By understanding the choices animals may make in social conflict situations, technicians can often decrease conflict, more humanely handle and restrain animals with less use of force, and be safer themselves. The most common agonistic behaviors technicians are likely to see in a veterinary medical context are described in following sections.

Escape, Avoidance, or Attempts To Do So

Many animals initially try to avoid conflict. Animals may try to get away or struggle to avoid restraint. Sometimes, it may be better to allow the animal to avoid conflict rather than escalating forceful restraint. Backing off, giving the animal a chance to calm down and then trying other techniques are safer choices for the technician and less stressful for the animal. Allowing avoidance to "work" for the animal is usually not as bad as forcing the issue and escalating the situation until the animal and possibly the technician are out of control.

Submissive Behavior

Dogs who show submissive behaviors (Figure 14-12) when threatened are not dangerous to handle. They are acquiescing, or "giving in." Technicians should reinforce submissive behaviors and also consider trying to appear less threatening.

Cats and other species of animals that do not live in structured social groups typically do not show submissive behaviors. When cats cannot avoid conflict, they typically become defensively threatening or aggressive (Figure 14-13). Cats may sometimes be fearful without being threatening (Figure 14-14).

Threatening Behavior

The goal of threats is to warn, not to harm or hurt. Many behaviors that are commonly referred to as "aggression" are more accurately categorized as threats. These include baring teeth, growling or hissing, lunging, barking, scratching, and attempts to bite or inhibited bites. Animals who "air-snap" or bite without injury are being threatening. It's generally not true that a technician can avoid a bite by being quicker than the animal. Rather it's usually the case that the animal was never intent on biting, only on threatening. Threats can be either offensive or defensive. An offensive threat is accompanied by the body postures seen in Figures 14-15 and 14-16. Defensive dogs and cats are shown in Figures 14-13 and 14-17. Animals are much more likely to be defensive in a veterinary context. This means they are both fearful and threatening. Defensive animals don't take the initiative to charge their opponents and won't bite if left alone. Offensive animals can lunge, charge, and chase their targets.

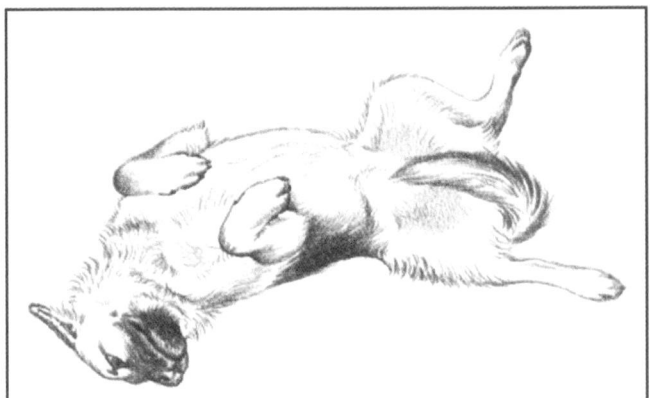

Figure 14-12 Submissive dog. Canine submissive postures and behaviors include rolling over or crouched body posture, avoidance of eye contact, low tail carriage, ears back, whining, and/or a submissive grin. (Used by permission from the ASPCA, New York.)

Aggressive Behavior

Aggressive behavior harms the opponent. Threats and aggression can overlap. An animal may initially respond to a threat by showing threatening body postures and may eventually bite or snap. While a bite attempt that never touches the opponent is clearly a threat, a bite that leaves a red mark, indentation, bruise, or other minor injury is in an area of transition between a threat and aggression. As with threats, most aggressive behavior that technicians will see in the veterinary context is likely motivated by a perceived need for self-defense. This is why it's so important for technicians to use the proactive, nonthreatening techniques to be discussed to prevent patients from becoming fearful and therefore defensive.

Using Puppy and Kitten Classes to Socialize Young Animals to the Veterinary Clinic

Puppy and kitten socialization classes, which have already been mentioned, are one way to help create positive expectations and associations with the veterinary clinic. These socialization classes can help young animals become familiar with the sights, sounds, and smells of the clinic under enjoyable conditions. During class, young animals can be put on the scales, an examination table, and subjected to brief handling procedures paired with treats and petting. This allows them to become somewhat familiar with staff and with the physical environment. When they come for their next appointment, they will be entering a familiar environment, expecting the same sorts of pleasant experiences they had during class, and will therefore be easier to handle.

When difficult-to-handle adult animals are identified, technicians can suggest that veterinarians encourage socialization visits. Owners are asked to bring the patient

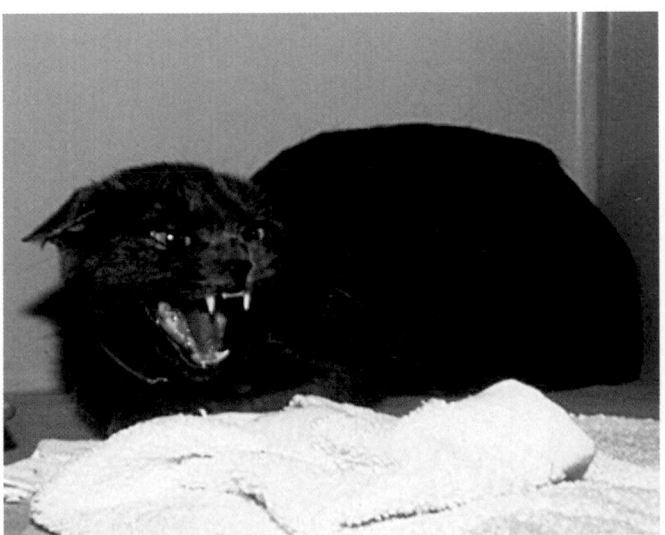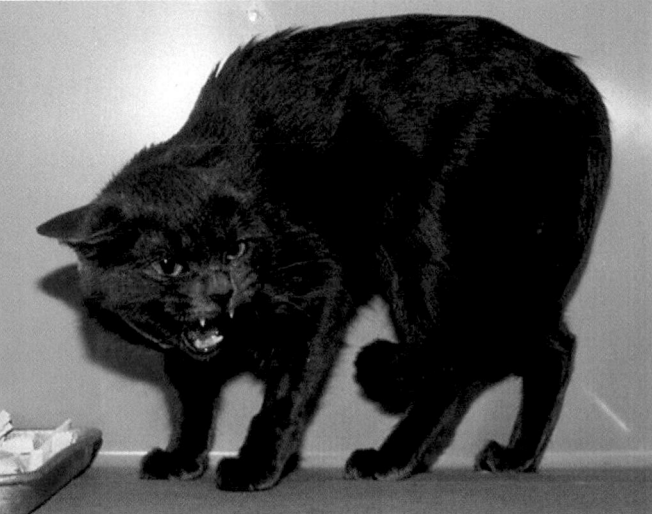

Figure 14-13 Defensively threatening cats. Feline defensive postures and behaviors include hissing, ears back or flattened to the side, baring teeth with an open mouth, rolling over or upright posture with arched back, tucked tail.

in for a brief visit during which only "good things" happen. Perhaps the animal is petted, given a tidbit, and placed on the scale. With each succeeding socialization visit, staff handles the animal a bit more and creates situations the animal might experience during an examination.

Using Behavior Assessments

Technicians should be aware of the results of patients' behavior assessments (Boxes 14-12 through 14-15) before handling them. By being forewarned about what a pet doesn't like done, how the pet reacts to everyday handling, and whether the pet has shown aggressive or threatening behavior under certain circumstances, the technician can be better equipped to prevent the patient from becoming fearful and stressed.

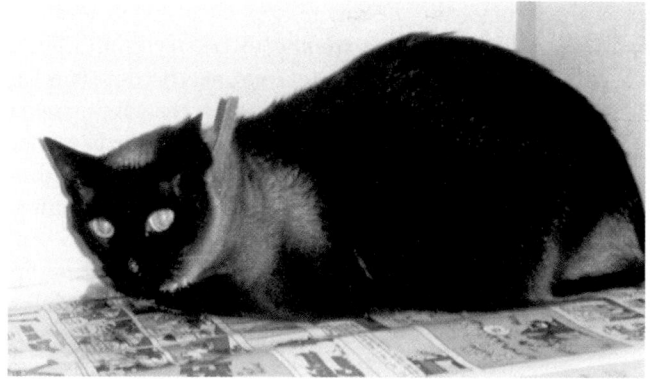

Figure 14-14 Fearful cat. Feline fearful postures include crouched body carriage, tail and feet tucked under body, and dilated pupils.

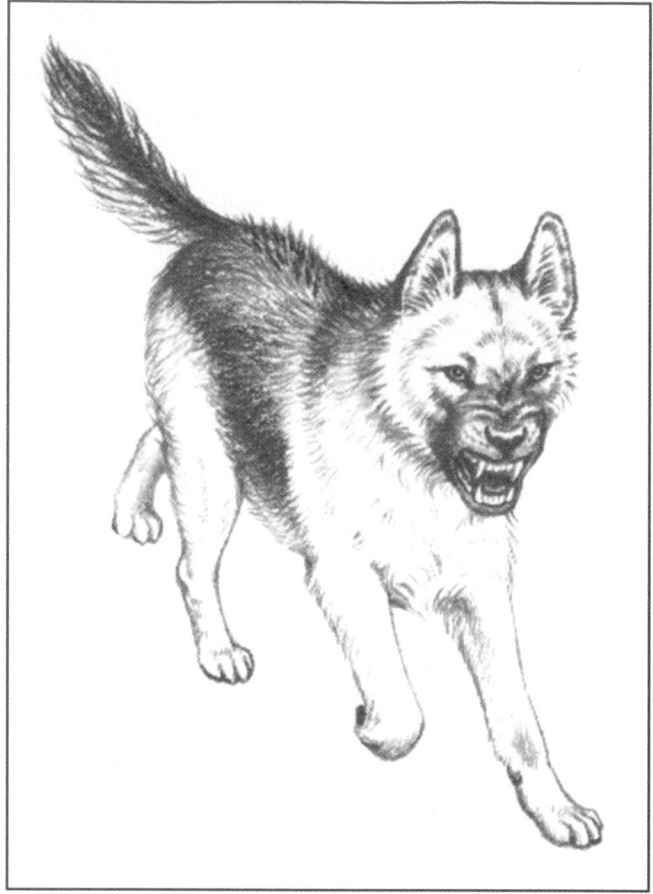

Figure 14-15 Offensively threatening dog. Canine offensive threats include upright ears, tail carried high, direct stare, piloerection, baring teeth with vertical lip retraction, stiff upright body carriage, and barking or growling. (Used by permission from the ASPCA, New York.)

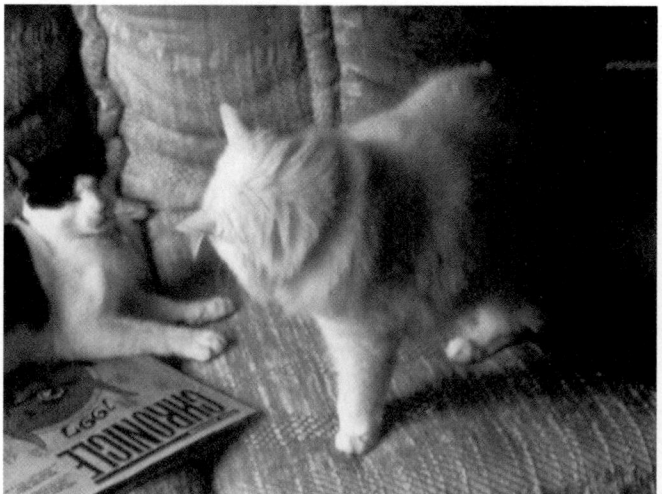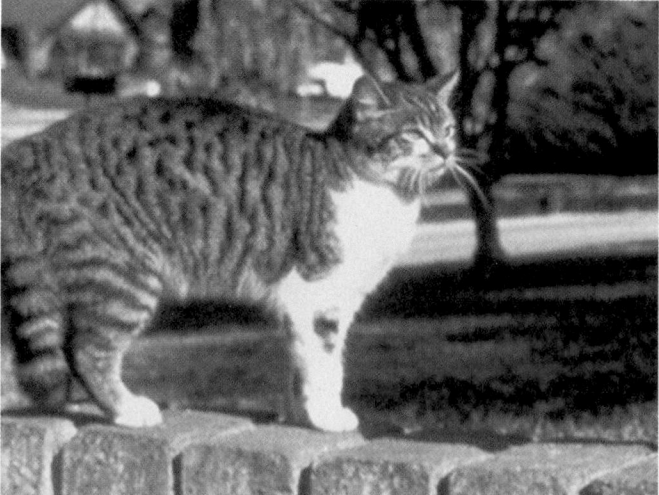

Figure 14-16 Offensively threatening cats. Feline offensive threats include a stiff upright posture, direct stare, ears upright, piloerection, tail stiff and held straight down. The tabby cat on the right has a slight arch to its back, indicating a small defensive component to its behavior.

Establish a Positive Expectation in the Waiting Area

The emotional reactions patients have in the waiting or reception area will affect their arousal level when they are examined. If experiences in the waiting area increase patients' arousal, patients will be more difficult to handle. Such experiences, particularly with cats, are common triggers for aggression later redirected toward technicians. Technicians can assess the waiting area from the patients' point of view. What do the animals see and hear when they first enter the door to the veterinary clinic? Do staff approach too quickly? Is a dog close enough to sniff and frighten a cat in a carrier or to lunge at another dog?

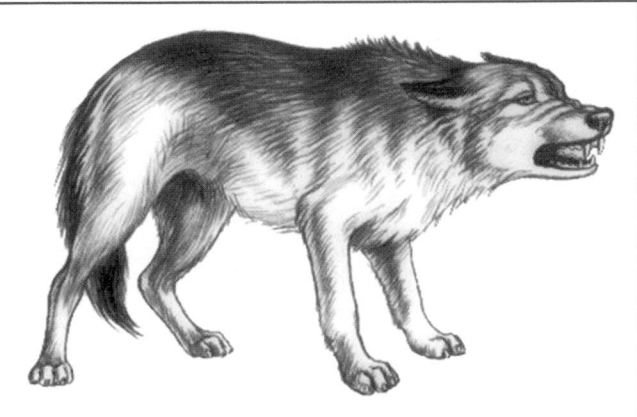

Figure 14-17 Defensively threatening dog. Canine defensive threats include avoidance of eye contact, crouched posture, ears back, tail down, teeth bared with horizontal retraction of the lips, barking or growling. (Used by permission from the ASPCA, New York.)

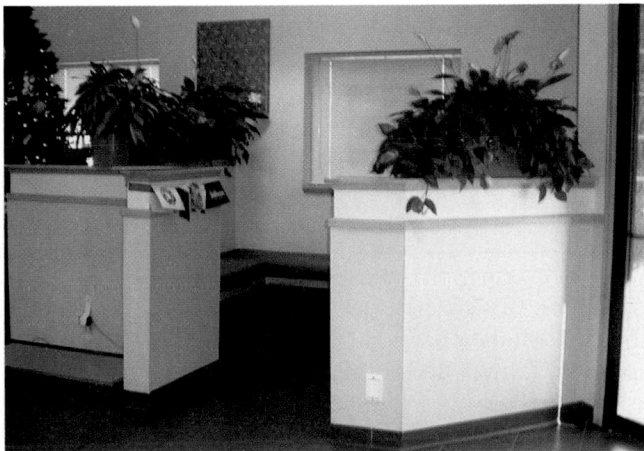

Figure 14-18 Cubicle in a veterinary clinic reception area. The cubicle creates social distance between patients, creates a barrier from the entrance, and helps to keep patients' arousal levels low.

Manage the Environment

Animals who are upset or overly excited should be moved out of the waiting area as quickly as possible. This not only helps to lower their arousal but also prevents them from agitating other patients. Technicians can move these animals into an examination room as soon as possible or even an office area if an exam room is not available. See-through cat carriers such as wire crates should be covered immediately so cats feel safer. If the clinic's location and weather permit, technicians can suggest that owners leave patients in the car until their appointment time or take dogs for a walk around the building or parking area.

Structural barriers such as half-walls (Figure 14-18), which create individual cubicles, are helpful additions to reception areas. Plants or other inanimate objects can be used to block patients' views of one another. Chairs can be arranged to create more space between patients and to minimize face-to-face encounters. Ideally, cats and dogs should have separate entrances, or at least be segregated into different sections of the waiting area.

Interactions With Staff: Greetings

Technicians must know how to approach patients in a nonthreatening way. The behaviors most people use to greet dogs are all, to the dog, offensive threats. These postures are listed in the left-hand column of Table 14-1 and illustrated in Figure 14-19. Cats also tend to perceive these postures as threatening.

Technicians must develop the habit of using non-threatening behaviors when greeting patients. In general, these are the opposite of the behaviors described previously and are listed in the right-hand column of Table 14-1 and illustrated in Figure 14-20.

Rather than invading the animal's personal space, when possible, technicians can allow the pet to approach them

Table 14-1	POSTURES TO AVOID WHEN APPROACHING FEARFUL OR UNFAMILIAR DOGS
Postures to Avoid	**Appropriate Postures**
Direct eye contact	Look at the floor, off to the side, or above the dog's head
Frontal approach	Turn the side of the body toward the dog or approach at a slight angle rather than head on
Reaching toward or over the dog's head or neck	Allow the dog to approach, let the dog sniff a hand held at the side of the body, pet the dog from under the chin
Leaning forward, over the dog's body	Bend at the knees, or stand straight up

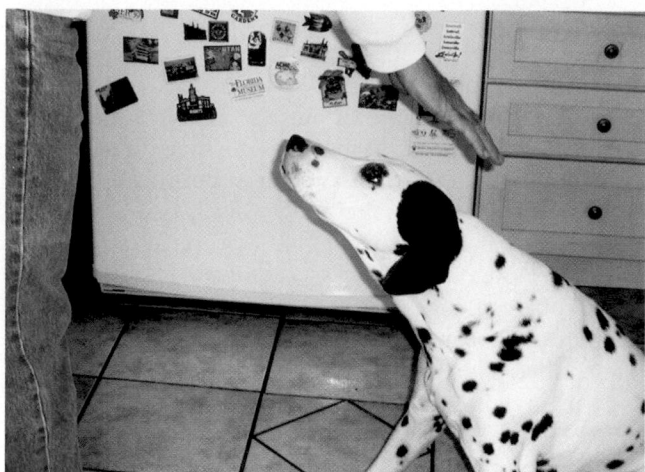

Figure 14-19 Threatening-appearing greeting. Person is reaching over dog's head, facing dog, and leaning over dog.

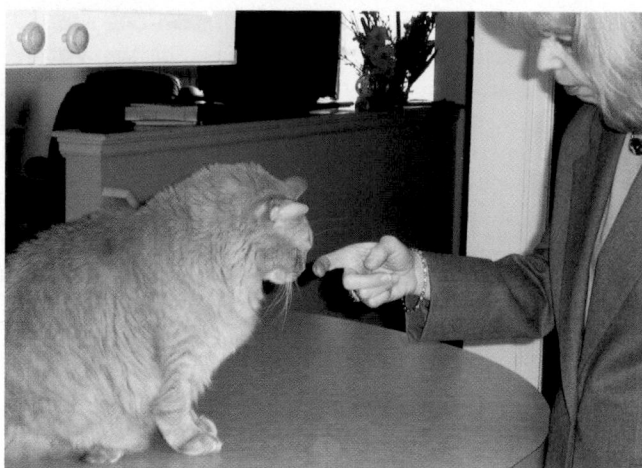

Figure 14-21 Friendly cat greeting person. Cat is sniffing the person's finger, similar to how it would sniff the nose of another cat.

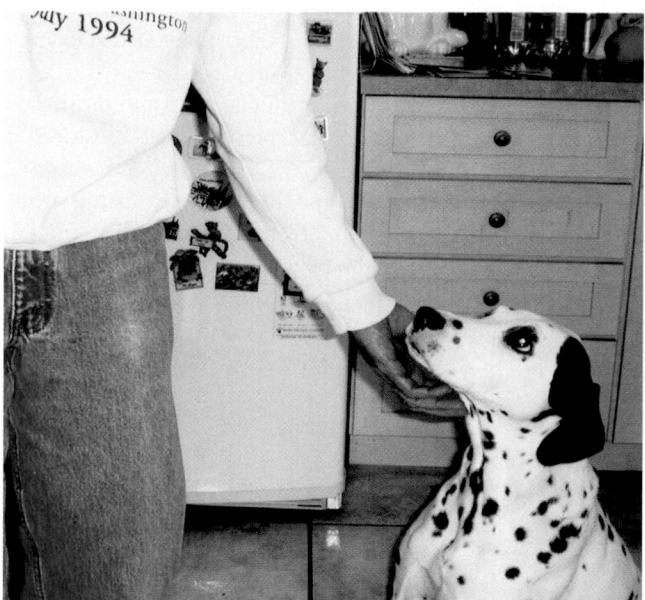

Figure 14-20 Nonthreatening greeting. Person has turned side of body toward dog, is not bending at the waist, and is petting dog under chin.

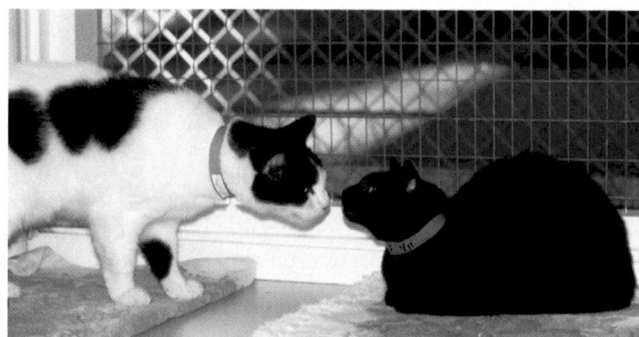

Figure 14-22 Friendly cat-to-cat greeting by sniffing noses.

the head, particularly by an unfamiliar person. Instead, technicians can rub cats on their scent glands located on their cheeks and in front of their ears (Figure 14-23).

TECHNICIAN NOTE
Most cats do not like to be stroked and patted in the same way dogs do.

Because cats are extremely sensitive to odors, technicians should wash their hands before greeting a cat, and consider spraying Feliway (Abbott Laboratories) on their hands as well. Feliway is a synthetic analog of the cat's facial pheromones and is said to have a calming effect on cats when they are in unfamiliar surroundings. Feliway can also be sprayed on an examination table or in a holding cage before the cat is placed in it. (This product has received mixed reviews and may work best to *prevent* the cat from becoming aroused, rather than to calm it once aroused.)

rather than vice versa. These nonthreatening behaviors make an immediate, significant, observable difference in patients' behaviors.

Before petting a cat, the technician should first allow the cat to sniff either a finger or an inanimate object such as a pen (Figure 14-21). This mimics a typical friendly cat-to-cat greeting of sniffing noses (Figure 14-22). Many cats do not liked to be stroked down their backs or patted on

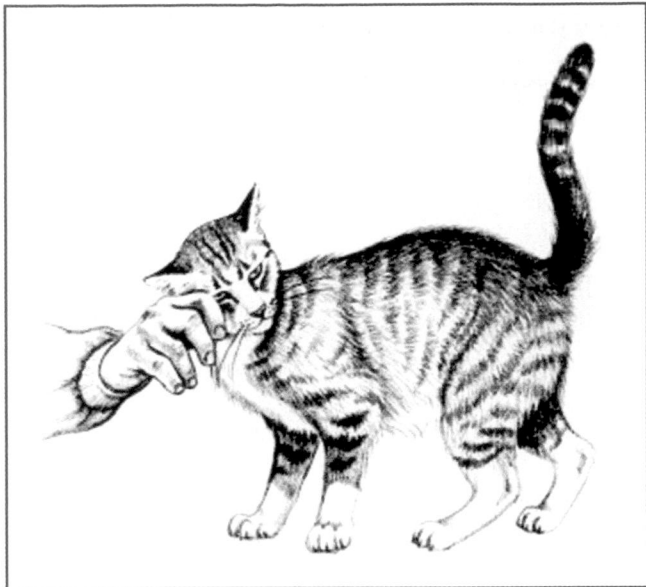

Figure 14-23 Recommended way to pet an unfamiliar cat. (Used by permission from the ASPCA, New York.)

Interactions With Staff: Use of Treats

Fearful or Threatening Animals

When patients are highly aroused and are displaying fearful, threatening, or aggressive behavior, technicians should try to decrease their emotional arousal. This may require more than just assuming the nonthreatening postures described previously. Technicians should also try offering the animal something that will elicit a more relaxed, friendly, or happy emotional reaction. For many animals, this means food or toys. Technicians and other staff members can offer patients small, highly palatable tidbits (assuming this will not interfere with the reason for the visit) from an open palm, not feeding from the fingers, while assuming other nonthreatening postures illustrated in Figure 14-20. An animal who refuses tidbits is likely very stressed or anxious. This reaction should be noted and shared with other staff who will be handling the patient.

If the animal attempts to avoid the technician (backs away, attempts to hide), displays fearful body postures (Figures 14-14 and 14-24), or displays threatening behaviors (Figures 14-13 and 14-15 to 14-17), the treat or toy should be dropped near the animal or into the carrier, with no other attempts at interaction. When time allows, multiple repetitions from the same person and from more than one staff member will help the animal generalize a more positive reaction before being examined.

Technicians need not worry that giving a treat to an animal that is fearful or threatening will reward these behaviors. Such behaviors are motivated by emotional arousal. Treats and toys serve to improve the animal's emotional reaction through classical conditioning. To better understand this phenomenon, refer to Box 14-16.

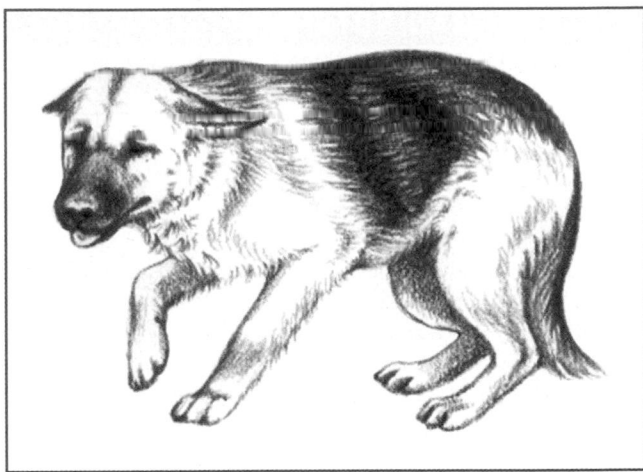

Figure 14-24 Fearful dog. Canine fearful postures overlap with submissive postures and can also include shaking, urination or defecation, shedding, panting, and dilated pupils.

Box 14-16 HOW CLASSICAL CONDITIONING WORKS TO CHANGE EMOTIONAL STATES

Emotions are not very amenable to reinforcements and punishments (operant conditioning). Thus reassuring a fearful animal does not make it more fearful (reward the fear). Consider the following example:

- Being cut off in traffic by another driver triggers an angry reaction.
- Whenever this occurs, your passenger gives you $10.
- After many repetitions, you are likely to be less angry about being cut off and may even look forward to the event, anticipating another $10.
- The $10 has made you less angry, not more.

Pairing the $10 (a pleasant event) with being cut off by another driver (an unpleasant event) is classical counterconditioning. In classical conditioning, an animal learns the association between two events, a phenomenon first illustrated by Ivan Pavlov.

Unruly Dogs

For unruly dogs, a more assertive approach can be used (facing the dog, making eye contact), and the dog can be required to sit, go down, or perform any trick it knows (e.g., shake hands) before receiving the tidbit. The tidbit can be used to lure the dog into a sit or down position if necessary. Any undesirable behavior (jumping up, barking) should be ignored (no verbal correction, turning away from the dog, moving out of its reach, breaking eye contact). Attempting to push the dog away or touching her to "help" her into the desired position (sit, down) will usually be counterproductive and can even be dangerous. If the dog jumps up, it is *never* appropriate to step on the dog's feet, squeeze the paws, or knee her in the chest.

✎ TECHNICIAN NOTE

Fearful or aggressive animals tend to respond better if they are allowed to approach a person, rather than the other way around.

Creating a Good First Impression in the Examination Room

Fearful and threatening patients respond better if they are allowed to approach a person, rather than the other way around. With dogs, the technician and/or the veterinarian should enter the examination room first, so the dog is coming into their space rather than vice versa. If the technician has already placed a problem dog in the examination room, one strategy might be for the technician to take the dog out of the room to the scale to be weighed. While the dog is gone, the veterinarian can enter the room and sit down. Fearful dogs may tolerate handling better if they are examined on the floor rather than the table. Both dogs and cats may be more comfortable on a nonslip surface, so technicians can place a rug or mat on either the floor or the examination table to provide better traction.

✎ TECHNICIAN NOTE

If the dog is intimidated and frightened by being on the examination table, the technician can try conducting the procedure on the floor.

Keeping Cats Calm

Before the cat and owner are brought to the examination room, Feliway can be applied to the examination table. Before attempting to take the cat out of the carrier, the technician should assess the cat's arousal level. What does the cat do if the carrier is moved, if the cat is touched with a pen or other harmless object (not a finger!) through the wires or air holes of the carrier? Is the cat vocalizing? Does the cat appear relaxed, friendly, fearful, or defensive, based on the illustrations of cat body postures in this chapter?

If the cat is significantly stressed or aroused, when possible, it may be better to delay handling and examinations until the cat is calmer. The carrier, with its door left open, can be put directly in a holding cage with a towel draped across the cage door, creating a quiet, dark hiding place for the cat.

Removing Cats From Carriers

If the cat resists coming out of the carrier, rather than reaching in and pulling her out, the technician can either take the top off the plastic carrier or tilt the carrier so that the cat slides out. Once the cat is on the examination table, the technician can greet the cat, using the procedures previously described.

Observe Body Postures Carefully

In addition to offensive and defensive postures, technicians should look for warning signs listed in Boxes 14-17 and

---

Box 14-17 WARNING SIGNS STRESSED CATS MAY DISPLAY

- Twitching, swishing tail
- Head turns; intention movements
- Rapid change of ear carriage
- Freezing
- Tense body
- Paws, tail tucked in
- Hiding
- Dilated pupils

Box 14-18 WARNING SIGNS STRESSED DOGS MAY DISPLAY

- Displacement (irrelevant) behaviors, such as frequent yawning, licking of the lips, grooming, or sleeping
- Ambivalent behaviors—alternating between different motivational states, such as fear and friendliness or submission and defensive threat
- Redirected behaviors—behaviors directed at other animals or people not directly involved with the animal; redirected aggression is particularly dangerous for others in the area if a dog is aggressively motivated but cannot get to the original target

---

For additional information on observing and interpreting canine and feline body postures, the videotape *Canine behavior: body postures,* available from ACT Programs, 918 N. Elm, Denton, TX 76201, 800-357-3182, is an excellent resource.

14-18, which include displacement behaviors. Displacement behaviors (yawning, grooming, lip licking) are conflict behaviors. They are normal behaviors but are displaced out of their expected context and indicate that an animal is stressed and unsure about how to respond.

A lack of friendly behaviors is also of concern. This pattern easily goes unnoticed, or the significance of their absence is not realized. Technicians should be cautious of animals that stare or watch them closely without any other behavioral responses (e.g., no tail wags, no avoidance responses, no fearful or threatening behavior). Before approaching or handling a dog in the examination room, technicians should ignore the dog, observe the dog's body postures and how he reacts to movements (e.g., shifting positions on the chair, reaching for something, standing up). These observations allow technicians to assess the dog's social behavior and emotional state before attempting any interaction. Technicians should avoid walking directly toward the owner and/or the dog.

Take a Preventive (Proactive) Approach Rather Than a Reactive One

Because initial friendliness is not always predictive of how an animal is going to react to restraint and handling,

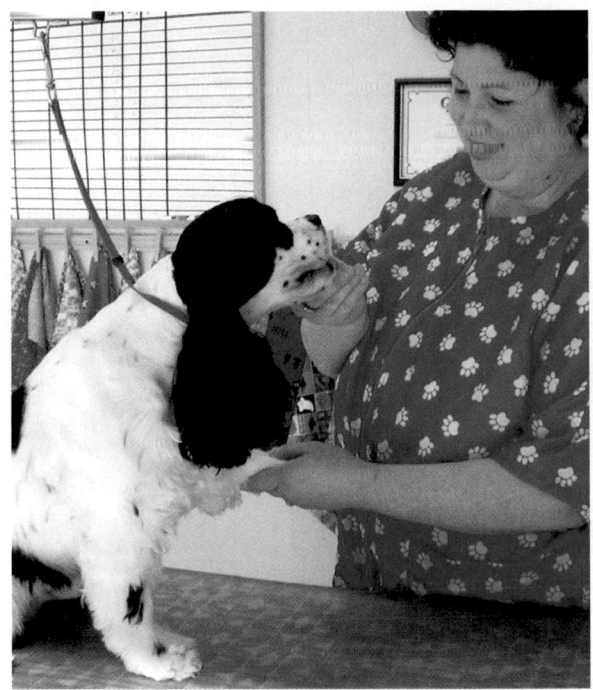

Figure 14-25 Pairing touching and holding paw with a treat for the dog. (Used by permission from the ASPCA, New York.)

the technician should not assume an animal will be tolerant and should not move too quickly when initiating handling procedures. Erring on the side of caution is better than being bitten. To continue to help animals maintain relaxed, friendly attitudes about the upcoming examination, the technician can offer a tidbit with one hand (Figure 14-25) while doing one of the following:

- Touching the pet's collar
- Touching or reaching toward the pet's feet
- Touching an ear
- Running a hand down the patient's back

Pairing the touch of potentially sensitive areas with something positive for the patient can help decrease fear or anxiety. Although it could be argued that this requires additional staff time, it may require less time for one technician to conduct these proactive handling exercises than the three or more staff members who might be required to restrain patients that become unmanageable.

Create a Protocol for Handling Exercises To Be Practiced at Home

For patients who, from past experience, are known to be threatening, aggressive, or generally difficult to handle, technicians can give clients a step-by step plan to accustom their animals to basic handling procedures. Initial steps in this process would be similar those listed in the previous section. As the pet begins to become more comfortable, owners can gradually do more—hold a paw rather than

just touching it, squeeze the foot, and so on, while pairing these procedures with something the pet enjoys.

Dealing With Threatening and Aggressive Animals

There are two issues in threatening situations: the technician's safety and well-being and the animal's safety and well-being. Good behavior skills should minimize the occurrence of those situations in which emergency restraint must be used for safety reasons.

When handling animals, it is best to assume an attitude of cautious calm (Hetts, 1999), as follows:

- Respect the animal and its ability to injure, without being overly fearful.
- Although a knowledge of breed *tendencies* is helpful, be careful that breed *biases* do not result in approaching or handling the animal in a manner that could be counterproductive.
- Have confidence in your ability to accurately observe, interpret, and react accordingly to the animal's body postures and other communication signals without being overconfident or feeling invincible.
- Know what can be done to avoid being bitten or getting in a confrontation with the animal.
- Know when to back off (or use proper restraint) if you do not think you can accurately interpret the animal's intentions or when you realize the animal will bite if you persist. If the situation permits (e.g., if the procedure does not need to be performed immediately), it may be most helpful to put the animal in a cage, cover the front with a towel, and allow the pet to calm down.
- Avoid taking the animal's behavior personally and becoming angry, frustrated, and impatient. Another technician or staff member may be better able to handle the pet. Certain animals and certain people have personality conflicts, just as people do.

The minimal amount of physical restraint necessary for the technician's safety is the maximum that should be used. For example, if a dog or cat tries to bite, it is usually appropriate to stop and muzzle it rather than increasing the level of physical restraint. Additional information on animal restraint can be found in Chapter 1.

The goal of restraint and force is to keep personnel safe while they are performing necessary procedures. It is *not* to "teach the animal a lesson" or "show him who's boss." The technician should keep in mind that using physical force may allow one to do what needs to be done at the time, but the price may be creating an animal who becomes increasingly difficult or even impossible to handle during future visits. This may happen after only *one* bad experience. If the owner is present, it may also cost the practice a client.

The recent case of a veterinarian who was charged (and later acquitted on appeal) with cruelty to animals for hitting a dog in the face when it tried to bite him has made it

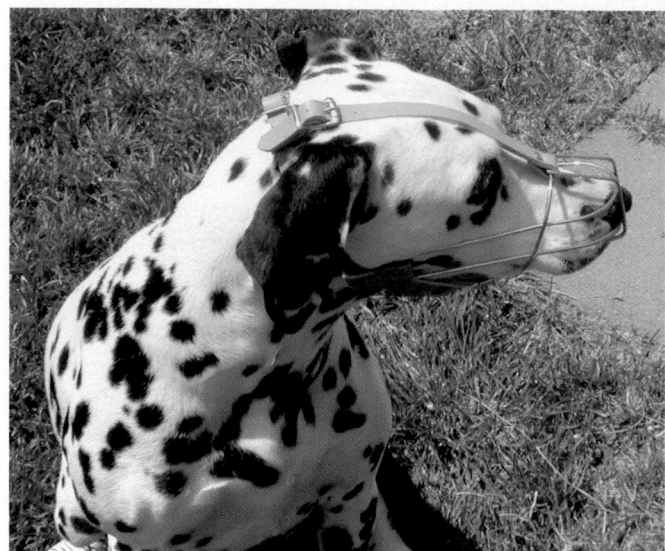
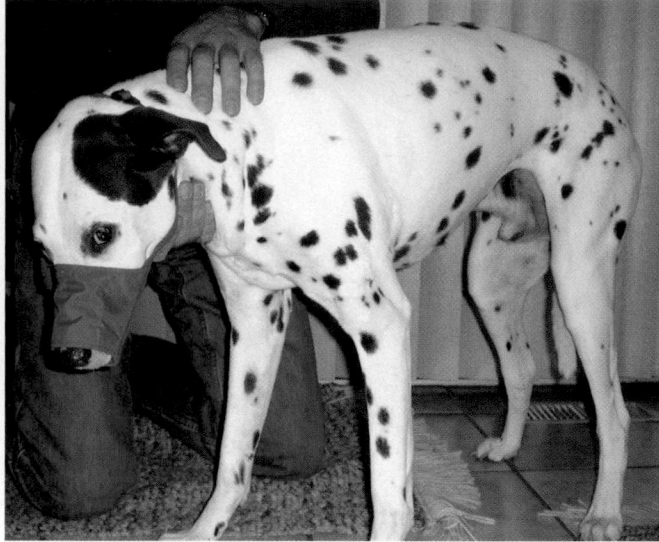

Figure 14-26 Dogs wearing wire basket (**A**) and nylon sleeve (**B**) muzzles.

clear that the issue of animal handling and restraint is an important one, not only to the veterinary profession but to the public as well (Nolen, 2000). Rather than increasing the level of interactive, social restraint, technicians may want to use appropriate equipment that can be less intimidating to the animal and safer for technicians and other staff. Examples of such equipment are described in the following sections.

Muzzles

Rather than struggling to control a pet with increased force because of concern that the animal might bite, a muzzle can be applied (Figure 14-26). With a muzzle on the animal, the technician will be less concerned with the need for tight restraint, and the animal may calm down if it is less tightly restrained. Technicians can also educate owners on how to accustom their pets to tolerate a muzzle for short periods. The practice can consider selling muzzles to ensure client compliance. With this proactive approach, owners can muzzle their animals immediately before entering the veterinary hospital.

Gentle Leaders

Some dogs are intimidated when wearing a Gentle Leader (Premier Pet Products). This has been referred to as a calming effect, but a better term is probably behavioral suppression. Other dogs, however, become somewhat panicked when the Gentle Leader is first put on and try frantically to remove it. Technicians should encourage owners to use a Gentle Leader as standard practice, in place of choke chains or pinch collars. This recommendation can be made during puppy class or the dog's first wellness examination. When dogs are accustomed to the Gentle Leader (Figure 14-27), technicians can easily use it to have greater control of dogs in the clinic.

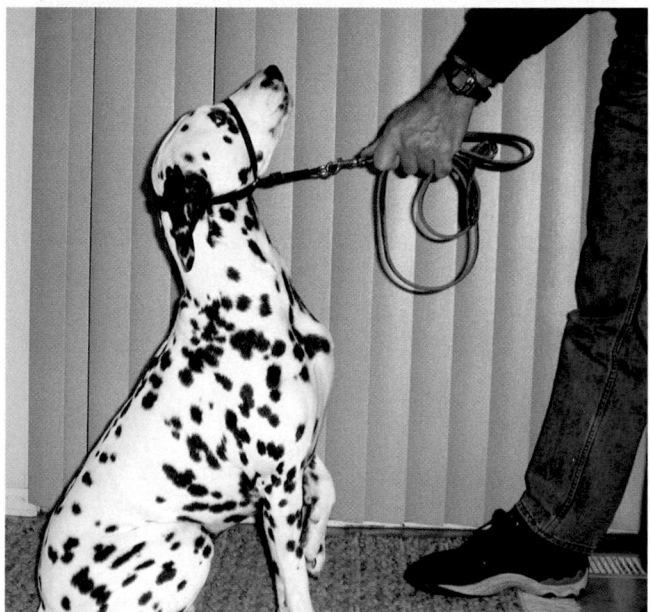

Figure 14-27 Control of the head with a Gentle Leader (Premier Pet Products, Inc).

Cat Bags

When possible, fractious cats should first be given a chance to calm down, as explained earlier. If the aggressive cat is still in a carrier, another option is to put the opening of the carrier directly into a large canvas cat bag. Some cats will crawl into the bag because it appears to be a darker, safer hiding place than the carrier. The cat can then be handled through the zippered opening of the bag. Some cat bags with frames (Figure 14-28) allow the cat to be put into the bag directly from a standard cage.

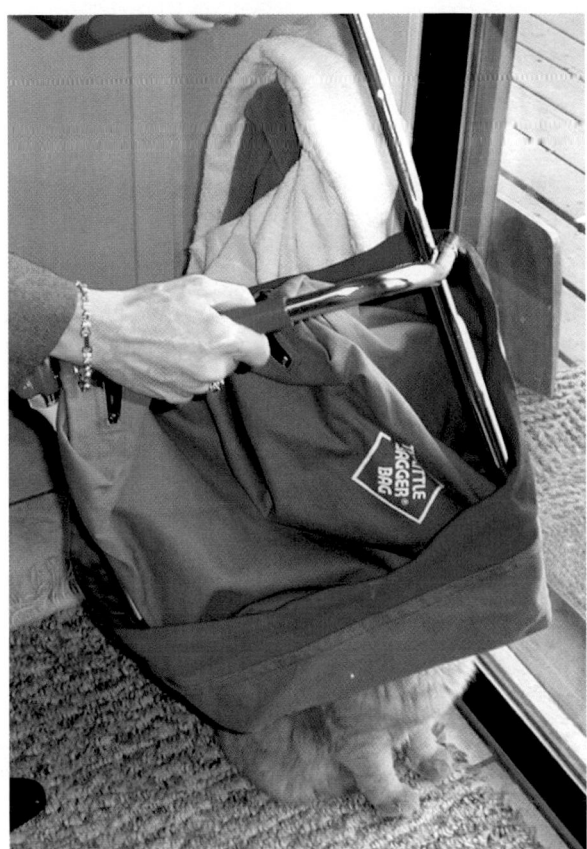

Figure 14-28 Cat Bagger (available from ACES, Inc) with frame being held over a cat.

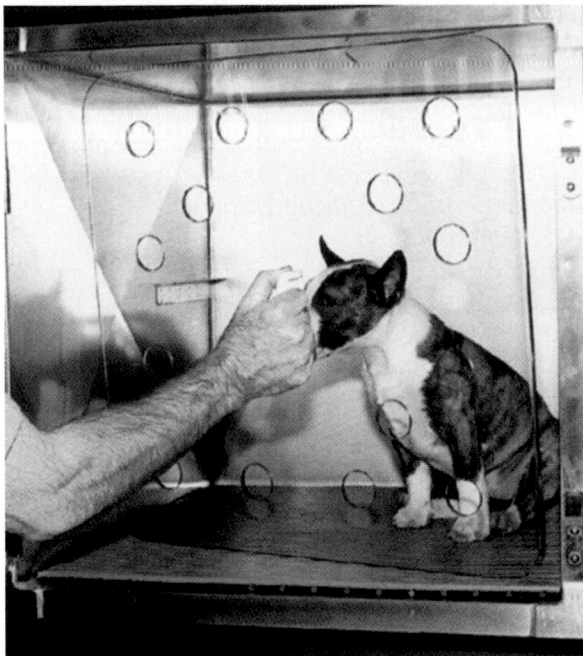

Figure 14-29 Plexiglas shield (available from ACES, Inc.) being used to push a dog to the back of the cage. Injections can be given through holes in the shield.

Plexiglas Shield

If the cat is in the larger cage, a Plexiglas shield (Figure 14-29) can be used to push and hold the cat to the rear of the cage if an injection is the only or first treatment that needs to be administered. This avoids having to handle the fractious cat at all until it is medicated. (Bag and shield are available from ACES, 800-338-ACES; Crestline, Calif.)

Towels

One of the best and easiest tools to use when handling cats is simply a large, thick towel (Figure 14-30). Holding the towel high, to partially block the cat's view of the technician's face, makes the technician appear less threatening.

PROBLEM RESOLUTION COMPONENT

Problem resolution is not something to be taken lightly or attempted with an off-hand, "try this, try that" approach. Behavioral problems should be approached in a systematic way: analysis of the behavior, creation of a behavior modification plan, and follow-up. Attempting to intervene with a behavioral problem without knowing the cause or motivation for the behavior can be just as disastrous as attempting to treat a medical condition without a diagnosis. For example, surgery would not be considered for a limping

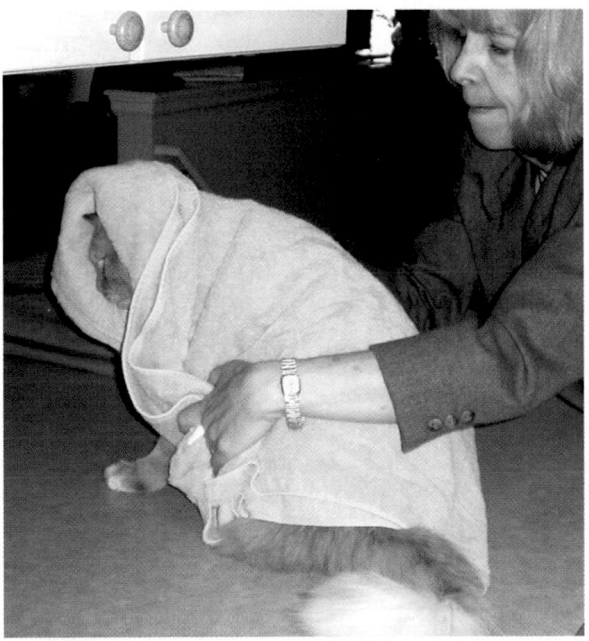

Figure 14-30 Using a towel to handle a cat.

dog until it was determined why the dog was limping; similarly, an antibark collar should not be recommended for a barking dog until the reason for the barking has been determined.

Technicians should always look to the veterinarian for guidelines regarding their role in providing problem resolution information to clients. Owners often ask technicians questions about their pets' behavior even before they ask the veterinarian. Both veterinary technicians and veterinarians should be aware of the disadvantages to jumping into problem solving without adequate preparation.

Dangers of Problem Solving Without Adequate Preparation

Attempting to problem solve without being prepared is not helpful to the technician, the client, or the pet. Behavioral consulting requires knowledge about animal behavior and animal learning, having sufficient time to obtain a behavioral history and explain detailed recommendations to clients, and being available to follow up after the initial consultation. Attempting to problem solve without sufficient preparation can have the following unwanted consequences.

Owners' Frustration

Behavioral problems are frustrating, and many pet owners can quickly lose patience. If owners are investing their time to implement recommendations yet see no results, their frustration level may quickly increase. In one case an owner was advised to confine her cat in a large crate with litterbox, food, and water for 1 month to "retrain" the cat to use the litterbox. The cat, of course, used the box reliably while confined. On being released from confinement, the cat walked over to the other side of the room and urinated on the carpet. Both the owner and the cat were frustrated, and the cat was surrendered to an animal shelter. What makes cases like this sad is that most litterbox problems can be resolved with proper intervention.

Technicians' and Practice's Credibility

If clients discover from other sources that the information the veterinary technician provided was not accurate, appropriate, or helpful, they may lose faith in the technician and the veterinary practice. Consider this example. An owner's dog was barking excessively when left home alone. The owner was told to sneak back and throw a can of coins at the dog to reprimand the barking. When the problem was later diagnosed as separation anxiety and the owner told that this approach would probably exacerbate the problem and increase the dog's anxiety, she no longer trusted the veterinarian who gave her inappropriate information and took her dog to another practice instead.

Liability for Injuries

A technician who advises a pet owner to handle his or her pet in a certain way that elicits an aggressive response from the animal may be legally liable for injuries that result. In one case, an owner was advised to give her dog a scruff shake when it did not obey her commands. When her dog failed to get off the bed when told to, she grabbed the dog by the neck as instructed, and the dog promptly bit off her finger. The owner sued the trainer who had given this instruction, and the case was settled out of court in her favor.

Worsening Problems

A playful kitten was pouncing on its owner's ankles as he sat in a chair. He was told to grab the kitten by the scruff of the neck, throw her into a room by herself, and leave her there for several hours. The kitten did not learn to stop pouncing on the owner's ankles. Instead, she learned that whenever her owner reached for her, she needed to defend herself. She began to hiss, scratch, and bite whenever the owner tried to touch her. The problem had escalated from simple play-motivated aggression, which might well have resolved on its own, to a much more difficult, defensive-aggressive behavior problem.

Self-Assessment

As technicians work with the veterinarian to determine what their role in problem resolution will be, the self-assessment questions in Table 14-2 may help guide decisions. Can the technician correctly analyze the reason or motivation for the behavior by knowing what questions to ask in a thorough behavioral history? If the technician cannot answer yes to most of the questions in Table 14-2, then problem solving may not be an appropriate role at this time.

> **✎ TECHNICIAN NOTE**
>
> Typically, veterinarians want to evaluate the potential that medical causes might be contributing to the pet's behavioral problem before making a referral.

Referring Behavior Cases

When to Refer

Technicians are often put in the role of referring clients to behavioral consultants or dog trainers without sufficient direction from the veterinarian. Veterinarians and technicians should work together to develop guidelines for when it is appropriate for a technician to make the referral. Technicians should not take it upon themselves to make the referral without these guidelines. For example, owners often call the veterinary practice for advice when a cat is urinating outside the litterbox, a dog has bitten a neighborhood child, or a dog is lifting his leg on the furniture. It should be the veterinarian's decision as to whether the pet should be seen at the clinic before the owner is referred for a behavioral consultation, either in-house or to an outside consultant. Typically, veterinarians want to evaluate the potential that medical causes might be contributing to the pet's behavioral problem before making a referral. Many behavioral consultants will not accept a referral until this has been done.

Type of Referral

For dogs, the first decision that needs to be made is whether the referral should be for behavioral consulting or for obedience training. Obedience classes are helpful when dogs are unruly and not responsive to verbal directions from

Table 14-2 SELF-ASSESSMENT BEFORE PROBLEM SOLVING

Question	Case Example
Can I take a behavioral history about this problem? Do I know what questions to ask to determine the type of problem that is causing the behavioral symptom?	Excessive barking can be caused by separation anxiety and territorial behavior (among other things). Can I obtain a behavioral history that will distinguish between these two problems?
Will my recommendations for resolving the problem address the specific type of problem rather than merely treating the symptom? If not, is there a rationale that makes the symptomatic approach appropriate?	Constructing a higher fence to resolve an escaping problem is a symptomatic treatment. The reason for escaping is ignored. If the higher fence keeps the dog in the yard without additional problems, this may be sufficient. However, if the escaping is motivated by separation anxiety, other symptoms of the problem are likely to be seen. Can I determine when a symptomatic approach is appropriate and when it is not?
Am I familiar with a variety of possible problem resolution methods, only a few of which are based on aversive techniques?	One approach to destructive chewing is to give off-limits items an unpleasant taste. Am I familiar not only with other ways of discouraging unacceptable chewing but also with even more ways to *promote* acceptable chewing behavior?
Do I have the time to complete all the components of a behavior case that includes analysis (diagnosis), treatment (devising and explaining a plan), and following up?	Obtaining a history and explaining a treatment plan to an owner may require several hours, certainly more than 10 or 15 minutes. Follow-up contacts can occur over several months. Can I realistically expect to have sufficient time to handle the case properly?

From Hetts, S: *Pet behavior protocols: what to say, what to do, when to refer,* Lakewood, Colo, 1999, AAHA Press.

the owners. Jumping up, door dashing, pulling on the leash, and not coming when called are all examples of undesirable behaviors that can be improved through a good obedience class. Obedience classes, however, do not resolve problems such as separation anxiety, excessive barking, house soiling, destructive behavior, or aggression. These types of problems require behavioral consultations that include analysis and subsequent modification of the problem behavior. When the decision is made to refer a cat for a behavioral problem, obviously, the owner should be referred to a behavioral consultant knowledgeable and experienced in cat behavior.

Evaluating Behavioral Consultants and Dog Trainers

Technicians can be very helpful to the veterinary practice by assisting with the evaluation of behavioral consultants and dog trainers the practice may be considering for use as referral resources. Veterinarians know that clients' experiences with referrals, both good and bad, will reflect directly back on the veterinary practice. Because there is such great variation in the qualifications and methods of behavioral consultants and dog trainers, it is incumbent on the veterinary practice to evaluate the credentials and competency of the people to whom it refers clients. This can be a time-consuming process, but one that can benefit greatly from using the skills of trained technicians.

The technician who has been given the assignment of gathering information about individuals in the community who offer behavioral consulting services should know that anyone can use the professional titles of animal behaviorist, behavioral consultant, dog behaviorist, cat behaviorist,

and so on, regardless of background and training. There are also no restrictions against nonveterinarians using the title behavior specialist. Although there is a veterinary board specialty in behavior and the Animal Behavior Society professionally certifies academically trained behaviorists who meet its criteria, relatively few individuals are certified in this manner, and it is likely that one is not located near a particular veterinary practice. Because some certified consultants provide behavioral consultations by telephone, access to one is always an option, regardless of the location of the veterinary practice. In addition, many people with a wide variety of backgrounds who are not certified offer behavioral consulting services. Obtaining information about the consultant's educational and experiential background and observing a consulting appointment are critical tasks the veterinary practice can assign to the technician before agreeing to refer its clients to a noncertified consultant. Veterinarians can then make informed decisions about which professionals are best qualified to provide consulting services to the practice's clients.

The Association of Pet Dog Trainers, through the Certification Council of Pet Dog Trainers, certifies trainers who have passed an examination and meet other criteria. The Association of Pet Dog Trainers promotes the use of dog-friendly training methods.

Technicians can be designated to observe several obedience classes and, ideally, participate in the class with a dog, before the veterinary practice agrees to refer clients to any given trainer. Box 14-19 provides recommendations for assessing behavior consultants and trainers. Websites

---

Box 14-19 GUIDELINES FOR EVALUATING A DOG TRAINER OR BEHAVIORAL CONSULTANT

FINDING AND WORKING WITH DOG TRAINERS

Look for trainers who rely on teaching methods that use positive reinforcement for the right response rather than punishing the wrong one.

Observe an obedience class without your dog. Are the dogs and people having a good time? Talk with a few participants, and see if they are comfortable with the trainer's methods. If someone will not let you sit in, do not enroll.

Do not allow trainers to work with your dog unless they tell you first exactly what they plan to do.

Do not be afraid to tell a trainer to stop if she or he is doing something to your dog you do not like.

If a trainer tells you to do something that you do not feel good about, do not do it! Do not be intimidated, bullied, or shamed into doing something that you believe is not in your dog's best interest.

Avoid trainers who offer guarantees about results. They are either ignoring or do not understand the complexity of animal behavior.

Avoid trainers who object to using food as a training reward. Food is an acceptable positive reinforcement training tool.

Avoid trainers who use *only* choke chains. Head collars are humane alternatives to choke chains and pinch collars.

Look for trainers who treat both people and dogs with respect, rather than an "I'm the boss" attitude.

FINDING AND WORKING WITH BEHAVIORAL CONSULTANTS

Look for academic training in the science of animal behavior, as well as hands-on experience.

Certification by a professional organization tells you the individual has met the requirements for education, experience, and professional ethics.

Look for people who recognize the importance of *you* working through the problem with your pet rather than sending it somewhere to be "fixed."

Membership in a professional organization suggests communication with colleagues and a means to keep current on new information.

Ask for professional references, such as former clients, colleagues, or veterinarians who refer cases.

A knowledge of positive reinforcement methods, behavior modification techniques such as counterconditioning and desensitization, how to use food rewards appropriately, and humane products such as head collars is a must.

Look for people who treat you with respect and are not abrupt and abrasive.

Avoid people who guarantee problem resolution. Animals are complex, and no one knows everything there is to know about them.

Avoid quick fixes. This approach does not do justice to you, your pet, or the problem.

---

of the various certifying bodies are listed in Box 14-3. Professional standards for dog trainers can be obtained from the Delta Society (see Box 14-3).

How to Make the Referral

If technicians will be making the referral to a dog trainer or behavioral consultant, such referrals must be conducted in a professional manner. A good guideline is to consider how a referral to a medical specialist is made. When a client is referred to a veterinary oncologist, technicians or veterinarians do not say "Try calling these people and see if they can give you a few tips for dealing with your pet's cancer." This sounds ludicrous, but in reality, this is similar to what many clients are told when they are referred to a behavior consultant. When a referral is made to a behavior consultant, clients should first be told what to expect from the referral. From previous evaluation of the consultant or trainer, the technician will know what kinds of services are offered and what fees are charged. Provide the client with this information rather than referring the client for "tips" or "advice." It frustrates the client and the behavioral consultant if the client expects a "25 words or less" solution free of charge. How the technician makes the referral will have a significant impact on clients' perceptions of behavioral consulting and how likely they will be to follow through with an appointment. If clients get the impression that this is a trivial referral, they are also unlikely to take it

seriously or believe that a behavioral consult can successfully help them change their pets' behavior. Similarly, clients will not take the importance of training classes seriously if the suggestion is made in an offhand manner, rather than emphasized as an important component of a behavior wellness program. A technician might say "Your pet needs to see a behavior consultant, because her problem requires more care than we can provide. Please call Dr. X at this number to set up an appointment. Dr. X will need to interview you at length and probably observe your pet as well. You can expect to pay between $A and $B for his services. We know Dr. X and we recommend him highly. I'll call you in a week to see when your behavior consultation is scheduled."

SUMMARY

This chapter has discussed the important role that technicians can play in making behavior wellness care an integral part of the practice of veterinary medicine. A focus on behavior wellness rather than on resolving complex behavioral problems makes sense for technicians and the veterinary practice. It also fills a need for pets and their owners that is too often going unmet. More effective promotion of how to create desirable behavior patterns and early detection of problems when they do occur have a great potential to keep pets out of animal shelters and prevent euthanasia for behavioral problems. Behavior wellness programs can be applied to any species of companion animal by inserting species typical behavioral information. It is hoped this chapter can motivate technicians to seek additional continuing education in animal behavior so they can make greater contributions to behavior wellness. Technicians interested in behavior should join the Society of Veterinary Behavior Technicians.

Recommended Readings and Literature Cited

Anderson RK, Line S, Jackson J: *Early learning for puppies—a program guide for humane societies and veterinary clinics,* Richmond, Va, 1999, Premier Pet Products.

Bateson P: How do sensitive periods arise and what are they for? *Anim Behav* 27: 470-486, 1979.

DiGiacomo N, Arluke A, Patronek G: Surrendering pets to shelters: the relinquisher's perspective, *Anthrozoos* 11:41, 1998.

Hetts S: *Pet behavior protocols: what to say, what to do, when to refer,* Lakewood, Colo, 1999, AAHA Press.

Hetts S, Estep DQ: *Canine behavior: I. Body postures II. The behaviorally healthy dog,* Denton, Texas, 1999, Animal Care Training, Inc (videotapes).

Hetts S, Heinke ML, Estep DQ: Behavior wellness concepts for general veterinary practice, *JAVMA,* 4:506-513, 2004.

Karsh EB, Turner DC: The human-cat relationship. In Turner DC, Bateson P, editors: *The domestic cat: the biology of its behaviour,* New York, 1988, Cambridge Univ Press, pp 159-177.

New JC et al: Moving: characteristics of dogs and cats and those relinquishing them to 12 US animal shelters, *JAAWS* 2:83, 1999.

Nolen RS: New Jersey veterinarian acquitted of cruelty conviction, *JAVMA* 216:1888, 1894, 2000.

Patronek GJ, Dodman NH: Attitudes, procedures, and delivery of behavior services by veterinarians in small animal practice, *JAVMA* 215:1606, 1999.

Patronek GJ et al: Risk factors for relinquishment of dogs to an animal shelter, *JAVMA* 209:572, 1996a.

Patronek GJ et al: Risk factors for relinquishment of cats to an animal shelter, *JAVMA* 209:582, 1996b.

Price G: President's message, *Newsletter for the Society of Veterinary Behavior Technicians* 9:1, 2001.

Salman MD et al: Human and animal factors related to the relinquishment of dogs and cats in 12 selected animal shelters in the United States, *JAAWS* 1:207, 1998.

Scarlett JM et al.: Reasons for relinquishment of companion animals in US animal shelters: selected health and personal issues, *JAAWS* 2:41, 1999.

Scott JP, Fuller JL: *Genetics and the social behavior of the dog,* Chicago, Ill, 1965, Univ Chicago Press.

Waring GH: *Horse behavior,* ed 2, Norwich, NY, 2003, Noyes Publications.

Wood F: Boost your passive income, *Vet Econ* 1997.

15

Companion Animal Clinical Nutrition

MARY TEFEND • SUSAN A. BERRYHILL

INTRODUCTION

Nutrition plays a critical role in the health of companion animals. The responsibility of the veterinary technician to educate clients about proper nutrition is therefore key in promoting the quality and longevity of a pet's life. Communication between the technician and client should include a discussion of the diverse nutritional needs of healthy companion animals and simple instructions regarding the frequency of feedings and the type and amount of food to offer. When appropriate, indications for therapeutic diets in clinically ill animals should also be discussed. Veterinary technicians who provide this level of nutrition counseling increase the quality of care provided to patients, help establish a valuable personal and professional bond with clients, and increase profitability for the practice.

Research in nutrition, particularly during the past decade, has greatly enhanced our understanding of what companion animals require in a balanced diet. Commercial diets are now formulated to help prevent nutritional deficiencies, boost the immune system, improve cognitive health, and help slow the aging process. Because obesity is now commonplace among pets, the veterinary technician should be prepared to discuss weight management regimens as well as other nutrition-based wellness programs.

Nutritional support is particularly important in times of illness and injury. The technician should be able to assist in assessing the hospitalized patient's body condition and daily energy requirements and help administer specialized feedings. Failure to recognize or address a patient's metabolic needs may have negative consequences and may adversely affect patient outcome. ■

OVERVIEW OF NUTRITIONAL OBJECTIVES AND PRINCIPLES

The goal of feeding companion animals is to maximize the length and quality of the animals' lives by reducing nutritional risk factors. For example, the veterinary professional will correlate diet with the life stage of the animal, so that an adult dog is fed an adult maintenance food and not a food formulated to meet the needs of a puppy. The nutritional goals for companion animals may therefore differ sharply from those for food animals, because the goal in meat production is to encourage rapid weight gain and not necessarily longevity.

Energy is essential for sustaining life in all animals. It is derived from components of food and food mixtures known as the diet. These energy-producing components include carbohydrates, fats, and protein. Water, vitamins, and minerals are also essential for life, because they are important in many biochemical reactions; however, they cannot be broken down to produce energy directly. The components of food that produce energy such as carbohydrates, fats, and protein and the components of food that do not produce energy such as water, vitamins, and minerals are all called nutrients. A nutrient can be defined as any substance that when ingested supports life (Figure 15-1). In addition, nutrients are divided into six categories: proteins, fats, carbohydrates (which are energy producing), water, vitamins, and minerals (which are not energy producing).

> ### TECHNICIAN NOTE
> Nutrients are divided into six categories: proteins, fats, carbohydrates (which are energy producing), water, vitamins, and minerals (which are not energy producing).

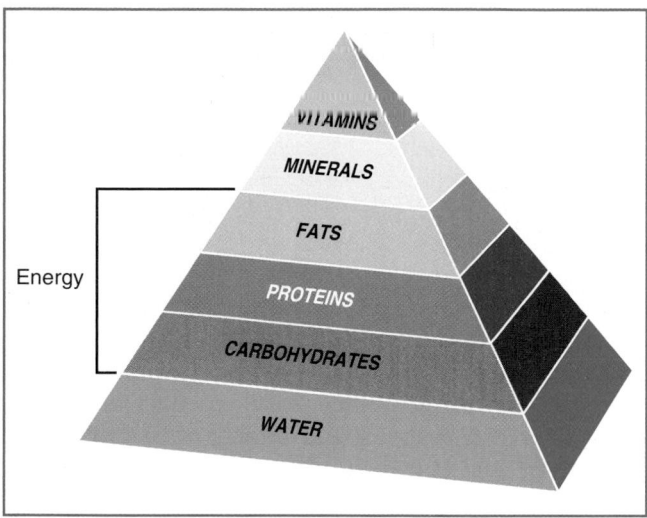

Figure 15-1 Six basic classes of nutrients are important for life sustenance. Carbohydrates, fats, and proteins may be used for energy but also serve as structural components.

Box 15-1 CARBOHYDRATES

SOLUBLE
Starches
Sugars

FIBER
Pectin
Lignin
Cellulose
Mucilage
Gum

ENERGY-PRODUCING NUTRIENTS

Carbohydrates can be further broken down into simple sugars, fats into triglycerides, and protein into amino acids. The digestion, assimilation, and metabolism of each of these nutrients produce chemical energy that is stored in the atomic bonds of "storage molecules" such as adenosine triphosphate. Storage molecules are portable and can be moved to any portion of the cell where energy is needed to complete an important job. In the case of adenosine triphosphate, the energy is stored in the bond that holds the last phosphate atom. When the phosphate atom breaks off, energy is released when the bond is broken. The energy can then be used to carry out a cellular process. Much of the energy that is gained from food is used to maintain and repair cell structures, such as the cell wall and the cytoskeleton. Animals that are growing, reproducing, exercising, or healing from an injury have a higher degree of cellular activity than animals that are not engaged in these activities. These animals therefore have higher energy (nutritional) demands. Heat production, muscle contraction, and the synthesis of new tissue are additional examples of cellular activity that requires energy.

As mentioned, carbohydrates provide the body with energy. Consumption of carbohydrates in excess of the body's immediate energy needs results in its storage as glycogen or conversion to fat. Carbohydrates include sugars, starches, and fibers.

Sugars are numerous and include simple sugars such as monosaccharides and disaccharides, or more complicated sugars. Multiple sugars can bond and link to form complex sugar polymers. Polymerized sugars include starch and fiber. Simple sugars and complex sugars are broken down

(catabolized) to provide energy, which is stored in the form of adenosine triphosphate. The type of polymer that is formed depends on the sugar template and the type of polymer bonds in the molecule. Glycogen is an animal-specific starch and can quickly depolymerize into units of glucose. Stores of glycogen therefore provide a rapid supply of glucose to tissues when sugar is in immediate demand. Most of the glycogen in the body is stored in the liver and in muscle tissue.

Insoluble fibers are referred to as complex carbohydrates such as cellulose and lignin, and they make up the structural elements of grass, plants, and wood. In the plant kingdom, starches and fibers are numerous and diverse (Box 15-1). Sources of starch include corn, wheat, rice, barley, oats, and potatoes.

Fiber differs from starch in that fiber is indigestible by the monogastric stomach and small intestine, which lack the enzymes needed to decompose them. However, fermentation of fiber does occur in the large intestine of some simple-stomached animals. The primary function of fiber in companion animals is to increase bulk and water content of the intestine. This effect finds applications in reducing caloric density for weight control foods while maintaining satiety. Some metabolic and gastrointestinal (GI) tract transit disorders also respond to increased levels of fiber in the food. For example, fiber is an important part of the diet for dogs with diabetes mellitus, because it helps to stabilize blood sugar levels by extending the time that nutrients are absorbed.

Fiber is digestible by bacteria and protozoan microbes in the rumen, cecum, and large intestine of grazing animals. Short-chain fatty acids result from fiber digestion, which in turn are transformed into glucose. Thus fiber serves as a major energy source for grazing animals.

The role of fiber in the diet is generally dependent on the physiology of the animal's digestive tract. In most species, fiber assists in regulating bowel function. In addition, the products of microbial fermentation (of fiber) play an important role in maintaining normal colonic function by decreasing pathogenic intestinal bacteria and may play a part in preventing intestinal cancer.

Box 15-2 ESSENTIAL FATTY ACIDS

CATS	DOGS
Linoleic	Linoleic
Alpha-linolenic	Alpha-linolenic
Arachidonic	

LIPIDS AND FATTY ACIDS

Lipids that are solid at room temperature are referred to as fats, whereas lipids that are liquid at room temperature are referred to as oils. Lipids are classified as dietary fats. Dietary fats are primarily made up of units called triglycerides, composed of three fatty acids held together by a molecule of glycerol. Fatty acids are the primary components of vegetable and animal fats.

The type of fatty acid primarily determines the structure and characteristic of fat. There are several families of fatty acids, named according to the position of the first double bond. Fatty acids with no double bonds in the primary hydrocarbon chain are referred to as saturated. Subsequently, a fatty acid with one double bond is called monosaturated, and a fatty acid with more than one double bond is called polysaturated.

The type and distribution of constituent fatty acids determine the physical, nutritional, and biologic characteristics of the fat and oil. Lipids have one to three molecules of fatty acids, are highly digestible, and have twice the caloric density of a similar quantity of carbohydrate or protein.

Fat also facilitates digestion. The length of the carbon chain backbone identifies a fatty acid as long-chain, medium-chain, or short-chain. Short-chain fatty acids (1 to 8 carbon atoms in length) from rumen fluids and gases are important sources of energy for grazing animals. Long-chain fatty acids (12 to 20+ carbon units) are the most common components of dietary fats and oils in companion animals.

The primary function of fat and fatty acids is multifold. They serve as principal sources of energy, provide palatability and texture to food, and most importantly, supply essential fatty acids and act as carriers for the fat-soluble vitamins (A, D, E, and K).

Essential fatty acids are polysaturated, long-chain fatty acids that are necessary for normal body function. Mammals cannot synthesize essential fatty acids; therefore fatty acids must be obtained from food. There are three known essential fatty acids: linoleic, α-linoleic, and arachidonic acids. Linoleic and α-linoleic acids are the parent compounds

from which more complex essential fatty acids are made (Box 15-2).

The essential fatty acids serve many important functions. They play integral roles in kidney and reproductive function, cell membrane formation, and prostaglandin production. Signs of deficiencies in essential fatty acids include alopecia, dull hair coat, anemia, and hepatic lipidosis.

Amino Acids and Protein

An amino acid is defined as any organic compound containing both an amino and a carboxyl group. Amino acids occur naturally in plant and animal tissue and are the chief constituents of protein. Proteins are long chains of amino acids held together by peptide bonds. There are roughly 22 known amino acid groups, but amino acids can be arranged in many different ways, with each arrangement having unique properties and characteristics. Amino acids are considered the building blocks of plant and animal protein.

Proteins are essential to all living cells. Functions include the regulation of metabolism, cell membrane construction, muscle fiber formation, and tissue growth and repair. Proteins also serve as enzymes, hormones, and antibodies.

Amino acids are classified as either essential or nonessential. Essential amino acids (Box 15-3) are substances that cannot be synthesized in the body in adequate quantities and therefore must be supplemented in the diet. Nonessential amino acids can be synthesized from other sources. Both are of equal importance in physiologic processes. Note that in the cat, taurine is an essential amino acid. Taurine deficiency in the cat results in retinal degeneration, reproductive insufficiency, and impaired immune function and has been linked to dilated cardiomyopathy.

The quantity and distribution of essential amino acids in a protein are important features determining a protein's biologic quality. All proteins are not of equal worth, and an

Box 15-3 ESSENTIAL AMINO ACIDS

- Arginine
- Hiotidino
- Isoleucine
- Leucine
- Lysine
- Methionine
- Phenylalanine
- Throonino
- Tryptophan
- Valine
- Taurine (essential in cats only)

ideal protein contains the essential amino acid distribution profile that exactly meets a specific requirement. In other words, the biologic value of a protein is determined by the extent to which it can be used for the growth and maintenance of normal body systems. Animal proteins generally have a higher biologic value than plant-based proteins.

Protein-containing ingredients are added to most commercial pet foods to supply the necessary amino acids. Protein digestibility and amino acid composition must be considered in any dietary analysis. Digestibility is an important consideration because the ease of digestion aids in absorption. Easily digestible proteins are of high nutritional value; consequently, smaller amounts are added to the diet to meet an animal's amino acid requirement. Thus, as protein quality is increased, the amount of protein needed decreases. The quality of the protein is often the limiting factor in the amount that must be fed to meet daily requirements.

An improper balance of amino acids can decrease protein quality. Even if digestibility is high, the correct balance of amino acids must be present to classify a protein as high in biologic value. Pet food companies will often mix animal and plant substances to provide multiple protein sources to improve the overall quality of the food by providing a wide amino acid profile. In addition, an individual amino acid may be added to the diet if the main protein source is limited to ensure a high biologic value. High-quality protein is especially needed during periods of growth, physical exertion, pregnancy, and lactation and for the repair of damaged tissues.

Amino acids are not stored in the body as fat and carbohydrates are. If the animal is unable to consume the required levels of amino acids (e.g., during starvation), breakdown of protein in the viscera and skeletal muscle will occur. The breakdown of skeletal muscle and visceral protein provides amino acids for energy. The breakdown of circulating and structural protein into glucose is called gluconeogenesis.

Muscle mass will decrease over time if nutritional needs are not met. Other signs of protein deficiency include weight loss, dull hair coat, anorexia, immunodeficiency, poor mentation, generalized edema, and death. Note that a deficiency of even a single essential amino acid can result in anorexia.

Cats are specifically adapted to high-protein, low-carbohydrate diets and depend on gluconeogenic amino acids as a major source of energy. Continuous protein catabolism limits the cat's ability to conserve protein, leading to higher requirements than those found in the dog. Dentition patterns of the cat further demonstrate carnivorous eating behaviors; cats have curved and tapered teeth suitable for tearing the flesh of their prey.

Dietary protein in excess of the body's requirement is converted to fat and stored as adipose tissue. Although the cat must consume twice as much as protein as the dog, feeding a food with proper levels of protein is essential. Metabolism of excess amino acids increases liver and kidney workload by increasing the processing and excretory requirements for the urea and organic acid waste by-products.

Protein Requirements

Clients often inquire about the best protein intake for animals. Crude protein quantity (on the label) is the usual concern, and clients assume that more is better. However, a high protein number is not always the defining criterion for food quality. Chemical analysis for crude protein measures only total nitrogen content. Unfortunately, the essential-to-nonessential amino acid profile, protein digestibility, and amino acid bioavailability may or may not be measured or stated on the label. It is best to contact the manufacturer directly to obtain this information. Lower quantities of a higher biologic quality protein usually represent a higher-quality food, and thus, a more appropriate nutritional objective.

> **✏ TECHNICIAN NOTE**
> The quality of the protein is often the limiting factor in the amount that must be fed to meet daily requirements.

NON–ENERGY-PRODUCING NUTRIENTS

WATER

Although water does not produce energy, it is considered the most important nutrient. Water is essential for almost every chemical reaction, such as the digestion (hydrolysis) of carbohydrates, proteins, and fats. Other functions of water in the body include transport of solutes and gases, temperature regulation, lubrication of joints and eyes, and electrolyte balance. Water is the largest and heaviest component of the body, making dehydration a common threat to sick patients unwilling or unable to eat and drink.

> **✏ TECHNICIAN NOTE**
> Minerals are inorganic chemicals that are an important part of a balanced diet. More than 18 mineral elements are believed to be essential for mammals.

MINERALS

Minerals are inorganic chemicals that are an important part of a balanced diet. More than 18 mineral elements are believed to be essential for mammals. Minerals are divided into two groups, macrominerals and microminerals. Macrominerals are required in relatively large amounts, whereas microminerals are required in very small amounts and are therefore also known as trace elements.

Macrominerals

Macrominerals include calcium, phosphorus, magnesium, sodium, potassium, chlorine, and sulfur (Table 15-1).

Calcium and phosphorous are constituents of bone and structural proteins. They sustain the structural rigidity of bones and teeth and participate as cofactors and catalysts in many biochemical reactions. Calcium is also a necessary ingredient in normal blood clotting, nerve transmission, and muscle function.

Phosphorus is also an important macromineral and is a major constituent of bone and muscle formation, energy production, and reproduction. Deficiencies impair growth and normal physiologic processes (Table 15-2). The ratio of calcium and phosphorus is of great clinical significance and should be maintained at 1:1. Imbalance of this ratio, such as an increase of phosphorus to calcium, can lead to serious bone malformation. However, nutritional excesses are far more common than deficiencies.

Calcium deficiency results in nutritional secondary hyperparathyroidism, in which there is increased bone resorption to restore circulating calcium levels. As a result, growing animals have skeletal deformities and lameness. Calcium deficiency frequently develops when inappropriate homemade foods are prepared for dogs, cats, and reptiles. Conversely, high levels of calcium and phosphorus are also harmful. Developmental skeletal diseases such as wobbler syndrome, hip dysplasia, and osteochondrosis are thought to be associated with high calcium/phosphorus ratios. Feeding vitamin-mineral supplements or dairy products and overfeeding a growth diet may create a nutritional excess of calcium, phosphorus, or both.

Concentrations of all macrominerals in the diet are of fundamental importance. Minerals circulate as cation (positive charge) or anion (negative charge) electrolytes and play important roles in the osmotic fluid balance, nerve conduction, muscle contraction, blood clotting, blood pH buffering, and numerous other physiologic processes (Table 15-2). Examples of macrominerals include potassium, sodium, chloride, and magnesium. Deficiencies of macrominerals are uncommon in animals fed a standard commercial diet but can occur in cases of anorexia, starvation, chronic diseases, and dietary insufficiency. Excess macromineral intake can result from feeding large amounts of supplements, such as bone meal, or a diet limited to meat. Owner supplementation leads to excess total intake when most commercial diets are already adequate in macrominerals. The technician most commonly encounters this situation among well-intentioned, but uninformed, purebred animal hobbyists.

Macrominerals are measured in the diet as a percentage (%), whereas microminerals are expressed in parts per million (ppm). When feeds are evaluated as potential sources of minerals, it is best to consider not only the amount of mineral contained in the food but also how much the mineral can be used by the animal. Mineral availability in the diet depends on solubility, metabolic interactions with other nutrient compounds, signalment of the animal, and the animal's ability to store the mineral. Animals consuming meat, for example, will consume much higher levels of minerals than animals consuming plant-derived food substances.

> **✏ TECHNICIAN NOTE**
>
> Minerals are divided into two groups: macrominerals and microminerals. Macrominerals are required in relatively large amounts, whereas microminerals are required in very small amounts and therefore are also known as trace elements.

Microminerals

Trace elements or microminerals are nutrients that are required in relatively small amounts but are nevertheless

---

Table 15-1 MINERAL CATEGORIES

Macrominerals*				Microminerals†	
Sodium and chloride	NaCl	Zinc	Zn	Copper	Cu
Potassium	K⁺	Selenium	Se	Iron	Fe
Phosphorus	P	Manganese	Mn	Boron	B
Magnesium	Mg²⁺	Iodine	I	Molybdenum	Mo
Calcium	Ca²⁺	Fluorine	F	Cobalt	Co
Sulfur	S	Chromium	Cr		

*Measured in %.
†Measured in ppm or mg/kg.

Table 15-2 MINERAL FUNCTIONS AND EFFECTS OF DEFICIENCY AND EXCESS

Mineral	Function	Deficiency	Excess
Calcium	Constituent of bone and teeth, blood clotting, muscle function, nerve transmission, membrane permeability	Decreased growth, decreased appetite, decreased bone mineralization, lameness, spontaneous fractures, loose teeth, tetany, convulsions, rickets (osteomalacia: adults)	Decreased feed efficiency and intake, nephrosis, lameness, enlarged costochondral junctions, adverse effect on bone and cartilage maturation
Phosphorus	Constituent of bone and teeth; muscle formation; fat, carbohydrates; and protein metabolism; phospholipid and energy production; reproduction	Decreased appetite, decreased feed efficiency, decreased growth, dull hair coat, decreased fertility, spontaneous fractures, rickets	Bone loss, urinary calculi, decreased weight gain, decreased feed intake, calcification of soft tissues, secondary hyperparathyroidism
Potassium	Muscle contraction, transmission of nerve impulses, acid-base imbalance, osmotic balance, enzyme cofactor (energy transfer)	Anorexia, decreased growth, lethargy, locomotive problems, hypokalemia, heart and kidney lesions, emaciation	Rare Paresis, bradycardia
Sodium chloride	Osmotic pressure, acid-base balance, transmission of nerve impulses, nutrient uptake, waste excretion, water metabolism	Inability to maintain water balance, decreased growth, anorexia, fatigue, exhaustion, hair loss	Occurs only if there is inadequate good-quality water available; causes thirst, pruritus, constipation, seizures, and death; chronic amounts may complicate hypertension
Magnesium	Component of bone, intercellular fluids, neuromuscular transmission, active component of several enzymes, carbohydrate and lipid metabolism	Muscular weakness, hyper-irritability, convulsions, anorexia, vomiting, decreased mineralization of bone, decreased body weight, calcification of aorta	Urinary calculi
Iron	Enzyme constituent: activation of O_2 (oxidases, oxygenases), O_2 transport (hemoglobin, myoglobin)	Anemia, rough hair coat, listlessness, decreased growth	Anorexia, weight loss, decreased serum albumin concentrations, hepatic dysfunction, hemosiderosis
Zinc	Constituent or activator of 200 known enzymes (nucleic acid metabolism, protein synthesis, carbohydrate metabolism), skin and wound healing, immune response, fetal development, growth rate	Anorexia, decreased growth, alopecia, parakeratosis, impaired reproduction, vomiting, hair depigmentation, conjunctivitis	Relatively nontoxic Reported cases of Zn toxicity from consumption of die cast Zn nuts or pennies
Copper	Component of several enzymes (oxidases), catalyst in hemoglobin formation, cardiac function, cellular respiration, connective tissue development, pigmentation, bone formation, myelin formation, immune function	Anemia, decreased growth, hair depigmentation, bone lesions, neuromuscular, enzootic ataxia, aortic rupture, reproductive failure	Hepatitis, increased liver enzyme activity
Manganese	Component and activation of enzymes (glycosyl transferases), lipid and carbohydrate metabolism, bone development (organic matrix), reproduction, cell membrane integrity (mitochondria)	Decreased growth (rare in dogs and cats), impaired reproduction	Relatively nontoxic
Selenium	Constituent of glutathione peroxidase and iodothyronine-5-deiodinase, immune function, reproduction	Muscular dystrophy, reproductive failure, decreased feed intake, subcutaneous edema, renal mineralization	Vomiting spasms, staggered gait, salivation, decreased appetite, dyspnea, "garlicky" breath, nail loss
Iodine	Constituent of thyroxine and triiodothyronine	Goiter, fetal resorption, rough hair coat, enlarged thyroid glands, alopecia, apathy, myxedema, lethargy	Similar to deficiency, decreased appetite, listlessness, rough hair coat, decreased immunity, decreased weight gain, goiter
Boron	Regulates parathyroid hormone, influences metabolism of Ca^{2+}, P, Mg^{2+}, and cholecalciferol	Decreased growth, decreased hematocrit, hemoglobin, and alkaline phosphate values	Similar to deficiency

From Hand MS et al, editors: *Small animal clinical nutrition*, ed 4, Topeka, 2000, Mark Morris Institute.
Ca, Calcium; *P*, phosphorus; *Mg*, magnesium; *Zn*, zinc.

essential for normal health in companion animals. Important microminerals include iron, manganese, copper, iodine, and selenium. Dietary requirements for these minerals are expressed in parts per million (or milligrams per kilogram of body weight) instead of the percentage amounts for macrominerals (Table 15-1).

The micromineral iron is a central component of the hemoglobin and myoglobin molecules, which carry oxygen in blood and muscle, respectively. Iron is also important in the enzymatic processes of cellular respiration. Most commercial pet foods have high concentrations of iron because of their meat content. Consequently, iron deficiency is not common among healthy animals fed standard commercial diets but can be seen in animals with chronic blood loss such as those with hookworm infestations. A microcytic, hypochromic anemia results when iron stores become depleted. Nursing pediatric patients are particularly susceptible to anemia because milk is low in iron.

Other micromineral constituents are chromium, fluoride, nickel, molybdenum, silicon, vanadium, and arsenic. Such trace elements play roles in cell membrane function, tooth and bone development, growth, and reproduction. The amounts required in the diet are low, and deficiencies are rarely seen in animals fed a balanced diet. Dietary excesses of trace elements can be toxic. The proportion of microminerals ingested must be appropriate or pathologic conditions can result.

Both microminerals and macrominerals can interact with one another. These interactions tend to be of two types, either antagonistic or synergistic. Antagonistic interactions are defined as the presence of one mineral reducing the transport or efficacy of the other. Synergistic interactions are two minerals acting in a complementary fashion by either enhancing biologic function or sparing the other mineral. Most mineral interactions are antagonistic and occur through a number of different mechanisms (e.g., during processing, digestion, storage, or transport or in the excretory pathway). Even a marginal deficiency of one vitamin can alter the efficacy of another.

> **✏ TECHNICIAN NOTE**
>
> The micromineral iron is a central component of the hemoglobin and myoglobin molecules, which carry oxygen in blood and muscle, respectively.

VITAMINS

Vitamins are organic compounds necessary for normal physiologic function. Most vitamins cannot be synthesized in the body and therefore must be present in the diet. Vitamins are classified as either fat-soluble (vitamins A, D, E, and K) or water-soluble (B complex vitamins and vitamin C). Because of such differences in solubility, vitamins are absorbed in the body through a variety of means.

> **✏ TECHNICIAN NOTE**
>
> Vitamins are classified as either fat-soluble (vitamins A, D, E, and K) or water-soluble (B complex vitamins and vitamin C).

Fat-soluble vitamins require bile salts and fat clusters for passive absorption through the wall of the duodenum and ileum. In contrast, water-soluble vitamins are absorbed via active transport. Water-soluble vitamins are poorly stored in the body, with excesses lost via the urinary tract. Consequently, frequent intake is critical. On the other hand, fat-soluble vitamins are stored in lipid deposits in all tissues and are therefore required in smaller daily doses. Because of such different absorptive and storage patterns, deficiencies and toxic effects vary among fat-soluble and water-soluble vitamins.

Vitamins are not energy nutrients, and not all types are essential for every species. In addition, intake in excess of requirements does not improve performance. In fact, oversupplementation with fat-soluble vitamins may lead to toxic syndromes (Table 15-3). Conversely, water-soluble vitamins are depleted faster because of limited storage capability, making toxic effects less likely than deficiency.

All commercial pet foods contain vitamins. However, in practice, patients can be presented with vitamin deficiencies. For example, cats fed home-cooked diets rich in polyunsaturated fatty acids (found in fish) are at risk of developing a deficiency of vitamin E. The deficiency causes painful inflammation of adipose tissue and is commonly known as yellow fat disease or pansteatitis.

Vitamin K deficiency is also clinically observed. Vitamin K plays a critical role in the coagulation of blood, and deficiencies result in clotting abnormalities and hemorrhage. Warfarin, found in rodent poison, interferes with the availability of vitamin K and causes fatal hemorrhaging in mice and rats. Cats that consume warfarin-poisoned rodents can become poisoned themselves and may bleed to death without emergency supplementation of vitamin K.

> **✏ TECHNICIAN NOTE**
>
> Vitamin K plays a critical role in the coagulation of blood, and deficiencies result in clotting abnormalities and hemorrhage.

Certain vitamins, such as vitamins C and E, are antioxidants and help free the body of the damaging effects of free radicals. Supplementation of these vitamins above the normal daily requirements can therefore be beneficial. Antioxidants function by stabilizing free radical molecules, which otherwise would have destructive interactions with surrounding tissues. In this way, antioxidants help to restore damaged tissues. Nutritional antioxidants in canine foods help protect immune function and improve cognitive function in senior dogs.

Breakthrough research in the field of animal nutrition has also improved senior pet foods by the addition of multiple

Table 15-3 VITAMINS

Vitamin	Function	Deficiency	Toxic Effects
Vitamin A	Component of visual proteins, differentiation of epithelial cells, spermatogenesis, immune function, bone resorption	Anorexia, retarded growth, poor hair coat, weakness, increased cerebrospinal fluid pressure, eye disorders, aspermatogenesis, fetal resorption	Cervical spondylosis (cat), retarded growth, anorexia, erythema, long-bone fractures
Vitamin D	Ca^{2+} and P homeostasis, bone mineralization and resorption, insulin synthesis, immune function	Rickets, osteoporosis, osteomalacia	Hypercalcemia, calcinosis, lameness, anorexia
Vitamin E	Biologic antioxidant, maintains membrane integrity	Sterility (males), steatitis, anorexia, dermatosis, immunodeficiency, myopathy	Minimally toxic, increased clotting time reversed with vitamin K
Vitamin K	Allows blood clotting protein formation	Prolonged clotting time, hemorrhage, hypoprothrombinemia	Minimally toxic, anemia (dogs), none described in cats
Vitamin B complex	Multiple metabolic reactions, component of energy-producing biochemical reactions that produce energy and allow proper function of tissues and organs	Retarded growth, diarrhea, emaciation, ataxia, anemia, dermatitis	Low toxicity, except niacin in the cat, which can cause convulsions and death
Vitamin C	Synthesized from D-glucose in dogs and cats; synthesis of collagen proteins and carnitine, biologic antioxidant	Deficiency symptoms have not been described in normal dogs and cats	None described in dogs and cats
Choline	Component of membranes, neurotransmitter	Fatty liver (puppies), thymus atrophy, decreased growth rate, anorexia	None described in cats or dogs None described in cats and dogs
Carnitine (vitamin-like nutrient)	Transports long-chain fatty acids into the cell	Hyperlipidemia, cardiomyopathy, muscle asthenia	

From Hand MS et al, editors: *Small animal clinical nutrition*, ed 4, Topeka, 2000, Mark Morris Institute.
Ca, Calcium; *P*, phosphorus.

antioxidant agents and omega-3 fatty acids to support cell membranes, protect against free radical damage, and help improve skin and coat condition. In addition, antioxidant additives in pet foods may be a natural alternative to synthetic preservatives and improve palatability.

There are vitamin-like compounds that exhibit properties similar to those of vitamins but are technically not classified as true vitamins. These include carnitine, carotenoids, and bioflavonoids. Their functions include the metabolism of fatty acids, support of electron transport, and antioxidant capability.

NUTRIENT TERMS

The terms nutrient, ingredient, formula, and nutrient profile are easily confused and sometimes used interchangeably. Nutrients are fundamental energy and metabolic substrates classified as essential or nonessential. Ingredients are the raw materials used in food compounding. The formula selects and apportions ingredients for a particular diet type. The nutrient profile describes the resulting quantitative distribution of the individual nutrients within the finished formula. These definitions are important to understand and distinguish from one another, because clients easily confuse them.

Many pet food companies advertise their product as being "unique" or including fine ingredients. In this way, clients are led to believe that the product has a superior nutrient profile as compared with other brands. Although a listing of ingredients can be useful in evaluation of a pet food, the nutritive value cannot be identified solely on the basis of an ingredient statement. Analysis of a particular food can give an indication of its nutrient content and the availability of a particular nutrient, but it is the absorptive capability of the nutrient (combined with availability) that determines nutritional value. In other words, digestibility of a food is a measure of its biologic availability. A balanced diet should supply all the key nutrients and energy needed to meet the daily requirements of the animal at its particular stage of life.

Feeding a food with higher digestibility may allow animals to consume less of a particular food. Consequently, feeding highly digestible foods may be more economical than feeding a less expensive food with lower digestibility. In addition, because more of the food is biologically usable, there is less waste to clean up in the yard! Digestibility of a food is determined by a mathematical equation comparing the amount of a nutrient in the food and the amount of the same nutrient in the feces (Box 15-4). Above-average

---

Box 15-4 OBESITY-PRONE DOG BREEDS

- Beagle
- Labrador
- Sheltie
- Cocker spaniel
- Golden retriever
- Cairn terrier
- Scottish terrier
- Dachshund
- Basset hound
- Cavalier King Charles spaniel

Box 15-5 FEEDING DO'S AND DON'TS

DO'S
Provide fresh water.
Feed for control of calorie intake.
Feed for ideal weight and body condition.
Feel but do not see ribs.
Provide a consistent food, and ritualize the time and place of feeding.
Use life-stage feeding concepts by correlating diet to pet's life stage.
Feed treats with nutrient profile and caloric density considerations.

DON'TS
Provide stagnant or frozen water.
Allow excess calorie consumption.
Feed obesity-prone dogs on an ad lib or free choice basis.
Rotate flavors or brands on a frequent basis.
Make rapid transitions.
Use growth/lactation foods for adult maintenance.
Supplement a balanced/high-quality food.
Allow competitive eating.

---

digestibility can be defined as protein, fat, carbohydrate, and energy digestibility more than or equal to 85%, 90%, 90%, and 85%, respectively. Foods higher in fiber will be lower in digestibility.

Palatability of a food involves sensory factors such as taste, smell, color, and even texture (Box 15-5). Palatability is an essential component of an animal's behavior toward a particular food type, and first impressions are generally important. Sensory components such as smell can entice an anorectic patient to eat, particularly if the food is warm and strong smelling.

Additives are nonenergy, nonnutrient substances purposely added to foods to enhance color, flavor, texture, and stability. Preservatives are defined as substances capable of inhibiting food-deteriorating microbes. Protection against microbes can also be achieved by both physical and chemical means, such as dehydration (dry foods), heat (moist and dry foods), and chemical treatments (semimoist and some dry foods). Many preservatives are organic acids, and their salts are added to retard oxidation, discoloration, and spoilage.

Humectants are preservative additives that bind to water to inhibit mold and fungal growth. Other chemical agents such as antioxidants can inhibit oxidation of fatty acids and fat-soluble vitamins, which keeps them from becoming rancid and losing potency. Antioxidants such as vitamins C and E are natural preservatives.

✏ TECHNICIAN NOTE

Additives are nonenergy, nonnutrient substances purposely added to foods to enhance color, flavor, texture, and stability.

PET FOOD EVALUATION

Many clients will ask for recommendations regarding the best food to feed their pets and will inquire about the many differences in commercial brand foods. Other owners will ask about the suitability of home cooking or about supplementing an existing diet with table food. Note that although various homemade foods can be suitable for daily maintenance, most commercial pet foods are superior in nutrient content, convenience, cost, and overall quality.

Nutritional terms commonly used in commercial pet foods include phrases such as complete and balanced. A complete diet contains nutrients with appropriate bioavailability, and a balanced diet provides the proper amount and nutrient ratio needed for a 24-hour period. When these two types of diets are combined, both the nutrient and energy requirements of the animal are fulfilled. If nonenergy nutrients are in proper concentration to the energy density of the food, the diet is also considered balanced. Complementary diets combine two or more food sources to improve outcome. For example, a small amount of a canned dog food mixed with dry food increases palatability for many dogs.

Other nutritional terms include all-purpose and special purpose. All-purpose foods are marketed under the premise that one particular diet type meets nutritional demands at every life stage. Such diets are typically found in grocery stores to target the uninformed consumer and are generally sold as off-brand or generic foods. Formulated for the growth and lactation periods of companion animals, such diets are not appropriate for the other stages of life. In other words, all-purpose foods provide nutrients in excess of what is required by the adult or geriatric animal.

✏ TECHNICIAN NOTE

All-purpose foods typically provide nutrients in excess of what is required by the adult or geriatric animal.

Special-purpose foods provide specialized nutrition for individual needs. Special-purpose foods are designed for animals with specific nutritional needs such as the obese or obese-prone animal, the working dog, or the sick and injured pet. Special-purpose foods are often sold in veterinary hospitals, where clients are educated about which diet is most beneficial for the individual needs of their pets.

NUTRIENT CONTENT AND FORMS OF PET FOOD

Commercial pet foods are prepared with varying amounts of water. Three basic forms are available to the consumer: dry, semimoist, and moist. Dry foods typically have 9% to 11% water. Semimoist foods have 25% to 35% moisture, and moist foods, which are the most palatable to dogs and cats, contain 70% to 83% moisture (Figure 15-2). Nutrient profiles vary with each type of food so that both high-quality and low-quality foods can be found in every form. Thus the quality of a diet is not related to the percentage of moisture it contains.

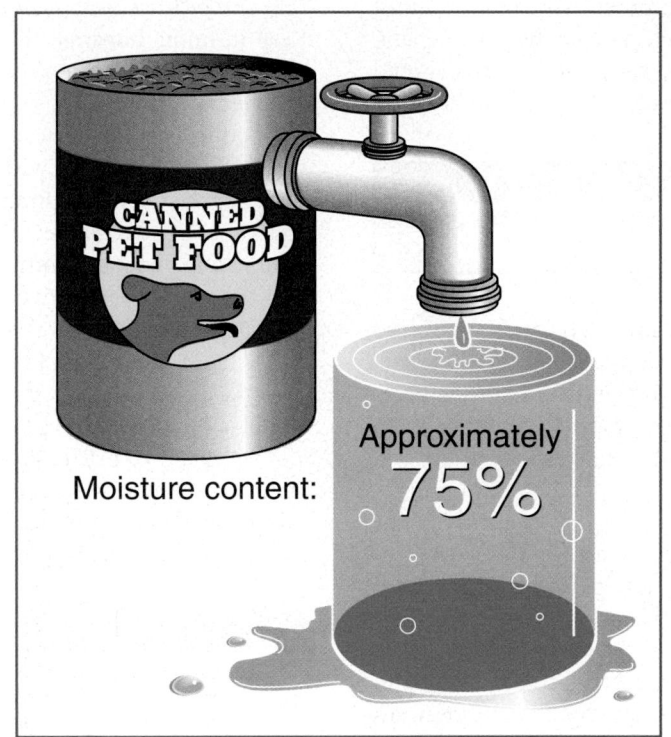

A

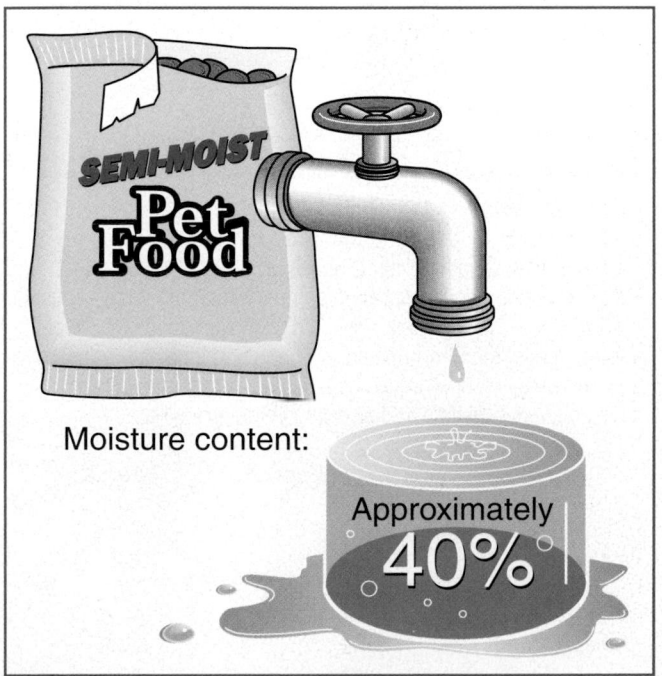

B

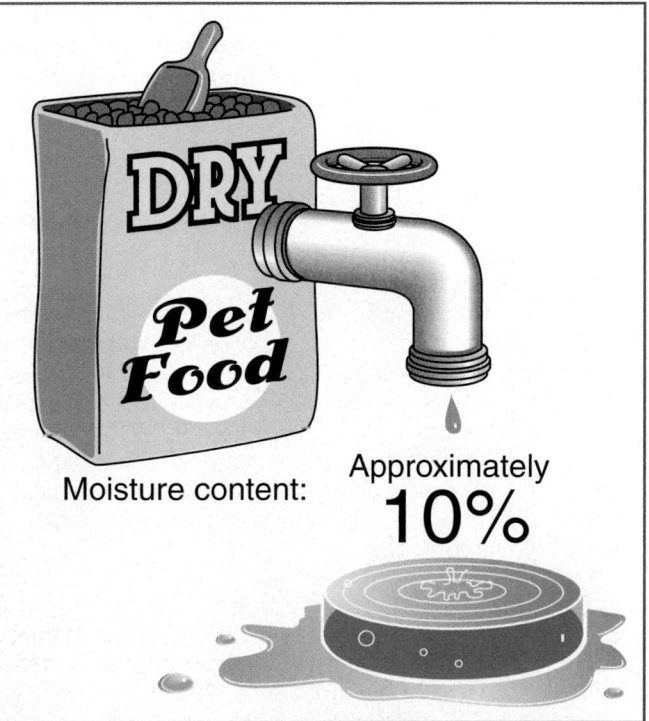

C

Figure 15-2 **A,** Moisture content in canned pet food. **B,** Moisture content in semimoist pet food. **C,** Moisture content in dry pet food.

TECHNICIAN NOTE

The quality of a diet is not related to the percentage of moisture it contains.

Dry foods characteristically have lower amounts of protein, fat, and minerals on a weight-per-volume basis than most moist foods. In addition, dry foods are produced with higher caloric density and typically cost less than most moist foods. Dry foods may also provide a dental hygiene benefit, although neither dry foods nor hard baked treats should replace regular dental prophylaxis.

TECHNICIAN NOTE

Neither dry foods nor hard baked treats should replace regular dental prophylaxis.

When dry pet food is made, raw ingredients are mixed and moistened into dough. The dough is kneaded, cooked, and processed via extrusion. Extrusion uses high temperatures to fully cook and shape kibble, which leads to digestibility and palatability. It is the most common method of making dry and semimoist diets, and it is important in killing the microorganisms that may be carried in the raw materials.

Although dry pet foods are less palatable than moist forms, they have the advantage of having a lower true cost (Box 15-6). True cost of feeding is the cost of feeding a pet per day or cost per year. This important concept needs to be explained to the pet owner, because there are significant differences between dry and canned food. Evaluating both types of food on a cost-per-pound or a cost-per-calorie basis may result in an economically sound decision. For example, dry foods cost approximately one third as much as moist

foods on a cost-per-calorie basis. In general, dry pet foods are the predominant source of calories for companion animals in North America. In addition to being cost effective, dry foods are convenient and easy to use and allow the owner to leave food out for extended periods. In this way, the pets may eat on an ad lib basis.

Water may be added to create a "gravy" that improves the acceptability of a dry pet food. In addition, palatability may also be improved by mixing dry food with canned food. Keep in mind, however, that if dry food is moistened with water and left outside in high temperatures, bacterial proliferation is possible.

Foodborne illnesses can be avoided by ensuring consumption of moist food within a few hours. Certain bacteria (e.g., *Bacillus cereus*) are found in soil, grains, cereal products, and other foods. These bacteria may be found in small numbers in dry pet foods and are normally of no health significance. However, they can rapidly increase in numbers when moisture levels are raised (e.g., addition of water or moist foods to dry pet food) at room temperature. These bacteria can produce a potent toxin that causes vomiting and diarrhea. Therefore pet owners should be warned not to add water to dry pet foods and leave them exposed to high ambient temperatures for prolonged periods. Dry pet foods mixed with water or moist foods are usually safe if they are consumed within a few hours.

TECHNICIAN NOTE

Dry food moistened with water and left outside in high temperatures can cause bacterial proliferation and consequent foodborne illnesses. Ensure consumption of moist food within a few hours.

Semimoist and soft-dry foods have a moisture content ranging from 25% to 40% and are composed of a meat and

---

Box 15-6 COST OF FEEDING

The cost of feeding on a per-day basis is a better measure of value than the unit cost of the can or package.

Pet owners usually compare the cost of pet foods on the price per unit (e.g., price per bag or price per can) rather than the true cost of feeding (cost per day or cost per year). It is easy to compare the price per unit when evaluating two different pet foods, but more difficult to compare the true cost of feeding. The following example demonstrates that veterinarians and their health care team members need to discuss the true cost of feeding with pet owners when clients are concerned about the price of a particular food.

MOIST CAT FOOD

A 4.5-kg, 3-year-old neutered male cat is diagnosed with lower urinary tract disease caused by struvite urolithiasis. A moist veterinary therapeutic food (Food A) is recommended to help prevent further episodes of struvite urolithiasis. The cat's owner is

concerned about the "high cost" of the veterinary therapeutic food but would be willing to use Food A if it costs the same as what she now feeds her cat (Food B, a gourmet grocery brand). This calculation shows that the veterinary therapeutic food costs markedly less to feed than the cat's current food. By feeding a therapeutic food formulated to prevent feline lower urinary tract disease, reoccurrence may decrease and the owner may have additional savings in decreased veterinary bills.

	Food A	Food B
Cost/can	.99	.50
Size of container	156 g	100 g
Cost/gram	.006	.005
Feeding amount (300 kcal)	285 g	350 g
Cost/day	$1.28	$1.75
Cost/year	$468	$639

cereal mixture extruded into small, attractive shapes. Artificial flavors provide a sweet, savory flavor yielding high palatability. Humectant preservatives and cellophane wrapping provide reasonable shelf life and convenience to the pet owner. Antimicrobial additives help prevent spoilage and bacterial proliferation. Semimoist foods have readily available soluble sugars and simple carbohydrate sources, which are not recommended for the diabetic animal or any other animal in which blood sugar needs to be regulated.

Soft-dry foods are the combined result of semimoist and dry products. Such hybrid mixes provide the advantages of dry food enhanced with the palatability found in semimoist foods.

> **TECHNICIAN NOTE**
>
> Semimoist foods have readily available soluble sugars and simple carbohydrate sources not recommended for the diabetic animal or any other animal in which blood sugar needs to be regulated.

Canned or moist foods are typically 70% to 83% water and have three forms: a ration loaf, an all-meat appearance, or processed meats and flours bound into a jellied matrix by gums or alginates. The high palatability of canned foods results from a high content of water, protein, and fat and the inherent flavor of animal source tissue. Moist foods require portion-controlled feeding to prevent overconsumption, because most pets prefer canned products to dry food. Most moist foods in North America are sold as complete diets, with all nutrients present.

Moist foods are preserved with heat sterilization and vacuum techniques to ensure an anaerobic environment. Enamel liners insulate the product and provide excellent nutrient stability. Shelf life ranges from 12 to 18 months, provided that care is taken to store products at normal temperatures. Palatability may decrease toward the end of the shelf life.

Moist foods have a low caloric density. Moist foods are expensive on a per-calorie basis, because fresh and frozen meat by-product ingredients are more costly than equivalent meals and flours. In addition, higher packaging costs correspond to a higher daily feeding cost to the pet owner.

The use of moist foods in combination with dry foods is an acceptable practice to increase palatability and control cost. Note that as the ratio of moist food increases in a mix, the palatability and percentage of fat and protein calories usually increase as well.

> **TECHNICIAN NOTE**
>
> The use of moist foods in combination with dry foods is an acceptable practice to increase palatability and control cost.

Treats are small food rewards that the pet owner may give as a training aid or to reinforce love or affection. Commercially prepared treats or snacks should not be given in excess because such a practice could interfere with normal appetite or dietary balance and may contribute to obesity (Tables 15-4 and 15-5). Chocolate is not recommended because it is toxic in high concentrations. Because treats may be a substantial source of calories and protein for some pets, it is important for the technician to inquire about the use of treats when completing the patient's history. This is particularly important if the pet has diseases that require

Table 15-4 NUTRIENT CHARACTERISTICS OF HUMAN SNACK FOODS*

Food	Serving Size	kcal/Serving	kcal/g	Protein (g)	Fat (g)	Sodium[†]
Cow's milk (3.5%)	1 C = 244 g	150	0.6	8	8	122/81
Whole egg (boiled)	1 egg = 50 g	79	1.6	6.1	5.6	69/87
Ice cream (vanilla, 10% fat)	1 C = 133 g	266	2.0	4.8	14.3	116/43
American cheese	1 oz	93	3.3	5.6	7	337/362
Cottage cheese (low fat, 2%)	1 C = 226 g	203	0.9	31	4.4	918/452
Gelatin	1 C = 280 g	162	0.6	3.2	0	108/67
Hot dog	8/lb = 57 g	180	3.2	6.9	16.3	585/325
Bologna (beef)	1 slice = 23 g	72	3.1	2.8	6.6	226/313
Big Mac	1 sandwich = 200 g	570	2.9	24.6	35	979/172
Peanut butter (smooth)	2 T = 32 g	188	5.9	9	5.4	234/124
Popcorn (w/ butter)	3 C = 37 g	192	5.2	2.8	11.5	273/142
Corn chips	1 oz	153	5.5	1.7	8.8	218/142
Potato chips	1 oz	148	5.3	1.8	10.1	133/90
Pretzels	1 oz	110	3.9	3.0	1.2	543/493

All values from Pennington JAT: *Food values of portions commonly used*, ed 15, New York, 1989, Harper & Row.
C, Cup; T, tablespoon.
*Metabolizable energy for humans.
[†]Sodium content per serving/sodium content per 100 kcal.

Table 15-5 DOG AND CAT TREATS

Treat	Manufacturer	Weight (g/treat)	Calories (kcal/ML)	Protein (g)	Fat (g)	Fiber (g)	Calcium (mg)	Phosphorus (mg)	Potassium (mg)	Sodium (mg)	Magnesium (mg)
DOG TREATS											
Milkbone (small)	Nabisco	5	16	1.1	0.3	0.1	71	54	30	21	7
Beggin Strips Orginal Bacon Flavor	Purina	10.3	29	1.7	0.6	0.1	44	49	33	65	11
Bonz	Purina	20.4	66	3.1	1.3	0.3	241	155	86	53	24
Purina Biscuits (medium)	Purina	10.2	37	2.5	1.3	0.2	114	106	91	29	21
Meaty Bone (medium)	Heinz	18.2	64	2.3	1.8	0.4	8	55	71	116	20
100% Natural Treats	Heinz	7.6	26	1.3	0.5	0.1	17	49	48	41	15
Snausages (beef flavor)	Heinz	6.6	17	1.5	0.6	0.1	61	46	98	44	7
Pup-Peroni Jerky Snack Sticks	Heinz	6.6	21	1.8	1	0.1	55	44	59	73	7
Original Jerky Treats	Heinz	6.8	22	2	1.3	0.1	35	35	71	140	7
Fiber Formula Biscuits (medium)	Stewart	10.1	26	1.5	0.3	1.7	63	37	NA	7	NA
Science Diet (adult maintenance)	Hill's	5	17	1.1	0.5	0.2	29	29	29	11	4
Science Diet (light)	Hill's	5	15	0.8	0.3	0.6	29	29	38	11	7
Science Diet (senior)	Hill's	5	16	0.8	0.4	0.4	30	27	28	7	5
Prescription Diet	Hill's	5	15	0.8	0.3	0.8	28	21	36	5	6
CAT TREATS											
Pounce (with tuna)	Heinz	1.5	3.7	0.32	0.13	0.01	13.5	11.3	1:1.2	9.2	1.2
Pounce Hairball Treatment	Heinz	1.0	2.9	1.7	0.4	0.2	2	6	7	5	0.6
Whisker Lickin's (Kluckers)	Purina	1.1	3	0.32	0.12	0.01	9	10.7	1:0.84	6.2	0.7

From Hand MS et al, editors: *Small animal clinical nurition*, ed 4, Topeka, 2000, Mark Morris Institute.
ME, Metabolizable energy; *NA*, not applicable.

dietary restrictions such as diabetes mellitus, urolithiasis, cardiac and renal insufficiency, and obesity. Commercial treats are not subject to testing, as are pet foods. Nutritional excesses are common in many commercial pet food treats.

The use of supplements should not be confused with the use of treats. Although treats are nutritionally trivial when used in small amounts, a supplement is generally administered to correct a nutritional deficiency. Routine use of supplements is not necessary if the pet is provided with a balanced commercial pet food.

HOME-PREPARED DIETS

Many dog and cat owners prefer to prepare homemade foods, despite the fact that most commercial foods are easier to use, are less expensive, and provide a better nutritional balance. Formulation of a home-prepared diet requires detailed knowledge of specific nutrient need, nutritional value of the ingredients, any possible dietary interactions, and possible deterioration of nutrients during cooking and storage, as well as consideration of the time and effort required in making such a diet. It is imperative that the owner follow a veterinarian-approved recipe so that a balanced diet is provided.

It is possible to achieve the same nutrient balance with a homemade food as with a commercially prepared food. However, it is still important for the client to understand that homemade recipes are not tested or evaluated, as are commercial pet foods. Pet owners interested in feeding a homemade diet should consult with a competent veterinarian, or preferably, a board-certified veterinary nutritionist to obtain a balanced recipe. Veterinarians and technicians together should provide pet owners with recommendations or provide guidelines for assessing homemade foods. In addition, owner compliance should be regulated by the veterinary professional, and diets should conform to the animal's needs.

✎ TECHNICIAN NOTE

Pet owners interested in feeding a homemade diet should consult with a competent veterinarian, or preferably, a board-certified veterinary nutritionist to obtain a balanced recipe.

Most homemade recipes have been crudely balanced by using the average nutrient content of specific foods and computer formulation. Unlike commercial foods, few of the numerous published homemade recipes for dogs and cats have undergone tests to document performance over sustained periods, including tests for palatability, digestibility, and safety. Therefore veterinarians and veterinary technicians should obtain dietary histories and provide patient monitoring on a regular basis for pets fed homemade foods.

The veterinary technician should help evaluate the patient on a homemade diet by noting body weight, body condition score (BCS), and activity level and by conducting a thorough physical exam. Veterinary technicians should be willing to assess an existing homemade food recipe, offer nutritionally adequate recipes, and make appropriate formula substitutions for clients. Taking the time to counsel clients about different homemade diets will prevent common problems and increase client compliance.

Many homemade diets contain excessive protein and are deficient in calories, calcium, vitamins, and minerals. Most formulations for dogs use staples such as carbohydrates and meat sources containing more phosphorous than calcium, often exceeding the animal's nutritional requirements. Homemade feline foods are often deficient in fat and have low energy density. In addition, no single supplement can be added to meet the mineral and vitamin requirements found in most commercially prepared foods.

Home-Prepared Diet Analysis

Homemade formulations can be checked for nutritional adequacy and adjusted by using the following "quick check" guidelines:

- *Do five food groups appear in the recipe?*
  - ✓ A carbohydrate/fiber source from a cooked cereal grain or potato
  - ✓ A protein source (preferably of animal origin; if multiple sources of protein are used, at least one source should be of animal origin)
  - ✓ A fat source
  - ✓ A source of minerals, particularly calcium
  - ✓ A multivitamin and trace mineral source
- *What are the type and quantity of the primary protein source?*
  - ✓ The overall protein quality in a homemade food can generally be improved by using an animal-source protein. Skeletal muscle protein from different animal species has very similar amino acid profiles; therefore there is no great advantage to feeding one meat source over another. Note that any cooked animal protein source should provide most of the essential amino acid requirements.
- *Is the primary protein source lean or fatty?*
  - ✓ The fat content of different cuts of meat varies. When the specified protein source is lean, an additional animal or vegetable fat source should comprise 2% to 5% of the formula to ensure that energy density requirements are met.
  - ✓ *Is the carbohydrate source a cooked cereal or potato? Is it present in an amount greater than or equal to that of the meat source?*
  - ✓ The carbohydrate/protein ratio should be approximately 1:1 to 2:1 for cat foods and 2:1 to 3:1 for dog foods.
- *Is a source of calcium and other minerals provided?*
  - ✓ A homemade food is almost never balanced in minerals; most homemade foods require a calcium supplement.

• *Is a source of vitamins and other nutrients provided?*

✓ Supplements providing vitamins, microminerals, fatty acids, taurine, and other specific nutrients of concern for cats and dogs should be used in homemade recipes. Owners should consult their veterinarians for proper supplement ratios.

Specific instructions as to feeding and storing homemade foods are of utmost importance. Most homemade foods lack preservative agents and are high in moisture content; consequently, such foods are very susceptible to bacterial growth. Pet owners should be advised to refrigerate or freeze homemade foods and monitor food for color and odor changes. Patients that eat homemade foods should be brought in for regular veterinary examinations and nutritional reviews (at least two visits per year). The technician should ask the client to record and submit a 3- to 5-day food history as part of the evaluation.

> **✎ TECHNICIAN NOTE**
>
> The veterinary technician should help evaluate the patient on a homemade diet by noting body weight, BCS, and activity level and by conducting a thorough physical exam.

Cooking techniques used by the owner providing a homemade diet need to be reviewed. Although cooking improves digestibility of starch in the carbohydrates, longer periods of cooking may depreciate vitamin concentration and cause protein denaturation of meat sources.

Increased digestibility and caloric density have an inverse relationship to the amount of feces produced from consumption of both homemade diets and commercially prepared foods. Many owners may be concerned with the volume and firmness of feces excreted by their pet. Notice in Figure 15-3 that the quantity and texture characteristics of feces relate to the amount and digestibility of dry matter eaten.

Ingredients for both homemade foods and commercially prepared foods are packaged to provide useful information, some of which is legally required. Labels should identify both product and target species.

PET FOOD LABELS

The pet food label represents a contract between the manufacturer and the consumer. The Association of American Feed Control Officials (AAFCO) establishes standards for label information and the description of ingredients on pet foods sold in the United States. The AAFCO ensures that adequate information is communicated to the consumer about the food product. The Association is made up of representatives from a wide range of professional organizations including the American Veterinary Medical Association, the American Animal Hospital Association, and the Pet Food Institute. Pet food labels provide useful information that enables both the veterinarian and the pet owner

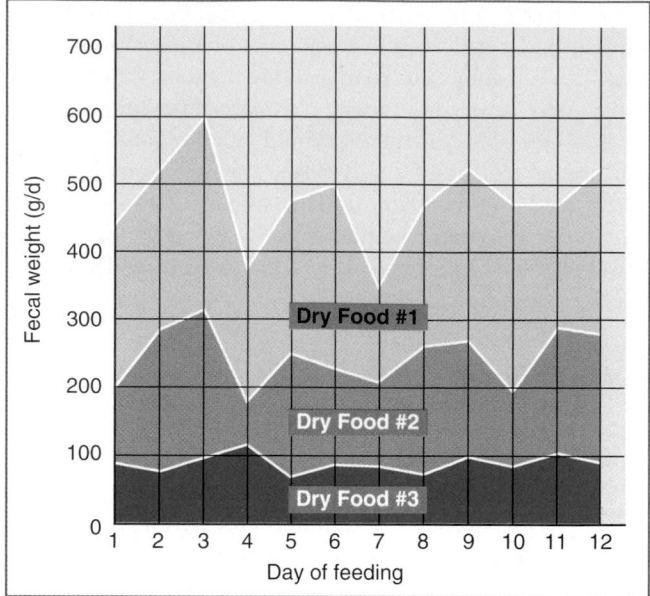

Figure 15-3 Increased digestibility and caloric density have an inverse relationship to fecal volume. Food 1 was a lower-energy food and produced voluminous stool volume with difficult cleanup characteristics. Food 3 featured high digestibility and was energy dense, and stool cleanup was quick and nonmessy.

to make decisions about what to feed and how frequently to feed it. It should be noted that in the United States, health claims on pet food labels, or in accompanying literature, are subject to Food and Drug Administration investigation. Pet food labels are required to state the following:

✓ Net weight

✓ Product designator (e.g., cat food)

✓ Name and address of the manufacturer or distributor

✓ Guaranteed analyses in percentages for crude protein, fat, fiber, and moisture

✓ A list of ingredients in descending order of predominance by weight

✓ Nutritional adequacy statement

✓ Feeding guidelines

Many labels contain more information than what is listed here. Feeding instructions, calorie content, and a statement that the diet is complete and balanced with respect to a particular life stage are all additional statements commonly found on pet food labels (Figure 15-4).

The nutritional adequacy statement on pet food labels may vary. Nutritional adequacy statements may include terms such as totally nutritious or complete and balanced. According to AAFCO regulations, the nutritional adequacy of a food only requires recommended levels of essential nutrients at two different life stages, growth and reproduction. Statements such as "formulated to meet the AAFCO dog food nutrient profile" (or similar wording) only indicate laboratory analysis for a minimal chemical content. Such testing is not an animal feeding performance trial and says nothing about adequacy, bioavailability, or excesses.

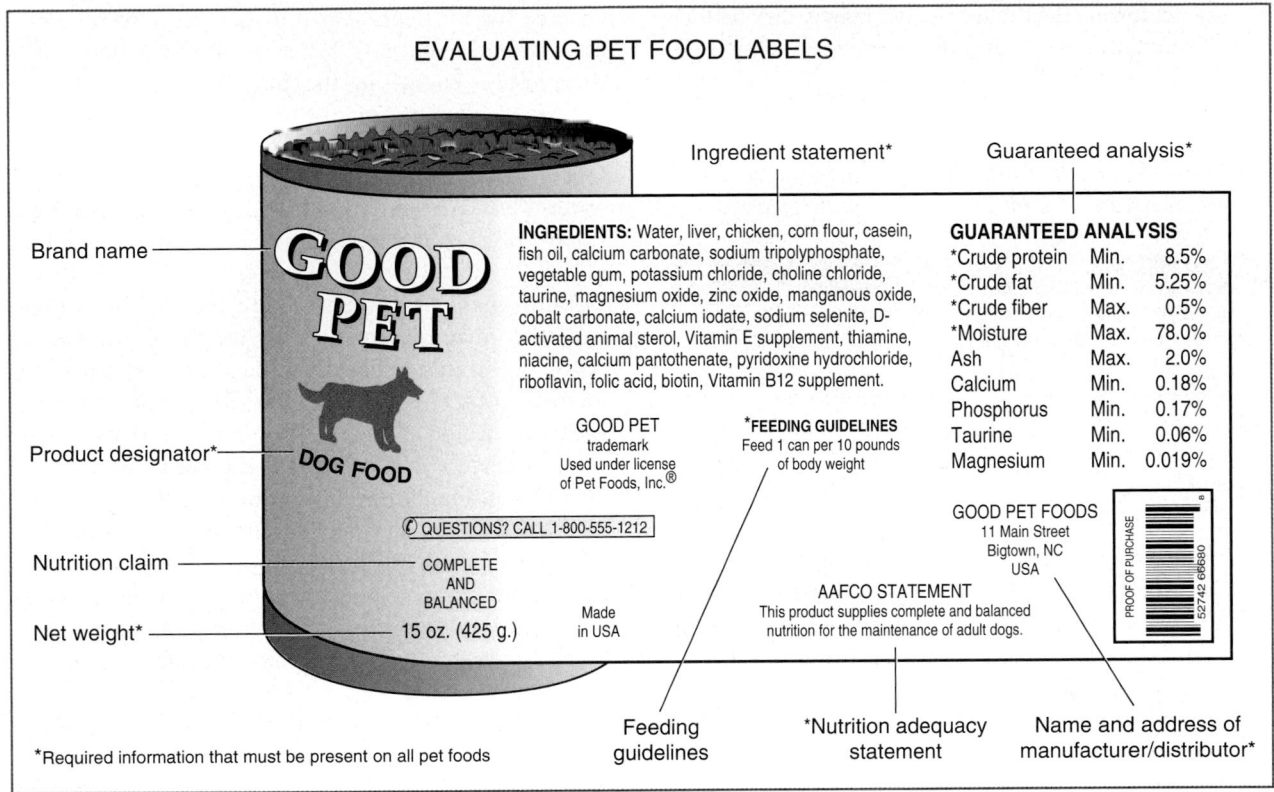

EVALUATING PET FOOD LABELS

Ingredient statement*

Guaranteed analysis*

Brand name

GOOD PET

DOG FOOD

INGREDIENTS: Water, liver, chicken, corn flour, casein, fish oil, calcium carbonate, sodium tripolyphosphate, vegetable gum, potassium chloride, choline chloride, taurine, magnesium oxide, zinc oxide, manganous oxide, cobalt carbonate, calcium iodate, sodium selenite, D-activated animal sterol, Vitamin E supplement, thiamine, niacine, calcium pantothenate, pyridoxine hydrochloride, riboflavin, folic acid, biotin, Vitamin B12 supplement.

GUARANTEED ANALYSIS
*Crude protein	Min.	8.5%
*Crude fat	Min.	5.25%
*Crude fiber	Max.	0.5%
*Moisture	Max.	78.0%
Ash	Max.	2.0%
Calcium	Min.	0.18%
Phosphorus	Min.	0.17%
Taurine	Min.	0.06%
Magnesium	Min.	0.019%

GOOD PET
trademark
Used under license
of Pet Foods, Inc.®

*FEEDING GUIDELINES
Feed 1 can per 10 pounds
of body weight

GOOD PET FOODS
11 Main Street
Bigtown, NC
USA

PROOF OF PURCHASE
52742 66680

Product designator*

© QUESTIONS? CALL 1-800-555-1212

Nutrition claim

COMPLETE
AND
BALANCED

Made
in USA

Net weight*

15 oz. (425 g.)

AAFCO STATEMENT
This product supplies complete and balanced
nutrition for the maintenance of adult dogs.

Feeding
guidelines

*Nutrition adequacy
statement

Name and address of
manufacturer/distributor*

*Required information that must be present on all pet foods

Figure 15-4   A pet food label is the contract between the manufacturer and the consumer. A label provides information required by law and may have optional information, such as a statement of calorie content, the universal product code, batch information, or a freshness date.

The AAFCO establishes minimal standards for testing new pet food products. These protocols are used by pet food manufacturers during feeding trials to substantiate the nutritional adequacy of their products. The *AAFCO Animal Feeding Test Statement* (Figure 15-4), which is required on food labels, lets the consumer know that the product was used in animal feeding tests and that it performed at acceptable levels. Consequently, the veterinary technician should recommend feeds to clients that have the "feeding test" information on the label and not the foods with the "formulated" statements, if given a choice. Nutritional adequacy statements are not needed on treats or snacks intended for intermittent feeding.

There are no governmental requirements in Canada for substantiation of nutritional claims on pet food labels. Rather, pet foods that meet nutrient standards and pass digestibility feeding trials are given special seals of certification by the Canadian Veterinary Medical Association.

Evaluating Pet Food Labels

Although there is substantial information on pet food labels regarding food quality, there are also some pitfalls to be examined and considered. For example, percentages listed in the guaranteed analyses state only maximal and minimal levels and do not reflect the exact amounts of each nutrient. In addition, because pet food labels represent a legal contract between the manufacturer and consumer, the guaranteed nutrient levels are conservative and may be far different from those determined by the actual analysis. The manufacturer can often supply a more reliable source of data.

> ### ✎ TECHNICIAN NOTE
> The ingredients on labels are listed by weight, with the heaviest ingredients first and the lightest ones last. This often means that water-containing ingredients are listed before drier ingredients, even though a dry ingredient may make up a larger portion of the food on a weight-per-volume basis.

Ingredient Percentages

Percentage rules for listed ingredients are important to note when a diet is analyzed for nutritional need. According to AAFCO rules, when a label statement identifies only one ingredient, at least 70% of the total product must consist of that named ingredient (e.g., beef). If any modifying words accompany the named ingredient, the amount of the named ingredient that must be present declines to 10% for moist foods and 25% for dry foods (e.g., chicken *dinner,* fish *entree,* liver *stew*). In addition, if a named ingredient is modified by the word *with* (e.g., with beef), the total portion of the named ingredient declines to 3%. Further, if the term *flavor* is used (e.g., cheese flavor), the named flavor must be detectable only by the animal. The designator *food* (e.g., dog food) means that there are no rules regarding minimal content of ingredients. Indirectly, the technician may gather further quality information about a product by understanding these nuances of pet food labeling.

Percentage rules also apply to moisture content. In the United States, the maximum moisture content is 78%; pet foods may exceed this amount if the label includes the words *stew, gravy,* or *juice* or the phrase *contains milk replacer.*

✎ TECHNICIAN NOTE

Patient assessment and daily feeding performance analysis will provide more insight into an animal's well-being than the most informative of pet food labels.

MARKET CATEGORIES

Understanding market objectives for a product may assist with some aspects of assessing a food's quality. Grocery brands are generally well-recognized pet foods sold in grocery stores with large-scale advertisement and distribution. Most grocery brands are all-purpose foods, balanced for the growth or lactation life stages (see the discussion of pet food evaluation). "Premium" grocery bands are specific-purpose food types generally designed with a more nutritional focus than traditional grocery brands. Other food types include "gourmet" foods to sell the consumer on increased palatability for finicky pets.

Generic (white label) and private label (a grocery chain's own brand) foods are made at contract feed mills by using least-cost formulation methods. Private label brands are common in large supermarket settings and pet retail outlets. Markets emphasize low cost and high palatability and generally sell on anthropomorphic appeal. Flavor, shape, color, ingredient, and brand name proliferation characterize these products, allowing them to engage the largest amount of shelf space.

Specialty brand pet foods are often sold in veterinary hospitals, pet superstores, and regular stores. Often called premium or super premium foods, they generally stress better-quality ingredients with exceptional nutritional focus. Although differences in nutritional philosophy may be noted among different manufacturers, these brands are consistent in the overall objective of emphasizing a philosophy of optimum nutrition. These specialty brand foods typically use the life stage and special needs approach, with a general aim at disease prevention.

COMPANION ANIMAL NUTRITION

ENERGY REQUIREMENTS

An estimate of the energy requirement of an animal is needed to determine how much food to feed. If you recall from the discussion of energy-producing nutrients in this chapter, the nutrients that provide energy include protein, carbohydrates, and fats. When these nutrients are burned, they release energy in the form of heat. Each nutrient releases a different amount of heat, which is measured in kilocalories or Calories. A kilocalorie is the amount of heat (energy) needed to raise the temperature of 1 kilogram of water 1° C. With this in mind, the energy requirements (food!) of an animal would be calculated and expressed in kilocalories.

Daily energy requirements are the number of calories needed to maintain an animal's weight. Obviously, an increase in the animal's exercise, lactation, and growth would increase energy requirements; whereas a decrease in these activities would lower energy requirements. Increased energy demands over and above the needs for maintenance are called production energy requirements.

Predictive equations are useful in calculating nutrient requirements, but judging the body composition and condition of the animal is also important in determining the caloric needs of the animal. Body condition can be assessed by feeling the ribs with flat palms. Ideally, the ribs should be felt but not seen (Figure 15-5).

Body condition scoring gives the veterinary professional an estimate of an animal's body composition. The BCS can be used to subjectively assess a pet's fat stores and muscle mass. Note that the body condition scoring system was developed with regard to both age and species.

NUTRITIONAL ASSESSMENT

A thorough nutritional assessment consists of a patient's history and a physical examination including body weight, BCS, and hydration status. The primary goal of nutritional assessment is to identify the dietary needs of the patient. In the course of a disease or treatment process, a patient's nutritional needs can change, and these changes need to be monitored regularly and discussed with the pet owner.

A baseline nutritional assessment should be made on admission to the hospital and then followed by serial assessments throughout the course of the hospitalization (see the discussion of clinical nutrition). The veterinary technician is particularly well positioned to identify baseline data and ongoing changes in nutritional status, because the technician typically spends a great amount of time with hospitalized patients. Nutritional intervention is crucial to recovery and survival, particularly with the critically ill patient, and appropriate consideration as to the type and route of nutrition should be given on the basis of the underlying disease process or diagnosis (see the discussions of routes of feeding and tube selection).

✎ TECHNICIAN NOTE

A thorough nutritional assessment consists of a patient's history and a physical examination including body weight, BCS, and hydration status.

BODY CONDITION SCORING SYSTEM

Body condition assessment will assist the veterinary technician in determining if the puppy or kitten is growing appropriately and if the correct amount of food is being offered. Proper growth can reduce risk for obesity and growth related skeletal disease.

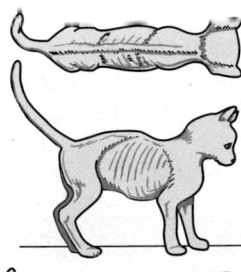
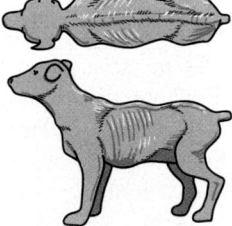
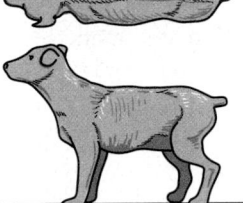

1. VERY THIN

The ribs are easily palpable with no fat cover. The tailbase* has a prominent raised bony structure with no tissue between the skin and bone. The bone prominences are easily felt with no overlying fat. In animals over six months, there is a severe abdominal tuck when viewed from the side and an accentuated hourglass shape when viewed from above.

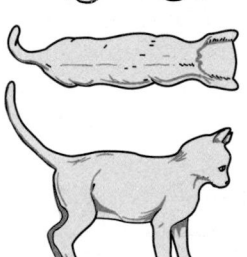
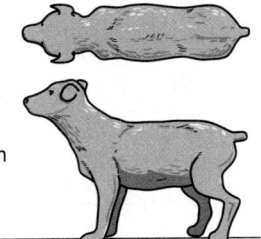

2. UNDERWEIGHT

The ribs are easily palpable with minimal fat cover. The tailbase* has a raised bony structure with little tissue between the skin and bone. The bony prominences are easily felt with minimal overlying fat. In animals over six months, there is an abdominal tuck when viewed from the side and a marked hourglass shape when viewed from above.

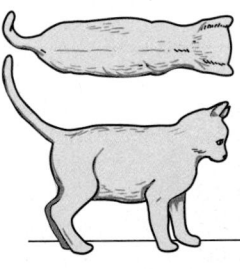
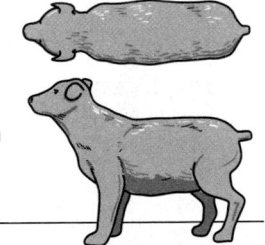

3. IDEAL

The ribs are palpable with a slight fat cover. The tailbase* has a smooth contour or some thickening and the bony structures are palpable under a thin layer of fat between the skin and the bone. The bony prominences are easily felt with a slight amount of overlying fat. In animals over six months, there is an abdominal tuck when viewed from the side and a well proportioned lumbar waist when viewed from above.

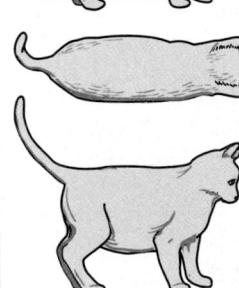
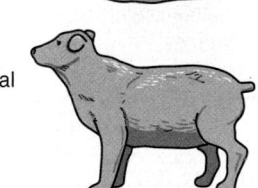

4. OVERWEIGHT

The ribs are difficult to feel with moderate fat cover. The tailbase* has some thickening with moderate amounts of tissue between the skin and bone. The bony structures can still be felt. The bony prominences are covered by a moderate layer of fat. In animals over six months, there is little or no abdominal tuck or waist when viewed from above. Abdominal fat apron present in cats.

5. OBESE

The ribs are very difficult to feel under a thick fat cover. The tailbase* appears thickened and is difficult to feel under a prominent layer of fat. The bony prominences are covered by a moderate to thick layer of fat. In animals over six months, there is a pendulous ventral bulge and no waist when viewed from the side. The back is markedly broadened when viewed from above. Marked abdominal fat apron present in cats.

*Tailbase evaluation is done only in dogs.

Figure 15-5 Body conditioning scoring system.

FEEDING NORMAL DOGS

Dogs are typically omnivores and exhibit eating behaviors similar to those of their relatives, the wolf (*Canis lupus*) and the coyote (*Canis latrans*). Dogs are opportunistic eaters, predators, and scavengers and have developed anatomic and physiologic traits that allow for the digestion of a variety of foods. Although dogs are omnivorous, pet food advertising emphasizes the carnivorous aspects of the canine diet ("meatier is better"). Many domesticated dogs eat vegetables, grains and pastas, meat, processed foods, various dairy products, and fruit. Some pet owners complain that their dogs eat grass and feces as well, though such behavior is natural. Application of cayenne pepper or hot sauce to feces has been helpful in reducing this objectionable behavior of dogs.

Because dogs range in size, age, and activity level, nutritional energy requirements are calculated based on the animal's metabolic body weight, or the weight of actively metabolizing tissue. Variations in body composition and breed are also considered. In addition, nutritional requirements should be based on a dog's particular life stage to achieve biologic performance and overall good health (Table 15-6).

The amount of food needed to meet the nutritional requirements of healthy dogs is calculated from the energy value of the food (see the discussion of energy-producing nutrients). Note that although most commercially prepared foods contain the nutrients essential for a particular life stage, each companion animal should be evaluated individually because of differences in both activity and environment. Regular weighing and body condition scoring will enable the technician to provide general feeding recommendations. If treats or table scraps are added to the staple diet, their energy content must also be taken into account when the technician calculates the amount of food to give.

The frequency of feeding normal dogs may vary. Most adult dogs in the maintenance life stage can obtain daily energy requirements by eating once a day, or two to three times a day to coincide with family meal times. Feeding dogs in the late evening should be avoided so that the owner is not inconvenienced by having to take the dog outside to eliminate in the middle of the night. In addition, large meals should be avoided before exercise, particularly in large-breed dogs, so that the risk of gastric dilation and torsion is minimized.

TECHNICIAN NOTE

Large meals should be avoided before exercise, particularly in large-breed dogs, so that the risk of gastric dilation and torsion is minimized.

CANINE PEDIATRIC NUTRITION

Milk provides a complete food source for neonates; it contains water, protein, fat, vitamins, and minerals. Colostrum is the key nutritional factor immediately after birth. Owners should ensure that the dam is producing colostrum and that the puppies are consuming it. This is particularly pertinent if the bitch delivered the puppies via cesarean section.

Table 15-6 NUTRIENT GUIDELINES FOR WELLNESS*

Life Stage	Energy kcal ME/g	Protein	Fat	Fiber	Calcium	Phosphorus	Sodium
				Dry Matter			
DOG							
Growth/reproduction	3.5-5.0	22-35	10-25	5 max	0.7-1.7	0.6-1.3	0.35-0.6
Large-breed growth	3.0-4.0	22-35	8-12	10 max	0.7-1.2	0.6-1.1	0.3-0.6
Adult maintenance	3.5-4.5	15-30	10-20	5 max	0.5-1.0	0.4-0.9	0.2-0.4
Obesity prone	3.0-3.5	15-30	7-12	5-17	0.5-1.0	0.4-0.9	0.2-0.4
High energy	>4.5	22-34	26 min	5 max	0.5-1.0	0.4-0.9	0.2-0.5
Geriatric†	3.5-4.5	15-23	7-15	10 max	0.5-1.0	0.2-0.7	0.15-0.35
CAT							
Growth/reproduction	4.0-5.0	35-50	18-35	5 max	0.8-1.6	0.6-1.4	0.3-0.6
Adult maintenance	4.0-5.0	30-45	10-30	5 max	0.5-1.0	0.5-0.8	0.2-0.6
Obesity prone	3.3-3.8	30-45	8-17	5-15	0.5-1.0	0.5-0.9	0.2-0.6
Geriatric†	3.5-4.5	30-45	10-25	10 max	0.6-1.0	0.5-0.7	0.2-0.5

Max, maximum; *min*, minimum; *C*, cup.

*Nutrients are expressed as % dry matter. Energy is expressed as kcal metabolizable energy (ME) per gram dry matter.

†Older animals require frequent body condition scoring. Feed intake adjustment may be required to maintain an ideal body condition because some older individuals tend to be heavy and others tend to lose weight.

Average Caloric Content of Pet Foods
Dog food (generic, private label, grocery)
- Dry — 350 kcal/C
- Soft-moist — 275 kcal/C
- Canned — 500 kcal/14- to 15-oz can

Cat food (generic, private label, grocery)
- Dry — 300 kcal/C
- Soft-moist — 250 kcal/C
- Canned — 180 kcal/5.5- to 6.5-oz can

Colostrum provides fluid for vital postpartum circulatory expansion and carries protective maternal antibodies, which are absorbed through the intestines of the puppies.

Most puppies are healthy and capable of active nursing. Ensure that the mothers are lactating well and are attentive to their litters. In general, no assistance is needed from the technician or owner. Exceptions may include extremely small, toy-breed puppies for which frequent, assisted hand feedings may be needed to prevent hypothermia and hypoglycemia.

Technicians should advise clients to weigh their puppies if there is concern about poor milk production by the dam or inadequate consumption of milk by the pups. Examination and expression of the mammary glands is also helpful in assessment of milk production. Regular checks are important to ensure good milk flow and to allow early detection of mastitis or other mammary gland complications.

The normal growth rate for puppies is 2 to 4 g/day per kilogram of anticipated adult weight. Weight gain below this rate, especially when puppies are restless and seem to be hungry, is generally a sign that the puppies are not receiving adequate amounts of milk.

> **✎ TECHNICIAN NOTE**
>
> The normal growth rate for puppies is 2 to 4 g/day per kilogram of anticipated adult weight.

FEEDING ORPHAN PUPPIES

Neonatal puppies that are unable to nurse should be fed a canine milk replacement formula. Canine milk is higher in protein and lower in lactose than bovine milk; consequently, water—and not cow's milk—should be used to mix the replacement formula.

The orphan formula dose is initially 15% of the puppy's weight per day divided into several doses. The process of feeding puppies can be facilitated by using a syringe and a flexible, rubber feeding tube (Figure 15-6). Small amounts of food should be given incrementally until the puppies become content. Satiation is often indicated when the puppies become quiet and fall asleep. If there is adequate nursing vigor, a pet nurser system may be used. Before the litter of puppies is discharged, the veterinary technician should pretest the flow rate from each of the nipples, and give explicit instructions for keeping the system clean. When the puppy reaches 2 to 3 weeks of age, the food dose should approximate 25% of the body weight divided into four to six daily feedings. Monitoring weight gain by the use of a gram scale is a good way to evaluate food intake.

Low birth weight is correlated with an increase in mortality rate. Puppies with low body weights are more prone to hypoglycemia, hypothermia, and sepsis. The bitch should also be monitored for behavior changes toward any particular pup, because the bitch may shun hypothermic and ill puppies. Because body fat is generally low in puppies in general, the environment should be kept between 84° and 90° F. The use of heating pads is recommended, but only if both mother and pups have adequate space in which to crawl away from the heat source if necessary.

Urination and defecation should be monitored in the pediatric animal as well. Normally, the mother's licking and washing of the anogenital region stimulates elimination; a Q-tip or moist cotton ball can be used to simulate the mother's tongue. Monitor for diarrhea and recognize that infant stool is normally very loose but should never be watery.

> **✎ TECHNICIAN NOTE**
>
> The orphan formula dose is initially 15% of the puppy's body weight per day divided into several doses.

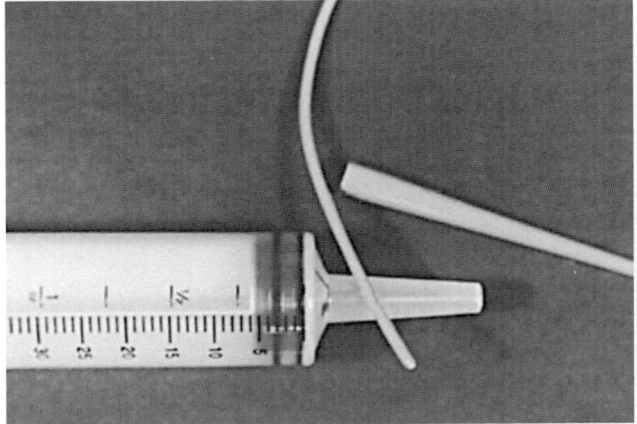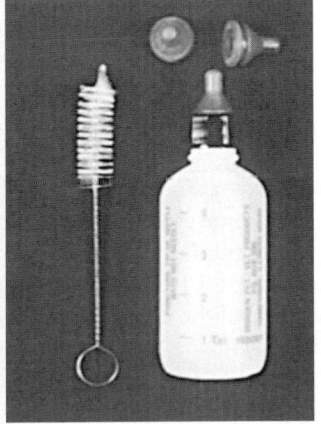

Figure 15-6 **A,** Orphan puppies and kittens are raised on species-specific milk replacement. Tube lavage with a flexible feeding tube and a catheter-tip syringe is an easy and safe technique for feeding neonatal puppies and kittens. **B,** Pet nursers are used in neonates with adequate sucking vigor. Always test the flow and temperature of formula in advance and sanitize equipment between uses.

WEANING PUPPIES

Peak lactation occurs at 4 weeks, and weaning concludes at 6 to 8 weeks. Begin introducing puppies to semisolid gruel made from 2 parts of water to 1 part high-quality, dry canine growth/lactation pet food. Three weeks of age is a suitable time to introduce a semisolid gruel, except in toy breeds and weak animals, which need more time before being offered solid food. Gruel can be finely chopped or mashed and placed in a shallow bowl for easy consumption. This serves as an important transition food and acclimates puppies to eating solid food. At 5 weeks of age, puppies are reducing their intake of mother's milk and are consuming larger amounts of gruel. The ratio of water can be reduced as the puppies are slowly moved from a semisolid to a solid food. After weaning, the ability of pups to digest lactose becomes less efficient. Consequently, it is important to avoid feeding weaned dogs large quantities of milk, which might cause diarrhea.

FEEDING GROWING DOGS

Proper nutrition for growing dogs is essential for normal growth and development. Excessive intake, however, can lead to medical complications. Overfeeding, for example, can result in obesity in small breeds and rapid growth rates in large-breed dogs. Inciting stress on the juvenile skeleton by overfeeding in the large breeds can cause abnormalities such as osteochondritis, hip dysplasia, panosteitis, and wobbler syndrome. Nutritional requirements change rapidly during a puppy's growth, with growth rates varying among breeds. Nutrient guidelines for small- and medium-breed versus large- and giant-breed dogs are listed in Table 15-6. Supplements are generally not needed if the puppies are fed name-brand commercial diets.

Most growing puppies eat four or five times daily during the postweaning period, or until about 10 weeks of age. Meal frequency should be cut to three meals a day until they have reached approximately 50% of their adult body weight, or approximately 4 months of age. Technicians should advise pet owners to feed small meals several times a day and not allow the puppies continuous access to food, because many puppies will overeat when fed ad lib.

GROWING CONCERNS FOR LARGE-BREED DOGS

Calcium and dietary fat are key nutrients for growing puppies. Unfortunately, some growth-type pet foods contain excessive amounts of calcium even at appropriate levels of dry matter intake. A study of two populations of Labrador retriever puppies examined the effects of nutritional excess. One group ate ad lib, and the second group was limited to 75% of the ad lib quantity. Serial pelvic radiography for 2 years showed significant reductions in hip laxity in the meal-limited group.

To help control the risk of abnormal orthopedic development in large- and giant-breed puppies, experts recommend that the calorie content be less than that for smaller breeds and contain no more than 12% fat on a dry matter basis.

FEEDING ADULT DOGS

The primary objective in feeding the adult dog is to find the maintenance energy requirement and proper food dose to maintain the ideal body composition. Recommended nutrient guidelines for adult dogs can be found in Table 15-6. Note that in the adult dog, ad lib feeding is commonly associated with overconsumption and obesity.

The amount of feed needed to meet energy requirements is based on the energy value of the food. Activity levels also vary among dogs and should be taken into consideration when a feeding protocol is compiled. In addition, environment plays a key role in energy expenditure. Regular weighing

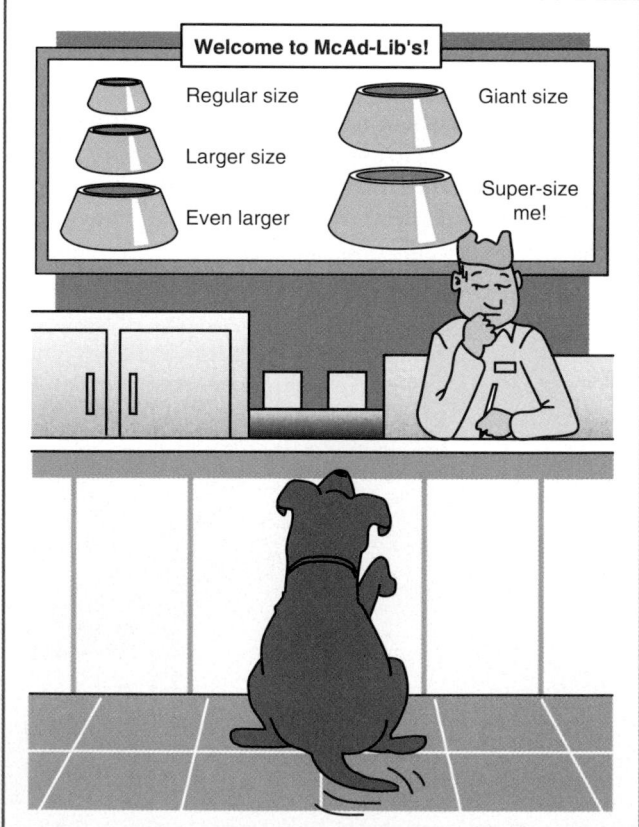

Figure 15-7 Ad lib feeding means an excess of food, at all times, for self-feeding.

and body condition scoring will allow both technician and owner to assess the adequacy of feeding. Note that after an animal has been spayed, energy requirements may be decreased 10%; consequently, adjustments in diet may be necessary to prevent weight gain.

Feeding each pet separately is best whenever possible (Figures 15-7 to 15-9). In the time-restricted method, feed each dog from one to three times daily with ad lib consumption for 5 to 15 minutes. If the dog consistently leaves a little food in its dish and also maintains an ideal body condition, the conclusion must be that the animal is self-regulating its food intake at its energy requirement.

Time-restricted feeding works well for many dogs and their owners; however, some dogs ravenously overeat during the allotted time. In dogs that overeat, try volume-restricted meal feeding by serving a calculated food dose. To determine the daily volume, divide the energy requirement by the food's caloric density. Then feed one half to one third of the daily volume two or three times per day. An average caloric density guideline for pet foods is listed in Table 15-6. Other aids for calculating how much food to feed are the feeding instructions found on the pet food label, food dose calculators, and technical information from manufacturers.

Maintenance pet food is recommended for the average house pet who is 1 to 7 years of age.

Table foods should be eliminated or used in moderation (10% or less). Fat trimmings quickly unbalance a bare diet and lead to finicky behavior and a predisposition to obesity. Avoid feeding animal bones because sharp fragments may wedge between teeth, lacerate the esophagus, or cause GI obstruction or constipation. Nylon bones and chew toys are safer substitutes for natural bones but still cause problems in some individuals. Table 15-6 lists guidelines for assessing pet foods used in life-stage feeding.

It is best for each dog to be fed individually; however, because of time and labor costs, this may be impractical in animal colonies and kennels. Refer to Box 15-7 for the Do's and Don'ts of Feeding. Problems associated with group feeding include anorexia in the timid animal and overconsumption in the aggressive or dominant dog. In addition, it is common for the boarded animal to be stressed or compromised and to stop eating as a result. Late detection of anorexia may lead to significant medical consequences for animals that do not have adequate intake. Technicians should frequently assess the appetite of boarding animals and feed on an individual basis.

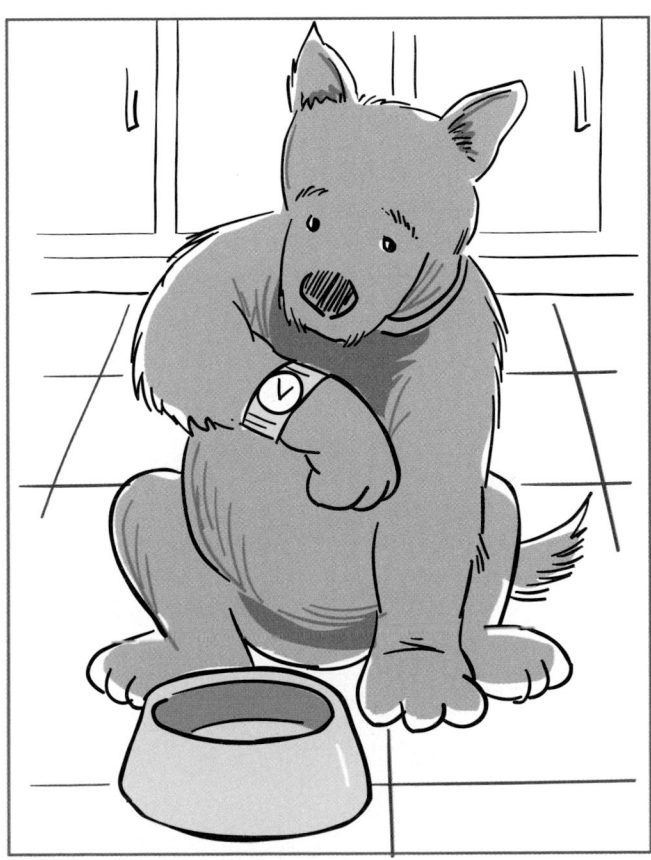

Figure 15-8 Time-controlled feeding provides an unrestricted food quantity in a set period.

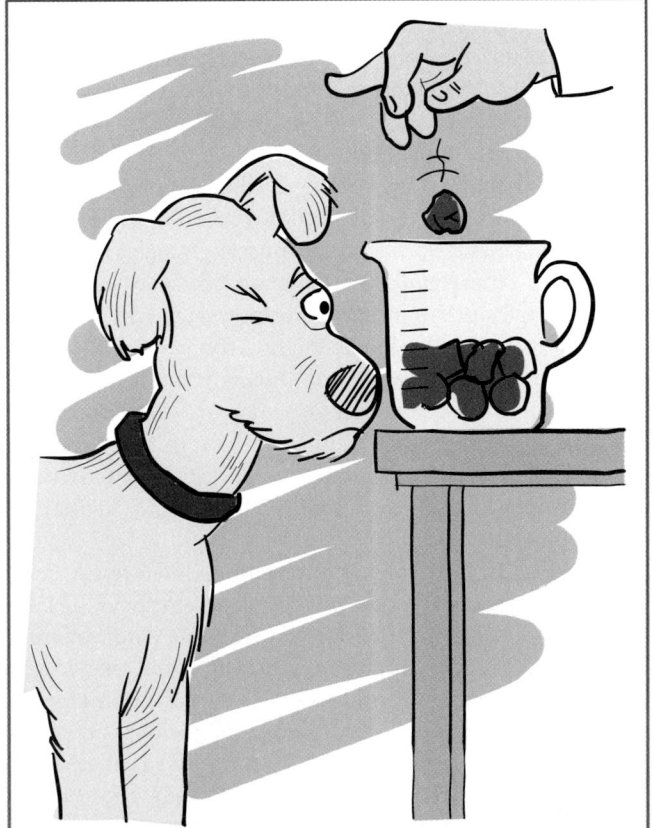

Figure 15-9 Portion-controlled feeding involves the measurement of pet food and providing it in a quantity that maintains optimum body condition.

Box 15-7 FOOD DIGESTIBILITY

Nutrient food−Nutrient feces
Nutrient food × 100% = % Nutrient digestibility

TECHNICIAN NOTE

Avoid feeding animal bones because sharp fragments may become wedged between teeth, lacerate the esophagus, or cause GI obstruction or constipation. Nylon bones and chew toys are safer substitutes for natural bones, but they may still cause problems in some individuals.

FEEDING ADULT DOGS WITH INCREASED ENERGY NEEDS

Increases in physical activity require extra energy to support increased muscle action. Diet and feeding protocols vary according to training schedules and amount of work performed. Supplying extra energy to working dogs by using pet foods with increased fat, caloric density, and digestibility will allow optimal performance. In addition, feeding diets with extra energy content allows dry matter intake and gastric fill to remain at familiar, nonexcessive levels. Increasing the quantity or frequency of a regular food is a secondary option to increase performance.

The specific nutrient composition of diets for working dogs varies and depends on the type of activity performed. In general, staples include fats and carbohydrates for intense muscular exercise. Note that in the sprinting or racing dog, short and intense bursts of energy are required and are typically obtained from readily available muscle glycogen stores. Large quantities of carbohydrates may be useful, because this may help maximize muscle glycogen reserves.

On the other hand, diets high in carbohydrates may be counterproductive in other working dogs and may even reduce athletic performance. High-carbohydrate diets may lead to lactic acid accumulation during prolonged exercise, resulting in muscle fatigue and/or damage. Therefore dogs engaged in activity that requires endurance may benefit from higher-fat diets, because their muscle activity is powered primarily by aerobic fatty acid oxidation (approximately 70% to 90%).

Animals can be aerobically conditioned before extensive fieldwork. Aerobic training increases the efficiency of fatty acid metabolism in the muscles and the cardiovascular system. Such aerobic conditioning spares the rate of glycogen consumption in muscles and increases the capacity for work. At the start of aerobic conditioning, technicians can advise clients to slowly convert the dog to a more calorie-dense food and suggest feeding the majority of daily calories after completion of training to help prevent hypoglycemia. This is particularly pertinent in hunting dogs.

Unfortunately, most clients feed the calorie-dense food before work or training. Subsequently, after digestion of such a meal, insulin is released as a result of glucose absorption, allowing for a high rate of glucose transfer into the cells. If the animal simultaneously begins hard work, the combination of the two glucose-consuming activities may precipitate hypoglycemia. If working dogs show consistent signs of hypoglycemia, even after conditioning, they may be fed 10% to 15% of the daily calorie dose as a light feeding at 2-hour intervals during work. Clients should also be reminded of the importance of adequate water intake throughout the work period.

FEEDING DURING PREGNANCY AND LACTATION

During lactation, proper nutrient intake is directly linked to successful milk production (Figure 15-10). Technicians should recommend a growth/lactation formula to meet the increased requirements. Lactation markedly increases energy, protein, and mineral requirements; nutrient requirements during lactation are greater than at any other adult life stage. After whelping, the bitch returns to her regular body weight and eats to meet increased needs (Figure 15-11). Expect food intake to rise rapidly by 50% the first week and by 200% to 400% by the fourth week of lactation. Free choice food should be available to the bitch. Water intake should also be monitored, because water is the most important nutrient during lactation. After whelping, energy requirements return to maintenance levels in approximately 8 weeks. Frequent physical examinations should be performed to maintain normal health and to assess adequacy of diet.

Key nutritional factors in the lactating bitch include highly digestible protein, increased concentrations of fat (in proportion with other nutrients), 10% to 20% soluble carbohydrates, and approximately two to five times more calcium than during the maintenance life stage (Table 15-7). Supplements are generally *not* needed for normal animals when high-quality pet foods are used.

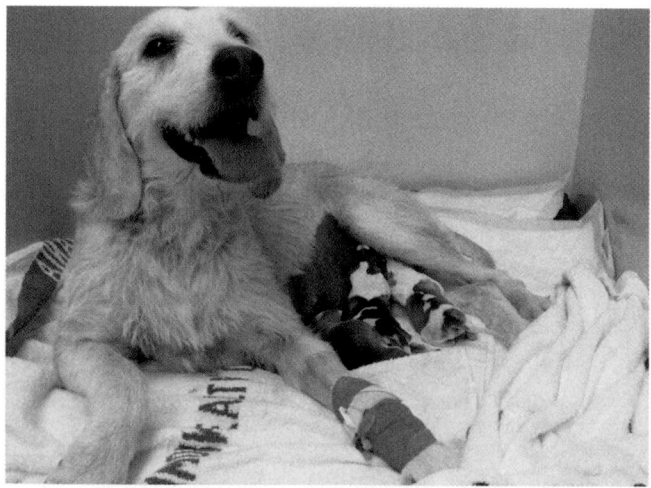

Figure 15-10 Mom and newborn puppies.

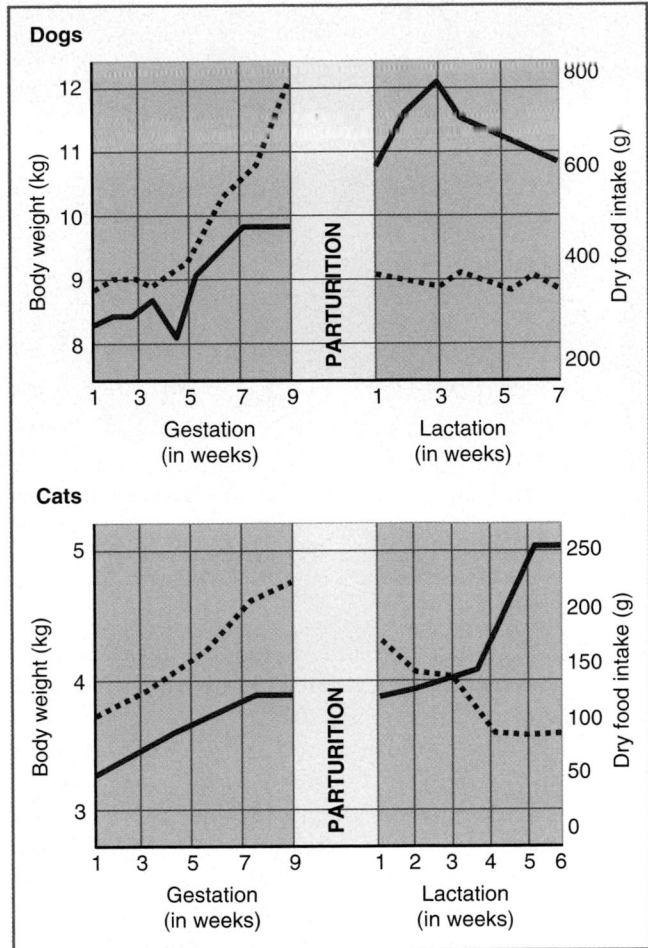

Figure 15-11 The pattern of normal weight gain during gestation and loss in the postpartum and lactation periods differs between cats and dogs. *Solid line* indicates food intake. *Dashed line* indicates body weight.

FEEDING METHODS DURING WEANING

Food intake should be terminated for 24 hours to help the bitch slow and stop milk production. Restricting food will reduce nutrients needed for milk production, resulting in mammary gland reduction. Technicians should advise clients not to allow any puppies to nurse, because such practices do not alleviate mammary gland engorgement and may stimulate milk production.

Food intake for the bitch can be resumed with maintenance foods at one third of the customary maintenance level. On the second day, two thirds of the normal feeding dose is recommended, with full intake on day 3. Because lactation quickly ceases as a result of acute calorie deprivation, the bitch will more readily reject the puppies' attempts to continue to nurse.

OBESITY-PRONE ANIMALS

DEFINITION, CAUSES, AND HEALTH RISKS OF OBESITY

The incidence of obesity in companion animals is almost epidemic. Canine and feline obesity estimates are approximately 25% and can vary within age-groups. Recent studies

---

Table 15-7 KEY NUTRITIONAL FACTORS FOR REPRODUCTION

Factors	Recommended Levels in Food (Dry Matter)	
	Gestation/Lactation*	Lactation†
Energy density (kcal ME/g)‡	3.5-4.5	4.5-5.0
Energy density (kJ ME/g)‡	14.6-18.8	16.7-20.9
Crude protein (%)	22-32	25-35
Crude fat (%)	10-25	≥18
Soluble carbohydrates (%)	≥23	≥23
Calcium (%)	≤5	≤5
Phosphorus (%)	0.75-1.5	1.0-1.7
Ca/P ratio (%)	1:1-1.5:1	1:1-2:1
Sodium (%)	0.35-0.60	0.35-0.60
Chloride (%)	0.50-0.90	0.50-0.90
Digestibility	Above average	Above average

From Hand MS et al, editors: *Small animal clinical nutrition*, ed 4, Topeka, Kan, 2004, Mark Morris Institute.

*Gestation for all bitches and for lactation of bitches with four or fewer puppies.

†Lactation for bitches with litters of more than four puppies. Some giant-breed bitches may need this type of food during gestation to maintain body weight, particularly during late pregnancy.

‡If the caloric density of the food is different, the nutrient content in the dry matter must be adapted accordingly.

by the American Veterinary Medical Association estimate that approximately 28 million dogs and cats are overweight or obese (Box 15-8) (Jewell, 2000).

Among dogs and cats, certain factors contribute to clinical obesity, including genetic background, high-calorie diets and snacks, physical inactivity, presence of endocrine or neuroendocrine disorders, and gonadectomy. By definition, obesity means a body composition with a ratio of too much fat to lean tissue, or body weight 15% to 20% greater than optimal (Figure 15-12).

Early detection in breeds that are prone to obesity is important in preventing and treating the condition. Veterinary technicians can play a vital role in recommending feeding regimens, exercise strategies, and educating the client on the health risks of obesity. Routine weighing, body condition scoring, and counseling of clients during routine examinations can further benefit patient health.

TECHNICIAN NOTE

Canine and feline obesity estimates are approximately 25% and can vary within age-groups.

A primary cause of obesity is overfeeding during growth life stages. A positive calorie balance during juvenile growth may induce increased numbers of fat cells (hyperplasia). Once formed, these fat cells are present for life and certain minimal volumes of triglyceride. Thus they can shrink but cannot disappear. (Crane, 1991). Therefore a lifelong predisposition for excess weight develops. Adipocyte hyperplasia is prevented by using meal feeding (as opposed to ad-lib feeding) for puppies, kittens, and foals.

Overeating during maintenance life stages is another factor contributing to obesity. Consuming more energy than is expended can lead to excess body fat. In addition, feeding the picky eater table food and other diets high in fat contributes significantly to obesity. Excess dietary fat is typically stored as body fat, with storage capabilities almost limitless. Volume-restricted meals and the elimination of calorie-rich treats is recommended to prevent obesity. Adult pets can be fed high-fiber, low-fat treats if providing snacks is important to the pet owner.

A third cause of obesity is genetic predisposition. Evidence has linked genetic inheritance with resting metabolic rates (Crane, 1991). Breeds at greater risk include the Labrador retrievers, Cairn terriers, Cocker spaniels, long-

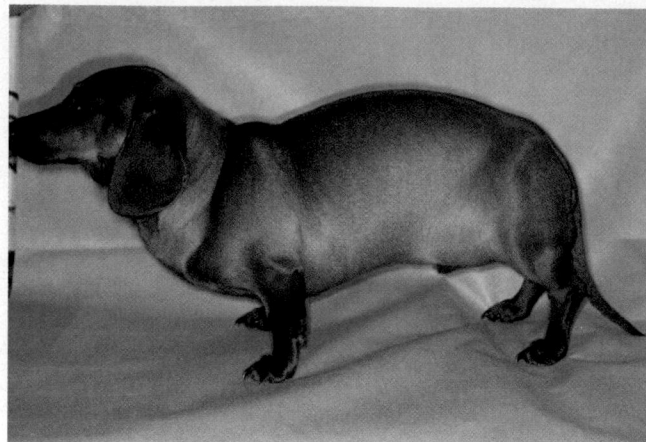

Figure 15-12 Obese dachshund. Once formed, fat cells are present for life, though they can shrink. Animals that eat too much as juveniles experience fat-cell division and are subsequently predisposed to excess weight gain throughout their lives.

haired Dachshunds, Shetland sheepdogs, Basset hounds, and Beagles. Mixed-breed cats tend to be more overweight than purebred cats (McIntosh, 2000).

Another cause of obesity is a declining lean body mass and declining activity level during normal aging processes. Decreases in energy requirements may be considered in a geriatric feeding program (Markham and Hodgkins, 1989). As pets become older and less active, lean body mass is reduced. Goals for maintaining optimal nutrition in the geriatric animal include avoiding food types with excessive protein, phosphorus, and sodium chloride. Refer to the discussion of feeding the geriatric pet in this chapter.

Competitive eating may also provoke obesity. Multi-animal households or other group-feeding situations may necessitate volume-restricted feeding and separation of the competitive individuals during feeding.

Surgical neutering of males and females can also alter metabolism, deregulate satiety, and increase the desire to feed. The technician may recommend less calorie-dense foods concurrent with suture removal after neutering, particularly in obesity-prone breeds.

HEALTH RISKS OF OBESITY

The health risks of obesity are numerous. Among the most common are the following:

- ✓ Coronary heart disease
- ✓ Type 2 diabetes and insulin resistance
- ✓ Hypertension
- ✓ Pulmonary disorders
- ✓ Liver, kidney, and gallbladder disease
- ✓ Colon, ovarian, endometrial neoplasia
- ✓ Musculoskeletal diseases including joint stress, hip dysplasia, and osteoarthritis
- ✓ Muscular injuries including cranial cruciate ligament rupture

In addition, obese patients have a high risk for complications during anesthesia and are typically exercise and heat intolerant. Obese patients with ailments such as asthma, elongated soft palates, or laryngeal paralysis are even further compromised and often have higher mortality rates. In addition, obesity is a predisposing factor for hepatic lipidosis in cats and is associated with some endocrine diseases, such as hyperadrenocorticism, hypothyroidism, and diabetes mellitus. Thus chemistry and endocrine profiles, in the obese animal, can be particularly important in identifying compounding disorders. Because obesity is such a common disease among pets, clients should be made aware of the many health risks associated with it. Obesity-related disorders can be prevented or delayed with proper feeding and exercise regimens.

✎ TECHNICIAN NOTE

Obese animals have a high risk for complications during anesthesia and are often intolerant of exercise and high ambient temperatures.

DIAGNOSIS AND TREATMENT OF OBESITY

Assessment of obesity among dogs and cats can be accomplished by examining the quantity of subcutaneous fat deposits visually and by palpation over the ribs, groin, and tail head. Radiographs of the abdomen and thorax will also reveal fat accumulations. Weighing the animal indirectly measures body composition and using ideal weight tables for preanesthesia calculations is useful. Body condition scoring (Figure 15-5) is a visual and useful method for combining various assessment criteria into an opinion regarding the pet's body composition and relative fatness. The dietary history should always be included in the patient history.

Specific treatment for obesity requires teamwork among the owner, the veterinarian, and the technician. In general, dietary recommendations include feeding calorie-restricted, low-energy foods. Certain food types with increased dietary fiber provide satiety and aid in weight reduction. In addition, feeding a diet high in fiber can reduce total energy intake and improve blood glucose and lipid levels. Clients should be continually reminded of the benefits of weight control, because the process can be both slow and frustrating. The veterinary technician can be a critical support person for the pet owner who is enforcing a pet weight reduction program at home. The technician should recommend to the owner a realistic time frame for weight loss so that frustration is minimized and the weight reduction goal is more likely to be reached and maintained. An important part of a pet weight reduction program is the restriction of supplemental calories in the form of treats, including both human snack foods and commercial pet treats (Tables 15-4 and 15-5). This concept must be especially stressed to the owner who is easily influenced by a begging pet with a plaintive expression.

FEEDING THE GERIATRIC ANIMAL

The definition of geriatric, as it pertains to the dog, is not precise because of breed variability. In general, toy and small-sized breeds are geriatric at 9 years, medium-sized dogs at 8 years, and large and giant breeds as early as 6 years of age.

Geriatric pets undergo physiologic changes similar to those experienced by elderly humans. Older animals, for example, have a higher incidence of multiple organ failure, benign and malignant tumor formation, osteoarthritis, dental disease, and loss of hearing and vision. Unfortunately, no specific diet or nutrient formula can delay the onset of disease or slow down the aging process. However, the dietary practices in the first three fourths of an animal's life can have an impact on the nutritional consequences manifested in the last part of its life (Burkholder, 1999).

Nutritional recommendations for the geriatric pet should be influenced by individual body condition and health history. The ideal goal in geriatric animals is maintenance of optimal weight. Commercially available senior diets should be evaluated and only recommended based on the status of the animal. Dietary modifications should be considered if a particular disease state could be ameliorated by the absence or presence of a particular nutrient. Pet foods specifically intended for seniors emphasize moderate energy density with good palatability and reductions of some excess nutrients that are found in all-purpose pet foods.

Age-related behavioral changes such as disorientation, changes in interaction with the owner, disturbances in sleep, and loss of bladder or bowel control may be ameliorated by diets enhanced with antioxidant formulations (Head and Zicker, 2004). Specific therapeutic diets that may help combat the signs of brain aging and improve the learning ability of senior dogs are now available. Exclusive blends of antioxidants and other nutrient formulations help protect against free radical damage, improve cell membrane health, and optimize senior health.

Calorie control may begin or be continued in some older animals. However, blanket feeding recommendations based solely on age, without consideration of the individual, are unwise. For example, although many geriatric animals have a propensity to put on weight, there are many that lose weight. Weight loss may be a symptom of systemic illness, dental or oral pain, a failing sense of smell, or heightened finicky tastes or fixed food addictions.

RENAL DISEASE

As animals age, many of their organ systems function less efficiently. Chronic progressive renal disease, for example, is common in older dogs and cats. Unfortunately, there is no "quick fix" for chronic renal failure. However, dietary adjustments can slow down the progression of renal aging and prolong the life of a beloved pet.

Progressive loss of renal function can ultimately reduce the animal's ability to excrete phosphorus, urea, and other by-products of protein metabolism. Controlling excesses of intake during the geriatric periods does no harm, even in the absence of clinical signs of renal failure. Therefore the recommendation to avoid excessive protein, phosphorus, and sodium chloride seems medically prudent. In addition, cats with renal insufficiency have elevated potassium requirements. Commercial prescription diets are designed with these goals in mind and are readily available from a veterinarian.

FEEDING CATS

Cats are not "small dogs" and are physically, physiologically, and behaviorally made to be solo-hunting, carnivorous predators. Protein metabolism is unique in cats; typically, cats require a higher amount of protein in their daily diet as compared with dogs (see discussion of amino acids and protein).

Key nutritional factors for feeding cats include higher percentages of total dietary calories from an ideal protein source (biologic value of 100%), or approximately 8% in adult cats as opposed to roughly 4% in adult dogs. Carbohydrate metabolism is limited because of low liver glucokinase activity, making the feline liver unique in energy metabolism. In general, cats require high-protein, low-carbohydrate foods. Feeding dog food to cats for convenience or economy is ill advised because of the different nutritional composition. Feeding dog food to a cat will not specifically provide the required amount of fat and protein.

In addition, taurine is an eleventh essential amino acid in cats. It is absent in dog food. The Association of America Feed Control Officials has determined that dry feline foods must contain 1000 mg of taurine per kilogram and canned feline foods must contain 2000 mg of taurine per kilogram to prevent diseases associated with deficiencies. Most feline foods are now appropriately supplemented with taurine. Other feline-specific requirements include vitamin A, niacin, and pyridoxine. In addition, arachidonic (fatty) acids are not synthesized in the cat; consequently, arachidonic acids are required in the feline diet.

Although calculating energy requirements for cats in differing life stages can be useful, each pet should be examined individually, and nutritional recommendations should be made based on signalment, BCS, activity level, and medical and dietary histories. The technician should consider the influence diet has on oral health and the role that the texture of food can play in preventing dental disease. The palatability and acceptability of a particular food type is often influenced by offering foods at body temperature, particularly to hospitalized or ill felines (see discussion of clinical nutrition).

FELINE PEDIATRICS

Adequate colostrum intake for all kittens is critical and should be monitored immediately after birth. Like puppies,

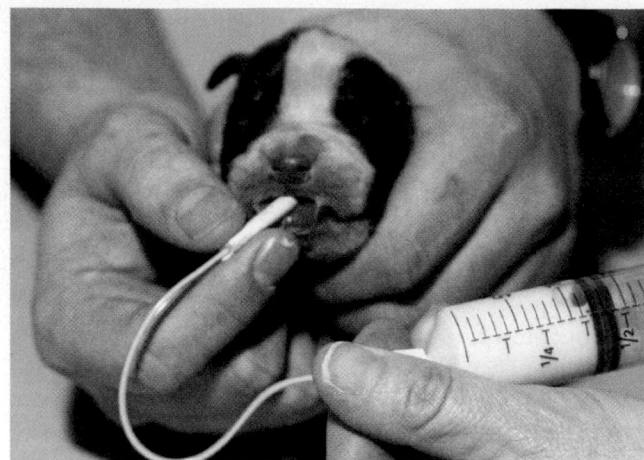

Figure 15-13 Tube feeding a neonate. Orphaned kittens can be given milk replacer by tube lavage.

orphaned kittens can be given milk replacer by tube lavage or pet nurser systems (Figure 15-13). It is important to ensure the correct placement of a gastric tube to prevent pulmonary aspiration. Stable environmental factors for pediatric felines are similar to those for pediatric canines; warm, dry bedding is paramount. Heating pads should cover only half the box so that kittens and mother can crawl away from the heat source if they become too warm. In addition, orphaned kittens may need assistance in urination and defecation, similar to orphaned puppies (see discussion of feeding orphaned puppies).

Kittens weigh between 85 and 120 g at birth and gain an average of approximately 100 g per week (McCune, 2003). Similar to canine pediatric care, the use of gram scales to monitor weight as an indicator for proper nutrient intake is recommended. Caloric needs for most puppies and kittens are 22 to 26 kcal per 100 g of body weight for the first 3 months of life. Feedings should be scheduled at least four times a day. In general, male kittens grow faster than females.

Formula should be warmed to about 100° F (37.8° C) before feedings. The initial feedings should have less volume (but not frequency) than those suggested on the lable. Over the next several days, gradually increase the volume of formula to the amount recommended on the label. Subsequent increases will be needed based on weight gain and satiation. Formula should be prepared according to label instructions, and all feeding equipment must be cleaned immediately after use.

Kittens are weaned later than puppies—generally at 7 to 9 weeks. Growth-sustaining kitten foods are fed two or three times daily until the kittens are 10 months of age.

✏️ **TECHNICIAN NOTE**

Kittens are weaned later than puppies—generally at 7 to 9 weeks.

ADULT CATS

During the adult maintenance life stage, it is recommended to feed a consistent diet and use a feeding schedule to eliminate finicky behavior and food aversion. The technician may encounter owners that vary food types in response to the great variety of cat food flavors on supermarket shelves. Providing a variety of flavors is unnecessary, and a transient "newness" factor can temporarily increase food intake and lead to weight fluctuations.

Most cat owners tend to feed ad lib. When allowed continuous access to food, cats usually eat small, frequent meals throughout the day. A common belief is that cats are better than dogs at maintaining their body condition. However, results of the latest epidemiologic studies no longer support this idea. When offered a highly palatable, high-fat diet, cats fed ad lib tend to overeat, especially if they are neutered or lead a sedentary lifestyle. A survey of 500 practitioners showed that while most clients were aware of the potential for weight gain in their neutered cats, only 10% of the veterinarians recommended that the cats be switched to a low-fat diet (Biourge, 2001).

Commercial feline treats are usually nutritionally synonymous with dry cat food (Table 15-5). As such, they are appropriate to be used as treats, but only if given in moderation. Some cat owners prefer "natural" treats, such as raw or cooked poultry necks, oxtails, or liver. Although little harm results from the use of these treats in moderation, finicky behavior and subsequent nutritional imbalance are potential hazards. Specifically, liver contains an inverted calcium/phosphorus ratio (1:17) and potentially toxic levels of vitamin A (hypervitaminosis A) can occur with long-term consumption.

Hairballs occur commonly in cats because of their meticulous grooming habits and the sharp barbs on their tongues, which increase the apprehension and consumption of hair. Hairballs are periodically regurgitated from the oropharynx or esophagus or vomited from the stomach. Occasionally, hairballs pass into the intestinal tract where they are voided in the feces. Owners may observe periodic gagging, retching, and regurgitation or vomiting of hair and mucus. Hairballs are often tubular and usually do not contain food or bile. Although hairballs do not usually cause significant clinical disease, they can be of concern to the owner. Many laxatives, lubricants, treats, and foods are available for routine management of these problems. Laxatives and lubricants should be used intermittently because large daily doses may interfere with normal digestion and nutrient absorption. Several complete and balanced moderate-fiber foods are now available for control of hairball problems in cats.

FEEDING CATS DURING GESTATION AND LACTATION

During the reproductive life stage, energy and nutrient requirements must support both queen and offspring during pregnancy, lactation, and milk production. At peak lactation, energy and nutrient requirements can be three to four times normal maintenance. Because providing larger amounts of food may not be feasible, owners can feed a diet that is more energy and nutrient dense, with increased digestibility to reduce bulk. It is important to advise clients that supplementation with vitamins and minerals is not necessary, as long as the queen is fed a balanced diet.

There are significant differences in food intake between the bitch and the queen during the initial stages of lactation (Figure 15-11). As a solitary hunter, the queen hunts less during the early part of lactation and uses the body fat stored during gestation to support her milk production. The practical significance here is that clients may question low food consumption in their new mother cats. Such clients can be advised that the queen will eat heavily, as expected, by the third week of lactation.

FEEDING GERIATRIC CATS

Evaluation of the geriatric individual is crucial in determining an appropriate food that will maintain a proper body weight and still provide adequate nutrient levels. In selecting the optimal diet for an older cat, overall health must be considered. Food intake should be monitored in association with changes in weight. Hyperthyroidism, for example, is characterized by chronic weight loss despite a ravenous appetite. Water intake should be noted, because increased frequency of drinking and urination may also be symptomatic of disease.

No single food can meet the needs of every geriatric cat. Dietary modification can help to optimize health in the healthy cat and to modulate disease in cats as they age. Significant protein restriction is not recommended in the healthy geriatric cat because of the high protein requirements in felines (see discussion of amino acids and proteins). Moderate restriction of protein is recommended for the cat with evidence of chronic renal failure (see discussion of clinical nutrition). Commercial diets with balanced nutrient contents for optimizing the health of the elderly cat are available. Oral hygiene is an important factor in feline geriatrics; routine dental examinations should be performed to ensure that there is no tooth pain and that food can be apprehended and chewed.

Similar to geriatric canine nutrition, certain dietary adjustments can help improve clinical signs or even slow progression of disease (see discussion of feeding the geriatric animal). The best diet, however, should be based on the individual cat's clinical signs, BCS, laboratory results, and stage of disease.

FELINE OBESITY

Feline obesity, like canine obesity, is a common nutritional problem. One important role of the technician is to educate the client and to encourage participation in weight reduction programs. A detailed dietary history is helpful for calculating the amount of food that will be offered during

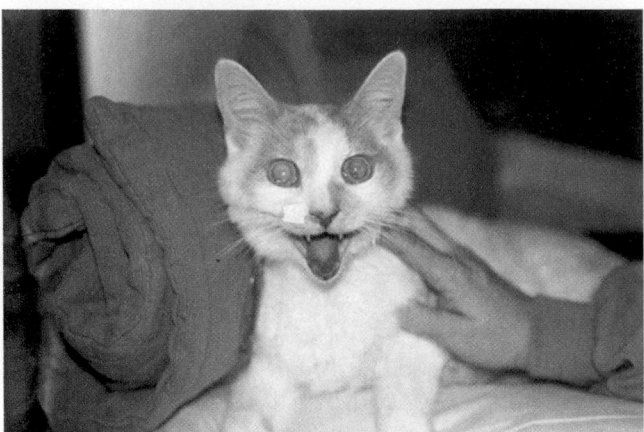

Figure 15-14 Fasting in obese cats has been associated with the accumulation of lipids in the liver, which in turn causes icterus.

a calorie-restricted diet. Fasting in obese cats is not recommended, because fasting has been associated with the accumulation of lipids in the liver. This can become pathologic over a 5- to 6-week period, and it mimics idiopathic feline hepatic lipidosis (Figure 15-14).

Obesity can be prevented if the veterinarian and the technician provide nutritional counseling during routine yearly examinations. In addition, owners of cats that are presented for gonadectomy should also be counseled as to the amount of food to be given after surgery to prevent excessive weight gain. Dietary therapy should only be instituted after a complete physical examination, biochemical profiling, and compilation of medical history. The client should be instructed to gradually introduce a new food over a period of 7 days. Obese cats that are given a new diet all at once may become anorexic.

Statistics show that cats being fed high-fat (±20%) premium and super-premium diets are two to three times more likely to become overweight. Conversely, cats being fed a diet containing around 10% fat are 50% less likely to be overweight. Dietary recommendations for feline obesity include feeding multiple small meals throughout the day to optimize digestive and absorptive energy expenditure. Traditionally, diets are composed of low-calorie, high-fiber substances. Recommendations for calorie restriction range from 50% to 80% of maintenance calories to achieve optimum weight (Burkholder, 2000).

Advanced nutritional technology has recently yielded prescription diets for overweight cats, as well as dogs. Such diets contain low-carbohydrate, high-protein formulas clinically proven to alter a cat's metabolism for effective weight loss. Addition of L-carnitine helps the feline patient lose weight while maintaining lean muscle mass and decreasing accumulation of fat in liver cells.

FELINE UROLITHIASIS AND LOWER URINARY TRACT DISEASES

The two most common calculi that occur in cats are struvite and calcium oxalate calculi, both of which can lead to lower urinary tract diseases. The amount and balance of mineral elements in the diet of a cat can have significant effects on the formation of urinary calculi. Other important factors in calculi formation include urinary pH, urine concentration, and high dietary magnesium levels.

Certain feline diets are formulated to induce acidic urine because of the addition of acidifiers such as methionine, ammonium chloride, and phosphoric acid. Struvite crystal formation is not possible at a urine pH below 6.5. Particular animal proteins and corn glutens found in feline diets can also promote acidic urine, as opposed to diets composed of vegetable proteins and mineral salts such as calcium carbonate, which promote the formation of alkaline urine.

Urine acidification is not without potential toxic effects. Excessive acidity can overpower the ability of the kidneys to excrete proteins and induce uncompensated metabolic acidosis. Consequently, chronic acidosis in cats can increase urinary potassium losses and could potentially slow growth, increase urine calcium excretion, and promote bone demineralization.

Acidifiers can also be toxic. Acidifying diets are recommended to safely prevent and manage struvite-related lower urinary tract disease. Technicians should consult with the veterinarian before recommending any acidifying diets. These diets are not recommended for kittens, because they are not formulated for growth and may interfere with bone formation.

Acidifying diets may also be contraindicated in the older cat; older felines are at higher risk for calcium oxalate urolith formation and renal insufficiency. No diet will promote the dissolution of calcium oxalate uroliths, but for the purpose of minimizing the risk of crystal formation, diets for mature and older cats should be formulated to induce higher urinary pH. Maintaining urine acidity (pH 6.2 to 6.4) and keeping magnesium intake at nonexcessive levels are prudent risk control measures for struvite crystalluria. Maintaining a more alkaline urine pH (6.4 to 6.8) while avoiding excess calcium, sodium, and magnesium is a prudent risk control measure for calcium oxalate crystalluria. It is also beneficial to increase the cat's water consumption. Feeding a canned food will decrease the cat's urine specific gravity and increase the overall volume of urine, thus decreasing the possibility of crystal formation.

Note that the main difference between canine and feline urolithiasis is that struvite uroliths are usually associated with urinary tract infections in the dog. Feline struvite uroliths are generally sterile. Bacteria such as staphylococci and other urease-producing organisms generally create an alkaline environment, which enhances the formation of struvite and other uroliths. Antibiotic therapy is therefore only recommended in patients with a positive urine culture.

✎ TECHNICIAN NOTE

Important factors that influence calculi formation include urinary pH, urine concentration, and high dietary magnesium levels.

It is an oversimplification to state that controlling urine mineral concentrations or pH always controls feline lower urinary tract disease (FLUTD). FLUTD syndrome is multifactorial; not all causative agents or combinations of contributory factors are presently known. The term idiopathic FLUTD is used in cats when there is no known cause. Potential causes of idiopathic FLUTD include viral infection, stress, and neurogenic inflammation. Idiopathic FLUTD is not well understood; however, water seems to be a key factor in controlling the recurrence of the disease. Canned and other high-moisture foods increase total urine volume and are the preferred products for cats with idiopathic FLUTD.

> **✎ TECHNICIAN NOTE**
>
> The FLUTD syndrome is multifactorial, and not all causative agents or combinations of contributory factors are presently known.

CLINICAL NUTRITION

Nutritional support during times of stress, disease, or injury has provided the hospitalized animal a greater chance for recovery. Failure to consider nutrition as an important therapeutic strategy to improve health can have tremendous negative consequences.

Clinical nutrition is a veterinary medical subspecialty with the objective of modifying the cause, progression, or end-stage effects of illness by applying specific nutrient profiles. Numerous nutrient profiles support various prophylactic and therapeutic applications in small animal patients and are summarized in Table 15-8, which provides a general guide for dietary therapy based on disease history.

NUTRITIONAL ASSESSMENT OF THE HOSPITALIZED PATIENT

The primary goal of nutritional assessment is to identify which patients are at risk for malnutrition. Because altered nutritional status is associated with adverse clinical outcomes, it is paramount to address the nutritional needs early in *every* hospitalized patient, particularly the critically ill or injured. Although clinical status alone may dictate the need for nutritional intervention, a thorough nutritional assessment consists of evaluating both clinical and biochemical data, including patient history, and a thorough physical exam including body weight and body condition scoring. A baseline nutritional assessment should be followed by serial assessments throughout the course of hospitalization.

The veterinary technician is in a crucial position to identify baseline data and ongoing changes in nutritional status, because the technician spends the most time with the patient. Baseline data include such physical exam findings as weight, BCS, hydration status, cardiopulmonary sounds,

body temperature, and a nutritional background on the patient. The owner or referring veterinarian must be questioned as to when the last complete meal or nutritional support was given, because intake is often impaired days before the initial visit to the veterinarian. Nutritional intervention is crucial to recovery and survival, and appropriate consideration as to the type and route of nutrition should be given based on the underlying disease process or diagnosis.

> **✎ TECHNICIAN NOTE**
>
> A thorough nutritional assessment consists of evaluating both clinical and biochemical data, including patient history and findings from a thorough physical exam including body weight and body condition scoring, hydration status, and cardiopulmonary sounds.

PATIENTS AT RISK FOR MALNUTRITION

Any patient that is anorexic or that has not had food or water for 3 days or longer is at risk for malnutrition. However, animals in danger of nutritional insufficiency include those with increased metabolic stress levels such as patients undergoing surgery, dehydrated patients, patients with sepsis, burn victims, patients with trauma or head injuries, patients with respiratory difficulties, and those with chronic vomiting or diarrhea.

In the healthy pet, short-term food deprivation results in quick adaptive mechanisms to maintain blood glucose levels. The body mobilizes its own tissue reserves to provide nutrients for basic physiologic processes while lowering the metabolic rate to reduce energy expenditure. Within a few days, fat becomes the major source of fuel. Unfortunately, not all cells can utilize fat stores; the brain, kidneys, and red blood cells require a continuous supply of glucose for energy. Tissue proteins are utilized to provide amino acids for glucose conversion.

In the ill or injured animal, such adaptive mechanisms are altered. During the initial shock of injury or illness, tissue perfusion is provided by intravascular fluid shifts in a compensatory fashion according to the severity of the patient's condition. Often, the initial metabolism is lowered as a result. After such fluid shifts are corrected and hemodynamic stability returns, the metabolism is accelerated to support healing and resistance to infection.

Hypermetabolic states increase both the resting energy expenditure and the rate of oxygen consumption. Hypermetabolic states result from increased catecholamine releases in order to increase fuel production. Unfortunately, the increased metabolic rate and subsequent catabolism rapidly exacerbate weakness in patients without nutritional support. Even more serious is the loss of visceral proteins such as serum proteins, immunoglobulins, and leukocytes needed to maintain immunocompetence to fight infection. The animal's nutritional requirements shift from those of an omnivore to those of an obligate carnivore requiring higher amounts of protein and fat. Chronically ill or injured patients not receiving nutritional support can experience a

Table 15-8 SUMMARY OF SMALL ANIMAL CLINICAL NUTRITION*

Disease	Objectives	Considerations	Product	Comments
Allergy, food				
Dog	Reduce antigen ingestion	Novel highly digestible protein source or protein hydrolysate Reduce total protein content Simplify food Distilled H$_2$O	Prescription Diet[†] Canine d/d or Canine z/d	8 to 10-wk trial period Avoid treats, snacks, access to other food sources, chewable medications, supplements
Cat		Same as dog except Control Mg^{2+} intake Provide taurine Control urine pH	Prescription Diet Feline d/d or Feline z/d	
Anemia	Support RBC production	↑ Iron, cobalt, and copper ↑ B complex vitamins ↑ Protein	Prescription Diet Canine p/d Feline p/d	Cat foods are suitable for dogs in acute care settings
Anorexia	Prevent protein/caloric malnutrition Stimulate appetite	Establish fluid/electrolyte balance Acid-base balance ↑ Protein and fat ↑ Micronutrients	Prescription Diet Feline/Canine a/d Canine p/d Feline p/d	
Ascites	Reduce fluid retention	Restrict sodium chloride	Prescription Diet Canine h/d, k/d Feline h/d, k/d	h/d = marked salt restriction k/d = moderate salt restriction
Bone loss and fracture healing	Correct deficiency of energy and protein	↑ Protein ↑ Energy Avoid supplementation	Prescription Diet Canine p/d Feline p/d	Extra dietary calcium does not increase rate of fracture healing
Cancer	Increase longevity and quality of life	↓ Soluble carbohydrate ↑ Fat and omega-3 fatty acids ↑ Arginine	Prescription Diet Canine n/d Canine/Feline a/d	Use in conjunction with chemotherapy or other forms of cancer therapy
Colitis	Normalize gastrointestinal motility Rebalance microflora Provide local healing factors	Feed small meals 3-6 times/day Control dietary antigens Vary levels of dietary fiber	Prescription Diet Canine w/d, i/d, d/d Feline w/d, d/d	
Constipation	Normalize gastrointestinal motility Maintain stool water Maintain stool bulk	>10% fiber	Prescription Diet Canine w/d Feline w/d	No table scraps or bones Increase exercise Encourage water intake Cats: keep litter box clean
Copper storage disease	Restrict copper intake	<1.2 mg copper/100 g dry diet	Prescription Diet Canine l/d	No table scraps or treats
Debilitation	Restore tissue, plasma, and nutrients	↑ Protein ↑ Fat ↑ Macronutrients and micronutrients	Prescription Diet Canine/Feline a/d	Assist feed if needed

Mg, Magnesium; *RBC*, red blood cell.

*Nutrients in table are expressed on a dry weight basis.

†Other North American therapeutic brands with wide distribution include CNM (Purina), VMD, Medi-Cal, and IVD Select Care (Heinz), Eukanuba Veterinary Diets (Iams), and Waltham Veterinary Diets (Mars)

Table 15-8 SUMMARY OF SMALL ANIMAL CLINICAL NUTRITION—CONT'D

Disease	Objectives	Considerations	Product	Comments
Developmental orthopedic disease	Reduce rapid growth	↓ Fat and energy density ↓ Calcium	Prescription Diet Canine p/d Large Breed	Avoid calcium-phosphorus supplements
Diabetes mellitus	Even rate of glucose absorption Consistent caloric intake	>10% fiber ↓ Soluble carbohydrates	Prescription Diet Canine w/d Feline w/d	Weigh animal frequently and note in medical record
Feline urolithiasis (struvite): Treatment	↑ Urine volume ↓ Urine pH (5.9-6.1) Restrict Mg^{2+}, Ca^{2+}, PO_4	↑ Caloric density ↓ P and Ca^{2+} Mg^{2+} >20 mg/100 Kcal ↑ Na^+	Prescription Diet Feline s/d	Dissolution is complete 1 mo after negative radiographs Recurrence is high if prevention is not implemented
Prevention	Maintain physiologic levels of urinary solutes and urine pH ↑ Caloric density	Urine pH (6.2-6.4) Mg^{2+} >20 mg/100 Kcal (0.1% DMB) ↓ P	Prescription Diet Feline c/d-s	In obesity, use calorie-restricted diets that maintain urine pH 6.2-6.4 (Prescription Diet w/d is suggested)
Feline urolithiasis (calcium oxalate): Prevention	↑ Urine volume ↓ Urinary Ca^{2+}, oxalate ↑ Urine pH	Urine pH (6.2-6.4) ↓ Protein ↑ Nonprotein calories ↓ P, Ca^{2+}, Na^+ Mg^{2+} <20 mg/100 Kcal	Prescription Diet Feline c/d-oxl	Monitor urinary crystalluria
Vomiting	Minimize gastric secretion Gastrointestinal rest	↑ Digestibility ↑ Caloric density	Prescription Diet Canine i/d Feline i/d	Frequent, small meals
Diarrhea, acute	Normalize gastrointestinal tract motility and secretion	Withhold food for 1-2 days Feed small amounts 3-6 times/day ↓ Fiber ↓ Sugar ↑ Digestibility	Prescription Diet Canine i/d Feline i/d	Electrolyte disturbances and dehydration are common
Eclampsia	Provide Ca/P in correct quantity and ratio prepartum	High digestibility of diet Balanced minerals/vitamins	Prescription Diet Canine p/d Feline p/d	Avoid supplementation
Flatulence	Decrease aerophagia Avoid food fermentation	Avoid milk or milk products Feed small meals 3-6 times/day ↑ Caloric density	Prescription Diet Canine i/d Feline i/d	Feed in a flat, open dish Avoid vitamin or fatty acid supplementation Separate competitive eaters
Gastric dilatation/bloat (postoperative)	Prevent gastric distension	Avoid exercise before and after feeding ↑ Digestibility of diet Small, frequent feedings	Prescription Diet Canine i/d	Diet form or type is NOT related to risk of occurrence or recurrence

Ca, Calcium; *DMB*, dry matter basis; *Mg*, magnesium; *Na*, sodium; *NH4*, ammonium; *P*, phosphorus; *PO*, phosphate; *RBC*, red blood cells.

Continued

Table 15-8 SUMMARY OF SMALL ANIMAL CLINICAL NUTRITION—CONT'D

Disease	Objectives	Considerations	Product	Comments
Renal failure	Reduce signs of uremia Slow progression of disease	↓ Protein (↑ biologic value of protein) ↑ Nonprotein calories ↓ Phosphorus and sodium Increase B complex vitamins	Prescription Diet Canine k/d Canine g/d Canine u/d Prescription Diet Feline k/d Feline g/d	Small meals 4-6 times/day Conversion to a protein-restricted diet may take 7-10 days Water available at all times
Canine urolithiasis (struvite): Treatment	↑ Urine volume ↓ Urine pH Restrict Mg^{2+}, NH_4^+, PO4	↓ Protein ↓ PO_4, Mg^{2+} ↑ Na^+ ↓ Urine pH (5.9-6.1)	Prescription Diet Canine s/d	Evaluate and treat urinary tract infection Average duration of stone dissolution is 36 days; follow-up via radiography
Prevention	Maintain physiologic level of urinary solutes and urine pH	Control protein excess ↓ Ca^{2+}, P, Mg^{2+} ↓ Sodium mildly ↓ Urine pH (6.2-6.4)	Prescription Diet Canine c/d	Monitor urine sediment for crystalluria and infection
Canine urolithiasis (ammonium urate): Prevention		↓ Protein ↑ Nonprotein calories ↓ Nucleic acids ↓ Ca^{2+}, P, Mg^{2+}, Na^+ ↑ Urine pH (6.7-7.0)	Prescription Diet Canine u/d	Drugs plus diet may be successful treatment Monitor urinary crystalluria Prevention may require long-term drug treatment
Canine urolithiasis (calcium oxalate and cystine): Prevention	↓ Urinary concentration of calcium oxalate or cystine	↓ Protein ↑ Nonprotein calories ↓ Ca^{2+}, P, Na^+, Mg^{2+} ↑ Urine pH (6.1-7.0)	Prescription Diet Canine u/d	Treatment by surgical removal Prevention by dietary management with or without drugs

Na, sodium; *P,* phosphorus; *Ca,* calcium.

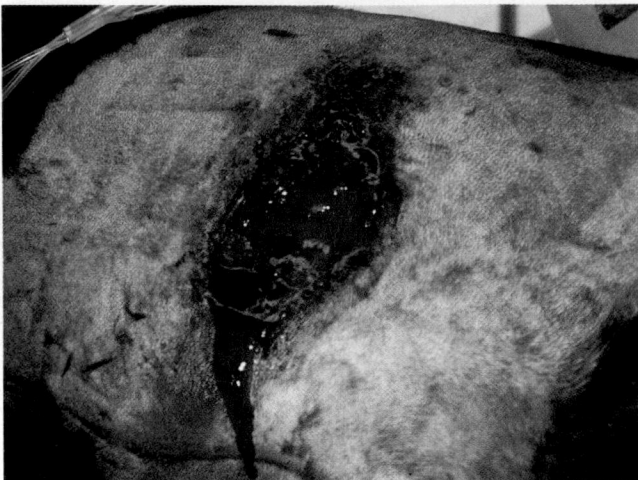

Figure 15-15 Undernourished patients are three times as likely to have major surgical complications such as wound dehiscense and poor healing.

> **Box 15-9** BENEFITS OF NUTRITIONAL SUPPORT IN THE DEBILITATED ANIMAL
>
> **PROTEIN**
> Helps maintain lean body mass
> Provides amino acids to support metabolism
> Promotes wound healing
> Enhances immune function
> Provides a source of fuel for muscle
>
> **FATS**
> Primary source of energy
> Provide essential fatty acids
> Modulate immune function
> Promote wound healing
>
> **VITAMINS AND MINERALS**
> Enhance cellular and humoral immunity
> Enhance the ability to taste and smell
> Provide antioxidants

cumulative tissue protein depletion state termed protein-energy malnutrition or PEM, which can have an adverse effect on recovery.

Undernourished patients are three times as likely as well-nourished patients to have major surgical complications. Wound dehiscence, decubital ulcers, sepsis, and pulmonary complications such as pneumonia are secondary to poor nutritional status (Figure 15-15). Pediatric patients are especially susceptible to malnutrition and often present with dangerously low blood glucose levels. In addition, the technician must always remember to monitor the appetite of healthy patients in boarding kennels, because they often become too stressed to eat and may go unnoticed until clinical signs are present.

Indications for nutritional support include recent weight loss of more than 10%, absent or poor food intake for more than 2 days, acute illness or injury, acute muscle wasting, and heavy GI or urinary system losses of protein or electrolytes. In addition, specific nutritional support is indicated if physical changes are accompanied by hypoalbuminemia, a BCS below the optimum value of 3, or surgical intervention or hospital procedures that may result in a reduction of oral intake over 3 to 5 days.

> **TECHNICIAN NOTE**
>
> Monitor the appetite of patients in boarding kennels, because they can become too stressed to eat and may go unnoticed until clinical signs are present.

FEEDING HOSPITALIZED SMALL ANIMAL PATIENTS

Patient Selection for Assisted Feeding

The technician frequently uses subjective global assessment (SGA) to determine nutritional status. SGA takes into consideration the dietary history, the body's condition scoring system (Figure 15-5), and the current morbidity index of the illness or injury. Body scoring is done by physical examination, with 0 = cachexia and 5 = obesity. Albumin and total protein levels and other markers for malnutrition decline with energy deprivation and protein-calorie malnutrition. However, these objective indicators change too slowly to be functional prognosticators, and the use of SGA permits functional, early clinical recognition of nutrient depletion and negative nitrogen balance. The most important outlook for the hospital is an awareness of the critical "need to feed" and the need to do so early. Taking steps to ensure that an animal feeds early in the course of treatment reduces catabolism and improves responses to virtually all other therapy.

The technician assesses daily needs and progress in conversation with both the veterinarian and other technicians by means of both patient progress notes and patient rounds. The clinical signs, the patient's desire and ability to eat, and the response to therapy can all change rapidly. Benefits of nutritional support in the debilitated animal are listed in Box 15-9.

ROUTES OF FEEDING

Enteral Versus Parenteral

The enteral route is the preferred method of feeding whenever possible, because this is the safest and least expensive route for providing nutrition. Enteral nutrition may be defined as the use of the upper alimentary tract (mouth, esophagus, stomach, and small intestine) for assisted feeding. There are four separate enteral feeding methods: coax feeding, appetite stimulation with drugs, forced oral feeding, and various tube administration techniques. Options for enteral feeding are listed in Table 15-9.

Table 15-9 OPTIONS IN ENTERAL FEEDING

Feeding Method	Objective	Technique	Advantage	Disadvantage
Owner hand feeding	Overcome partial anorexia	Hospital visit; bring favorite foods	Familiarity with food preferences should be explored	No effect in full anorexia
Temptation	Overcome partial anorexia	Use an unfamiliar food with strong odor	New odor may stimulate food exploration	No effect in full anorexia
Force feeding pet foods	Overcome partial anorexia	Bolus of moist food; mouth held to force swallowing	Food is complete and balanced	High handling stress Probably limited calorie intake
Forced feeding (calorie pastes)	Overcome partial anorexia	Administer flavored pastes from tube	Moderate handling stress	Pastes not complete food Limited calorie intake Severe protein restriction
Assisted feeding	Achieve full caloric intake Overcome partial anorexia	Oral syringing of specific formula	User and patient friendly Moderate handling stress High calorie intake Food given at rate for comfortable swallowing	Learned aversion if nauseous
Orogastric	Achieve full calorie intake	Intubate esophagus/stomach	Rapid administration No tube clogging Best for short-term use	High handling stress Intolerance to repeated feedings
Nasoesophageal	Bypass oral cavity and swallowing Achieve full caloric intake	Indwell 6-10 Fr. tube in nostril	Ease of intermediate use	Sedation/topical anesthesia Liquid food only
Pharyngostomy	Bypass oral cavity and swallowing Achieve full caloric intake	Indwell 16-28 Fr. tube in pharynx	None	General anesthesia required Mechanical interference with laryngeal function Possible gagging and vomiting Possible esophagitis
Esophagostomy	Bypass oral cavity and swallowing Achieve full caloric intake	12-18 Fr. tube in left lateral cervical esophagus	Easy to maintain and install Easy to "eat around the tube" Minimal risk of esophageal stricture	General anesthesia required
Gastrostomy	Bypass proximal gastrointestinal tract for full or partial caloric intake	16-28 Fr. tube placement at laparotomy Percutaneous endoscopic placement Nonendoscopic placement	Well-tolerated long term Effective and efficient	General anesthesia required Gastrocutaneous fistula forms in 5 days Wait 24 hr to use
Gastroduodenostomy	Bypass stomach	Duodenum cannulated via tube gastrostomy	Achieve full caloric intake	Loss of mechanical and chemical phases of gastric digestion May require endoscopic equipment
Jejunostomy	Bypass stomach and duodenum	10 Fr. tube through submucosal tunnel Anchor bowel and tube to body wall	Achieve full or partial caloric intake Predigested foods required to maximize nutrient delivery and minimize digestive work	Water transfer to gut lumen may cause cramping and diarrhea

Oral supplementation is recommended for the patient that can eat and has both normal digestion and absorption but simply cannot consume the amounts of calories and protein required. Examples include the orthopedic patient or burn victim, patients with mild anorexia, geriatric patients, and patients simply stressed from hospitalization. Enteral tube feedings are generally reserved for the patient who has digestive or absorptive capabilities but is unwilling to be or cannot be fed by mouth. Examples include patients with mandibular or maxillary fractures, oral tumors, megaesophagus, or laryngeal or pharyngeal weakness and patients that become too stressed to be force-fed. In addition, those patients that have profound cachexia or weakness may benefit from tube feeding until they are strong enough to consume their daily requirements without assistance.

The location and type of feeding tube depends on both the length of time feedings are anticipated and the type of injury or illness (see discussion of tube selection). Enteral feeding tubes commonly used in veterinary medicine include nasogastric, esophageal, nasoesophageal, gastronomy, and jejunal tubes. Nursing responsibilities usually include tube insertion (if surgery is *not* required), maintenance of the tube, and administration of the feedings.

Prevention of complications associated with each particular tube, including assessment of the patient during feeding, is vital to patient recovery. Other nursing responsibilities include daily bandage changes to inspect the insertion site for infection or migration and frequent flushing of the tube to prevent clogging. It is important to monitor for delayed gastric emptying of the feeding tube by aspirating the stomach contents before subsequent feedings (see discussion of administration techniques and tube selection).

TUBE SELECTION

A variety of enteral tubes can be used for patients who have at least some digestive and absorptive capabilities but are unwilling or unable to consume food by mouth. The location and type of feeding tube depends on the length of time feedings are anticipated, as well as the type of injury or illness. Types of intubation include nasogastric, nasojejunal, esophageal, pharyngeal, jejunal, and GI.

Nasogastric, nasojejunal, and jejunostomy tubes are most often used when there is danger of pulmonary aspiration, because the pyloric sphincter provides a barrier, which appears to lessen the risk of regurgitation and aspiration. Jejunostomy tubes also have the added advantage of being able to bypass an upper GI obstruction. Advantages of these tube types include ease of insertion, low cost, variability in size and length of the tubes, radiopaque insertion stylets, and fenestrated ends to facilitate ease of nutritional delivery. Disadvantages include limitations as to the type of diet administered; generally, the tube diameter is significantly smaller than other feeding tubes, and the use of thick enteral substances may precipitate clogging.

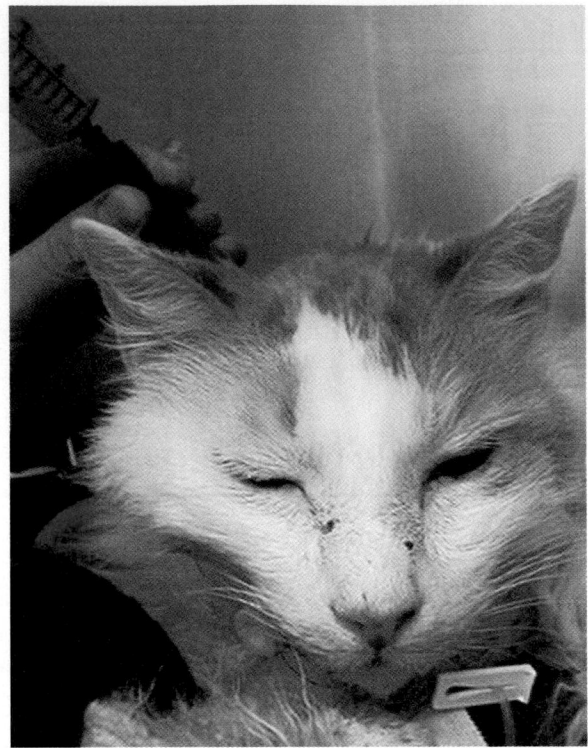

Figure 15-16 Feeding via an esophagostomy tube is well tolerated in cats.

Nursing responsibilities often include tube insertion (nasogastric and nasojejunal) in which proper techniques are critical. Technicians are often required to ensure patency after tube placement by radiographic examination. Before food administration, the tube should always be aspirated for negative pressure and proper gastric emptying to prevent gastric distension. Suturing is recommended in lieu of tissue glue, because nasal and skin erosion can occur.

Other types of enteral devices include pharyngeal, esophagostomy, and GI tubes. Usually intended for the patient requiring long-term nutritional support, these types of feeding tubes have the general disadvantage of the need for local anesthesia. Relatively inexpensive, these specialty tubes generally require the same type of nursing care as other enteral feeding tubes. A wide range of diet formulations can be used because of the ease of administration, facilitated by larger tube diameters (Figures 15-16 and 15-17). In addition, placement of such long-term enteral devices allows the patient to be discharged sooner, because clients can often administer prepared diets at home with minimal effort.

Regardless of tube type, careful attention to both tube maintenance and administration of feeding solutions can prevent many complications. Maintenance of the tubes requires regular irrigation to maintain patency, particularly after feedings. Canned loaf diets should be blenderized and strained, particularly with smaller-diameter tubes (see discussion of administration techniques). Moist

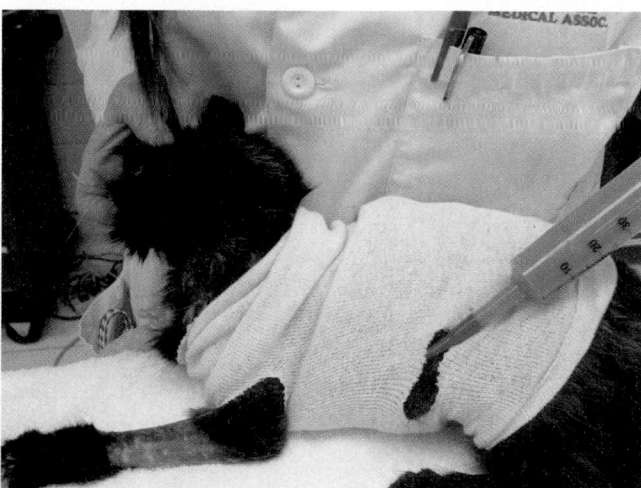

Figure 15-17 Gastronomy tube feeding of an anorectic cat. A larger range of diet formulations can be used because of the ease of administration, facilitated by larger tube diameter.

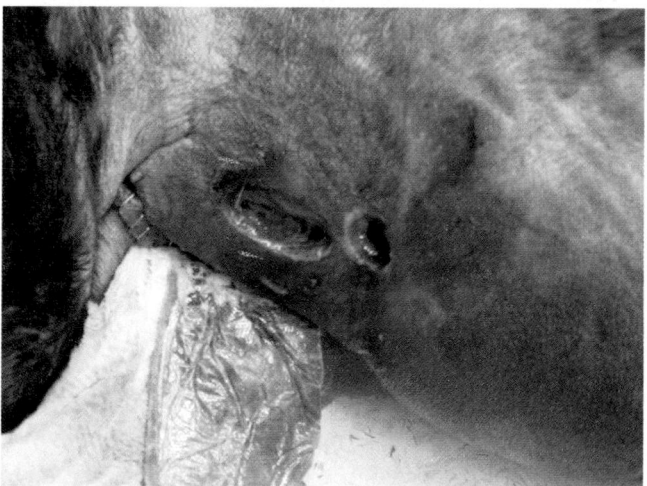

Figure 15-18 Tube migration of J tube.

homogenized foods may need to be mixed with water to pass through small-diameter tubes. Aseptic techniques in handling during both tube placement and diet delivery can help prevent many complications. The skin around the tube should be cleaned and inspected for fluid leaks at least daily, and the tape or bandage around the tube should be changed daily. The tube should be marked with permanent marker where it enters the skin in order to monitor correct placement. Tube migration can cause peritonitis or severe local infection (Figure 15-18). Application of a light bandage or dressing around most feeding tubes is recommended to keep the entry site clean.

Enteral feeding is more efficient, safer, and cheaper than parenteral nutrition (PN). Therefore feeding by mouth or tube is used whenever possible and as long as the GI tract can absorb nutrients. Enteral nutrition is contraindicated when GI secretory rest is required and when there is a high risk of vomition and aspiration (i.e., uncontrolled nausea).

FEEDING SCHEDULES AND ENTERAL ADMINISTRATION TECHNIQUES

Proportions of fat, carbohydrate, and protein in foods fed to hospitalized patients should be similar to that which the liver is estimated to be using from body stores. By the fifth day of food deprivation or later, patients should receive the majority (more than 50%) of their calculated resting energy requirement (RER) as fat. For dogs, use a food that provides protein of at least 4 to 6 g/100 kcal; for cats, use a food that provides at least 6 to 8 g/100 kcal.

In general, most food types are diluted in water, particularly if administered through a feeding tube. In addition, when a feeding tube is used, blenderizing and straining loaf products or adding water to moist homogenized products will facilitate easier flow and will yield fewer complications with clogging.

Feeding schedules are recommended as follows:

- ✓ **Day One:** Dilute one third of food with two thirds water
- ✓ **Day Two:** Dilute two thirds of food with one third water
- ✓ **Day Three:** Give full food amount

The amount fed should be divided into portions and fed every 4 to 8 hours or fed continuously by fluid pump. Patient response to feeding is important to note. Initially, the animal may feel slight discomfort with administration but will adapt after several feedings. Food should be warmed to room temperature and should be fed slowly over several minutes. After feeding, the tube should be flushed with water to prevent obstruction.

Patient response to feedings is important during administration. Signs of discomfort during feeding such as restlessness, salivation, abdominal bloating, or vomiting can indicate improper tube position. Other common but serious complications of tube feedings include pulmonary aspiration, diarrhea, constipation, tube occlusion, peritonitis from improper tube position, and delayed gastric emptying. Such complications can be prevented by checking tube placement before feeding, measuring gastric residue before each feeding, monitoring gastric tubes for migration during daily bandage changes, and evaluating both diet type and concurrent medications to determine the cause of diarrhea or constipation.

Bacterial contamination can also occur during enteral tube use. It is important to use clean techniques during tube placement and handling, to keep opened containers of formula refrigerated and discard them after 48 hours, and to routinely change enteral bags and administration lines every 24 hours. If constant-rate infusions are required, the administration bag should contain only a few hours of solution at a time to ensure stability.

The technician must also carefully monitor all assisted feeding methods for the stress associated with restraint

---

ENTERAL FEEDING WORKSHEET

1. Calculate resting energy requirement (RER)

   RER = (70) × (kg)$^{0.75}$

   $70 \times$ [Body weight (kg)]$^{0.75}$ = [RER (kcal/day)]

2. Choose a veterinary-specific critical care formula

3. Calculate volume of diet required

   [Name of diet choosen]

   [RER (kcal/day)] ÷ [Kcal/ml] = [ml formula/day]

4. Number and volume of feedings

   [ml formula/day] ÷ [Number feedings/day] = [ml formula/feeding]

Figure 15-19 Calculations for the daily food dose are done by dividing the patient's kilocalorie requirement by the energy content in kilocalories per milliliter of the food (see Table 15-10). The daily amount (milliliters) of food is usually divided into small portions that are given frequently.

---

and monitor all feeding tubes for mechanical blockage or kinking, particularly with small-bore tubes. Capping the tube prevents air from entering the catheterized viscus between uses. It is preferable for the same person to feed, because this may allow quicker notation of flow and resistance changes in the tube.

Gastric motility should be monitored, and depending on the type of tube used, the contents of the stomach should be aspirated before feeding. If more than one third of the previous feeding remains in the stomach, the subsequent feeding should be skipped. If two consecutive feedings are missed, pharmacologic agents may be instituted by the veterinarian to promote gastric motility. Feces should be analyzed for normal composition.

The stomach capacity of dogs and cats varies. In general, the stomach volume of the dog is approximately 90 ml/kg. However, the amount fed typically should not exceed 50 ml/kg. In the cat, the general stomach capacity is 100 ml/kg, and the amount fed should never exceed 45 ml/kg.

Tube placement should always be confirmed with a radiograph to prevent airway complications. In the sick or debilitated animal, coughing may not be present if a tube is inadvertently placed into the trachea. In this way, a "silent" aspiration may occur in critically ill or weak patients. The technician should monitor the patient for increased lung sounds, areas of dullness on auscultation of the lungs, coughing, and fever. If such clinical signs are present, feedings should be discontinued, and oxygen should be supplied immediately. The patient may benefit from partial PN or total PN while recovering from aspiration pneumonia.

FOOD SELECTION

Consider physical form and other nutritional characteristics before selecting a feeding product. For example, oral calorie paste supplements are extremely deficient in protein, and meat baby foods are neither complete nor balanced. In addition, dextrose additives do not provide adequate calorie concentrations and are devoid of protein. Table 15-10 summarizes the nutrient profile of selected enteral products used in small animal patients.

CALCULATING NUTRIENT REQUIREMENTS AND FOOD SELECTION (Figure 15-19)

1. Calculate RER as follows:
   RER = 30 × (Body weight in kg) + 70
   For animals <2 kg or >45 kg use:
   RER + 70 × (Body weight in kg)$^{0.75}$
2. Calculate illness energy requirement (IER):
   IER = RER × Illness factor
3. Calculate amount of food required:
   Food amount (ml) = IER ÷ Caloric density of selected food (kcal/ml)

✎ TECHNICIAN NOTE

Upright feedings are recommended for patients at risk of aspiration.

Table 15-10 COMPOSITION OF ENTERAL VETERINARY FORMULAE

Product	Caloric Content (kcal/g)	Protein Content (g/100 kcal)	% Protein Calories	% Fat Calories	% CHO Calories
VETERINARY PRODUCTS (CANNED)					
Prescription Diet					
Feline p/d*	0.8	10.1	36	56	8
Feline k/d*	0.8	6.0	23	49	28
Feline c/d-s*	0.6	9.9	36	43	21
Feline 1/d	1.05	7.2	25	45	30
Canine k/d†	0.6	3.1	11	48	41
Canine p/d†	0.8	1.9	23	51	26
Canine n/d†	0.8	7.8	27	57	16
Canine i/d†	0.7	5.8	23	30	47
Canine/Feline a/d	1.3	8.8	35	53	12
Purina CV-Formula Feline	1.4	8.7	32	50	18
Eukanuba Maximum Calorie Canine/Feline	2.0	7.4	29	66	5
Select Care Canine Development	0.9	8.0	28	30	42
Select Care Feline Development	1.0	10.4	36	54	10
VETERINARY PRODUCTS (LIQUID/PASTE)					
CliniCare Canine	1.0	5.5	20	55	25
CliniCare Feline	1.0	8.6	30	45	25
CliniCare RF Feline	1.0	5.6	22	57	21
NutriCal paste	4.6	0.3	1	62	37
HUMAN POLYMERIC FOODS					
Jevity	1.1	4.2	17	29	54
Pulmocare	1.5	4.2	17	55	28
Osmolite HN	1.1	4.2	17	29	54
Sustacal	1.0	6.1	24	21	55
HUMAN MONOMERIC					
Peptamen	1.0	4.4	16	33	51
Vital HN	1.0	4.1	15	9	74
SUPPLEMENT					
Promod (protein)	1.5 Kcal/ml	23.6	0	0	0
Casec (protein)	4.0	30.7	0	100	0
MCT oil (medium triglycerides)	8.3 Kcal/ml	0	0	100	0
Vegetable oil	8.5 Kcal/ml	0	0	100	0
Baby food (turkey)	1.0	14.6	58	42	0

CHO, Carbohydrate.
*1/2 Can (202 g) + 3/4 C (170 ml) water.
†1/2 Can (209 g) + 3/4 C (170 ml) water.

Disease factors for determining energy requirements in dogs and cats are suggested as follows:

Cage rest	1.1
Surgery, trauma, cancer, sepsis	1.2-1.5
Severe burns, head trauma, ventilator patients	1.7-2.0

Most hospitalized veterinary patients have metabolic rates very near their RER. Therefore initially feeding patients at RER is a logical and safe recommendation. Regular nutritional assessment of the patient is strongly recommended to adjust initial feeding rates (see discussion of nutritional assessment of the hospitalized patient).

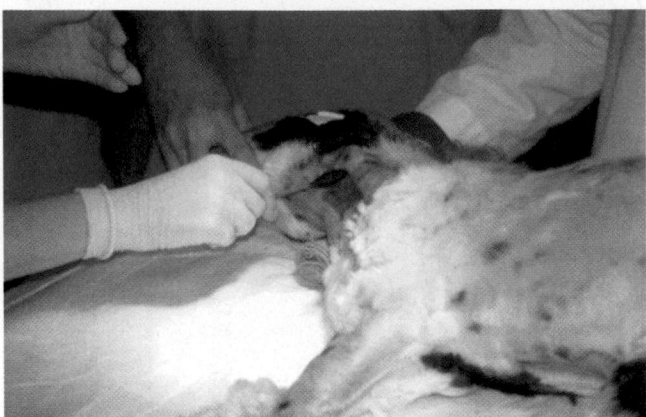

Figure 15-20 Central venous catheter preparation. Administration of PN is typically made through a central venous catheter, which can remain in place for a prolonged period.

✎ **TECHNICIAN NOTE**

Parenteral nutrition refers to the delivery of nutrients intravenously.

PARENTERAL NUTRITION

PN refers to the delivery of nutrients intravenously. Candidates for PN include patients who are unable to digest or absorb nutrients via the GI tract and those that have uncontrolled vomiting. Examples include patients with severe pancreatitis, inflammatory bowel disease, and peritonitis and patients that have undergone intestinal surgery and require bowel rest.

PN is a compounded solution containing electrolytes, amino acids, and lipids in a standard crystalloid suspension. Calculations are based on the patient's RER, disease history, protein levels, and hydration status. PN solutions can also be obtained from human hospitals and independent pharmaceutical companies, although concentrations of each nutrient must still be calculated.

Administration of PN is achieved through a central or peripheral catheter. However, administration is typically through a central venous catheter to prevent such common complications as phlebitis and infection. In addition, if long-term parenteral nutritional support is anticipated, central venous catheters made of polyurethane are recommended, because they need not be removed at a predetermined time.

PN is expensive and requires strict antiseptic technique in catheter placement (Figure 15-20). Nursing management of catheters carrying hyperosmolar solutions containing amino acids warrants special focus, because the solution type is an excellent medium for bacterial colonization. Sterile technique and catheter care should be the same for ANY type of fluid administration, regardless of PN administration, but a sterile protocol should be strictly enforced for patients receiving PN.

Catheter care includes use of strict sterile technique during insertion, including proper skin preparation, placement of a sterile underwrap over the insertion site, and strict aseptic technique of intravenous tubing and administration bags. The patients intravenous lines should not be disconnected from the bag of nutritional supplement. If diagnostic testing or frequent walking is necessary, the intravenous lines and administration bags should accompany the patient. Intravenous injections should follow sterilization of the port. If a multilumen catheter is placed, proper identification to each port is necessary, with one line dedicated to the total PN solution only (usually the proximal port).

Laboratory analysis during administration of PN is important in order to monitor electrolytes, presence of lipemia, liver disease, coagulopathies, and thrombocytopenia, as well as signs of infection or patient compromise. Drug administration or drug additions a parenteral solution are not recommended.

Maintaining enterocyte function is important to reduce complications of PN such as bowel atrophy and bacterial translocation. Combined enteral and parenteral feeding has been recently recommended to prevent intestinal mucosal deterioration and intestinal hypertrophy and to facilitate healing by promoting intestinal growth. Therefore a small portion of enteral feeding to support the bowel during administration of PN is encouraged.

✎ **TECHNICIAN NOTE**

Candidates for PN include patients that are unable to digest or absorb nutrients via the GI tract and those that have uncontrolled vomiting.

NUTRITIONAL CONSIDERATIONS FOR THE CRITICAL PATIENT

Critical illness is associated with an increase in metabolism to provide energy for immune responses and healing. This hypermetabolic process is an effort by the body to mobilize its supply of circulating nutrient substrates, such as glucose and amino acids. Unfortunately, this mobilization occurs at the expense of body tissue and function at a time when protein synthesis demands are also high. The body becomes dependent on its protein stores to provide gluconeogenesis, because glucose is desperately needed as a fuel source. Consequent loss of protein results in weight loss and alternations in protein homeostasis. Loss of lean body mass is associated with patient morbidity and death, and it is crucial to be able to recognize symptoms of nutritional insufficiency.

In the critically ill or injured patient, the hypermetabolic state continues as the body attempts to heal itself. As a result, a patient's RER and oxygen demands are increased (see discussion of patients at risk for malnutrition). Clinical signs of such metabolic events include tachycardia, tachypnea, transient hyperglycemia, and the eventual net breakdown of skeletal muscle protein and the mobilization of body fat.

Unexplained weakness or dull mentation often accompanies the nutritionally starved critically ill patient (Figure 15-21). Dull mentation and weakness are often a reflection of the loss of skeletal muscle mass from altered protein

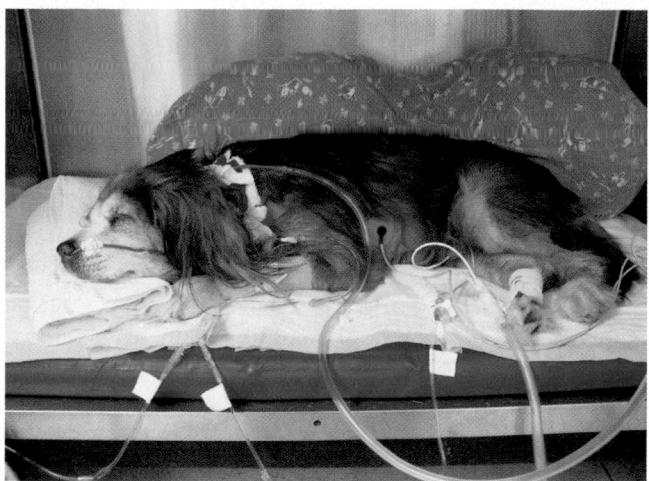

Figure 15-21 Critical patient with unexplained weakness. Note that the various administration lines are clearly labeled.

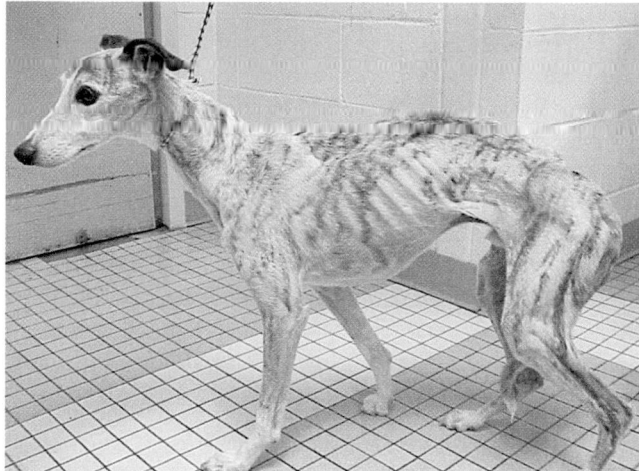

Figure 15-22 A 7-year-old castrated male whippet presented with chronic diarrhea and weight loss.

homeostasis. Because patients are using protein reserves from multiple body organs, without nutritional support, organ dysfunction is an eventuality. Obese and overweight critical patients can also develop malnutrition in spite of excessive amounts of fat reserves. The overweight patient's nutritional needs may also be overlooked because the signs of muscle weakness and muscle wasting are less obvious. Thus all critically ill patients, regardless of body weight, need the same degree of nutritional assessment and monitoring.

> ### ✎ TECHNICIAN NOTE
> Dull mentation and weakness often reflect the loss of skeletal muscle mass from altered protein homeostasis.

Respiratory function deteriorates as intercostals and diaphragmatic muscles waste as a result of poor nutritional support, exacerbating poor ventilation and hypoxia. Chronic hypoxia results in pneumonia and atelectasis. Increased respiratory effort and increased respiratory rate are often present in the critically ill patient, requiring tremendous amounts of energy. In addition, the critically ill patient is often recumbent. Recumbent patients have the greatest risk of respiratory insufficiency because nutritional uptake is generally poor, with muscle fatigue and muscle wasting further complicating recovery. Recumbent patients with muscle wasting are prone to megaesophagus and aspiration pneumonia. Limb edema can be present, suggesting hypoproteinemia.

Kidney function can also deteriorate as decreased urea concentration in the renal medulla reduces the kidney's ability to concentrate urine. Poor nutrition can cause decreased muscle function, leading to decreased motility and malabsorption in the GI tract. Even cardiac muscle can be weakened by the increased demand for oxygen consumption as a result of the hypermetabolic state caused by injury or illness.

In essence, no organ is spared in the critically ill patient with malnutrition. The interrelationships of organ function and nutrition are complex and delicate. Although no single measurement or observation can define the degree of nutritional insufficiency, being conscious of the nutritional need for patient maintenance is an important step in providing good patient care.

Routine laboratory tests can also provide additional evidence of nutritional insufficiency in the critically ill patient. Tests of immune function such as lymphocyte count are important, as well as the hematocrit and reticulocyte count if anemia is present. In addition, serum albumin is important to measure in nutritionally challenged patients. Any abnormal lab findings can also be due to several underlying disease processes that are complicated by poor nutrition.

> ### ✎ TECHNICIAN NOTE
> Poor nutrition can cause decreased muscle function, leading to decreased motility and malabsorption in the GI tract.

SMALL ANIMAL NUTRITION

Case Example

A 7-year-old castrated male whippet, named Dash, was presented to the veterinarian because of chronic diarrhea and weight loss over an 8-week period (Figure 15-22).

On physical exam, a BCS of 1 was observed, with a grade III/VI systolic heart murmur. Lab results showed a mild anemia (hematocrit of 35%, normal 37%-55%), lymphopenia (452, normal 1000-4000), panhypoproteinemia (albumin 1.8, normal 2.6-3.5, globulins 1.3, normal 3.6-5.0), and a possible urinary tract infection with rods identified on the urine sediment despite negative urine culture results. Chest radiographs showed mild to moderate left-sided heart enlargement. No significant findings were identified on abdominal radiographs or abdominal ultrasound examination. Bile acid results were unremarkable. Results are most consistent with a severe protein-losing enteropathy or other small-intestinal diseases such as exocrine pancreatic insufficiency (EPI), small-intestinal bacterial overgrowth, or lymphangiectasia. Intestinal biopsy was recommended to the owner. Pancreatic function tests (TLI) later revealed a diagnosis of EPI. Ultrasound examination of the heart revealed mitral insufficiency. Treatment included antibiotics, PN administration, enzyme replacement therapy, and a restricted diet on discharge from the hospital. Combined enteral and parenteral feeding was implemented to prevent intestinal mucosal deterioration and intestinal hypertrophy and to facilitate healing by promoting intestinal growth.

Discussion of Case

Restriction of dietary fat is recommended for such small-intestinal diseases as EPI. Chronic diarrhea occurred as a result of interference with normal digestion and absorption of nutrients. Nutrients can be retained within the intestinal lumen, exerting an osmotic effect and leading to the retention of water and diarrhea, often referred to as osmotic diarrhea. Although osmotic diarrhea is most commonly seen with nutritional overload, it is also associated with deficiencies of digestive enzymes such as those found in EPI. EPI is a disease of maldigestion caused by a lack of digestive enzymes. Digestion of fat is significantly impaired.

Diet plays a fundamental role in the management of EPI. Recommended dietary treatment includes the following:

✓ Restriction of dietary fat
✓ Moderate to high quantities of good-quality protein
✓ Highly digestible carbohydrates such as rice
✓ Avoidance of dietary fiber
✓ Supplementation of water-soluble vitamins such as B complexes and folate

Note that severe protein deficiency can further compromise a diseased intestinal tract. Protein-enriched foods are critical in the management of such diseases. In addition, because protein plays a key role in dietary sensitivity (because most allergens are proteins), sources of dietary protein should be limited to one or two ingredients not normally associated with sensitivity reactions.

Carbohydrate digestion can be impaired with EPI; therefore highly digestible carbohydrates are recommended in the diet. Simple sugars such as lactose should be avoided because the enzymes required for digestion may be insufficient.

Fiber is contraindicated in EPI, because it may interfere with pancreatic enzyme activity. Although fiber may improve fecal consistency, it may interfere with digestion and absorption, thereby further compromising the patient. In addition, increased intestinal permeability may accompany low blood protein levels, because intestinal pore size becomes large and fluid filled, allowing proteins to escape, creating protein-losing enteropathies and diarrhea.

NUTRITION OF SMALL AND EXOTIC PETS

FEEDING PET BIRDS

Nutritional disease is common in pet birds. Box 15-10 lists human foods that can add diversity to the diet of companion birds. Box 15-11 lists nutritional deficiencies of birds and the resulting conditions.

Dietary-induced diseases frequently occur in psittacine and passerine bird species because of their diverse nutrimental requirements. Unfortunately, each species of bird has differences in nutritional demands, with few data to determine specific quantities or qualities of diet. All-seed diets (particularly diets composed of only one seed type, such as millet or sunflower) and diets supplemented with fruits, vegetables, and other human foods are often thought to be complete diets for birds. Such practices lead to feeding and nutritional disorders.

Small birds have high metabolic rates and high-energy requirements; therefore a continuous supply of food should be available. However, most commercially available seeds are deficient in certain limiting nutrients (e.g., specific amino acids, vitamins, trace minerals, and macrominerals, such as calcium and sodium). In addition, seeds are not the primary or natural diet of most species of companion birds. Natural diets contain a wide variety of insects, fruits, and seeds; captive birds are commonly fed seed diets. In addition, seed diets consist primarily of sunflower seeds, which are high in fat but low in calcium and vitamin A, perpetuating obesity and/or nutritional deficiencies.

✐ TECHNICIAN NOTE

Small birds have high metabolic rates and high-energy requirements; therefore a continuous supply of food should be available.

Box 15-10 FEED DIVERSITY FOR COMPANION BIRDS

- Cheerios
- Pellets, crumbles, crimps
- Cooked vegetables
- Bananas
- Peanut butter

Box 15-11 NUTRITIONAL DEFICIENCIES TYPICALLY FOUND IN COMPANION BIRDS

- Vitamin A (squamous metaplasia, hyperkeratosis)
- Iodine (hypothyroidism)
- Vitamin E (encephalomalacia)
- Zinc (failure to thrive)
- Selenium (muscular dystrophy)

Perhaps the most common cause of dietary-induced diseases in companion birds is the practice of adding fruits and vegetables sold for human consumption to commercially prepared foods or supplemented seed mixtures. The most readily available fruits and vegetables contain primarily water, carbohydrates, and fiber. They are severely deficient in protein, vitamins, and minerals when compared with the nutrient recommendations for psittacine and passerine birds.

Fruits and vegetables primarily dilute key nutrients present in nutritionally balanced commercially prepared foods. Birds often preferentially eat fruits and vegetables because of their high water content instead of dry extruded or pelleted foods and seed mixtures. In fact, birds often select food items based on water content, texture, color, or taste, rather than nutrient content, resulting in very imbalanced nutrient intakes.

Captive birds also develop nutritional deficiencies by habitually selecting specific food items from a variety of offerings. Because malnourished birds often tend to overeat the food items presented to them, it is unclear whether this is a cause or an effect of malnutrition. Unfortunately, such eating behavior leads to the popular misconception that birds are able to preferentially balance their diets.

TECHNICIAN NOTE

Each species of bird has its own unique nutritional requirements.

All birds do have similar nutritional requirements, including proteins and amino acids, carbohydrates, fats, vitamins, inorganic elements, and water. Different species require different amounts of these substances.

Proteins required by companion birds are composed of approximately 20 amino acids. Ten of these amino acids are essential: arginine, histidine, isoleucine, leucine, lysine, methionine, phenylalanine, threonine, tryptophan, and valine. In the infant bird, glycine (or serine) and proline are of utmost importance. In the United States, methionine and lysine are often absent in the diet. Evidence suggests that increased protein may be needed during certain points in the reproductive cycle. In the wild, insects supply these increased needs. It is difficult for bird owners to meet these special needs by feeding only seed mixtures.

White worms (*Enchytraes* larvae) are available commercially and can be kept for long periods, much like earthworms, in a cool, damp moss and leaf litter substrate. These worms are especially useful to provide when parent birds are brooding and feeding their young. Ant pupae, which bird fanciers have relied on heavily for avian diets, are now available commercially in large outlets and by mail order. Water shrimp (*Daphnia* spp.) are relished by some species and greatly enhance red pigments in their plumage. Aphids that feed on members of the rose family concentrate the same pigments and may be more appropriate for small passerine birds. Moth larvae, commonly known as wax worms, and beetle larvae, called mealworms, supply extra protein and fat, especially at the onset of the breeding season. Care should be taken to restrict the intake of these insects, or birds will rapidly gain weight and become obese.

TECHNICIAN NOTE

Care should be taken to restrict the intake of certain insects, or birds will rapidly gain weight and become obese.

Foods appropriately balanced in carbohydrate, protein, fats, vitamin, mineral, and water content are essential for all birds. Stewardship of confined birds must address good nutrition at several levels: the daily satisfaction and health of the bird as well as the long-term contributions to growth, maturation, defense against disease, and reproductive health (the hallmark of good nutrition).

The major benefits of commercially prepared foods are nutrient balance and convenience. Manufacturers commonly formulate commercial foods by using sound scientific principles according to established nutrient recommendations. Although adherence to these recommendations and ingredient quality may vary among manufacturers, an extruded or pelleted diet supplies all the nutrients in one particle. Such formulations help prevent alteration of nutrient balance by uninformed owners who feed imbalanced seeds or human foods or by birds that consume different quantities of imbalanced foods that are fed separately.

A potential disadvantage of feeding commercial foods is that testing protocols for nutritional adequacy have not yet been established for avian foods, as they have been for commercial canine and feline foods. Nevertheless, the probability of producing a nutritional imbalance by feeding a commercial avian food is significantly less than when seeds or human foods are prepared by uninformed owners.

Although seeds are a popular, convenient, and inexpensive method of providing nutrients to companion birds (Figure 15-23), they are not necessarily the best or even the most natural food for pet birds. The types of seeds present in most commercial mixes are not native to areas where most pet bird species originate.

TECHNICIAN NOTE

Although well-balanced seed mixtures supply essential nutrients, they are rarely sufficient to meet all of the nutritional needs of pet birds.

A well-balanced seed mixture can supply essential nutrients such as fats, carbohydrates, and some minerals. However, seeds are rarely if ever an appropriate sole nutritional source because they provide inadequate levels of protein, vitamins, and minerals. Commercially available seed mixtures vary greatly in type and quality. Individual seed types are also sold in most stores; thus formulating seed mixtures is a common practice. Unfortunately, the availability of individual seed types promotes nutrient imbalance

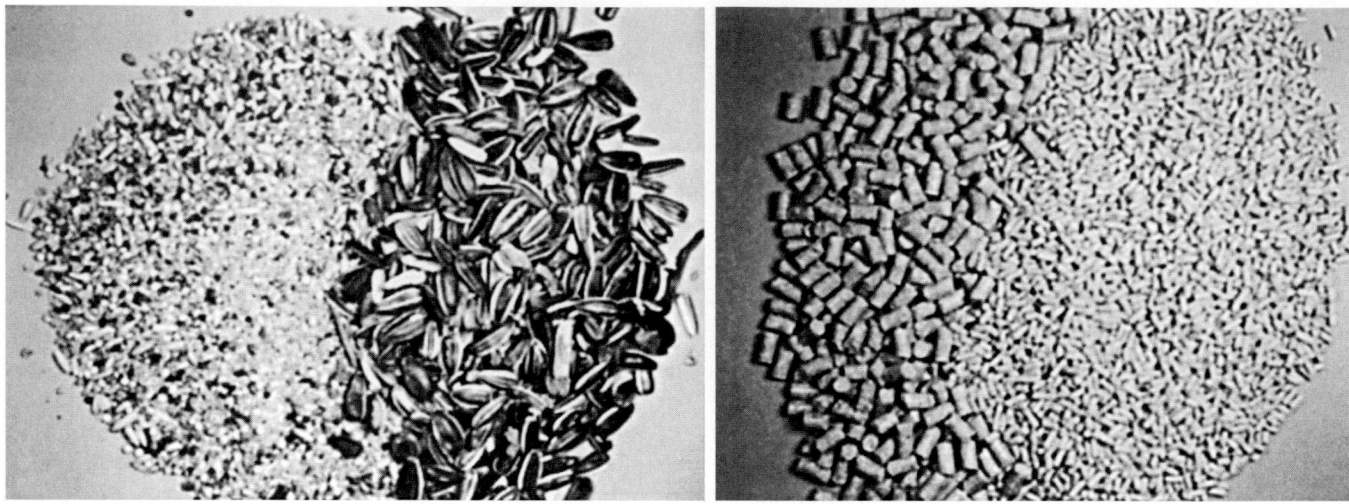

Figure 15-23 **A,** Seeds are an important part of many avian diets. However, high-oil seeds and nuts, such as sunflower seeds and peanuts, may cause addictions and nutritional imbalance. Oil seeds are deficient in protein relative to calorie content and in calcium and micronutrients. **B,** Complete and balanced avian foods are available as fortified seed mixtures and extruded and pelleted foods.

when uninformed owners create a mixture based primarily on the price and physical appearance of the seeds. Thus creation or use of homemade seed mixtures should be discouraged.

A wide variety of homemade mixed-food diets have been suggested as alternatives for birds that will not accept commercially prepared foods or seed mixtures even with added fruits and vegetables. These diets can result in excellent feathering and appropriate body mass for the species, with no discernible signs of nutritional deficiency, if they are prepared carefully from scientifically developed recipes. These diets often contain varying amounts of ingredients such as seeds, nuts, cooked eggs, low-fat yogurt or cheese, vegetables, fruits, grains, bread, pasta, multigrain cereals, legumes, seed mixes, pelleted or extruded psittacine diets, vitamin supplements, and calcium supplements (Table 15-11). When birds are being introduced to a new homemade diet, have the client offer a mixture containing all the ingredients at one time. This practice usually prevents preferential selection of certain ingredients. Although larger parrots have difficulty eating small seeds such as milo or oat groats, a seed mixture containing 30% hulled safflower, 30% milo, 30% oats, and 10% peanuts works well for smaller birds.

Insoluble and soluble mineral grit are often given to birds as a dietary supplement. Insoluble grit (quartz or silica) remains in the gizzard where it may facilitate mechanical digestion. Soluble grit (oyster shells or cuttlefish) is completely digested and supplies a source of such minerals as calcium and phosphorus. However, be advised that oversupplementing mineral grit can be harmful to caged birds and may lead to gizzard impaction.

> ✎ **TECHNICIAN NOTE**
> Oversupplementation of mineral grit can be harmful to caged birds.

Although homemade mixed-food diets may provide adequate nourishment, most companion bird owners are unwilling to devote the time necessary to adequately prepare these diets. In addition, owners must be willing to regularly observe which food components are being consumed to prevent birds from developing or reverting to preferential selection of specific ingredients.

Although feeding a well-balanced diet is essential, it is easy to overlook the single most important dietary component: water. Water makes up more than 50% of a bird's body weight. Because birds have no sweat glands, water intake plays an important role in thermoregulation. Breeding females may require increased amounts of water for egg production and for heat regulation while incubating eggs.

Although some foods are high in water content, others are dry and require the bird to have free access to water for efficient digestion and absorption. Some avian species are more physiologically adept at extracting water from their foods. As a general rule, birds should never go for more than a few hours without access to fresh clean water. Studies have shown that canaries will die within 48 hours if water is withheld.

Water should be provided in containers that are easily accessible but not in a location that will allow feces, feathers, or food particles to accumulate. For this reason, water bowls should be attached to the wall of enclosures, near or above food bowls. In addition, large water bowls should be discouraged because they may invite bathing.

> ✎ **TECHNICIAN NOTE**
> Water should be provided in containers that are easily accessible but not in a location that will allow feces, feathers, or food particles to accumulate.

Table 15-11 Suggested Diet for Maintenance of Adult Caged Birds

	Canary	Budgerigar	Cockatiel	Conure	Amazon/ African Gray Parrot	Macaw/ Cockatoo
OFFER DAILY						
Whole-grain bread cubes or primate biscuit	1/4 T	1/2 T	1 T	1 1/2 T	2 T	4 T
Fresh dark green or yellow vegetables	1/2 T	1 T	2 T	4 T	3 T	1/2 C
Protein source (cheese, hard-cooked eggs, meat, mature legumes)	1/4 Size of pea	1/2 Size of pea	Size of pea	1/4 t	1/2 t	1 T
Dry seeds (two 15-min periods) (surflower)	0	0	1 T	2 T	2 T	4 T
Small seeds (canary, niger, poppy, rape, millet, safflower, hemp)	Ad lib	Ad lib	Ad lib	Ad lib	Ad lib	Ad lib
2 TO 3 TIMES WEEKLY						
Fruit (cantaloupe, apricot, apple)	1/8 t	1/8 t	1 t	1/12 Apple	1/12 Apple	1/6 Apple
Citrus fruit	0	0	0	1/12 Orange	1/12 Orange	1/6 Orange
Fresh corn on the cob	3 or 4 Kernels	1/8 Piece	1/2 Piece	1/2 Piece	1/2 Piece	1 Piece
Peanuts	0	0	0	1	2	4
ADD TEMPORARILY FOR NEW BIRDS						
Vitamin A (from 10,000 IU capsule)	1 Drop/wk	2 Drops/wk	3 Drops/wk	1 Drop/day	1-2 Drops/day	4 Drops/day
Yogurt	Drop	Few drops	1/4 t	1/4 t	1/2 t	1
ALWAYS AVAILABLE						
Calcium/mineral supplements (cuttlebone, mineral treat block, oyster shell, calcium lactate)						

Modified from Harrison GI, Harrison LR: *Clinical avian medicine and surgery*, Philadelphia, 1986, WB Saunders.
C, Cup; *T*, tablespoon; *t*, teaspoon.

RABBITS

Dietary requirements vary according to the age and use of a rabbit. For example, a balanced mixture of timothy grass, grass hay, and vegetables is the best diet for most pet rabbits, whereas show and production rabbits typically do better on a commercially produced alfalfa meal–based pellet diet. In general, however, rabbits are herbivores with high fiber requirements.

The best pet rabbit diet is an alfalfa-based pellet with a hay supplement given on a daily basis. "Treats" of fresh greens or other vegetable supplements are encouraged only as occasional rewards. Foods recommended include carrots, small pieces of ripe banana, rice cakes, dry wheat bread, and dandelion leaves. It is important to remove any uneaten portion, because spoilage can cause GI upset.

Regular feeding schedules are important to the rabbit. Because rabbits are nocturnal in nature and consume most of their feed during the night, hay should be given in the morning, and pellets with grains in the afternoon or evening. Adequate fresh water is essential to ensure proper feed intake. Water delivery systems can be superior to water bowls, which may tip or become contaminated with feces. Application of syrup or molasses to the tip of the waterspout may induce use and encourage water consumption.

> ### 🖉 TECHNICIAN NOTE
> Rabbits are nocturnal and consume most their feed during the night; hay should be given in the morning, and pellets with grains in the afternoon or evening.

Other components of rabbit nutrition include vitamin supplementation. Vitamin A deficiency can result in infertility and other reproductive complications, central nervous system defects, and increased neonatal mortality rates. Most fresh alfalfa pellets contain adequate vitamin A to prevent such deficiencies; adding a supplement to a diet already rich in vitamin A can cause excesses with consequences just as harmful. Technicians should advise rabbit owners to buy fresh alfalfa pellets and monitor appetite.

All commercial feeds should have a mill location and date of manufacture clearly printed on the bag; feeds should be purchased within 90 days of production. Feeds older than 6 months have poor nutritional quality. In addition, feeds that contain antibiotics are generally not recommended. Antibiotics may disrupt the balance of intestinal flora, resulting in diarrhea, anorexia, or death.

Pellets high in calcium or excessive vitamin D can occasionally produce chalky white or cream-colored urine. Termed dystrophic calcification, excess calcium causes urinary lithiasis or excessive excretion of calcium "sand," and may even cause calculi to form in the kidneys and ureters. Although rabbits have unusual calcium metabolism, dietary management to regulate calcium intake includes feeding alfalfa-based diets without additional calcium supplementation. Normal urine color in the rabbit varies from straw to a reddish brown.

> ### 🖉 TECHNICIAN NOTE
> Dietary management to regulate calcium intake includes feeding alfalfa-based diets without additional calcium supplementation.

GUINEA PIGS

Guinea pigs are notoriously fastidious eaters. They are herbivores with normal coprophagic behavior. Any abrupt changes in feed or feeding systems can result in a refusal to eat or drink for extended periods.

Recommended diets include food types with increased fiber, because insufficient levels can cause cecal impaction and fur chewing, resulting in the formation of hairballs. Diets should be composed of freshly milled guinea pig feed found in most pet or grocery stores, supplemented with a good quality hay to satisfy fiber requirements. Because of specific nutrient and vitamin requirements, guinea pigs *should not* be fed rabbit or any other diet designed for another species. Guinea pigs should also be given access to hard food diets that promote gnawing, because malocclusion can prevent eating and drinking.

Guinea pigs lack an enzyme in the glucose to the vitamin C pathway, thus requiring a daily dietary ascorbic acid supplement. Commercially prepared guinea pig diets generally contain minimal vitamin C concentrations, and concentrations are depleted with a shelf life of more than 3 months. Fresh fruit can be used to supplement commercial diets, but abrupt changes in diet should be avoided to prevent GI upset.

Absolute requirements of 10 mg/kg of ascorbic acid per day are recommended, with increases up to 30 mg/kg per day during pregnancy. If supplementation is not provided in the feed, 1 g/L may be added to the water, or one small handful of cabbage or kale or one fourth of an orange may be given daily. Clinical signs of vitamin C deficiency include alopecia, anorexia, dehydration, poor wound healing—and eventually—periodontal disease including brown discoloration of teeth and temporomandibular joint inflammation.

Fresh water is essential to the guinea pig and should be provided daily. Water bottles or other water delivery systems are recommended to prevent water contamination or spillage. Note that because guinea pigs have a propensity for chewing and gnawing, water valves should be located outside the cage to prevent destruction.

> ### 🖉 TECHNICIAN NOTE
> Guinea pigs lack an enzyme in the glucose to the vitamin C pathway and thus require a daily dietary ascorbic acid supplement.

HAMSTERS

Hamsters are omnivores and should be provided with hard food, such as an occasional dog biscuit, in their diets to promote gnawing and chewing to prevent malocclusion and overgrowth of teeth. Dietary recommendations include pelleted diets or mixes designed for hamsters, supplemented with treat foods such as washed vegetables, seeds, fruits, crackers, and cooked meat. Food should be given at night, because hamsters are typically nocturnal. Stale food should be removed from the cage, because hoarding is a common social behavior.

Water should also be provided either in a heavy bowl or in a water delivery system to prevent contamination and spillage.

GERBILS

Gerbils are herbivorous or graminivorous. In the wild, gerbils typically eat plants, seeds, and insects. Commercial pelleted foods designed for gerbils are available, although adult gerbils can be fed a good-quality rat or mouse diet. Note that gerbils will preferentially eat sunflower seeds and ignore other dietary ingredients, resulting in obesity and possible calcium deficiency. Technicians should advise gerbil owners to avoid mixes containing large amounts of sunflower seeds.

Gerbils typically eat frequent small meals, up to eight times a day. Weight loss will occur if food supplies are limited. Diets should be supplemented with green vegetables, fresh fruit, and hard food or pieces of wood to prevent tooth malocclusion.

Although gerbils can conserve water very efficiently, fresh water should be provided on a daily basis. Heavy water containers or water delivery systems are recommended to prevent contamination and spillage.

> ✎ **TECHNICIAN NOTE**
>
> Gerbils typically eat frequent small meals, up to eight times a day. Weight loss will occur if food supplies are limited.

RATS AND MICE

Both rats and mice are omnivorous. Commercially available pellet-based diets supply most known nutritional requirements, although it is generally recommended to supplement diets with small amounts of apples, tomatoes, or biscuits. "Treats" may be given to encourage handling but should be used sparingly to prevent obesity. Fresh water should be supplied in sipper bottles on a daily basis.

CHINCHILLAS

Chinchillas are hindgut fermenters, meaning they have complex digestive systems for fermenting fiber in the food.

Inappropriate diets (such as foods devoid of fiber) can cause diarrhea, constipation, bloat, or rectal prolapse. Recommended diets include mainly grasses and seeds, supplemented with small quantities of dried fruits, nuts, carrots, and green vegetables or green grass. Commercially prepared diets are available specifically for chinchillas, although rabbit or guinea pig foods are suitable. Hard foods or pieces of wood should be available to prevent malocclusion.

Chinchillas should be provided with a dust bath for grooming needs. It is recommended to allow bathing for only short periods in the day; keeping dust baths in the cage may result in fecal contamination. Daily fresh water is also necessary and should be provided either in a heavy bowl or in a water delivery system.

FERRETS

Ferrets are typically carnivores, with general requirements of roughly 30% protein and 25% fat in a daily diet. High-fiber diets are *not* recommended. Pelleted commercial ferret diets are available, although high-quality dry cat foods can be substituted. Commercial diets may occasionally be supplemented with mice or chicken heads to provide required protein. Small amounts of apples, cooked meat, or dried fruits can also be offered, although consistency in diet is generally recommended because a ferret may resent dietary changes. Body weight may have seasonal fluctuations, and the summer and autumn are months associated with possible weight reduction. Fresh water should be provided on a daily basis.

FEEDING CAPTIVE REPTILES

CHELONIANS

Land tortoises are predominantly herbivores but will occasionally eat insects and small rodents. In captivity, diets should primarily consist of vegetables (mainly dark leafy greens, grasses, and weeds), some fruits, and limited quantities of high-protein foods. Typical tortoise diets include the following substrates:

- ✓ **85% Vegetables** such as collards, radish and turnip greens, dandelions, kale, cabbage, bok choy, broccoli, cauliflower, summer and winter squash
- ✓ **10% Fruit** such as grapes, apples, oranges, pears, peaches, plums, dates, melons, strawberries, raspberries, mangos, and tomatoes
- ✓ **>5% High-protein foods** such as dry maintenance dog food, parrot chow, cereals, mice, scrambled eggs

Successfully caring for captive tortoises depends heavily on varying the diet. A shallow water dish should be provided to allow consumption, although caution should be taken not to overfill it with water, because tortoises and box turtles cannot swim and will drown if submerged. The water should be changed daily, because turtles may defecate in the water dish.

Sunlight or ultraviolet light should be provided to allow cholecalciferol (vitamin D) synthesis for shell formation and repair and to stimulate appetite and basking behavior. Multivitamins containing vitamin D may be added to the diet every 1 to 2 weeks.

Aquatic turtles need a variety of foods to achieve a balanced diet. The majority of the diet should consist of whole animals such as mice, earthworms, chopped goldfish or guppies, and slugs. Small amounts of insects such as crickets, mealworms, flies, and grasshoppers can also be offered. Feeding of meats such as hamburger or shellfish is not recommended. Vegetables, such as dark leafy greens, cabbage, or romaine lettuce, can also be offered in small amounts. Commercial diets are available in floating stick forms, but keep in mind that supplementation with natural foods such as earthworms and small fish is also recommended. Some tropical fish foods can also be used to provide variation in diet. Note that aquatic turtles will only feed if they are in the water.

The most common nutritional deficiency in captive turtles is vitamin A deficiency. Clinical signs include respiratory tract infections, edematous eyes, urogenital tract obstructions, and beak overgrowths. Hypovitaminosis A can be prevented by providing a proper diet that supplies beta-carotene, found in such foods as earthworms, small fish, and green leafy vegetables.

> 🖉 **TECHNICIAN NOTE**
>
> Successfully caring for captive tortoises depends heavily on varying the diet.

SNAKES

Snakes are carnivores and need to be fed a varied diet. Specific dietary needs depend on the species of snake, although staples generally include rodents. The size of the rodent fed should be about the same diameter as the snake's body and about one eighth the length. Typical rodents used for snake food include rabbits, rats, mice, gerbils, chickens, lizards, and other snakes. It is usually prudent to feed frozen or freshly killed rodents to prevent injury or infection caused by prey bites to the snake.

Most species of snake are fed once every 1 to 2 weeks, but the size of prey and frequency of feeding depends on both the time of year and the signalment of the snake. If the snake is fed more than once a week, the environment needs to be warm enough to facilitate digestion. The incidence of nutritional deficiency in the captive snake is rare, because most snakes are fed whole prey. Note that because snakes eat infrequently, inappetence or weight loss may go undetected. Periodic weighing is recommended to

prevent nutritional deficiency. Although water requirements are low, water should be supplied on a daily basis.

LIZARDS

Most captive lizards are omnivorous, eating such foods as mealworms, crickets, locusts, and silkworm larvae. Most insects are calcium deficient, however, and the insects themselves should be fed nutritional supplements to pass on to the lizard. Lizards in the wild are primarily carnivorous, eating invertebrate or vertebrate prey. In general, captive lizards require vitamin and mineral supplementation with an emphasis on a variety of foods. Juvenile lizards should be fed one to two times a day, and adults should be fed two to three times per week. Most lizards are diurnal and require day feedings and time to bask in natural or ultraviolet light.

Herbivorous lizards, such as the green iguana, require a varied diet to ensure an adequate nutritional balance. Recommended foods for herbivores include leafy greens (romaine lettuce and collard greens), mustard greens, and clover. Vegetables are also adequate dietary substances, including green beans, okra, carrots, and squash. It is important, however, to note that certain vegetables such as spinach, cabbage, peas, and potatoes contain substances that bind calcium and other trace minerals, inhibiting their absorption. Alfalfa rabbit pellets can also be fed to the common iguana.

Commercially prepared diets are available, with additional supplementation unnecessary if the captive lizard is fed a diet based primarily on such purchased food. Homemade diets of vegetables and fruits should always be supplemented with appropriate vitamins and minerals. Technicians can advise lizard owners to purchase a quality reptile vitamin, containing vitamin D_3, which should be administered one to two times a week if a good diet is provided.

> 🖉 **TECHNICIAN NOTE**
>
> Captive lizards require vitamin and mineral supplementation with an emphasis on a variety of foods.

Common iguanas also require protein for normal growth and development. Juvenile iguanas in captivity generally need more protein and calcium than adults do. Common protein sources include dog food, monkey biscuits, and tofu. Owners should use dog food sparingly because of the high purine content. Cat food is not recommended. Protein substances can be blenderized or grinded and sprinkled on vegetables.

Water should be provided in a bowl for bathing and drinking. Note that some lizards, such as the chameleon, will only drink water in the form of droplets on plants. Therefore it is important to spray or mist the tank several times a day. In addition, most lizards should be sprayed with water or allowed to bathe to prevent skin problems associated with low humidity.

AMPHIBIANS

Amphibians include such pets as frogs, toads, salamanders, and newts. Most adult amphibians are carnivores, eating live prey when not in a captive environment. Captive amphibians may adapt to eating dead prey or meat; raw meat must be supplemented with calcium, at a recommended dose of 10 mg per gram of meat (McCune, 2003). In general, captive amphibians should be fed two to three times a week.

Frogs and toads eat a diet based primarily on insects, such as crickets, mealworms, and fruit flies. Salamanders eat earthworms, slugs, and other insects. Owners should be encouraged to replicate the natural environment of each species of amphibian to ensure food consumption and longevity.

EQUINE NUTRITION

NUTRIENTS FOR HORSES

Nutrients of concern for horses are water, energy, protein, calcium, phosphorus, and vitamin A. Although all animals require access to good-quality water on an ad lib basis, this is especially true for an animal capable of copious sweating (Carson, 1993). Hot, exhausted horses should rest and perhaps consume some hay while cooling. A waiting period of 30 minutes should occur before a horse is allowed to drink water after heavy exercise.

Horses evolved eating grass and other range forages. Not surprisingly, grass and hays serve well as a foundation for feeding all horses. Good-quality grass or legume hay, free-choice water, calcium, phosphorus as needed, and trace-mineralized salt are the only foods needed by adult horses during the maintenance life stage.

TECHNICIAN NOTE
Good quality grasses and legume hay are crucial for the adult horse.

Grain and protein meal concentrates balance forages during periods of higher-than-maintenance nutrient demand. Unfortunately, some horse feeding programs overlook quality forages and focus on elaborate programs of concentrate supplementation. The technician attending performance horses will also encounter a wide variety of owner- and trainer-selected supplements. These are diverse and may well match the current nutritional fad; note that time-proven horse feeding programs emphasize simplicity and quality forage feeds.

Equine food dose calculations are based on the horse's weight. One simple and frequently used method is calculation of the amount of feed per 100 lb of horse. Therefore a horse weight tape is a simple and inexpensive tool worth having and using to measure girth circumference to estimate

Table 15-12 ESTIMATING HORSE WEIGHT

Girth Circumference		Body Weight	
(in)	(cm)	(lb)	(kg)
64.5	163.8	800	363.6
67.5	171.5	900	409.1
70.5	179.1	1000	454.5
73.0	185.4	1100	500.0
75.5	191.8	1200	545.5
77.5	196.9	1300	590.9

body weight (Table 15-12). For example, a 6-year-old, 1000-lb light-breed gelding is at rest in a backyard paddock. The animal receives only 1 hour per week of light work. This horse is considered to be at maintenance activity, requiring 1.5% of the horse's body weight per day as dry matter (Figure 15-24). This means that 15 lb of a good-quality hay will suffice in addition to salt and water. If a 6-inch hay "flake" weighs 5 lb, then feeding three per day (one in the morning and two in the evening) can be suggested as a food dose. Figure 15-25 summarizes different dry matter intake levels for various activity and physiologic states. Note that feedstuffs should still be weighed to ensure accurate proportions.

As in small animals, equine overfeeding is a common problem. Routine body condition assessments should be included in all horse examinations. Note that some hays or hay-grain combinations require calcium and phosphorus supplementation. Most commonly, a source of phosphorus is added only when a good legume hay is the sole source of nutrition. Powdered mineral supplements are often mixed with hay or loose rock salt and provided as part of the diet. Loose rock salt should be a 50:50 mix of dicalcium phosphate and salt. Nutrient intake objectives and feeds to meet these can be found in Table 15-13.

TECHNICIAN NOTE
Routine body condition assessments should be included in all horse examinations.

The microminerals zinc, manganese, iron, copper, cobalt, and sometimes iodine are found in trace-mineralized salts. Salt blocks are generally *not* useful for the sick or depressed horse; in addition, blocks are generally for rough-tongued animals such as the deer.

Routine horse feeding problems include overgrazed pastures, ingestion of sand and weeds, underfeeding as a result of poor-quality forage, excessive grain consumption, too fine a grind pelleted feeds, various nutrient imbalances, and toxic supplementation. In addition, molasses or other sweet feeds should be used sparingly because of their high potassium content. Unfortunately, horses are not routinely or easily weighed in the typical setting, and changes in

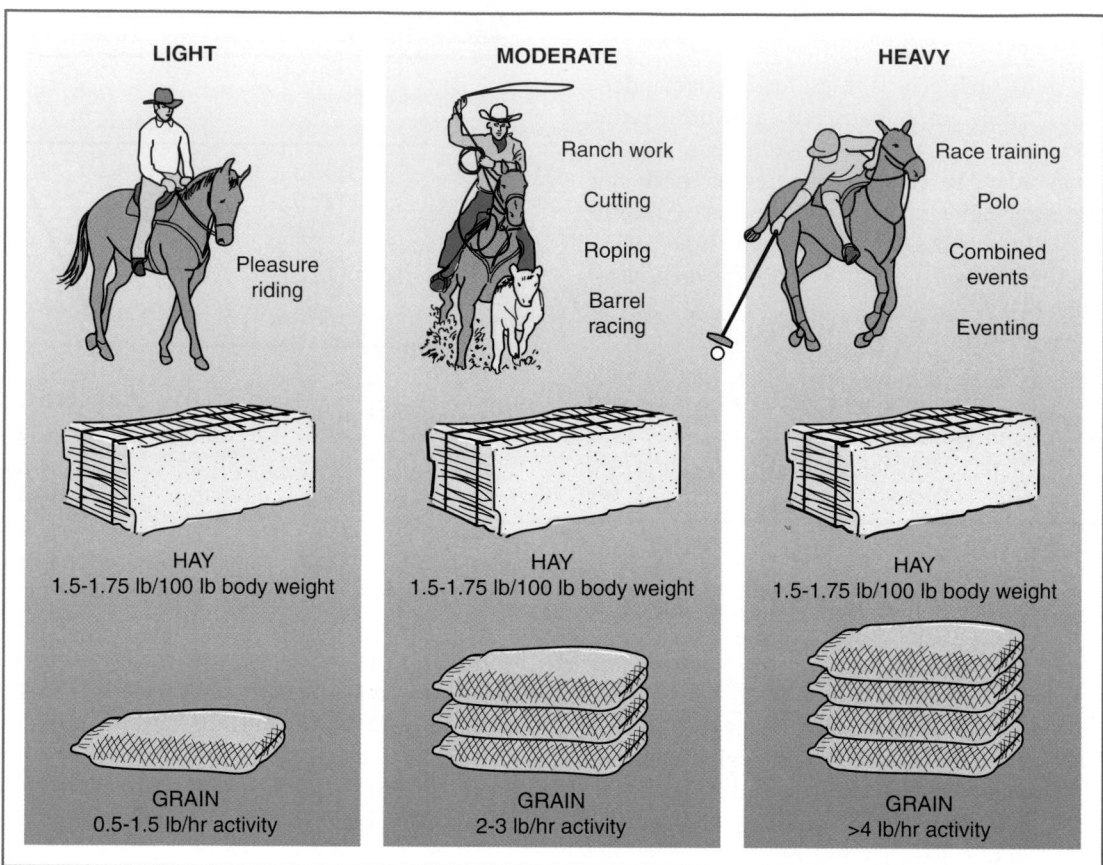

Figure 15-24 Adjusted feeding based on an activity level. Maintenance feed levels can be based per 100 lb of weight. Supplemental feeding over maintenance should be based on the level and duration of work.

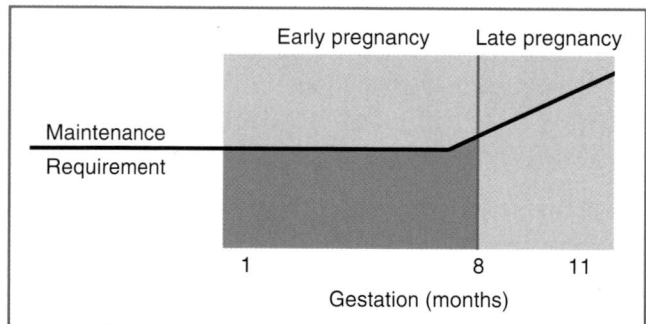

Figure 15-25 Early gestation is not "eating for two," and the mare should be fed for maintenance. In the last trimester of pregnancy, requirements for energy, protein, and minerals increase.

condition may be insidious. Accidental engorgement of grain may precipitate colic or founder with morbid or even tragic results. In general, daily grain ingestion of more than 6 lb increases the incidence of founder and colic.

FEEDING SICK HORSES

Hospitalized horses develop the same protein-calorie deficits, hypermetabolic stress, and catabolic wasting states as small animals. These have identical negative clinical effects, and early interventional feeding is vital in equine critical care. Major GI tract (colic) surgery is especially challenging in the perioperative period. The animal needs a diet rich in protein, calories, and micronutrients despite reduced GI motility. The veterinarian will focus closely as to when GI motility returns in order to support the sick horse. Often, homogenized, moistened alfalfa pellet mashes are high-protein, high-energy, and nonirritating formulas designed for replenishing nutrients. Such diets may be given as slurries through nasogastric tubes and are often enriched with nutriment modules. Liquid enteral formulas based on mare's milk replacement and commercial equine critical care formulas are available and well tolerated. Formulas should be given in small frequent feedings via indwelling nasogastric tubes.

ASSESSING FORAGES AND GRAINS FOR HORSES

The veterinary technician can assess the quality of water, pastures, and hays (Figure 15-26). A feed-bunk rule for horses is not to exceed a 50:50 ratio of concentrate to roughage. Oats and corn are the two most common feeds, and noting their relative energy content is important. Oats

Table 15-13 Nutrient Supply for Horses*

Age	Energy	Protein	Vitamins and Minerals	Comments
Nursing foals	Supplement mare's milk	>16%	Ca²⁺ >0.85% P>0.5% Cu >25 mg/kg Vitamin A 50 IU/kg BW	At 2-3 mo of age, begin 1 lb if foal is very thin concentrate mixture/mo of age/day Adequate Ca²⁺, P, trace minerals in grain mix If creep feeding, mix 50:50 chopped hay to grain Wean at 4 mo
Weaning	Adequate to feel but not see the ribs	15%	Ca²⁺ 0.7% P 0.4% Vitamin A 50 IU/kg BW	Dry matter intake = 3% of BW Free-choice good roughage and trace mineral salt 1 lb concentrate mix/mo of age/day: 7-9 lb mix
Yearling	Adequate to feel but not see the ribs	13%	Ca²⁺ 0.5% P 0.3% Vitamin A 50 IU/kg BW	Dry matter intake = 2.5% BW Free-choice good roughage, trace mineral salt 1 lb concentrate mix/mo of age/day: 7-9 lb max Feed as mature horse at 90% of mature weight
Adult *Maintenance*	Adequate to feel but not see the ribs	8.5%	Ca²⁺ 0.3% P 0.2% Vitamin A 50 IU/kg BW	Dry matter = 1.5% BW 1½-1½ lb roughage/100 lb BW Free-choice trace mineral salt
Adult *Working* Light (pleasure ride)	Add 0.5-1.5 lb of grain/hr of activity/day	8.5%	Ca²⁺ 0.3% P 0.2% Vitamin A 50 IU/kg BW	Amortize grain supplement over the week
Moderate (ranch work, roping, cutting, jumping, barrel racing)	Add 2-3 lb grain/hr of activity/day	8.5%-10%	Ca²⁺ 0.3% P 0.2% Vitamin A 50 IU/kg BW	
Heavy (race training, polo)	Add 4 or more lb of grain/hr of activity/day	8.5%-10%	Ca²⁺ 0.3% P 0.2% Vitamin A 50 IU/kg BW	Dry matter = 1.75% BW
Adult reproduction *Mares*	Feed at maintenance until late pregnancy	8.5%-10%		
Late pregnancy	Needs 20% more energy	11%	Ca²⁺ 0.5% P 0.35% Vitamin A 50 IU/kg BW	Feed 1½-1¾ lb grass hays/100 lb BW with addition of ½-¾ lb grain or concentrate mix/100 lb BW Free-choice trace mineral salt-mineral Ca²⁺/P mix
Last 3 wk of pregnancy	Needs 30% more energy		Needs 100%, more Ca²⁺ and P Vitamin A 60 IU/kg BW	1¾-2 lb legume hay/100 lb BW Free-choice trace mineral salt-mineral Ca²⁺/P mix
Lactation	Allow 75% energy increase at peak lactation	14%	Ca²⁺ 0.5% P 0.35% Vitamin A 60 IU/kg BW	Dry matter = 1.75%-2.0% BW free-choice grass hay Add 1½-2 lb/100 lb BW of concentrate Add Ca²⁺/P mix and trace mineralized salt At weaning, stop concentrate; return to maintenance forage
Stallions	Feed for maintenance			

BW, Body weight; *Ca*, calcium; *Cu*, copper; *P*, phosphorus.
*Free-choice, potable water should be available at all times.

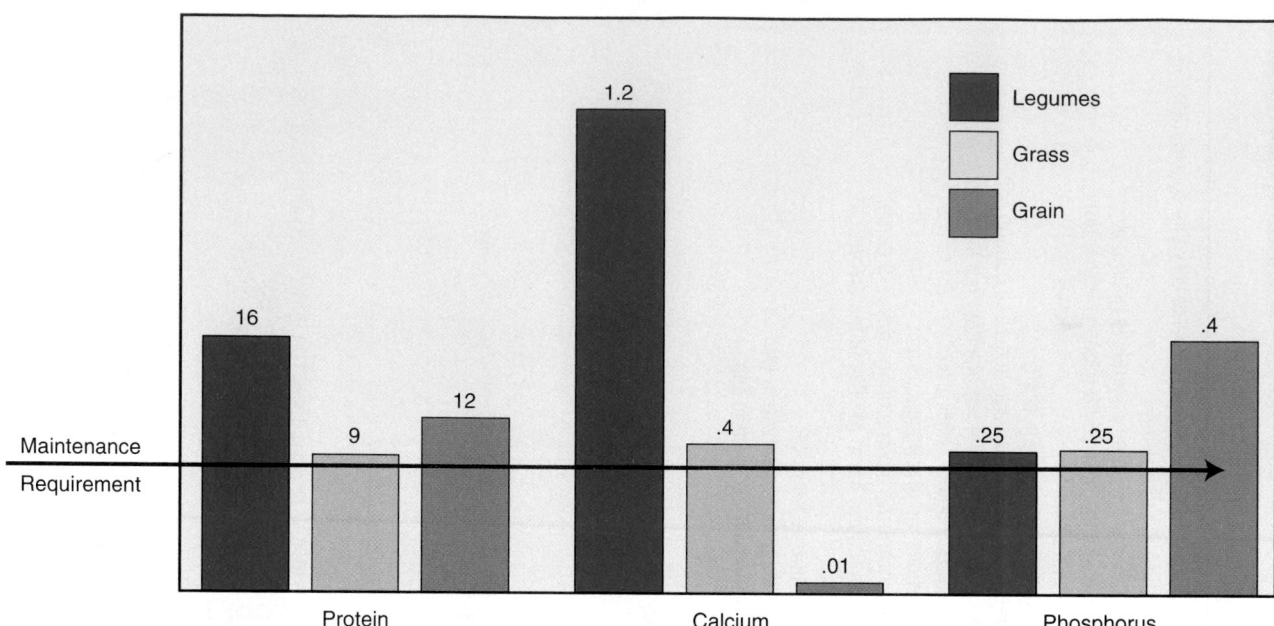

Figure 15-26 High-quality grass and legume hays, water, and salt suffice for equine maintenance. However, a source of supplemental phosphorus benefits some hay and can be provided as mineral mix.

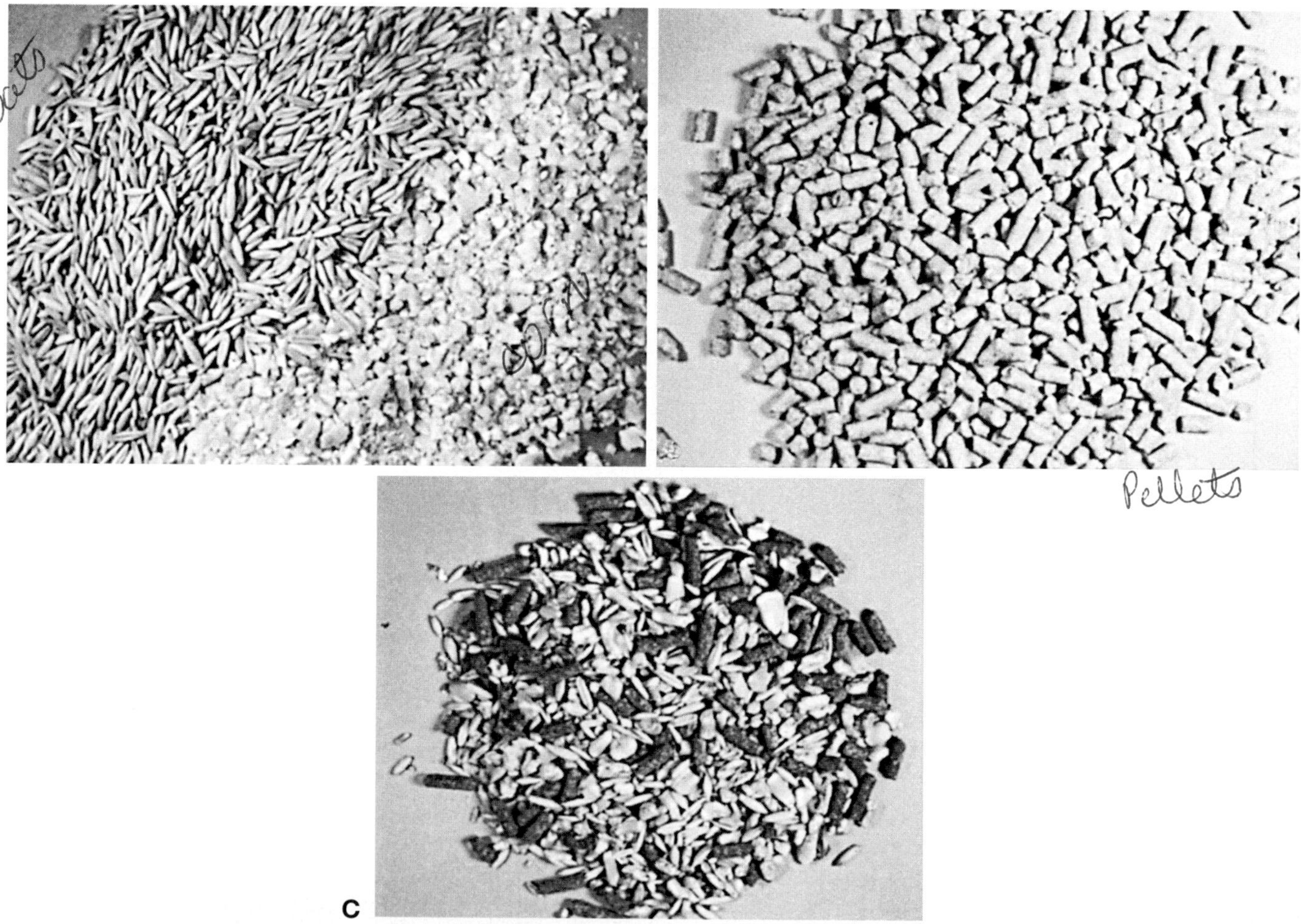

Figure 15-27 **A,** Grain and protein-meal concentrates complement the forage foundation of equine feeds. Concentrates are needed when significantly more energy or protein is required. Oats *(left)* and corn are two popular concentrate grains. On an equal volume basis, corn provides twice the energy of oats. This difference should be made clear to owners who usually feed by volume (coffee can) and may switch between the two grains. **B,** Pelleted horse foods are an expensive convenience but may lack the chewing or gastrointestinal fullness effects associated with long-stem roughage. Some horses chew or gnaw wood when consuming only complete foods. **C,** Complete horse feeds may be mixed from grain, forages, and mineral mixes and then pelleted or extruded. Complete feed can be used as a hay supplement or as the total diet when hay is unavailable.

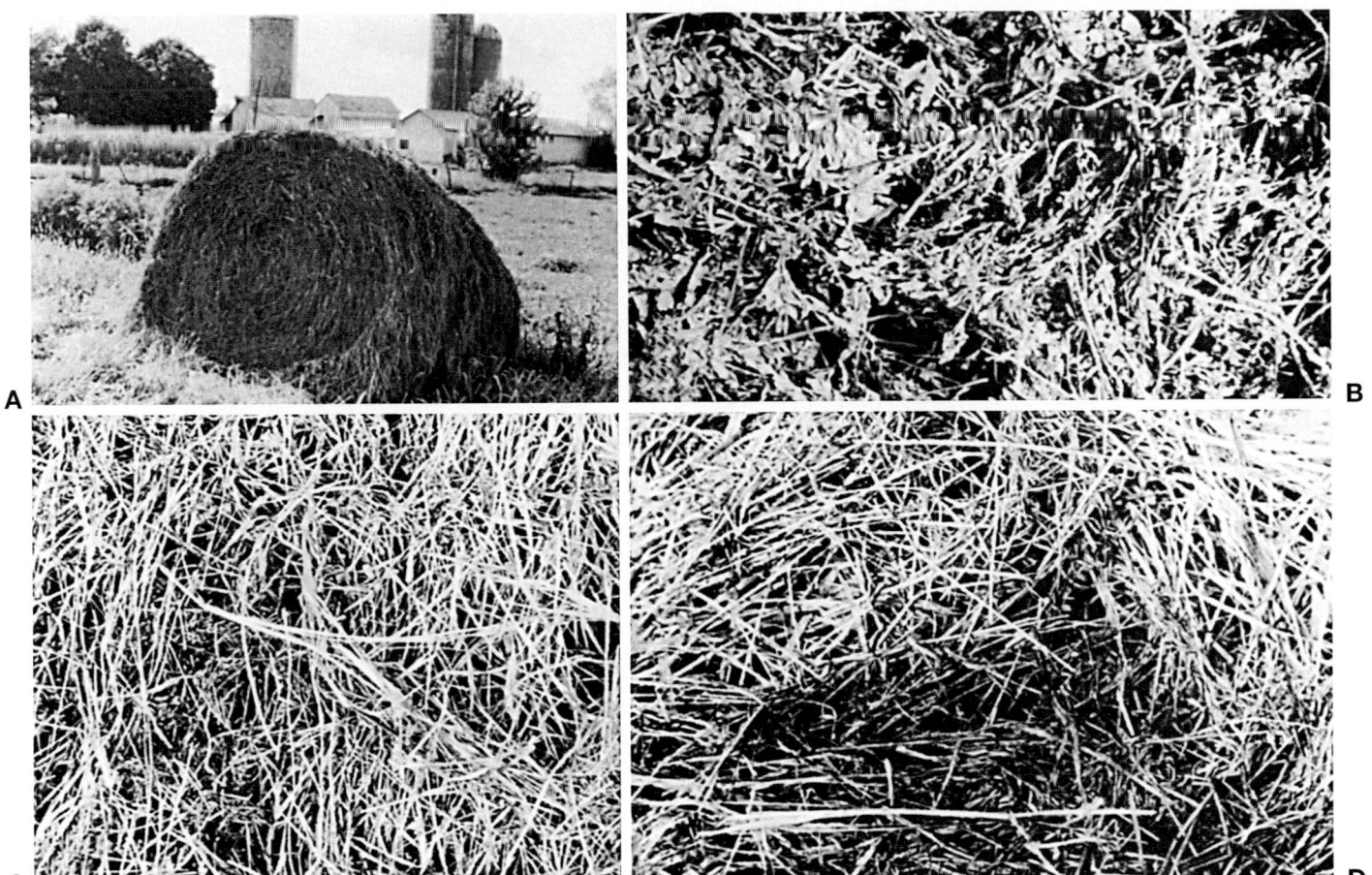

Figure 15-28 A laboratory analysis for protein, energy, and macrominerals gives objective guidelines to forage quality and is available from agricultural extension services. Hay quality depends on the species of forage (legume vs. grass), maturity, cutting number, curing, handling, storage (**A**), and age when fed. **B,** High-quality alfalfa hay is not overmature and has a high proportion of leaves to stems. Leaves contain two thirds of the energy and three fourths of the protein. Flexible, tender stems, light green color, and absence of molds and dust are seen in good legume hay. **C,** Poor-quality alfalfa hay has reduced leaf numbers and tough stems. Seed heads in a grass hay and flowers in alfalfa hay indicate overmaturity at the time of cutting. **D,** A hay contaminated by mold *(dark areas)* is usually unpalatable and possibly dangerous.

are generally digested easily with less resultant cecal pH changes. Various horse grains, mixed concentrate supplements, and several totally complete extruded or pelleted horse feeds will be encountered on horse calls (Figure 15-27). If horses consume only complete extruded or pelleted feeds, adequate roughage intake may be an issue. A minimum of 10% to 15% of long-stem fiber sources in the diet is recommended. The sudden onset of fence chewing suggests the need for at least some long-stem or coarse chopped hay, particularly if only a complete pelleted food is used.

Forage quality varies greatly by soil quality, species of grass, season of year, rainfall, overgrazing, pasture rotation, weed control, and the presence of toxic weeds. Laboratory analysis of forages for moisture, energy, protein, fiber, and macrominerals and micronutrients is fundamental in assessing roughage nutrient content. Hay analysis is performed at little or no cost by regional agriculture extension services. When hay analysis is unavailable, one can make some conclusions about hay quality from a physical inspection. Observe the leafiness and the leaf/stem ratio; this is important because two thirds of the energy and three fourths of the protein are found in leaves (Figure 15-28). Smaller and more flexible stems suggest the correct maturity for grass and legume hays. Fully developed seed heads in grass hay and flowers in alfalfa may indicate overmaturity. Greenness (chlorophyll and beta-carotene); presence of weeds, mold, or foreign material; rain damage; poor curing; and mechanical mishandling are other qualities to be checked in visual forage assessment.

TECHNICIAN NOTE

Forage quality varies greatly by soil quality, species of grass, season of year, rainfall, overgrazing, pasture rotation, weed control, and the presence of toxic weeds.

ACKNOWLEDGMENT

The authors and editors wish to acknowledge the exceptional contributions of Drs. Philip Roudebush and Stephen W. Crane and Sheila R. Grosdidier, RVT, whose original contributions served as the foundation for the material appearing in this edition. Drs. Pugh, Lawhorn, and Stanton from the Department of Clinical Sciences at Auburn University are also acknowledged for recommending current therapies in equine nutrition.

References

Biourge V: Feline nutrition update, 2001, http:www.vin.com/VINDBPub/SearchPB/Proceedings/PR05000/PR00119.htm.

Carson TL: Water quality for livestock. In Howard JL, editor: *Current veterinary therapy: food animal practice*, ed 3, Philadelphia, 1993, WB Saunders.

Crane SW: Occurrence and management of obesity in companion animals, *J Small Anim Pract* 32:275, 1991.

Head E, Zicker SC: Neutraceuticals, aging, and cognitive dysfunction. In *The veterinary clinics: small animal practice*, St. Louis, 2004, WB Saunders.

Hillyer, Quesenberry: *Ferrets, Rabbits, and Rodents, Clin Medicine and Surgery* 1997, WB Saunders.

Markham RW, Hodgkins EM: Geriatric nutrition, *Vet Clin North Am* 19:165, 1989.

McCune S: Nutrition. In: *Veterinary nursing*, ed 3, 2003, Butterworth-Heinemann.

McDonald ML et al: Essential fatty acid requirements of cats: pathology of essential fatty acid deficiency, *Am J Vet Res* 45:1310, 1984.

Mumma RO et al: Toxic and protective constituents in pet food, *Am J Vet Res* 47:1633, 1986.

Recommended Reading

Bonagura JD: *Current veterinary therapy*, XIII, Philadelphia, 2000, WB Saunders.
  Management of anorexia, pp 69-74
  Nutritional assessment of pet food labels, pp 74-80
  Parenteral nutrition products, pp 80-84
  Mechanical devices for percutaneous placement of gastrostomy tubes: use of Eld applicator, pp 94-97
  Refeeding syndrome, pp 87-89
  Microenteral nutrition, pp 136-140
  Hypoallergenic diets for dogs and cats, pp 530-536
  Essential fatty acids, pp 538-542
  Esophageal feeding tubes, pp 597-599
  Dietary sensitivity, pp 632-637
  Nutritional management of diarrheal diseases, pp 653-658
  Nutritional management of liver disease, pp 693-697
  Nutritional management of heart disease, pp 711-716
  Summary of dietary recommendations in urinary diseases, pp 841-846

Hand MS et al, editors: *Small animal clinical nutrition*, ed 4, Topeka, Kan, 2000, Mark Morris Institute.
  Small animal clinical nutrition: an iterative process, pp 1-19
  Nutrients, pp 21-107
  Introduction to commercial pet foods, pp 112-126
  Making commercial pet foods, pp 127-146
  Pet food labels, pp 147-161
  Making pet foods at home, pp 163-181
  Food safety, pp 183-198
  Health maintenance programs for dogs and cats, pp 201-211
  Normal dogs, pp 213-260
  Normal cats, pp 291-347
  Assisted feeding in hospitalized patients: enteral and parenteral nutrition, pp 351-399
  Obesity, pp 401-430
  Dental disease, pp 475-504
  Developmental orthopedic disease of dogs, pp 505-521
  Renal disease, pp 563-594
  Feline lower urinary tract disease, pp 689-718
  Feeding small exotic mammals, pp 943-960
  Feeding reptiles, pp 961-977
  Feeding passerine and psittacine birds, pp 979-991
  Neonatal, pediatric and orphaned puppy and kitten care, pp 1012-1019
  Comparative analysis of milks and milk replacers, pp 1064-1072
  Feeding orphaned and injured birds, mammals, amphibians and reptiles, pp 1101-1121

Lewis LD: *Equine clinical nutrition: feeding and care*, Philadelphia, 1995, Williams & Wilkins.

Robinson NE: *Current therapy in equine medicine*, ed 4, Philadelphia, 1997, WB Saunders.

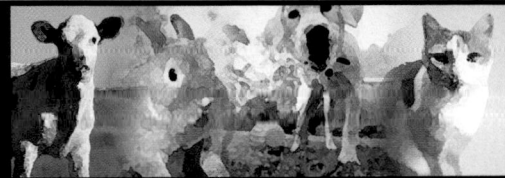

Large Animal Clinical Nutrition

WILLIAM D. SCHOENHERR

INTRODUCTION

Optimal nutrition has often been identified as the most expensive element in achieving full productivity and profitability in livestock (Ensminger, 1990). The veterinary technician must have a strong fundamental knowledge of nutrient needs and be able to identify potential for problems and increase the client's understanding of essential feeding philosophies. The client who has the greatest need for this type of information is not the large intensive livestock farmer who normally has feeds professionally formulated for optimum production. Most often, the questions will be from clients who run small operations, have family members raising livestock for 4-H or Children's club's (e.g., as future Farmers of America) projects, or possess a "hobby farm." With these needs in mind, this chapter focuses on common nutritional problems and sound principles to help the veterinary technician provide meaningful, relevant information.

Various nutritional disorders can be very similar to a vast array of diseases and may not be easily identified by the livestock producer as a nutritional disorder until the problem becomes chronic and additional assistance is sought. Therefore it is essential to get a complete history, including a detailed feeding regimen, on any livestock patient who is exhibiting signs of illness.

Dramatic enhancements have occurred in large animal nutrition, including studies that have increased understanding of the specific nutrient needs of livestock to maximize the genetic potential for efficient production, successful breeding, and generation of high-quality, lean meat. Future research will continue to improve our understanding of animal physiology and lead to improvements in livestock production (Table 16-1). ■

NUTRIENTS

Nutrients are ingested to support life. Livestock producers want to obtain the most desirable results from the nutrients their animals consume at an economical rate and with an advantageous financial return. Ingested nutrients are either retained by the animal or excreted in the urine and feces. Retained nutrients are used for a wide array of body functions, such as homeostasis; replenishment and development of tissues; reproduction; and milk, wool, and meat production.

Maintenance nutrient requirements (MNRs) are the levels of nutrients needed to sustain body weight without gain or loss (Box 16-1). The MNR is the minimum level of dietary need; usually the vast percentage of published requirements are higher than this standard. As a general rule, one half of consumed and absorbed nutrients are used to fulfill MNRs. Individual variation results in fluctuation from this standard; be sure to evaluate need against all information to achieve most accurate results.

Feeding standards are available listing the amounts of nutrients required by different species for specific productive purposes, such as maintenance, growth, finishing, lactation, work, wool, or eggs. The most widely used feeding standards in the United States are those published by the National Research Council (NRC), and they are established for beef cattle, dairy cattle, sheep, goats, swine, and poultry (see Recommended Reading). Periodically, the feeding standards are updated and published by a committee appointed by the NRC.

✑ TECHNICIAN NOTE

MNRs are the level of nutrients needed to sustain body weight without gain or loss.

Table 16-1 FEEDING PROBLEMS IN RUMINANTS

Disease	Symptoms	Cause	Prevention	Comments
Bloat	Distension of the left flank and then the right flank Hypersalivation Profuse burning ↑ Froth or gas accumulation in the rumen Respiratory distress Cyanosis Death	↑ Change in pasture with heavy fertilizer Genetics Bacterial overgrowth Overeating	Feed coarse grasses or dry forage before turnout to quick-growing pastures. Avoid straight pastures. Keep stock on pasture continuously rather than sporadically. Allow full access to water and salt.	Watch legume exposure for all ruminants.
Enterotoxemia (overeating disease)	Death is often the first symptom Circling Progressive weakness Head butting Convulsions	Often occurs in faster-growing juveniles *Clostridium perfringens* Excess consumption of high-energy feeds or lush pasture or heavy milk supply	Vaccinate with *Clostridium perfringens* type D for lambs and types C and D for breeding ewes.	Applies primarily in sheep and goats; sometimes cattle. If outbreak occurs, consider enterotoxemia antiserum for 21-day protection in lambs.
Fescue toxicosis (fescue foot)	↓ +/- Lameness Necrosis of tail end Milk production Abortion	↑ Change in parasitized animal ↑ In malnourished animal Endophyte fungus *Acremonium coerophalum*	Avoid heavy parasitism and malnutrition. Use fungus-free fescue seed for planting.	Applies for cattle and sheep mostly. Highest occurrence is in fall and winter in all fescue pasture.
Grass tetany (hypomagnesemia)	Disorientation Paddling Convulsions Muscle twitching	Most common in cows 4 yr and older ↑ Occurrence during early lactation in heavy milking cows Pastures with ↓ Mg²⁺ and ↑ K⁺ and ↓ Ca⁺ availability	Start providing Mg²⁺ 30 days before high-risk times. ↑ Mg²⁺ in lactating and older cows and ewes Highest risk is during spring, winter, and fall. Molasses supplement with Mg²⁺ may be required.	Stress front weather, movement, or environment increases risk.
Milk fever (parturition, paresis, or hypocalcemia)	↓ Appetite Nervous behavior Collapse Wrenching of head toward back	Postcalving in high-producing cows ↓ Blood Ca²⁺	Feed ↑ P, ↓ Ca²⁺ 14 days before parturition. Feed balanced Ca²⁺/P rations. Vitamin D intake provided 1 wk before parturition. Avoid obesity.	Watch Ca²⁺ and P levels in dry periods.
Displaced abomasum	↓ Appetite ↓ Milk production Diarrhea, discolored feces	Pregnancy Lack of bulk in diet Sudden jarring of fresh cows Poor muscle tone Mycotoxin exposure	Avoid acidosis or alkalosis. Eliminate or reduce moldy or mycotoxin-laden feeds.	Occurs most frequently in high-producing, heavily fed dairy cattle near parturition.

Table 16-1 FEEDING PROBLEMS IN RUMINANTS—CONT'D

Disease	Symptoms	Cause	Prevention	Comments
Ketosis	Occurs: 14-50 days after parturition in cattle 2 wk before parturition in sheep ↓ Milk production ↓ Appetite Sugary-acid breath ↓ Body weight Frequent urination Trembling Collapse	↑ Chances in multiple births with ewes and does Rapid loss of body fat and low availability of carbohydrates in diet	Maintain lean body condition and avoid excess fat. ↑ Energy intake before parturition and ↓ after parturition. Avoid sudden changes in the physical nature of the feeds.	Ewes are at risk before lambing. Cows are typically at risk after calving.
Thiamine-deficiency polio	Decreased vision Incoordination Acute death Excitable	Thiamine deficiency Overgrazing Feeding lambs in rich pasture	Cause not fully discovered. ↓ Grain intake while ↑ roughage quality, 1 wk before. ↑ Animals' intake of high-energy diets.	Occur primarily in feedlot and young cattle under 2 yr old. Goats may be affected while nursing young.
Rickets	In young animals, enlarged joints Painful gait Leg bowing	Incorrect Ca^{2+}, P, vitamin intake	Provide balanced Ca^{2+}, P, and vitamin D diets.	
Urinary calculi Urolithiasis Water belly	Difficult urination Bloody urine Kicking at abdomen Rupture of bladder	↑ Increase in feedlots High K^+ consumption, ↑ P, ↓ Ca^{2+} Vitamin A deficiency Excess silicate intake	Provide readily available water Balance P/Ca^{2+} ratio. Avoid vitamin A deficiency. ↑ Salt availability. Balance ratios.	Males have ↑ risk.
White muscle disease	Irregular gait Hunched-back appearance Heart irregularities Death	Selenium deficiency Geographic distribution: ↓ Se in many areas of United States and Canada	↑ Se to dietary intake in known deficient areas.	Most commonly occurs in most rapidly growing individuals in flock or herd.

From Naylor JM et al: *Large animal clinical nutrition*, St Louis, 1991, Mosby; McDonald P et al: *Animal nutrition*, New York, 1995, Longman Scientific and Technical; Maynard LA et al: *Animal nutrition*, ed 7, New York, 1979, McGraw-Hill; Ensminger ME et al: *Feeds and nutrition*, Clovis, Calif, 1990, Ensminger Publishing.

Box 16-1 ELEMENTS THAT INFLUENCE NUTRIENT REQUIREMENTS OF LIVESTOCK

- Body size
- Health status
- Stress
- Environment
- Exercise
- Behavior
- Genetics
- Reproductive status
- Gender
- Breed

Box 16-2 RELATIVE IMPORTANCE OF LIVESTOCK FEEDS (% OF TOTAL TONNAGE FED)

- Pasture/grasslands 40.0%*
- Corn 23.3%
- Hay 12.2%
- Grains/high-protein feeds 16.9%
- Silage/miscellaneous 7.6%

From the U.S. Department of Agriculture (USDA) Economic Research Service, 1983-1984.
*Varies significantly by season and pasture quality.

Digestion (the process of protein, carbohydrate, and fat breakdown into absorbable nutrients) is accomplished by both chemical and physical methods. It is essential to remember that it is not the alfalfa hay, corn, or oats that is actually used by the cells of livestock but rather the digested and absorbed nutrients, such as amino acids, sugars, fatty acids, minerals, and vitamins, that present at the cellular level. The quality, quantity, and cost of nutrients that can be provided by the feedstuff are of primary importance when choosing ingredients for farm animal feeding.

PROTEIN

Protein is the principal constituent of organs and soft tissues. It is constructed of building blocks called *amino acids* that are linked together in a chain. The arrangement of amino acids in the chain and the length of the chain are two factors that help to determine the composition of the protein. There are 10 essential and 12 nonessential amino acids. Essential amino acids must be supplied in the diet because the animal body cannot synthesize them fast enough to meet its requirement. Amino acids consist of nitrogen, carbon, oxygen, and sulfur. The deconstruction or deamination process releases these elements into the body system and results in either their elimination from the body or their use as energy.

> **TECHNICIAN NOTE**
>
> Protein is a common component of plants, with highest constituency in the seed and leafy portions.

Animal feeds (Box 16-2) are identified often by crude protein content, but the measurement rarely illustrates the quality or utilization potential of the protein. A feed can possess a high protein content, yet the *biologic value* of that protein is low. Protein biologic value is the percentage of true absorbed protein that is available for productive body functions. Conceptually, it is the "amino acid grade card," since it defines the available amino acids. In general, proteins of animal origin have greater biologic value than do proteins of plant origin. The higher the biologic value, the better is the protein used for productive purposes. Protein quality is also measured as *protein efficiency ratio,* which is the number of grams of body weight gain per unit of protein consumed (McDonald, 1995).

Animal and plant proteins vary greatly in their distribution of amino acids and biologic value. When combined in correct proportions with other protein (e.g., animal protein), proteins that individually have very poor biologic value (e.g., corn) may yield a biologic value similar to that of a single high-quality protein. The quality of proteins depends on disallowing overprocessing of feeds, overheating in storage, and form of the feed (Nash, 1985) (Figure 16-1).

USE BY RUMINANTS

Rumen digestion facilitated by microbes has the ability to convert most feed protein into peptides and amino acids, many of which are further degraded into ammonia, organic acids, and carbon dioxide. The ammonia released on microbial degradation of feed protein will be removed from the rumen by absorption through the rumen wall or used by the microorganisms for synthesis of microbial protein. Microbial protein synthesized by the microorganisms results in a fairly constant protein quality supply to the lower digestive tract. The protein quality from moderate to poor feeds will usually be improved by rumen metabolism, whereas the opposite may occur with high-quality protein feeds. The rumen microbes also have the ability to convert nonprotein nitrogen sources into microbial protein. Typical nonprotein nitrogen sources include urea, ammonium salts, ammoniated by-products, or free amino acids and are best used judiciously because an excess or an imbalanced intake can be toxic (Church, 1984).

FATS

Fats provide dietary energy; serve as a source of heat, insulation, and protection for the animal body; and provide essential fatty acids. Fat has 2.25 times more energy per gram than protein or carbohydrates. Fats also aid the absorption of fat-soluble vitamins. Linoleic, linolenic, and arachidonic fatty acids are considered essential, even though linoleic acid is capable of being converted to arachidonic acid. However, the process to make these conversions is arduous and inefficient, and as such, arachidonic acid should be considered conditionally essential (McDonald, 1995).

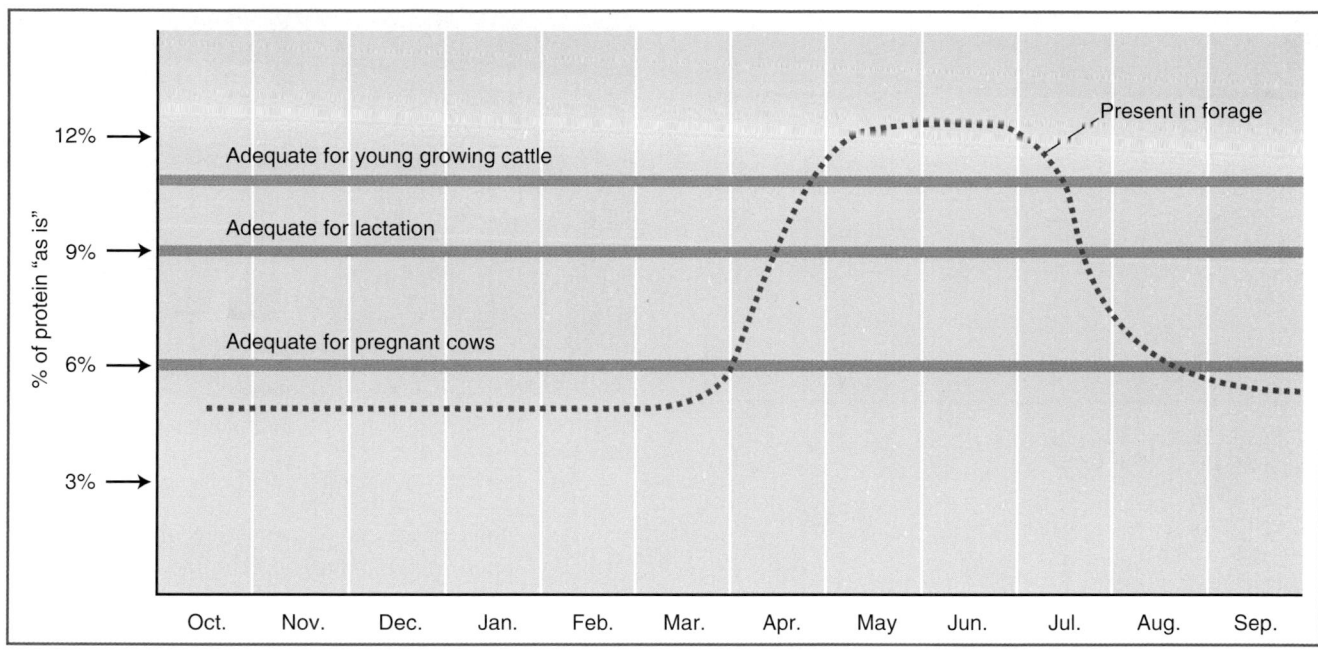

Figure 16-1 Nutrient content of forage varies with pasture quality and season.

✏ **TECHNICIAN NOTE**

Fat has more energy per gram than all other nutrients.

CARBOHYDRATES

Carbohydrates (Box 16-3) are the primary energy source in livestock rations. They are less expensive and more readily available than proteins or fats. Most feedstuffs of plant origin are high in carbohydrate content, especially cereal grains. Carbohydrates must be broken down into simple sugars for absorption from the digestive system. This requires digestive enzymes generated by the host or by microflora inhabiting the digestive system of the host. The carbohydrate-splitting enzymes are effective in splitting most complex carbohydrates into simple sugars except those with the beta linkage, as found in cellulose (fiber). Microflora in the rumen of ruminants and the cecum of some nonruminants, such as the horse or rabbit, produce an enzyme so that these species can use fiber for energy. Carbohydrates are commonly categorized into animal feeds as concentrates (grains, high-starch compounds) and forages (grass, hays, legumes). There are no minimum or maximum requirements for carbohydrates; rather, intake is defined in conjunction with energy need.

✏ **TECHNICIAN NOTE**

Carbohydrates are the primary energy source in livestock rations.

Box 16-3 CATEGORIES OF CARBOHYDRATES

- *Fiber-forages:* Structural carbohydrates, cellulose, hemicellulose
- *Sugars (molasses, growing plants):* Glucose, sucrose, fructose
- *Starches:* Stored carbohydrates, grains

FEEDSTUFF ENERGY

The largest function of feed is to provide energy for body processes. Total digestible nutrients (TDNs), gross energy, digestible energy, metabolizable energy, and net energy are all different measures of feed energy value.

TDN is a general measure of the nutritive value of a feed. Digestibility coefficients are used to compute the content of total digestible nutrients. The usefulness of TDN as a measure of feed energy is limited in that it does not take into account energy losses in urine, combustible gases, and heat. The discrepancies can be large for forage-based feeds, because they tend to overestimate the energy available for productive purposes. TDN is expressed as a percentage of the ration or in units of weight and not as an actual caloric number.

Gross energy (GE) is the total energy (Box 16-4) potentially available in a feed consumed by an animal. All energy values used in the following scheme are expressed in kilocalories (kcal) or megacalories (Mcal) per unit of weight. During digestion and absorption, a portion of the GE escapes the body in the form of undigested food residue in the feces. Subtraction of the energy lost in the feces from the consumed GE accounts for energy that was digested and

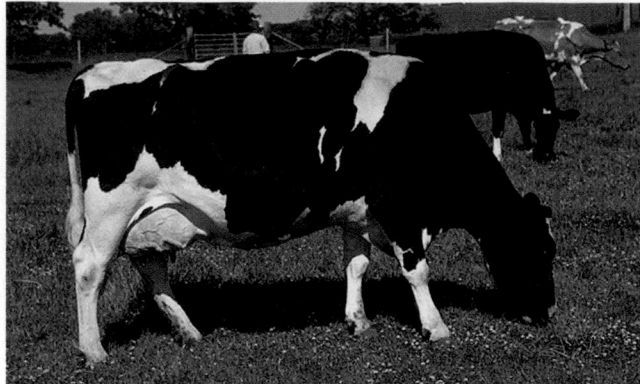

Figure 16-2 Holsteins are the predominant breed in the dairy industry.

many metabolic processes. Minerals are divided into two categories: microminerals and macrominerals (Box 16-5). The list of minerals and vitamins and their functions are given in Tables 16-2 to 16-4.

WATER

Water is the cheapest and most abundant nutrient. It makes up 65% to 85% of an animal's body weight at birth and 45% to 60% of body weight at maturity. Water is derived metabolically from the breakdown of organic nutrients in the animal tissues or drinking water or obtained from foodstuffs. Because water is the largest constituent of the animal, deprivation of water of only a few percentages of body weight is life threatening. Clean, fresh water should be readily available to maintain a zero water balance (Table 16-5).

⬛ TECHNICIAN NOTE
Water is the cheapest and most abundant nutrient.

DAIRY CATTLE

The dairy industry is successfully using many different production systems. Systems are based on geographic area and feedstuff availability. The traditional pasture system continues to be used in areas with readily available land, whereas dry lot systems are more popular in urban and suburban areas (Figure 16-2).

Regardless of the dairy production system, two feeding programs predominate. Total mixed ration (TMR) is the practice of weighing and blending all feedstuffs into a complete ration. Each bite consumed by the cow contains all the required levels of nutrients needed. The other program is a forage and grain diet fed separately. The animals are provided hay free choice at all times, silage is offered once or twice per day, and feed concentrates are fed twice daily.

Feeding, more than any other single factor, determines the productivity of lactating dairy cows. Feed represents

absorbed, or *digestible energy (DE)*. The measurement of DE uses the same elements as TDN and gives similar energy values to feed. Energy that is digested and absorbed by the body is not used with 100% efficiency; a portion of the absorbed energy is lost in the urine and as combustible gases. Accounting for these energy losses leads to a step beyond DE or TDN, *metabolizable energy (ME)*. The energy values for ME are used widely in the formulation of swine and poultry feeds. One further refinement in this energy scheme is accounting for heat lost from the body during metabolism of the nutrients. *Net energy (NE)* represents the actual portion of energy available to the animal for use in maintaining body tissues or during pregnancy or lactation. NE values are used extensively in the beef, dairy, and sheep industry.

MINERALS AND VITAMINS

Minerals and vitamins are needed in small amounts compared with other nutrients but play integral roles in

Table 16-2 MACROMINERALS FOR FOOD ANIMALS

Minerals	Use	Toxicity	Deficiency	Sources
Calcium	Nerve transmission Clotting cascade Cardiac function Muscle contraction Milk production	Calcium kidney stones ↑ Calcium deposition into soft tissue ↑ Blood calcium level ↓ Absorption of Zn, Mg, Fe, Cu	↓ Quality of bone/teeth ↓ Milk production Osteomalacia Osteoporosis Hypocalcemia (tetany) Rickets	Alfalfa Milk Fish by-products Soybean meal Bone meal Dicalcium phosphate supplement
Phosphorus	Milk secretion Building muscle Teeth/bone development Acid-base balance Protein metabolism	↓ Absorption of Ca Urinary stones if Ca low	Similar to Ca Osteomalacia Rickets Hematuria Pica ↓ Breeding ↓ capability	Meat meals Soybean oil meal Wheat bran Bone meal Monosodium phosphate supplement
Sodium	Muscle contraction Absorption of carbohydrates Part of sweat and bile Osmotic pressure Acid-base balance Water balance	↑ Toxicity with ↓ H_2O intake Staggering Blindness Hypertension Neurologic disorders	↓ Breeding capability Cravings: urine drinking ↓ Growth rate ↓ Milk production Weight loss ↓ Appetite	Molasses Meat by-products Salt/mineral blocks Monosodium glutamate supplement
Potassium	Heart function Insulin secretion Acid-base balance Muscle development	↓ Heart rate ↓ Mg use Exaggerated when ↓ Mg and H_2O restricted	↓ Growth Excess NaCl depletes K Irregular gait Pica ↓ Weight	Molasses Forages Soy by-products Carrots Potassium gluconate supplement
Chlorine	Water balance Osmotic pressure Acid-base balance HCl production in stomach	↑ When water is restricted Rare	↓ Appetite ↓ Growth Alkalosis ↓ Respiratory rate Muscle cramps Convulsions Alfalfa	Meat meals Molasses Salt blocks (NaCl) Potassium chloride supplement
Magnesium	Cellular energy metabolism Alkalinizer Nerve impulse relaxant Bone and teeth	Rare	↑ Grass tetany ↑ Body temperature Respiratory rate Hypersalivation Death	Meat/bone meal Molasses Wheat bran Alfalfa supplements
Sulfur	Carbohydrate metabolism Insulin production Hair and wool production	Hydrogen sulfide gas production	↓ Growth ↓ Hair/wool production	Meat meal Yeast Whey Supplements

about 50% of the total cost of milk production. Therefore a good feeding program is necessary for profitable milk production. Nutrient requirements for lactation are large and often several times the MNR (Figure 16-3 and Tables 16-6 to 16-8). Water is also important for dairy cows (Boxes 16-6 and 16-7).

TECHNICIAN NOTE

Feed represents 50% of the total costs of milk production.

ENERGY

Carbohydrates (forage, concentrate) are the major energy source for lactation, followed by fats and proteins. Carbohydrates constitute 50% to 80% of energy on a dry matter basis of many forages and grains. Forages possess a significant fiber content that is broken down by the microbial population in the rumen and used as energy.

Although the rumen capacity of the dairy cow is considerable, she cannot eat sufficient forage to meet her extensive nutrient needs during lactation. Estimated daily intake for

Tables 16-3 Microminerals for Food Animals

Minerals	Use	Toxicity	Deficiency	Sources
Zinc	Skin Hair Bone maintenance Synthesis of protein Development of 　reproductive organs	↓ Growth Anemia Bone changes ↑ Appetite Stiff gait	↓ Growth ↓ Appetite Bone irregularities ↓ Wound healing Wool and hair loss Parakeratosis	Meat meal Corn gluten or germ meal Wheat by-products 　supplements
Selenium	Vitamin and sparing-tissue 　damage Fatty acid oxidation	Weight loss Blind staggers Lameness Anemia Paralysis	White muscle disease 　(sheep) Liver necrosis (pigs)	Poultry/fish meals Wheat by-products Cereals Oil seed meals
Manganese	Bone/cartilage growth Clotting cascade Metabolism of nutrients	Nontoxic	↓ Growth Lameness Reproductive disorders	Wheat Grass/alfalfa/hay Corn Sorghum supplements
Iodine	Hormone production Influence growth Muscle tissue development Milk production Nutrient metabolism	Horse: Hyperparathyroidism Goiter ↓ Utilization of iodine	↓ Hair quality ↓ Growth Reproductive problems Abortion	Molasses Meat/bone meal Oats Wheat Iodized salt Soybean meal
Fluorine	Bone Teeth	↓ Feed use ↓ Hair/wool quality Deformed teeth/bone	Rare	Fish meals Present in most foods
Chromium	Synthesis of some fatty acids ↑ Insulin use Stabilizes DNA and RNA	Rare	Hyperglycemia glucosuria ↓ Fat metabolism	Wheat Potatoes Corn Vegetable oil Supplements
Copper	Pigment of hair/wool Reproduction Skeletal structure Hemoglobin construction Absorption of iron	Although rare, sometimes 　seen in sheep ingestion 　of copper foot bath Gastroenteritis Hypersalivation ? Appetite Thirst	Swayback (lambs) ↓ Wool quality Lameness Anemia Diarrhea	Safflower oil Molasses Grass hays Cotton seeds Mineral mix
Iron	Hemoglobin production Muscle oxygenation Enzyme activation	Irregularity in red blood 　cell production Reproductive disorders	Anemia Pica Diarrhea ↓ Hair coat quality ↓ Iron in milk	Fish/meat meals Safflower Alfalfa Corn gluten meal Supplements
Silicon	Skeletal development	Calculi formation	Skeletal abnormalities	Meat by-products Grains
Molybdenum	Metabolism of fats, 　carbohydrates, proteins Growth promotion Enamel production	Diarrhea ↓ Weight ↓ Hair quality ↓ Reproduction	Rare	Grass/alfalfa/hay Meat meal Corn Oats Wheat
Cobalt	Formation of vitamin B_{12}	Rare	↓ Skin/hair coat quality Abortion ↓ Milk ↓ Appetite	Soybean meal Meat/poultry meal Corn Wheat Molasses

Table 16-4 VITAMINS FOR LIVESTOCK

Water soluble	Function	Toxicity	Deficiency	Sources
B COMPLEX				
Biotin	Metabolism of carbohydrates, fats, proteins Enzyme activities	No known toxicity	↓ Growth ↓ Hair quality Lameness ↓ Reproduction	Young grasses Safflower meal Soybean meal supplements
Thiamine (vitamin B_1)	Coenzyme of energy metabolism Peripheral nerve function Maintenance/assistance of appetite	No known toxicity	Heart irregularities ↓ Body temperature	Wheat Millet Oil seed meals Oats Supplements
Pyridoxine (vitamin B_6)	Nitrogen metabolism Fat and carbohydrate metabolism	Nontoxic	Anorexia ↓ Growth Eye discharge Anemia	Green pastures Meat/fish meals Corn gluten meal Safflower meal Alfalfa
Cobalamin (vitamin B_{12})	Red blood cell formation Maintenance of nerve tissue DNA synthesis	Nontoxic	↓ Coordination (blackleg: pigs) ↓ Reproduction	Fish/meat meals Whey Brewer's yeast supplements
Niacin	Growth ↓ Cholesterol levels Release of energy from fats, proteins, carbohydrates	Nontoxic	↓ Growth ↓ Appetite Diarrhea Unthriftiness	Wheat barley Yeast supplements
Folic acid	Construction of hemoglobin Manipulation of protein Choline synthesis	Nontoxic	Anemia Diarrhea ↓ Growth	Soybean meal Alfalfa Wheat Meat/fish meal Supplement
Pantothenic acid	Metabolism of fats, protein, carbohydrates Hemoglobin production Maintenance of normal blood levels	Nontoxic	Neurologic disorder Goose stepping (swine) ↓ Hair quality Enteritis	Wheat bran Alfalfa Safflower meal Supplements
Riboflavin (vitamin B_2)	Metabolism of amino acids and fatty acids Retinal pigment Adrenal function	Nontoxic	↓ Growth Moon blindness (horses) Anemia Unthriftiness ↓ Reproduction (swine)	Alfalfa Green pastures Sweet/white clover Supplements
Vitamin C	Absorption of iron Metabolism of folic acid Antioxidant Teeth/bone integrity	Rare in food animals	↓ Wound healing Hemorrhage Enlarged joints Ulcerated gums	Green pastures Hay Potatoes

---

Box 16-6 FACTORS AFFECTING WATER INTAKE

- Dry-matter intake
- Reproductive status
- Activity
- Type of feeding regimen
- Environment
- Weight
- Age
- Rate of gain

Box 16-7 IMPORTANCE OF WATER

- For digestion, absorption, and utilization of nutrients
- For production requirements
- Watering methods
  - Free water always available
  - Twice daily watering
- Cleanliness
  - Water heaters in winter to prevent freezing
  - Troughs kept clean

Table 16-5 WATER CONSUMPTION GUIDELINES

Species	Weight (lb)	Consumption (gal/day)	Species	Weight (lb)	Consumption (gal/day)
SWINE			**CATTLE**		
Pigs	30-125	0.3-2.0	Calves	100-200	1.2-2.5
Feeder pigs	126-200	2.0-3.2		201-400	2.5-4.9
Finisher pigs	201-250	3.2-4.0	Developing steers/heifers	401-600	4.5-6.2
Sow/boar maintenance	150-400	1.3-3.5		601-800	6.0-8.2
	401-600	3.5-5.2		801-1000	8.0-9.8
Sow: late gestation	250-400	4.5-5.0	Finishing steers		
	401-600	5.0-7.5	Pasture	1001-1200	8.5-10.2
Sow: lactation	250-400	5.5-6.5	Maintenance	800-1000	3.6-4.6
	401-600	6.5-9.8		1001-1200	4.4-7.2
				1201-1400	5.0-7.2
SHEEP				1401-1600	6.0-9.0
Lambs	20-50	0.4-0.6	Cows: late gestation	800-1000	4.4-5.5
Feeder lambs	50-110	0.5-1.4		1001-1200	5.3-6.6
Finisher lambs	111-125	1.4-1.8		1201-1400	6.4-7.9
Ewes: grain and hay intake*				1401-1600	7.7-9.5
Maintenance	150-300	0.3-1.2	Beef cows/heifer lactation	800-1000	6.7-15.6
Lactation	150-300	0.5-2.4		1001-1200	8.3-18.8
Rams: grain and hay intake	150-300	0.3-2.0		1201-1400	10.0-21.8
				1401-1600	11.7-25.0
			Dairy cows/heifer peak lactation[†]	800-1000	14.8-20.6
				1001-1201	18.5-24.3
				1201-1400	22.5-28.8
				1401-1600	28.0-32.2
				1601-1800	30.5-36.0

*Intake is influenced dramatically by factors found in table. Table is intended as a guideline.
†Dairy cattle intake varies on milk production more than beef cattle.

Table 16-6 DAILY FEEDING CONSIDERATIONS IN DEVELOPING FEMALE DAIRY CATTLE*

Weight (lb)	NE (Mcal)[†]	Total Crude Protein (%)	Minerals[‡]	
			Ca^{2+}	P
200-399	6.4-11.5	16-18	15-18	9-15
400-599	11.5-15.4	12-16	18-23	13-15
600-799	15.4-19.5	12-14	23-24	15-17
800-999	19.5-23.9	12-14	24-26	17-18
1000-1199	23.9-28.4	12-14	26-28	18-19
1200-1399	28.4-33.8	12-14	28-30	19-21

*Ranges shown in table are to be used as guidelines, recognizing that variations can occur as a result of breed, milk production levels, butter fat content, rate of gain, and lactation cycle.
†Net energy (NE) expressed in megacalories (Mcal).
‡Ca^{2+}/phosphorus ratio needs to be maintained from 0.43% to 0.66%; levels above 0.95% to 100% can result in decreased performance and metabolic abnormalities.

forages is based on body weight and forage quality. A guide for estimating consumption of forage (dry matter basis) fed on a free-choice basis is in Box 16-8 and Table 16-9.

If cows are allowed to consume all the forage they want, they will not have sufficient rumen capacity to consume enough concentrate to meet the energy requirements needed for lactation. In general, most dairy farmers try to feed forage at a rate of 1.75% of body weight. The concentrate fed with the forage will vary with the kind of forage offered (a high-protein concentrate will be needed with a low-

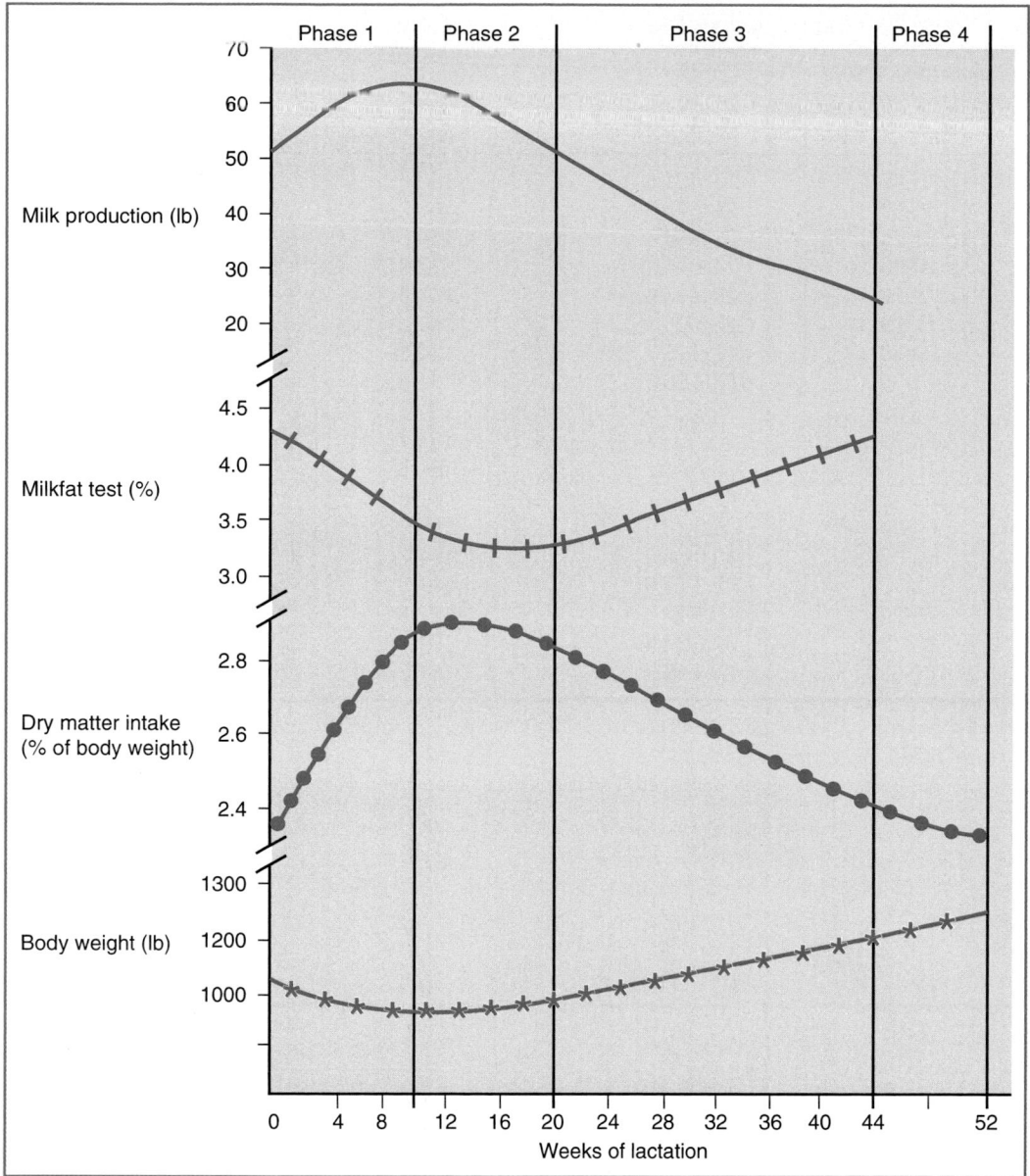

Figure 16-3 Milk production varies during a typical 52-week production phase. Disparity is also observed in milk fat content, dry matter intake requirements, and body weight.

Box 16-8 FACTORS AFFECTING DRY-MATTER INTAKE

- Stage of lactation
- Body condition
- Quality of feed
- Environment
- Size of cow
- Milk production
- Feeding regimen
- Age

protein forage) and the availability and cost of the feedstuffs. The concentrate provides more energy and usually is higher in protein than the forage. Fat utilization varies with age, environment, and reproductive status. Fat intake during lactation can be 5% to 6% of total energy intake. Excessive dietary fat intake can negatively affect rumen microbial activity, depressing fiber utilization (Shirley, 1986).

PROTEIN

Restriction of protein or energy during lactation can lead to reduced milk production and increased reproductive problems. Protein is supplied by the forage or concentrate and should be added at levels to ensure that minimum

Table 16-7 DAILY GUIDELINES FOR LACTATING DAIRY COWS*

Weight (lb)	Milk Yield (lb)	NE (Mcal)[†]	Total Crude Protein (%)	Minerals[‡]	
				Ca^{2+}	P
800	15-45	13.1-21.6	12-16	40-77	25-49
	45-60	21.6-25.8	16-17	77-96	49-61
	61-75	25.8-34.0	16-18	96-115	61-78
1000	20-40	14.9-20.3	12-16	44-70	29-44
	41-70	20.3-25.6	16-18	70-114	44-73
	71-90	25.6-36.3	16-18	114-146	73-86
1200	20-40	17.0-23.7	12-16	50-81	33-52
	41-60	23.7-30.3	16-18	81-110	52-70
	61-80	30.3-37.0	16-18	110-139	70-87
1400	50-75	27.7-35.7	15-17	95-131	62-83
	76-100	35.7-43.7	16-18	131-165	83-104
	101-125	43.7-51.7	16-18	165-200	104-126
1600	60-90	31.0-40.0	15-17	108-146	69-92
	91-120	40.0-48.3	16-18	146-184	92-116
	121-150	48.3-57.0	16-18	184-221	116-137
1800	60-90	40.9-44.6	16-18	121-164	78-104
	91-120	44.6-54.4	16-18	164-207	104-131
	121-150	54.4-64.1	16-18	207-249	131-157

This table is designed to be used only as a guideline. Feed to maintain body condition. Table assumes a 4% milk fat content of lactation.
[†]Net energy (NE) measured in megacalories (Mcal).
[‡]Mineral values assume that balance has been established. Variations occur with breed, lactation phase, milk yield, and age.

Table 16-8 DAILY NUTRIENT CONSIDERATIONS FOR DAIRY CATTLE*

Weight (lb)	ME[†] (Mcal)	Total Crude Protein (g)	Minerals (g)[‡]		Vitamins (1000 IU)	
			Ca^{2+}	P	A	D
FEMALES: 60 DAYS BEFORE GESTATION						
800-1000	13.8-16.4	850-925	24-30	16-18	30-35	12-14
1000-1200	16.4-19.2	925-1000	30-35	18-22	35-42	14-17
1200-1400	19.2-21.5	1000-1100	35-42	22-26	42-48	17-19
1400-1600	21.5-23.6	1100-1200	42-45	26-30	48-56	19-22
DAIRY BULLS						
1000-1300	14.3-17.8	775-900	16-20	10-12	17.00-21.00	2.7-3.3
1301-1500	17.8-19.7	900-1000	20-24	12-15	21.00-25.25	3.3-3.9
1501-1700	19.7-21.6	1000-1125	24-28	15-18	25.25-29.50	3.9-4.6
1701-1900	21.6-23.5	1125-1225	28-32	18-20	29.50-33.75	4.6-5.3
1901-2100	23.5-25.3	1225-1325	32-36	20-22	33.75-38.00	5.3-5.9
2101-2300	25.3-27.0	1325-1425	36-40	22-25	38.00-42.50	5.9-6.6
2301-2500	27.0-28.8	1425-1520	40-44	25-28	42.50-46.60	6.6-7.3
2501-2700	28.0-30.4	1520-1610	44-48	28-30	46.60-50.90	7.3-7.9
2701-2900	30.4-32.1	1610-1700	48-52	30-32	50.90-55.10	7.9-8.6

*Ranges shown in table are to be used as guidelines, recognizing that variations can occur because of milk production levels, butter fat content, rate of gain, and lactation cycle.
[†]Metabolizable energy (ME) measured in megacalories (Mcal).
[‡]Ca^{2+}/phosphorus ratio needs to be maintained from 0.43% to 0.66%; levels above 0.95% to 100% can result in decreased performance and metabolic abnormalities.

Table 16-9 FORAGE QUALITY

Forage Quality	Daily Intake (% Body Weight)
Excellent	3.0
Good	2.5
Average	2.0
Fair	1.5
Poor	1.0

protein requirements are met (Tables 16-6 to 16-8). Protein intake that exceeds the requirement is used as energy at a premium value. Protein is an expensive nutrient and is not an economic source of energy. Most cows are fed a high-protein legume hay, such as alfalfa, and grain, which should supply most or all the protein needs during lactation. Nonprotein nitrogen supplied as urea also can be an effective feedstuff to supply protein equivalents in dairy rations. The use of animal protein sources derived from ruminant species *is not allowed* in dairy rations in order to prevent the possible transmission of bovine spongiform encephalopathy (BSE).

MINERALS AND VITAMINS

Milk is composed of 0.7% minerals on a dry weight basis. The average cow will lactate 140 lb of mineral as a portion of the milk produced per year. Balanced mineral intake is essential; mineral requirements for lactation are given in Tables 16-6 to 16-8.

Rumen microorganisms can synthesize the water-soluble vitamins, whereas vitamin K is the only fat-soluble vitamin readily synthesized by microorganisms. The supplementation of water-soluble vitamins or vitamin K normally is not necessary in rations for ruminants.

Forages of good quality and properly harvested normally contain adequate levels of vitamin E and the precursor of vitamin A, carotene. Vitamin A is stored for extended periods in the body. Vitamin D is synthesized through ultraviolet radiation by the skin or added to a dairy ration as sun-cured forage or a vitamin supplement.

Although water-soluble vitamins are synthesized by the rumen microflora, some evidence indicates that supplemental thiamin, choline, and niacin may be beneficial in cows undergoing heavy stress or various disease states. Daily requirements for vitamins for lactating dairy cows are found in Table 16-8.

DAIRY CALVES

Newborn calves require the mother's colostrum within the first 72 hours of life to acquire energy and maternal immunity from disease. Peak benefits of colostrum intake are realized within the first 24 hours postpartum. Optimally, the first milking colostrum should be given to the calf at 10% to 12% of the calf's weight with at least one half administered within 4 to 6 hours after birth. Colostrum can

be successfully frozen and used at a later date as well as diluted equally with water should diarrhea occur because of the richness of the colostrum. The initial sucking of the calf will create a bypass of the rumen, allowing the milk to go directly into the abomasum. This ability will decrease as the calf ages and the rumen becomes functional. Calves normally start on milk replacers and then are offered calf starters within the first week of life. Calf-starter rations are commonly fed until about 3 months of age at a rate of 5 to 7 lb of calf starter per day. During the first week of life, a forage source should be added to diet selection as well as free-choice water. Calves are typically weaned at 4 to 8 weeks of age and accustomed to solid food.

BEEF CATTLE

Feeding represents almost three fourths of the cost of production of beef cattle (Neumann, 1977). Beef producers control their profitability by obtaining optimal nutrient intake with least cost feed formulation. Profitability hinges on the ability to balance utilization of resources, such as pasture and feedlot, with the production of high-quality finishing animals generated by the breeding herd. Beef production usually is divided into two primary areas: cow-calf production and finishing cattle.

✎ TECHNICIAN NOTE
Feeding represents 75% of the cost of beef cattle production.

COW-CALF PRODUCTION

A live calf from each cow each year should be the goal of the profitable cow-calf producer. Nutrition has a large impact on the beef breeding herd. Cows gaining weight just before and during the breeding season have a shorter period between calving and the first estrus period and typically have higher conception rates.

Energy
Carbohydrates are the major energy source for beef cows, followed by proteins and fat. Forages commonly fed to beef cows possess a significant fiber content that is broken down by the microbial population in the rumen and used as energy.

✎ TECHNICIAN NOTE
Carbohydrates are the major energy source for beef cows.

Feeding beef cows can be very economic because high-quality forage or pasture can supply all energy needs with no need for energy supplementation from grains or fats (Figure 16-4). In the summer, pasture normally will supply adequate energy for the cow. If pasture is inadequate,

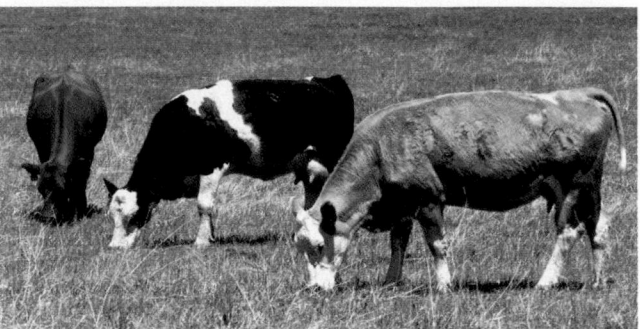

Figure 16-4 Beef cows are used predominantly in pasture production systems. Good pasture rotation management ensures optimal nutrition for grazing animals.

Box 16-9 TYPICAL GRAIN: NUTRITIONAL OVERVIEW

- 20% (or less) protein
- 18% (or less) crude fiber
- Variable moisture
- 85% (or less) carbohydrate
- 6% (or less) fat
- 75%-80% total digestible nutrients (TDNs)

---

supplemental energy should be provided in the form of silage or hay. In the winter, pregnant cows are fed wintering rations (a combination of forages, grain, and a protein source supplemented with vitamins and minerals) to meet energy needs with minimal weight gain (Box 16-9). Cows in good condition are more tolerant to the stresses of winter and require less maintenance energy per unit of weight than do cows in poor condition.

Protein

Most pasture, silages, and forages contain adequate levels of protein to meet the needs of the breeding cow. If low-grade roughages (e.g., cobs, straw, stalks) are fed over extended periods of time, the ration must be supplemented daily with 1 to 1.5 lb of a 35% to 45% crude protein supplement. A review of deficiency and toxicity signs can be found in Boxes 16-10 and 16-11. The use of animal protein sources derived from ruminant species *is not allowed* in beef breeding herd rations. This is to prevent the possible transmission of BSE.

Minerals and Vitamins

Mineral supplementation will be necessary and is usually offered on a free-choice basis when animals are on pasture (Figure 16-5). Trace-mineral salt blocks and granular salt are popular methods of offering minerals and salt to animals on pasture. Good-quality pasture and roughages are adequate in vitamins A and E with ample levels to meet the needs of breeding cows. Supplemental vitamin A should be provided when low-grade roughages or long-stored hays

---

Box 16-10 SIGNS OF UNDERNUTRITION

- ↓ Growth
- ↓ Hair/skin quality
- Skeletal irregularities
- ↓ Reproductive capabilities
- ↓ Immune function
- Death

Box 16-11 PROTEIN DEFICIENCY AND TOXICITY IN CATTLE

- Deficiency
- ↓ Appetite
- Weight loss
- ↓ Growth
- ↓ Reproductive capability
- ↓ Milk production
- Toxicity
- Ammonia: Avoid >40% excess protein or nonprotein nitrogen (NPN) intake.

Box 16-12 FEEDING CONSIDERATIONS FOR CALVES

DAIRY CALVES
Days 1-3: Obtain colostrum from dam.
Days 4-7: Transition to milk replacer or other liquid feed; begin offering starter and free-choice water.
Days 5-84: Starter and free-choice water through weaning; begin offering forage.

BEEF CALVES
Ensure calf nurses within 2 hr of birth to obtain vital colostrum.
Ensure that calf continues to thrive and that cow does not show signs of mastitis or decreased milk production.

ORPHANS
Can sometimes be grafted to another cow.
Ensure that colostrum has been administered.
Feed like dairy calves.

---

are used as a major source of energy in wintering rations. There are mineral mixes that contain a stabilized form of vitamin A.

CALVES

The basic food for calves consists of the mother's milk (Box 16-12) plus access to pasture or forage fed to the cows. Many cow-calf producers offer calves a highly palatable creep feed to supply additional nutrients, leading to improved weaning weights and decreased weight loss by nursing cows. Creep-fed calves will weigh an extra 30 to 50 lb by weaning

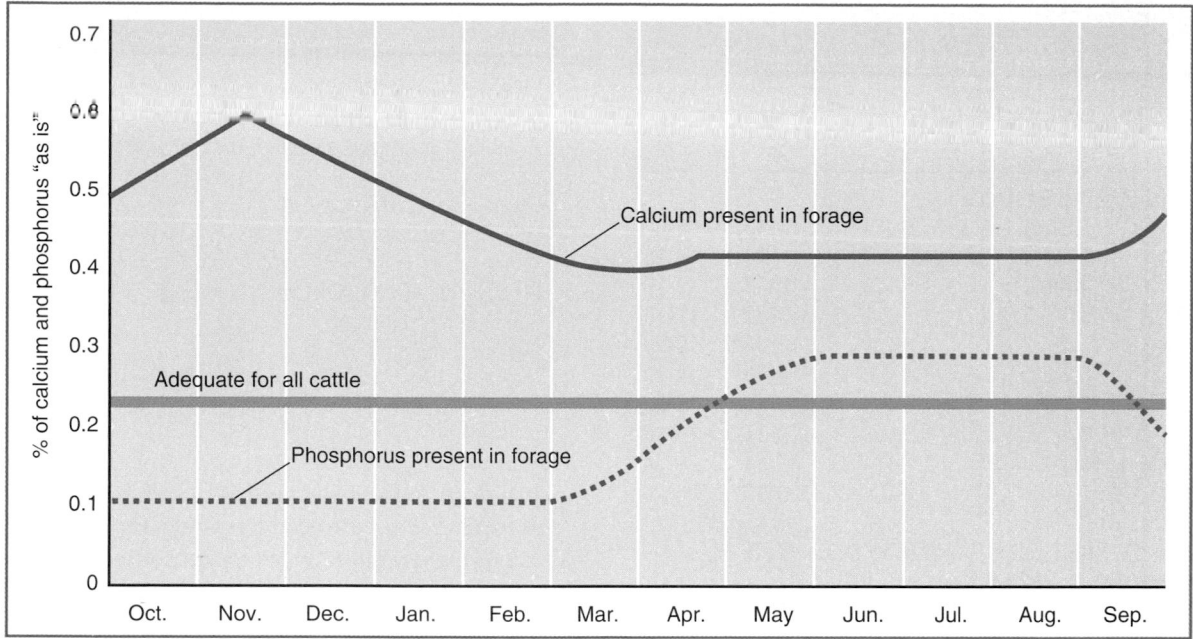

Figure 16-5 Calcium and phosphorus availability varies greatly during the seasons of the year and should be supplemented if inadequate amounts are present in livestock forage sources.

time. The greatest response to creep feeding is found when pasture is inadequate or quality is poor. Beef calves generally are weaned at 7 to 8 months of age.

> **TECHNICIAN NOTE**
> Creep-fed calves can weigh 30 to 50 more pounds by weaning time.

FINISHING CATTLE

The *finishing* of cattle refers to the time in the growth phase of growing cattle when they are fed to produce beef that is desirable to the food consumer. Most finished cattle are between 1 and 2 years of age and weigh more than 1000 lb. The goal of the finishing feeding program is to maintain maximum feed intake and gain without causing digestive upsets (Table 16-10).

Energy

High-energy diets are used to increase weight gain, improve the carcass characteristics, and decrease the cost of energy compared with diets high in fiber. Total dry feed intake commonly will be 2% to 3% of the animal's body weight. The feed contains high levels of grains to supply readily available energy (Figure 16-6). Cattle fed these rations are more prone to develop digestive upset (rumen acidosis), founder, or liver abscesses and require more attention and management to avoid these problems.

Protein

Protein requirements (9% to 14%) are greatly affected by age, size of animal, and growth rate. Young cattle require

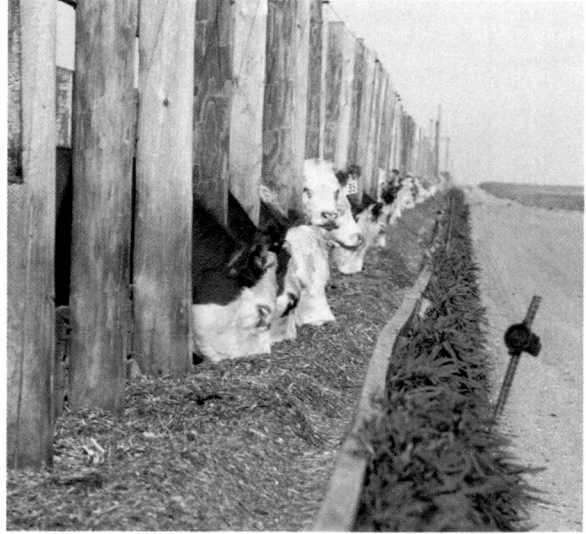

Figure 16-6 Large quantities of forage and grain are ingested by finishing cattle on a daily basis and are paramount to fulfillment of energy requirements.

higher levels of protein (as a percentage of the diet) than do older cattle. Protein sources cost more than feed grains, but experienced finishing cattle producers know that a protein deficiency is more expensive than a slight protein excess in the ration. When protein is deficient, energy is not well used, and performance suffers.

Supplemental protein for finishing cattle can be provided by natural protein sources or nonprotein nitrogen (e.g., urea). Nonprotein nitrogen sources are used most efficiently by cattle consuming relatively high levels of grain. A normal

Table 16-10 Daily Nutrient Considerations for Beef Cattle*

Weight (lb)	Net Energy (NE; Mcal)	Total Protein (lb)	Minerals (g) Ca²⁺	P
GROWING/FINISHING†				
300-400	3.0-3.6	0.75-1.5	10-42	6-8
401-500	3.7-4.4	0.90-1.9	11-40	8-18
501-600	4.4-5.0	1.0-2.0	12-38	9-19
601-700	5.0-5.6	1.1-2.1	13-36	11-19
701-800	5.6-6.2	1.3-2.1	14-34	12-20
801-900	6.2-6.8	1.4-2.2	15-33	14-20
901-1000	6.8-7.3	1.5-2.3	16-37	16-22
1001-1100	7.3-7.5	1.6-2.3	19-35	18-23
1101-1200	7.5-7.8	1.7-2.4	20-34	20-24
1201-1300	7.8-8.4	1.8-2.4	20-32	20-24
YEARLING HEIFERS, EARLY TO LATE GESTATION				
700-800	8.0-8.6	1.3-1.6	19-28	19-22
801-900	8.6-9.1	1.4-1.7	21-28	15-19
901-1000	9.1-9.8	1.5-1.7	20-23	14-20
1001-1100	9.8-10.3	1.5-1.7	23-25	18-20
1101-1200	10.3-10.8	1.6-1.8	25-27	20-21
1201-1300	10.8-11.4	1.6-1.8	26-28	21-23
1301-1400	11.4-12.0	1.8-2.0	26-28	23-24
LACTATING COW/HEIFER				
800-900	10.0-14.0	2.0-2.4	23-35	19-20
901-1000	10.4-14.5	1.9-2.5	24-36	19-20
1001-1100	11.0-15.0	2.0-2.6	25-38	20-22
1101-1200	11.5-15.5	2.0-2.7	27-39	22-23
1201-1300	12.0-16.2	2.1-2.3	23-41	23-25
1301-1400	12.5-17.0	2.2-2.9	30-42	25-26
BREEDING BULLS				
1300-1500	9.3-10.3	2.0-2.2	23-31	22-25
1501-1700	10.3-11.3	1.7-2.2	23-31	22-25
1701-1900	11.3-12.3	2.0-2.2	26-29	26-29
1901-2100	12.3-13.3	2.0-2.3	27-33	27-33

From National Research Council: *Nutrient requirements of beef cattle*, ed 8, Washington, DC, 1990. National Academic Press.
*Values represent guidelines, and individual variations dictate the constant appraisal of body condition to ensure desirable results.
†Assumes medium- to large-frame steers.

range of urea intake for many finishing rations is 0.10 to 0.15 lb per animal per day. The use of animal protein sources derived from ruminant species *is not allowed* in finishing cattle rations to prevent the possible transmission of BSE.

Minerals and Vitamins

Calcium is often added to the high-grain diets fed to finishing cattle. Generally, when forage (especially legumes) constitutes more than 25% of a finishing ration, additional calcium is not required. Grain contains adequate levels of

Box 16-13 Salt Use in Cattle

RULE 1: SUPPLY
3-5 lb in each spring and summer month
1-1.5 lb in each fall and winter month

RULE 2: AVAILABILITY
Make salt available at all times.

RULE 3: ROTATION
Continue to rotate salt.
Manger throughout pasture.

phosphorus to meet the needs of finishing cattle. Finishing rations are balanced to contain a calcium/phosphorus ratio of 2:1 or higher. Salt is added to diets or fed on a free-choice basis to finishing cattle to meet the sodium requirement (Box 16-13). The less forage that is formulated into the diet, the more need there is for trace-mineral supplementation.

High-quality forages contain adequate amounts of vitamin A precursors and vitamin E. Generally, finishing rations are supplemented with 20,000 to 30,000 IU of vitamin A daily because they contain high levels of grain. Vitamins E and D are added to finishing rations when the feed ingredients are devoid of these vitamins or the production practices merit their inclusion (Table 16-10).

SHEEP

Feeding represents the single largest cost of production for all types of sheep operations. Sheep producers control their revenue by offering feeds that support optimum production, are cost effective, and minimize nutrition-related problems. Sheep production is divided into two principal areas: the breeding flock and lamb production.

BREEDING FLOCK

Ewes are the foundation of the sheep operation; they produce lambs and generate wool (Box 16-14). These two cash crops can be influenced greatly by feeding management. The mature ewe (3 to 8 years of age) needs only sufficient feed to maintain her normal weight from the time her lambs were weaned until 15 weeks (21-week gestation) into her next pregnancy, assuming not much weight was lost during lactation. Pasture is adequate to meet her nutrient needs during this period of production (see Figures 16-1 and 16-5 for reviews of nutrient composition of pasture).

Energy

The energy requirements of the ewe largely depend on the stage of the reproductive cycle (Box 16-15). During the first two thirds of the pregnancy, energy requirements are close

Box 16-14 COMMON SHEEP BREEDS

WOOL BREEDS
Rambouillet
Merino
Debouillet
Columbia
Targee

MEAT BREEDS
Suffolk
Dorset
Hampshire
Shropshire
Southdown
Oxford

COMBINATION BREEDS
Polypay
Texel
Tunis
Leicester
Cheviot

Box 16-15 ENERGY INTAKE VARIABLES IN SHEEP

- Breed size
- Gender
- Reproductive status
- Weaning age
- Multiple birth
- Age
- Environment
- Stress
- Shearing
- Forage quality

Box 16-16 ADVANTAGES AND DISADVANTAGES OF PASTURE FEEDING LIVESTOCK

ADVANTAGES
- Provides exercise.
- Uses land unsuitable for other purposes.
- Decreases diseases transmitted through close contact with other animals.
- Decreases feed costs.
- Good-quality pastures can provide quality feedstuffs.

DISADVANTAGES
- Depends on soil quality (deficiencies result in poorer quality pasture).
- Large acreage often needed to support animal's energy requirements.
- Land may be made valuable for other uses.

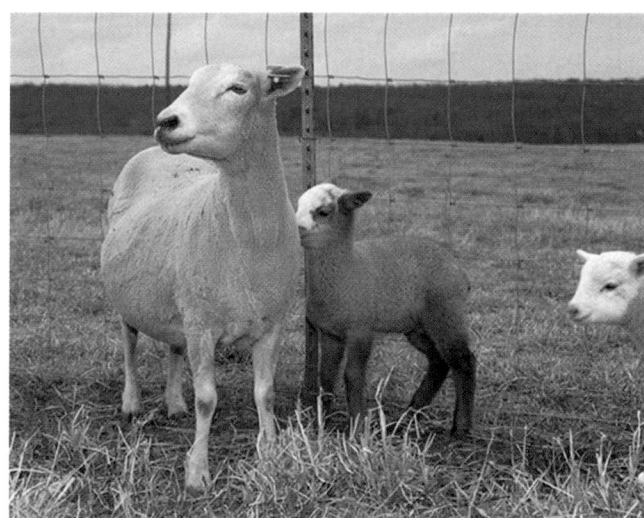

Figure 16-7 Ewes are the foundation of the sheep operation. Good feeding management ensures healthy lambs and first-class wool production.

to those required for MNR, and good pasture or hays can supply all the energy needs (Box 16-16). In the last trimester, energy requirements increase, and forages must be supplemented with grains. Poor care during the last trimester of pregnancy leads to lambing problems, lower wool output, and depressed milk production. A common problem attributed to poor nutrition in ewes is lambing paralysis or ketosis. Feeding inadequate forages with little or no grain can create a deficiency of usable carbohydrates during the last trimester of pregnancy in ewes carrying twins or triplets and can lead to paralysis and coma in the mother. Prevention is the least expensive route to avoid pregnancy disease in the breeding flock. Energy requirements are highest during lactation and proportional to the number of lambs the ewe is nursing (Figure 16-7 and Table 16-11).

> ✎ **TECHNICIAN NOTE**
>
> A common problem attributed to poor nutrition in ewes is lambing paralysis or ketosis.

Protein

Adequate protein intake ensures good wool production and reproductive function (Box 16-17 and Table 16-11). The most limiting amino acid for the maturation of wool is methionine; protein ingested by the breeding flock must contain adequate levels of this amino acid. Most pasture, silages, and forages contain adequate levels of protein and amino acids to meet the needs of the breeding flock. If low-grade roughages (e.g., cobs, straw, stalks) are fed over extended periods of time, the ration must be supplemented daily with a protein supplement or a nonprotein nitrogen source (Box 16-18). The use of animal protein sources derived from ruminant species *is not allowed* in ewe rations to prevent the possible transmission of BSE.

Table 16-11 DAILY NUTRITIONAL CONSIDERATIONS IN SHEEP

Weight (lb)	ME (Mcal)*	Daily Consumption (as fed) (lb/day)	Total Crude Protein (lb/day)	Minerals (g)		Vitamins	
				Ca²⁺	P	A (1000 IU)	E (IU)
WEANED LAMBS TO FINISHING							
20-40	1.3-2.6	1.2-2.9	0.35-0.45	4.9-6.5	2.2-2.9	.47	12
41-60	2.6-3.2	2.9-3.4	0.45-0.48	6.5-7.2	2.9-3.4	.95	24
61-80	3.2-3.8	3.4-3.7	0.48-0.51	7.2-8.6	3.4-4.3	1.40	21
81-100	3.8-4.0	3.7-4.1	0.51-0.53	8.6-9.4	4.3-4.8	2.30	25
101-Finish	4.0-4.2	3.8-4.1	0.53	8.2-9.4	4.5-4.8	2.80	25
EWE LAMBS							
Early							
80-100	2.9-3.0	3.4-3.7	0.35-0.36	5.2-5.5	2.7-2.8	3.0-3.1	21
101-120	3.0-3.1	3.7-3.9	0.35-0.36	5.2-5.5	2.8-3.0	3.1-3.4	22
121-140	3.1-3.2	3.7-3.9	0.35-0.36	5.5	3.0-3.3	3.4-3.7	24
141-160	3.1-3.3	3.9-4.1	0.35-0.36	5.5	3.3-3.4	3.4-3.7	26
Late							
80-101	5.0-5.4	3.7-3.9	0.41-0.44	6.4-7.8	5.0-5.4	3.1-3.9	22
101-120	5.4-5.8	3.0-4.1	0.44-0.45	7.8-8.1	5.4-5.8	3.9-4.3	24
121-140	5.8-6.2	4.1-4.4	0.45-0.48	8.1-8.2	5.8-6.2	4.3-4.7	26
141-160	6.2-6.3	4.4-4.7	0.46-0.48	8.1-8.2	6.2-6.3	4.3-4.7	27
Lactation							
80-100	2.9-3.0	5.1-5.7	0.67-0.71	8.4-8.7	5.6-6.0	4.0-5.0	32-34
101-120	3.0-3.1	5.7-6.1	0.71-0.74	8.7-9.0	6.0-6.4	5.0-6.0	34-36
121-140	3.1-3.2	6.1-6.7	0.74-0.77	9.0-9.3	6.4-6.9	6.0-7.0	36-38
Ewes: Maintenance to Early/Mid							
110-130	2.4-2.6	2.4-2.9	0.21-0.27	2.0-3.2	1.8-2.5	2.35-2.80	18-20
131-150	2.6-2.7	2.5-3.1	0.27-0.29	2.5-3.5	2.4-2.9	2.80-3.30	20-21
151-170	2.7-2.9	2.9-3.7	0.29-0.31	2.8-3.8	2.4-3.3	3.30-3.75	21-22
171-190	2.9-3.1	3.0-3.9	0.31-0.33	2.9-3.9	2.8-3.4	3.75-4.25	22-24
Ewes: Late Gestation (Last 30 Days)/Lactation							
100-130	4.0-6.0	4.1-5.9	0.43-0.45	5.6-6.9	4.8-5.2	4.25-5.10	24-27
131-150	4.2-6.6	4.4-6.1	0.45-0.47	6.9-9.1	5.2-6.6	5.10-5.95	26-28
151-170	4.4-7.0	4.7-6.3	0.47-0.49	7.6-9.5	6.6-7.4	5.95-6.80	28-30
171-190	4.7-7.5	4.9-6.6	0.49-0.51	8.5-9.6	6.8-7.8	6.80-7.65	30-33

*ME (metabolizable energy) is measured in megacalories (Mcal); 1 Mcal = 1000 kilocalories.

Box 16-17 VARIABLES IN PROTEIN REQUIREMENTS OF SHEEP

- Breed size
- Reproductive status
- Age
- Body condition
- Ratio of protein to energy
- Nonprotein nitrogen availability

Minerals and Vitamins

Trace-mineral salt blocks and granular salt represent popular methods of offering minerals and salt to ewes on pasture. Sheep store copper quite well in various organs and tissues and develop toxicity symptoms to copper more rapidly than other livestock. Care should be taken to avoid exposing sheep to high levels of copper in their trace-mineral source.

Good-quality pasture and roughages are adequate in vitamins A and E with ample levels to meet the needs of the breeding flock. Supplemental vitamin A should be provided when low-grade roughages or long-stored hays are used as a major source of energy in wintering rations (Table 16-11).

Box 16-18 FEEDING GUIDELINES FOR NONPROTEIN NITROGEN (NPN) USE IN SHEEP

- Balance NPN within total nutritional profile. Feed continuously after 3- to 6-wk transition.
- Avoid sporadic availability.
- Maintain nitrogen/sulfur ratio at not more than 10:1.
- Restrict use to not more than 1.0% dry matter, with one third of total nitrogen ration as NPN.
- Avoid excess intake and possible toxicity.
- Watch NPN levels when they coincide with high roughage intake.

From Ensminger ME et al: *Feeds and nutrition*, Clovis, Calif, 1990, Ensminger Publishing; Maynard LA et al: *Animal nutrition*, ed 7, New York, 1979, McGraw-Hill; McDonald P et al: *Animal nutrition*, New York, 1995, Longman Scientific and Technical; Naylor JM et al: *Large animal clinical nutrition*, St Louis, 1991, Mosby.

Box 16-19 MILK REPLACEMENT FOR LAMBS

OPTIMAL REQUIREMENT
25% to 30% fat
20% to 25% protein derived from milk product
<30% lactose derived from milk product

FEEDING
Provide ration immediately.
Ration should be 20% to 24% protein, high in vitamins and minerals, well balanced, and ground fine.
NOTE: Avoid cow's milk (too high in lactose).

From Ensminger ME et al: *Feeds and nutrition*, Clovis, Calif, 1990, Ensminger Publishing; Maynard LA et al: *Animal nutrition*, ed 7, New York, 1979, McGraw-Hill; McDonald P et al: *Animal nutrition*, New York, 1995, Longman Scientific and Technical; Naylor JM et al: *Large animal clinical nutrition*, St Louis, 1991, Mosby.

LAMBS

Lambs must be nursed with colostrum milk within the first hour after birth to improve survivability. Colostrum milk provides immunologic protection and energy for the newborn lamb. The lamb must consume at least 6 to 8 oz of colostrum to receive immunologic protection. Lambs are weaned successfully at 8 weeks of age or earlier.

TECHNICIAN NOTE
Lambs must receive colostrum within the first hour after birth to have immunologic protection.

Lambs also can be successfully weaned from their mother at 1 day of age and offered a milk replacer (Box 16-19). They should be weaned from the milk replacer at 3 to 4 weeks of age and transitioned to a high-quality, palatable solid feed. Postweaning rations (until lambs reach 50 lb) should be high-quality protein (16% to 20% crude protein), high energy, and well fortified with vitamins and minerals.

Grower (50 to 85 lb) and finisher (more than 85 lb) rations for lambs are normally formulated to contain 15% to 16% and 13% to 14% protein, respectively. A simple ration of shelled corn, long alfalfa hay, and supplement (protein, calcium, vitamins, trace minerals) can be fed to growing-finishing lambs (Figure 16-8). Research does not clearly indicate the need for vitamin additions to rations for early lambs, but it has become a common practice to fortify the rations with vitamins A, D, and E (Table 16-11).

Large, fast-growing lambs are susceptible to overeating disease (enterotoxemia), which can cause death. This disease is caused by toxins produced by *Clostridium perfringens* and appears to be related to overeating by lambs of a ration high in grain. A vaccination with bacterin or toxoid can be used for lambs older than 2 months of age and will virtually eliminate symptoms of overeating disease.

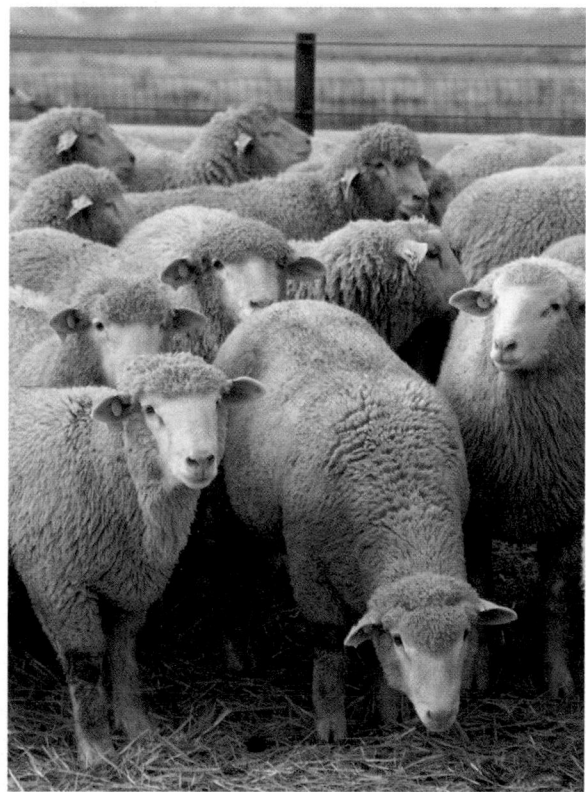

Figure 16-8 Optimal feed regimens in sheep will provide excellent results.

SWINE

The swine industry has changed dramatically over the past 30 years. Most pigs are raised in confinement to reduce labor requirements for the owner and to improve the environment for the animal. The genetic base of the swine industry has changed to a more prolific breeding herd and

Table 16-12 COMPLETE FEED RATION CONSIDERATIONS IN SWINE

Stage Weight	Protein (%)	Complete Ration Fed (lb)	Comments
Weaning pigs (12-20 lb)	20-24	Free feed	Use if weaned early and transitioning to solid feed.
Starter pigs (up to 40 lb)	18-20	Free feed	
Feeder/finisher pigs			
(40 lb to 220-250 lb finishing weight)	13-18	Free feed*	May be limited in feed after 125 lb.
Gilts and sows			
Breeding/maintenance	11-14	4-6	Increase amount to maintain body condition and last
Gestation	11-14	4-6	month of gestation through weaning.
Lactation	14-20	10-15	
Boars	14-16	4-7	Increase in breeding season.

*See text on feeding methods.

better-muscled, faster-growing offspring. Feed still constitutes 60% to 70% of the cost of raising swine. Few swine are grazed on pasture; most are fed complete high-grain rations in self-feeders or are limit fed if in the breeding herd. The production of pigs normally is divided into three distinct areas: the breeding herd, starter pigs, and growing-finishing pigs.

> ✏ **TECHNICIAN NOTE**
> Feed constitutes 60% to 70% of the cost of raising swine.

BREEDING HERD

For profitable production of swine, the sows must be bred, gestate 114 days, nurse a litter for 21 to 35 days, rebreed within 10 days after weaning, and continue the cycle for five to seven litters. Nutrition plays a key role in allowing this to occur, especially during lactation (Table 16-12).

Energy

After breeding and for the first two thirds of gestation, energy intake is limited to 6000 to 7000 kcal ME (metabolizable energy) per day. The total amount of feed is increased during the last third of gestation, providing 9000 to 10,000 kcal ME per day, which contributes additional energy to the developing fetuses during this last stage of gestation. Overfeeding energy during gestation has a direct negative impact on lactation feed intake, which can impair lactation performance.

In lactation, the goal of the swine producer is to encourage as much energy intake by the lactating female as possible (15,000 to 20,000 kcal ME per day). Sows are often fed twice per day to ensure fresh feed and improved energy intakes. Frequently, fat is added to the lactation ration to improve palatability and energy density. Sows peak in milk production between the second and third weeks of lactation, and they should be full fed to support the production of milk. A rule of thumb for feeding lactating

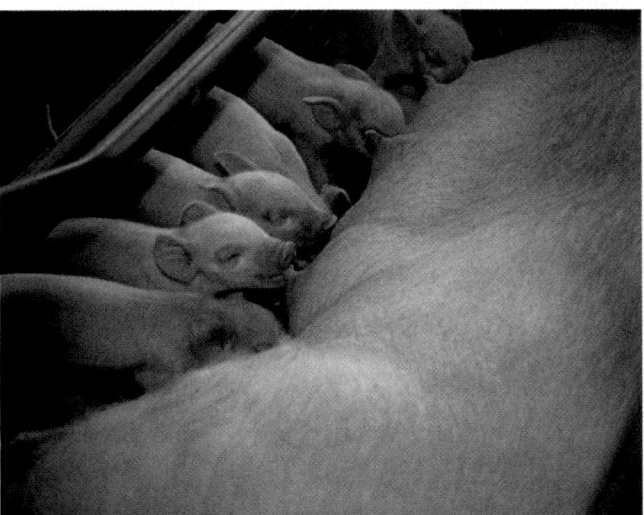

Figure 16-9 Sow nursing piglets in containment of farrowing pen.

sows is to offer 4 to 5 lb of the base ration plus 1 additional pound for every pig nursing (Figure 16-9).

> ✏ **TECHNICIAN NOTE**
> Sows are often fed twice daily to ensure adequate energy intake.

Protein

The protein requirements during gestation are relatively low (11% to 12% crude protein, 0.5 lb of protein per day). The development of the fetuses and reproductive tissue requires small amounts of protein each day.

During lactation, sows require higher levels of protein intake to support milk production (2 to 3 lb of protein per day), which is accomplished by feeding a ration with a higher protein content at a greater intake level. Sows not fed adequate levels of protein or energy during lactation will support milk production with loss of body tissue stores.

Box 16-20 Prevention of Iron-Deficiency
Anemia in Baby Pigs

- Allow access to soil that has not been in contact with other pigs.
- Inject 100-200 mg iron before 72 hr of age.
- Paint sows' teats lightly with iron solution periodically.
- Encourage prestarter ration creep feeding early.
- Provide iron supplementation in creep feeder.

Sows can lose more than 100 lb in weight during lactation if not fed proper amounts of energy or protein.

Minerals and Vitamins

Minerals and vitamins need to be supplemented throughout the life of pigs. The breeding herd is normally fed diets fortified with the minerals calcium, phosphorus, salt, zinc, iron, copper, iodine, selenium, and manganese. Calcium and phosphorus are kept in a balance of 1:1 to 2:1 for all stages of production. Low levels of calcium and phosphorus in the breeding herd rations can lead to fractures and lameness in the female.

Sow's milk is virtually devoid of iron, and anemia of nursing pigs will occur unless they are supplemented with another source of iron (Box 16-20). The two most common ways to supply additional iron are as follow:

1. Injection of iron (150 to 200 mg) as iron dextran or other iron–carbohydrate complexes at 3 days of age
2. Oral iron solution given at 3 days of age or swabbed onto the dam's udder several times during lactation

The vitamins supplemented in breeding herd diets are the fat-soluble vitamins A, D, E, and K and the water-soluble vitamins thiamin, riboflavin, niacin, pantothenic acid, B_6, B_{12}, choline, biotin, and folic acid. Adequate additions of these vitamins ensure proper development of the fetus in gestation and milk production in lactation (Box 16-21).

> ✎ **TECHNICIAN NOTE**
>
> Sow's milk is devoid of iron, and nursing pigs will develop anemia unless they are supplemented with iron.

STARTER PIGS

Pigs are commonly weaned at 3 to 5 weeks of age and remain in the starter phase until they weigh 40 to 50 lb (Figure 16-10). The earlier the age at weaning, the more complex is the ration required to help in the transition from mother's milk to solid food. Starter diets (20% to 24% protein) are very complex and nutrient-dense complete feeds and therefore often purchased from a commercial feed manufacturer. The highest-quality ingredients are used to make starter diets and include milk products, fish meal, spray-dried

Box 16-21 Orphan Piglet Feeding

HOMEMADE REPLACER
32 oz whole cow's milk
Water-soluble antibiotics
1 raw egg
16 oz half-and-half

DIRECTIONS FOR FEEDING PIGLETS
Give 2 oz per feeding per piglet every 3 hr.
Feed in a shallow, clean feeding pan.
Be sure that all piglets are eating.
Give iron supplementation as needed.
Start creep feeding at 7 days of age.

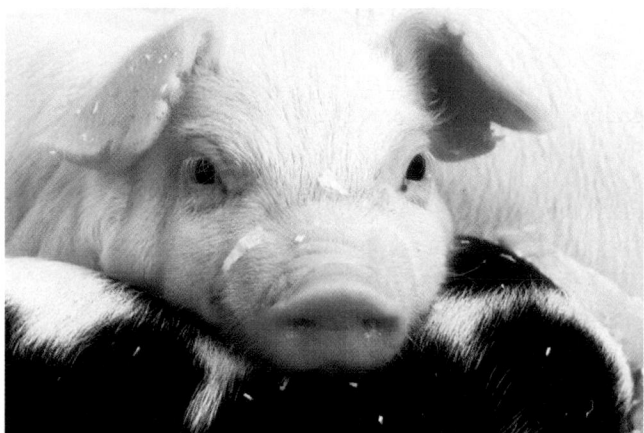

Figure 16-10 Young pigs need to be kept in a clean, dry, draft-free environment for optimal health and growth.

blood products, oats, corn, and fat. Vitamin and mineral supplementation levels are high in starter diets. These feeds typically are pelleted and quite costly (Table 16-12).

As the pig ages, the complexity and nutrient density of the starter ration decrease, leading to a lower-cost formula. In the last 2 or 3 weeks of the starter period, crude protein decreases to 18% to 20%, and the diet is often offered as a ground feed.

GROWING-FINISHING PIGS

Growing-finishing diets have been modified to complement the changes in the genetic base of modern swine. The leaner pigs require higher levels of protein and consume less energy than previous generations (Table 16-12).

Energy

Complete grower-finisher rations are based on cereal grains and frequently have fat added to increase caloric intake. Fibrous feed ingredients often are not used or are used sparingly to prevent depressions in caloric intake. Corn, wheat, sorghum, and barley are the more popular cereal

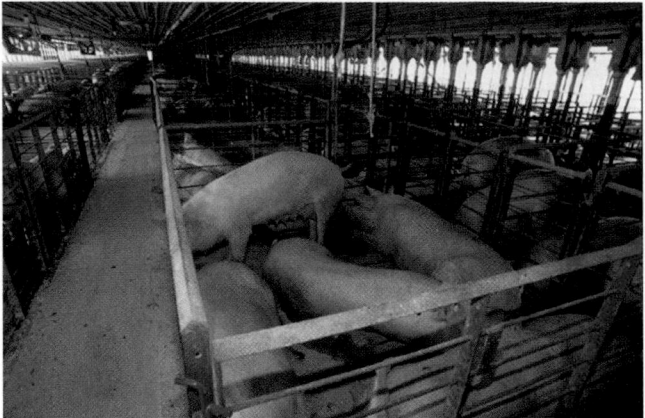

Figure 16-11 Grower–finisher pigs are fed large quantities of complete rations to obtain the most desirable carcass quality.

grains used to supply energy and comprise 60% to 85% of the ration.

Protein

Contemporary swine nutrition concentrates not on the protein content of feeds but on the amino acid levels. Lysine typically is the first limiting amino acid in swine formulas. Amino acid levels decrease as a percentage of the diet throughout the growing-finishing phase.

Amino acid levels are matched to muscle growth throughout the growth period to maximize lean tissue growth. Underfeeding of amino acids depresses muscle deposition, and overfeeding amino acids leads to excess, which is costly.

Typical protein sources in growing-finishing diets are soybean meal, meat and bone meal, and synthetic amino acids. When protein sources are expensive, synthetic amino acids can replace a portion of the protein source with no loss in performance. The most commonly available synthetic amino acids are lysine, methionine, threonine, and tryptophan (Figure 16-11).

Minerals and Vitamins

Growing-finishing swine are fed diets fortified with the minerals calcium, phosphorus, salt, zinc, iron, copper, iodine, selenium, and manganese. Calcium and phosphorus are kept in a balance of 1:1 to 2:1 throughout this period. Deficiencies of phosphorus will depress growth performance as the animal grows.

Riboflavin, niacin, pantothenic acid, and vitamin B_{12} are the water-soluble vitamins most likely to be deficient in swine diets formulated with grains and plant protein. The fat-soluble vitamins A, D, E, and K also should be added to growing-finishing rations.

References

Church DC: *Livestock feeds and feeding,* Corvallis, Ore, 1984, O and B Books, pp 19-31, 89-93, 189-234.

Ensminger ME: *Swine science,* Danville, Ill, 1990, Interstate Printers and Publishing, pp 416-441, 506-534.

McDonald P et al: *Animal nutrition,* ed 7, New York, 1995, Longman Scientific and Technical Publishing, pp 91-134.

Miller ER et al: *Swine Nutrition,* Boston, 1991, Butterworth-Heinemann, pp 483-558.

Nash MJ: *Crop conservation and storage,* Oxford, England, 1985, Pergamon Press, pp 85-101.

Neumann AL: *Beef cattle,* New York, 1977, John Wiley & Sons, pp 187-221.

Shirley RL: *Nitrogen and energy nutrition of ruminants,* Orlando, 1986, Academic Press, pp 54-79.

Recommended Reading

Cunha TJ: *Swine feeding and nutrition,* New York, 1977, pp 201-208.

Garmsworthy PC: *Nutrition and lactation in the dairy cow,* London, 1988, University Press, pp 246-254.

Haresign DJ: *Recent developments of pig nutrition,* London, 1985, Butterworth, pp 368-386.

Jones DH, Wilson AD: Nutritive quality of forage. In Hacker ED, editor: *The nutrition of herbivores,* Sydney, 1982, Academic Press, pp 106-119.

Kruesi WK: *Sheep raiser's manual,* Charlotte, Vt, 1985, Williamson Publishing, pp 23-26, 67-72, 90-111.

Linciciome DR: *Sheep: applied and basic research information,* Scottsdale, Ariz, 1983, International Goat and Sheep Research, pp 85-99.

Lloyd LE et al: *Fundamentals of nutrition,* ed 3, San Francisco, 1978, WH Freeman & Sons, pp 456-501.

Machlin LJ: *Handbook of vitamins,* New York, 1984, Marcel Dekker, pp 29-54.

Maynard LA et al: *Animal nutrition,* ed 7, New York, 1979, McGraw-Hill.

Menzies CS: *United States sheep and goat industry,* Ames, Iowa, 1982, CAST Report, pp 12-31.

National Research Council: *Nutrient requirements for beef cattle,* ed 7, Washington, DC, 2000, National Academic Press.

National Research Council: *Nutrient requirements for dairy cattle,* ed 7, Washington, DC, 2001, National Academy Press.

National Research Council: *Nutrient requirements for sheep,* ed 6, Washington, DC, 1985, National Academy Press.

National Research Council: *Nutrient requirements for swine,* ed 10, Washington, DC, 1998, National Academic Press.

Naylor JM, Ralston SL: *Large animal clinical nutrition,* St Louis, 1991, Mosby, pp 21-42, 460-468, 267-274.

Pond WG: *Swine production and nutrition,* Westport, Conn, 1984, AVI Publishing, pp 91-96.

Taylor RE: *Beef production and the beef industry,* Minneapolis, 1984, Burgess Publishing, pp 389-404.

Tribble LG, Stansbury WF: *Swine report,* Dallas, 1985, Texas Technical University.

Webster J: *Calf husbandry: health and welfare,* London, 1984, Collins, pp 71-78.

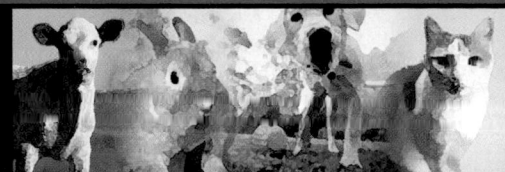

17

Animal Reproduction

Carlos R.F. Pinto • Bruce E. Eilts • Dale L. Paccamonti

INTRODUCTION

The events that occur in the process of reproduction in domestic animals are elegant processes of checks and balances that ultimately result in the birth of a newborn, which carries the genes for the next generation. This chapter provides a generic overview of female and male reproductive events, followed by more in-depth reviews of the most important aspects of reproduction in the canine, feline, equine, bovine, swine, ovine, caprine, and camelid.

There are two embryologic tubular systems present in the early embryo that will become either the male genitalia or the female genitalia. If an animal has XY chromosomes, it will become a male, and one tubular system (wolffian) will persist. The female tubular system regresses, and the wolffian system becomes the epididymis and vas deferens. If an individual has an XX karyotype, the other tubular system (müllerian) will persist and develop into a female reproductive system. The müllerian system becomes the uterine tubes, uterus, cervix, and anterior vagina. Because there are two systems, many potential abnormalities can occur when sections of the systems fail to regress or fail to develop fully. An example of embryonic malformation would be the hermaphrodite, which has developed both male and female gender organs.

In both the male and female, the brain is the initiator of the reproductive cycle. Neural input from higher brain centers results in the release of gonadotropin-releasing hormone (GnRH) from neurons in the hypothalamus into the hypophyseal-portal vessels. The GnRH then enters the anterior pituitary, causing release of the gonadotropins, follicle-stimulating hormone (FSH), and luteinizing hormone (LH). ■

FSH and LH are large, complex hormones that are stored within granules inside cells in the anterior pituitary. These hormones are glycoproteins, a complex of carbohydrates and proteins. Because the gonadotropins are extremely large and complex, they cannot be synthesized in the laboratory. The complexity and protein nature of the gonadotropins make them antigenic, and exogenous administration of these drugs derived from other species can induce antibody formation.

GENERAL FEMALE REPRODUCTION

THE ESTROUS CYCLE

The normal stages of reproduction are proestrus (the time leading to estrus), estrus (the time of mating), and diestrus (the time when pregnancy is being established). In most species, pregnancy is the normal event that ensures species survival. However, if pregnancy does not occur, the female will return to a sexually active state to entice mating with a male. If pregnancy is not established, the events will recur, thus forming a cycle of proestrus, estrus, diestrus, proestrus, estrus, diestrus, and so forth. The other normal events in the reproductive life of an animal are puberty, the time of first ovulation, pregnancy, and anestrus, a time when the animal is not undergoing any reproductive events. The name given to these recurring events is the *estrous cycle*. (Note that *estrus* is spelled *estrous* when it is an adjective, as in estrous cycle.)

The beginning of an estrous cycle in most females starts with GnRH from the hypothalamus, causing the release of FSH from the anterior pituitary (Figure 17-1). The FSH is released into the bloodstream and is carried to the ovaries where it initiates its follicle-stimulating action, causing the growth of ovarian follicles. Ovarian follicles are structures on the ovary that contain the egg, or oocyte (Figure 17-2). All the oocytes that a female will ever have are present on the ovary at birth, and most of the follicles contain no fluid. Some follicles are selected to grow and start to develop fluid around them (an antrum) in a process that is independent from FSH stimulation. Once a follicle has reached the antral stage, action of the FSH causes rapid growth of the follicle. The follicle wall is composed of two layers, the thecal cell layer and the granulosa cell layer. As the follicle grows, it produces the steroid hormone estrogen. Estrogen is the hormone that causes the characteristic behaviors and sexual receptivity when the female is in estrus. The oocyte within the follicle also begins to mature, so it will be ready for fertilization after ovulation. As the follicle grows and reaches maturity, the granulosa cells also produce a protein hormone called *inhibin*. Inhibin inhibits further FSH release, so that only a species-specific number of follicles are chosen for final growth and maturation (depending on the species, this may be one or more).

TECHNICIAN NOTE

Estrogen causes the female to become sexually receptive to the male.

The estrogen surge produced by the developing follicle stimulates the release of GnRH from the hypothalamus, which causes release of LH from the anterior pituitary. At the ovary, LH causes the mature follicle to ovulate. Ovulation is the release of the oocyte into the oviduct. After ovulation the follicle transforms into a corpus luteum, or yellow body. The corpus luteum (Figures 17-2 and 17-3) has been transformed by the LH surge to produce only progesterone, the hormone that maintains pregnancy.

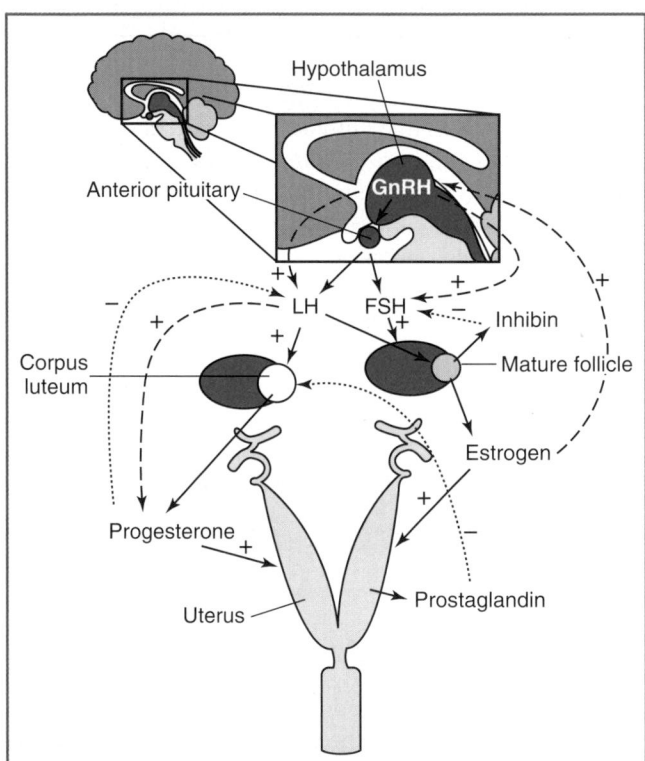

Figure 17-1 The general hormonal control of female reproduction: Pulsatile GnRH causes FSH to be released from the anterior pituitary. FSH causes follicular growth and maturation, where estrogen is produced. Inhibin from the follicle feeds back on the anterior pituitary and causes less FSH to be released. A surge of estrogen from the follicle causes GnRH release from the hypothalamus, which causes an LH surge. LH causes ovulation of the follicle and the formation of a corpus luteum, which produces progesterone. If a pregnancy signal is not secreted by the early embryo (bovine, equine, ovine, caprine), prostaglandin is released from the uterus, goes to the corpus luteum, and causes luteolysis (luteal death). The cycle then starts over with follicular growth.

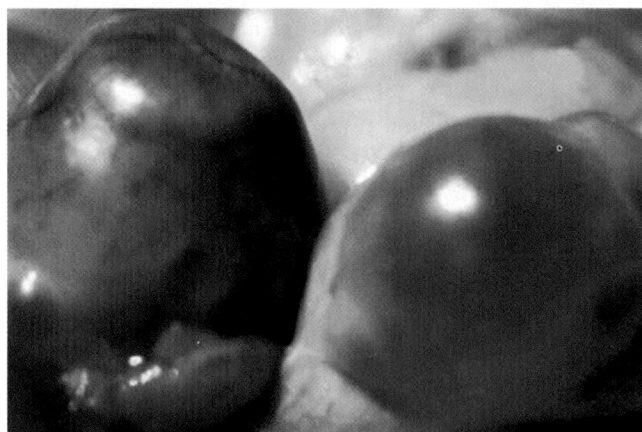

Figure 17-2 A bovine corpus luteum and follicle on the ovaries.

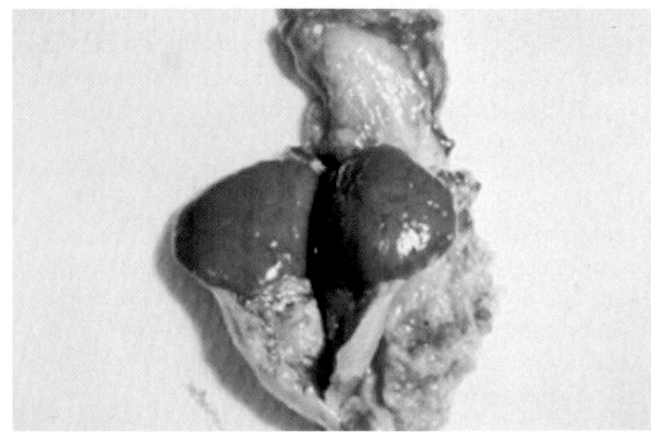

Figure 17-3 A cut section of a bovine corpus luteum.

Pregnancy actually begins in the oviduct. The oviduct is often called the *uterine tube* and consists of three segments: the infundibulum, the ampulla, and the isthmus (Figure 17-4). When ovulation occurs, the oocyte is picked up by the dilated end of the oviduct called the *infundibulum*. The oocyte is then transported through the ampulla to the junction of isthmus and ampulla. In most species, this is where fertilization occurs. Fertilization is the joining of the oocyte, which has half the chromosome complement, with the sperm cell, which has the other half of the chromosome complement, thus forming the embryo that has both the maternal and paternal chromosome complements. The embryo normally stays within the oviduct for several days before it moves into the uterus.

If the oocyte is not successfully fertilized, the corpus luteum still develops and maintains progesterone production for a time that is consistent within each species. This time of progesterone domination is called *diestrus*. It is the early embryo in most species that signals to the uterus/ovary that pregnancy has been established. If the signal for pregnancy is not received by the uterus, most species (not the dog and cat) will initiate an ending of diestrus, so the animal can return to estrus and have another chance to become pregnant. In most species this occurs when the hormone prostaglandin is released from the uterus. Prostaglandin is a small molecule derived from arachidonic acid. When prostaglandin is released, it binds to receptors on the corpus luteum and lyses it. Because the corpus luteum is the source of progesterone, after the corpus luteum is destroyed by prostaglandin, progesterone concentrations in the blood fall. When progesterone is not present, there is a rise in FSH that allows new follicles to grow. This time of growing follicles after the death of the corpus luteum is called *proestrus*. As the animal enters proestrus the follicles grow, estrus follows, the LH surge causes ovulation, and a corpus luteum forms. Therefore the animal has estrous cycles until pregnancy is established.

Once the embryo is in the uterus, it must establish itself as a viable pregnancy before prostaglandin destroys the corpus luteum. Different species have different mechanisms to do this. Each species appears to have a relatively unique substance produced by the early embryo that prevents the corpus luteum from being destroyed by prostaglandin released from the uterus. Dogs and cats appear rather unique in that their corpora lutea (plural for corpus luteum) appear to have preprogrammed life spans without any endogenous destruction by prostaglandins if they are not pregnant.

As pregnancy progresses the early embryo changes from an embryonic disk and a yolk sac of nutrients to a more complex structure that includes the embryo or fetus and placenta. After all the bodily organs are formed, the embryo is called a *fetus*. The placenta forms from specialized cells on the embryo. These cells develop into the chorion and allantois. The amnion is a fluid-filled sac that immediately surrounds the fetus, whereas the chorion and allantois fuse to form the chorioallantois. Therefore the fetus has two fluid-filled sacs surrounding it (Figure 17-5). The chorion attaches to the uterus and has the function of transferring nutrients from the uterus to the fetus. The structure of the placenta varies from species to species (Figures 17-6 and 17-7). The ruminants have many individual attachment areas called *placentomes*. Dogs and cats have a zone of the placenta that attaches to the uterus. Horses and pigs have a more generalized attachment (diffuse) of the placenta to the uterus. In some species, such as the ewe and horse, the placenta produces the progesterone that maintains the pregnancy instead of the corpus luteum.

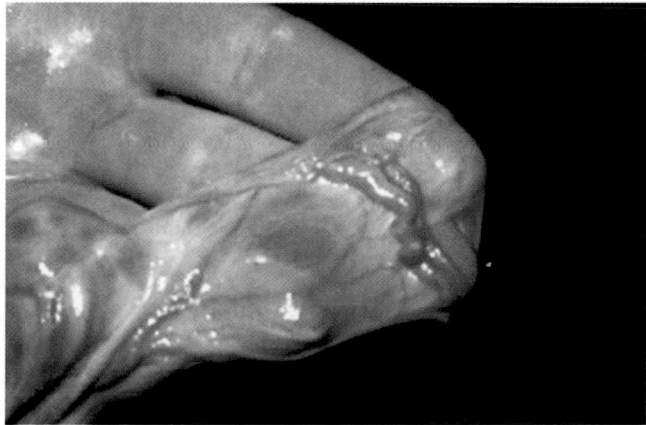

Figure 17-4 A bovine oviduct showing the fingers inserted in the infundibulum.

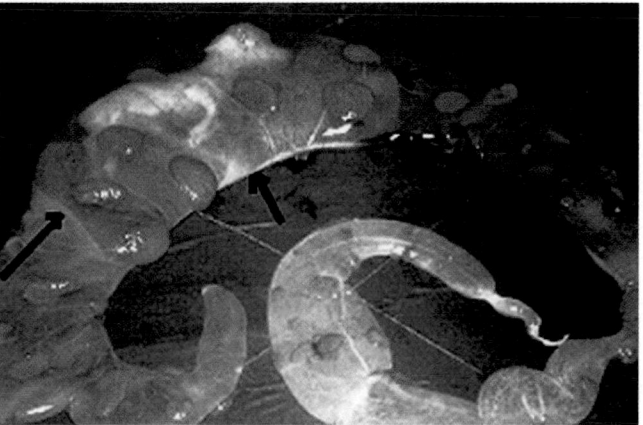

Figure 17-5 A bovine fetus within the amnion *(arrows)*, which is within the chorioallantois.

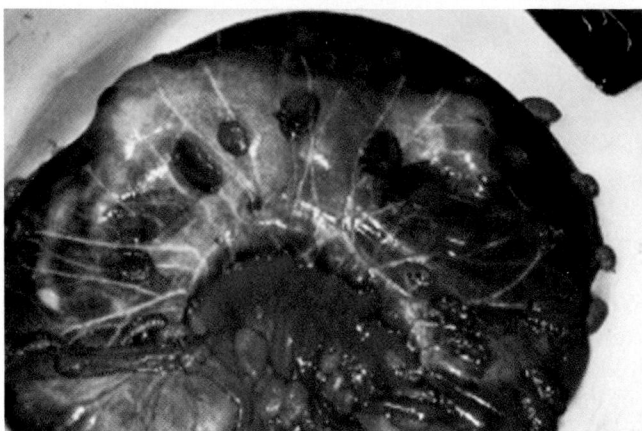

Figure 17-6 Cotyledons on the bovine chorioallantois.

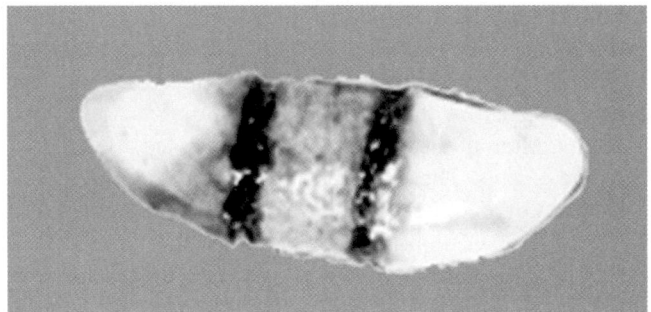

Figure 17-7 A canine puppy with the zonary placenta surrounding it.

✎ TECHNICIAN NOTE

Parturition is the act of giving birth.

Parturition is the act of giving birth. The only domestic species in which the entire parturition mechanism is completely understood is sheep; other species are hypothesized to be similar. As gestation progresses, the fetal hypothalamus and pituitary mature enough to cause the fetal release of corticotropin-releasing hormone from the hypothalamus, which causes the fetal adrenal to produce high concentrations of cortisol. The high cortisol concentrations cause a change in placental production of progesterone to estrogen and a release of prostaglandin from the uterus. These hormones cause the cervix to dilate and the uterus to contract, thereby forcing the fetus out. Parturition is normally divided into three stages: I, II, and III. Stage I is the preparatory stage. Maternal pelvic ligaments relax and the cervix softens, preparing for delivery. Behaviorally, the female becomes restless and prepares to give birth. The expulsion of the fetus is stage II (Figure 17-8). Stage III is the expulsion of the placenta. The timing of the events of parturition varies by species. A summary of the length of the estrous cycle and the length of gestation is found in Table 17-1.

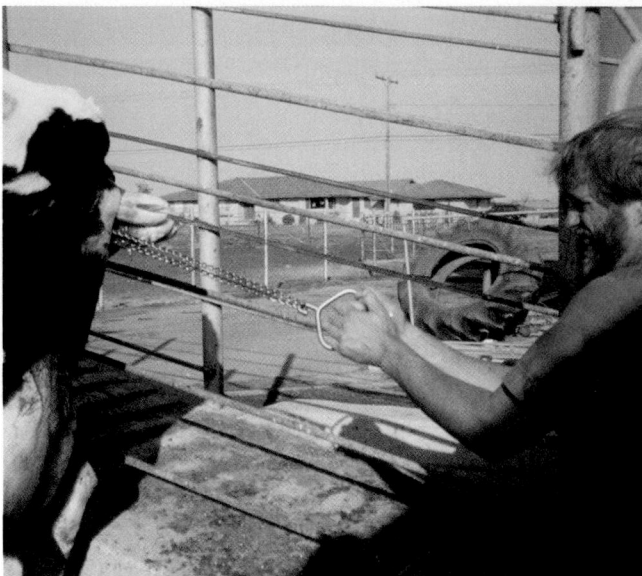

Figure 17-8 Chains placed around the legs of a bovine calf in a normal delivery position.

CANINE REPRODUCTION

The estrous cycle of the bitch has four phases: proestrus (9 to 10 days average), estrus (9 to 10 days average), diestrus (57 to 58 days average), and anestrus (2 to 5 months average) (Figure 17-9). Interestrus consists of diestrus and anestrus combined and therefore usually lasts 4 to 7 months. Interestrus periods of less than 4 months are associated with infertility.

During proestrus, the bitch is attractive to male dogs but will not allow mating. The vulva appears swollen, and a serosanguineous discharge is present. Estrogen, which is rising during proestrus, causes the epithelial cells in the vagina to cornify. Vaginal cytology is a common tool used to follow a bitch's cycle. To prepare a vaginal cytology slide, moisten a long cotton swab and pass it through the vulva and vestibule (Figure 17-10). The canine vagina is nearly vertical at the entrance. To get a swab into the cranial vagina once past the vulvar lips, direct the swab nearly vertical (toward the anus) until it will go no further. Redirect the swab horizontally, and twirl it to obtain a sample. Roll the swab on a slide, and stain the slide using a modified Wright's or Giemsa stain. Noncornified cells have a rounded cytoplasm and a large stippled nucleus. Cornified cells have a more angular-shaped cytoplasm, and the nucleus is either pyknotic or not apparent. The percentage of cornified cells increases approximately 10% per day, reaching 90% to 100% (full cornification) by the onset of estrus (Figure 17-11).

✎ TECHNICIAN NOTE

The vaginal cytology is 100% cornified during estrus in the bitch.

Table 17-1 Summary of the Lengths of the Estrous Cycle and Gestation Periods in Domestic Animals

Species	Puberty	Estrous Cycle Length	Estrus Duration	Ovulation	Optimal Breeding (Fresh/Frozen)	Gestation
Canine (dog or bitch)	6 months	No true cycle (Estrus is 2 times/year.)	9 days	2-4 days after onset of cytologic estrus	Days 3 and 5 or 4 and 6 after LH peak/day 5 or 6 after LH peak	57 days from first day of cytologic diestrus or 65 days from ovulation or 65 days from LH peak
Feline (cat or queen)	6-12 months	Seasonally polyestrous and depends on whether ovulation occurs	8 days	Induced ovulators after coitus	After third day of estrus and >2 hours apart for at least 3 breedings	65 days
Equine (horse or mare)	18 months	Seasonally polyestrous, 21 days (Diestrus is consistently 15 days.)	4-7 days	1-2 days before end of estrus	(Within 48 hours of ovulation) At ovulation	330 days, variable
Bovine (cow)	12 months	21 days	12-18 hours	12-18 hours after end of estrus	12 hours after end of estrus	283 days
Caprine (goat or doe)	6-9 months	Seasonally polyestrous, 21 days	24-36 hours	24-30 hours after onset of estrus	18-24 hours after onset of estrus	150 days
Ovine (sheep or ewe)	6-9 months	Seasonally polyestrous, 17 days	24-48 hours	24-30 hours after onset of estrus	12-30 hours after onset of estrus	150 days
Porcine (pig or sow)	5-6 months	21 days	2 to 3 days	Day 2 of estrus	24 and 36 hours after onset of estrus (12 and 24 in gilts)	114 days
Llama	10-12 months	Induced ovulators	1-36 days (induced ovulators)	Induced ovulators	Induced ovulators	344 days
Alpaca	10-12 months	Induced ovulators	1-36 days (induced ovulators)	Induced ovulators	Induced ovulators	344 days

ESTROUS CYCLE IN THE DOG

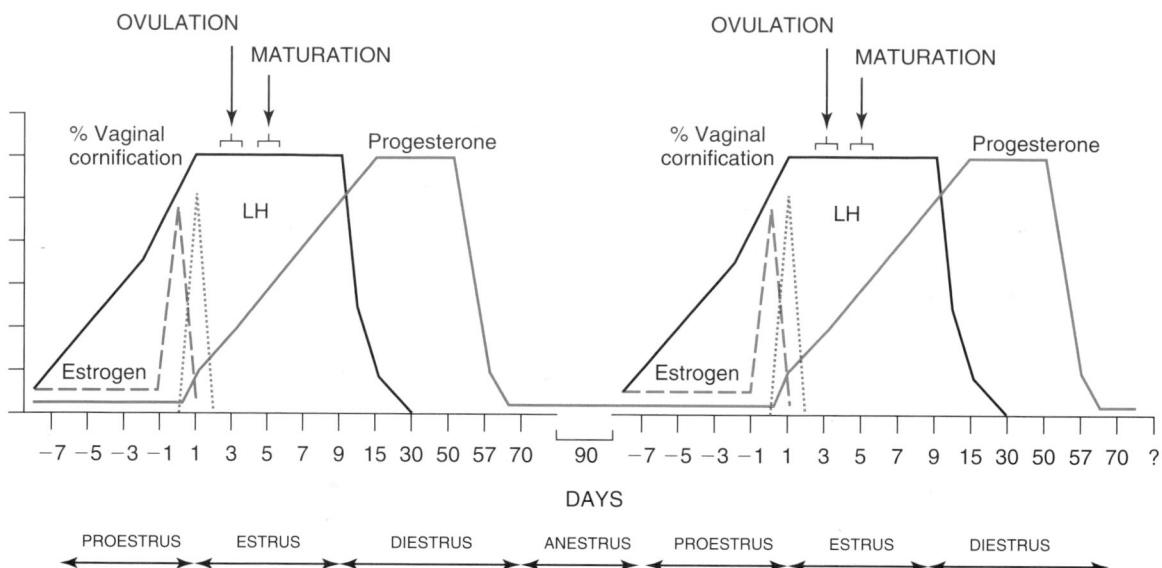

Figure 17-9 The canine estrous cycle. Proestrus lasts about 9 days. During proestrus the vaginal cornification increases about 10% per day, and estrogen peaks at the end of proestrus. There is 100% vaginal cornification throughout a 9-day estrus. At the beginning of estrus the LH peaks. At the same time the LH peaks, progesterone starts to rise. About 2 days after the LH peak, ovulation occurs, followed by a 2- to 3-day maturation of the oocytes. At the start of diestrus, the vaginal cornification abruptly declines to less than 50% cornified. Diestrus lasts about 57 days and is characterized by high progesterone. At the end of diestrus, progesterone declines and the bitch enters a 90- to 150-day anestrus. The cycle then starts over again.

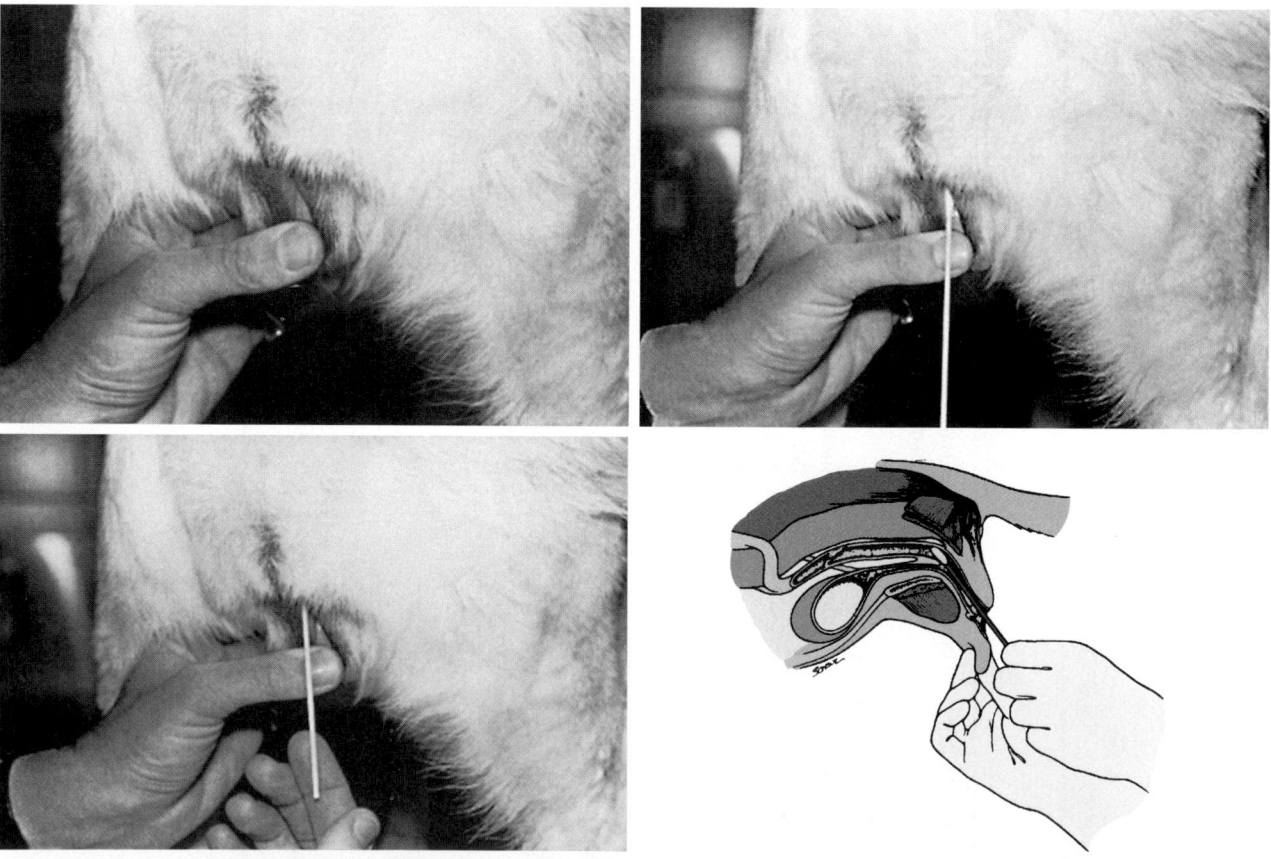

Figure 17-10 Vaginal cytology preparation. (From Feldman EC, Nelson RW, editors: *Canine and feline endocrinology and reproduction,* ed 2, Philadelphia, 1987, WB Saunders.)

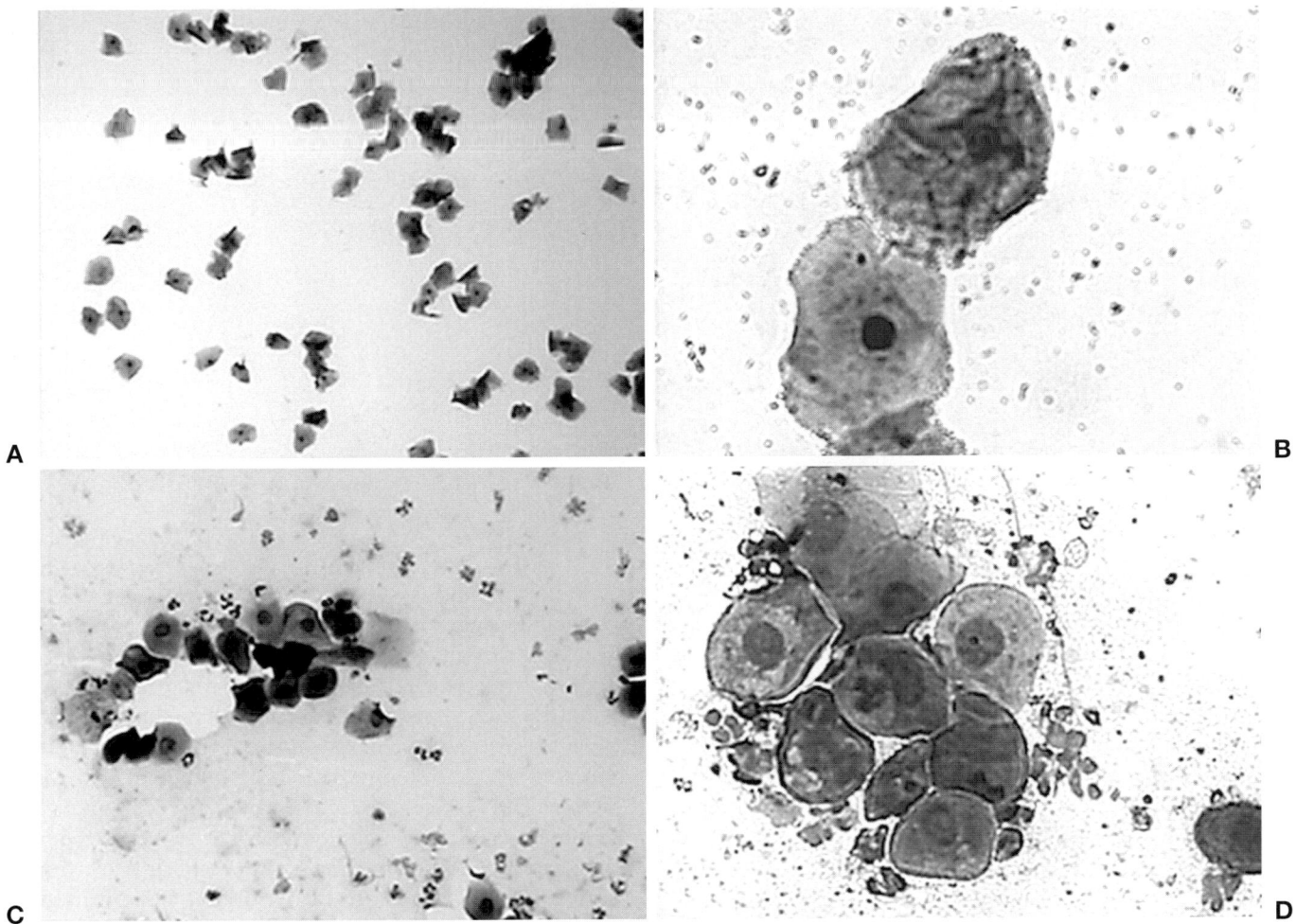

Figure 17-11 A low-power (**A**) and a high-power (**B**) view of a vaginal cytology sample of a dog in estrus. A low-power (**C**) and a high-power (**D**) view of a vaginal cytology sample of a dog in diestrus.

Estrus is the period of receptivity when the bitch will allow mating. During estrus, the vulvar swelling typically decreases slightly, and the bloody discharge changes to a straw color, although a bloody discharge may continue throughout estrus. Vaginal cytology is fully cornified, and the background of the slide is clear. No white blood cells should be present. Occasionally, bacteria may be seen on the slide.

The end of estrus, or the first day of diestrus, is typified by an abrupt decline in the percentage of cornified cells. This day is important to detect because whelping can be accurately predicted from day 1 (D1) of diestrus. Day 1 of diestrus also correlates well with the LH peak (8 days before D1) and ovulation (approximately 6 days before D1).

To maximize fertility, viable sperm must be present when the oocyte is ready to be fertilized. If the male is readily available, mating every other day is usually practiced. If performing artificial insemination and male availability is not limited, breeding three times per week (e.g., Monday, Wednesday, Friday) for as long as the vaginal cytology is fully cornified provides equally good results. However, when the number of breedings is reduced to one or two during a single estrus, such as with frozen or fresh cooled semen, timing insemination to coincide with ovulation becomes critical. Ovulation occurs approximately 2 days after the LH surge. The bitch ovulates immature oocytes that require 2 to 3 more days for maturation. Mature oocytes are then viable for another 2 to 3 days. Therefore the fertile period is 4 to 8 days after the LH surge, with peak fertility occurring 5 to 6 days after the LH surge.

TECHNICIAN NOTE

The bitch ovulates immature oocytes that require 2 to 3 more days for maturation.

To best estimate the day of ovulation, hormone assays should be used. Vaginal cytology does not give a very precise prediction of ovulation. The LH peak may occur anywhere from the same day of, or up to 2 days after, full cornification. Unlike most species, serum progesterone rises before ovulation in the bitch. Therefore progesterone is useful to predict

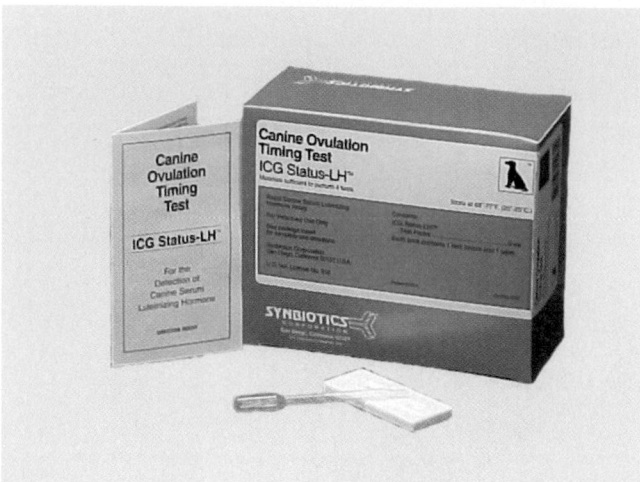

Figure 17-12 A commercially available kit to perform qualitative LH analysis.

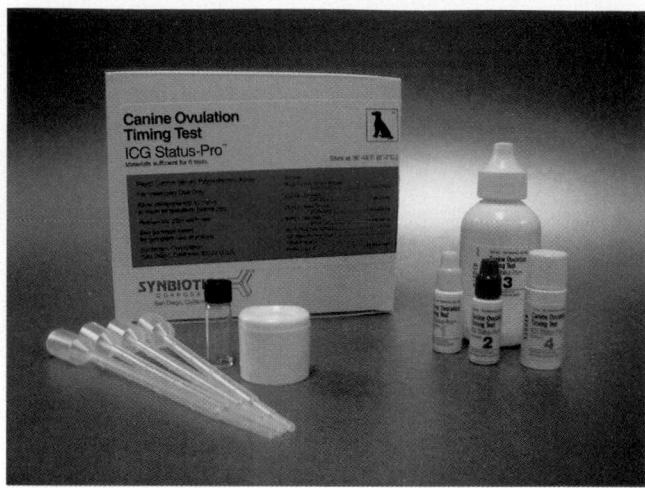

Figure 17-13 A commercially available kit to perform semiquantitative progesterone analysis.

the LH surge because the increase in serum progesterone is closely associated with the LH peak. Before the LH surge, serum progesterone is less than 1 ng/ml. On the day of the LH surge, serum progesterone rises to 1.5 to 2.0 ng/ml (2 ng progesterone = 3.18 nmol progesterone) and after that continues to rise during diestrus or pregnancy. By identifying this initial rise in progesterone, the day of the LH surge can be estimated and insemination performed during the period of peak fertility. Although LH can be measured semiquantitatively with in-house test kits (Figure 17-12), the peak only lasts 1 day, so serum must be tested daily. Progesterone assays provide some advantages because after the initial rise (on the same day as the LH surge), progesterone continues to rise, so the day of initial rise can be estimated even if a day is missed. Ovulation occurs 2 days after the LH rise and is associated with a progesterone concentration of 5 ng (15.90 nmol)/ml.

In-house, semiquantitative kits for progesterone analysis are available (Figure 17-13). The in-house tests are easy to perform, and results are available in about 20 minutes. Some aspects of the tests require attention to detail to achieve meaningful results. The kits need to be at room temperature before use, and the manufacturers recommend the kits be placed at room temperature for approximately 2 hours before use. If the test is run using a cold kit, results will be incorrect, often giving a false-high progesterone. Blood should be allowed to clot at a cool temperature (in the refrigerator), and cells should be separated from serum or plasma as soon as possible (within 20 minutes of collection is the manufacturer's recommendation). If serum is allowed to remain in contact with the red blood cells, progesterone will be bound by them and test results will be artificially low. Hemolyzed or lipemic samples may also cause erroneously low results. Serum samples may also be frozen for analysis later. If a laboratory is available that can give rapid turnaround time and provide quantitative results, this is

preferable when breeding with frozen semen or any time breedings are limited.

If only two breedings are to be performed, such as with fresh cooled semen, insemination should be performed on either days 3 and 5 or days 4 and 6 after the LH peak or initial rise in progesterone, keeping in mind that viability of fresh chilled semen is reduced and timing of insemination is more critical. The viability of frozen semen is reduced even further and timing is even more critical. When frozen semen is used, usually a single surgical insemination is conducted. Insemination with frozen semen should be performed on day 5 or 6 after the LH peak or initial rise in progesterone or 3 days after a progesterone level of 5 ng (15.90 nmol)/ml. Insemination with frozen semen is performed either surgically or by a transcervical endoscopic method. It is beneficial to continue to monitor vaginal cytology and identify Day 1 of diestrus (D1), which usually occurs 8 days after the LH peak or 6 days after ovulation. Significant variations of the first day of diestrus from this expected time frame are associated with decreased fertility.

> **TECHNICIAN NOTE**
>
> The fertile period is best identified using hormone assays for LH or progesterone.

VAGINAL CULTURES

Vaginal cultures can be taken from the bitch for various reasons including prepubertal or postpubertal vaginitis, postparturient discharge, discharges during pregnancy, postabortion discharge, and prebreeding in normal or infertile bitches. Vaginal cultures are best performed with a guarded swab to avoid contamination as the culture swab is passed through the vestibule. If a culture is to be performed

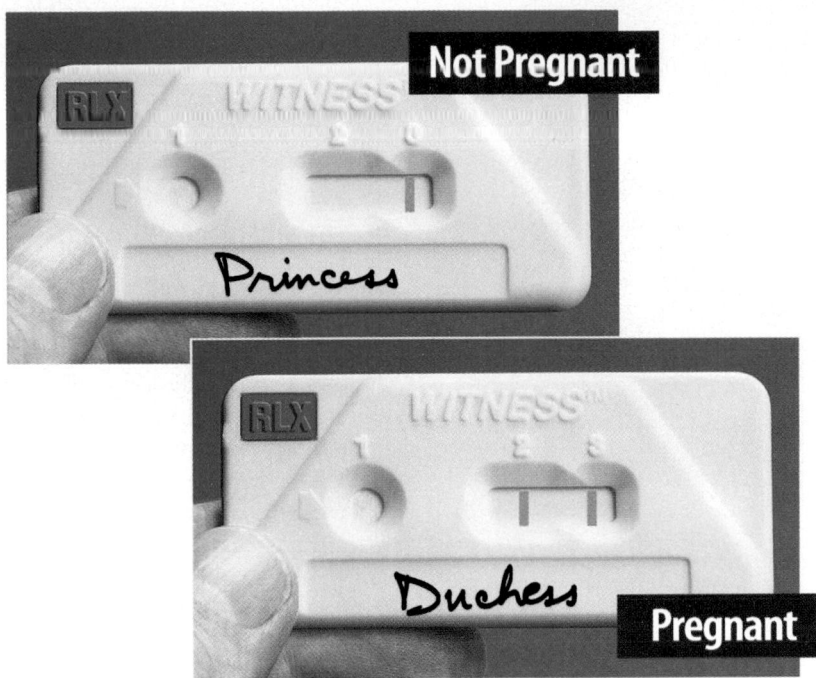

Figure 17-14 A commercially available kit to measure canine relaxin to determine pregnancy in a bitch.

as part of a prebreeding examination, and the client needs a negative culture before breeding, then the performance and interpretation of the culture become critical. Bacteria, including mycoplasma, can be cultured from the vagina of the majority of fertile and infertile bitches. Once a culture has been obtained, it must be interpreted. If the culture was obtained as part of a workup for a clinical problem, a pure culture is probably significant. However, a vaginal culture as part of a prebreeding examination, and in the absence of clinical signs, often produces results of little significance.

PREGNANCY DIAGNOSIS

Pregnancy diagnosis can be performed by palpation, hormone assay, ultrasonography, or radiography. Palpation can be performed during a 7- to 10-day window beginning around day 21 after D1. After approximately day 30 post-D1, the embryonic vesicles become confluent and the ability to diagnose pregnancy by palpation is lost until late in gestation. Ultrasound can be used after approximately day 20 post-D1, possibly earlier, depending on the machine and probe used, until parturition. Radiography can be used after day 45 post-LH (day 37 post-D1). An in-house assay for relaxin is available and is reliable after about day 28 post-LH (day 20 post-D1) (Figure 17-14). When pregnancy testing, it is very helpful to know the day of progesterone rise or day 1 of diestrus to be able to estimate gestation length. Whereas gestation length seemingly can be as short as 55 days or as long as 70 days when timed from breeding, it is a reliable 57 to 58 days when timed from day 1 of diestrus. Because

a bitch is receptive to the male for 9 or 10 days, timing from breeding is quite variable, resulting in errors (false-negative results) when examining for pregnancy or predicting whelping.

> ### TECHNICIAN NOTE
> Pregnancy diagnosis can be performed by palpation, hormone assay, ultrasonography, or radiography.

PARTURITION AND DYSTOCIA

Stage I of whelping averages 6 to 12 hours but can be as long as 36 hours. The bitch is usually restless and may show nesting behavior. She often appears nervous, pants, and may tremble or shiver. Body temperature drops to 99° F about 24 hours before stage II in approximately 85% of bitches. This temperature drop is related to the abrupt decline in progesterone and can be useful for the dog owner to signal that whelping is imminent. To be reliable, the temperature should be taken at the same time each day, preferably in the morning before any activity. Stage II, when the bitch pushes the puppies out, lasts approximately 20 to 60 minutes per puppy (Figure 17-15). However, no more than 2 hours should elapse between each delivery. Stage II usually lasts a total of 3 to 6 hours but may be as long as 24 hours total. The presentation of the puppies is 60% anterior in the bitch. A blackish-green discharge is normal during parturition and comes from the site of placental attachment to the uterus.

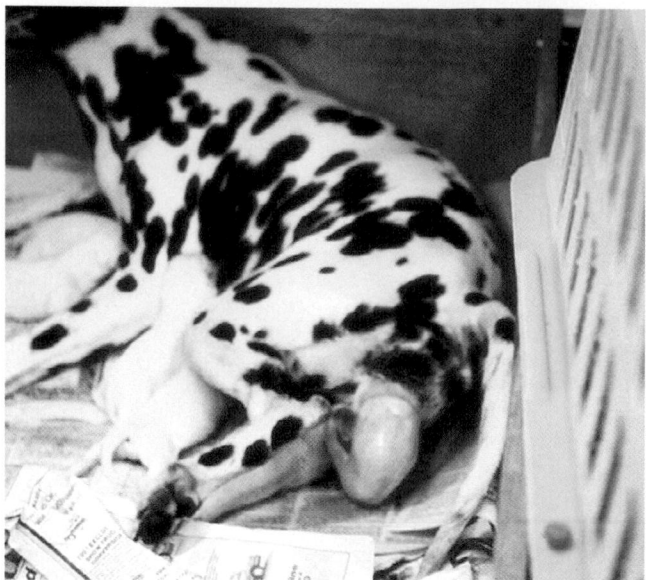

Figure 17-15 A puppy being delivered during a normal canine parturition.

Guidelines for recognizing dystocia (difficult birth) are strong continual contractions for 30 minutes without progress; weak, infrequent contractions for 2 hours without progress; or a prolonged interval between puppies. If any of these criteria is met, veterinary examination is warranted. Ultrasound can be used to assess fetal viability, but radiography is the only reliable method to accurately determine the number of pups in utero, their relative size, and their position.

POSTPARTUM PROBLEMS

The bitch has the longest postpartum uterine involution period of the domestic species. A nonodorous hemorrhagic vulvar discharge is normal for 8 to 10 weeks after whelping and does not indicate metritis. Clients are often concerned when a bloody discharge persists for that length of time but should be reassured that it is normal. When the discharge persists for a prolonged period, such as 12 weeks or more, the bitch is considered to have subinvolution of the placental sites (SIPS). Treatment in these cases can be medical (ergonovine), surgical (ovariohysterectomy), or conservative (monitoring).

Indications that a bitch is suffering from postpartum problems include signs of discomfort, such as crying and whining, by the pups caused by the lack of attention from the dam. Metritis is characterized by a foul-smelling vaginal discharge. Retained placenta results in a green discharge. Clinical signs of mastitis in the dam include fever, lethargy, and swollen mammary glands. The glands may be discolored as well. In many cases of metritis or mastitis, the pups will need to be hand fed or at least supplemented.

Eclampsia, or hypocalcemia, is characterized by tremors and excitation and is more common in smaller breeds. It most commonly occurs in the postpartum period. It is a true emergency. Hyperthermia and convulsions may require sedation or short-term anesthesia in addition to calcium treatment.

PSEUDOPREGNANCY

All bitches experience a 57- to 58-day period of elevated serum progesterone after estrus, whether pregnant or not. As progesterone declines at the end of a nonpregnant diestrus, many bitches, even if not pregnant, will experience mammary development, lactation, and maternal behavior. Clients may be concerned that the bitch is uncomfortable, or the behavioral changes may be unacceptable. With time, clinical signs will fade, and the bitch will return to normal. Alternatively, hormonal treatment with mibolerone or cabergoline can be used. Treatment with a progestogen, such as megestrol acetate, is contraindicated because signs of pseudopregnancy will return when therapy is halted.

Pyometra (uterine infection) can be a life-threatening situation in the bitch. It is progesterone related, usually occurring during diestrus, and may follow inappropriate estrogen therapy. The bitch may have a vaginal discharge depending on whether the cervix is open or closed. A bitch with pyometra is often lethargic, depressed, and febrile and exhibits polyuria and polydipsia. A leukocytosis is found on complete blood count (CBC). Palpation or ultrasonography reveals an enlarged, fluid-filled uterus. If the breeding potential of the bitch is to be preserved, medical treatment with prostaglandin, cabergoline, and antibiotics is indicated; otherwise, surgical treatment (ovariohysterectomy) is usually recommended.

✎ TECHNICIAN NOTE

A bitch with pyometra is often lethargic, depressed, and febrile and exhibits polyuria and polydipsia.

MISMATING

It is not unusual to have a client bring in a dog that has been bred accidentally or escaped while in estrus and request that she be "mismated" (aborted). In the past, few options were available other than estradiol cypionate (ECP), ovariohysterectomy, or allowing her to whelp. The use of ECP is not without risks. If given late in estrus or at the beginning of diestrus, there is a significant risk of pyometra. Another very serious potential complication with the use of ECP is aplastic anemia. Further, many bitches presented for mismating may actually not have been bred or will not become pregnant. In one report, more than half of the bitches presented for pregnancy termination were not pregnant and therefore would have been treated needlessly.

For these reasons, and the availability of suitable alternatives, the use of ECP for mismating is no longer recommended. In many cases, the preferred method is to wait until such time as pregnancy diagnosis can be performed. If the bitch is pregnant, therapeutic options include prostaglandin, cabergoline, bromocriptine, or dexamethasone.

Prostaglandin effectively terminates pregnancy and is safe in dogs if used properly. Prostaglandin should be given subcutaneously, rather than intramuscularly. Further, a single dose will be ineffective in lysing the corpora lutea, so multiple small doses are used, usually two or three times per day for 5 to 7 days. Side effects include vomiting, diarrhea, and urination. An uncommon complication is cardiovascular collapse. Therefore an intravenous catheter is often recommended during the initial phases of treatment in case fluid therapy is necessary.

An alternative to prostaglandin is cabergoline (or a related compound, bromocriptine). Both are dopamine agonists, and administration will result in progesterone decline and pregnancy loss. Bromocriptine may be associated with vomiting, whereas cabergoline causes few side effects.

Dexamethasone is an attractive alternative to the previously mentioned drugs. It is administered orally, so it can be given at home. With any of these drugs, it is important to monitor pregnancy loss and continue therapy until abortion is complete. In addition, if the pregnancy is advanced when therapy is begun, it is important to inform the client that fetal discharge may be observed.

BRUCELLOSIS

Canine brucellosis, although typically thought of as a disease characterized by abortion and infertility, may manifest itself in a variety of ways. Although usually considered a venereal disease, *Brucella canis* is also spread through oronasal routes. Aborted fetuses and vaginal discharges are rich sources of *B. canis* organisms. Infected males shed the organism in their urine in addition to their semen. Transmission can occur between adult dogs in the absence of aborted material or sexual contact.

Because *B. canis* is an intracellular organism, the disease is extremely difficult to treat effectively and cures are nearly impossible to achieve. No treatment has been found that is 100% effective in achieving a cure, although serum titers may decrease. Because of the nature of the disease and the potential for spread, euthanasia is commonly recommended for breeding animals in a kennel situation. A less drastic choice for pets is neutering and antibiotic therapy, although persistent infection is still likely.

Because of the finality of neutering or euthanasia, a correct diagnosis is imperative. Unfortunately, many testing methods result in a high incidence of false-positive results and can be regarded as screening tests only. For example, antibodies against antigens of *Pseudomonas aeruginosa*, *Bordetella bronchiseptica*, and some *Staphylococcus* spp. can cause a false-positive result in a brucellosis test. Therefore

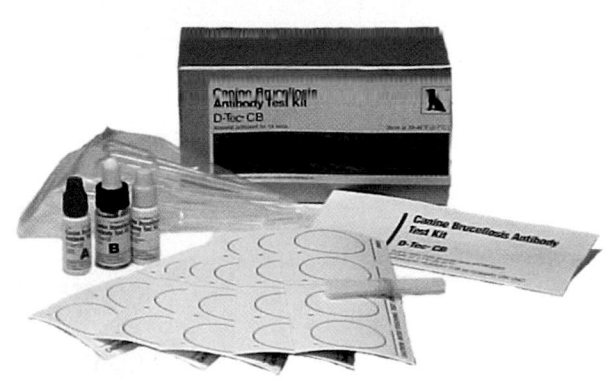

Figure 17-16 A commercially available kit to check for *Brucella canis*.

a positive reaction on a screening test does not mean a dog is infected but does suggest the need for further, more definitive diagnosis.

The in-house screening test (D-Tec CB, Synbiotics) is very rapid and very sensitive. False-positive results are very common (20% to 50% of positive dogs do not have brucellosis, and some breeds, such as English sheepdogs, have exceptionally high false-positive rates) (Figure 17-16). A negative result is highly accurate, provided infection did not occur within 3 to 4 weeks before testing. Screening tests can give a false-negative result when a dog is infected for less than 4 weeks or is chronically infected and has recently received antibiotic treatment. If a dog is positive on the in-house test, samples should then be submitted to a diagnostic laboratory for further testing with a more specific test.

🖉 TECHNICIAN NOTE

Although false positives are common with in-house *Brucella canis* screening, false negatives are rare.

FELINE REPRODUCTION

Although most species have a spontaneous LH surge that causes ovulation during every estrous cycle, the queen must have vaginal stimulation to induce an LH surge. The queen is therefore an induced ovulator. Because the queen does not necessarily ovulate during each estrous cycle, there are unique aspects in the queen's estrous cycle that are not seen in other species. When a queen comes into estrus, there are three potential outcomes after estrus: the queen can ovulate and become pregnant, the queen can ovulate and not become pregnant, or the queen may not ovulate (Figure 17-17). Each of these outcomes results in a different

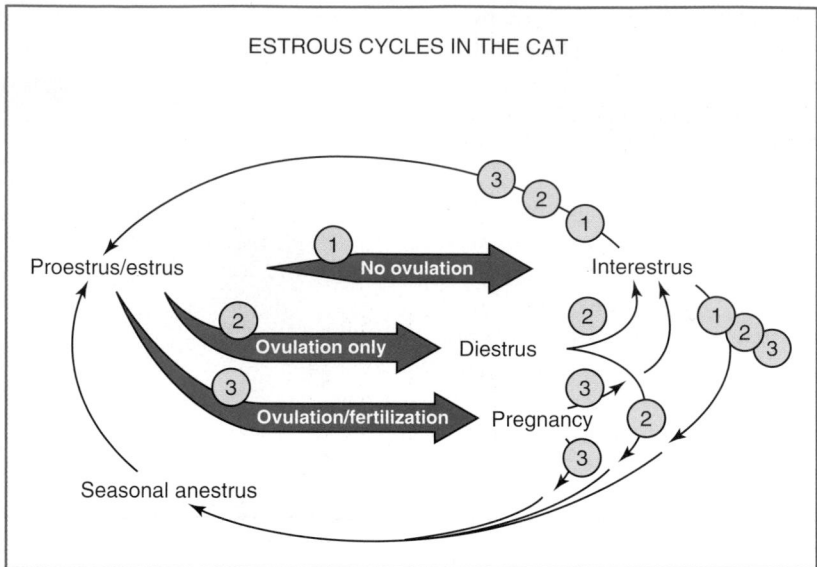

Figure 17-17 The feline estrous cycle. Depending on the season and whether ovulation occurs, the queen can do one of six things on entering an 8-day estrus. *1,* If ovulation is not induced, the queen can go into a 2- to 14-day interestrus or seasonal anestrus. *2,* If the queen ovulates but is not pregnant, a 36-day diestrus followed by either a 2- to 14-day interestrus or seasonal anestrus can occur. *3,* If the queen ovulates and is pregnant, a 65-day pregnancy followed by either a 2- to 6-week interestrus or seasonal anestrus may occur.

series of subsequent events and time sequences for return to estrus. The outcomes also depend on the season of the year, because queens are seasonal breeders.

> **TECHNICIAN NOTE**
> The queen is an induced ovulator.

SEASONALITY

Most queens have estrous cycles during the spring and are considered long-day breeders. This may be masked by the fact that most domestic cats are kept indoors under artificial lighting. The artificial lighting may be sufficient to stimulate estrous cycles all year long. The season and effect of artificial lighting must always be taken into account when discussing the queen's estrous cycle.

ESTROUS CYCLE

Proestrus in the queen is only 1 to 3 days long and may not be apparent. Estrus in the queen lasts 8 to 10 days, and the queen shows very distinctive outward signs of estrus. These signs include rolling and assuming an exaggerated lordosis when petted. The lordosis results in an elevation of the queen's hindquarters. These signs are so intense that many queens in estrus are presented for neurologic problems. Unlike other species that automatically enter a diestrus period of progesterone domination after estrus, the queen must have adequate vaginal stimulation to ovulate. The vaginal stimulation must come after the third day of estrus,

and there must be multiple stimulations at least 2 to 3 hours apart to induce an LH rise of sufficient magnitude and duration to cause ovulation. Even if breeding does occur, vaginal stimulation will not necessarily be adequate to elicit a sufficient LH rise to cause ovulation.

If the queen ovulates and becomes pregnant, the gestation period is 63 to 66 days after mating. After parturition the queen undergoes an anestrous period of variable duration. Anestrus is a time when nothing is happening on the ovaries and the queen does not come into estrus. Postpartum anestrus may be as short as 2 weeks or as long as 6 weeks. Depending on the season and/or lighting conditions, the queen may then return to proestrus or go into seasonal anestrus.

If a queen is bred, ovulates, but does not become pregnant, a diestrus (or pseudopregnancy) of approximately 40 days follows the estrus. During diestrus the queen has a high concentration of progesterone in the blood that is produced by the corpora lutea on the ovaries that prevents the return to estrus. These corpora lutea apparently have a finite life span and cannot be lysed with exogenous prostaglandin. After a nonpregnant diestrus, a short anestrus occurs. This anestrus is approximately 2 weeks long. Again, depending on the season and/or lighting conditions, the queen may return to proestrus or enter a seasonal anestrus.

If the queen is not bred or is bred and has insufficient stimulation to cause an LH surge, ovulation will not take place. If there is no ovulation, the follicles on the ovary regress. At this time there are no structures on the ovaries (follicles or CLs), so this is called *anestrus.* This is a transitory anestrus, so a better term is *interestrus.* Depending on the season and/or lighting conditions, the interestrus may be 3 to 14 days or may extend into a long seasonal anestrus.

Pregnancy can be diagnosed in the queen 16 to 30 days postcoitus by abdominal palpation, after 14 days postcoitus to term by ultrasound, and after 43 days by radiography. Palpation must be done within a time frame because the gestational sacs are too small before day 16 and they become too confluent after day 30 to distinguish. Ultrasound can detect if the fetus is alive by seeing the fetal heartbeat, but it is difficult to count the number of fetuses and to estimate their size. Radiography is the best method to count the number of concepti and to estimate their size, but fetal mineralization of the skeleton must be adequate to detect them radiographically.

COMMON REPRODUCTIVE PROBLEMS

Queens are generally very fertile and have few infertility problems. Because most pet queens have ovariohysterectomies performed at an early age, few of these queens are seen for reproductive problems.

The most common questions arise from the clinical signs that accompany estrus in the queen and irritate the owner. Queens that have not undergone ovariohysterectomy are often presented for prolonged estrus. Although cystic ovaries do occur in queens, they are not often the cause of the prolonged estrus. More commonly, a queen with persistent estrus is undergoing normal estrus, with a very short 1- to 2-day interestrus, followed by another estrus. This makes it seem like the queen is in constant estrus, when in fact there are normal periods of estrus and interestrus occurring. Treatment for this condition is either ovariohysterectomy or induction of ovulation.

Ovulation can be induced by vaginal stimulation with a cotton swab, glass rod, or thermometer. The stimulations must meet the same criteria as breeding to be effective: the vaginal stimulation must come after the third day of estrus, and there must be multiple stimulations at least 2 to 3 hours apart to induce an LH rise sufficient to cause ovulation. An alternative to vaginal stimulation is the administration of GnRH or human chorionic gonadotropin (hCG). The GnRH will cause an endogenous release of LH from the anterior pituitary, thereby resulting in ovulation. The drug hCG has LH action and will directly cause ovulation. After ovulation induction, estrus will not be shortened; however, the queen will then enter diestrus and interestrus phases, so estrus will not recur for approximately 2 months. There are no drugs approved to control the estrous cycle in the queen.

Another common complaint is the queen that comes into estrus after ovariohysterectomy. It is important to document the presence of extra ovarian tissue by hormone analysis. This is most easily done using the same techniques to induce ovulation. If the queen goes out of estrus and has high progesterone, then extra ovarian tissue must be sought surgically. If not, then the adrenals may be the source of the estrogen causing the signs of estrus.

Parturition in the queen (queening) can last as long as 36 hours. The following criteria can be used to diagnose dystocia (abnormal birth): 20 minutes of intense labor with no kitten, 10 minutes of intense labor when a kitten is present, acute depression, or the presence of fresh blood for more than 10 minutes. If any of these criteria is noted, it is advised that the queen be examined. Although most queens do not have problems queening, an examination and radiographs will help rule out if a cesarean delivery is required.

The normal postpartum discharge is red-black, non-odorous fluid that can be seen as long as 3 weeks after queening. If the queen appears depressed or the kittens are dying, the queen should be examined for mastitis or metritis.

Pyometra in the queen presents with similar signs as seen in the bitch, including depression and vaginal discharge. Bitches with pyometra tend to be older, whereas queens can be any age.

EQUINE REPRODUCTION

Mares are seasonally polyestrous, meaning that during the breeding season they cycle repeatedly. The natural breeding season centers around the period of long day length. Under natural conditions, mares begin cycling in late March or early April and continue until September or October. Some mares may continue to cycle year round. In the northern hemisphere, many breed associations have designated January 1 as the birth date for all horses born in a given year. This means that a horse born in January and a horse born in June will both be considered 1 year old the following January when they are actually 12 months and 7 months old, respectively. This is a large difference for horses competing as 2 year olds. Therefore there is a great deal of pressure to have foals born early in the season (January or February). Unfortunately, many mares are not cycling at this time. The most cost-effective method to stimulate earlier cyclicity is to "trick" the mare into perceiving that the days are lengthening by providing artificial lighting and mimicking a 16-hour daylight period. This should be started by December 1 to get the most benefit. A 200-watt bulb in a

12- × 12-foot stall is sufficient. For an outdoor situation, eight 1000-watt metal halide flood lights at a height of 20 feet will provide sufficient light for an 84- × 66-foot paddock. Artificial lighting should be added in the evening, rather than in the morning. Turning the lights on earlier in the morning is less effective than leaving them on later in the evening.

During the breeding season, the mare's estrous cycle averages 21 to 22 days in length. Diestrus, the period when a corpus luteum is present and producing progesterone, is a consistent 15 days in length, based on hormone levels (Figure 17-18). During this time, the mare will tease "out," resisting the stallion's advances by kicking, squealing, pinning her ears back, and clamping her tail between her legs. Based on behavioral signs, diestrus is shorter (approximately 14 days) because she does not tease out until 1 day or so after ovulation. Estrus, or the period of receptivity, is shown by teasing "in." The mare squats, urinates, lifts her tail, and "winks" (everts her clitoris) on approach of the stallion.

> **TECHNICIAN NOTE**
> Estrus, or the period of receptivity, is shown by teasing "in."

Between the noncycling period (anestrus) and the cycling period, a period called *transition* occurs. Transition varies in length and is characterized by irregular periods of estrous behavior but without ovulation. A mare may exhibit estrous behavior for 2 or 3 days, then stop for a few days, and then begin again. Alternatively the mare may exhibit estrous behavior continuously without ovulation for 3 weeks or more. Although follicles may be present during these periods, they do not ovulate. The transitional period is a physiologically normal occurrence. Although cyclicity can be induced earlier in the year, a transitional period will still precede the onset of cyclicity. Awareness of this can help to reduce needless breedings and help mare owners understand this sometimes aggravating period. Administration of altrenogest, a synthetic progestogen, will stop the estrous behavior and is often used during transition.

During the breeding season, the duration of estrus is variable (4 to 7 days). Estrus tends to be shorter near the peak of the breeding season (June) and longer farther away from June, such as March or September. Follicular development can be monitored by palpation per rectum and ultrasonography during estrus to decide optimal breeding time.

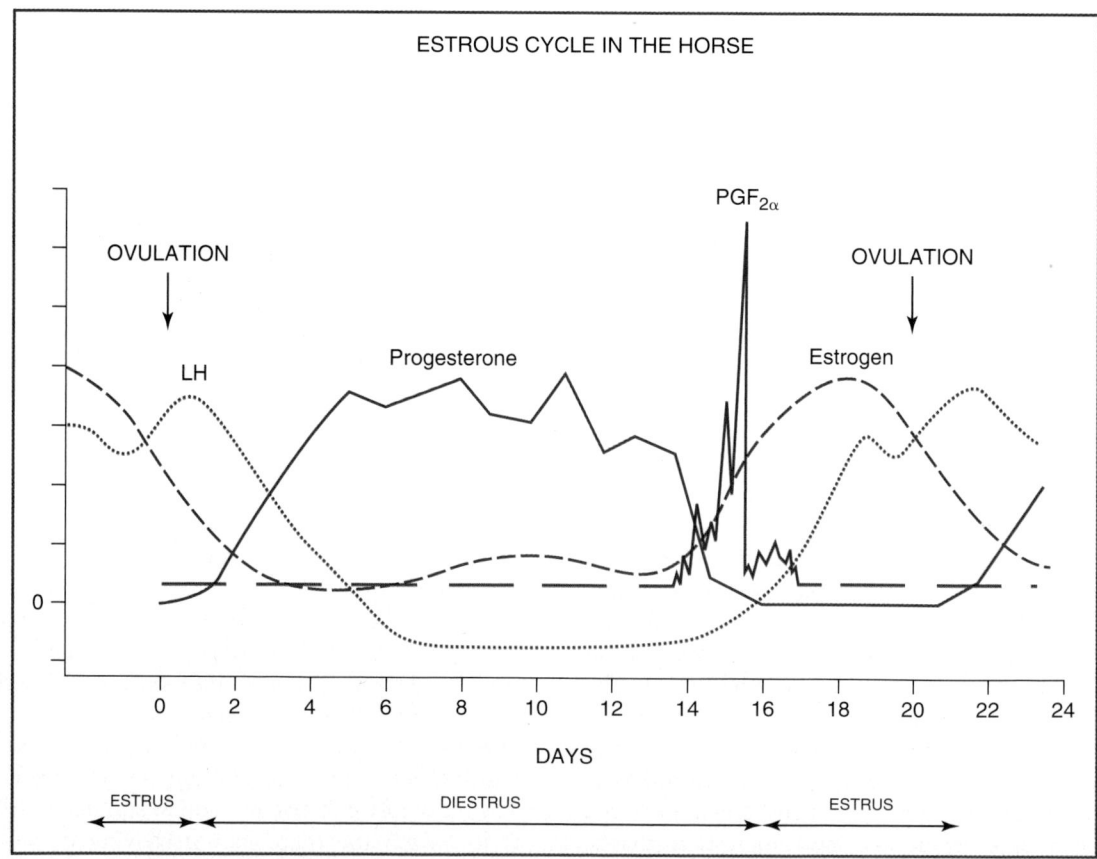

Figure 17-18 The equine estrous cycle. Estrus is 4 to 7 days long, and LH peaks after ovulation. Diestrus begins around 2 days after ovulation. Progesterone is high throughout a 14- to 15-day diestrus. If a pregnancy signal is not secreted by the early embryo by day 14 to 16, prostaglandin is released from the uterus, goes to the corpus luteum, and causes luteolysis (luteal death). The cycle then starts over.

BREEDING SOUNDNESS EXAMINATION

Breeding soundness examinations are commonly performed at the sale or purchase of a mare or when a mare fails to become pregnant after breeding. A typical breeding soundness examination consists of rectal palpation, ultrasonography, vaginal speculum examination, uterine culture/cytology, and a uterine biopsy. During the ultrasonographic examination, structures on the ovaries, and more importantly, features of the uterus can be observed. Fluid-filled structures such as follicles (Figure 17-19) and endometrial cysts will be black. Corpora lutea have a variable appearance, ranging from a rather homogeneous gray to a "spider web" trabecular pattern with a brighter thick-walled circumference. An important indication of the stage of the estrous cycle is the ultrasonographic appearance of the uterus. During diestrus it has a homogeneous hyperechoic appearance, but in estrus it has a very characteristic appearance caused by edema in the endometrial folds. It has been described as looking like the spokes of a cartwheel, a sliced orange, or pizza (Figure 17-20).

Vaginal speculum examination, uterine culture/cytology, and uterine biopsy are performed aseptically. First wrap the tail with a clean tail wrap or gauze. Prepare a clean bucket with clean water and add small (approximately 10 cm × 10 cm) pieces of cotton. Rather than placing disinfectant in the bucket, it is preferable to place the soap on the cotton itself before scrubbing the vulva, thereby leaving clean water to rinse the vulva. Otherwise, disinfectant residues may remain on the vulva and be carried into the vagina, with a potential spermicidal or tissue-irritating effect. Cleansing of the perineal area should be done using the "clean hand–dirty hand" technique. One hand (the clean hand) is used to retrieve clean pieces of cotton from the bucket. The cotton is then transferred to the other hand (the dirty hand), which is then used to scrub the perineal area. This method keeps the bucket with clean water and cotton from being contaminated. The vulvar labia should be scrubbed in a manner similar to that for surgical preparation, i.e., from the center of the area being cleaned to the perimeter, and repeated until clean. Check the inside of the labia during the procedure to be sure no feces have entered as a result of the palpation and ultrasonography procedures.

> ### ✐ TECHNICIAN NOTE
> All vaginal procedures in mares should be performed aseptically.

A vaginal speculum examination can discern trauma to the cervix; discharge emanating from the uterus, cervix, or vagina; urine pooling in the cranial vagina; and other conditions associated with subfertility. After aseptically preparing the vulva, a small amount of sterile lubricant is placed on the end of a speculum, the labia are parted, and the speculum is placed into the vagina. A light source is then used to look through the speculum and examine the vagina and cervix (Figure 17-21).

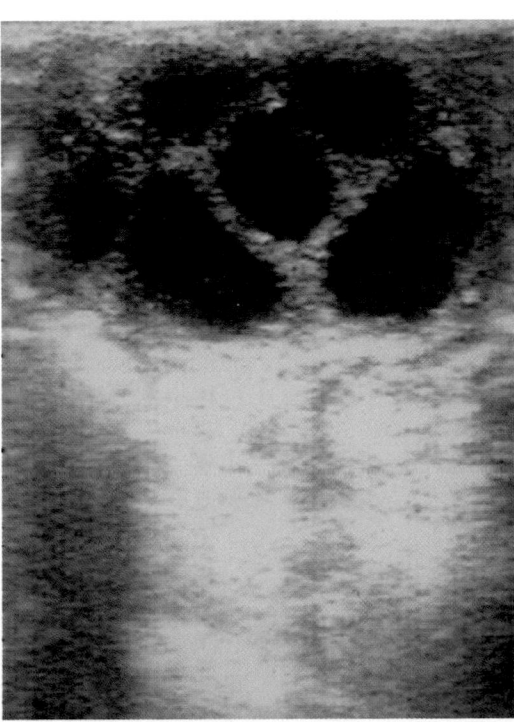

Figure 17-19 An ultrasound image of the black appearance of multiple follicles on an equine ovary.

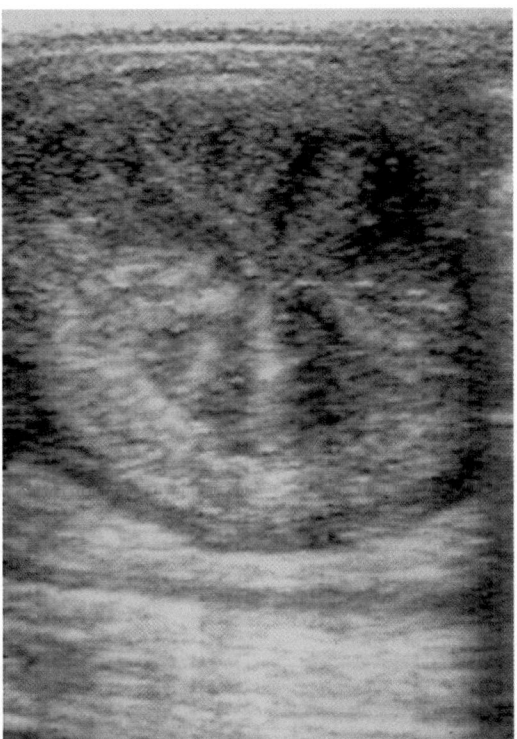

Figure 17-20 The "sliced-orange" ultrasonographic appearance of the uterus of a mare in estrus.

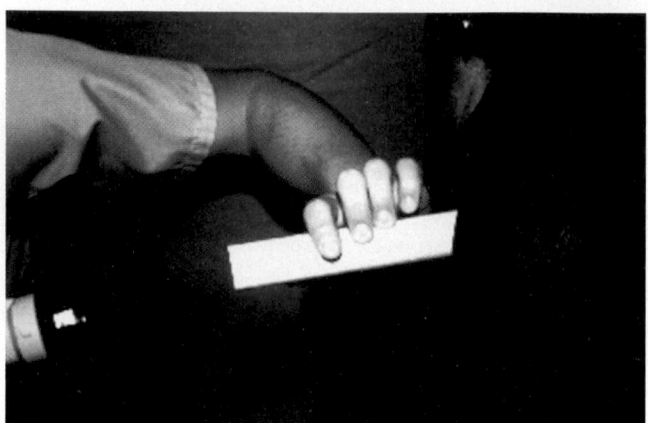

Figure 17-21 A vaginal speculum examination being performed on a mare using a disposable speculum.

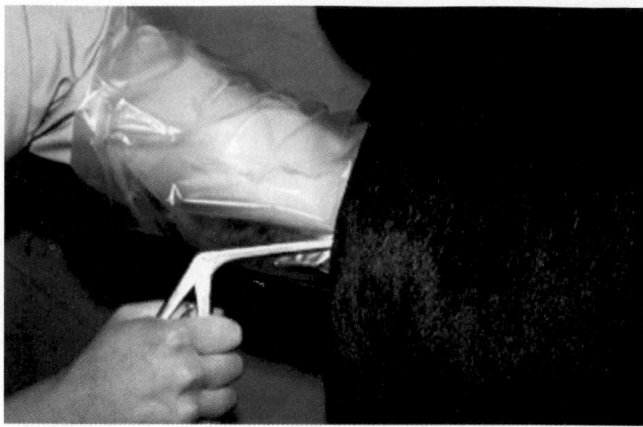

Figure 17-22 A uterine biopsy instrument being inserted through the vagina and cervix into the uterus.

The next procedure usually performed is a uterine culture/cytology. The importance of performing a cytologic examination in conjunction with the culture cannot be overstated. Without a cytologic specimen, it is impossible to differentiate between an infectious process and a contaminant resulting from improper sampling or mare preparation. When obtaining a culture/cytology specimen, only guarded swabs should be used. After aseptically preparing the vulva, a sterile sleeve is used to introduce the culture/cytology instrument into the vagina, through the cervix, and into the uterus. After the swab is withdrawn, the sample can be used to prepare a cytology specimen. Stain the cytology slide using a modified Wright's or Giemsa stain. The slide should contain numerous epithelial cells and be examined for inflammatory cells, primarily neutrophils. A positive cytology slide will contain numerous inflammatory cells, whereas a negative slide will not. Bacteria isolated from a culture with a negative cytology finding can be considered contaminants. In fact, an argument can be made to not submit the culture if the cytology slide is negative. However, if the cytology slide is positive, not only do culture results reveal the causative agent but also sensitivity results aid in making a therapeutic choice. Excess lubricant used during the procedure can interfere with interpretation by staining darkly and obscuring the field.

> ✎ **TECHNICIAN NOTE**
>
> Endometrial cytology should always be performed in conjunction with an endometrial culture to aid in interpretation of results.

The next, and often final, step in the breeding soundness examination is to obtain an endometrial biopsy. Again, as with the previous procedures, it is done in an aseptic manner. The closed instrument is carried into the uterus, wearing a sterile sleeve (Figure 17-22). The instrument is held in the uterus while the hand is withdrawn and placed

in the rectum. The instrument is then opened to permit endometrial tissue to enter the jaws and then closed to snip off a piece of endometrium. The tissue is next placed in fixative and processed through a laboratory.

BREEDING MANAGEMENT

Monitoring follicular development by palpation and ultrasonography per rectum allows the mare to be inseminated close to ovulation. This has numerous benefits including making sure that sperm are present when the oocyte is released, minimizing overuse of a stallion, and reducing the number of times a mare is bred during an estrus. Reducing the number of breedings per estrus becomes more important as a mare's fertility declines. When breeding a mare with fresh cooled or frozen semen, daily, or even more frequent, examinations are usually performed. With fresh cooled semen use, the semen is usually ordered after a follicle reaches 35 mm in diameter, and semen is shipped overnight to the mare's location. With frozen semen, the semen is stored in liquid nitrogen and insemination must occur within 24 hours before to within 6 hours after ovulation.

After a mare is bred, an ultrasonographic examination is usually preformed the following day (possibly sooner or later depending on the mare and the particular situation) to confirm that ovulation has occurred and to examine the uterus for the presence of fluid. Failure of a mare to clear the fluid from her uterus after breeding has been associated with decreased fertility and is the reason for many postbreeding treatments.

Artificial Insemination (Uterine Infusion)

Breeding a mare by artificial insemination (AI) is a relatively simple procedure. It is an aseptic procedure, and the same procedure is used for uterine infusion as for AI. A sterile sleeve is donned and a sterile pipette carried through the vagina and cervix into the uterus. The semen or intrauterine medication is then deposited directly into the uterus.

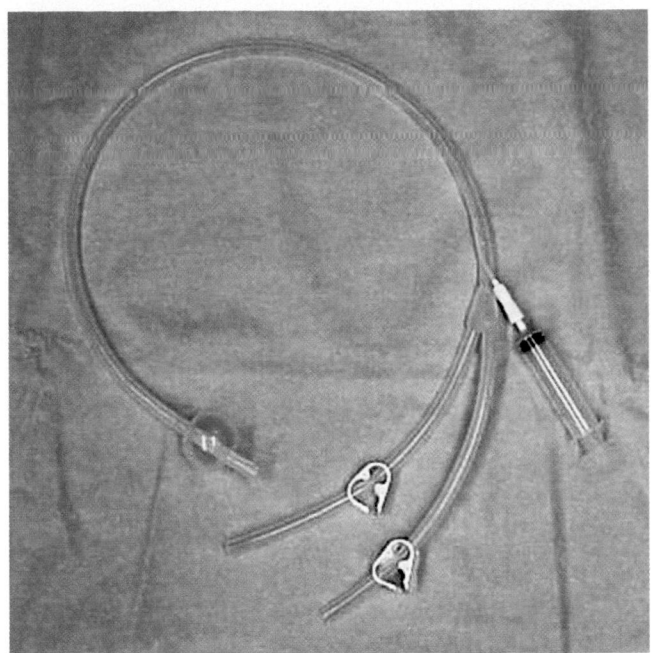

Figure 17-23 A large-bore catheter used to lavage a mare's uterus.

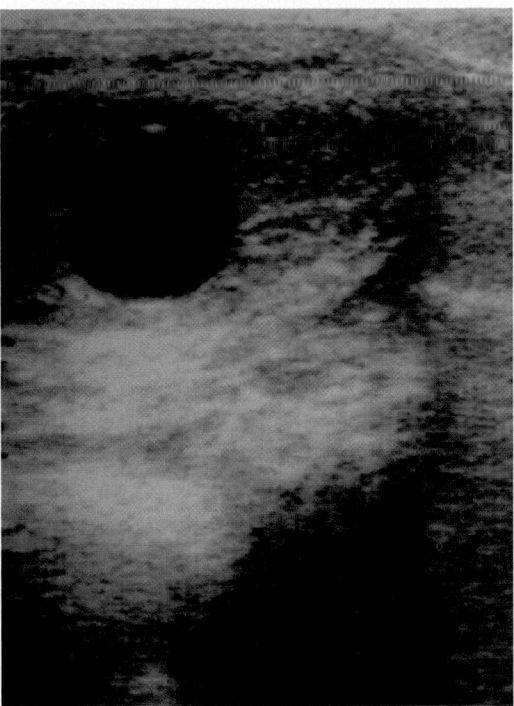

Figure 17-24 An ultrasound image of a 14-day pregnancy in an equine uterus.

Postbreeding Treatments

If fluid is detected in the uterus by ultrasonography 8 hours or more after breeding, treatment to aid uterine clearance is indicated. Oxytocin or cloprostenol are the two most commonly used drugs to stimulate uterine clearance.

In addition to oxytocin or cloprostenol injections, common postbreeding treatments include intrauterine infusion of antibiotics and uterine lavage. Intrauterine infusion and lavage are performed in the same aseptic manner using sterile equipment as artificial insemination.

Uterine lavage is performed using a large-bore catheter with an inflatable cuff (Figure 17-23). The catheter is placed in the uterus, and the cuff is inflated and seated against the internal cervical os to provide a good seal. Sterile saline, usually 1 L at a time, is infused into the uterus and then retrieved. This is repeated until the saline retrieved is clear. This procedure helps to clear the uterus of debris.

PREGNANCY

Diagnosis

Pregnancy diagnosis is usually done with the aid of ultrasonography 2 weeks after ovulation. With experience the characteristic ultrasonographic appearance of the conceptus at various stages can be easily recognized and used to evaluate its growth and health (Figure 17-24). The term *conceptus* refers to everything derived from the fertilized ovum, including the fetal membranes and fluids as well as the embryo or fetus. Fetal sexing is most commonly performed between 60 and 70 days by identifying the position of the genital tubercle.

TECHNICIAN NOTE

Pregnancy examination in the mare is usually performed 14 days after ovulation with the aid of ultrasonography.

Hormonal methods for pregnancy diagnosis exist. They can be useful in cases where rectal palpation is not feasible, such as with very small miniature horses or wild, fractious mares. Pregnant mares will test positive for equine chorionic gonadotropin (eCG), formerly called *pregnant mare serum gonadotropin* (PMSG), from 35 days until approximately 120 days of gestation. False-positive results happen if fetal death occurs during that period. Another hormone used for pregnancy testing is estrone sulfate. The benefit of estrone sulfate, compared with eCG, is that it is produced in high quantities by a viable fetoplacental unit beginning around 60 days of gestation. If the pregnancy is lost, estrone sulfate drops off rapidly, so false-positive results are uncommon. Progesterone cannot be used to test for pregnancy because it is elevated during diestrus in nonpregnant mares as well as during gestation in pregnant mares.

Vaccinations

Equine herpesvirus can be a significant cause of abortion in horses. Vaccines are available, and a good program consists of vaccination at 5, 7, and 9 months of gestation. Either a killed or modified live vaccine may be used. Repeated vaccinations at these intervals are necessary each time a mare is pregnant in order to provide good protection. In addition, it is advisable to minimize stress and is important to keep pregnant mares separated from new additions to the herd or horses that have a lot of outside contact.

It is also recommended to give an annual booster for flu, encephalitis (Eastern, Western, West Nile), and tetanus at 10 months' gestation. This practice will help ensure good-quality colostrums and increase the level of protection provided to the foal by passive transfer of antibodies through the colostrums. Additional information on preventive health programs is found in Chapter 11.

> ### TECHNICIAN NOTE
> An annual booster vaccination given to the mare at 10 months' gestation can improve the quality of the colostrums and enhance the foal's immunity.

Induction of Parturition

Gestation length in mares is generally quoted as 330 to 340 days. However, there is a wide variation in normal gestation length, ranging from 320 to 400 days. It is important to remember that the fetus determines gestation length. For this reason, chemical induction of parturition based on gestation length alone is risky and can result in the birth of premature foals. The decision to induce parturition is based on the following criteria:

1. Gestation length greater than 330 days
2. Relaxation of pelvic ligaments
3. Presence of colostrums in the udder
4. Relaxation or softening of the cervix
5. Most importantly, milk calcium more than 400 ppm with milk potassium higher than sodium

The electrolyte changes are very well correlated with fetal maturity and are the best way to assess readiness for birth. Calcium can be measured with a water hardness test kit, but be sure to use one that measures only calcium, not just divalent cations. Magnesium, another divalent cation present in colostrums, rises slowly as parturition approaches and can interfere with interpretation of the results. Milk calcium greater than 400 ppm and potassium less than sodium can occur in cases of placentitis or twins, so induction of parturition should not be considered unless potassium is greater than sodium, along with the increase in calcium.

PARTURITION

Parturition is a very rapid process in horses. In the normal course of events, as the mare begins labor (stage I) she will lie down, get up, roll, and so forth. During these maneuvers, the foal is getting into the correct position. Finally at the end of stage I, the chorioallantois ruptures ("water breaks"), signaling the onset of stage II. Usually within 10 minutes a bluish white membrane (amnion) appears at the vulvar

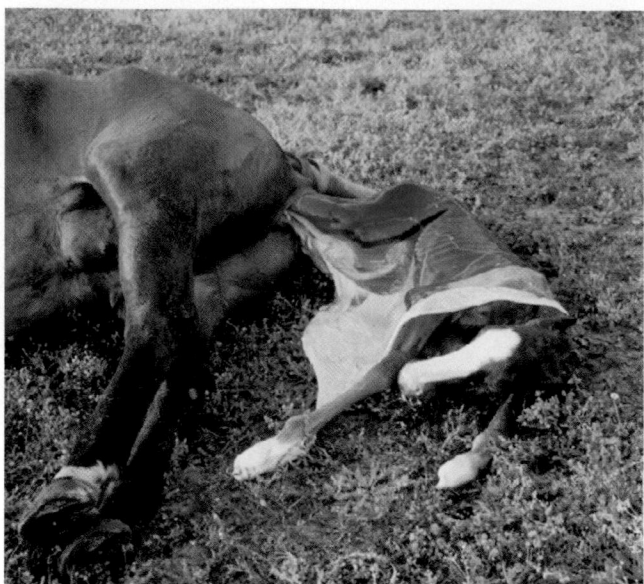

Figure 17-25 A foal being delivered by a mare.

opening. Within another 10 minutes the feet will protrude through the vulva, still within the amnion. After another 10 minutes the head protrudes and delivery will be completed soon thereafter (Figure 17-25).

> ### TECHNICIAN NOTE
> Parturition is a very rapid process in horses.

A red membrane protruding from the vulva, the chorioallantois, is an indication of premature placental separation, or "red bag" (Figure 17-26). This is an emergency, and the chorioallantois must be ruptured manually and delivery assisted or the foal will quickly die.

If the guidelines for the time frame of delivery are not being met, examination for possible dystocia is indicated. It is critical to perform any obstetric manipulations in as clean a manner as possible and with sufficient good-quality obstetric lubricant. Failure to adhere to guidelines of strict cleanliness and ample lubrication invites complications in the postpartum period and can compromise future fertility.

POSTPARTUM PROBLEMS

Mares do not experience postpartum problems as commonly as cows, but when they do, they can be life threatening. A retained placenta for more than 6 hours' duration deserves veterinary attention. Various methods, such as large-volume saline distension or oxytocin therapy, can be used to stimulate placental release. Manually detaching the placenta should not be done because of the potential for causing damage to the uterus and hemorrhage. Systemic antibiotics, anti-inflammatories, and tetanus toxoid are usually administered in cases of retained placenta more than 6 hours in duration.

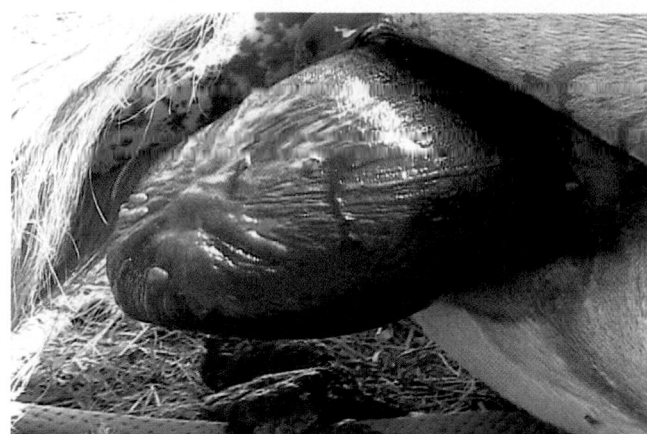

Figure 17-26 Premature placental separation ("red bag") during parturition in the mare. The chorioallantois is observed protruding through the vulvar opening.

✎ TECHNICIAN NOTE

A retained placenta for more than 6 hours' duration deserves veterinary attention.

A prolapsed uterus is a true emergency and must be dealt with as quickly as possible. Unfortunately, even with proper treatment, mortality can approach 50%. The mare should be restrained and the uterus protected from trauma until the veterinarian arrives.

The clinical signs of postpartum hemorrhage due to a ruptured uterine artery, usually either into the broad ligament or the abdomen, include signs of abdominal pain and pale mucous membranes. Mares exhibiting such signs in the postpartum period should be kept calm and quiet and be confined to a stall until examined by a veterinarian.

Postpartum metritis, often a sequela to retained placenta or contamination during obstetric procedures, can lead to septicemia and laminitis. As a result, treatment should not be delayed in a postpartum mare that has a foul-smelling vaginal discharge or is febrile or depressed.

HORMONE USE IN MARES

Prostaglandin

Prostaglandin $F_{2\alpha}$, and its analog cloprostenol, can be used to lyse a corpus luteum and return a mare to estrus. It is effective beginning about 5 or 6 days after ovulation, when the corpus luteum has matured sufficiently to respond. Mares will return to estrus in 2 to 7 days after prostaglandin administration. Prostaglandin should not be used to induce parturition because of the high incidence of premature placental separation, dystocia, and fetal death.

Human Chorionic Gonadotropin

Human chorionic gonadotropin (hCG) is used to induce ovulation in mares that have a follicle 35 mm or larger.

Doses commonly used range from 2000 to 3500 IU given intravenously, and ovulation can be expected to occur in 36 to 40 hours in approximately 80% of mares. Although concerns about antibody production have been expressed, no correlation between antibodies and failure to induce ovulation has been shown. Nevertheless, some mares fail to ovulate after receiving hCG repeatedly.

Deslorelin

An alternative to hCG for ovulation induction is an analog of GnRH, deslorelin (Ovuplant, Fort Dodge Animal Health). Ovulation occurs within approximately the same time frame as with hCG. However, deslorelin appears to be more effective on slightly smaller (30-mm) follicles than hCG, and failure of the mare to ovulate is reportedly less common.

Progestins

Altrenogest (Regu-Mate, Intervet) is a progesterone-like compound that is administered orally. It is used primarily for pregnancy maintenance and estrous cycle control. Its use for pregnancy maintenance is empiric in that true progesterone deficiency as a cause of pregnancy loss has not been documented. However, anecdotal reports of mares failing to maintain pregnancy unless supplemented with altrenogest are not uncommon. Because the fetoplacental unit eventually takes over progestogen production, altrenogest therapy can usually be discontinued at about 4 months' gestation.

The other reason to use altrenogest is estrous cycle control. Altrenogest mimics progesterone in the mare. Therefore, mares given altrenogest act as if they are in diestrus. Altrenogest can be used for estrus synchronization in embryo transfer programs and to manipulate the estrous cycle to prevent or control the onset of estrus in performance mares. Altrenogest is also used in mares in late gestation when there is concern about possible impending abortion. Through its action, uterine motility is inhibited, thereby supporting maintenance of pregnancy.

Oxytocin

A common cause of infertility is persistent mating-induced endometritis. An inflammatory response to sperm cells normally occurs after breeding, whether by natural service or artificial insemination. This inflammatory response is necessary to remove excess semen and debris and to prepare the uterus for pregnancy. Uterine clearance mechanisms, such as uterine motility and lymphatic drainage, are critical in this process. Infertility results when uterine clearance mechanisms fail and fluid remains in the uterus after breeding. Ultrasound examination 12 hours or more after breeding should reveal no fluid in the uterus. If fluid is still present, oxytocin therapy (20 IU intravenously or intramuscularly) should be instituted. Oxytocin is very effective in aiding uterine clearance and can be given as often as every 2 or 3 hours.

Oxytocin is also the only drug available to safely and reliably induce parturition. If the mare has met the criteria and is ready to give birth, a small dose (10 IU intravenously) of oxytocin is sufficient to initiate parturition. Lower doses result in a more natural process, whereas higher doses result in a faster and more forceful delivery.

Domperidone

Domperidone is a dopamine antagonist used to alleviate the effects of fescue toxicosis and stimulate lactation. It has also shown some promise to stimulate cyclicity in mares with lactational anestrus and may be beneficial in hastening the onset of cyclicity in the spring, but this has not yet been well documented.

BOVINE REPRODUCTION

The cow is a nonseasonal polyestrous species, meaning that cows have estrous cycles all year around. The entire estrous cycle averages 21 days long, but it can be as short as 18 days and as long as 24 days (Figure 17-27). Estrus lasts 18 to 20 hours but may be shorter in hot, humid weather because of heat stress. Estrus is the time the cow is in "standing heat" and will stand with all four legs firmly braced to be mounted by a bull or another cow. Ovulation occurs 12 to 18 hours after the end of estrus. Estrus is followed by metestrus, which is 3 to 5 days long and is the time of luteal development. A bloody discharge from the vulva may be noticed in nearly half of all cows and heifers 1 or 2 days after they are in estrus. This is no indication of fertility or infertility but merely a sign that the individual was in estrus 1 or 2 days earlier. During metestrus, a corpus hemorrhagicum (CH) is formed at the site of ovulation. This structure will develop into a corpus luteum over the next few days. However, during metestrus the CL is not yet mature and not yet susceptible to the luteolytic action of prostaglandin. The next phase is called *diestrus* and lasts from day 5 or 6 until day 17 of the estrous cycle and is the time that the mature corpus luteum ("yellow body") is present and producing progesterone. During diestrus there are waves of follicular growth that are important in understanding a cow's response to estrous cycle synchronization. At the end of diestrus, if an embryo is not present in the uterus to provide a pregnancy signal, the uterus releases prostaglandin that lyses the corpus luteum, resulting in a decline of progesterone, and the cow returns to proestrus.

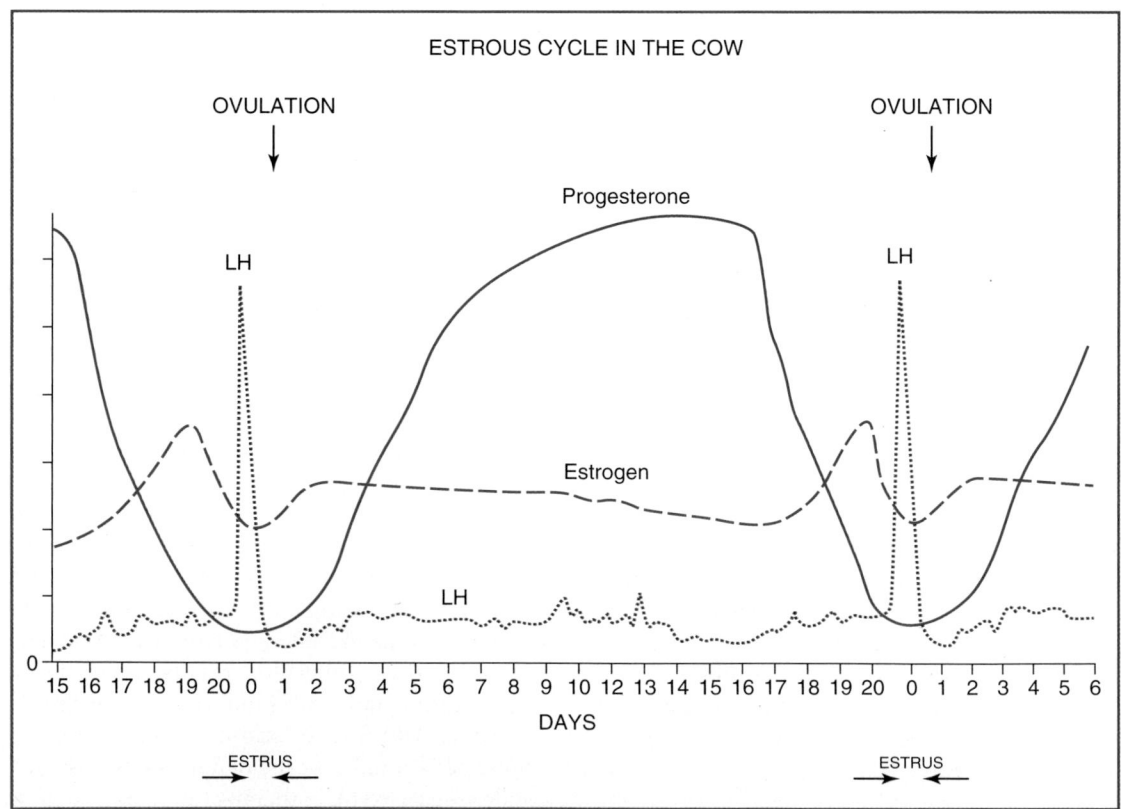

Figure 17-27 The bovine estrous cycle. Estrus is 12 to 18 hours long, and LH peaks during estrus. Diestrus lasts until about day 17, and progesterone is high throughout diestrus. If a pregnancy signal is not secreted by the early embryo by day 16 or 17, prostaglandin is released from the uterus, goes to the corpus luteum, and causes luteolysis (luteal death). The cycle then starts over.

BOVINE PREGNANCY DIAGNOSIS

Various methods of pregnancy diagnosis exist, but the most commonly employed is rectal palpation. An experienced person can diagnose pregnancy by 30 days' gestation. Ultrasonography is becoming more popular for pregnancy diagnosis. Machines have become more affordable, and accurate pregnancy diagnosis can be performed by 24 days or earlier in some cases. Fetal viability can be assessed and fetal sexing is possible between 55 and 70 days.

TECHNICIAN NOTE

Various methods of pregnancy diagnosis exist, but the most commonly employed is rectal palpation.

Progesterone tests should not be regarded as pregnancy tests. Although a progesterone test can detect the presence of a corpus luteum, many scenarios exist where a corpus luteum is present and progesterone is high but the cow is not pregnant.

BREEDING/ARTIFICIAL INSEMINATION

Most dairy cattle, and increasing numbers of beef cattle, are bred by artificial insemination. There are numerous advantages to artificial insemination, with rapid genetic improvement being the primary one. However, the need for estrus detection in order to time insemination is a major drawback. Fortunately, cows, especially dairy cows, exhibit "standing heat" when in estrus, and observation of this behavior is the best method of estrus detection. "Teaser" bulls, bulls that have been surgically altered to prevent vaginal penetration with the penis and have had vasectomies to render them sterile, can be used to help with estrus detection.

Estrus synchronization, through the use of hormones, also helps improve estrus detection. Many schemes have been devised using prostaglandin to lyse the corpus luteum. Other schemes use progestogen to mimic the luteal phase and suppress follicular growth. An ear implant, Synchro-Mate B, containing the progestogen named norgestomet, has been successfully used for years in cattle but it is no longer available in the United States as of the time of the writing of this chapter. Recently, an intravaginal device has been approved for synchronization of estrus in dairy heifers and for synchronization of return to estrus in lactating dairy cattle. The product is called EAZI-BREED CIDR and contains 1.38 grams of progesterone in silicone molded over a nylon spine. EAZI-BREED CIDR is the first and only approved source of progesterone for use in dairy cattle. EAZI-BREED CIDR can be used in association with prostaglandin $F_{2\alpha}$ ($PGF_{2\alpha}$). Another popular method for synchronization of estrus involves an injection of GnRH at random stage of the estrous cycle, followed by an injection of $PGF_{2\alpha}$ 7 days later, followed by a second injection of GnRH 48 hours later and insemination 16 to 18 hours after that.

ABNORMALITIES OF THE ESTROUS CYCLE

Anestrus

The most common reason for failure of a cow to show estrus is pregnancy, whether as a result of poor record keeping or an unknown visit by a neighboring bull. For this reason it is always advisable to have a cow examined for pregnancy before attempting to "bring her into heat" with prostaglandin. After calving, a period of postpartum anestrus is common. This period is usually shorter for dairy cows (2 to 4 weeks depending on nutrition and environmental conditions) than for beef cows. Beef cows nursing calves have a longer period of postpartum anestrus, usually 45 to 90 days. The postpartum anestrus period in beef cattle is prolonged if the cows are not in good body condition when they calve.

Pathologic reasons for anestrus include pyometra, luteal cysts, and follicular cystic degeneration. Pyometra may be caused by a number of factors, including trichomoniasis, bovine viral diarrhea (BVD) virus and postpartum uterine infection. It is characterized by a pus-filled uterus and a persistent corpus luteum. Treatment consists of simply administering prostaglandin, although two injections, 24 hours apart, may be needed to improve response.

Luteal cysts arise from follicles that fail to ovulate but do form luteal tissue. Progesterone is elevated, and a period of prolonged diestrus results. Treatment consists of prostaglandin injection. Follicular cysts result from follicles that fail to ovulate and do not form luteal tissue. Progesterone is low, and although some cows may exhibit persistent or frequent estrus, anestrus is much more common. Treatment consists of GnRH or hCG administration.

ABNORMALITIES OF PREGNANCY

Uterine Prolapse

Uterine prolapse is easily recognized by the presence of the mucosal, or inner, surface of the uterus, with its characteristic caruncles, hanging from the vulva (Figure 17-28). It is more common in dairy than beef cattle. It occurs in the immediate postpartum period and is often associated with hypocalcemia or dystocia. Uterine prolapse should be considered an emergency, and the uterus should be replaced to its normal position as soon as possible. Uterine prolapse is not hereditary and is not considered to be likely to recur.

Vaginal Prolapse

Although seemingly similar to uterine prolapse, vaginal prolapse is actually quite different. This is a hereditary problem. Therefore, affected individuals should not be kept as breeding stock. It occurs under conditions associated with elevated estrogen, most commonly seen during late gestation, although it may also be associated with cystic follicular

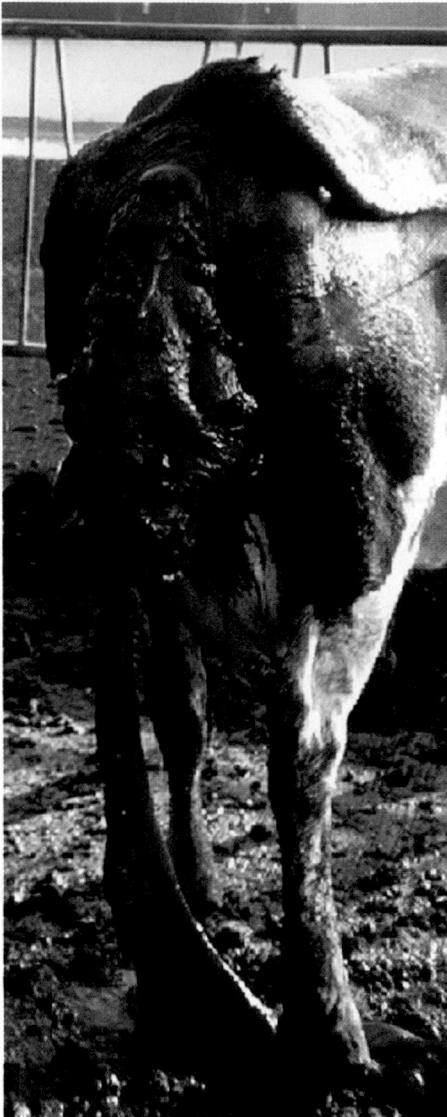

Figure 17-28   A bovine uterine prolapse. Note the caruncles on the exposed interior uterine surface.

degeneration or ingestion of certain plants. Typically the affected animal will be a beef cow or heifer, in late gestation, and the vagina, and maybe also the cervix, will be protruding from the vulva. Various methods have been described to treat the condition, but all consist of cleaning the exposed tissue, replacing it, and preventing recurrence. It must be remembered that in most cases the cow will not have calved yet, so care will need to be taken to monitor her to reduce the chance of dystocia and mortality.

Dystocia

Dystocia is much more common in cattle than in mares. It is most commonly caused by fetal/maternal disproportion in size. Uterine torsion is also a fairly common cause of dystocia. As with mares, cleanliness and lubrication are essential for successful management of dystocia.

Milk Fever

Milk fever, or parturient hypocalcemia, most commonly occurs during the postpartum period although it may also occur during parturition. It is more common in dairy cattle than beef cattle. The incidence is increased when cattle are fed high levels of calcium prepartum. This condition should be viewed as an emergency and is treated by slow intravenous infusion of calcium gluconate. Milk fever is characterized by flaccid paralysis.

SWINE REPRODUCTION

PUBERTY

Gilts usually reach puberty at 4.5 to 6 months of age. Social environment and nutrition are important factors determining the onset of cyclicity in gilts. Onset of puberty is commonly seen in gilts weighing 82 kg or more. Direct contact between boars and gilts is very important in swine reproduction. Boars have pheromone-secreting salivary glands that sexually stimulate female pigs. This "boar effect" (stimulating or detecting estrus) is even more evident if mature, experienced boars are used. Daily exposure of 5- to 6-month-old gilts to a mature boar will hasten the onset of cyclicity. Season probably influences the onset of puberty, because gilts born in the fall start to cycle earlier than their spring-born counterparts. In addition, all factors that contribute to good management, such as number of gilts per pen, adequate physical space per gilt, ambient temperature, and health status (diseases, parasites) in general, will ensure that gilts reach puberty around 5 to 6 months of age.

Pharmacologic agents can also induce puberty. Fertile estrus and ovulation can be induced using exogenous gonadotropins. Equine chorionic gonadotropin in association with hCG is effective in inducing estrus in gilts. These two gonadotropins are marketed in a combination to induce estrus and ovulation. Estrogen administration is also effective but does not yield as reliable results as the eCG-hCG combination. GnRH is very effective, but it is expensive and needs to be delivered in a pulsatile fashion (every hour for 3 to 4 days), making this difficult to be done in a commercial unit.

ESTROUS CYCLE

Domestic pigs are nonseasonal polyestrous animals. Female pigs exhibit estrus at 21-day intervals after they reach puberty. Longer estrous cycles, such as 26 days, have been associated with early embryonic mortality.

During proestrus, follicular development intensifies as the corpora lutea in the nonpregnant pig start to regress around day 15 of the estrous cycle. Initial behavioral signs of estrus are not always easily recognized. They include increased restlessness, reduced appetite, mounting other animals, homosexual behavior (malelike sexual activity), and lordosis. Lordosis occurs when pressure is applied on the pig's back by someone sitting on it and the female pig stands still, quiet, and passive, assuming a mating position. The vulva swells and becomes more pink and moist. A cloudy mucous discharge may be present during this phase.

Estrus is the period when the female pig is responsive to the boar's approach. If male and female are put together during this stage, they start to show a precopulatory behavior (foreplay) that includes sniffing each other and head-to-head contact; the male starts to compulsively follow the female pig and initiate mounting attempts. Courtship culminates with the female pig standing still and allowing the boar to mount. The duration of estrus can be variable among individuals of different breeds or age or during different times of the year (longest in summer and shorter in winter). Estrus lasts on average 40 to 60 hours (2 to 3 days), but it can vary from 1 to 4 days. Ovulation usually takes place during the second day of estrus (36 to 44 hours after the onset of estrus), and mated females reportedly ovulate 4 hours before unmated female pigs. Follicular rupture of all follicles present in the ovary (10 to 20) may take 1 to 9 hours.

Diestrus is behaviorally characterized by a lack of sexual receptivity and lasts for 18 days if the female pig is not pregnant. Anestrus is mainly seen when sows are lactating.

PREGNANCY

Deposition of semen in pigs is intracervical. The presence of cartilaginous rings in the sow's cervix in association with the fibroelastic spiral tip (corkscrew) of the boar's penis provides a natural and strong lock of the penis inside the cervix. Subsequently, during mating, strong contractions of the cervix are potentiated by oxytocin release in response to coitus. Several billion sperm cells are released during coitus in an average of 200 to 250 ml of semen. Uterine contractions allow a controlled number of sperm cells to reach the oviduct, where fertilization occurs. It seems that a minimum number of four embryos must be present in the uterus to cause appropriate maternal recognition of pregnancy. The average length of gestation is 114 days (3 months + 3 weeks + 3 days). Piglets are born weighing on average 1.4 to 1.6 kg. A tail-first presentation is not abnormal. Interval time between piglets averages 10 to 15 minutes. Intervals greater than 20 minutes are associated with an increasing number of stillbirths. All fetal membranes should be delivered in 4 to 6 hours.

Control of Farrowing

Farrowing can occur at any time of the day or night. Each sow may take several hours to deliver all the piglets and fetal membranes. It is important to assist sows during delivery because early detection and correction of potential problems during farrowing prevent piglet losses. Assistance during farrowing can be facilitated by pharmacologically inducing parturition. Accordingly, prostaglandin adminis-

Table 17-2 HORMONES USED IN SWINE REPRODUCTION

Desired Effect	Drug	Regimen
Induction of puberty	P.G. 600	5 ml IM
	eCG/hCG	400-1000 IU/200-1000 U IM
Estrus/ovulation	P.G. 600	5 ml IM
	eCG/hCG	500-1000 IU/500-1000 U IM
	Regu-Mate	15 mg/gilt/day for 18 days orally
Abortion	PGF$_{2\alpha}$	10 mg Lutalyse or 500 µg Estrumate 12-45 days after breeding

eCG, Equine chorionic gonadotropin; *hCG*, human chorionic gonadotropin; *IM*, intramuscularly; PGF$_{2\alpha}$, prostaglandin.

tration after day 112 of gestation will induce parturition in 20 to 30 hours. Combining prostaglandin with oxytocin or xylazine will help to improve the precision of response to prostaglandin administration.

PHARMACOLOGIC CONTROL OF THE ESTROUS CYCLE

Exogenous hormones can be used to alter or manipulate the estrous cycle in pigs. Estrus and ovulation can be induced by different means either in cycling pigs or in early pregnant pigs to synchronize estrus (Table 17-2).

P.G. 600 contains 400 IU of eCG and 200 units of hCG. It can be used to induce estrus in prepubertal gilts or in sows showing anestrus after weaning. It can also be used in cycling sows after day 16 of the estrous cycle. The administration of P.G. 600 will cause estrus and ovulation in 3 to 5 days following treatment. Estrus/ovulation can also be induced by administration of eCG and hCG 2 days apart. Prostaglandin can be used to terminate pregnancy or diestrus only if given 12 days after ovulation. Before day 12, multiple injections (twice daily for 5 days) of prostaglandins are necessary to interrupt diestrus (short cycling) or to terminate pregnancy. Weaned sows usually show spontaneous signs of estrus in 11 to 12 days after weaning. Administration of P.G. 600 on the day of weaning will also induce estrus in 3 to 5 days. Sows that do not come into estrus in 2 weeks after weaning will show signs of estrus if P.G. 600 is administered.

ARTIFICIAL INSEMINATION

Artificial insemination with fresh or cooled semen is commonly performed in the swine industry. The boar is easily trained to mount a dummy and have semen manually collected. After collecting the sperm-rich portion of the ejaculate, semen is evaluated to determine its quality and how much extender to add. A sow should be inseminated with 3 to 4 billion sperm cells in a volume of 80 to 100 ml.

The number of total insemination doses will depend on the frequency of collection, age of boar, breed, and some individual variation. Farrowing rates from sows artificially inseminated are comparable to those observed in sows naturally mated. Artificially inseminating twice, 12 to 24 hours apart, is likely to improve pregnancy rates. In a commercial unit, heterospermic insemination (mixing semen from two or more boars) is sometimes used and reportedly increases pregnancy rates.

> **✎ TECHNICIAN NOTE**
>
> Artificial insemination with fresh or cooled semen is commonly performed in the swine industry.

PREGNANCY DIAGNOSIS

Ultrasonography procedures are used to diagnose pregnancy in pigs. Doppler and amplitude-depth ultrasound were the first methods to be employed and are accurate between 30 and 90 days of gestation. Real-time (B-mode) ultrasound is being used with more frequency in the swine industry as equipment cost decreases. Accuracy is greater than 90% if used after 20 days of gestation.

POSTPARTUM COMPLICATIONS AND DISEASES

Retained placenta is not a very common occurrence in pigs. Fetal membranes from all piglets are usually expelled after the last piglet is born. Manual examination of the birth canal is warranted if the placenta is not passed out after sows apparently deliver their last piglet.

Obstetric problems are also not very common, and the great majority of sows and gilts deliver without any technical or veterinary assistance. Nevertheless, persistent and forceful abdominal contractions without delivery of a piglet for longer than 1 hour suggest potential complications. A problem will be even more evident if it is accompanied by vaginal discharge but not expulsion of a fetus. An increased time interval between deliveries is also suggestive of dystocia. The reason may be a primary absence of uterine contractions (primary inertia) or secondary to the presence of either an oversized, malpositioned, or malformed fetus. Oxytocin can be administered for primary uterine inertia. Removal of piglets is also helpful for stimulating progression of delivery. Occasionally, a cesarean delivery is needed to deliver the piglets.

Prolapse of the uterus can occur during parturition or after all piglets have been delivered. Excessive straining or a large pelvic inlet may predispose to uterine prolapse. Uterine prolapse is likely fatal. Vaginal prolapse generally happens a few days before parturition. It requires veterinary intervention to reposition it, and sows should be watched for any problems during labor.

Metritis and mastitis are the main diseases of the postpartum period and consequently lead to a disturbance in milk production. Hypogalactia (low milk production) and agalactia (absence of milk production) are often associated with mastitis and metritis. Any signs of abnormal, fetid vaginal discharge or abnormal enlargement of the udder warrant veterinary assistance. Oxytocin can be used to stimulate milk letdown during treatment.

> **✎ TECHNICIAN NOTE**
>
> Metritis and mastitis are the main diseases of the postpartum period and consequently lead to a disturbance in milk production.

OVINE AND CAPRINE REPRODUCTION

SEASONALITY

Sheep and goats are seasonally polyestrous, short-day breeders. Estrous cycles start to occur in the late summer and autumn. The photo period is the primary environmental cue controlling seasonal breeding in the ewe. Exposure of sheep and goats to increasing or long day length induces anestrus, whereas short or decreasing day length initiates estrous cycles. Perception of the day length by the eye is signaled to the pineal gland, which will cause melatonin release. Melatonin will induce the secretion of GnRH and LH, which initiates cyclicity. Low ambient temperature also cues small ruminants to start to cycle. Sheep and goats kept in tropical or subtropical areas do not display marked seasonality and can cycle almost year-round.

The geographic origin of a specific breed influences the length of the breeding season. For example, some breeds have a 2- to 4-month breeding season and some cycle all year long. Suffolk and Suffolk crosses average 6 months of breeding season. Dorset and Finn sheep have extended breeding seasons (8 months), whereas Merino ewes cycle almost all year-round.

Dairy goats (Saanen, Toggenburgh) cycle from August to February in the northern hemisphere. Most meat or crossbred-type goats have a more extended breeding season and undergo anestrus in late spring and summer.

ESTROUS CYCLE

Ewes cycle regularly every 17 (range 14 to 19) days and does every 21 (range 18 to 22) days during the breeding season. During proestrus, ewes and does are not sexually receptive but attract the male's attention, and courtship is initiated.

Estrus lasts 24 to 48 hours in ewes and 24 to 36 hours in does. Estrogen causes the vulva to be edematous and moist. Does show overt signs of estrus more often than ewes. Accordingly, does may exhibit homosexual behavior, but ewes do not. Estrus detection is efficiently achieved using males that have undergone vasectomy. Both species actively seek the male as they advance into estrus. Multiple copulations during the same estrus are correlated with higher pregnancy rates. A cloudy vaginal discharge may be seen at the end of estrus and should not be mistaken for infectious vaginal discharge. Ovulation occurs 24 to 30 hours after the onset of estrus in both species. Diestrus lasts 15 to 17 days in ewes and 18 to 20 days in does.

BREEDING MANAGEMENT

Puberty of ewes occurs at 6 to 9 months, but it can be as late as 1 to 2 years of age depending on breed, nutrition, and time of birth during the year (e.g., lambs and kids born in the fall come into puberty later than spring-born offspring). Pubertal ewes and does should be bred only if they have attained 65% of their mature body weight. The male/female ratio should be 1:50 in natural breeding situations or 1:10 for synchronized breeding. Fresh or frozen semen can be used for artificial insemination. Deposition of semen can be intravaginal, intracervical, or intrauterine (Table 17-3). Laparoscopic procedures have become common practice in the sheep and goat industry.

PREGNANCY

Gestation lasts approximately 150 days in both species. Ewes are dependent on luteal function only during the first 2 months of gestation. Because maintenance of pregnancy in ewes is accomplished by placental hormones after day 50 of gestation, administration of prostaglandin after 2 months of gestation does not induce abortion or parturition. Does are dependent on luteal function throughout gestation, and prostaglandin administration interrupts pregnancy at any stage. Parturition can be safely induced by prostaglandin administration in goats after day 146 of gestation. Does go into labor an average of 28 to 36 hours after prostaglandin administration. Dexamethasone induces parturition in ewes within 36 to 48 hours if administered after day 144 of gestation. Twinning is very common, and lambs and kids should be standing within 15 minutes and nursing within 1 hour after being born.

RAM/BUCK EFFECT

Male pheromones produced under androgenic stimulation dramatically influence cyclicity in ewes and does. The introduction of a new, mature, odoriferous male during the transition from the anestrus season into the breeding season will induce estrus in most females. Ewes ovulate in 3 to 6 days, but the corpus luteum of this first cycle is short lived. After the second ovulation, regular cyclicity is established. The buck effect is more efficient in does inasmuch as cyclicity is regularly initiated with first ovulation.

> ### ✎ TECHNICIAN NOTE
> Male pheromones produced under androgenic stimulation dramatically influence cyclicity in ewes and does.

PHARMACOLOGIC CONTROL OF THE ESTROUS CYCLE

Intravaginal sponges delivering progestogen are used to synchronize estrus in ewes and does. Controlled intravaginal drug-releasing devices (CIDRs) are widely used internationally but are not yet commercially available in the United States. Recently, a vaginal sponge impregnated with flurogestone acetate (45 mg/sponge) has been approved by the Food and Drug Administration (FDA) for synchronizing estrus in cycling adult ewes during their normal breeding season. This vaginal sponge has not been approved for use in ewes that have not had lambs. Prostaglandin (extralabel use) is also used to synchronize estrus alone or in combination with progestogen.

PREGNANCY DIAGNOSIS

Pregnancy diagnosis can be performed by checking for returning to estrus, ballottement (palpation) of the fetus in the abdomen, or ultrasonography. Return to estrus can be observed by using a marking harness and crayon on the male (Figure 17-29). Doppler ultrasonography is 90% accurate after 75 days of gestation. Real-time (B-mode) ultrasonography using a 5-MHz probe is 100% accurate after 60 days.

PERIPARTURIENT PROBLEMS

Dystocia usually results from an abnormal fetal disposition or fetopelvic disproportion. It is important to recognize dystocia, because the cervix will close after 2 to 3 hours of

Table 17-3 ARTIFICIAL INSEMINATION (AI) BREEDING IN EWES

Method	Semen	Semen Dose (Number of Spermatazoa)	Lambing Rate (%)
Laparoscopic IU	Fresh or frozen	$20\text{-}40 \times 10^6$	40-100
Transcervical IU	Fresh or frozen	$50\text{-}100 \times 10^6$	30-80
Cervical	Fresh only	200×10^6	40-80
Vaginal	Fresh only	400×10^6	20-60

*Modified from Youngquist RS, editor: *Current therapy in large animal theriogenology*, Philadelphia, 1997, WB Saunders.
IU, Intrauterine.

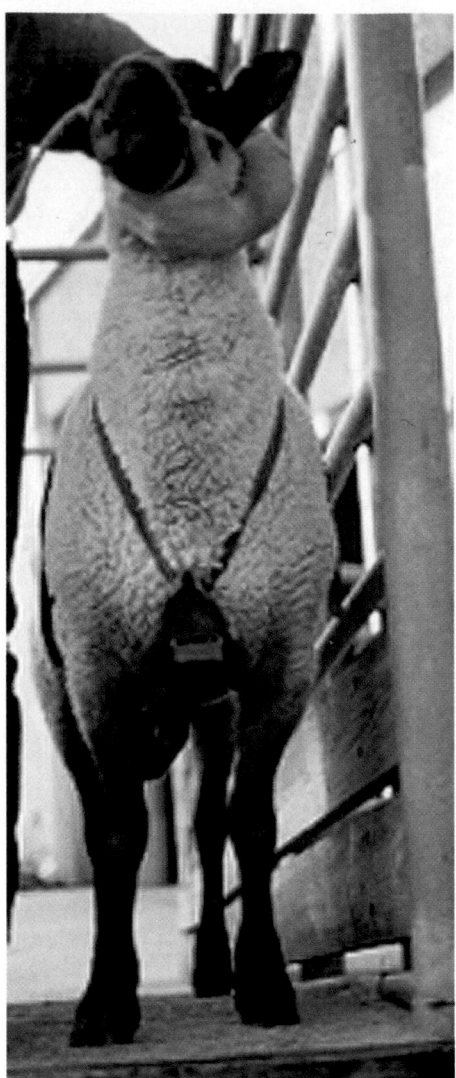

Figure 17-29 A ram fitted with a marking harness to detect estrus in ewes.

nonproductive labor. A cesarean delivery is the treatment of choice. *Ringwomb* refers to the failure of the cervix to dilate during parturition.

Pregnancy toxemia is a common problem seen in ewes in the last 6 weeks of gestation. It is associated with multiple fetuses and inadequate nutrition. Hypoglycemia in these cases may lead to neurologic signs and incoordination. Vaginal prolapse usually occurs in late gestation (3 to 6 weeks before parturition), and dystocia is likely to result in a cesarean delivery.

Hypocalcemia is a condition of pregnant ewes and does leading to cool extremities, failure of the cervix to dilate, and generalized weakness. Treatment is intravenous calcium administration. The hypocalcemic female should be examined 3 hours after calcium treatment. If no progress in delivery is observed, a cesarean delivery is indicated.

Pseudopregnancy is a common condition in goats. It is characterized by a collection of fluid inside the uterus without pregnancy (hydrometra). If not treated with prostaglandin, the natural expulsion of the fluid is called a *cloudburst*.

INFERTILITY

The natural absence of horns in goats is associated with abnormal sexual development. This condition is called *polled (hornless) intersex*. The polled condition is determined by an autosomal-dominant gene that is the same or very closed linked to a recessive gene causing infertility. Homozygous polled genes cause sex reversal in the female. Affected animals may be genetically female but exhibit male, female, or mixed characteristics and sexual behavior. The polled gene is dominant but, fortunately, the intersex condition is seen only in homozygous animals. Therefore this condition can be avoided by having at least one horned parent.

CAMELID REPRODUCTION

New world camelids include the llama, alpaca, vicuna, and guanaco. They developed from a common ancestry in South America before the arrival of Europeans. Many aspects of reproduction are similar, but there are differences that can be attributed to speciation.

ESTROUS CYCLES

Puberty occurs at 10 to 12 months of age when the animal reaches approximately 60% of the adult body weight. Although llamas have peak fertility during the summer, they cycle year-round. Environmental and endocrinologic factors responsible for the onset and cessation of sexual activity are not yet clearly defined.

TECHNICIAN NOTE
Camelids do not have regular estrous cycles. They are induced ovulators, similar to cats.

Camelids do not have regular estrous cycles. They are induced ovulators, similar to cats. Sexual receptivity can vary from 1 to 36 days. Coitus lasts 5 to 50 minutes with an average of 18 minutes. One mating is sufficient to induce ovulation, which occurs 1 to 3 days later. Delayed ovulation occurs in 30% and absence of ovulation in 10% of females after a single copulation. Treatment with hCG (500 to 700 IU) or GnRH (800 µg) is effective to induce ovulation. The use of a male that has had vasectomy is more effective to induce ovulation. The ovulatory follicle can be on either ovary, but the pregnancy is invariably in the left horn. Luteolysis is mediated by $PGF_{2\alpha}$. The CL remains functional throughout gestation. Prostaglandin $F_{2\alpha}$ can be used to induce parturition.

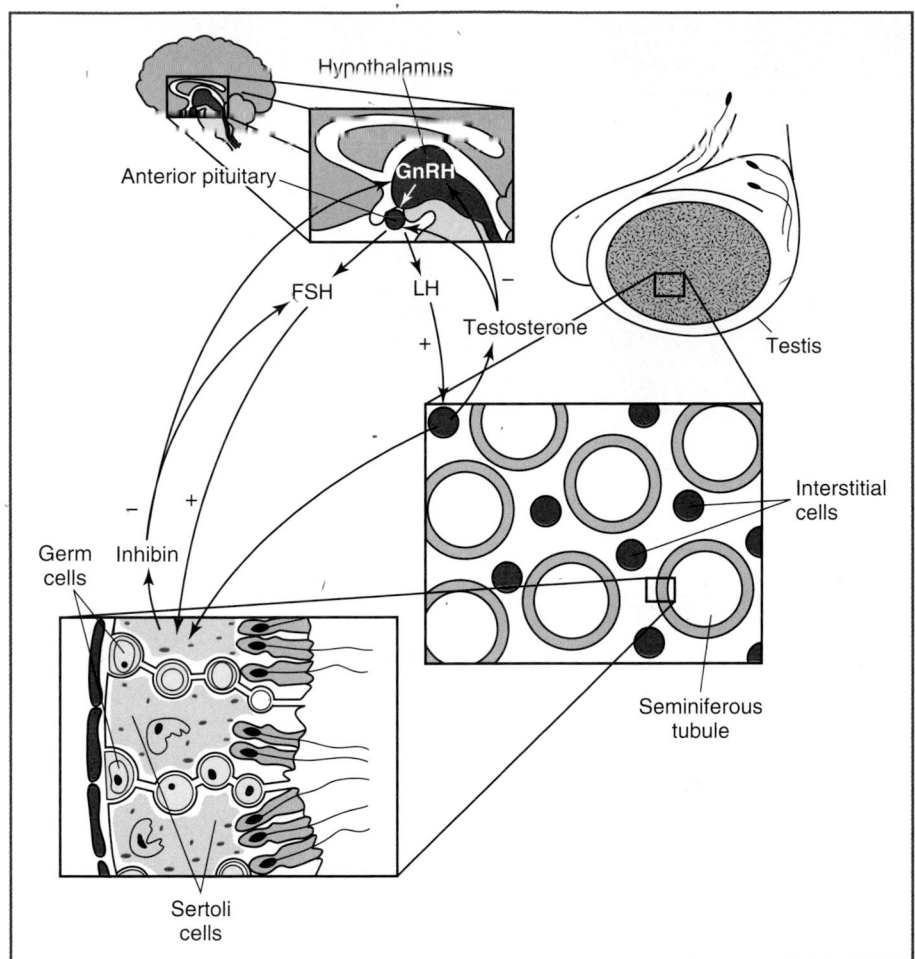

Figure 17-30 The general hormonal control of male reproduction: Pulsatile GnRH causes FSH to be released from the anterior pituitary. FSH causes increased sperm growth, maturation, and release. Inhibin from the Sertoli cells in the tubules feeds back on the anterior pituitary and causes less FSH to be released. GnRH secretion from the hypothalamus also results in LH release, which cause testosterone production by the interstitial cells of Leydig. The rise in testosterone causes less LH and GnRH to be released.

Gestation length averages 344 days (range 331 to 347 days). Parturition lasts 1 to 2 hours, and few complications occur. Approximately 90% of crias (baby camelids) are born between 7:00 AM and 1:00 PM.

GENERAL MALE REPRODUCTION

The male differs greatly from the female in the production of gametes. Whereas in the female only 1 to 10 oocytes ovulate during an estrous cycle, males are continually producing and excreting millions of sperm cells. Testicular anatomy differs significantly from ovarian anatomy. The testis is made up of many tubules, each of which connects to a central collecting duct. Between the tubules are the interstitial cells, which continually produce testosterone (Figure 17-30). Each tubule is lined by primordial germ cells (very immature

sperm cell precursors) and Sertoli cells. The Sertoli cells surround all the developing sperm cells, leaving them with no other contact to the body. This is critical in that the developing sperm are recognized as a foreign substance to the male and would be destroyed by the immune system if they were not protected. As the sperm cells mature, they leave their attachment to the Sertoli cell and are moved through the tubules.

The entire testis is covered by a tight capsule, the tunica albuginea (Figure 17-31). The paired testes are contained within the scrotum. The scrotum maintains the testes at a lower body temperature than the rest of the body. If the testes are not kept at a lower temperature, sperm cell production will cease. However, even though sperm cell production ceases, the interstitial cells still produce testosterone. A common example of these consequences is in a cryptorchid animal. A cryptorchid animal has one or both of the testes retained in the abdomen. If the testes are in the abdomen, the animal is sterile but will still show masculine behavior because testosterone is still produced by the testes.

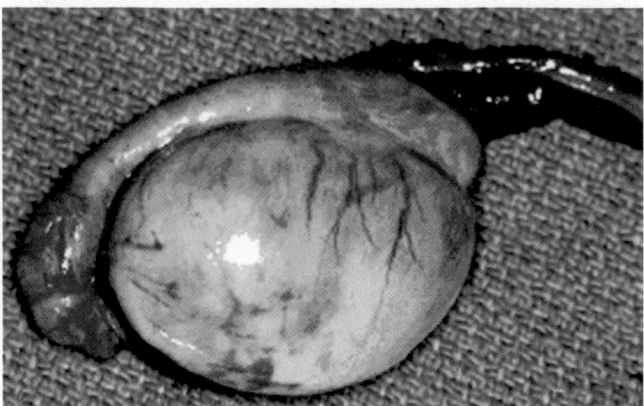

Figure 17-31 A canine testis showing the capsule surrounding the testicular tissue.

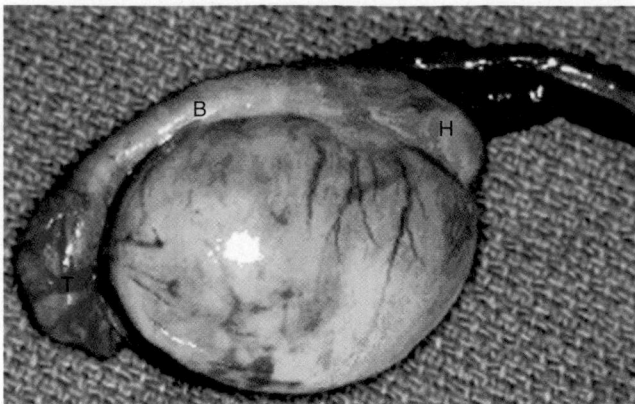

Figure 17-32 Lateral view of the right canine testis and epididymis with the, *H,* head, *B,* body, and, *T,* tail of the epididymis.

✐ TECHNICIAN NOTE

If the testes are not kept at a lower temperature, sperm cell production will cease.

Although the anatomy of the testes differs from that of the ovary, the control of sperm cell production is quite similar to that of oocyte production; however, it is more continuous and does not occur in cycles. In the male, LH from the anterior pituitary causes an increase in testosterone production (Figure 17-30). As testosterone production rises, it causes a decrease in GnRH and LH release. The decreased GnRH and LH release causes less testosterone to be produced. As less testosterone is produced, it follows that more GnRH and LH are produced, thus resulting in a balanced feedback mechanism and a relatively constant testosterone production. Testosterone is essential for the production of sperm cells. If testosterone is not present, sperm cells will not be produced. The concentration of testosterone within the testis is 10 times that in the systemic circulation. Administration of testosterone decreases endogenous testosterone production because of the negative feedback on the anterior pituitary and hypothalamus. This will result in lower testosterone concentrations within the testis. Because testosterone is needed for sperm cell production, the exogenous testosterone will eventually decrease sperm cell production.

The other hormone involved in sperm cell production is FSH. Just as in the female, FSH release is triggered by GnRH from the hypothalamus. The FSH acts on the Sertoli cell to increase the division of primordial sperm cells and to release more sperm cells that are embedded in the Sertoli cells. As sperm cell production rises, the hormone inhibin feeds back on the hypothalamus and anterior pituitary to decrease GnRH and FSH, respectively. This causes fewer sperm cells to be produced. As fewer cells are produced, the FSH will increase to produce more sperm cells, thereby keeping sperm cell production relatively constant. In general, FSH causes production of the gamete (oocyte in the female and sperm cell in the male), and LH causes production of the dominant hormone (progesterone in the female and testosterone in the male).

After the sperm cells are released, they move through the tubules and into the head of the epididymis. Within the epididymis, the sperm cells attain motility and the ability to fertilize. The movement through the epididymis to the tail of the epididymis is relatively constant and cannot be increased by increasing the number of breedings. The sperm cells are finally stored in the tail of the epididymis, where they are either ejaculated or voided in the urine if they are not ejaculated (Figure 17-32).

Ejaculation through the penis is the final process in sperm production and delivery. In most domestic species the penis comprises cavernous blood tissue surrounded by a firm covering, or tunic. An erection occurs when the male is sexually stimulated. During sexual stimulation, parasympathetic innervation causes blood flow increase into the cavernous portions of the penis. As blood flow increases to the penis, muscles around the proximal penis also contract to prevent blood outflow. Because the cavernous portions of the penis are contained within the tunic, the pressure increases, resulting in a penile erection. Any disruption of the cavernous tissue or the tunic can result in an erection failure.

During an erection the sperm cells in the tail of the epididymis are moved to the end of the ductus deferens into the ampullae in the process called *emission.* Once the sperm cells are present in the ampullae, the stimulation to the penis during mating causes ejaculation. Ejaculation is the forceful expulsion of the semen through the penis. The force comes from sympathetic nerves causing smooth muscle contractions in the urethra. During ejaculation the sperm cells are mixed with fluid from the accessory sex glands. The accessory sex glands include the ampullae, prostate, vesicular glands, and bulbourethral glands. Each species has one or all of these glands, and different glands have different clinical problems in each species. When the sperm cells are mixed with the accessory sex gland fluid, the result is now termed *semen*. Secretions from the accessory sex glands fluid add various components to the ejaculate, increase the volume, and stabilize the sperm cell membrane. Once the sperm cells enter the female reproductive tract, the sperm cell membrane undergoes a physical and biochemical change called *capacitation*. Capacitation is required before the sperm cells are capable of fertilization. In the uterus, the sperm cells are quickly moved to the oviduct, where fertilization occurs. Sperm cells are moved to the oviduct by uterine contractions.

✏ TECHNICIAN NOTE

Once the sperm cells enter the female reproductive tract, the sperm cell membrane undergoes a physical and biochemical change called *capacitation*.

CLINICAL EXAMINATION OF THE MALE

Depending on the species, evaluation of the male as a sound potential breeder may employ different techniques to collect semen and evaluate sperm output. Although semen collection procedures may differ among species, analysis of the semen is quite similar.

SEMEN ANALYSIS

When evaluating semen, it is important to have all equipment at 37° C. Sperm cells are very susceptible to cold shock and osmotic shock. Semen is best handled with a thin wooden stick, because the wood is thermoneutral and will not cold shock the sperm cells. The first step in semen analysis is to examine the motility. Motility will decline with time because of changes in the semen temperature and pH. Gross motility is examined by placing a drop of semen on a warm slide and examining it at ×10. The light on the microscope needs to be reduced greatly in order to see the cells. The sample is only evaluated for movement; however, the concentration can be estimated to help prepare other samples.

After the gross motility is evaluated, percent of progressively motile sperm is assessed. Individual motility slides are made by placing a drop of semen on the slide and then placing a coverslip over the sample. The sample should be evaluated at ×40. It is desirable to have approximately 10 cells per high-power field. If there are more cells, the motility cannot be estimated accurately. Motility is estimated by determining the percent of cells that move progressively across the field. Cells that swim in tight circles are not progressively motile. If more than 10 cells are seen per high-power field, the sample can be diluted. Dilution can be done

by placing a drop of warm saline on a slide and then placing a small amount of semen into the saline (concentrated bull and ram semen usually only requires a quick touch of the saline with a wooden stick dipped into the semen). If the cells were alive on the gross motility examination but are dead on the individual motility examination, then the saline should be suspected of being hypertonic. As saline remains opened, the water evaporates and increases the osmolarity of the solution. Replace the saline, and repeat the motility evaluation.

✏ TECHNICIAN NOTE

Sperm motility is the first parameter assessed because it can change quickly under adverse conditions.

Sperm morphology is generally examined after staining with an eosin-nigrosin stain (Lane Manufacturing). Slides are made by painting a line of the stain across one end of the slide. A small amount of semen is placed in the stain. A second slide is then used to push the stain across the length of the slide. The objective of making the slide is to have a very dark background to highlight the cells. If there are lighter and darker areas on the slide, it may be easier to find a more suitable area to examine the cells. To examine the morphology slide, always use ×100 (oil) magnification. Lower magnification will not allow adequate assessment of the sperm cells. A total of 100 cells are counted, and they are classified as normal or abnormal. A spermiogram can be performed to differentiate the different types of sperm abnormalities, which include proximal droplets, distal droplets, kinked tails, coiled tails, acrosome abnormalities, midpiece abnormalities, and misshaped heads.

✏ TECHNICIAN NOTE

Sperm morphology is assessed under high magnification (×100, oil).

Sperm concentration is also performed in situations where a physiologic ejaculate is obtained, such as with a stallion or dog. In those species in which the sperm cell output is estimated using scrotal circumference (SC), a sperm count is not done. The concentration of sperm is determined by diluting the sample 1:100 and then counting the diluted sample on a hemacytometer. The easiest way to make a 1:100 dilution is to prepare two tubes of 0.9-ml formal buffered saline. Add 0.1 ml of raw semen to the first tube, and mix. Take 0.1 ml of diluted semen from the first tube, and add it to the second tube. The second tube now has a 1:100 dilution. Place the 1:100 dilution on a hemacytometer, and count all the sperm cells in the middle big square surrounded by triple lines (it has 25 smaller squares). The total number of sperm cells counted and multiplied by 10^6 gives the concentration per milliliter. The volume of the sample multiplied by the concentration gives the total number of sperm cells in the ejaculate.

BULL, RAM, AND BUCK

The bull, ram, and buck have a fibroelastic penis that has a very low blood volume in the cavernous space, but it attains very high pressure. The stimulus for ejaculation in these species is temperature. When sensors on the penis encounter the correct temperature in the female vagina, the male ejaculates. It is important to note that even though there is no pain response on the penis, the temperature sensors may still be able to signal ejaculation. However, it is also difficult to ascertain whether the temperature sensors are functional. In order to obtain a physiologic ejaculate, an artificial vagina needs to be used to collect the semen. Most artificial vaginas consist of a hard shell with a rubber liner inserted. Warm water is placed between the rubber liner and the shell. The temperature of the water is critical in inducing ejaculation.

The animal is allowed to become sexually stimulated and mount an estrual female, restrained male, or immobile object; the collector then diverts the penis into the artificial vagina. Because this is not easy to do and most ruminants are not trained to breed an artificial vagina, most semen collections in the field are performed using an electro-ejaculator (Figure 17-33). An electroejaculator consists of a probe inserted into the rectum. On the ventral side of the probe are electrodes that stimulate the sympathetic and parasympathetic nerves. The probe is connected to a control box. The box controls how much stimulation the animal receives. The stimulation is very low at first and is gradually increased until the animal has an erection, protrudes the penis, and ejaculates. The ejaculate is then collected into a receptacle. Some machines have an automatic progression of power settings, whereas other machines have to be stepped up manually to control the power.

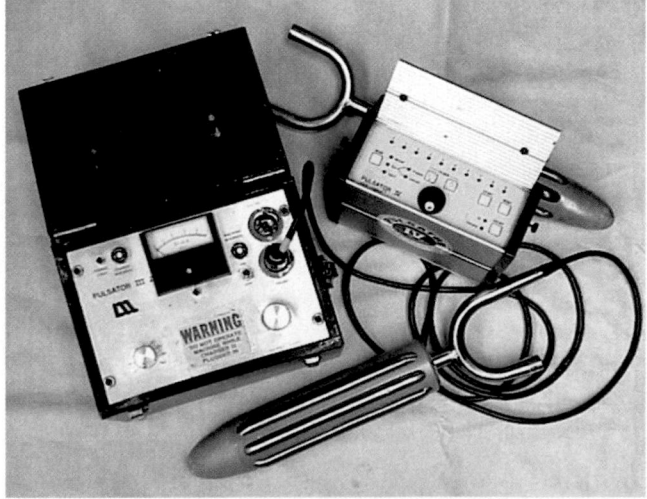

Figure 17-33 Two models of ruminant electroejaculators and two rectal probes.

Although commonly used, electroejaculation may be a painful process for the animal. As long as the power is applied, that animal will produce fluid (from the accessory sex glands), so the "ejaculate" is not truly physiologic. Because the ejaculate is not physiologic, other estimates must be used to estimate sperm output. Sperm output is generally estimated by measuring the SC. When measuring the SC, the testes and epididymides are also palpated for size and consistency. A normal bull testis has the consistency of a flexed human bicep. Standards have been set for the desired SC of different ruminant species of different ages.

> ### ✎ TECHNICIAN NOTE
> When measuring the SC, the testes and epididymides are also palpated for size and consistency.

In the ram it is very important to palpate the epididymides carefully because *Brucella ovis* causes infertility and epididymitis. In the bull a rectal examination is performed to evaluate the vesicular glands. Other body systems to evaluate are vision, teeth, and locomotion. The animal must be able to see, eat, and move around to be a successful breeder. Guidelines have been set by the Society for Theriogenology regarding the minimal criteria needed for an animal to be acceptable for breeding. Breeding soundness evaluation forms and criteria are available for veterinarians from the Society for Theriogenology (Figure 17-34).

Bulls commonly get seminal vesiculitis, and white cells will be seen in the semen. Other common problems in bulls are penile hematomas and preputial injuries (Figure 17-35). A penile hematoma usually occurs when a bull is breeding and the penis bends. This increases the pressure in the penis and causes a rupture of the penile tunic. The rupture almost always happens at the distal sigmoid flexure, and a blood clot forms. Preputial injuries are common in *Bos indicus* bulls. These bulls have a very redundant prepuce that often is everted or hangs out. When the prepuce is damaged, it swells and the bull cannot retract it. Conservative therapy is common in these cases, but a reefing surgery or a circumcision may be needed.

STALLION

Semen is collected most commonly with an artificial vagina (AV) (Figure 17-36). The temperature and pressure of the artificial vagina are the criteria that contribute to the stallion ejaculating. A final temperature of 45° C to 48° C is generally needed, and the pressure must be adequate. Some stallions prefer hotter and some colder; some prefer more pressure, and some prefer less pressure. Once the AV is prepared, the stallion is teased with an estrual mare until he attains an erection. The penis should be washed with clean warm water, avoiding the use of disinfectants because they can disrupt the normal commensal organisms on the penis and are spermicidal. If a mare is used for a mount, the stallion

Bull Breeding Soundness Evaluation

Guidelines Established by Society for Theriogenology
530 Church Street, Suite 700 • Nashville, TN 37219
Phone 615/344-3060 • FAX 615/254-7047 • www.therio.org

OWNER		CASE NO.	DATE
ADDRESS		BULL NAME	BREED
	ZIP	I.D. NO.	Brand ❏ Tattoo ❏ Ear tag ❏
TELEPHONE ( )		BIRTH DATE	AGE (MO.)
HISTORY: Previous BSE	DATE	CASE NO.	CLASSIFICATION

PHYSICAL EXAMINATION

Body condition score _____   Thin ❏   Moderate ❏   Good ❏   Obese ❏
Beef   1, 2, 3, 4, 5, 6, 7, 8, 9   Pelvic Ht. _____ Width _____ Area _____
Dairy   1, 2, 3, 4, 5

Feet/legs	❏
Eyes	❏
Vesicular glands	❏
Ampullae/prostate	❏
Inguinal rings	❏
Penis/prepuce	❏
Testes/spermatic cord	❏
Epididymides	❏
Scrotum (shape)	❏

Other

SCROTAL CIRCUMFERENCE (CM) _____ . _____

This bull has been examined for physical soundness and quality of semen only. Unless otherwise noted, no diagnostic tests were undertaken for libido, mating ability or infectious disease status of this bull.

Remarks and interpretation (diagnosis, prognosis, recommendations)

SEMEN EXAMINATION

Collection method: EE ❏   AV ❏   Massage ❏

Response: Erection ❏   Protrusion ❏   Ejaculation ❏

Semen characteristics		Ejaculate 1	Ejaculate 2
Motility	Gross (or) —— individual (%)		
% Normal cells			
% Primary abnormalities			
% Secondary abnormalities			
WBC, RBC, other			

CLASSIFICATION

Interpretation of data resulting from this examination would indicate that *on this date,* this bull is a:

❏ Satisfactory potential breeder

❏ Unsatisfactory potential breeder

❏ Classification deferred

Re-examination recommended on _____
DATE

Signed: _____
MEMBER—SOCIETY FOR THERIOGENOLOGY

Clinic:

Figure 17-34 Bull breeding soundness examination form. These forms are copyrighted and available from the Society for Theriogenology (Society for Theriogenology, PO Box 3007, Montgomery, AL 36109).

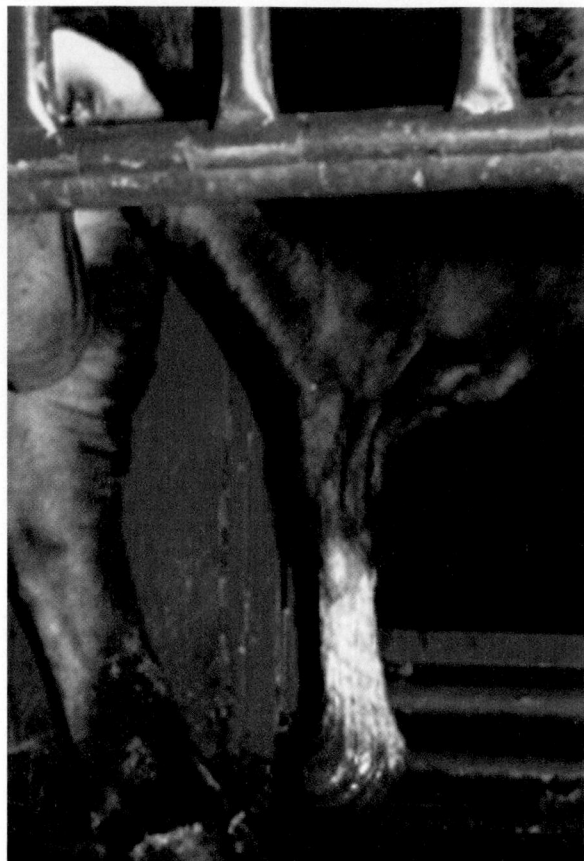

Figure 17-35 *Bos indicus* bull with a preputial prolapse.

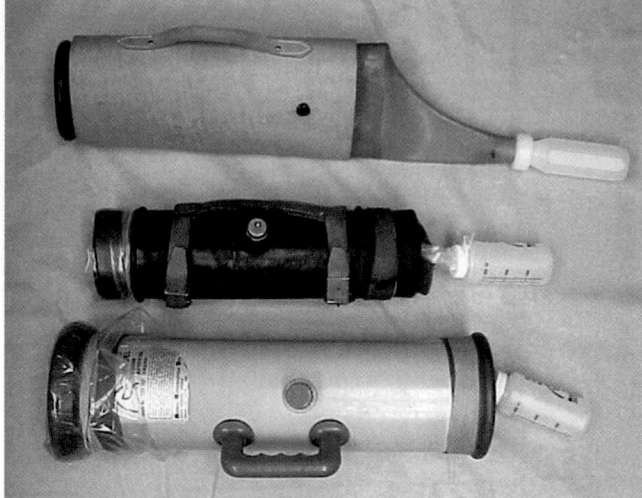

Figure 17-36 Three models of equine artificial vaginas. *From the top,* Missouri, Hannover, ARS/Colorado.

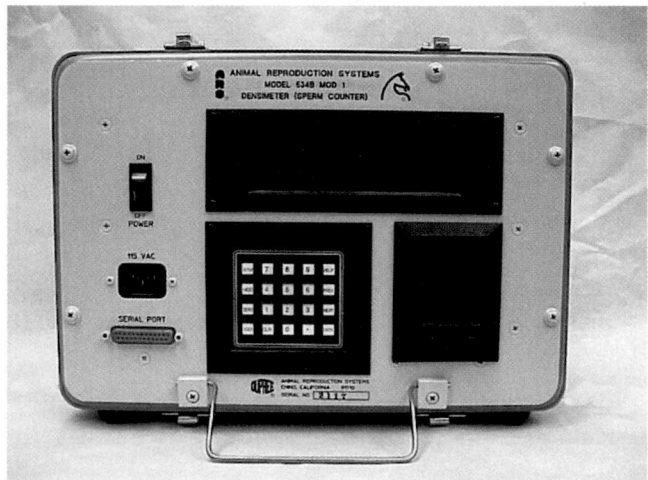

Figure 17-37 Densimeter used to measure the concentration of stallion semen.

is led to the side of the mare and allowed to mount. The stallion will then position himself on the mare. As the stallion begins to thrust, the penis is diverted into the AV, and the stallion allowed to thrust and ejaculate into the AV. As the stallion dismounts, the AV is held vertical to prevent semen from draining out the open end. Immediately after the dismount, the water in the AV should be drained out to prevent heat shock to the cells and to allow the semen to drain into the collection bottle.

✐ TECHNICIAN NOTE

Stallion semen often has a large gel fraction that must be removed before analysis can be performed.

Stallions can also be trained to mount dummies, or phantoms. A dummy allows collection of a stallion without an estrual mare present and is a safer way to collect semen. Stallion semen often has a large gel fraction that must be removed before analysis can be performed. This is usually done with an in-line filter attached to the collection bottle. Alternatively, the ejaculate can be filtered in the laboratory after collection. Motility and morphology assessments are performed the same as in other species. Stallion semen may be diluted and counted manually or using a densimeter.

A densimeter measures the amount of light that passes through the semen sample. The higher the concentration of cells, the less light passes through, the less the percent transmittance. Commercially available machines are calibrated to read out the sperm cell concentration based on internal calculations made from the percent transmittance (Figure 17-37).

If semen is being collected as part of a breeding soundness evaluation, two ejaculates are obtained, 1 hour apart. If the second sample has about half the number of sperm as the first ejaculate, the ejaculates can be considered representative. Stallions are also seasonal, and both sperm production and libido decrease in the winter when day length is short and increase in the summer.

The transport of cooled stallion semen is becoming more and more popular with certain breeds. Commercially available shipping containers cool the extended semen at a specific rate and keep it cool for up to 48 hours. Extenders are liquids added to the semen to help the longevity of shipped semen. Most extenders are made from skim milk and glucose and have some antibiotics added. When extending stallion semen, the final concentrations should be between 25×10^6 and 50×10^6 cells/ml; however, the final dilution ratio should be at least four parts of extender to one part of semen. If the semen cannot be extended to that concentration and ratio, the semen must be centrifuged and the resulting pellet resuspended to the desired 25 to 50 million/ml concentration. Many stallions, despite having semen that appears good, do not have semen that withstands even the best cooling and shipping procedures.

Stallions may have problems with decreased libido, hind limb lameness resulting in breeding difficulties, blood in the semen (hemospermia), or urine in the semen (urospermia). These may be challenging problems for the veterinarian to diagnose and treat. The most common breeding injury in the stallion is when the mare kicks the penis or scrotum. The sequela to a kick on the penis is often a hematoma. This is a large blood clot on the outside of the penile tunic, which results in paraphimosis (the penis will not go back into the sheath). If the scrotum is kicked, the testes can swell and be damaged by both the heat from the inflammation and pressure necrosis of the testicular parenchyma swelling within the confined testicular tunic. Conservative therapy for these conditions includes hydrotherapy and anti-inflammatories.

CANINE

Canine semen evaluation is performed as in other species, which includes motility, morphology, and a semen count. The main difference is the way the semen is collected. Dog semen is collected by manual massage of the penis. It is best to have an estrual bitch present when the collection is attempted. Once the dog is somewhat aroused, the prepuce is pushed caudal to the bulbus glandis with a rubber or plastic cone. Circumferential manual pressure is then applied proximal to the bulbus glandis. Pressure is applied while the dog ejaculates. The initial portion of the ejaculate is clear, followed by the sperm-rich fraction. The final portion of the ejaculate is the clear prostatic portion. Normally, it is not necessary to collect the prostatic fraction. It is common for the dog to step over the collector's hand during the collection process. The criteria for a dog to be a good potential breeder have been published by the Society for Theriogenology. The most common reproductive disorder in the dog is prostatitis. A dog with prostatitis will have white blood cells in the ejaculate and possibly show pain during ejaculation.

TECHNICIAN NOTE

The most common reproductive disorder in the dog is prostatitis.

TOM

It is very uncommon to collect semen from the tom. However, semen can be collected using a small AV or an electroejaculator. A tom must be extensively trained to use an AV and must be anesthetized to use an electroejaculator. This is why semen evaluations are rarely performed in the tom. One option is to use a vaginal swab to detect the presence of sperm cells in a queen that has just been bred. The tom will also have retrograde ejaculation into the bladder, so after breeding, a cystocentesis can be performed in an attempt to find sperm cells as another option. The most common causes of infertility in the tom are poor teeth (because the tom bites the queen's neck during breeding) and hair rings around the penis.

BOAR

Semen from the boar is collected by manual pressure of the distal penis. The boar is led to an estrual sow or can be trained to mount a dummy. As the boar mounts and extends the penis, the collector grasps the penis "backhand" such that the tip of the penis is grasped mainly with the little finger. It is the manual pressure that elicits ejaculation in the boar. The tip of the penis is diverted to an open container. The bottle should be covered with gauze or cheesecloth to filter out the gel fraction of the ejaculate. The boar takes approximately 10 to 20 minutes to ejaculate and will continue to ejaculate as long as pressure is applied to the penile tip (the collector's hand usually tires before the boar). The most common breeding problems in boars are bite wounds to the penis and infections of the preputial diverticulum.

CAMELIDS

Llamas and alpacas can have semen collected by electroejaculation or with an AV, or they can have semen recovered from the vagina of the female after natural mating. The AV is the best method to obtain a semen sample. The copulatory pattern of the llama is somewhat unique when compared with other domestic species. The female llama lies down, and the male llama will lie on top of the female during copulation. Copulation can take as long as 30 minutes, and the male may ejaculate several times. Semen is evaluated as with other species.

Recommended Reading

Knottenbelt DC et al: M. *Equine stud farm medicine and surgery,* Edinburgh, 2003, WB Saunders.

McKinnon AO, Voss JL, editors: *Equine reproduction,* Philadelphia, 1993, Lea & Febiger.

Root Kustritz MV, editor: *Small animal theriogenology,* St Louis, 2003, Butterworth-Heinemann.

Younquist RS, editor: *Current therapy in theriogenology,* Philadelphia, 1997, WB Saunders.

18

Care of Birds, Reptiles, and Small Mammals

THOMAS N. TULLY, JR.

INTRODUCTION

The veterinary field of exotic or nondomestic pet medicine is expanding; in the area of pet ownership and money, owners are willing to spend on their animals (Figure 18-1). Caged and aviary birds are now the third most common small animal pet. In the 2002 American Pet Products Manufacturers Association's (APPMA) National Pet Owners Survey reported that 6.9 million households owned a total of 19 million birds. Pet bird owners are utilizing veterinary care for their animals according to the 2002 American Veterinary Medical Association's *U.S. Pet Ownership and Demographics Source Book* (Wise, 2002). This chapter discusses avian and nondomestic pet species, with particular attention paid to the individual requirements of birds, reptiles, and small mammals. It is important to note that approximately 85% of the problems seen in exotic pet medicine result from the lack of basic husbandry information among pet stores, pet owners, veterinarians, and veterinary technicians. With increased veterinary public education, all species covered in this chapter will have a greater chance of living long and healthy lives. For handling and restraint of the animals described in this chapter, see Chapter 1. ■

TECHNICIAN NOTE

Approximately 85% of the problems seen in exotic pet medicine result from lack of information on the part of pet stores, pet owners, veterinarians, and veterinary technicians.

BIRDS

The veterinary technician may, on occasion, be involved in telephone communication with clients. When clients call regarding avian patients, it is important to instruct the owner in the following areas. Ask the owners to bring the bird in its own cage if at all possible. If the bird is larger and the cage cannot be transported, then the bird should be transported in a plastic small animal carrier. Small animal carriers work well for birds, particularly the carriers with the door in the front. Newspaper or a towel can be used as material to cover the bottom, which is easily cleaned when removed. Wooden dowels can be placed in the carrier as perches and secured in place with screws and washers from the outside. Owners should always be advised never to bring their bird to the clinic nonsecured; they should be in either a carrier or, if small, its cage. They should not clean the cage, except to empty the water dish to prevent it from spilling during the trip. A good evaluation of the bird's environment is helpful to the veterinarian, and clean papers and a clean cage do not provide that information.

TECHNICIAN NOTE

Owners should always be advised never to bring their bird to the clinic nonsecured; the bird should be in either a carrier or, if small, its cage.

All grit should be removed because some birds tend to gorge themselves on grit, particularly when ill. The cage should be covered with a towel or blanket to protect it from the weather, and the owner should be instructed to bring along any medication and vitamin supplements the bird is taking, as well as a sample of food. Most avian telephone inquiries should be considered emergencies because of most

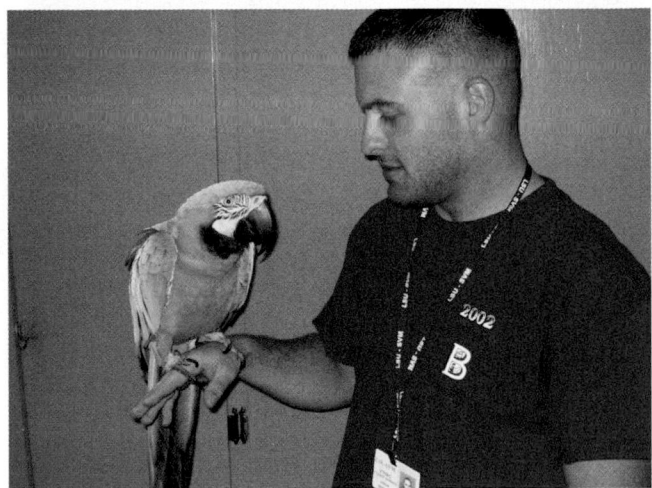

Figure 18-1 A bird is an attractive, popular companion.

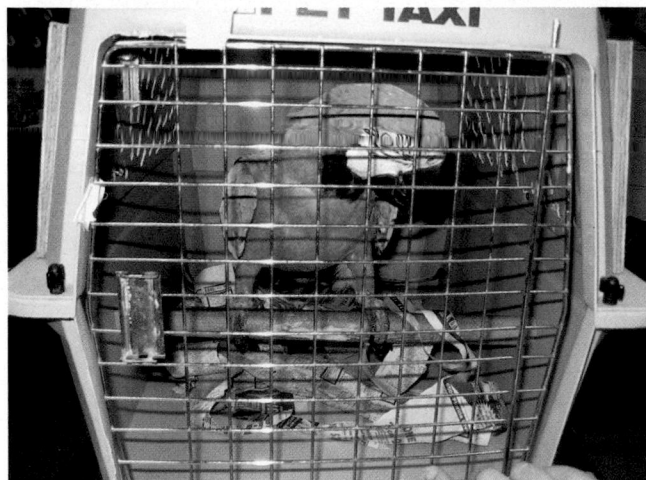

Figure 18-2 A pet carrier is recommended for transport of companion birds to the veterinary hospital.

Box 18-1 COMMON PET BIRDS

PSITTACINES	PASSERINES
Budgerigar	Canary
Cockatiel	Zebra finch
Amazon parrot	Java rice bird
Macaw	
Conure	
Lovebird	
African gray parrot	

---

owners' inability to note early signs of illness, the bird's inherent ability to mask clinical problems, and the rapid speed with which avian species succumb to disease.

TAKING THE CLINICAL HISTORY

The following is a suggested list of questions to ask the client regarding avian patients:

- What is the chief complaint?
- Obtain signalment (includes the species, gender, and age) (Box 18-1).
- *Origin:* Where was the bird obtained? How long has it been owned by the presenting party?
- *Environment:* What is the construction and design of the cage? Is it painted? If so, what type of paint has been used? What is the design and composition of the water and food bowls, substrate (newspaper, wood shavings, corncob, etc.), and perches? Where is the bird kept (indoors or outdoors)? In what room of the house is it kept (e.g., kitchen or garage where potential toxins may be located)? Is it close to a window? Are insecticides, household cleaners, or other chemicals used around the house in the vicinity of the cage? Is the bird allowed out

of the cage? If so, is it allowed to fly freely, and how well is it supervised?
- *Diet:* What is the bird being fed (e.g., seed, fruits, vegetables, grain)? How often is it fed? Are vitamins and minerals added to the food? How often is the water changed? How is the food prepared and stored?
- *Appetite:* Notes should be made regarding the bird's overall appetite and daily food consumption.
- *Feces:* Questions regarding consistency, color, and number of droppings per day are all important. The client should be asked whether feces have been previously submitted for parasite evaluation.
- *Cage mates:* Are there other animals in the collection in the same cage or in the household? If so, how many, what species, and what degree of contact do they have with the patient? Does the owner maintain a quarantine policy?
- *Molting cycle:* When did the bird go through its last general molt, and are there any abnormalities in the feather coat or feather growth?
- *Behavior:* What is the overall attitude and behavior, including voice quality and changes in vocalization? Have there been behavior-related problems in the past (e.g., feather picking, screaming, or other abnormal behavior)?
- *Previous medical history:* Has the bird been ill before? Is there a history of disease in other pets in the house? If so, what illnesses have been diagnosed and treated in the past? Have they been to a veterinarian before?

BEHAVIOR CONSIDERATIONS DURING THE EXAMINATION PROCESS

As recommended, all birds should present at the clinic in a carrier or cage (Figure 18-2). Although a carrier may be recommended, there are avian patients that will arrive unrestrained. However a bird enters the room, there should

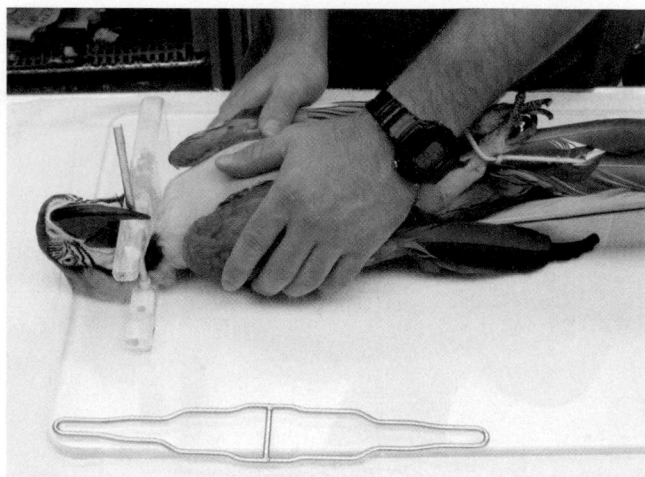

Figure 18-3 Once the bird is restrained, an avian exam board may be used to easily examine the patient and obtain diagnostic samples. Care should be made to prevent chest compression by the handler.

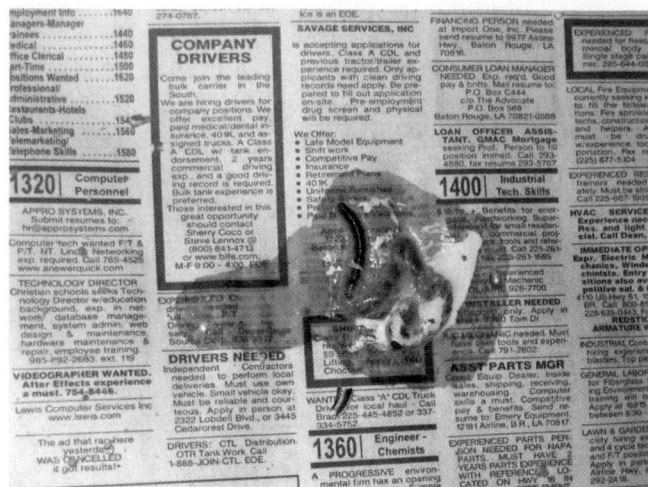

Figure 18-4 Normal psittacine stool. Note the dark solid feces, white solid urates, and liquid urine.

be an understanding that the patient is in an unfamiliar stressful environment. To reduce behavior complications that may arise as a result of the examination, certain considerations are recommended. Capture and restraint is necessary for examination, but pain and stress should be reduced as much as possible. To achieve this goal, capture and restrain should be accomplished using a towel that covers the hand being used to grasp the bird. The bird should be in a standing position with the towel in full view as the hand approaches the patient's head. Most birds will allow the hand within the towel to grasp behind the neck with very little resistance if the towel is slowly advanced in full view. All diagnostic testing materials and medication should be ready before the bird is restrained. Examination, diagnostic sample collections, treatment, and procedures must be performed quickly to reduce the stress and adverse psychological effects of the hospital visit (Figure 18-3). Once the examination is completed positive reinforcement of scratching the bird behind its head and communication will aid in transitioning the bird back to the owner.

If the avian patient has to be hospitalized, placing the bird's cage within a hospital cage will help with accommodation to the unfamiliar surroundings. If the cage is too big to place in the hospital cage, familiar food and toys will help promote psychological well-being. One point to emphasize to pet bird owners is that by returning their bird to its familiar home surroundings as soon as possible will not only help the animal's psychological comfort but possibly aid in healing.

SAMPLE COLLECTIONS AND DIAGNOSTIC PROCEDURES COMMONLY USED IN BIRDS

Diagnostic plans in avian species are no different from the clinical approach to other domestic pets. Evaluation of the stool is an important first step. The technician should become familiar with normal stool presentation to determine differences between polyuria (excessive urine output) and diarrhea (change in the fecal consistency and amount) (Figure 18-4). Fecal parasites may be detected on fresh smears with saline and a coverslip. This is the best method to check for protozoa, such as *Giardia*. Fecal flotation will bring some parasite ova to the surface (e.g., ascarids and *Capillaria*). Fecal sedimentation is an important procedure for diagnosis of flukes, which may be seen in wild avian species including raptors. Fecal specimens that are Gram stained are useful to determine the bacterial flora of the digestive tract. Most cage bird species have predominantly gram-positive organisms inhabiting the digestive system. Fecal Gram stains are only a preliminary diagnostic test and should be followed up with bacterial culture.

> ### ⬗ TECHNICIAN NOTE
> Most cage bird species have predominantly gram-positive organisms inhabiting the digestive system.

Cloacal Swab
A cloacal swab is often done on a psittacine species to determine the bacterial flora of the lower gastrointestinal tract. A cotton swab is moistened, inserted into the cloaca, and gently rotated. Cloacal swabs are useful for cytologic evaluations, looking for inflammatory cells, such as heterophils. They may also be used for culture and sensitivity tests and *Chlamydophila psittaci* or viral isolation.

Oral Examination and Crop Wash
The technician should become adept at assisting in the performance of oral examination and crop wash by the

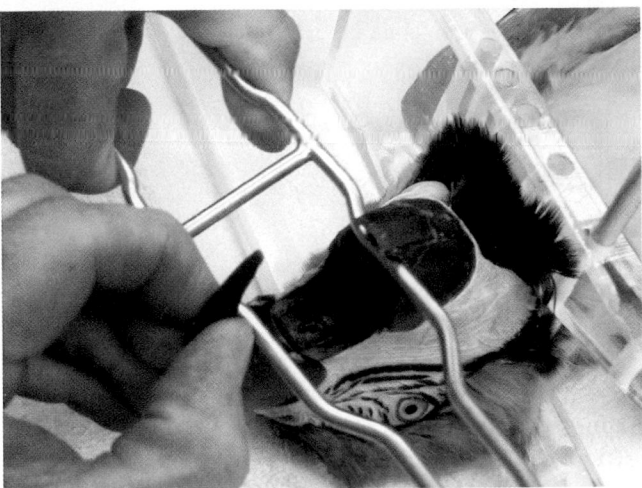

Figure 18-5 Oral examination demonstrating the use of a beak speculum on a macaw.

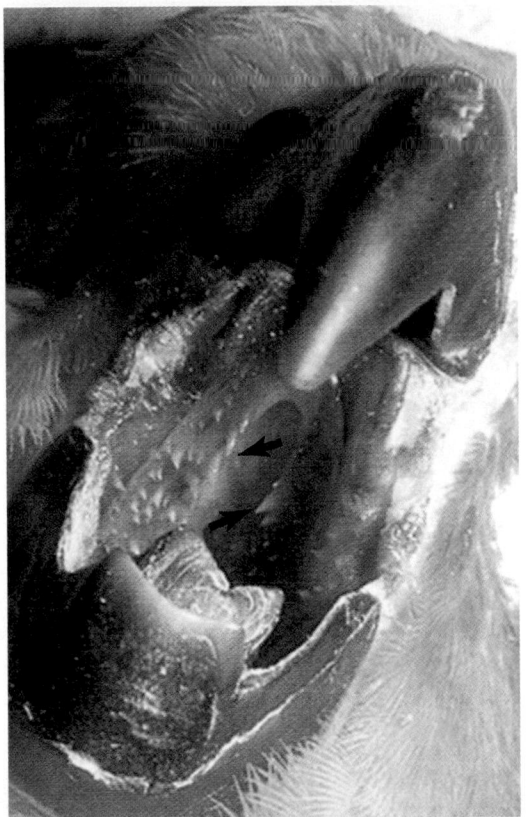

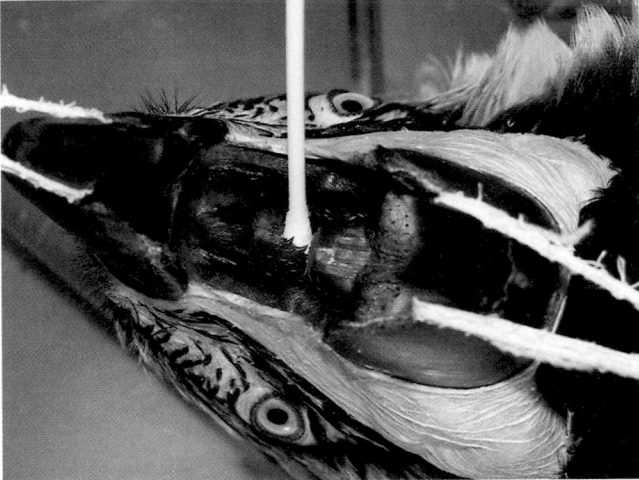

Figure 18-6 Culturette placement in the rostral aspect of the choana.

veterinarian. Good restraint technique is essential (see Chapter 1). An avian beak speculum is placed in the bird's mouth parallel to the commissure and then rotated to open the beak (Figure 18-5). A choanal culture should be taken when birds are exhibiting upper respiratory signs. The Culturette is placed in the rostral area of the choana to prevent cross contamination with flora in the oral cavity (Figure 18-6).

Another important diagnostic technique is the crop wash. The crop wash permits examination of the upper gastrointestinal tract. A sterile or clean tube is passed through the mouth into the crop or into the esophagus in those birds with an underdeveloped crop. A syringe of sterile saline is connected to the tube, and a simple flush is performed (Figure 18-5). Tubes may be made of plastic, rubber, or metal and have a ball tip (Figure 18-6). The crop wash is important for direct microscopic examination to check for protozoans, such as *Trichomonas* or yeast *(Candida albicans)*, using a wet mount technique. Slides may be prepared for cytologic examinations with Diff-Quik stains or Wright's stain, looking for inflammatory cells, such as heterophils. A Gram stain is often done on crop wash samples from psittacine species, or the sample may be submitted for culture and sensitivity (see Chapter 8). A Culturette may be passed into a bird's crop for culture and sensitivity diagnostics. Care must be taken so the patient does not bite the Culturette and swallow it. Young psittacine species readily accept Culturettes into the crop through normal feeding responses.

Passing a tube into the crop of the psittacine bird is an important technique to learn because tube feeding is often necessary (Figure 18-7). The tube should be passed over the trachea at the base of the tongue down the esophagus and palpated in the crop at the level of the thoracic inlet. Food that is administered using a feeding tube must have a lower temperature than the bird being fed. Most psittacine species have a body temperature of 102° F to 104° F, so the food should be between 98° F and 101° F. The feeding formula must be thoroughly mixed before uptake into the syringe. Many baby birds develop thermal burns from hot feeding formula, usually on the weight-dependent ventral surface area of the crop. This injury can be prevented by careful preparation of the food by the attending technician. The one rule of thumb to remember when using a tube for either feeding or a crop wash is to try to pick a tube with a diameter larger than the glottis.

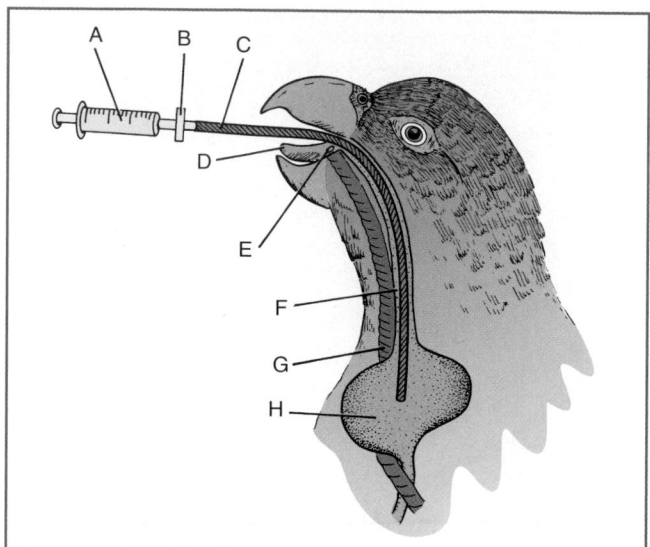

Figure 18-7 Proper tube placement for a crop wash or for tube feeding a bird. The bird's neck should be gently stretched. *A,* Syringe. *B,* Adapter, if necessary. *C,* Tube. *D,* Tongue. *E,* Tracheal opening. *F,* Proximal esophagus. *G,* Trachea. *H,* Crop.

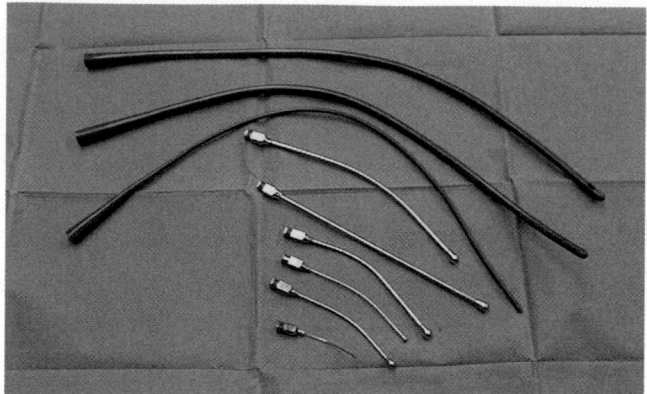

Figure 18-8 Various tubes used for tube feeding and crop washes.

> ✐ **TECHNICIAN NOTE**
>
> Thermal burns to the crop of young birds can be easily prevented by proper preparation of food and feeding at the recommended temperatures.

The glottis of the bird is located at the base of the tongue and is easy to visualize. The tube may be passed into the crop easily by positioning the tube in the side of the bird's mouth (Figure 18-8). The tube is easily palpated through the wall of the crop and the skin. While doing a crop wash or tube feeding, the handler should watch the back of the bird's mouth to ensure that food or water does not begin to accumulate. If the crop is overfilled, the bird may aspirate. If the crop overfills, put the bird down and let it attempt to clear its airway. The bird itself has a better chance of clearing its airway than does the technician or veterinarian using cotton-tipped applicators. Never handle a bird after placing oral medications into the crop or filling the crop unless the bird is experiencing respiratory difficulty.

> ✐ **TECHNICIAN NOTE**
>
> Never handle a bird after placing oral medication into the crop or filling the crop unless the bird is experiencing respiratory difficulty.

Blood Work

Blood work is an important part of the diagnostic examination in avian species. Common venipuncture sites include the basilic vein, right jugular vein, and medial metatarsal vein, but other sites may be used depending on avian species and experience of the phlebotomist. Each has its own advantage and disadvantages, and the veterinarian and technician will tend to develop their own sites of preference, but the right jugular vein is the recommended site for most, if not all, psittacine species.

The right jugular vein is large and easily found in most birds on the right dorsolateral aspect of the neck. However, it is highly mobile and therefore difficult to stabilize. In most birds the right jugular vein is located in a featherless tract lateral to the trachea. With minimal practice and proper restraint, it becomes an easy procedure to perform. An avian restraint board is recommended for blood collections from larger psittacine patients (see Chapter 1). Small psittacine and passerine patients can be handheld when blood is being drawn for diagnostic tests.

In general, the basilic vein is accessible but difficult to completely immobilize in the psittacine patient, because of the tremendous strength of the pectoral muscles (Figures 18-9 and 18-10).

The medial metatarsal vein is easy to immobilize and secure, even on an awake fractious patient. However, if large volumes of blood are to be collected, the medial metatarsal vein may not be a good choice in psittacine patients.

A toenail-clipping blood sample may be obtained, but it is painful to the patient and often causes lameness for several days following the procedure. It may result in a poor blood flow, low yield, and invalid results.

The blood may be collected in syringes, microhematocrit tubes, or blood collection tubes from the hub of the needle. A 3-ml syringe with a 26-gauge needle should be used in most avian patients. In extremely small psittacine and passerine patients a 1-ml syringe with a 30-gauge needle may be used. The technician should learn to proficiently perform a complete blood count (CBC) on avian blood.

Radiography

Radiography is an important diagnostic tool in avian patients. Typically, lateral and ventrodorsal views of the whole body or selected extremities may be taken (Figure 18-11). Technique charts must be developed based on the

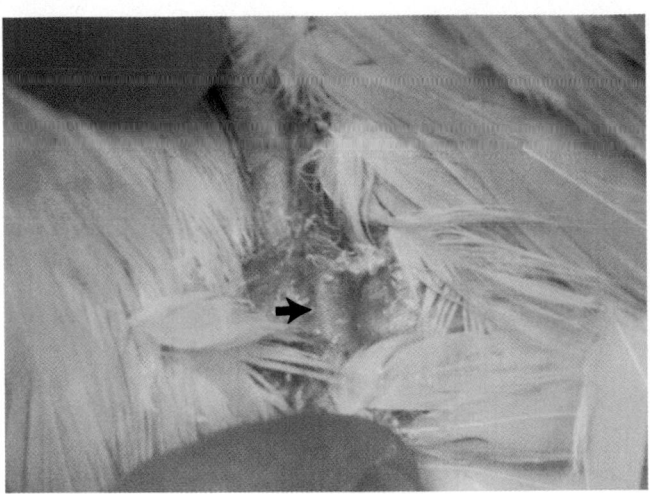

Figure 18-9 Location of the basilic vein (black arrow). Ventral view of humerus, radius, and ulna.

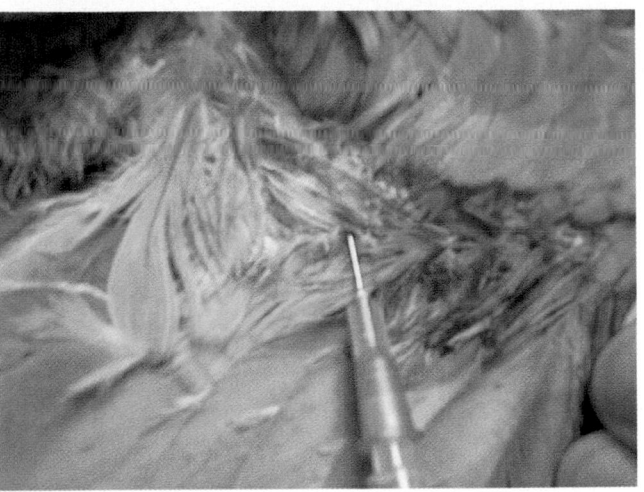

Figure 18-10 Intravenous injection using the basilic vein of a blue and gold macaw.

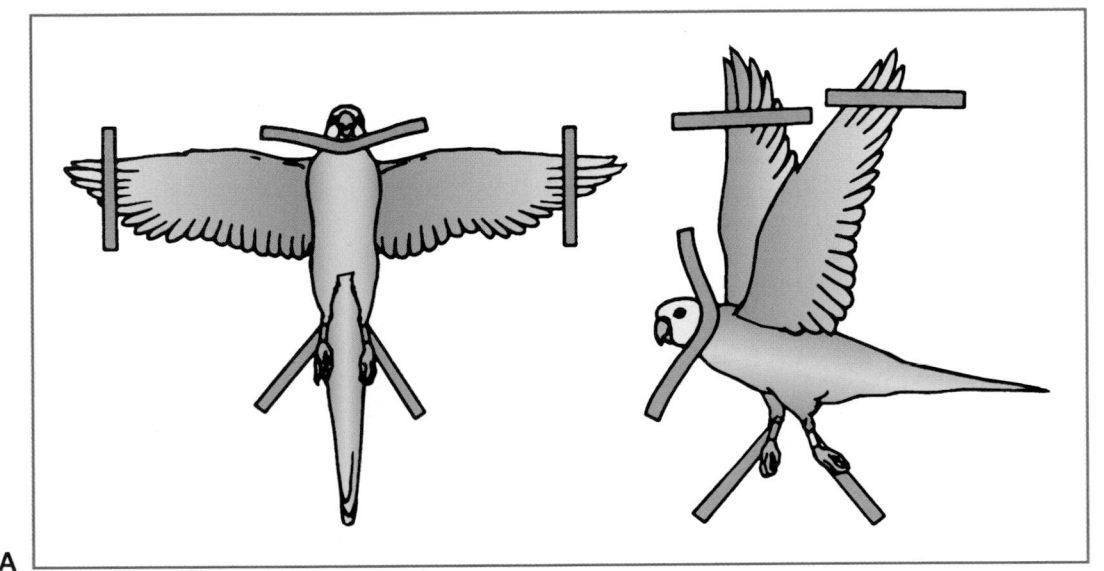

A   B

Figure 18-11 Positioning of a budgerigar for radiographs using masking tape. **A,** Ventrodorsal and, **B,** lateral positions.

equipment available. Contrast films may be made with standard contrast agents, including iohexol and barium sulfate. Because good positioning and absence of motion are important to high-quality radiographs, it is generally recommended that all avian patients be sedated or anesthetized, except those who may be too ill. Proper positioning is important, and an avian restraint board is essential (Figure 18-12). Other diagnostic procedures, such as laparoscopy, endoscopy, tracheal or air sac washes, biopsies, cytologic examinations, and bone marrow aspirates, may be performed on the patient. The technician's role may be to secure the animal with good restraint during these more sophisticated procedures.

HUSBANDRY AND TREATMENT IN THE HOSPITAL

Generally speaking, drugs administered in the food or water will not reach adequate therapeutic levels. This is an unreliable way to administer most medications because of the inconsistent intake of water by most birds. Direct oral absorption is inconsistent with tablets, but most liquid suspensions tend to work well. Injections of drugs into birds are best done in the large pectoral muscle mass. Drugs injected into the caudal half of the animal (e.g., the legs) may result in the agent being absorbed into the bloodstream and shunted toward the kidneys by way of the renal portal system. Therefore, potentially nephrotoxic drugs, such as

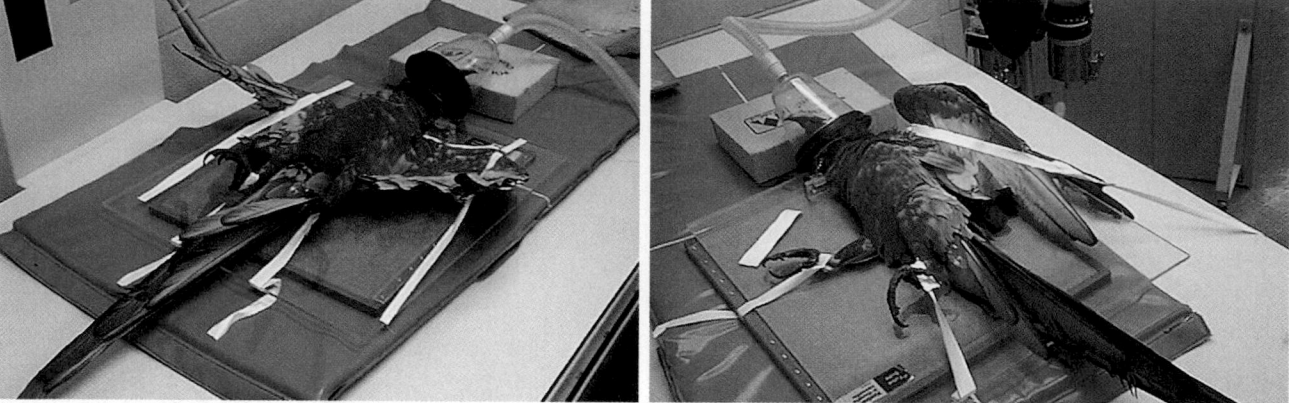

Figure 18-12 Ventrodorsal (**A**) and, lateral (**B**) positioning of a macaw with the use of adhesive tape. The bird is on an Plexiglas avian restraint board for uniform positioning of patients. A face mask is used for the administration of inhalant isoflurane anesthesia.

aminoglycosides, should never be administered by injection into the legs except in ostriches, emus, and rheas.

> **TECHNICIAN NOTE**
>
> Injections of drugs into birds are best done in the large pectoral muscle mass.

Common procedures that the veterinary technician often performs are nail trims and clipping of the wing feathers. Figure 18-13 illustrates one technique for clipping the flight feathers of pet birds. Both wings should be clipped for a symmetric effect, but there are many different feather clip variations that owners request. Typically the primary flight feathers are cut for heavier birds and both the primary and secondary feathers for lighter birds to achieve maximum flight restriction. If only one wing is clipped, the bird cannot control its flight and will be prone to injury. Feather clipping is flight restriction, not prevention. Find out what the owner wants to achieve through the feather trim and how the owner wants the feathers clipped. No trim technique will prevent the bird from flight. In the end, both the owner and technician or veterinarian has to be happy with the look and flight restriction of the trim.

Trimming nails in larger psittacine species should be done with a Dremel Motor Tool (Dremel, Inc., Racine, Wisconsin). For small psittacine species and passerines, human nail clippers or an electrocautery unit can be used. Cautery units can be used on the nails of birds of all sizes but work especially well on the smaller species (Figure 18-14). Grinding with a Dremel Motor Tool cauterizes as it reduces the length of the nails (Figure 18-15). Chemical cautery (as with silver nitrate sticks) should be available if bleeding occurs, especially in younger birds.

Dietary management and nutritional support are particularly important in the compromised avian patient. Table

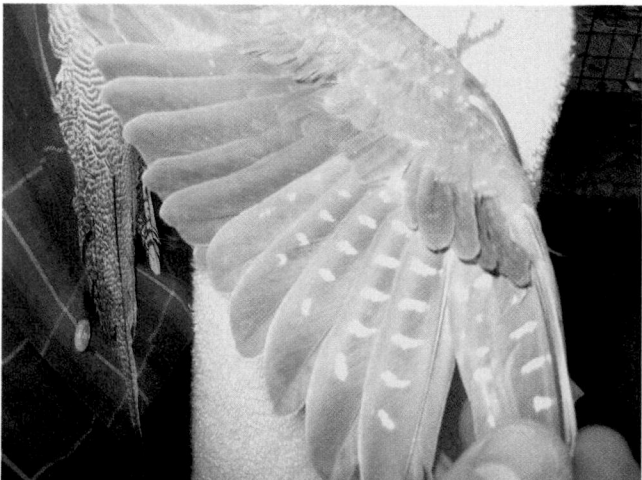

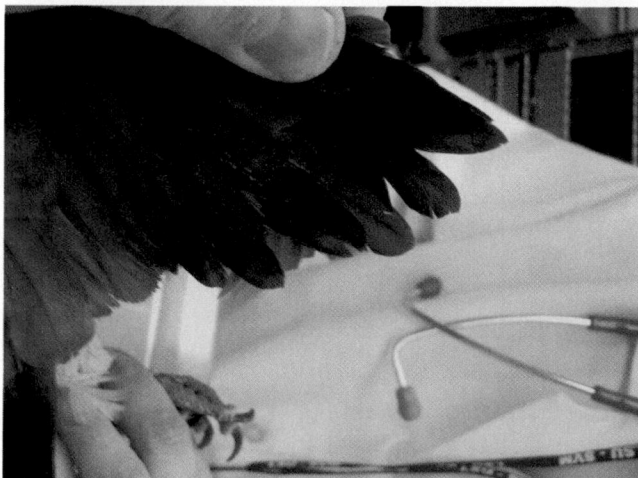

Figure 18-13 **A,** Ventral view of extended wing (when performing a proper feather trim, a symmetrical cut of the 10 outermost feathers are cut below the level of the dorsal coverts). **B,** Proper feather trim of wing on African gray parrot.

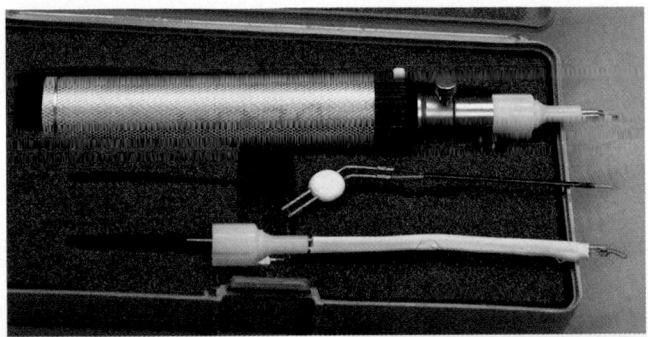

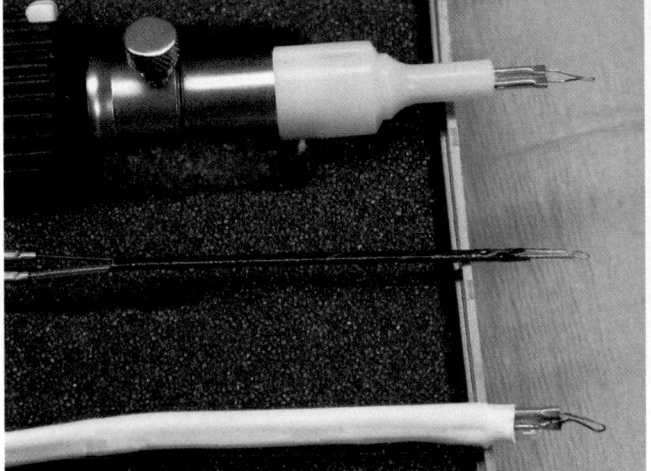
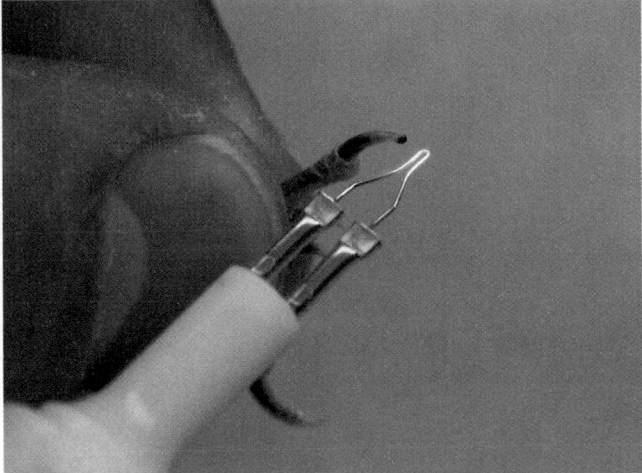

Figure 18-14 Electrocautery unit for trimming small birds' nails.

Table 18-1 RECOMMENDED PSITTACINE DIET

Food Group	What It Supplies	What It Lacks
Cereals and grains, 45%-50%	Proteins, fats, B vitamins	Vitamins A, D, and K and calcium (high phosphorus)
Vegetables, 45%-50%	Vitamins A and K, fiber, carbohydrates ± calcium	Protein, fats, vitamin D₃
Fruit, approximately 5%	Sugars, simple carbohydrates	Proteins, vitamins, minerals
Meats (in combination with dairy products), about 5%	Proteins, fats, calcium	

Mineral supplements (e.g., cuttlebone, oyster shell, mineral blocks, or avian vitamins) may be added to the above diets.
Commercial pelleted diets are primarily a cereal-and-grain–based diet with vitamin and mineral supplementation added.

18-1 provides the basic feeding guidelines for psittacine species and other seed-eating birds. It is important to remember to keep the cage as clean as possible. Food and water dishes should be cleaned at least daily and occasionally more often. Fresh fruits, vegetables, and meats should only be left in a food dish for short periods of time. Food consumption should be closely monitored. New foods should be introduced gradually, especially the pelleted avian diets.

Some foods may provide the bird a source of activity while eating, such as peeling vegetables, fruits, and nuts. Tube feeding in psittacine birds is an important nursing procedure. Generally, a commercially available cereal-based baby avian formula is recommended for hand-raising young psittacine species. Tube feeding should begin with small amounts frequently, which are then slowly increased in volume and decreased in time interval. The bird should be

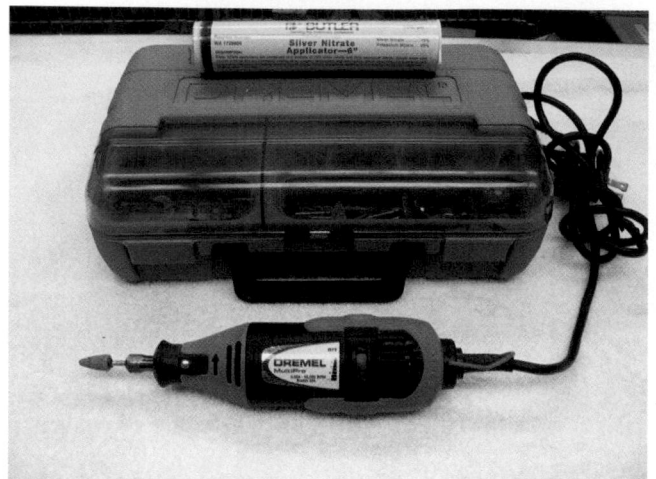

Figure 18-15 Motor tool for grinding larger birds' nails and grooming beaks.

weighed one or two times per day to chart weight gain. The crop should be monitored for prompt emptying, and the stools should be examined for consistency. The basal metabolic rate (BMR) may be calculated as a rough approximation of energy requirements. The normal BMR for a nonpasserine species, such as parrots, is approximately 79 × body weight (in kilograms). This should be doubled for an ill bird. For passerine species, 130 times the body weight raised to the power of 0.7 should be used. For carnivorous birds, such as raptors, a high-quality canned cat food, such as Control Diet (C/D) (Hill's Pet Products) may be used to meet their energy requirements.

Hospital facilities should be appropriate for the species being housed. Bird cages should be in a separate room, if possible, to minimize the stress of sounds and sights of other species. Isolation of birds also prevents contamination of potentially pathogenic bacteria. For example, most psittacine birds have a predominantly gram-positive gut flora. Housing birds near animals with gram-negative gut flora, such as dogs, cats, reptiles, and carnivorous birds, could result in gram-negative enteric infections. A visual barrier should be provided for the bird, such as a cage cover or hide box in the cage. Large parrots may do well in standard dog or cat cages if adequate perches and water and food bowls are provided. Alternatively, Plexiglas custom cages are an excellent alternative and easily cleaned. Perches should be disposable, simple to disinfect, and sized according to the individual patient. An isolation area should be available for avian psittacosis suspects. Again, cleanliness is one of the most important details in the hospital.

Temperature control is important, particularly with sick birds. In general, birds will tolerate cold better than heat. Sudden changes in temperature and drafts should always be avoided. Sick birds have difficulty maintaining and regulating their own body temperature, as do birds with poor feather coats, oil-damaged feathers, or plucked feathers. Therefore these birds should be kept warm but not hot.

Temperatures between 80° F and 90° F are best. The bird should be observed for signs of heat stress or shivering. Common signs of heat stress in avian patients are panting, wings extended, flushed (reddish) facial patches on macaws, and depression. An environmentally controlled cage or unit should be available for the intensive care avian patients.

ZOONOSES AND COMMON CLINICAL PROBLEMS

Although zoonotic diseases are discussed in Chapter 34, one disease, *Chlamydophila psittaci*, should be mentioned here because it is commonly diagnosed in pet bird species. Therefore a sick bird that presents with nonspecific clinical illness (e.g., signs of diarrhea, vomiting, or just not doing well) should be considered for differential diagnosis of avian chlamydiosis. Patients that have recently been through quarantine or pet shops and exposed to other birds are most suspect.

Avian chlamydiosis is a disease transmissible to humans, caused by the bacterium *C. psittaci*. Those patients suspected of potentially being infected with *C. psittaci* should be treated with appropriate antibiotics. The bird should be isolated, gloves and masks should be used, and feces should be disposed of through cleaning of the cage and bagging the disposable substrate. Transmission is primarily through respiratory inhalation of the infectious elementary body. Psittacosis is a potentially fatal disease in humans. Many wild birds may carry *C. psittaci* organisms without showing clinical signs. It is important that the veterinary technician working with birds become familiar with this disease.

REPTILES

It is estimated that there are 9 million pet reptiles in the United States according to the AAPMA 2003/2004 pet survey. Although the number of pet reptiles does not match dog and cat populations, there is a significant population of animals that require veterinary health services. The diversity of reptile species maintained in captivity requires owner education in health, nutritional, and environmental management (Box 18-2). With excellent owner care, most reptile species live long, healthy lives. In many cases, it is the responsibility of the technician to handle and collect diagnostic samples and educate the owner about their captive reptile.

Once a veterinary hospital decides to treat reptiles, there are a few pieces of specialized equipment needed to provide an adequate hospital environment and aid the technician and veterinarian. Required medical equipment includes an electronic gram scale, an incubator, heating pad, tuberculin and microliter syringes, exotic animal formulary (see Recommended Reading), microhematocrit tubes, snake cloacal probes, and metal feeding tubes (Figures 18-16 to 18-18). Common material used on turtle shell repair includes epoxy, resin, and fiberglass patches. There has been a move away from using epoxy resins, dental acrylics, and

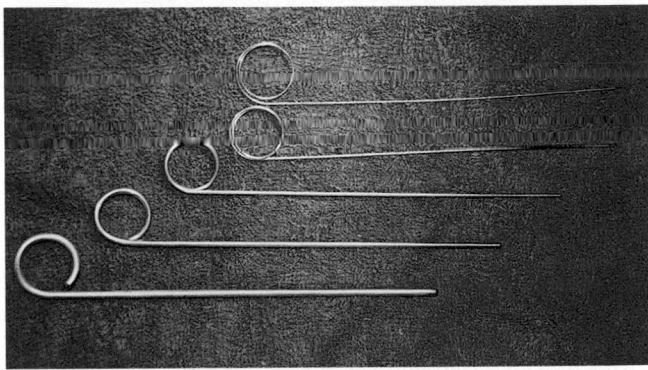

Figure 18-16 Snake cloacal probes for sexing.

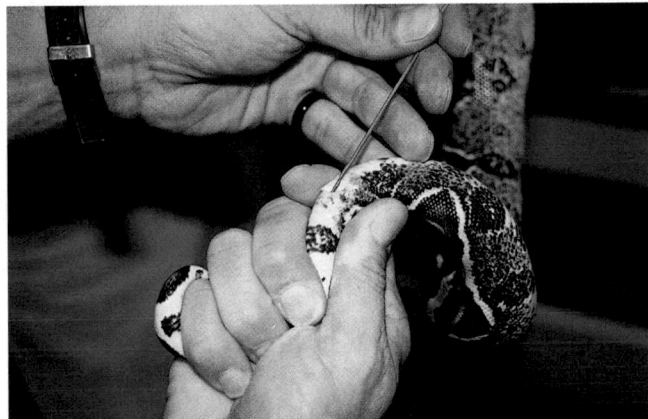

Figure 18-17 Snake being sexed with cloacal probe.

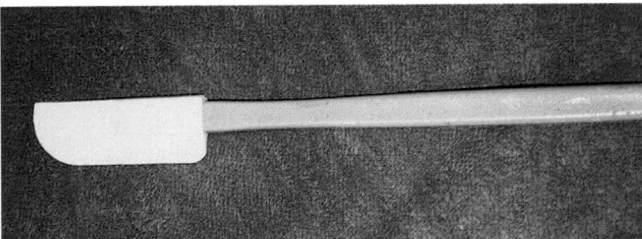

Figure 18-18 A spatula is often used as a reptile oral specula.

patches on turtle shell repair and toward fracture fixation using cerclage wire and open wound healing. We have found that a combination of both the cerclage fixation of fragments and protection of the fracture site with epoxy resin lead to faster healing and release. Surgical equipment used for reptiles but available in most exotic animal practices includes a Dremel Motor Tool, stainless steel suture material, transparent surgical drapes, and a magnifying surgical headset.

Reptile housing equipment must be adaptable to the different species that may be hospitalized. Examples of hospital caging and equipment include fluorescent light tubes (regular and full spectrum), humidifier, fiberglass cages, small aquaria with secure ventilated tops, a heated room, or heat lamps and pads. To aid in capture and restraint, a snake hook, tongs, Plexiglas tubes, and pole snare should be available. As with other exotic species, proper restraint reduces stress to the client, animal, and health care personnel. Once a practice is properly equipped and personnel are trained, interesting patients and cases will begin to receive quality health care.

TAKING THE CLINICAL HISTORY

The following is a list of questions to ask clients regarding reptile patients:

- *Chief complaint:* Why does the owner want the pet examined?

- *Signalment* (including the species as specifically as possible): What is the age and gender of the animal, and how long has the client owned the animal?
- *Origin:* Where did the animal come from?
- *Environment:* Factors such as cage design, construction materials, substrates, perches, or branches are of critical importance in determining the health of these species. Temperature and humidity, as well as photo period and exposure to sunlight or full spectrum artificial light may have a significant impact on the animal's health. The owner should be questioned as to where the cage is kept in the house, as well as the type of heat source used and the usual temperature gradient within the cage. For

aquatic species, questions pertaining to water quality control, filter systems used, sources of water, and frequency of water change are important. Owner need to list types of cleaning agents and disinfectants being used and the frequency of use.

- *Food:* How often is food offered? How much is consumed? What is the source of the food? How is the food stored, and how is it presented to the animal?
- *Water:* How often is the water cleaned or changed? How is it offered to the animal? If a water bowl is used, how large is it? For many species, it is important to offer water in a bowl large enough for the animals to completely submerge.
- *Feces:* How often does the animal defecate in relation to feeding? What are the color and consistency of the stool? Has the owner submitted a fecal sample previously for parasite evaluation?
- *Cage mates:* Does the client have other animals in his or her collection or in the same cage? If so, what species are they, and where are they kept: Does the owner maintain a quarantine policy? If so, for how long?
- *Behavior:* What are the current attitude and behavior of the patient, and have there been any recent changes?
- *Shedding:* For lizards and snakes, how often does the animal shed? When was the last period of shedding or ecdysis?
- *Previous medical history:* Has the animal been ill previously? If it has, it is important to get the owner to describe its illness and any treatments that were done. It is often helpful to include the attending veterinarian's name. Have other animals in the collection ever been ill?

SAMPLE COLLECTION AND DIAGNOSTIC PROCEDURES

Diagnostic approaches in reptiles are often similar to those of other small animal species. As with any diagnostic procedure, ability through experience and confidence determines who will collect the sample needed from the patient. Any of the procedures listed in this section can be mastered by the technician who has the proper sampling equipment and desire.

Colonic Wash

Fecal samples may be collected and examined for gastrointestinal parasites. A fresh sample should be examined under a wet mount, and fecal flotation and sedimentation should be evaluated. If a fecal sample is not available at the time of the examination, specimens may be collected by performing a colonic wash; this is done by passing a lubricated tube or catheter through the cloaca into the colon. A syringe of sterile saline is attached, and a typical flush is performed. The volume of saline is recommended at a volume of 1% or less of the animal's weight. Samples may then be examined for parasites or parasite eggs or prepared for cytology or culture and sensitivity tests.

Bone Marrow

Large lizards, crocodilians, and some other chelonians yield adequate diagnostic bone marrow specimens from their femoral cavities (Frye, 1995). Bone marrow from turtles and tortoises may also be obtained by drilling a hole between the outer and inner layers of the bony shell and using a biopsy needle (Vim-Silverman, Becton-Dickinson Primary Care Diagnostics) to obtain the sample (Frye, 1995). The hole should be patched with epoxy or acrylic resin (Frye, 1995). Snake diagnostic bone marrow specimens may be obtained from the marrow cavities in their ribs.

Stomach Lavage

To examine the upper gastrointestinal tract, especially for identification of cryptosporidiosis, a stomach wash is often performed. This procedure is well tolerated by most reptiles and is a quick and easy procedure to execute in the clinic. A lubricated soft rubber catheter is advanced through the mouth into the stomach after premeasuring alongside the animal. The stomach area is in the midcranial body area, and this location should be used as a reference point for tube placement length. A syringe containing sterile isotonic saline is attached to the catheter, and a simple flush is performed after agitating the stomach with external palpation. Samples obtained are used for direct microscopic examination for parasites, to prepare slides for cytology, or to perform Gram stains for culture and sensitivities.

Urine Samples

Urine samples may be collected from those species that produce a large volume of urine. Many turtles and lizards have urinary bladders. All reptiles have a cloaca into which the reproductive, gastrointestinal, and urinary tracts empty. A routine urinalysis may be performed on fresh urine samples. A cystocentesis may be performed on turtles by advancing a needle cranial to the hind limb. Turtles will typically void when stressed; thus handling the patient may yield a urine sample. Green-stained solid urates rehydrated with saline may reveal amoebic cysts or fluke ova when examined under a microscope.

BLOOD SAMPLES

Blood collection in reptiles varies considerably, depending on the species. Do not withdraw more blood than is necessary. If you are not sure of the volume needed, contact your diagnostic laboratory. Direct cardiocentesis and venipuncture using the ventral and lateral caudal veins, jugular, brachial, popliteal, periorbital, pterygopalatine, and dorsal postoccipital sinuses can be used depending on the species and size of the animal (Frye, 1995). Toenail clipping is not recommended for blood sample collection because of the inability to obtain reliable hematologic results from this site.

Venipuncture techniques in snakes depend on the experience of the handler. Sites that are often used include

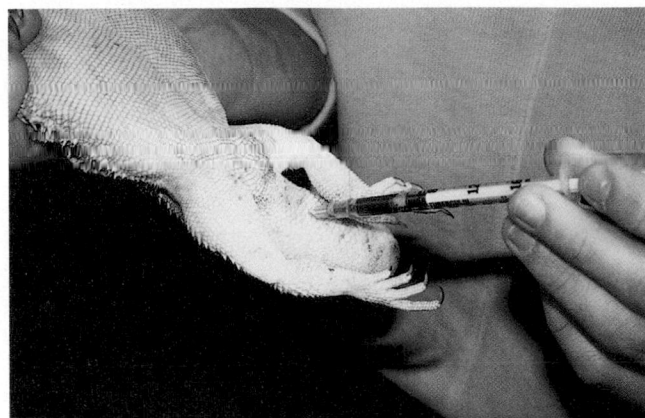

Figure 18-19 Restraint of a bearded dragon for venipuncture using the tail vein.

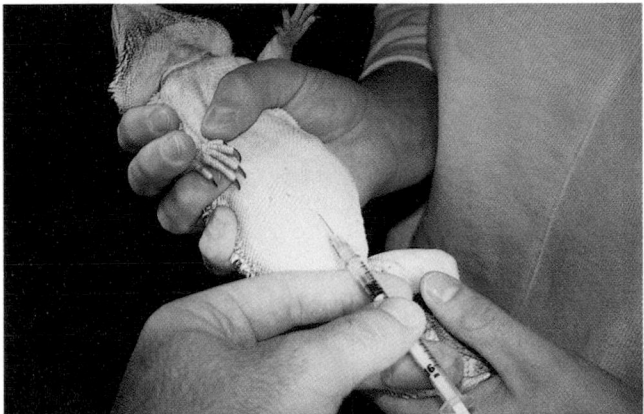

Figure 18-20 Venipuncture from the ventral abdominal vein.

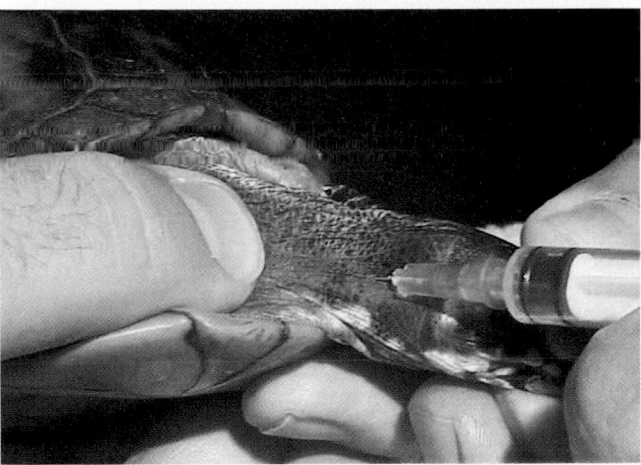

Figure 18-21 Jugular venipuncture in a box turtle. The jugular veins are located dorsally at the 10 o'clock and 2 o'clock positions.

the caudal or coccygeal vein of the tail, cardiac puncture, and the ventral abdominal vein or palatine vessels. For blood collection at any site, good restraint of the patient is necessary. For lizards, the caudal tail vein is often most accessible; however, cardiac puncture and the ventral abdominal vein may also be used (Figures 18-19 and 18-20). In turtles, large jugular veins are present and are easily used for venipuncture sites (Figure 18-21).

In large crocodilians, turtles, and tortoises, the occipital sinus or the caudal tail vein may be used. The site chosen will depend on the veterinarian and the technician and their experience with the particular species being tested. In small lizards, the peribulbar and retrobulbar plexuses may be used for blood samples by inserting a heparinized microhematocrit tube between the eyelids and directing it to the inner edge of the orbit. Rotating the tube will damage the plexus, yielding enough blood to fill the collection device.

RADIOGRAPHY

Radiography often is useful to aid in the diagnosis of reptile patients. For many species, radiographs may be taken on

unsedated animals by restraining them in shallow boxes, acrylic tubes, or canvas bags. It is important to remember to take at least two views. With turtles a third (frontal) view should also be taken. Contrast studies may be done, and barium sulfate is easily administered; however, gastrointestinal transit times are long, and it may take 1 week to complete a gastrointestinal barium study. Various other diagnostic procedures may be used, according to the preference of the veterinarian. The technician's knowledge of restraint and reptile behavior will aid in any immobilization process.

HUSBANDRY IN THE HOSPITAL

Reptiles require a controlled microenvironment in a hospital setting. It is important to remember that temperature and humidity are important because these animals are poikilothermic; that is, they depend on their environment to regulate their body temperature. A temperature gradient should be provided whenever possible by using a thermostat at each end of the cage, resulting in a cooler end and a warmer end. For most species, temperatures should not exceed 32° C (90° F) or dip below 24° C (75° F). Humidity is the other important environmental consideration that is determined by species-specific requirements. In general the majority of captive reptile species accommodate well in humidity ranges of 50% to 70%. The technician must remember that jungle species usually require a higher humidity while desert species do better in lower humidity ranges.

🔷 TECHNICIAN NOTE

In general the majority of captive reptile species accommodate well in humidity ranges of 50% to 70%. The technician must remember that jungle species usually require a higher humidity while desert species do better in lower humidity ranges.

It is important that hospitalized reptiles are maintained at the upper end of their temperature gradient during convalescence to aid in recovery. For many species, a variety of aquaria are sufficient for short-term hospitalization. Any substrate used should be one that is easily cleaned and disinfected or disposable, such as newspaper. It is important to house reptiles separately from psittacine birds, in particular, to avoid contamination of birds from the normal gram-negative flora of most reptiles. Cages should be provided with hide boxes or areas of seclusion, as well as perching for some species, such as iguanas and some snakes.

> ✏ **TECHNICIAN NOTE**
>
> It is important that hospitalized reptiles are maintained at the upper end of their temperature gradient during convalescence to aid in recovery.

Tube feeding is an important technique for the veterinary technician to learn. Supplemental feed administration using a tube is easily accomplished, even by technicians without much experience with reptiles. A tube should be well lubricated and then passed the distance necessary to place it in the stomach. The glottis of reptiles is adjacent to the base of the tongue and is easily avoided. The glottis of snakes may actually be extended by the animal outside the mouth to accommodate large prey items. The tube is gently passed all the way to the stomach, and food injected. Fluids may also be administered by this route. For patients that are anorectic, supplemental tube feeding may be accomplished by using a blended formula of food that is appropriate for the species being cared for. There are also commercial critical care supplements (Walkabout Farm, Pembroke, Virginia) available that can be tube fed to herbivorous, carnivorous, and insectivorous species after reconstitution with water. Dietary references for reptile species are listed in Recommended Reading. It is imperative that the technician become familiar with proper reptile diets to maintain healthy animals and supplement sick patients.

Injections given to reptiles are usually performed on the cranial half of the animal's body, primarily the epaxial muscles and the muscles of the forelimbs (e.g., *biceps brachii* and long heads of the *triceps brachii*) (Figure 18-22). This is due to the renal portal system that routes blood from the caudal third of the body through a capillary network into the kidneys before returning it to general circulation. It is important to refrain from giving nephrotoxic drugs in the caudal third of the reptile patient's body. Injection sites are easily found in all reptile species, either in the forelimbs or in the epaxial musculature of the snake. Oral medications are easily given using a stomach tube. Liquids are preferred over tablets, which are not consistently absorbed.

> ✏ **TECHNICIAN NOTE**
>
> It is important to refrain from giving nephrotoxic drugs in the caudal third of the reptile patient's body.

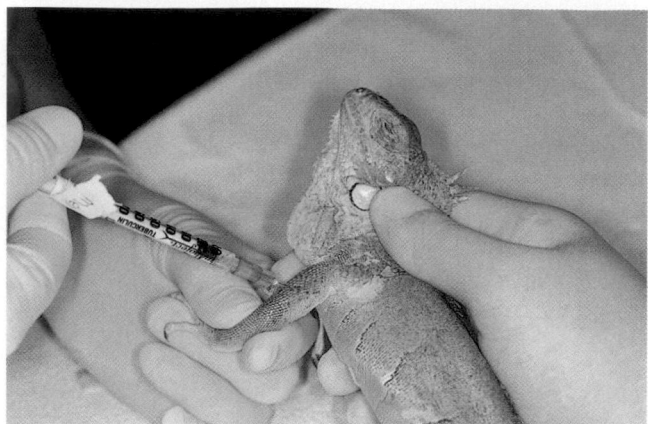

Figure 18-22 Injection into the forelimb of an iguana.

Dietary requirements vary tremendously from species to species and may be an important factor in the disease of the patient. Dietary deficiencies are not commonly seen in snakes, which eat a whole-animal diet; however, a variety of dietary deficiencies are commonly seen in lizards, turtles, and crocodilians. One of the most common is metabolic bone disease. Metabolic bone disease is caused by inappropriately low calcium intake, low vitamin D_3 intake, or excessive phosphorous intake (Figure 18-23). This may be prevented by a suitable diet and exposing the animal to ultraviolet light, either naturally or artificially. It is essential that reptiles, especially lizards, have full-spectrum light available during normal daylight hours. Sunlight through glass does not provide the needed light supplementation due to the blocking ability of glass; direct sunlight or the appropriate artificial lighting is needed. Animals with metabolic bone disease must be treated very gently because their bones are subject to pathologic fractures. Vitamin A deficiency is commonly seen in turtles and tortoises and usually manifests itself by overgrown beak, palpebral edema, and conjunctivitis. This underscores the importance of thoroughly researching the dietary history of the reptile patient.

> ✏ **TECHNICIAN NOTE**
>
> It is essential that reptiles, especially lizards, have full-spectrum light available during normal daylight hours.

SKIN

There are clinical dermatologic diseases noted in reptilian species as in other animals. Proper diagnostic techniques are needed to identify the problem to implement the appropriate treatment.

Skin specimens may be cultured for bacterial and fungal organisms. For fungal identification, dermatophyte test medium (DTM) fungal growth medium or Sabouraud's

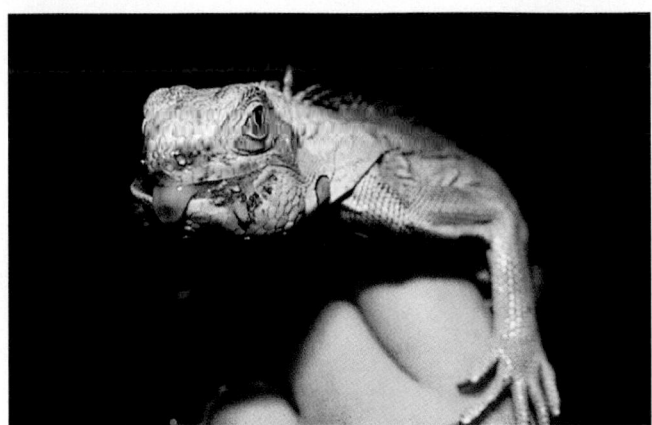

Figure 18-23 Metabolic bone disease in a lizard caused by an improper diet.

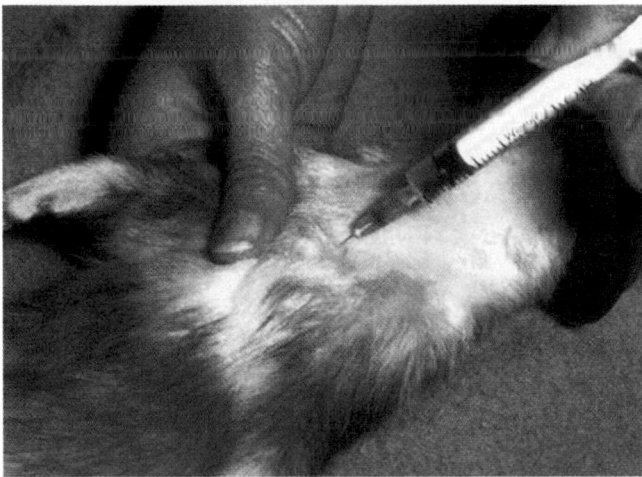

Figure 18-24 Cranial vena cava venipuncture of an anesthetized ferret with its head in an anesthetic mask.

culture media may be used. Bacterial organisms may be isolated on blood agar or subcultured in a thioglycollate-containing medium. Samples for skin culture may be taken using cotton-tipped Culturettes or by using pieces of the affected skin, scales, or dermal scutes.

FECES

Fecal material can be very useful in diagnosing parasite infestations, bacterial infections, pancreatic enzyme levels, and the presence of blood in the gastrointestinal tract. The fecal specimen should be as fresh as possible. If a fresh voided sample is not available, then fecal material may be removed from the terminal alimentary tract by gentle palpation or by the insertion of a fecal extractor or cotton-tipped applicator stick through the cloacal vent (Boyer, 1998). The aid of a warm water enema may stimulate defecation in difficult cases. As with the colonic wash, an enema of 1% or less of the animal's body weight is recommend as the fluid volume to use for most captive reptile species.

SPUTUM

To obtain a sample of sputum, insert a cotton-tipped applicator into the discharge. Roll the sample applicator across a microscope slide, add a drop of coloring agent, apply a coverslip, and examine for parasite ova (Boyer, 1998). Common parasites diagnosed in sputum samples are *Rhabdias* spp., *Entomelas* spp., and *Stronglyloides stercoralis*. When handling diagnostic samples, proper hygiene is essential because of the zoonotic potential of many animal diseases and parasites.

ZOONOSES AND COMMON CLINICAL PROBLEMS

The technician should be aware of common zoonotic infections and clinical problems associated with reptiles (see Chapter 35).

SMALL MAMMALS

FERRETS

Ferrets have been gaining in popularity as a companion animal. As ferrets gain popularity they are also seen with increasing frequency in veterinarians' offices; thus it is imperative that technicians become familiar with these pets.

Ferrets do not have retractable claws, but they do have a vascular "quick" delineation that can be used as a point to trim. Small nail trim scissors or human nail clips are recommended for ferret nail trims. If bleeding occurs after a nail trim, silver nitrate sticks can be used for chemical cautery. Ferret nails are sharp, and owners often request nail trims to blunt the claws.

When obtaining sample collections of blood, physical restraint alone is often inadequate. Chemical restraint therefore is commonly employed. Blood samples are drawn from the jugular vein, the cranial vena cava, or the cephalic vein. To draw samples of blood from these sites, the animal's head must be securely restrained and grasped around the neck with thumb and fingers resting on the mandibles. To position an animal for jugular venipuncture, it is often best to stretch the animal out, using the other hand to grasp the hind limbs. The ferret's thick skin and subcutaneous fat make blood collection from the jugular vein difficult. To draw adequate blood samples, the cranial vena cava may be preferred (Figure 18-24).

TECHNICIAN NOTE

The ferret's thick skin and subcutaneous fat make blood collection from the jugular vein difficult. To collect adequate blood samples, the cranial vena cava may be preferred.

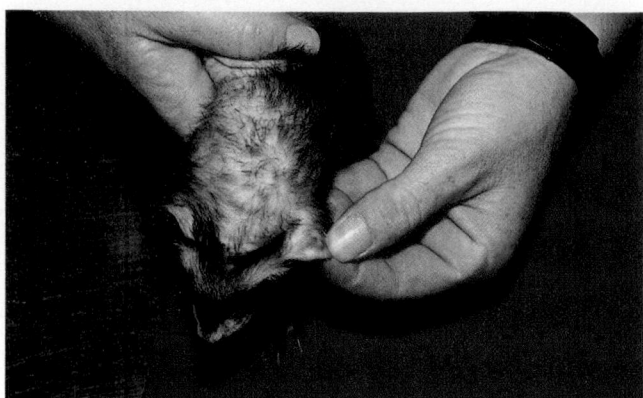

Figure 18-25 A tattooed dot indicates this is an early spay/neuter/descented ferret.

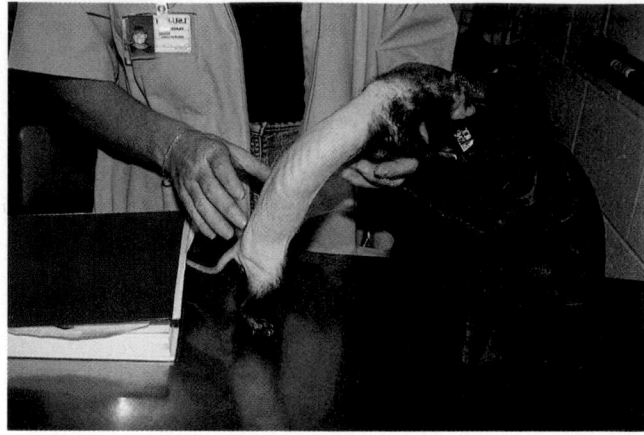

Figure 18-27 Hair loss in a ferret due to adrenal gland disease.

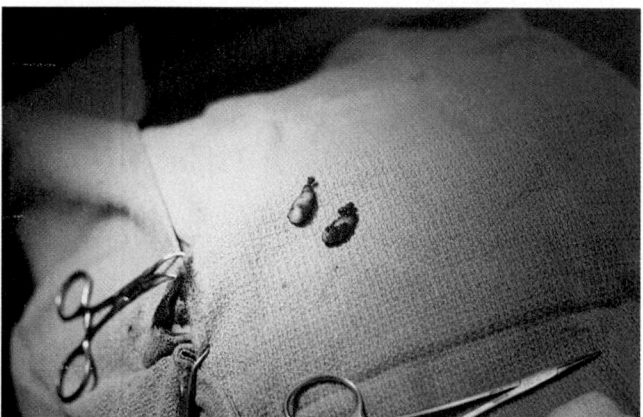

Figure 18-26 Anal sacs removed from a ferret.

Ketamine hydrochloride or gas anesthetic agents such as halothane or isoflurane may be used for chemical restraint. When using gas anesthesia, an induction chamber is recommended for induction. The patient may be removed from this chamber as it loses the ability to right itself. Anesthesia may then be continued with the use of a face mask. Sample collection on the anesthetized animal is much easier, safer, and less stressful to the animal. Urine may be obtained by cystocentesis because the bladder is easily palpated. If desired, for prolonged anesthesia, ferrets are easily intubated with small standard endotracheal tubes or Cole tubes.

Strategies for treating ferrets in the clinic revolve around the handler's ability to restrain the animal and perform the treatment in the most efficient and quickest manner possible. For giving drugs, Nutrical, dairy products, and sweets are useful in bribing animals and in hiding medications. Most ferrets will do almost anything for yogurt or ice cream. Liquid medications are much easier to administer than pills.

A potentially fatal common clinical problem of the ferret is estrogen toxicity in females as a result of prolonged estrus. Female ferrets are induced ovulators and occasionally will not cycle out of heat unless bred. These animals then become severely anemic and thrombocytopenic because of the toxic effects of estrogen on the bone marrow. Ferrets often present with signs of lethargy, dyspnea, petechial hemorrhages, vomiting, and diarrhea. This is best treated by prevention and client education. Female ferrets not intended for breeding should be spayed before their first heat. Since most ferrets in the United States have been spayed and descented prior to purchase, this is not a concern with most owners. Ferrets that have been spayed/neutered and descented by a breeding facility at an early age will have one or two tattooed blue dots on the surface of the pinna (Figure 18-25). When an owner talks of descenting a ferret, the procedure involves surgically removing the two anal scent glands of the animal. The two anal scent gland openings are located at the 4 and 8 o'clock position when the anal mucocutaneous junction is slightly everted (Figure 18-26). Most ferrets have had the anal scent glands removed prior to purchase (look for the ear tattoo) but still have a musky odor. Shampooing the ferret on a regular basis will reduce the musky smell but not eliminate the odor. Ferret-specific shampoo and cologne products are recommended and can be purchased at most large retail pet outlets.

TECHNICIAN NOTE

Ferrets that have been spayed/neutered and descented by a breeding facility at an early age will have one or two tattooed blue dots in the inside surface of the pinna.

Clinical signs similar to those of prolonged estrus include hair loss and a swollen vulva, which may be caused by adrenal hyperplasia (Figures 18-27 and 18-28). Female ferrets that have been spayed at an early age are extremely susceptible to this clinical condition. An adrenal hyperplasia workup should be performed on an older spayed female ferret exhibiting signs of vulvar swelling. Adrenal hyperplasia can be treated by a partial adrenalectomy and/or administration of therapeutic agents (e.g., leuprolide acetate). Response to therapy and surgery has been varied.

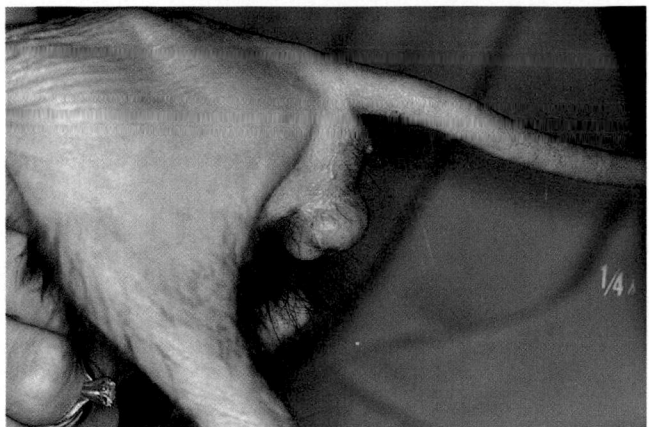

Figure 18-28 Swollen vulva in ferret due to adrenal gland disease.

Ferrets are susceptible to human influenza, and therefore clients should be counseled when members of the family have influenza the ferret should not be handled. Human influenza in a ferret must be differentiated from canine distemper and bacterial pneumonia, to which ferrets are also susceptible. Both present with similar signs of respiratory disease: nasal and ocular discharges, coughing, and sneezing. The ferret with influenza will, in most cases, recover from the infection on its own in 5 to 10 days. Topical antihistamines and decongestants may be of benefit. The nonvaccinated ferret will not survive a canine distemper infection, and signs usually progress to severe dyspnea, anorexia, and sometimes involvement of the central nervous system.

> ### 🖋 TECHNICIAN NOTE
> A potentially fatal common clinical problem of the ferret is estrogen toxicity in females caused by prolonged estrus.
>   The nonvaccinated ferret will not survive a canine distemper infection.

Parasites are a problem that must be understood by the ferret owner. Heartworm prevention is required in animals that are maintained in an outdoor enclosure where they are exposed to mosquitoes. Fleas commonly plague ferrets, even if maintained within a household setting. Feline flea control products are generally safe to use on flea-infested animals. Ear mite treatment and control and heartworm prevention are also important issues that need to be addressed with the owner (see Chapter 7).

Ferrets are also fond of chewing on objects, preferably soft rubbery toys, and should be watched closely for foreign body ingestion. A ferret that presents with signs of anorexia should be considered to have a potential gastrointestinal obstruction. Toys for ferrets should be limited to objects they cannot bite or "ferret tubes" in which they can crawl. Ferrets have very strong jaws and sharp teeth; therefore there are few leather or rubber objects that they cannot bite and eventually swallow. There are also many reports of various neoplastic diseases in ferrets, including insulinomas,

osteomas, lymphosarcomas, and fibrosarcomas. If a ferret presents depressed or moribund, a blood serum glucose test should be performed because of common hypoglycemia.

Ferrets should be vaccinated for canine distemper using the PUREVAX ferret canine distemper vaccine (Merial, Duluth, Georgia). The American Ferret Association, Inc. (AFA), recommends that 1 ml of the vaccine be injected subcutaneously in healthy ferrets at 8, 11, and 14 weeks of age and then annually. If the ferrets are over 14 weeks of age or with an unknown or outdated vaccine history, a series of two vaccines should be given 2 weeks apart then annually on the anniversary of the first booster. In cases were kits are exposed, the vaccine may be given as young as 6 weeks of age. Ferrets are not susceptible to feline panleukopenia and therefore should not be vaccinated. In many jurisdictions ferrets are required to have a rabies vaccine and tag, although they are often not required to wear the tag. It is unlikely that an indoor ferret will be exposed to the rabies virus, but the IMRAB-3 rabies vaccine (Rhone Merieux, Inc., Athens, Georgia) will protect the ferret in the event of exposure and support its quarantine if a person is bitten. The AFA recommends that all ferrets be vaccinated against the rabies virus. Other preventive medicine measures regarding ferrets include good dental care and surveillance for gastrointestinal parasites. Ferrets are strict carnivores and should be feed a diet that meets their unique nutritional requirements. There are a number of commercially available diets that will provide the proper nutrition for the pet ferret. If the ferret diets are not available, a high-quality cat food may be used. Although a cat food diet may be slightly low in protein requirements for the pregnant or lactating ferret, few problems have been reported in ferrets eating high-quality cat food diets.

> ### 🖋 TECHNICIAN NOTE
> Ferrets should never be vaccinated against canine distemper using a vaccine of ferret cell origin.

Administration of fluids in a ferret that is <5% dehydrated may be administered *per os* or subcutaneously, whereas an indwelling intravenous catheter should be placed in any animal that is >5% dehydrated. Subcutaneous fluids may be administered in the subcutaneous space between the shoulder blades. The cephalic and lateral saphenous veins are routine sites for intravenous catheter placement.

Fecal samples are often voluntarily given by patients prior to or during an examination. If a fecal sample needs to be obtained, a lubricated small feline fecal loop will often provide a sufficient sample for test evaluation.

RABBITS

The rabbit is not a rodent but rather a lagomorph of the family Leporidae. Rabbits may be housed indoors or

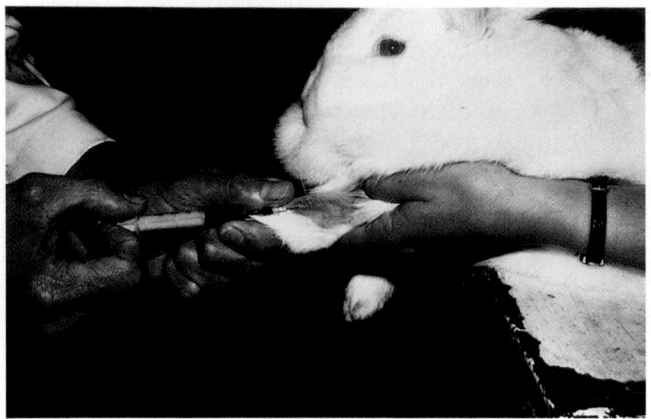

Figure 18-29 Blood collection from cephalic vein of rabbit.

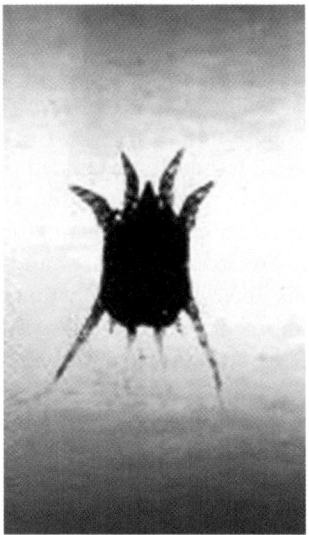

Figure 18-30 Microscopic view of *Psoroptes cuniculi*, the rabbit ear mite.

outdoors and fed primarily a grass-based diet (Oxbow Enterprises, Murdock, Nebraska) with supplemented grass-based pellets. Rabbits come in many sizes, ranging from the Flemish Giant (6 to 7.5 kg) to the Dutch and Polish breeds (1 to 2 kg). If proper husbandry practices are maintained, a pet rabbit should live a long, healthy life (5 to 6 years). Rabbits are sensitive to extreme hot and cold conditions, but primarily heat.

Rabbits defend themselves by using their long incisors to bite and by kicking with the hind legs. When kicking, their sharp claws can seriously injure the handler. Owners often inquire about "declawing" their rabbit, but this surgical procedure is strongly discouraged. To sex the rabbit, stretching the perineum while the animal is in dorsal recumbency will reveal the anogenital area. Males have a round urethral opening; females have a slit opening.

The rabbit that is a candidate for anesthesia should have food withheld for 8 to 12 hours and be free from respiratory disease. Some breeds of rabbits have atropinesterase, which inactivates atropine. Atropine may be given subcutaneously as a preanesthetic to decrease salivation. If a rabbit has atropinesterase, it may be necessary to increase the dose of atropine. Rabbits are seldom intubated during anesthesia because they rarely regurgitate and are extremely difficult to intubate. Recommended endotracheal tubes in rabbits have inside diameters of 2 to 4 mm. A medium laryngoscope or rigid endoscope will aid in passing the tube into the rabbit's glottis to near the thoracic inlet. Do not use a topical anesthetic on rabbits to prevent laryngospasm.

> **✏ TECHNICIAN NOTE**
>
> Rabbits are seldom intubated during anesthesia because they rarely regurgitate and are difficult to intubate.

Injectable anesthetic agents used in rabbits include ketamine, xylazine, and acepromazine; isoflurane is the inhalation anesthetic agent of choice. The movement of the nictitating membrane over approximately one third of the cornea, a respiratory rate of 18 to 24 respirations per minute, abdominal musculature relaxation, and the loss of the ear, mouth, toe pinch, and palpebral reflexes indicate a suitable plane of surgical anesthesia in the rabbit.

By placing a rabbit in dorsal recumbency and gently stroking its ventrum, one causes hypnosis to occur. Hypnosis is a good restraint for injections and radiographic procedures.

When giving intravenous injections to rabbits, the dorsal surface of the ear should be shaved to expose the marginal ear vein. Visibility of this vein will increase if alcohol is rubbed on the area. The central artery of the ear or the cephalic or lateral saphenous vein can also be used for bleeding (Figure 18-29). Cardiac puncture for blood collection should be used only under strict professional supervision and only as a last resort in the clinical setting. The lateral saphenous vein, which is located higher on the leg than in dogs, may be used to place an indwelling catheter.

Rabbits are affected by a number of infections and parasitic organisms. A pet rabbit may be presented for hair loss caused by self-trauma, nutritional deficiencies, bacterial dermatitis (*Pasteurella multocida*, *Pseudomonas aeruginosa*, *Staphylococcus aureus*, and *Fusobacterium*), or parasites (ear mite *Psoroptes cuniculi* [Figures 18-30 and 18-31], fur mite *Cheyletiella parasitovorax*, and rabbit lice *Haemodipsus ventricosus*]. Flea prevention and control is also needed for rabbits, especially animals that are maintained outside (see Chapter 7). Ulcerative lesions on the ventral surface of the rear hocks are usually due to poor husbandry or environmental pressures. Fungal organisms that have been noted to cause dermatopathies in rabbits are *Microsporum gypseum* and *Trichophyton mentagrophytes*.

An anorexic pet should be examined for malocclusion, hair balls, trauma, dietary change, stress, dysbiosis, or poor feed. Heat stress (stroke) is common when adequate cooling is not provided in the summer. Diarrhea may be caused by colibacillosis, rotavirus infections, *Clostridium* infections,

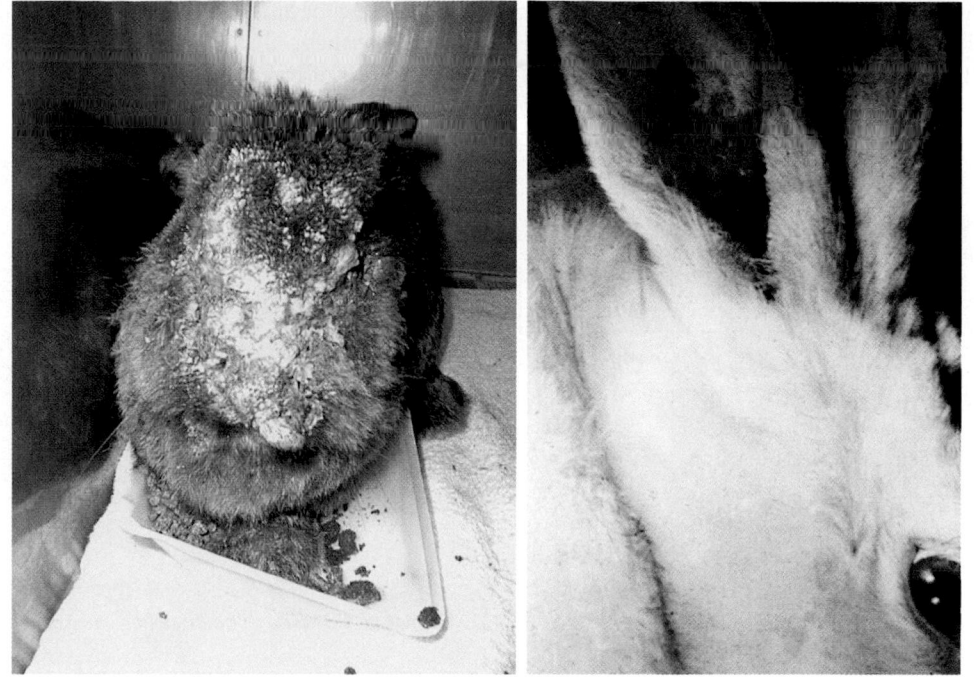

Figure 18-31 **A,** Rabbit exhibiting severe clinical signs of *Psoroptes cuniculi* infestation, extending to the face. **B.** *P. cuniculi* infestation in external ear canal of rabbit.

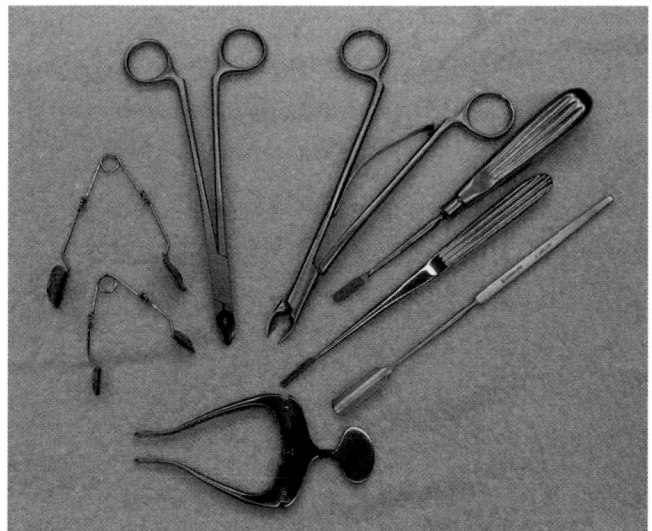

Figure 18-32 Rabbit dental instruments.

mucoid enteropathy, antibiotic intake, or Tyzzer's disease *(Bacillus piliformis)*. A high-fiber diet, which includes timothy hay, has been shown to improve digestive tract function and reduce incidence of hair balls.

One of the main disease problems in rabbits is *Pasteurella multocida* infection (snuffles). Clinical signs include nasal discharge, torticollis, abscesses, conjunctivitis, and respiratory distress. Venereal spirochetosis should always be considered when rabbits are exhibiting infertility. *Eimeria stieda* is a hepatic coccidium that may affect attitude and eating habits.

Rabbits are territorial and fight when sexual maturity is reached or a male is placed in a female's cage for breeding. Neutering or ovariohysterectomy is recommended to prevent unwanted offspring.

Malocclusion often leads to elongated incisors and sharp enamel points on the molars. Rabbit-specific dental instruments should be used (Jorgensen Laboratories, Loveland, Colorado) to reduce teeth fracture and other complications associated with dental procedures (Figure 18-32). Most teeth-trimming procedures are done under general anesthesia, particularly when a Dremel Motor Tool is used. Gingival, lingual, and buccal lacerations are the primary complications when trimming molars. To access the oral cavity when trimming molars a nose cone is used to maintain gas anesthesia, and buccal specula are recommended.

RODENTS

Rodent species commonly presented to the veterinary hospital include guinea pigs, hamsters, gerbils, rats, and to a lesser extent mice. Although all of these animals are rodents, each species has particular anatomic characteristics, dietary requirements, and diseases.

ANTIBIOTICS IN RODENTS

Care must be taken when prescribing antibiotics to rodents. Guinea pigs, rabbits, and hamsters are extremely sensitive to the penicillin class of antibiotics, which may cause severe intestinal flora changes (dysbiosis); penicillins, streptomycin, and dihydrostreptomycin are drugs that may cause this problem. Tetracyclines work well in cases that require antibiotic therapy. An exotic animal formulary is essential to an exotic animal practice to obtain specific information and dosage.

✎ **TECHNICIAN NOTE**

Guinea pigs, rabbits, and hamsters are extremely sensitive to penicillin antibiotics.

ANESTHETICS IN RODENTS

Ketamine hydrochloride, pentobarbital sodium, and thiamylal sodium are injectable anesthetic agents that may be used in rodents. Isoflurane is the anesthetic agent of choice, providing quick induction and recovery while providing an adequate plane of anesthesia. Chapter 19 discusses anesthesiology.

ANTIPARASITIC AGENTS IN RODENTS

Carbaryl powder, dichlorvos, and ivermectin can be used to treat ectoparasites. Dichlorvos, thiabendazole, and ivermectin are adequate to treat internal parasites. See Chapter 7 for additional information on parasitology.

ZOONOTIC DISEASES

Some of the zoonotic diseases found in rodents are listed in Chapter 35.

GUINEA PIG

The cavy, or guinea pig, is a rodent related to porcupines and chinchillas. Guinea pigs have a long gestation that leads to birth of large, precocious young. The most common guinea pig species kept as pets are the English or American, Abyssinian, and Peruvian long hair (Figures 18-33 and 18-34). The guinea pig has open-rooted teeth that may become maloccluded (Figure 18-35). The overgrown teeth

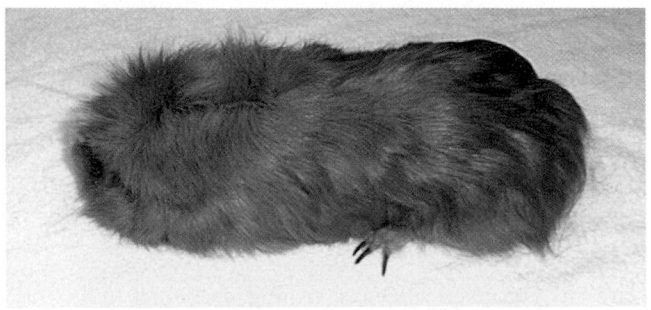

Figure 18-33 An Abyssinian guinea pig.

will irritate the gingiva, causing excessive salivation. Although the female has only two mammary glands, it can successfully raise litters of three or more offspring.

A female guinea pig that is bred past 7 or 8 months of age may have trouble separating the pubic symphysis, causing a nondeliverable dystocia. Fat pads may also occlude

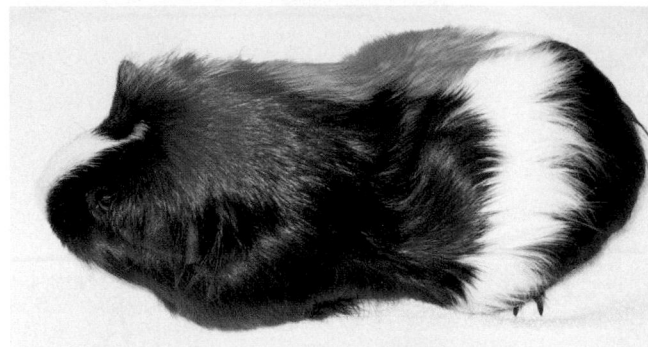

Figure 18-34 The English guinea pig, a common house pet.

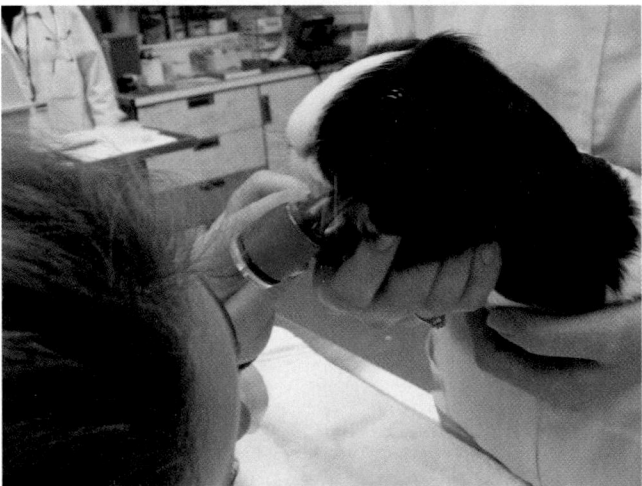

Figure 18-35 An otoscope with a disposable head may be used to examine a guinea pig's premolars and molars.

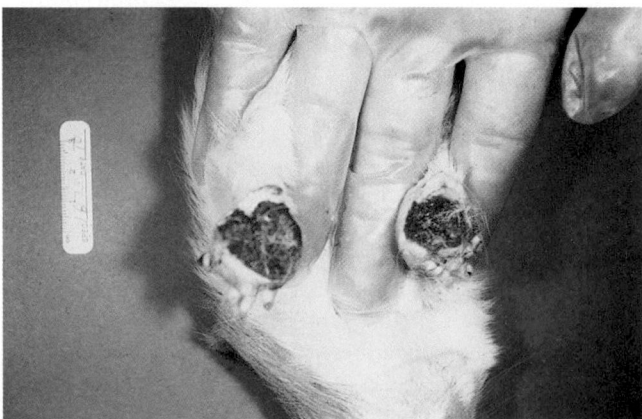

Figure 18-36 Footpad dermatitis is a common problem that affects guinea pigs.

the pelvic canal, complicating parturition. These problems usually lead to dystocia or death. If the sow is experiencing dystocia, a cesarean retrieval of the young can often save the babies. Food preferences are established within a few days after birth for the young. Hand-rearing of the young requires regular stimulation of the anus for defecation and urethral opening for urination as with most neonatal mammals. Females usually allow foster nursing of other young.

Guinea pigs rarely become excited or bite when handled. Through their gentle nature, they become conditioned to their surroundings. However, if a group is contained in an enclosure, subordinate animals may be traumatized (as by hair loss and bite wounds) by dominate cage mates.

Footpad dermatitis resulting in ulcers may develop on animals placed on wire (Figure 18-36). Metal, plastic, and glass make excellent cages for guinea pigs. Substrate may be paper (shredded), wood shavings, or hay. Chewing their substrate is a vice commonly associated when animals develop submandibular abscesses. Hard fibrous splinters penetrate the oral mucosa, inoculating the tissue with bacteria (usually *Streptococcus zooepidemicus*) that develop into abscesses. Changes in the substrate may be indicated to stop this problem, although it may be difficult to find an adequate alternative substrate, which must have absorptive qualities for the opaque, pale yellow, crystalline urine.

The feed and water are best placed in bowls that cannot be chewed (e.g., stainless steel or ceramic crocks). A vitamin C supplementation may be added to the water, such as Tang (General Foods Corp.). The food should be a freshly milled complete guinea pig ration. Storage in a freezer or refrigerator will extend the life of the food. All food and water containers should be placed above the substrate to prevent soiling.

Unlike other pet rodents, guinea pigs require dietary vitamin C supplementation. Vitamin C is highly unstable in the feed, especially when exposed to heat. Use of old feed is one of the primary reasons vitamin C deficiencies are seen.

TECHNICIAN NOTE

Unlike other pet rodents, guinea pigs require dietary vitamin C supplementation.

The cavy requires 0.5 mg/kg body weight dietary ascorbic acid per day because it lacks ʟ-gulonolactone oxidase. Published dosages of vitamin C for guinea pigs are 1 to 30 mg/kg intramuscularly twice daily or 200 to 400 mg/L in drinking water (freshly mixed daily). Guinea pigs *must* be fed species-specific food within 90 days of milling. Fruit and vegetable supplementation is discouraged because of the possibility of disturbing the normal gut bacterial flora.

To sex a guinea pig, the handler must observe the urethral orifice and anus. The male has no break in the ridge between the openings, whereas the female has a shallow U-shaped break.

One boar will service up to 10 sows beginning at 8 weeks of age. The sow becomes sexually mature around 5 to 6 weeks of age. Gestation length is on average 63 to 68 days, with litter size ranging from one to six precocious offspring.

HAMSTER

The golden hamster is a native of Syria and comes in many different color varieties (Figure 18-37). Cheek pouches that extend along the head and neck to the proximal dorsum of the back serve as a food transportation device. Along the caudal lateral abdominal region lie the flank glands. A dark brown patch of skin on each side delineates these sebaceous glands that are used to mark territory and in mating rituals (Figure 18-38).

Hamsters have a tendency to bite and are good at chewing through cage material. To accommodate the animal's physical nature, an exercise wheel should be placed in the cage.

Female hamsters often attack newly introduced males and females. Hamsters live 18 to 24 months, have a gestation length of 16 days, and produce about five offspring. Young hamsters are weaned in 20 to 25 days. If disturbed, the female may cannibalize her litter or hide them in her cheek pouches. When the young are hidden in the cheek pouches, they may suffocate. Hamsters can be picked up by the nape skin at the base of the neck or by cupping the hands under the hind limbs.

TECHNICIAN NOTE

Hamsters live, on average, 18 to 24 months and have a gestation period of 16 days.

There are several commercially available hamster habitats. An aquarium with a mesh top may be used to house a hamster, with hardwood shavings being the substrate of choice. Aromatic shavings such as cedar or pine may cause ocular and respiratory irritation, severe dermatitis, and

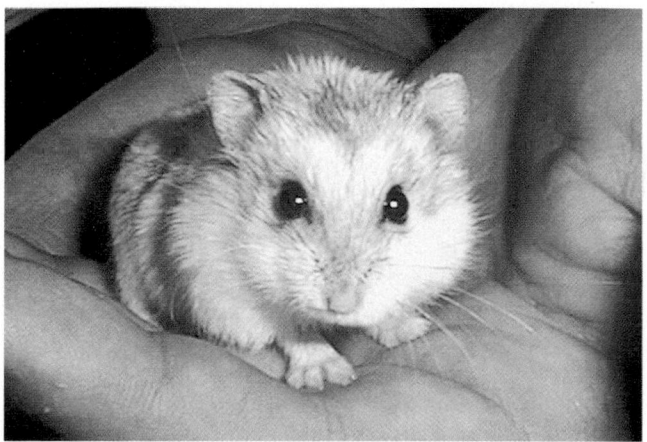

Figure 18-37 Siberian dwarf hamsters are popular pets.

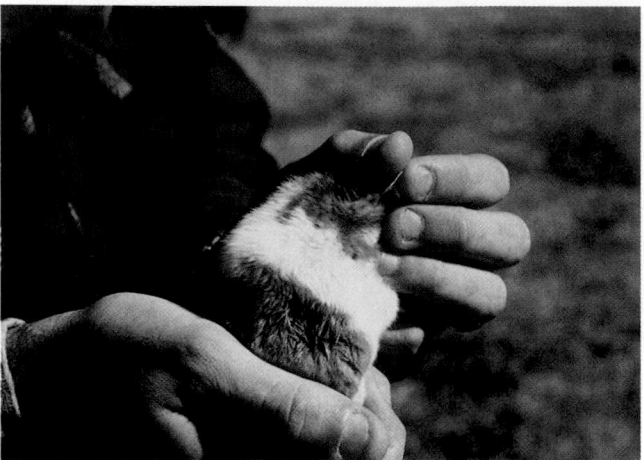

Figure 18-38 Flank glands on hamsters, noted in this figure by the moistened area in the caudodorsal region of the animal.

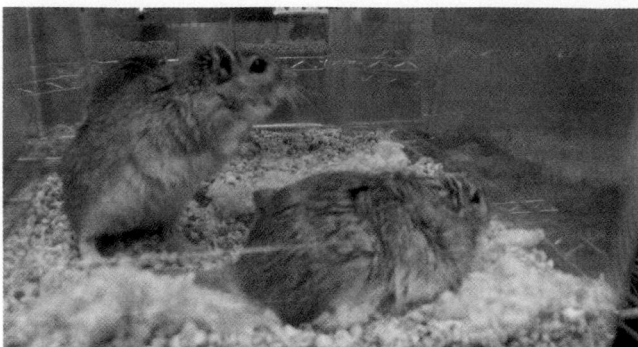

Figure 18-39 Young gerbil.

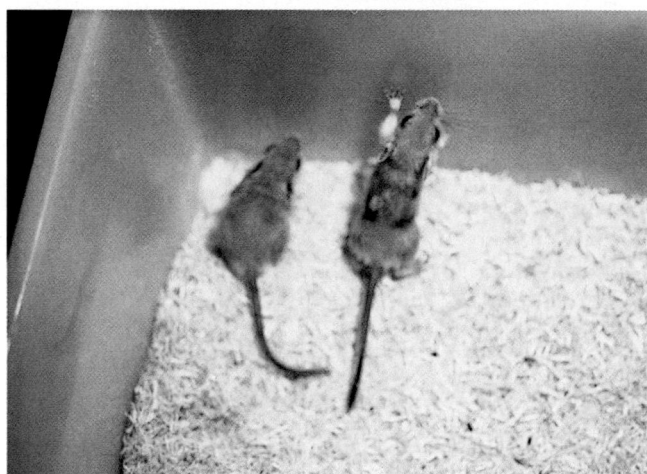

Figure 18-40 Typical small rodent cage containing gerbils.

allergic reactions. Sipper bottles are perfect for water dispensing, and nonchewable bowls should be used for food containers or food should be placed on the floor of the enclosure. All food and water access should be made available to the young.

Males have a greater anogenital distance than females. Hamsters may be mated monogamously or in a harem. It is important that females with young are not disturbed so that cannibalism and abandonment of the litter do not occur.

Wet tail is a general term to describe diarrhea in the hamster. Bacterial infections, cestodiasis, and antibiotic administration are a few causes of diarrhea in these rodents.

GERBIL

The Mongolian gerbil is a popular pet native to Mongolia and northeastern China. It is an active burrowing animal adapted to desert environments. Gerbils have a midventral pad consisting of sebaceous glands used in territorial marking.

TECHNICIAN NOTE

Under no circumstances should gerbils be grabbed by the tail. As a defense mechanism the tail skin will deglove, necessitating a tail amputation.

The gerbil has a life span of 3.5 years, with a gestation length of 25 days without lactation and 24 to 48 days with lactation. The litter sizes average five offspring that wean in approximately 25 days (Figure 18-39). Certain gerbil lines are prone to epileptiform seizure activity. Gerbils are friendly rodents that may be housed in hamster units (Figure 18-40). These animals are good at escaping; therefore the cage should be designed to prevent chewing.

The gerbil's diet may be similar to that of the hamster, and water can be supplied in a sipper bottle. Sexing is accomplished by measuring the urogenital distance. The male has a much longer distance than the female. Males aid in the care of the young.

Gerbils commonly present with a nasal dermatitis caused by a bacterial infection initiated by their burrowing activity. Topical antibiotic treatment is recommended for resolution of this infection.

Tyzzer's disease may be diagnosed in gerbils and is caused by *Bacillus piliformis*. Dietary change and colibacillosis also cause diarrhea in these animals.

MOUSE

Mice are small rodents that are used most often in the research setting but are maintained as pets. Mice are usually aggressive and bite. They are territorial animals and quickly develop a hierarchy when placed in groups (Figure 18-41). These small animals require small amounts of food and water but are escape prone and may develop an unpleasant odor.

Common clinical conditions affecting mice include ectoparasites, neoplasia, and trauma. Most mice have a life span of 2 years and are prone to geriatric disease conditions

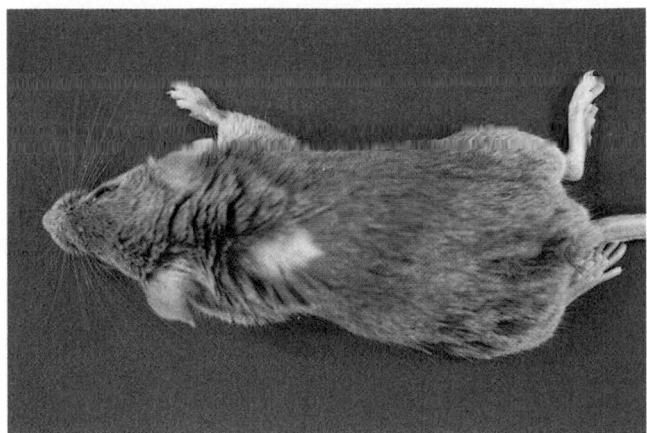

Figure 18-41 Trauma (cage mate–inflicted hair loss) on a mouse. This is commonly referred to as *barbering*.

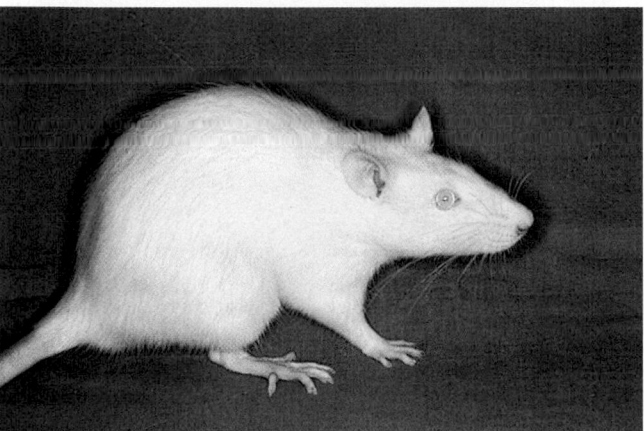

Figure 18-42 Rats make one of the best companion animals of all rodent species.

within a relatively short time of ownership. One of the most common geriatric disease conditions is neoplasia. Tumors of various types have been identified in mice, making the education of owners particularly important to aid in early detection and treatment.

Housing should be similar to that of gerbils and hamsters. Hardwood shavings or chips are recommended instead of the aromatic softwood chips (cedar and pine) because of potential liver damage and epithelial damage.

Housing should be cleaned regularly to prevent odor and health problems. Pelleted rodent feed and fresh water in sipper bottles are recommended to be supplied free choice.

Male mice have a greater urogenital distance than females. Female mice become sexually mature at 50 days of age and are best bred in the harem scheme, with one male combined with 2 to 6 females.

RAT

Rats are clean and unassuming and can be trained to be good pets (Figure 18-42). These animals may live up to 3 years or longer and become sexually mature at 1.5 to 2 months of age.

As with mice, rats are relatively short-lived, predisposing them to geriatric diseases. Rats are also very susceptible to neoplasia, particularly mammary gland tumors. In addition, *Mycoplasma* spp. respiratory infections are commonly diagnosed and clinically may appear as dyspnea with signs of nasal discharge. The nasal discharge is commonly tinged with a red color due to the pigment of the harderian gland secretions. Enrofloxacin and tetracycline have been used to treat *Mycoplasma* spp. infections in rats.

✎ TECHNICIAN NOTE

Rats seldom bite, but caution must be used in a stressful situation.

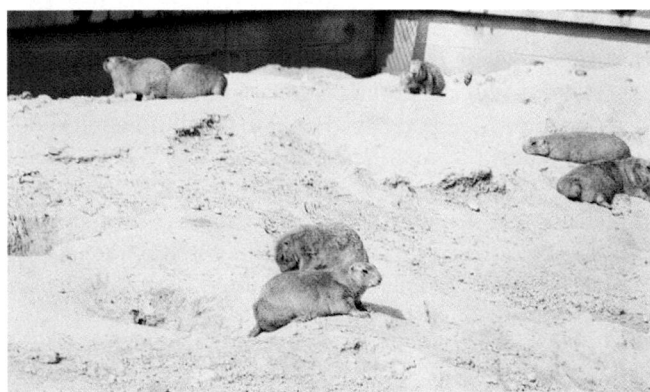

Figure 18-43 Sociable prairie dogs are not recommended as a companion animal.

Commercial rodent cages can be obtained for proper housing. Substrate should be similar to that of other rodents.

Males have a longer anogenital distance than females. The gestation length is 22 days, and nesting material should be provided before birth.

PRAIRIE DOGS

The black-tailed prairie dog (*Cynomys ludovicianus*) may present to a veterinary clinic even though it is illegal to keep wild North American species as pets. Wild prairie dogs may carry *Hantavirus*, rabies, ectoparasites, *Salmonella* spp., the plague bacteria, monkey pox, and other zoonotic agents (see Chapter 35). Some prairie dogs have been raised in captivity and are therefore less likely to carry dangerous zoonotic diseases. Nevertheless, it is recommended that all prairie dogs remain where they belong, in their natural habitat (Figure 18-43).

Prairie dogs may live up to 10 years and can survive on rodent chow and timothy grass hay. They are, however,

- 3 teaspoons high-quality cat or kitten chow
- 1 teaspoon fruit/vegetable mix
- 4-8 small meal worms or 2-3 small crickets

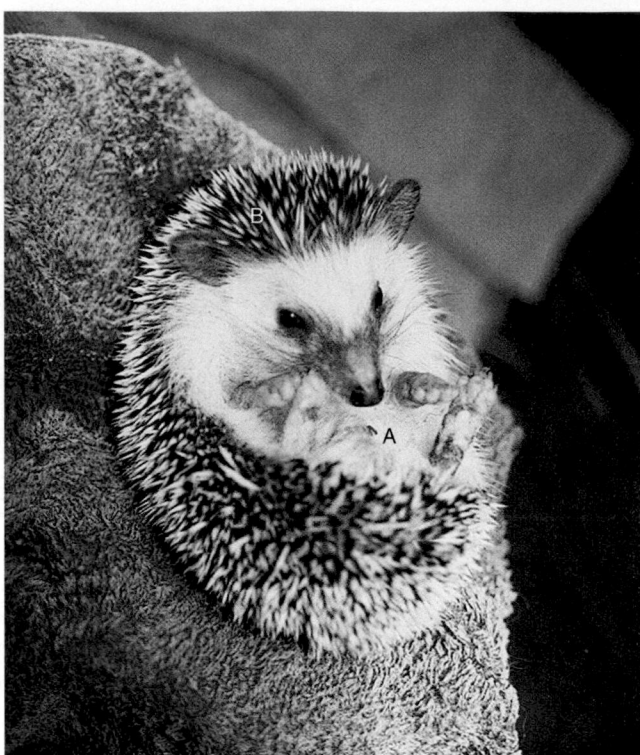

Figure 18-44 *A*, The ventral surface of hedgehogs is devoid of spines. *B*, The dorsal aspect, as noted with this pet in its enclosure, is covered with sharp spines.

susceptible to obesity, making it essential to monitor food intake, especially in adult animals. Digging and tunneling are important parts of their daily activity. The provision of deep bedding therefore enables this type of exercise and allows them to hide and feel secure. Prairie dogs can be managed much like rats in regard to their management and care. The scrotal sac is the identifying characteristic of male prairie dogs when sex determination is required. Venipuncture is best accomplished using the lateral saphenous or cephalic vein. Jugular venipuncture or cranial vena cava collection should only be attempted when the patient is under general anesthesia.

Common disease problems identified in captive prairie dogs are obesity, respiratory disease, malocclusion, infectious pododermatitis, trauma, and neoplasia. The most difficult situation to overcome for most prairie dogs raised in captivity is obesity. Obesity usually complicates concurrent disease states, making it difficult at times to differentiate the primary disease problem from complications caused by excess body fat.

HEDGEHOGS

The African hedgehog *(Atelerix albiventris)* has become an increasingly popular pet in recent years. These nocturnal spinal animals often adapt best to captivity when left alone. Hedgehogs like to hide, like dark quite areas, and will burrow to escape. Hedgehogs may be maintained much like rodents. For example, enclosures that are 20 gal or larger and lined with an absorbable paper bedding make excellent habitats.

The life span of hedgehogs is 3 to 5 years. The most common disease conditions are neoplasia and external parasites. Yearly physical examinations are needed for teeth cleaning, nail trimming, and tumor checks. Hedgehogs are not rodents and rely on an insectivore/omnivore diet such as the one listed in Box 18-3.

One feature of hedgehog medicine is hedgehog patients must be anesthetized simply to be examined. The spines are very sharp, so caution must be taken during handling; gloves are necessary, particularly before anesthesia (Figure 18-44).

Blood collection sites are cranial vena cava, jugular vein, cephalic vein, and lateral saphenous vein, with the cranial vena cava being the site of choice. Common diseases diagnosed in hedgehogs are neoplasia, obesity, otitis externa,

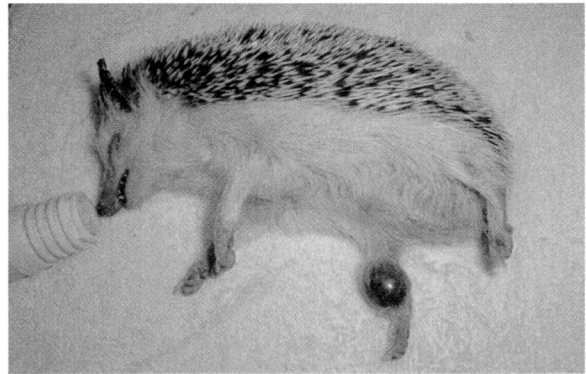

Figure 18-45 This hedgehog has a tumor on its rear leg. Tumors are common in hedgehogs.

dermatitis, external parasites, and respiratory disease (Figure 18-45).

SUGAR GLIDERS

Sugar gliders are nocturnal marsupials from Australia (Figure 18-46). As with hedgehogs, they are unusual pets with unique qualities that should be considered carefully by a potential owner before a purchase is made. They are

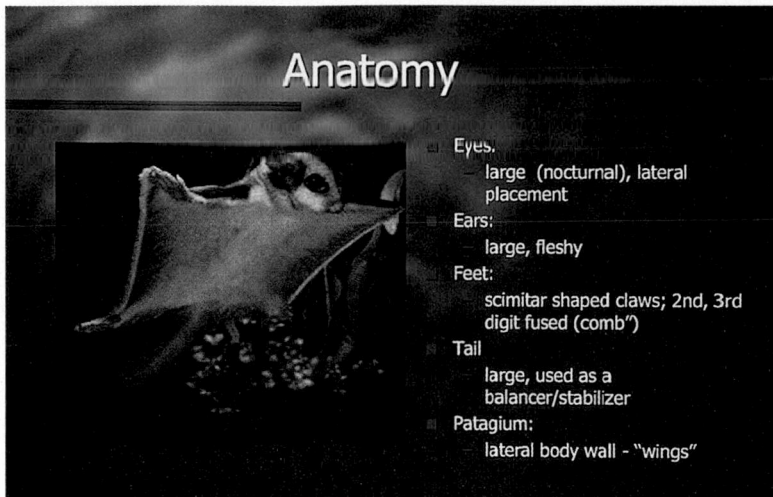

Figure 18-46 A sugar glider with its skin stretched out, giving it the ability to "fly" and also its name.

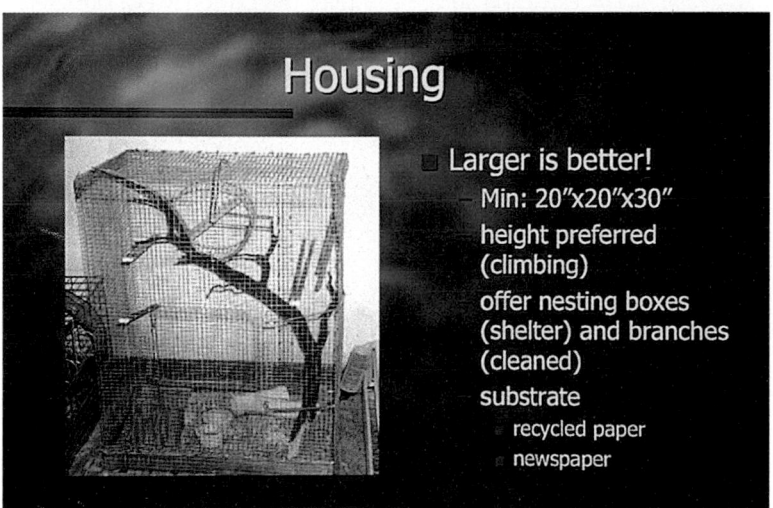

Figure 18-47 A typical sugar glider enclosure.

very social animals. If maintained as a single pet, a glider will require additional attention from the owner to meet its psychological needs. In addition, their nocturnal habits give rise to much activity throughout the night, which can be annoying to those who wish to sleep.

Housing needs to be a tall wire enclosure with fresh branches and places to hide, such as a bird box (Figure 18-47). The wire mesh should have spacing no more than 1-inch square to prevent escape. The bottom tray should be lined with shredded paper or pelleted paper products for easy cleaning and optimum absorption of urine, food, and water.

Malnutrition (e.g., hypocalcemia, hypoglycemia) is one of the most common disease conditions diagnosed in sugar gliders. There are commercial pelleted glider diets available, but they are not actively marketed in most areas. One source of information worth exploring is the Internet. Websites

Box 18-4 Daily Sugar Glider Diet

• Zoo-formula insectivore diet
• Equal amounts:
  • Chopped apple
  • Grapes
  • Carrot
  • Sweet potato
  • Hard-cooked egg yolk
• 10-12 small meal worms
• Dust food and insects with vitamin mineral powder

that focus on these animals can be found via most search engines. An example of a complete sugar glider diet is listed in Box 18-4.

REFERENCES

Boyer TH: *Essentials of reptiles a guide for practitioners*, Lakewood, Colo, 1998, American Animal Hospital Association, pp 7-21.

Frye FL: *Reptile clinicians handbook*, Malabar, Fla, 1995, Krieger, pp 70-100.

Wise JK: *U.S. pet ownership and demographics sourcebook*, Schaumburg, Ill, 2002, American Veterinary Medicine Association, pp 1-113.

RECOMMENDED READING

Campbell TW: *Avian hematology and cytology*, ed 2, Ames, 1995, Iowa State University Press.

Carpenter JW, Mashima TY, Rupiper DJ: *Exotic animal formulary*, ed 2, Philadelphia, 2001, WB Saunders.

Fox JG: *Biology and diseases of the ferret*, ed 2, Philadelphia, 1998, Lippincott, Williams & Wilkins.

Tully TN, Mitchell MA, editors: *Semin Avian Exotic Pet Med*, Philadelphia, WB Saunders (published quarterly).

Harcourt-Brown F: *Textbook of rabbit medicine*, Oxford, 2002, Butterworth-Heinemann.

Harkness JE, Wagner JE: *The biology and medicine of rabbits and rodents*, Philadelphia, 1995, Lea & Febiger.

Johnson CA, Harrison LR: *Exotic companion medicine handbook for veterinarians*, Lake Worth, Fla, 1996, Wingers Publishing.

J Avian Med Surg, Lawrence, Kan, Association of Avian Veterinarians, Allen Press (published quarterly).

J Herpetological Med Surg, Lawrence, Kan, Association of Reptilian and Amphibian Veterinarians, Allen Press (published quarterly).

J Zoo Wildlife Med, Lawrence, Kan, American Association of Zoo Veterinarians (published quarterly).

Lewington JH: *Ferret husbandry, medicine and surgery*, Edinburgh, Butterworth-Heinemann.

Mader DR: *Reptile medicine and surgery*, Philadelphia, 1996, WB Saunders.

Quesenberry KE, Carpenter JW: *Ferrets, rabbits and rodents clinical medicine and surgery*, ed 2, Philadelphia, 2004, WB Saunders.

Spadafori G, Speer BL: *Birds for dummies*, Foster City, Calif, 1999, IDG Books.

Tully TN, Lawton MPC, Dorrestein GM: *Avian medicine*, Oxford, 2000, Butterworth-Heinemann.

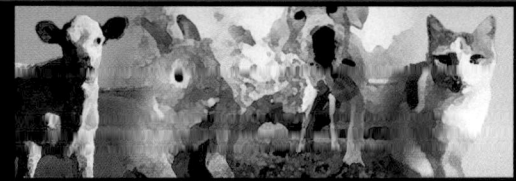

19

Veterinary Anesthesia

GLENN PETTIFER

INTRODUCTION

In a single veterinary practice, some form of anesthesia is used almost every day. In its many forms, anesthesia is used to provide chemical restraint, the alleviation of pain during surgical procedures, muscle relaxation for surgery, and an increase in safety associated with animal handling. Some animals may need only mild sedation for minor diagnostic procedures, while others will require general anesthesia during surgical procedures. Less commonly, general anesthesia can be used for the control of seizure activity or as a component of a humane euthanasia procedure.

Veterinary technicians contribute substantially to all areas of the practice of veterinary medicine, but it is in the administration of anesthesia that the technician plays a particularly important and valuable role. In many practices the veterinary technician is responsible for the supervised administration of anesthesia and monitoring of animals during surgery. Thus an individual who is knowledgeable and comfortable with the administration of anesthesia is an extremely valuable asset to veterinarians, their practices, and their animals. ■

DEFINITIONS

Anesthesia comes from the Greek work for "insensibility," and it is generally used to describe the loss of sensation to all or part of the body. *Local anesthesia* refers to loss of sensation in a particular part of the body, for example, what we commonly experience when the dentist "freezes" a tooth. *General anesthesia* refers to drug-induced unconsciousness that is controlled and reversible. Injectable or inhaled drugs may produce general anesthesia. *Tranquilizers* are drugs that reduce anxiety and promote relaxation. *Sedatives* are drugs that lessen excitement, produce central nervous system depression, and promote drowsiness. *Analgesia* refers to the absence of pain.

CONCEPT OF BALANCED ANESTHESIA

In the past, the components of general anesthesia (unconsciousness, muscle relaxation, analgesia) were frequently accomplished by the administration of a large dose of a single drug. While this practice accomplished the objective of producing general anesthesia, the large doses of these single drugs were also associated with more profound, unwanted, negative side effects. In most cases, this practice has evolved into the administration of smaller doses of a number of drugs that individually target specific components of the anesthetic state. In doing so the negative side effects associated with the administration of a high dose of a single drug can be avoided.

As an example, consider the general anesthesia required for ovariohysterectomy in a dog. A less sophisticated anesthetic technique for this procedure could involve the mask induction of anesthesia with an inhalant anesthetic and maintenance of the animal on the inhalant for the duration of the surgery. This type of procedure would be associated with a high degree of stress for the animal (and anesthetist) because of the struggling during the induction period and excitement during the recovery period. High doses of the inhalant would be needed to provide sufficient anesthesia for the surgical period, and once the anesthetic is discontinued, there would not be any drug left for the postoperative control of pain. In contrast, a *balanced anesthetic* technique includes the administration of a tranquilizer or sedative in combination with an appropriate analgesic (acepromazine and morphine, for example) prior to the induction of anesthesia. Induction of anesthesia is performed with a single dose of an injectable anesthetic (thiopental, for example), and anesthesia is maintained with an inhalant anesthetic (isoflurane, for example). With this balanced technique, the administration of a sedative prior to the induction of anesthesia decreases the stress associated with the induction process and reduces the amount of drug required for induction as well as the amount of inhalant required for maintenance of anesthesia. The administration of morphine prior to the induction of anesthesia ensures that the analgesic properties of morphine are active prior to the surgical insult. This *preemptive* administration of analgesics has, in most cases, been shown to provide analgesia that is more effective than that produced when the analgesic is administered after the surgery (when the animal is in pain). Preanesthetic administration of morphine also reduces the dose of both the induction drug and the inhaled anesthetic that is used for maintenance of anesthesia during the surgery. The inclusion of an injectable induction drug in the anesthetic protocol serves to reduce the stress associated with the induction of general anesthesia and provides for an induction that is typically much smoother than a mask induction. Thus this technique of balanced anesthesia provides for an anesthetic period characterized by calmer inductions and recoveries, less stress for the animal, better pain control, and fewer negative side effects that may be seen when large doses of a single drug are used alone.

TECHNICIAN NOTE

Balanced anesthesia refers to the administration of a number of drugs that target different components of the anesthetic process. Such a technique avoids the use of a large dose of a single drug that is associated with a higher incidence of negative side effects.

PROCESS OF GENERAL ANESTHESIA

The process of anesthesia can be divided into six different stages:

1. Equipment preparation
2. Preanesthetic assessment, stabilization, and protocol selection
3. Premedication
4. Induction
5. Maintenance
6. Recovery

ANESTHETIC EQUIPMENT

It is normally the responsibility of the veterinary technician to maintain equipment used for anesthesia in a veterinary practice. Schedules for specific equipment maintenance tasks will vary from practice to practice; however, a routine, documented system of equipment maintenance should be

established. Equipment maintenance duties will include stocking of both equipment and drugs, appropriate cleaning of those components that require routine cleaning, and routine assessment of the safe functioning of anesthetic vaporizers and machines.

For any anesthetic procedure the basic equipment and supplies include needles, syringes, intravenous catheters, tape for securing catheters, heparinized saline (2 IU/ml of heparin per milliliter of 0.9% saline), a variety of sizes of endotracheal tubes, laryngoscope, lubricant for the endotracheal tubes, ophthalmic lubricant, an oxygen source, a method for delivering oxygen, an apparatus for manual ventilation (i.e., an Ambu bag or anesthesia machine), and a selection of anesthetic drugs. If gas anesthesia is used in the practice, an anesthesia machine, appropriate breathing systems, and a selection of rebreathing bags and face masks should be available. Finally, an emergency drug box (discussed under Anesthetic Emergencies) should be readily available during any procedure that involves anesthesia.

TECHNICIAN NOTE

It is normally the responsibility of the veterinary technician to maintain the equipment used for anesthetic procedures. A documented system of routine maintenance should be established.

CATHETERS

Intravenous administration equipment and catheters are presented in Chapter 3. A dependable venous access should be available in all anesthetized animals. Such access can be provided by an intravenous catheter, or for short-term procedures a butterfly needle may be appropriate (Figure 19-1). An intravenous catheter provides a route for the administration of fluids during the anesthetic period, the administration of additional anesthetic drugs (especially important when injectable anesthetic techniques are used) and for the administration of drugs required during an anesthetic emergency such as cardiopulmonary arrest. Continuous intravenous access provided by a hypodermic needle attached to a syringe that is taped to the limb of the animal is an unreliable access to the vascular space. This type of access is associated with complications such as the loss of access and the subsequent subcutaneous, rather than intravenous, administration of drugs.

ENDOTRACHEAL TUBES

The endotracheal tube serves to connect the anesthetic breathing circuit to the animal's airway. Although it is not essential to place an endotracheal tube when only injectable anesthesia is used, tubes must be available for those instances when respiratory arrest dictates the need for assisted ventilation and delivery of oxygen or when the risk of regurgitation and aspiration is increased (as in animals who have not adequately fasted, who have a history of

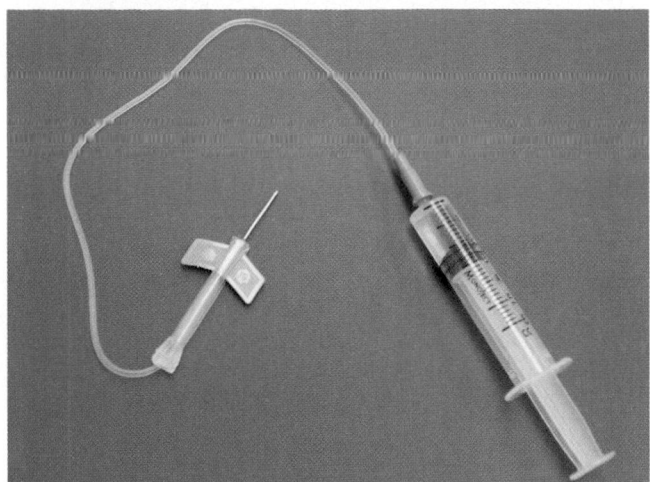

Figure 19-1 In situations where an intravenous catheter has not been placed, a butterfly needle may be used for the short-term administration of injectable anesthetics.

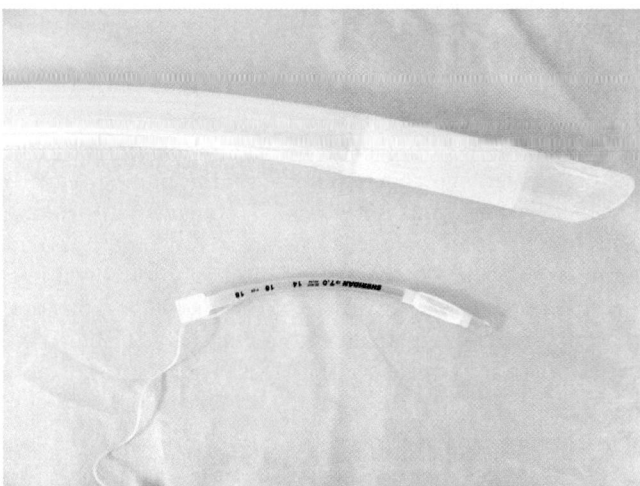

Figure 19-3 Large animal endotracheal tube (30 mm ID) used for horses and large ruminants. A 7.0-mm-ID tube used in small animals is shown for comparison.

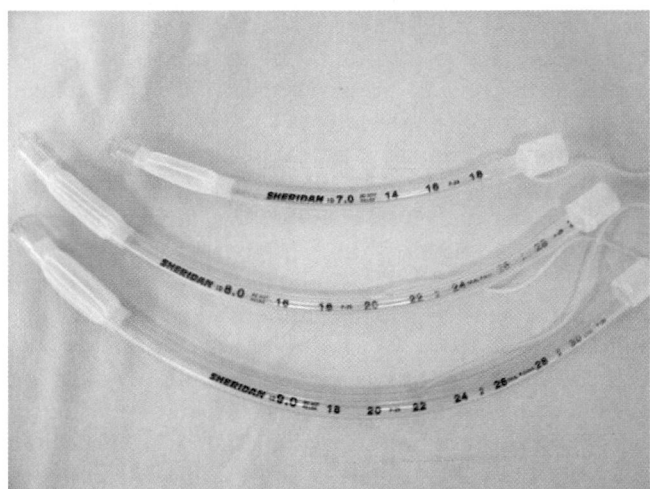

Figure 19-2 Endotracheal tubes used in small animals, small ruminants, and swine.

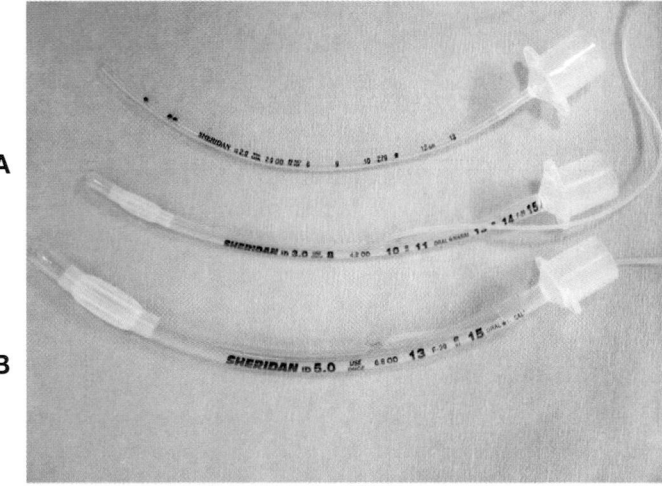

Figure 19-4 Uncuffed *(A)* and cuffed *(B)* endotracheal tubes for use in small animals. Uncuffed tubes are used in very small mammals (puppies, kittens, ferrets, rabbits), reptiles, and birds.

vomiting, or who are pregnant). Some veterinarians prefer to place an endotracheal tube routinely during injectable anesthesia as a precautionary measure. Routine placement of endotracheal tubes, even during injectable anesthesia, ensures that animals receive supplemental oxygen throughout the anesthetic period. As well, the risk of complications arising when an animal does become apneic during the procedure is reduced.

Cuffed endotracheal tubes are most commonly used in veterinary practice (Figure 19-2). They provide an effective seal within the airway, thereby preventing aspiration and facilitating effective ventilatory support. Cuffed endotracheal tubes are available in a wide variety of sizes. They are classified according to the internal diameter (ID) of the tube. Sizes of 2.5 to 14 mm ID are appropriate for dogs, cats, swine, and small ruminants and sizes of 16 to 30 mm ID are used for large ruminants and horses (Figure 19-3). Uncuffed endotracheal tubes are used in very small animals (i.e., kittens, puppies, ferrets) because they preserve a larger airway diameter. They are also used in birds because the complete tracheal rings in birds make the trachea less compliant when the endotracheal tube cuff is inflated (Figure 19-4).

TECHNICIAN NOTE

Uncuffed endotracheal tubes are used in very small animals (i.e., kittens, puppies, ferrets), reptiles, and birds.

LARYNGOSCOPES

Laryngoscopes facilitate the placement of an endotracheal tube (intubation), and their routine use reduces the risk of complications during endotracheal intubation. Although the use of a laryngoscope should be routine, it is particularly beneficial when intubating small ruminants, swine, cats, and brachycephalic breeds of dogs (i.e., bulldogs). A laryngoscope should be used for intubation of any animal that has upper airway obstruction. Laryngoscopes consist of a battery-containing handle with a detachable blade. There are a variety of blade sizes and shapes (Figure 19-5).

ANESTHETIC MACHINES

The anesthetic machine is a highly sophisticated piece of equipment that is designed to vaporize the liquid anesthetic and deliver the anesthetic vapor safely and at a known, accurate concentration. Although the design of these machines is complex and the number and types of machines and vaporizers is varied, they do have some common design principles (Figures 19-6 and 19-7). An understanding of these design principles is essential for the proper maintenance of anesthetic machines and the safe, effective delivery of inhaled anesthetics.

Conceptually, it is useful to think of the anesthetic machine as a mixing machine that mixes the carrier gas with the anesthetic vapor in a controlled manner, delivers oxygen to the animal, removes exhaled carbon dioxide, provides a mechanism to assist or control the animal's ventilation, and provides a mechanism for the scavenging of waste anesthetic gases.

The carrier gas is most commonly oxygen, although nitrous oxide is sometimes used as an additional carrier gas that provides some level of supplemental analgesia. Nitrous oxide is never administered as the sole carrier gas. These gases are supplied in cylinders compressed to a high pressure to allow the storage of high volumes of gas. Cylinders are color coded according to their contents and are classified by letter according to their size. Oxygen-containing cylinders may be white or green (United States), and those containing nitrous oxide are blue. Associated with the compressed gas cylinder is a pressure gauge. For an oxygen-containing cylinder, the pressure reading on the gauge reflects the amount of gas remaining in the cylinder. Regardless of its size, a full oxygen tank will read a pressure of approximately 2200 psi. This pressure decreases proportionately as the tank empties. Thus a standard E type cylinder attached to an anesthetic machine reading a pressure of 2200 psi will contain approximately 700 L of oxygen. As oxygen is removed from the cylinder and the pressure drops, so will the volume of gas remaining in the cylinder. At a pressure of 1100 psi (one half the original pressure), the cylinder will contain one half of its initial volume or 350 L (Figure 19-8).

Gas from the cylinder passes through a pressure regulator that reduces the pressure of the gas as it enters into the anesthetic machine. At this low pressure, the gas then flows through the flowmeter, which, when open, delivers a known amount of gas per unit time (ml/min) to the vaporizer and breathing circuit (Figure 19-7). Most anesthetic machines will include an oxygen flush valve. The oxygen flush valve delivers high flows of oxygen (35 to 75 L/min) to the fresh-gas outlet, bypassing the vaporizer and quickly filling the breathing system with pure oxygen (Figure 19-7). The flush valve may be used to quickly decrease the concentration of anesthetic gas in the breathing circuit. Flushing the breathing circuit with pure oxygen can produce a rapid decrease in anesthetic depth or facilitate recovery from anesthesia. Since the gas delivered to the breathing circuit is only oxygen, the oxygen flush valve should not be used to inflate the rebreathing bag unless a decrease in depth of anesthesia is desired. The oxygen flush valve should not be engaged when the pop-off valve is closed or when a non-rebreathing system is used because of the danger associated with delivering high volumes of gas that create excessive airway pressure.

Vaporizers convert a volatile liquid inhaled anesthetic into a vapor that is combined with the carrier gas and then delivered to the breathing circuit. Vaporizer classification and construction is complex (see Recommended Reading). Most vaporizers currently in use provide precise vapor concentrations according to the settings on the vaporizer, regardless of temperature and incoming gas flow rate. Such vaporizers are known as *precision vaporizers* (Figures 19-7 and 19-9). Nonprecision vaporizers deliver anesthetic

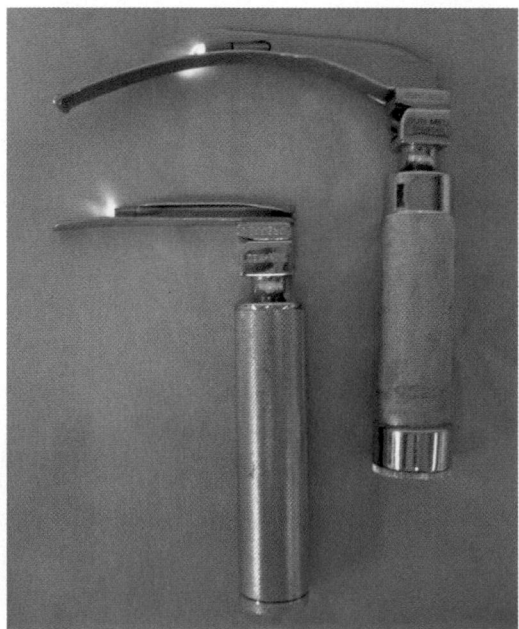

Figure 19-5 Laryngoscopes used in veterinary anesthesia. Their use facilitates endotracheal intubation in most animals but is particularly beneficial when intubating small ruminants, swine, cats, brachycephalic breeds of dogs, and animals with upper airway obstructions.

vapor without producing a precise vapor concentration. In addition, their output varies with temperature, gas flow rate through the vaporizer, and the animal's rate and depth of ventilation (Figure 19-7) Although nonprecision vaporizers are less expensive and have been widely used in veterinary medicine, newer precision vaporizers are preferred because of their ability to deliver a known concentration of anesthetic vapor regardless of variations in gas flow rate, temperature, and ventilation.

Vaporizers may be located outside of the breathing circuit (out-of-the-circuit) or in the breathing circuit (in-the-circuit) (Figure 19-5). Out-of-the-circuit vaporizers are generally of the precision type, and in-the-circuit vaporizers are nonprecision type.

BREATHING SYSTEMS

Fresh, mixed gas leaves the mixing portion of the anesthetic machine through the fresh-gas port (common gas outlet) (Figures 19-6 and 19-7). Fresh gas then enters a breathing circuit that is attached to the animal, either by a direct connection to the endotracheal tube or by a face mask.

The circle breathing circuit is the most commonly used breathing circuit in veterinary anesthesia (Figure 19-7). Three sizes of circle breathing systems are available: pediatric (<7 kg), standard adult circle (7 to 135 kg), and large animal (>135 kg). These circuits differ in internal diameter and volume. As the name implies, gases move in a circular fashion through the circuit. Because of this, the animal rebreathes some previously exhaled gases. This circular movement of the gases within the circuit is accomplished by the inclusion of one-way valves in the circuit that direct the flow of gases. Because the buildup of exhaled carbon dioxide in the circuit would be detrimental to the animal, carbon dioxide is removed by soda lime or barium hydroxide lime contained in the absorbent canister. Most absorbent granules contain an indicator dye that becomes visible as the absorbent granules are exhausted. Strong, persistent color change in

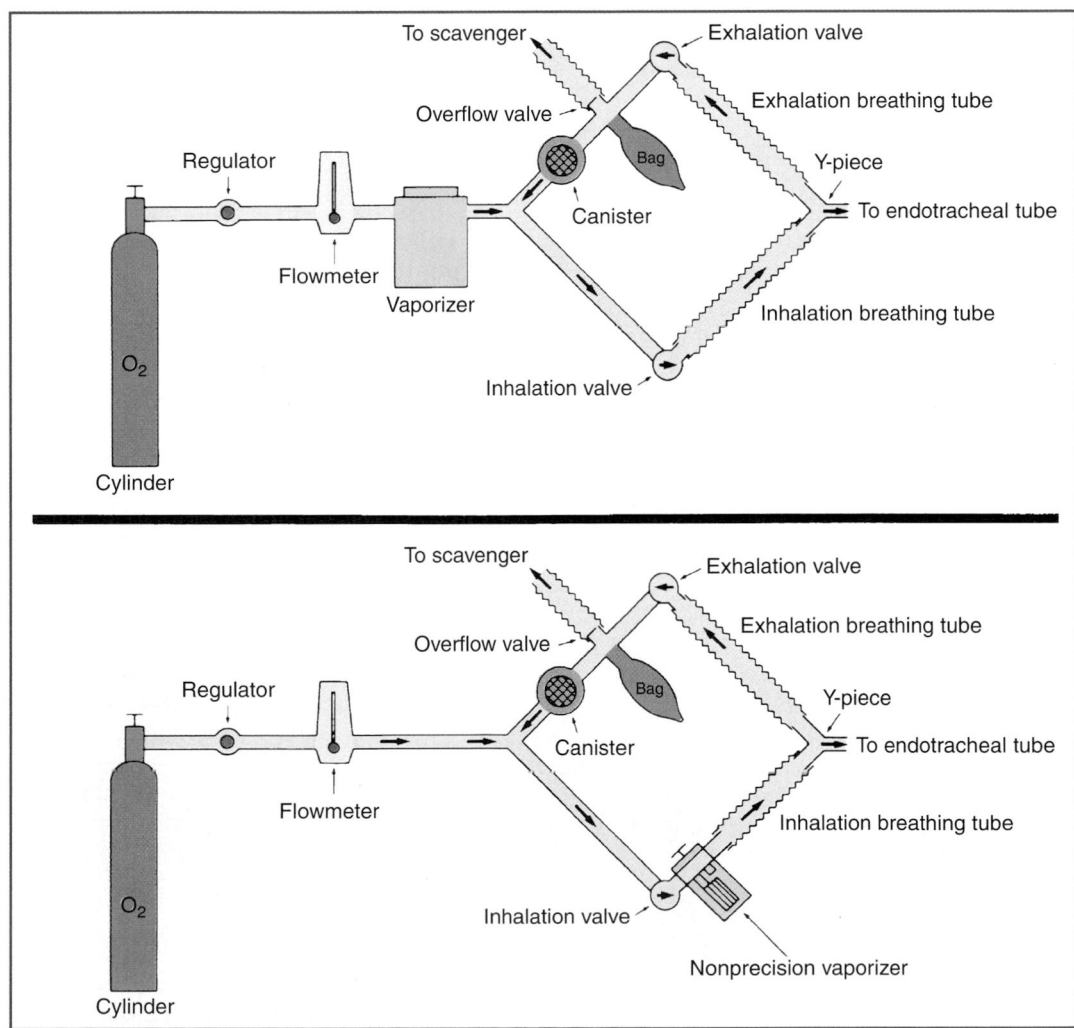

Figure 19-6 Basic design and components of a gas anesthetic machine, circle breathing system, out-of-the-circuit precision vaporizer (**A**) and in-the-circuit nonprecision vaporizer (**B**).

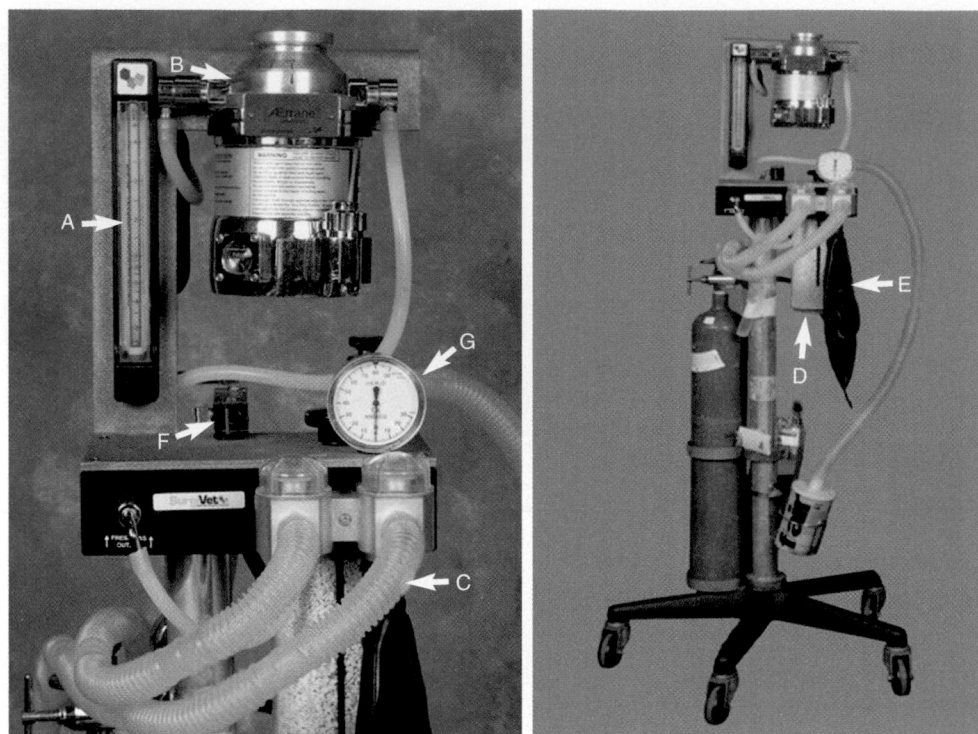

Figure 19-7 Standard anesthetic machine. Individual components are identified. *A,* Flowmeter; *B,* vaporizer; *C,* circle breathing circuit, *D,* soda lime canister; *E,* rebreathing bag; *F,* oxygen flush valve; and, *G,* pressure manometer.

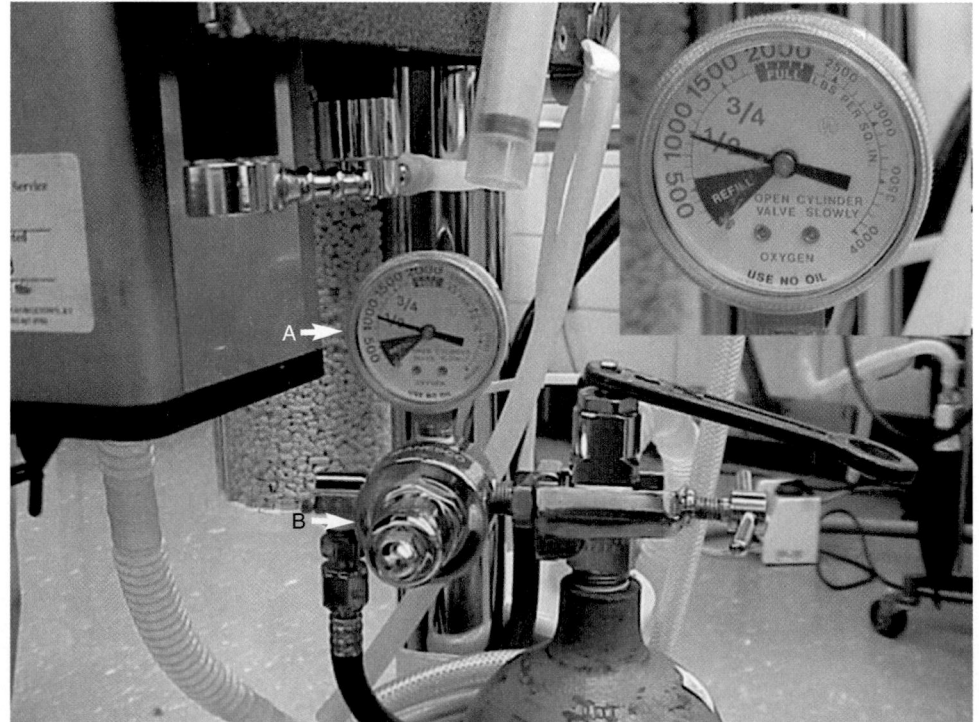

Figure 19-8 Pressure gauge *(A)* and regulator *(B)* attached to a green E cylinder containing oxygen. Inset shows the pressure regulator reading 1000 psi. Using this value, the volume of gas remaining in the cylinder can be determined. (See text for complete description.)

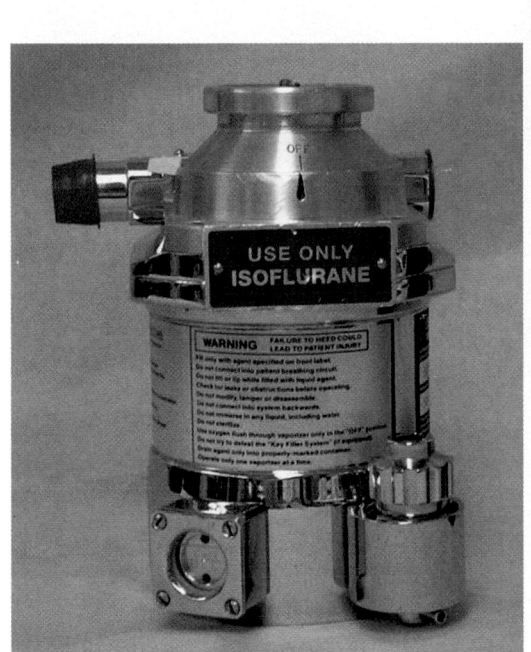
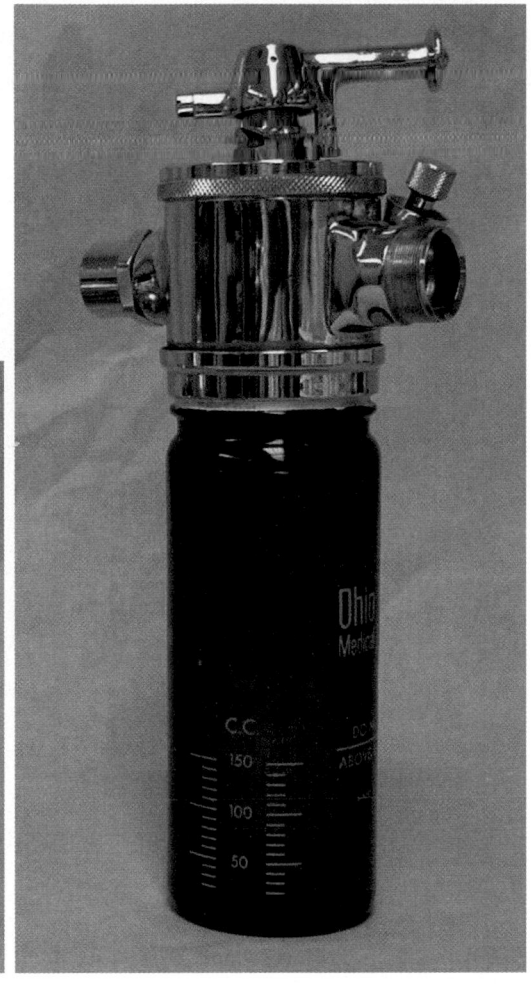

A   **B**

Figure 19-9 Precision (**A**) and nonprecision vaporizers (**B**).

the absorbent granules indicates the need for fresh granules (Figure 19-10). Absorbent granules also demonstrate a texture change from soft to hard as they become exhausted. Although the standard circle breathing circuit has separate inspiratory and expiratory limbs that maintain the appearance of a circle, the Universal F circuit is a circle breathing circuit with a coaxial design. The Universal F circuit is similar to the Bain nonrebreathing circuit in appearance but very different in its design principles (Figure 19-11).

The circle breathing circuit contains a rebreathing bag that supplements the inspiratory demands of the animal (Figure 19-7). The rebreathing bag may also be used to provide manual ventilation. Selection of the appropriate size of rebreathing bag is made by multiplying the animal's tidal volume (10 ml/kg) by a factor of 6. Rebreathing bags available for animals less than 135 kg include 0.5-, 1-, 2-, 3-, 5-, and 6-L sizes, and for animals more than 135 kg, the bags include 15-, 20-, and 30-L sizes.

The fresh-gas flow rates used with a circle breathing circuit vary. A flow rate that just meets the animal's metabolic oxygen needs (small animal, 4 to 10 ml/kg/min; large

animal, 2 to 3 ml/kg/min) is used with a closed circle system. With this type of flow rate, the pop-off valve is closed, and fresh-gas flow rates are adjusted to meet the metabolic oxygen consumption of the animal. This consumption is reflected by a decrease in the volume of gas in the rebreathing bag. Use of this flow rate is economical, allows for the retention of more heat and humidity in the circuit, and is associated with less environmental pollution. Use of this flow rate requires particular vigilance to avoid the inadequate delivery of fresh gas. A semiclosed flow rate is defined by fresh-gas flows of three times the animal's metabolic oxygen needs (small animal, 30 ml/kg/min; large animal, 6 to 10 ml/kg/min). With this flow rate, the pop-off valve is open. Although these flow rates are less economical and result in more pollution, they may ensure greater animal safety. Regardless of the fresh-gas flow rate used during the maintenance period, flow rates for mask induction and for a short period following intubation and connection to the breathing system (2 to 5 minutes) should be increased (except for in-the-circuit nonprecision vaporizers) to facilitate delivery of anesthetic gas to the animal and to aid in denitrogenation of the animal. A rate of two to three

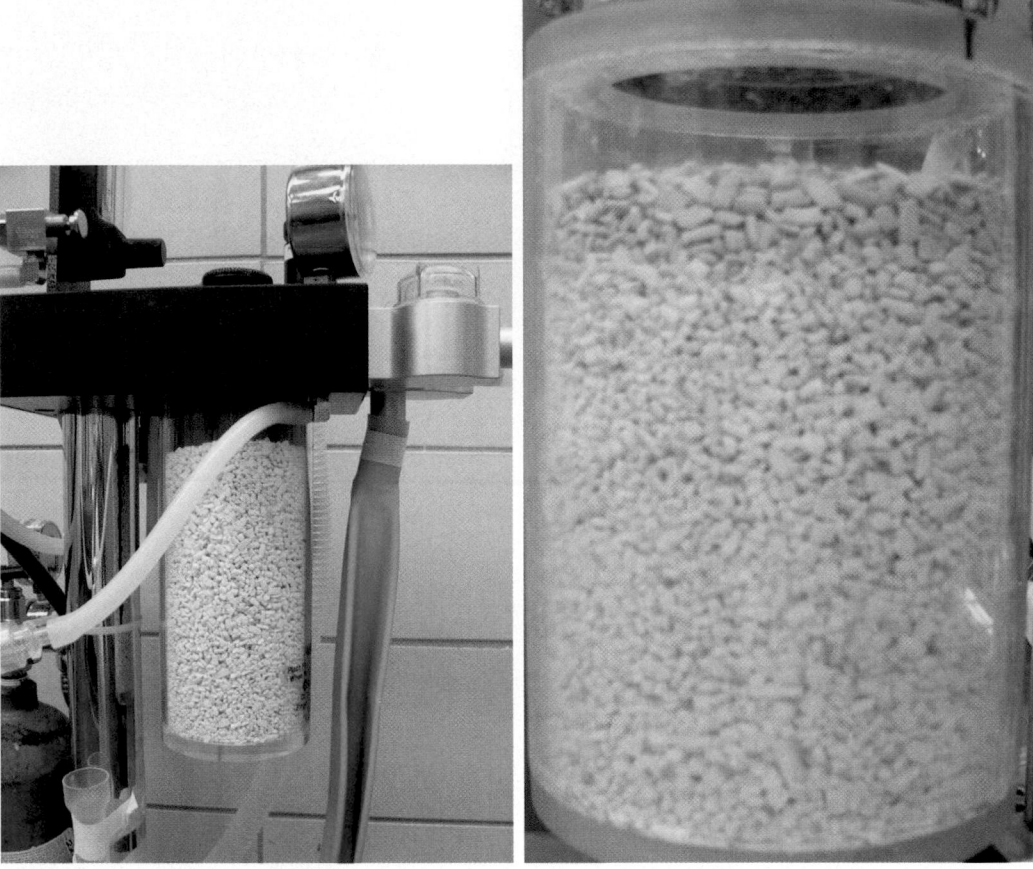

Figure 19-10 **A,** Soda lime granules in canister. **B,** The change in color of granules from white to purple indicates that the granules have exhausted their ability to remove carbon dioxide from the gas in the breathing circuit.

times the calculated maintenance flow rate will be adequate (100 ml/kg/min).

Nonrebreathing breathing circuits are also used in veterinary medicine for smaller animals (<5 to 7 kg). The particular design of nonrebreathing circuits allows for removal of exhaled gases by high fresh-gas flow rates negating the need for carbon dioxide absorbent. Their simple design reduces the resistance associated with breathing, hence their use with smaller animals. Nonrebreathing systems are not as economical as rebreathing systems because of the high fresh-gas flow rates that are used. These high fresh-gas flow rates also increase the pollution associated with waste gases, and they reduce the temperature and humidity of inspired gases. Flow rates vary according to the particular system but are approximately 100 to 300 ml/kg/min. A commonly used nonrebreathing system in veterinary medicine is the Bain coaxial system (Figure 19-12). An appropriate flow rate when using the Bain coaxial system is 150 to 200 ml/kg/min.

> ### ✎ TECHNICIAN NOTE
> The fresh-gas flow rate during induction and recovery using a circle breathing system is 100 ml/kg/min. During the maintenance of anesthesia, the flow rate may be reduced to 30 to 50 ml/kg/min.

In veterinary hospitals in which inhalation anesthetics are used, it is important to minimize exposure of personnel to waste anesthetic gases (see Chapter 36). Reduction of environmental pollution is facilitated by scavenging the waste gas exiting the pop-off valve, checking equipment frequently for leaks, and practicing techniques that minimize environmental pollution. The components of a scavenging system include a gas-capturing device, an interface, and a disposal system (Figures 19-7 and 19-13). Considerations that help to minimize waste-gas exposure include the following:

- Filling of vaporizers at the end of the workday when fewer people are present.
- Taking care to avoid spillage.
- Using low-flow techniques when possible.
- Recovering animals in well-ventilated areas, and leaving the animal attached to the breathing system as long as possible so that expired gases can be scavenged.
- Not turning on the vaporizer until the animal is connected to the machine.
- Using mask or chamber inductions only when considered necessary.
- Exhausting an induction chamber out of doors.

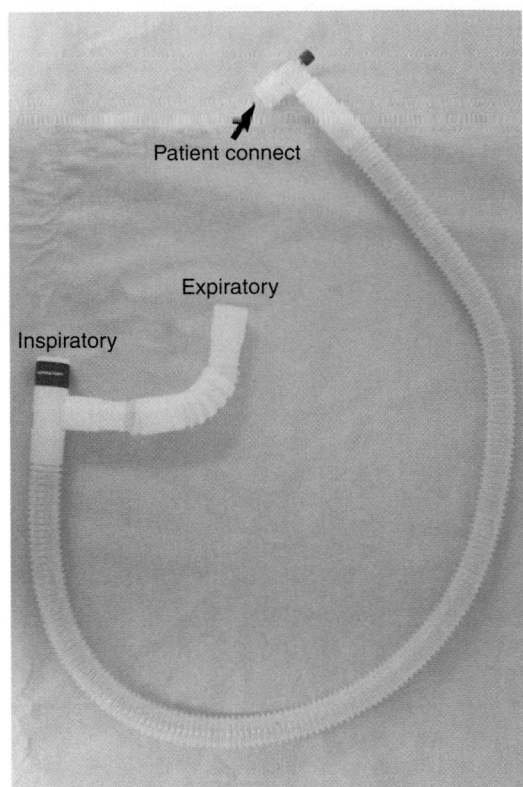

Figure 19-11 The universal F circuit is a coaxial circle system and should not be confused with a nonrebreathing Bain circuit (Figure 19-12).

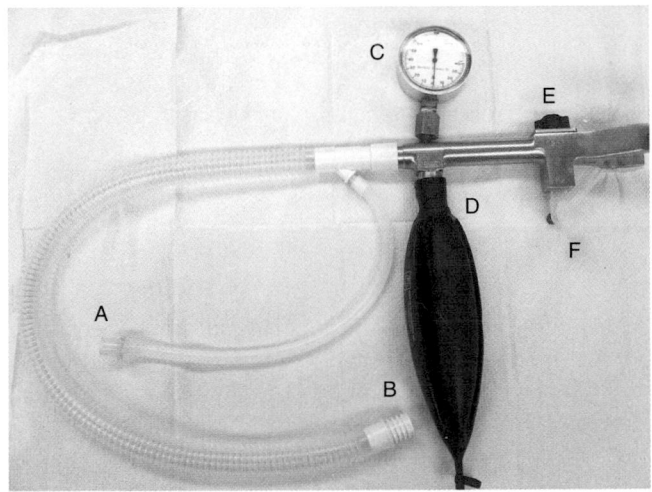

Figure 19-12 The Bain circuit is a nonrebreathing coaxial system. *A,* Connection to fresh-gas outlet on the anesthetic machine; *B,* patient connect; *C,* pressure manometer; *D,* reservoir or rebreathing bag; *E,* pop-off valve; and *F,* connection to scavenger hose.

⚕ TECHNICIAN NOTE

Unwarranted exposure to inhaled anesthetics can be reduced when vaporizers are filled at the end of the workday. Fewer people are present, and in the event of a spill, exposure time is reduced.

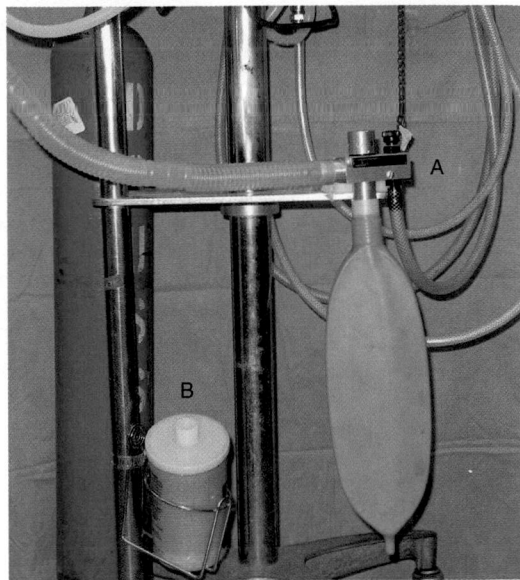

Figure 19-13 Examples of waste-gas scavenging systems. In locations where a central vacuum line is available, waste gas is scavenged through the pressure relief (pop-off) valve and drawn into the, disposal system *(A)* by vacuum. *B,* Charcoal absorbent canister is used to scavenge waste anesthetic gases when a central vacuum line is unavailable or passive scavenging is undesirable.

PREANESTHETIC ASSESSMENT, STABILIZATION, PROTOCOL SELECTION

PREANESTHETIC EVALUATION AND STABILIZATION

Prior to the induction of anesthesia in any animal, its medical and past anesthetic histories should be reviewed. A thorough physical examination must be performed, with special attention to the cardiovascular and pulmonary systems. For an otherwise healthy animal, the minimum laboratory database prior to general anesthesia usually includes packed cell volume (PCV), total protein concentration, and quick assessments of blood glucose and blood urea nitrogen levels (Table 19-1). Animals that are debilitated or have concurrent disease processes will require more extensive evaluation prior to the induction of anesthesia. In these cases, a complete blood count (CBC), serum chemistry panel, electrolyte concentrations, and urinalysis should be performed. An electrocardiogram should be obtained for traumatized or geriatric animals or those with evidence of cardiac abnormalities. Preanesthetic thoracic radiographs are indicated in animals with evidence of cardiac or pulmonary disease or those with a history of trauma.

The collection of much of the information outlined above will provide an assessment of the animal's ability to adequately respond to the depressive effects of anesthesia as well as its ability to eliminate the anesthetics. In addition, a thorough preanesthetic evaluation of an animal will

Table 19-1 Reference Values for Cardiovascular and Respiratory Parameters, Temperature, Packed Cell Volume, Total Protein, and Blood Gases in Common Domestic Animals

Component	Dog	Cat	Horse	Cow	Goat/Sheep	Pig
Heart rate (beats/min)	70-180	145-200	30-45	60-80	60-90	60-90
Respiratory rate (breaths/min)	10-40	20-40	8-20	20-40	15-40	10-40
Temperature						
(°F)	101-104	101-104	99.5-101.5	100.5-102.5	101-104	101-103
(°C)	38.3-40.0	38.3-40.0	37.5-38.5	38.1-39.2	38.3-40.0	38.3-39.5
Packed cell volume (%)	35-54	27-46	25-45	23-43	30-50	30-48
Total protein (g/dl)	5.7-7.8	6.3-8.3	6.0-8.5	6.7-8.6	6.3-7.1	6.0-7.5
Systolic arterial pressure (mm Hg)	110-160					
Diastolic arterial pressure (mm Hg)	70-90					
Mean arterial pressure (mm Hg)	80-110					
Arterial blood gas values						
pH	7.35-7.45					
$Paco_2$ (mm Hg)	35-45					
Pco_2 (mm Hg)	80-110					
HCO_3^- (mEq/L)	17-30	(mean = 24: higher values refer to horses and ruminants; lower values refer to dogs and cats)				
Total CO_2 (mEq/L)	18-31					
Base excess (mEq/L)	−4+4					

HCO_3^-, Bicarbonate; Pao_2, partial pressure of arterial oxygen; $Paco_2$, partial pressure of arterial carbon dioxide.

Table 19-2 American Society of Anesthesiologists Physical Status Classification

Classification	Definition	Example
I	Normal animal admitted for elective surgery	Elective castration
II	Animal with slight to moderate systemic disturbance	Obesity, dehydration
III	Animal with major systemic disturbance that limits activity but is not incapacitating	Heart disease, anemia, severe fracture
IV	Animal with very severe systemic disturbance that could lead to death if surgical or medical intervention is not applied	Frequent arrhythmias, ruptured bladder, internal hemorrhage, severe pneumothorax
V	Animal in a moribund state that will probably die despite surgical or medical intervention	Prolonged gastric dilation/volvulus, severe trauma with shock

increase the likelihood that a previously unrecognized pre-existing condition will be discovered and treated prior to any anesthesia associated with an elective procedure.

Any significant abnormalities that are discovered during the physical examination or from laboratory evaluation of the animal (i.e., dehydration, anemia, electrolyte or acid-base imbalance, respiratory embarrassment, cardiac arrhythmias) should be corrected prior to anesthetic induction.

Following the preanesthetic assessment of an animal, a physical status is assigned according to the criteria outlined in Table 19-2. The assignment of a physical status prior to anesthesia is a procedure developed by the American Society of Anesthesiologists (ASA). It is also used in veterinary anesthesia and serves as an aid in identifying the relative level of risk of the development of complications during the anesthetic period. Use of this classification system serves to direct protocol selection and is useful in communicating

with clients regarding the risk of anesthesia for their particular animal.

Prior to the induction of anesthesia, most animals should have food and water withheld. This fasting reduces the risk of regurgitation and the potential for aspiration of stomach contents during anesthesia, particularly during the induction and recovery periods. The recommended duration of this withholding varies from species to species. With the exception of cattle and small ruminants, food should be withheld for approximately 12 hours prior to the induction of anesthesia. Access to water should be denied for 8 to 10 hours prior to anesthesia. Cattle have relatively longer fasting times (36 to 48 hours for food, 12 to 24 hours for water) because of the large capacity of the rumen. Small ruminants should be fasted for 18 to 24 hours (8 to 10 hours for water) prior to anesthesia. Neonates, birds, and animals weighing less than 2 kg should not be fasted because of their limited glycogen stores and high metabolic rates. With these animals, fasting may induce hypoglycemia or dehydration in a short period of time.

PROTOCOL SELECTION: PHARMACOLOGY OF ANESTHETIC DRUGS

PREMEDICATION

The administration of preanesthetic drugs is an important part of safe animal management. Anticholinergics, tranquilizers, sedatives, opioids, and alpha$_2$ agonists, alone or in combination, are routinely used as preanesthetics in veterinary anesthesia. Preanesthetic drugs are used to aid in animal restraint prior to the induction of anesthesia, reduce anxiety, provide for preemptive analgesia, and decrease the amount drug required for the induction or maintenance of anesthesia. These drugs also help to produce safe, smooth, and uncomplicated induction, maintenance, and recovery periods. The use of combinations of tranquilizers, sedative, and opioids reduces the dose required for each individual component of the combination.

ANTICHOLINERGICS

Anticholinergics are administered prior to the induction of anesthesia to prevent bradycardia, excessive salivation and to reduce upper airway secretions. Atropine and glycopyrrolate are examples of anticholinergics that are routinely used in veterinary anesthesia. Although atropine is more economical, glycopyrrolate offers a longer duration of action, is less likely to promote cardiac arrhythmias, and produces less suppression of gastrointestinal motility. Glycopyrrolate appears to increase heart rate less than atropine. This property is beneficial in animals with heart disease in which the increase in myocardial oxygen consumption associated with a profound increase in heart rate could be detrimental. Glycopyrrolate, unlike atropine, does not cross the placental barrier; thus it has no effect on the fetus during cesarean delivery.

Although many veterinarians use anticholinergics as a routine part of a preanesthetic regimen, their use can be based on the needs of the individual animal and the associated procedure. The anticipated response to the anesthetics such as the development of bradycardia or excessive salivation or whether the procedure may increase vagal tone due to traction on abdominal organs or manipulation of the neck, throat, or eyes are all factors that indicate the need for the preanesthetic administration of an anticholinergic drug. Anesthetic drugs that promote bradycardia include opioids, alpha$_2$ agonists, barbiturates, and gas anesthetics. Dissociative agents, such as ketamine and tiletamine, may cause excessive salivation.

The use of anticholinergic agents is controversial in large animal species. They are not used routinely in horses because of the potential for gastrointestinal ileus and the subsequent development of colic. Glycopyrrolate is less likely to produce this effect, so it is used for the treatment of bradycardia

in anesthetized horses. In some cases the administration of anticholinergics is avoided in ruminants because of the potential for the development of more viscous secretions that may be more difficult to clear from the respiratory tract. Anticholinergic drugs may be used in swine in conjunction with drugs known to promote bradycardia or excessive salivation.

TECHNICIAN NOTE

When calculating drug doses, always double-check your calculations; double-check the label on the bottle from which you are drawing and the concentration of the drug in the bottle. Label all syringes to avoid medication administration errors.

TRANQUILIZERS AND SEDATIVES

These drugs are used to depress the central nervous system (CNS), to aid in restraint, and to reduce anxiety. Tranquilization or sedation can minimize stress during both induction and recovery, and it can reduce the requirements for drugs used for induction and maintenance of anesthesia.

Tranquilizers and sedatives used in veterinary medicine include phenothiazines (acepromazine), benzodiazepines (diazepam, midazolam, and zolazepam), and alpha$_2$ agonists (xylazine, medetomidine, detomidine, romifidine). Some of the opioids also produce sedation as a beneficial side effect of their administration.

Acepromazine calms animals and decreases motor activity; however, animals may be readily aroused by external stimuli, especially animals that are highly excitable or apprehensive. Acepromazine does not provide analgesia but enhances the analgesic effects of concurrently used drugs. Acepromazine has a long duration of action (2 to 4 hours) and is dependent on metabolism by the liver; thus acepromazine should be avoided in animals with liver disease and in geriatric and pediatric animals. The most prominent side effect of acepromazine is hypotension that is a result of vascular dilation. Other side effects and contraindications are presented in Table 19-3.

Drugs in the benzodiazepine class produce less profound sedation than that observed with either acepromazine or an alpha$_2$ agonist. Occasionally, their administration to dogs, cats, or horses results in excitation rather than sedation. Benzodiazepines are most commonly used in combination with other premedications (e.g., opioids) or in combination with ketamine to counteract the muscle rigidity produced by this drug. Benzodiazepines produce minimal cardiovascular depression so they are useful in geriatric or pediatric animals and animals with heart disease. Benzodiazepines have anticonvulsant activity and are useful in animals with a history of seizures or any neurologic disorder. Diazepam is usually used intravenously because its carrier, propylene glycol, causes pain when given intramuscularly. Midazolam is water soluble and may be used intramuscularly, subcutaneously, or intravenously.

Table 19-3 SIDE EFFECTS OF DRUGS USED FOR PREMEDICATION AND INDUCTION OF ANESTHESIA

Drug	Cardiovascular	Pulmonary	Adverse Effects	Contraindications
PREMEDICATIONS				
Acepromazine	Hypotension Antiarrhythmic	Minimal	Penile paralysis (stallions) Lowers seizure threshold Promotes hypothermia	Liver disease History of seizures Dehydration Hypovolemia Shock Heart disease Geriatric patients Pediatric patients
Diazepam/midazolam	Minimal	Minimal	Hypotension if injected too rapidly (diazepam) Irritation following IM administration (diazepam)	Should not use alone because excitement is possible
Xylazine/detomidine/ medetomidine/romifidine	Bradycardia Conduction disturbances Hypotension Arrhythmias with halothane anesthesia in dogs and cats	Respiratory depression	Impaired thermoregulation Hyperglycemia Profound muscle relaxation may exacerbate upper respiratory abnormalities	Heart disease Geriatric patients Pediatric patients Ruminants require low doses
Opioids	Minimal Bradycardia that is responsive to anticholinergic administration	Respiratory depression	Impaired thermoregulation (panting in dogs) Hyperresponsive to external stimuli Excitement in cats (dose dependent) and horses (pure agonists)	Use with tranquilizer or sedative in horses and cats
INDUCTION DRUGS				
Barbiturates	Myocardial depression Arrhythmias Hypotension	Respiratory depression (apnea)	Excessive salivation Laryngospasm Tissue necrosis with perivascular injection	Heart disease Liver disease Geriatric patients (use lower doses) Pediatric patients (use lower doses) Sight hounds *Obese animals* (dose on lean body weight)
Ketamine/tiletamine	Increase in heart rate and blood pressure Some direct myocardial depression	Minimal Apneustic breathing May cause apnea when given IV	Profuse salivation Muscle rigidity when used alone Convulsions with high doses	Never use alone except in cats Must have good sedation before administration in horses Animals with seizure history
Propofol	Myocardial depression Hypotension	Apnea	Heinz body anemia with repeat administration (5-7 days) in cats	None
Guaifenesin	Minimal	Minimal	Tissue necrosis with perivascular injection	

IM, Intramuscular; *IV*, intravenous.

Xylazine, detomidine, medetomidine, and romifidine are alpha₂ agonists that provide excellent sedation, muscle relaxation, and analgesia. Because of the profound cardiovascular effects that include bradycardia, conduction disturbances, and myocardial depression, alpha₂ agonists should be used only in healthy dogs and cats. Despite the profound bradycardia that can be produced by these drugs, the use of an anticholinergic is best avoided in favor of the titration of a reversal agent to elevate the heart rate. Thermoregulation is impaired for several hours following xylazine administration, so extremes in environmental temperature must be avoided. Requirements for maintenance of anesthesia with inhalation agents are greatly reduced (by 50% or more) when an alpha₂ agonist is used for premedication, so close attention to the degree of sedation prior to anesthetic induction is required. Xylazine, detomidine, and romifidine are commonly used in horses. Ruminants are particularly sensitive to the effects of alpha₂ agonists necessitating the use of much lower doses (roughly $^1/_{10}$ the dose used in horses) (Table 19-4). Reversal agents for alpha₂ agonists include yohimbine, tolazoline, and atipamezole.

OPIOIDS

Opioids are used to provide both analgesia and sedation. In horses, opioids are used in conjunction with a tranquilizer or sedative because the sole administration of pure opioids such as morphine or oxymorphone can produce excitement. Opioids promote anticholinergic-responsive bradycardia, but depression of cardiac contractility is minimal. The most significant side effect of opioid administration is respiratory depression. This depression renders the animal less sensitive to the accumulation of carbon dioxide in its blood and is manifest as hypoventilation or, in its most extreme form, apnea. Ventilatory support may be required to counteract this effect. Since opioid-induced respiratory depression can occur during the preanesthetic or recovery periods, it is important to monitor any animal that has received an opioid throughout the entire anesthetic period.

Thermoregulation is impaired by opioids delaying the return of a normal body temperature following anesthesia. Animals that have received opioids may be hyperresponsive to external stimuli, particularly noise. Such stimulation should be kept to a minimum. The effects of opioids may be reversed with pure antagonists (naloxone, diprenorphine) or mixed agonists/antagonists (butorphanol) (Table 19-4).

✐ TECHNICIAN NOTE

An induction protocol should facilitate the smooth transition from consciousness to unconsciousness and provide adequate muscle relaxation for an atraumatic endotracheal intubation.

N-Methyl-D-aspartate ANTAGONISTS (DISSOCIATIVE DRUGS)

N-Methyl-D-aspartate (NMDA) antagonists are most commonly used as part of an induction or maintenance protocol. In cats they may be used alone as a premedicant to produce immobilization for intravenous catheter placement or to facilitate induction of general anesthesia.

INDUCTION DRUGS

Induction drugs are used to facilitate the smooth and rapid transition from consciousness to unconsciousness for the maintenance of general anesthesia. Alternatively, these drugs may be used to maintain anesthesia for short periods of time where the use of inhaled anesthetics is unwarranted or impractical.

Ultra-Short-Acting Barbiturates

The most commonly used ultra-short-acting barbiturate is thiopental (Table 19-5). It may be used without preanesthetic medication to produce rapid loss of consciousness; however, it is safer to use premedications to facilitate intravenous injection and to reduce the dosage required to achieve unconsciousness. The degree of respiratory depression associated with barbiturate administration depends on the dosage and rate of administration. One should be prepared to intubate and provide ventilatory support when this drug is used.

Detrimental cardiopulmonary effects are more likely to occur when large doses are administered rapidly and when higher concentrations are used. Although solutions up to 10% are used in large animals, it is preferable to use a 2% to 2.5% solution in small animals. The more dilute solutions will reduce the likelihood of adverse effects and cause less tissue necrosis if accidental perivascular injection occurs. If accidental perivascular administration occurs, 2% lidocaine diluted 1:9 with sterile saline should be infiltrated into the injection site. Barbiturates are metabolized by the liver and should be avoided in animals with liver disease. Repeated bolus doses to maintain anesthesia with barbiturates are not recommended because these drugs have a cumulative effect and repeated administration will contribute to a rough, prolonged recovery.

Sight hounds (greyhounds, Irish wolfhounds, whippets) are unable to metabolize thiobarbiturates effectively, resulting in a prolonged recovery. An alternative induction method for sight hounds is propofol (4 to 6 mg/kg).

Propofol

Propofol is a nonbarbiturate, intravenously administered anesthetic agent that produces a rapid loss of consciousness for induction of anesthesia (Table 19-5). The drug is noncumulative and is rapidly cleared from the body. Propofol produces a smooth, rapid recovery and may also be used for maintenance of anesthesia by infusion (0.15 to 0.4 mg/kg/min) or repeated bolus doses. The major side effects are transient apnea and cardiovascular depression. Titrating the induction dose slowly to the desired level of anesthesia may reduce induction apnea. Propofol is formulated in a milky white emulsion containing soybean oil, egg lecithin, and glycerol. This formulation supports bacterial growth

Table 19-4 Dosages* (mg/kg) of Commonly Used Anesthetic Agents for Premedication and Chemical Restraint

Agent	Dog	Cat	Horse	Cow	Goat/Sheep	Pig
ANTICHOLINERGICS						
Atropine	0.02-0.04	0.02-0.04	—	0.04 (max 20 mg)	0.04	0.04
Glycopyrrolate	0.01-0.02	0.01-0.02	—	—	—	0.003
TRANQUILIZERS						
Aceptromazine	0.01-0.1	0.01-0.1	0.02-0.05	0.02-0.05	0.02-0.05	0.1-0.4
Diazepam	0.1-0.5	0.1-0.5	0.05-0.02	0.5-1.0	0.5-1.0	0.5-0.1
Midazolam	0.05-0.04	0.1-0.3	—	—	—	0.2-0.5
SEDATIVES						
Xylazine	0.3-1.1	0.3-1.1	0.3-1.1	0.02-0.11	0.02-0.1	0.5-4.0
Detomidine	—	—	0.01-0.04	—	—	—
Medetomidine	0.05-0.04	0.05-0.04	—	—	—	0.03-0.08
Romifidine	—	—	0.003-0.08	—	—	—
OPIOIDS						
Hydromorphone	0.1-0.2	0.1-0.2	—	—	—	—
Oxymorphone	0.05-0.1	0.05-0.1[†]	0.01-0.04[†]	—	—	0.15
Butorphanol	0.3-0.4	0.2-0.4	0.04-0.1	0.03-0.04	0.02-0.04	0.2-0.4
Morphine	0.5-1.0	0.05[†]-0.2[†]	0.04-0.1[†]	—	—	0.4-0.1
Meperidine	3-5	3-5	0.2-0.4[†]	2-4	—	—
Pentazocine	0.2-0.4	0.1	0.5-1.0	—	—	—
Buprenorphine	0.01-0.04	0.005-0.04	0.005-0.03	—	—	—
NEUROLEPTANALGESIC COMBINATIONS						
Acepromazine	0.05-0.1	0.05-0.1	—	—	—	—
Oxymorphone	0.1-0.2	0.05-0.1	—	—	—	—
Acepromazine	0.05-0.1	0.05-0.1	0.02-0.05	—	—	—
Butorphanol	0.2-0.4	0.2-0.4	0.02-0.04	—	—	—
Xylazine	0.22	0.22	0.5-1.0	0.02-0.05	0.02-0.05	—
Butorphanol	0.11-0.22	0.22-0.44	0.02-0.04	0.02-0.04	0.02-0.04	—
Medetomidine	0.01-0.02	0.01-0.02	—	—	—	—
Butorphanol	0.2	0.2	—	—	—	—
REVERSAL AGENTS						
Yohimbine[‡] (alpha$_2$ antagonist)	0.1-0.2	0.1-0.2	0.75-0.15	0.1-0.2	0.1-0.2	0.1-0.2
Tolazoline (alpha$_2$ antagonist)	0.2-1.0	0.5-2.0	4.0	2.0-3.0	2.0	2.0
Atipamezole (alpha$_2$ antagonist)	0.2-0.4	0.2-0.4	—	—	—	—
Naloxone (opioid antagonist)	0.04	0.04	0.005-0.02	0.002-0.03	0.002-0.03	0.04

*Most drugs may be administered either intravenously or intramuscularly. When administering a drug intramuscularly, the higher dosage of a given range is used.

[†]Use opioids only in conjunction with a tranquilizer or sedative.

[‡]Administer yohimbine to effect in large animal species. Calculate recommended dose and administer slowly until the desired effect is observed.

necessitating special handling procedures for this drug. According to manufacturer recommendations, once a propofol vial is opened, the remainder should be drawn into sterile syringes; each syringe should be prepared for single animal use only. Unused propofol should be discarded within 6 hours.

Propofol (1%) and thiopental (2.5%) can be used in combination (1:1, vol:vol) as an induction drug This

combination also results in significant bacteriostatic activity that is not seen with the propofol formulation alone.

Etomidate

Etomidate is a nonbarbiturate, noncumulative sedative-hypnotic administered intravenously for the induction of anesthesia (Table 19-5). An expensive induction drug, its use in veterinary medicine is limited to high-risk animals

Table 19-5 DOSAGES (mg/kg)* FOR DRUGS USED FOR INDUCTION OR SHORT-TERM MAINTENANCE OF ANESTHESIA

Agent	Dog	Cat	Horse	Cow	Goat/Sheep	Pig
Thiopental	8.8-13	8.8-13	6.6-11	4.4-11	4.4-11	8.8-13
Propofol	2-6	2-6	1-3	—	—	—
Etomidate	0.5-2.0	—	—	—	—	—
Guaifenesin	44-88	—	66-132	66-132	66-132	44-88
Ketamine	—	2.2-18	—	—	2.2-6.6	2.2-6.6
Telazol	2.2-11†	2.2-11†	—	4.4-11	2.2-11	4.4-11†
Guaifenesin/thiopental	3.3-88	—	44-88	44-88	—	33-88
	2.2-6.6	—	2.2-6.6	2.2-6.6	—	2.2-6.6
Guaifenesin/ketamine	33-88	—	44-88	44-88	44-88	—
	1.1	—	1.1-1.5	0.6-1.1	0.6-1.1	—
Acepromazine/ketamine	0.11	0.22†	—	—	—	0.44†
	11.0	4.4-11†	—	—	—	2.2-6.6†
Xylazine/ketamine	0.66-1.1†	0.66-1.1†	1.1	0.044-0.088†	0.044†	2.2-4.4†
	2.2-11†	4.4-22†	2.2	2.2-6.6†	2.2-6.6	2.2-11†
Diazepam/ketamine	0.25	0.25	—	—	0.25-0.55	0.22-0.44
	5.0	5.0	—	—	4.4	4.4
Xylazine/telazol	0.44†	0.66†	1.1	0.022-0.11†	0.044-0.088†	0.66-1.1†
	6.6†	2.2-6.6†	1.1-2.2	2.2-6.6†	2.2-6.6†	4.4-6.6†
Xylazine/guaifenesin/ketamine	(See Boxes 19-1 to 19-5 giving specific species protocol.)					

*Dosage is for intravenous use unless otherwise designated.
†Indicates protocols that may be used intramuscularly in some species.

that can benefit from the cardiovascular stability afforded by this drug. The side effects associated with etomidate include pain on injection, myoclonus, vomiting, excitement, and suppression of cortisol secretion. Myoclonus can be reduced with appropriate premedication.

NMDA Antagonist (Dissociative) Combinations

NMDA antagonists (ketamine, tiletamine) produce immobilization and analgesia (Table 19-5). Swallowing and ocular reflexes remain intact, and muscle tone is increased. These drugs may be administered intramuscularly or intravenously; however, intramuscular administration requires higher dosages and results in a prolonged recovery. Intramuscular administration is most commonly used in cats, small ruminants, and swine and is never used in horses.

Concurrent administration of an anticholinergic agent may be needed in some species (cats, dogs, swine) to reduce the excessive salivation associated with the administration of an NMDA antagonist. Although some direct depression of cardiac function occurs, an increase in sympathetic tone can compensate for this by increasing heart rate and arterial blood pressure. This effect on heart rate and blood pressure offers an advantage over the thiobarbiturates for use in unstable animals or some animals with heart disease. Since elimination of ketamine depends on both liver metabolism and renal excretion, high dosages should be avoided in animals with liver or kidney disease.

Ketamine, combined with a benzodiazepine, is an alternative method of induction for sight hounds. Telazol is a commercially produced combination containing equal parts of zolazepam (benzodiazepine) and tiletamine (NMDA antagonist) that may be used for both induction and maintenance of anesthesia. Although approved only for intramuscular use, intravenous administration of very low dosages provides an effective method for the induction of anesthesia as well as short-term injectable anesthesia (Table 19-5).

Guaifenesin

Guaifenesin is an intravenously administered central-acting muscle relaxant that potentiates the effects of preanesthetic and anesthetic drugs, allowing for lower dosages of either of these drugs. Guaifenesin is used in large animals as part of both induction and maintenance protocols (Table 19-5). Cardiopulmonary effects are minimal, and there is a wide margin of safety. Excessive dosages may result in muscle rigidity of the forelimbs and neck and an apneustic breathing pattern. Administration is best performed through an indwelling venous catheter because large volumes must be administered (usually as a 5% solution) and perivascular injection can cause tissue necrosis.

TECHNICIAN NOTE

Mask induction of anesthesia with an inhaled anesthetic should be reserved for high-risk patients that are adequately sedated. This technique greatly increases waste-gas contamination.

ANESTHETIC MAINTENANCE

The maintenance of anesthesia is most commonly accomplished with inhaled anesthetics; however, effective maintenance of anesthesia for short periods may be achieved using various combinations of the induction drugs discussed above.

INHALED ANESTHETICS

Inhaled anesthetics are most commonly used for the maintenance of anesthesia; however, they may be used for the induction of anesthesia (mask or chamber) in animals where induction of anesthesia with an injectable drug is impossible or contraindicated. Inhaled anesthetics used in veterinary medicine include isoflurane, halothane, sevoflurane, and methoxyflurane. The use of methoxyflurane has greatly decreased because of several undesirable effects that include significant hepatic metabolism and the associated production of metabolites that are toxic to the renal system, prolonged recovery, and a lack of availability. Sevoflurane has been introduced recently into the practice of veterinary anesthesia and generally has properties similar to those of isoflurane. In some situations sevoflurane provides a more rapid induction or recovery than observed with isoflurane.

Inhaled anesthetics produce general anesthesia that includes unconsciousness and muscle relaxation and are suitable for use in all species. Inhaled anesthetics provide more rapid control of changes in the depth of anesthesia and a more rapid recovery than seen with injectable anesthetics. These drugs produce profound effects on cardiopulmonary function and animals must be closely monitored throughout the anesthetic period.

Some properties of the inhaled anesthetics must be understood in order to gain an appreciation both for the function of anesthetic vaporizers and the way that the inhaled anesthetics behave in the body (Table 19-6). The vapor pressure of an inhaled anesthetic determines the maximum concentration that may be achieved in the carrier gas (oxygen) at any given temperature. Methoxyflurane has a low vapor pressure (23 mm Hg) and will only reach a maximum concentration of 3.5% at room temperature. In contrast, halothane and isoflurane, both with vapor pressures of approximately 240 mm Hg, can reach a maximum concentration of approximately 32% at room temperature. This means that a precision vaporizer (see discussion of equipment) that delivers a precise concentration of anesthetic gas is safer and helps to avoid potentially lethal concentrations of isoflurane and halothane. Although the use of halothane, isoflurane, and sevoflurane in nonprecision vaporizers has been reported, methoxyflurane is most commonly used in this type of vaporizer.

Solubility refers to how the anesthetic vapor distributes itself between the blood and gas phases. Solubility determines the speed of induction and recovery from anesthesia with a particular inhaled anesthetic. Methoxyflurane has a very high solubility in the blood and other tissues that delays the development of an effective level of anesthetic gas in the blood. This effective level of anesthetic vapor in the blood is required for the gas to pass into the brain in quantities sufficient to render the animal unconscious. The high solubility of methoxyflurane is associated with inductions and recoveries that are slow in comparison to those associated with the other inhaled anesthetics. The other inhaled anesthetics are much less soluble than methoxyflurane making induction and recovery with any of these drugs much faster than that observed with methoxyflurane. The blood:gas solubility coefficients of common inhaled anesthetics are presented in Table 19-6.

Minimum alveolar concentration (MAC) is the minimum concentration of anesthetic in the alveolar gas that prevents a response in 50% of animals exposed to a surgical stimulus. MAC is a measure of anesthetic potency and is used as a guide to support the delivery of an appropriate concentration of an anesthetic for surgical procedures. The MAC values have been determined for the commonly used gas anesthetics for many animal species (Table 19-6). Since MAC defines the level of anesthesia required to prevent only 50% of animals from responding to surgical anesthesia

Table 19-6 PHYSICAL CHARACTERISTICS AND MINIMUM ALVEOLAR CONCENTRATIONS (MAC) FOR INHALED ANESTHETICS USED IN VETERINARY MEDICINE

Inhalant	Vapor Pressure	Blood:Gas Solubility Coefficient	MAC Values (%)			
			Dog	Cat	Horse	Pig
Isoflurane	240	1.46	1.3	1.6	1.31	1.45-1.75
Halothane	243	2.54	0.8-0.9	0.8-1.2	0.88	0.9-1.25
Sevoflurane	157	0.68	2.10-2.36	2.6	2.31	1.97-2.66
Methoxyflurane	23	15.0	0.23	0.23	0.28	†

*Due to the slow induction and recovery phases, methoxyflurane is not used routinely in large animals.
†Not available.

and practitioners require almost 100% assurance of anesthesia, multiples of MAC are used to determine appropriate vaporizer settings (concentrations). For most procedures in most species, 1.5 to 2.0 times MAC is adequate to maintain a surgical plane of anesthesia. Anesthetic induction is usually accomplished at anesthetic concentrations of 2.0 to 3.0 times the MAC for that anesthetic. The MAC level of an anesthetic is not absolute. Several factors can decrease the MAC for an inhaled anesthetic: age (older animals require less), hypothermia, administration of other depressant drugs (e.g., opioids, tranquilizers), and concurrent diseases such as septicemia.

The inhaled anesthetics cause dose-dependent depression of cardiac function, with isoflurane and sevoflurane having the least effect at clinically relevant concentrations. All anesthetic gases cause some respiratory depression, and ventilation should be monitored and assisted when appropriate (see Ventilatory Support). Halothane has the additional undesirable characteristic of "sensitizing" the heart to catecholamines, which can result in the development of arrhythmias. Methoxyflurane is less likely to induce arrhythmias, and isoflurane and sevoflurane do not have this effect. Isoflurane and sevoflurane, although more expensive than halothane, are the safest and most versatile inhaled anesthetics.

✐ TECHNICIAN NOTE

Ideally, all anesthetized animals should be intubated so that the airway is protected and maintained. Intubation greatly facilitates the administration of supplemental oxygen during injectable anesthesia.

MONITORING DURING ANESTHESIA

Monitoring during the perianesthetic period is an essential component of any anesthetic procedure. Chemical restraint and general anesthesia can profoundly depress the physiological functioning of both normal and debilitated animals. Changes can occur relatively quickly in the anesthetized animal, so frequent monitoring (at least every 5 minutes) should be employed.

The anesthetic record is a concise method for recording the time of administration and doses (in milligrams) of anesthetic drugs that are administered (Figure 19-14). The anesthetic record is also used to record the parameters measured during the anesthetic period (heart rate, respiratory rate, blood pressure, etc.). The anesthetic record is a legal document that prompts the anesthetist to evaluate and record the animal's vital signs at regular intervals. Recording parameters at regular, frequent intervals permits not only the detection of marked changes in any parameters but also the recognition of more gradual changes that occur over a period of time (trends). Gradual changes may go undetected when parameters are not recorded over time. The anesthetic record also provides information about an animal's response to anesthesia and anesthetic drugs as an aid in planning subsequent anesthetic procedures.

Monitoring includes both the manual assessment of physical parameters such as heart rate, respiratory rate, temperature, eye reflexes and muscle tone and the more technical assessment of blood pressure, cardiac rhythm, hemoglobin saturation with oxygen, and end-expired carbon dioxide levels. More invasive monitoring may involve an assessment of arterial blood gas values, direct arterial blood pressure, and central venous pressure. Monitoring during the anesthetic period focuses on the cardiovascular, pulmonary, and central nervous systems since these systems are most likely to be affected by anesthesia or surgery. The preanesthetic physical status of the animal (see Preanesthetic Evaluation and Stabilization), the anesthetic protocol, the intended procedure, and its duration will determine the sophistication of the monitoring techniques used.

Cardiovascular system monitoring involves an integrated assessment of heart rate and rhythm, pulse quality, capillary refill time (CRT), and mucous membrane color. Heart rate and rhythm may be assessed by auscultation or with an esophageal stethoscope in small animals (Figure 19-15). Palpation of a peripheral pulse may be easier to perform than auscultation during the surgical procedure. This provides a method of counting the pulse rate as well as an assessment of pulse strength or quality. Peripheral pulses may be palpated over the femoral, dorsal metatarsal, digital, and lingual arteries in dogs; the femoral artery in cats and swine; the facial, transverse facial, submandibular, and lateral metatarsal arteries in horses; and the auricular, digital, coccygeal, and dorsal metatarsal arteries in ruminants.

Monitoring cardiac rhythm is accomplished with a continuous electrocardiogram (ECG). The ECG determines both rate and cardiac rhythm. In small animals, lead II is most frequently monitored. In large animals, a base-apex lead placement is used. Lead placement for a base-apex ECG (right arm over heart, left arm over jugular furrow, and left leg over point of shoulder) will yield a large positive R wave. It is important to remember that a normal ECG only indicates electrical activity in the heart. It does not yield information regarding myocardial contractility or tissue perfusion. The capillary refill time (CRT) (normal = 2 seconds) is employed as a rough, insensitive assessment of peripheral perfusion and pulse quality.

✐ TECHNICIAN NOTE

The vital signs of anesthetized animals should be monitored every 5 minutes, and all data should be recorded in the anesthetic record.

Arterial blood pressure may be measured directly or indirectly. Indirect methods include the oscillometric and ultrasonic Doppler methods. Both of these indirect methods require the placement of an inflatable cuff over a peripheral artery. Relatively easy to use compared to the direct method, these methods yield values that are less accurate than those

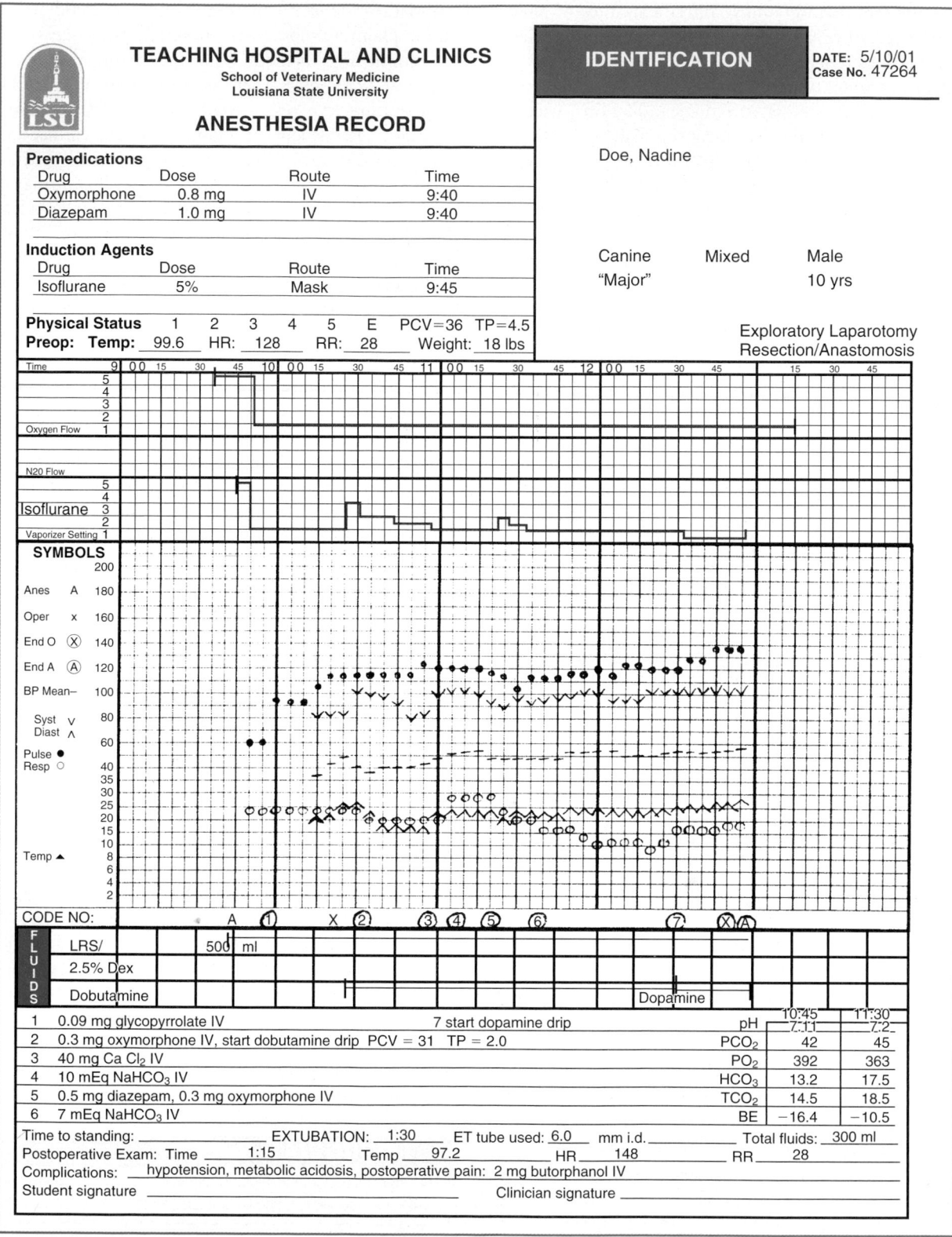

Figure 19-14 An example of an anesthetic record used to record drug administration, heart and respiratory rates, direct arterial blood pressure, arterial blood gases, and other significant treatments or events during an anesthetic period.

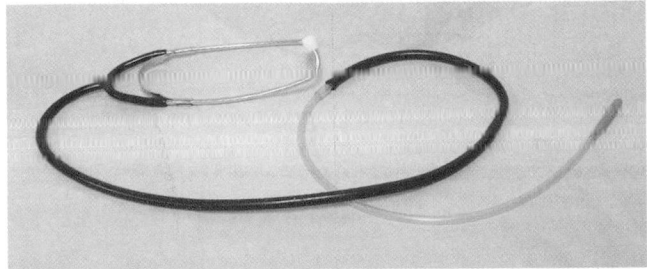

Figure 19-15 An esophageal stethoscope is a relatively simple device that allows auscultation of heart sounds during anesthesia.

obtained with direct pressure measurement (Figures 19-16 and 19-17).

For direct pressure monitoring, a catheter is placed in a peripheral artery and connected via heparinized saline-filled tubing to a pressure transducer. Direct methods require more technical skill and knowledge of the equipment. A pressure transducer connected to an appropriate monitor provides measures of the mean, systolic, and diastolic arterial pressures. Direct blood pressure monitoring is beneficial in high-risk animals of all species. Direct blood pressure monitoring is used more frequently in anesthetized

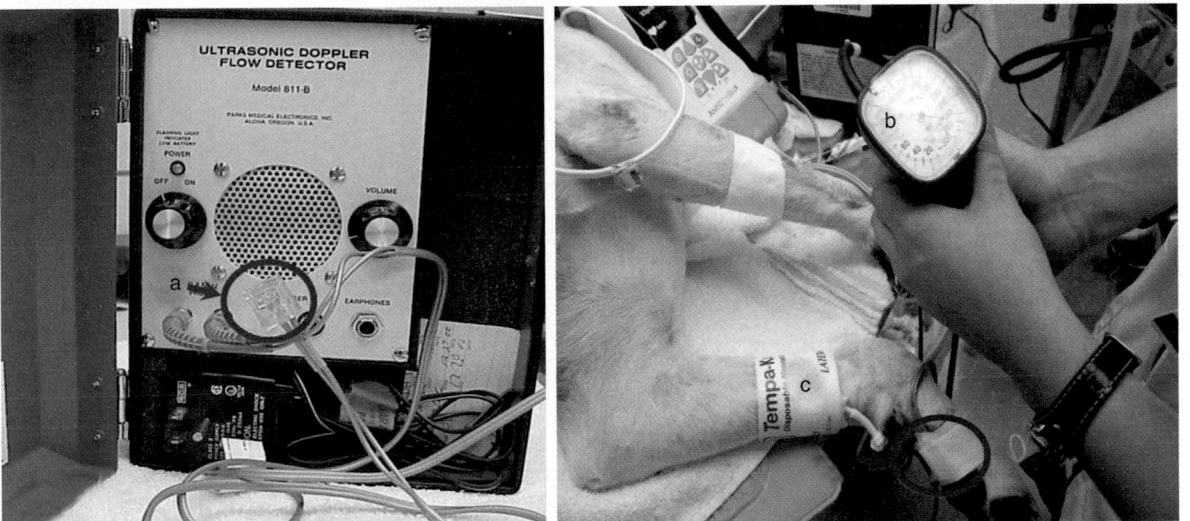

A **B**

Figure 19-16 **A,** Doppler ultrasound unit for the indirect measurement of blood pressure. **B,** The ultrasound probe *(a)* is placed over a peripheral artery, and a sphygmomanometer *(b)* and cuff *(c)* are used to determine the systolic blood pressure.

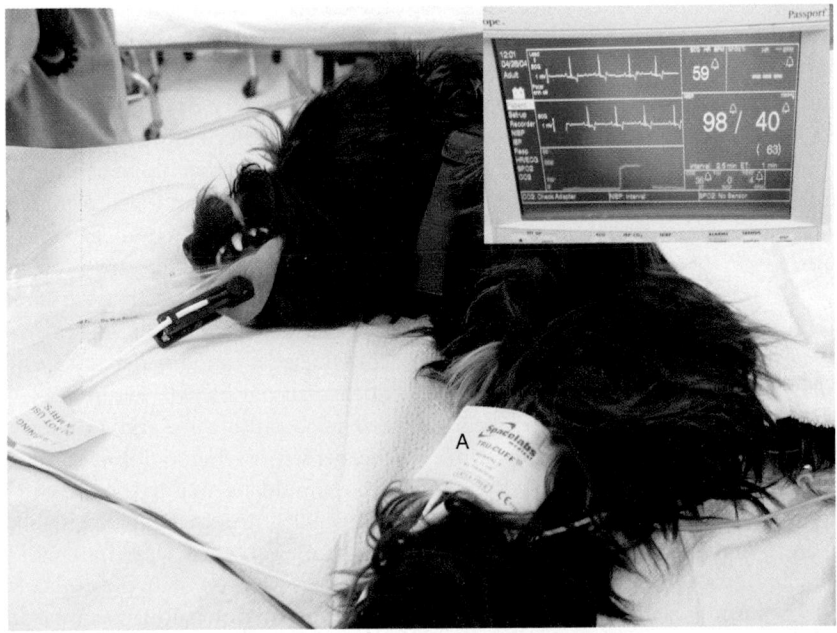

Figure 19-17 An oscillometric blood pressure measurement unit indirectly determines blood pressure by detecting changes in pressure oscillations in the, *A,* inflated cuff as it is deflated. The pressure oscillations are converted into values for systolic, diastolic, and mean blood pressure that are displayed on the monitor screen *(inset).*

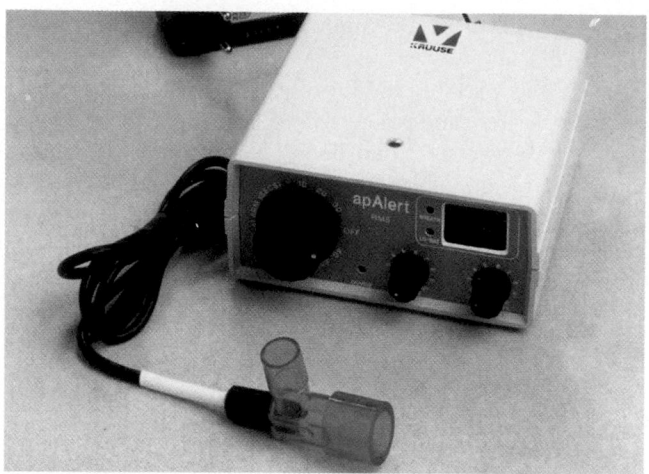

Figure 19-18 Apnea monitor detects changes in the temperature of the gas moving past the probe. The monitor creates an audible signal for every breath and can be set to alarm if a breath has not occurred within a specified period of time.

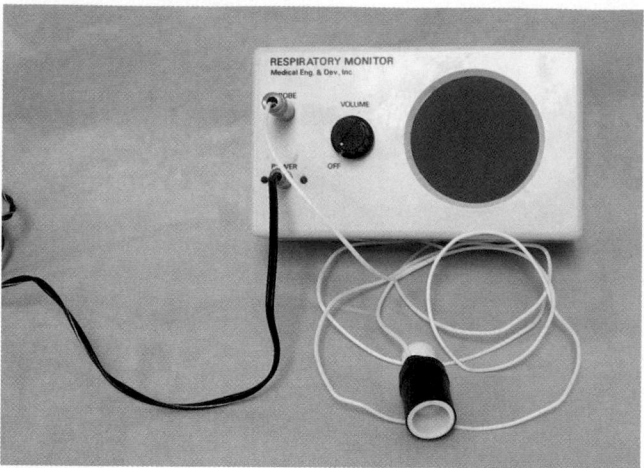

Figure 19-19 A respiratory monitor that detects the flow of air created by each breath. The flow is converted into an audible signal. Unlike the apnea monitor, this monitor gives information about the duration of the flow of respiratory gas past the monitor probe that is located in the breathing circuit.

horses during inhaled anesthesia as an accurate method of determining arterial blood pressure. Prolonged hypotension is of particular concern in anesthetized horses because of its contribution to the development of postanesthetic myopathy. Normal values for arterial blood pressure are listed in Table 19-1.

During anesthesia, the *pulmonary system* is monitored by assessing respiratory rate, rhythm, depth, the amount of hemoglobin saturated with oxygen (SpO_2), arterial blood gas tensions, and the amount of carbon dioxide in the expired gas ($ET-PCO_2$).

Respiratory rate, rhythm, and depth are very crude assessments of the adequacy of ventilation and oxygenation. Sudden changes in the ventilatory pattern may signal the need for intervention. As an example, the onset of apnea during anesthesia may indicate excessive anesthetic depth. An increase in respiratory rate following the beginning of surgery may indicate an anesthetic level that is too light for the intended procedure. The degree of collapse of the rebreathing bag provides a crude estimate of the depth of respiration and tidal volume.

Respiratory rate may be monitored with an apnea monitor that produces an audible "beep" following expiration (Figure 19-18). It is set to alarm when a specific time period has passed without a detected expiration. The sensing portion of the monitor is placed between the endotracheal tube and the breathing circuit where it detects changes in the temperature of gases flowing past it. On expiration, there is an increase in the temperature of the gas that is detected by the sensor. It is important to note that the apnea monitor makes no assessment about the quality of the breath. Thus a breath of inadequate tidal volume is detected in the same manner as a larger, more adequate breath. The apnea monitor may be particularly useful in small animals and birds whose respirations may be difficult to assess by

observing either chest wall excursions or movement of the rebreathing bag. Some apnea monitors may lack the sensitivity required to detect the expiratory flow of very small animals. Another respiratory monitor (Figure 19-19) converts the movement of air past the airway sensor into an audible signal that is amplified by the monitor speaker.

Arterial carbon dioxide ($PaCO_2$) and oxygen (PaO_2) partial pressures provide the most accurate method of determining adequacy of ventilation. Patient-side blood gas analyzers are being used more frequently in veterinary anesthesia, but their cost remains prohibitive in some practices. Arterial blood gas analysis requires the collection of an arterial blood sample that is most commonly taken from the dorsal metatarsal artery in dogs, submandibular or facial artery in horses, and the femoral artery in cats. It is essential when handling an arterial blood sample for blood gas analysis that all air bubbles are removed prior to analysis. Contamination of the sample with room air will alter the carbon dioxide and oxygen levels that are reported by the analyzer. Two patient-side blood gas analyzers are shown in Figure 19-20.

Pulse oximetry is a noninvasive method of monitoring both pulse rate and the percentage of oxygenated hemoglobin in the arterial blood (Figure 19-21). Most pulse oximeters provide a pulse wave and a digital display of pulse rate and the percent of hemoglobin saturated with oxygen (SpO_2). SpO_2 should be maintained above 95% in animals. Values below 90% are associated with an arterial oxygen partial pressure (PaO_2) of less than 60 mm Hg, a value that is indicative of severe hypoxemia. Several sources of error including hypotension, tachycardia, hypothermia, movement, and poor probe positioning can create measurement error when using a pulse oximeter. These sources of error should be considered when interpreting SpO_2 derived from

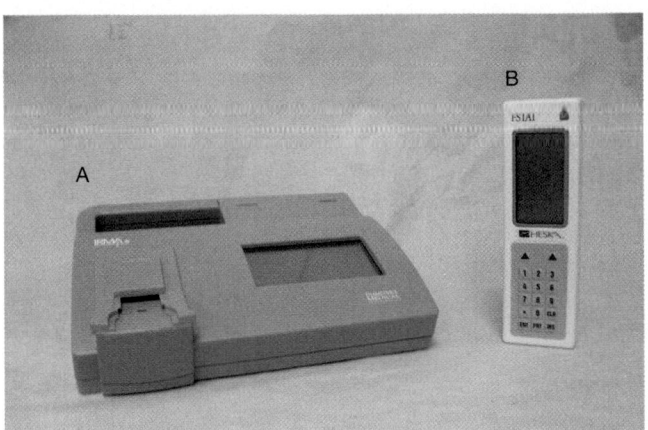

Figure 19-20 Patient-side or portable blood gas analyzers such as the IRMA *(A)* (ITC Edison, NJ) or I-STAT *(B)* (Heska Corp., Ft. Collins, Colo.) are compact and easy to use.

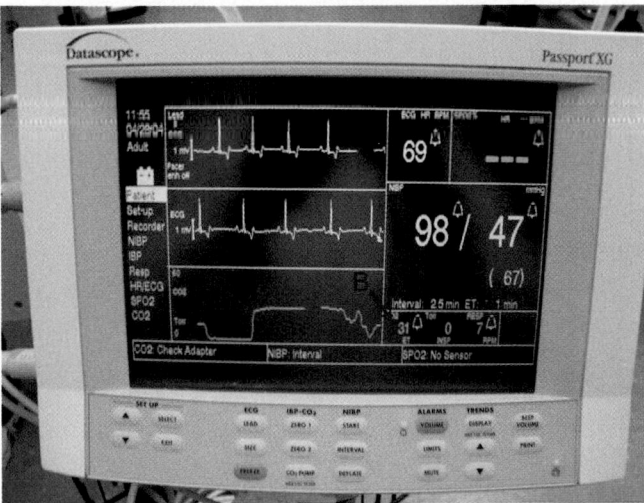

Figure 19-22 Multifunction monitor showing capnograph display *(A)* and $P_{ET}CO_2$ *(B)*.

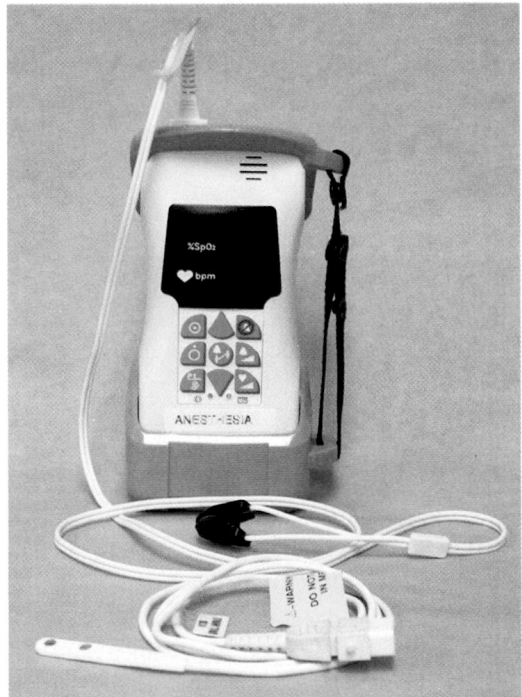

Figure 19-21 Pulse oximeter shown with two different probes. The reflectance probe in the foreground may be placed in the esophagus or rectum in animals where the use of the tongue probe is difficult.

a pulse oximeter. Sites for probe placement in animals include the tongue, lip fold, toe web, ear, skinfolds, vulva, and nasal septum. A reflectance probe that may be used in the rectum and esophagus or laid flat against a mucous membrane is also available (Figure 19-21).

Capnometry provides a noninvasive method for monitoring respiratory rate and adequacy of ventilation (Figure 19-22). The capnometer yields an assessment of the partial pressure of carbon dioxide in the end-tidal (at the end of expiration) gas (ET-P_{CO_2}). The capnometer attaches to

the animal's endotracheal tube and also reports the respiratory rate. The ET-P_{CO_2} is a close estimate of the amount of carbon dioxide in the blood (Pa_{CO_2}) and should be maintained between 35 and 40 mm Hg. As a general rule, ET-P_{CO_2} tends to underestimate Pa_{CO_2} by 5 to 10 mm Hg. An increase in ET-P_{CO_2} usually indicates hypoventilation and the need for ventilatory assistance (see Ventilatory Support).

Most anesthetics are potent respiratory depressants and apnea after the induction of anesthesia is common. Ventilation should be supported at this time (two to four breaths per minute) to ensure adequate delivery of oxygen and anesthetic gas until spontaneous ventilation returns (see Ventilatory Support). It is important to ensure that assisted ventilation during this time is not overly aggressive. Excessive ventilation may reduce the animal's carbon dioxide level below the point that triggers spontaneous ventilation.

> ✎ **TECHNICIAN NOTE**
> The use of monitoring devices during the anesthetic period does not replace frequent, careful assessment of an anesthetized animal by the veterinary anesthetist.

Central nervous system monitoring yields information regarding the depth of anesthesia and includes assessment of the position of the eye in the orbit and the strength of eye reflexes. In light and medium levels of surgical anesthesia in dogs and cats, the eyeball is generally turned downward, the eyelids are closed, and the palpebral reflex (blinking response to stimulation of the lateral or medial canthus) is sluggish. In horses, nystagmus (eyeball movement) and lacrimation (tearing) are signs of light anesthesia. In cattle, the eyeball rotates from a central position to a ventromedial position when surgical anesthesia is reached. Although eye position can be helpful, there is considerable species variability, and it should not be used exclusively as an indicator of anesthetic depth. The degree of muscle relaxation (e.g., jaw tone), absence of voluntary movement, and response to stimulation also aid in the evaluation of anesthetic depth. In some species, loss of the anal reflex is a crude indicator of excessive anesthetic depth.

VENTILATORY SUPPORT

Since general anesthesia depresses respiratory function, ventilatory support may often be necessary. Ventilatory support is particularly indicated in animals with pulmonary and pleural cavity disease, abdominal distention, or diaphragmatic hernia. Obese or debilitated, weak animals may also require ventilatory support. Ventilation is an absolute requirement in animals undergoing a thoracotomy and in those animals receiving neuromuscular blocking drugs.

ASSISTED VENTILATION

The technique of assisted ventilation involves closing the pop-off valve and compressing the rebreathing bag so that gas within the breathing circuit is gently forced into the airways and lungs of the animal. When performing assisted ventilation, care must be taken to ensure that the pop-off valve is opened following the administration of each assisted breath. Most anesthesia machines are equipped with a pressure manometer that measures the pressure in the breathing system. During assisted ventilation, a peak inspiratory pressure (PIP) (the pressure on the manometer at the end of inspiration) of 20 to 25 cm H_2O for small animals and 25 to 30 cm H_2O for large animals is frequently associated with the delivery of an adequate tidal volume. Higher pressures may be needed in animals with open thoracic cavities or those with primary lung disease. Continuous ventilatory support is normally not required in healthy animals undergoing routine surgical procedures. A "sigh" (a breath of a tidal volume that is greater than the normal tidal volume and associated with slightly higher PIPs) can be delivered once every 5 to 10 minutes in an attempt combat atelectasis in these animals.

MECHANICAL VENTILATION

Mechanical ventilators are most commonly used during prolonged, perhaps more complicated, procedures and where ventilatory support is absolutely indicated (Figure 19-23). The indications for mechanical ventilation [also known as *intermittent positive-pressure ventilation* (IPPV)] include the following:

- Prolonged apnea
- Evidence of severe hypoventilation (marked decrease in respiratory rate, increase in ET-P_{CO_2} or Pa_{CO_2})
- Intrathoracic surgery
- Intraoperative use of neuromuscular blocking agents

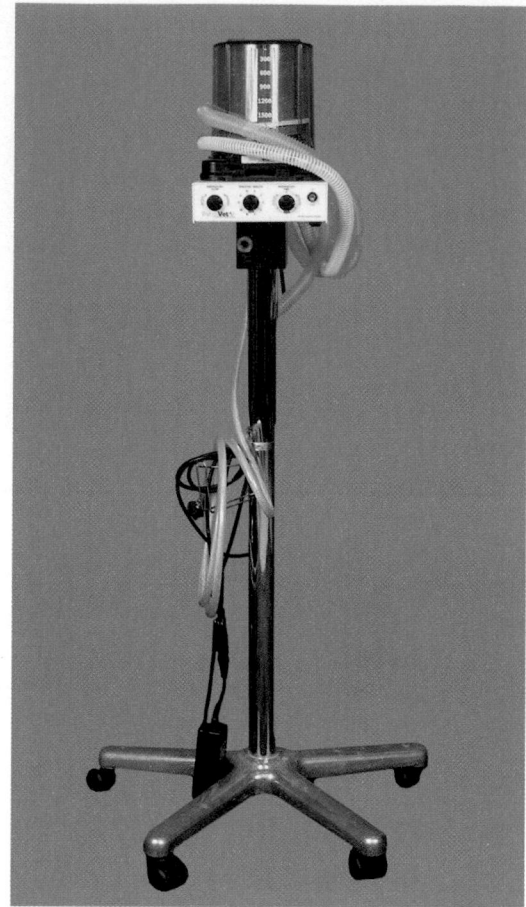

Figure 19-23 Example of a mechanical ventilator commonly used in veterinary anesthesia.

- Prescribed need for hyperventilation in cases of elevated intracranial pressure following head trauma
- Unstable plane of anesthesia due to inadequate uptake of inhaled anesthetics IPPV does have a significant, negative effect on cardiovascular performance because of reduced venous return to the heart during positive pressure inspiration. These effects may be reduced by ensuring adequate intravascular volume, the use of positive inotropes (dopamine, dobutamine, and ephedrine, for example), and delivering IPPV according to the following guidelines:
  1. *Tidal volume* is the volume of gas delivered during each ventilatory cycle. The tidal volume is 15 to 20 ml/kg for small animals and 10 to 15 ml/kg for large animals. This volume is higher than the actual tidal volume of the animal to allow for expansion in the breathing system and airway during positive pressure ventilation.
  2. *Inspiratory time* is the time taken for one inspiration. It should be approximately 2.0 seconds (longer in large animals). The inspiratory/expiratory (I/E) ratio is the ratio of the inspiratory time to the expiratory time. The normal I/E ratio should be approximately

1:2 (therefore, the normal expiratory time would be 4 seconds). Inspiratory times shorter than expiratory times help to minimize the negative cardiovascular effects of positive pressure ventilation. The peak inspiratory pressure is influenced by both the tidal volume and inspiratory time. A value of 15 to 20 cm H_2O will expand the lungs of most small animals. Higher PIP values (20 to 30 cm H_2O) are normally required for the mechanical ventilation of large animals.

3. The recommended respiratory rate during IPPV is 8 to 14 breaths/min for dogs and cats and 6 to 12 breaths/min for large animals. When small tidal volumes must be used (i.e., animals with abdominal distention, diaphragmatic hernia), the respiratory rate should be increased to compensate for the reduction in tidal volume.

SPECIAL ANESTHETIC TECHNIQUES

NEUROLEPTANALGESIA

Neuroleptanalgesia is produced by the administration of a combination of a tranquilizer or sedative with an opioid. The administration of this drug combination produces a state of profound central nervous system depression and analgesia (Table 19-4). Animals may become unconscious but remain responsive to external stimuli. The administration of this drug combination produces more profound analgesia and sedation than is the case when either agent is administered alone. The combination may provide adequate analgesia and restraint for procedures such as radiography, wound debridement, suturing of minor skin lacerations, or ear treatment.

EPIDURAL ANALGESIA/ANESTHESIA

Epidural drug administration provides a method of complete anesthesia (when local anesthetics such as lidocaine and bupivacaine are administered) or supplemental intra- and postoperative analgesia (when opioids are administered). Alpha$_2$ agonists and NMDA antagonists may also be administered epidurally (Chapter 20). The site of injection is at the lumbosacral intervertebral space for small animals, small ruminants, and swine and at the first intercoccygeal space in horses and cattle.

The epidural administration of local anesthetics produces total analgesia and muscle relaxation in the caudal portion of the body. This facilitates surgery of the hind limbs, perineal region, and abdomen. The cranial extent of the analgesia produced with this technique varies from animal to animal so that supplementary anesthesia may become necessary for some animals.

This technique is associated with less cardiovascular depression than general anesthesia and can be an ideal component of an anesthetic protocol for high-risk cases or cesarean section. Side effects may include hypotension because of the vasodilation produced by the epidural administration of local anesthetics. Ensuring the animal is adequately volume expanded prior to anesthesia may reduce epidural associated hypotension. In the very rare instance, respiratory arrest may occur if cranial migration of an excessive dose of the local anesthetic occurs following lumbosacral administration. For this reason, animals receiving local anesthetics epidurally should never be placed in a head-down position. Acute or delayed respiratory depression may occur in animals following the epidural administration of opioids. The epidural administration of morphine has been associated with urinary retention and pruritus.

The dosage is approximately 1 ml/4.5 kg of 2.0% lidocaine or 0.5% bupivacaine. The durations of effect of epidurally administered lidocaine or bupivacaine are 60 to 90 minutes and 4 to 6 hours, respectively. The dosage should be reduced by 50% if cerebrospinal fluid is observed in the hub of the needle during placement of the epidural. Pregnant and obese animals require a dose reduction of 10% to 20%. Epidural administration of preservative-free morphine (0.1 mg/kg) provides analgesia lasting 10 to 18 hours. Morphine may be administered alone for intraoperative or postoperative analgesia or in combination with a local anesthetic agent for the immediate local anesthesia. The analgesic effects of epidural morphine may extend as far forward as the forelimbs. Morphine administered epidurally at the coccygeal space has been shown to be effective for managing pelvic limb and abdominal pain in horses and cattle. Contraindications for epidural injection include animals with sepsis, clotting abnormalities, or severe dermatitis over the injection site.

PROTOCOL SELECTION AND PREPARATION OF EQUIPMENT

PROTOCOL SELECTION

Selection of an anesthetic protocol is based on many factors: the animal's temperament and physical status, the intended procedure, available drugs, the familiarity of personnel with those drugs, and the amount of assistance available for the procedure. Some commonly employed protocols for the common domestic species are listed in Boxes 19-1 to 19-5.

EQUIPMENT PREPARATION

A successful anesthetic procedure is the result of many important factors. Foremost among these is the thorough planning of the procedure and identification of the anticipated equipment needs. Complications may arise very quickly during anesthesia, and the easy availability of equipment required for a successful intervention is essential.

Box 19-1 EXAMPLES OF PROTOCOLS USED FOR CHEMICAL RESTRAINT AND GENERAL ANESTHESIA IN DOGS

PROTOCOL FOR ASA STATUS I AND II ANIMALS

Premedication	Acepromazine: 0.05-0.1 mg/kg IM
	or
	Medetomidine: 5-10 µg/kg IM
	and one of
	Hydromorphone: 0.1 mg/kg IM
	or
	Butorphanol: 0.2-0.4 mg/kg IM
Induction	Thiopental: 8-10 mg/kg IV
Maintenance	Halothane, isoflurane, or sevoflurane

PROTOCOL FOR ASA STATUS III-V ANIMALS

Premedication	Midazolam: 0.1 mg/kg IM
	Hydromorphone: 0.1 mg/kg IM
Induction	Propofol: 2-4 mg/kg IV to effect
	or
	Mask induction or diazepam (0.25 mg/kg) + ketamine (5 mg/kg) mixed together and administrated IV.
Maintenance	Isoflurane or sevoflurane

INJECTABLE PROTOCOLS FOR SHORT-DURATION ANESTHESIA

1. Medetomidine　10-20 µg/kg IV
   Ketamine　5-10 mg/kg IV
2. Propofol administered IV to effect.
3. Diazepam (0.25 mg/kg) + ketamine (5 mg/kg) mixed together and administered IV.

IV, Intravenously; *IM*, intramuscularly.

Box 19-2 EXAMPLES OF PROTOCOLS USED FOR CHEMICAL RESTRAINT AND GENERAL ANESTHESIA IN CATS

PROTOCOLS FOR ASA STATUS I AND II ANIMALS

Premedication	Medetomidine: 10-20 µg/kg IM (depending on temperament)
	and one of
	Hydromorphone: 0.1 mg/kg IM
	or
	Butorphanol: 0.2 mg/kg IM
	In a particularly fractious cat, ketamine 10 mg/kg IM may be added to provide more profound restraint.
Induction	Thiopental: 5-10 mg/kg IV
	or
	Diazepam (0.25 mg/kg) + Ketamine (5 mg/kg) mixed together and administered intravenously.
Maintenance	Halothane, isoflurane, or sevoflurane

PROTOCOL FOR ASA STATUS III-V ANIMALS

Premedication	Midazolam: 0.1 mg/kg IM
	Buprenorphine: 10-20 µg/kg
Induction	Mask induction with isoflurane or sevoflurane.
	or
	Diazepam (0.25 mg/kg) + Ketamine (5 mg/kg) mixed together and administered intravenously.
	or
	Propofol: 2-4 mg/kg IV
Maintenance	Isoflurane or sevoflurane

INJECTABLE PROTOCOLS FOR SHORT-DURATION ANESTHESIA

1. Butorphanol (0.44 mg/kg) + Telazol (6-11 mg/kg). Mix and administer IM.
2. Medetomidine (10-20 µg/kg) + Butorphanol (0.2 mg/kg) + Ketamine (10-15 mg/kg). Mix and administer IM.

IV, Intravenously; *IM*, intramuscularly; *SC*, subcutaneously.

Box 19-3 EXAMPLES OF PROTOCOLS USED FOR CHEMICAL RESTRAINT AND GENERAL ANESTHESIA IN HORSES

STANDING CHEMICAL RESTRAINT

1. Xylazine: 0.5-1.0 mg/kg IV
   Butorphanol: 0.02-0.04 mg/kg IV
            Administer xylazine first.
2. Detomidine: 0.02-0.04 mg/kg IV

PROTOCOL FOR INDUCTION OF ANESTHESIA PRIOR TO MAINTENANCE WITH AN INHALED ANESTHETIC

Premedication   Xylazine: 0.5 mg/kg IV
         Butorphanol: 0.02-0.04 mg/kg IV
         Administer xylazine first.
Induction   Diazepam: 0.05 mg/kg IV
         Ketamine: 2.2 mg/kg IV

INJECTABLE PROTOCOL FOR INDUCTION AND SHORT-DURATION ANESTHESIA

Premedication and *induction*   As described above

Maintenance   Mix 1000 mg of ketamine and 500 mg xylazine in 1 L of 5% guaifenesin. Administer intravenously at a rate of approximately 2.2 ml/kg/hr.

IV, Intravenously.

Box 19-4 EXAMPLES OF PROTOCOLS USED FOR CHEMICAL RESTRAINT AND GENERAL ANESTHESIA IN RUMINANTS

CATTLE

Protocol for Induction of Anesthesia Before Maintenance With an Inhaled Anesthetic

Premedication   Xylazine: 0.02-0.05 mg/kg IV/IM
Induction   To 1 L of 5% guaifenesin, add approximately 2000 mg of thiopental or ketamine. Administer intravenously until animal is recumbent.
Maintenance   Halothane or isoflurane

Injectable Protocol for Induction and Short-duration Anesthesia

To 1 L of 5% guaifenesin, add 1000 mg ketamine and 100 mg xylazine. Administer mixture at a dosage of 0.55 ml/kg for the induction of anesthesia and approximately 2.2 ml/kg/hr for maintenance.

SHEEP AND GOATS

Protocol for Induction of Anesthesia Before Maintenance With an Inhaled Anesthetic

Premedication   Butorphanol: 0.1-0.2 mg/kg IM
         Xylazine: 0.02-0.05 mg/kg IM
Induction   Thiopental: 10-15 mg/kg IV
Maintenance   Halothane or isoflurane

Injectable Protocol for Induction and Short Duration Anesthesia

To 1 L of 5% guaifenesin, add 1000 mg ketamine and 100 mg xylazine. Administer mixture at a dosage of 0.55 ml/kg for the induction of anesthesia (sheep may require up to 1.2 ml/kg) and approximately 2.2 ml/kg/hr for maintenance.

IV, Intravenously; *IM,* intramuscularly.

A routine anesthesia preparation checklist should be developed. Use of such a checklist will serve to assist in the organization of the equipment required for a successful anesthetic procedure. For a routine anesthetic procedure, the following equipment preparations should be carried out:

- Organize intravenous catheterization supplies; appropriate catheters, tape, heparinized saline, and antiseptic solutions for sterile preparation of the skin site.
- Organize equipment for endotracheal intubation; appropriately sized tubes that have been checked for cuff leaks, laryngoscope, stylet and topical anesthetic spray (if needed), an oral speculum for cattle, gauze or tape to secure the tube in place, sterile lubricant to facilitate passage of the tube into the trachea, and a syringe to inflate the endotracheal tube cuff.
- Prepare the anesthesia machine, and select a breathing system according to the animal's size (see selection criteria under Anesthesia Equipment):
  - Check to ensure the vaporizer contains enough liquid anesthetic for the procedure. (Vaporizers should be filled at the end of the day to decrease exposure of personnel to anesthetic gases.)
  - Check the oxygen supply.
  - Evaluate soda lime absorbent, and refill if exhausted.
- Turn on flowmeter to check for free movement of the flow indicator.
- Perform a high-pressure leak test on the breathing system: Close pop-off valve, and pressurize the breathing system to 20 to 30 cm H_2O (on the pressure manometer) using the oxygen flush valve. This may be accomplished by placing your thumb over the animal connection. The system should maintain pressure if no leaks are present. Leaks of 300 ml/min (determined by dialing the flow required to maintain pressure in a system with a minor leak) or less are considered acceptable. Leaks above this must be identified and corrected prior to the use of an anesthetic machine. If the leak cannot be identified, the machine must be taken out of service until a more exhaustive search for the leak can be performed.
- Connect the breathing system (at the pop-off valve) to the waste-gas scavenging system.
- Calculate the appropriate fresh-gas flow rates.

Box 19-5 EXAMPLES OF PROTOCOLS USED FOR CHEMICAL RESTRAINT AND GENERAL ANESTHESIA IN SWINE

Premedication	Xylazine: 0.05-1.0 mg/kg IM Ketamine: 5.0 mg/kg IM
Induction and *Maintenance*	Mask with isoflurane or sevoflurane, then intubate and maintain on inhaled anesthetic.

INJECTABLE PROTOCOL FOR INDUCTION AND SHORT-DURATION ANESTHESIA

Premedication	Use above protocol for chemical restraint required for intravenous catheterization.
Induction and *Maintenance*	In 1 L of 5% guaifenesin, add 1000 mg ketamine and 1000 mg xylazine. Use 0.05-1.0 mg/kg (depending on degree of sedation from premedication) IV for induction and 2.2 ml/kg/hr for maintenance.

IV, Intravenously; *IM,* intramuscularly.

- Organize fluids for administration, and calculate the appropriate administration rate (see below).
- Calculate doses for all drugs and draw up these drugs. Remember to double-check your calculations and dispensing. Label all syringes.

ENDOTRACHEAL INTUBATION

Endotracheal intubation techniques vary depending on the species and intended procedure. Several principles should be remembered when performing intubation in any species:

- Test the endotracheal tube cuff for leaks prior to use.
- Have two or three tube sizes readily available.
- For cats, dogs, small ruminants, and swine, position the animal in sternal recumbency so that the head and neck are extended in a straight line (Figure 19-24). This position offers the best visualization of the larynx for successful intubation. Some anesthetists prefer to perform endotracheal intubation in swine with the animal in dorsal recumbency. Horses are usually intubated while positioned in lateral recumbency with the head, neck, and back placed in as straight a line as possible to facilitate introduction of the tube into the larynx (Figure 19-25). Adult cattle are most safely intubated when they are maintained in sternal recumbency following the induction of anesthesia (Figure 19-26). This positioning minimizes the risk of regurgitation and aspiration of rumen contents.

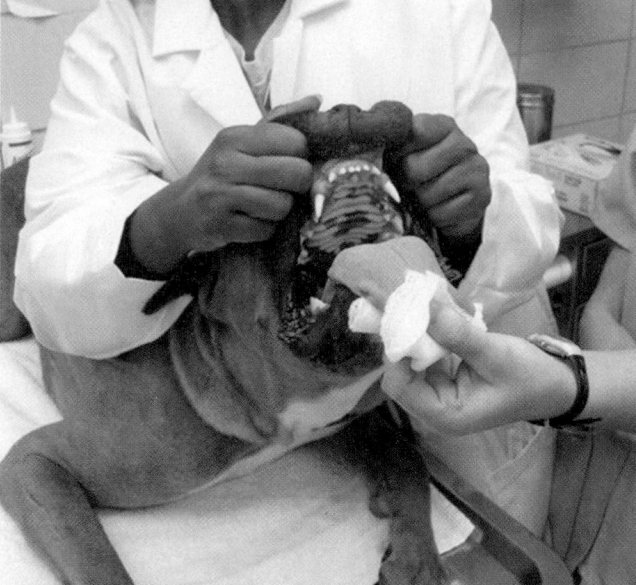

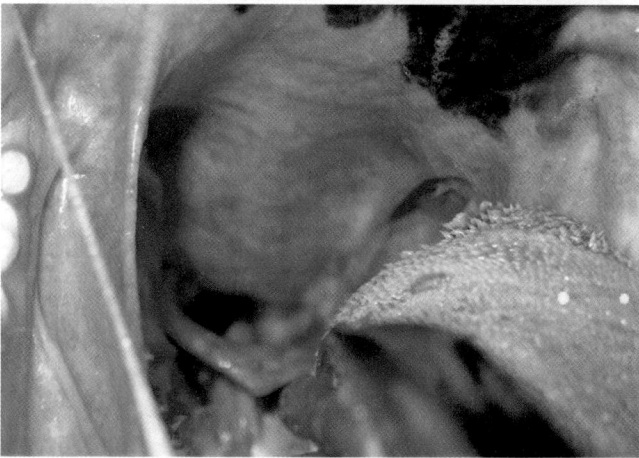

Figure 19-24 **A,** Endotracheal intubation in the dog and cat is best accomplished with the animal in sternal recumbency. **B,** The larynx is best visualized with the aid of a laryngoscope. Once intubation is completed, the laryngoscope is used to verify the correct placement of the endotracheal tube.

Nasotracheal, rather than orotracheal, intubation may also be indicated for procedures involving the oral cavity. Nasotracheal intubation is especially useful in foals and may be performed in an awake foal with minimal sedation to facilitate a rapid induction with inhalation anesthetics.

- A stylet with an atraumatic tip may be necessary in some situations. A rigid stylet will provide support for very flimsy tubes and will facilitate proper placement. In species such as small ruminants, swine, and cats, an atraumatic stylet such as a dog urinary catheter will facilitate introduction of the tube into the larynx. Visualization of the larynx is poor in small ruminants and swine because of their narrow oral cavity. In these species, use of both a laryngoscope and stylet facilitates

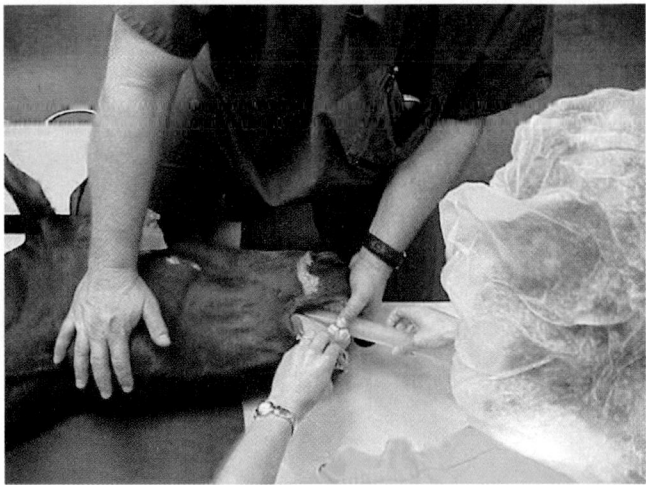

Figure 19-25 Endotracheal intubation in the horse is accomplished using a blind intubation technique.

intubation. In adult cattle, a nasogastric tube placed in the trachea by digital palpation serves as a flexible stylet over which the endotracheal tube may be passed. Use of a wire or any sharp instrument as a stylet should be avoided as these instruments may induce tracheal trauma and even rupture.

- Conservative use of a topical local anesthetic agent in the laryngeal area is useful in species that are prone to laryngospasm during intubation (cats, swine, and small ruminants). Laryngeal desensitization is effectively performed using 0.1 ml (cats) and 0.2 to 0.5 ml (other species) of 2% lidocaine deposited on the larynx with a syringe. When lidocaine is deposited on the larynx, it is important to allow an adequate period of time (30 to 60 seconds) for the drug to take effect. Commercial topical benzocaine preparations (e.g., Cetacaine) should be avoided in cats because of reports of methemoglobinemia associated with its use.
- Adequate anesthetic depth and muscle relaxation are important for successful intubation. This will avoid unnecessary laryngeal trauma and excessive autonomic nervous system stimulation that may give rise to cardiac arrhythmias. Animals that cough, gag, or visibly react to attempts at endotracheal intubation are too light and require administration of a supplemental dose of the induction drug.
- The endotracheal tube should be long enough to reach midway between the larynx and carina so that accidental dislodgment does not occur. It should not be too long because this can increase the risk of placing the end of the endotracheal tube in a single bronchus (endobronchial intubation). Excessive tube length that extends beyond the oral cavity constitutes apparatus dead space (space within the anesthetic breathing system in which expired gases may accumulate). An increase in dead space in a breathing system will lead to hypercapnia.

- Proper tube placement may be assessed by (1) visualization of the tube passing between the arytenoid cartilages (not applicable in horses and cattle), (2) condensation of respiratory gases on the inside of the tube with expiration, (3) only one tubular structure (trachea) palpable in the neck region, (4) auscultation of lung sounds during assisted ventilation, and (5) a normal capnograph waveform.
- Once the endotracheal tube is properly placed, the animal may be connected to the anesthetic machine and the oxygen flowmeter turned on. The vaporizer should not be turned on until the endotracheal tube cuff is properly inflated. Failure to do so will result in anesthetic gases escaping around the endotracheal tube and unnecessarily exposing personnel to anesthetic gases. The cuff of the endotracheal tube is inflated to the proper level by closing the pop-off valve, delivering a breath, and inflating the endotracheal tube cuff until the sound of gas escaping around the tube disappears.
- Once a leak-free system has been established by properly inflating the cuff of the endotracheal tube, the vaporizer may be turned on to the appropriate level.
- Following endotracheal intubation, the tube should be secured in place. This is accomplished by tying gauze tightly around the tube and then securing it around the head (cats, brachycephalic breeds) or to the upper or lower jaw. In large animals, the tube can be secured in place by wrapping tape around the tube and then the muzzle of the animal.

> **✎ TECHNICIAN NOTE**
>
> The risk of complications associated with a difficult endotracheal intubation can be reduced by the administration of oxygen using a face mask for a period of 5 minutes prior to the induction of anesthesia.

FLUID ADMINISTRATION DURING ANESTHESIA

Routine fluid administration during anesthesia assists in counteracting the relative reduction in circulating blood volume that occurs as a result of the vasodilation that often accompanies anesthesia. The intravenous catheter used for fluid administration also provides venous access for the intraoperative delivery of routine and emergency drugs (e.g., antibiotics, inotropic agents) and short-term injectable anesthesia. Fluid imbalances throughout the anesthetic period may occur because of blood loss, the drying of exposed tissues, ongoing urinary loss, dry inhaled gases, and the removal of effusions. Guidelines for fluid administration during anesthesia and surgery include

- The fluid type administered most commonly during anesthesia and surgery is an isotonic crystalloid solution,

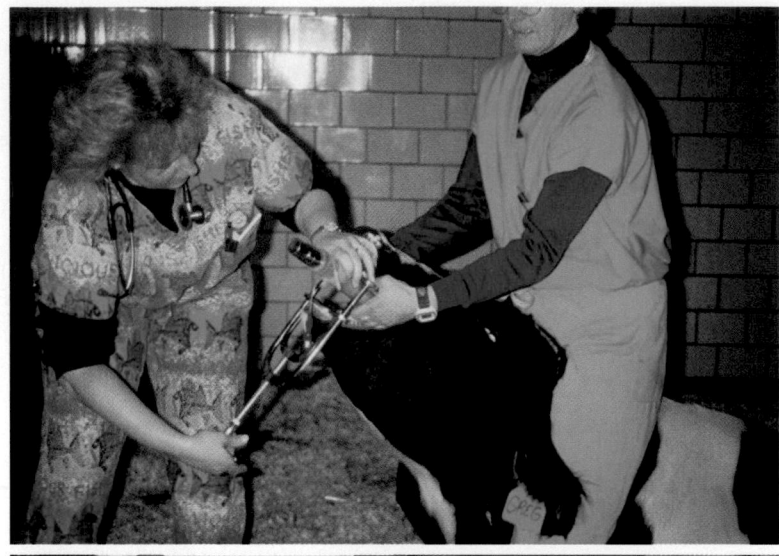

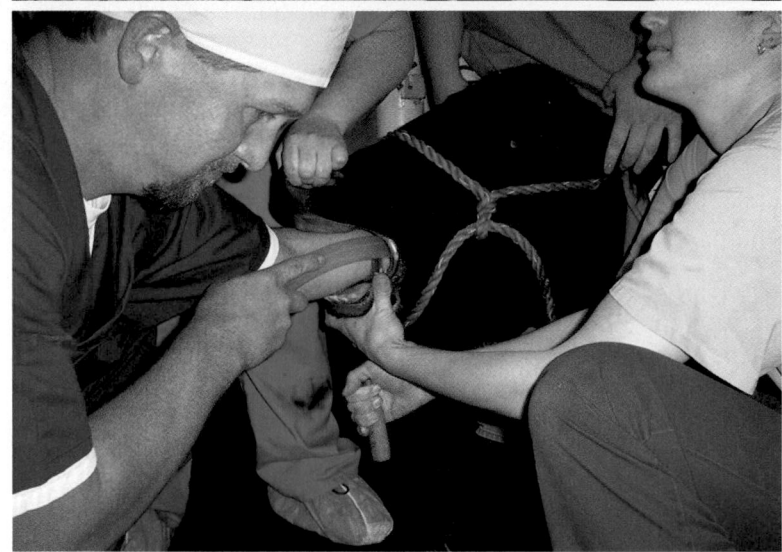

Figure 19-26 **A,** Endotracheal intubation in the cow is performed with the animal in sternal recumbency to reduce the risk of regurgitation and aspiration of rumen contents. (Courtesy of Dr. Victoria Lukasik, Southwest Veterinary Anesthesiology.) **B,** In larger ruminants, the endotracheal tube is introduced manually. To avoid aspiration of rumen contents during transport and positioning of the animal, the endotracheal tube should be correctly in place and the cuff inflated before any manipulations. (Courtesy of Dr. J. Ko, Oklahoma State University.)

such as lactated Ringer's or Normosol-R. For neonates (<1 month of age), very small animals, and birds, a 5% dextrose solution or lactated Ringer's with 5 or 10 ml of 50% dextrose per 100 ml of Ringer's solution for dextrose concentrations of 2.5% or 5.0%, respectively, may be administered.

- For healthy animals during routine procedures intravenous fluids are normally administered at a rate of 5 to 10 ml/kg/hr. The following modifications may apply:
  - Increasing the administration rate in animals with preexisting dehydration, excessive intraoperative blood loss, or hypotension

- Decreasing the administration rate in animals that have significant cardiac or renal disease that limit their ability to tolerate excessive fluid administration (Animals with preexisting anemia or hypoproteinemia should not receive excessive volumes of fluids because of the possibility of further dilution of the hematocrit or plasma proteins.)
- Quantified blood lost during surgery should be replaced at a volume of three times the approximate loss in addition to the basic fluid rate during anesthesia. When blood loss is significant, the PCV and total protein should be monitored to avoid excessive dilution. An

acute fall in PCV below 20% should be treated with packed red cells or whole blood. Total protein should not fall below 3.5 g/dl because of the increased risk of developing pulmonary edema

INDUCTION AND MAINTENANCE

Guidelines for induction and maintenance are as follows:

- Following induction and endotracheal intubation, the animal is connected to the breathing circuit and the endotracheal tube cuff is inflated as outlined above. Once the endotracheal tube cuff is appropriately inflated, turn the vaporizer to the appropriate induction setting. Fresh-gas flow rate during this induction period (approximately 3 to 5 minutes) using a circle system should be 100 ml/kg/min.
- Assess the depth of the animal.
- Assess pulse rate and quality.
- Assess ventilation. If the animal is apneic or the rate is slow, assist ventilation at two breaths per minute. Remember that excessively aggressive ventilation will decrease the animal's carbon dioxide below the level that will stimulate it to breathe spontaneously.
- Apply ophthalmic ointment to protect the cornea from drying during the anesthetic period.
- Following the initial induction period, reduce vaporizer settings and fresh-gas flow rates (from 100 ml/kg/min to 30 to 50 ml/kg/min) to the appropriate maintenance levels.
- Set appropriate intravenous fluid administration rates.
- Following induction and assessment of the animal, place the appropriate monitoring equipment.
- Record all pertinent information in the anesthetic record, and begin recording vital signs every 5 minutes (Figure 19-12).
- When using injectable techniques in horses and adult cattle, procedures should be limited to 30 to 60 minutes. An oxygen source should be available for the insufflation of oxygen (15 L/min) to prevent the development of hypoxia that occurs as a result of hypoventilation and atelectasis. In small animals anesthetized with an injectable protocol, the anesthetic period should also be limited to 1 hour. During procedures for which anesthesia is produced with injectable drugs alone, oxygen should be administered through a face mask or, more ideally, an endotracheal tube.
- During long procedures, check the vaporizer liquid level periodically during the anesthetic period. If the vaporizer needs to be filled during the anesthetic period, this may be carried out by turning off the vaporizer, leaving the fresh-gas flow on and filling the vaporizer. After filling the vaporizer, remember to close the filling port before the vaporizer is turned back on. Failure to do so will result in anesthetic liquid being forced out of the vaporizer when the vaporizer is turned on and carrier gas entering the vaporization chamber.

PADDING AND POSITIONING OF THE ANIMAL

Proper padding and positioning depend on the procedure to be performed and the particular species.

- Dogs, cats, neonates of all species, and all other small species should be placed on a covered circulating warm water heating pad, circulating water blanket, or forced warm air blanket to minimize hypothermia. Careful attention must be paid to the temperature of supplemental heat-source devices. Heat sources that are too hot can lead to thermal burns in anesthetized animals.
- When securing limbs to the surgery table, do not apply ties too tightly and do not apply excessive traction on the limbs. Both actions may result in neurologic damage, and the latter may impede ventilatory effort.
- Ensure that the head and neck are positioned to avoid kinking of the endotracheal tube or disconnection from the breathing system.
- Ensure that appropriate expansion of the thorax is not compromised.
- For horses and adult cattle, adequate padding, such as a thick foam or water-filled pad is essential for prevention of the development of postoperative myositis and neuropathy. For procedures in the field, a grassy area offers the best padding. The down eye should be protected and the head padded if possible.
- For horses and cattle in lateral recumbency, the most dorsal forelimb and hind limb should be supported so that they are parallel to the table surface (Figure 19-27).
- Always remove the halter from horses during general anesthesia to avoid damage to facial nerves by the metal connectors.
- Ruminants should be placed in right lateral recumbency *when possible* so that the rumen is on the up side. During

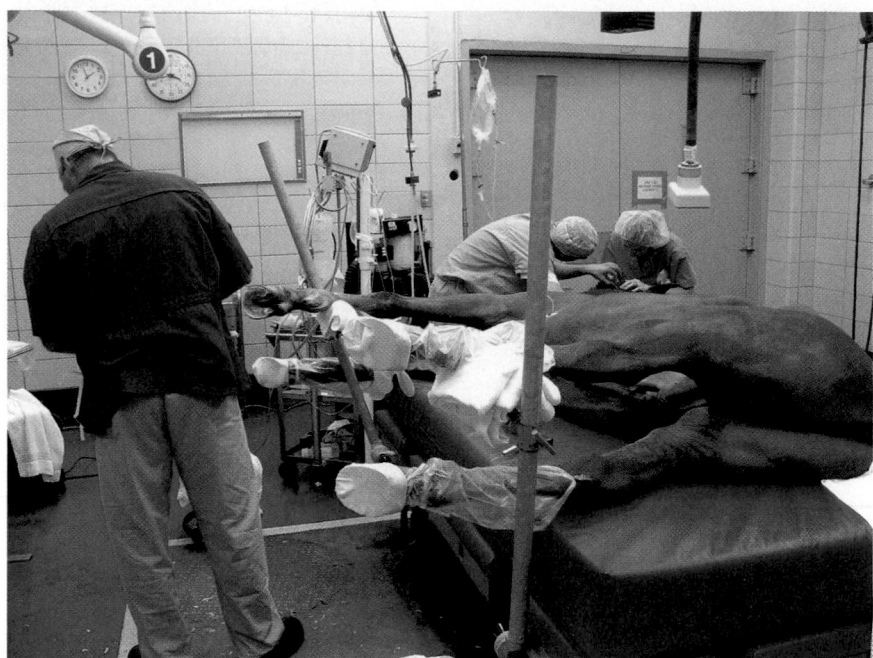

Figure 19-27 Careful attention to positioning of the limbs of a horse during general anesthesia is essential. Improper limb positioning can lead to postanesthetic lameness and myopathy. Here the upper limbs of the horse are supported by limb supports. Also note the thick padding on which the horse is placed.

lateral recumbency, the neck should be elevated with a soft pad so the head angles downward to promote flow of saliva and regurgitated rumen contents out of the oral cavity.

- Because of the high incidence of regurgitation in mature ruminants, an endotracheal tube should be placed and the cuff inflated (even if injectable anesthetics are used) before positioning the animal (especially in dorsal recumbency).

RECOVERY

Guidelines for recovery from anesthesia vary according to species.

DOGS AND CATS

- Ensure adequate attention has been paid to the ongoing need for analgesia in the immediate postoperative period. Supplemental analgesics should be administered prior to recovery from anesthesia.
- Turn off the vaporizer, increase the oxygen flow rate to 100 ml/kg/min and flush the breathing circuit (unless a nonrebreathing circuit is being used where the flow rate used during recovery will be the same as that used during induction and maintenance). Maintain oxygen administration as long as possible. Continued administration of oxygen during the recovery period prevents the development of hypoxemia in a

hypoventilating animal. Oxygen supplementation also offsets the increase in oxygen consumption that is associated with shivering in the hypothermic animal. Continued administration of oxygen during the recovery period with the anesthetic machine also provides a method for scavenging expired anesthetic gases during the recovery period.

- As the animal's depth of anesthesia lightens, deflate the endotracheal tube cuff. If the animal is at risk for regurgitation, the cuff should be left inflated as long as possible. The endotracheal tube may be removed once the animal's pharyngeal reflexes have returned. This is indicated by the return of normal swallowing. In animals that have regurgitated during the anesthetic period, the oral cavity should be suctioned and flushed with saline and the endotracheal tube withdrawn with the cuff partially inflated. The endotracheal tube should remain in place as long as possible in animals that are at risk for airway obstruction (brachycephalic breeds).
- Providing a quiet environment facilitates a smooth recovery. Excessive stimulation of an animal during recovery will lead to a more excited recovery.
- Most animals are hypothermic following general anesthesia and require supplemental heat sources during the recovery period. Hot water bottles, heating pads, or a circulating water blanket may be used. With the exception of forced-air warming blankets, external heat sources should not be placed directly on the animal's skin.
- Some animals may need continued intravenous fluid therapy (e.g., animals with renal disease, dehydration).

The daily maintenance fluid administration rate is 60 ml/kg/24 hr.
- During recovery, check the animal frequently until it can maintain sternal recumbency, has stable cardiovascular and respiratory parameters, and is within 1 to 2 degrees of normal body temperature.

HORSES

- When inhalation anesthesia is used, the horse should be placed in a padded dark room and allowed to recover unassisted. The horse may be extubated with the cuff deflated when swallowing is observed or earlier as the situation dictates. During recovery, the horse's airway can be maintained by replacing the endotracheal tube with a smaller uncuffed tube that is placed nasotracheally following removal of the endotracheal tube. Alternatively, some anesthetists will secure the original endotracheal tube in place with tape and remove it once the horse has recovered from anesthesia and is standing.
- Oxygen should be insufflated at a rate of 15 L/min through either the nasotracheal or endotracheal tube for as long as possible or until the animal is standing.
- For recoveries in the field, the halter should be replaced so the animal can be assisted during recovery. The eyes should be covered to minimize external stimulation until the horse attempts to stand.
- In horses in which an excited or rough recovery is anticipated, the administration of a sedative such as xylazine or a tranquilizer such as acepromazine in low doses may serve to sedate the horse until it is ready to rise unassisted.

RUMINANTS

- If inhalation anesthesia is used, 100% oxygen should be administered until extubation.
- Ruminants should be positioned in sternal recumbency as soon as possible to promote eructation and minimize the chance of regurgitation.
- Extubation should be performed with the cuff inflated only after swallowing is observed.
- A stomach tube should be passed to decompress the rumen if bloat has developed intraoperatively.
- Ruminants generally recover smoothly from general anesthesia, and minimal assistance is required.

SWINE

- Oxygen administration should continue until extubation.
- Extubate with the cuff deflated (unless there is evidence of regurgitation) when swallowing is observed.
- Position the animal in sternal recumbency as soon as possible, and allow the animal to recover in a cool and quiet environment.

TECHNICIAN NOTE
Regardless of the species of animal that is anesthetized, the recovery process is improved if the animal recovers in a quiet environment without excessive external stimulation. Careful monitoring during the recovery process and attention to the animal's need for postoperative analgesia are important parts of the recovery process.

POSTOPERATIVE ANALGESIA

Any procedure considered to be painful to humans should be considered painful to animals; if there is any doubt whether an animal is in pain, it should be treated (see Chapter 20 for signs of pain in animals and an approach to evaluation). In large animals, nonsteroidal antiinflammatory drugs, such as phenylbutazone or flunixin meglumine, are most commonly used. In small animals, opioids, such as hydromorphone, butorphanol, morphine, or buprenorphine, are most frequently used for the control of postoperative pain (see Chapter 20). Buprenorphine offers the advantage of prolonged duration of effect (8 to 12 hours). Nonsteroidal antiinflammatory drugs are also used as a component of an effective postoperative pain management strategy.

An alternative to systemic opioid administration is epidural administration, offering the advantages of longer duration of action and elimination of side effects such as respiratory depression and bradycardia. Preservative-free morphine (0.1 mg/kg) diluted to a volume of 1 ml/5 kg with sterile saline provides postoperative analgesia lasting 12 to 18 hours. Butorphanol (0.2 mg/kg), oxymorphone (0.1 mg/kg), and buprenorphine (0.003 to 0.005 mg/kg) may also be used epidurally, but the duration of action of these drugs following epidural administration is similar to that seen with systemic administration.

ANESTHETIC EMERGENCIES

The most extreme form of an anesthetic emergency during the anesthetic period is cardiopulmonary arrest (CPA). CPA most often occurs in high-risk, unstable animals that succumb to the depressive effects of anesthesia. CPA may occur at any time during the anesthetic period. Cardiopulmonary resuscitation (CPR) is divided into four phases: readiness and prevention, recognition and basic cardiac life support, advanced cardiac life support, and post-resuscitation care.

READINESS AND PREVENTION

A clearly defined protocol for the treatment of CPA should be present in any setting where anesthesia is administered. A readily accessible location for the administration of CPR should be identified and stocked with all of the necessary

Box 19-6 READINESS CHECKLIST FOR
CARDIOPULMONARY RESUSCITATION

- Well-lighted area with adequate workspace
- Emergency drugs (Table 19-8)
- Endotracheal tubes (in order and cuffs checked for leaks)
- Tie gauze for endotracheal tubes, syringe for inflating cuffs
- Two long urinary catheters for oxygen insufflation
- Tracheostomy tubes (sterile pack for tracheostomy procedure)
- Laryngoscopes (functioning)
- Face masks
- Method for artificial ventilation (anesthetic machine or Ambu bag)
- Oxygen source
- Needles and syringes
- Suction device
- Intravenous catheters; intravenous fluids (crystalloids and colloids)
- Fluid administration sets
- Electrocardiogram
- Doppler blood flow detector (charged)
- Defibrillator (internal and external paddles and contact solution)
- Clippers

IV, Intravenously; *IM,* intramuscularly.

emergency equipment and drugs (Box 19-6). All of the staff members involved in resuscitation efforts should have an assigned role. It is extremely valuable for personnel assigned to the CPR team to stage mock drills that allow the team to practice their approach to CPR and identify areas where it can be improved.

The prevention of CPA involves the recognition of animals that are at a high risk of experiencing CPA and initiating any possible treatments that may reduce that risk. Central to risk reduction are appropriate preanesthetic stabilization of the animal, appropriate protocol selection, and monitoring throughout the anesthetic and recovery periods. A variety of clinical signs may signal an impending CPA: cyanosis, marked changes in respiratory function such as apnea, tachypnea, dyspnea, and marked abdominal effort associated with breathing. Impending cardiovascular collapse may be indicated by acute bradycardia, tachycardia, diminished or absent pulses, hypotension, pale mucous membranes, and increased capillary refill time. Hypothermia can increase the risk of CPA in an unstable animal by contributing to the development of bradycardia and excessive anesthetic depth. A body temperature less than 30° C (86° F) predisposes to life-threatening ventricular arrhythmias. The possible causes of and treatments for some more commonly encountered anesthetic-related problems are presented in Table 19-7.

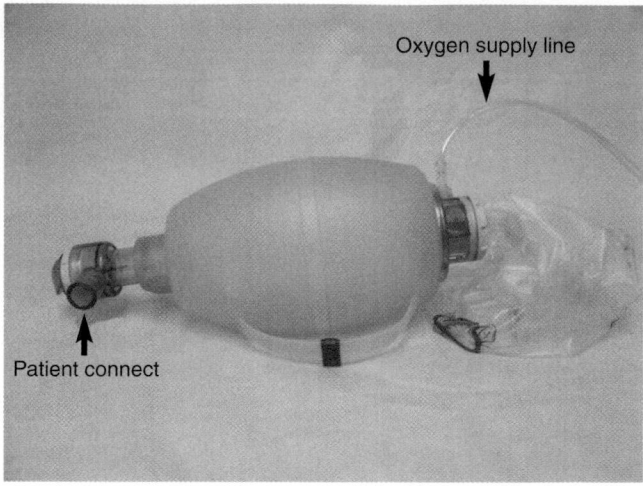

Figure 19-28 Ambu bag is used to ventilate and deliver oxygen to a patient that is intubated but not connected to an anesthetic machine.

RECOGNITION AND BASIC CARDIAC LIFE SUPPORT

Early recognition of CPA is critical to successful resuscitation. The likelihood of recognition of impending collapse is increased when appropriate monitoring is performed throughout the anesthetic and recovery periods. Once CPA in an anesthetized animal has been identified, the following should be performed:

- Stop delivery of anesthetic to the animal. Turn off vaporizer, and increase fresh-gas flow rate (100 ml/kg/min for a circle breathing system; 200 ml/kg/min for Bain circuit).
- If a circle system is being used, the oxygen flush valve should be used to flush the system.
- In most cases, the fluid administration rate should be increased (shock rate of fluid administration is 90 ml/kg/min). Not all animals benefit from aggressive fluid administration during CPR. Dehydrated animals or those that have experienced significant blood loss require volume replacement.
- Reverse any anesthetics, such as opioids or alpha₂ agonists.
- Basic cardiac life support techniques should be initiated concurrently and include the following:
  - *Airway.* If the animal is not already intubated, an endotracheal tube should be placed. If the animal is already intubated, the tube should be checked for proper placement and patency. If endotracheal intubation is impossible, a long catheter placed in the trachea may be used to deliver oxygen until intubation is possible. In cases involving severe upper airway obstruction, a tracheostomy may be indicated if endotracheal intubation is impossible.
  - *Breathing.* Ventilate the animal with 100% oxygen using the anesthesia machine rebreathing bag or an Ambu bag (Figure 19-28). The rate of ventilation

Table 19-7 DIAGNOSES

Abnormality	Potential Causes	Treatment

Bradycardia	Excessive anesthetic depth
	Drugs: opioids, xylazine, gas anesthetics
	Hyperkalemia
	Vagal reflex (intubation, oculocardiac reflex)
	Visceral manipulation
	Hypothermia
	Terminal stages or hypoxia
	Exogenous and endogenous toxemias
		1. Correct underlying cause
		2. Administer anticholinergic
		3. Administer sympathomimetic
		   Dopamine: 2-10 µg/kg/min*
		   Dobutamine: 2-10 µg/kg/min*
		   Ephedrine: 0.05-0.5 mg/kg bolus*
		   Isoproterenol: 0.5-0.2 µg/kg/min*

Tachycardia	Drugs: ketamine, thiobarbiturates, anticholinergics, sympathomimetics Hypokalemia Hyperthermia Inadequate anesthetic depth Hypercapnia, hypoxemia Anemia, hypovolemia Hyperthyroidism, pheochromocytoma Anaphylaxis	1. Correct underlying cause

Hypotension	Hypovolemia (i.e., blood loss)
	Sepsis
	Shock
	Drugs (thiobarbiturates, inhalant)
		1. Reduce inhaled anesthetic concentration
		  • Administer supplementary analgesic if required to allow reduction in inhalant concentration
		2. Increase fluid administration rate (bolus 10 ml/kg)
		3. Administer sympathomimetic
		   Dopamine: 2-40 µg/kg/min*
		   Dobutamine: 2-20 µg/kg/min*
		   Ephedrine: 0.055-0.55 mg/kg bolus (small animals),* 0.022 mg/kg bolus (horse)*

Apnea	Drug effects Deep anesthesia Hypothermia Hyperventilation Aminoglycoside administration	1. Correct underlying cause
Tachypnea	Pain Hypercapnia Hyperthermia Metabolic acidosis	1. Correct underlying cause

IV, Intravenously.

*These drugs may cause cardiac arrhythmias. Monitor electrocardiogram during administration.

should be approximately 20 breaths/min performed simultaneously with chest compressions. Recent research has demonstrated that for the first few minutes of CPR, effective ventilation can occur solely as a result of chest compressions. Thus in situations where the number of personnel is limited, ventilation should not be performed at the expense of the immediate initiation of cardiac compressions.

• *Circulation.* When a pulse or heartbeat cannot be detected, external cardiac compressions should be initiated. The goal of these compressions is to maintain adequate blood flow to the brain and heart until cardiac function can be restored. In most animals, compressions are performed with the animal in right lateral recumbency, at the level of the costochondral junction between the fourth and eighth ribs. A rate of 80 to 120 compressions per minute is used. In barrel-chested dogs, compressions may be more effectively delivered with the animal in dorsal recumbency. Abdominal wrapping or interposed rhythmic abdominal compressions may help to improve forward blood flow.

ADVANCED CARDIAC LIFE SUPPORT

Drugs

The preferred route for administration of drugs during CPR is central venous. Because many animals will not have

Table 19-8　DRUG DOSAGES AND DEFIBRILLATOR SETTINGS FOR USE DURING CARDIOPULMONARY RESUSCITATION

Drug	Dosage	Indication	Comments
Epinephrine	0.02-0.2 mg/kg (SA) 0.001-0.005 mg/kg (LA)	Initiate heartbeat Increased contractility Improve blood flow during CPR Increase heart rate	Repeat q3-5 min
Atropine	0.04 mg/kg (SA) 0.01 mg/kg (LA)	Increase heart rate Treat asystole	
Lidocaine	1.0-2.0 mg/kg (SA) 0.5-1.0 mg/kg (LA)	Treat ventricular arrhythmias	
Prednisolone sodium succinate	5-10 mg/kg (SA) 1.0-2.0 mg/kg (LA)	Shock and ischemia Prevention of cerebral edema	
or Dexamethasone sodium phosphate	2.2-4.4 mg/kg		
Sodium bicarbonate	0.5-1.0 mEq/kg/every 5 min of CPA	Metabolic acidosis	Use after 10 min of arrest or with preexisting acidosis
Calcium carbonate	10 mg/kg (SA) 2.2 mg/kg (LA)	Treatment of arrhythmias associated with hyperkalemia Hypocalcemia	Has been incriminated in reperfusion injury
Hypertonic saline	2-4 ml/kg	Rapid volume expansion	Use with concurrent isotonic fluid administration
Furosemide	1-2 mg/kg	Pulmonary and cerebral edema	Monitor hydration status following administration
Mannitol	0.5-1 mg/kg	Cerebral edema	Monitor hydration status following administration
Doxapram	1.0-4.0 mg/kg (SA) 0.2 mg/kg (LA)	Central respiratory stimulation	Contraindicated in hypoxemia
Oxyglobin	10-30 mg/kg	Acute or chronic anemia	Colloidal properties similar to hetastarch
Hetastarch (6% solution)	10-20 ml/kg/24 hr	Rapid volume expansion	May produce alterations in coagulation when given at high doses
Debrillation 　External 　Internal	 3-5 J/kg 0.2-0.3 J/kg	Treatment of ventricular fibrillation	

CPR, Cardiopulmonary resuscitation; *LA*, large animal; *SA*, small animal.

a central venous access, peripheral venous access may be used instead. Intratracheal administration is a more effective route than peripheral venous for most resuscitation drugs (epinephrine, lidocaine, atropine). For intratracheal administration, the dose should be double that of the intravenous dose and diluted in 3 to 10 ml (depending on animal size) of sterile saline. The drug is delivered through the endotracheal tube and followed with several large ventilations to aid in delivering the drug to the pulmonary vasculature. The intraosseous route (via the tibial tuberosity, greater tubercle of the humerus, trochanteric fossa of the femur, wing of the ilium) may also be used for fluid and drug administration if venous access cannot be obtained. The intraosseous route is typically used in very small animals in which venous catheterization is difficult, if not impossible. The types, dosages, and indications for use of drugs commonly employed during CPR are presented in Table 19-8.

Electrocardiogram/Defibrillation

A continuous ECG should be displayed during CPR. This is essential for the prompt recognition and treatment of the type of cardiac arrhythmia that accompanies (or may be responsible for) the CPA. Three of the most common arrhythmias observed during CPA are ventricular asystole, ventricular fibrillation, and electromechanical dissociation. Examples of these rhythms are presented in Figure 19-29. Each rhythm type requires specific treatments (Table 19-9).

Fluid Therapy

Appropriate fluid therapy during CPR is a component of successful resuscitation. It is not appropriate to solely increase the fluid administration without attention to a calculated dose. In most cases an isotonic, polyionic solution such as that administered during anesthesia and/or surgery is appropriate. Dextrose-containing solutions should not

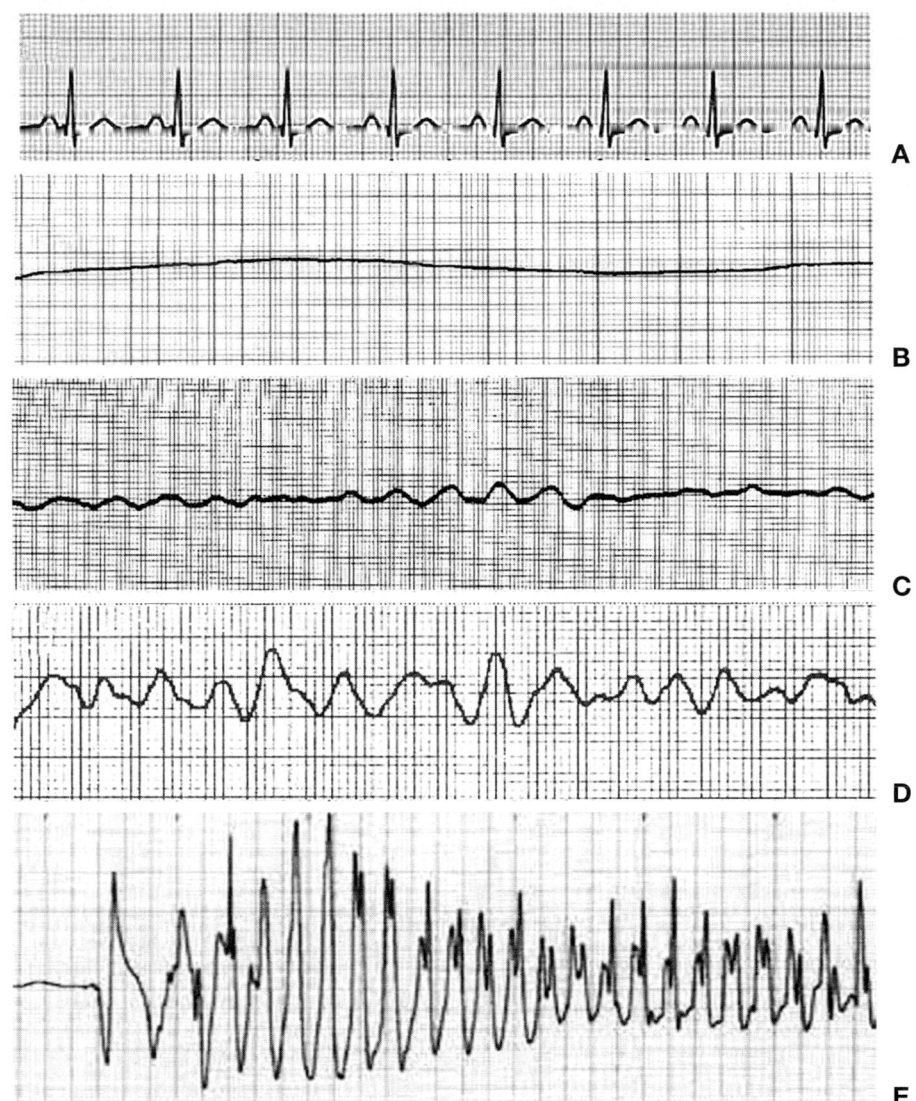

Figure 19-29 Electrocardiogram tracings demonstrating the different arrhythmias observed most frequently during cardiopulmonary arrest. **A,** Electromechanical dissociation (EMD) presents a normal tracing but no palpable pulse associated with the electrical activity. **B,** Ventricular asystole presents no electrical activity in the heart (flat ECG). **C,** Fine fibrillation. **D,** Coarse fibrillation. **E,** Ventricular tachycardia.

be administered during CPA because of their potential for exacerbating cerebral damage following successful resuscitation efforts. In most cases a dosage of 70 to 90 ml/kg/hr is appropriate for fluid resuscitation during CPR. This is generally administered for a period of 15 minutes. The animal is reevaluated and fluid administration is adjusted or continued at that rate as indicated. Solutions containing large-molecular-weight sugarlike molecules (dextran, hetastarch) may also be administered to promote rapid volume expansion. Hypertonic saline of 3% to 7% (4 ml/kg) has also been shown to be of benefit during CPR. In cases where blood loss has been significant and replacement of that blood is indicated, fresh whole blood or components may be administered. Commercially prepared hemoglobin-based oxygen carrying solutions (Oxyglobin, Biopure) may also be administered.

Internal Cardiac Massage

Internal cardiac massage is indicated when external resuscitation efforts have not established effective circulation within 3 minutes. Internal cardiac massage is performed through a thoracotomy incision at the left fourth or fifth intercostal space. Internal cardiac massage should be performed immediately in very large or barrel-chested animals or in animals with fractured ribs or pneumothorax that will prevent effective external compressions.

POSTRESUSCITATIVE CARE

Unstable animals may suffer arrest again following successful resuscitative efforts. Careful monitoring of the ECG, blood pressure, pulse quality, respiratory pattern, body temperature, and CNS (pupillary responses, mentation, seizure

Table 19-9 RECOMMENDED TREATMENT PROTOCOLS FOR DIFFERENT TYPES OF ARRHYTHMIAS ASSOCIATED WITH CARDIOPULMONARY ARREST

Arrhythmias	Treatment	Dosage
Ventricular asystole	Epinephrine	0.02-0.2 mg/kg IV or IT
	Atropine	0.044 mg/kg IV or IT
	Prednisolone sodium succinate (Solu-Delta-Cortef)	22 mg/kg IV
	Sodium bicarbonate (if >10-15 min)	1.0 mEq/kg IV
Ventricular fibrillation	Precordial thump (if defibrillator not available)	
	Epinephrine	0.2 mg/kg IV or IT
	Defibrillate	See Table 19-8
	Defibrillate	Double original dose
	Lidocaine	2.2 mg/kg IV or IT (cats: 0.5 mg/kg)
	Sodium bicarbonate (if >10-15 min)	1.0 mEq/kg IV
Electromechanical dissociation	Epinephrine	0.2 mg/kg IV or IT
	Prednisolone sodium succinate (Solu-Delta-Cortef)	22 mg/kg IV
	Or	
	Dexamethasone sodium phosphate	2.2 mg/kg IV
	Sodium bicarbonate	1.0 mEq/kg IV

IV, Intravenous administration; *IT*, intratracheal administration, double the recommended intravenous dose.

activity) is essential for several hours after the primary event. Postresuscitation neurologic damage may become evident 24 to 48 hours after the arrest, so serial neurologic examinations should be performed. Oxygen therapy should be continued for a period of time, particularly in those animals that demonstrated decreased cardiopulmonary function.

ACKNOWLEDGMENT

The author wishes to acknowledge the extensive contribution of earlier editions of this chapter written by Dr. Janyce L. Cornick-Seahorn in the preparation of this edition.

Recommended Reading

Dorsch JA, Dorsch SE: *Understanding anesthesia equipment,* ed 4, Baltimore, 1999, Williams & Wilkins.

Muir WW, Hubbell JAE, editors: *Equine anesthesia monitoring and emergency therapy,* St Louis, 1991, Mosby.

Muir WW, Hubbell JAE, editors: *Handbook of veterinary anesthesia,* ed 3, St Louis, 2000, Mosby.

Seymour C, Gleed R, editors: *Manual of small animal anaesthesia and analgesia,* United Kingdom, 1999, British Small Animal Veterinary Association.

Thurmon JC, Tranquilli WJ, Benson GJ, editors: *Lumb & Jones' veterinary anesthesia,* ed 3, Baltimore, 1996, Williams & Wilkins.

Pain Management

GLENN PETTIFER

INTRODUCTION

The veterinarian and veterinary technician together have an obligation to recognize and alleviate animal pain. This task is difficult, for only human patients can point to their specific source of discomfort and describe it. We must assume that veterinary patients experience pain under any circumstance in which humans would feel pain. There are, in fact, many similarities between animals and humans in the anatomic and chemical pathways of pain perception. Differences that do exist are generally attributed to alternative pathways for pain and not the absence of them. For many years there has been an erroneous but well-meaning belief that pain in animals is beneficial and that it provides a constant reminder to the patient to avoid movement that might cause further injury. This line of thought is illogical in that uncontrolled pain may lead to prolonged hospitalization, poor wound healing, and an increased rate of complications and mortality in both animals and humans. It has now become widely acknowledged that the recognition and alleviation of pain in animals is the essence of good patient care. In many practice situations, it is the veterinary technician who engages in the majority of the patient contact and pain assessment while providing nursing care and carrying out prescribed treatments. Thus the veterinary technician plays a very valuable, central role in the management of animal pain. ■

DEFINITIONS

The International Association for the Study of Pain (IASP) has defined *pain* as "an unpleasant sensory and emotional experience associated with actual or potential tissue damage, or described in terms of such damage." This definition demonstrates that there are both objective and subjective components to the experience of pain and that pain is a psychobehavioral and sensory experience that arises from the activation of nociceptors and nociceptive pathways. A *nociceptor* is a receptor that is preferentially sensitive to a noxious (damaging to tissue) stimulus or to a stimulus that would become noxious if prolonged. The distinction is made between *nociception* and *nociceptive pathways* that are located in the periphery and spinal cord and *pain* which requires perception. Normally when we speak of the events taking place in the periphery and the spinal cord, we refer to *nociception*, saving the use of the word *pain* to describe an event that involves perception of nociceptive stimulation. *Analgesia* is the absence of pain in response to stimulation that would normally be painful. *Allodynia* is the production of pain due to a stimulus that does not normally provoke pain. *Hyperalgesia* refers to an increased response to a stimulus that is normally painful. *Peripheral sensitization* refers to the reduction in activation threshold of peripheral nociceptors due to exposure to a number of chemical substances that arise as a result of tissue damage. In addition, the development of *peripheral sensitization* is also aided by initiation of activity in silent nociceptors that normally demonstrate little activity, except in the presence of local inflammation. *Central sensitization* refers to changes in the receptive field properties of neurons located in the spinal cord (dorsal horn), a reduction in the activation threshold of these neurons, and the inclusion of input from receptors that are normally not involved in the transmission of nociceptive information. Changes in the receptive field properties of these neurons are reflected in the observation of the development of an area of heightened sensitivity in the tissues adjacent to the primary site of injury. This area is referred to as the *zone of secondary hyperalgesia*. Central sensitization is produced, in part, by changes in the membrane excitability of dorsal horn neurons. This change

The authors acknowledge and appreciate the original contribution of Jill Sackman, whose work has been incorporated into this chapter.

in excitability is associated with the development of a condition known as *wind-up*. Wind-up is produced following repeated, low-frequency input from nociceptors. Input from nociceptors summates, creating increasingly longer and longer depolarizations of neurons in the spinal cord. Wind-up is mediated by *N*-methyl-D-aspartate (NMDA) receptors and other neurotransmitters.

ORGANIZATION OF NOCICEPTIVE PATHWAYS

PERIPHERAL NERVOUS SYSTEM

The transmission of a noxious stimulation involves activation of specialized receptors (nociceptors) and peripheral nerves in the traumatized tissue. This information transmitted by the nociceptors and peripheral nerves is then conducted through the spinal cord to multiple areas in the brain. When a noxious or potentially painful stimulus occurs, a chain of events that lead to the sensation of pain is initiated. The degree of tissue sensitivity to pain is directly related to the density of nociceptors in that tissue. Nociceptors respond to noxious or traumatic stimuli by converting the chemical, mechanical, or thermal insult into nerve impulses. These impulses are conducted from the peripheral tissue to the spinal cord and brain. Tissues containing a high density of nociceptors include skin, periosteum, joint capsule, muscle, tendon, cornea, dental pulp, and arterial wall.

> ✎ **TECHNICIAN NOTE**
> Tissues containing a high density of nociceptors include skin, periosteum, joint capsule, muscle, tendon, cornea, dental pulp, and arterial wall.

Peripheral nerves that transmit the nociceptive information to the central nervous system vary in size and in the speed with which they conduct that information in the form of electrical impulses. Nerve fibers with a myelin sheath (*A delta fibers*) are larger and conduct pain much more rapidly than the smaller unmyelinated ones (*C fibers*). Evidence indicates that A delta and C nerve fibers are capable of producing two distinct sensations of pain. Most painful events initially produce a sharp prickling pain followed by a dull burning sensation. The fast-conducting A delta fibers appear to be responsible for the rapid initial sharp sensation. The subsequent burning or throbbing pain involves conduction by the slower C fibers.

Some of the most intensely painful sensations result from chemical injury such as that associated with inflammation. Chemical substances such as prostaglandins, histamine, and proteolytic enzymes are produced by the body in association with tissue inflammation. In fact, these substances are so potent that they not only stimulate pain receptors but can actually alter their function and activity, producing peripheral sensitization that can result in allodynia and hyperalgesia (see Definitions). One of the most important classes of chemical mediators of pain formed during inflammation is the metabolic products of arachidonic acid. This group of metabolites includes the prostaglandins and leukotrienes. Prostaglandin production from arachidonic acid is blocked by nonsteroidal antiinflammatory drugs (NSAIDs). Aspirin, phenylbutazone, flunixin meglumine, carprofen, ketorolac, and deracoxib are examples of NSAIDs used in clinical veterinary practice.

> ✎ **TECHNICIAN NOTE**
> Some of the most intensely painful sensations result from chemical injury, such as that associated with inflammation.

CENTRAL NERVOUS SYSTEM

The pathways involved in the transmission of nociceptive information in the central nervous system (CNS) are considerably more complex than those in the periphery. Nerve fibers transmitting nociceptive information from the peripheral nerves enter the spinal cord through the dorsal nerve roots. Once the fibers have entered the spinal cord, they may associate with several types of neural hormones (e.g., substance P, somatostatin, cholecystokinin) that play a role in suppressing or augmenting the transmission and subsequent experience of pain.

Once the impulse reaches the spinal cord, nerve fibers segregate into neural tracts, which carry specifically grouped fiber types (Figure 20-1). The spinothalamic tract is important in the transmission of pain impulses through the spinal cord and to the brain. The nerve fibers or axons, which travel in the *spinothalamic tract*, terminate in several areas of the thalamic area of the brain and brainstem. The fibers terminating in the thalamus are involved in the perception and conscious discriminatory aspects of pain, including location, nature, and intensity.

Pain Localization

The localization of pain to a particular area of the body is the responsibility of the CNS. Pain can be poorly localized because sensory nerve fibers may be present in low densities in the peripheral tissue or because pain pathways frequently branch and converge, making it difficult for the brain to localize the sensation. For example, the pain resulting from gastroesophageal acid reflux in humans is felt as a diffuse burning sensation only vaguely localized to the sternum. A dull, poorly defined burning sensation is felt instead of well-localized pain, partly because of the poor sensory innervation of internal organs. Noxious stimulation of tissues with a high density of pain receptors, such as the skin, is generally much more precisely localized than that stimulation associated with internal organs.

In clinical practice, pain associated with the viscera of the thorax and abdomen is often used to help diagnose disease. The experience of pain associated with visceral tissues is

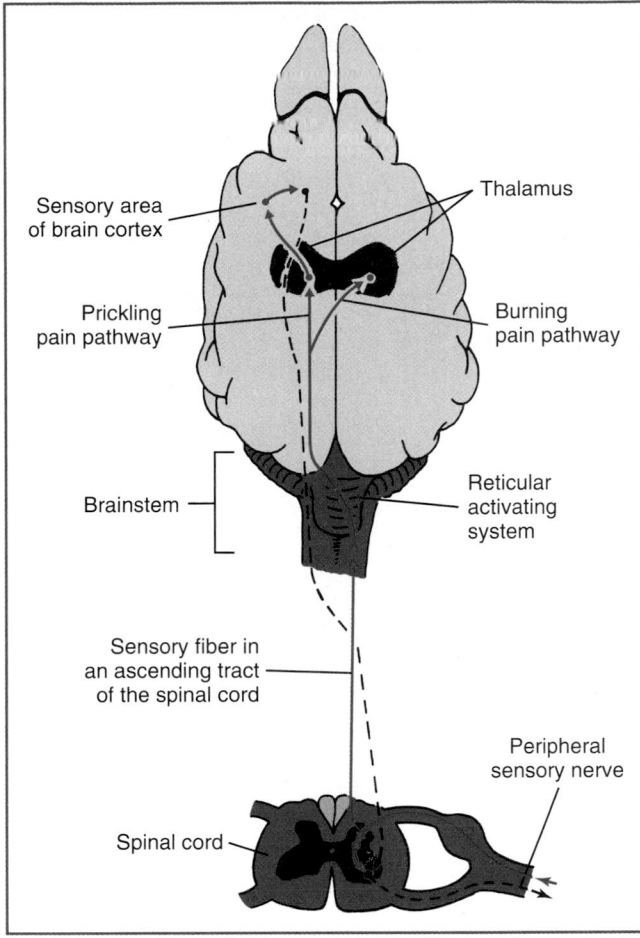

Figure 20-1 Transmission and segregation of nerve fibers carrying nociceptive impulses within the central nervous system.

different from surface or somatic (e.g., skin) pain. Somatic pain from the skin is highly localized because of the large number of pain receptors present in this area. By contrast, viscera such as the bladder or intestinal tract are poorly innervated. Because of this poor visceral innervation, abdominal and thoracic pain often occurs only following extensive, diffuse irritation. Common causes of visceral pain include leakage of damaging substances (e.g., bile, gastric acid) from the gastrointestinal tract leading to peritonitis or distention of the intestinal tract that occurs with an intestinal obstruction or gastric torsion.

RECOGNIZING PAIN IN ANIMALS

PROBLEMS WITH EVALUATION

Recognizing pain and anxiety in animals is critical before appropriate analgesic therapy can be initiated. Animals experiencing pain may exhibit specific behavior patterns that arise as a result of secondary stimulation of the autonomic nervous system. The response of the autonomic nervous system to pain and stress forms the basis of the classic fight-

Table 20-1 COMMON CLINICAL SIGNS OF PAIN OR DISTRESS	
System	**Signs**
Cardiovascular	Elevated heart rate and blood pressure, decreased peripheral circulation, prolonged capillary refill, cool extremities (ears, paws)
Respiratory	Rapid, shallow breaths, panting
Digestive	Weight loss, poor growth (young), vomiting, inappetence, constipation, diarrhea, salivation
Musculoskeletal	Unsteady gait, lameness, weakness, tremors, shivering
Urinary	Reluctance to urinate, loss of house training
Laboratory findings	Neutrophilia, lymphocytosis, hyperglycemia, polycythemia, elevated cortisol, elevated catecholamines

or-flight reaction. Autonomic nervous system stimulation results in the release of epinephrine and norepinephrine (catecholamines) from the adrenal glands, resulting in elevated heart rate, blood pressure, and respiratory rate and pupillary dilation (mydriasis). However, the fight-or-flight response is not unique to painful situations. It may occur in purely stressful situations such as restraint or manipulation. Because of its nonspecific nature, it is not possible to use autonomic stimulation as the sole criterion for pain evaluation. In addition to catecholamines, cortisol is released in response to pain and anxiety. Cortisol, like catecholamines, is released nonspecifically in response to stressful situations. Nonspecific physiologic signs that animals in pain may exhibit include neutrophilia and lymphocytosis (secondary to elevated endogenous catecholamines), hyperglycemia (especially in cats), and polycythemia (secondary to splenic contraction).

✎ TECHNICIAN NOTE

The recognition of pain and anxiety in animals is critical before appropriate analgesic therapy can be initiated.

SIGNS OF PAIN AND DISTRESS: ANIMAL VARIABILITY

Common physiologic responses to pain include increased heart rate and blood pressure, pupillary dilation, increased respiratory rate, and arousal (Table 20-1). These signs are not absolute, however; some animals may demonstrate a reduction in heart rate in response to pain. It is essential for the veterinary staff to be aware of normal physiologic values, typical physical appearance, and behavior patterns for each species and breed seen in the practice. Behavioral responses to pain and anxiety vary not only by species involved but also between breeds and even among individuals. As an example, the behavioral response that a stoic hound might exhibit to postoperative pain will be considerably different from that of the nervous toy breeds of dogs. The veterinary staff is more likely to become aware of the pain and anxiety experienced by the toy breed than those experienced by the less vocal hound. Further, behavioral responses to pain may vary between individuals or even families within a breed, making generalizations about signs of discomfort extremely difficult.

CLINICAL EVALUATION OF PAIN

In many cases, an animal initially reacts to a painful situation by retreating in an attempt to remove itself from the source of discomfort. If this reaction fails to bring relief, the animal may rely on other behavioral responses, such as vocalization, increased attempts to escape, pacing, guarding, sleeplessness, and aggression (Table 20-2). In horses, sweating, kicking, pawing, lip curling, and rolling are commonly exhibited with abdominal pain. More stoic species of animals such as cattle may only exhibit bruxism (teeth grinding) in response to pain. Animals that are experiencing acute postoperative or traumatic pain may also respond by biting, licking, or scratching at the source of discomfort. Chronic, low-grade pain in animals is often associated with prolonged hospitalization, radiation, and chemotherapy. Severe osteoarthritis may be manifested by failure to groom, lack of interest in surroundings, reluctance to move, anorexia, weight loss, constipation, and dysuria. Animals experiencing chronic pain may be withdrawn and quiet, unlike the seemingly "energized" state observed in animals experiencing acute pain. It is important to remember that *not all signs of pain may be present at one time* and *no single sign is a reliable indicator of the level of pain.* It is also important to note that animals may demonstrate a very different set of behaviors in the presence of an observer than they will when alone. Recent evidence indicates that dogs experiencing post-operative pain demonstrate significantly fewer pain-related behaviors in the presence of an observer than they do when alone.

> ### ✎ TECHNICIAN NOTE
> It is important to remember that not all signs of pain may be present at one time, and no single sign is a reliable indicator of the intensity of pain. Painful animals may not demonstrate the same behaviors while being observed that they do when alone.

CONTROL OF PAIN IN ANIMALS

Pain assessment in animals is an area of clinical practice to which veterinary technicians can contribute significantly. The veterinary technician is often the one involved most closely with the minute-by-minute treatment and monitoring of postoperative surgical and intensive care patients. The observant technician can contribute a great deal to pain relief by learning to recognize the clinical signs of discomfort in patients.

ENVIRONMENT AND NURSING CARE

The importance of good nursing care, particularly in the treatment of postoperative pain, cannot be overemphasized. Environmental factors often affect the emotional component of pain perception in both humans and animals. Keep the surroundings as familiar as possible to the animal, including providing toys or blankets from home or visits by owners in patients hospitalized for a long time. When possible, animals will often recover better at home from noncritical illnesses if owners are able to provide good nursing care. Recovery areas should be quiet and located away from busy areas with loud animal and human noise. Try to provide as stress free an environment as possible.

Table 20-2 POSTOPERATIVE PAIN EVALUATION

Type of Surgery	Signs of Pain	Suspected Pain Level	Duration
Head, ear, oral, dental	Rubbing; shaking; salivating; reluctance to eat, swallow, or drink; irritability; vocalizing	Moderate to high	Intermittent
Ophthalmologic	Rubbing, vocalizing, reluctance to move	High	Intermittent to continual
Orthopedic	Guarding, aggression, abnormal gait, self-mutilation, reluctance to move, dysuria, constipation	Moderate	Intermittent
Abdominal	Guarding, splinting, abnormal posture, vomiting, inappetence	Mild to moderate	Intermittent
Cardiovascular/thoracic	Changes in respiratory rate and pattern, reluctance to move, vocalizing	Moderate to high	Continual
Perirectal	Licking, biting, scooting, self-mutilation, constipation	Moderate	Intermittent

From Johnson JM: *Compend Contin Educ Pract Vet* 13:804, 1991; Wright EM, Marcella KL, Woodson JF: *Lab Anim* 14:20, 1985; and author's clinical experience.

During patient recovery, interaction with humans may also help to relieve stress and anxiety. Talking to an animal, stroking, and petting can help to reduce restlessness, rapid breathing, increased heart rate, and other signs of discomfort. Also remember that an animal's pain may be greatly exacerbated by frequent moving, monitoring, or administration of medications. Prepare a dry, comfortable, warm area for the patient. Schedule treatments and monitoring so that the animal is moved and disturbed as little as possible.

ANALGESIC DRUGS

Two main types of analgesics are often considered in the control of pain in animals: nonnarcotic NSAIDs and narcotics. The clinical indications for each of these families of drugs are often very different. Likewise, their mechanism of action and adverse effects also differ significantly.

The narcotic (opioid) analgesics are the most commonly used analgesics postoperatively. NSAIDs are predominantly employed for mild to moderate chronic pain associated with the musculoskeletal system. Finally the use of tranquilizers along with analgesic drugs to treat the anxiety often associated with pain and distress in companion animals is discussed.

OPIOIDS

Narcotic drugs (opioids) are the oldest and most extensively studied analgesic drugs available. The analgesic effect of narcotics is due to their interaction at specific opioid receptors located within the CNS and elsewhere in the body. Opioid receptors are present in the brain, spinal cord, and, as discovered more recently, in peripheral tissues such as the synovium, lung, and the surface of immune cells. With this wide distribution of opioid receptors, drugs that stimulate the opioid receptor (agonists) can be administered at many different sites.

Two of the five main receptor types are used in clinical pain management (mu and kappa). This historical classification of opioid receptor types has been replaced more recently by an alternative classification that is based on the genetic sequence associated with each receptor type. In this classification the mu receptor is now referred to as the OP_3 receptor and the kappa receptor is referred to as the OP_2 receptor. Each receptor produces a slightly different response when stimulated by an opioid drug (Table 20-3). For example, the OP_3 (mu) receptor subtype will cause respiratory depression, sedation, euphoria, and addiction when a drug stimulates it. Stimulation of the OP_2 (kappa) receptor, produces analgesia and sedation without the drug addiction response.

Opioids referred to as *pure agonists* are substances that exert their effects by only stimulating opioid receptors. An example of a pure agonist is *morphine*. Opioid *antagonists* bind at opioid receptors but block or fail to elicit a response.

The antagonists bind the opioid receptors and compete with the agonists, such as morphine, for the opioid receptor. The antagonists are often referred to as *narcotic reversal agents* because of their ability to reverse the effects of the opioid agonists by displacing them at the receptor level. The classic opioid antagonist is *naloxone*.

In addition to the pure opioid agonists and antagonists, there is a third category, the *mixed agonist/antagonist*. These substances have been synthesized to act like agonists at some of the opioid receptors and antagonists at others. An example of this class of drug is *butorphanol*. Butorphanol acts like naloxone at the mu (OP_3) receptor but has agonistic activity at the kappa (OP_2) receptor. This mixed effect allows butorphanol to be a good analgesic without having the addictive properties of morphine. The antagonistic activity of butorphanol can also be used to reverse an excessive dose of morphine while maintaining some analgesia produced by kappa (OP_2) agonism.

In general, the narcotic drugs produce minimal cardiovascular effects and are safe in patients with cardiac disease. They are known to produce bradycardia and can produce hypotension if they stimulate the release of histamine (morphine, meperidine), particularly when administered intravenously. Their effects on the respiratory system include respiratory depression (decreased rate and tidal volume) and a decreased sensitivity of the respiratory center to increasing levels of carbon dioxide. This effect is particularly important in the postoperative period when opioid administration may depress ventilation profoundly enough to produce hypoxemia. Narcotics can also cause salivation, nausea, vomiting, and nonpropulsive intestinal motility (segmental contractions). Along with their analgesic effects, these drugs will produce sedation and in some animals dysphoria (hallucinations), although the dysphoria is a dose-related effect.

The narcotic drugs are extensively metabolized by the liver and excreted in the urine. Animals with liver disease or neonates with poorly developed hepatic metabolism require reduced dosages of narcotics to avoid prolonged drug effects.

Table 20-3 RECEPTOR ACTIVITY OF OPIOID DRUGS

Drug	Receptor Activity	
	Mu (OP_3)	Kappa (OP_2)
Agonist opioids: fentanyl, morphine, meperidine, oxymorphone	Agonist	Agonist
Butorphanol	Weak antagonist	Agonist
Pentazocine	Weak antagonist	Agonist
Buprenorphine	Weak agonist	Antagonist
Nalorphine	Weak agonist	Antagonist
Naloxone	Antagonist	Antagonist

Morphine

Morphine is considered to be the prototypic narcotic analgesic. It is the opioid to which the potency of other opioids is compared. The *potency* of a drug refers to the amount of drug that is required to produce a desired effect. For example, if drug A is given at a dosage of 1 mg/kg to achieve a desired effect and it only takes a dosage of 0.1 mg/kg of drug B to produce the same effect, then drug B is 10 times more potent than drug A. In the clinical setting, the potency of a drug is of little consequence as long as the appropriate dose can be administered conveniently.

Two advantages of morphine are analgesia and sedation. The effects of morphine are reversed with narcotic antagonists, such as naloxone. Adverse effects of morphine administration include depression of the respiratory and central nervous systems.

> **✏ TECHNICIAN NOTE**
>
> Morphine is considered to be the prototypic narcotic analgesic.

As with most of the narcotics, morphine is metabolized by the liver and excreted through the kidneys. Care should be taken when administering morphine to animals with renal or hepatic compromise, because drug elimination may be prolonged. Morphine produces excitation when administered alone to horses. Because of this, it should always be administered with an appropriate sedative. In the past, there has been concern that cats are sensitive to the excitatory effects of morphine. Clinically, this appears to be a dose-related effect that is not frequently observed when clinically appropriate doses are administered. Morphine is effective against moderate to severe pain. As with all analgesic drugs, it has its most profound effect when given before the pain-eliciting insult. Morphine is relatively inexpensive making it one of the most cost-effective narcotic analgesics. In addition to subcutaneous and intramuscular routes of administration, morphine is frequently administered epidurally for long duration postoperative analgesia. Morphine is also administered intraarticularly in combination with a local anesthesia to provide analgesia for arthroscopic procedures.

Fentanyl

Fentanyl is a synthetic opioid with approximately 100 times the potency of morphine and 500 times the potency of meperidine. Fentanyl acts rapidly after intravenous or intramuscular injection. Profound analgesia and respiratory depression develop within 6 to 8 minutes after injection. Auditory sensitization and alterations in the thermoregulatory center that lead to panting also occur frequently. Bradycardia is commonly produced, frequently necessitating the concurrent use of atropine or glycopyrrolate. Extreme caution should be used if fentanyl is administered concurrently with barbiturates (e.g., thiamylal, thiopental) because bradycardia, hypotension, and respiratory depression can be difficult to reverse.

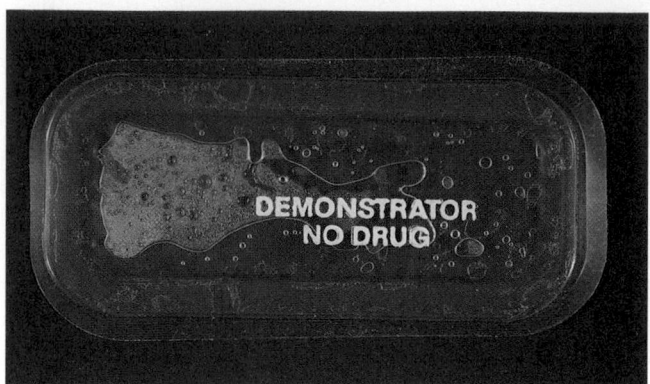

Figure 20-2 A transdermal patch used to deliver fentanyl. Fentanyl patches are used for long-term administration of fentanyl. One patch contains enough fentanyl for approximately 72 hours.

Fentanyl has a short duration of action, with peak effects lasting for only 30 to 45 minutes. Although fentanyl is an excellent analgesic for moderate to severe pain, the utility of the administration of a single dose is limited by this short duration of effect. Consequently, fentanyl is frequently administered as a continuous rate intravenous infusion either as an adjunct to inhalant anesthesia, as part of a total intravenous protocol for general anesthesia, or as an infusion for the management of postoperative pain.

Transdermal Administration of Fentanyl

Another method that is used to provide a continuous infusion of fentanyl is the transdermal patch. The transdermal fentanyl patch has become quite popular in veterinary medicine because of the relative ease of use of this delivery system. The transdermal patch is composed of a drug reservoir that is sandwiched between an impermeable backing and a permeable skin-contacting membrane (Figures 20-2 and 20-3). Transdermal fentanyl patches have been used clinically in a variety of species (dogs, cats, pigs, horses, goats). There is some variability in the uptake and/or delivery of fentanyl from the patch, so clinical results may be unpredictable. For all species, there is some delay in the time between application of the patch and when therapeutic plasma levels of fentanyl are reached. When treating cats, the patch should be applied 12 to 16 hours before the intended surgery. In dogs, a period of 24 hours is required to achieve steady-state levels of fentanyl in the blood. Patches are designed to deliver fentanyl for approximately 72 hours. Hypothermia and anesthesia can reduce the amount of fentanyl that is taken up from the patch, so one should not assume that an animal that is receiving fentanyl transdermally would not require supplemental analgesia in the immediate perioperative period. Patches are available in 25, 50, 75, and 100 μg/hr concentrations. A patch with 2.5 mg of fentanyl is designed to release 25 μg/hr. Dosage guidelines are presented in Table 20-4. Patches should never be cut to reduce the delivery rate; however, exposing only half of the patch when administering fentanyl transdermally to

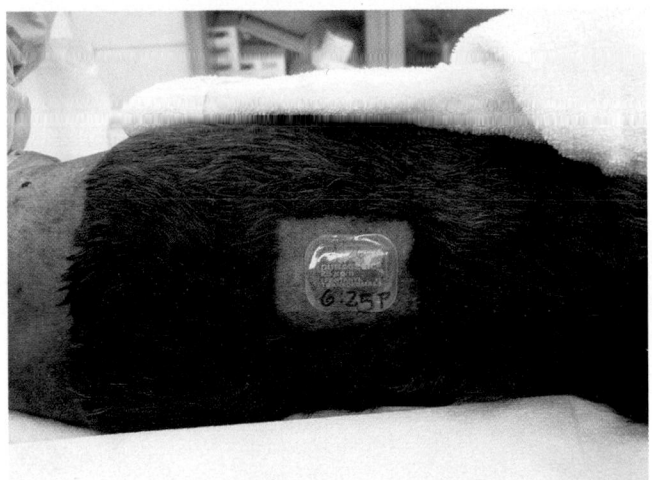

Figure 20-3 A transdermal delivery system for fentanyl ("fentanyl patch") in place on the dorsum of a dog. Note the date and time of placement of the patch are written on the patch. When using these patches, care must be taken to avoid applying external heat sources (i.e., heating blankets) directly to the patch. The application of heat to the patch will cause an increase in the release of fentanyl from the patch potentially resulting in an overdose.

Table 20-4 DOSE GUIDELINES FOR TRANSDERMAL FENTANYL IN DOGS AND CATS

WEIGHT	PATCH SIZE
3-10 kg	25 µg/kg
10-20 kg	50 µg/kg
20-30 kg	75 µg/kg
>30 kg	100 µg/kg

cats provides adequate analgesia following a routine ovariohysterectomy.

> **TECHNICIAN NOTE**
>
> Transdermal patches should never be cut or altered in any way that will increase the rate of release of drug from the patch. Doing so can result in the administration of an overdose of drug with potentially fatal consequences.

Hydromorphone and Oxymorphone

Oxymorphone and hydromorphone are semisynthetic narcotic analgesics that are approximately 10 times more potent than morphine. Their duration of action is from 4 to 6 hours. Side effects are similar to those of morphine, although oxymorphone and hydromorphone typically produce less vomiting than morphine. Other reported side effects associated with the administration of either of these drugs include auditory sensitization, bradycardia, and panting. Both of these drugs are excellent for moderate to intense pain.

> **TECHNICIAN NOTE**
>
> Hydromorphone and oxymorphone are considered excellent analgesics for moderate to intense pain.

Epidural Administration of Opioids

Because of significant success with the epidural administration of opioids in humans, much attention has been focused on their use in companion animals. The technique of epidural administration involves the use of either a spinal needle or epidural catheter that is placed in the space around the dura mater. For many of the drugs that are administered epidurally, a dose lower than the dose that is used systemically may be used. This reduced dose decreases the incidence and intensity of side effects. When morphine is administered epidurally, the duration of the clinical effect is much longer than the duration of clinical effect following systemic administration. The onset and duration of action of epidurally administered opioids varies markedly among drugs depending on their molecular weight, ionization, and lipid solubility. Lipid-soluble drugs such as fentanyl have a rapid onset of action and very short duration, whereas water-soluble morphine has a delayed onset and long duration.

Morphine is the opioid used most frequently for epidural administration in animals. Administered this way, morphine is used to provide postoperative analgesia after pelvic or hind limb soft-tissue or orthopedic surgery. Intraoperative anesthesia may be augmented by adding a local anesthetic (bupivacaine or lidocaine) to the morphine. Epidurally administered morphine has also been used to provide analgesia following abdominal surgery or for chronic pain management (Figures 20-4 and 20-5). The dose of epidural morphine (preservative-free drug) commonly used in most species is 0.1 mg/kg. The latency of onset is approximately 30 to 60 minutes, and the duration of analgesia is 12 to 18 hours.

MIXED-ACTION AGONIST/ANTAGONIST NARCOTIC ANALGESICS

Butorphanol

Butorphanol belongs to a group of synthetic analgesics with both agonist and antagonist properties. Butorphanol is considered to be a weak antagonist at the mu (OP_3) receptor but a strong agonist at the kappa (OP_2) receptor. Butorphanol is three to five times more potent an analgesic than morphine. It is important to keep in mind that this does not mean that butorphanol is a better analgesic, rather that it requires less butorphanol to achieve similar clinical effects. However, clinical experience with butorphanol does not support this equivalency of clinical effect. The antagonist activity of butorphanol is nearly 50 times less than that

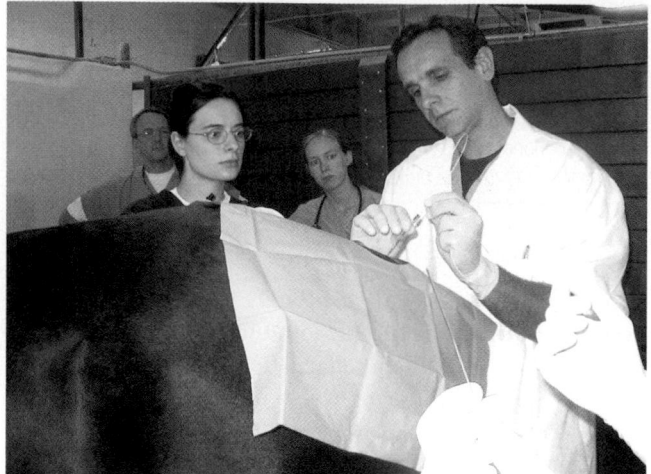

Figure 20-4 Long-term epidural administration of morphine may be achieved by placing a catheter in the epidural space. Here the catheter is being introduced into the epidural space through a Tuohy needle at the first intercoccygeal space. Strict asepsis must be observed during this procedure and when administering drugs through the catheter.

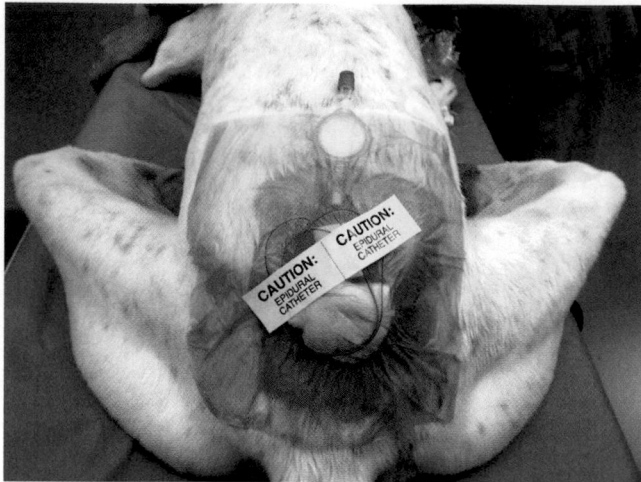

Figure 20-5 Epidural catheters may be placed for the long-term administration of analgesic drugs to dogs, cats, and other companion animal species. Care must be taken to prevent contamination of the catheter or the insertion site.

of naloxone. The respiratory depression produced by butorphanol is similar to that of morphine; however, butorphanol reaches a ceiling effect beyond which higher doses fail to increase the depression. Butorphanol is also a well-recognized antitussive and has been used as an antiemetic in cancer patients. The antagonistic properties of butorphanol are sometimes used to reverse excessive doses of mu agonists. The advantage of using butorphanol to reverse mu agonists is that some analgesia is provided by the butorphanol-mediated kappa agonism after the mu agonism is reversed. This is not the case when mu agonists are reversed with naloxone. Similar to other narcotics, butorphanol is metabolized by the liver and has a plasma half-life of 3 to 4 hours in dogs, although the duration of clinical effect does not appear to be this long.

Butorphanol appears to act as an acceptable analgesic for mild to moderate pain in the dog, cat, and horse. Butorphanol is a Schedule IV substance.

Buprenorphine

Buprenorphine is classified as an agonist/antagonist, but its most significant effect is as a partial agonist at the mu opioid receptor. Its effect at the kappa receptor is relatively minimal. This drug also differs from butorphanol in that its association and dissociation with the mu opioid receptors occurs very slowly. Because of its slow receptor association and dissociation it may take up to 60 minutes after intravenous injection for buprenorphine to take effect. It has the potential for duration of effect of 8 to 12 hours, but the clinical effect is rarely greater than 6 hours. Because buprenorphine binds tightly to the opioid receptor, its effects can be difficult to reverse with naloxone. An important adverse effect following injection of buprenorphine is

its delayed respiratory depression. It has been recommended that animals given buprenorphine be observed closely for at least 2 hours after administration. Buprenorphine is 300 times more potent than morphine and is effective only for mild to moderate pain.

NARCOTIC ANTAGONISTS

Relatively minor structural changes to opioids can convert a drug with primary agonist activity to one with antagonist action. Narcotic antagonists allow for the quick reversal of a narcotic overdose and its associated side effects.

Naloxone

Naloxone is a pure antagonist with 50 times the reversal potential of butorphanol. Naloxone is regarded as a pure competitive antagonist at all the opioid receptors and is not regulated by the Controlled Substances Act. The dosage for naloxone is 0.02 to 0.04 mg/kg. The intravenous route of administration is the preferred route for immediate effect of the drug.

In patients with respiratory depression, an increase in respiratory rate occurs 1 to 2 minutes after naloxone administration. The sedative, cardiovascular, and analgesic effects of the opioids are also rapidly reversed. Antagonist effects will last for 1 to 4 hours, depending on the initial dose given. When naloxone is being used to reverse a pure agonist, repeat administration may be necessary since many of the narcotics will last longer than naloxone. At low doses, naloxone has a high binding affinity for the mu receptor, which is responsible for respiratory depression and sedation; much higher doses are needed to antagonize the kappa receptor.

Nalorphine

Nalorphine is a morphine derivative that is classified as a partial agonist, but it reverses the effects of many opioids. Nalorphine is a Schedule III drug, which means that it is less addictive than a Schedule II drug, such as morphine. In the presence of narcotic agonists, nalorphine acts as a partial antagonist. Like butorphanol, nalorphine may be used alone for sedation and analgesia. The drug has the advantage of having less CNS and respiratory depression than the pure agonists.

MANAGEMENT OF CONTROLLED SUBSTANCES

Controlled substances, as defined by the Controlled Substances Act of 1970, include opioids (narcotics), barbiturates, hallucinogens (ketamine), amphetamines, and other addictive or habituating drugs. This act regulates the manufacturing, distribution, and dispensing of controlled substances. The licensed veterinarian wishing to prescribe or maintain controlled drugs must register with the U.S. Drug Enforcement Agency (DEA).

Controlled substances must be kept in a locked cabinet or safe with attachment to a concrete floor. Strict inventory, including patient/client name and volume dispensed, is required by law.

Controlled drugs are listed in five different schedules (C-I, C-II, C-III, C-IV, C-V). *Schedule I* drugs have a high abuse potential and are not currently accepted in the United States for treatment. Examples include heroin, lysergic acid diethylamide (LSD), mescaline, and marijuana. *Schedule II* drugs have a high abuse potential and can produce severe psychic and physical dependence in humans. Examples include morphine, meperidine, oxymorphone, and pentobarbital. *Schedule III* drugs have less abuse potential than those in schedules I and II. Abuse of these drugs leads to moderate or low physical dependence. Examples include preparations with low levels of morphine as well as nalorphine, ketamine, and barbiturates. *Schedule IV* drugs are considered to have a low abuse potential and include phenobarbital and diazepam (Valium). Additional information on controlled substances may be found in Chapter 21.

NONSTEROIDAL ANTIINFLAMMATORY DRUGS

INFLAMMATION

NSAIDs exert their analgesic effects in the peripheral tissues primarily by blocking the production of prostaglandins. Prostaglandins are normally produced in tissues as a result of tissue damage and inflammation.

Tissue inflammation is the result of a series of events that are mediated by substances such as vasoactive amines (histamine, serotonin), leukocyte products (lymphokines, oxygen radicals, interleukins), and substances that are formed from the metabolism of arachidonic acid (prostaglandins, leukotrienes). Arachidonic acid, a phospholipid, is present in cell membranes. When it is released, it can be metabolized to form prostaglandins and leukotrienes (Figures 20-6 and 20-7).

Inflammation begins with local tissue injury. Vasoactive substances released from both blood cells (leukocytes, platelets) and cells in the peripheral tissue result in the production of pain, heat, and swelling. Fluid exudation from capillaries can cause swelling and pain secondary to the pressure exerted on local nerve endings. Along with the vascular changes, neutrophils and monocyte-macrophages migrate to the injured tissue to ingest and destroy foreign material. During this process, toxic oxygen radicals and enzymes are released into the local tissues, further exacerbating the inflammatory process.

NSAIDs control pain by inhibiting *cyclooxygenase,* a major enzyme in the arachidonic acid pathway leading to the production of prostaglandins. Cyclooxygenase also converts arachidonic acid to thromboxane (causes platelet aggregation) and prostacyclin (inhibits platelet aggregation). An important point to remember is that by blocking cyclooxygenase, NSAIDs inhibit the production of the prostaglandins involved in inflammation as well as those involved in regulating such important functions as renal blood flow and gastric secretion.

MECHANISM OF ACTION

Recent research has shown why some NSAIDs produce more gastrointestinal adverse effects than others. There are two isoforms of cyclooxygenase (COX): COX-1, the constitutive gastroprotective form, and COX-2, the inducible form associated with inflammation. Some NSAIDs are more COX-2 selective than others. The current thought is that drugs with higher levels of COX-1 inhibition result in greater gastrointestinal injury although there may be a protective role for the COX-2 enzyme in the maintenance of gastrointestinal integrity. Pharmaceutical research has recently been directed toward developing COX-2–selective NSAIDs that have fewer gastrointestinal and renal complications.

SALICYLATE ANALGESICS

Salicylate analgesics were first introduced into clinical medicine in the late nineteenth century. Salicylates commonly used in veterinary practice include aspirin and bismuth subsalicylate. Salicylates are effective in relieving pain

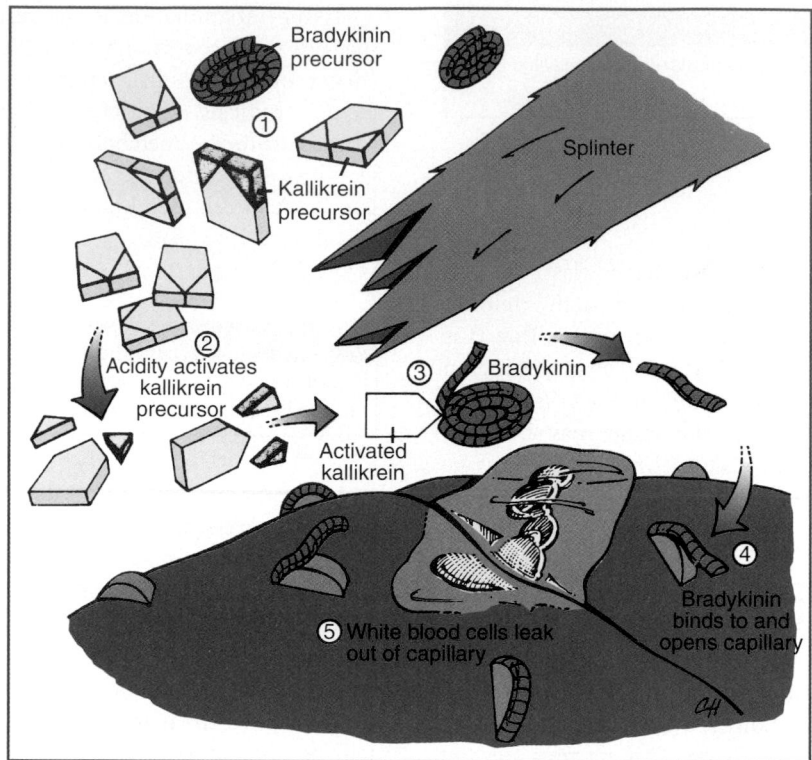

Figure 20-6 The inflammatory process involves the generation of many substances responsible for causing pain and swelling.

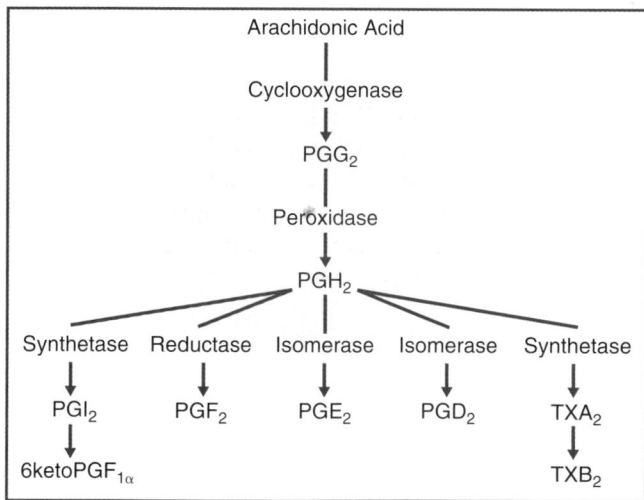

Figure 20-7 Many different prostaglandins are generated enzymatically after the release of arachidonic acid from damaged cell membranes.

associated with peripheral inflammation, such as muscle and joint disease, but have virtually no effect on deep or visceral pain. Salicylates have antipyretic effects because of their ability to reduce the prostaglandin-induced fever response. Aspirin, like other NSAIDs, inhibits the generation of thromboxane and thus decreases platelet aggregation.

Salicylates are readily absorbed through the gastrointestinal tract and quickly enter synovial fluid, peritoneal fluid, milk, saliva, and placental membranes. These drugs are metabolized in the liver by the enzyme glucuronyl transferase. Once processed in the liver, metabolic by-products are excreted through the kidney. The drug half-life of salicylates is higher in cats than in dogs because the cat has considerably lower levels of hepatic glucuronyl transferase and subsequently a decreased ability to metabolize the drug.

Clinical use of aspirin has centered on the management of inflammatory (e.g., rheumatoid arthritis) and degenerative joint diseases. Aspirin may be used in the cat as long as it is administered no more often than every 36 to 48 hours.

Clinical signs of toxicity associated with salicylates, as well as other more potent NSAIDs, include nausea and bloody vomitus (hematemesis) associated with gastric ulceration, renal disease, and bleeding tendencies secondary to platelet aggregation inhibition. Gastrointestinal ulceration is the most commonly encountered adverse reaction secondary to NSAID use in the dog and horse. Ulceration occurs secondary to direct irritation of the drug on the gastric mucosa and, importantly, secondary to prostaglandin inhibition. Prostaglandins produced by the gastric mucosa are normally involved in increasing gastric mucus and bicarbonate production, thus helping to coat the stomach lining, neutralize acid produced, and protect the mucosa from irritation. Prostaglandins are also involved in decreasing the volume and acidity of gastric secretion. By inhibiting prostaglandin production, NSAIDs contribute to decreased gastrointestinal protective mechanisms and predispose an individual to ulcer formation.

PROPIONIC ACID DERIVATIVES

Carprofen

Carprofen is a reversible inhibitor of COX-1 and COX-2. In dogs, carprofen is 90% absorbed after oral administration and has a mean half-life of approximately 8 hours after a single dose. Effective analgesic and antiinflammatory effects of carprofen have been established through subjective clinical trials, objective gait analysis, and force plate examinations. Carprofen is considerably more potent for management of signs of chronic pain than aspirin. Studies involving more than 450 dogs have been performed to evaluate the safety and efficacy of carprofen. The number of reports of adverse events has been minimal. The most common adverse events have been vomiting, lethargy, and anorexia. Recently, isolated drug-induced hepatotoxicity has been identified in dogs not previously showing signs of liver disease. Most animals recovered with supportive therapy after drug administration was discontinued. The Labrador retriever appears to be at increased risk. It has been recommended that evaluation of both renal and hepatic function be performed in dogs before administering carprofen. Carprofen is available in oral and injectable formulations and is currently approved for the control of pain and inflammation associated with osteoarthritis in dogs and the control of postoperative pain associated with soft-tissue and orthopedic surgeries in dogs.

Deracoxib

Deracoxib is a member of the coxib class of NSAIDs. It is available in an oral formulation and is approved for use in the control of pain associated with osteoarthritis and for the control of postoperative pain associated with orthopedic surgery. At clinical doses, deracoxib does not inhibit the production of COX-2, however; the clinical significance of this effect is not known. The major route of elimination of deracoxib is by hepatic biotransformation and the majority of deracoxib is excreted in the feces as parent drug or metabolites.

Naproxen

There are a considerable number of propionic acid derivatives on the market, most of which act by inhibiting cyclooxygenase. Naproxen, an NSAID, has effective antiinflammatory, analgesic, and antipyretic properties and is an effective cyclooxygenase inhibitor. Naproxen has approximately 20 times the potency of the related drug ibuprofen. In humans, naproxen has been used successfully to treat degenerative joint disease as well as posttraumatic soft-tissue injury.

The toxicity of naproxen is similar to that of other nonsteroidal drugs. Gastrointestinal ulceration leading to perforation and peritonitis has been reported. Because naproxen has a long duration of action in the dog, it can be administered once daily. Because of the convenience of a single dose per day, naproxen has gained some popularity in treating pain related to orthopedic conditions. The use of naproxen should be limited to dogs in which salicylates do not control pain. If clinical signs of gastric upset occur, administration should be discontinued immediately. In horses, naproxen is administered twice daily and is very effective for soft-tissue inflammation.

Ibuprofen

Ibuprofen was the first phenylpropionate to be marketed in the United States and has been used successfully to treat rheumatoid arthritis and osteoarthritis in humans. In humans, ibuprofen is considered to have less of an analgesic effect than aspirin; however, it is preferred in many cases because it appears to be associated with a lower incidence of gastric bleeding.

The most common form of ibuprofen is available without prescription as 200-mg tablets under a wide variety of proprietary names.

Studies on ibuprofen use in the dog indicate that gastric irritation and repeated vomiting began after 2 to 4 days of administration and continued several days after the drug was discontinued. These studies indicate that dogs are more sensitive than humans to ibuprofen's gastric-irritating effects. Ibuprofen offers no advantage over other NSAIDs, and because of significant gastrointestinal irritation, its use in the dog is not recommended.

> **✐ TECHNICIAN NOTE**
>
> Ibuprofen offers no advantage over other NSAIDs. Because of significant gastrointestinal irritation, its use in the dog is not recommended.

Ketoprofen

Ketoprofen is a propionic acid NSAID approved for use in humans and horses. It is a strong cyclooxygenase inhibitor and is subsequently a powerful analgesic and antiinflammatory drug. While not approved for use in dogs and cats in the United States, it is recommended for the control of postoperative and chronic pain in dogs and cats in Europe and Canada.

In a multicenter clinical trial, ketoprofen used intravenously at 2 mg/kg exhibited a potent analgesic effect in the management of pain in horses with colic. An excellent response was obtained in 89.5% of the horses, without any local or general side effects noted. Ketoprofen may be administered daily for up to 5 days in horses.

FENAMIC ACIDS

Meclofenamic Acid

Meclofenamic acid inhibits cyclooxygenase and may also block cell surface receptors for prostaglandins. The drug has gained popularity for treating musculoskeletal pain that is refractory to aspirin. Toxic side effects have been observed in dogs and include diarrhea, vomiting, and gastrointestinal ulceration.

Meclofenamic acid is frequently used in dogs when aspirin therapy has failed to relieve pain associated with chronic degenerative joint diseases, such as elbow and hip dysplasia. In horses, meclofenamic acid is used for musculoskeletal pain.

Flunixin Meglumine

Flunixin meglumine is an NSAID with both analgesic and antipyretic activity. Like other NSAIDs, flunixin inhibits the enzyme cyclooxygenase, blocking the production of prostaglandins. Flunixin is considered to be one of the most potent cyclooxygenase enzyme inhibitors available. The analgesic potency of flunixin is greater than that of phenylbutazone, meperidine (narcotic), or codeine (narcotic).

Flunixin is recommended for relief of persistent, severe inflammation and pain associated with degenerative joint disease that is unresponsive to milder NSAIDs, such as aspirin. Because flunixin is a potent inhibitor of prostaglandin synthesis, it also frequently causes severe gastrointestinal ulceration and bleeding. Flunixin is particularly useful for visceral analgesia in horses. Toxicity in horses is rare; it appears to have a wider margin of safety than phenylbutazone.

OXICANS
Meloxicam

Meloxicam is another COX-2 preferential NSAID. It is available as an oral liquid suspension and as an injectable formulation. It is approved for use in the United States in the control of pain and inflammation associated with osteoarthritis in dogs. In some countries, meloxicam is approved for use in the treatment of mastitis and noninfectious locomotor disorders in pigs and for the treatment of inflammation associated with acute mastitis in cattle.

PYRAZOLONE DERIVATIVES
Phenylbutazone

Phenylbutazone has analgesic, antiinflammatory, and antipyretic properties similar to those common to the salicylate analgesics. As a member of the pyrazolone family, it has been associated with significant toxic effects in humans and, less commonly, in animals. Phenylbutazone in humans is known to cause fatal blood disorders (agranulocytosis). Prolonged use in the dog has also led to similar blood diseases.

Clinically, phenylbutazone has been used in the dog for treatment of painful arthritis and skeletal muscle disease and is considered to inhibit cyclooxygenase activity more effectively than aspirin but less effectively than meclofenamic acid and naproxen. Phenylbutazone is known to cause gastrointestinal ulceration, renal and hepatic disease, and, rarely, bone marrow suppression with prolonged use. Phenylbutazone is commonly used in horses for the control of musculoskeletal and visceral pain. The drug has a narrow margin of safety and, when compared to flunixin meglumine and ketoprofen, was found to cause a higher incidence of gastrointestinal ulceration. Certain pony breeds (Shetland and Welsh crosses) have been shown to exhibit acute toxicity to phenylbutazone. Lower daily dosage (4.4 mg/kg once daily

for 4 days and then every other day) has been recommended for ponies.

TREATMENT OF GASTROINTESTINAL ULCERATION

Adverse drug reactions are common with the use of NSAIDs, especially when used long term and at high doses for musculoskeletal pain. Gastric ulceration, nausea, vomiting, and diarrhea commonly occur in dogs given NSAIDs. Gastric ulceration, weight loss, and inappetence occur in horses receiving NSAIDs long term. Several options have been suggested for the prophylaxis and treatment of ulcers associated with NSAID administration. Mucosal-adherent sucralfate binds to mucosal defects, providing a barrier to gastric acid, and may accelerate healing. The H_2-receptor antagonists cimetidine, ranitidine, and famotidine and the proton pump inhibitor omeprazole are also commonly used. Misoprostol, a prostaglandin analog, has been shown to diminish gastric ulceration in dogs by providing the cytoprotective effects that NSAIDs reduce by blocking natural prostaglandins.

PSYCHOTROPIC DRUGS

TRANQUILIZERS

Animals experiencing pain and anxiety occasionally benefit from the effects of tranquilizers used in conjunction with analgesic drugs. Tranquilizers provide sedation, some muscle relaxation, and anxiolysis. It is important to remember that *tranquilizers provide no analgesia* and that *it is inappropriate to use these drugs alone for postoperative pain control.* The phenothiazines (e.g., acetylpromazine, chlorpromazine, promazine) are used extensively for their sedative effects. Other useful tranquilizers include the benzodiazepines diazepam and midazolam. The use of tranquilizers after surgery should be limited to providing sedation and relaxation to animals with pain-related distress and apprehension. Combining narcotics with low doses of tranquilizers often provides effective control of pain after surgery in anxious patients.

ALPHA$_2$-ADRENERGIC AGONISTS
Xylazine

Xylazine binds at alpha$_2$ receptors in the CNS, causing its sedative and analgesic effects. Many of the side effects of xylazine are secondary to its binding at peripheral alpha$_2$ receptors. Peripheral alpha$_1$-receptor stimulation causes vasoconstriction with an increase in arterial blood pressure. This increase in blood pressure may be associated with bradycardia. Xylazine administration is frequently associated with second-degree atrioventricular block. Xylazine can also cause smooth muscle relaxation and vomiting. One significant advantage of xylazine is that its effects may be reversed with the antagonists yohimbine, atipamezole, tolazoline, or idazoxan.

Xylazine hydrochloride is a potent visceral analgesic in the horse, but it may be less effective for peripheral pain.

Xylazine has been used to provide analgesia in the dog and cat, however; the use of xylazine in small animal species has been replaced with the use of the more specific alpha$_2$ agonist medetomidine. Medetomidine is an effective analgesic for minor procedures.

Detomidine

Detomidine is a sedative-analgesic originally developed for horses and cattle. Detomidine is more potent than xylazine and has greater central alpha$_2$-adrenoreceptor specificity.

Detomidine has similar cardiovascular effects to xylazine when administered intravenously at 10 to 60 µg/kg. Sedation and analgesia are of a longer duration than xylazine. Administration of detomidine with opioids eliminates the excitation seen in horses when opioids are given alone. The combination of detomidine and butorphanol gives effective sedation and analgesia; detomidine (10 to 15 µg/kg intravenously) precedes butorphanol (20 to 30 µg/kg intravenously).

CORTICOSTEROIDS

Corticosteroids principally act by dampening the fire of inflammation and not by eliminating the cause of it. Significant impairment of wound healing and masking of the underlying disease can occur with the prolonged administration of high doses of corticosteroids.

Useful corticosteroids for treatment of inflammation include the short-acting cortisone, hydrocortisone, prednisone, and prednisolone. The antiinflammatory effects of prednisolone and prednisone are approximately five times greater than those of cortisone. Corticosteroids are frequently used as short-term (3 to 5 days) antiinflammatory drugs in the treatment of acute exacerbations of chronic musculoskeletal pain (e.g., osteoarthritis of the elbow or hip). Corticosteroids should not be used with NSAIDs because of an increased risk of gastrointestinal ulceration.

LOCAL ANESTHETICS AS SELECTIVE NERVE BLOCKS

The use of local anesthetics to selectively block peripheral nerves prevents the transmission of nociceptive information from the periphery to the spinal cord. In cases where the analgesia is required for the treatment of pain associated with surgery and general anesthesia, selective nerve blocks may be used in combination with other analgesics (i.e., opioids). In some cases local anesthetic selective nerve blocks are often used in conjunction with sedation. In dogs, selective blocking of intercostal nerves before chest wall closure after thoracic surgery has been shown to provide analgesia equal to that of systemic morphine. The technique involves injecting 0.5% bupivacaine into the intercostal nerves as they pass behind the head of the ribs for two to three rib spaces in front of and behind the thoracotomy incision. A maximum total dosage of 4 to 5 mg/kg in dogs and 2 to 3 mg/kg in cats should be used. Complete blocking

of the intercostal nerves with bupivacaine will provide analgesia for 4 to 5 hours. Selective intercostal nerve blocks have a distinct advantage in not producing the respiratory depression that is occasionally seen with the administration of narcotics.

Recently, analgesia in dogs for thoracotomy-associated pain has been achieved by instilling 0.5% bupivacaine, 1.5 mg/kg, through chest tubes placed during surgery. The analgesia provided is considered to be equal to either systemic morphine or intercostal nerve block. The technique involves instilling the appropriate dose of bupivacaine through the chest tube followed by flushing the tube with 5-ml sterile physiologic saline. The dog is then rolled on its back and slightly tilted to the incision side for 10 to 15 minutes. This technique allows the local anesthetic to block the nerve roots at the site of the incision.

Local nerve blocks are also used for injection of transected nerves following thoracic or pelvic limb amputation. Significant postoperative pain is often associated with cut nerve fibers following limb amputation. Analgesia may be provided by injecting 0.5% bupivacaine (0.5 ml per nerve, not to exceed 4 to 5 mg/kg in the dog) into the nerve stump before wound closure. Local nerve blocks may also be used as part of a pain management strategy for the treatment of pain associated with onychectomy in the cat.

TREATMENT OF PAIN IN DOGS AND CATS

The first step in the management of pain in animals is recognizing the behavioral and physiologic signs associated with significant discomfort. Recognize that abnormal respiration, rapid heart rate, aggression, and changes in appetite and grooming behavior can all be associated with pain. It is critical to remember that no single sign is definitive in determining whether an animal is experiencing discomfort. It is helpful to remember, when clinical signs are confusing, that if the patient experienced a procedure that would be painful to a human, it is likely that it was painful to the animal.

Good nursing care is critical in the management of pain. Providing clean, dry, comfortable bedding in an area free from noise and confusion goes a long way in relieving the distress and anxiety associated with pain. Many patients will benefit from gentle human contact, such as talking and petting. Avoid excessive movement and treatments in patients recovering from a painful surgery.

✎ TECHNICIAN NOTE

When administering any of the NSAIDs, always be aware that they can cause gastric upset, vomiting, and ulceration.

When one is selecting an analgesic drug for the treatment of pain (Tables 20-5 to 20-9 and Box 20-1), animals should

Table 20-5 NARCOTIC ANALGESICS USED IN DOGS

Drug	Potentcy	Dose	Analgesic Duration (hr)	Comments
Morphine	1	0.25-1.0 mg/kg IM, SC Epidural: 0.1 mg/kg	4 10-14	Causes respiratory depression and vomiting; elevates intracranial and intraocular pressure; metabolized by liver
Oxymorphone/ hydromorphone	10	0.005-0.2 mg/kg IM, SC, IV Epidural: 0.1 mg/kg	6 10	Causes respiratory depression, auditory hypersensitivity, and altered thermoregulation; metabolized by liver
Butorphanol	5	0.2-0.6 mg/kg IM, SC, IV	2-4	Agonist/antagonist; antitussive, antiemetic; ceiling on respiratory depression
Buprenorphine	25-50	0.005-0.02 mg/kg IM, SC, IV	6-12	Agonist/antagonist; prolonged ($\geq$30 min) time from administration to onset of action; long duration; difficult to reverse with naloxone
Fentanyl	100	0.04-0.08 mg/kg IM, SC, IV	2	Causes respiratory depression, auditory sensitization, decreased cardiac output, bradycardia; metabolized by liver
Nalorphine	0.8	11-22 mg/kg IM, SC, IV	2-3	Agonist/antagonist
Naloxone		0.04 mg/kg IM, SC, IV; may be repeated as necessary	2	Pure opiate antagonist; GABA-receptor antagonist

GABA, Gamma aminobutyric acid; *IM,* intramuscularly; *IV,* intravenously; *SC,* subcutaneously.
*Morphine is used as a standard of potency.

Table 20-6 NARCOTIC ANALGESICS USED IN CATS

Drug	Potency	Dose	Analgesic Duration (hr)	Comments
Morphine	1	0.1-0.5 mg/kg IM, SC	4	Overdose causes excitation; causes respiratory depression, emesis; elevates intraocular pressure; metabolized by liver
Oxymorphone/ hydromorphone	10	0.1 mg/kg IM, SC, IV	6	May cause ataxia; overdose causes excitation; causes respiratory depression, auditory hypersensitivity, altered thermoregulation; metabolized by liver
Butorphanol	5	0.4-0.8 mg/kg IM, SC, IV	2-4	Analgesia for visceral pain lasts longer than for somatic pain
Buprenorphine	25-50	0.005-0.02 mg/kg IM, SC, IV	6-12	Agonist/antagonist; prolonged (>30 min) time from administration to onset of action; long duration; difficult to reverse with naloxone
Naloxone		0.04 mg/kg IM, IV; may be repeated as necessary	2	Pure opiate antagonist; GABA-receptor antagonist

GABA, Gamma aminobutyric acid; *IM,* intramuscularly; *IV,* intravenously; *SC,* subcutaneously.
*Morphine is used as a standard of potency.

be divided into at least two categories: those with acute pain resulting from surgery and those experiencing chronic, low-grade pain, frequently of musculoskeletal origin. Patients experiencing acute pain generally benefit the most from short-term opioid analgesics. When anxiety, as demonstrated by excessive vocalization, is involved with acute pain, low doses of tranquilizers may be added to opioid analgesics.

Remember that tranquilizers alone have no analgesic effect. Patients with musculoskeletal pain often benefit from the use of one of the NSAIDs. When administering any of the NSAIDs, always be aware that they can cause gastric upset, vomiting, and ulceration. Patients with existing kidney disease may also experience a worsening of their condition when given NSAIDs.

Table 20-7 ANTIINFLAMMATORY DRUGS USED IN DOGS

Drug	Dose	Frequency (hr)	Comments
Aspirin	10-25 mg/kg PO	8	Induces gastric ulceration Decreases platelet aggregation
Phenylbutazone	10-25 mg/kg PO	8-12	May cause agranulocytosis Induces gastric ulceration
Carprofen	0.5 mg/kg PO	12	Induces gastric ulceration Hepatic toxicosis (idiosyncratic)
Flunixin meglumine	0.5-1.0 mg/kg IM, IV	24; 3-dose maximum	Induces gastric ulceration
Naproxen	3 mg/kg PO	24	Induces gastric ulceration
Meclofenamic acid	1.1 mg/kg PO	24	Induces gastric ulceration

IM, Intramuscularly; *IV,* intravenously; *PO,* orally.

Table 20-8 DRUG THAT PROVIDE VISCERAL ANALGESIA IN HORSES

Drug	Recommended Intravenous Dose (mg/kg)
NARCOTIC AGONISTS	
Morphine	0.02-0.04
Meperidine	0.2-0.4
Oxymorphone	0.01-0.02
MIXED AGONIST/ANTAGONISTS	
Butorphanol	0.02-0.05
Pentazocine	0.4-0.8
NONSTEROIDAL ANTIINFLAMMATORIES	
Ketoprofen	2
Flunixin meglumine	0.6-1.1
ALPHA$_2$ AGONISTS	
Xylazine	0.3-0.5
Detomidine	0.005-0.02

Table 20-9 ANTIINFLAMMATORY DRUGS USED IN HORSES

Drug	Recommended Dose (mg/kg)
Aspirin	15-100 PO, every 12 hr
Flunixin meglumine	0.25-1.1 PO, IM, IV, every 8-24 hr
Meclofenamic acid	2.2 PO, every 24 hr
Naproxen	10 PO, every 12 hr
Phenylbutazone	2-4 PO, every 12-24 hr
Sodium hyaluronate	10-40 mg/joint intraarticularly every 7 days
Polysulfated glycosaminoglycans	250 mg/joint intraarticularly every 7 days 500 mg IM every 5 days

IM, Intramuscularly; *IV,* intravenously; *PO,* orally.

TREATMENT OF PAIN IN HORSES

The relief of pain in horses with gastrointestinal or musculoskeletal pain is important both for the comfort of the patient and to minimize injury to attending personnel. Technical staff must be aware that analgesics may mask many important clinical signs, including heart and respiratory rates, which are used for monitoring colic patients or lameness associated with musculoskeletal injury. In both cases, worsening of the condition may occur in the face of improving clinical signs. Analgesic therapy should be tailored to each case based on a thorough knowledge of the potency, mechanism of action, and drug side effects.

ANALGESICS IN THE TREATMENT OF COLIC

Colic produces many behavioral and cardiovascular changes that are frequently used to assess the severity and prognosis of the disease. Pain associated with gastrointestinal injury is most frequently related to abdominal visceral distention, obstruction, and torsion, along with the release of inflammatory mediators, such as histamine, serotonin, kinins, prostaglandins, and leukotrienes. Severe colic can cause such extreme pain that both the horse and attending technical staff may be at risk of injury. NSAIDs, narcotics, and tranquilizers are all used to control pain associated with colic (Table 20-7). In experimental equine models, xylazine was found to produce the most pronounced visceral analgesia for the longest period of time.

TECHNICIAN NOTE

In experimental equine models, xylazine was found to produce the most pronounced visceral analgesia for the longest period of time.

Box 20-1 SUGGESTED POSTOPERATIVE ANALGESICS FOR DOGS AND CATS

ABDOMINAL SURGERY
Morphine
Butorphanol
Oxymorphone

Suggestions
- May add low doses of tranquilizers to opioids for additional sedation.
- Opioids cause respiratory depression and are metabolized slowly in patients with liver disease.

THORACIC SURGERY
Intercostal nerve block with bupivacaine
Intrapleural nerve block with bupivacaine
Morphine
Butorphanol
Oxymorphone

Suggestions
- Use low doses of opioids with local nerve blocks for additional pain control.
- May add low doses of tranquilizers for additional sedation.
- Opioids cause respiratory depression; use with caution in patients with respiratory disease.

OPHTHALMIC SURGERY
Butorphanol
Oxymorphone

Suggestion
- May add low doses of tranquilizers for additional sedation.

ORTHOPEDIC/NEUROSURGERY
Morphine
Butorphanol
Oxymorphone

Suggestions
- Butorphanol and morphine may not provide enough analgesia for severe postoperative pain.
- May add low doses of tranquilizers for additional sedation.
- By 24 hr after operation, NSAID may be tried in place of opioids; be alert for gastric ulceration.

NSAID, Nonsteroidal antiinflammatory drug.

Visceral analgesia is immediate in onset after xylazine administration. Xylazine causes sedation characterized by lethargy, drooping and extension of the neck, and ataxia. Heart and respiratory rates are significantly depressed. Xylazine also depresses intestinal motility, which may contribute to postoperative ileus. Butorphanol produces visceral analgesia and is second to xylazine in potency. The combination of xylazine (1.1 mg/kg intravenously) followed by butorphanol (0.1 mg/kg intravenously) produces excellent analgesia. Morphine, meperidine, and oxymorphone produce visceral analgesia that is highly variable and often inferior to that of xylazine and butorphanol. Flunixin meglumine is also recommended for alleviation of colic pain and is widely considered the best NSAID for this purpose. Flunixin is also effective in preventing the clinical signs of endotoxemia.

ANALGESICS FOR THE TREATMENT OF MUSCULOSKELETAL PAIN

NSAIDs are extremely useful in the treatment of musculoskeletal pain in the horse (Table 20-9). This group of drugs provides analgesia when inflammation contributes significantly to pain. Examples include acute laminitis, joint sprains, severe muscle and tendon injuries, and chronic degenerative joint disease. The NSAID used most frequently in the horse is phenylbutazone. Drug actions and side effects for the nonsteroidal group in horses are similar to those described for the dog and cat.

TECHNICIAN NOTE
The NSAID used most frequently in the horse to control musculoskeletal pain is phenylbutazone.

A miscellaneous group of agents used for modifying the disease process in degenerative joint disease includes sodium hyaluronate and polysulfated glycosaminoglycans. The mechanism of action of these drugs is variable, but all are aimed at returning the synovial joint to normal. Individual responses are variable and depend on the level of disease present. The intraarticular dose for hyaluronate is between 10 to 40 mg per joint. The dose may be repeated at weekly intervals. PS-GAGs are given at 250 mg per joint intraarticularly on a weekly basis. Alternatively, PS-GAGs may be given at 500 mg intramuscularly for 4 days for a total of seven treatments. The PS-GAGs have an advantage over hyaluronate in that they inhibit enzymes involved in cartilage degradation. Use of PS-GAGs is contraindicated in cases of infectious arthritis.

Recommended Reading

Carroll GL: *Small animal pain management,* Lakewood, Colo, 1998, AAHA Press.

MacPhail CM et al: Hepatocellular toxicosis associated with administration of carprofen in 21 dogs, *J Am Vet Med Assoc* 212:1895, 1998.

Mathews, K. Management of pain, *Vet Clin North Am Small Anim Pract* 30:4, 2000.

Sackman JE: Pain and its management, *Vet Clin North Am Small Anim Pract* 27:1487, 1997.

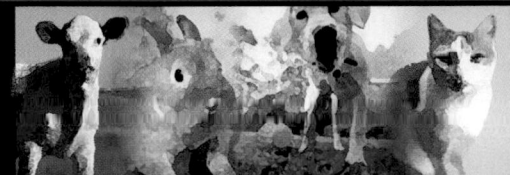

Pharmacology and Pharmacy

MARVENE AUGUSTUS • SONYA BREMER BOSS

INTRODUCTION

In most practices, the technician shares the responsibility of administering drugs, which may range from the simplest chewable tablet to a gaseous anesthetic. As new drugs and strategies are applied to veterinary care, the role of the technician becomes increasingly sophisticated. The technician must have some knowledge regarding mechanisms of drug actions, therapeutic uses, and potential side effects. Verification that the drug and dosage are correct is a major responsibility of the technician. For this reason the technician should be familiar with the dosage forms of drugs, able to recognize common medications, and translate drug dosages into the appropriate number of tablets or volume of drug for the individual patient. It is essential that the technician understand federal and state laws that regulate drug acquisition and distribution.

This chapter is intended to provide the technician with minimal knowledge of drug laws, inventory control, and calculation of dosages. Other chapters in this book will address drug classes with their pharmacology specifically. There are several good books written primarily to veterinary technicians dedicated entirely to the subject of drugs and should prove helpful for these with greater interest in veterinary therapeutics.

Controversial issues relating to the practice of pharmacy are briefly discussed in this chapter. ■

PHARMACOLOGY

GENERAL PRINCIPLES

DEFINITIONS

A *drug* is defined as any chemical agent that affects living processes. These agents may be used to prevent, diagnose,

or treat diseases. *Pharmacology* is a broad term defined as the study of drugs. Aspects of pharmacology include the history and source of drugs *(pharmacognosy)*; physical and chemical properties of drugs and effects and actions of drugs on living organisms *(pharmacodynamics)*; characteristic ability of living organisms to absorb, distribute, metabolize, and excrete drugs *(pharmacokinetics)*; therapeutic uses of drugs *(pharmacotherapeutics)*; and *toxicology*, the study of the symptoms, mechanisms, treatments, and detection of biological poisoning. Toxicology has a set of related terms itself that need to be defined in order to better understand the study of pharmacology.

Therapeutic drug monitoring deals with the proper timing of blood samples drawn to determine the serum concentration of a drug. This value must be compared to reported levels in consideration of the pharmacokinetics properties of the drug being measured.

Half-life is the time required for the serum concentration of a drug to decrease by 50%. It shows the intradose fluctuation of a drug and is useful in estimating the time a drug concentration should approach zero. Half-life is most helpful in determining optimal dosing schedules of oral agents and the time required to reach *steady state*.

Steady-state serum concentrations are values that recur with each dose and represent a state of equilibrium between the amount of drug administered and the amount being eliminated in a given time interval. It takes five half-lives to reach steady state after dose adminisitration has begun.

> ### TECHNICIAN NOTE
> *Steady state* is a state of equilibrium between the amounts of a drug administered and eliminated in a given time interval.

Peak serum concentration is the point of maximum concentration of drug on the time-versus-serum-concentration curve.

Trough serum concentration is the minimum drug serum concentration (Figure 21-1) during a given dosage interval.

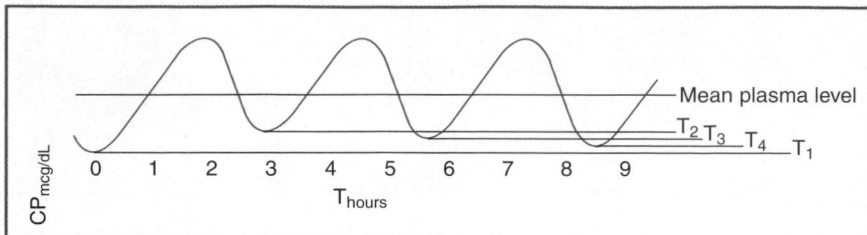

Figure 21-1 Illustration of trough levels after continuous doses of medications.

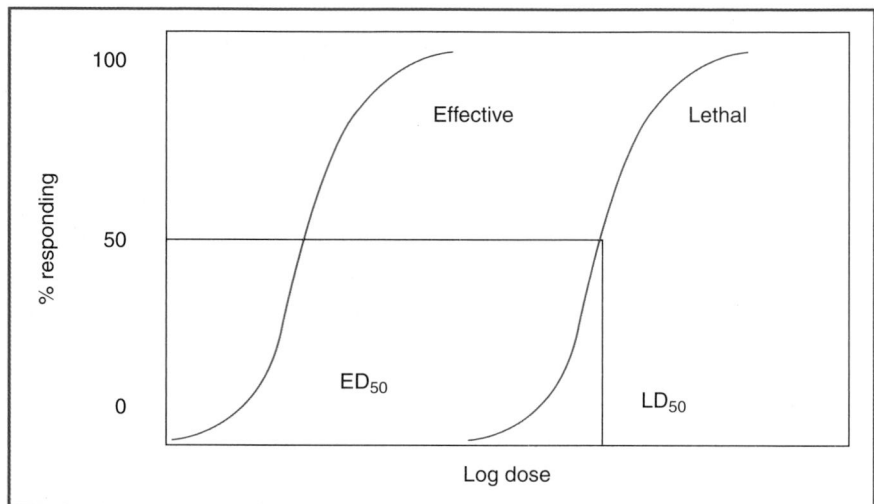

Figure 21-2 Illustration of toxic dose and therapeutic window.

Therapeutic window (range) is a range of a drug serum concentration associated with a high degree of efficacy and a low risk of undesired dose-related adverse reactions. Correct timing is important for sample collection. Steady-state concentrations should be achieved because low readings may cause premature and erroneous dose increases.

Toxic dose is a dose greater than the upper limit of the therapeutic range (Figure 21-2) that causes poisonous or toxic symptoms.

Therapeutic index is the ratio between the toxic dose and therapeutic dose of a drug used as a measure of the relative safety of the drug for a particular treatment. A drug that has a narrow therapeutic index may cause toxic results with small changes in doses. These drugs require constant monitoring so that the dose of drug can be adjusted as necessary to ensure uniform and safe results. These ranges should only be used as guides because there are differences among patients in the manner in which drugs are distributed and are available at the receptor site. Some patients may achieve adequate relief of symptoms before the drug level is within therapeutic range and may experience toxic symptoms when drug level is within the target range. Other patients may see toxic symptoms before adequate levels are achieved. Examples of drugs with narrow therapeutic windows are digoxin, theophylline, warfarin, phenobarbital, and levothyroxine.

LD_{50} is the dose of drug that kills 50% of the animals tested (LD = lethal dose). It is a standardized measure for expressing and comparing the toxicity of chemicals (Figure 21-2).

ED_{50} is the minimum dose of drug required to cause the desired effect in 50% of the test subjects.

PRINCIPLES RELATING TO DRUG ACTION

The pharmacokinetic factors of a drug are absorption, distribution, metabolism, and excretion (ADME). These factors determine how the drug enters the body, reaches the site of action, and is removed from the body.

> **✎ TECHNICIAN NOTE**
>
> Pharmacokinetic factors include absorption (how the drug enters the body), distribution (how the drug reaches the target tissue organs), metabolism (how the drug is chemically altered), and excretion (how the drug is removed from the body).

DRUG ABSORPTION

For drugs to exert an effect, they must reach their site of action *(target tissue)*. For some drugs, a simple topical application accomplishes this. Most drugs, however, must cross several barriers of cell membranes to produce the desired action. Cell membranes also must be crossed for the subsequent deactivation and elimination of the drug from the body. *Absorption* is defined as the uptake of substances into or across tissues.

Drugs with systemic actions that are administered orally must cross the gastrointestinal lining of the stomach or small intestine to be effective. Absorption of drugs from the gastrointestinal tract will be influenced by several factors. To pass through the membrane lining of the gastrointestinal tract, a drug must dissolve to some degree in oil (lipid soluble) because the membranes contain a high concentration of lipid (fat). Ionic (charged) forms of drugs do not easily pass through these membranes, whereas the nonionic forms of drugs pass more easily. Most drugs are weakly acidic or basic and have some lipid-soluble properties. The stomach is a highly acidic environment. The weakly basic drugs that are highly ionized (charged) in the acidic stomach will not be readily absorbed until they are farther down the digestive tract in the small intestine, because it is basic in nature. In the small intestine, the weakly basic drugs exist in an un-ionized form, which permits easier transport across the lipid membrane. Drugs that are weak acids are un-ionized in the acidic stomach diffuse more easily through the lipid membrane. They are rapidly absorbed from the stomach and therefore expected to exert their action more quickly than weakly basic drugs. Most drugs with poor lipid solubility cannot pass through cell membranes. Drugs such as the antimicrobial aminoglycosides (e.g., gentamicin) have poor lipid solubility and therefore are inadequately absorbed and ineffective after oral administration.

Stomach contents may inactivate or trap certain drugs. The volume of stomach contents also may delay absorption, thus delaying action. In ruminants, one is confronted not only with slow absorption from dilution but also with the effect of the action of the ruminal microorganisms on certain susceptible agents. Common drugs of plant origin, such as digoxin and atropine, are ineffective in the ruminant when administered orally because of digestive microorganisms.

Drugs that are administered by intradermal injection are deposited into the outer layer of the skin and are primarily used for diagnostic purposes, as in allergy and tuberculosis. The volume is less than 0.5 ml. The drug produces a local effect. Drugs that require injection *subcutaneously* or *intramuscularly* must be absorbed from the injection site to exert their action. The subcutaneous route is appropriate for small drug volumes (less than 1 ml) and drugs intended to be absorbed slowly. Because of limited blood flow, subcutaneous drug administration results in a more sporadic absorption compared with those drugs injected intramuscularly. Insulin and heparin are examples of drugs that are administered subcutaneously. In animals that are highly dehydrated, there is a restricted blood flow at body surfaces, so subcutaneous administration is not usually recommended.

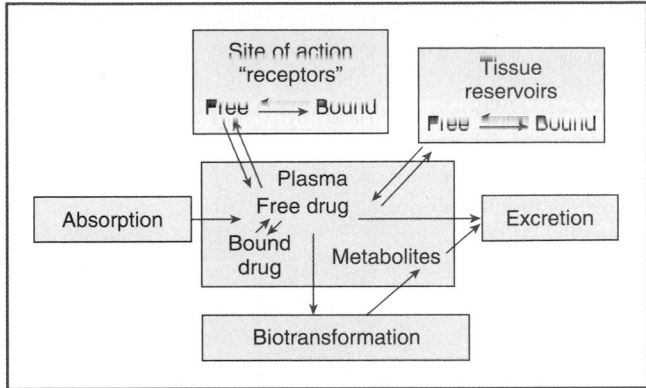

Figure 21-3 Schematic depicting fate of drug on administration.

Intramuscular injection is appropriate when a larger volume of drug must be administered. Absorption from the intramuscular site is faster than that from subcutaneous sites because muscles are better supplied with blood vessels than the skin.

Procaine penicillin is an example of a drug to be injected in the muscle.

Absorption from the subcutaneous or intramuscular site can be hastened by applying heat or massage to the site to accelerate blood flow. Applying ice packs at the injection site to decrease blood flow can slow absorption.

Drugs that are introduced into the vascular system (*intravenous*) will not go through an absorption phase. These drugs are placed directly into the plasma compartment and take effect immediately.

DRUG DISTRIBUTION

Drug distribution is the dispersion of the drug that is systemically available from the intravascular (within the vessels) space and the extravascular (outside the vessels) fluids and tissues to the target receptor sites.

Figure 21-3 depicts the distribution of drugs after administration. Drug concentration is a dynamic process that continually varies at different sites until it is virtually all excreted. Generally, another dose is administered before the complete removal of the previous dose, so the effective tissue levels (site of action) may be maintained. High lipid solubility and low protein binding are favorable characteristics indicative of the ability of a drug to diffuse through membranes. Drug transport into tissues involves passage through lipid-containing membranes. Diffusion is a difficult process for water-soluble compounds.

Most drugs in the bloodstream bind in varying degrees to plasma proteins such as albumin. Only the unbound drug *(free drug),* which may be as little as 10%, is available to diffuse into tissues and produce biologic effects. As a rule, drugs bound to albumin or other proteins remain in the blood because these proteins do not diffuse through capillary walls. Drug binding to albumin is a reversible process. Protein binding serves as a reservoir site because the drug becomes available as the plasma concentration of the free drug is reduced. Equilibrium is maintained at all times between protein-bound and free drug in the blood. A common form of drug interaction occurs when a second drug has a stronger affinity for the plasma protein. The first drug is replaced and becomes free to exert its effects in a greater concentration at its site of action.

Accumulation of drugs may occur in various body compartments, such as fat, muscle, and liver, prolonging the effects of the drug as it is released from these storage sites. The potential of a drug to accumulate at these different sites will vary greatly among drugs, depending on their physiochemical properties. For example, a highly lipid-soluble drug, such as thiopental, will accumulate in body fat. This accounts for the slow recovery of obese dogs from barbiturate anesthetics compared with leaner dogs, such as the greyhound.

Although all the aforementioned distribution sites of a drug are important, the amount of drug reaching its site of action is of primary concern. The place at which a drug interacts with cellular components to exert its effect is called a *receptor.* There are numerous sites throughout the body. Some sites are specific for certain drugs, whereas others are general and may respond or interact with several types of drugs.

> **TECHNICIAN NOTE**
>
> Receptor is the place in the body at which a drug exerts its effect.

The ability of a drug to bind to a specific receptor determines the biologic activity of the drug. The interaction of a drug with a specific receptor is similar to a lock-and-key fit (Figure 21-4). Only a certain critical portion of the drug is usually involved in binding with the receptor. Drugs that have similar critical portions but differ in other parts of the biologic molecule might be expected to have similar biologic activity.

A drug, in interacting with its receptor, may mimic the action of a natural body substance *(transmitter).* For example, acetylcholine is a natural transmitter that is secreted at terminal nerve endings, causing muscle contraction. A drug (bethanechol chloride) that is chemically similar to acetylcholine produces similar effects. Such drugs that directly produce the normal function of the receptor are termed *agonists.*

DRUG METABOLISM

For free drugs to be removed (cleared) from the blood, they must be excreted directly without change or metabolized *(biotransformed).* *Biotransformation* is the ability of a living organism to modify the chemical structure of drugs so that they are no longer active *(inactive metabolites).* The liver is the principal organ responsible for biotransformation, but some of the activity may occur in the kidneys, brain, lungs, small intestine, and other organs.

> **TECHNICIAN NOTE**
>
> The liver is the principle organ responsible for biotransformation.

Simple changes in the drug molecule, such as the removal or addition of certain atoms, may completely inactivate the drug. Through the mammalian enzyme system, potentially toxic compounds are changed into water-soluble compounds, which are more easily eliminated from the body by the kidneys. One means of removing many of the lipid-soluble drugs is through *conjugation.* This process involves

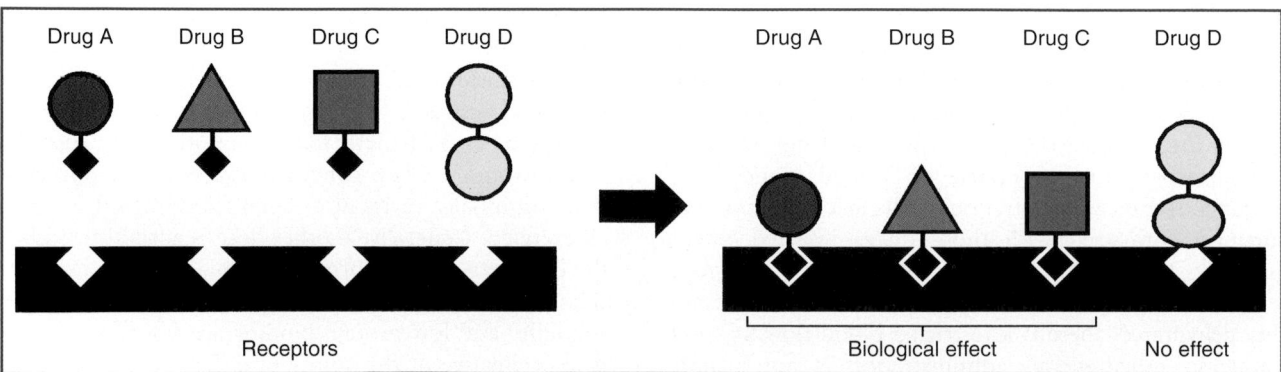

Figure 21-4 Lock-and-key fit between drugs and receptors through which they act.

the attachment of various endogenous substances to the drug. An example is the attachment of glucuronic acid to aspirin. After conjugation, the aspirin complex is much more water soluble, making it more readily excreted by the kidney. Cats are deficient in the enzymes required to conjugate drugs with glucuronic acid. This accounts for the relatively longer action of certain drugs in cats compared with most other mammalian species that do not have this deficiency.

Other common biotransformations of drugs by the liver include *hydroxylation* and *acetylation*. Biotransformation often inactivates drugs, but it does not always produce inactive products. Drugs such as codeine, diazepam, and amitriptyline are changed by the liver into metabolites that also exert a pharmacologic effect. These are called *active metabolites.*

In older animals or animals with hepatic disease, the ability of the liver to biotransform drugs may be impaired. Newborns less than 30 to 60 days of age are generally not capable of metabolizing many drugs because their liver enzyme system is not yet fully developed. To avoid drug toxicity, it might be necessary to reduce the drug dosage, increase the interval between doses, or switch to a drug that is not metabolized by the liver.

A few drugs are administered in an inactive form and do not become active until they are biotransformed by the liver; these are called *pro drugs* [i.e., angiotensin-converting enzyme (ACE) inhibitor *enalapril* must be converted by the liver to enalaprilat before it will exert any biologic activity].

Bacteria may carry out some biotransformation within the colon. This process may limit absorption of the drug from the bowel after oral administration, or it may help to eliminate drugs from the blood after parenteral administration.

EXCRETION

The kidneys eliminate (excrete) most drugs or their metabolites, although some may be removed via the bowel or lungs or in some other minor way in limited amounts. The removal of drugs from the blood by the kidney is somewhat complex and will vary from drug to drug. One route of elimination involves the liver and kidney. Biotransformation of drugs by the liver tends to form more polar compounds, which can be more efficiently excreted by the kidneys. For example, chloramphenicol is metabolized by the liver to chloramphenicol glucuronide. In this form the drug cannot be reabsorbed via the kidney tubules from the urine back into the blood and therefore is excreted in the urine.

The pH of the urine will also influence excretion of drugs. Urine pH is normally basic, so drugs that are weakly acidic will exist in the ionized state and be more readily excreted. The weakly basic drugs will be in an un-ionized state and more apt to be reabsorbed back from the urine. For example, the elimination of aspirin, a weak acid, is enhanced in more

basic urine. The reverse is true of weak bases in acidic urine. Ammonium chloride can be used to produce more acidic urine, and sodium bicarbonate can be used to produce basic urine.

> **TECHNICIAN NOTE**
>
> The pH of the urine will influence excretion of drugs.

Some drugs are not extensively metabolized by any organ in the body and are excreted unchanged in the urine. Some are excreted through passive diffusion into the glomerular fluid and are not reabsorbed to any significant degree and therefore enter the urine. Other drugs are actively secreted by specific systems in the renal tubules, which leads to more rapid drug elimination.

Drugs that are excreted by the kidney will accumulate in the body when there is a loss of kidney function. Creatinine (a natural waste product) levels in the blood are sometimes measured to determine the extent of renal damage so the dose of various drugs can be adjusted accordingly. Kidney function declines with age, even in the healthy animal. Elderly animals may show a reduced ability to excrete drugs in their urine. Certain drugs, such as the aminoglycosides, may directly damage the kidney (nephrotoxicity) and ultimately interfere with their own excretion.

> **TECHNICIAN NOTE**
>
> Loss of kidney function causes drugs to accumulate in the body if the drug is excreted by the kidney.

Another route of drug excretion involves uptake by the liver, release into the bile, and elimination in the feces. Drugs in the bile enter the small intestine, in which they may be reabsorbed into the blood, returned to the liver, and secreted again into the bile. This process is called *enterohepatic circulation.* The drugs that are reabsorbed and resecreted will persist in the body much longer than the drugs that remain in the lumen of the intestine and pass out with the feces.

DOSAGE FORMS

To administer drugs through the various routes, manufacturers have produced products in different formulations to accomplish the desired effect. For oral administration, there are not only traditional tablets and capsules but also chewable, flavored tablets to encourage animal acceptance and ease in owner administration. Care must be taken in dogs and cats with food allergies when considering the use of chewable flavor tablets. Many tablets are beef-based and can cause adverse drug reactions in animals allergic to beef. Because of an undesirable flavor or high alcohol content, animals may not readily receive oral liquids developed for human use. Liquids specifically flavored and designed for dogs, cats, and exotics reduce stress for both client and patient during administration. Some cats are very hard to administer drugs orally. Compounding pharmacists can incorporate the drug into a gel that is placed on the outer or inner ear or a place with the least amount of hair. The advantages of using this dosage form are good absorption, high serum blood levels, and avoidance of the hepatic first-bypass effect. The two drugs that are currently available for this dosage form are methimazole and amitriptyline.

Equine owners often cannot administer many drugs to horses orally due to a disagreeable taste or odor and amount to administer. Some crushed tablets and powders can be mixed with molasses or other suitable compounds and then mixed with the animal's grain ration. Veterinary drug manufacturers have formulated granules and pellets for ease in oral administration. Oral paste forms, though somewhat more expensive, have gained popularity because of convenience to the owner and receptiveness of the animal.

Injectable drugs are frequently available in solutions or suspensions ready for use. Special buffers to maintain pH or absence of oxygen are required because of the instability of some components. Instability of some drugs may require a dry lyophilized powder be mixed with a diluent *(reconstituted)* such as sterile water or saline just prior to use.

Some vials of drugs in solution are designed for "single use only" because the preparation may not have a preservative or the drug is highly susceptible to oxygen in the air. Certain vaccines or intravenous products may advise on their labeling that unused portions be discarded.

A variety of other dosage forms exist for use in veterinary medicine, such as ophthalmic ointments, solutions, or suspensions; topical sprays, cream, ointments, and lotions; and otic drops. Most are designed for a local effect, although occasionally there may be sufficient absorption from the application site to produce some systemic side effect. Another dosage form that is gaining popularity is the transdermal patch. It is designed for local application to produce systemic results. *Duragesic* (Fentanyl) patches were introduced to veterinary medicine to control postsurgery pain. Compounding pharmacists are able to make a transdermal patch for any drug except antibiotics. The molecules of the antibiotics are too large and will not pass through the lipid biolayer.

TECHNICIAN NOTE

A transdermal patch is designed to apply topically but produce systemic results.

Intrauterine administration of some antibacterials is not uncommon in mares, cows, and other breeding stock. Antibiotics are also formulated for intramammary infusion for milk-producing animals. Some of these products are used to prevent (prophylactic) infections at the end of the milking period only. These agents are designated for use in dry cows and usually have a longer duration of action. Other mastitis preparations are for use in lactating cows to treat an infection during the milking period and for a time after the last treatment. The withdrawal time (usually 36 to 72 hours) will vary with the drug and formulation and is stated on the product label.

ROUTES OF ADMINISTRATION

Several methods are available for administering drugs to animals (Chapter 3). Each route of administration has advantages and disadvantages. The route selected will depend on a number of factors, including the patient's size, disease state, temperament, and unique species characteristics; the characteristics and commercial formulation of the drug; and the expertise and knowledge of the individual administering the drug. The cost of drugs should be a factor in the selection of a route of administration when all other clinical factors have been considered.

ORAL ADMINISTRATION

Oral administration is one of the most convenient methods used by clients and animal health personnel for giving drugs. Tablets and capsules are fairly economical and provide accurate and uniform doses. Oral liquids offer some convenience, but the amount of active ingredient administered may vary from dose to dose, depending on measurement or the animal's acceptance. Administration of oral liquids by force in cats usually results in an undesirable salivary gag reflex episode. Oral paste forms for horses and food-producing animals have gained popularity because of their ease in administration. The acceptance of oral granules and powders, although variable among animals, offers convenience for administering doses to larger species. Drugs formulated for mixing in the animal's drinking water are least desirable because water consumption is highly variable and unpredictable. However, when dealing with large numbers of sick animals in flocks or herd, the use of water mixes may be the only economic and feasible method of treatment. For small birds, medicated drinking water is sometimes used to avoid the stress that occurs with other methods.

Absorption of drugs administered orally depends on a number of factors. Even when accurate doses are give, the actual amount of drug absorbed may vary, altering the expected therapeutic response. Most medications that can be administered orally can also be administered via feeding tube. It is preferred to give liquids by tube; however, some solid medications can be finely crushed and mixed with sufficient liquid to ensure complete passage of the drug into the stomach. Before administration of any drug via tube, make sure the tube is correctly placed.

PARENTERAL ADMINISTRATION

Parenteral administration of drugs is usually accomplished by subcutaneous, intramuscular, intradermal (Figure 21-5),

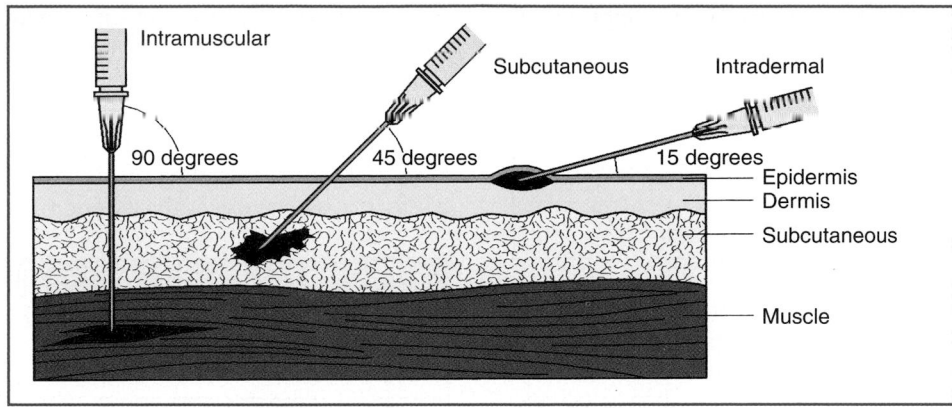

Figure 21-5 Comparison of angle of injection and location of medication deposit for IM, SC, and ID injections.

or intravenous injections. Parenteral administration of drugs requires sterile technique to reduce the possibility of introducing infection into the animal. (See Chapter 3.)

An *intradermal injection* is made just below the outer layer of skin *(epidermis)*. This route of administration is used for allergy testing and giving local anesthetics. The volume of drug injected is small, usually less than 0.5 ml.

Subcutaneous injections are common in veterinary medicine because they are less painful to the animal and are easily administered. Some drugs cannot be given in this way because tissue irritation or sloughing may occur. Many vaccines are given subcutaneously, but some require intramuscular injection to produce the desired immune response.

Increased risks are inherent in the intramuscular administration of drugs. One must ensure the drug will not be injected into a vein or an artery by accident. The potential also exists for injecting the drug in or near a major nerve fiver, which could cause paralysis. One must have knowledge of the location of major nerves to avoid accidental damage.

When giving drugs subcutaneously or intramuscularly, only a limited amount can be administered at the injection site. Multiple sites may be used for some preparations, but the absorption may be more erratic.

The absorption from an intramuscular or a subcutaneous injection site is primarily through simple diffusion. A number of factors will influence the rate of diffusion from the site. Of primary importance is capillary circulation in the area. Because circulation is limited at subcutaneous sites, compared with intramuscular sites, one would expect a lower absorption and longer action for drugs given subcutaneously.

Label directions should be followed regarding route of administration when administering drugs by injection. There may be a few exceptions for preparations where sufficient experience exists for administration by routes other than those stated on the label. In most cases, however, there is a definite reason why the recommended route is stated. For example, antibiotics given by subcutaneous injection may not produce adequate blood levels to destroy microorganisms.

For intravenous administration, one must not only know the location of the larger veins that are used but also possess some skill in placement of the needle or catheter within these blood vessels. An immediate effect can be obtained from drugs administered intravenously without the delay of absorption encountered with other administrative routes. This route may also be used when larger volumes are required. Even certain irritating compounds can be given intravenously if they are given slowly, allowing adequate blood dilution.

Although intravenous administration has advantages, it also has risks. Highly irritating drugs, such as *phenylbutazone, sodium thiopental,* and *triple sulfa,* can severely damage blood vessels and surrounding tissue if injected outside the vein *(perivascularly).* Injecting certain drugs too rapidly may lead to untoward effects, including circulatory collapse and death. Some drugs may irritate vein walls, stimulate vasoconstriction, and raise the pressure inside a blood vessel until it ruptures. Drugs that leave the vein and leak into the soft tissue that surrounds the vein and cause tissue damage are *vesicants.* The leakage of intravenous drugs from the vein into the surrounding tissue is called *extravasation.* Once extravasation has occurred, damage can continue for months and involve nerves, tendons, and joints. It may cause full thickness skin loss above the area of injury and may require skin grafting. Delayed treatment to the area may result in surgical debridement, skin grafting, and even amputation. Injury from extravasation can occur with any medication that is highly acid, basic, or cytotoxic or has a high osmolarity. Drug items noted for extravasation are cytotoxic agents (cancer drugs), intravenous nutrition, and solutions of calcium, potassium, bicarbonate, and 10% dextrose.

In order to avoid extravasation, great care must be taken to assure the veins are intact with a good blood flow since drugs may leak from sites of previous or recent punctures or occluded veins. Insertion site should not be distal to a recent venipuncture or an extremity with compromised circulation.

The first line of treatment is to remove as much of the offending fluid as possible. One method reported has been to dilute the infiltrated fluid with saline. Small surgical incisions are made around the area and then suctioned with a *liposuction device*. Application of dimethyl sulfonate (DMSO) has been used topically on the area to reduce inflammation. Hyaluronidase has been used with great success because it can work for a wide variety of fluids. It is injected into the area via a catheter or using small injections. An enzyme degrades hyaluronic acid (involved with the inflammatory process) and then enhances absorption of the extravasated fluid.

To treat tissue damage in most injuries, regular assessment of the site is all that is necessary. To facilitate healing to injuries leading to necrosis, use the following wound care principles:

1. *Remove* necrotic tissue.
2. *Eradicate* infection.
3. *Absorb* excess exudates.
4. *Obliterate* damaged space.
5. *Maintain* a moist wound surface.
6. *Insulate* the wound.
7. *Protect* the wound from further trauma or bacteria.

NEUROPHARMACOLOGY

Many different classes of drugs affect the nervous system, even though they are used for a variety of therapeutic uses. Some drugs will cause a direct effect, and others will alter functions of the nervous system as a side effect. The *central nervous system* (CNS) includes the brain and spinal cord. Its function is to monitor, convey, and process signals from receptors throughout the body.

Neurons (nerve cells) relay information from the CNS to the rest of the body. They use neurotransmitters (NTs) to contact neurons and other cells. A *neurotransmitter*, a chemical substance released from the axon terminal of a presynaptic neuron or excitation *(stimulation)*, diffuses across the synaptic cleft to either excite or inhibit the target cell *(receptor)*. Most neurons make only one kind of NT. The receptor recognizes only one specific NT and initiates a cellular response to it. The binding of the NT to its receptor is reversible. The stimulation of the cell is terminated when the NT is degraded or removed away from the receptor.

The nervous system is divided according to general function. The two primary divisions of the CNS are the *autonomic*

nervous system, or involuntary system, and the *somatic* (motor) *nervous system,* or voluntary system. The somatic system initiates muscle contraction by both conscious and unconscious control. The autonomic system innervates involuntary activities of the body. Although both systems have efferent fibers leading from the CNS, the focus of this discussion is on those of the autonomic nervous system.

AUTONOMIC NERVOUS SYSTEM

The role of the autonomic nervous system is to monitor and control internal body functions, such as digestive processes, blood volume, cardiac output, and kidney function.

For impulse transmission to occur between nerves or between nerves and effector site (e.g., muscles, glands, organs) a small amount of NT must be released by the efferent nerve (Figure 21-6). Two major NTs exist in mammals: *acetylcholine* (Ach) and *norepinephrine* (NE). Ach is released into the synapse. Ach that diffuses into opposing membranes is degraded into acetate and choline by the membrane-bound enzyme acetylcholinesterase. Ach that diffuses into the blood is degraded by nonspecific cholinesterase in the blood and tissues. Enzymes deactivate NE, but *reuptake* of NE by the nerve that released it occurs as well, and the NT is again stored in the granules.

The autonomic nervous system is subdivided into the *sympathetic* and *parasympathetic* nervous systems. Both

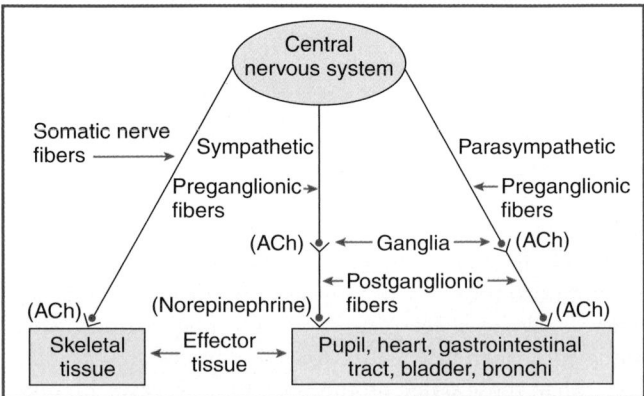

Figure 21-6 Schematic of efferent fibers showing sites of neurohumoral transmitters.

divisions commonly act on a given organ, but they produce opposite responses. NE is the predominant NT in the sympathetic system, and Ach is the principal NT of the parasympathetic system. Ach is also the transmitter substance found at the ganglia and at the neuromuscular junction in the somatic nervous system.

Within the sympathetic nervous system, at least three different types of receptors exist (alpha, beta$_1$, and beta$_2$), with others being postulated. All theses receptors may be found within the same effector tissue, and response to the transmitter will therefore vary, depending in large part on the type of receptor that is predominant at the site as well as on the amount of transmitter substance present. The general responses of various effector tissues to normal sympathetic and parasympathetic stimulation are listed in Table 21-1. This antagonism allows full control of organ function according to body requirements. It should be noted that sympathetic response is a *fight-or-flight* response in that the animal's heart rate increases, bronchioles are dilated for better ventilation, and blood vessels to the heart and skeletal muscle dilate to increase blood supply. In the parasympathetic response the heart rate slows, bronchioles constrict to restrict airways, and blood vessels constrict in the heart and skeletal muscle.

Drugs affecting the autonomic nervous system may mimic or block all or selected effects of the NT, or they may alter the synthesis, storage, release or degradation, and uptake of the transmitter. The classification of these drugs is difficult, not only because there are so many different types of action possible but also because most drugs possess more than one specific action. Drugs are generally classified based on their primary or predominant action.

Cholinomimetic (cholinergic or parasympathomimetic) *agents* are drugs that mimic the stimulatory effects of Ach. Cholinomimetic drugs can be further divided into muscarinic and nicotinic agents. Receptor sites that are found to be postganglionic in the effector tissue may be stimulated by a naturally occurring alkaloid, *muscarine*. Most other Ach receptor sites, including end plates of muscle, may be stimulated by *nicotine*. *Anticholinergic* (cholinergic blocking or parasympatholytic) *agents* are those that are capable of blocking Ach effects. They can also be subdivided according to the site or sites blocked.

Sympathomimetic (adrenergic) *agents* and *sympatholytic* (adrenergic blocking) *agents* are those drugs that mimic or block, respectively, the effects of NE. These agents also are further classified by the particular receptor that they stimulate or block.

AUTONOMIC DRUGS

Cholinomimetic Agents

Ach is not effective systemically as a drug because it is rapidly hydrolyzed by the enzyme acetylcholinesterase at the receptor site. Only an Ach ophthalmic formulation is available for immediate constriction of the pupil during eye surgery.

Bethanechol is similar in structure to Ach and mimics much of its pharmacologic action. Bethanechol is sufficiently different from Ach in that it can resist hydrolysis by the cholinesterase enzymes; therefore it is a fairly long-acting drug. It is used as a smooth muscle stimulant. When given orally, indications for bethanechol use include gastric atony or stasis and urinary retention when there is no obstruction.

Adverse reactions to bethanechol in small animals are mild and may include vomiting, diarrhea, salivation, and anorexia. Arrhythmias, hypotension, and asthma are most likely to occur in overdosage.

Several drugs are able to bind with the cholinesterase enzyme, preventing it from breaking down Ach. This not only allows Ach to act longer but also creates increased concentration, resulting in exaggerated effects. Theses agents are toxic (some related compounds were used as nerve gases in World War II), and their therapeutic usefulness is limited to a few unique medical problems. In veterinary medicine, the use of cholinesterase inhibitors is primarily for treatment of parasites—both internal and external.

Cholinesterase inhibitors (anticholinesterases) are divided into three groups on the basis of reversibility: truly reversible (short acting, 5 minutes), edrophonium chloride; reversible (long acting, 30 minutes to 4 hours), physostigmine, pyridostigmine, and neostigmine; and irreversible, organophosphates and echothiophate iodide.

Table 21-1 PARTIAL LISTING OF GENERAL RESPONSES SEEN AT EFFECTOR SITES

Effector Tissue	Sympathetic Stimulation (Dominant Receptor Type)	Parasympathetic Stimulation
Pupil	Dilated	Constricted
Glands		
Salivary	Scanty viscous secretion	Copious secretion (watery)
Gastrointestinal tract	—	Increased
Bronchioles	Dilated	Constricted
Heart		
Rate	Accelerated	Slowed
Contractile force	Increased	Decreased
Blood vessels		
Muscle (skeletal)	Dilated	—
Heart	Dilated	—
Skin	Constricted	Dilated
Gastrointestinal tract		
Muscle wall	↓ Peristalsis and tone	↑ Peristalsis and tone
Sphincter	↑ Tone	↓ Tone
Urinary bladder		
Wall	Relaxed	Contracted
Sphincter	Contracted	Relaxed

Edrophonium chloride is a drug used to diagnose myasthenia gravis, a disease of the nerves and muscles that is characterized by weakness and marked fatigue of skeletal muscles. Edrophonium chloride induces an immediate improvement, although it is of very short duration. The longer-acting agents *physostigmine, pyridostigmine*, and *neostigmine* are used to treat the disease in humans. Myasthenia gravis is a disease with a poor prognosis. It is a condition that is very expensive to treat; therefore treatment is rare in veterinary medicine.

A common veterinary use of injectable neostigmine is in the treatment of ruminal atony or gut stasis. Neostigmine is relatively short acting (2 to 4 hours), but its stimulatory effects may be beneficial in returning the rumen and gastrointestinal tract to normal peristaltic activity after surgery. This agent is sometimes employed to treat urinary retention because of its stimulatory effects on smooth muscle in the urinary bladder.

Neostigmine and physostigmine can also be used to treat atropine intoxication and to reverse the affects of certain neuromuscular blocking agents (e.g., tubocurarine, gallamine, pancuronium) used during surgery.

> **✎ TECHNICIAN NOTE**
> Neostigmine and physostigmine can be used to treat atropine intoxication.

Symptoms of overdose of the anticholinesterase agents include gastrointestinal effects (nausea, vomiting, diarrhea), salivation, sweating, respiratory effects (increased bronchial secretions, bronchospasms, pulmonary edema), ophthalmic effects (miosis, blurred vision, lacrimation), cardiovascular effects (bradycardia or tachycardia, hypotension, cardiac arrest), muscle cramps, and weakness.

Other cholinesterase inhibitors are available only as ophthalmic preparations to treat glaucoma. Glaucoma is a disease complex that is characterized chiefly by a increase in intraocular pressure that may lead to blindness if left untreated. The anticholinesterase agents reduce the intraocular pressure by lowering the resistance to outflow of the aqueous humor.

Anticholinergics

As mentioned previously, nicotinic receptors are predominantly at the end plates of skeletal muscle and autonomic ganglia. Muscarinic receptors are predominant in smooth muscle, heart, and glands. Some drugs have the capability of stimulating both types of receptors to varying degrees, whereas other drugs are capable of blocking both sites in varying degrees. Furthermore, some drugs may block the nicotinic effects at the skeletal muscle and not at the autonomic ganglia.

Drugs that inhibit the action of Ach at the muscarinic sites (antimuscarinic drugs) are used widely in veterinary medicine; the most popular drug in this class is atropine. Atropine is a belladonna alkaloid found in nature and commonly incriminated in plant poisoning. Other belladonna alkaloids, such as homatropine and scopolamine, are commercially available and have a slight difference in action.

Because anticholinergic drugs exhibit their usefulness in inhibiting the action of Ach by competing at a number of sites, their potential for correcting a disorder or altering a response is significant. One can rarely choose a single site for the therapeutic action without concomitant side effects occurring at other muscarinic sites. There have been numerous compounds synthesized in attempts to reduce certain unwanted actions and enhance desired effects. The success of such efforts has been limited, depending somewhat on the unique response of the individual patient.

The significant responses that are seen with therapeutic doses of atropine and related drugs are nearly the opposite of parasympathetic stimulation (Table 21-1). The pharmacologic effects of atropine are dose related. Low doses will produce decreased salivation and bronchial secretions. Dilation of the pupil and increased intraocular pressure and heart rate are experienced with moderate systemic doses. High doses decrease motility and tone of the gastrointestinal and urinary tracts.

The antimuscarinic drugs are frequently used before and during surgery in small animals to reduce or prevent secretions of the respiratory tract and to reduce bradycardia (decreased heart rate). Atropine and its analogs have been used in combination with other drugs to treat diarrhea (see later discussion of antidiarrheal agents).

Atropine is indicated in eye examinations and some ophthalmic surgery in which dilation of the pupil is desired. Atropine is long acting; therefore some of the shorter-acting mydriatics (dilating agents), such as tropicamide, are used. One of the most important uses of antimuscarinic drugs is to block spasms of the small ciliary eye muscles, thereby alleviating the associated pain.

Another significant use of atropine is as an antidote for organophosphates and other anticholinesterases found in many insecticides or parasiticides. Muscarine toxicity from poisonous mushrooms is also treated with atropine.

> **✎ TECHNICIAN NOTE**
> Atropine is an antidote for organophosphates and other anticholinesterases. It is contraindicated in the horse except for life-threatening organophosphate toxicity.

Atropine must be used with caution because of potential side effects, which are merely extensions of the pharmacologic effects. Some clinicians believe atropine is contraindicated in the horse except for life-threatening organophosphate toxicity because the decreased peristaltic activity in the lengthy gut of the horse leads to gas and toxin complications. Atropine can increase ocular pressure and is therefore contraindicated in the treatment of animals with certain types of glaucoma.

Neuromuscular Blockers

Neuromuscular blockers (NMBs) act at the junction of the nerve and skeletal muscle to paralyze skeletal muscle. These compounds are classified according to their onset and duration of action. Older agents, such as, d-*tubocurarine*, *succinylcholine, gallamine*, and *pancuronium* are still available commercially. Newer agents like *vecuronium* and *atracurium* are widely used in veterinary medicine.

Some NMBs have been used in darts to capture animals, but their use is dangerous because respiratory paralysis occurs. The main clinical use of NMBs is as an adjuvant in surgical anesthesia to obtain relaxation of skeletal muscle, particularly of the abdominal wall, and in orthopedic surgery. These agents are selectively used in veterinary medicine. Guaifenesin, another type of muscle relaxant, is commonly used in equine and bovine surgery to selectively depress transmission of nerve impulses at the internuncial neurons of the spinal cord, brainstem, and subcortical regions of the brain. Symptoms of NMB overdose include increased risks of hypotension, histamine release, and prolonged muscle blockade.

Sympathomimetics

The sympathetic nervous system is extensively involved in regulating a number of body functions, including heart rate, blood pressure, bronchial airway tone, body temperature, carbohydrate and fatty acid metabolism, and appetite. Although NE is the primary transmitter substance, epinephrine is released from the adrenal gland when an animal is stressed through physical, psychological, or other stimulatory means.

> ### ✎ TECHNICIAN NOTE
> Epinephrine is released from the adrenal gland when an animal is stressed.

Because the NE molecule can be modified extensively and still possess some type of stimulatory properties, numerous agents are commercially available. Manufacturers seek a molecule that produces a desired response and eliminates or reduces all the other adrenergic effects. NE possesses only alpha effects and has limited therapeutic use in the treatment of certain hypotensive shock conditions.

Epinephrine has several therapeutic applications in veterinary medicine, although the actual frequency of use is limited. Clinical applications include the following:

- Allergic reactions (often lifesaving in the face of shock)
- Bronchospasm (provides rapid relief)
- Cardiac effects (sometimes used in specific heart disorders)
- Local hemostasis [may be used in dilute solution (1:100,000 to 1:20,000) to control surgical bleeding in highly vascular tissue]
- Prolongation of the effects of local anesthetics (even though there may be undesirable systemic effects from epinephrine if overused)

Isoproterenol, which has few alpha effects but powerful beta effects, is useful as a bronchodilator in respiratory disorders and as a cardiac stimulant in certain heart conditions. Isoproterenol is available in many preparations for humans that are designed for inhalation use or as tablets for under the tongue *(sublingual)*. Only the short-acting injectable form has application in veterinary medicine.

Epinephrine and NE are not available in oral forms because both are destroyed by stomach acid. In addition, both drugs are relatively short acting when given by injection. Epinephrine and phenylephrine hydrochloride are also commercially available as ophthalmic preparations. They cause the pupil to dilate, but unlike atropine, they directly stimulate those muscles of the eye controlled by sympathetic nerves. This mydriatic effect is useful in selected cases of glaucoma as well as in ophthalmic examinations.

Symptoms of toxicity include arrhythmias, pulmonary edema, dyspnea, vomiting, headache, and sharp rises in systolic, diastolic, and venous blood pressures.

Sympatholytics

Many chemicals interfere with the function of the sympathetic nervous system. Some agents act by interfering with the synthesis, storage, and release of the transmitter substance. Others interfere with the ability of receptors to interact effectively with NTs. Some blocking agents are specific in their action; for example, prazosin hydrochloride is specific in blocking the alpha receptors. Other agents (e.g., the phenothiazine tranquilizers, such as *acepromazine*) are nonselective in activity, blocking alpha and beta$_1$ receptors. (See Chapter 19 on information about preoperative drugs and drugs used in anesthetic emergencies.)

Alpha-Adrenergic and Beta-Adrenergic Blocking Agents

The alpha-adrenergic blocking agents, as phenoxybenzamine, prazosin, and hydralazine cause vasodilation and are used mainly in animals for lowering blood pressure or improving blood flow in certain vascular diseases.

Phentolamine, an expensive, injectable alpha blocker, is used to diagnose adrenal gland tumors and during surgery to control abnormally high blood pressure. Adverse effects seen with use of alpha$_1$-adrenergic blocking agents include first-dose syncope, transient lethargy and dizziness, nausea, vomiting, diarrhea, and constipation.

> ### ✎ TECHNICIAN NOTE
> Phentolamine is used to diagnose adrenal gland tumors and during surgery to control abnormally high blood pressure.

Beta-adrenergic blocking agents, such as propranolol and atenolol, are therapeutically useful as antihypertensive agents and in the treatment of certain heart arrhythmias.

Betaxolol and timolol are two beta-adrenergic blocking agents that are widely used in veterinary ophthalmology.

After topical application to the eye, each reduces both elevated and normal intraocular pressure with or without glaucoma. Overuse of beta-adrenergic blocking agents results in symptoms of hypotension, bradycardia, bronchospasm, depressed consciousness to seizures, hypoglycemia, respiratory depression, and atrioventricular block.

Tranquilizers

Tranquilizers are drugs that act on the CNS to produce a calmness of mind or detached serenity without loss of consciousness or marked depression. Their use in veterinary medicine is to modify the behavior of the animal to make it more manageable or less responsive to external stimulation.

Phenothiazines

Phenothiazine was originally used in veterinary medicine as an anthelmintic. Derivatives of the drug (chlorpromazine and acepromazine) have been synthesized to enhance the sedative effects of phenothiazine. Some of the derivatives are used as antihypertensive agents because they exhibit peripheral alpha-adrenergic blocking activity and cause vasodilation. The exact mechanism of action for sedation is unknown, but phenothiazines block postsynaptic dopamine receptors. These drugs have found usefulness as antihistamines, antiemetics, and anti–motion sickness agents.

The phenothiazine tranquilizers are used as preanesthetics by "taking the edge off" the animal and enhancing or prolonging the effects of certain anesthetics. Some side effects to be aware of when administering the phenothiazines include a drop in blood pressure, paralysis of the retractor penis muscle in horses, and lowering of the seizure threshold in dogs.

> ### ✎ TECHNICIAN NOTE
> Phenothiazine tranquilizers are used to "take the edge off" the animal and to enhance the effects of some anesthetics.

Alpha₂ Agonists

Although xylazine, detomidine, and medetomidine in the strictest sense may not be classified as tranquilizers, their sedative and analgesic properties are useful for chemical restraint, especially in the horse. Detomidine is approved for use only in the horse and has little application in other species. It appears to differ slightly from xylazine by producing greater analgesia and sedation. Although it is dose dependent, the duration of action of detomidine is longer than xylazine.

Both xylazine and detomidine are commonly used in combination with other sedatives, tranquilizers, and anesthetic agents. The effects of these drugs in combination are greatly potentiated and must be used with caution. Common side effects seen in the horse include muscle tremors, partial A-V block, bradycardia, respiratory changes, sweating, penile prolapse, increased intracranial pressure, or decreased mucociliary clearance.

Xylazine is used widely in cattle, although the U.S. Food and Drug Administration (FDA) has not currently approved it for use in food-producing animals. The popularity in ruminants results from its excellent anesthetic properties. Ruminants are sensitive to xylazine, requiring approximately one tenth the dose (based on body weight) used in horses. Adverse effects in cattle include ruminal atony, intestinal stasis, salivation, hypothermia, diarrhea, bloating, ataxia, and regurgitation with aspiration pneumonia.

Although xylazine is approved for the management of hyperexcitable behavior in the cat and dog, it is not widely used in these species. Vomiting is a common side effect seen in the dog and frequently in the cat soon after administration. A single episode usually occurs, but the use of antiemetics may delay this phenomenon. Xylazine is frequently used as an emetic when an emetic effect is desired (e.g., emptying stomach before surgery). Gaseous extension with use may occur in dogs making radiographic interpretation difficult. Movement in response to sharp auditory stimuli may be observed. Increased urination may occur in cats following the use of xylazine.

Yohimbine is an alpha₂-adrenergic receptor antagonist that competitively blocks and antagonizes CNS depression or sedation and the bradycardia and respiratory depression caused by xylazine.

Antipamezole hydrochloride, a synthetic alpha₂-adrenergic antagonist, reverses the effects of medetomidine hydrochloride in dogs.

The use of propofol in veterinary medicine for induction in high-risk patients, such as those with compromised organ systems, is rapidly gaining popularity. It is used mainly for sedation/relaxation of 5 to 10 minutes in duration because it is rapidly metabolized. Because propofol can cause respiratory depression, its use should be restricted to situations where controlled intubation is available. Propofol may cause increased vasodilation and negative inotropy (weakening the force of muscular contraction) when used in conjunction with preanesthetic agents, such as acepromazine or opiates. Animals with preexisting cardiopulmonary disease, in shock, or suffering from trauma should be of particular concern. Propofol-induced bradycardia may be exacerbated in animals receiving opiate premedication especially when anticholinergic agents are not given concurrently.

Drugs that inhibit the hepatic P-450 enzyme system and other basic lipophilic drugs may increase recovery times associated with propofol. Cats with liver disease as a preexisting condition may be susceptible to longer recovery time.

> ### ✎ TECHNICIAN NOTE
> Propofol is useful for induction in high-risk patients. It should be used in situations with controlled intubation because of its ability to cause respiratory depression.

Anticonvulsants

Of the several different causes of seizures (convulsions) in dogs, only about two thirds can be controlled by the various anticonvulsant drugs. Benzodiazepine derivatives may be the most popular injectable drug for use during seizures or in other emergency situations. This benzodiazepine agent depresses the subcortical levels of the CNS, thus exhibiting sedative, skeletal muscle relaxant, and anticonvulsant properties. Diazepam is relatively short acting (30 minutes to $2^1/_2$ hours). Phenobarbital sodium is also available for injection when a longer effect (4 to 6 hours) is required.

Midazolam, an imidazobenzodiazepine, exhibits similar pharmacologic actions as other drugs in its class. The unique characteristic of being lipid soluble at body pH gives it a very rapid onset of action after injection. It can be used as a premedication before surgery alone or in combination. When combined with potent analgesic/anesthetic drugs like ketamine or fentanyl, midazolam produces conscious sedation. Intracarotid artery injections must be avoided. Midazolam should be used very cautiously in animals that are comatose, in shock, or have significant respiratory depression. Use in the first trimester of pregnancy should only occur when the benefits clearly outweigh the risks associated with the use. This drug should be used in an inpatient setting only or with direct professional supervision.

Adverse effects seen with benzodiazepine use include muscle fasciculations, weakness, and ataxia in the horse at sedative doses; irritability, possible development of hepatic failure, and aberrant demeanor in cats; and CNS excitement in the dog.

BARBITURATES

Phenobarbital is a barbiturate with CNS effects. The mechanism of action of this group of drugs is not quite understood, but they have been shown to inhibit the release of Ach, NE, and glutamate. Phenobarbital tends to depress motor activity without causing excessive sedation, which makes it a good anticonvulsant agent. One major side effect of this drug is dose-dependent respiratory depression.

✐ TECHNICIAN NOTE

Major side effect of phenobarbital is dose-dependent respiratory depression.

An effective and inexpensive agent used to treat epilepsy (status epilepticus) and seizures caused by acute encephalitis or meningitis in dogs is oral phenobarbital. For some cases that are uncontrolled by phenobarbital, oral administration of potassium bromide has been effective. (Potassium bromide is not available in a commercial formulation. Authorization may be obtained from the FDA to compound preparations for treatment of refractory cases.)

ANALGESICS, ANTIPYRETICS, AND ANTIINFLAMMATORY AGENTS

Analgesics are agents that alleviate pain. Although local as well as general anesthetics inhibit the sensory perception of pain, analgesics are generally considered to increase the threshold of pain in the pain perception areas of the brain. Antiprostaglandins (e.g., aspirin, flunixin) inhibit the biosynthesis of these natural pain-producing substances and are also considered analgesics. (See Chapter 20 for additional information on opioids.)

OPIOID ANALGESICS

The naturally occurring narcotics (e.g., morphine, codeine) as well as synthetic narcotics (e.g., hydrocodone, meperidine) are the most potent analgesics. These agents stimulate the *mu*-opioid receptor and are thought to have some activity at the *delta*-opioid receptor. Although these addictive agents are used for severe postsurgical or posttrauma pain in dogs and horses, their more common use is as an anesthetic or preanesthetic agent.

The pharmacologic effects differ somewhat among the various narcotics, but most will produce the following:

- CNS depression in the dog, monkey, and human
- CNS stimulation (excitement) in the cat and horse
- Cough sedation in the dog and human
- Respiratory depression (panting may initially be seen)
- Increased tone of intestinal smooth muscle, causing constipation
- Effects of these drugs are reversed by narcotic antagonists, such as naloxone.

Unfortunately, narcotic analgesics are fairly short acting in the dog and the horse (2 to 4 hours). Gut stasis in the horse is a concern when considering opioid analgesics. The opioid analgesics have questionable efficacy in the ruminant.

The agonist activity of the synthetic opioid *butorphanol* is thought to be exerted at the *kappa* and *sigma* receptors. Butorphanol, a morphine congener, has shown promise in dogs as a longer-acting (4 to 8 hours) analgesic. Adverse effects seen in dogs include sedation (occasionally), ataxia, and anorexia or diarrhea (rarely). Transient ataxia and sedation may occur in the horse at usual doses. Butorphanol is used in horses as an effective analgesic, although its stimulatory effects must be suppressed by the concurrent use of depressant drugs, such as xylazine. Butorphanol is approved by the FDA for use as an antitussive in dogs.

Gaining popularity in veterinary medicine for pain relating to surgery is *fentanyl*. Fentanyl shares the actions of the opioid agonists; the same precautions should apply. One advantage of using fentanyl is that it is marketed in a transdermal patch system for pain management that delivers continual analgesia for about 72 hours.

Hydrocodone bitartrate is a phenanthrene-derivative opioid agonist that exhibits the characteristics of other opiate agonists. It is used in veterinary medicine mainly as an antitussive agent. The mechanism is thought to be a result of direct suppression of the cough reflex on the cough center in the medulla. Hydrocodone is more sedating than codeine, but not as constipating.

OPIOID ANTAGONISTS

The opioid antagonists reverse the pharmacologic effects of narcotics and have no analgesic activity. *Naloxone* appears to be the only true antagonist because it possesses no other apparent pharmacologic effect at usual doses. (It reverses the majority of effects associated with high-dose opiate administration—respiratory and CNS depression.)

> ✎ **TECHNICIAN NOTE**
>
> Effects of opioids may be reversed with the use of narcotic antagonist naloxone.

Although narcotic antagonists are used commonly in human addicts to reverse overdoses of self-administered narcotics, their principal use in veterinary medicine is to reverse the sedative and quieting effects of analgesics used for temporary restraint. Dogs receiving narcotic sedation for minor procedures (e.g., radiographs, suture removal) are easily "reversed" with naloxone; the animal is almost immediately alert. The duration of action of naloxone is shorter than that of most narcotics, and generally the effects of the unmetabolized analgesic are inadequate to cause the animal to return to its sedated state.

CORTICOSTEROIDS

Corticosteroids are extremely active compounds that have numerous pharmacologic effects on all organ systems. They have been used in an attempt to treat practically every malady that afflicts animals. They are valuable in the treatment of certain conditions; however, there are significant risks when one considers the potential adverse effects.

Because corticosteroids are naturally occurring body substances (cortisol is derived from the adrenal gland), one indication for the use of steroids would be replacement therapy to correct a deficiency. Such a deficiency is relatively rare. Most steroids used in veterinary medicine are given for their antiinflammatory effect; the mechanism for the antiinflammatory response is complex. They suppress the tissue swelling and pain that normally follow injury. Because inflammation is common in a variety of diseases, there is extensive use, perhaps overuse, of these agents.

Steroids also possess antiimmunologic effects, altering the immune response of the body. Therefore, they are used in certain allergic diseases because they reduce the hypersensitive and allergic reactions of the patient. Immunizations generally should not be given during corticosteroid therapy because of the potential for inadequate immune response.

> ✎ **TECHNICIAN NOTE**
>
> Immunizations should not be given during corticosteroid therapy because of potential for inadequate immune responses.

Common side effects seen with the long-term use of steroids include gastrointestinal bleeding; increased susceptibility to infections or wounds that will not heal; potassium loss, causing irregular heartbeats, muscle cramps, and weakness; sodium and water retention (edema or ascites); muscle weakness resulting from protein breakdown; and behavioral changes. The primary adverse effects associated with long-term administration, especially if given at high doses or on an alternate-day regimen, are generally manifested as symptoms of hyperadrenocorticism (Cushing disease).

Dexamethasone is one of the most popular steroids used in veterinary medicine; it is fairly long acting (more than 48 hours). *Prednisolone* and *prednisone* are used interchangeably and are available in tablet form. *Triamcinolone* and *betamethasone* are also used extensively in veterinary medicine.

Steroids are found in various dosage forms, including ophthalmic, otic, topical, injection, and oral. It should be noted that long-term use of these steroids as ophthalmic or topical agents may lead to some of the systemic toxic effects previously mentioned.

NONSTEROIDAL ANTIINFLAMMATORY DRUGS

To avoid side effects inherent to steroids, other agents possessing antiinflammatory action have been synthesized. These are called *nonsteroidal antiinflammatory agents* (NSAIDs). NSAIDs exhibit antipyretic, analgesic, and antiinflammatory activity. The major mechanism of therapeutic effect is believed to be the result of inhibition of prostaglandin synthesis. Many inhibit both COX-1 and COX-2 isoenzymes. *Phenylbutazone,* one of the original members of this group of compounds, remains one of the most widely used agents in equine medicine. Phenylbutazone is not frequently used in small animals, although there is a label claim for use in dogs. Dogs metabolize phenylbutazone rapidly, which makes it difficult to maintain therapeutic levels of the drug. Cats metabolize the drug slowly and thus become prone to its toxic effects. Blood dyscrasias have been reported in several species receiving phenylbutazone. The drug has the potential for reducing the effects of other drugs metabolized by the liver because it increases the hepatic microsomal enzymes necessary to deactivate these drugs.

Flunixin has gained popularity not only for its antiinflammatory effects but also for its ability to reduce gastrointestinal pain in horses and ruminants. Although not approved for food-producing animals, flunixin appears to be the best analgesic available for ruminants, providing relatively long, effective relief.

Ketoprofen and *carprofen* are propionic acid derivatives structurally related to ibuprofen and naproxen. Ketoprofen has been approved for use in the horse to alleviate inflammation and pain associated with skeletal disorders. Carprofen has been approved for dogs only to relieve pain and inflammation associated with osteoarthritis.

Oral administration of the NSAIDs is apparently irritating to the gastrointestinal tract, and may cause ulceration in the mouth, stomach, or intestines. Newer generation NSAIDs (*etodolac, meloxicam, deracoxib,* and *tepoxalin*) are gaining in popularity because of once-a-day dosage and decreased adverse effects on the gastrointestinal (GI) tract.

DIURETIC AND CARDIOVASCULAR DRUGS

Fluid and electrolyte imbalances and their treatment are discussed in Chapter 25. The function of the kidney and its role in maintaining proper fluid volume and electrolyte concentration are also mentioned. Blood is initially filtered in the kidney, and most of the filtrate is reabsorbed from the kidney tubules back into the blood. Most diuretic drugs affect the reabsorption process, preventing the reabsorption of some sodium and water from the filtrate. As a result, urinary output and sodium excretion are increased.

DIURETICS

Diuretic drugs are used primarily to relieve edema (the presence and abnormally large amounts of fluid in the intercellular tissue spaces of the body) associated with diseases of the kidney, heart, or liver. Although there are numerous diuretic agents, *furosemide* appears to be the most routinely used diuretic in veterinary medicine. Furosemide is a loop diuretic that inhibits primarily reabsorption of sodium (Na^+) and Chloride (Cl^-) in the kidney. It is commercially available in convenient forms for oral and injectable administration is small and large animals. Besides being potent and effective in most cases, furosemide is rapid acting and usually produces diuresis within 5 minutes when given intravenously.

Furosemide can cause a "wasting" of potassium, so serum potassium levels should be monitored for animals that take furosemide. Potassium supplementation may be indicated during furosemide therapy.

TECHNICIAN NOTE

Loop diuretics can cause "potassium wasting." Serum potassium levels should be monitored; potassium supplementation may be indicated.

Occasionally, when renal blood flow is inadequate because of trauma or shock, furosemide or similar diuretics are ineffective in altering tubular reabsorption. In such cases, an osmotic diuretic such as *mannitol*, which is poorly absorbed from the renal filtrate, is used to produce diuresis. Animals that have been hit by cars may be likely candidates to receive mannitol. Crystallization may occur if the solutions are at low temperatures in concentrations greater than 15%. It is important to dissolve crystals before administering.

CARDIAC GLYCOSIDES

Cardiac (heart) drugs are probably the most potent and hazardous group of drugs used in medicine because of their effects on such a vital organ. Any carelessness in calculation, administration, or observation of the patient may lead to death. The dosage for these drugs should be individualized through frequent and careful monitoring to ensure the desired therapeutic response and avoid or minimize toxic effects.

The heart performs a relatively simple function (to circulate blood) and is essential to life. The heart consists primarily of *myocardium* (muscle), valves, and some specialized impulse-conducting nodes and fiber. Even though the heart has the ability to compensate for certain defects, disorders left untreated reduce the quality of life with severe disability, leading to premature death.

Significantly severe defects in the valves can only be treated surgically. Medical therapy is available for the treatment of a weakened myocardium and conductance disorders (*arrhythmias*).

The normal healthy heart can increase its output readily when demands, such as increased exercise, are placed on it. This increased cardiac output is a result of either an increased heart rate or an increase in the volume of blood pumped per beat (*stroke volume*), but usually it is a combination of both. Heart muscle weakened with age does not contract as fully and therefore can lead to reduced output. Because the body cannot tolerate much decrease in cardiac output, the heart rate will increase slightly, and the heart will become enlarged because the myocardium will thicken in an attempt to improve contractility. *Congestive heart failure* is the condition of an enlarged heart with poor myocardium contractility.

Various glycosides found in the leaf of the *digitalis* plant have been found to be useful in the treatment of congestive heart failure. *Digoxin* is one of the glycosides that is commonly used in veterinary medicine. Digoxin is unique in that it not only improves the inotropic ability (contractility) of the myocardium but also reduces the demand of heart for energy and oxygen. It also decreases the conduction of certain impulses within the heart and therefore decreases the heart rate. It is used for treatment of atrial fibrillation, an arrhythmic disorder of the heart.

Digoxin dosage is very critical. Toxic effects of the cardiac glycosides are seen at doses close to the therapeutic dose (narrow therapeutic window) and therefore complicate its use. Owners should be aware of signs of toxicity, which include vomiting, diarrhea, loss of appetite, and depression. Associated with these symptoms are a decreased heart rate and drug-induced arrhythmias.

Further complications to digoxin therapy are witnessed in animals with reduced liver or kidney function, as is common to the older animal. Good client compliance and close monitoring are essential in digoxin therapy because of the toxicity possibilities. The drug is available as an oral tablet, oral liquid, and injection.

Animals that are concurrently using a diuretic may have low serum potassium levels and are more susceptible to digoxin toxicity.

Although the cardiac glycosides are effective by injection in horses and cattle, and to some extent orally in horses, it is not feasible to use theses drugs to treat congestive heart failure (CHF) because of the long-term nature of the disease. These drugs are commonly used in dogs and cats. There is adequate absorption of digoxin from the gastrointestinal tract in these species; however, it may differ somewhat among animals and can be influenced by feeding times.

ANTIARRHYTHMIA DRUGS

Arrhythmias of the heart fall into several categories and require skilled clinicians and electronic instrumentation for proper diagnosis and treatment. Some minor cardiac arrhythmias are likely to correct themselves and may be left untreated. The use of antiarrhythmic drugs in veterinary medicine is usually limited to treatment of those arrhythmias that are life threatening and require immediate attention.

Calcium channel blockers provide the veterinarian with an efficacious weapon in the treatment of certain cardiovascular disorders. This group of drugs has a low incidence of side effects. Of the numerous agents, *diltiazem* has surfaced as the most commonly used agent to treat supraventricular tachyarrhythmias in dogs and cats. It is used in the treatment of hypertrophic cardiomyopathy in cats. Diltiazem acts as an antihypertensive agent through arteriolar dilation, but the benefit of this action is not fully known.

Three older commonly used antiarrhythmic drugs are *quinidine, procainamide,* and *lidocaine.* Their more ordinary uses are only mentioned because detailed discussion is beyond the scope of this chapter. Quinidine is used in horses and large dogs for the treatment of supraventricular and ventricular arrhythmias. Other uses include treatment of atrial fibrillation and atrial flutter. Procainamide is related chemically to *procaine,* and it is used in the treatment of ventricular extrasystoles and tachycardia, atrial arrhythmias, ectopic contraction and tachycardia, flutter, and fibrillation. Lidocaine, although used primarily as a local anesthetic, has therapeutic application in the treatment of ventricular tachyarrhythmias. Clinical monitoring and electronic evaluations should accompany the use of these drugs.

All antiarrhythmia drugs are toxic to the heart and may produce their own serious arrhythmias. In addition, in the horse quinidine can produce urticarial wheals, gastrointestinal disturbances (e.g., anorexia, colic, diarrhea), erythema, and edema of nasal mucosa with dyspnea and laminitis. Signs of quinidine toxicity in the dog include vomiting, depression, incoordination, and convulsions. Procainamide toxicities are exemplified in dogs by a loss of appetite, vomiting, and serious immunologic reactions with long-term use. A serious decrease in blood pressure may occur when procainamide is given intravenously. Lidocaine is not effective orally and has brief action when given intravenously. In large doses, lidocaine can produce a drop in blood pressure.

ANGIOTENSIN-CONVERTING ENZYME INHIBITORS

Vasodilatory drugs, or angiotensin-converting enzyme (ACE) inhibitors, prevent the conversion of angiotensin I to angiotensin II (a potent vasoconstrictor). The drugs compete with angiotensin I for the active site of ACE. In veterinary medicine, this group of drugs is primarily used to treat canine congestive heart failure. *Captopril* was the first agent in this class to be commercially available. Treatment presented risks, such as renal failure. Other ACE inhibitors have been synthesized; they are *pro-drugs* because they require a functioning liver to convert them to the active metabolite. *Enalapril* is commercially available with label indication for use in veterinary medicine. Other ACE inhibitors that are in use are human-labeled *benazepril hydrochloride,* and *ramipril.*

The side-effect profile of the second generation of ACE inhibitors has improved, and the dosage schedule is one or two times per day, which should help with client compliance.

Hydralazine is a phthalazine derivative antihypertensive/vasodilating agent. The main use of hydralazine is an afterload reducer for the adjunctive treatment in CHF in small animals, particularly if the primary cause is mitral valve insufficiency. It is usually administered in cases where enalapril is not effective in clinically improving dogs with mitral valve insufficiency. Hydralazine should be given with a diuretic because of the sodium and water retention associated with its use.

AGENTS USED TO TREAT PARASITISM

TREATMENT OF INTERNAL PARASITISM

Anthelmintics (wormers) are an extremely important group of drugs in veterinary medicine. The presence of internal parasites in an animal can shorten its life span or reduce the quality of life. It can contribute to considerable economic loss in food-producing animals. Although several different parasites are capable of infecting each species, most parasite infections can be effectively prevented or treated with proper care and medication. Current anthelmintics are much improved because they are more effective in eradicating the parasite and less toxic to the host. In addition, dosage forms such as pastes or chewable tablets are now available. These formulations are much more easily administered, which reduces stress to the animal and client.

There are a vast number of anthelmintics currently available; however, this discussion is limited to a select, popular few. Specific parasite information is given in Chapter 7.

PIPERAZINE

Piperazine is an older, safe drug used for the eradication of roundworms (ascarids) in dogs, cats, horses, swine, and poultry. Because most of the newer anthelmintics are either more efficacious against ascarids than piperazine or have a broader spectrum of anthelmintic activity, piperazine has lost much of its popularity. Once commercially available as a single-ingredient product for large animal use, it is now more frequently found in combination with other anthelmintics to broaden the spectrum or increase efficacy. Piperazine salts block neuromuscular transmission of the nematode, resulting in paralysis in the gastrointestinal tract and passive removal from the body by peristalsis. Piperazine is considered to be a safe drug to use, even during pregnancy and concurrent gastroenteritis; however, in horses with heavy manifestations of ascarids, rupture or blockage of the intestine is possible due to the rapid death and detachment of the worm.

BENZIMIDAZOLES

Benzimidazoles are a large class of anthelmintics. They inhibit the enzyme fumarate reductase and thereby interfere with parasitic carbohydrate metabolism. *Thiabendazole, oxibendazole, mebendazole, albendazole, parbendazole, fenbendazole, cambendazole,* and *oxfendazole* are safe and effective agents against several gastrointestinal parasites. They are formulated primarily for large animals to eradicate strongyles, pinworms, and ascarids in the horse and roundworms as well as several other parasites in cattle, sheep, swine, and goats. Albendazole shows activity against liver flukes. Fenbendazole and mebendazole are available for use in small animals to eradicate roundworms, hookworms, whipworms, and some tapeworms, although neither is effective for the common *Dipylidium* tapeworm. Adverse effects are not usually seen at recommended doses of benzimidazoles.

ORGANOPHOSPHATES

Trichlorfon, coumaphos, and dichlorvos are a group of agents that bind irreversibly to cholinesterase in the parasite, leading to Ach "poisoning" of the parasite. These drugs would also be toxic to the host, but they are selectively formulated to be poorly absorbed from the gastrointestinal tract of the animal. Precautions must be taken so animals dewormed with organophosphates are not exposed to other organophosphates, cholinesterase inhibitors, pesticides, or muscle relaxants, such as succinylcholine, until a few days after treatment. There is potential danger to humans in administration of these agents.

Common toxic signs of organophosphate poisoning (e.g., widespread parasympathetic stimulation) include miosis, salivation, breathing difficulties, vomiting, defecation, and muscle fasciculation. *Atropine* is used as a specific treatment to block the muscarinic effects. *Pralidoxime* (2PAM) is an expensive product for humans and may be used in severe cases of organophosphate poisoning to reactivate the cholinesterase enzyme.

TECHNICIAN NOTE
Pralidoxime (2PAM) is used in severe cases of organophosphate poisoning to reactivate the cholinesterase enzyme.

The organophosphates are fairly effective in treatment of a number of principal parasites in horses, cattle, swine, sheep, dogs, and cats. With the potential toxicity of the organophosphates, many are being replaced with safer agents. The use of organophosphates is no longer professionally accepted; however, they are still obtainable.

TETRAHYDROPYRIMIDINES

Pyrantel and *morantel* are two drugs in the tetrahydropyrimidine class. These drugs act as a cholinergic agonist and depolarize neuromuscular junctions. They are effective against the adult nematodes but are not active against larvae form.

Morantel is an analog of pyrantel that is safer and more effective in sheep and cattle than pyrantel. It is available only as a feed additive.

Pyrantel is widely used in horses for ascarids, strongyles, and pinworms. In dogs, pyrantel is used in the prevention and treatment of hookworms, and ascarids. Tetrahydropyrimidine products are safe and nontoxic to all species at the recommended therapeutic doses. There is no contraindication for use of these agents with other cholinergic drugs.

IMIDAZOTHIAZOLES

Two popular drug agents, *febantel* and *levamisole* are in the broad category of imidazothiazoles. Febantel is approved by the FDA for use in a number of species against parasites. It is only commercially available in the combination product (Drontal, Bayer). It has only been recognized to treat the most common equine parasites except bots and is reported to be very safe in pregnant mares.

Levamisole has broad anthelmintic activity in a large number of hosts, including sheep, cattle, pigs, horses, chickens, dogs, and cats. Use and FDA approval are limited primarily to food-producing animals. Although levamisole is relatively safe, some signs of toxicity occur similar to those of organophosphate poisoning. The toxic doses are only one or two times the therapeutic dose. Muzzle foam may be seen in ruminants after oral administration, but it usually disappears within a few hours. Transitory excitement has been seen in horses after treatment.

> ✎ **TECHNICIAN NOTE**
>
> Toxic doses of levamisole are only one to two times the therapeutic dose.

MILBEMYCINS

The *milbemycins* are macrocyclic lactones that act by interfering with the chloride-channel-mediated neurotransmission in the parasite, thereby resulting in its paralysis and elimination.

Moxidectin is an oral dewormer and boticide for horses and ponies at least 4 months old. The label claims that one dose of the drug will suppress strongyle egg production through 84 days. *Doramectin* is an injectable drug marketed as a single dose for control of a wide range of roundworms and arthropod parasites in cattle and swine.

IVERMECTINS

The ivermectins enhance the release of gamma-aminobutyric acid (GABA), which paralyzes nematodes by blocking neurotransmission at excitatory motor neurons. *Ivermectin* has demonstrated effectiveness in a number of species against a wide variety of internal and external parasites. In cattle, swine, sheep, and goats, injectable ivermectin is used to treat infestations by numerous gastrointestinal roundworms, lung worms, cattle grubs (cattle only), sucking lice, and mites. The paste and oral liquid forms of ivermectin have been approved for treatment of infestations by large and small strongyles, pinworms, and bots, as well as for other equine parasite infestation. It is also approved for the treatment of ascaridiasis, although for some stages it may be less effective than desirable.

Ivermectin has been approved for use in dogs and cats only for heartworm prevention; however, it has also been used at higher doses for treatment of other canine parasite infestations, including scabies. In certain dogs (most pure collie breeds) that are inherently sensitive to ivermectin, toxicities, sometimes fatal, have occurred with higher doses. Except for these unique toxicities, ivermectin has proved to be safe in other breeds and species when given at therapeutic doses. Overdose may manifest clinically as blindness, ataxia, and even death.

AGENTS USED IN HEARTWORM TREATMENT AND PREVENTION

There is considerable risk involved in the treatment of heartworms; therefore the American Veterinary Medicine Association (AVMA) Council on Veterinary Service established guidelines suggesting that first adult heartworms and then the microfilariae (the larvae forms of the tissue filarial) be eliminated. The adult worms usually stay in tissues, such as the heart, but the microfilariae migrate throughout the host. Heartworm disease is primarily seen in dogs; however, cats may also become infected. Dogs subject to infestation or reinfestation must be found free of microfilariae and adult heartworms before being placed on a preventive heartworm regimen.

> ✎ **TECHNICIAN NOTE**
>
> Dogs subject to infestation must be found free of microfilariae and adult heartworms before being placed on a heartworm prevention program.

Melarsomine dihydrochloride is an arsenic agent used in treatment of heartworm disease caused by immature to adult infections. Dogs are at risk for posttreatment pulmonary thromboembolism; therefore, they should be exercise restricted after treatment. The site of administration is critical for this drug, and it should be given only by deep intramuscular injection into the epaxial muscle. Adverse reactions observed with melarsomine dihydrochloride treatment include abdominal hemorrhage and pain, discolored urine, hematuria, tachypnea, disorientation, restlessness, and icterus. Melarsomine overdosage may show signs of arsenic toxicity. Dimercaprol (BAL) is an antidote for arsenic toxicity and may reduce signs of toxicity in overdoses. Coadministration of BAL may reduce the efficacy of melarsomine dihydrochloride.

> ✎ **TECHNICIAN NOTE**
>
> Dimercaprol (BAL) is an antidote to arsenic toxicity.

Microfilariae ingested by mosquitoes from infected animals molt in the mosquitoes and are then introduced back into other animals when another blood meal is taken. It is these reintroduced microfilariae that molt again into larvae and become adult heartworms. Drugs used for heartworm prevention, such as *diethylcarbamazine* (DEC), *ivermectin*, *milbemycin*, and *moxidectin*, act by killing the tissue-migrating larvae. To review the heartworm life cycle, see Chapter 7.

DEC should be administered daily at the beginning of mosquito season and continued for 2 months after the season is over. If ivermectin or milbemycin is used, it should be given within 1 month of the initial exposure and then once monthly. The final dose is given within 30 days of the last exposure. If more than 45 days elapse between doses, animals should be retested for heartworms before restoration of preventative therapy. In mild climates where mosquitoes prevail year round, prophylactic treatment must be administered for the lifetime of the dog.

Although relatively nontoxic at the low dose used for heartworm prevention, DEC is somewhat irritating to the gastric mucosa. Oral administration is therefore recommended immediately after a meal to reduce nausea and vomiting. These adverse effects are usually seen only with the higher doses of DEC that are sometimes used to treat ascarids.

Milbemycin and ivermectin are available as once-per-month heartworm preventatives. Milbemycin (Interceptor, Novartis) and ivermectin/pyrantel (Heartgard Plus, Merial Ltd.) have the added protection against adult hookworms caused by *Ancylostoma caninum*. Ivermectin toxicities (although rarely observed at the low-dose heartworm preventative level) unique to collie breeds are not seen with milbemycin.

✎ TECHNICIAN NOTE
Ivermectin toxicities are unique to some collie breeds.

Moxidectin (Pro-Heart, Fort Dodge) activity results in paralysis and death of the affected parasites at the tissue larvae stage. Not only is moxidectin indicated for heartworm prevention use in dogs 6 months and older, but also treatment of existing larvae and adult hookworm infections. Moxidectin is the first antimicrofilaria that is injectable and provides 6 months of continuous protection in one dose. It should be administered by a Doctor of Veterinary Medicine (DVM). Professional administration avoids the need of the owner to remember when the dose is due.

ANTICESTODAL DRUGS
Anticestodal drugs kill and/or facilitate expulsion of tapeworms. The original drugs used were agents that temporarily paralyzed the tapeworms, causing them to lose their attachment to the gastrointestinal tract. Even when these drugs contained purgative properties (causing the emptying, cleansing, or evacuation of the bowels) or were given with harsh laxatives, reattachment of a number of tapeworms was likely to occur. This treatment was stressful to the host because its ineffectiveness required repeated dosages. Newer drugs, although more expensive, kill the tapeworm and have replaced most other anticestodal drugs on the market.

After oral administration, *praziquantel* is widely distributed throughout the body, which makes it unique in its effectiveness against various stages of tapeworm development, including the adult stage. In addition, it is nontoxic and has a wide margin of safety. It can also be given by injection.

Epsiprantel has proven to be safe and effective. Unlike praziquantel, only trace levels of it are absorbed after oral administrations, and it remains at the site of action within the gastrointestinal tract. Exact mechanism of action has not been determined; however, this drug exerts its action directly on the tapeworm causing disruption of attachment to the host. The worm is vulnerable to digestion by the host animal.

DRUGS USED TO TREAT GIARDIASIS
Giardia canis is a protozoan that may produce chronic diarrhea in dogs. Treatment with *metronidazole* is usually effective. In general, the toxicity is low; few adverse effects are reported during or after the 5-day treatment period.

Giardiasis is also found in cats, but clinically it is usually not a problem (its diarrhea-producing role is not known). For treatment in the cat, metronidazole is given in a dosage regimen similar to that used in dogs. The margin of safety in cats is much narrower. Overdosing must be avoided because it may lead to death.

Investigations show that *Giardia* with presenting diarrhea may be successfully treated with an alternating "7 days on/7 days off" regimen of *fenbendazole*. Label claim to this indication has not been made.

EXTERNAL PARASITE TREATMENT
Chlorinated Hydrocarbons
Various chlorinated hydrocarbon compounds (e.g., *lindane* and *methoxychlor*) were once popular and marketed in several different formulations for a variety of uses in a number of species. The compounds were effective and possess rapid knockdown capability, with some having residual effects for several days. The long-lasting residual properties posed a threat as environmental hazard, and as a result, many of these types of products have been banned. Although the degree of toxicity will vary among the various chlorinated hydrocarbons, they should all be treated with caution and used as advised on the container label. Some diluted aqueous suspensions and powders may be applied directly to livestock. Signs of toxicity include vomiting, weakness, and other CNS effects, such as tremors, incoordination, convulsions, coma, and respiratory failure. Young, debilitated, or lean animals are more susceptible to the toxic effects. There is no specific antidote for chlorinated hydrocarbon toxicity. The animal should be removed from further exposure and given supportive treatment such as barbiturates to control seizures, if necessary.

✎ TECHNICIAN NOTE
There is no specific antidote for chlorinated hydrocarbon toxicity.

Organophosphates
Organophosphates *(ronnel, coumaphos, trichlorfon, malathion)* are formulated specifically for the treatment of

external parasites. As with chlorinated hydrocarbons, a number of preparations exist, such as sprays, dips, foggers, pour-ons, and pest strips. These compounds have good insect-killing ability, but residual effects are related to the vehicle used to apply the agent. Topical application of these preparations permits significant absorption through the skin to produce signs of toxicity. Signs and treatment of toxicity are the same as those mentioned in the discussion of organophosphates used for internal parasitism treatment. Persons applying these agents should avoid getting them in their eyes or on their skin. The use of disposable gloves and eye protection is recommended. Prolonged breathing of spray mists should also be avoided.

Pyrethrins

Pyrethrum flowers (chrysanthemums) have been used as insecticides for centuries. Formulations for animal use are reported to be nontoxic to mammals as well as having little effect on the environment. Some toxicity has occurred in cats.

Pyrethrins are marketed in numerous formulations for convenient use. Most have chemicals, such as piperonyl butoxide, added to potentiate their killing power. Also, microencapsulation has significantly increased the residual activity of these compounds that were known initially for their quick "knockdown" effect.

Permethrin, a synthetic pyrethroid, is formulated and used similarly to the natural pyrethrins.

Miscellaneous Agents

Several manufacturers have marketed new once-per-month flea control products. *Lufenuron* is a benzoyl-phenyl-urea derivative classified as an insect development inhibitor. The product does not kill adult fleas but instead safely and effectively controls flea populations by breaking the life cycle at the egg stage. Preexisting flea populations may continue to develop and emerge after flea treatment, so noticeable control may not be seen for several weeks after dosage. Lufenuron is available in tablet formulation for dogs and oral liquid and injectable formulation for cats over 6 weeks of age.

Imidacloprid is a flea adulticide formulated for topical application. It is classified as a nitroguanidine and acts as an NT blocker in the insect. Imidacloprid will kill fleas within 1 day of treatment. The disadvantage with this product is that shampooing may shorten the duration of flea protection. The product is considered safe for dogs and cats over 4 months of age.

Fipronil is classified as a phenylpyrazole and acts as a GABA inhibitor. It is a topical formulation for control of fleas by killing adult fleas. There is product label claim for killing all stages of brown dog ticks, American dog ticks, lone star ticks, and deer ticks. After application, the animal can be handled immediately and shampooed the following day. Fipronil is safe for dogs and cats 8 weeks of age and older.

Moxidectin is an endectocide of the milbemycin class used to treat infections caused by internal and external parasites in cattle.

Selamectin, a member of the avermectin class, is a once-per-month topical treatment for dogs and cats 6 weeks of age and older. Selamectin kills adult fleas and prevents flea eggs from hatching for 1 month. It is indicated for the prevention and control of flea infestations, prevention of heartworm disease, treatment and control of ear mite infestation, treatment and control of sarcoptic mange, control of tick infestation in dogs, and treatment of intestinal hookworm and roundworm infection in cats.

ANTIMICROBIAL AGENTS

Initially, *antibiotics* (antimicrobials) were defined as substances produced by microorganisms, which in low concentrations destroy or inhibit growth of other species of microorganisms. Many of these substances may be produced totally or in part through chemical synthesis. Because antibiotics have the potential to cure life-threatening infections, they are one of the most popular and useful groups of drugs in veterinary medicine.

It is important to know the characteristics and uses of the various antibiotics and have a proper understanding of the principles of antibiotic therapy (chemotherapy). It is beyond the scope of this chapter to present a thorough discussion of chemotherapy; however, some basic principles are discussed. Not all microorganisms are harmful or disease producing (pathogenic). Many bacteria normally found in the gastrointestinal tract, mucous membranes, and skin are helpful to their host. They compete with invading harmful pathogens and keep them from proliferating, thereby preventing progression to a disease state.

Each antibiotic is effective against specific groups of microorganisms. Some antibiotics are bacteriocidal (destroy bacteria), and some are bacteriostatic (inhibit growth); some may be both, depending on the concentration of the antibiotic (Box 21-1). The various species of bacteria that are affected by the antibiotic are known as the *spectrum*.

Box 21-1 ANTIBACTERIAL ACTION AT USUAL SERUM CONCENTRATIONS

BACTERIOSTATIC
Chloramphenicol
Tetracyclines
Erythromycin
Sulfonamides
Lincomycin

BACTERICIDAL
Penicillin
Aminoglycosides
Cephalosporins
Trimethoprim-sulfa combinations
Quinolones

Broad-spectrum antibiotics are those that are effective against a wide range of microorganisms, both gram positive and gram negative.

One method of classification of bacteria is to determine their tendency to absorb dye (gentian violet) into their cell wall. Those absorbing stain are referred to as *gram positive* (dark blue cell walls), and those that do not absorb the stain are known as *gram negative* (light pink cell walls) (Box 21-2).

For an antibiotic to be effective, it must be able to reach the site of infection in a sufficient concentration to exert its effect on the microorganism. In addition, the antibiotic concentration must be maintained or reached frequently over a period of time to completely destroy all bacteria or inhibit bacterial growth and provide time for the natural defense mechanisms of the body to eradicate the pathogen.

> **✎ TECHNICIAN NOTE**
>
> For an antibiotic to be effective, it must reach the site of infection in a sufficient concentration to exert an effect on the microorganism.

The length of antibiotic therapy may vary, depending on factors such as the site of infection, the microorganism, and the duration of infection. When antibiotics are prescribed, the treatment is usually for a minimum of 5 days. Although improvement may be seen with inadequate antibiotic therapy, it is an unwise practice to stop treatment until the total regimen has been given. Microorganisms exposed to subtherapeutic antibiotic levels may develop resistance to that particular antibiotic, which will then be ineffective even when given at high doses. Bacteria can not only develop resistance to several antibiotics but also pass resistance on to other species of bacteria. Multiple antibiotic-resistant bacteria is also a serious problem if resistance is developed in a hospital or clinic. Nosocomial (originating in hospitals) infections from resistant bacteria can be treated with only the most potent and expensive antibiotics. Nosocomial infections are discussed in Chapter 8.

The choice of antibiotic is obviously critical to successful therapy. The microorganism must be sensitive to the antibiotic chosen. A sample from the site of infection (blood, urine, or tissue) should be collected for culture and antibiotic sensitivity testing to determine the causative organism and the effective antibiotics (see Chapter 8). This is not always economically or clinically feasible, so potentially effective antibiotics are frequently just chosen (empiric treatment). Empiric treatment usually includes agents effective against gram-positive, gram-negative, fungal, and viral infections. In selecting an antibiotic, one tries to choose an agent that is most likely to be effective against the pathogen and least likely to disturb normal, nonpathogenic bacteria. Even the narrow-spectrum antibiotics are effective against a number of types of bacteria, both pathogenic and nonpathogenic. Destruction of the nonharmful bacterial flora may allow a second pathogen to manifest and proliferate.

> **✎ TECHNICIAN NOTE**
>
> Destruction of nonharmful bacterial flora may allow a second pathogen to proliferate.

Administered antibiotics that are not effective may actually worsen the disease by destroying nonpathogenic bacteria that are actively competing with the pathogen. Indiscriminate use of broad-spectrum antibiotics eventually leads to resistant strains, ineffective antibiotic use, and expensive, perplexing therapeutic problems.

PENICILLINS

The discovery of penicillin in 1920 has dramatically changed the outcome of many life-threatening infections. The basic penicillin molecule (Figure 21-7) has been continuously manipulated and changed to produce a number of improved penicillins with unique characteristics.

Penicillin G (benzylpenicillin), the first clinically used penicillin, is still used extensively in large animals in its procaine salt form. *Procaine penicillin G* is poorly soluble and is released slowly from its site of injection, providing adequate penicillin levels to allow once-daily dosage;

> **Box 21-2** COMMON ANIMAL PATHOGENS
>
> **GRAM-POSITIVE ORGANISMS**
> *Streptococcus* spp.
> *Staphylococcus* spp.
> *Clostridium perfringens*
> *Corynebacterium* spp.
>
> **GRAM-NEGATIVE ORGANISMS**
> *Escherichia coli*
> *Proteus* spp.
> *Pseudomonas* spp.
> *Klebsiella* spp.
> *Salmonella* spp.
> *Brucella*
> *Vibrio*
> *Pasteurella* spp.

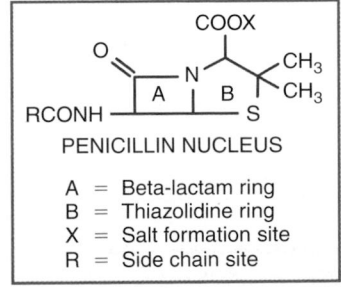

A = Beta-lactam ring
B = Thiazolidine ring
X = Salt formation site
R = Side chain site

Figure 21-7 Penicillin nucleus.

however, twice-daily dosage is usually recommended. Penicillin G is effective when given orally, but high doses must be administered because only approximately one fourth of it is absorbed from the gastrointestinal tract. Most of the antibiotic is destroyed by stomach acid, so it should *not* be given directly after feeding, when stomach acid is greatest.

Penicillin acts by blocking bacterial cell wall synthesis in the final stages of replication. Without a cell wall, the bacteria swell and cannot function properly, and some *lysis* (rupturing) may occur. New infections in their high-log growth phase are therefore most susceptible to penicillin. Penicillin has no direct effect on mammalian cells because they do not have cell walls.

> ### ✎ TECHNICIAN NOTE
> Infections in the high-log phase are more susceptible to penicillin.

Penicillin G is effective against most of the gram-positive microorganisms, including many of the streptococcal and staphylococcal species. Some staphylococcal species have the ability to produce penicillinase, an enzyme that hydrolyzes the lactam ring and thus renders the penicillin inactive. At high doses, penicillin G is effective against a few gram-negative species.

One alteration of the penicillin molecule was to make it more resistant to hydrolysis by stomach acid. For example, amoxicillin and a specific beta-lactamase inhibitor, potassium clavulanate, is a combination product prepared to resist the action of penicillinase. Table 21-2 provides some comparison among various commercially available penicillins. From side-chain alteration of the molecule emerged penicillins that are effective against a wide variety of microorganisms. Some of the penicillins available for human use have a broad spectrum of activity and are the most important potent antibiotics for use against many gram-negative organisms that may be resistant to most other antibiotics.

There is documentation that some patients that are sensitive to the penicillins are also sensitive to another class of antibiotics, cephalosporins (cross-sensitivity). In general, the penicillins are safe. Allergic reactions, such as skin rashes, fever, urticaria, salivation, cutaneous edema, and other hypersensitivities, may occur and lead to justifiable concern.

AMINOGLYCOSIDES

Aminoglycosides (*streptomycin, neomycin, kanamycin, amikacin, gentamicin*) have a fairly broad spectrum but are used primarily for their activity against gram-negative organisms. Aminoglycosides are not adequately absorbed when administered orally, but they may be used orally for intestinal tract infections or "sterilization" of the gastrointestinal tract before surgery. Aminoglycosides exert their action by interfering with bacteria protein synthesis. Although toxicity may vary among agents, all are potentially *ototoxic* (affecting hearing and balance) as well as *nephrotoxic* (renal toxicity). Neuromuscular blockage is also an adverse effect that is manifested by apnea and progressive paralysis of skeletal muscle. When aminoglycosides are administered to animals with preexisting renal damage, the patient must be closely monitored because potential for toxicity is much greater.

> ### ✎ TECHNICIAN NOTE
> All aminoglycosides are potentially ototoxic and nephrotoxic and may cause neuromuscular blockage.

Table 21-2 COMPARISON OF PENICILLIN PRODUCTS

Penicillin	Acid Stable	Resists Penicillinase Hydrolysis	Spectrum, Comments
Penicillin G	No	No	Mostly gram positive
Penicillin V	Yes	No	Mostly gram positive, less effective than penicillin G against some species
Procaine penicillin G	NA*	No	Same as penicillin G
Dicloxacillin, oxacillin	Yes	Yes	Mostly gram positive
Ampicillin, hetacillin	Yes	No	Mostly gram positive plus *Escherichia coli, Proteus mirabilis*, and a few other gram-negative organisms
Amoxicillin	Yes	No	Spectrum similar to ampicillin, better absorbed
Carbenicillin	Yes†	No	Gram positive plus several gram negative, including *Pseudomonas aeruginosa* (oral form effective only in urinary tract infections)
Azlocillin, mezlocillin, piperacillin	NA	No	Broadest-spectrum penicillins effective against most gram-negative organisms, including *Klebsiella* spp.

*NA, Not applicable (no oral forms).
†Indanyl sodium salt for oral use.

Resistance, toxicity, and expense are major considerations in the selection of these agents. Resistance demonstrated by organisms may be to a particular aminoglycoside or, commonly, to several aminoglycosides within this class (cross-resistance).

Neomycin is nephrotoxic and therefore finds its use primarily in topical or ophthalmic preparations. Kanamycin, gentamicin, and amikacin are commercially available as veterinary products. Although expensive for humans, other aminoglycosides are finding use in veterinary medicine for highly resistant organisms that are not susceptible to other antibiotics.

Aminoglycosides are frequently used simultaneously with some of the newer penicillins or cephalosporins to treat stubborn gram-negative infections. Because the combinations are more effective than the use of either agent alone, the activity of the combination is called *synergism*. The use of aminoglycosides and chloramphenicol together is contraindicated because it is an antagonistic combination, resulting in decreased antibacterial action.

CEPHALOSPORINS

Cephalosporins (*cephalexin, cefadroxil, cephradine, cephapirin, ceftiofur*) are somewhat chemically similar (Figure 21-8) to the penicillins and share a similar mechanism of action and spectrum. Cephalosporins are not destroyed by penicillinase-producing bacteria, although some resistance exists to them.

The cephalosporins are subclassified primarily by spectrum into first, second, third, and fourth generations. Only minor differences exist in the spectrum of the first generation; all are effective against most gram-positive bacteria and several gram-negative species. The second generation has a somewhat broader spectrum, displaying activity against most *clostridial species* and adds more gram-negative coverage and less gram-positive coverage. Although *Pseudomonas aeruginosa* is not susceptible to the first- or second-generation cephalosporins, it may be treated with the third-generation cephalosporins. Severe infections, such as *Pseudomonas* infections, are usually treated with a combination of antibiotics to ensure eradication and limit the possibility of developing resistance. The fourth-generation

cephalosporin, cefepime, can be compared to the third generation but is more resistant to some chromosal beta-lactams like those produced by *Enterobacter*.

The cost of the cephalosporins limits their use in veterinary medicine. Even with the availability of veterinary cephalosporin and generic products for humans, cost remains a major concern when considering second- and third-generation cephalosporins.

The cephalosporins have a low incidence of adverse effects. Long-term use of excessively large doses may lead to some complications similar to those of other antibiotics, including possible allergic reactions or overgrowth of nonsusceptible bacteria or fungi, leading to intestinal pain, bloating, and diarrhea.

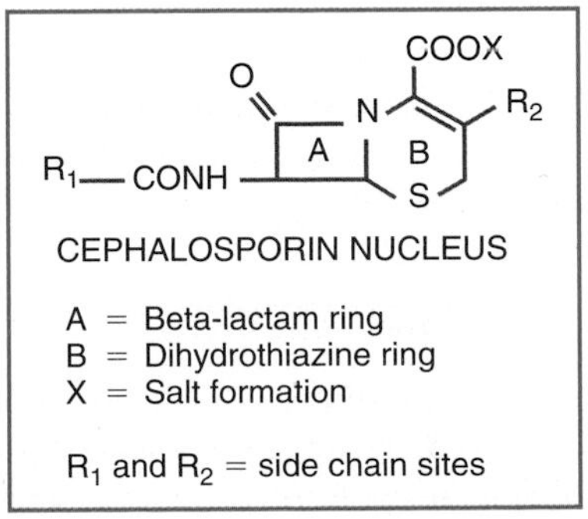

QUINOLONES

Quinolones constitute a class of antibiotics finding extensive use in veterinary medicine for treatment of a wide variety of organisms, including *P. aeruginosa*. *Enrofloxacin* is approved primarily for urinary, skin, and respiratory infections in dogs and cats, but it is also being used to treat bone and other infections in several additional species. There is a subcutaneous injection approved for cattle not intended for food to treat bovine respiratory disease (BRD) associated with *Pasteurella haemolytica*, *Pasteurella multocida*, and *Haemophilus somnus*.

Enrofloxacin seems to be well tolerated, and few side effects have been noted in animals. It is contraindicated in puppies during the rapid growth phase because it can induce abnormal cartilage formation, leading to weakness or lameness. This potential adverse effect discourages the use of enrofloxacin in other young animals as well as in adult horses. Although bacterial resistance to enrofloxacin is not yet common, indiscriminate use to treat routine infections is likely to produce resistant strains, making this very valuable drug worthless.

CHLORAMPHENICOL

Chloramphenicol (CHPC) use in humans is limited to a few specific infections because of a rare but potentially fatal occurrence of irreversible aplastic anemia. Personnel who handle CHPC and administer it to animals should use care, avoiding direct contact with the drug. Although some blood dyscrasias have been seen in animals, particularly in neonates, the condition is usually reversible by withdrawal of the drug.

CEPHALOSPORIN NUCLEUS

A = Beta-lactam ring
B = Dihydrothiazine ring
X = Salt formation

R_1 and R_2 = side chain sites

Figure 21-8 Cephalosporin nucleus.

> **TECHNICIAN NOTE**
>
> CHPC causes reversible blood dyscrasias. Personnel who handle or administer CHPC should use care and avoid direct contact.

CHPC is an important antibiotic in veterinary equine medicine. Although CHPC is bacteriostatic, it has a fairly broad spectrum of activity. It is rapidly distributed to most body compartments and tissues in adequate therapeutic concentrations. A small amount of CHPC is excreted unchanged in the urine, but most undergoes biotransformation in the liver to the inactive glucuronide conjugate.

Other adverse effects include anorexia, diarrhea, vomiting, and depression, as well as other rare but severe effects. CHPC in combination with other antibiotics is usually contraindicated. It interacts with several specific drugs or groups of drugs, including anticonvulsants, penicillins, phenylbutazone, and lincomycin.

Florphenicol is a broad-spectrum, primarily bacteriostatic antibiotic with a range of activity similar to that of CHPC against many gram-negative and gram-positive organisms. It does not carry the risk of inducing blood dyscrasias.

TETRACYCLINES

Oxytetracycline and *tetracycline* are practically used interchangeably because of a similarity in spectrum and pharmacologic properties. One tetracycline, doxycycline, has gained acceptance for use in small animals. It requires less frequent dosage and penetrates the CNS better than other tetracyclines.

These bacteriostatic agents affect the vital protein synthesis of the microorganism. Although the tetracyclines possess a relatively broad spectrum of activity, the development of resistant organisms has been a factor limiting their use. Through more judicious use of these agents, less-resistant strains are being encountered.

The absorption of tetracyclines from the gastrointestinal tract is adequate but is decreased in the presence of food, milk, or antacids. Some injectable preparations use propylene glycol as a solvent and are not recommended for intramuscular use because they are painful. When given intravenously, the tetracycline must be injected slowly because the solvent and drug may exert a blocking effect on the heart, causing the animal to temporarily collapse. Other injectable preparations contain povidone or similar agents, which reduce intramuscular irritation and eliminate the cardiac problem. The intramuscular product formulated for extended action must not be given intravenously.

Out-of-date or improperly stored tetracyclines should never be administered because they form nephrotoxic products.

> ✎ **TECHNICIAN NOTE**
> Tetracyclines form complexes with calcium in developing bones and teeth and should not be given to young animals.

Tetracyclines are relatively inexpensive and widely used, especially in food animals. The tetracyclines are also commonly used at low levels as a livestock feed additive to increase weight gain and decrease liver abscesses. This practice promotes the development of resistant strains of bacteria, rendering the tetracycline useless for treatment even when given at therapeutic levels.

Although popular, the tetracyclines have toxicities. A common toxicity is the intestinal problems associated with disruption of the natural intestinal flora, including the possibility of superinfection by resistant organisms. Hypersensitivity reactions of rashes, fever, and liver damage may also occur with use of tetracyclines. The tetracyclines form complexes with calcium in developing bones and teeth; they should not be given to pregnant or young animals because tooth discoloration, increases in dental caries, and temporary suppression in bone growth may occur.

MISCELLANEOUS ANTIBIOTICS

Erythromycin and *tilmicosin* are classified as macrolide antibiotics because of their high molecular weight. Their spectrum of activity is similar to that of penicillin; therefore they are commonly used instead of penicillin against penicillinase-producing microbes. Erythromycin does not alter intestinal flora extensively, but gastrointestinal effects such as vomiting and diarrhea have been observed.

Tilmicosin is a macrolide used to treat bovine respiratory diseases, including those caused by *Mycoplasma*. A distinct advantage of tilmicosin is its long half-life, which allows a single-dose treatment. Tilmicosin must only be administered by subcutaneous or intramuscular injections because fatalities have been reported with intravenous dosage. Deaths have been reported after the use of tilmicosin in swine, horses, and nonhuman primates. The drug must be handled with extreme caution and administered in accordance with the detailed label instructions.

> ✎ **TECHNICIAN NOTE**
> Fatalities have been reported with IV use of tilmicosin; therefore it must be administered subcutaneously or intramuscularly only.

Azithromycin is a long-acting macrolide administered orally that is used to treat *Chlamydia* infections of the eye.

Lincomycin is in the class lincosamide. It has a spectrum of activity similar to erythromycin and is particularly effective against *Staphylococcus* and *Streptococcus* spp. It has been useful when resistant strains or hypersensitivities to other antibiotics exist. Favorable results have been reported in the treatment of bone infections and various skin disorders (pyoderma) with lincomycin. The drug is concentrated and excreted in the bile. Lincomycin causes severe intestinal flora disturbances in horses, hamsters, and rabbits, so it should be avoided in these species.

OTHER ANTIMICROBIAL AGENTS

In addition to the antibiotics discussed, other chemical agents exist that are effective against certain strains of microorganisms. The sulfa drugs were the first antimicrobial agents to be used systemically in the treatment of bacterial infections.

SULFONAMIDES

Numerous sulfonamides (*sulfamethazine, sulfadiazine, sulfadimethoxine*) have been formulated. Their value and use have declined with the discovery of newer antibiotics, however, a few sulfonamides remain useful for certain conditions. These agents are relatively inexpensive, which makes them attractive for use is large animals for herd or flock treatment. The sulfonamides are particularly useful in the treatment of various infections of the respiratory system and urinary tract, bacterial diarrhea, foot rot, and coccidial infections. Unfortunately, bacterial resistance to the sulfonamides limits their effectiveness. A toxicity seen with the original sulfonamides was crystalluria, a condition in which insoluble crystals formed in the urine, causing renal damage. Because the solubility of one sulfonamide is independent of other sulfonamides, the formulation of triple sulfa was developed to avert crystalluria. More soluble sulfonamides are also available, thereby further reducing concern. It is important that animals receiving sulfonamide have adequate water available.

> ✎ **TECHNICIAN NOTE**
>
> It is important that animals receiving sulfonamides have adequate water available.

The intravenous preparations of sulfonamides have a high (basic) pH and are therefore damaging to tissue when inadvertently given *perivascularly* (in spaces around blood vessels). In addition, the intravenous preparations should be given slowly to avoid acute toxicity demonstrated by CNS effects, such as salivation, vomiting, diarrhea, weakness, ataxia, and convulsions.

TRIMETHOPRIM-SULFONAMIDE COMBINATIONS

Effective antibacterials being used are combination products of one part *trimethoprim* and five parts *sulfadiazine* or *sulfamethoxazole*. *Ormetoprim with sulfadimethoxine* is a comparable combination with similar use and actions. These combinations block two essential sequential steps in the replication process of the bacteria, resulting in a synergistic antibacterial action. The combinations are effective against a wide range of organisms, but not *Pseudomonas*.

Undesirable side effects seen with these combinations are infrequent. Although vomiting may occur, diarrhea is seldom seen. Animals that are deficient in folic acid may be prone to develop blood disorders, as has been reported in humans.

NITROFURANS

The nitrofurans (*nitrofurazone, nitrofurantoin, furazolidone*) have been replaced, to a great extent by newer, more effective, and safer antibacterials. These synthetic agents have a fairly broad spectrum of activity, but they are not effective against *Pseudomonas*.

Except for topical application, use in food-producing animals is strictly forbidden by the FDA because of carcinogenic properties.

Nitrofurantoin is sufficiently absorbed and has some use in small animals in the treatment of urinary tract infections. Nausea and vomiting, which are common adverse effects, can be reduced by administering nitrofurantoin with food or using the macrocrystal human preparations.

ANTIFUNGAL AGENTS

Numerous topical agents are available to treat fungal infections of the skin (*dermatomycosis*). *Griseofulvin* is administered orally; it has no antibacterial activity, but inhibits the growth of various skin fungi. It is an expensive product and is not usually the first-line choice unless the infection is widespread.

The treatment of systemic fungal infections (e.g., *cryptococcosis, blastomycosis, histoplasmosis*) is usually expensive, requiring lengthy treatment with limited success. *Amphotericin B,* an antibiotic used for various fungal infections, is toxic, causing kidney and liver damage and CNS abnormalities. A newer formulation of amphotericin B in a lipid complex suspension eliminates some toxic effects experienced with the original solution. *Nystatin,* another antibiotic, is relatively nontoxic but has a narrow spectrum of activity. Nystatin has activity against a variety of fungal organisms, but is used systemically to treat oropharyngeal and GI *Candida* infections.

Ketoconazole, an expensive antifungal agent, has proven to be effective against a variety of fungal infections. Ketoconazole causes hepatotoxicity (liver damage), so liver enzymes should be monitored during therapy. *Itraconazole* is a newer agent that is efficacious against a variety of fungal infections and is less hepatotoxic than ketoconazole and more expensive.

> ✎ **TECHNICIAN NOTE**
>
> Ketoconazole causes hepatotoxicity, and the liver functions should be monitored during use.

HORMONES AND SYNTHETIC SUBSTITUTES

The thyroid gland is controlled primarily by the amount of *thyroid-stimulating hormone* released from the pituitary gland. When stimulated, the thyroid gland releases thyroid hormones consisting primarily of *thyroxin*. Because the thyroid hormones affect the metabolism of carbohydrates, protein, and fats, thyroid-deficient (hypothyroid) animals show signs of lethargy, reduced alertness, increased body weight, poor hair coat, and other related signs. Insufficient amounts of iodine in the diet can result in inadequate production of thyroid hormones. Such hormone deficiencies can be treated with desiccated thyroid because it is effective orally. *Sodium levothyroxine* may be the most popular agent for the treatment of hypothyroidism. *Sodium liothyronine*, the other active component of desiccated thyroid, is also available commercially.

Feline hyperthyroidism is treated with *methimazole*. It interferes with iodine incorporation into tyrosyl residues of thyroglobulin, thereby inhibiting the synthesis of thyroid hormones.

INSULIN

Insulin is normally produced and released by islet cells of the pancreas. This hormone is necessary to facilitate the use of food by the body, especially sugar. Insulin enhances the absorption of glucose in most cells of the body. Animals with inadequate insulin will have abnormally high blood glucose levels (hyperglycemia) and other associated metabolic disorders. Dog and cat insulin are thought to resemble more closely to porcine than beef insulin. Insulin injection (regular *Iletin*) is a solution of dissolved insulin crystals, which accounts for its immediate action and short duration. There are other insulin preparations that are intermediate acting (approximately 24 hours) to long acting (approximately 36 hours). *Isophane insulin suspension* (NPH), an intermediate-acting insulin, tends to be widely used in small animal medicine.

Protamine zinc insulin (PZI) may take 1 to 4 hours for onset of action to occur. The effect of PZI peaks between 5 and 20 hours after dosage and may persist up to 30 hours. Dogs are generally controlled with once-a-day dosage. In cats, PZI insulin will begin to decrease blood sugars in about 1 to 3 hours and has its peak effect in 4.5 to 10 hours. The duration of action may be 12 to 30 hours. Nearly all cats require twice-daily dosage for good control.

With the emergence of recombinant products it may be difficult to obtain insulin of animal origin. Animals that were originally administered insulin from animal sources may need to have dose adjustments if switched to recombinant products. Any change in insulin should be made cautiously and under the medical supervision of the veterinarian.

> ✎ **TECHNICIAN NOTE**
> Dose adjustments may be needed if animals are switched to recombinant products from insulin of animal origin.

Overdoses of insulin produce hypoglycemia, which, if severe, can lead to coma and death. Treatment of hypoglycemia consists of administration of intravenous dextrose.

If an animal develops hypersensitivity (local or systemic reaction) or should develop insulin resistance, a change in type or species of insulin should be tried.

OXYTOCIN

Oxytocin is a hormone released at the end of pregnancy to stimulate uterine contractions during parturition and induce milk letdown. The synthetically produced oxytocin is destroyed in the GI tract and must be administered parenterally. It is beneficial during delayed parturition, for aiding milk letdown, and treatment of postpartum retained placenta and metritis.

PROSTAGLANDINS

Prostaglandins (PGs) are found in many mammalian tissues and have been shown to have a wide variety of effects on a number of body systems, including the CNS, cardiovascular, urinary, gastrointestinal, and reproductive systems. Commercially available PGs such as *dinoprost* and *cloprostenol* are used because of their effects on the reproductive system.

In cattle, the PGs can be used to regulate the heat cycle, so breeding and consequent calving times for a herd can be planned. PGs are approved by the FDA to abort feedlot heifers. For certain conditions in mares, PGs can effectively restore the normal heat cycle so that the animals can be bred.

Pregnant women should not handle these agents because they are abortifacients. Bronchospasm is another serious adverse effect in animals and humans that may occur as a result of contact with the product. Consequently, PGs should not be handled by asthmatics or used in animals with respiratory diseases.

> ✎ **TECHNICIAN NOTE**
> PG are abortifacients and cause bronchospasms. They should not be handled by pregnant women or asthmatics or used in animals with respiratory disease.

GASTROINTESTINAL DRUGS

ANTIEMETICS

Certain species, such as horses, rabbits, and rodents are unable to vomit, but protracted vomiting may become a problem in dogs, cats, and other species.

The vomiting reflex may be stimulated through at least four different pathways. For example, chemical substances in the blood (bacterial toxins or certain drugs) may mediate vomiting via the chemoreceptor trigger zone (CTZ) pathway (medulla of brain). Vomiting arising from movement of the head (motion sickness) is transmitted through another pathway (cortex of the brain). In selecting an antiemetic agent, it is desirable to know the underlying cause of vomiting and the pathway involved because some antiemetic drugs are specific in their site of action. Vomiting may be a symptom of a disease state, so initial attention should be directed to treatment of the primary disease.

Although independent of their antihistaminic activity, a few of the antihistamines (e.g., *dimenhydrinate, cyclizine, clemastine, and meclizine*) and *scopolamine* are effective in preventing vomiting induced by motion sickness. The principal side effect of the antihistamine is drowsiness, which may be desirable in pets that are traveling.

A number of phenothiazine tranquilizers (*chlorpromazine, prochlorperazine,* and *triflupromazine*) are classified as broad-spectrum antiemetics that control vomiting by blocking the CTZ at low doses and at the emetic center (in the medulla of the brain) at higher doses. Although these agents have the potential of producing a number of adverse effects, the risk of toxicity is low because of the low dose and short duration of therapy. Some potent broad-spectrum, human antiemetics (e.g., *haloperidol and metoclopramide*) are finding use in veterinary medicine.

Metoclopramide is a unique pharmacological agent. Besides its potent antiemetic property, especially in drug-induced emesis (e.g., cancer chemotherapy), metoclopramide is also a peristaltic stimulant, increasing gut motility. It has been used for gastric stasis in a number of species, including horses and cattle. In addition, to facilitate radiological examination of stomach or small intestine, metoclopramide may be used to stimulate gastric emptying and intestinal transit of barium in cases where delayed emptying interferes. Reflux esophagitis in dogs and cats has also been treated with metoclopramide.

Cisapride (Propulsid, Janssen) is not classified as an emetic; however, it is very useful as an equine gastrointestinal prokinetic agent (increases motility) in reflux conditions.

EMETICS

Agents to induce vomiting are used clinically as a rapid means of eliminating certain poisons or to remove food from the stomach before induction of general anesthesia. A once common emetic used in veterinary medicine is *apomorphine*. Although still commercially available, it is extremely expensive and difficult to obtain. Apomorphine stimulates the CTZ and may be administered orally, intramuscularly, intravenously, or via the conjunctival sac of the eye. Because apomorphine depresses the emetic center, repeated dosage is not recommended when the initial dose is ineffective. Apomorphine should not be given to cats because it produces extreme excitement. *Xylazine,* a sedative analgesic, can be used as an emetic because of the routine vomiting it produces in the cat.

Ipecac, once used commonly in cats and occasionally in dogs, has the disadvantage of having to be administered via a stomach tube because of taste. In addition, its effects may be somewhat sporadic; toxic effects, including death, may be induced with ipecac in cats. However, ipecac syrup remains a popular, convenient emetic for children for the removal of accidentally ingested, noncorrosive poison.

ANTIDIARRHEAL AGENTS

Diarrhea, like vomiting, may only be a symptom of an underlying problem. Ideally, it is best to identify the specific problem and correct it. Current trends are not to slow the gut but to allow it to remain active to remove any present toxins or irritants. Most small animals with diarrhea recover regardless of therapy. Persistent diarrhea not only may be offensive to pet owners but also may require supportive treatment, such as electrolyte and fluid replacement. Anticholinergics, such as the various belladonna alkaloids (*atropine, homatropine,* and *scopolamine*), have historically been used to treat diarrhea. Although *peristalsis* (propulsive intestinal contractions) is reduced, a minimal antidiarrheal effect results. The value of anticholinergic use is questionable because they have adverse effects such as increased heart rate, dryness of mouth, and diarrhea from gut paralysis.

Opiates, including opium tincture, morphine, codeine, and similar derivatives, such as diphenoxylate, are unique in that they increase rhythmic segmentation contraction, which resists intestinal flow and decreases peristalsis. In addition, the opiates increase the tone of the various sphincters and valves in the gastrointestinal tract, which further delays movement of the contents. The commercial product *diphenoxylate hydrochloride with atropine sulfate* (Lomotil, Searle) is effective in treating diarrhea in dogs.

The use of antidiarrheal opiates in cats is controversial because this species may react with excitatory behavior. Opiate antidiarrheals should be used with caution in patients with head injuries or increased intracranial pressure and acute abdominal conditions, such as colic, because the opiates may obscure diagnosis or clinical course of the condition. Opiate antidiarrheals should be used with extreme caution in patients with hepatic disease and CNS symptoms of hepatic encephalopathy because hepatic coma may result.

The use of opiates in animals with acute diarrhea that may be bacterially induced may enhance bacterial proliferation, delay the disappearance of the microbe from the feces, and prolong the febrile state. Acute overdoses of the opiate antidiarrheals could result in central nervous, cardiovascular, or respiratory system toxicity.

Another over-the-counter preparation that is extensively used in veterinary medicine is the human product *loperamide.* Loperamide is a synthetic piperidine derivative that slows intestinal motility through a direct effect on the nerve endings and/or intramural ganglia of the intestinal wall. In animals, loperamide does not have analgesic activity, even in extremely high doses. Loperamide is available in tablet, capsule, and oral liquid formulations.

Bismuth subsalicylate is thought to have weak antibacterial properties as well as being a protectant and antiendotoxic. Popular thought suggests the compound is cleaved in the small intestine into bismuth carbonate and salicylate. The bismuth carbonate is responsible for the protective, antiendotoxic, and weak antibacterial properties.

The salicylate component has antiprostaglandin activity, which may contribute to its effectiveness and reduce symptoms associated with secretory diarrheas. In humans, the preparation is used for other gastrointestinal symptoms (e.g., indigestion, cramps, and gas pains) and in the treatment and prophylaxis of traveler's diarrhea.

CATHARTICS (LAXATIVES)

There are relatively few clinical reasons to use cathartics in veterinary medicine. Occasionally, an older animal may have constipation, but usually alteration of the diet will correct the problem. Another indication might be for the treatment of hair balls in cats. After bowel or anal surgery, stool softeners may reduce stress at the surgery site until healing takes place. Cathartics as well as enemas may also be used before gastrointestinal tract radiographic examinations, proctoscopy, or elective surgery. One of the most legitimate uses of cathartics is in treating food animals and horses suffering with over ingestion of concentrated carbohydrates, such as grain. There are a few other unique circumstances in which the use of cathartics is appropriate; however, one is discouraged from overuse because it leads to dependence.

Cathartics increase the motility of the bowel by directly stimulating the smooth muscle or indirectly activating receptors through increased bulk. The irritant laxatives, which directly increase bowel motility, include (1) *emodin*, found in cascara sagrada, aloe, and senna; (2) *sodium ricinoleate*, a digestive end product of castor oil; and (3) *danthron*, a synthetic compound. Bulk-producing cathartics include (1) indigestible materials, such as psyllium seed, methyl cellulose, mineral oil, and white petrolatum, which not only increase bulk but lubricate and soften the fecal mass; (2) saline cathartics, such as magnesium sulfate, sodium sulfate, magnesium oxide, and phosphate salts, which draw water into the bowel; and (3) stool softeners, such as docusate sodium and dioctyl calcium sulfosuccinate. These are surface-active agents like soap that increase bulk through water retention and lubricate and soften the fecal mass.

The cathartics as a group are relatively safe for short-term use, although some may be harsh and cause cramping and diarrhea. Chronic use of the petrolatum-type cathartics may lead to deficiencies in fat-soluble vitamins because of absorption interference.

ULCER MANAGEMENT DRUGS

Gastric ulceration and subsequent blood loss appear to be related to acid damage commonly associated with high doses of corticosteroids or NSAIDs as well as to certain medical disorders. Several methods are currently available for treatment and prevention.

Antacids were initially used, but they required round-the-clock administration every 2 to 3 hours to truly be effective. A major advancement in human medicine for ulcer management was the introduction of cimetidine, a histamine$_2$ receptor antagonist. Although these agents are not approved for veterinary use, cimetidine, ranitidine, and others are used to block the acid-producing effects of histamine on the gastric parietal cells.

Sucralfate in an acid environment forms an ulcer-adherent complex providing a protective, Band-Aid-like barrier for the damaged mucosa. Sucralfate also inhibits pepsin activity.

Omeprazole is an agent that acts directly on the parietal cell, blocking acid secretion. Omeprazole (Gastrogard, Merial) is an oral gel that is indicated for treatment and prevention of recurrence of gastric ulcers in horses and foals 4 weeks of age and older. *Misoprostol* not only blocks gastric acid secretion but also appears to enhance natural gastromucosal defense mechanisms.

PHARMACY

DRUG LAWS

STATE LAWS

Most state pharmacy laws are primarily concerned with the distribution of drugs within the state. These laws specify who is authorized to prescribe and dispense legend drugs, the licensing of distributors, records required, and certain processing standards.

Because state laws are unique to each state, it is the responsibility of those practicing veterinary medicine to know the laws that apply to them. State laws work in conjunction with federal laws. Sometimes state laws are more restrictive than federal laws; in such cases, one should comply with the state law.

FEDERAL LAWS

Although the Food, Drug, and Cosmetic Act of 1938 has been amended numerous times, it is still the basic federal law governing drugs in the United States. This law assures the public that drugs have been prepared through approved manufacturing standards and are safe as well as effective for the claims made. The Durham-Humphrey Amendment (1951) restricted the availability of certain drugs to prescription through licensed practitioners. This class of drugs, referred to as *prescription drugs* or *legend drugs*, is deemed unsafe for lay medication, even with clear and precise label directions.

✎ TECHNICIAN NOTE

FDA restricts legend drugs to prescription through a licensed practitioner.

Veterinary labeled prescription drugs bear the legend, "Caution: Federal law restricts this drug to use by or on the order of a licensed veterinarian." Human labeled prescription drugs bear the legend, "Caution: Federal law prohibits dispensing without a prescription." Commercial packagers may elect to utilize the *Rx* symbol on the label copy to denote drug product status as a legend drug instead of the written caution.

The FDA has the responsibility for determining the marketing status of a drug, whether or not it is possible to prepare adequate directions for use under which a layperson can use the drug safely and effectively. Nonprescription or *over-the-counter* (OTC) drugs may be sold directly to clients but must bear extensive labeling, which includes warnings as well as instructions for proper use.

The American Veterinary Medical Association has approved the following guidelines regarding the use and distribution of veterinary drugs:

1. A prescription drug can be dispensed only by or upon the lawful written order of a licensed veterinarian within the course of his/her professional practice where a valid veterinarian-client-patient relationship (VCPR) exists.
2. All veterinary prescription drugs must be properly labeled when dispensed.

> **TECHNICIAN NOTE**
>
> A prescription drug can be dispensed to a client only where a VCPR exists.

VETERINARIAN-CLIENT-PATIENT-RELATIONSHIP

A VCPR exists when *all* of the following conditions have been met:
1. The veterinarian has assumed the responsibility for making clinical judgments regarding the health of the animal(s) and the need for medical treatment, and the client has agreed to follow the veterinarian's instruction.
2. The veterinarian has sufficient knowledge of the animal(s) to initiate at least a general or preliminary diagnosis of the medical condition of the animal(s).
3. The veterinarian is readily available for follow-up evaluation, or has arranged for emergency coverage in the event of adverse reactions or failure of the treatment regimen.

LABEL REQUIREMENTS

Labeling requirements vary between states but may include:

- Name, address, and telephone number of clinic
- Name of client
- Animal identification
- Species of animal
- Date

- Prescribing veterinarian
- Name of medication
- Quantity of medication dispensed
- Adequate directions for proper administration of medication
- Number of authorized refills
- Prescription transaction number (optional)

Auxiliary labels may also be required to caution or inform the client. Examples include "shake well," "keep refrigerated," "do not use after (date)," "poison," "external use only," and "for veterinary use only." It is the responsibility of the veterinarian to inform clients to whom prescription drugs are delivered or dispensed about appropriate handling and storage.

The ultimate responsibility for any medication dispensed through a veterinary practice lies with the authorizing veterinarian. In some states, the technician may be allowed to assist the veterinarian by typing labels, counting or pouring, attaching labels, and pricing. The technician *should not issue or refill medications without the veterinarian's approval.* For most medications, this would be in violation of the federal law.

Readily retrievable dispensing records may be required by some states in order to safeguard the public's health. Accidental ingestion of prescription drugs by animals and small children is not uncommon. Proper records can provide attending physicians with the name and the amount of medication dispensed, so appropriate treatment can be provided.

> **TECHNICIAN NOTE**
>
> Readily retrievable dispensing record may be required in order to safeguard the public's health.

The Federal Poison Prevention Packaging Act passed in 1970 requires pharmacists and physicians to dispense medications intended for oral human use in childproof containers. AVMA recommends that prescription drugs to companion animal owners be placed in child-resistant containers. Certain states mandate the use of such. Veterinary clinics failing to use such a safeguard would be highly vulnerable to legal action in a case of accidental poisoning.

CONTROLLED SUBSTANCES

The Controlled Substances Act of 1970 reduced drug abuse by defining certain legal and illegal acts regarding substances of high abuse potential. It established and authorized the Drug Enforcement Administration (DEA) to enforce this law. The law is designed to provide an approved means for proper manufacture, distribution, dispensing, and use of controlled substances through licensing of legitimate handlers of these drugs. This "closed" system has been effective in reducing widespread diversion of these drugs

Table 21-3 SCHEDULE OF CONTROLLED SUBSTANCES

Schedule	Abuse Potential	Dispensing Limits	Distribution Restrictions	Schedule Examples	Comments
I	High	Research use only	DEA form C-222 required	LSD, heroin	No accepted medical use
II	High	Requires written prescription, no refills	DEA form C-222 required	Oxymorphone, sodium pentobarbital injection	Abuse may lead to severe dependence
III	Less than I and II	Oral or written, refills up to five times within 6 mo	DEA registration number	Hycodan, Tylenol with codeine, anabolic steroids	Abuse may lead to moderate dependence
IV	Low	Oral or written, refills up to five times within 6 mo	DEA registration number	Diazepam, phenobarbital	Abuse may lead to limited dependence
V	Low	No DEA limits	DEA registration number	Lomotil, Robitussin AC	Lowest potential for abuse

into the illicit market. Controlled substances are classified into five classes (schedules) according to their use or abuse potential (Table 21-3).

All veterinarians using these drugs in the course of their practice are required to have a DEA license number. Those who engage in administering or dispensing controlled substances in Schedules II, III, IV, and V are required to keep record of such transactions for 2 years. Receiving record for reports of controlled substances received must also be kept for 2 years.

> **TECHNICIAN NOTE**
>
> All veterinarians using controlled drugs in the course of their practice are required to have a DEA license number.

In addition, practitioners who handle controlled substances are required to take an initial inventory at the opening of business of all controlled substances. Biannual inventories are required after the initial inventory. Records for receipts and dispensing of Schedule II substances must be kept separate from all other records. When records for Schedules III, IV, and V drugs are incorporated with other drugs, they should be identified with a red *C* in the lower right-hand corner of the record. All controlled substance records must be "readily retrievable." Each commercial container of a controlled substance shall have printed on the label the symbol designating the schedule in which such is listed (CII). The word *Schedule* need not be used.

> **TECHNICIAN NOTE**
>
> All controlled substance records must be "readily retrievable."

Acquisition and distribution of controlled substances should be monitored by maintenance of a perpetual inventory (Figure 21-9) for each product stored in the practice. Drugs in Schedule II must be ordered on a DEA Form C-222 and completed when drugs are received.

A perpetual inventory is a "checkbook" balance system that provides an up-to-date balance of each drug. It is easier to reconcile inventory when this system is used.

It is best that those persons responsible for handling controlled substances be familiar not only with federal laws governing them but also with state laws, which may be more strict. Agencies such as the State Board of Pharmacy or the local DEA office are quite helpful in answering questions concerning compliance.

The law states that, "A practitioner who has controlled substances stored in his office or clinic must keep these drugs in a securely locked, substantially constructed cabinet or safe." A secure area is usually interpreted as a double-locked container that cannot be picked up and moved. Examples would be a locked metal box stored inside a floor safe or an attached locked wall cabinet. The responsibility for access to controlled substances should be restricted to only one or two people in the practice. Practitioners experiencing theft or significant loss of controlled substances must report such loss to the DEA regional office and the local police department when the loss is discovered.

> **TECHNICIAN NOTE**
>
> Controlled substances should be stored in a securely locked, substantially constructed cabinet or safe.

A government publication entitled the *Act of Physician's Manual: An Information Outline on the Controlled Substances 1970* is an excellent guide for proper handling of controlled substances. This government manual may be obtained free by request from the following:

US Department of Justice
Drug Enforcement Administration
1465 I Street, NW
Washington, DC 20537

CONTROLLED DRUG INVENTORY

Date	Dept. Rm No.	Vendor	Invoice No./ Control No.	Quantity Received	Quantity Issued	Balance on Hand	RPh	Date	Dept. Rm No.	Vendor	Invoice No./ Control No.	Quantity Received	Quantity Issued	Balance on Hand	RPh
			BEGINNING BALANCE →→→		→→→	20	MA								
1/2/04	SAICU		108221		1	19	MA								
1/7/04	SAICU		108236		1	18	SB								
1/9/04		M/D	9162710	25		43	MA								
1/10/04	63415		108376		1	42	MA								
1/13/04	64489		108389		1	41	SB								
1/15/04	64285		108401		1	42	MA								

FENTANYL TRANSDERMAL 75 MCG/HR (DURAGESIC)

Figure 21-9 Controlled drug inventory form.

EXPIRATION DATES AND DISPOSAL OF DRUGS

EXPIRATION DATES

The concept behind expiration dates is that the prescriber and consumer can be confident the potency of the drug remains unaffected during the time of use. The expiration date guarantees if the drug is stored properly as instructed by the manufacturer, no toxic by-products accumulate prior to completion of drug regimen.

Some manufacturers first began putting expiration dates on drugs in the 1960s. Although it was not required, FDA began to mandate this practice in 1979 in order to set uniform testing and reporting guidelines.

The expiration date is set by the manufacturer after stability studies have been submitted to FDA. This date is required in all labeling and should be clearly expressed as month, day, and year (i.e., 1/5/04 = January 5, 2004) and not as a code.

> **✎ TECHNICIAN NOTE**
>
> Expiration dates are set by the manufacturer and should be clearly expressed on labels as month, date, and year or month and year.

If this date is stated only in terms of month and year, according to U.S. Pharmacopeia (USP), the product becomes expired the last day of the stated month (i.e., 3/04 = March 31, 2004).

If a drug has not been stored properly and the integrity of the product has been compromised, the product's safety and effectiveness is questioned and should not be used. If a bottle of pills is wet or has been kept in a room with extremely high humidity and temperatures, the medication may go bad before its expiration date. Freezing temperatures may also ruin a drug's effectiveness. If capsules are sticking together or the shiny coat of a tablet is rubbing off in your hands, the drug may be degrading because it is stored in a place that is too humid. If a solution changes color or consistency, the product is light sensitive and has been stored under direct light. It should not be used even if the expiration date has not passed.

Drugs regulated by Environmental Protection Agency (EPA) (i.e., Advantage, Bayer Animal Health) have no labeled expiration dates. The required shelf life is a minimum of 5 years.

Homeopathic medicine is medication that works with your whole body to restore your health and is made from all natural substances. Unlike *synthetic* or man-made drugs, they never lose their potency or efficacy because all of the components are natural and not combined with any unnatural substances that will expire. If exposed to very strong scents, left out in extreme heat or cold for a period of time, or contaminated by returning pills back to the bottle after they have been handled, they may be ineffective. If this happens, it is better to throw the product away. Do not reuse the bottle; send them to a recycling center. Homeopathic medicines are exempt from labeling laws that require expiration dates.

> **✎ TECHNICIAN NOTE**
>
> Homeopathic medicines are exempt from labeling laws that require expiration dates.

Commercially prepared products that are reconstituted (mixed with a diluent) prior to administration or repackaged must be labeled with an appropriate period limiting the time of use. If products are compounded, the compounder must establish an expiration date and appropriate withdrawal times for food-producing animals.

DISPOSAL OF DRUGS

Regardless of how well managed inventory control is, every facility will have drugs expire or unwanted drugs that need disposal. EPA states that a drug product only becomes outdated when the decision is made to discard it. While flushing was once, and in many instances still is, the most commonly used method of disposing left-over and expired medications, there are environmental concerns resulting from hormones and antibiotics contaminating drinking water supplies.

The Department of Environmental Quality (DEQ), EPA, FDA, and local boards of pharmacy have established guidelines to regulate drug disposal.

All drugs for discard are to be separated from usable stock and clearly marked as "outdated."

Medications that can be returned for credit are sent back to the manufacturer, distributor, or *reverse distribution company* (RDC)—a company that serves as liaison between purchaser and vendor for credit. The purchaser will need to establish an account with the RDC of their choice before any drugs are sent to them.

When using an RDC, make sure it is understood which items were purchased or received using special programs so that problems won't be incurred in getting credit at the correct price. Understand that their fee for this service comes off the top, so that your credit for returns will be less than the statement.

Items that are unacceptable for credit may also be discarded through the RDC on a "by-the-pound" basis. In most instances, this is determined after the medications reach the company. As an alternative, those items that are not accepted for credit may be destroyed through some waste disposal companies.

Open containers may be placed in the Biological Waste Collection Containers for disposal. Prior arrangements must be made with the companies for destruction of medications.

DEA regulates the disposal of controlled drugs. In no case should controlled drugs be forwarded to the DEA. The procedures established shall not be construed as altering, in any way, state laws or regulation for disposal of controlled substances.

The only approved method of disposal of controlled substances by DEA is through the hire of an RDC. The registrant (clinic) should complete a C-II Request Form (disposition and reporting form for expired Schedule II pharmaceuticals) from the RDC. This will list all C-II drugs that will need disposal, including partial containers. After completing the form and sending it back to the RDC, the registrant will receive the triplicate form C-222 (U.S. Official Order Forms—Schedules I and II). The registrant now becomes the supplier and will keep the suppliers copy (now in brown color). The blue copy (purchaser's copy) and green copy (DEA copy) are included in the box of drugs to be sent to RDC. The green copy is then forwarded to DEA by the RDC.

> **✎ TECHNICIAN NOTE**
>
> DEA only approves disposal of controlled substances through use of a reverse distribution company.

An inventory should be taken of all controlled drugs in Schedules III to V. The registrant should submit a written or type written list of every item for disposal to the RDC. A copy of the list should be filed with the registrant.

After receipt and disposal of all drugs, the RDC will send the following records to the registrant as necessary:

1. C-II manifest (DEA Form #41—Registrants Inventory of Drugs Surrendered)
2. Returnable manifest (credit listed)
3. Nonreturnable manifest (drugs destroyed)

All records pertaining to disposal of drugs should be kept for 2 years as required by DEA.

Used drug containers should be disposed of properly to reduce the risk of environmental contamination with chemicals. Always use the manufacturer's label recommendation for disposal of empty or partial containers. Unused products should not be dumped down a drain, a toilet, or on the ground. Disinfectants should be added to unused portions of live or modified live vaccines to reduce accidental exposure to disease.

Disposal of medical wastes may be regulated by your state. Contact the agency in your state that oversees the disposal of medical waste. A list of agencies can be found at the following EPA Web site: www.epa.gov/epasewer/osu/stateweb.htm

MATERIAL SAFETY DATA SHEETS

The U.S. Occupational Safety and Health Administration (OSHA) under the authorization of the U.S. Department of Labor set forth standards for current practice relations and requirements. The OSHA Act of 1970 was enacted to ensure the safe and healthful working conditions for working men and women (see Chapter 36). The law was based on the simple concept that every employee has the basic "right to know" the potential hazard of any substance in the workplace. Employees also need to know what protective measures are available to prevent adverse effects from occurring. Along with the federal government, the U.S. chemical industry developed a chemical identification system. It requires a paper document to accompany every chemical shipped, used, or stored. These paper documents are called *Material Safety Data Sheets* (MSDSs) and are sent to users such as industries, hospitals, universities, clinics, and others when the chemicals are sent. The company that produces the chemicals writes the MSDS. Every drug and pharmaceutical aid has a MSDS. A file of these fact sheets must by maintained in the veterinary practice and be accessible to every employee.

> **✎ TECHNICIAN NOTE**
>
> OSHA requires a file of MSDSs because every employee has a need and right to know the hazards and identities of the chemicals he or she is exposed to when working.

The essential parts to a MSDS are as follows:

1. *Name, address*, and *telephone number* of manufacturer or supplier
2. *Chemical name* as it appears on the container's label: common name; scientific name: trade name or brand name that the manufacturer uses; synonyms for the mixture or chemicals
3. For hazardous ingredients, the MSDS should list
   a. The *permissible exposure level* (PEL): amount of an air contaminant a worker can be exposed to four 40-hour work weeks over a working lifetime (30 years), without suffering adverse drug reaction
   b. The *threshold limit value* (TLV): amount of a substance in the air nearly everyone can be exposed to daily without adverse drug reactions
4. *Physical properties:* vapor pressure; specific gravity; appearance and odor; solubility; boiling point; melting point; freezing point; vapor density; evaporation rate.
5. *Potential for fire and explosion data:* flash point (when will a fire start and what should be done about it); flammability or explosive limit [lower explosive limit (LEL) and upper explosive limit (UEL)]—numbers used to describe the range in which fire or explosion can occur; extinguishing media required to put out class A, B, C, and D fires.
6. *Health hazards:*
   a. Body entry by inhalation, ingestion, or transdermally
   b. The short-term (acute) and long-term (chronic) harmful effects

c. Carcinogenicity (cancer producing), corrosive, or sensitizer (an allergen or irritant that after an initial sensitizing exposure, produced atopic or contact dermatitis), irritant, target organ effector

7. *Reactivity*: conditions under which a chemical reaction will occur either by itself or with other materials, e.g., whether the chemical bonds are strong or weak and make the substance stable or unstable, incompatibility with other substances storage compatibilities, whether the substances will break down under conditions and release toxic or flammable vapor or gas, or whether *hazardous polymerization* can occur (a chemical reaction that can cause a fire or explosion and possibly release hazardous gases)

8. *Spill or leak procedures*: precautions for disposal of released substances taken during handling and storage

9. *Special precautions*: respiratory protection, ventilation, protective clothing and gear, and hygiene practices

10. *Special precautions*: first-aid in case of exposure

MSDSs are written for:
- Employees who may by exposed to hazard at work
- Employers who need to know proper methods of storage, etc.
- Emergency responders such as firefighters, hazardous material crews, emergency medical technicians, and emergency room personnel

MSDS are not intended for consumers. It reflects the hazard of working with a material in an occupational fashion. Employees must have ready access to MSDSs while in the workplace. MSDSs must be on hand for every hazardous chemical known to be present in the workplace in such a manner that employees may by exposed under normal conditions for use or in a foreseeable emergency.

CALCULATIONS

There is no need to fear calculations involved in the dose and the compounding of medications. Most are simple arithmetic. A methodical approach to each problem will simplify the concept and minimize the risk of error. Remember the following:

- If you are transferring data from a reference source, double-check what you have written down.
- Write down every step; express all quantities in the same system of units.
- Do not take short cuts; you are more likely to make a mistake.
- Try not to be totally dependent on your calculator. There is something to be said for common sense. Have an approximate idea of what the answer should be, and then if you happen to hit the wrong button on the

calculator, you are more likely to be aware that an error has been made.
- Finally, always double-check your calculations. There is frequently more than one way of doing a calculation; so if you get the same answer by two different methods, the chances are your answer is correct. Alternatively, try working the problem in reverse to see if you get the starting numbers.

EXPRESSION OF CONCENTRATION

The metric system is the International System of Units (SI) for weight, volume, and length. The basic unit for weight is gram (g), while the basic unit for volume is the liter (L), and the basic unit of length is the meter (m). The prefix *milli-* indicates one thousandth (10^{-3}) and *micro-*, one millionth (10^{-6}).

In some countries, the avoirdupois system (pounds and ounces) is still used in commerce and daily life. The apothecary system of volume (pints and gallons) is still a common system for commerce and household measurement. One should be aware of these systems in order to avoid serious errors in interpretation of prescriptions. It is important to be able to change between the systems (Box 21-3).

Examples of unit conversions:

1. Express 70 grains in metric units (to two decimal places).
   You know: 1 grain (gr) = 64.8 milligrams (mg).
   Let Y = Unknown number of milligrams.

   Therefore: $\dfrac{60 \text{ mg}}{1 \text{ grain}} = \dfrac{Y \text{ mg}}{70 \text{ grains}}$

   $Y = \dfrac{60 \text{ mg}}{1 \text{ grain}} \times 70 \text{ grains}$

   $Y = \textbf{4200 mg.}$

   To change the units to grams:
   You know: 1 gram (g) = 1000 mg
   Let X = Unknown number of grams.

   Therefore: $\dfrac{1 \text{ gram}}{1000 \text{ mg}} = \dfrac{X \text{ g}}{4200 \text{ mg}}$

   $X = \dfrac{1 \text{ g}}{1000 \text{ mg}} \times 4200 \text{ mg}$

   $X = \textbf{4.20 g}$ (to two decimal places)

2. Sulphacetamide eye drops contain 200 drops in a 10-ml bottle. Calculate the volume of one drop.
   You know that 200 drops = 10 ml (20 drops = 1 ml).
   Let y = volume of one drop.
   Therefore, $y/1$ drop = 10 ml/200 drops = **0.05 ml**.

EXPRESSION OF STRENGTH

Ratio is the relative magnitude of two like quantities.
Ratio strength is the expression of a concentration by means of a ratio, for example, 1:10.

Box 21-3 MATHEMATICS CONVERSION CHART

ABBREVIATIONS
Weight
grain = grain
gram = g
kilogram = kg
milligram = mg
microgram = μg
pound = lb

Volume
cubic centimeter = cm³
drop = gtt
gallon = gal
liter = L
milliliter = ml
ounce = oz
pint = pt
quart = qt
tablespoon = tbsp
teaspoon = tsp
unit = unit

CONVERSIONS
Weight Conversions
1 g = 1000 mg
1 mg = 1000 μg
1 g (mass) = 1 ml (volume)
1 kg (mass) = 1 L (volume)
1 lb = 16 oz
1 lb = 454 g
1 grain = 60 mg

Volume Conversions
1 L = 1000 ml
1 L = 32 oz
1 ml = 1 cm³
1 drop = 0.05 ml
1 ml = 15-16 drops
1 tsp = 5 ml
1 tbsp = 15 ml
1 oz = 30 ml
1 gal = 3785 ml
1 pt = 473 ml
1 qt = 960 ml

Percentage strength is a ratio of parts per hundred, for example, 10%.

Thus 1:10 = 1 part in 10 parts total volume of solution.

If 1 ml of glucose is in 10 ml of solution, the ratio is 1:10. Therefore, 10 ml of glucose is in 100 ml of solution. This can be expressed as a percentage; so it is equivalent to a 10% volume/volume (vol/vol) solution. The same concept applies whether the expression is % volume/volume (vol/vol), % weight/volume (wt/vol), or % weight/weight (wt/wt).

TECHNICIAN NOTE
The ratio 1:10 does not mean 1 ml of glucose and 10 ml of water. It means 1 ml of glucose and 9 ml water (1 ml of glucose in 10 ml total volume of solution).

1. Express 0.1% wt/wt as ratio strength.
   You know 0.1% = 0.1 g/100 g.
   Let Y = total parts.
   Therefore, 0.1 g/100 g = 1 part/Y parts.
   $Y = 100 \times 1/0.1 = 1000$.
   The ratio strength = 1:1000.
2. Express 1:2500 as percentage strength.
   You know that percentage is a ratio of parts/100 parts.
   Let Y = percentage strength.
   Therefore, 1 part/2500 parts = Y parts/100 parts.
   $Y = 1 \times 100/2500 = 0.04\%$.
3. Express 1 part per million (ppm) as percentage strength.
   You know that ppm is another expression of ratio strength (ppm = 1 part per million = 1:1,000,000).

Let Y be the percentage strength.
Therefore, 1 part/1,000,000 = Y parts/100 parts.
$Y = 1 \times 100/1,000,000 = 0.0001\% = 1 \times 10^{-4}\%$.

Percentage weight in weight (wt/wt) is the number of grams of an active ingredient in 100 g (solid or liquid).

4. How many grams of a drug should be used to prepare 200 g of a 5% wt/wt solution?
   You know 5% = 5 g/100 g.
   Let Y = the weight of the drug needed.
   Therefore, $Y/200 = 5$ g/100 g
   $Y = 5 \times 200/100 = 10$ g.

Percentage weight in volume (wt/vol) is the number of grams of an active ingredient in 100 ml of liquid.

5. If 6 g of iodine are in 240 ml of iodine tincture, calculate the percentage of iodine in the tincture.
   You know that % weight in volume is part (g)/100 ml.
   Let Y = percentage of iodine in the tincture.
   Therefore, $Y/100$ ml = 6 g/240 ml.
   $Y = 6 \times 100/240 = 2.5\%$ wt/vol.

Percentage volume in volume (vol/vol) indicates the number of milliliters of an active ingredient in 100 ml of liquid.

6. If 20 ml of Betadine are mixed with water to make 60 ml of solution, what is the percentage of Betadine in the solution? You know that % volume in volume

is part (ml)/100 ml. Let Y be the percentage of Betadine in the solution.

Therefore, Y/100 ml = 20 ml/60 ml.

$Y = 20 \times 100/60 = 33\%$ vol/vol.

7. Express 15 g of dextrose in 300 ml of solution as a percentage, indicating wt/wt, wt/vol, or vol/vol.

You know that weight (g)/volume (ml) is expressed as % wt/vol.

Let Y grams be the weight of dextrose in 100 ml.

Therefore, Y/100 ml = 15 g/300 ml

$Y = 15 \times 100/300$ ml = 5% wt/vol.

8. What is the percentage of sodium chloride in the following syrup?

Sodium chloride 10 g

Dextrose 420 g

Water q.s. ad 1000 ml

You know that percentage is the number of grams (wt) of sodium chloride in 100 ml (vol) of syrup.

Therefore, Y/100 ml = 10 g/1000 ml.

$Y = 10 \times 100/1000 = 1\%$ wt/vol.

CALCULATING THE STRENGTH OF A DRUG SOLUTION

The following basic equation is used to calculate the concentration of a liquid dosage form:

Concentration (g/ml) = Mass (g)/Volume (ml)

If you know any two of these quantities, the third can be found.

Example 1: What is the strength of a 1-L solution containing 50 g of drug?

You know

1. Volume of solution (1 L = 1000 ml)
2. Mass of drug (50 g)

Solution:

Substitute all known quantities in the equation. Solve for the unknown:

Concentration (g/ml) = 50 g/1000 ml = 5 g/100 ml 100% = 5% solution.

Manipulation of this equation is frequently used for finding the quantity (mass) of a given volume of drug solution at a known concentration:

Mass (g) = Volume (ml) × Concentration (g/ml)

Example 2: How much drug is needed to prepare 4 oz of a 2% solution?

You know

1. Volume of solution (4 oz = 120 ml)
2. Concentration of solution (2% = 2 g/100 ml)

Solution:

Substitute all known quantities in the equation. Solve for the unknown:

Mass (g) = 120 ml 2 g/100 ml = 2.4 g

The original equation is also used to find out the total volume of drug solution that can be prepared at a desired concentration with a given quantity of drug:

Volume (ml) = Mass (g)/Concentration (g/ml)

Example 3: How much of a 10% solution can be prepared with 15 g of drug?

You know

1. Concentration of desired solution (10% = 10 g/100 ml)
2. Mass of drug (15 g)

Solution:

Substitute all known quantities in the equation. Solve for the unknown:

Volume (ml) = 15 g/10 g/100 ml = 150 ml

CALCULATING THE STRENGTH OF DILUTED SOLUTIONS

A basic equation can be used to solve problems for dilution stock (concentrated) solutions. [A more concentrated (stronger) solution can never be made from a diluted (weaker) solution without adding pure drug.]

Concentration of desired solution × Volume of desired solution = Concentration of stock × Volume of stock

Knowing any three of these quantities, one can solve for the unknown.

Example 1: Prepare 2 qt of a 1:1000 solution from a 20% solution.

You know

1. Concentration of desired solution (1:1000 = 1 g/1000 ml)
2. Volume of desired solution (2 qt = approximately 2000 ml)
3. Concentration of stock (20% = 20 g/100 ml)

Solution:

Substitute all known quantities in the equation. Solve for the unknown:

Volume of stock solution (ml) × 20 g/100 ml = 2000 ml × 1 g/1000 ml = 10 ml

Example 2: How much of a 1% solution can be prepared from 6 ml of a 5% solution?

You know

1. Concentration of desired solution (1% = 1 g/100 ml)
2. Volume of stock (6 ml)
3. Concentration of stock (5% = 5 g/100 ml)

Solution:

Substitute all known quantities in the equation. Solve for the unknown:

Volume of desired solution (ml) × 1 g/100 ml = 5 g/100 ml × 6 ml = 30 ml

CALCULATING DRUG DOSAGES

A drug dosage is expressed as units or mass of drug per body weight (BW) of the patient. The usual dosage for human drugs is based on the ideal BW of 140 lb (70 kg). There is no ideal BW in veterinary medicine because of the variety of species and breeds of animals. The usual drug dose for animals is based on BW expressed in pounds or kilograms.

The following equation is used for calculating the quantity of drug to be administered based on BW:

$$\frac{\text{BW} \times \text{Dosage}}{\text{Concentration of drug}} = \text{Volume of drug (dose)}$$

Example 1: An 88-lb dog is to receive a drug dosage of 25 mg/kg of BW. How many milliliters of the supplied drug at 50 mg/ml are required?
1. Drug dosage (25 ml/kg of BW)
2. Animal's body weight (88 lb = 40 kg)
3. Concentration of drug solution (50 mg/ml

Solution:

Substitute all known quantities in the equation. Solve for the unknown:

Volume of drug = 40 kg × 25 mg/kg / 50 mg/ml = 20 ml (dose)

The dosage of highly toxic drugs such as *antineoplastic* (anticancer) agents is calculated on the basis of body surface area (BSA). BSA is difficult to calculate. Nomograms and charts (Table 21-4) have been constructed to help relate BW to BSA. BSA is expressed in square meters (m^2).

To determine dosage based of BSA, modification of the previous equation will enable this:

$$\frac{\text{BSA (m}^2) \times \text{Drug dosage}}{\text{Concentration of drug}} = \text{Volume of drug}$$

Example 2: A 44-lb dog is to receive a dosage of 0.2 mg/m^2. What volume of a drug should be given at a concentration of 1 mg/ml?

You know
1. BSA (44 lb = 20 kg = 0.74 m^2)
2. Drug dosage (0.2 ml/m^2)
3. Concentration of drug solution (1 mg/ml)

Solution:

Substitute all known quantities in the equation. Solve for the unknown:

Volume of drug solution = 0.74 m^2 × 0.2 mg/m^2/1 mg/ml = 0.148 ml

CALCULATING INFUSION RATES

Many drugs must be administered intravenously by slow infusion rather than as a rapid bolus injection. Large volumes of fluids are also given by intravenous infusion. Disposable intravenous sets and infusion pumps are used to deliver intravenous fluids at a steady rate over a period of time.

Table 21-4 CONVERSION TABLES FOR WEIGHT (KG) TO BODY SURFACE AREA (M₂)

Dogs				Cats	
kg	M²	kg	m²	Kg	m²
0.5	0.06	33	1.03	2.0	0.159
1	0.10	34	1.05	2.5	0.184
2	0.15	35	1.07	3.0	0.208
3	0.20	36	1.09	3.5	0.231
4	0.25	37	1.11	4.0	0.252
5	0.29	38	1.13	4.5	0.273
6	0.33	39	1.15	5.0	0.292
7	0.36	40	1.17	5.5	0.311
8	0.40	41	1.19	6.0	0.330
9	0.43	42	1.21	6.5	0.348
10	0.46	43	1.23	7.0	0.366
11	0.49	44	1.25	7.5	0.383
12	0.52	45	1.26	8.0	0.400
13	0.55	46	1.28	8.5	0.416
14	0.58	47	1.30	9.0	0.432
15	0.60	48	1.32	9.5	0.449
16	0.63	49	1.34	10	0.464
17	0.66	50	1.36		
18	0.69	52	1.41		
19	0.71	54	1.44		
20	0.74	56	1.48		
21	0.76	58	1.51		
22	0.78	60	1.55		
23	0.81	62	1.58		
24	0.83	64	1.62		
25	0.85	66	1.65		
26	0.88	68	1.68		
27	0.90	70	1.72		
28	0.92	72	1.75		
29	0.94	74	1.78		
30	0.96	76	1.81		
31	0.99	78	1.84		
32	1.01	80	1.88		

Calculations of infusion rates can be found by using the following equations:

Rate (drops/min) = **Total volume to be administered (ml)/Total time of infusion (hr)** × **Conversion of hours to minutes (1 hr/60 min)** × **Calibrated IV set (drops/ml)**

Example 1: If 500 ml of a solution is to be infused over 6 hours, what is the correct infusion rate (drops/min) if the set delivers 10 drops/ml?

You know
1. Drops/min calibration of intravenous set (10 drops/ml)
2. Volume of solution to be infused (500 ml)
3. Hours of infusion (6 hr)
4. Conversion of hours to minutes (1 hr/60 min)

Solution:

Substitute all known quantities in the equation. Solve for the unknown.

Rate (drops/min) = 500 ml/6 hr × 1 hr/60 min × 10 drops/ml = 13.89 drops/min

Example 2: If a drug is to be infused at a dosage rate of 2 µg/kg/min into a 50-lb animal, what rate (ml/hr) should a pump be set on for a drug concentration of 400 mg in 250 ml of dextrose 5%?

You know

1. Dosage rate = 2 µg/kg/min
2. Weight of patient = 50 lb (22.73 kg)
3. Concentration of drug solution 400 mg/250 ml = 1.60 mg/ml

$$
\begin{aligned}
\text{Constant rate infusion (ml/hr)} = &\ \text{Dosage rate (µg/kg/min)} \\
&\times \text{weight (kg)} \\
&\times \text{conversion of min to} \\
&\ \text{hour (60 min/1 hr)} \\
&\times \text{conversion of µg to mg} \\
&\ (1\ \text{mg}/1000\ \text{µg})/ \\
&\ \text{concentration (mg/ml)}
\end{aligned}
$$

Solution:

Substitute all known quantities in the equations. Solve for the unknown:

Constant rate infusion (ml/hr) = 2 µg/kg/min × 22.73 kg = 45.46 µg/min

45.46 µg/min × 60 min/1 hr = 2727.6 µg/hr

2727.6 µg/hr × 1 mg/1000 µg = 2.72 mg/hr

2.72 mg/hr/1.60 mg/ml = 1.70 ml/hr

INVENTORY CONTROL

The maintenance of an active working inventory requires both planning and continuous monitoring. Failure to keep abreast of use and needs results in shortage, inefficient use of time, increased costs, and added stress. The time invested to maintain appropriate levels of stock is therefore beneficial to the overall operations of the practice.

Veterinary technicians who demonstrate interest in an active inventory may find themselves acquiring an increasing role in inventory control and maintenance. Assuming this additional responsibility not only increases employee value in the practice but also adds to job satisfaction.

Ideally, the quantities of each item stocked should be as small as possible without running out between reasonable ordering periods. Because it is worse to have a shortage of certain items than to have extra, most practices lean toward a higher inventory than actually required. *Inventory turnover* (the number of times per year an item is bought and sold) should be at least four to six times per year. Some items, such as pet food, may turn over 12 to 14 times per year. With the assistance of a computer, monitoring of daily usage, and keeping helpful records, the average turnover rate can usually be increased. The higher the turnover, the lower the investment in the item. Drug ordering can become a full-time duty if care is not given to organization and planning.

> **✎ TECHNICIAN NOTE**
>
> Inventory turnover (the number of times per year an item is bought and sold) should be at least four to six times per year.

INVENTORY MAINTENANCE

The primary disadvantage of having a large inventory is the expense of having working capital tied up in drugs and supplies. A large inventory makes switching to equivalent products difficult, even at a cheaper price. There is great potential for product outdates, breakage, spoilage, and obsolescence when the inventory is large. Some states have an inventory tax that provides added incentive for keeping working stock to a minimum.

Occasionally, there is some justification for increasing the purchase of certain products. The "savings" claimed through many of the deals offered by vendors should be approached with caution. Unless one can accurately predict the use of certain products, quantity buying is difficult to justify. To participate in most marketing promotions, a significant financial commitment is usually required. Before entering into these agreements, one should truly determine whether the products offered are desirable and will be used within a reasonable period and whether the savings really merit the capital commitment.

Processing small orders is costly because the time commitment required to process the order is not much different from that of a larger order with several items. One is justified in increasing quantities on these small orders, especially if the items are inexpensive, to reduce ordering frequency and cost of acquisition. Some vendors charge handling fees if the total order is below a minimal required dollar amount or volume.

Availability of replacement goods is a factor that will affect the inventory turnover. With some items, one may be able to accurately predict monthly use and maintain a few weeks' supply. Unfortunately, the use of most items cannot be readily anticipated, which results in larger inventory requirement, especially if delivery time cannot by predicted.

PROCUREMENT

Veterinary Suppliers

One may purchase supplies through veterinary wholesale suppliers (distributors) or directly from manufacturers. Distributors may specialize in one class of items, such as surgical supplies or bulk pharmaceuticals. Some wholesale suppliers may offer a complete line of products, ranging from buckets to gas machines.

One advantage in dealing with wholesalers is the ability to reduce the number of small orders that would be required in purchasing from several individual vendors. A few manufacturers only sell their products directly to veterinarians rather than distributors. *Compendium of Veterinary Products* (see Recommended Reading) offers a complete reference to veterinary pharmaceutical companies and their product lines.

Veterinary Practices

It is an excellent idea to establish and maintain a good working relationship with another practice in the area. In a crisis, you can borrow items from that practice to see you through the emergency. Borrowing seldom-used items in an emergency is encouraged rather than stocking them. However, your practice is expected to order the item and return it. Thus, inventory of seldom-used items should be maintained elsewhere and record keeping is not necessary. Purchasing some items from another practice may be helpful, especially for expensive, short-dated items.

Several large buying groups have been established by some practices to increase their purchasing power and decrease costs.

Pharmacies and Drug Wholesalers

Using the services of a retail pharmacy is nearly essential to the practice of quality veterinary medicine. Veterinarians have need for various human products that are not obtainable through veterinary suppliers. Retail pharmacies may not stock many injectable products, but they can help with most ophthalmic and oral products and some topical preparations. In some locations, a human drug wholesaler may deal directly with the small, individual practitioner. Most, however, do not welcome these small accounts and will serve only as a distributor for hospitals and pharmacies. The veterinary practitioner must make arrangements with pharmacists to obtain human products for practice or client use. Most pharmacists welcome this opportunity to serve the veterinarian.

Human Hospitals and Hospital Suppliers

A local human hospital may be a valuable resource for the veterinary clinic. Federal laws restrict hospitals with special buying privileges from selling to anyone outside their institution. As a result, it may be difficult for veterinarians and their clients to obtain some of the more potent, expensive, or rarely used medical supplies, except in an emergency. Practicing veterinarians should make human hospital contacts to determine the local availability of human drugs and supplies. The hospital's library and clinical laboratory may also provide some welcome assistance.

Local hospital suppliers will stock items such as syringes, needles, cotton balls, tongue depressors, and other disposable supplies. Although veterinarians do not routinely purchase from the local hospital, do not overlook them as an immediate source in times of shortages.

Other Sources of Suppliers

In addition to bulk chemicals, major chemical suppliers will stock glassware, balances, disposable beakers, brushes, carboys, and other laboratory and clinic supplies and equipment that would be useful in a veterinary practice. Most of these suppliers are located in metropolitan areas and have addresses and telephone numbers listed in the telephone directory.

Numerous mail order suppliers exist that provide not only pharmaceuticals but also a wide variety of veterinary products and equipment. The quality of product and service may vary greatly among these outlets. Of major concern is the return policy for handling inferior or unacceptable items.

Feed stores and lay veterinary drug outlets can be used for an occasional urgently needed item. One may at times also want to take advantage of certain specials offered through these suppliers.

ORGANIZING THE PHARMACY

A comprehensive list of all activities conducted in the pharmacy should be prepared whether planning a major hospital complex or rearranging a small portion of a hospital. Activities related to the pharmacy include storage (refrigeration, security), ordering, receiving, cleanup, dispensing, withdrawal and administration of medication, compounding and manufacturing, product information, and so forth. In the design, the location of each activity must be determined, and each activity should be coordinated with other areas when required. Although most areas will be multifunctional, some activities may be unique and have their own special requirements.

Regulating agencies require that refrigerators that store vaccines and biologicals should be kept at 40° C. Minor fluctuations in temperature may occur. A daily temperature log must be maintained (Figure 21-10). Personal foodstuffs should not be stored in the refrigerator designated for pharmacy use.

> ## ⌦ TECHNICIAN NOTE
> Refrigerators should be kept at 40° C. Personal foodstuffs should be stored separately.

A detailed list of functions pertaining specifically to the pharmacy inventory should include the following:

- *Ordering* requires a telephone, desk, file, and calculator
- *Receiving* should be near an outside door and requires temporary counter or floor space.
- *Returns* require space for holding broken items, outdated items, and damaged items.
- *Storage* areas must be adequate for working and backup stock. Refrigeration for perishable items and security for volatile hazardous bulk materials.
- *Pricing* involves the use of a computer or price book, markup schemes, record, and a collection of material safety data sheets (MSDS) for all products.

REFRIGERATOR / FREEZER TEMPERATURE MONITORING CHART

Refrigerator Location: _____ Month: _____ Year: _____

Used for (√ One):   ❏ Medications   ❏ Staff   ❏ Nourishment   ❏ Other:_____

Freezer in Use: ❏ Yes   ❏ No

Refrigerator Acceptable Range: 35-40 Degrees Fahrenheit or 2-8 Degrees Centigrade

Freezer Acceptable Range: Less than 0 Degrees Fahrenheit or Less than -18 Degrees Centigrade

** *IF THE TEMPERATURE FALLS OUTSIDE OF THE ACCEPTABLE RANGE, NOTIFY SUPERVISOR IMMEDIATELY AND RECORD ALL CORRECTIVE ACTION TAKEN ON THIS FORM.*

Date	Refrigerator	Freezer	Initials	Cleaned	Thawed	Corrective Action Taken	Initials
1							
2							
3							
4							
5							
6							
7							
8							
9							
10							
11							
12							
13							
14							
15							
16							
17							
18							
19							
20							
21							
22							
23							
24							
25							
26							
27							
28							
29							
30							
31							

PF-IC-1049 (Rev. 07/02)

Figure 21-10 Refrigerator/freezer temperature monitoring chart.

In addition, consideration should be given to the movement of items to areas of use for dispensing. Monitoring of inventory levels of all items is a much-needed function to ensure an adequate supply on demand without shortages.

ARRANGEMENT OF INVENTORY

Working inventory should be placed on shelves in an organized fashion. One method is to arrange items by dosage form. Categories would include the following:

- Oral solids (tablets, capsules)
- Oral liquids
- Oral miscellaneous (boluses, powders, pastes)
- External liquids
- External miscellaneous (sprays, powders, ointments, creams)
- Ophthalmic drugs (ointments, suspensions, solutions)
- Small-volume injectables
- Large-volume injectables
- Mastitis preparations
- Miscellaneous, such as chemicals for compounding

Each section should be further arranged, perhaps by generic name, brand name, or more common name used by individuals in the practice. One may wish to make exceptions for items that are popular, but they should be limited.

A different type of arrangement would be to group items by their most common therapeutic use. Classification would be similar to that in the discussion of drugs found in the first portion of this chapter:

- Analgesics
- Anesthetics
- Antibiotics
- Anticonvulsants
- Antiinflammatory drugs
- Antineoplastic agents
- Cardiovascular drugs
- Diuretics
- Fluids and electrolytes
- Gastrointestinal drugs
- Hormones and related substances
- Other antibacterial drugs
- Parasiticides
- Tranquilizers
- Vitamins

Each drug class could then be further divided into more specific uses, such as GI drugs divided into antiemetics, emetics, and antidiarrheals. Some classes may have only two or three items. Disadvantages of using this system are the poor use of shelf space and the possibility of gallon jugs ending up next to ampules.

Another arrangement is to group items by company or vendor. This method may be acceptable for backup stock because it is helpful when preparing orders. In an active inventory there may be poor use of shelf space. Perhaps the greatest disadvantage is trying to recall the last supplier for rarely used items. Another disadvantage is purchasing generic items from multiple vendors, which may lead to multiple locations of the same item and duplicate stock.

Pharmacy organization is desirable and has advantages, primarily by assisting each individual in locating items. The best method of organizing stock is probably a combination of these various arrangements. Each practice should design its own method. In addition to the methods listed, placement of selected items in areas where they are frequently used should be considered.

COMPOUNDING

Compounding is the preparation of a drug product by mixing legally, obtainable ingredients and/or appropriate vehicles that have not been listed as an unapproved drug for animals by the regulatory action of FDA, USDA, or EPA. When drug products are compounded, distributed, and used, there is a possibility of harm to public health and animals if there is no adequate and well-controlled safety and effectiveness data and when there is no adherence to the good manufacturing practices (GMP). Death or animals that do not do right may result when these compounded drugs are used.

Federal and state laws permit compounding because it sometimes provides value to patients. The practice of veterinary medicine continues to require medications to treat or prevent diseases and requires dosages for different animal species for which there are no commercially prepared, FDA-approved products currently available or efficacious. Concentrations, dosage forms, or combinations of medications that are unavailable can be compounded. Compounding can be used to prepare products that are hard to acquire or are temporarily unavailable from their manufacturer. Pharmacies require a written prescription specifying that the product can be compounded for a specific patient. Veterinarians may compound medicaments for their own patient use. Whether compounding is done at the local clinic or in a pharmacy, a recipe is provided so that other pharmacists or veterinarians can provide refills of the same recipe.

The veterinarian who compounds or makes the decision to use a compounded product must assume the responsibility for the safety of animals as well as wholesomeness of foods of animal origin.

✐ TECHNICIAN NOTE

The veterinarian who prescribes a compounded product must assume the responsibility of safety to animals and wholesomeness of foods.

Both the pharmacist and veterinarian who compound must use professional judgment that is consistent with proper pharmaceutical and pharmacological principles when compounding medications. The following points must be considered:

- The stability of the active ingredients must be known.
- The physical and chemical compatibility of the ingredients must be known.
- The pharmacodynamic compatibility of the ingredients must be known.
- The inactive ingredients and diluents must be of known compositions and not contaminated with harmful substances or agents or unapproved sources.
- The prepared medication must be properly labeled before dispensing.
- Compounded medications must not be advertised or displayed to the public.

When compounded medications are used, appropriate records must be maintained. When compounded products are used in food-producing animals, appropriate residue tests, when available and practical, and other procedures for assuring volatile residue avoidance should be instituted.

> **✎ TECHNICIAN NOTE**
>
> Compounded products for food-producing animals require testing for volatile residues.

In the July 14, 2003, *Federal Register,* the FDA released a revised Compliance Policy Guide (CPG) section 608.400 entitled "Compounding of Drugs for Use in Animals" (61FR34840). The purpose of the guide is to ensure that the agencies enforcement policy regarding the compounding of drugs intended to use in animals is consistent, to the extent practical, with its policy regarding the compounding of drugs intended for use in humans. The FDA does not make a distinction between compounding and manufacturing or other processing of drugs for use in animals rather than in humans. It does acknowledge the use of compounding within certain areas of veterinary practice. Regulations specifically permit compounding of products from approved animal or human drugs under conditions set forth in 21CFR 530.13. The activity of compounding is not the subject of this guidance.

Veterinarians and pharmacies that are engaged in manufacturing and distributing unapproved new animal drugs in a manner that is clearly out of bounds of the traditional pharmacy or veterinary practice violate the act.

The three restrictions set for compounding by FDA are:

- The drug product must not be identified by the FDA as a drug product that presents demonstrable difficulties for compounding in terms of safety or effectiveness.
- In states that have not entered into a "memorandum of understanding" with the FDA addressing the distribution of "inordinate amounts" of compounded drugs in interstate commerce, the pharmacy, pharmacist, or physician compounding the drug may not distribute compounded drugs out of state in quantities exceeding 5% of that entity's total prescription orders.
- The prescription must be "unsolicited" [section 353a(a)], and the pharmacy, licensed pharmacist, or licensed physician compounding the drug may "not advertise or promote the compounding of any particular drug, class of drug, or type of drug." The pharmacy, licensed pharmacist, or licensed physician may, however, "advertise and promote the compounding service" they provide (*Thompson v. Western States Medical Center* [section 353a(c)]).

Generally, FDA will defer to state authorities regarding the day-to-day regulation of compounding of animal and human drugs that are intended to be used in food-producing animals. When the scope and nature of activities raise concern associated with manufacturing resulting in significant violation of the new drug, adulteration, or misbranding provisions of the Food, Drug and Cosmetic Act, FDA has determined it will seriously consider enforcement action. In determining whether to initiate such action, the agency will consider whether the veterinarian or pharmacist engages in any of the following acts:

- Compounding of drugs for use in situation (1) where the health of the animal is not threatened and (2) where suffering or death of the animal is not likely to result from failure to treat
- Compounding of drug in anticipation of receiving prescriptions, except in very limited quantities in relation to the amounts of drugs compounded after receiving prescriptions issued within the confines of a valid VCPR
- Compounding of drugs that are prohibited for extralabel use in food-producing or non–food-producing animals, under 21 CFR 530.41(a) and (b), respectively, because the drugs present a risk to the public health
- Compounding finished drugs from human or animal drugs that are not the subject of an approved application, or from bulk drug substances, other than those specifically addressed for regulatory discretion by the FDA, Center for Veterinary Medicine, e.g., antidotes (Inquiries about compounding from unapproved drugs or bulk drug substances should be directed to CVM, Division of Compliance, 301-827-1168.)
- Compounding from approved human drugs for which FDA has implemented a restricted distribution system
- Using commercial-scale manufacturing equipment for compounding drug products
- Compounding drugs for third parties who resell to individual patients, or offering compounded drug products at wholesale to other state licensed persons or commercial entities for resale
- Failing to operate in conformance with applicable state law regulating the practice of pharmacy

- Compounding of drugs for use in animals where an approved new animal drug or approved new human drug used as labeled or in conformity with 21 CFR Part 530 will, in the available dosage form and concentration, appropriately treat the condition diagnosed
- Compounding from a human drug for use in food-producing animals if an approved animal drug can be used for the compounding
- Instances where illegal residues occur in meat, milk, eggs, honey, aquaculture, or other food-producing animal products and such residues were caused by the use of a compounded drug
- Labeling a compounded drug with a withdrawal time established by the pharmacist instead of the prescribing veterinarian
- Labeling of compounded drugs without sufficient information, such as withdrawal times for drugs for food-producing animals or other categories of information that are described in 21 DFR 530.12

The foregoing list of factors is not intended to be all-inclusive. Other factors may be appropriate for consideration in a particular case.

While many veterinarians say that in some cases the use of bulk drugs is medically necessary, the FDA regulations forbid the use of bulk drugs. The revised guide provides a list of bulk substances for compounding and subsequent use in animals to which the FDA will not normally object.

- Ammonium molybdate
- Ammonium tetrathiomolybdate
- Ferric ferrocyanide
- Methylene blue
- Picrotoxin
- Pilocarpine
- Sodium nitrite
- Sodium thiosulfate
- Tannic acid

NUTRACEUTICALS

In the past, owners chose animal products on the basis of packaging designs, advertising claims, cost, and convenience. Today, they are taking proactive movements and assuming greater responsibility for the health of their animals. Owners are feeding with highly digestive, energy-dense foods and specialty treats so that the animals will feel and look better. The owners are now turning to nutritional supplements that offer more natural benefits than the synthetic products available.

Every animal, depending on the condition, temperament, age, and lifestyle has unique nutritional requirements. Today's trends suggest that animals cannot get optimal care with conventional medicine or nutrition alone. A combination of both seems to promote the best health care. There

is no doubt that nutraceuticals are impacting the world. With the cost of medical care continually increasing there is public demand to take a look at alternative medicine.

While drugs are toxic substances designed to force the body to "fix" things that have gone wrong, nutraceuticals support the body in healing "itself" and working to prevent things from going wrong. They are used to correct underlying imbalances while keeping internal organs healthy.

WHAT ARE NUTRACEUTICALS?

Nutraceuticals are a new class of substances having effectiveness in the body that is similar to that of pharmaceuticals. They are not herbs, vitamins, minerals, or food. They are more than food, and somewhat less than a drug. They are highly specialized chemicals derived from plants (phytochemical) in the form of supplements.

> **TECHNICIAN NOTE**
> Nutraceuticals are not herbs, vitamins, minerals, or food but chemicals from plants in the form of supplements.

Nutraceuticals are nondrug substances that are produced in a purified or extracted form from foods (although they are not associated with food) and administered to patients to provide an agent required for normal body structure and function, with the intent of improving the health and well-being of animals. They are effective because they interact with specific chemical receptors within the body and, in a pharmacodynamic sense, are drugs themselves.

Nutraceuticals are used to modify many conditions in the body. Popular categories and their uses include glucosamine/chondroitin sulfate (joint health), antioxidants (free-radical damage), and omega-3 fatty acids (allergies and skin dysfunctions).

As medications, nutraceuticals have side effects and interact with medications and foods. They can be contraindicated in certain conditions or disease states. Some nutraceuticals are naturally toxic to certain species and breeds of animals.

Many products will benefit animals if intelligently and judiciously used under the guidance of a licensed veterinarian.

REGULATIONS OF NUTRACEUTICALS

The use of nutraceuticals has increased even though most are unproven and uncontrolled. Most do not meet USP standards. None require the scrutiny of the FDA because it considers nutraceuticals as dietary supplements, not drugs. Pet products are regulated under the auspices of specific animal regulatory agencies.

Preparations of nutraceuticals do vary widely between manufacturers. There is no mechanism to establish the effectiveness of levels of products consumed or support label claims. There are no guarantees that the product is stable enough to withstand extreme temperatures or prolonged storage. There is no supportive documentation of stability of raw ingredients. In addition, some nutraceuticals are poorly manufactured. Some may be contaminated with bacteria or heavy metals. A number of side effects have been identified but not passed on to the consumer.

There is truly a need for some level of government to regulate the safe use of nutraceuticals as effective dietary supplements for animals as well as accurate function claims.

> ✏ **TECHNICIAN NOTE**
> There are no government regulations on nutraceuticals.

MATTERS OF PUBLIC CONCERN

Before purchasing pet supplements, owners need to make sure the products are truly helpful, safe, and effective. They need to make sure the products have undergone many of the same scientific and clinical evaluations that are now required of human products.

INTERNET PHARMACY

The Internet is rapidly transforming the way we live and shop in all sectors of the economy. In the area of health care, it permits individuals to obtain medical information to help them understand health issues and treatment options for themselves and their animals. The Internet allows consumers to shop online for health care products and get prescriptions filled.

There are great benefits as well as challenges that the Internet presents when consumers use it to shop. One of the greatest benefits of shopping online to fill prescriptions is the ease with which consumers can comparison shop. Many pharmacies offer price comparisons between its charges and that of other legitimate pharmacies, which helps to stretch the health care dollar. Some Internet pharmacies sell drugs for less than traditional "brick-and-mortar" pharmacies, which is most important for people who love their animals but have limited income.

Legitimate online pharmacies offer valuable health care information in searchable format. Drug prices and drug information are accessed by the Web site. It may be requested by E-mail. Consumers do not have to wait on the phone for an answer or travel to the pharmacy to get it!

There is convenience and flexibility to ordering and receiving medications without leaving home, which is a tremendous time-saver. For the pet owner who has limited time, online prescriptions allow for the convenience of shopping 24 hours a day. This is especially valuable to homebound pet owners for whom a trip to the pharmacy may be difficult.

Online pharmacies provide more privacy than traditional pharmacies. Sometimes consumers are too embarrassed to purchase certain items or health care products from the local pharmacy. They may find greater anonymity by ordering online where staff may not be able to put "face to name."

CONCERNS ABOUT ONLINE SITES

As beneficial as computer technology is, the Internet also creates a new market place for illegal activity such as the sale of unapproved new drugs and dispensing prescription drugs without a valid prescription. Consumers may encounter difficulties in identifying illegitimate sites.

One problem found with illegitimate online pharmacies is that they open and close on a daily basis. One company may have many URLs or Web addresses, and they frequently sell customer links. Many customers are unable to contact the pharmacy because phone lines are disconnected or there is no answer.

Often consumers experience nondelivery of medications ordered, and they face credit card charges that these illegitimate pharmacies refuse to remove. Genuine risks exist when foreign drugs are dispensed.

Medications dispensed that are considered unsafe for laypersons to administer without monitoring by a licensed veterinarian are called *legend drugs* (they bear the "caution," which restricts the use of the drug). In order for the veterinarian to write a prescription, he should have established a valid VCPR with the animal and its owner. This cannot be done online. Because online pharmacies only provide a questionnaire to be completed, the physical examination (PE), a requirement of VCPR, cannot be done. When a VCPR is established without the PE, inappropriate medications can worsen an underlying, undiagnosed, serious disease state. When pharmacies do not employ licensed professionals, the animal's life may be threatened because the pharmacy may not sell the right drug.

Illegitimate online pharmacies use patient questionnaires and fee-based cyberspace consultations. They will sell legend drugs and controlled drugs without a consult. It is no longer legal to sell controlled drugs over the Internet.

> ✏ **TECHNICIAN NOTE**
> Controlled drugs cannot be sold over the Internet.

Many illegitimate sites will use drugs from foreign countries. FDA generally prohibits the importation of foreign-made versions of prescriptions medications that are commercially available in the United States. Genuine risks exist when foreign drugs are dispensed. The safety and efficacy of these medications cannot be guaranteed. Online pharmacies may dispense expired, subpotent, contaminated or counterfeit product; the wrong or contraindicated product, incorrect dose, or medications without adequate directions for use.

The prescription order should come directly from the prescriber to be valid—not the patient. Online sites that do not protect the integrity of the original prescription or do not verify the authenticity of the prescription may be in violation of the law.

REGULATIONS

The challenge for regulatory agencies concerning online prescriptions is to make sure that protection for consumers is just as strong as that for consumers when they purchase drugs at their corner pharmacy.

FDA has actively engaged a number of states in jointly pursuing illegal Internet sales. Regulation is primarily the jurisdiction of each State Board of Pharmacy with some federal insight. Most states protect their citizens by licensing "out-of-state" pharmacies to ship medications in their jurisdiction. National Association of Boards of Pharmacy (NABP) does not regulate online pharmacies.

Verify Internet Pharmacy Practice Sites (VIPPS) is a voluntary certification. The program offers an accompanying seal of approval that identifies to the public those online pharmacy sites that are appropriately licensed and are legitimately operating over the Internet. Those approved sites have successfully completed a rigorous criteria review inspection.

The value of the VIPPS program is to provide members of the public a means to assure themselves that the Internet pharmacy they choose is a bona fide, fully licensed facility exercising competent Internet/interstate pharmacy practices. Regulations that apply to traditional brick-and-mortar mail-order pharmacies apply to online pharmacies.

VIPPS-certified pharmacies are required to offer customers free phone consultation with a registered pharmacist and may offer free ask-a-pharmacist E-mail service.

VIPPS has a mechanism in place to report errors made by its certified pharmacies. They are to document, track, and analyze the types of error to determine what went wrong and to make suggestions to prevent recurrences.

ADVICE FOR CONSUMERS

- Suspect the pharmacy if it will dispense medications without requiring a hard copy of the prescription to be mailed in.
- Suspect the pharmacy if it dispenses prescription medications and does not contact the prescriber to obtain a valid verbal prescription.
- Suspect the pharmacy if it will dispense medications solely based on a consumer questionnaire without a preexisting VCPR with a prescriber on site.
- Suspect the pharmacy if it does not have a toll-free number and street address posted to the Web site.
- Suspect the Web site if the pharmacy merely has an E-mail feature as the sole communication between consumer and facility. Legitimate Web sites allow you to contact the pharmacist.
- Avoid the Web site if it does not advertise the availability of a registered pharmacist for consultation.
- Avoid a pharmacy that does not have policies in place that address different issues.
- Always look for the Verify Internet Pharmacy Practice Sites (VIPPS) seal of approval!

RECOMMENDED READING

Baumgartner K, Hoffman D, editors: *Controlled substances handbook*, Washington, DC, 1998, Government Information Services.

Bonagura JD, editor: Small animal practice. In *Kirk's current veterinary therapy*, ed 14, Philadelphia, 2005, WB Saunders.

Compendium of Veterinary Products, ed 7, Port Huron, Mich, 2003, North American Compendium.

Hardarman JG et al: *The pharmacological basis of therapeutics*, ed 9, New York, 1995, McGraw-Hill.

Physician's desk reference, ed 57, Montvale, NJ, 2003, Medical Economics Co.

Plumb DC: *Veterinary drug handbook*, ed 4, White Bear Lake, Minn, 2002, PharmaVet Publishing.

USP DI: *Drug information for the health care professional*, ed 23, vol 1, Englewood, Colo, 2003, Micromedex.

Veterinary pharmaceutical and biologicals, ed 12, Lenexa, Kan, 2001, Veterinary Healthcare Communications.

22

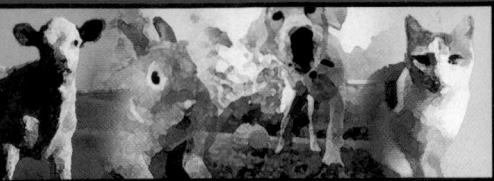

Surgical Instruments and Aseptic Technique

Jacqueline R. Davidson • Daniel J. Burba

INTRODUCTION

The veterinary technician may need to assist the veterinarian with many aspects of surgery. The technician may need to prepare the patient for surgery, act as a circulating nurse in the operating room, and take responsibility for the care, cleaning, packing and sterilization of the instruments. The technician is often responsible for ordering surgical instruments and implants, so familiarity with this equipment is essential. In addition, the principles of aseptic technique should be second nature. The technician may need to alert the veterinarian to potential problems with aseptic technique and may be required to "scrub in" to assist with surgical procedures. A surgical assistant can be of great value by anticipating which instruments the surgeon will need and by aiding in tissue retraction and hemostasis. The technician is an invaluable part of the surgical team and can greatly enhance the quality and efficiency of surgical procedures. ∎

INSTRUMENTATION

Thousands of different surgical instruments are available, and new instruments are continually being designed to increase the efficiency and ease of performing surgery. The surgical technician must know the purpose of each instrument in order to anticipate when it will be used and must understand how to handle and care for it.

✎ TECHNICIAN NOTE

Each instrument is designed for a specific purpose such as cutting, holding, clamping, or retracting.

GENERAL SURGERY INSTRUMENTS

SCALPEL

The scalpel is the best instrument for incising tissues with minimal trauma. A variety of disposable blades are designed to fit several different scalpel handles (Figure 22-1). The *Bard-Parker no. 3 handle* uses detachable blade nos. 10, 11, 12, and 15 and is the most useful for small animal surgery. The *Bard-Parker no. 4 handle* is larger and uses detachable blade nos. 20, 21, and 22. This handle is most commonly used for large animal surgery.

BIOMEDICAL LASERS

Surgical lasers may be used to cut or ablate (destroy) tissue. There are many different types of lasers. The most commonly used in veterinary medicine are carbon dioxide (CO_2) and neodymium:yttrium-aluminum-garnet (Nd:YAG) lasers. Advantages of incising tissue with a laser include some hemostasis and possibly less postoperative swelling and pain as compared with cutting with a scalpel blade. Disadvantages include delayed wound healing and safety issues associated with the use of lasers. Special glasses must be worn by everyone in the room, and care must be taken to avoid ignition of combustible materials. Smoke evacuators and laser-safe surgical masks should be used to reduce the amount of particulate debris inhaled from the smoke plume.

ELECTROSURGERY

Electroscalpels can be used to cut or coagulate tissue and help to minimize bleeding. They work by passing a high-frequency alternating electrical current through the tissue (Figure 22-2, *A*). Cutting or coagulation can be performed through the same handpiece, and the surgeon can activate

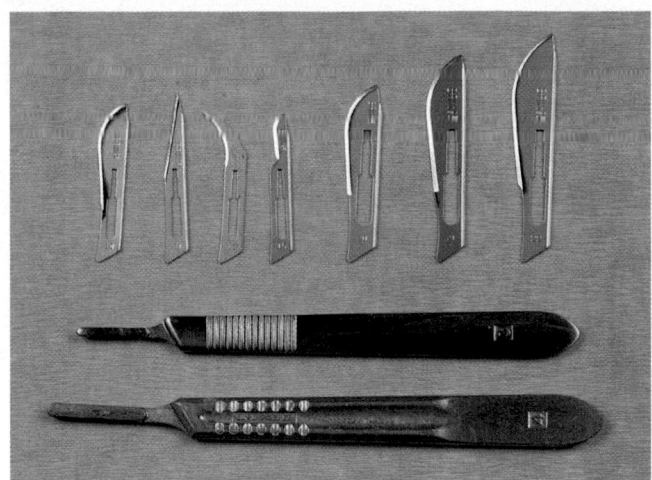

Figure 22-1 Scalpel handles and attachable surgical blades. Surgical blade nos. 10, 11, 12, and 15 fit the Bard-Parker no. 3 scalpel handle and surgical blade nos. 20 to 22 fit the Bard-Parker no. 4 handle. The no. 3 handle and no. 10 blade are commonly used in small animal surgery. The no. 4 handle and no. 20 blade are commonly used in large animal surgery.

it by a switch on the sterile handpiece or by a foot switch (Figure 22-2, *B*). However, the power level must be adjusted by a nonsterile technician. In *monopolar electrosurgery*, current passes from the handpiece (Figure 22-2, *C*) through the patient to a metal ground plate (Figure 22-2, *D*) that is placed under the patient. Poor contact between the patient's skin and the ground plate can burn the patient at the site of the ground plate. In *bipolar electrosurgery*, the current passes between two tips on the handpiece (Figure 22-2, *E*), which grasp the tissue. No ground plate is needed for bipolar electrosurgery.

SCISSORS

Specific scissors are designed to cut tissue, suture, wire, or bandage material (Figure 22-3). There are many types of dissecting scissors, made for precise cutting and dissection of tissue. *Operating scissors* vary by the type of blades (straight or curved), the type of points (blunt-blunt, blunt-sharp or sharp-sharp), and the cutting edge of the blades (plain or serrated). *Mayo dissecting scissors* are heavy scissors used for cutting tough tissue such as heavy connective tissue. The blades may be straight or curved. *Metzenbaum dissecting scissors* are fine, curved scissors used for cutting delicate tissue such as fat or thin muscle. Metzenbaum scissors are preferred for most soft tissue dissection. They should never be used for cutting suture because this dulls their edges and causes the blades to separate and lose their effectiveness. Stitch scissors or *Littauer suture removal scissors* are used to cut all sutures except wire sutures. *Wire-suture-cutting scissors* can cut wire suture. *Lister bandage scissors* are available to cut bandage material. One blade of the Lister scissors has a blunt end to facilitate sliding under a bandage without

poking the skin. To prolong the life of any scissors, it should be used only for its intended purpose.

NEEDLE HOLDERS

Needle holders are designed for holding curved suture needles during suturing and for performing instrument suture ties. *Mayo-Hegar* and *Olsen-Hegar* needle holders are two commonly used needle holders (Figure 22-4). The Olsen-Hegar needle holder has built-in suture scissors, which negates the need for an assistant to cut suture. It allows the surgeon to work alone and cut suture without switching instruments. The potential disadvantage of this needle holder is that the suture may be accidentally cut during suture placement.

Needle holders consist of a set of jaws, a hinge or box lock, and handles with a ratcheted locking device (Figure 22-5). The size and design of these components vary greatly depending on their intended use. The jaws commonly have tungsten carbide inserts that provide excellent grip. The tungsten carbide insert is hard, resistant to wear, and can be replaced when worn, thereby prolonging the life of the instrument. Worn inserts can result in improper closure of the jaws or sharp edges that inadvertently cut suture. Needle holders are available in different sizes, depending on the needle sizes they are designed to hold. Improper use of needle holders (such as using a needle holder that is too small for the size of the needle or using the needle holder to bend or twist wire) may not only damage the jaws but may also spring the box lock and ratchet.

THUMB FORCEPS

Thumb forceps are special tissue forceps designed to hold and easily release tissue with a simple finger motion (similar to tweezers). They have a spring action and the jaws are opposed by compressing the two metal handles together. Several different jaw surfaces are available and are designed for use with various tissues (Figure 22-6, *A* to *C*). *Brown-Adson thumb forceps* have multiple intermeshing teeth with a broad tip, providing good tissue and needle handling. They are commonly used during suturing and wound closure. *Rat-tooth thumb forceps* have large interdigitating teeth and are primarily used for skin or fascia. *Adson thumb forceps* have delicate intermeshing teeth ("rat toothed") that provide a good, atraumatic grasp of delicate tissues. They are

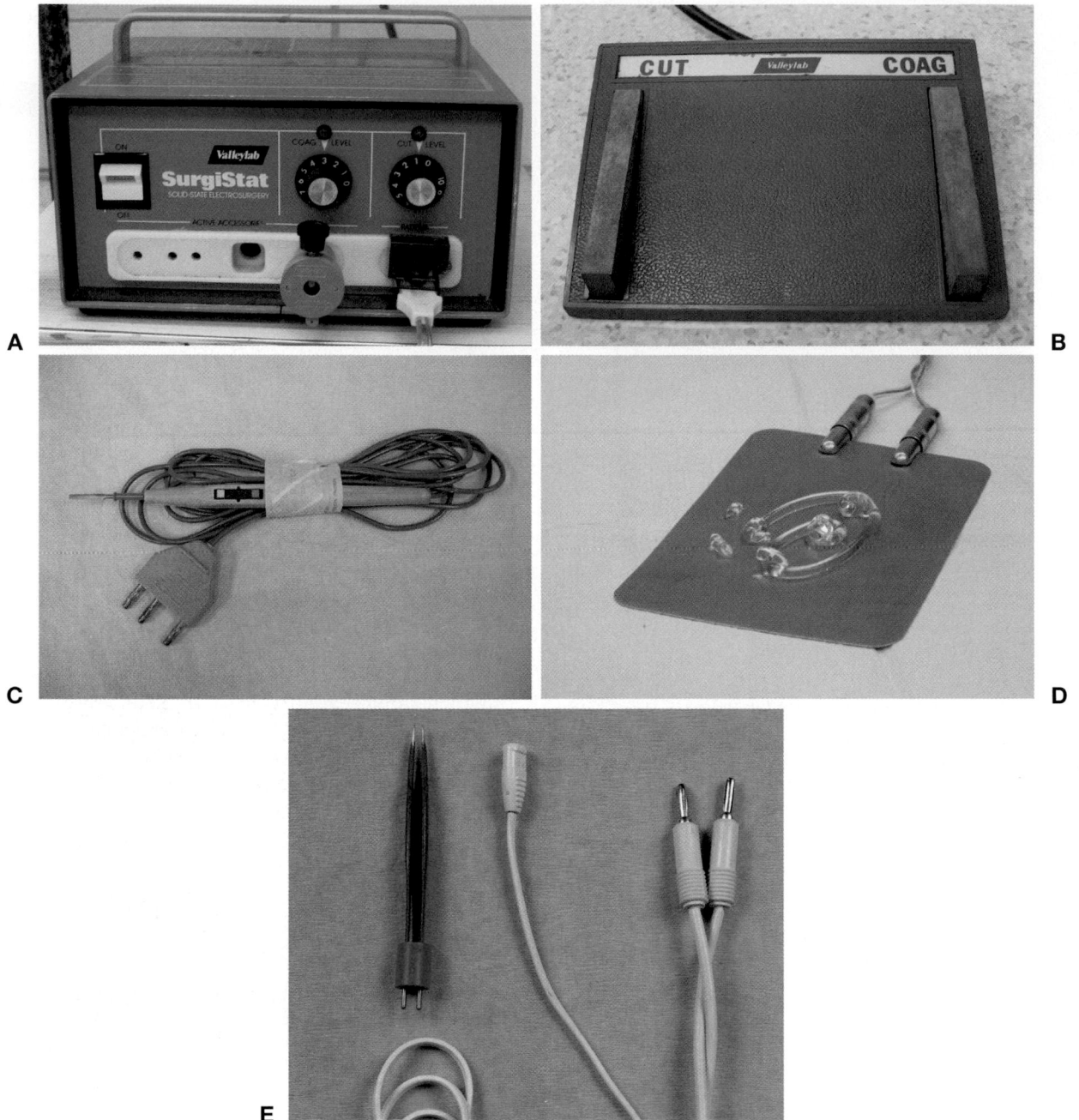

Figure 22-2 Electrosurgical equipment. **A,** Settings on electrosurgical unit are adjusted by nonsterile technician. **B,** Electrosurgical foot switch is placed near surgeon's foot. **C,** Monopolar electrosurgery handpiece. If the handpiece has a cutting/coagulation button, a foot switch is not needed. The handpiece is sterilized and given to the surgeon. The surgeon passes the end of the cord to a nonsterile assistant who plugs it into the electrosurgical unit. **D,** Ground plate on surgery table with gel to improve skin contact when the animal lies on it. Good contact is important for proper function. **E,** Bipolar handpiece is sterilized for use. A nonsterile foot switch is needed for activation.

commonly used during dissection. Cooley and *DeBakey thumb forceps* have long, narrow jaws with multiple delicate sets of teeth that are especially good for vascular surgery. *Russian thumb forceps* have a broad curved surface good for needle handling but are traumatic when used to hold tissues. *Dressing thumb forceps* do not have teeth and are used for applying and removing dressings. They are not designed to grasp tissue and are undesirable for this use because the surgeon must squeeze hard and crush the tissue in order to grasp it. Thumb forceps are available in a variety of sizes depending on the intended surgery. For example, thoracic forceps have very long handles to enable the surgeon to reach tissues deep within the chest, but these same forceps would be too cumbersome and awkward to use on the skin.

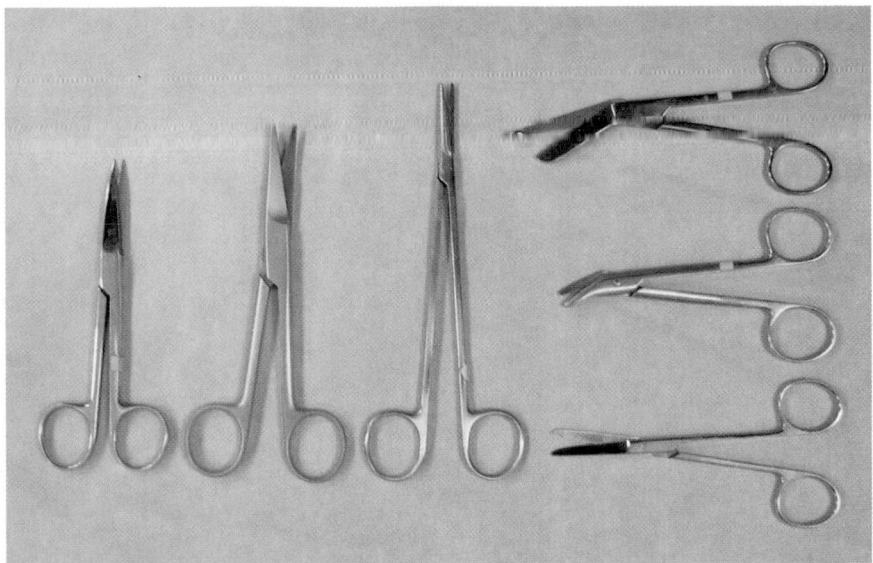

Figure 22-3 Scissors. *Left to right:* Sharp-sharp operating scissors, Mayo dissecting scissors, and Metzenbaum dissecting scissors. *At right, from top to bottom:* Lister bandage scissors, wire-suture-cutting scissors, and Littauer suture removal scissors.

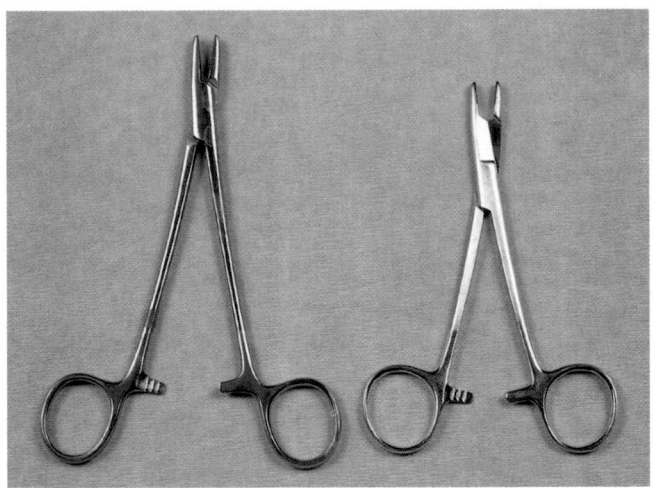

Figure 22-4 Needle holders. Mayo-Hegar needle holder *(left)*, Olsen-Hegar needle holder *(right)*.

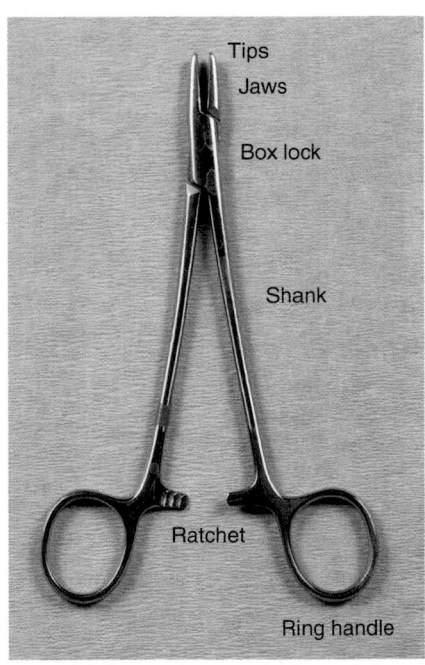

Figure 22-5 Basic components of a surgical instrument.

> ✐ **TECHNICIAN NOTE**
>
> Thumb forceps are commonly used in the surgeon's nondominant hand to hold tissues while dissecting or suturing.

TISSUE FORCEPS

Tissue forceps are locking instruments that clamp tissues (Figure 22-7, *A*). Different teeth patterns allow them to grip various types of tissues without slipping. *Allis tissue forceps* securely grasp tissue but also crush it (Figure 22-7, *B*). Therefore, they are considered to be traumatic and should only be used on tissue that is being removed. *Babcock forceps* are shaped similarly to the Allis forceps but are less

traumatic because they have a smoother grasping surface and less tip compression (Figure 22-7, *B*). The Doyen intestinal tissue forceps (Figure 22-7, *A*) is a more delicate instrument used to occlude and hold intestine. The disadvantage of less traumatic tissue forceps is that they are less secure on the tissues.

> ✐ **TECHNICIAN NOTE**
>
> Tissue forceps are used to clamp and hold tissues with a self-locking mechanism.

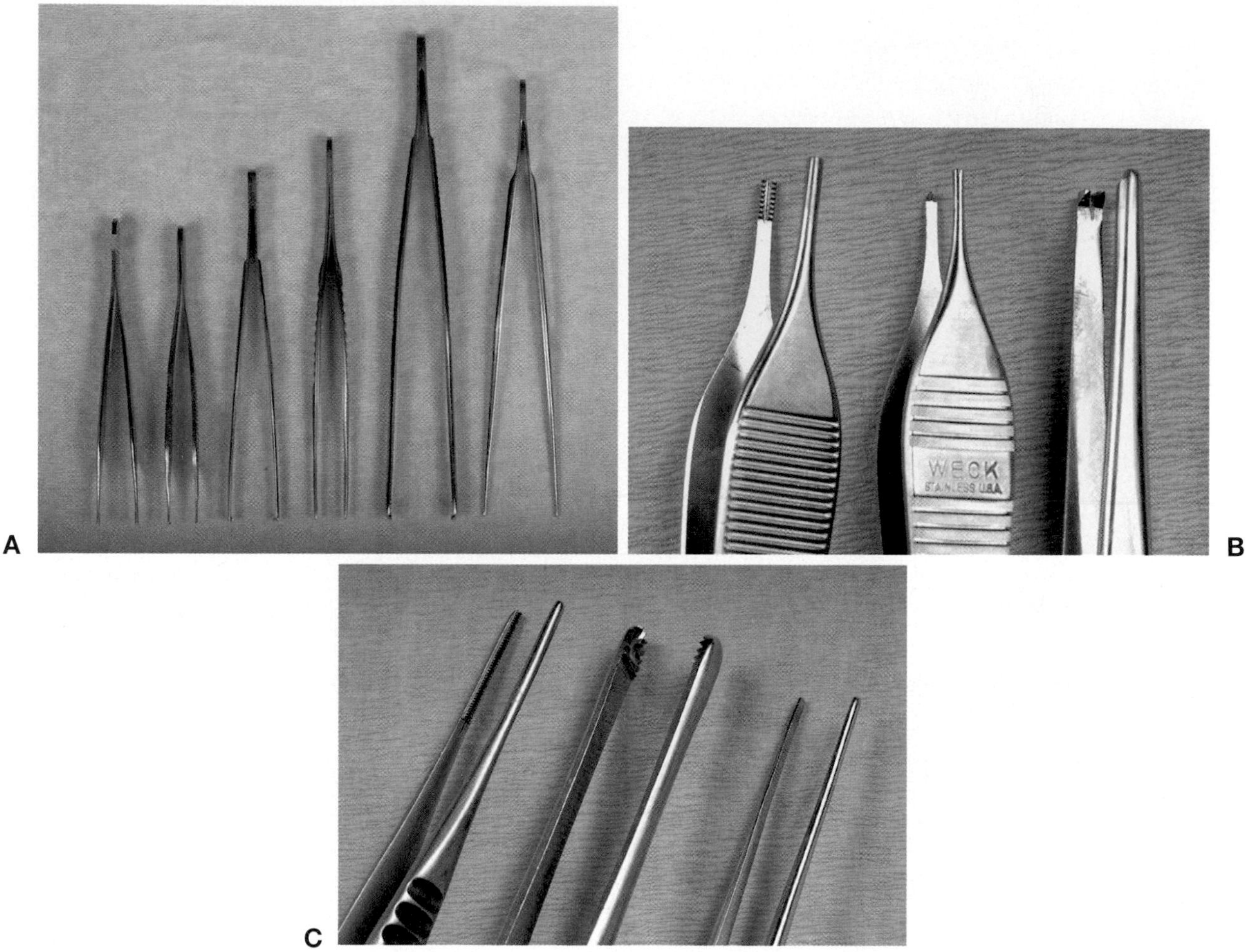

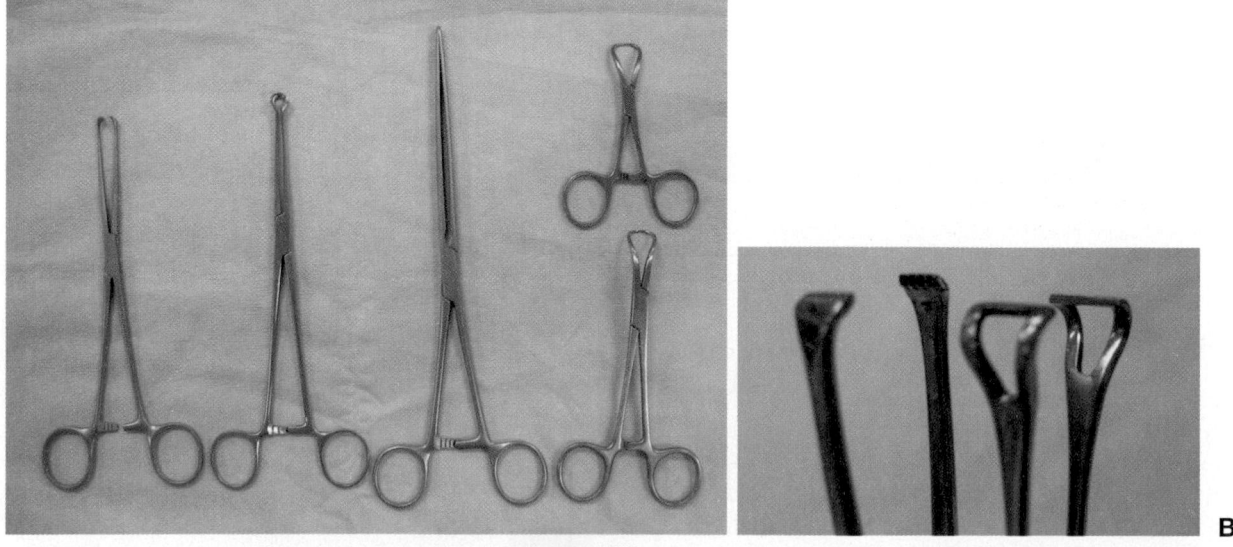

Figure 22-6 Thumb forceps. **A,** *Left to right:* Brown-Adson thumb forceps, Adson thumb forceps, rat-tooth thumb forceps, DeBakey vascular thumb forceps, Russian thumb forceps, dressing thumb forceps. **B,** Close-up of tips *(left to right):* Brown-Adson thumb forceps, Adson thumb forceps, rat-tooth thumb forceps. **C,** Close-up of tips *(left to right):* DeBakey vascular thumb forceps, Russian thumb forceps, dressing thumb forceps.

Figure 22-7 Tissue forceps. **A,** *Left to right:* Allis tissue forceps, Babcock tissue forceps, Doyen intestinal tissue forceps, Backhaus towel clamps (two sizes). **B,** Close-up of tips: Allis tissue forceps *(left)*, Babcock tissue forceps *(right)*.

Towel clamps are forceps used to attach towels and drapes to the patient. These forceps have pointed tips that curve and join like ice tongs. They are available in different sizes (Figure 22-7, *A*). *Backhaus towel clamps* and *Roeder towel clamps* are two common designs. The Roeder towel clamp has a metal bead or ball stop attached to the jaws that prevents deep tissue penetration and prevents the towel from slipping toward the box lock of the forceps.

HEMOSTATIC FORCEPS

Hemostatic forceps are tissue forceps used to stop bleeding by crushing blood vessels (Figures 22-8 and 22-9). They are available in different sizes and may be straight or curved. Most hemostatic forceps have transverse grooves on the inside surface of the jaws to better grasp the tissue. *Halsted mosquito hemostats* are small and designed to occlude small

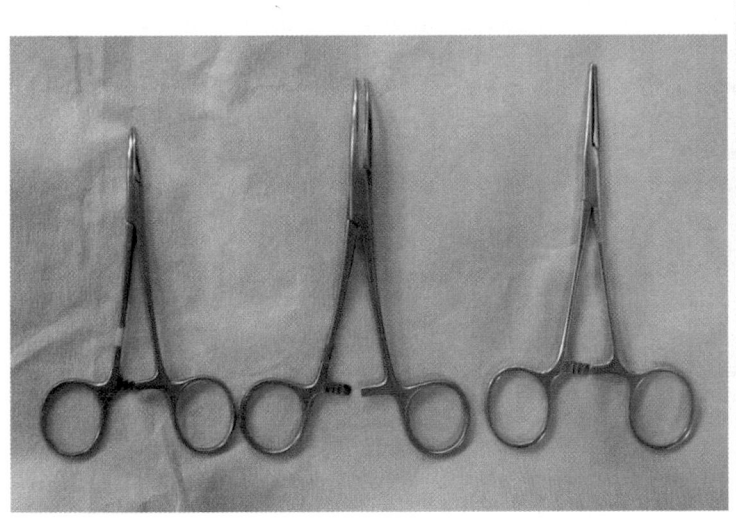
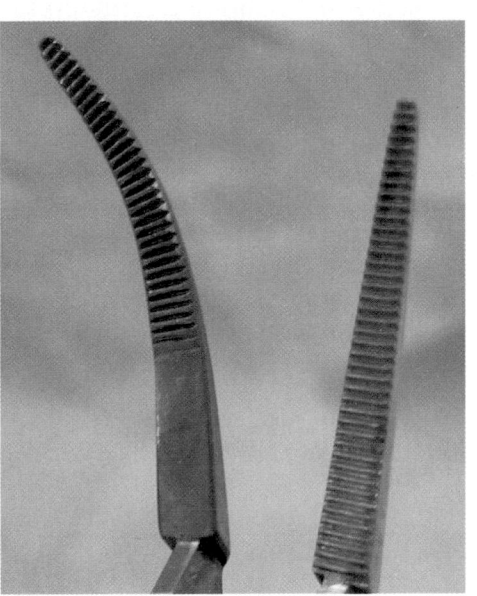

Figure 22-8 Hemostatic forceps. **A,** *Left to right:* Halsted mosquito hemostatic forceps, Kelly forceps, Crile forceps. **B,** Close-up of jaws: curved Kelly *(left),* straight Crile *(right).*

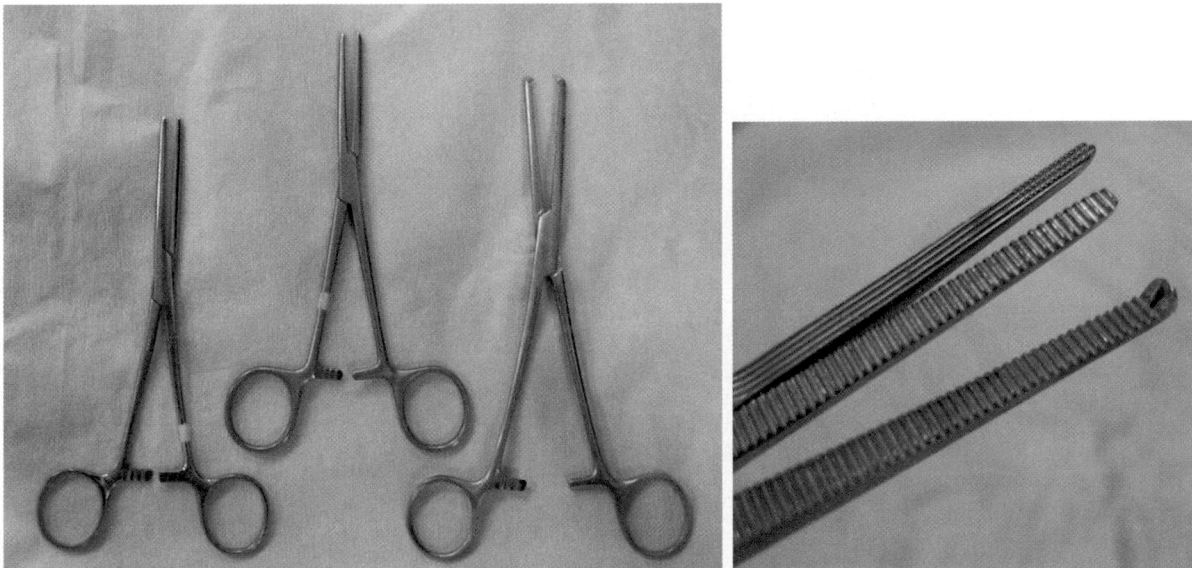

Figure 22-9 Hemostatic forceps. **A,** *Left to right:* Rochester-Carmalt forceps, Rochester-Pean forceps, Rochester-Ochsner forceps. **B,** Close-up of jaws *(left to right):* Rochester-Carmalt forceps, Rochester-Pean forceps, Rochester-Ochsner forceps.

vessels (Figure 22-8, *A*). When using hemostatic forceps, the tips of the forceps should be used to grasp only as much tissue as necessary. *Crile forceps* and *Kelly forceps* (Figure 22-8) are larger hemostatic forceps and are used on larger vessels. The jaws of the Crile forceps are transversely grooved for entire length, but only the distal halves of the Kelly forceps are grooved. *Rochester-Pean forceps* are large, transversely grooved forceps that are used to clamp tissue bundles and large vessels (Figure 22-9). *Rochester-Ochsner forceps* are similar to the Rochester-Pean forceps but have interdigitating teeth at the tips (Figure 22-9) that aid in grasping the tissue. Rochester-Oschner forceps are used most commonly in orthopedic or large animal surgery. *Rochester-Carmalt forceps* are large crushing forceps with longitudinal grooves and cross-grooves at the tip to provide more traction (Figure 22-9). These forceps are used for clamping across tissue containing vessels. The Rochester-Carmalt forceps are commonly used to crush the vessels of the ovarian pedicle or the body of the uterus during an ovariohysterectomy (spay) operation. When clamping across vessels, the forceps should be applied with the concave surface facing upward to facilitate tying the ligature. Refer to Chapter 23 for more information on the use of hemostatic forceps.

> ✎ **TECHNICIAN NOTE**
>
> Hemostatic forceps are used to clamp, crush, and hold blood vessels with a self-locking mechanism.

RETRACTORS

Properly placed retractors do not interfere with the surgery, yet provide good visibility of the surgical site and allow more room for the surgeon to work. Retractors may be handheld or self-retaining. A surgical assistant is needed to maintain the position and tissue tension of a handheld retractor. The *Army-Navy retractor* and the *Senn retractor* are double-ended handheld retractors commonly used to retract skin, fat, or muscle (Figure 22-10). The Army-Navy retractor has smooth blades, while the Senn has one smooth blade and one blade with three sharp or blunt prongs. The *malleable retractor* is made of thin metal that is easily bent to the desired shape (Figure 22-10). It is commonly used to retract abdominal organs. The *Snook ovariohysterectomy hook* is a specialized type of handheld retractor used to expose the horn of the uterus during an ovariohysterectomy (Figure 22-10). The *Hohmann retractor* consists of a single blade and a handle that are used to lever tissues out of the way for better visibility (Figure 22-10). It is used almost exclusively in orthopedic surgery and can provide good visibility in certain joint surgeries.

> ✎ **TECHNICIAN NOTE**
>
> Retractors rather than hands are used to retract tissues and provide good visibility of the surgical site.

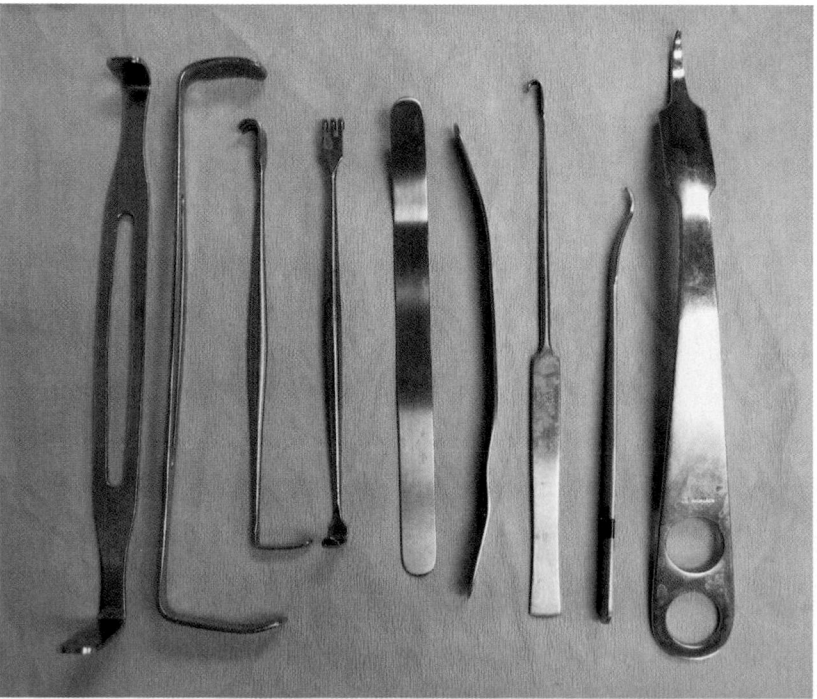

Figure 22-10 Handheld retractors. *Left to right:* Two Army-Navy retractors, two Senn retractors, two small malleable retractors, Snook ovariohysterectomy hook (spay hook), two Hohman metractors (different sizes).

Self-retaining retractors are maintained in the desired position by some type of locking mechanism on the retractor handle. The advantage of the self-retaining retractors is that the surgeon and the assistant have their hands free for other tasks. The *Balfour retractor* provides increased exposure of the abdominal cavity (Figure 22-11). The two wire-like blades are used to distract the abdominal incision and the solid spoon-like blade is hooked onto the sternum to distract it cranially. The *Finochietto rib spreader* retracts the ribs to expose the surgical field within the thoracic cavity (Figure 22-11). The ratcheted part of the retractors is positioned at the dorsal aspect of the thoracic incision so that it does not interfere with the surgeon. *Gelpi retractors* and *Weitlaner retractors* (Figure 22-12) are self-retaining retractors commonly used for muscle retraction, especially in orthopedic and neurologic surgery. Refer to Chapter 23 for more information on retraction techniques.

SUCTION TIPS

Several different suction tips are commonly used (Figure 22-13). The *Poole tip* is used primarily in the abdominal or thoracic cavity because it has an outer sleeve with small holes to prevent tissue, such as fat, from becoming entrapped in the tip. The *Frazier tip* is most commonly used in orthopedic and neurologic surgery. The *Yankauer tip* is a general-purpose suction tip. The suction tip is attached to a long, sterile suction tube. The other end of the suction tube is connected to a nonsterile suction canister. Refer to Chapter 23 for more information on the use of suction.

STAPLING EQUIPMENT

Several different surgical stapling devices are available for an array of purposes (Figure 22-14). There are many advantages to using stapling devices in both large and small animal surgery. Stapling devices provide an easier and faster alternative to hand suturing. Some stapling devices also cut tissue after stapling. The staplers are named by an abbreviation of their designed function (Table 22-1). A number may be used after the name thoracoabdominal stapler (TA) or gastrointestinal stapler (GIA) to indicate the length of the row of staples (e.g., a TA 30 places two rows of staples 30 mm long).

MICHEL SKIN CLIPS

Drape material is often attached to the incised skin edge during surgical procedures to minimize contamination of the surgical field by the surrounding skin. The use of Michel skin clips is one method of attaching the drape to the wound edges (Figure 22-15). One end of the Michel clip-applying-and-removing forceps grips the clip. When the handles are squeezed, the clip bends to pinch the edges of the drape and the skin together. The other end of the forceps has jaws that remove the clip by bending it backward and disengaging it from the incision edge. There are alternatives to Michel clips including the use of suture, "scalp clips," towel clamps, and adhesive drapes.

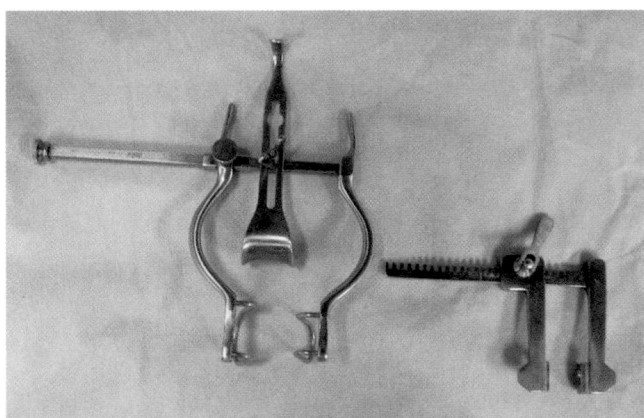

Figure 22-11 Self-retaining retractors. Balfour abdominal retractor *(left)*, Finochietto rib retractor *(right)*.

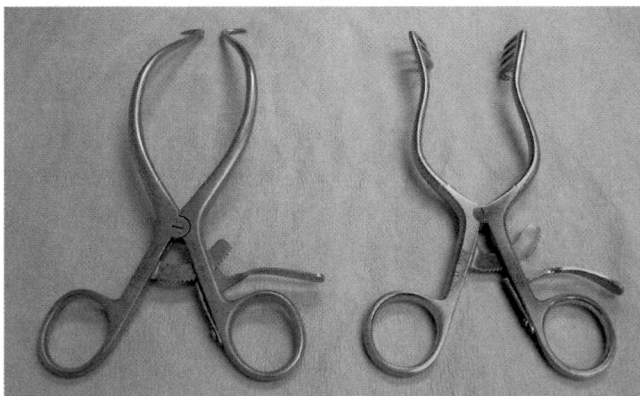

Figure 22-12 Self-retaining retractors. Gelpi retractor *(left)*, Weitlaner retractor *(right)*.

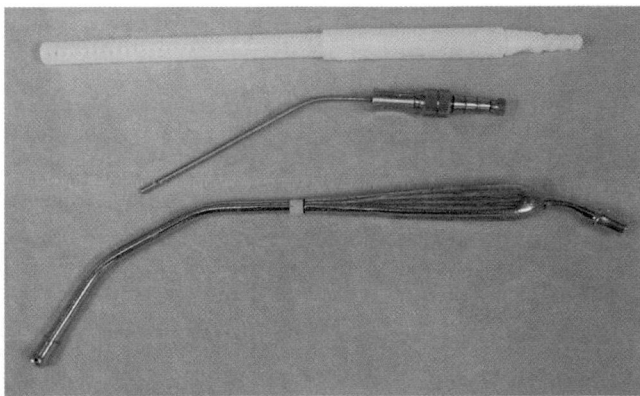

Figure 22-13 Suction tips. *Top to bottom:* Poole, Frazier, Yankauer. The suction tip is attached to a sterile hose. The surgeon hands the other end of the hose to a nonsterile assistant in order to plug it into the suction unit.

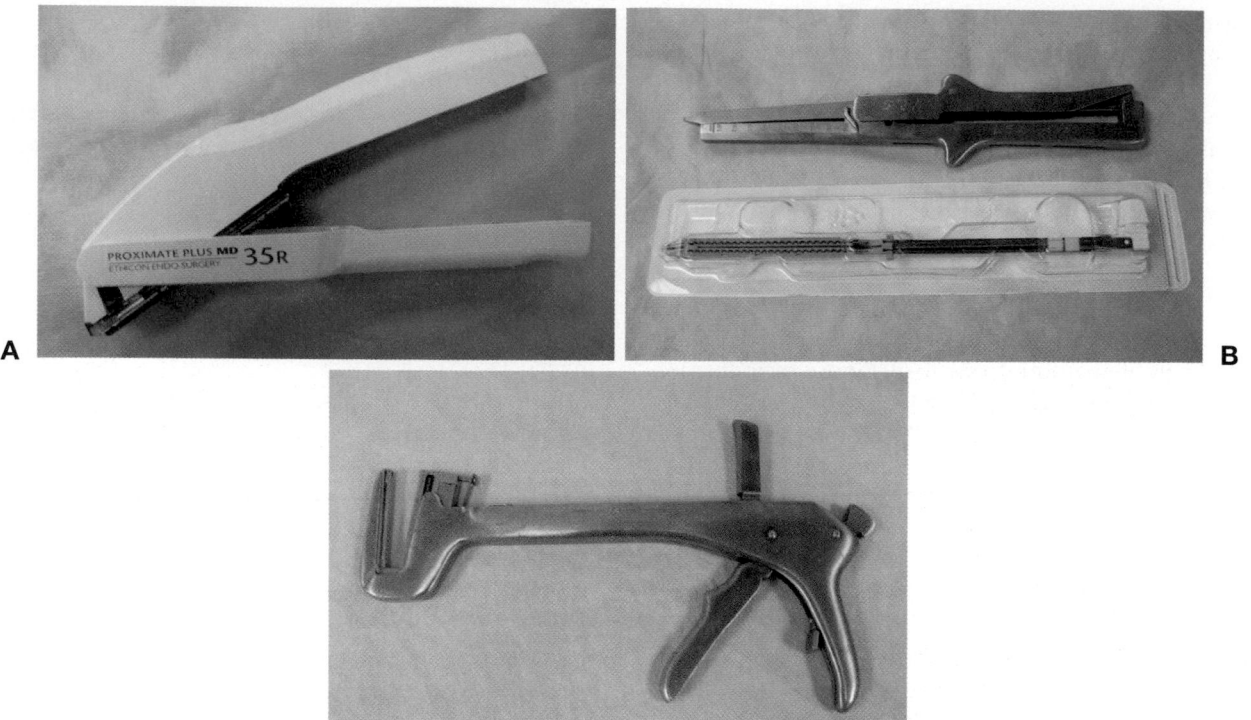

Figure 22-14 Surgical stapling equipment. **A,** Surgical skin stapler applies a single staple with each squeeze of the trigger (staple guns commonly hold 25 to 35 staples). **B,** Gastrointestinal stapler (GIA). Cartridge of staples are for one-time use, and are purchased in presterilized package. **C,** Thoracoabdominal stapler (TA). Staple cartridges are purchased as for GIA. Shown here with staple cartridge in place.

Table 22-1 STAPLING EQUIPMENT

Name	Derivation of Name	Common Use	Comments
TA	Thoracoabdominal	Lung resection	Places double or triple row of staples.
GIA	Gastrointestinal anastomosis	Gastrointestinal resection and anastomosis	Places four rows of staples, and cuts between the middle two rows.
EEA	End-to-end anastomosis	Gastrointestinal anastomosis	Staples two intestinal segments together in a circular manner with a functional lumen.
Skin and fascial stapler		Skin or fascia closures	Places a single staple.
LDS	Ligate-and-divide stapler	Blood vessel ligation	Places two staples on a vessel, and cuts between them.

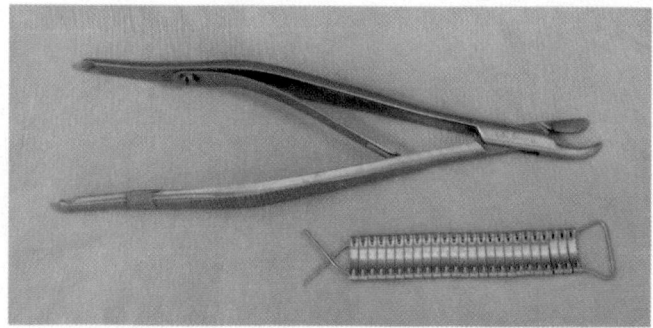

Figure 22-15 Michel skin clips and Michel clip forceps.

OPHTHALMIC INSTRUMENTS

Ophthalmic surgery requires the use of delicate instruments that must be handled carefully. Basic ophthalmic instruments include specialized scalpels, scissors, thumb forceps, needle holders, and retractors (Figure 22-16).

ORTHOPEDIC INSTRUMENTS

RONGEURS

Rongeurs have sharp cupped tips that are used to cut small pieces of dense tissue such as bone, cartilage, or fibrous tissue (Figure 22-17, *A*). Rongeurs have a double-action or

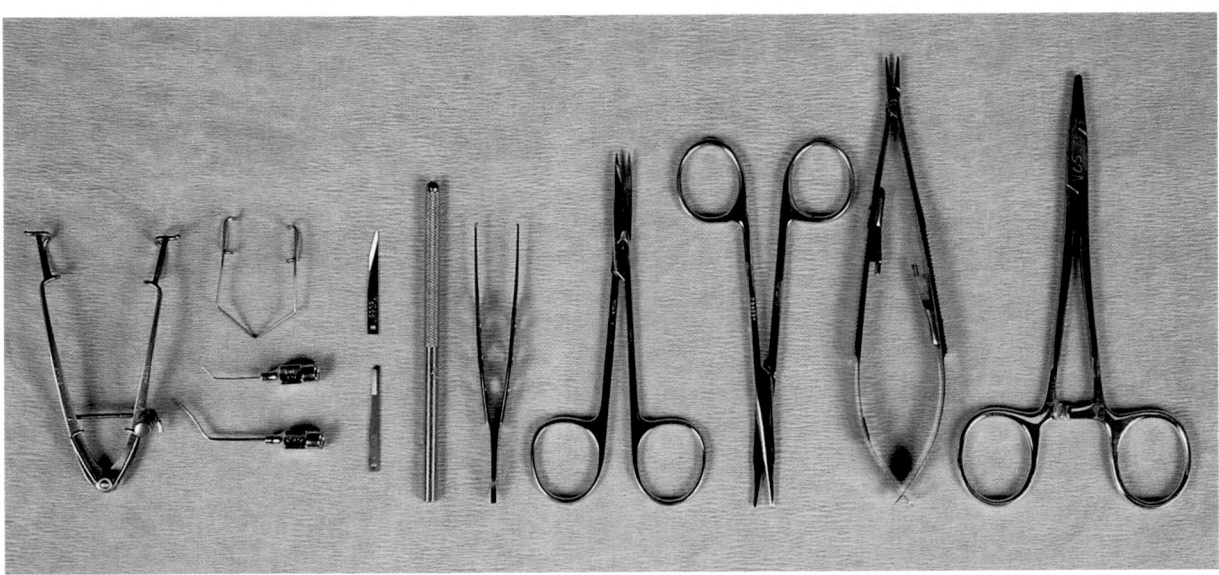

Figure 22-16 Common ophthalmic instruments. *Left to right:* Lid speculum, small lid speculum *(above)* and lacrimal cannulas *(below)*, beaver blade handle with no. 64 and 65 surgical blades, Bishop-Harmon thumb forceps, iris scissors, tenotomy scissors, Castroviejo needle holder, and Derf needle holder.

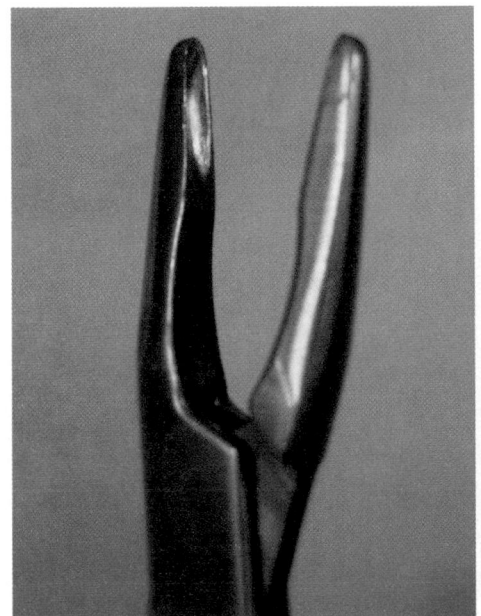

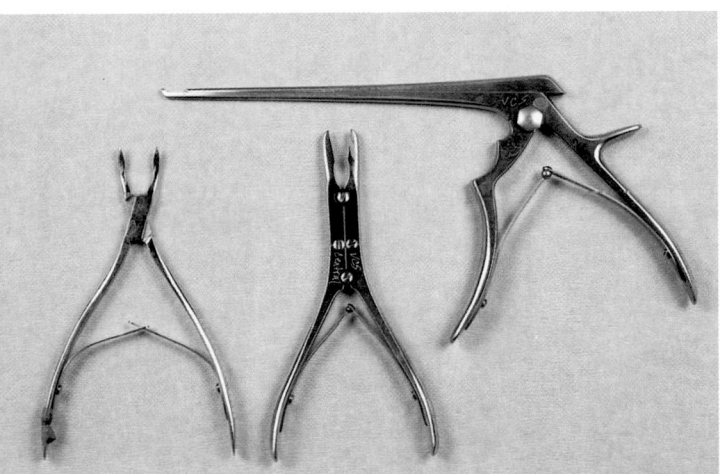

A   **B**

Figure 22-17   Rongeurs. **A,** Close-up of tips. **B,** *Left to right:* Single-action rongeur, double-action rongeur, Kerrison rongeur.

single-action mechanism (Figure 22-17, *B*). Double-action rongeurs have a smooth cutting action and are mechanically stronger than single-action rongeurs, but they are also larger. Double-action rongeurs are preferred for removing large amounts of dense tissue. Single-action rongeurs are more commonly used in confined areas, as in removing bone to perform spinal surgery. Kerrison rongeurs have a gun-shaped appearance and are useful for spinal surgery. Bone-cutting forceps are similar to rongeurs but have paired chisel-like tips. They are used for cutting bone and should not be mistaken for wire cutters (Figure 22-18).

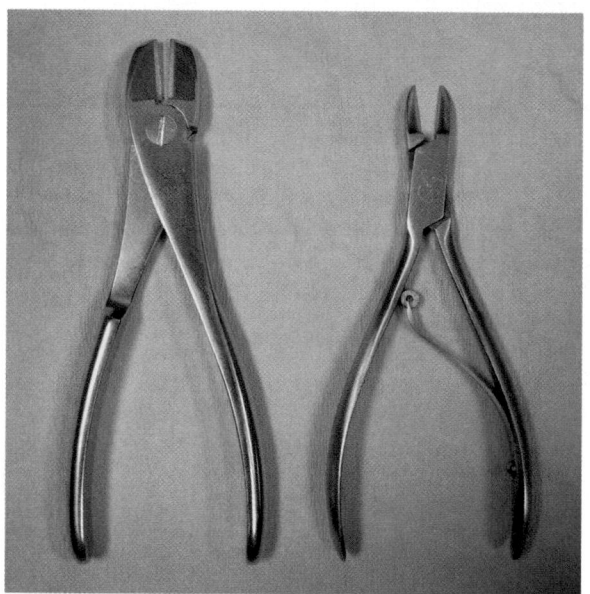

Figure 22-18 Wire cutters *(left)* and bone cutters *(right)*. They look similar but should not be confused. Bone cutters have finer jaws.

BONE-HOLDING FORCEPS

Bone-holding forceps are designed to hold bone and bone fragments in alignment while orthopedic implants (screws, pins, wires or plates) are applied (Figure 22-19). Most bone-holding forceps are self-retaining. *Kern bone-holding forceps* has a ratcheted handle that allows it to be clamped securely on the bone. The *self-retaining bone-holding forceps*, also known as *speed locks*, has a nut that tightens against one handle to squeeze the handles together.

CURETTES

Curettes are used to scrape hard tissue such as bone or cartilage. Curettes are designed with a small cuplike structure at one or both ends of a handle (similar to an ice cream scoop). The cup has a sharp cutting edge and is available in various sizes (Figure 22-20). A common use of bone curettes is to retrieve cancellous bone from the medullary cavity (tibia, humerus, ilium) for use as a bone graft. Cancellous bone grafts are often used during fracture repair.

PERIOSTEAL ELEVATORS

Periosteal elevators are instruments that are used to pry periosteum or muscle from the bone surface. They have a bladelike structure at one or both ends of a handle. The blades have sharp or blunt edges and are available in various sizes (Figure 22-21).

OSTEOTOMES AND CHISELS

Osteotomes and chisels are used to cut bone. Osteotomes and chisels are used by pounding on the flared end of the

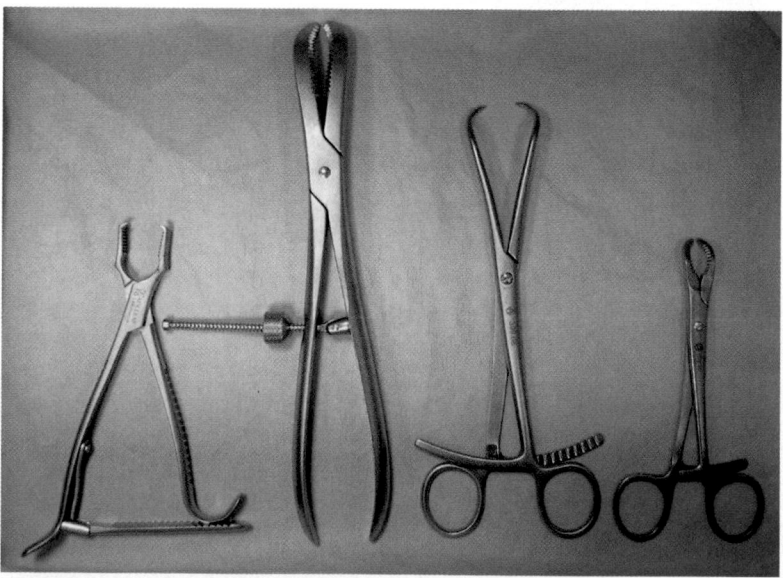

Figure 22-19 Bone-holding forceps. *Left to right:* Small Kern forceps, large speed-lock forceps, large point-to-point forceps, small clamshell forceps.

handle with a mallet (Figure 22-22, *A*). The cutting edge of the osteotome is tapered on both sides, while the chisel is tapered only on one side (Figure 22-22, *B*).

GIGLI WIRE

Gigli wire is used to cut bone by placing the wire around the bone and drawing it back and forth in a sawing fashion.

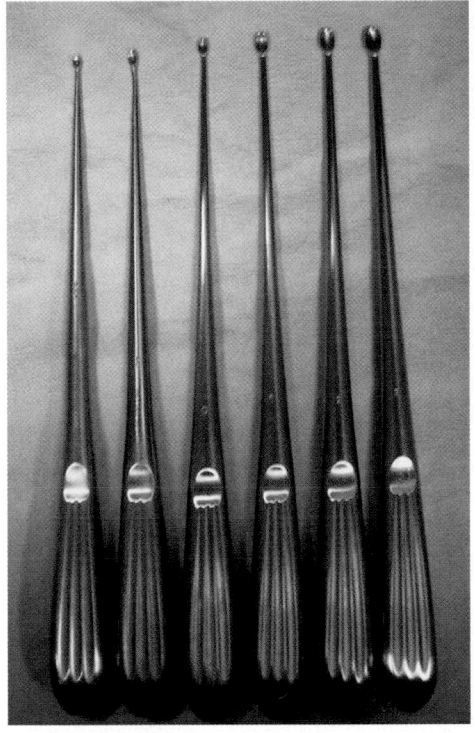

Figure 22-20 Bone curettes of various sizes.

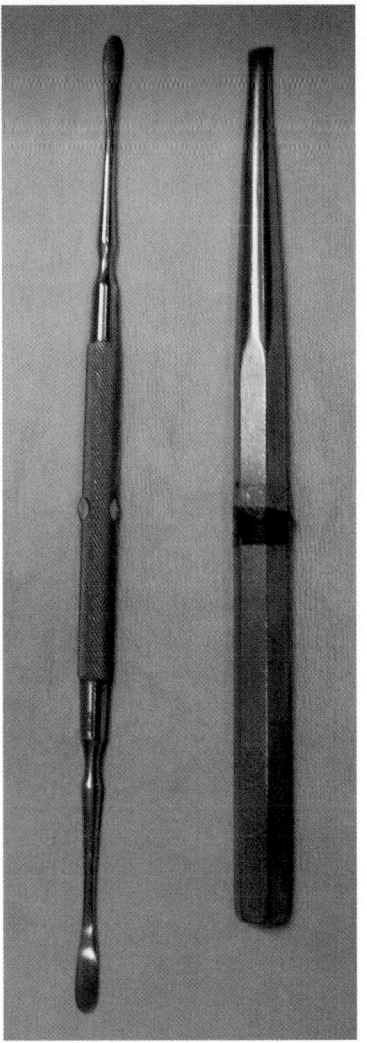

Figure 22-21 Periosteal elevators. Freer elevator and ¹/₄-inch Key elevator.

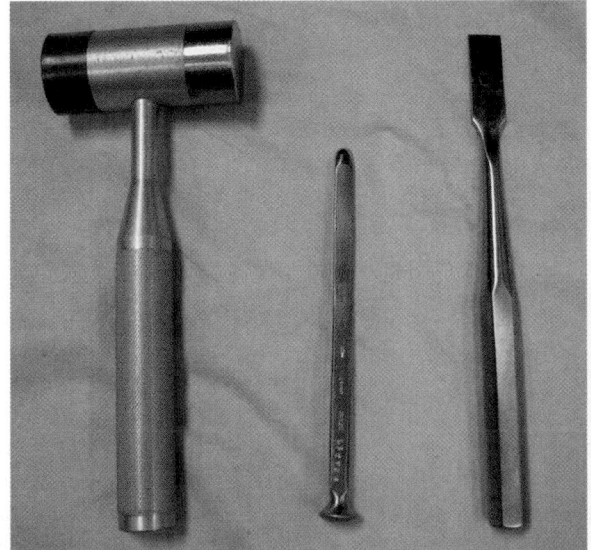

A

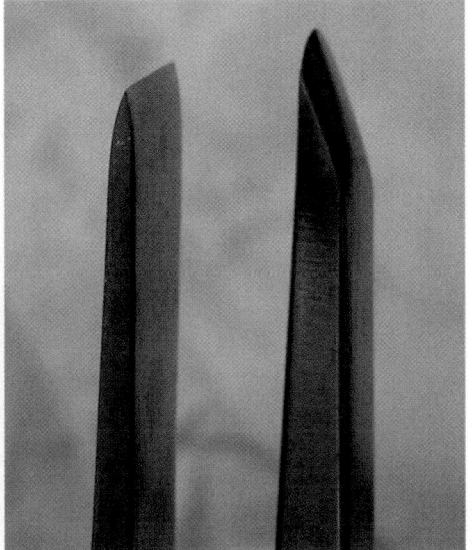

B

Figure 22-22 **A,** Mallet, chisel, and osteotome. **B,** Osteotome *(left)* and chisel *(right)*.

Figure 22-23 Michel trephine.

T-shaped handles hook onto the wire to give the surgeon a firm grasp of the wire.

TREPHINES

Trephines are T-shaped tubular instruments with a cylindrical cutting blade (Figure 22-23). Trephines are usually used to remove a core of bone for biopsy.

POWER EQUIPMENT

Some power equipment is commonly used in orthopedic and neurologic surgery. Although some drills are electric or battery powered (Figure 22-24, *A*), many orthopedic drills and saws are powered by nitrogen gas that is supplied via a sterile hose (Figure 22-24, *B* and *C*). The Hall air drill is a specialized high-speed burr that grinds bone (Figure 22-24, *D*). It is most commonly used for spinal surgery.

ORTHOPEDIC IMPLANTS

Orthopedic surgery sometimes involves the use of various products that are placed in or around the bone and left in place permanently or for an extended period of time. Metal implants are usually made of stainless steel alloy, cobalt-chromium alloys, or titanium. Of these three types, titanium is the most resistant to corrosion and has the best fatigue life. It is also the most expensive.

Table 22-2 COMMONLY USED ORTHOPEDIC WIRE SIZES

Guage	Inches	Millimeters
22	0.025	0.64
20	0.032	0.81
18	0.040	1.02

BONE PINS

Bone pins vary in diameter, length, and the type of points. *Steinmann pins* are smooth, stainless steel pins ranging in diameter from $^1/_{16}$ to $^1/_4$ inch. Three different types of pin points are available, including chisel, trocar, or threaded trocar. Some pins have threads, similar to a screw. A power drill or a Jacobs hand chuck is required to insert the pin into bone, and a pin cutter is necessary to cut it to the proper length (Figure 22-25). Steinmann pins may be called *intramedullary* (IM) *pins* because they are often placed in the medullary cavity of long bones for fracture fixation. Kirschner wires (K-wires) are similar to Steinmann pins but smaller and can be used to pin small bone fragments. The available sizes are 0.035-inch, 0.045-inch, and 0.062-inch diameter.

INTERLOCKING NAILS

Interlocking nails are similar to intramedullary pins but have preplaced holes through the pin that allow screw placement. Interlocking nails have more rigid fixation than IM pins. Equipment is similar to that required for pins, but specialized equipment is needed for screw placement.

ORTHOPEDIC WIRE

Stainless steel orthopedic wire is supplied on spools (Figure 22-26). The common sizes used in small animal surgery are 22 gauge, 20 gauge, and 18 gauge (Table 22-2). It is most commonly applied in a cerclage fashion by encircling the bone or bone fragments and twisting the ends in a "twist-tie" manner. Orthopedic wire is often used for fracture repair in combination with pins or bone plates.

EXTERNAL FIXATORS

External fixation is a means of stabilizing fractures using pins placed through the skin and bone. The pins are held rigid by a metal or acrylic connecting bar that is attached to the pins several centimeters from the skin (Figure 22-27). The metal apparatus uses special clamps to attach a metal connecting bar to the pins. Acrylic (methyl methacrylate) connecting bars are often made from dental acrylics or hoof-wall-repair acrylics because they are less expensive than surgical grades of acrylic. The acrylic connecting bar

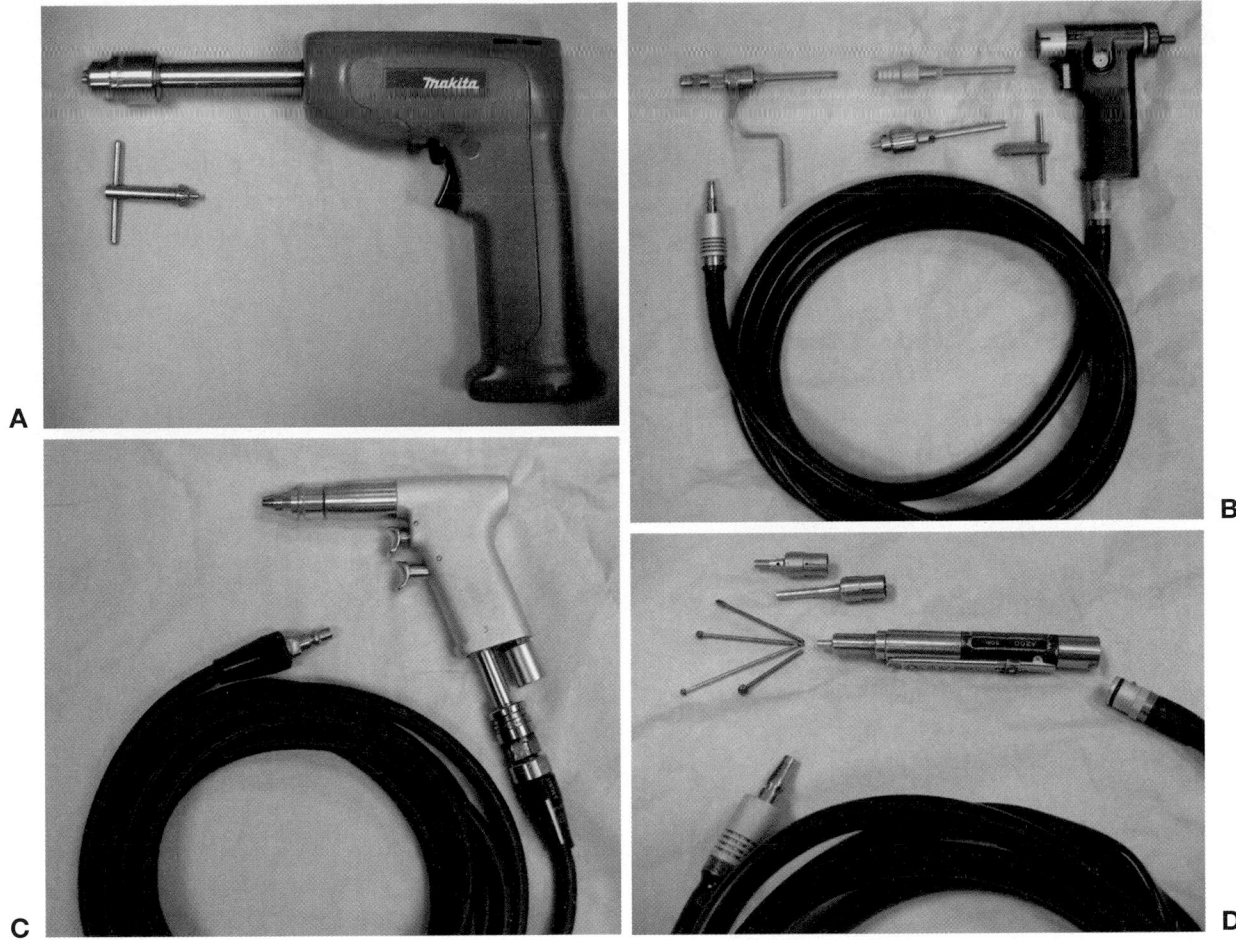

Figure 22-24 Power equipment. **A,** The Makita drill is an example of a battery powered drill. **B,** The 3-M mini driver is powered by a tank of pressurized nitrogen gas. It has an attachment for K-wires, and quick-release or chuck attachments for drill bits. **C,** The ASIF drill is also powered by nitrogen gas. **D,** The Hall air drill has various sizes and shape of burrs, and two different length burr guards.

is more versatile and lighter than the metal apparatus. Ring fixators use special wires instead of pins in the bone. Several metal rings encircle the limb and are fixed in alignment using rods. Each bone wire is clamped to one of the rings.

BONE SCREWS

The two basic screw types are cortical and cancellous screws. Cortical screws are fully threaded screws that are designed for dense (cortical) bone. Cancellous screws are either partially threaded or fully threaded and are made with wider threads in order to have better grip in the softer cancellous bone (Figure 22-28).

The general steps of screw placement include drilling a hole in the bone, measuring the hole with a depth gauge to determine the proper screw length, using a bone tap (a screwlike instrument with sharp threads) to cut a screw path in the bone, and inserting the screw with a specialized screw driver. Bone screws may be used alone or in conjunction with a bone plate or interlocking nail.

Bone screws are named by both the screw length and thread diameter (in millimeters). Commonly used screws in small animal surgery are 2.7- and 3.5-mm-diameter cortical screws and 4.0-mm-diameter cancellous screws. All of these screws have hexagonal heads and are driven by the same hexagonal screwdriver. Smaller screws (1.5- and 2.0-mm diameter) have cruciate heads and require a small, cruciate screwdriver. Larger screws (4.5-, 5.5-, and 6.5-mm diameter) are used in large animal surgery. These screws use a large hexagonal screwdriver.

BONE PLATES

There are many different types of bone plates (Figure 22-29). Bone plates are named by the number of screw holes and by the screw diameter size that best fits the plate. For example, a seven-hole, 3.5-mm plate would use seven, 3.5-mm-diameter screws. Bone plates must be bent to match the curve of the bone and fastened to it with bone screws. Instrumentation required to apply a bone plate is highly

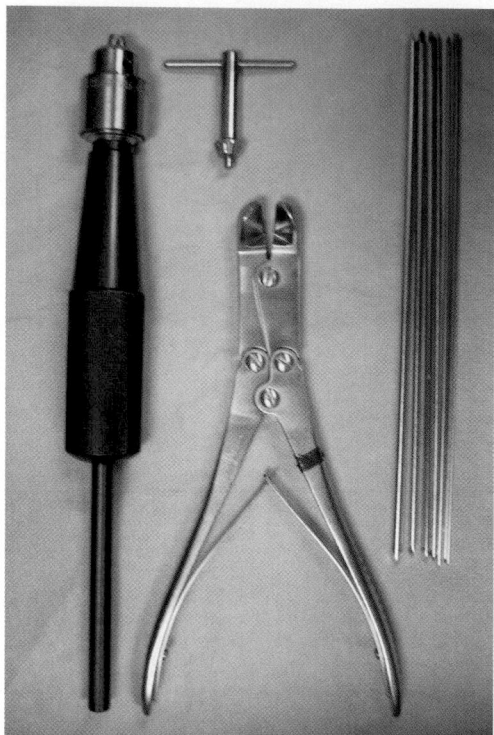

Figure 22-25 Jacobs hand chuck, key, pin cutter, and various sizes of Steinmann pins and K-wires.

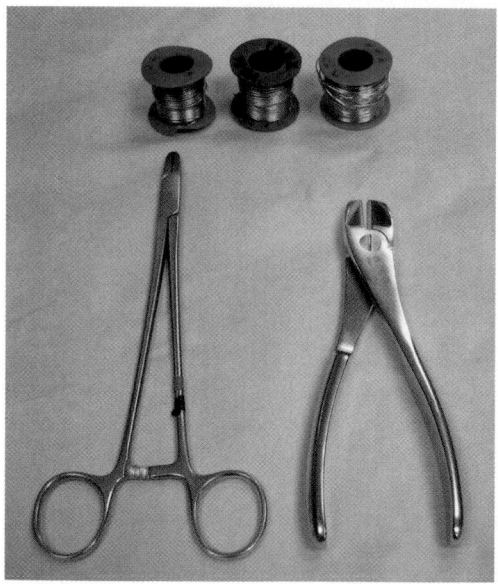

Figure 22-26 Orthopedic wire, wire twisters, wire cutters. Wire twisters look similar to needle holders but are more rugged and designed to withstand higher forces.

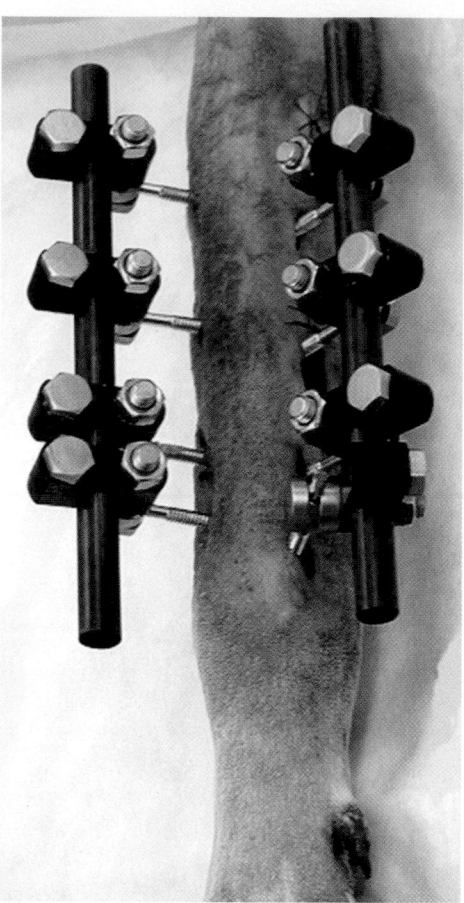

Figure 22-27 An external fixator on the radius of a dog. Pins that penetrate the skin and bone are fixed to bars using special clamps. (Courtesy Dr. James Toombs.)

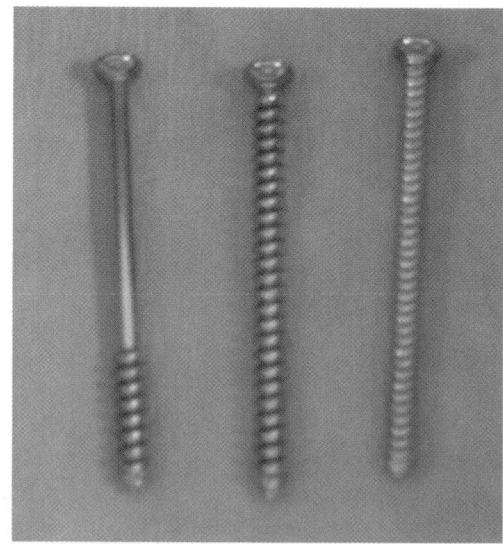

Figure 22-28 Bone screws. *Left to right:* Partially threaded cancellous screw, fully threaded cancellous screw, and fully threaded cortical screw.

specialized and includes drills, drill bits, drill guides, depth gauges, bone taps, tap sleeves, screws, screwdrivers, and plate benders (Figure 22-30). Although bone plating is more complex than other types of orthopedic fixation, plate fixation is much more stable in most cases.

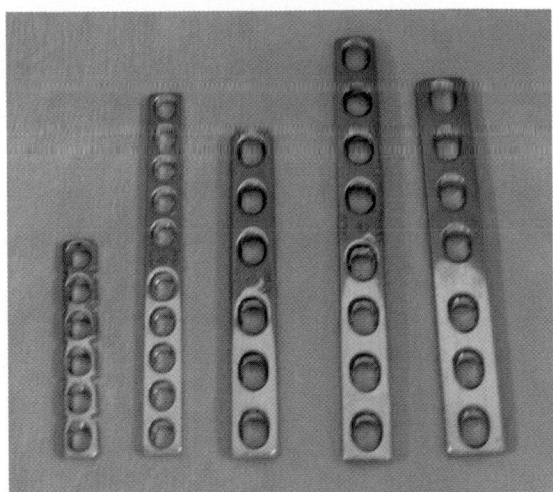

Figure 22-29 Various sizes of bone plates.

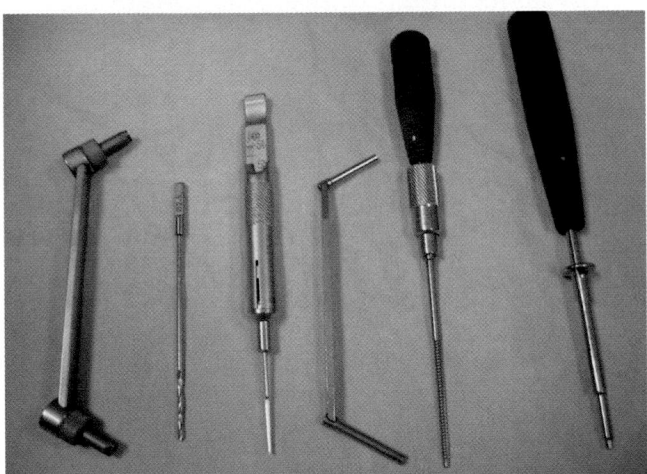

Figure 22-30 Bone plating equipment. *Left to right:* Drill guide, drill bit, depth gauge, tap sleeve (to prevent soft tissues from being caught on the bone tap), bone tap, and screwdriver.

TOTAL HIP PROSTHESIS

Replacement of the hip joint with a prosthesis may be done in some dogs with severe arthritis. This procedure is done by highly trained veterinary surgeons and requires much specialized orthopedic equipment in addition to the prosthesis itself. The femoral prosthesis consists of a long stem that fits inside the proximal femur and a ball that replaces the femoral head. A special cup replaces the acetabulum.

ARTHROSCOPIC INSTRUMENTS AND EQUIPMENT

The arthroscope is used as a diagnostic and surgical tool in veterinary surgery. It is used mostly to examine various joints of the horse, including the scapulohumeral,

humeroradial, carpal, fetlock, distal interphalangeal, coxofemoral (foals only), stifle, and tarsocrural. It is also used to examine various joints in the dog. Arthroscopy is used primarily to remove osteochondral chip fragments and osteochondritic lesions on the articular surface in joints of young horses and dogs. The arthroscope has been used to visualize intraarticular fractures for lag screw fixation, such as third carpal bone slab fractures in horses, as well as meniscal and cruciate injuries in dogs. The arthroscope has also been used to perform tenoscopy of the digital flexor tendon sheath and sinuscopy of the paranasal sinuses through trephined holes in the facial bones overlying the sinuses of horses. Most of the equipment used in veterinary arthroscopy has been adapted from human arthroscopy. New technology is constantly being developed that will no doubt influence the veterinary field. This section is intended to allow the veterinary technician to become more familiar with the instruments and techniques of arthroscopy.

ARTHROSCOPE

There is a selection of different arthroscopes that have been developed with various diameters and viewing angles. For example, there is a 5-mm-outer-diameter (OD) arthroscope with either a 10-, 25-, or 70-degree lens angle; a 4-mm OD with a 10-, 30-, 70-, or 110-degree lens angle; a 2.7-mm OD with a 5-, 30-, or 70-degree lens angle; and a 1.9-mm OD with a 5- or 30-degree lens angle. A 4-mm OD, 25- or 30-degree angled lens scope is generally used by most equine surgeons (Figure 22-31), whereas a 2.7-mm-OD, 30-degree angled lens scope is commonly used for canine arthroscopy. Most arthroscopes have a television camera permanently coupled to it, which allows the surgeon to view the joint on a television monitor (Figure 22-32). A television monitor has the advantage of a larger image. This greatly improves visualization of the intraarticular space compared with direct viewing through the eyepiece of the arthroscope. This method also provides better aseptic technique, because the surgeon's face is not near the surgical field and an assistant can operate the camera-scope unit, allowing the surgeon more freedom. A monitor also allows several people to observe the procedure simultaneously, and a videotape record can be made for future replay.

ANCILLARY ARTHROSCOPIC EQUIPMENT

Along with the arthroscope come various instruments used to introduce the scope into the joint. Stab incisions are made in the skin, over the joint space once the site is surgically prepared, through which the arthroscope and hand instruments will be inserted once the animal is positioned for surgery.

Sharp Trocar and Sleeve

A pointed instrument called a *sharp trocar* is inserted inside a hollow, cannula-type instrument called the *sleeve* (Figure

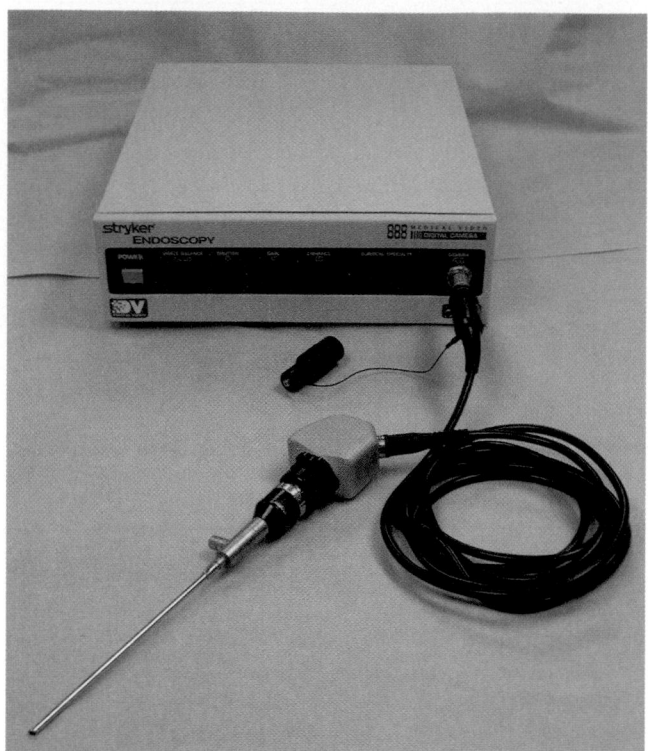

Figure 22-31 Television camera and 4-mm-OD arthroscope.

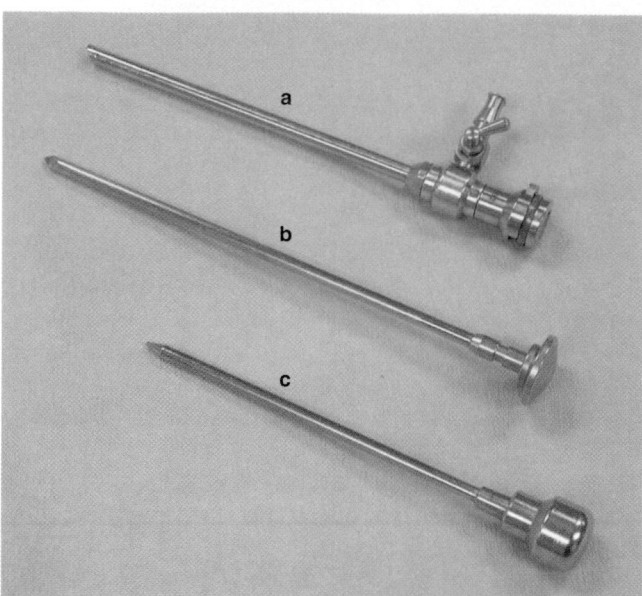

Figure 22-33 The sharp trocar *(b)* fits inside the arthroscope sleeve *(a)*. The unit is used to penetrate the fibrous joint capsule through a stab incision in the skin. The conical obturator *(c)* replaces the sharp trocar in the sleeve once the fibrous joint capsule is penetrated.

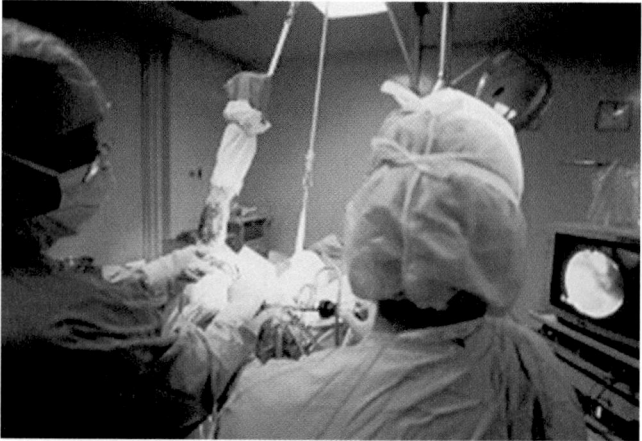

Figure 22-32 Most arthroscopic procedures are viewed on a television monitor.

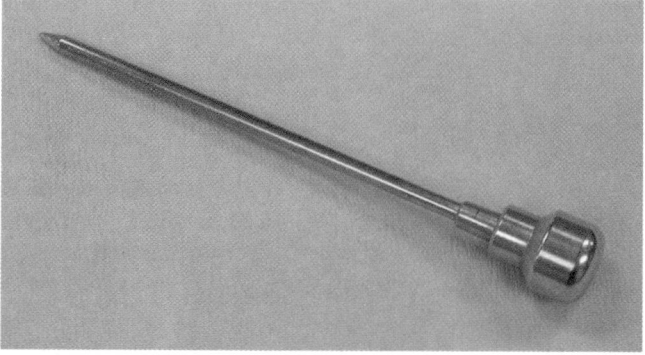

Figure 22-34 The conical obturator replaces the sharp trocar in the sleeve and is used to penetrate the synovial membrane portion of the joint capsule and advance the sleeve further into the joint.

22-33). The trocar and sleeve unit are used to penetrate the fibrous portion of the joint capsule through a stab incision.

Blunt Obturator

Once the sharp trocar has penetrated the fibrous joint capsule, the sharp trocar is replaced with a conical (blunt) obturator (Figure 22-34), which is used to penetrate the synovial membrane of the joint capsule and advance the sleeve into the joint space with less risk of damaging the articular cartilage. At this point the obturator is withdrawn from the sleeve. The joint space is distended with a

sterile balanced electrolyte solution (fluids) before placement of the sleeve in the joint, so a rush of fluids through the barrel of the sleeve will occur as the obturator is being removed. The obturator is replaced with the arthroscope (Figure 22-35), which is designed to lock onto the sleeve once it is slid into position in the sleeve.

Light Cable, Light Projector, and Television Camera

Once the arthroscope is positioned in the joint a fiber-optic light cable (Figure 22-36) is attached directly to the optical light port on the arthroscope (Figure 22-37). A high-intensity

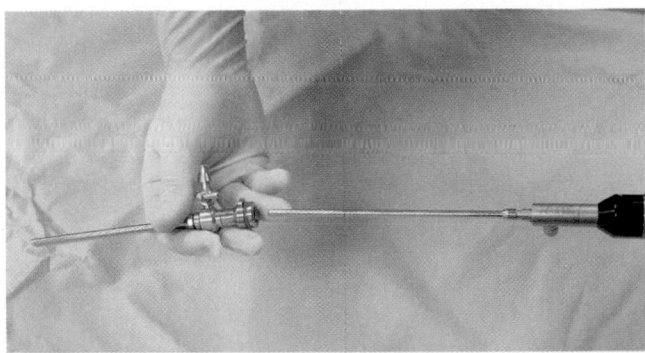

Figure 22-35 Once the sleeve is in position in the joint, the obturator is removed and the arthroscope is placed into the sleeve.

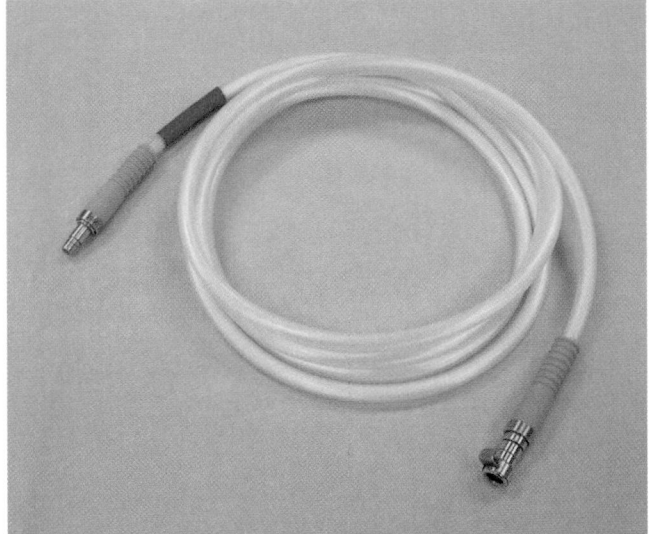

Figure 22-36 Fiber-optic light cable. It should be handled very carefully to avoid damaging the optic fibers.

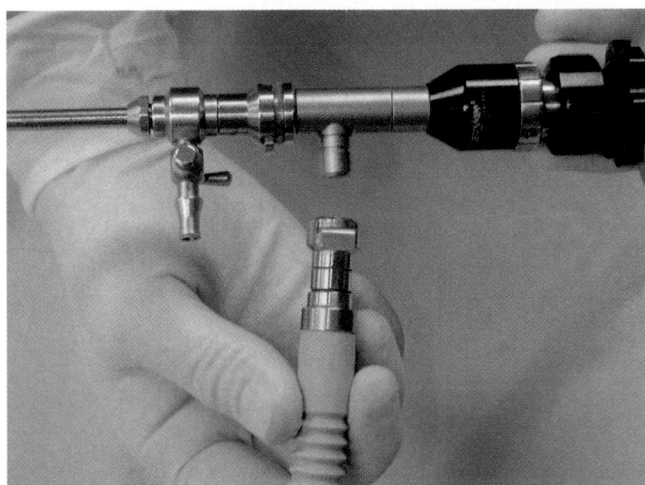

Figure 22-37 The fiber-optic light cable attaches to the light port of the arthroscope.

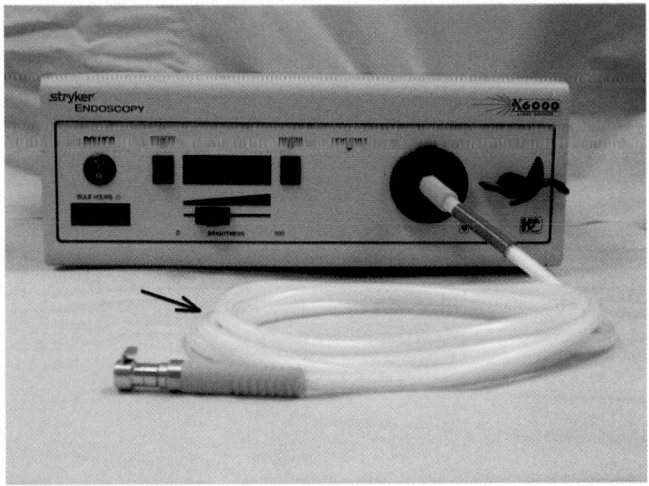

Figure 22-38 Light projector is designed to project light through a fiber-optic light cable *(arrow)* of the arthroscope.

light generated from a specially designed light projector is fed through the fiber-optic cable and through the arthroscope to illuminate the joint space (Figure 22-38).

FLUID DELIVERY SYSTEMS

Fluids, usually a balanced electrolyte solution, are infused into the joint under pressure to maintain distention of the joint capsule, which is essential for visualization of the intra-articular space. Gas insufflation, using carbon dioxide or nitrous oxide, has also been used as a method of distending the joint. However, a special system with a pressure-regulating device is required. One disadvantage of gas is that it does not allow for lavage of the joint space if osteochondral chip fragments become detached in the joint. The fluids are infused into the joint space through the sleeve, around the arthroscope. The sleeve has at least one stopcock that is used as an ingress port to connect a sterile fluid line (Figure 22-39).

Pressurized Bag System

Various systems are available to deliver fluid to the joint. One system is a pressurized bag design. A pneumatic pressure cuff is slipped around a bag containing sterile fluids. The cuff is inflated with air, which squeezes the fluid bag, thus pressurizing the fluids (Figure 22-40). The amount of pressure is regulated by the amount of cuff inflation.

Automated Pump System

Another type of system uses a motorized pump to regulate the fluid rate through the fluid lines connected to the arthroscope. One example of this type of system is the Hydroflex (Devol Inc.) (Figure 22-41). The pressure and fluid volume going into the joint are automatically regulated within the fluid pump. This automated pressure-sensitive pump system regulates the pressure via a pressure feedback control. This

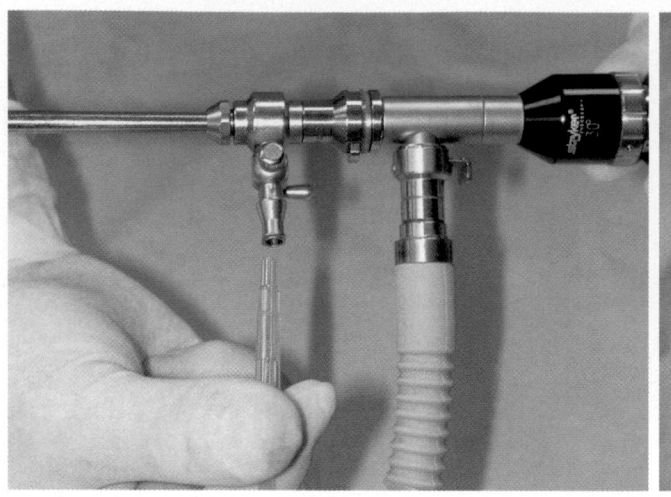
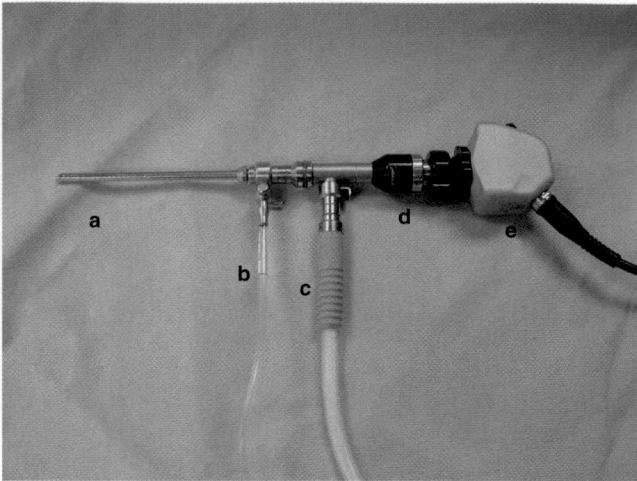

A

B

Figure 22-39 **A,** The fluid line is connected to the stopcock of the arthroscope. **B,** Arthroscopic sleeve *(a),* fluid line *(b),* light cable *(c),* arthroscope *(d),* and camera *(e).*

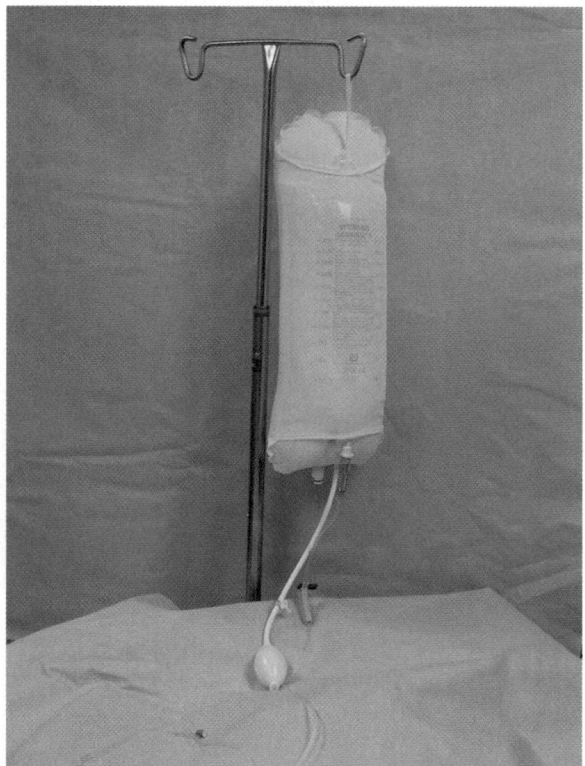

Figure 22-40 Pressurized bag of fluids can be used to distend a joint during arthroscopy.

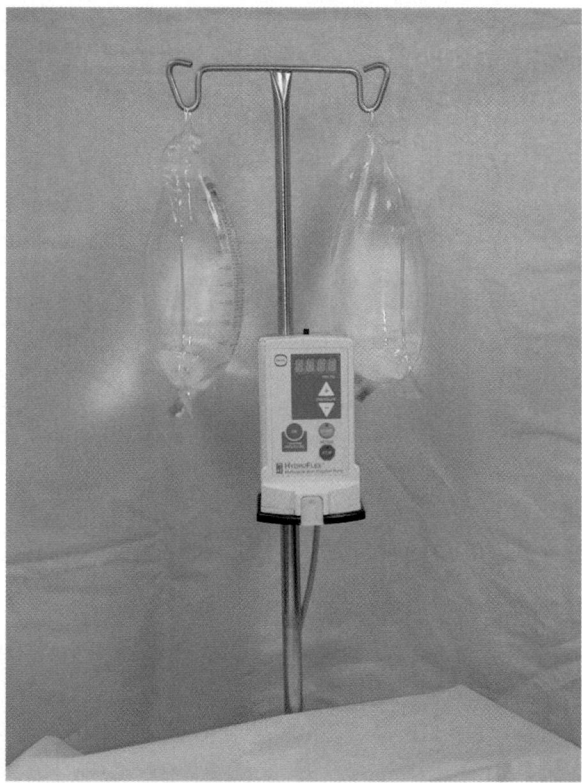

Figure 22-41 Automated fluid pressure pump can be used to infuse sterile fluids into a joint during arthroscopy. The pressure within the joint is automatically regulated by the pump.

allows the pump to maintain a preset pressure in the joint without the surgeon having to adjust the fluid pressure.

HAND INSTRUMENTS FOR ARTHROSCOPIC SURGERY

Numerous hand instruments of various types are available or have been adapted for arthroscopy. They are used to remove or retrieve osteochondral chip fragments, debride articular cartilage or subchondral bone, or probe cartilage or cartilage lesions. The instruments are inserted into the joint through a separate stab incision, and the arthroscopic operation is performed via a technique called *triangulation.* Only the most commonly used instruments are discussed here.

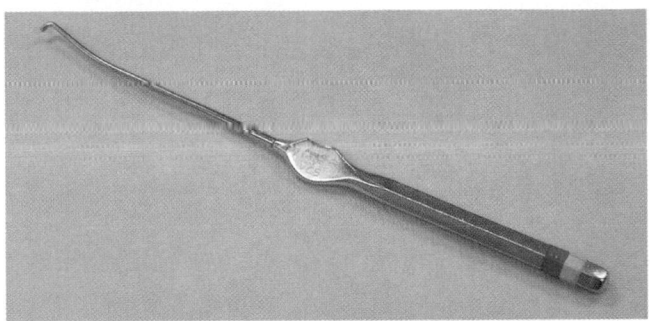

Figure 22-42 Blunt arthroscopy probe.

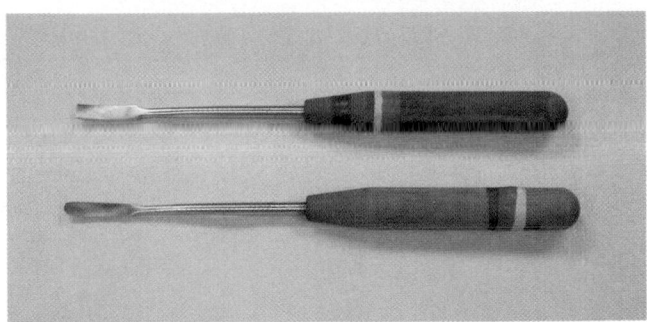

Figure 24-44 Elevator and osteotome used in arthroscopy.

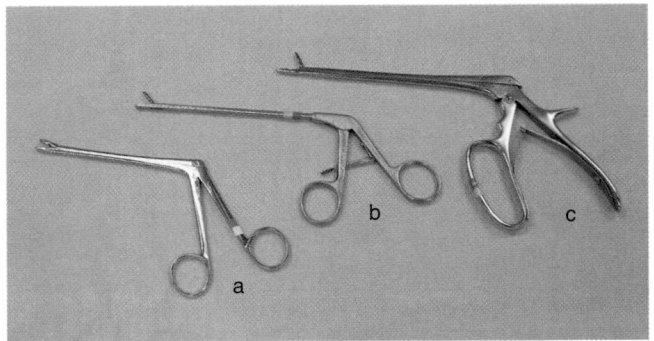

Figure 22-43 Rongeurs used in arthroscopy: Love and Gruenwald *(a)*, grasping forceps *(b)* and Ferris Smith *(c)*.

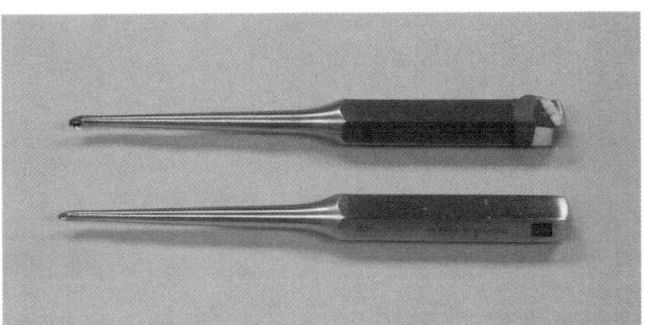

Figure 22-45 Small cupped bone curettes used in arthroscopy.

Blunt Probe

The blunt probe is used to probe a site in the joint to determine such aspects as cartilage integrity or the extent of a cartilage lesion (Figure 22-42).

Rongeurs and Grasping Forceps

Various types and sizes of rongeurs have been adapted for use in arthroscopy. These instruments have a beveled edge along cupped jaws to cut the attachments of an osteochondral chip fragment as it is being removed (Figure 22-43). Forceps are used to retrieve loosely attached fragments (Figure 22-43).

Elevators and Osteotomes

These instruments have small beveled heads that are designed to cut or break down the attachments of an osteochondral chip fragment and elevate it from the parent subchondral bone bed (Figure 22-44).

Curettes

Curettes are inserted into the joint to debride a defect left in the articular cartilage or subchondral bone after removal of an osteochondral chip fragment or osteochondritic lesion (Figure 22-45).

Motorized Burrs

Motorized burrs are often referred to as a *motorized arthroplasty system*. The system consists of a small rounded burr attached to a power-driven shaft. The burr and shaft are enclosed in a sleeve, with a portion of the burr protected to prevent inadvertent damage to surrounding articular cartilage (Figure 22-46). This instrument is also used to debride a defect left in the articular cartilage or subchondral bone after removal of an osteochondral chip fragment or osteochondritic lesion. The speed of rotation of the burr can be adjusted, and the burr is usually operated at several thousand revolutions per minute. Most systems operate with an on/off foot-pedal switch for the surgeon.

INSTRUMENT PACKS

Most veterinary hospitals organize their surgical instruments into several different instrument packs based on the type of surgical procedure. Surgical pack organization is dependent on the type of practice and surgeries performed, but some examples are as follows: general packs for soft tissue surgeries, bone packs for orthopedic surgeries, emergency packs for emergency and minor procedures, and

Table 22-3 SMALL ANIMAL INSTRUMENT PACKS

Soft Tissue/General Pack	Emergency Pack	Orthopedic Pack
No. 3 scalpel handle	No. 3 scalpel handle	Army-Navy retractors
Brown-Adson thumb forceps	Brown-Adson thumb forceps	Senn retractors
Adson thumb forceps	Needle holder, Olsen-Hegar	Rongeurs
Needle holder, Mayo-Hegar	Mayo scissors, curved	Large Kern bone-holding forceps
Mayo scissors	Mosquito hemostats (3 curved, 3 straight)	Small Kern bone-holding forceps
Metzenbaum scissors	Crile or Kelly forceps (1 curved, 1 straight)	Bone curette
Wire-suture scissors	Allis forceps	Periosteal elevator
Mosquito hemostats (4 curved, 4 straight)	Towel clamps (4)	Steinmann pins (5/64, 3/32, 7/64, 1/8, 9/64,
Crile forceps (1 curved, 1 straight)	Towels (4)	5/32, 3/16, 1/4)
Carmalt forceps (2 curved)	Sponges(standard count)	Kirschner wire (0.035, 0.045, 0.062)
Allis forceps (2)	Sterilization indicator	Jacobs chuck and key
Ovariohysterectomy hook (Snook hook)		Roll 18-gauge stainless steel wire
Towel clamps (8)		Roll 20-gauge stainless steel wire
Towels (6)		Roll 22-gauge stainless steel wire
Stainless steel bowl		Metal ruler
Sponges (standard count)		Michel clips and applicator
Lap sponges (2)		Sterilization indicator
Sterilization indicator		

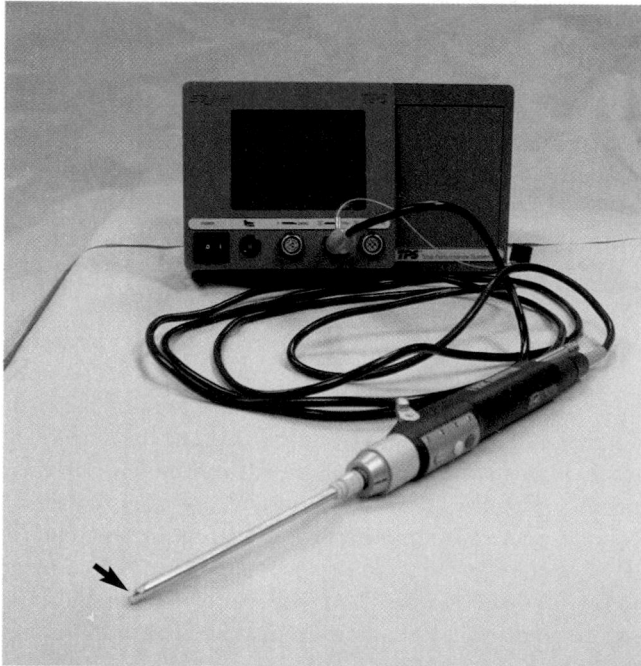

Figure 22-46 Motorized arthroplasty system with burr attachment *(arrow).*

Table 22-4 LARGE ANIMAL STANDARD AND EMERGENCY PACKS

Standard Pack	Emergency Pack
No. 3 scalpel handle	No. 3 scalpel handle
No. 4 scalpel handle	No. 4 scalpel handle
Rat-tooth thumb forceps (3)	Rat-tooth thumb forceps
Adson thumb forceps (3)	Brown-Adson thumb forceps
Needle holders (2)	Needle holder
Mayo scissors (1 curved, 1 straight)	Mayo scissors (1 curved, 1 straight)
Operating scissors (sharp-sharp)	Mosquito hemostats (2 curved, 2 straight)
Metzenbaum scissors (1 curved, 1 straight)	Allis tissue forceps (2)
Bandage scissors	Towel clamps (4)
Mosquito hemostats (4 straight, 4 curved)	Towel
Kelly or Crile forceps (2 straight, 2 curved)	Sponges (standard count)
Ochsner forceps, 15-cm (1 curved, 1 straight)	Sterilization indicator
Allis tissue forceps (2)	
Towel clamps (16)	
Towels (4)	
Saline bowl	
Sponges (standard count)	
Sterilization indicator	

neurologic packs for spinal surgeries (Tables 22-3 and 22-4). A pack system helps to organize the instruments so that the most commonly used instruments are readily available and infrequently used instruments are not contaminated and resterilized unnecessarily. For example, all commonly used instruments for spinal surgery are in one pack, so it is opened, used, cleaned, sterilized, and repacked only when necessary. Infrequently used instruments are typically

wrapped individually. Large and bulky instruments are also packed separately. In addition, some commonly used instruments (e.g., scalpel handle, hemostats, thumb forceps, scissors, needle holders, sponges) may be wrapped individually to

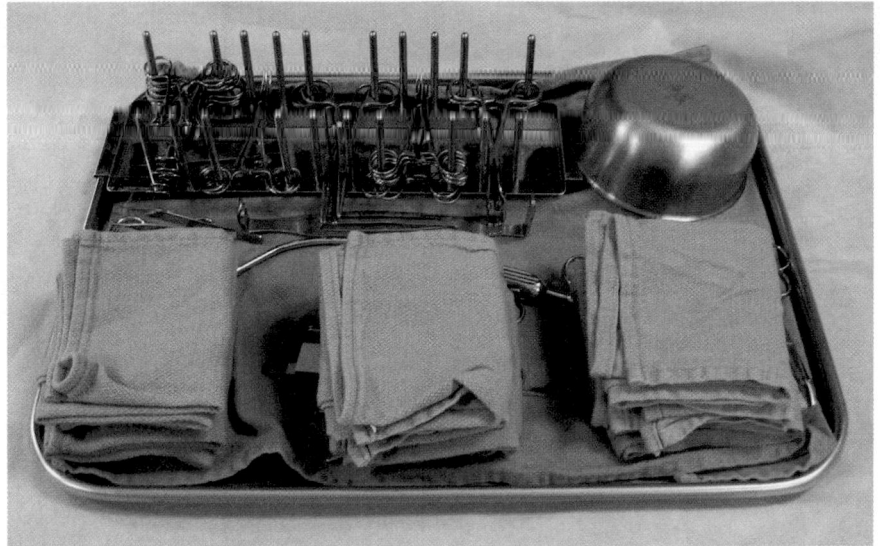

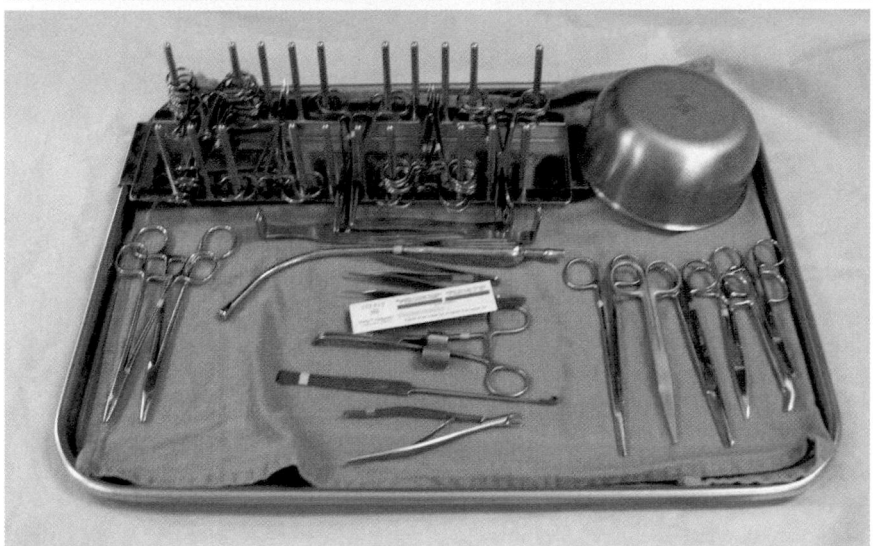

Figure 22-47 **A,** Properly organized instrument tray. **B,** Same tray but towels have been removed.

provide access to an additional instrument without having to open an entire instrument pack.

Each type of pack should be organized such that items are always placed in the same location on the tray (Figure 22-47). This makes it easier to inventory the instruments and facilitates finding the instruments quickly during surgery. Sponges may be counted at the beginning and end of each surgery to be sure none has been left in the patient.

INSTRUMENT CARE

Most surgical instruments are made of stainless steel, which is rust resistant and retains a sharp edge. The two common instrument finishes are polished or satin. The polished finish is durable but tends to reflect light, which may impair the surgeon's vision. The satin or dull finish was developed to eliminate glare, but it is less resistant to spotting and discoloration.

Good quality instruments are expensive but will last for years if treated properly. All instruments should be handled gently and delicate instruments should be separated from the general instruments before cleaning. Multiple-component instruments should be disassembled prior to cleaning. Power equipment should be cleaned separately to ensure that water does not get inside the components.

Immediately after use, instruments should be rinsed with cold water to prevent blood and organic debris from drying in the serrations, hinges, box locks, or ratchets. Distilled or deionized water is preferable to tap water to prevent staining or corrosion of the instruments. If there will be a delay before final cleaning, the instruments can be immersed in water containing an instrument detergent. Each instrument is scrubbed with a soft brush in warm water using a neutral pH instrument detergent. Abrasive cleaning agents should never be used on surgical instruments. An ultrasonic (high-frequency sound) cleaner (Figure 22-48) is used after manual cleaning to remove tightly bound soil or clean areas

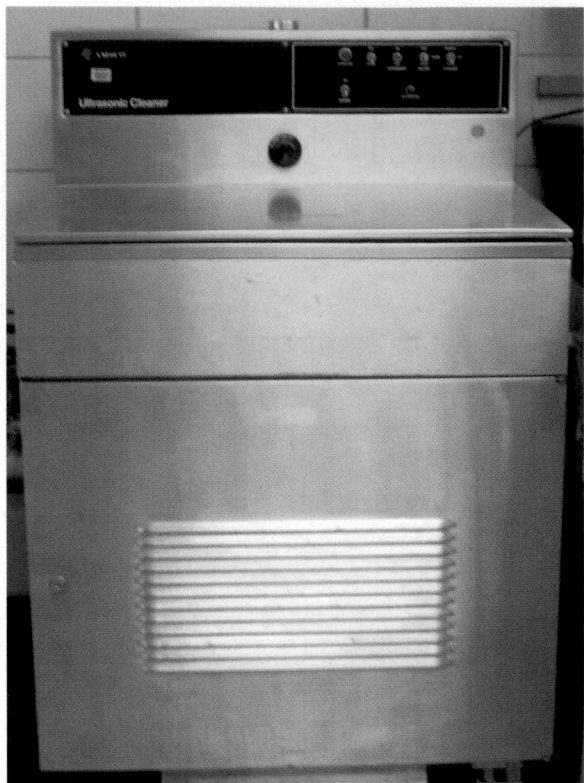

Figure 22-48 Ultrasonic cleaners are available in different sizes and models. Follow manufacturer's recommendations regarding use.

that the brush cannot reach. Instruments should be placed in the ultrasound unit with the box locks open. Instruments of dissimilar metals (e.g., chrome and stainless steel) should not be put together in the ultrasound unit, as this may result in pitting of the instruments. Instruments should be thoroughly rinsed and air-dried (wiping instruments may leave lint residue) before autoclaving to prevent rust spots.

Instruments with a working action, such as a hinge or box lock, should be treated with an instrument lubricant or instrument "milk" after each cleaning. The recommended lubricants are water soluble, so thorough cleaning will remove all the lubrication. Instrument lubricants are not oily or sticky, inhibit rust formation, and do not interfere with steam sterilization. Working components of power equipment should also be lubricated to maximize efficiency and to prolong the working lifetime of the equipment. Before instruments are repacked for sterilization they should be thoroughly inspected for cleanliness, stiff or "frozen" hinges, improper jaw alignment, rust spots, and worn or broken parts. Defective instruments should be repaired or replaced.

DRAPES AND GOWNS

Surgical drapes and gowns may be paper or cloth. Paper drapes and gowns are designed to be disposable and should be used only once. They are bought prepackaged and sterilized for individual use. Cloth drapes and gowns are designed for repeated use, but they require washing after each use. Immediately soaking the cloth in cold water will prevent blood and other fluids from setting. All cloth drapes and gowns should be washed in a mild detergent and thoroughly dried prior to sterilization. They should also be inspected for holes or other signs of wear.

> ✎ **TECHNICIAN NOTE**
> Accordion folding of drape allows easy unfolding and placement on the patient.

Cloth gowns must always be folded and packed in the same manner (Figure 22-49). This technique allows the sterile gown to be unfolded and put on without contaminating the exterior surface. Cloth drapes must also be folded and packed such that sterility can be maintained while they are unfolded and applied to the patient. "Accordion folding" allows easy unfolding and placement of the drape (Figure 22-50). Many specifically designed drapes are also available, including adhesive drapes, transparent drapes, fenestrated drapes, stockinettes, and compressive wraps. After the drapes and gowns have been properly folded, they are usually double-wrapped in muslin or a nonwoven barrier prior to sterilization (Figure 22-51).

ASEPTIC TECHNIQUE

Asepsis is a condition of sterility, where no living organisms are present. Aseptic technique includes all steps taken to prevent contamination of the surgical site by infectious agents. A thorough understanding of aseptic technique is required to properly sterilize the surgical equipment and clean the operating room. Certain principles of aseptic technique must also be followed when scrubbing the surgical site and placing sterile drapes on the patient. The technician may need to act as a circulating nurse by getting the patient in the operating room and opening sterile equipment for the surgeon. Additionally, the technician may be called upon to scrub in as a scrub nurse or surgical assistant to organize and pass instruments to the surgeon or to assist with the surgical procedure. A working knowledge of aseptic technique is necessary to perform these tasks correctly and also to monitor for inadvertent "breaks" in sterile technique.

Microorganisms must be introduced into the surgical site for infection to develop. The source of microorganisms includes exogenous and endogenous routes. Exogenous sources of contamination include the air, the surgical instruments and supplies, the patient's skin, and the surgical team. Endogenous contamination arises from within the patient and reaches the wound through the blood stream. Examples of endogenous sources are bacteria from gingivitis or dermatitis.

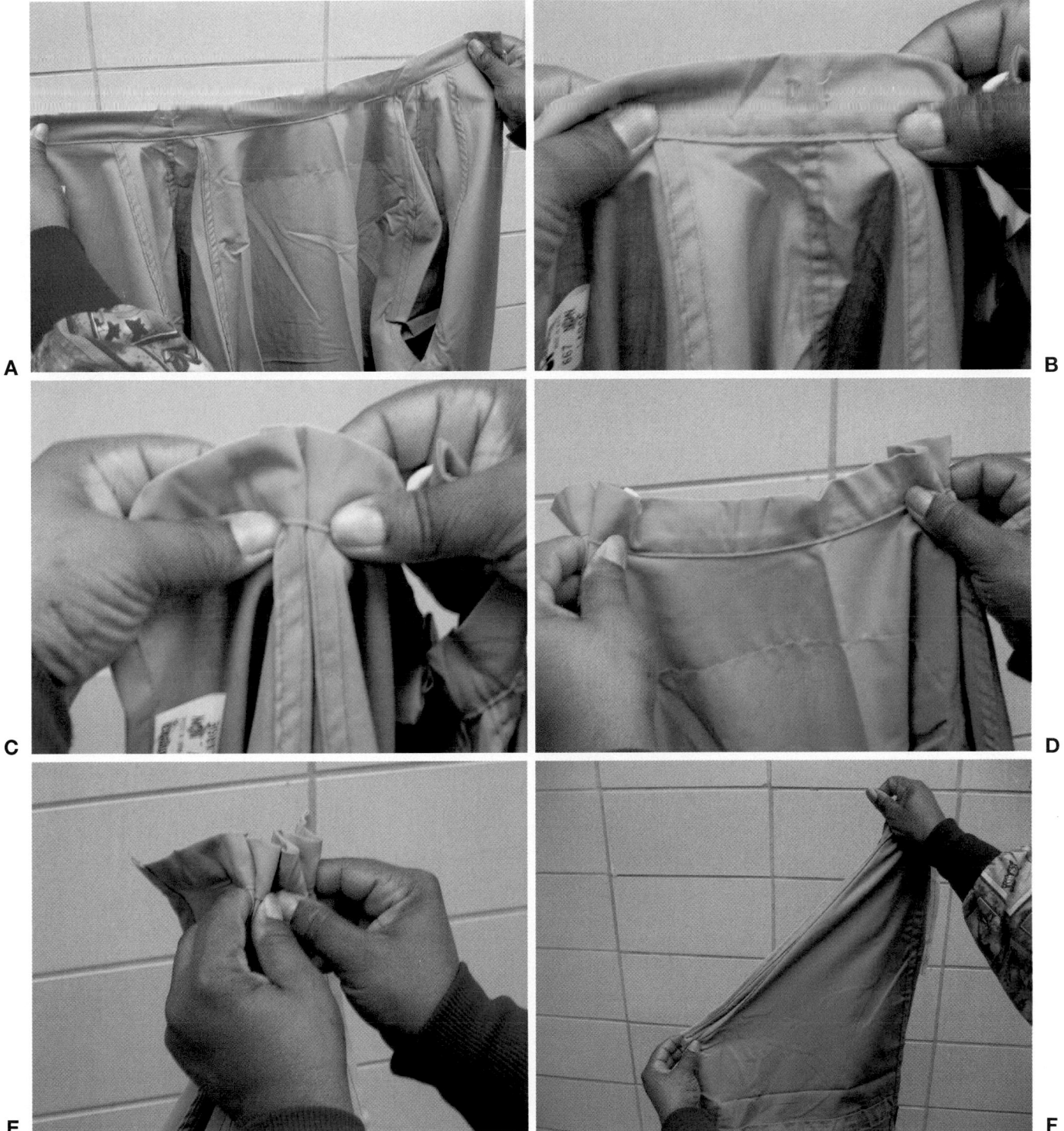

Figure 22-49 Method of folding a cloth surgical gown. **A,** The gown is held by the neck to see the shoulder seams on the inside of the gown. **B,** Close-up of the three seams of one shoulder. **C,** The gown is folded so the outer two seams of one shoulder are touching. **D,** The same fold is done with the other shoulder. **E,** The gown is folded so the seams of both shoulders are touching. **F,** The shoulders are held in one hand while the other hand aligns the armpit seams.

Continued

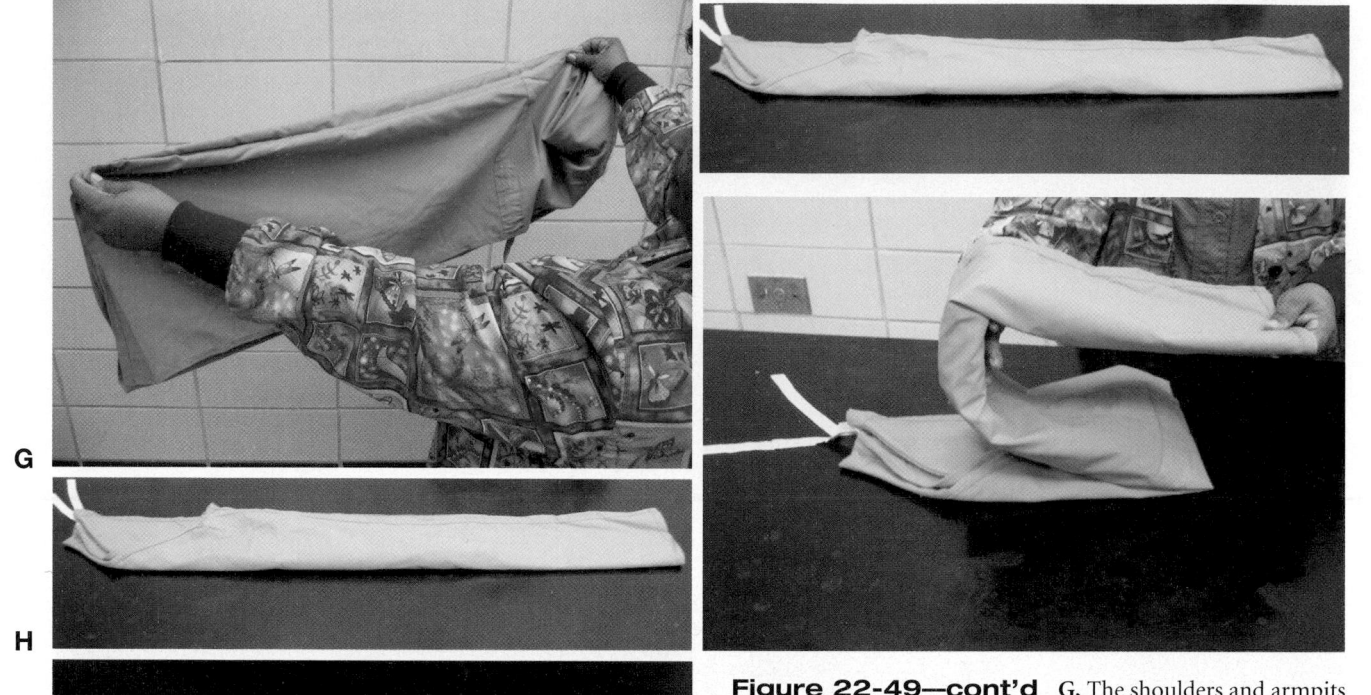

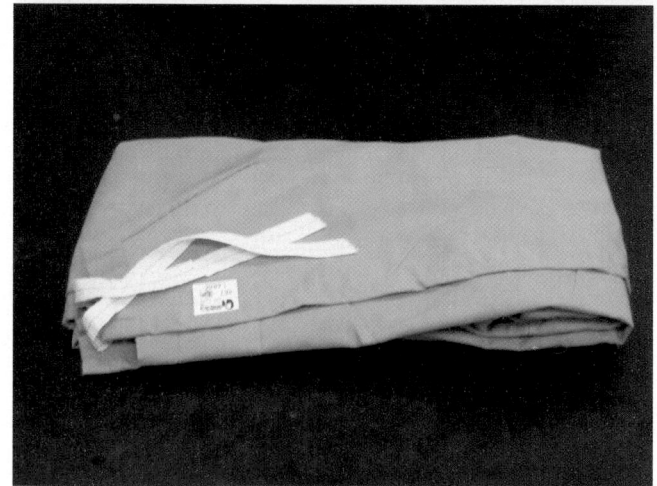

Figure 22-49—cont'd **G,** The shoulders and armpits are held in one hand while the other hand aligns the gown hem. **H,** The gown is laid flat on the table. (A tabletop method of folding is to first lay the gown open flat on the countertop with the outside of the gown facing up, sleeves on top. The side edges of the gown are each folded to meet near the middle, and then the gown is folded in half.) Only the inside surfaces of the gown are now exposed. **I,** The gown is folded in half lengthwise. **J,** The gown is folded in accordion fashion. **K,** The gown is laid on the table so the neck ties are uppermost. Proceed to Figure 22-51 to wrap the gown.

During every surgery, some bacterial contamination occurs at the surgical site. Whether the contamination progresses to an infection depends on many factors, including the general health of the patient, the degree of tissue damage in the wound, the virulence of the infectious agent, and the number of infectious agents. The factor over which the surgical team has the most control is the number of infectious agents that are introduced into the wound by an exogenous route. Strict adherence to the principles of aseptic technique will minimize exogenous wound contamination and prevent many infections from developing.

All procedures do not require the same degree of vigilance regarding aseptic technique. For example, the debridement of a cutaneous abscess is considered to be a contaminated or dirty surgery, so aseptic technique would not be strictly followed. The wound would be scrubbed, but surgical instruments may be disinfected (cold sterilization) rather than sterilized (steam autoclave or gas sterilization), and the surgeon may wear sterile gloves but forgo complete sterile surgical attire. It may be preferable for such a patient to remain outside the operating room to prevent contaminating it. In contrast, total hip replacement surgery involves the implantation of synthetic material and infection can be devastating to the success of the surgery. In such cases, the surgical team adheres strictly to aseptic protocol. The surgeon will determine the degree to which the principles of asepsis are to be followed for each case.

Sterilization is the destruction of all organisms and spores on an object. *Disinfection* is the destruction of the vegetative forms of bacteria but not the spores. Both sterilization and disinfection are used to prepare medical and surgical materials. The process used depends on the nature of the

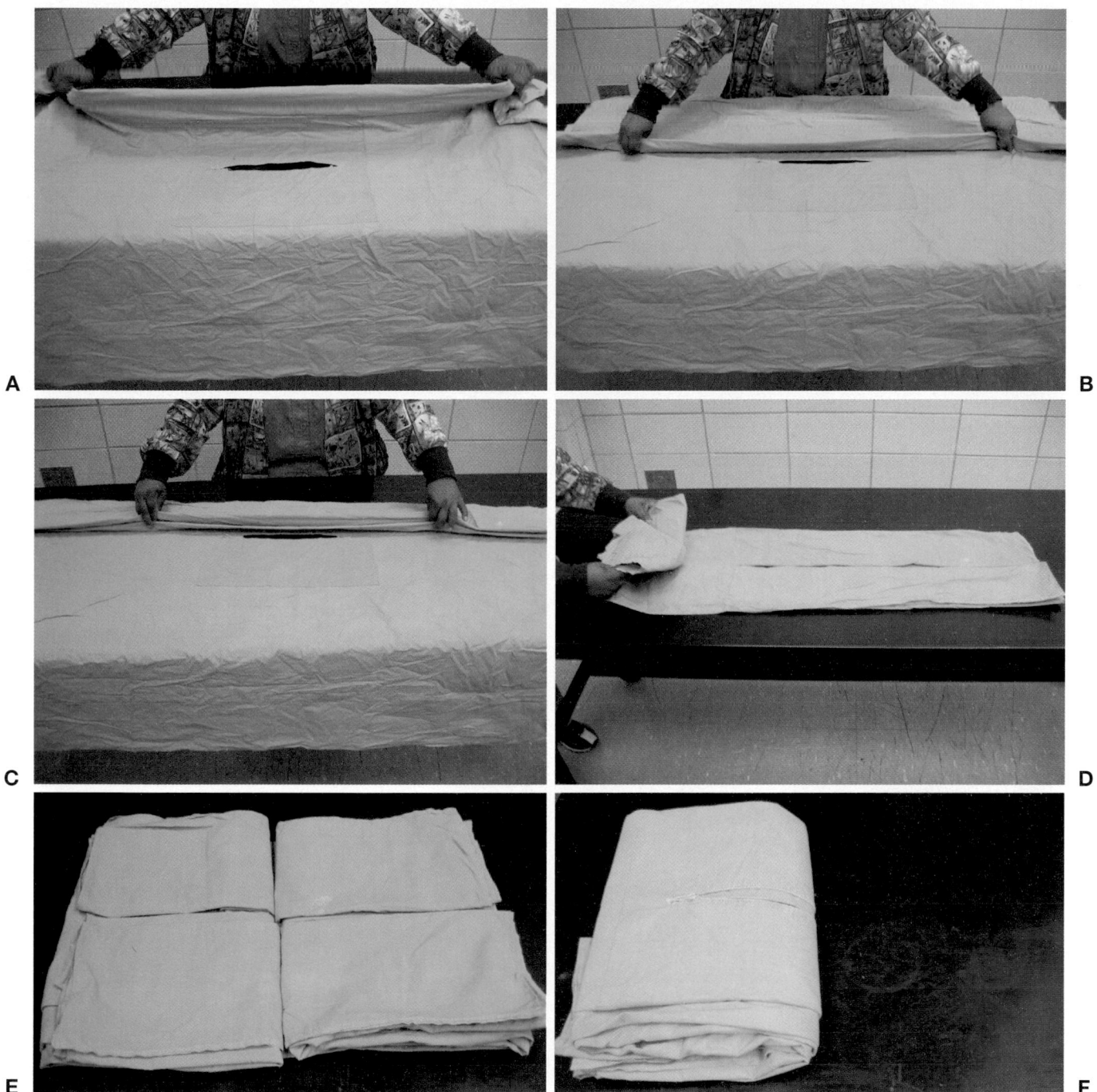

Figure 22-50 Cloth drapes are folded in accordion fashion so that they are easily unfolded onto the patient. **A** and **B,** A lengthwise fold is created in the drape (approximately 30 cm from the middle), and the folded edge is brought to the fenestration at the middle of the drape. **C,** This is repeated with a second fold, creating an accordion folding. Each section of folded drape is approximately 15 cm wide. **D,** The opposite side is folded in a similar manner. Then one end of the drape is folded to the center in accordion fashion. **E,** The opposite end is folded in the same manner. **F,** The drape is folded in half (half of the fenestration is visible), and it is ready to be wrapped as in Figure 22-51.

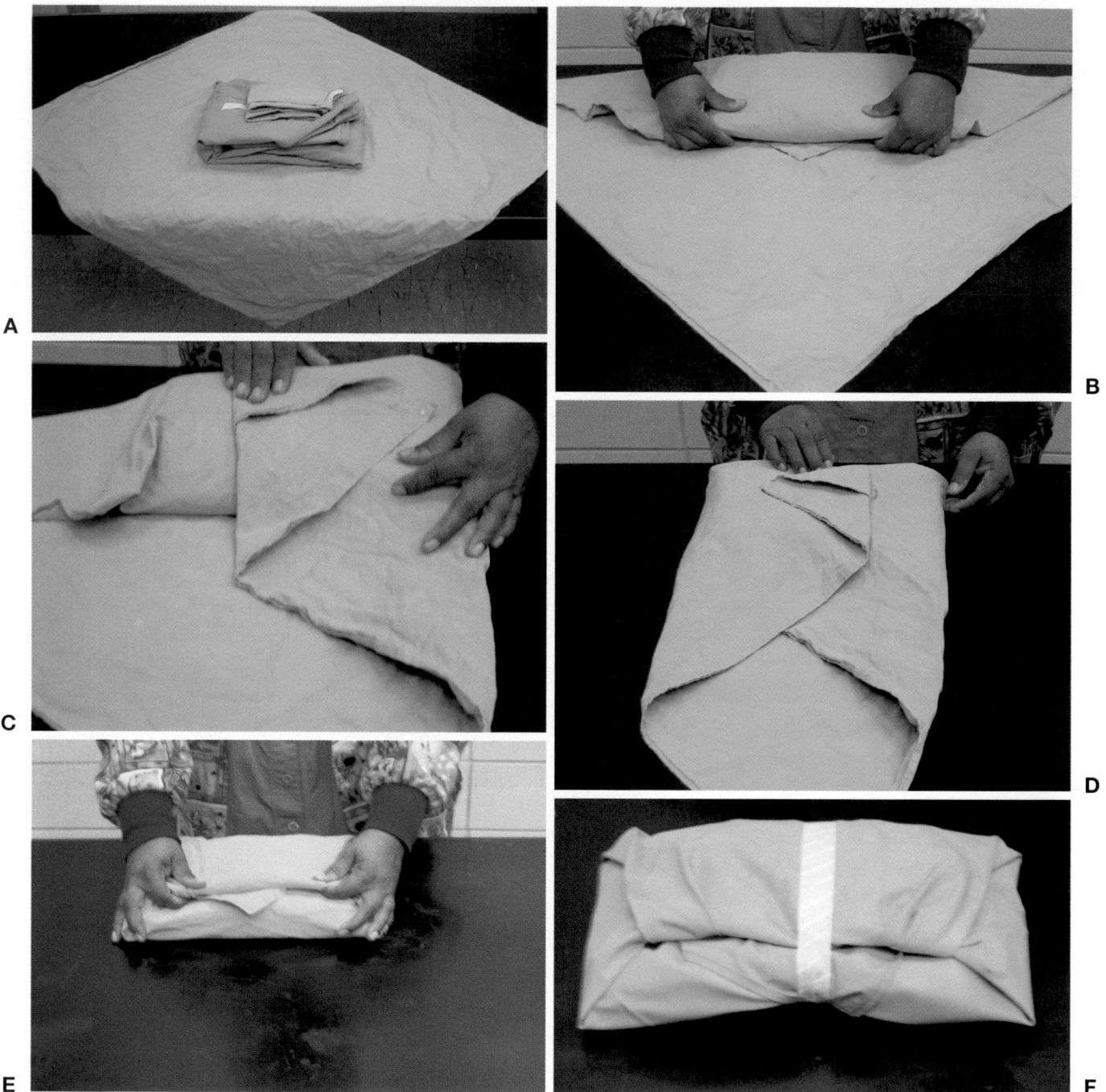

Figure 22-51 Wrapping a cloth drape or gown, or an instrument pack. **A,** The gown, along with an accordion-folded hand towel and sterilization indicator, is placed diagonally onto the drapes. **B,** One corner is folded over the entire pack and tucked under it, leaving the tip visible. **C,** An adjacent corner is folded over the end of the pack, and the tip folded back so the drape is flat on top of the pack. **D,** The opposite corner is folded the same way. **E,** The pack is turned around and the final corner is folded over the top of the pack and tucked under the folded drape edges, leaving the tip visible. **F,** The pack is then wrapped in a second layer in the same manner. The pack is secured with autoclave tape and is then labeled with contents, date, and the initials of the individual preparing the pack.

material and its intended use. Methods of sterilization and disinfection can be classified as either physical or chemical.

PHYSICAL METHODS OF STERILIZATION

The three general types of physical methods used for sterilization include filtration, radiation, and heat. Filtration and radiation are primarily used during the production and packaging of certain surgical products.

FILTRATION

Filtration is the use of a filter to separate particulate material from liquids or gases. Pharmaceuticals are commonly sterilized by filtration.

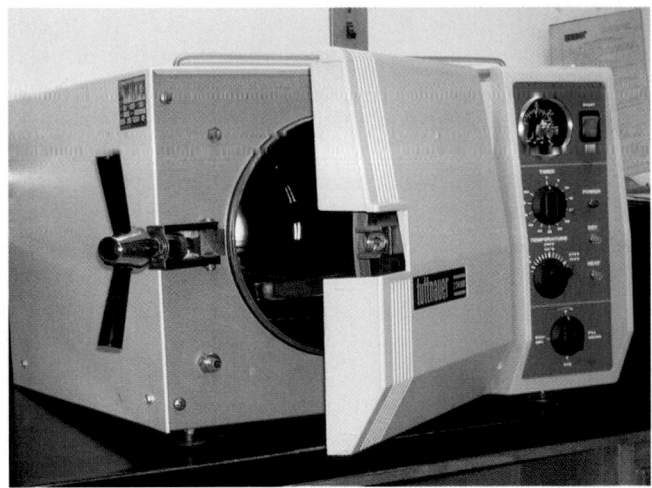

Figure 22-52 Autoclave. They are available in different sizes and models.

RADIATION

Some materials that would be damaged by other methods of sterilization can be safely sterilized by radiation. Radiation destroys microorganisms without causing any significant temperature elevation. Gloves and some suture materials are sterilized by radiation during the manufacturing process.

THERMAL ENERGY

The most common method used for sterilization is heat. The mechanism by which heat destroys microorganisms is not completely understood, but it is believed that death is the result of protein denaturation. This is probably a gradual process and may be reversible during the early stages of sterilization. The thermal susceptibility of microorganisms is influenced by several factors, including inherent resistance, individual variation, and age (young bacteria are more susceptible). There is no one temperature at which all microorganisms are killed instantly because death of bacteria and spores is a function of temperature and duration of heat.

The two basic types of heat sterilization are moist heat and dry heat. Dry heat is used to sterilize materials that cannot tolerate moist heat but can withstand high temperatures. Oils, powders, and petroleum products are most effectively sterilized by dry heat, whereas rubber, fabrics, and some metals may be damaged by the high temperatures. An advantage of dry heat is that it will not rust or corrode needles or sharp instruments. Dry heat is more difficult to control than moist heat, and the sterilization time is longer.

Both dry and moist heat destroy bacteria through protein denaturation; however, dry heat kills by protein oxidation, whereas moist heat kills by coagulation of critical cellular proteins. Moisture facilitates the coagulation of proteins; thus moist heat kills bacteria and spores at lower temperatures and shorter exposures than dry heat.

Moist heat sterilization is accomplished by either boiling water or by steam under pressure. Boiling water at ambient pressures is not a reliable means of sterilization because of its relatively low temperature. The bactericidal effect of boiling water can be enhanced by alkalinization with sodium hydroxide (0.1 g/dl) or sodium carbonate (2 g/dl). The addition of these agents reduces instrument corrosion, but they cannot be used with glassware or rubber goods. Boiling water probably results in disinfection rather than sterilization, and is rarely used.

The most common method of sterilization is saturated steam under pressure. Increased pressure causes steam to achieve a higher temperature. Materials to be sterilized in this manner must be penetrable by steam and not damaged by heat or moisture. Sterilizers that employ steam under pressure are called *autoclaves* (Figure 22-52).

Autoclave Sterilization

Autoclave sterilization is technique sensitive, so operating instructions accompanying the autoclave should be followed. An autoclave load is not sterile unless the steam has penetrated the packs completely so that all materials have been exposed to steam at the proper temperature and for the proper duration. Adequate steam penetration requires that the packs be properly prepared and loaded into the autoclave. The most common autoclaves are *gravity displacement* or downward displacement sterilizers, meaning the steam is introduced into the top of the chamber and forces the air to the bottom. In *prevacuum sterilizers*, a vacuum pump evacuates the air before the steam is introduced. This provides a more rapid and even penetration of steam than with gravity displacement, permitting higher temperatures and shorter time duration.

Proper pack preparation begins by checking that all materials are thoroughly clean and free from grease, oil, or protein residues. Complex instruments should be disassembled and any box locks should be open. Packs must be properly wrapped with steam-permeable wrappers, such as double-thickness muslin (thread count of 140 threads per 6.45 cm^2) or a nonwoven barrier (crepe paper or polypropylene fabric). Muslin wrappers can be washed and reused, but nonwoven barriers are designed for single use. Packs are usually wrapped in two layers of muslin or nonwoven wrappers. The external wraps are folded around a large pack in the same manner as described for drape and gown packs (Figure 22-51). Heat-sealable paper/plastic or plastic peel pouches may be used for individual instruments (Figure 22-53). Each pack must be labeled identifying the pack contents, the person who prepared it, and the date it was sterilized.

Materials need to be packed as loosely as is practical to assure good steam penetration. There should be 2.5 to 7.5 cm of space around each pack, and they should be arranged to allow steam to flow readily from top to bottom. For example, a large pack should not be placed on top of several small ones because it will block the flow of steam down to the smaller packs. Steam flow may be facilitated by positioning packs vertically (on edge). It is recommended that packs be no larger than 30 cm 30 cm 50 cm and weigh no more than 5.4 kg, depending on the type of material being autoclaved. In many practices, the pack size is limited by the size of the autoclave.

A number of minimum time-temperature standards have been established for routine sterilization of surgical packs. Exposure to saturated steam at 121°C (250°F) for 13 minutes is considered to be a safe minimum standard. Five to 10 minutes at 121°C will destroy most resistant microbes, and an additional 3 to 8 minutes provides a margin of safety. When the temperature in the exhaust line reaches the desired level, the entire contents of the sterilizing chamber have been exposed to steam, so this is the beginning of exposure time. The time required to reach the sterilizing temperature is referred to as the *heat-up time* and is extremely short (about 1 minute) in prevacuum and pulsing type sterilizers. Large linen packs require both a longer heat-up time and a longer exposure time. They should be saturated for 30 to 45 minutes at 121°C (250°F) in gravity displacement sterilizers and 4 minutes at 131°C (270°F) in prevacuum sterilizers.

Emergency sterilization, also called *flash* sterilization, is usually performed in prevacuum sterilizers. The recommended exposure time is 3 minutes at 131°C (270°F). The unwrapped instruments are placed in a perforated metal tray for sterilization and then carried to the operating room using detachable handles.

✎ TECHNICIAN NOTE

The safe minimal standard for autoclave sterilization is 121°C (250°F) for 13 minutes.

After sterilization, the autoclave door is unlocked and "cracked" open. If the autoclave door is opened wide, the cool outside air will condense the steam in the materials, making them soggy and promoting corrosion of metal instruments. About 10 minutes after cracking the door, the remaining moisture will have vaporized and escaped, leaving the contents thoroughly dry. Paper-wrapped products should not be left in the autoclave more than 15 to 20 minutes after cracking the door. If left too long, the heat will dry the paper, making it brittle and likely to crack and split when handled.

Sterilization Quality Control

The only assurance that sterilization has been achieved is through proper technique and the use of dependable sterilization indicators. Indicators should always be checked before using the materials.

There are four types of sterilization indicators used in autoclaves: (1) autoclave tape, (2) fusible melting pellet glass type, (3) culture tests, and (4) chemical sterilization indicators. These indicators are meant to be used combination because no one test alone can provide quality assurance of sterility.

Autoclave tape is useful for identifying packs and articles that have been exposed to steam, but it does not indicate whether the proper requirements of time, temperature, and steam have been met (Figure 22-54). The fusible melting pellet glass type indicates that a temperature of approximately 118°C (244°F) was reached, but does not indicate whether proper time or steam saturation was achieved. Culture test indicators are strips that contain a controlled-count spore population of some particular strain of

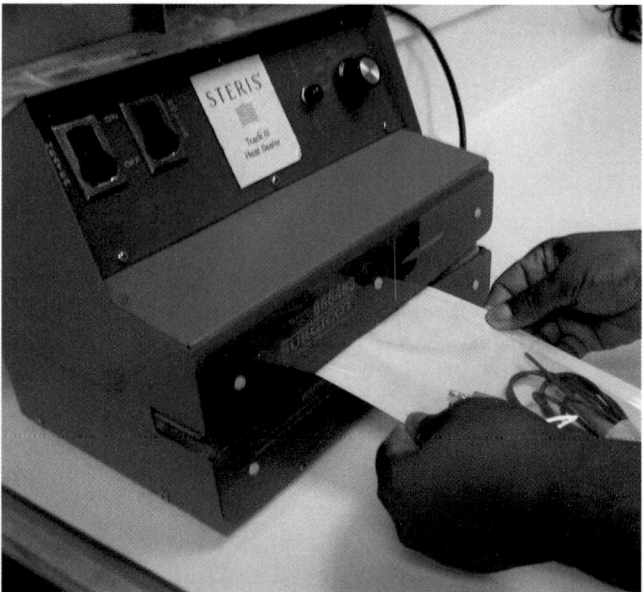

Figure 22-53 Individual instruments may be heat sealed in plastic/paper pouches in preparation for steam or chemical sterilization. The instrument should be positioned in the pouch so that the handle will be presented to the surgeon when the pouch is opened.

bacterium. This biologic challenge test is useful since it is the only test that proves microorganisms were killed. The disadvantages of this test are that the results are not immediately available and it does not assess steam penetration. Chemical sterilization indicators are available in many types, and they undergo color changes when subjected to saturated steam for adequate periods of time (Figure 22-55). Most practices will use a combination of autoclave tape on the outside of the pack and a chemical sterilization indicator within the center of the pack to assess sterility.

In the prevacuum sterilizers, an air removal test can be run daily to ensure that air is sufficiently removed from the autoclave. In gravity displacement sterilizers, temperature graphs can be kept as a record of autoclave performance. Therefore quality assurance occurs at two levels, one to ensure that the pack runs through a sterilization cycle and another to ensure that the autoclave system is working properly. Quality control is essential for any surgical practice, because failure to ensure proper sterilization can have far-reaching consequences.

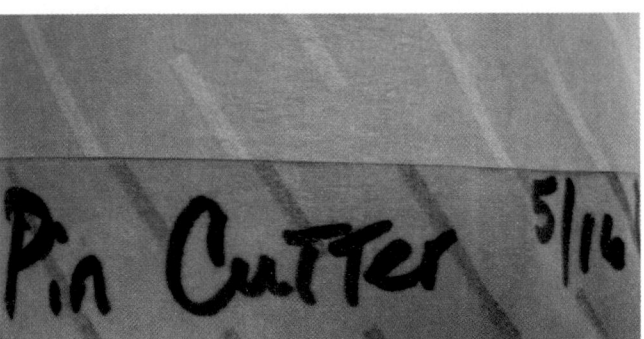

Figure 22-54 Autoclave tape before *(above)* and after *(below)* sterilization. Notice the appearance of the black stripes indicating exposure to steam.

> **TECHNICIAN NOTE**
>
> The four types of sterilization indicators are (1) autoclave tape, (2) melting pellet glass, (3) culture tests, and (4) chemical sterilization indicators.

Care and Handling of Sterile Packs

Sterile packs should be stored in a dust-free, dry, and well-ventilated area away from contaminated equipment. Closed cabinets provide a cleaner storage area than open shelving. Safe pack storage times are listed in Table 22-5. If a pack is dropped, the tape sealing the pack is broken, or the pack wrap becomes wet, punctured, or torn, the pack should be considered contaminated. If there is any doubt as to the sterility of an item, consider it to be nonsterile.

> **TECHNICIAN NOTE**
>
> Because of the high toxicity of ethylene oxide, it is being replaced by hydrogen peroxide gas plasma sterilization.

CHEMICAL METHODS OF STERILIZATION

Chemical sterilization is performed with certain liquids or gases. Liquid chemicals can be used for instrument sterilization. The most common agent used for liquid sterilization is glutaraldehyde. Gas sterilization is used for items that cannot tolerate the high temperatures or steam associated with autoclaving (some power equipment or plastic products). The most common agents used for gas sterilization are ethylene oxide and hydrogen peroxide gas plasma.

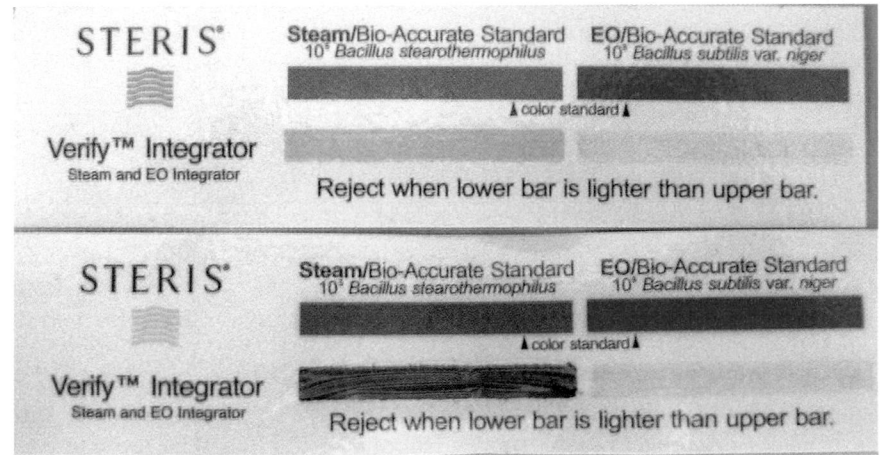

Figure 22-55 Chemical indicator strip to be placed inside pack. This strip can monitor steam *(left)* or gas *(right)* sterilization. Lower strip has been exposed to adequate steam, as indicated by the darkened bar.

Table 22-5 Safe Storage Times for Sterile Packs

Wrapper	Closed Cabinet	Open Cabinet
Single-wrapped muslin	1 week	2 days
Double-wrapped muslin	7 weeks	3 weeks
Single-wrapped crepe paper	At least 8 weeks	3 weeks
Single-wrapped muslin sealed in 3-mil polyethylene		At least 9 months
Heat-sealed paper and transparent plastic pouches		At least 1 year

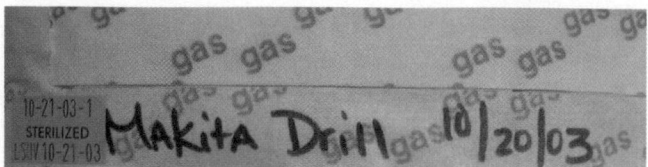

Figure 22-56 Gas tape before *(above)* and after *(below)* sterilization. Notice the change in color of the word *gas*, indicating exposure.

ETHYLENE OXIDE

Ethylene oxide is a colorless gas at room temperature. It is flammable, explosive, and toxic. It can cause skin burns, respiratory irritation, vomiting, headaches, and birth defects. (Refer to Chapter 36.) The manufacturer's guidelines should be followed carefully to avoid injury to hospital personnel and patients. Ethylene oxide penetrates paper and plastic film packaging. The item to be gas sterilized is wrapped in plastic packaging (polyethylene, polycoated paper, and Mylar) and heat sealed prior to sterilization (Figure 22-53).

Ethylene oxide destroys metabolic pathways within the cells by alkylation, and it is capable of killing all microorganisms. Effective sterilization with ethylene oxide is dependent on the concentration of gas, exposure time, temperature, and relative humidity. Ethylene oxide activity is enhanced by increasing the temperature or the gas concentration. Ethylene oxide sterilizers usually operate at temperatures between 21° C and 60° C (70° F and 140° F). The activity of ethylene oxide approximately doubles with each 10° C increase in temperature. Doubling the ethylene oxide concentration decreases the sterilization time by approximately one half. Moisture is necessary for the lethal action of ethylene oxide and optimal relative humidity for sterilization with ethylene oxide is 40%. Exposure time varies from 48 minutes to several hours, but 12 hours of exposure is commonly used when sterilizing at room temperature.

After ethylene oxide sterilization, materials should be quarantined in a well-ventilated area for a minimum of 7 days or in an aerator for 12 to 18 hours. Recommended aeration time varies with the type of material and other factors. Color-coded chemical sterilization indicators are commonly placed within the packs when using ethylene oxide sterilization (Figure 22-55). Biological indicators are available for ethylene oxide sterilization and are the only truly reliable test for sterility. Since results are unavailable for several days, biological indicators are most commonly used to evaluate the sterilization system and not individual packs. External tape can be used to indicate exposure to gas sterilization (Figure 22-56).

HYDROGEN PEROXIDE GAS PLASMA

Gas plasma sterilization has been replacing ethylene oxide because it is safer for the environment and personnel. It can inactivate mycobacteria, bacterial spores, fungi, and viruses and can be used to sterilize most items. Items that cannot be sterilized with this method include linen, wood or paper, endoscopes, some plastics, liquids, and tubes or catheters that are very long (>12 inches) or of small diameter (<3 mm). Items to be sterilized are wrapped in nonwoven polypropylene fabric or plastic (Tyvek-Mylar) pouches and placed in the sterilization chamber. A vacuum is drawn and hydrogen peroxide is injected and is vaporized. After 50 minutes, the pressure is lowered and radio waves are applied to the chamber, creating a gas plasma. This creates free radicals, which kill the microorganisms. The process takes about an hour and requires no aeration. A biological indicator is used to test for sterility, and a chemical indicator is used to show that hydrogen peroxide was present.

CHEMICAL DISINFECTION

A *disinfectant* is an agent that destroys bacteria or inactivates viruses. Disinfectants are chemical agents that are applied to inanimate objects to destroy the vegetative form of bacteria but not necessarily the spore forms. Disinfectants that are capable of destroying vegetative bacteria, plus spores, tubercle bacilli, and viruses may be used as chemical sterilizers.

Disinfection time is the time required for a particular agent to produce its maximum effect. It is influenced by many factors including the nature of the material being disinfected, the degree of soil and microbial contamination, and the concentration and germicidal potency of the disinfectant.

Antisepsis is the prevention of infection by inhibiting the growth of infectious agents. Antiseptics agents, such as iodine or chlorhexidine, are substances used on living tissue to effect antisepsis. A glossary of key terms used in describing aseptic technique may be found in Table 22-6.

Table 22-6 GLOSSARY OF KEY TERMS

Antiseptic	Agent capable of preventing infection by inhibiting the growth of infectious agents. This term is generally applied to living tissues.
Autoclave	Sterilizers that use saturated steam under pressure to achieve high temperatures for sterilization. Minimal exposure to saturated steam 13 min at 121° C (250° F).
Disinfectant	Agent that destroys or inhibits microorganisms. Typically refers to inanimate objects.
Ethylene oxide	Gas chemical sterilization agent used to sterilize objects that cannot withstand heat. A good exhaust system must be used.
Flash sterilization	Emergency sterilization in which object (instrument) is placed unwrapped in an autoclave and taken directly to the surgery following sterilization. Recommended exposure is 3 min at 131° C (270° F).
Sterilization	Destruction of all microorganisms. This term is generally applied to inanimate objects.

Table 22-7 COMMON ANTISEPTIC AND DISINFECTANT AGENTS

Agent	Examples	Common Uses	Spectrum of Activity	Residual Activity
Povidone-iodine detergent	Betadine scrub (Purdue-Frederick) (brown sudsy solution)	Preoperative scrubs	Bacteria, viruses, fungi, protozoa, yeast	4-6 hr, but inactivated by organic debris and alcohol
Povidone-iodine solution	Betadine solution (Purdue-Frederick) (brown solution)	Preoperative antiseptic application; wound lavage when diluted 1:100	Bacteria, viruses, fungi, protozoa, yeast alcohol	4-6 hr, but inactivated by organic debris and
Chlorhexidine detergent	Nolvasan scrub (Fort Dodge Laboratories) (blue solution), Hibiclens scrub (Stuart Pharmaceuticals) (pink solution)	Preoperative scrubs	Bacteria, viruses, fungi, yeast	2 days; not inhibited by organic matter or alcohol; less skin irritation
Chlorhexidine solution	Nolvasan solution (Fort Dodge Laboratories) (nonsudsy blue solution)	Preoperative antiseptic application; wound lavage when diluted 1:40.	Bacteria, viruses, fungi, yeast	2 days; bactericidal, but not cytotoxic in open wounds at diluted concentrations
Alcohol, isopropyl and ethanol	Many manufacturers	Surgical preparations; disinfection antisepsis; do not use in open wounds	Bacteria, some fungi	None
Phenol, hexachlorophene	PHisoHex scrub (Sanofi; Winthrop) (white)	Preoperative hand scrub	Bacteria (more effective against gram-positive than gram-negative species)	Up to 2 days
Phenol, glutaraldehyde		Cold sterilization; not intended for living tissues	Bacteria, viruses, fungi, yeast, spores	None; causes skin irritation

ANTISEPTIC AND DISINFECTANT COMPOUNDS

Iodine

Iodine compounds are effective antimicrobial agents but have limited activity against bacterial spores. Iodine solutions are used for surgical preparation, topical wound therapy, and joint and body cavity lavage (Table 22-7). Iodine compounds are available as aqueous solutions, tinctures, and iodophors. *Aqueous solutions* contain higher levels of free iodine than iodophors and therefore have greater bacteriocidal activity. However, aqueous solutions are also cytotoxic and cannot be used in living tissue unless they are greatly diluted. Aqueous iodine also stains materials and is corrosive to instruments.

Tincture of iodine is a solution of 2% iodine in 50% ethyl alcohol and is intended for use on intact skin. It is not commonly used in veterinary practices.

Iodophors contain iodine complexed with surfactants or polymers, so free iodine is slowly released. The adverse properties of staining and irritation are reduced, and delivery of iodine to the tissues is enhanced. *Povidone-iodine* is the most commonly used iodophor and is available as scrubs or solutions. Dilution of stock solutions (common dilutions include 1:10, 1:50, and 1:100) increases the bactericidal activity and decreases the cytotoxicity. The residual bactericidal activity (i.e., continued action when left on the skin) of povidone-iodine is 4 to 6 hours, but this is greatly diminished in the presence of organic matter.

Povidone-iodine is one of the most common surgical scrubs used in veterinary hospitals. Although it is a relatively safe skin preparation, there are several considerations regarding its use. Alcohol, lavage solutions, or organic debris such as blood will destroy residual bactericidal activity. Povidone-iodine can cause skin irritation or acute contact dermatitis in up to 50% of canine patients, and it may be a problem for some hospital staff. Rarely, individuals who have repeated contact with iodine scrub solutions may develop systemic iodine toxicity, resulting in metabolic acidosis and thyroid dysfunction.

> ### TECHNICIAN NOTE
> The two most commonly used antiseptic agents are povidone-iodine and chlorhexidine.

Chlorhexidine

Chlorhexidine is an antiseptic agent that is available in aqueous, tincture and detergent formulations. It is an effective antimicrobial agent with activity against bacteria, molds, yeasts, and viruses. Chlorhexidine has a rapid onset and a long residual activity that is not affected by alcohol, lavage solutions, or organic debris. It has become a popular surgical scrub because of its effectiveness and because it is nonirritating to the skin. In several human studies chlorhexidine has been found to be superior to povidone-iodine as a surgical hand scrub. The effectiveness of povidone-iodine and chlorhexidine is similar when used as surgical scrubs for canine surgery.

As a lavage solution for open wounds, chlorhexidine must be diluted 1:40 with sterile water or saline to produce a 0.05% solution. At this concentration, chlorhexidine has significant antibacterial activity with no cytotoxicity and is superior to povidone-iodine, saline, and other antiseptics. Higher concentrations can cause inflammation and cytotoxicity, so they are not recommended in open wounds. When chlorhexidine is mixed with electrolyte solutions

(such as lactated Ringer's solution), it will precipitate, but this does not affect antimicrobial activity and the solution can still be used for wound lavage.

> ### TECHNICIAN NOTE
> Chlorhexidine is an effective antimicrobial agent with rapid onset and long residual activity.

Alcohols

Alcohols are used as disinfectant and antiseptic agents. They are organic solvents that evaporate rapidly and leave no residue. Alcohols are bactericidal, but ineffective against spores and fungi. They have no residual effects and are inhibited by organic debris. Ethyl and isopropyl alcohols are more effective than methyl alcohol as disinfecting agents. Alcohols should never be used in open wounds because they are both painful and cytotoxic.

Phenols

Phenols (carbolic acid) have been used historically as both antiseptics and disinfectants, but phenols have been routinely replaced by newer, safer, and more effective agents. Hexachlorophene, a skin preparation, was one of the most popular phenols, but it has been replaced by povidone-iodine and chlorhexidine.

Quaternary Ammonium

Quaternary ammonium compounds are synthetic cationic detergents that act on cell membranes and are effective against bacteria, but not spores or some viruses. Very bland and nontoxic, these agents are quite popular. Benzalkonium chloride is the most commonly used quaternary ammonium compound and is used as a disinfectant.

Chloride

Chloride compounds were among the first agents to be used as medical disinfectants and found popularity for wound treatment in World War I as Dakin's solution. Antimicrobial chlorine compounds, specifically the hypochlorites, have broad bactericidal and virucidal activity but can be cytotoxic when improperly used on living tissues. Presently, sodium hypochlorite (bleach) is commonly used as a disinfectant in many hospitals.

Aldehyde

Formaldehyde and glutaraldehyde are the most commonly used aldehydes in veterinary medicine. They are both toxic and irritating, which restricts them from use on living tissues. They are very effective antimicrobial agents, but may require several hours of exposure time. Formaldehyde is commonly used in the preservation of tissue specimens. Glutaraldehyde is commonly used for chemical sterilization in cold trays and for endoscopic equipment.

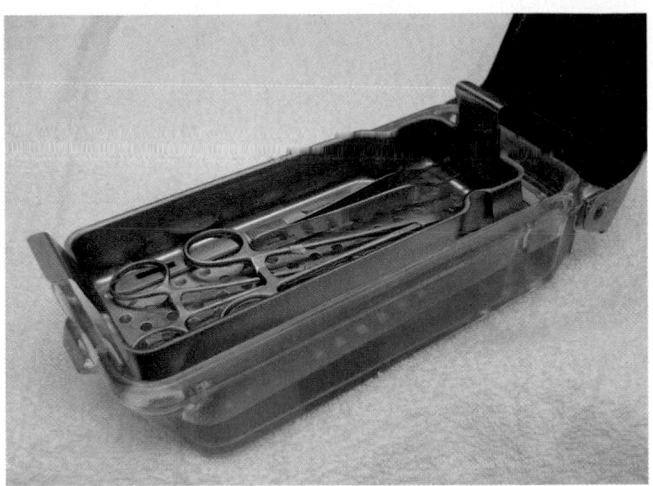

Figure 22-57 Cold sterilization tray. Instruments are kept submerged in disinfectant and retrieved by lifting the rack.

COLD STERILIZATION

Cold sterilization refers to soaking instruments in disinfecting solutions such as chlorhexidine or glutaraldehyde. Metal trays used to soak instruments in disinfectant are called *cold trays* (Figure 22-57). Since sterility cannot be guaranteed, cold-sterilized instruments should be used only for minor procedures (superficial lacerations, dental procedures) or for equipment that cannot tolerate other forms of sterilization such as endoscopic equipment. Exposure times should exceed 3 hours, and the equipment must be rinsed thoroughly before use.

> **TECHNICIAN NOTE**
>
> The arthroscope, fiber-optic light cable, and camera should never be steam sterilized.

STERILIZATION OF ARTHROSCOPIC EQUIPMENT

Most hand instruments and ancillary equipment can be steam sterilized. They can also be gas sterilized with ethylene oxide or cold sterilized using a glutaraldehyde-based solution (Cidexplus, Johnson & Johnson Medical Inc.). Cold sterilization affords the ability to use the equipment more than once in a single day, unlike steam and gas sterilization in most situations. The arthroscope, light cable, and camera can be gas sterilized or cold sterilized but *not* steam sterilized.

With cold sterilization, the instruments are soaked for a minimum of 20 minutes in the Cidexplus just before surgery. The electrical plug of the camera cable is not submerged in the cold sterilization solution, which would damage it. The end is draped out over the top of the container with the Cidexplus. The surgeon or assistant double gloves and removes the instruments from the solution.

The instruments are then placed in a sterile autoclave tray containing sterile water. Once the instruments have been submerged in the sterile water, each piece is gently agitated, individually removed from the tray, rinsed with sterile water by a scrub nurse or other assistant, and transferred to the instrument table. The surgeon or assistant removes his or her outer gloves and dries the instruments. It is important that the Cidexplus be thoroughly rinsed from the instruments. Glutaraldehyde can cause a chemical synovitis and is injurious to chondrocytes. A double rinse further reduces the amount of glutaraldehyde residue remaining on the instruments.

> **TECHNICIAN NOTE**
>
> Glutaraldehyde causes a chemical synovitis and is injurious to chondrocytes.

OPERATING ROOM PREPARATION

Operating room design is important for ease of cleaning. The operating room should be simple and uncluttered. Commonly used equipment and materials should be readily available, but excess stock should not be stored in the operating room. When additional equipment is needed, it is brought to the operating room by the circulating nurse.

Operating room cleanliness is essential for proper aseptic technique. A routine daily and weekly cleaning schedule should be established to keep the operating room clean and dust free. The surgery table should be cleaned and disinfected, and soiled areas of the floor should be cleaned and disinfected by damp mopping immediately after each surgery. It is preferable to perform thorough daily cleaning at the end of each day because cleaning creates airborne dust that takes several hours to settle. Buckets should be emptied and cleaned. The operating table and all equipment should be cleaned and wiped with a disinfectant solution. (The operating room is never dry-mopped or dusted because this produces excessive airborne dust.) The casters on equipment should be cleaned, and the entire floor should be mopped.

Once a week, the operating room should undergo a thorough cleaning in which movable equipment is removed and cleaned with a disinfectant solution. Permanent structures such as walls, air vents, window sills, light fixtures, and the surgical table should also be wiped clean. Cabinets should be emptied, washed and restocked. The operating room floor should be scrubbed and disinfected. Disinfectant can be applied with a mop, although this may actually spread dirt and microorganisms throughout the room. To avoid this, the mop head should be laundered daily and not stored in used disinfectant solution. The wet-vacuum method in which the clean floor is flooded with disinfectant solution and then vacuumed is superior to mopping.

Cleaning equipment used in the operating room should be kept separate from all other cleaning equipment.

Daily cleaning of the surgical preparation room is also important because this room is subject to continual contamination. Sinks and plumbing fixtures should be scrubbed. Buckets and vacuum canisters should be emptied. Furniture and cabinets should be wiped clean and the floor scrubbed. If there are holding cages in the preparation room, they should be cleaned and disinfected. All surgical preparation solutions and supplies should be replenished.

> ### ✏ TECHNICIAN NOTE
> Daily and weekly cleaning schedules should be established for the operating room.

PATIENT PREPARATION

SURGICAL CLIP

The surgical site is usually prepared after the animal is anesthetized. The hair is first clipped in the same direction as the hair growth. Then it is clipped against the direction of growth to achieve the closest shave possible (using a no. 40 clipper blade). A wide region of skin is clipped around the proposed surgical incision. A general rule is to shave at least 2 to 4 cm in every direction from the proposed incision, depending on the size of the animal and location of the incision. For abdominal procedures, the clip should extend several centimeters cranial to the xyphoid, caudal to the pubis, and lateral to the nipples. For orthopedic procedures, the entire circumference of the limb is clipped from the foot up onto the body. Long hair growing near the periphery of the clipped area should be cut short enough that it cannot hang over the clipped area. Sterile, water-soluble lubricant may be placed in open wounds before clipping around them. The lubricant will collect hair, allowing it to be rinsed away before the surgical scrub. Areas that appear to be infected should be clipped last so the clippers do not spread infected material. After clipping, a vacuum cleaner may be used to eliminate loose hairs on the skin. The surgical clip should be thorough but gentle. Unnecessary roughness will result in inflamed or traumatized skin, which can cause greater postoperative complications.

SURGICAL SCRUB

Initial skin preparation is done in the preparation room to remove gross contamination. Before scrubbing the abdomen of a male dog, the prepuce should be flushed with an antiseptic solution. Examination gloves are worn to decrease contamination from the hands. The surgical scrub is performed by alternating an antiseptic scrub (such as povidone-iodine or chlorhexidine scrub) with alcohol or

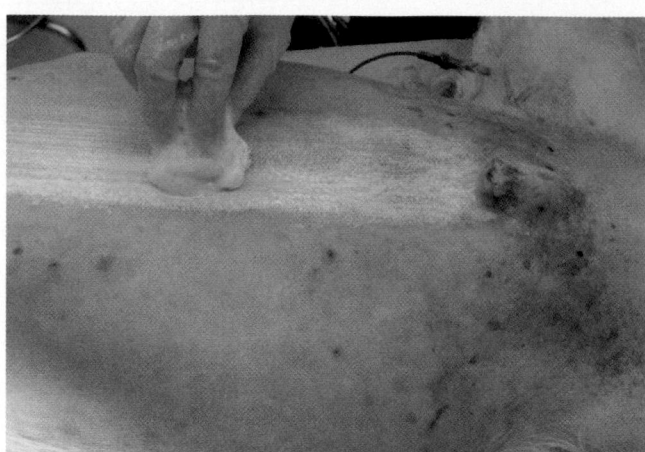

Figure 22-58 The surgical preparation should begin at the proposed incision site and should progress outward, never returning to the proposed incision line with the same gauze sponge. Gloves are worn during the preparation to decrease contamination from the hands.

sterile saline. (Remember not to use alcohols or detergents in open wounds, eyes, or mucous membranes.) Scrubbing should begin over the proposed incision site and extend outward in a spiraling pattern, never going back toward the center with the same gauze sponge (Figure 22-58). The sponge is replaced with a clean one and the process is repeated until no dirt is visible on the discarded sponges.

The sterile surgical scrub is done once the animal is properly positioned on the operating table. Sterile gloves should be worn and sterile sponges are used. If the sterile surgical scrub is performed by alternating povidone-iodine with alcohol, the total contact time of the povidone-iodine should be at least 5 minutes. After the final povidone-iodine scrub, a 10% povidone-iodine solution should be sprayed or painted on the skin. Alternatively, the sterile surgical scrub may be performed by alternating chlorhexidine gluconate with either alcohol or sterile saline. Either chlorhexidine or sterile saline may be left on the skin at the end of preparation. Both povidone-iodine and chlorhexidine are effective scrub solutions, but the contact time for chlorhexidine is less critical than for povidone-iodine.

> ### ✏ TECHNICIAN NOTE
> It is generally recommended that the surgical site be scrubbed and rinsed at least three times. The sterile scrub should provide at least 5 minutes of contact time for povidone-iodine. An antiseptic solution is often applied to the skin following the scrubs.

There are many modifications to the surgical preparation technique. For example, in preparation for feline orchiectomy (castration) the scrotal hair is plucked rather than clipped. Feline onychectomy (declawing), and tail docking and dewclaw removal of neonatal puppies are commonly performed without clipping the hair. The surgical site is soaked or gently scrubbed with detergent and swabbed with alcohol or antiseptic solution. Bovine and porcine castrations are performed without clipping the hair, and an alcohol or antiseptic wash is usually used. Equine castrations may be prepared with three thorough washes using dilute chlorhexidine or povidone-iodine solution.

PATIENT POSITIONING

There are several common positions in which to place an animal for surgery. The position of the animal is described by the region of the body that contacts the table. For example, right lateral recumbency means the animal is lying on its right side, dorsal recumbency means the animal is on its back, and sternal recumbency means the animal is on its belly. Maintaining patient positioning is facilitated by the use of adjustable surgical tables, portable tabletop V troughs, sand bags, or vacuum-activated "beanbags."

In orthopedic surgery the affected leg is often suspended from an overhead support or intravenous (IV) stand during skin preparation and initial surgical draping. The advantage of hanging the leg is that it allows aseptic preparation of the entire circumference of the limb, so the surgeon can manipulate it during surgery. To hang the leg, the distal limb is wrapped (using gauze or an examination glove covered with tape) to cover any unclipped areas, and strips of tape ("stirrups") are extended from the end of the foot. The leg is suspended by these stirrups (Figure 22-59). The entire limb circumference is clipped and scrubbed from the foot to the level of the inguinal or axillary region. The skin preparation usually extends to the dorsal and ventral midlines of the body.

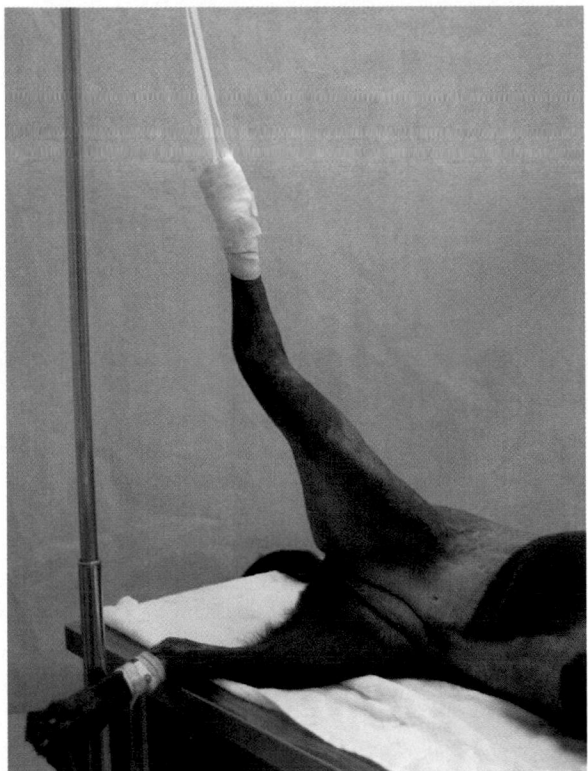

Figure 22-59 Hanging leg surgical preparation. This is commonly used for orthopedic surgeries of legs including the shoulder and hip. The operated limb is suspended by tape stirrups that cover all distal leg hair. The surgical scrubs are started at the highest aspect of the clipped leg and worked downward with gravity in a circular fashion. Note the wide area of skin preparation on the body. At surgery, the taped foot is wrapped in a sterile towel, and the stirrups are cut.

> ### TECHNICIAN NOTE
> The dorsal recumbent position is commonly used for abdominal surgical procedures.

SURGICAL TEAM PREPARATION

ATTIRE

Proper surgical attire, and proper scrubbing, gowning, and gloving procedures are important aspects of aseptic technique. Street clothing, especially shoes, are a major source of contamination and should not be worn into the operating room. Ideally, each person should have a pair of shoes designated for use only in the operating room. Also, disposable shoe covers may be worn in the operating room and discarded upon leaving the room. Lint-free scrub suits should be worn in the operating room. The shirt should be tucked into the pants to reduce the amount of skin debris dispersed into the room. Outside the operating room, scrub suits should be protected by a laboratory coat to reduce contamination.

During surgery, surgical caps and masks are worn by all people who are in the room. The surgical cap covers the hair to reduce airborne contamination. Different types of surgical head covers are available to cover short hair, long hair, or beards (Figure 22-60). The mask protects the wound from saliva droplets, primarily by redirecting air flow out the sides of the mask. Masks are effective for relatively short periods and should be changed between procedures.

> ### TECHNICIAN NOTE
> Anyone entering the operating room should wear a cap, mask, and scrub suit.

HAND SCRUB

Scrubbing of the hands and arms, followed by gowning and gloving, is performed by all personnel who will be in close proximity to the surgical site. Surgical gloves may have tiny holes, so they cannot be solely relied upon to prevent

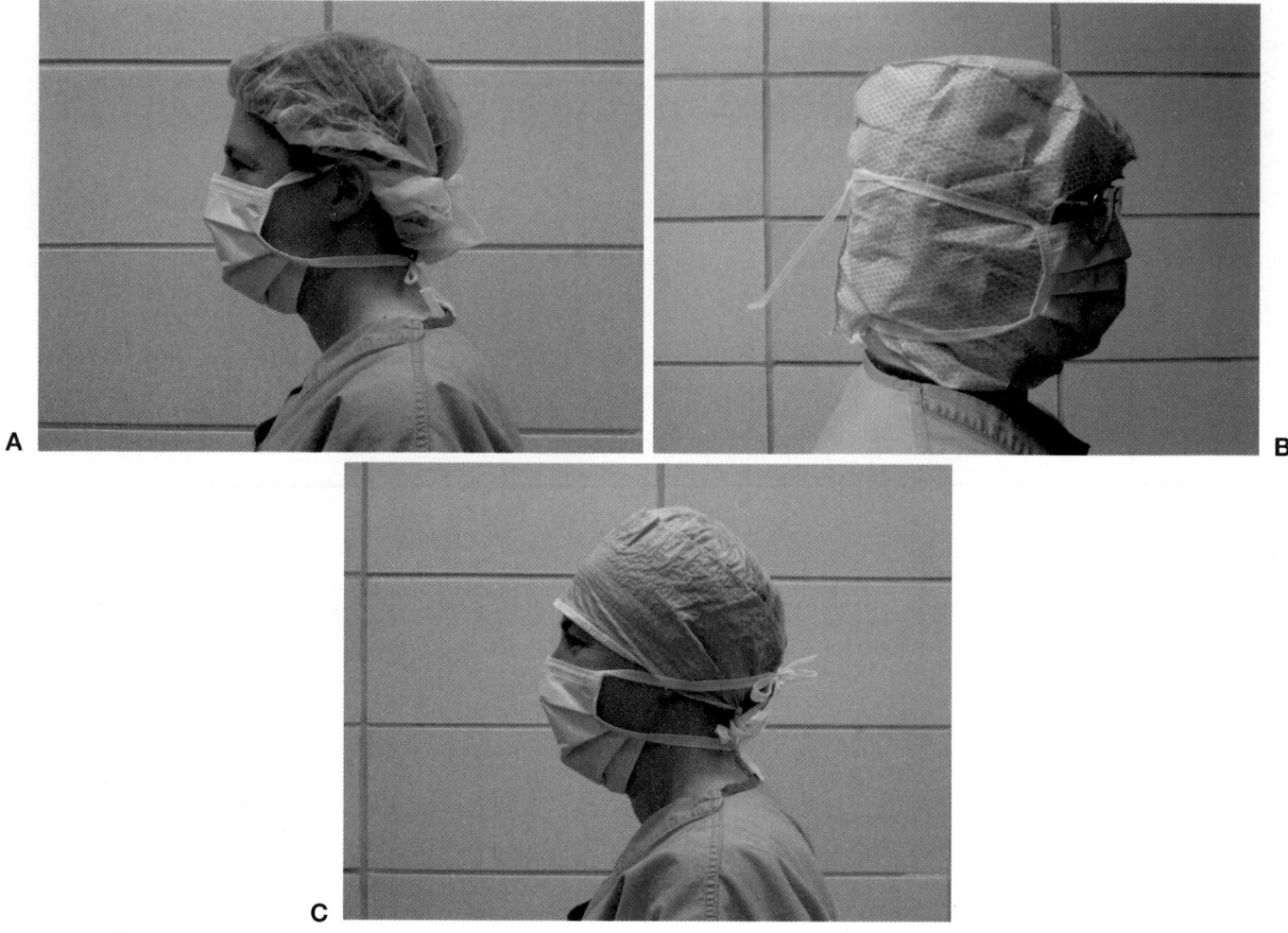

Figure 22-60 Surgical caps and masks. **A,** Bouffant head cover is used to cover long or short hair. **B,** Hoods are available for individuals with sideburns or a beard. **C,** A cap may be suitable to cover very short hair.

contamination from the hands. The purpose of scrubbing the hands and arms is to remove dirt and decrease the concentration of bacterial flora. The surgical cap and mask must be donned. The gown pack may be opened before scrubbing (Figure 22-61). All jewelry is removed from hands and arms before beginning the sterile hand scrub, and fingernails should be short and free of polish or artificial nails. Once the scrubbing has begun, the hands and arms should not touch nonsterile objects. If this occurs the scrub is started over.

While scrubbing, the hands are always held above the level of the elbows so the water drains off the elbows. Soap is applied to a sterile brush and a systematic scrub is begun. Scrub all four sides of each finger, with special attention to the fingernails (Figure 22-62, *A*). The back, both sides and the palm of the hand are scrubbed. Next, the wrist and forearm are scrubbed, working toward the elbow (Figure 22-62, *B*). After both hands and arms have been scrubbed, they are rinsed in running water (Figure 22-62, *C*). The entire scrub process is then repeated.

The two basic methods of surgical scrubs are the counted brush strokes and the timed. The counted brush stokes method is performed by counting the number of brush strokes used on each skin surface. Ten to twenty five brush strokes are made on each surface of the fingers, hands, and arms before rinsing. This is performed four times. The timed method is more commonly used. This is done by repeatedly scrubbing and rinsing for a set period of time. The initial scrub of the day should last about 5 minutes. For subsequent scrubs during the day, 2 to 3 minutes is adequate.

TECHNICIAN NOTE

The surgical hand scrub requires that all surfaces of the fingers, hand, and forearm be scrubbed. Skin-soap contact time should last 5 minutes.

GOWNING AND GLOVING

The hands and arms are thoroughly dried with a sterile towel (Figure 22-63) before gowning (Figure 22-64) and gloving.

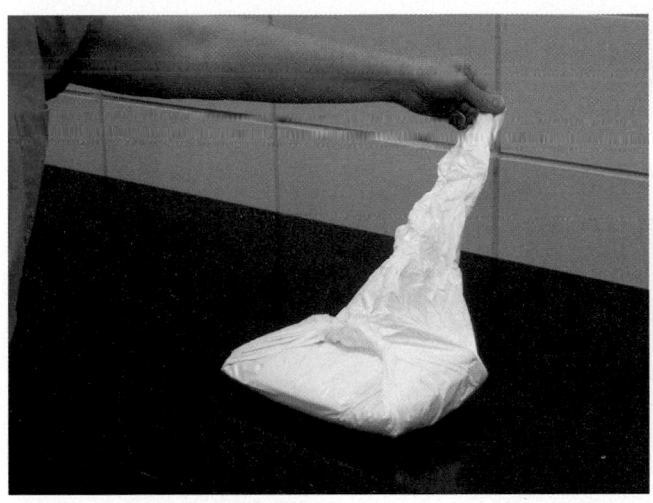
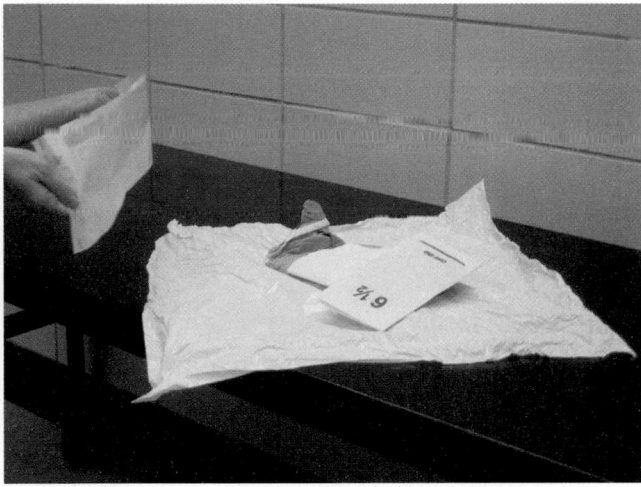

A   B

Figure 22-61 Open gown pack. **A,** The gown pack may be opened before scrubbing so the hand towel is available. When opening a pack always open the flap away from you first. Keep the arm off to the side, not directly over the pack. Then open the other three sides, touching only the corners of the wrap on the outside surface. **B,** The sterile gloves are opened onto the gown. With the package positioned at the edge of the sterile field, it is opened symmetrically. This gives the contents enough forward momentum to fall on the sterile field without having to reach over it.

The two methods for gloving yourself are *closed gloving* and *open gloving*. The risk of contamination is minimized with closed gloving (Figure 22-65) since the outside of the gloves never contacts skin. There is a much higher risk of contamination during open gloving (Figure 22-66), and it is generally reserved for minor procedures when a gown is not worn (e.g., sterile patient scrub, urinary catheterization). If it is necessary to replace gloves during surgery, it is preferable to have a nonsterile assistant remove the old gloves and simultaneously pull the gown sleeve so that the hands remain inside the sleeves (Figure 22-67). If the old gloves are removed in this manner, new gloves can be put on by the closed gloving method or by *assisted gloving* (Figure 22-68).

> ### ✎ TECHNICIAN NOTE
> The two methods of gloving yourself are *closed gloving* and *open gloving*. *Assisted gloving* requires the help of a sterile assistant.

MAINTAINING STERILITY

It is important for the entire surgical team to be conscious of sterility, even if they are not "scrubbed-in" (i.e., gowned and gloved). Nonsterile personnel should only touch nonsterile items or areas and should not lean over or reach across sterile fields. Those who are scrubbed-in should only touch sterile items or areas and should always face the sterile field. Only sterilized items can be placed on a sterile field. If anyone on the surgical team notices a potential source of contamination or "break" in sterile technique, it should be mentioned immediately so that steps can be taken to reduce the risk of further contamination. To reduce contamination, only essential personnel should be present in the operating room, and excessive movement should be avoided. Also, conversation should be kept to a minimum.

> ### ✎ TECHNICIAN NOTE
> Nonsterile personnel should not lean over or reach across sterile fields.

Scrubbed-In Personnel

The sterile area on a person is considered to be the front of the gown, from just below the shoulders (the neckline is not sterile) to the waist or the level of the table. The gown sleeves are also considered to be sterile. Note that the back of a gowned person is considered to be nonsterile, so it should not be turned to face any sterile field. Gloved hands may be rested on a sterile drape or clasped in front of the body in the zone between the shoulders and waist. The arms should not be folded across the chest because the armpit region is considered to be nonsterile, and the hands should not drop below waist level.

> ### ✎ TECHNICIAN NOTE
> After gowning and gloving, the sterile region is the front of the gown between the waist and just below the shoulders. The gown sleeves are also sterile, but not the back.

THE PATIENT

Sterile surgical drapes are used to maintain a sterile field around the surgical site. Draping is performed by personnel who have scrubbed-in. First, four small towels (cloth or paper) are placed to surround the area where the surgical incision will be. These are called *quarter drapes* and they are

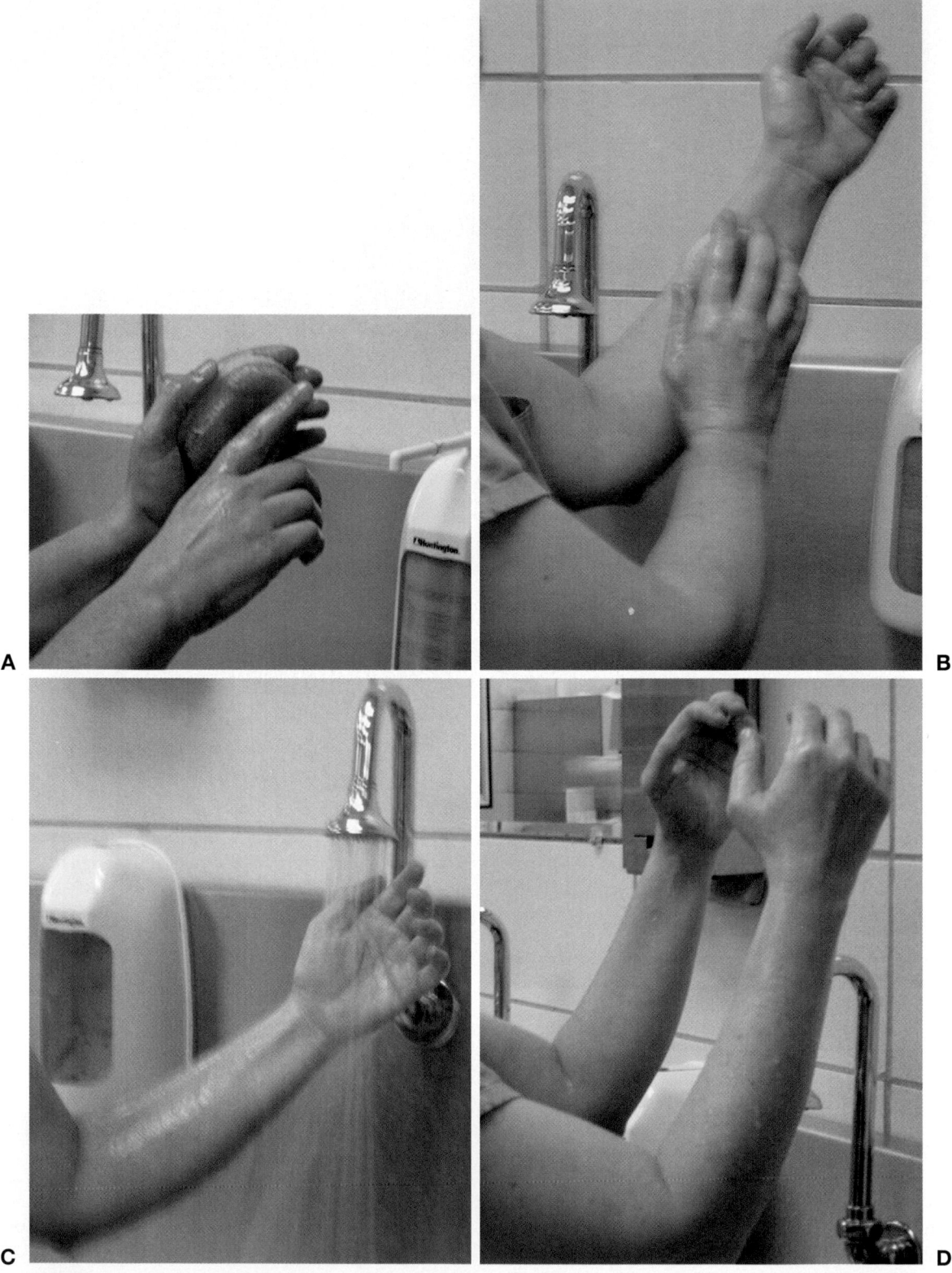

Figure 22-62 Surgical hand scrub. **A,** Imagine each finger as having a tip and four sides. Scrub each surface of each finger. Also scrub the palm, back and sides of the hand. **B,** Imagine the forearm as having four sides and scrub each side. **C,** After scrubbing both hands and arms, rinse the brush, hands, and forearms. The hands are always kept above the elbows. **D,** After the last scrub, drop the brush, rinse, and let the excess water drip off the elbows.

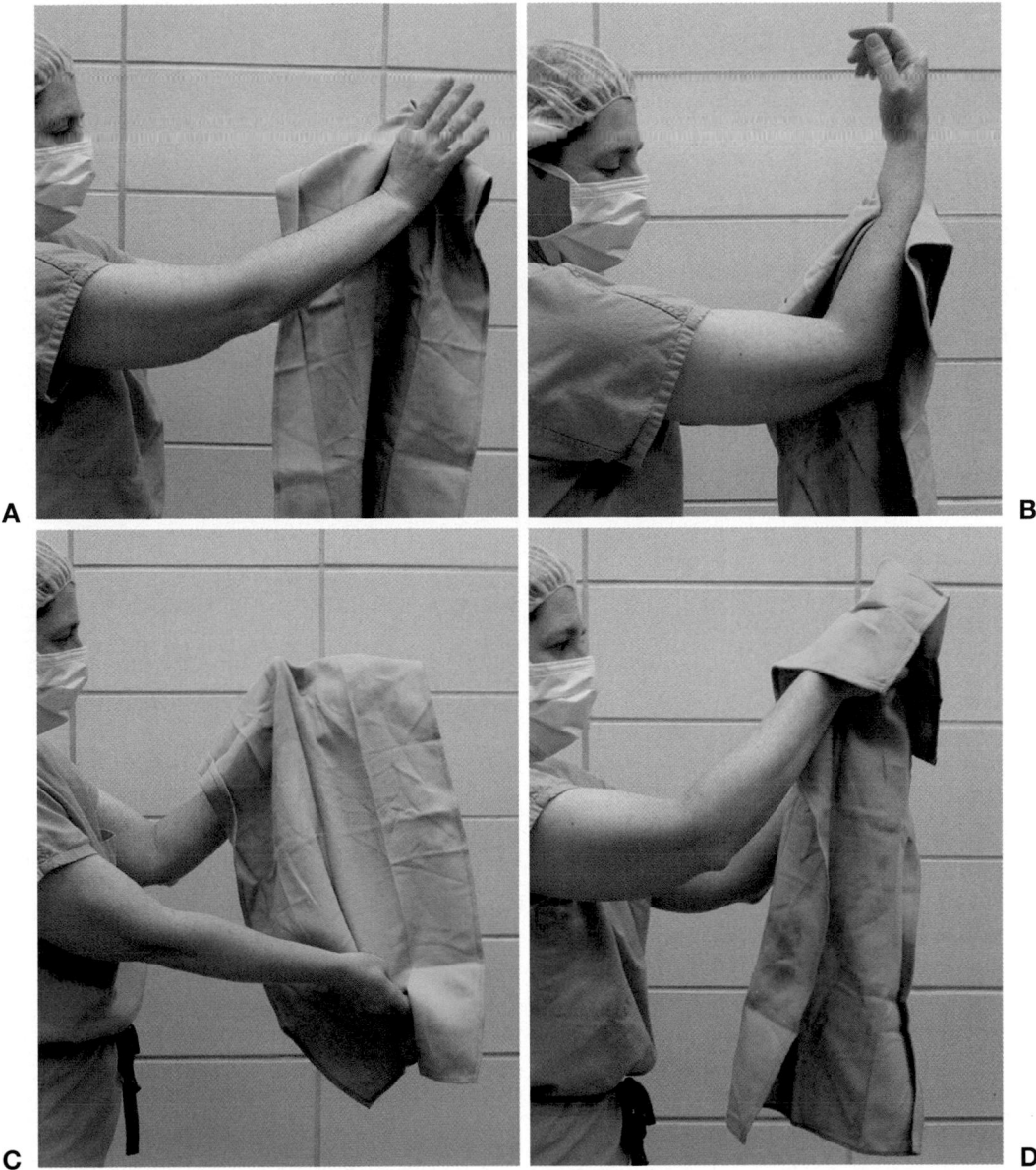

Figure 22-63 Towel dry. **A,** One hand is dried first, holding the towel away from the body. **B,** Move the towel down to dry the arm, using only the top end of the towel. **C,** The dry hand now grasps the dry end of the towel. **D,** The other hand and arm are dried. Note that the hands do not switch sides of the towel during the process.

secured to the skin using towel clamps. During this procedure, one must be careful not to brush the front of the surgical gown against the surgical table. Then a large drape is placed over the animal, surgical table, and instrument stand to provide one continuous sterile field. Cloth drapes have an opening or "fenestration," which is positioned over the surgical site. If a disposable paper drape is used, the appropriately sized hole may be cut after the drape has been placed.

If a limb has been suspended in preparation for an orthopedic procedure (as described under Patient Positioning), the quarter drapes are placed on the body, around the base of the limb. The distal limb is then held with a sterile wrap while a nonsterile assistant cuts the stirrups. The nonscrubbed, distal portion of the limb is covered with a sterile towel or sterile Vetrap. A sterile cotton stockinette or adhesive drape may be used to cover the entire leg. Finally, the limb is passed through a hole in the large sterile drape that covers the entire animal.

After draping is completed, sterile instrument packs, light handles, suture material and other sterile equipment may be opened. Draped tables and instrument trays are considered to be sterile only on the top of the draped surface, so if part of a sterile item slips below the level of the tabletop,

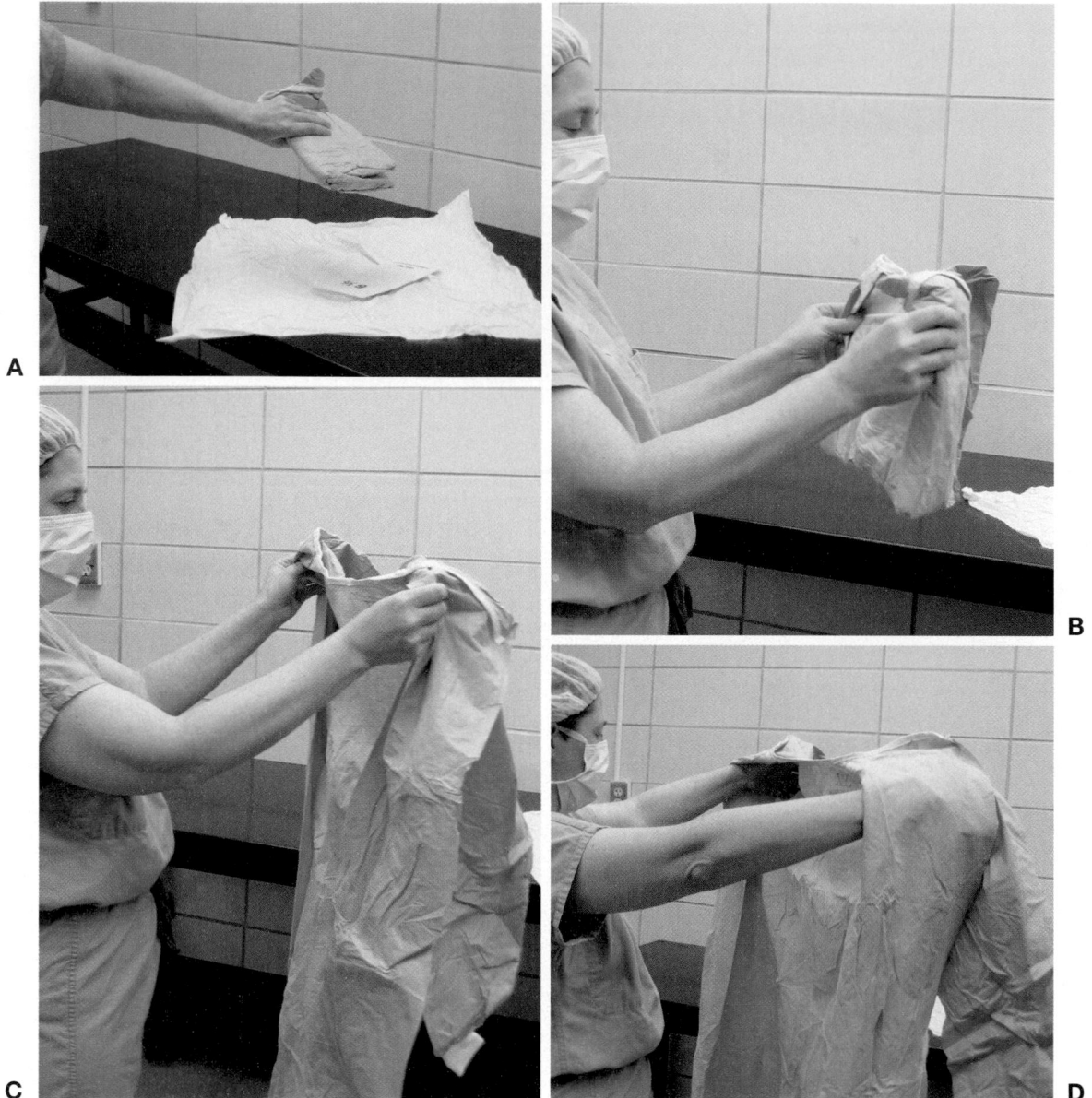

Figure 22-64 Gowning. **A,** The gown is picked up in its folded state. This same technique is used when picking up sterile folded towels or drapes. This reduces the risk of accidental contamination. **B,** Move to a spacious area to reduce the risk of contamination. **C,** The gown is held away from the body by the inside shoulder seams and allowed to unfold. **D,** The arms are slid into the sleeves, but the hands should not extend through the cuff openings.

it is considered to be contaminated and should no longer be touched by the surgeons.

TECHNICIAN NOTE

The *optimal* approach to draping includes isolating the surgical site with two layers of drapes: (1) four quarter drapes and (2) large drape that covers the entire animal and the instrument table.

OPENING STERILE ITEMS

Nonsterile assistants must open all sterile items for the surgeons. Nonsterile assistants can only touch the outside

of sterile packs and should never reach over a sterile field. Large or heavy packs, such as an instrument pack, may be set on a table to be opened. The four folded edges of the outer wrap are opened one at a time, while never extending the hand and arm over the top of the pack (Figure 22-61, *A*). If the pack can be placed on a Mayo instrument stand, this can be accomplished by moving around the stand and pulling each fold away from the center. The inner wrap may be opened by the surgeon or by a nonsterile assistant. Once the instrument tray is exposed, the surgeon can pick it up and set it on the draped instrument stand.

A smaller wrapped pack may be opened while holding it in one hand (Figure 22-69). As each corner of the pack is

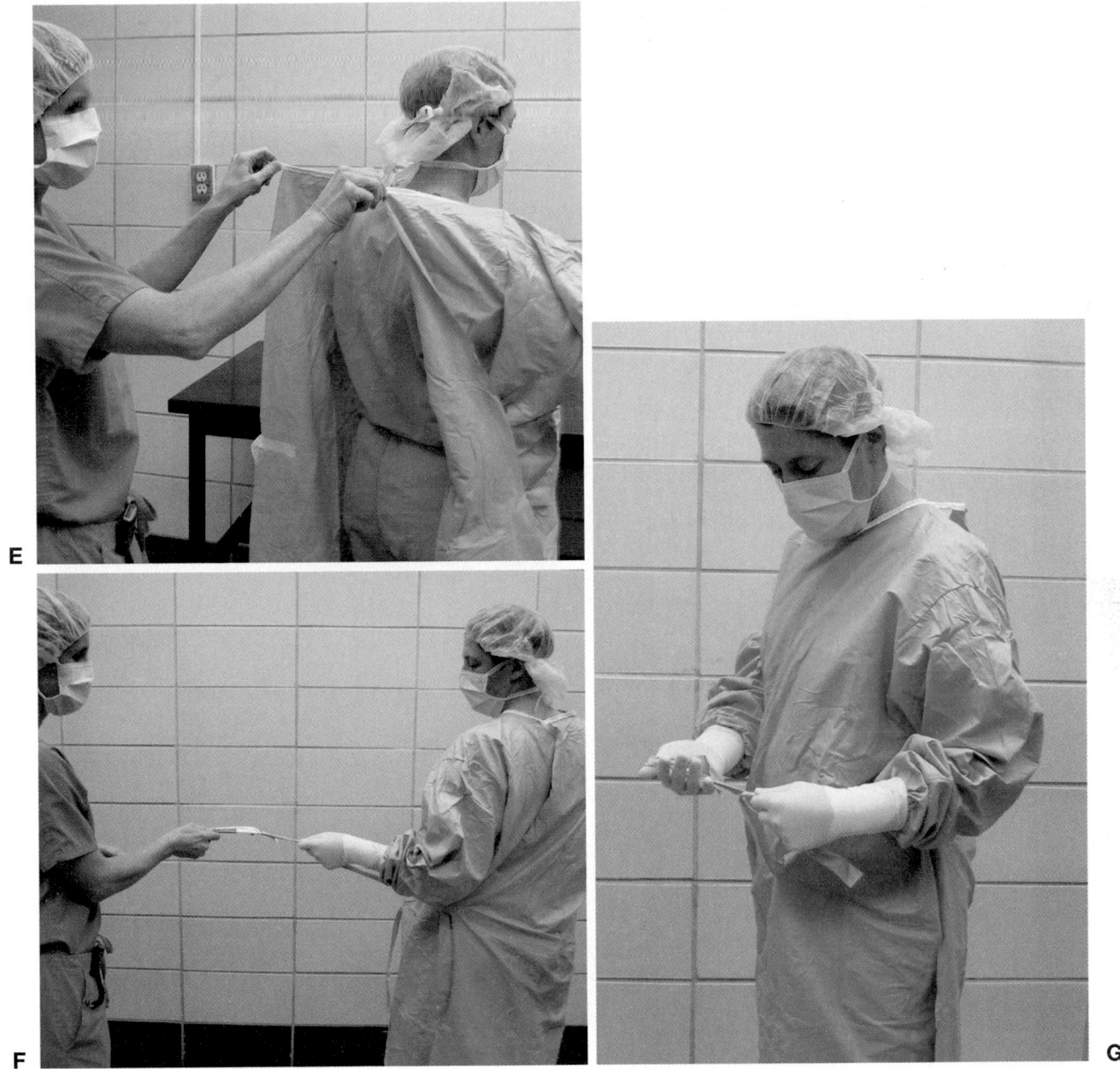

Figure 22-64—cont'd E, A nonsterile assistant pulls the gown over the shoulders and ties the back of the gown at the neck and waist. F, If the gown has a wraparound back, the last tie is performed after the surgeon has gloved. The surgeon hands the sterile tag to a nonsterile assistant. The assistant holds the end of the tag while the surgeon turns around, causing the gown to cover the surgeon's back. The surgeon takes the gown tie and pulls, releasing it from the tag that is still in the assistant's hand. G, The final tie is done in front by the surgeon.

unfolded, it is grasped by the hand that is holding the pack. This prevents the edges of the wrap from contaminating the contents of the pack. The exposed item may be grasped by the surgeon or carefully set on the sterile field.

To open a plastic/paper pouch, scalpel blade, or suture package the edges of the wrapper should be peeled back slowly and symmetrically, keeping the package opening directed away from the body. Some items may be dropped onto the sterile field, being careful not to lean or reach across the sterile field (Figure 22-61, *B*). If the item is small

or awkward to handle, the surgeon can grasp it with a gloved hand or sterile instrument. The item should not be allowed to touch the peeled edges of the pouch because the edges are considered contaminated.

Sterile saline may be poured into the sterile saline bowl. To avoid reaching over the sterile field with the saline container, the surgeon may hold the bowl away from the instrument tray or position it on the tray at the edge of the sterile field. The lip of the saline container should be a few inches above the rim of the bowl to reduce the risk of

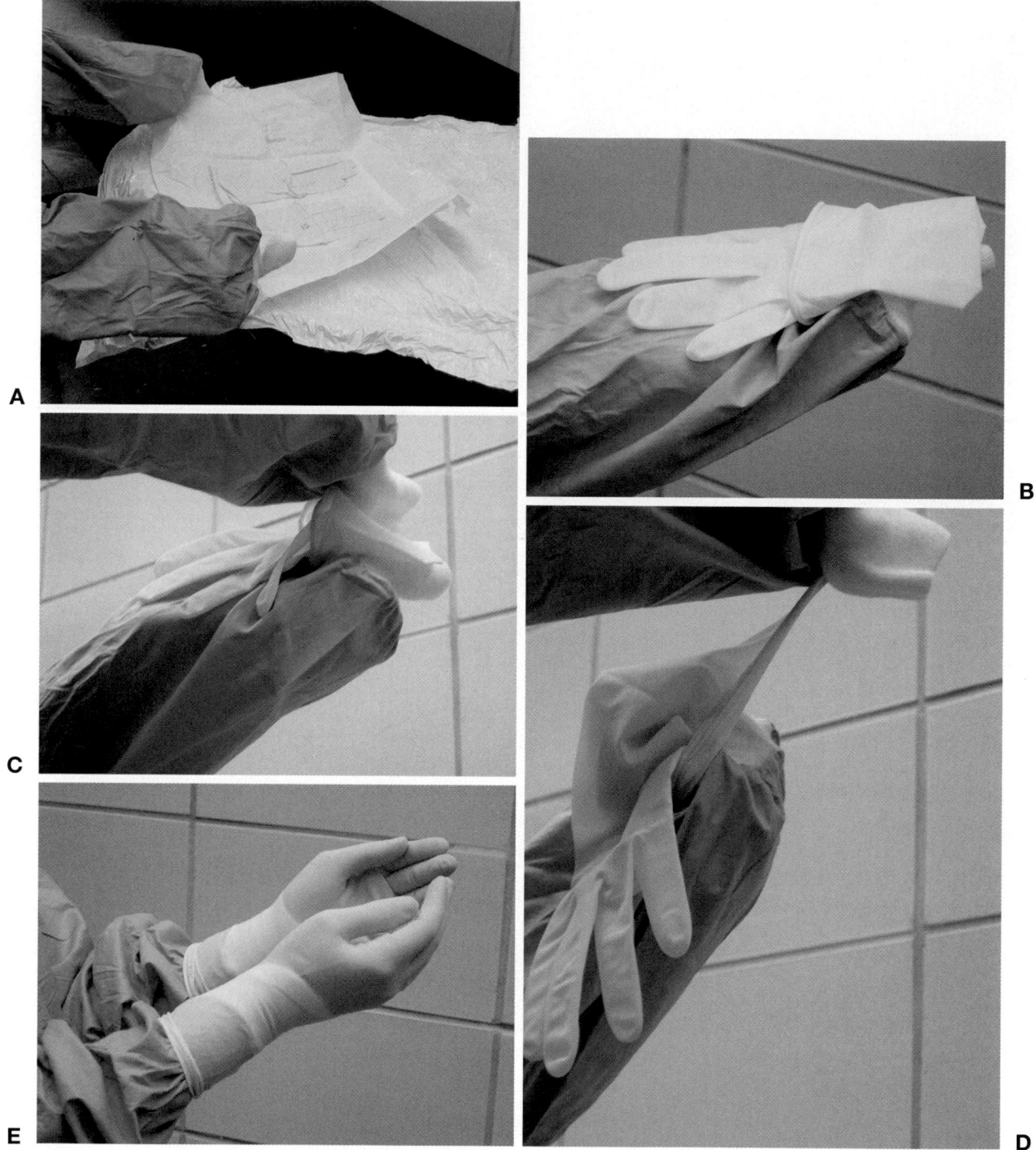

Figure 22-65   Closed gloving. **A,** The sterile pack is close to the table edge so that the surgeon can maintain some distance from the table to prevent contaminating the sterile gown. The sterile paper wrap containing the gloves is unfolded and one glove is picked up. It is easiest for most people to glove their nondominant hand first. The fingers must be kept inside the sleeves at all times during closed gloving. **B,** The glove is laid on the hand to be gloved, with the glove fingers pointing toward the elbow and the glove thumb lying against the sleeve. The edge of the glove cuff is grasped through the gown sleeve. **C,** The opposite side of the cuff is grasped in the other hand. **D** and **E,** The glove is pulled over the hand. Now the gown and glove cuff may be grasped together to pull the glove completely onto the hand. **E,** The opposite hand is gloved in a similar fashion. Once completed, the gown cuffs should be completely covered by the gloves.

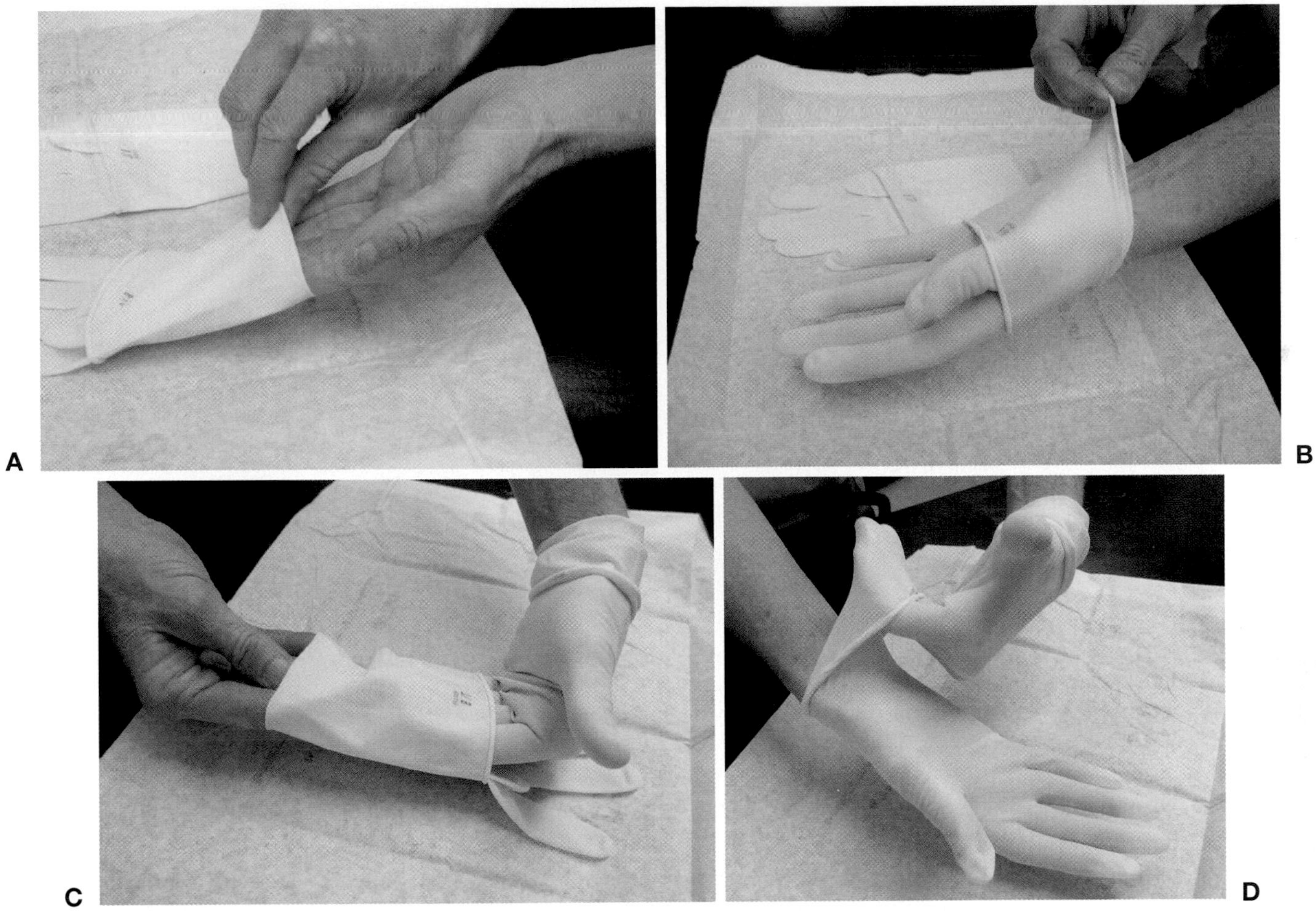

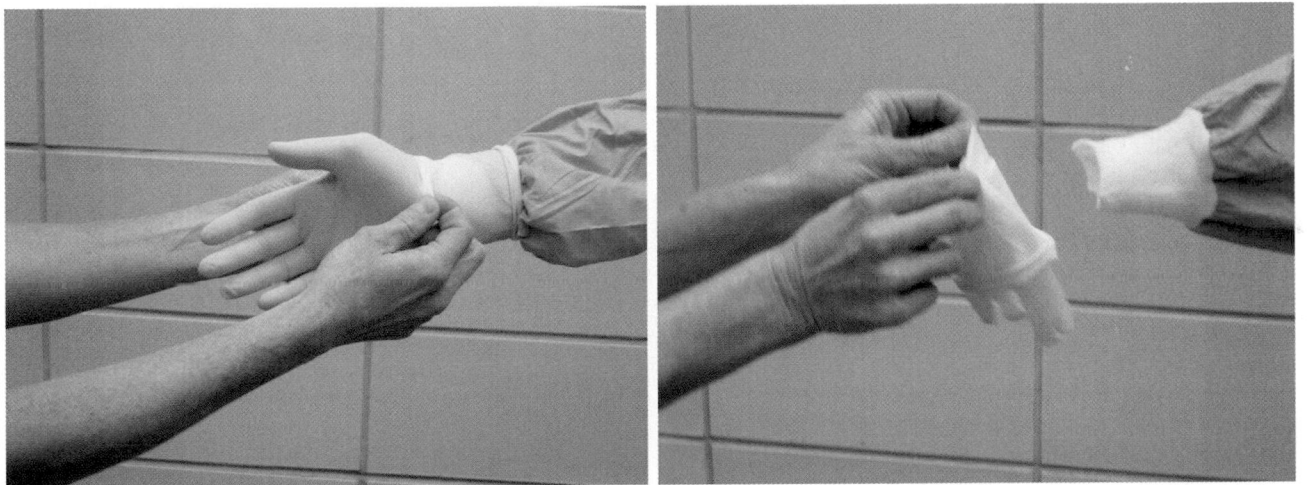

Figure 22-66 Open gloving. **A,** The glove pack is opened near the edge of a table. The hand is inserted into the glove opening, taking care not to touch the outside of the glove. The inside of the glove will not be sterile, so the cuff may be touched. **B,** The glove is pulled on by grasping the cuff fold with the other hand. The cuff will still be folded, but the glove is on well enough to allow use of the hand. **C,** The gloved hand is placed between the cuff and the palm of the glove to assist gloving the other hand. This protects the gloved hand from accidental contamination on the arm. **D,** The cuff can be unfolded. Now adjustments can be made to both gloves, taking care to touch only the sterile areas of the gloves.

Figure 22-67 Removing gloves aseptically. **A,** A nonsterile assistant grasps the glove and gown cuff together, without touching the gown sleeve. **B,** As the glove is removed the gown is pulled over the fingers. The gown cuff is considered contaminated. The surgeon can reglove, being careful not to contaminate anything with the gown cuff. It may be preferable to perform an assisted gloving as shown in Figure 22-68.

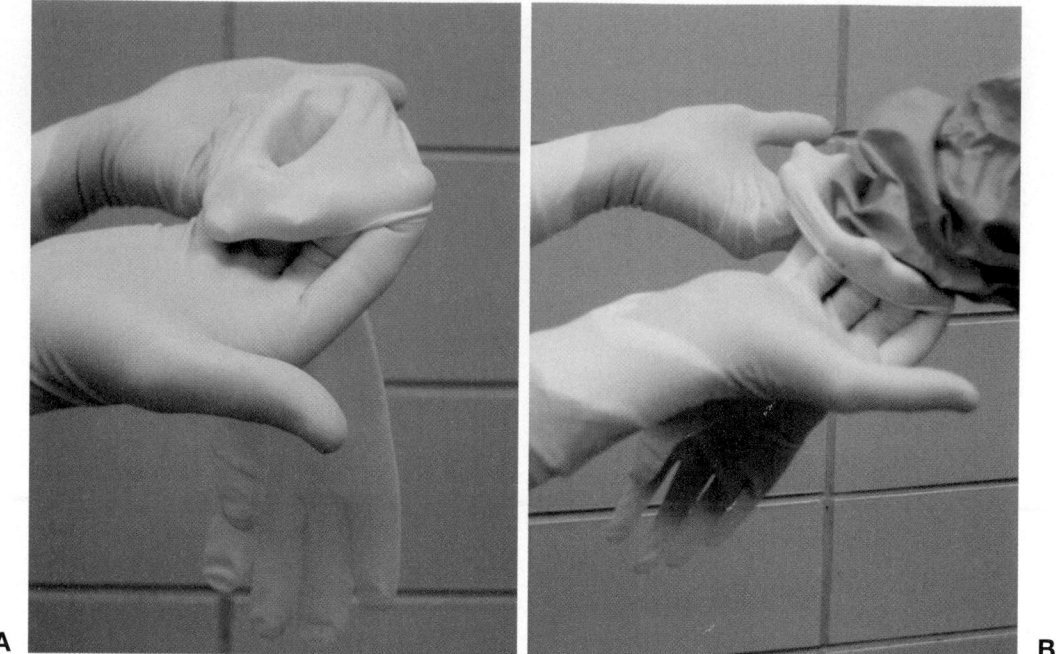

Figure 22-68   Assisted gloving. **A,** A sterile assistant picks up the appropriate sterile glove, holding it so the location of the glove thumb is apparent. The assistant hooks their fingers under the glove cuff and pulls to make the glove opening as large as possible. **B,** The surgeon slides their hand into the glove, while the assistant pulls the glove cuff up to be sure it covers the gown cuff before releasing.

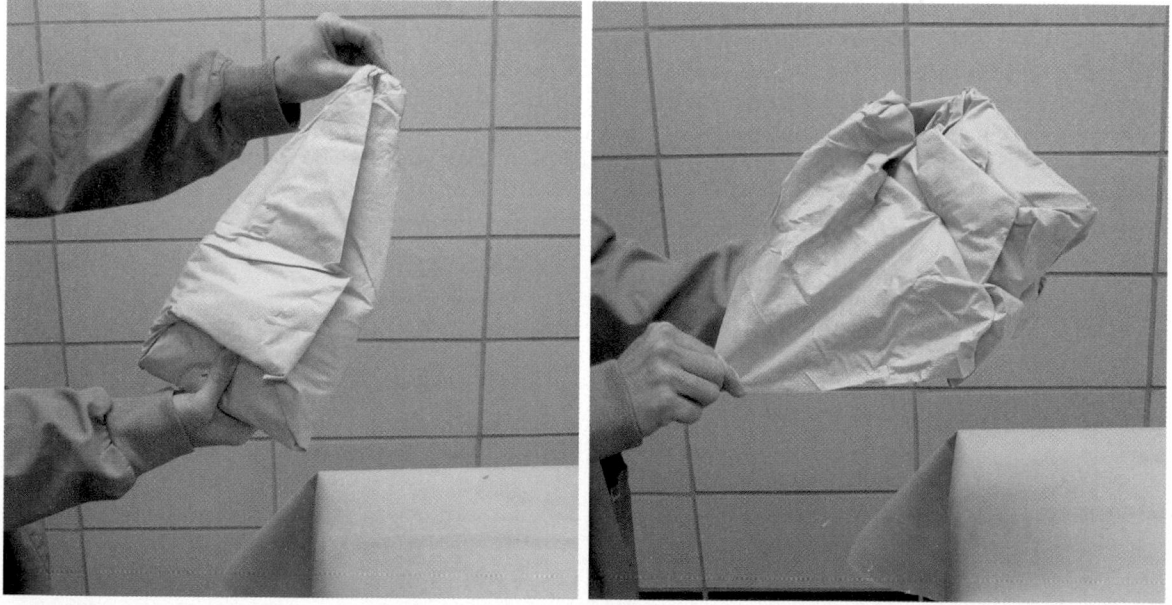

Figure 22-69   Opening sterile pack that can be held in one hand. **A,** Open the first flap away from you. **B,** As each flap is opened, it is held together with the hand holding the pack. After the fourth flap is pulled back and secured, the inner package may be grasped by the surgeon. Move the wrap down and toward you as the surgeon lifts the contents up and toward them. Alternatively, the package may be set on a sterile field, near its edge to avoid reaching over the field.

touching it, but not so high that the saline splashes as it is poured. If drapes or gowns (especially those made of cloth) become wet with saline or blood, they may no longer be impermeable to bacteria and are said to have "strike-through."

TECHNICIAN NOTE

If drapes or gowns (especially those made of cloth) become wet with saline or blood, they may no longer be impermeable to bacteria and are said to have "strike-through."

While opening a pack, make sure that the opening faces away from you.

Recommended Reading

Beale BS et al: *Small animal arthroscopy.* Philadelphia, 2003, WB Saunders.

Cockshutt J: In Slatter D, editor: *Textbook of small animal surgery,* ed 3, Philadelphia, 2003, WB Saunders, pp 149-155.

Hobson HP: In Slatter D, editor: *Textbook of small animal surgery,* ed 3, Philadelphia, 1993, WB Saunders, pp 179-185.

Lemarie RI, Hosgood G: Antiseptics and disinfectants in small animal practice, *Compend Cont Educ Pract Vet* 17:1339-1352, 1996.

McIlwraith CW: *Diagnostic and surgical arthroscopy in the horse,* ed 2, Philadelphia, 1990, Lea & Febiger.

Mitchell SL, Berg J: In Slatter D, editor: *Textbook of small animal surgery,* ed 3, Philadelphia, 2003, WB Saunders, pp 155-162.

Nieves MA, Wagner SD, in Slatter D: *Textbook of Small Animal Surgery,* ed 3, Philadelphia, 2003, Saunders, pp 185-198.

Pavletic MM: Surgical stapling, *Vet Clin North Am* 24:225-429, 1994.

Shmon C: In Slatter D, editor: *Textbook of small animal surgery,* ed 3, Philadelphia, 2003, WB Saunders, pp 162-178.

Tracy DL: *Small animal surgical nursing,* St. Louis, 2000, Mosby, pp 1-247.

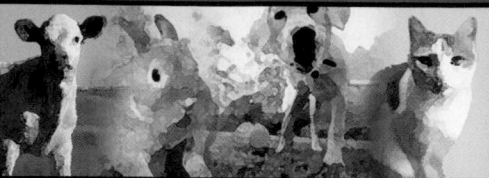

Surgical Assistance and Suture Material

SUSANNE K. LAUER

ROLE OF THE VETERINARY TECHNICIAN IN SURGICAL ASSISTANCE

Excellent support of a dedicated surgical technician can make a difference between successful surgical outcome and failure. The ideal surgical assistant "prethinks" and anticipates the surgeon's needs before the surgeon asks for it. Thus already on the day prior to surgery the surgical assistant generates a plan for the following day. As a rule of thumb sterile surgeries are performed first and more contaminated surgeries later throughout the day with the intent to prevent surgical infections. The surgical assistant verifies that the required instruments, implants, surgical and diagnostic supplies, medications, anesthetic equipment, and operating room are available and set up for surgery.

The surgical assistant supervises or performs preparation of the patient (see Chapter 22 for clipping, scrubbing, preoperative antibiotics) and positions the patient in an ideal secure position on the operating table according to the instructions of the surgeon. The surgical technician will then drape the patient for the surgeon and set up the instruments properly.

Intrasurgical assistance includes improving the surgeon's visualization by providing retraction and hemostasis in the surgical field, being familiar with the objectives of the technique, and manipulating the instrumentation and tissues into position for completion of the surgical task. The second charge of the technician is to protect the patient from hazards of surgery, such as infection, by maintaining an aseptic surgical field and expediting surgical completion by anticipating needs for proper instruments and suture readiness. Because the surgeon is often concentrating on the

surgical procedure, the technician must be constantly aware of the patient's anesthetic and cardiovascular status while assisting. After the surgery the assistant will help with bandaging and anesthetic recovery of the patient.

TECHNICIAN NOTE

The ideal surgical assistant anticipates the surgeon's needs before the surgeon asks for it and plans in advance.

PATIENT AND INSTRUMENT TABLES SETUP

POSITIONING OF PATIENT

Before sterile preparation is performed, the surgical patient is moved into the operating room and secured to the table. The surgical site must be accessible for the surgeon and the assistant standing (sitting) in a neutral position to prevent long-term health problems secondary to abnormal posture. Depending on the surgical procedure performed, the patient is placed in the appropriate position and secured with V-shaped troughs, ropes, towels, sandbags, and vacuum-activated positioning devices (Figure 23-1). The patient is placed on prewarmed water-circulating heating pads and covered with warm-air circulating blankets (see Chapter 24). Many surgeons prefer the warm-air circulation to be only activated after the patient is draped to prevent potential blowing of particles into the sterile surgical field. If the surgeon plans to use monopolar electrosurgery, the ground plate must be positioned in direct contact with the patient under the animal. Care must be taken that the securing devices do not restrict respiratory function or apply excessive pressure on peripheral nerves, vessels, or muscles. When extremities with intravenous/arterial catheters or

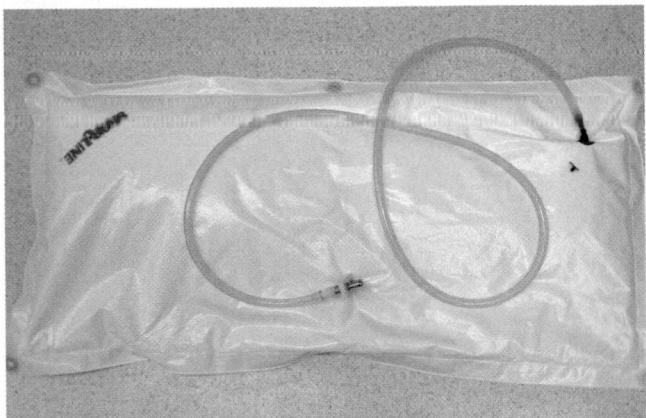

Figure 23-1 Vacuum-activated positioning device for accurate positioning of the patient on the table.

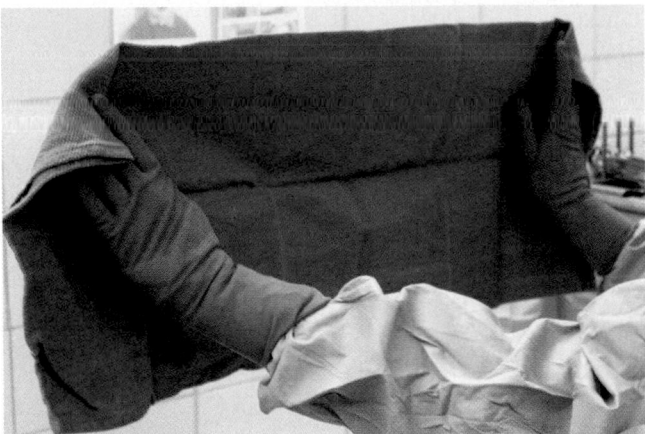

Figure 23-2 The drape is wrapped around the hands for protection of the sterile gloves.

blood pressure monitoring devices are tied to the table, rope tension or position often have to be adjusted to allow for adequate flow of fluids and correct measuring.

DRAPING

The function of draping is to separate the sterile surgical site from contaminated areas of the patient. Draping can only be performed by a sterile gloved and gowned member of the surgical team. Draping and instrument setup performed by the surgical assistant will speed up the procedure. Sterile quarter (field) drapes, Backhaus towel clamps, and large table covering drapes are opened on a sterile table by a nonsterile assistant. The first field drape is unfolded and an edge folded under toward the patient. Then the corners of the drape are wrapped around the hands to protect these from contamination (Figure 23-2). The drape is floated above the patient and placed in the appropriate position without dragging the sterile drape along the patient's contaminated body. This is easier if the table is positioned relatively low considering the height of the draping person. When applying the drapes, keep in mind that the undraped surgical table is not sterile and cannot be touched by the draping person. Therefore the draping assistant should stand at least 15 inches away from the table border and be constantly aware of her or his environment to avoid contamination of sterile hands and gown. The drape should only be adjusted minimally once it has been laid onto the patient. If the drape needs to be adjusted, it should only be moved in a direction away from the sterile surgical site and never toward the sterile site. Four quarter drapes are secured to each other and to the patient's skin with Backhaus towel clamps around the incision site (Figure 23-3). The Backhaus towel clamps are considered unsterile once they have penetrated the skin. If you need to remove towel clamps for readjustments, do not touch the contaminated tips; hand them off the table (to a nonsterile assistant) and utilize a new clamp. For final draping, a large fenestrated or unfenestrated drape is placed over the animal and the

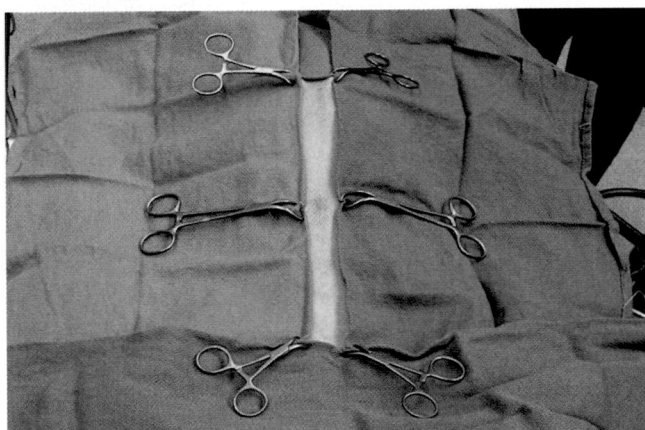

Figure 23-3 Four quarter drapes are secured with towel clamps approximate to the incision.

table (Figure 23-4). The fenestration is placed over the incision site or a slit is cut into the unfenestrated drape at the incision site (Figure 23-5).

For orthopedic or neurologic surgeries (especially when implants are placed or if lengthy surgery is expected), exposed aseptic skin in the fenestrated area can be covered with additional adhesive drapes (Ioban, 3M Healthcare, St. Paul, MN) (Figure 23-6, A and B). A spray adhesive should be evenly applied to the skin to augment the plastic's ability to remain in place throughout the surgery (Figure 23-6, C). Alternatively, sterile towels or drapes may be applied to the margins of the skin incision to protect the deeper incision. These towels may be attached with additional towel clamps spaced every 5 to 10 cm along the incision, with Michel clips (Figure 23-7) or by suturing the rolled edge of the towel or drape to the subcutaneous tissue with a simple continuous pattern of a strong, inexpensive suture material.

For orthopedic surgery, the limb is often enclosed in a sterile nonpermeable stockinette (General Econopak, Inc,

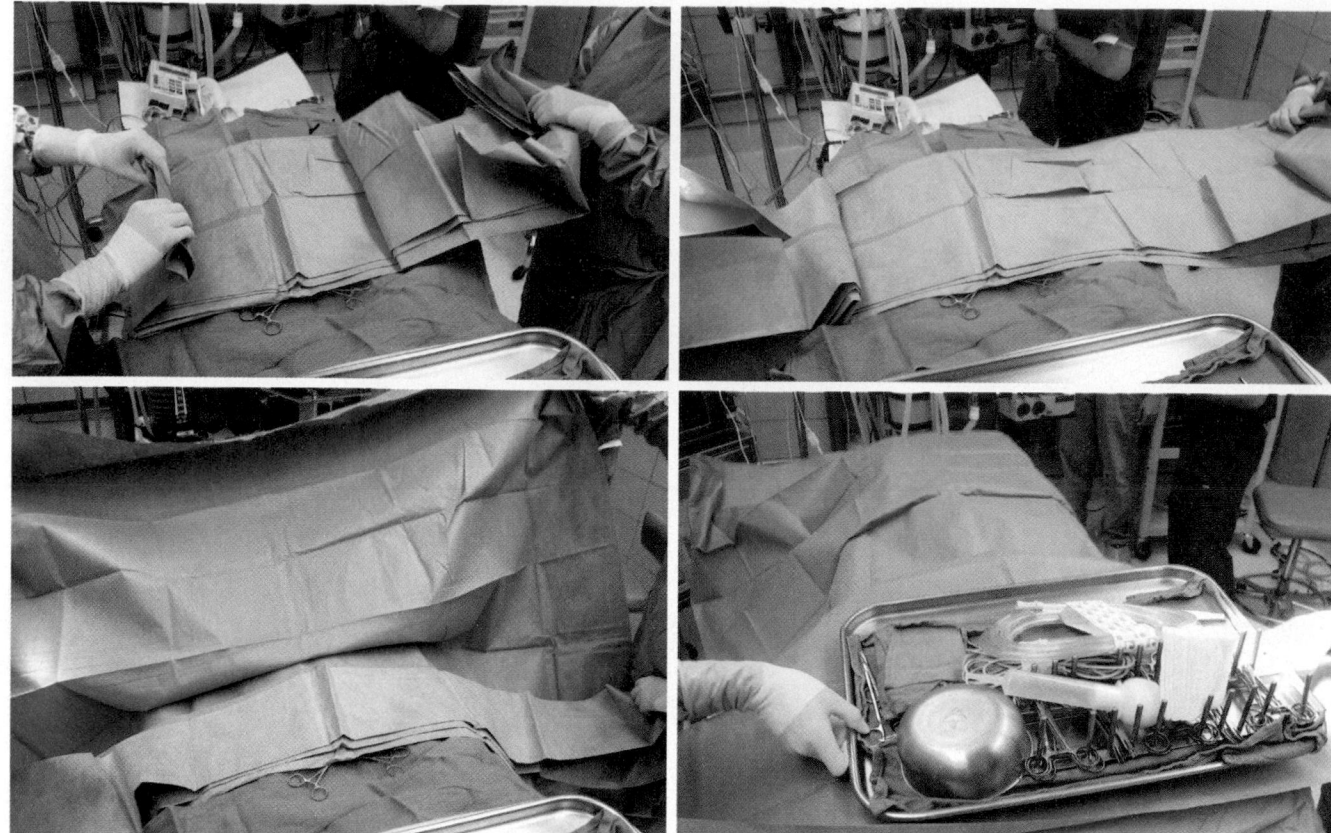

Figure 23-4 A large drape is placed over the four quarter drapes.

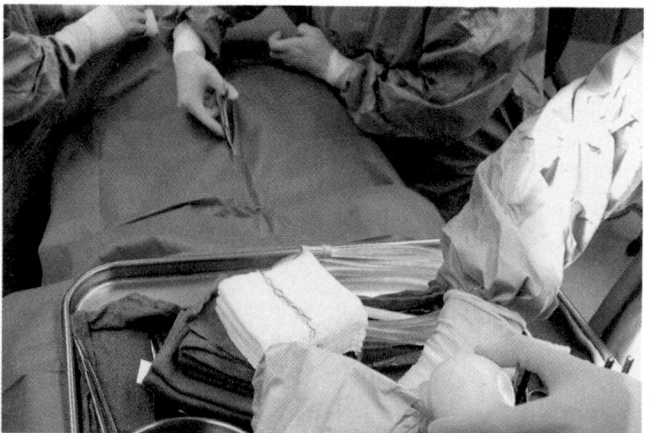

Figure 23-5 A fenestration is cut into the final drape to expose the incision site.

Philadelphia, Pa) to allow movement and manipulation and to limit exposed skin (Figure 23-8). The edges of the incised stockinette can be attached to the surgical incision as described above. The cut edge of the stockinette should be rolled under so that cut fragments of the stockinette material will not fall into the incision. The rolled-under stockinette is usually pulled over the skin edge and attached to the subcutaneous tissue to completely cover the cut skin

edge. This will also control much of the minor hemorrhage that occurs following skin incision.

> **⬛ TECHNICIAN NOTE**
>
> If Backhaus towel clamps are positioned directly in the corners (of a four-toweled drape set) to attach the drapes to each other, the edges of the drapes will lie flat and not bulge up.

INSTRUMENT SETUP AND HANDLING

After the patient is draped, instrument packs are opened on an adjacent table with sterile cover. Depending on the surgical procedure and surgeon's preference, the cover of the instrument table is continuous with the surgical field or remains as an isolated sterile isle that can be independently moved. Cautery and suction tubing are attached approximate to the incision site with specialized nonpenetrating towel clamps (Lorna or Edna clamps) or with Allis tissue forceps to the drape (Figure 23-9). The assistant decides which instruments from the pack are required by the surgeon and the surgical assistant for the procedure and places them according to surgeon's preference: instruments not required for the procedure (or may be used later) on the back side of the table, instruments directly required by the surgeon (scalpel, Mayo or Metzenbaum scissors) on the

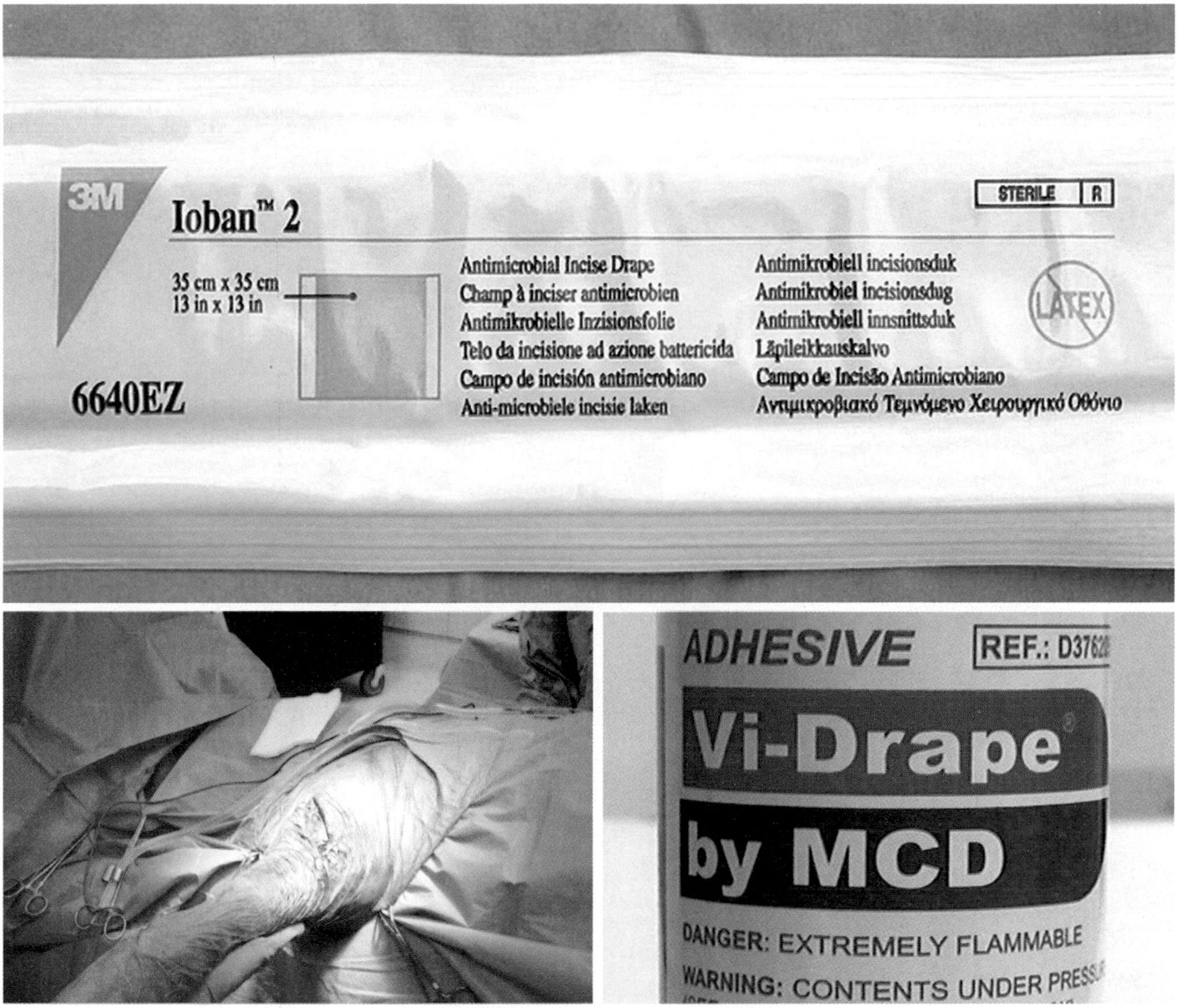

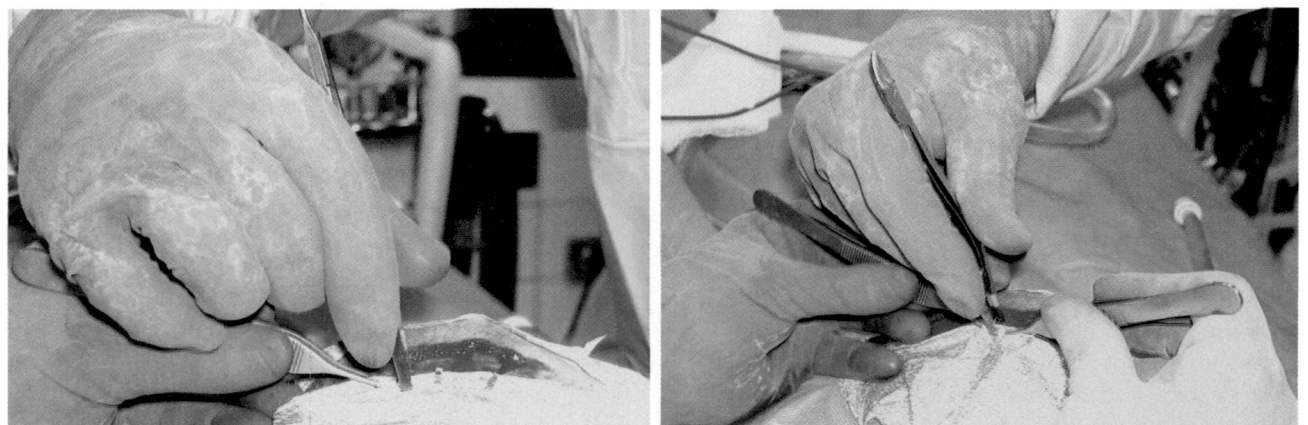

Figure 23-6 **A** and **B,** A sterile adherent plastic drape has been applied to the skin to minimize potential contamination. **C,** A spray adhesive is recommended to enhance adhesion of the plastic drape.

Figure 23-7 **A** and **B,** Towels or stockinettes can be attached to the skin with Michel clips.

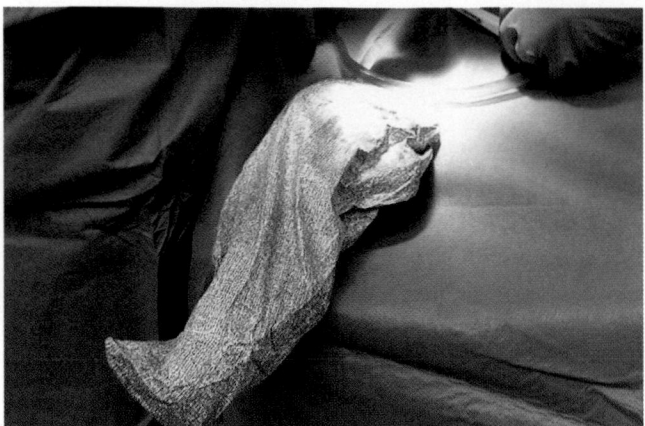

Figure 23-8 Nonpermeable stockinette to minimize contamination during orthopedic surgeries.

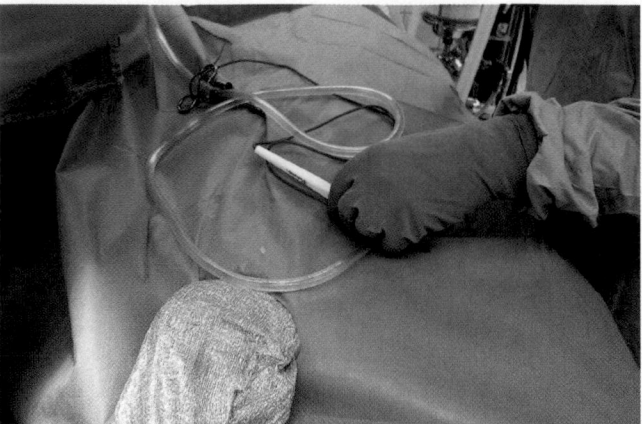

Figure 23-9 Cautery and suction are secured with Allis tissue forceps to the drape approximate to the surgical field.

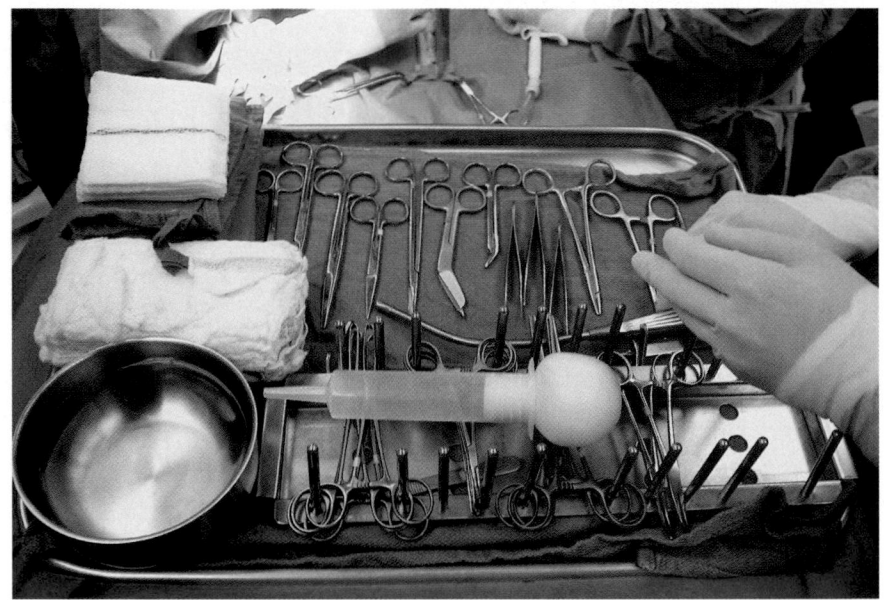

Figure 23-10 Example of a typical instrument arrangement.

surgeon's side, and instruments/material typically handled by the assistant (suture scissors, sutures, needle holders, hemostats) on the assistant's side (Figure 23-10). Blades are attached to the surgical knife handles (unless a disposable blade unit is used), and physiologic sterile saline is poured into a bowl for most surgeries. The saline bowl should be placed either inside a sterile tray or on waterproof drapings to prevent wicking from underlying nonsterile surfaces. Although no specific organizational scheme is universally used because of the variation in instruments and specialty equipment, the surgical assistant should be consistent in the general arrangement of the instrument stand. This will save time and effort for the assistant and speed up the procedure.

Special precautions are taken for oncologic and contaminated surgeries. Instruments utilized for manipulation of neoplastic or contaminated tissues are only placed in a so-called dirty corner on the table. In this way the other instruments are kept sterile and can be used for the remaining "clean" part of the surgical procedure. The surgeon might also consider changing gloves, suction devices, and potentially contaminated drapes and laboratory sponges during the course of surgery.

To be truly efficient and effective as a surgical assistant, the veterinary technician must be familiar with the procedure being performed. This allows readiness of proper instruments and supplies and minimizes the time spent explaining positioning and retraction. This may require maintenance of a card file detailing necessary equipment and a brief review of the operative technique for each procedure (Figure 23-11).

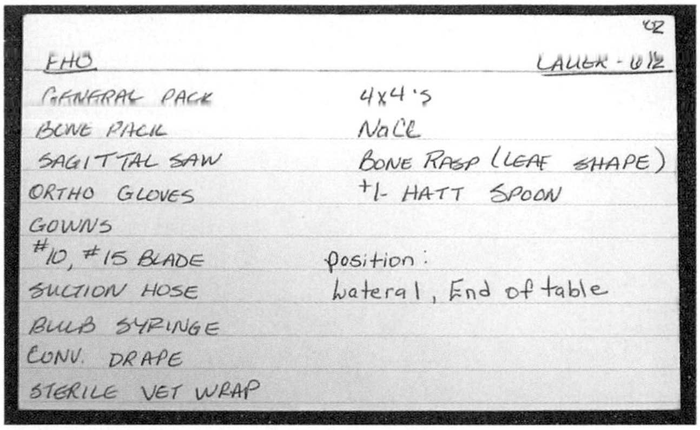

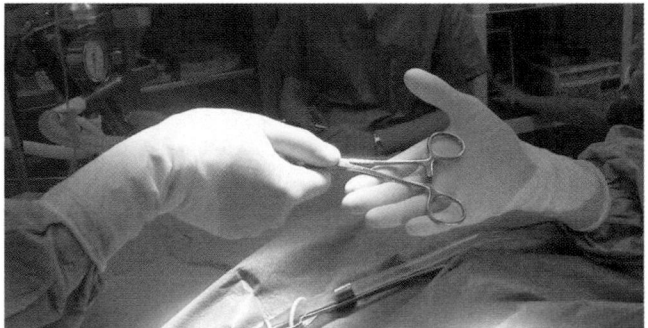

Figure 23-11 A technique card that is used to detail the necessary equipment for each surgical procedure.

![Instrument passing photograph]

Figure 23-12 Instruments are passed, ready for use, into the open hand of the surgeon.

Technicians should follow the progress of the procedure closely to anticipate the surgeon's needs. When passing instruments, the assistant should firmly "snap" the handle or handles into the open palm of the surgeon (Figure 23-12). This keeps the instrument firmly under control and in position for use. When the surgeon has finished with an instrument, it should be quickly wiped clean of blood and tissue and returned to its position on the instrument stand. Prolonged soaking of instruments in water (particularly saline) should be avoided because this ultimately causes corrosive damage to sharp cutting edges and hinges.

> ✎ **TECHNICIAN NOTE**
> Card files about surgical procedures and surgeons' preferences allow more efficient setup of the operating room.

STERILITY IN THE OPERATING ROOM

Maintaining sterility during surgery is a demanding task and requires the assistant being constantly aware of the operating room (OR) environment. Especially in the beginning of surgery, when nonsterile assistants still move around to open instrument packs, to adjust the table height, or to adapt anesthetic equipment, communication is important and position changes should be announced. The gowned and gloved sterile surgical team should primarily face the sterile field and must not touch or bend over nonsterile regions. The back of the surgical gown is always considered nonsterile, and only the front of the gown extending from below the shoulder level to the level of the surgical field is considered sterile. Therefore the assistant's hands must be positioned above the waist and below the shoulder. The sleeves of the gowns are considered sterile from 5 cm above the elbow to the level of the cuff (the stockinette cuff is not a bacterial barrier, and it is therefore considered nonsterile and should be always covered by the gloves). Clasping of the hands in front of the body is recommended, or the hands can be simply rested approximate to the incision site ready to assist. Unnecessary traffic and visitors in the surgery suite should be avoided, not only during the procedure but at all times, to help control dust and aerial contamination of the facility.

PROPER TISSUE-HANDLING TECHNIQUES

Surgical manipulation of each tissue by hands and instruments results in trauma. If the technician understands the general surgical principles of each body tissue system, he or she can minimize iatrogenic tissue injuries by simple routine actions and measures (such as handling the gastrointestinal track with saline-soaked sponges).

SKIN

The preparation of the patient's skin for surgery is described in Chapter 22. One must remember that preparation results in *aseptic* but not *sterile* skin. This means that the number of bacteria has been reduced below the number required to overwhelm the body's defense mechanism. However, with a depressed immune system or prolonged surgery, these resident bacteria can start to multiply and result in infection. Therefore the surgeon and assistant should avoid unnecessary direct handling of the skin.

The skin incision itself should be performed with a sharp scalpel blade (Figure 23-13). A scissors will crush and shear skin as it cuts. Skin is generally sensitive to this form of injury and will commonly react with severe swelling and scar formation. The skin is relatively thick and elastic; therefore it will also tend to force or "spring" the blades of the scissors apart, damaging the instrument. A sharp incision with a scalpel blade results in the least trauma, most rapid healing, and the least amount of scar formation but results in more hemorrhage compared to high-energy cutting incisions. Skin incision with high-energy cutting instruments (electrosurgical scalpel, plasma scalpel, and lasers) reduces resistance of wounds to infection and delays healing. Therefore after high-energy cutting, skin sutures or staples should remain in place 2 to 3 days longer compared

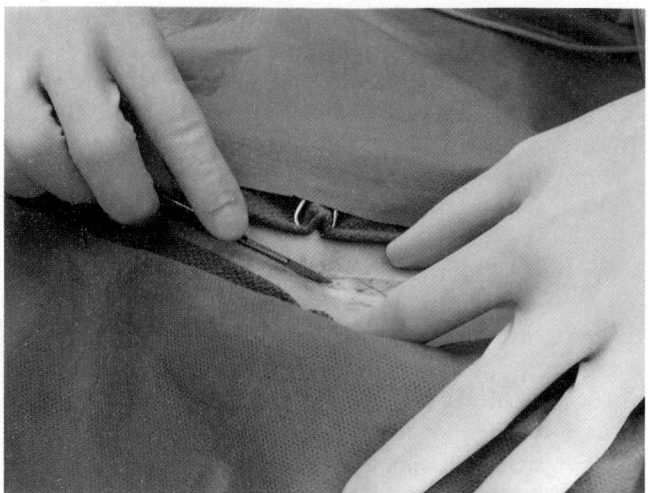

Figure 23-13 Skin incision with a scalpel blade results in rapid healing, with minimal trauma and scar formation.

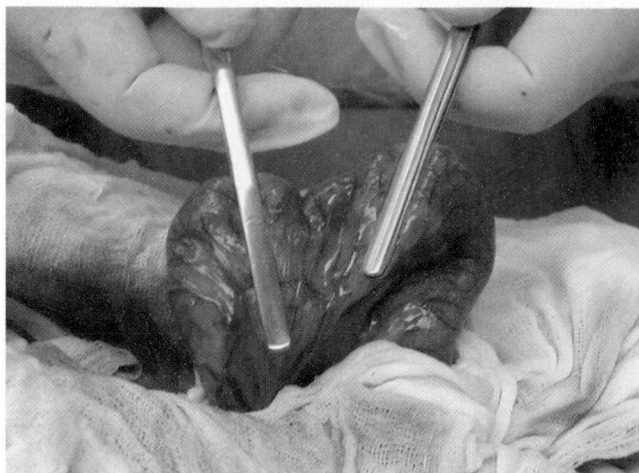

Figure 23-15 Use of Doyen intestinal forceps to prevent luminal content leakage during an enterotomy or a resection.

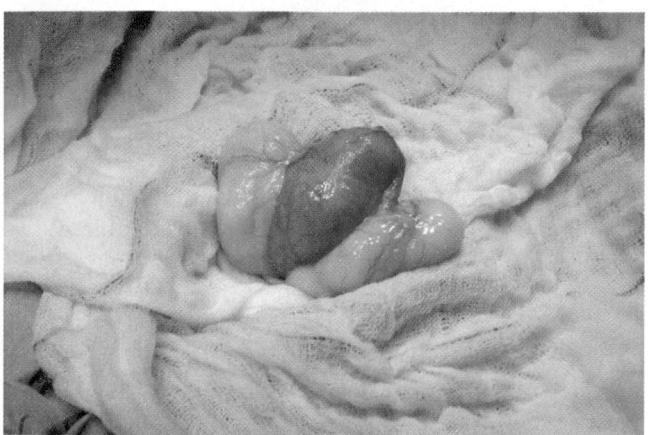

Figure 23-14 The bladder is isolated from the abdominal cavity with laboratory sponges prior to cystotomy.

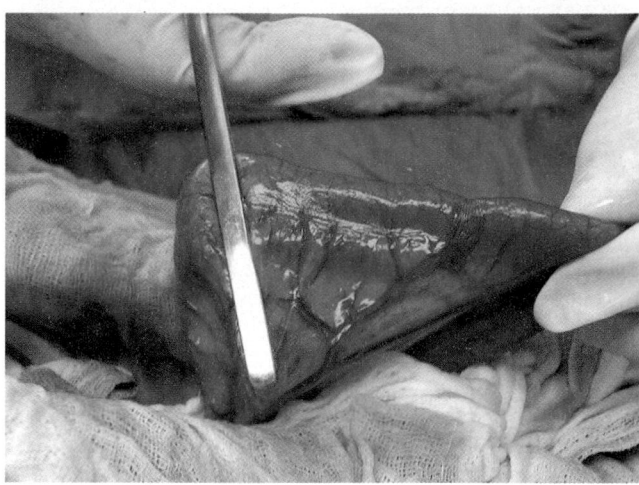

Figure 23-16 Area of intestinal damage from excessive tightening of a Doyen intestinal clamp.

to conventional scalpel incisions. The principles and use of the electroscalpel are discussed later under electrosurgery.

Skin edges can be controlled, rolled, and steadied with the thumb and index finger. Any instrument used to hold or manipulate skin should grip the tissue with teeth or hooks. Instruments that have smooth tips hold the tissue by pressure, which tends to crush skin and damage it in much the same way as scissors do. Traumatic surgical technique is known to contribute to postsurgical seroma formation.

✎ TECHNICIAN NOTE

Surgically prepared skin is *aseptic* and the number of bacteria on the skin has only been reduced below the number required to overwhelm the body's defense mechanism.

HOLLOW ORGAN SURGERY

Surgery of the hollow organs (i.e., stomach, intestines, bladder, esophagus) requires both complete control of luminal contents to avoid contamination and gentle handling to avoid iatrogenic damage to these delicate tissues. The surgical site is isolated from the body cavity with saline-moistened laparotomy sponges (Figure 23-14). Doyen intestinal forceps have thin bowed jaws with longitudinal grooves that prevent luminal content leakage when performing enterotomies or intestinal resections (Figure 23-15). The jaw tips make tissue contact, as soon as the ratchet's first teeth engage. Doyen intestinal forceps must not be overtightened or left in place too long, as this might result in excessive tissue damage (Figure 23-16). Many surgeons prefer the assistant to occlude the intestinal lumen by using moistened gloved fingers (Figure 23-17).

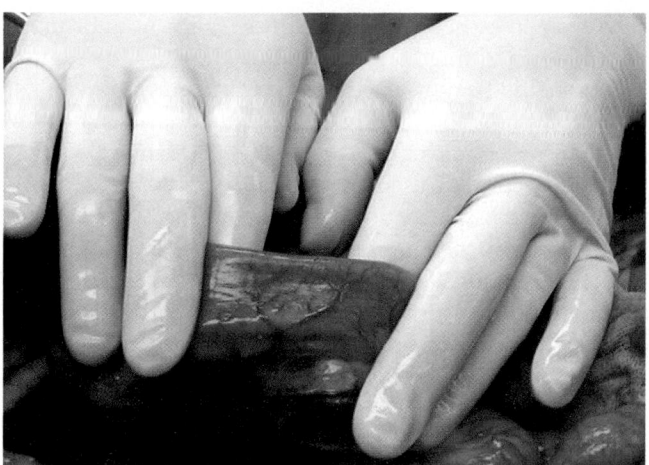

Figure 23-17 Use of moistened gloved fingers to occlude the intestinal lumen.

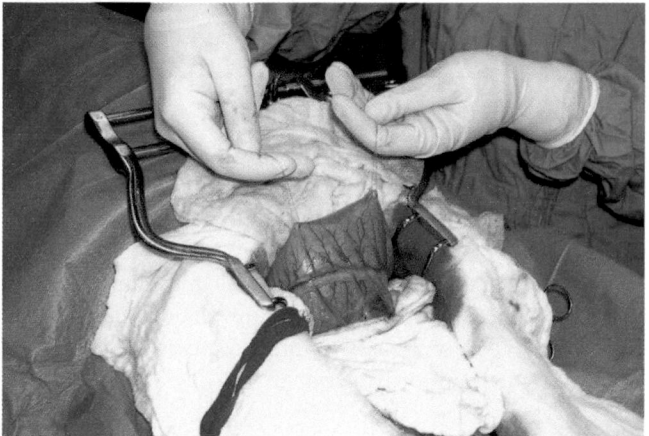

Figure 23-18 Stay sutures are passed through the outer layers of hollow organs. Both ends are held with a clamp. The assistant elevates the area of incision by applying traction to the stay sutures.

Large, hollow organs, such as the stomach or urinary bladder, often cannot be completely exteriorized. To avoid leakage of contaminated organ contents into the body cavity, the incisional region is elevated and stabilized with stay sutures. Stay sutures are simple loops of suture that pass through the holding layers of the viscus and are held together at their ends with a clamp (Figure 23-18). The surgical assistant applies controlled traction to the clamps to keep the incision in the desired location and elevated to avoid content leakage (Figure 23-19). Stay sutures are removed after the luminal incision has been closed.

✏️ **TECHNICIAN NOTE**

Instruments contaminated with luminal contents are only placed in a so-called dirty corner on the table. In this way the other instruments are kept sterile and can be used for the remaining "clean" part of the surgical procedure.

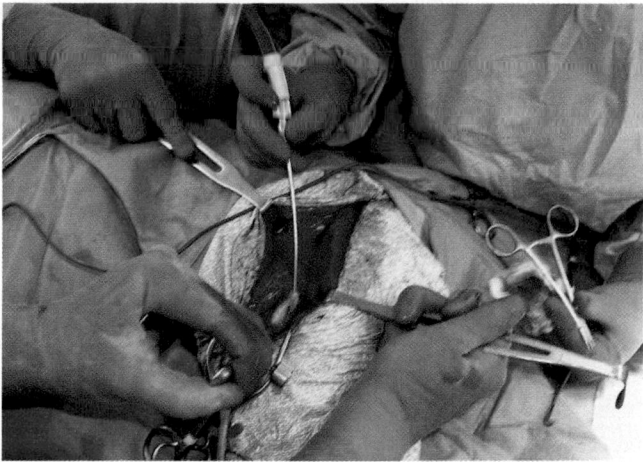

Figure 23-19 Exposure in the incision can be increased with hand retractors by the application of traction in one direction and countertraction in the opposite direction.

MUSCULOSKELETAL SURGERY

Surgery of the musculoskeletal system often requires surgical assistance. Muscle itself is highly vascular and has great healing ability. The natural blood supply of bone is compromised after fractures and healing only occurs if there is patent blood supply from the adjacent muscles. Consequently all efforts should be made to preserve soft tissue attachment to the bone as the assistant retracts and manipulates fractures. The assistant must also be cognizant of adjacent nerves and vessels and protect them from damage by bony fragments or the surgeon. Specifically, the radial, ulnar, and ischiadic nerves are often exposed during surgical approaches or course very closely to commonly occurring fractures. The surgical assistant must be familiar with the anatomic location of these major structures.

RETRACTION TECHNIQUES

Retraction of tissues is used to increase visibility and ease of manipulation in the incision. This can be accomplished with handheld retractors by which the assistant provides traction in one direction with one retractor and countertraction in the opposite direction with a second retractor (Figure 23-19). Retractors are available with various tips and blades to be used on different tissues. (Please see Chapter 22.) Care should be taken that retractors do not slide around or pull out of the incision, because this causes significant tissue trauma. Consequently, sharp-tipped retractors that maintain a grip on the tissue (without crushing) are often preferable to blunt-tipped retractors, particularly for muscle and skin retraction (Figure 23-20). Self-retaining retractors are also used to free the assistant for other duties (Figure 23-21, *A* and *B*). Excessive retraction for prolonged periods must be avoided with self-retaining instruments to prevent pressure-induced tissue damage.

Manual traction on adjacent tissues is often used to increase visibility or expose organs.

Visualization of the liver and the diaphragm can be significantly improved if the assistant carefully pulls up the sternum (Figure 23-22). Deep structures of the right abdominal cavity can be clearly visualized by retracting the proximal duodenum with mesoduodenum. If the abdominal viscera are positioned behind the mesoduodenum to the left, the right liver lobes, adrenal gland, kidney, and ureter are exposed (Figure 23-23). The left half of the abdominal cavity may likewise be visualized by retracting the abdominal viscera to the right, behind the mesocolon of the descending colon (Figure 23-24). The pancreas and portal vein are best exposed by gentle traction on the adjacent duodenum. As when using fingers for occluding the intestinal lumen, gloves should be moistened and excessive pressure avoided.

Nerves or large blood vessels are often retracted to improve visualization or to avoid potential damage. Careful blunt dissection is used to free the nerve or vessel from surrounding tissue. A broad, flat band, such as a Penrose drain or moistened umbilical tape, is passed around the structure (Figure 23-25), and the ends are clamped together much like a stay suture. The assistant can gently retract the nerve or vessel to one side, carefully avoiding entanglement with other instruments or equipment.

HEMOSTASIS

Hemostasis is a physiologic response to arrest bleeding. Various surgical techniques can be used to augment this physiologic clotting process. The surgical assistant should be able to perform or to assist with routine hemostatic procedures.

Excellent hemostasis is vital (1) to obtain optimal visibility at the surgical site, (2) to limit the volume of blood loss, and (3) to decrease risk of infection (extravasated blood is an ideal medium for bacterial growth).

SPONGE HEMOSTASIS

Low-pressure bleeding from small vessels can be controlled by sustained pressure through gauze sponges or similar

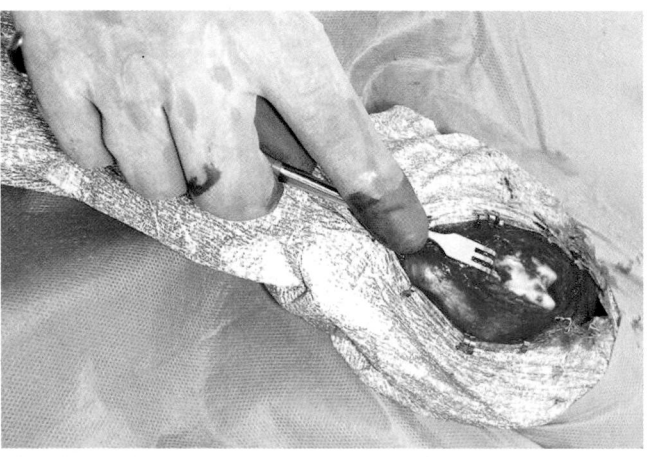

Figure 23-20 Use of a sharp-tipped, self-retaining retractor (Gelpi) to increase stifle joint exposure during an arthrotomy.

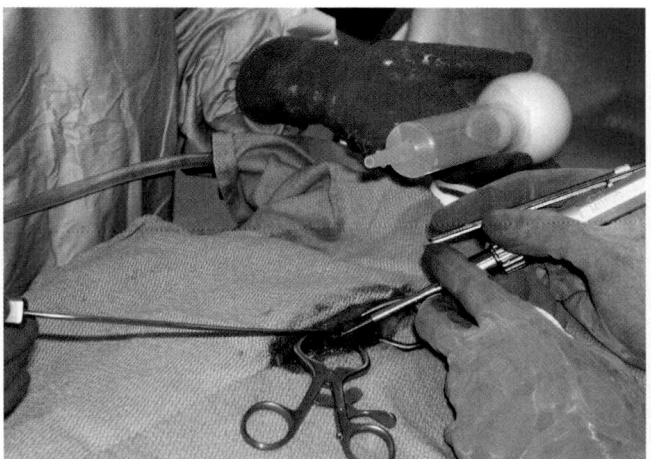 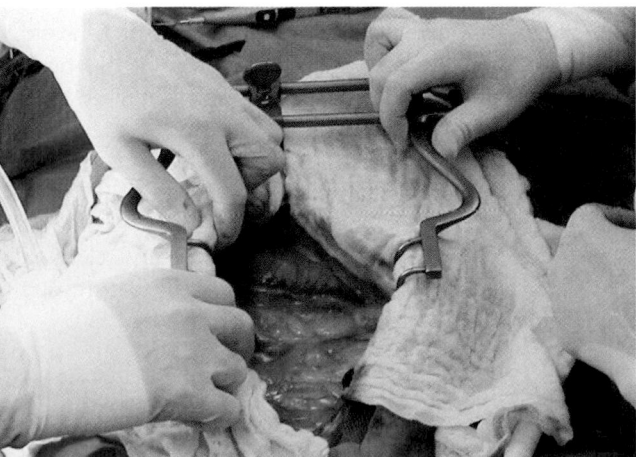

A   B

Figure 23-21 **A,** Self-retaining Gelpi retractors applied during a hemilaminectomy free up the hands of the assistant for suction and lavage while the surgeon removes bone with a drill. **B,** Placement of a blunt-tipped, self-retaining retractor (Balfour) in an abdominal incision verifying that abdominal organs are not entrapped.

material. The sponge should be applied with a blotting type of motion. A wiping motion (especially if sponges are not moistened with saline) will irritate tissue and will often renew bleeding by pulling the forming blood clots out of incised capillaries. The pressure apparently stops hemorrhage by collapsing the vessels until clotting can occur. With persistent hemorrhage, pressure may need to be sustained for up to 5 minutes to allow adequate coagulation.

✎ TECHNICIAN NOTE

Because any dry material is damaging to body tissues, slight moistening of sponges with saline before using them in the incision will reduce tissue trauma.

Sponge Complications

Gauze sponges left in the body after closing of the incision will cause severe inflammatory reaction, adhesions, and drainage. The abdominal and thoracic cavities are particularly hazardous locations for sponges to become lost. Consequently, many surgical assistants count sponges in such areas to make sure all sponges have been removed. Before surgery begins, sterile sponges are counted out in piles on the Mayo stand. Usually, two or three piles of 10 sponges are used to start. The total number is recorded, and all other sponges (e.g., those used for skin preparation) are removed from the area. If additional sponges are required during surgery, they are supplied in packs of 10, and their number is added to the total. The used sponges are saved in a separate pile and are counted at the termination of the procedure before the incision is closed. The number

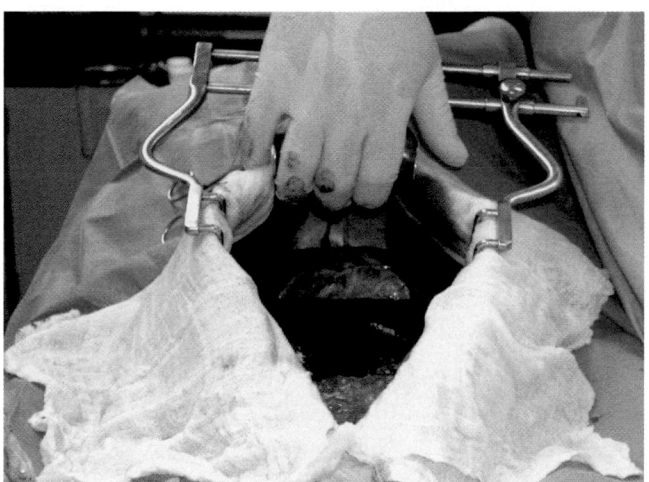

Figure 23-22 Gentle lifting of the sternum increases exposure of the diaphragm and liver during abdominal exploratory surgery.

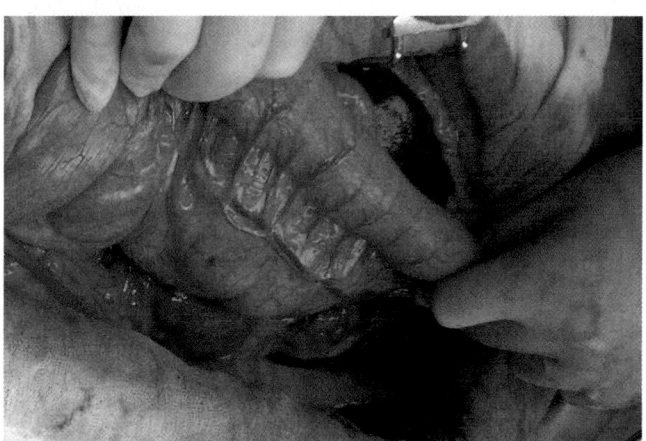

Figure 23-24 Retraction of the descending colon to the right exposes the left adrenal gland, kidney, and ureter.

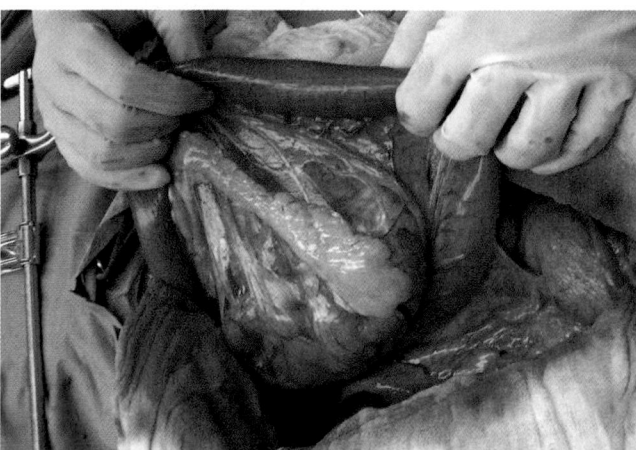

Figure 23-23 Retraction of the proximal duodenum/mesoduodenum to the left exposes the right adrenal gland, kidney, and ureter.

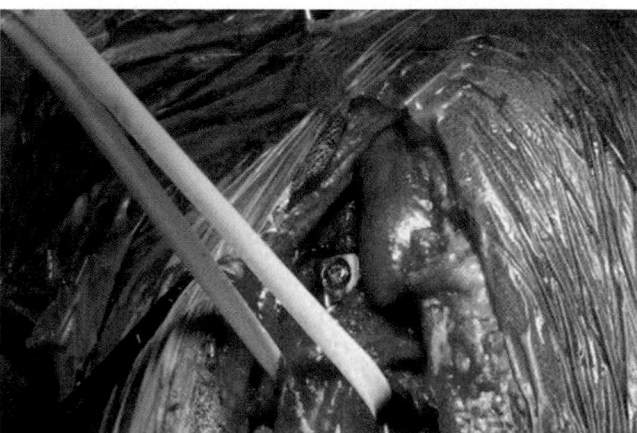

Figure 23-25 A Penrose drain is passed around the radial nerve and brachial muscle for atraumatic manipulation of the nerve during fracture repair with plate and screws.

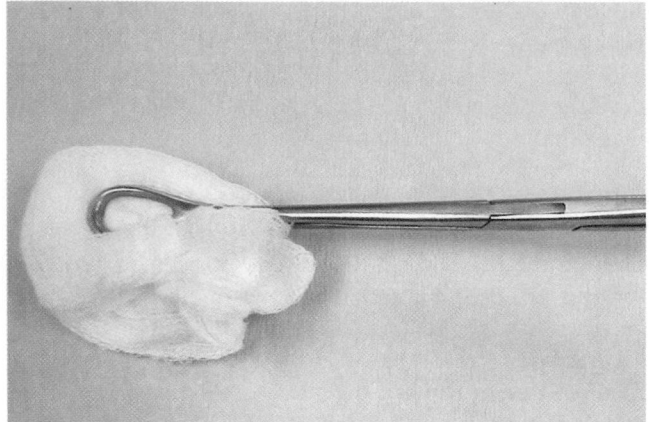

Figure 23-26 Gauze sponge held in a sponge forceps.

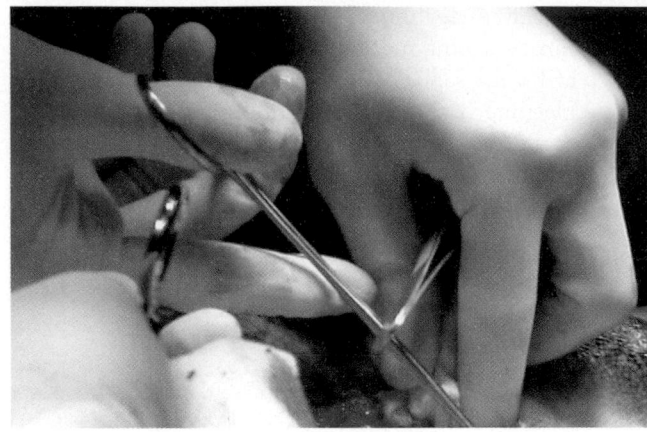

Figure 23-28 A hemostatic forceps is perpendicularly applied to the bleeding vessel with a minimal amount of adjacent tissue included.

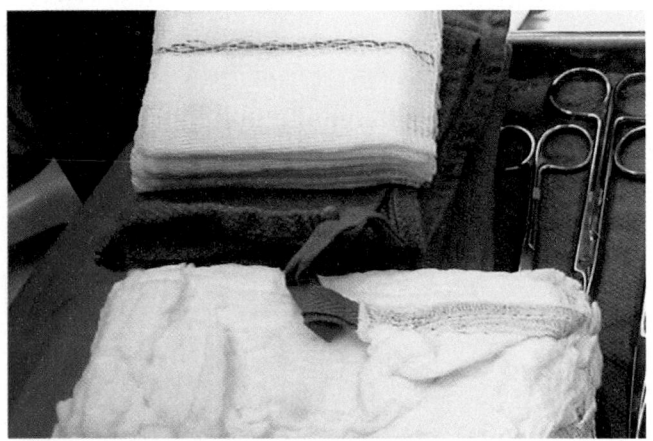

Figure 23-27 Laboratory sponges with tail and sponges with radiopaque markers can be used in deep incisions.

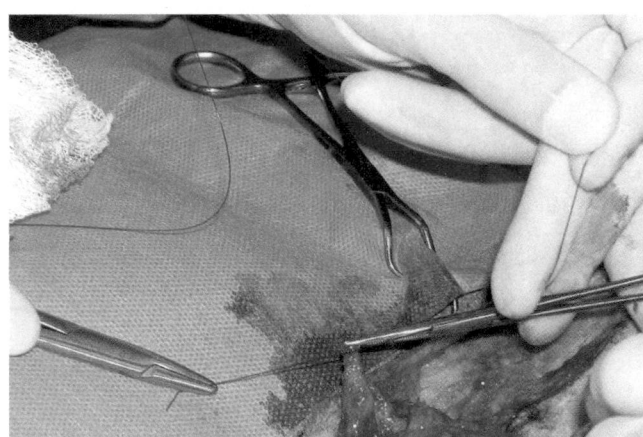

Figure 23-29 Lowering the handles of the hemostatic forceps raises the tips, forcing the ligation loop to form around the vessel.

of used sponges plus the remaining clean sponges must equal the total amount to account for all sponges. Additional precautions include use of sponges with radiopaque markers and never placing used or superfluous sponges approximate to the incision.

For particularly deep incisions, sponges may be held in a sponge forceps (Figure 23-26), or laboratory sponges can be used (Figure 23-27). The tape attached to the laboratory sponge is left extending out of the incision, and the sponge can then be easily removed by pulling on it.

HEMOSTATIC FORCEPS

Hemorrhage from slightly larger vessels can be occluded by clamping with a hemostatic forceps. When the vessel wall is crushed with the hemostatic forceps, the bleeding stops temporarily and the physiologic clotting mechanism is activated. The clamp should be applied perpendicular to the tissue surface and the bleeding vessel, with a minimal

amount of adjacent tissue being grasped in the tips of the clamp (Figure 23-28).

SUTURE LIGATION

A larger bleeding vessel that has been clamped can be ligated to achieve permanent hemostasis. After the suture material is passed around the vessel, the assistant lowers the handles of the clamp, which raises the tips (Figure 23-29). This causes the ligation loop to form around the vessel and not the instrument. As the first throw of the knot is pulled tight, the assistant releases the clamp. This allows the vessel to totally collapse, thus occluding the lumen. However, the assistant should return the vessel to its origin before releasing the clamp so that the knot is not snapped off the cut end of the vessel. After the surgeon finishes the knot, the assistant cuts off excessive suture, using the tips of the scissors. Care must be taken not to pull the ligature off the end of the vessel. Only enough material to secure the

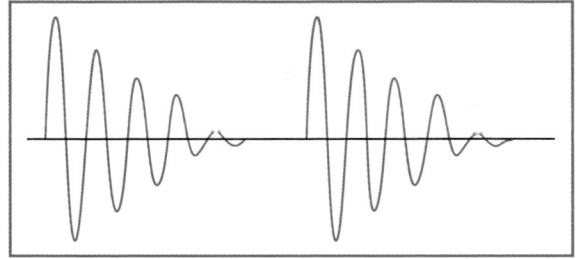

Figure 23-30 Diagram of the damped sine wave current, which causes coagulation.

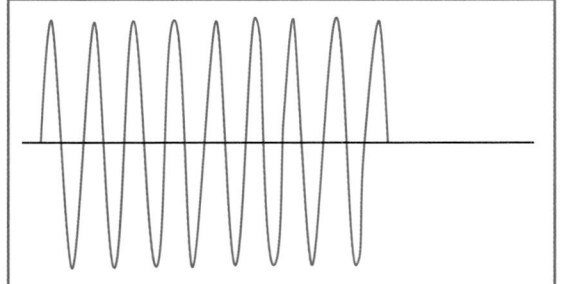

Figure 23-31 Diagram of the undamped sine wave current, which "cuts" tissues.

knot should be left. Arteries are commonly ligated twice, particularly if they are more than 2 mm in diameter.

ELECTROSURGERY

Electrocoagulation and Cutting Function

Electrosurgical units not only offer a means of stopping hemorrhage from an already cut vessel with electrocoagulation but also allow prevention of hemorrhage with an electroscalpel that coagulates as it cuts a vessel. Most electrosurgical units allow both coagulation and cutting depending on the waveform of the current selected.

Interrupted damped sine waves primarily result in coagulation, but they also allow for some cutting (Figure 23-30). The current causes protein coagulation of the blood elements within the blood vessel wall. Electrocoagulation should be used only on vessels smaller than 1.5 mm. As a rule of thumb, vessels with visible lumen should be ligated.

Continuous undamped sine waves primarily result in cutting associated with some minimal coagulation (Figure 23-31). Microcoagulation of the tissue proteins occur at a small point of contact.

Modulated pulsed sine waves allow simultaneous cutting and coagulation.

Monopolar and Bipolar Electrosurgical Modes

Most electrosurgical units allow both monopolar and bipolar modes of coagulation.

The monopolar mode is most commonly used in veterinary medicine and can be used for coagulation and/or

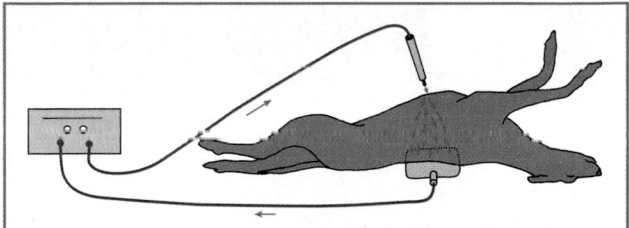

Figure 23-32 Diagram of electrical current passing from the handpiece, dispersing in the body, and returning to the generator via the ground plate.

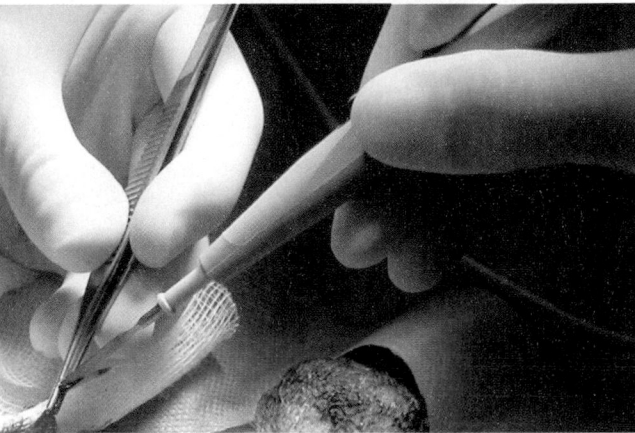

Figure 23-33 Application of current to a bleeding vessel by touching the handpiece to the Brown Adson forceps.

cutting. The current flows from a small handpiece (active electrode) through the animal's body and returns to the current generator via a ground plate (indifferent electrode) that is necessary to complete the electrical circuit (Figure 23-32). Direct maximal contact between the patient and the ground plate is important to prevent burns approximate to the ground plate. For hemostasis the current can be applied through a hemostatic forceps clamped on the vessel (Figure 23-33) or directly from the monopolar handpiece tip to the vessel. Monopolar electrocautery only works if all blood and fluid, which would dissipate the current, has been blotted away.

For a truly bloodless incision (modulated pulsed sine wave mode), the handpiece is held in a modified pencil grip perpendicular to the tissue surface. Because the electrode cuts whatever tissue is contacted, continuous visualization is indispensable when the electrode is activated. To avoid lateral heat damage to adjacent tissues, it has been recommended to move the instrument slowly at a speed of 7 mm per second (Figure 23-34).

Bipolar electrocautery utilizes a thumb forcepslike handpiece as active electrode (Figure 23-35). The vessel to be cauterized is grasped between the tips of the forceps, and the coagulating current runs from one blade to the other, not through the body (Figure 23-36). For effective use, a slight gap must remain between the tips when the

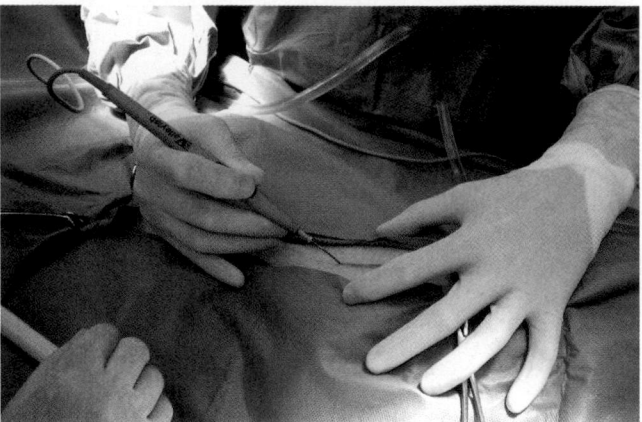

Figure 23-34 A bloodless incision can be obtained by blending cutting and coagulating currents.

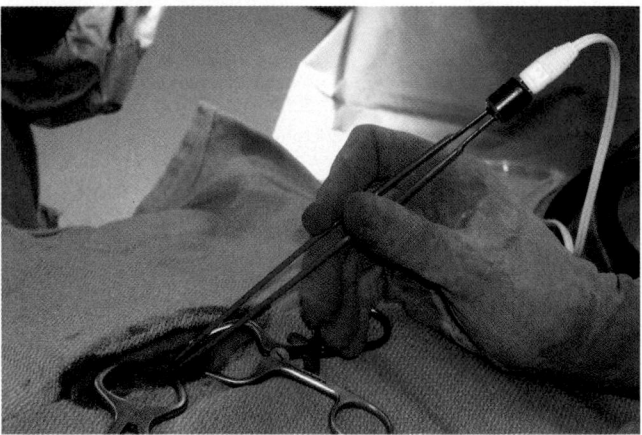

Figure 23-35 The thumb forcepslike handpiece used for bipolar cautery.

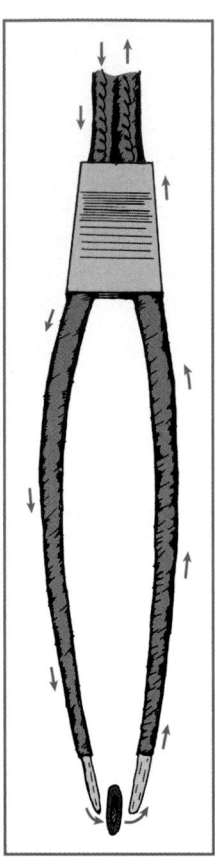

Figure 23-36 Diagram of the bipolar coagulation current as it passes from one tip of the handpiece to the other.

tissue is grasped. Because the short current pathway results in minimal damage to adjacent tissues, this form of electrocoagulation is particularly useful in microvascular, ophthalmic, and neurosurgery. In contrast to the monopolar mode, bipolar coagulation is only used for coagulation, but it has the advantage to function in a wet surgical field.

> ✎ **TECHNICIAN NOTE**
>
> Monopolar cautery only works in a dry surgical field, but bipolar coagulation also functions in a wet surgical environment.

The monopolar setup allows for cutting and/or coagulation, but the bipolar setup only allows for coagulation.

Battery-Powered Cautery Units
Disposable battery-powered cautery units can be used for hemostasis of very small vessels. Hemostasis is based on protein coagulation produced by a heated filament.

Carbon built up on the active tip of mono- and bipolar handpieces should be periodically removed by the assistant,

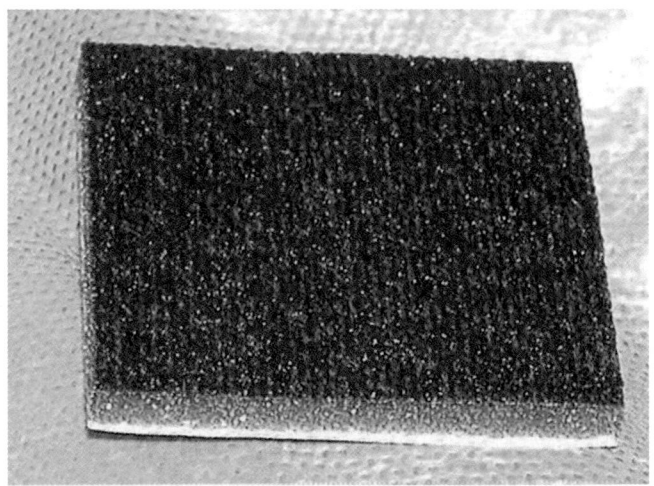

Figure 23-37 Buildup of protein on the handpiece tip, which prevents passage of current, can be removed with a scratch pad.

who scrapes it on a scratch pad (Figure 23-37) or with a hard metallic edge, such as the backside of a scalpel blade.

Safety With Electrosurgery
Electrosurgery will result in spark formation, and therefore it should not be used when explosive anesthetics, such as

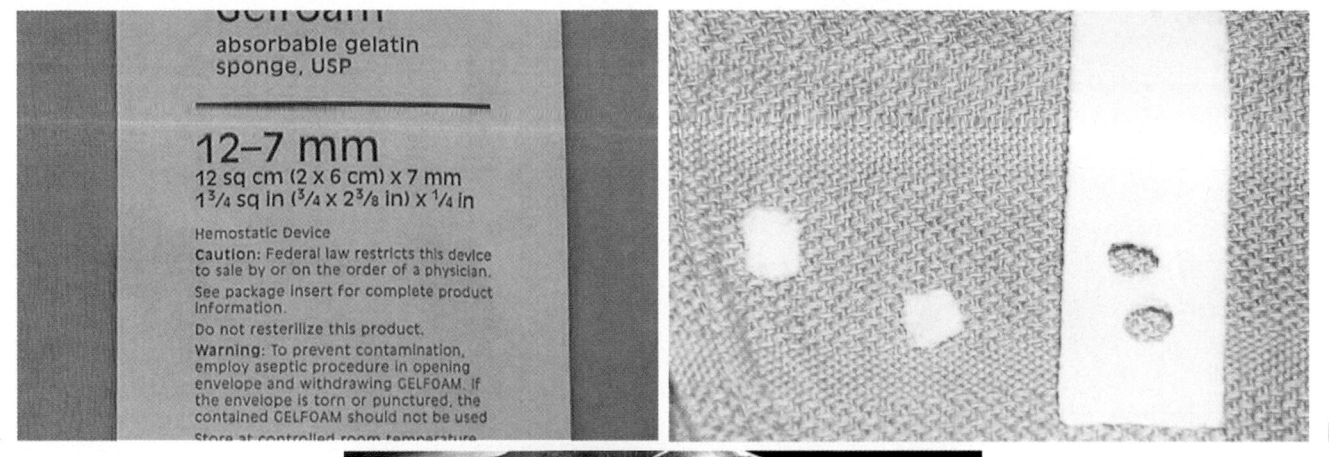

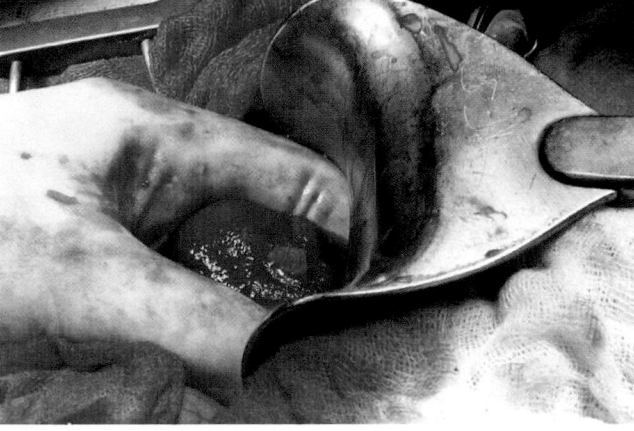

Figure 23-38 **A,** Biologic hemostatic agents, such as gelatin foam, promote coagulation and clot adherence. **B** and **C,** The foam is punched out of the sheet and placed in a bleeding liver biopsy site for hemostasis.

ether and cyclopropane, are present. Likewise, some antiseptic preparation materials (alcohol based) and adhesive agents are volatile and should be avoided or allowed to dry thoroughly before using electrosurgery. In order to avoid a burn at the point of current grounding, most electrosurgical units require generous application of conductive gel or fluid to provide good electrical contact between patient and ground plate. An electrical shock to hands holding the clamp or electrosurgical handpiece is usually caused by a hole in the glove. Regloving should alleviate the problem. Continued shocking reflects poor grounding or an equipment malfunction that should be checked by a qualified service representative.

TECHNICIAN NOTE

Electrosurgery should not be used in the presence of explosive anesthetics (ether) or alcohol-based antiseptic materials.

Tissue healing following the use of the electroscalpel has been shown to be significantly delayed. Likewise, the incidence of incisional infection is somewhat increased. Therefore techniques of asepsis and atraumatic tissue handling must be strictly adhered to when using electrosurgery.

HEMOSTATIC AGENTS

Absorbable hemostatic agents, such as gelatin sponges (Gelfoam, Upjohn), oxidized regenerated cellulose gauze (Surgicel, Johnson & Johnson), or bovine dermal collagen (Instat collagen absorbable hemostat, Johnson & Johnson), can be used to achieve hemostasis on tissues that tend to continually ooze or to pack small bleeding cavities (Figure 23-38).

Gelatin sponges are applied dry, soak up blood, and provide a lattice for the forming clot to adhere to. They are normally absorbed in 4 to 6 weeks but should not be used in infected areas.

Cellulose is a knitted material that only activates clotting of whole blood. Therefore it is not useful if oozing occurs in a serohemorrhagic environment.

Bovine collagen triggers clot formation via platelet aggregation and release of coagulation factors. Collagen's hemostatic capabilities are inactivated by autoclaving.

Bone wax is a nonabsorbable agent that is used during orthopedic (midfemoral amputation) and neurologic surgery to control bleeding from bone (Figure 23-39). Bone wax functions as a mechanical plug when pressed into bleeding bony surfaces. Keep in mind that it results in mild inflammation and should be used sparsely.

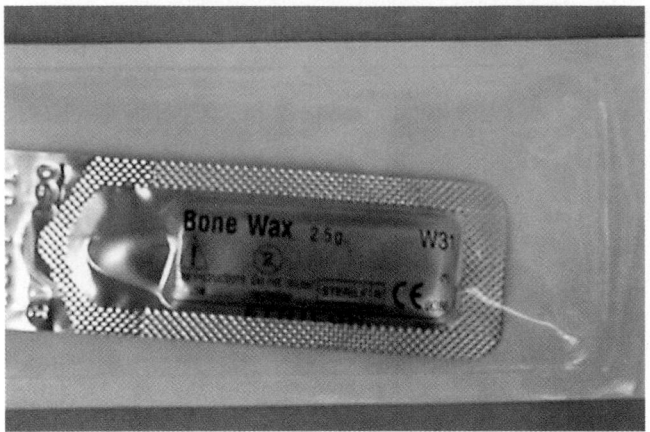

Figure 23-39 Bone wax is a nonabsorbable hemostatic agent used to control bleeding from exposed bone.

CHEMICAL CAUTERIZATION

Chemical cauterization by agents such as phenol, ferric subsulfate, and silver nitrate will achieve hemostasis by denaturing the proteins of the tissues they contact, thus sealing small blood vessels. However, these agents are difficult to apply without contacting and damaging adjacent soft tissues. This usually precludes their use in general surgery. However, silver nitrate is commonly used to stop nail bleeding when the nail bed has been cut during routing nail trimming.

VASCULAR CLIPS

Metal clips made of noncorrosive materials (Hemoclip, Weck Closure Systems) and the specialized forceps to apply them are available in a variety of sizes and designs (Figure 23-40). They are very effective and can be applied quickly to occlude vessels up to 5 mm in diameter in locations that are not accessible for ligation. Their use in veterinary surgery is becoming more widespread as their expense relative to convenience decreases. Vascular stapling devices that automatically occlude both sides of a vessel with small metallic staples, as well as divide it, are available (LDS, U.S. Surgical Corp.) and are commonly used in human surgery. Although the staple cartridges are expensive, the supplying company will often lease the application device.

INCISION IRRIGATION AND SUCTION

Incision irrigation and suction (lavage) serve four main purposes. The first is to physically dilute and remove bacteria carried into the incision from the skin or the air or from spillage from incising a contaminated or infected structure, such as the intestine. The body has a tremendous ability to resist infection from low numbers of bacteria. Consequently, lavaging the site after the initial skin incision,

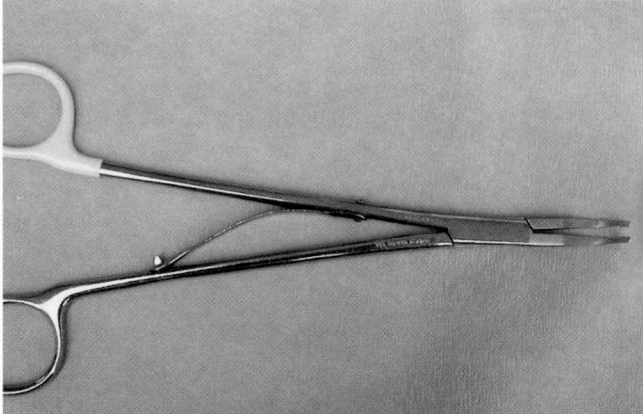

A

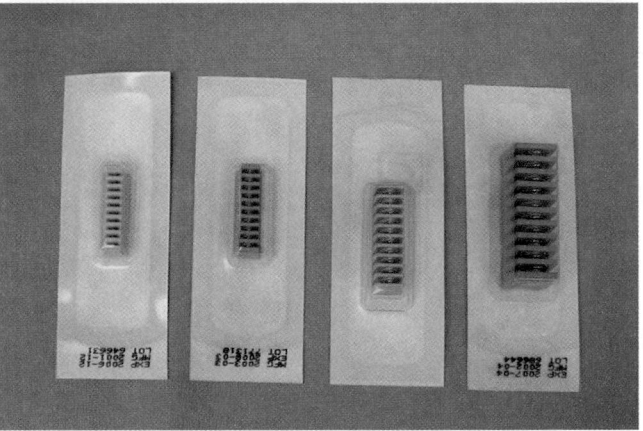

B

Figure 23-40 **A** and **B,** Metallic hemoclips with applicators are available in several sizes.

and periodically throughout the procedure to decrease bacterial numbers, will dramatically reduce the incidence of infection. Second, irrigation and suction are used to remove hemorrhage, increasing visibility at the surgical site. This makes both hemostasis and surgical manipulations easier to accomplish. Third, lavage keeps the tissues moist, particularly during longer procedures. If the tissues desiccate (dry out), cell damage and death occur. This decreases the rate of healing and increases the incidence of infection by devitalizing the natural cellular defense mechanisms. There is an old surgical saying that "moist tissues are happy tissues." Finally, lavage is used to dilute and remove irritating and degenerative material, such as urine, bile, or bony fragments. Although these materials will not cause infection, they can cause undesirable biologic reactions and should be removed.

LAVAGE FLUID

Many different fluids are used for lavage, but they all have common characteristics. The fluid should be a physiologically neutral, isotonic solution (i.e., buffered normal saline or lactated Ringer's solution), meaning it has the same pH (acidity) and osmolality (mineral concentration) as serum.

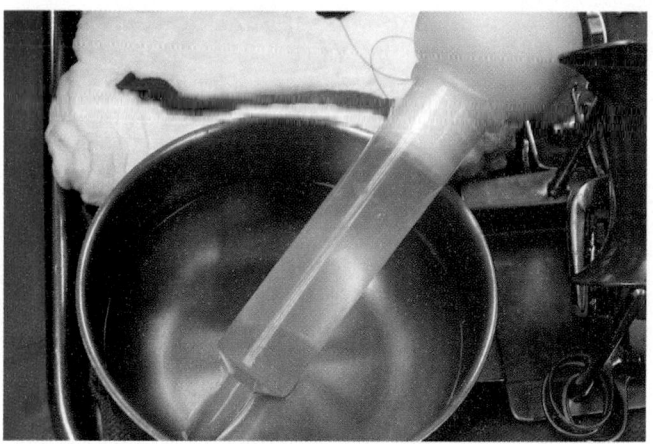

Figure 23-41 The saline bowl and bulb syringe are placed on a waterproof drape to avoid wick contamination after spillage.

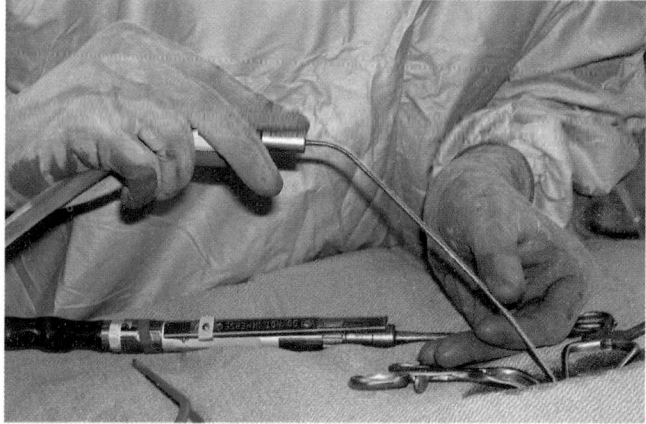

Figure 23-42 The single-orifice suction tip (Frazier) is used for precise control.

Excessively acid or basic fluids can promote bacterial growth and cause cell damage. Hypotonic (less concentrated) solutions, such as distilled or tap water, will be imbibed by the tissues, resulting in significant edema. Hypertonic (more concentrated) solutions, such as hypertonic saline will pull water out of tissues and result in dehydration. This reaction is occasionally used to reduce preexisting edema.

Antibiotic agents are rarely added to lavage solutions, as systemic administration of intravenous antibiotics in general provides higher antibiotic tissue levels than topical application. Antibiotic solutions (for example, tetracyclines) can be irritating to tissues when applied topically and result in chemical peritonitis or pleuritis. Antibiotic solutions should not be used with cancellous bone grafts, because the antibiotic will diminish the graft's biologic activity.

Diluted antiseptics like povidone-iodine and chlorhexidine hydrochloride have been used for lavage of wounds. Because these agents are irritating for synovium, pleura, and peritoneum, joints, thoracic cavity, and abdominal cavity are in general not lavaged with antiseptic solutions. The routine use of buffered normal saline is preferred.

LAVAGE TECHNIQUE

Irrigation solutions can be applied with a bulb syringe or a large syringe to obtain a hydraulic cleansing effect (Figure 23-41). They should be warmed to body temperature to avoid causing hypothermia. This is particularly important in very small or debilitated patients. Cloth drapes should not become excessively damp during surgery, since this will allow capillary movement of bacteria (wicking) from the underlying nonsterile area. Alternatively, waterproof draping materials, such as sterile baby crib sheets or diapers, may be used.

Suction of the surgical incision requires a suction tip, tubing, and a suction bottle. The suction tip may have a single orifice or multiple fenestrations. The single-orifice

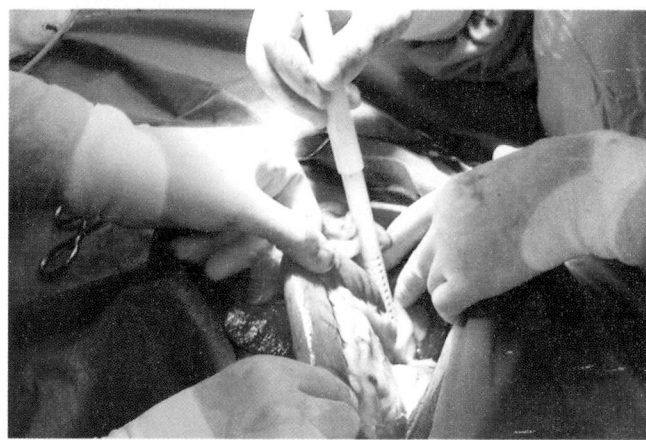

Figure 23-43 The multiple-fenestrated suction tip (Poole) is used to remove large volumes of fluids and to avoid omental occlusion.

tip (Yankauer or Frazier tip) is most useful in orthopedic surgery, neurosurgery, and general surgery in which the exposure is limited and relatively small amounts of liquid must be removed from very precise areas (Figure 23-42). The surgical assistant controls the strength of suction by occluding the vent hole in the handle of the suction tip. If the tip becomes plugged, it can be cleared by passing a stylet made of slightly smaller stainless steel wire.

The multiple-fenestrated tips (Poole tip) are used in thoracic and abdominal procedures in which large volumes of fluid are removed (Figure 23-43). Fenestrated tips also reduce the incidence of plugging with movable soft tissue, such as omentum and mesentery. The assistant can also use her or his hands as a barrier between the omentum and the suction tip to prevent plugging. Periodic suction of clean irrigation solution during the surgical procedure will reduce the incidence of suction tube plugging and make cleaning of the tube much easier.

SURGICAL DRAINS

Postoperative drainage of the surgical area may be indicated for several different reasons. Any incision that is thought to be infected should be allowed to discharge. This can be accomplished by leaving the wound open or by inserting a drain. A drain is also indicated when soft tissues cannot be opposed to obliterate dead space. Serum tends to accumulate in such spaces, and seromas (serum pockets under the skin) can develop if a drainage route is not established. Drains commonly used in veterinary surgery are classified as passive and active drain devices. The draining effect of passive systems is based on gravity, whereas active systems produce negative pressure (suction) resulting in drainage.

PASSIVE DRAINS

Soft, thin-walled, collapsible, latex rubber tubes named *Penrose drains* are most commonly utilized as passive drains in veterinary medicine. Passive drains made of stiffer polypropylene, Silastic, or red rubber tubes are rarely utilized. Discharge escapes by moving along the outside of the drain (Figure 23-44). Therefore the holes in the tissues through which the drain runs must be kept spread open and clean for the drain to work properly. Cleanliness is particularly important, because the hole and drain can act as an avenue for ascending infections.

ACTIVE DRAINS

Active (i.e., suction) drains are thick-walled tubes of rubber or Silastic. Suction is applied to the outside end of the drain, and discharges are pulled through the lumen of the tube. Multiple openings are present in the wall of the tube on the implanted end (Figure 23-45). Suction must be maintained

for this type of drain to work. Negative-pressure–activated devices are commercially available (Jackson Pratt, Allegiance) (Figure 23-46). A homemade device can be made from a large injection syringe, butterfly catheter, and a hypodermic needle (Figure 23-47).

Drains are foreign bodies and can be removed after 2 to 5 days when the discharge volume has decreased and becomes serosanguineous.

SUTURE MATERIAL

Suture is any material that holds tissues together until they heal. The use of suture has been documented since the first century AD. However, it was not until the advent of

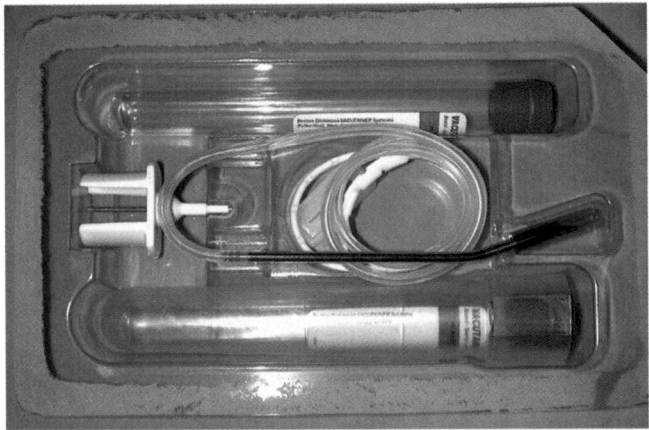

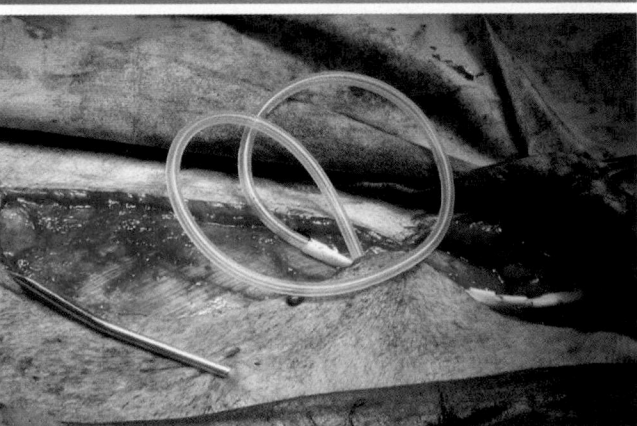

Figure 23-45 **A** and **B,** Multiple openings on the implanted end of a commercially available active suction drain (TLS) after mammary resection.

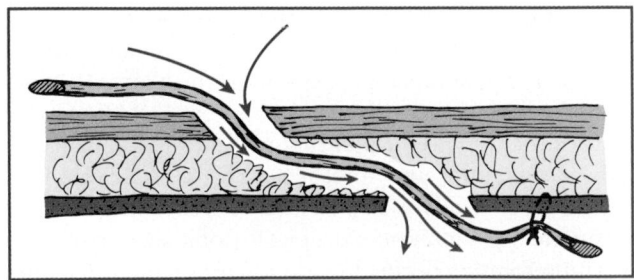

Figure 23-44 Diagram of discharge escaping around the outside of a Penrose drain.

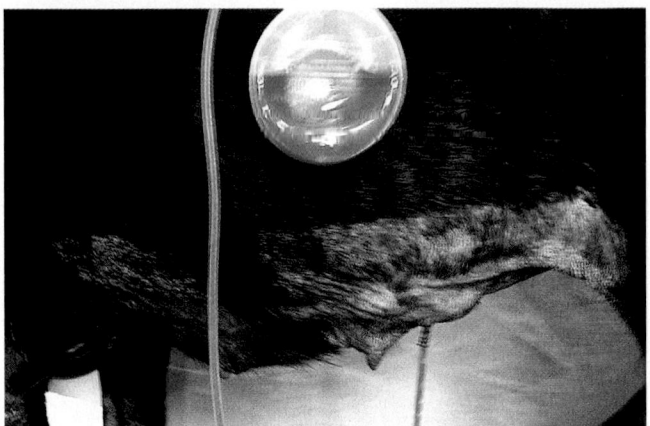

Figure 23-46 A commercially available negative-pressure-activated, constant-suction device (Jackson Pratt drain).

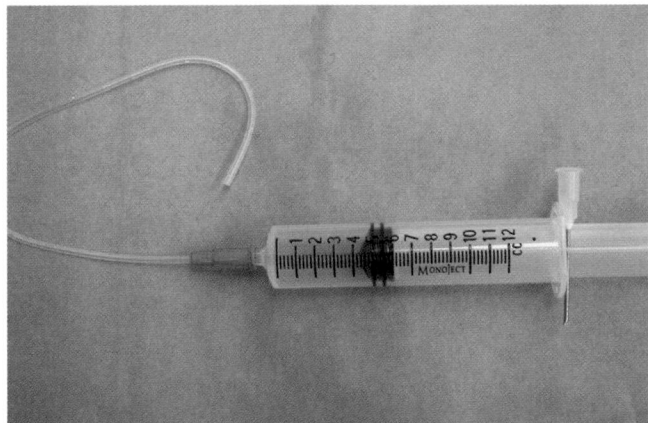

Figure 23-47 A homemade constant-suction device constructed from a large syringe, butterfly catheter, and hypodermic needle.

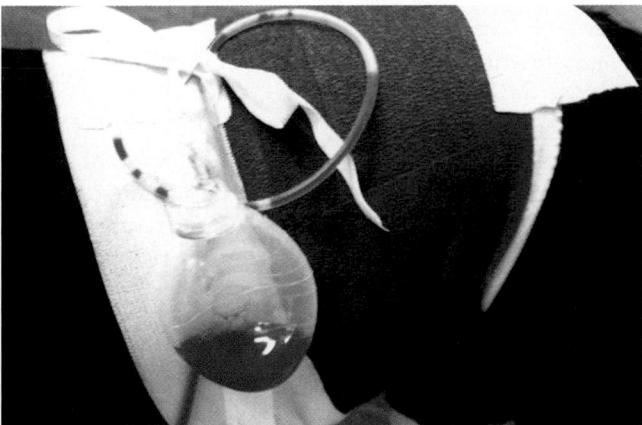

Figure 23-48 The exit point of the drain at the skin level should be always covered with a sterile dressing to minimize risk of infection along the drain. The dressing must be changed before strike-through occurs.

sterilization and aseptic technique that suture became commonly used. During the late 1800s and early 1900s, suture materials were derived mainly from natural sources. Synthetic suture materials first became available in the 1930s and are still being developed.

Some uses of suture include the following:

- Apposing the edges of an incision or wound
- Obliterating open space in which serum would tend to accumulate
- Tightening and stabilizing joints that have sustained ligament injury or have luxated
- Strengthening or replacing weakened tissues, as in hernias
- Ligating blood vessels or tissues that will be removed

QUALITIES OF THE IDEAL SUTURE MATERIAL

The ideal suture material would have the following qualities:

- Able to be used for any procedure with the same characteristics in all tissues.
- Is easily handled and tied by the surgeon.
- Causes minimal tissue reaction and does not support, spread, or sequester bacterial growth.
- Has high tensile strength in a small diameter, yet not cut through tissues.
- Knots securely with a minimum number of throws with small knot size.
- Is easy and economical to produce and sterilize.
- Does not induce allergic, electrolytic, or neoplastic changes.
- Holds tissues until healing occurs, then resorbs with minimum tissue reaction.

Obviously, no such suture material exists or probably ever will since several of these attributes are contradictory. Consequently, veterinary personnel must be aware of the advantages and disadvantages of all available sutures and choose the one most appropriate for the use at hand. The technician will need to become familiar with all sutures used by the surgeon.

SUTURE NOMENCLATURE

Suture material can be classified by a number of characteristics. Absorbable suture is broken down and resorbed by the body, resulting in a loss of tensile strength within 60 days. Consequently, it should be used in tissues that heal rapidly to adequate strength. Nonabsorbable suture does not significantly weaken with time. It is used in areas that heal slowly and are subject to disruptive stresses. Multifilament or braided suture material is made up of a number of very small elements that are braided or twisted together to form

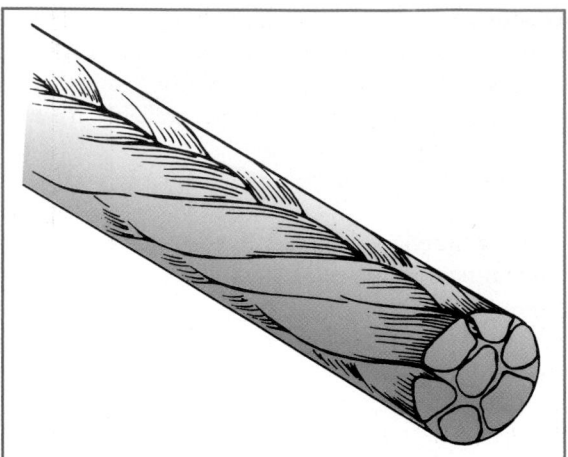

Figure 23-49 Constructed multifilament suture. (From Meeker MH, Rothrock JC: *Alexander's care of the patient in surgery,* ed 11, St Louis, 1999, Mosby.)

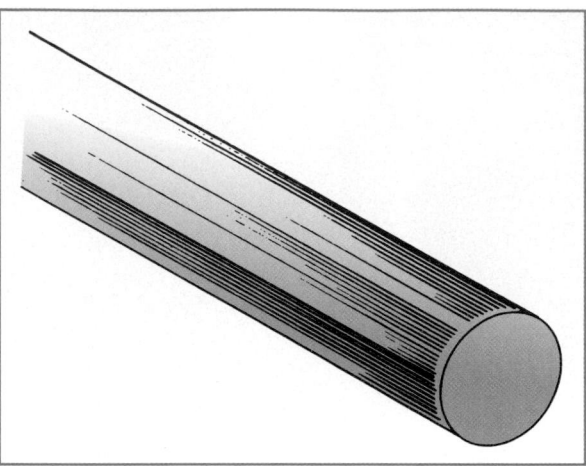

Figure 23-50 Monofilament suture. (From Meeker MH, Rothrock JC: *Alexander's care of the patient in surgery,* ed 11, St Louis, 1999, Mosby.)

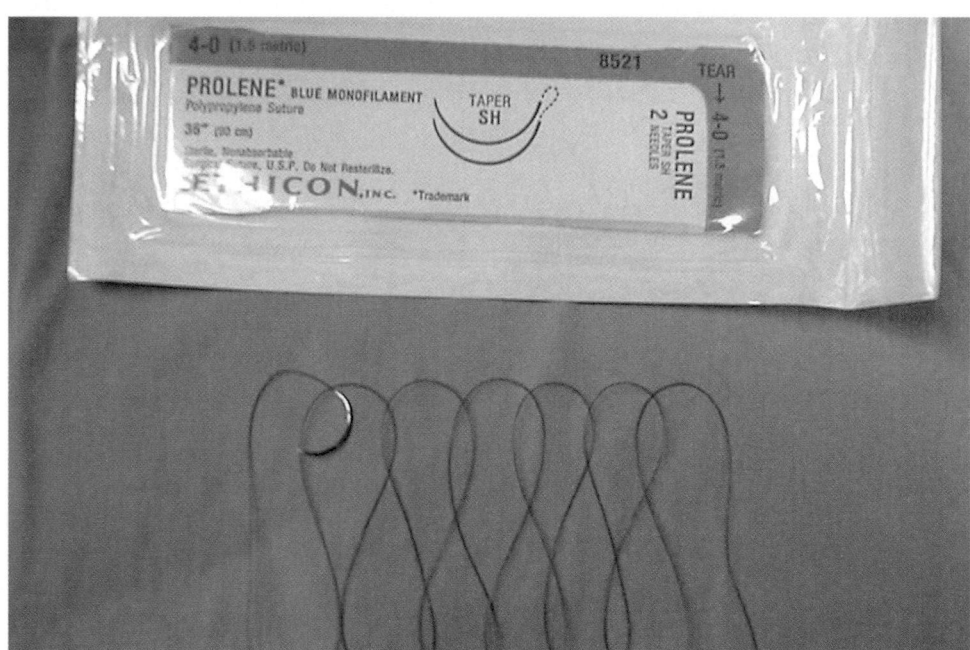

Figure 23-51 Memory is the tendency of suture to return to its package shape.

the desired diameter (Figure 23-49). Multifilament suture tends to be relatively strong, handles well, and has good knot-holding abilities. However, many braided sutures induce significant tissue reaction and can harbor bacteria, leading to intractable suture tract infections if they become contaminated. Moreover, most braided suture will exhibit capillary or "wicking" characteristics in which fluids travel along the length of the suture between the filaments. Therefore multifilament suture should not be used in hollow organs or in the skin when part of the suture is exposed to a contaminated environment and the wicking fluid can carry bacteria into the body. Monofilament suture (Figure 23-50) avoids the capillary problem and consequently has a lower

incidence of infection. It also has a low coefficient of surface friction, making it easy to generally pull through tissues. However, the low surface friction ("drag") results in poor knot security, necessitating many throws on each knot. Some monofilament suture also has a tendency to return to its original shape (called *memory*), resulting in poor handling characteristics (Figure 23-51).

> **✎ TECHNICIAN NOTE**
>
> Suture material can be classified as absorbable or nonabsorbable and monofilament or multifilament.

ABSORBABLE SUTURE MATERIAL

Surgical gut is collagenous protein obtained from the sub mucosal layer of sheep small intestine. It was originally known as *kit gut* (meaning fiddle string, because the material was used for stringed instruments). Over the years, the term *kit* was mistakenly changed to *cat*, resulting in the common misnomer *catgut*. When implanted in tissues, surgical gut incites an inflammatory reaction that ultimately resorbs the suture by phagocytosis. The severity of reaction, and consequently the rate at which the gut loses strength, can be decreased by tanning the material with chromic salts. Surgical gut has been classified into four groups: plain, mild, medium, and extra chromic, treated with resorption times of 10, 20, 30, and 40 days, respectively. Because surgical gut is broken down by phagocytosis, implantation in inflamed, highly vascular, or biologically active tissue will result in a faster rate of resorption. Medium chromic gut is relatively inexpensive and has predictable handling and knotting characteristics. However, its variability in rate of tensile strength loss, particularly in response to an inflammatory environment, should be considered and has led most surgeons away from its use for closure of support layers.

Other natural absorbable suture materials, such as collagen, kangaroo tendon, and fascia lata, have been developed but have shown few distinct advantages over surgical gut.

SYNTHETIC ABSORBABLE SUTURE MATERIAL

Synthetic absorbable sutures are in general broken down by hydrolysis and have been developed to avoid the variation of resorptive rates in inflammatory environments. Synthetic absorbable sutures can be principally subdivided in sutures retaining strength for more than 21 days (Dexon, Vicryl, Maxon, PDS and Polysorb) and sutures retaining strength for less than 21 days (Monocryl, Biosyn).

Polyglycolic acid (Dexon, Kendall) is a synthetic polyester polymerized from hydroxyacetic acid. It is produced in fine filaments that are braided into sutures of various sizes. Consequently, it has excellent handling and knot-holding characteristics. Dexon is broken down in the body by enzymatic hydrolysis, which does *not* induce a significant inflammatory reaction. Further, the rate of absorption is not affected by placement in an inflamed or infected environment. Dexon loses about 35% of its tensile strength in 14 days and 65% of its strength within 21 days. Some studies have shown that Dexon absorbs more rapidly in the presence of urine. Overall, it has a superior initial strength, but it loses its strength more rapidly than surgical gut.

Polyglactin 910 (Vicryl, Ethicon) is a coated multifilament suture consisting of a copolymer of lactic and glycolic acids. Its production and resorption processes are similar to those of Dexon. Vicryl also has a high initial strength that declines rapidly when implanted. Likewise, it has good handling qualities and knot security.

Polydioxanone (PDS, Ethicon) and polyglyconate (Maxon, Kendall) are newer synthetic polyester materials that are pliable enough to be produced and used in monofilament form. Consequently, they have significantly less tissue drag in placement. However, they do possess some memory characteristics and must have multiple throws to gain knot securely. The process of resorption is similar to that of the other synthetic absorbable materials. PDS retains 86% strength at 14 days and 69% strength at 42 days. Maxon retains 70% strength at 14 days and 45% at 21 days. Consequently, they are particularly useful in slow-healing tissues. Despite their absorbable classification, it takes about 180 days until PDS and Maxon are completely absorbed.

Polysorb (Kendall) is a multifilament glycoside/lactide copolymer with good knot-tying capabilities. Polysorb retains 80% strength at 14 days and 30% strength at 42 days. Although entirely absorbed at day 70, its bacterial wicking potential due to the braided characteristics should be considered.

Poliglecaprone (Monocryl, Ethicon) and Glycomer 631 (Biosyn, Kendall) are more rapidly absorbed monofilament sutures that can be used in situations where healing occurs more quickly. Their predictability has led to their replacing gut for many applications. Monocryl is not as strong as and Biosyn is as strong as PDS and Maxon.

Monocryl absorbs at a rate similar to medium chromic gut. Monocryl retains 60% to 70% strength at 7 days, 30% to 40% strength at 14 days, and 0% at day 21. The suture is absorbed between day 90 and 120. Biosyn consists of 60% glycoside, 26% trimethylene carbonate, and 14% dioxanone. Biosyn retains 75% strength at 14 days, 40% to 50% strength at 21 days, and 25% at 28 days. The suture is absorbed between day 90 and 120.

Vicryl and Dexon are more rapidly degraded in alkaline environment and dissolve faster in infected urine. Therefore PDS and Maxon have been recommended for closure of the bladder, as these sutures retain their strength in urine.

✏ TECHNICIAN NOTE

Absorbable sutures retain their tensile strength in tissues for several weeks, whereas nonabsorbable sutures last 60 days or more.

NONABSORBABLE SUTURE MATERIAL

Nonabsorbable suture retains its tensile strength for more than 60 days. It can be organic fiber, metallic, or synthetic and will be described according to origin.

Silk is one of the first and still most commonly used organic nonabsorbable materials. It is obtained from the cocoon of the silkworm and is braided or twisted into multifilament strands. It has excellent handling and knotting qualities and is commonly used in cardiovascular surgery. However, it can induce a severe soft-tissue reaction, allow capillary migration of contamination (wicking), and serve as a nidus for infection. Despite its nonabsorbable classification, the inflammatory reaction usually results in complete loss of tensile strength within 6 months.

Cotton and linen are natural fibers that are also used to make suture. They both increase slightly in strength when wet but otherwise behave very much like silk. They have seen limited use in veterinary surgery.

Metallic sutures have been used since the fourteenth century, when the biologically nonreactive nature of gold was first described. Stainless steel is the major metallic suture in use today. It is biologically inert and will not support bacterial growth. Also, steel retains its high tensile strength when implanted. Consequently, it is particularly useful in infected wounds or tissues that are expected to be stressed while healing slowly. Stainless steel suture is available in monofilament and multifilament forms. The major disadvantage of steel is its poor handling quality and its tendency to kink. Silver, aluminum, and tantalum sutures have some limited use in human surgery.

SYNTHETIC NONABSORBABLE SUTURE MATERIAL

Polyamide (Nylon, Ethicon) is a polymerized plastic that is available as suture in both monofilament and braided forms. It does not cause tissue reaction when implanted, but it gradually loses its tensile strength over several years. It is somewhat stiff and slippery, and it has significant memory, making handling and knot security exacting. Monofilament nylon is typically used for skin sutures that are removed.

Polypropylene (Prolene, Ethicon; Surgipro, Kendall) is a synthetic plastic that is similar to nylon. However, polypropylene does not weaken with time, making it useful when permanent suture support is needed.

Polybutester (Novafil, Kendall) is a similar synthetic suture that is much more elastic. This means it can stretch and return to its original length without breaking, making it useful for repairing ligaments and other structures that must stretch under weighted motion.

Polyester fibers (Mersiline, Ethicon; Ti-cron, Kendall) are braided to form a strong noncapillary suture. Handling quality is good, but five or six throws are required for good knot security. It also has significant tissue drag and induces just slightly less tissue reaction than silk. Some manufacturers coat the polyester fibers with Teflon (Tevdek and Polydek, Deknatel) or silicone (Ti-cron, Kendall) to reduce drag and reaction. However, chronic infection and draining fistulae remain common complications of polyester use.

Polymerized caprolactum (Supramid, S. Jackson; Braunamid, Vetcassette II, B. Braun Melsungen AG) is made of synthetic fibers coated with a smooth plasticlike material. It has high tensile strength and does not induce a significant tissue reaction. As the outer sheath of these sutures often breaks, the underlying multifilament fibers allow bacterial migration. Therefore these sutures should not be used below the skin level, as they predispose to fistulation and infection.

Table 23-1 Limits on Suture Diameter

| Size | Millimeters | | Limits on Knot-Pull Tensile Strength | |
	Minimum	Maximum	kg	lb
7-0	0.025	0.064	0.06	0.125
6-0	0.064	0.113	0.16	0.35
5-0	0.113	0.179	0.32	0.7
4-0	0.179	0.241	0.68	1.5
3-0	0.241	0.318	1.13	2.5
2-0	0.318	0.406	1.18	4.0
1-0	0.406	0.495	2.50	5.5
1	0.495	0.584	3.40	7.5
2	0.584	0.673	4.80	9.0
3	0.673	0.762	5.22	11.5

From US Pharmacopeial Convention: United States pharmacopeia, ed 16, Rockville, Md, 1960, The Convention.

SUTURE SIZE AND STRENGTH

✎ TECHNICIAN NOTE
Oversized sutures do not strengthen a wound and may lead to overtightening and strangulation of tissues.

The size or diameter of suture has been classified by the U.S. Pharmacopeia. Table 23-1 lists the established limits of surgical gut from 7-0 (pronounced "seven ott" or "seven zero") to no. 3. Other suture materials use the same sizing limits and have extended down to an 11-0 nylon for microvascular anastomosis and up to no. 7 stainless steel for orthopedic use. The appropriate-sized suture for each procedure needs to be no stronger than the tissue on which it is used. Oversized sutures do not strengthen a wound and may lead to overtightening and strangulation of tissues. In addition to suture tensile strength, knot security should be considered when selecting suture size. Because the knot is the strength-limiting area of most suture and the relative knot security decreases as suture size increases, smaller suture offers a mechanical advantage. This is particularly true of the synthetic monofilament sutures, which have a low coefficient of friction (slippery). Besides untying, knotting decreases a suture's strength by converting the longitudinal tensile force into a shearing force that collects at the base of the knot, at which point strands cross and angle. The process of tying the knot also weakens suture by abrading its surface as strands cross. This is particularly true of surgical gut sutures and braided sutures. Excessive suture material should be cut off, leaving the ends just long enough to secure the knot on buried sutures. Of course, this length varies with surface friction and knot security. In general, multifilament and metallic sutures can be cut off quite close to the knot (about 2 mm). Monofilament sutures

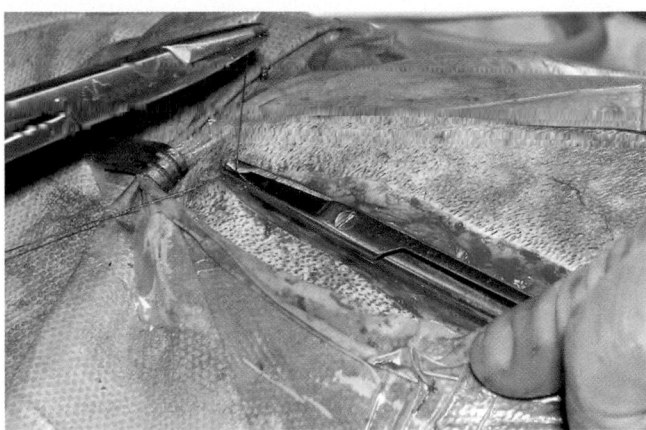

Figure 23-52 Monofilament sutures with memory and polyester sutures need to have 3 to 4 mm left to prevent knot untying.

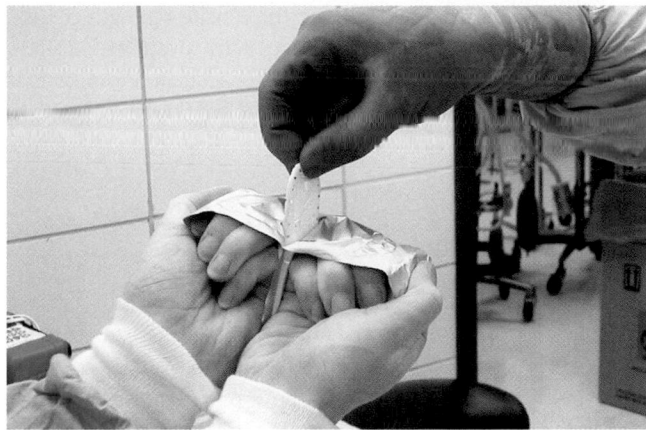

Figure 23-53 Peeling back the outer covering of a prepackaged suture material.

with memory and polyesters need to have 3 to 4 mm left to prevent knot untying (Figure 23-52). Skin sutures usually have about 0.5- to 1.0-cm tails to aid in easy removal.

SUTURE REACTION

As previously noted, some suture materials induce more tissue reaction than others. In descending order of reactiveness, surgical gut is most reactive, followed by multifilament natural fiber, synthetic multifilament suture, synthetic monofilament suture, and finally metallic suture. Recognizing a suture's reactivity becomes particularly important when suture reaction might affect function of the tissue, as in neurosurgery or cardiovascular surgery.

Tissue reaction also impedes healing of normal tissue. The presence of infection or contamination has a much greater effect on the more reactive sutures. For example, the inflammatory process associated with infection will often phagocytose surgical gut at an increased rate, leading to resorption before healing and wound dehiscence. Likewise, the presence of silk has been shown to increase the incidence of infection 10,000-fold in contaminated incisions. Finally, nonabsorbable suture, such as silk or polyester, may cause ulceration of the gastrointestinal tract or serve as the nidus for stone formation in the urinary bladder or gallbladder if it penetrates the lumen of those hollow organs.

PREPARATION OF SUTURE MATERIAL

Several methods are used by suture producers to sterilize various suture materials. Many prepackaged sutures are sterilized by gamma irradiation. Ethylene oxide is used on those products that will not tolerate irradiation. Prepackaged suture material has a sterile shelf life that varies as denoted by the expiration date printed on the package. Consequently, expiration dates should be periodically checked and stock rotated when new supplies arrive. Steam sterilization (autoclaving) can be used on some materials, with variable damaging effects. The following describes the effects of autoclaving:

I. Severe damage, destroys tensile strength.
   A. Surgical gut
   B. Polyglycolic acid (PDS)
   C. Polyglactin (Vicryl)
II. Mild damage, reduces tensile strength.
   A. Silk
   B. Linen
   C. Cotton
III. Tolerates at least three autoclavings without loss of tensile strength.
   A. Polyester
   B. Nylon
   C. Polypropylene
   D. Metallics

Sutures that can be steam sterilized are sometimes bought in bulk and are sterilized in the practice. When preparing such suture, an appropriate number of strand lengths (usually 30 to 60 cm) should be cut and coiled or loosely wound around a card or sponge. This will avoid repeated autoclaving, which will damage even the most steam-tolerant material.

Prepackaged suture material is opened (by a nonsterile assistant) onto the instrument tray by peeling back the outer packaging (Figure 23-53). The surgical assistant opens the inner pack by tearing off one end and grasping the suture end or swaged needle with needle holders as directed on the package. Before use, the suture should be stretched slightly to overcome memory but not snapped because this commonly leads to contamination of the suture end. Any excessive preserving fluid should be wiped off. The tissue drag of many sutures (particularly the synthetic multifilaments) can be reduced by moistening with sterile saline. However, this will reduce the tensile strength of silk, and surgical gut will imbibe water to swell and soften. Multifilament suture strands tend to accumulate blood as they pass through tissue and should be wiped off with a moistened sponge between use.

SUTURE NEEDLES

Suture needles vary considerably in shape, point design, method of attachment to the suture (eye), and size. The size and shape of the needle are determined by the thickness of tissue being sutured and the depth of the incision (Figure 23-54, *A*). Straight needles are usually used superficially in very accessible locations where the needle can be manipulated with the fingers. Curved needle types are manipulated with needle holders. One-fourth ($^1/_4$) circle needle are commonly utilized in ophthalmologic surgery, whereas three-eighth ($^3/_8$) and one-half ($^1/_2$) circle needles are most popular in general surgery.

The point design varies with the toughness of tissue being sutured (Figure 23-54, *B*). Skin, eye tissues, and some tough facial tissues are sutured with a cutting-edged needle. Cutting needles have two or three opposing cutting surfaces. Regular cutting needles have a third cutting surface on

the inside curvature resulting in a "cut-out" effect. Reverse cutting needles have the third cutting surface on the outside curvature resulting in a more robust design with less cut-out effect. Reverse-cutting needles (K needles) are therefore preferred by some surgeons, as they do not bend or break as easily. The cut-out effect makes passage of the needle and suture easier, but a true incision that can leak is created. Therefore cutting-edged needles should not be used when an air-tight or watertight suture line is required. Taper needles do not actually cut tissue but spread it open around the needle and following suture. This spreading effect avoids hemorrhage and results in a sealed suture line. Taper needles and reverse-cutting needles are used in suturing most hollow organs.

The needle can be attached to the suture by three different methods (Figure 23-54, *C*). Single-eyed needles have one hole in the head of the needle. The eye should be single threaded, since double threading leaves a large bulk of suture around the shank, which will cause excessive tissue drag and damage as the needle is passed. A curved needle is threaded from within the curve so that the short end of the suture falls away from the outside curve. About 10 cm of suture should be pulled through the eye. These steps will help to prevent the suture from pulling out of the eye during suturing. Spring or French-eyed needles have a complete eye and

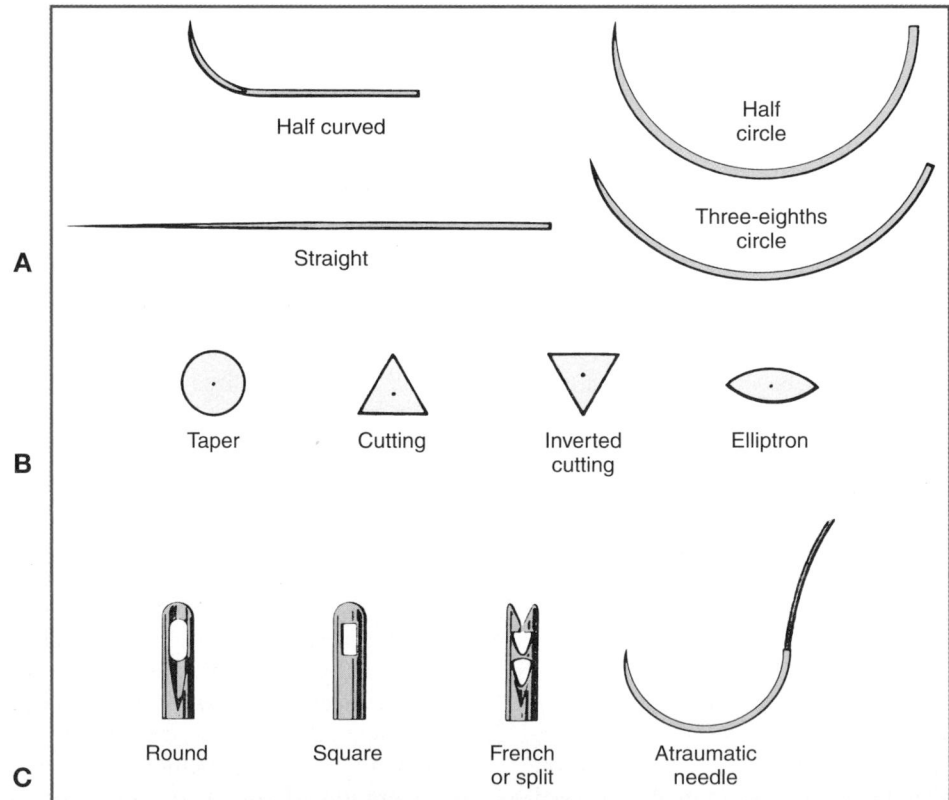

Figure 23-54 **A,** The size and shape of the needle are chosen according to the thickness of the tissue. **B,** The needle point design is determined according to the toughness of the tissue on which it is used. **C,** The needle is attached to the suture either by threading through an eye or by being swaged. (Courtesy Sherwood Davis & Geck, Milford, N.J.)

an incomplete "spring" eye. Suture is threaded through the complete eye and is then forced back through the spring eye, which grips the suture end.

Eyeless or swaged needles are attached directly to the end of the suture by the factory. The surgeon draws a single strand through the tissue and automatically uses a new sharp needle with every strand. Therefore swaged needles are the most atraumatic and most popular surgical needles in veterinary practice.

TECHNICIAN NOTE

Cutting-edged needles should not be used when an airtight or watertight suture line is required (lung, urinary bladder, intestine, etc.).

ACKNOWLEDGMENT

The author also wishes to acknowledge the work of Erick L. Egger in editions one through five of this book.

Recommended Reading

Evans HE, Christenson GC: *Miller's anatomy of the dog,* ed 3, Philadelphia, 1993, WB Saunders.

Slatter D: *Textbook of small animal surgery,* ed 3, Philadelphia, 2002, WB Saunders.

24

Small Animal Surgical Nursing

Loretta J. Bubenik

INTRODUCTION AND GENERAL PRINCIPLES

The veterinary technician's role in surgical assistance is an important part of hospital and patient management. Preoperative, intraoperative, and postoperative responsibilities should be considered for a successful outcome. The surgical patient must undergo preoperative assessment including examination and laboratory evaluation. In addition, the patient must undergo the appropriate restraint and preparation for surgery. Surgical assistance during the procedure includes patient monitoring and surgeon assistance. In the postoperative period patient monitoring and assistance are still very important for the patient well-being. Duties of the veterinary technician include appropriate animal restraint; appropriate sample collection and diagnostic evaluation; administration of sedation, anesthesia, and pain medication; appropriate patient preparation and positioning for surgery; aseptic patient and instrument handling; patient monitoring; direct surgical assistance; instrument preparation; and operating room preparation. Patient restraint, anesthesia, pain management, aseptic technique, and instrumentation are discussed in Chapters 1, 19, 20, and 22. This chapter will focus on familiarizing the technician with specific surgical procedures and highlighting technician responsibilities in the pre-, intra-, and postoperative period.

Many operative procedures require the assistance of a veterinary technician. A working knowledge of common surgical procedures will help make the veterinary technician proficient at surgical assistance. Procedures that often require such assistance include orthopedic surgery (retraction, reduction, traction, countertraction), open chest procedures (artificial ventilation, retraction), and complicated abdominal procedures (diaphragmatic hernia repair, renal surgery, tumor resection). An understanding of aseptic technique, a familiarity with surgical instrumentation, and a working knowledge of the specific surgical procedure are prerequisites for proper intraoperative assistance. Surgical assistance is discussed in Chapter 23.

Small animal surgical nursing includes many aspects of the primary care of the veterinary surgical patient. This chapter deals primarily with the postoperative care and evaluation of patients by the veterinary technician. In addition, the more commonly performed small animal surgical procedures are discussed, with emphasis on the role of the veterinary technician. ■

PREOPERATIVE PATIENT ASSESSMENT

The veterinary surgical patient should undergo a complete preoperative assessment. It is important to know what the primary problem is so that specific needs can be anticipated. Elective surgical procedures will not require the same demands that emergency or urgent surgical procedures will. Eating, drinking, urination, and defecation habits of the animal should be ascertained by the owner. An animal that has not been eating or drinking will likely require rehydration before anesthesia and surgery. Rehydration may then necessitate a blood or plasma transfusion in some animals since dilution of the cell volume occurs with rehydration. Fluids should not be withheld to prevent anemia. If the animal has eaten the day of scheduled surgery, then the procedure will have to be delayed to decrease the risk of aspiration (inhalation of stomach contents into the trachea and lungs). The animal should not have food for at least 12 hours prior to anesthesia, water is OK. Emergency surgeries will have to be performed whether the animal has eaten or not, but owners should be warned of the increased risk of aspiration. Temperature, pulse rate/quality, respiration rate/character, capillary refill time, mucous membrane color, body weight, and demeanor should be assessed prior to surgery. Abnormalities should be brought to the attention of the surgeon

Preanesthetic screening will depend on the animal condition and reason for surgery. Specifics of this are covered in Chapter 19. From a nursing standpoint, it is important to discuss with the surgeon what diagnostics are appropriate prior to surgery and ensure that they are performed in a timely manner. Diagnostics might include blood work such as packed cell volume, total plasma protein concentration, blood urea nitrogen concentration, blood glucose concentration, complete blood count, complete biochemical analysis, and heartworm test; blood gas analysis; electrocardiogram; radiographs; fine-needle mass aspiration; fecal analysis; and/or urinalysis. Abnormalities detected on the preanesthetic screen should be brought to the attention of the surgeon.

SURGICAL PREPARATION AND ANIMAL POSITIONING

It is the veterinary technician's responsibility to inquire about the surgical procedure to be performed and what instrumentation will be required. The technician should have all the necessary equipment readily accessible and prepared for use. The operating room should be clean and anesthesia equipment checked and ready for use. A circulating heated water blanket should be placed on the operating table, turned on, and covered with a towel so that it is warm by the time the patient is positioned on the table. A heated water blanket should also be set up in the recovery cage (or the warmed blanket from the operating table can be placed in the cage with the animal). Hair clippers and skin cleansing solutions should be made available for use as well.

Inadequate patient preparation or inappropriate positioning can hinder surgical technique and/or result in wasted time spent correcting deficiencies. Aseptic protocol should always be followed with patient preparation, patient draping, and surgical instrument handling. The hair should be liberally clipped around the surgical site and the skin cleansed appropriately (Chapters 22 and 23). The veterinary technician should be familiar with the type of surgery being performed so that animal preparation is consistent and adequate.

PERIOPERATIVE ANTIBIOTICS

Prophylactic antibiotics are used to decrease the rate of infection in clean or clean-contaminated surgeries. Using antibiotics to treat active infection is an entirely different scenario. Antimicrobial prophylaxis will not entirely eliminate infections associated with a surgical procedure.

Antibiotics should never be given indiscriminately to animals undergoing surgery. All antibiotics have potential side effects, and there use also increases surgery cost. More importantly, indiscriminant use of antibiotics contributes to the development of resistant strains of bacteria (hospital "superbugs") that are very difficult to treat.

✎ TECHNICIAN NOTE

Antibiotics should never be given indiscriminately to animals undergoing surgery since this contributes to the development of resistant strains of bacteria (hospital "superbugs") that are very difficult to treat.

INDICATIONS FOR PROPHYLACTIC ANTIBIOTICS

- Operative time is over 90 minutes. Open surgical wounds are constantly being exposed to bacteria from the animal's skin, the operative team, and the air. The longer the wound is open, the higher the chance of infection. Prolonged anesthesia also increases the risk.
- The patient is at increased risk of infection. Things that might increase the risk of infection include immunosuppressive drugs (steroids), Cushing disease, some cancers, chemotherapy or radiation therapy, FeLV/FIV positive, or any other immunosuppressive factor.
- A hollow viscus is to be entered [i.e., gastrointestinal (GI) tract, urinary bladder]
- The incision is to involve an area that is difficult to aseptically prepare (such as a toe or ear).
- Orthopedic implants are being placed.
- Joint procedures are long and aggressive, or certain joint procedures require multiple entrances into the joint (arthroscopy).
- Consequences of infection could be devastating, such as total hip replacement or spinal fracture.
- Prophylactic antibiotics are not recommended for short, clean surgical procedures like simple mass removal, osteochondritis cartilage flap removal, ovariohysterectomy, castration, and simple biopsy.

Therapeutic drug levels must be present in the wound fluid (serum) at the time of surgical incision or the antibiotics will not be effective. They should be given at least 20 minutes before the surgical incision is made. Antibiotics given 3 or more hours prior to the procedure select for resistant bacteria. Therapy delayed more than 3 to 5 hours after contamination is infective. There is no advantage to continuing antibiotics beyond 6 to 24 hours after surgery unless treating an active infection or a break in sterile technique occurred during surgery. The appropriate antibiotic should be broad spectrum, achieve good tissue concentrations, and have minimal side effects. The veterinarian in charge should be questioned as to what antibiotic is appropriate for what surgical procedure and when antibiotic prophylaxis is needed. If a break in sterile technique occurred, the animal has an active infection, or the risk of infection is still a major postoperative concern, then antibiotics are continued in the postoperative period according to the manufacturer's dosing recommendations and under the supervision of the veterinarian in charge.

MONITORING

Intra- and postoperative monitoring are critical to proper surgical nursing care. Chapter 19 covers anesthetic monitoring in detail, and the reader should refer to that chapter for further information. Some important components of patient monitoring as they pertain to surgery and recovery after surgery will be covered here.

The postoperative phase is a critical transition period from general anesthesia to consciousness and continual monitoring should be provided until the animal is safely extubated, normothermic, and in sternal recumbency. Surgical manipulation can result in several potential problems including blood loss, hypothermia, pain, and cardiac and respiratory problems. The veterinary surgical technician must be prepared to deal with changes in animal status and address issues as the need arises. During surgery, a surgical plane of anesthesia is crucial to appropriate surgical technique and animal well-being, and careful monitoring in the perioperative period might alert the observer to potential fatal complications.

> ### ✐ TECHNICIAN NOTE
> One abnormal sign at one given time is not enough to diagnose a significant problem. All indicators (temperature, pulse, respiration, mucous membranes) should be evaluated serially to determine a trend in the patient's condition. It is this trend that will determine the severity of the postoperative problem and dictate the appropriate treatment.

Patient monitoring does not stop once the animal is recovered from anesthesia. As long as the animal is hospitalized, vital signs, behavior, appetite, and the surgical incision should be evaluated. Depending on animal status, daily or more frequent observation of these parameters is performed. Abnormalities should be reported to the veterinarian in charge.

BLOOD LOSS

Many procedures can result in substantial blood loss as a complication, or blood loss could be due to the inherent nature of the procedure. A packed red blood cell volume (PCV) and total plasma protein concentration (TP) should always be assessed prior to surgery to obtain a baseline value. Preoperative anemia should be brought to the attention of the veterinarian in charge. If substantial blood loss occurred during surgery, another PCV/TP should be assessed postoperatively. It can be very difficult to determine if an animal

is hemorrhaging or has lost a substantial amount of blood immediately postoperative since a painful, recovering animal can have very similar clinical signs. Temperature, heart rate, pulse quality, respiration, and character of mucous membranes should be examined periodically during and after surgery. Animals with substantial blood loss may experience continued hypothermia or a drop in body temperature, rapid heart rate with weak peripheral pulses, rapid respiratory rate, and pale/white mucous membranes. Abnormalities should be promptly reported to the veterinarian in charge. Other signs include abdominal enlargement if intra-abdominal hemorrhage occurs, incision swelling or oozing of blood and dyspnea and decreased ventral lung sounds if intrathoracic hemorrhage occurs.

Besides PCV and TP determination, abdominocentesis (aspiration of fluid from the abdomen), thoracocentesis (aspiration of fluid from the thoracic cavity), or fine-needle aspiration beneath the incision can be performed when the patient is suspected of having substantial bleeding. It must be kept in mind that PCV and TP may not drop immediately in the hemorrhaging patient and that volume equilibration must occur before the drop is seen. However, if the sampled fluid has a PCV nearly equal to the systemic PCV and clinical signs are consistent, substantial hemorrhage should be suspected. Treatment strategies include crystalloid fluid bolus, colloidal fluid administration, blood transfusion, oxygen carrier fluid administration (Oxyglobin), pressure bandages, and/or reoperation with ligation of bleeding vessels. The treatment of choice depends on the animal's status and ability to maintain stability. The reader should review the clinical signs and treatment strategies for various types of shock as discussed in Chapter 26.

HYPOTHERMIA

Hypothermia is defined as a subnormal body temperature. Once an animal is anesthetized, its body temperature begins to drop. It is very important to monitor body temperature throughout general anesthesia and during recovery. All surgical patients should be placed on a heated, circulating water blanket covered with a towel to help maintain body temperature, especially small dogs and all cats. Although rare, if the body temperature rises above normal during the procedure, the heat source can be turned off. Small animals become hypothermic quickly when placed under general anesthesia, especially if a body cavity is opened. It is important to remember that the more surface area exposed (i.e., large incision exposing the abdominal organs), the faster and lower the body temperature is expected to drop. If the exposed area is moist, then evaporative cooling occurs as well. Mechanisms to maintain body temperature include placing animals on heated, circulating water blankets; wrapping paws and the body in plastic wrap to prevent heat loss (Figure 24-1); wrapping warm water bottles (or gloves filled with warm water) with towels and placing them next to the animal; covering areas not involved in the surgical

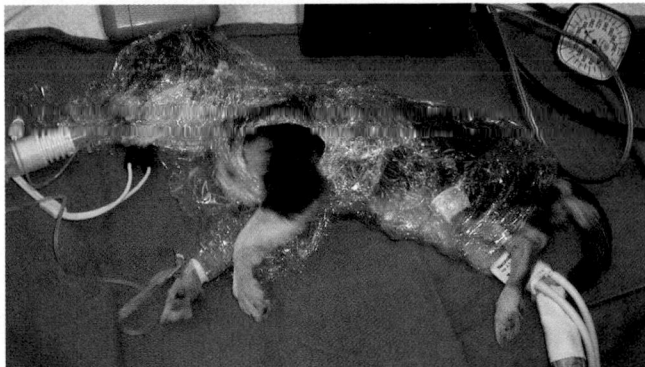

Figure 24-1 One method of heat retention during surgery is to wrap the animal in plastic. This works very well for small dogs and cats.

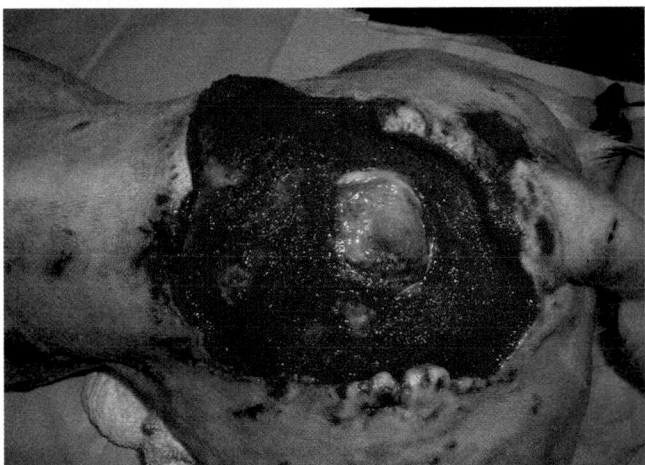

Figure 24-2 The area of denuded skin over the rump of this dog is a result of a thermal burn sustained from an electric heating pad used to maintain body temperature during ovariohysterectomy.

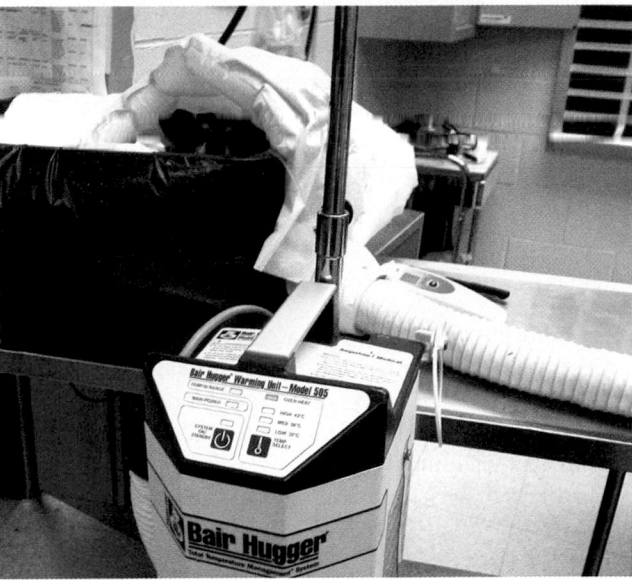

Figure 24-3 Blankets that blow warm air and warm water baths can be used to bring the body temperature up quickly. Notice the dog placed under the blue hot air blanket in a well constructed water bath.

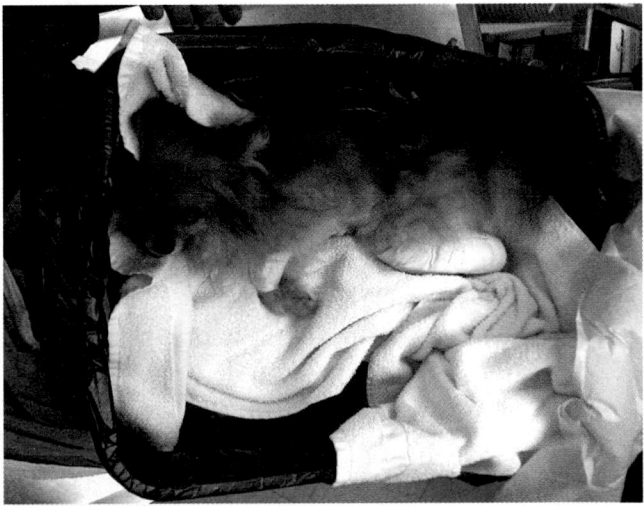

Figure 24-4 This is a close-up of a water bath. A large container is filled with warm water and covered with thick plastic and a towel. The dog or cat is placed on the towel in the container and is allowed to sink down into the warm water with the plastic preventing soaking. The animal must be monitored carefully to prevent accidental puncture of the plastic and drowning.

procedure with insulated blankets; and using a Bair Hugger (Arizant Healthcare, Inc.) (warm air blanket) on areas not involved in the surgical procedure. Heat lamps are not recommended as they can cause thermal burns, especially in an anesthetized patient that cannot respond to painful, concentrated heat. Also, it must be remembered that electric heating pads should never be used to warm anesthetized animals. Electric heating pads concentrate heat and cause thermal burns (Figure 24-2). The veterinarian is liable for burns caused by electrical heat units as it is a known cause of thermal skin injury during anesthesia.

After surgery, the patient is placed in a warm area to recover with a heated circulating water blanket. If the patient is severely hypothermic, a Bair Hugger and/or warm water bath can be used to raise the temperature quickly (Figure 24-3). A warm water bath is made by filling a large, deep pan, big enough to place the entire animal in, 3/4 full with warm water, placing a thick garbage bag over the pan and water, and placing a towel over the garbage bag where

the animal is to be placed (similar to a heated water bed). The animal is placed in the water bath allowing the warm water to "wrap" around the animal while the plastic prevents soaking. The animal must be monitored closely to prevent accidental puncture of the plastic and drowning (Figure 24-4). Only small dogs and cats can be warmed in this way.

Body temperature should show a steady rise as the animal recovers. When the animal's temperature approaches 100° F, heating sources can be discontinued, but the animal should be kept covered and body temperature should be reevaluated periodically to ensure it returns to and remains normal. If the temperature remains low or continues to fall, it may be an indication of a potential problem and the veterinarian in charge should be alerted. Heat should be reapplied if the animal's body temperature begins to drop.

PAIN

Intra- and postoperative pain assessment is important for patient well-being and health. During surgery, increases in heart rate, respiratory rate, and blood pressure and lightening of the anesthetic plane can indicate the animal is painful. As the animal is recovering, painful animals, among other things, may vocalize, have elevated heart and respiratory rates, thrash, bite or chew at the surgery site, and/or become aggressive. Other signs of pain include a disinterest in the environment, crying upon manipulation, insomnia, and lack of appetite (Figure 24-5). It should be remembered that changes in vital signs can mean numerous things, e.g., elevated heart rate could also signify substantial blood loss. The animal should be carefully evaluated by the technician and surgeon prior to drug administration. It is best not to allow the animal to become painful before giving pain medication. If an incision was made, pain is going to be experienced by the animal. It is up to the veterinary technician to decide how much pain a particular procedure might cause. Very painful procedures include fracture repair, amputation, declaw, joint surgery, and any major abdominal procedure. Moderately painful procedures include minor abdominal procedures (spay, cystotomy) and simple body wall hernia repair. Mildly painful procedures might include simple mass removal or biopsy. It can be very difficult to determine how painful an animal is since animals respond so differently to pain. Some animals may act very painful after spay while others may not, even though they are both likely experiencing pain. When in doubt, it should be assumed the patient is having some degree of postoperative discomfort.

Pain treatment is accomplished in several ways, and it depends on the animal, availability of pain medications, and the type of procedure that was performed as to what sort of regime is chosen. Most soft tissue surgical pain will last 4 to 5 days after surgery. For bone and joint procedures, this should be extended 4 to 5 days. It is best to preemptively manage pain rather than wait for the animal to show pain before administration of pain medication. If the animal is allowed to become painful before administration of pain medication, then the pain is harder to treat and may not be relieved by the medication administered (see Chapter 20). Pain medication should be administered prior to surgery in the premedicants, and they should be continued throughout the surgical procedure and then into the postoperative period according to the dosing regimen for the particular drug being used. A wait-and-see attitude should never be adopted since this allows the animal to become painful before treatment is given.

> ### ✎ TECHNICIAN NOTE
>
> The animal should not be allowed to become painful before the medication is given. Pain medication should be administered at dosing intervals appropriate for the medication being administered, not as needed.

Another misconception that should be avoided is that animals will stay quiet and calm if they are painful, so avoidance of pain medication is a form of treatment. You would never be treated that way in a hospital and veterinary patients should not be treated that way. This is an ethical dilemma many veterinarians and technicians must face.

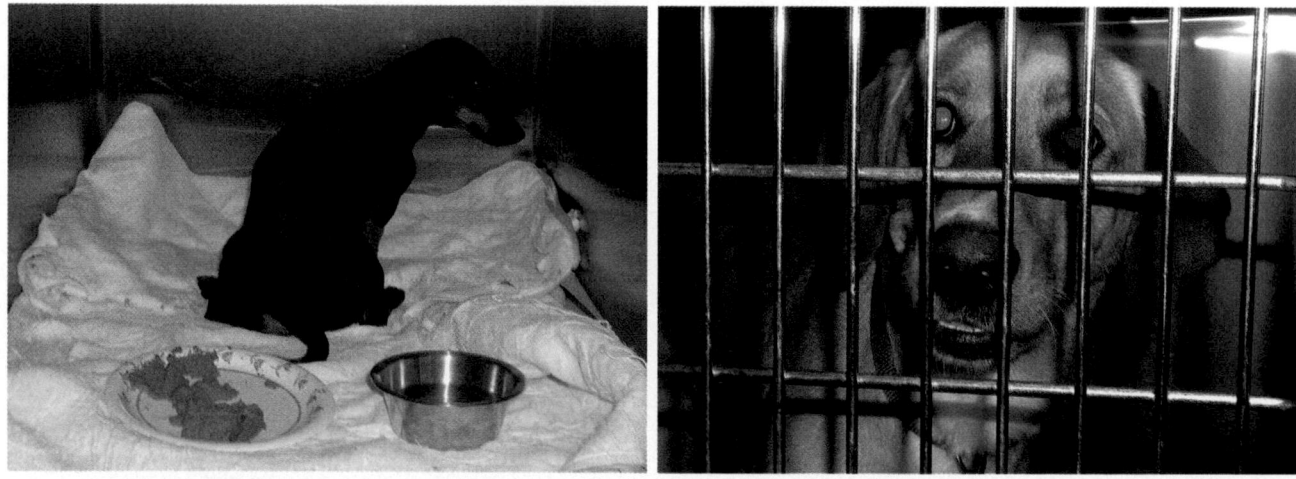

Figure 24-5 Note how the dog in **A** does not turn to face the door even when it is opened. Also note the full food dish in the front of the cage. This is a dog suffering from severe spinal pain and is uninterested in her environment. Comfortable animals are often interested in their surroundings and will come to the cage door to greet you. In spite of her tibia fracture, the dog in **B** is more than willing to interact with those around her.

An appropriately managed patient will likely sleep for several hours after surgery, should be comfortable when manipulated, should be alert and interested in its environment when aroused, and will likely be willing to eat and drink.

INCISION EVALUATION

Visual and palpable inspection of the surgical wound should be made daily. (See Chapter 4 for detailed information on wounds and healing.) The surgical incision is usually left uncovered after surgery. Ointments and creams (even antibiotic topicals) should not be placed on the incision since this can cause irritation and components of the ointment can delay wound healing. The incision can be covered with an adhesive or a wrap bandage for the first few days after surgery to keep the incision clean and absorb seepage.

Abnormalities that can occur in the early postoperative period (1 to 3 days) include redness, swelling, drainage, and dehiscence (wound breakdown). An incision should be evaluated with respect to the type of surgical procedure performed on the patient. Elective operations, such as ovariohysterectomy and castration, can be expected to produce mild redness and swelling with no drainage from the incision site (Figure 24-6). However, if the wound was contaminated (e.g., laceration, perianal wound) or if the surgical exposure was extensive, the incision is expected to be somewhat swollen, reddened, and warm to the touch and have mild to moderate drainage in the first 24 to 48 hours postoperatively (Figure 24-6). Swelling secondary to surgical trauma will usually resolve within 3 to 7 days after surgery. However, *seromas* (serum accumulation under the incision) and *hematomas* (blood accumulation under the incision) may persist for weeks.

Surprisingly, most animals will not lick or chew at the surgical incision. Animals will usually lick or chew at the incision only if the character of the incision is irritating.

Contributors to incision irritation include sutures placed too tight, traumatic tissue handling, suture reaction, tension on the suture line, clipper burn, prepping irritation, incision infection, and seroma formation. Only rarely will an animal chew the sutures because they are bored. Using appropriate suture technique will minimize incision self-trauma. However, if an animal begins to traumatize the incision via licking or scratching, an Elizabethan collar, bandage, neck brace, T-shirt, and/or chemical restraint should be used to protect the incision.

Seromas can form if extensive surgical dissection occurred beneath the incision, tissue planes could not be or were not adequately closed, or excessive motion occurs at the incision site. Seromas are recognized as localized areas of fluctuant swellings that are not usually painful or warm to the touch (Figure 24-7). Seromas will usually resolve without treatment. Warm compresses, hydrotherapy, and bandaging may aid in resolution. If the seroma is very large and/or is causing impairment, drainage is warranted. Drainage should be performed aseptically and an active, closed drain should be placed. It is important to keep animals calm in the postoperative period to decrease chance of seroma occurrence. Hematomas are treated the same way.

✎ TECHNICIAN NOTE

Repeated aspiration of seromas can result in infection and should be avoided. If an area must be aspirated, it should be aseptically prepared prior to aspiration. Suspected abscesses should be aseptically aspirated for cytology and culture, but there is no reason to aspirate a suspected seroma unless for the purpose of treatment, which is rare.

If incision swelling occurs 4 to 6 days postoperative, is warm to the touch, or is associated with an elevated body temperature, reddened, and/or draining, the possibility of infection or cellulitis (infection along tissue planes) must be considered (Figure 24-8). Abscess/infection or cellulites must be treated by drainage, warm compresses, and systemic

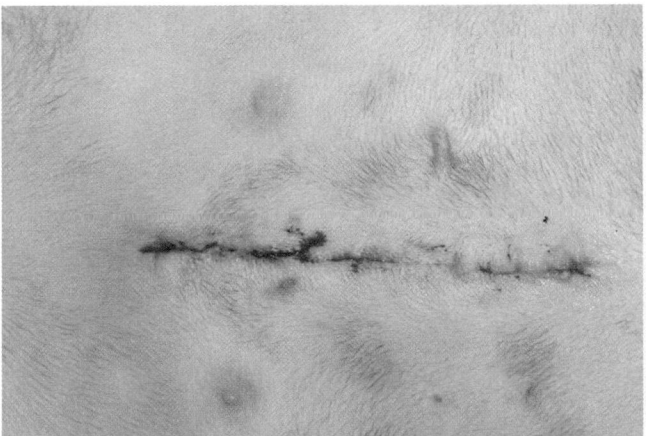
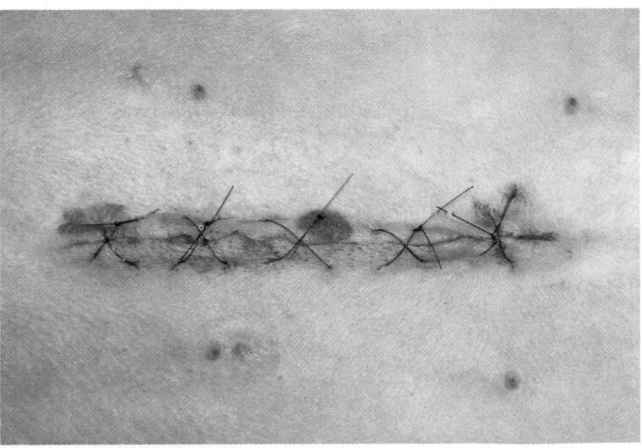

A **B**

Figure 24-6 These photographs were taken 4 hours after surgery. **A** shows a celiotomy incision following routine ovariohysterectomy, whereas **B** shows a celiotomy incision following severe traction on the skin during surgery for exposure. Note the minimal redness, swelling, and drainage from incision **A** compared with incision **B**.

antibiotics. Some infected incisions can be flushed and managed with an active, closed suction drain, but others will require open wound management. (See Chapter 4 for details on infected and open wound management.)

Wound dehiscence is defined as the separation of all layers of an incision or wound. Early recognition is imperative in any wound but especially in abdominal and thoracic

incisions. Dehiscence is most often due to technical error in suture technique, but incision complications can also play a role. Things that will contribute to wound dehiscence include using inappropriate suture to close a wound, inappropriate suturing technique, tension on the incision line, incision infection, seroma formation, or disease/drug therapy leading to delayed wound healing. Rarely would an animal self-mutilate an incision and cause dehiscence (see above).

Early detection of surgical incision problems is of paramount importance to help prevent more serious complications. If dehiscence is suspected, the reason for dehiscence should be ascertained. If the external suture layer (skin) is dehiscing and it is only partial, conservative management may be possible. The open portion of the wound will heal by second intention. However, the open wound will likely need to be bandaged and the animal placed in an Elizabethan collar to prevent licking of the open wound and further dehiscence. If the phase of healing is early (first few days after surgery), cleansing and closure of the incision may be necessary depending on the degree of dehiscence. Dehiscence of deeper layers can be more serious and should be brought to the attention of the veterinarian in charge as soon as possible, especially if the incision involves the abdominal or thoracic cavity. Complete dehiscence of an abdominal wound can result in evisceration (exposure) of

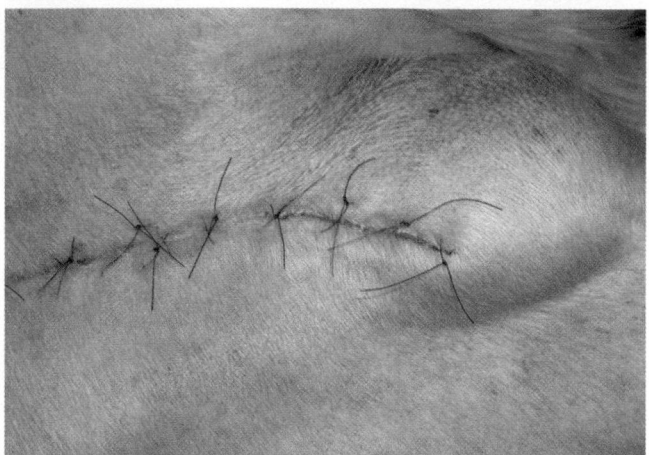

Figure 24-7 Note the swelling beneath the incision on cranial thigh of this dog. The swelling was nonpainful, and the dog's vital signs were normal. The swelling was diagnosed as a seroma.

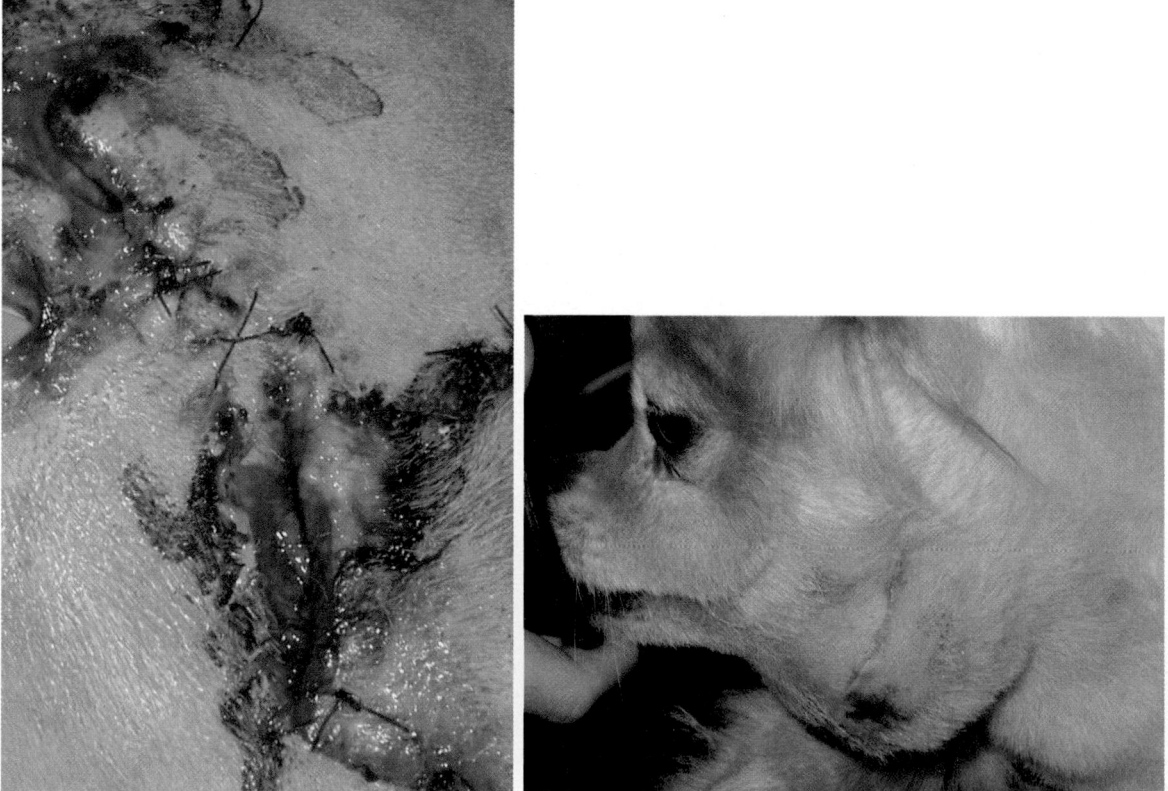

A   **B**

Figure 24-8 Incisional infection is recognized by drainage, redness, swelling, fever, dehiscence, and/or abscess formation. Notice the purulent discharge and partial dehiscence of the incision in **A**. **B** shows an abscess that recently ruptured.

the abdominal organs, with subsequent contamination and infection (Figure 24-9). Complete dehiscence of a thoracic wound will result in a *pneumothorax* (air within the chest causing collapse of the lungs), a problem that may result in sudden death.

> ### ✎ TECHNICIAN NOTE
>
> Dehiscence of an abdominal wound or thoracic wall can result in life-threatening complications. The veterinarian should be alerted immediately of impending complications.

Suture removal is commonly performed by the veterinary technician. The procedure is usually performed 10 to 14 days after surgery, as this is the approximate time that the wound is beginning to strengthen (see Chapter 4). If internal sutures were placed in the dermis with the external skin sutures, then external suture removal can be performed in 5 to 7 days since the internal suture layer will hold the incision closed while healing continues. The incision should be inspected carefully for adequate healing prior to removal. A healed incision is usually confluent, slightly raised, and whitish in color and has no gaps between skin edges (Figure 24-10). An appropriately healed incision should not be draining, severely reddened, or severely swollen. However, if complications were encountered, then some reddening, swelling, and excessive scarring is expected. Incisions that are swollen, draining, reddened or have obvious separation should be inspected by the veterinarian in charge before suture removal.

Skin sutures are usually easy to remove in the calm patient. Suture scissors are simple to use and allow removal with minimal discomfort. The suture should be grasped with thumb forceps or your finger. Gentle traction is placed on the suture and the suture is cut near the skin surface (Figure 24-11). The suture is manually pulled out of the skin after cutting. If metal staples were placed, then a staple remover should be used to allow removal with minimal discomfort (Figure 24-12).

BANDAGE CARE

If a bandage was placed, then the limb in which the bandage was placed should be monitored carefully. The bandage should be kept clean and dry. A plastic bag should be placed over the bandage when walking the animal outside and removed once back inside. The plastic will prevent the bandage from getting wet, but it should not be left in place since moisture will accumulate under the plastic if left on for extended periods of time. The animal's toes should be checked twice daily for swelling or coldness as long as a limb bandage is in place. This is especially important

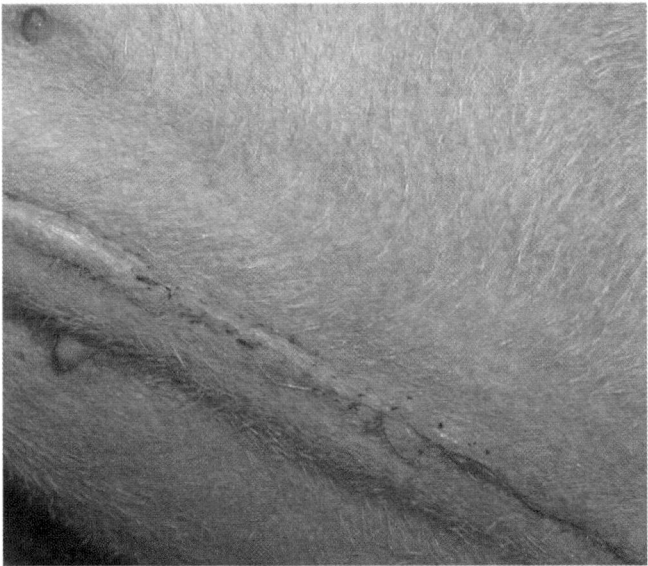

Figure 24-10 Healed incision. Note that the incision is not red, swollen, or draining. The skin edges are apposed, and the scar is slightly raised. This photo was taken 12 days after surgery.

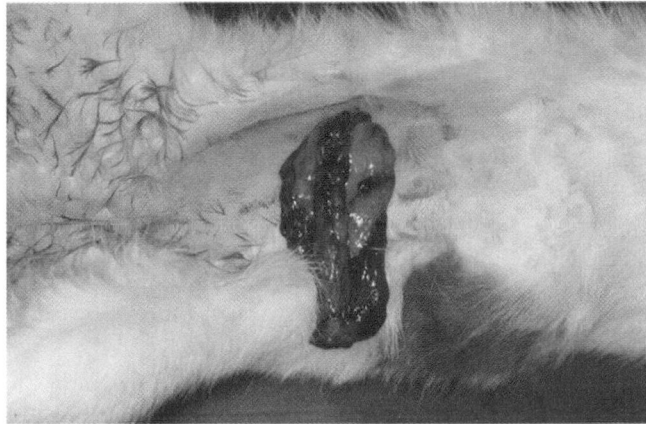

Figure 24-9 Complete dehiscence of an abdominal incision. Note the intraabdominal contents protruding through the incision.

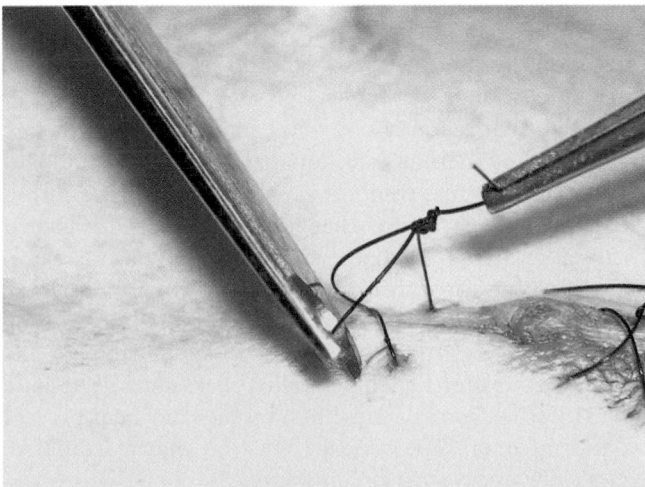

Figure 24-11 Suture removal. The suture is grasped with forceps or fingers and gently tensioned. It is cut with suture scissors near the skin and then pulled with slow, steady traction until it is completely removed.

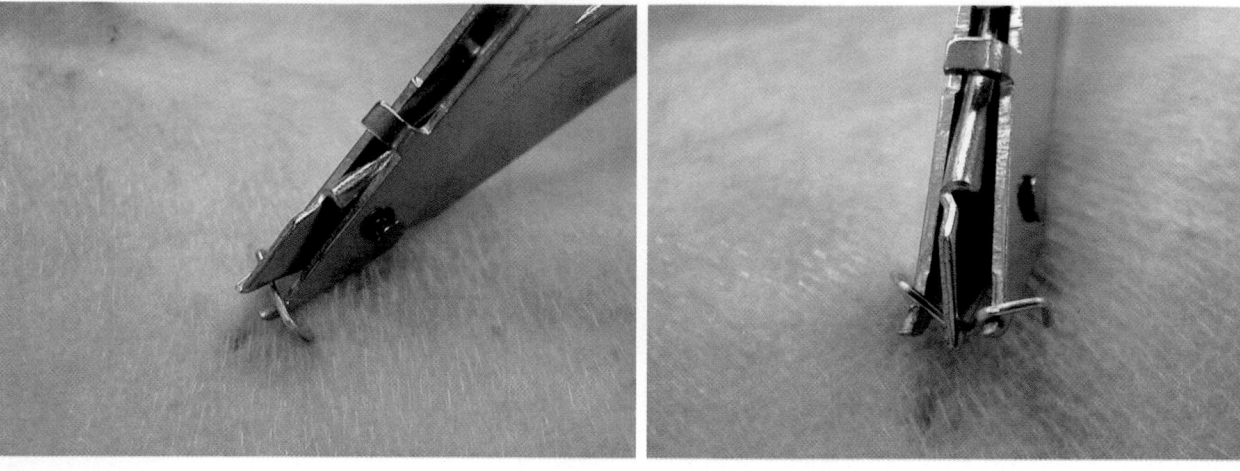

A   **B**

Figure 24-12 Staple removal. Staple remover is used. **A,** Staple remover is slipped under the staple. **B,** Staple remover is closed, causing the staple to be folded at its mid section and the teeth on either end of the staple to be dislodged from the skin.

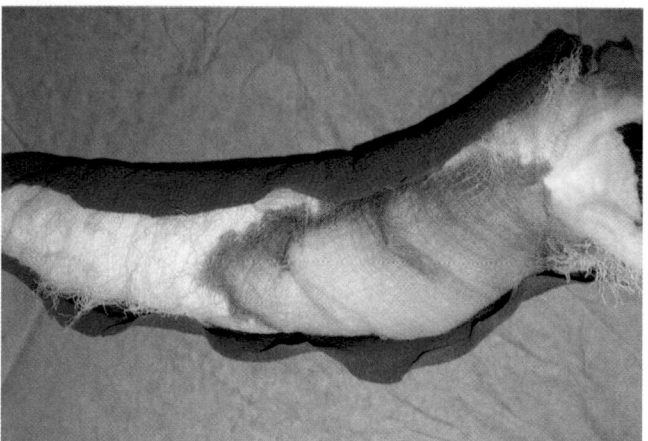

Figure 24-13 Strike-through. Notice red-tinged fluid seeping through the bandage from the wound bed.

immediately after placement. Swollen toes might be an indication the bandage is too tight. If the bandage gets wet, dirty, has an odor, or the toes become swollen or cold, it should be changed. A soiled, wet bandage can lead to sore formation and incision infection. Bandages placed too tight can result in vascular compromise to the skin with death and sloughing. Bandages are changed at intervals designated by the veterinarian in charge and depending on the reason for placement. Bandages covering open wounds will have to be changed daily. Some wounds drain excessively causing serum to seep through the bandage and extend to the external environment. This is called *strike-through* (Figure 24-13). Strike-through must be prevented to help prevent wound infection. The bandage must be changed multiple times a day under such circumstances.

DRAIN CARE

Drains are placed to collect fluid under a wound (surgical incision). They are often placed when large amounts of

tissue are resected (mammary chains, amputation, large skin masses) or when a large amount of drainage is expected (a contaminated/infected wound). If a drain is placed, the drain exit site should be kept covered with a bandage. Additionally, the animal should be placed in an Elizabethan collar to prevent premature removal or drain breakage by the patient. Active drains (drains that are sealed to the environment and actively collect fluid from the wound into a reservoir) should be emptied as needed (Figure 24-14). Passive drains (drains that provide an exit port for fluid to the external environment) should be avoided due to risk of ascending bacterial infection and difficult maintenance due to constant drainage of fluid through the drain exit site, but they are placed under some circumstances (Figure 24-14). If passive drains are used, the bandage should be changed frequently to prevent strike-through. Drains are removed when the amount of drainage has substantially decreased. Some drainage is expected as long as a drain is in place due to tissue irritation by the drain, but it should be minimal.

✎ TECHNICIAN NOTE

Some drainage is expected as long as a drain is in place due to tissue irritation by the drain, but it should be minimal.

RESTRAINT

Animal restraint is important for appropriate surgical technique. Naturally, the animal will have to be manually restrained during the preoperative examination and sample collection; however, surgical restraint involves sedation and/or general anesthesia. The type of surgical procedure dictates whether simple sedation or general or local anesthesia will be required. The specifics of anesthetic drug administration are covered in Chapter 19 and should be reviewed. Appropriate protocol should be discussed with the

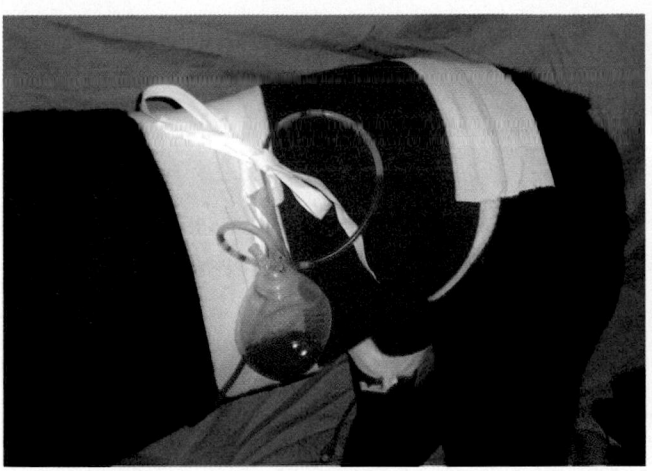
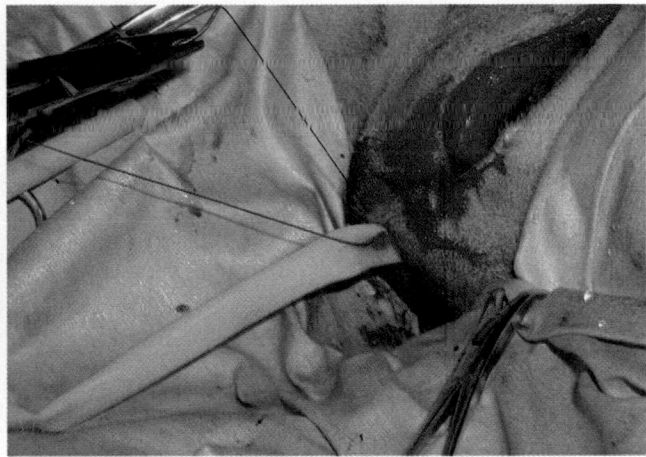

Figure 24-14 Drains. **A,** Active drains actively suck fluid from the wound bed into a sealed reservoir. **B,** Passive drains are placed under incisions and just provide surface area for fluid to drain from the wound with gravitational forces. In photo **B** the wound is being closed over a rubber drain (yellow). The incision and drain will be bandaged afterward.

surgeon prior to surgery so that preparation of the animal and the operating room can be initiated.

All animals should be well controlled after surgery to minimize complications. The length and severity of confinement depend on the type of procedure performed. Animals undergoing routine sterilization or simple mass removal usually require 10 to 14 days of restricted activity, whereas animals undergoing orthopedic surgery will likely require 6 to 8 weeks of confinement. No animal should be allowed free roam immediately after surgery. Additionally, self-trauma should be avoided.

Besides crate, leash, and room confinement, chemical agents and mechanical devices can also be used for restraint. Tranquilizers and noxious-tasting substances are commonly used chemical restraints. Tranquilizers must be used with caution since they can have undesirable side effects. They are not meant to be used long term. Phenothiazine derivatives (acepromazine) are commonly used tranquilizers in veterinary medicine, but alpha$_2$ adrenergic agonists, benzodiazepines, and cyclohexamines are also used (see Chapter 19 for more information on drugs used for sedation). Appropriate crate or room confinement usually will suffice without the addition of tranquilization.

Noxious-tasting agents are used to prevent animals from licking or chewing and they must also be used with discretion. Some commonly used substances include Bandguard Cream (Schering-Plough), Bitter Apple (Grannick's), Tabasco, and various thumb-sucking preparations. The agent can be impregnated into bandage material, and some can be placed directly on the skin around the incision. These agents should never be placed directly on the incision since they can burn, irritate the incision, and have the potential to delay wound healing.

Mechanical restraint devices include the Elizabethan collar, the body brace, the side bar, hobbles, and various bandages. These devices are used to limit motion, prevent licking and chewing, and prevent weight bearing. The assembly,

materials necessary, specific indications, contraindications, and complications have been adequately described elsewhere (see Chapter 4 and Recommended Reading) and are beyond the scope of this chapter. A properly selected, constructed, and applied device will be well tolerated by the patient and effective for its desired purpose.

COMMON SURGICAL PROCEDURES

The veterinary technician must have a working knowledge of common surgical procedures in order to properly prepare the patient preoperatively, act as an efficient surgical assistant, and manage the immediate and long-term postoperative care. The remainder of this chapter reviews common small animal surgical procedures performed in veterinary practice. A brief description of the procedure, with emphasis on the role of the veterinary technician, will be given.

TECHNICIAN NOTE

The veterinary technician must have a working knowledge of common surgical procedures in order to properly prepare the patient preoperatively, act as an efficient surgical assistant, and manage the immediate and long-term postoperative care.

ELECTIVE VERSUS NONELECTIVE SURGERY

Surgical procedures are divided into elective and nonelective. Elective procedures are performed at the veterinarian and owner's convenience, usually in healthy patients.

Spay, castration, and declaw are examples of such procedures. Some procedures must be done to improve the animal's quality of life, but are not necessarily urgent, like stifle stabilization for cranial cruciate ligament rupture, correction of patella luxation, and cancer resection. For these procedures, if animals are not ideal candidates for surgery at the time of presentation, surgery can be delayed. However, ideally surgery would be performed at some point to alleviate the animal's clinical signs or to decrease chance of tumor spread. Nonelective surgical procedures must be done urgently. These are usually emergency procedures performed on compromised animals.

TAIL DOCKING ON PUPPIES

DEFINITION

Tail docking refers to partial amputation (removal) of the tail.

INDICATIONS

Tail docking in young puppies is specifically performed for aesthetic reasons. Dog breeders have traditionally developed breed standards by alteration of the breed character with surgery. Tails are docked according to breed standards set forth by the American Kennel Club.

PREOPERATIVE CONSIDERATIONS

The dam can get upset as puppies are removed from her and from the nest for the procedure. Some dams will even become aggressive. Care must be taken with removal and replacement of the puppies from the nest. If the dam becomes too upset, it may be necessary to place her in another room while the procedure is performed on the puppies. Alternatively, some dams are more comfortable being in the same room with the puppies.

Tail docking should be performed during the first week of life (3 to 5 days of age). At this age, the procedure can be performed without general anesthesia and is minimally traumatic to the dam and puppies. It must be remembered that puppies of this age are immunogenetically naive. It is important to perform the procedure in an area where the puppies will not be exposed to a high concentration of infectious agents.

TECHNIQUE AND INTRAOPERATIVE CONSIDERATIONS

The puppy should be cradled in the palm of both hands, with the hind limbs held between the index and middle fingers and the tail directed toward the surgeon. The surgical site is prepared using aseptic technique. The desired length of remaining tail is marked, and the skin of the tail is retracted craniad (toward the base of the tail). The tail is amputated with a pair of scissors, bleeding is controlled with electrocautery or pressure, and the skin is released, allowing it to retract over exposed bone. One simple interrupted absorbable suture is placed to appose the skin edges.

POSTOPERATIVE CONSIDERATIONS

The puppies should be returned to the mother as soon as hemorrhage is controlled. The surgical site should be monitored for the first few hours for excessive bleeding. During the week following surgery, the tail should be monitored for drainage, redness, and swelling daily. The suture remains until it is absorbed or licked out by the mother. Complications are not expected following tail docking but may include hemorrhage and infection. In some animals, too much skin is removed during the amputation. Those animals may have chronic wound healing problems and bone exposure at the amputation site. Revision of the surgery site may be necessary to correct the problem.

DEWCLAW REMOVAL ON PUPPIES

DEFINITION

The claws located on the medial aspect of the forelegs and hind limbs are known as *dewclaws*. Dewclaw removal is amputation of the claw.

INDICATIONS

Dewclaws are commonly removed from the forefeet and hind feet of purebred dogs for aesthetic reasons and from hunting dogs because they may be torn as the dog runs over terrain densely covered with shrubs. It should be remembered that in certain breeds (e.g., Great Pyrenees, Newfoundland) the presence of dewclaws is necessary for proper show quality.

PREOPERATIVE CONSIDERATIONS

The preoperative considerations are the same as those described above.

TECHNIQUE AND INTRAOPERATIVE CONSIDERATIONS

Dewclaws should be removed during the first week of life (3 to 5 days). Removal is generally performed at the same time as tail docking most breeds. The surgical site is prepared aseptically. The puppy is cradled in the palm of one hand, and the extremity is extended with the other hand. Scissors are used to amputate the claw. Hemorrhage is controlled with electrocautery or pressure. The skin edges may be left to heal by second intention or apposed with one absorbable suture.

POSTOPERATIVE CONSIDERATIONS

The puppies are returned to the mother immediately. The surgical site should be monitored for the first few hours for excessive bleeding. During the week following surgery, the amputation site should be monitored for drainage, redness, and swelling daily. Complications are not expected following tail docking but may include hemorrhage and infection.

TAIL DOCKING AND DEWCLAW REMOVAL IN THE ADULT

Tail docking and dewclaw removal should ideally be done within the first week of life if it is being performed for aesthetic purposes. In some instances, adult dogs are presented for one or both procedures.

INDICATIONS

Indications for tail docking or dewclaw removal in the adult dog include aesthetics, trauma, infection, and neoplasia.

PREOPERATIVE CONSIDERATIONS

One must consider the reason for tail or claw amputation before patient prepping and performance of the procedure. If it is being done to treat cancer, acceptable tumor-free margins should be taken with the removed tissue, and the appropriate amount of tissue must be prepared before surgery. Removed tissues will have to be placed in formalin at a 1:10 ratio for eventual histopathologic evaluation. If trauma is the reason for the procedure, the patient may have to be stabilized before surgery can safely be performed. If amputation is being performed as a treatment for infection, then the veterinary technician should have culture swabs available so that the veterinarian can obtain appropriate cultures at the time of surgery.

TECHNIQUE AND INTRAOPERATIVE CONSIDERATIONS FOR DEWCLAW REMOVAL

The patient must be placed under general anesthesia. The surgical site is clipped and prepared using aseptic technique, and an elliptical incision is made at the base of the dewclaw. The dewclaw is dissected free and is transected at the carpometacarpal joint in the front paw or the tarso-metatarsal joint in the hind paw. Hemorrhage is controlled with suture, electrocautery, and/or direct pressure. The skin edges are apposed with suture. The paw is usually bandaged to prevent swelling and self-trauma.

TECHNIQUE AND INTRAOPERATIVE CONSIDERATIONS FOR TAIL AMPUTATION

The tail should be clipped and hung from an intravenous stand. The skin should be prepared using aseptic technique. If the tail is to be amputated near the base, the rump adjacent to the tail base must also be clipped and aseptically prepared. A tourniquet may be placed at the base of the tail to help control hemorrhage and is placed before the animal is draped for surgery. The tail is amputated at the desired location by skin incision and disarticulation of the caudal vertebra at the appropriate site. The skin incision is made a centimeter or two distal to the expected amputation site to ensure adequate skin coverage of the stump. Blood vessels are identified and ligated. The skin edges are sutured over the remaining vertebrae, and the tourniquet is removed.

POSTOPERATIVE CONSIDERATIONS

The surgical sites should be monitored for hemorrhage, swelling, drainage, redness, evidence of self-trauma, and dehiscence. Elizabethan collars should be placed on those animals attempting to traumatize the surgical site. Bandages placed on the foot should be maintained as previously discussed. If placed, skin sutures are removed in 10 to 14 days. Pain medication is generally needed for 4 to 5 days following the procedure. Complications are rare for these procedures even in adult animals.

FELINE ONYCHECTOMY

DEFINITION

Onychectomy (declawing) is removal of the claw and its associated third phalanx.

INDICATIONS

Onychectomy is an elective procedure to prevent scratching of owners and household items. Most veterinarians recommend declawing the front feet only. This does not significantly impair the cat's ability to climb trees or defend itself from intruders. Onychectomy is often performed at the same time as castration or ovariohysterectomy.

PREOPERATIVE CONSIDERATIONS

Onychectomy is a very painful procedure. Preoperative analgesics should be administered.

TECHNIQUE AND INTRAOPERATIVE CONSIDERATIONS

The cat is placed under general anesthesia. The feet are surgically scrubbed but need not be clipped unless the patient is a long-haired breed. If laser is to be used during the procedure, then alcohol should not be used to prepare the toes since it is flammable and likely to ignite when the laser beam strikes the soaked area. The nails are left long to aid in nail manipulation during the procedure (Figure 24-15). A tourniquet is usually placed to control hemorrhage during the procedure. It should be placed over the foot prior to aseptic preparation, but tightened when the surgeon is ready to perform the procedure. The tourniquet should *always* be placed distal to the elbow to prevent nerve damage (Figure 24-16). The radial nerve is more superficial just proximal to the elbow and can be permanently damaged if the tourniquet is tightened over that area (Figure 24-16). The tourniquet should only remain in place for no more than 1.5 hours. The veterinarian should be alerted as that time approaches so the tourniquet can be removed.

Three techniques can be used to remove the claws. The Rescoe (nail trimmer technique), scalpel blade, and the CO_2 laser techniques are all effective means to perform the

procedure. For the Rescoe technique, a Rescoe nail trimmer is positioned snugly onto the dorsal surface of the toe between the second phalanx and third phalanx. During positioning of the nail trimmer, the claw should be pulled cranially. As little skin as possible should be excised. The cutting edge of the Rescoe nail trimmer is positioned at the cranial edge of the foot pad. As the cutting edge is advanced, the pad is moved caudally while rotating the nail dorsally and caudally. The third phalanx is then excised by the Rescoe nail trimmer. Care is taken to avoid cutting the foot pad. Each nail is amputated in a similar fashion. A portion of the third phalanx is usually left behind with this technique, but the entire germinal layer is removed to prevent regrowth of the nail. The blade technique amputates the entire third phalanx using a no. 12 scalpel blade. The phalanx is disarticulated dorsolaterally first by cutting through the collateral ligaments, then the nail is cut away from the underlying tissue and digital pad. The pad is moved out of the way while the nail is being removed to avoid inadvertent laceration.

The laser technique is very similar to the blade technique except that it uses laser energy to dissect the third phalanx free from the second phalanx instead of a sharp edge. The surgical site usually does not bleed with the laser technique, so a tourniquet is not necessary. If a laser is being used, the technician should ensure that plenty of saline-soaked sponges are available to cover the remainder of the cat's foot, instruments, and surgeons fingers to absorb extraneous laser energy and prevent iatrogenic laser burns. It is best to use instruments approved for laser surgery to prevent reflected laser beams from inappropriately penetrating objects and tissues. Everyone in the room should wear safety glasses to prevent inadvertent ocular damage. The technician should be familiar with laser safety prior to its use.

One to two sutures are often placed to oppose the skin edges after nail removal. Surgical glue (cyanoacrylic tissue adhesive) is used instead of sutures in some instances. If surgical glue is used, it should never be placed on the exposed bone of the second phalanx or dropped inside the

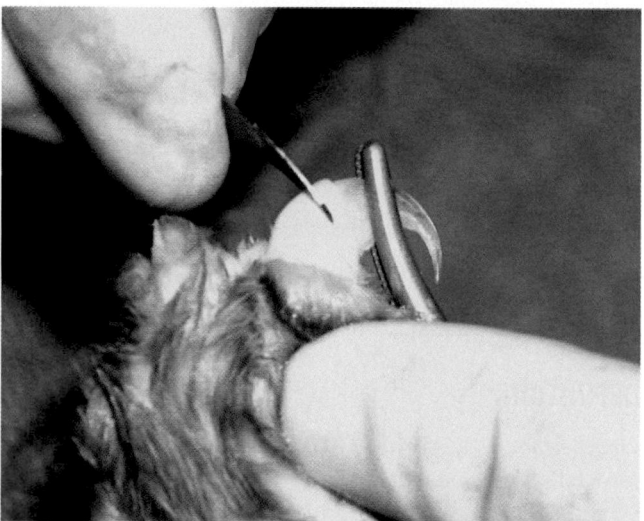

Figure 24-15 Declaw. The nail is not trimmed before surgery to aid in nail manipulation.

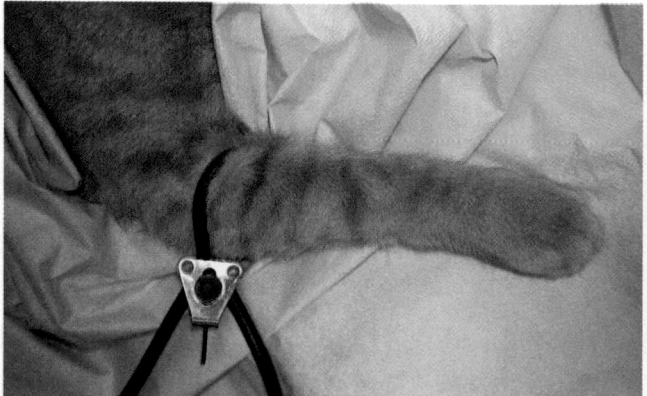
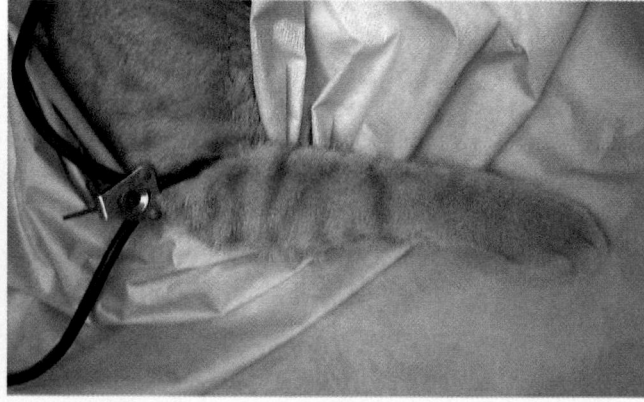

A   B

Figure 24-16 Declaw. A tourniquet should always be placed, distal to the elbow (**A**) rather than, proximal to the elbow (**B**) to help prevent permanent radial nerve damage.

void (wound) created by removal of the third phalanx (Figure 24-17). Instead, the wound should be manually closed and a drop of glue placed only on the skin edges of the closed wound (Figure 24-17). Dropping glue into the wound can cause chronic lameness and foreign body reaction. Some veterinarians do not oppose the skin edges with anything other than a bandage.

> ### ✎ TECHNICIAN NOTE
>
> Do not place tissue glue into the open wound formed after the claw is removed. The wound should be manually apposed, and the glue placed only on the skin edges. Placing surgical glue internally can result in chronic lameness and foreign body reaction.

After surgery, the paws are bandaged snugly with strips of tape and a gauze sponge. The sponge is placed over the excised digits. Strips of tape are placed longitudinally along the leg and distally around the paw. Tape is then placed circumferentially around the paw up to the elbow. Care is taken to lay tape on the leg and not to pull too tightly. The tourniquet is removed as soon as bandaging is complete. Bandages placed too tight can result in vascular compromise to the foot with skin sloughing.

POSTOPERATIVE CONSIDERATIONS

Onychectomy is painful. Pain medication should be administered to all cats in the postoperative period. It is appropriate to administer a pure opioid agonist for the first 24 hours after surgery. (See Chapter 20 for details on the administration, advantages, and disadvantages of specific pain medications). A fentanyl patch will often work well. It can be placed the day before surgery to allow the fentanyl to take effect and will last up to 3 days postoperative. Alternatively, injectable pain medication can be given intermittently. Some nonsteroidal antiinflammatory drugs can also be used in cats; however, care must be taken to avoid

overdosage. A wait-and-see attitude regarding pain medication for this procedure is not acceptable. Instead, medication should be given at the appropriate dosing intervals for at least 4 to 5 days postoperative.

The bandages are kept on for 24 hours, but no longer. After surgery, litter should consist of shredded paper or pellets to prevent accumulation of clay or sand in the surgical wounds with resultant irritation and infection. Normal litter should not be reintroduced until 10 days after surgery. The paws should be monitored for hemorrhage, swelling, drainage, and redness. Cats will be fairly sensitive on the front legs after surgery, but this should start improving within 2 weeks of surgery. If sutures were placed, suture removal is generally not necessary since the cats will remove them on their own.

> ### ✎ TECHNICIAN NOTE
>
> The bandage from an onychectomy should be removed within 24 hours. The cat should remains in the hospital until the bandages are removed.

Most cats allow removal of the bandages by carefully cutting the bandage apart longitudinally and gently peeling it off the leg. If the cat is intractable, the bandage may be cut, and the cat returned to its cage. The cat will then remove the bandage on its own. In severely intractable patients, a light dose of a tranquilizer may be necessary to remove the bandages safely. Cats are monitored carefully for 8 to 12 hours after bandage removal for hemorrhage. Rebandage with prolonged hospitalization will be necessary if hemorrhage occurs.

Onychectomy complications can be divided into those that occur in the early postoperative period and those that occur in the late postoperative period. Early complications include loose bandages and postoperative bleeding. Cats should be checked frequently for evidence of loose, bloody bandages or complete bandage removal and severe hemorrhage. In the event of hemorrhage, the paws should be rebandaged snugly. Late complications include regrowth of

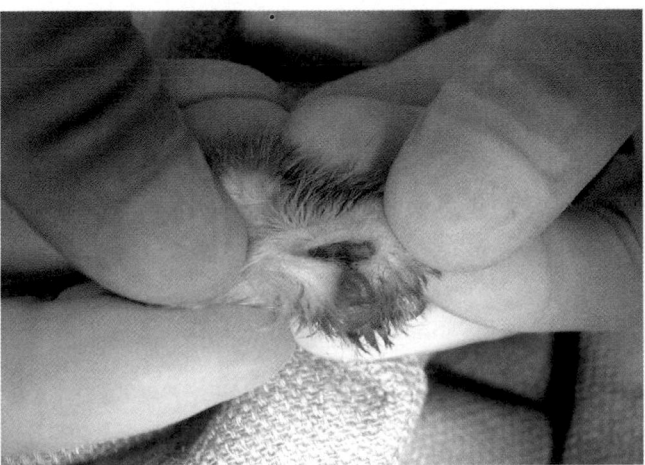
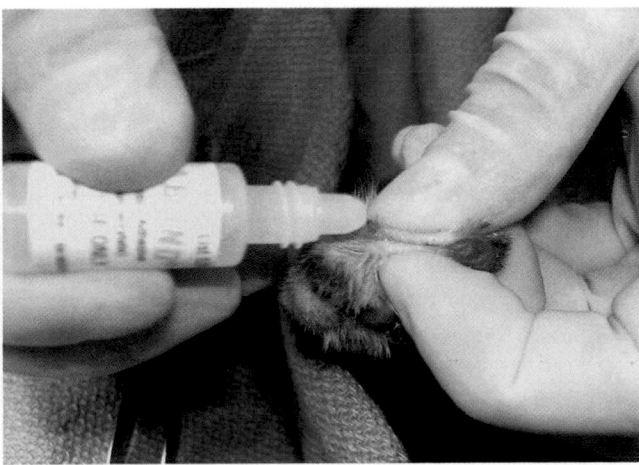

A   B

Figure 24-17 Declaw. When applying tissue adhesive to a wound, **(A)**, the glue should never be placed inside the wound created from removing the claw. **B,** The wound should be manually closed and the glue placed along the skin edges.

the claws, chronic lameness, or both. Claw regrowth requires reoperation and removal of remaining germinal epithelium. Chronic lameness without evidence of regrowth may be seen with incomplete removal of the phalanx or cut foot pads. For this reason, it is essential that the pads be preserved during the operative procedure. Other complications include radial nerve damage secondary to tourniquet placement and skin sloughing secondary to tight, prolonged bandage placement.

CELIOTOMY

DEFINITION

Celiotomy (laparotomy) is a surgical incision into the abdominal cavity. There are several locations in which the incision can be made: ventral midline, paramedian, paracostal, parapreputial, and flank (Figure 24-18). The most commonly used incision site is ventral midline.

INDICATIONS

A celiotomy is performed for both elective and nonelective procedures. Some of the common elective procedures include ovariohysterectomy, organ biopsy, cystotomy, planned cesarean delivery, intestinal surgery, gastric surgery, and retained abdominal testicles. Some common nonelective procedures include emergency cesarean delivery, gastric dilation and volvulus (bloated, twisted stomach), intussusception, gastrointestinal foreign bodies, ruptured spleen, penetrating foreign bodies (e.g., knife wound, arrow wound, bullet wound), severe abdominal bleeding, and diaphragmatic hernia. In some instances, the patient is presented for an unknown abdominal problem. These patients may need elective or nonelective celiotomy, referred to as an *exploratory celiotomy*. Exploratory celiotomy is often performed for abdominal masses of unknown origin and to obtain biopsies for disease diagnosis.

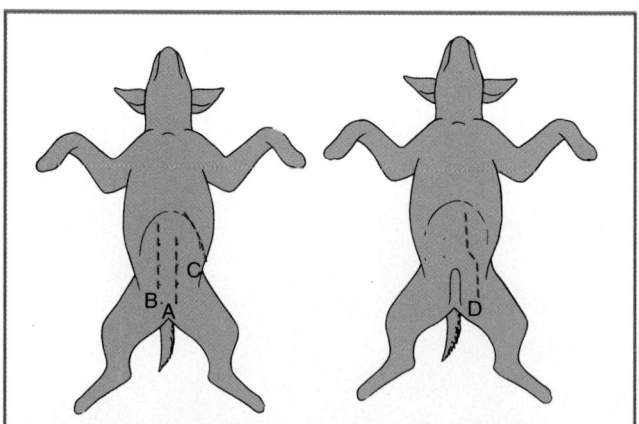

Figure 24-18 Locations for celiotomy incisions. *A*, Ventral midline. *B*, Paramedian. *C*, Paracostal. *D*, Parapreputial.

PREOPERATIVE CONSIDERATIONS

Animals should always be clipped widely for abdominal incisions. At times the incision must be extended, and an inappropriate prep will hinder surgical exposure. Animals undergoing abdominal incision due to illness or trauma may have to be stabilized before anesthesia is administered. If biopsies or cultures are to be taken, the veterinary technician should make sure that culture supplies and tissue sample cups with formalin are available.

TECHNIQUE AND INTRAOPERATIVE CONSIDERATIONS

For ventral midline celiotomy, the patient is placed in dorsal recumbency. Larger dogs should be placed in a V-trough to help stabilize them in that position (Figure 24-19). Smaller dogs and cats can be placed on moldable beanbags or sandbags. The abdomen is widely clipped from 2 cm cranial to the xiphoid cartilage to 2 cm caudal to the pubis. The skin is aseptically prepared for surgery.

The various incisions (paramedian, paracostal, etc.) are all slight variations of the ventral midline incision and are less commonly used (see Figure 24-18). For this reason, emphasis will be given to the ventral midline incision.

The line of the incision is from the xiphoid process to the pubis. The length used varies with the type of procedure (see specific procedures). A surgical sponge count is performed prior to entry into the abdominal cavity. The incision is made with a scalpel blade or electrocautery in the cutting mode. The incision is carried through the subcutaneous tissue to the level of the linea alba, which is elevated with forceps to pull it away from the underlying abdominal viscera. This will prevent the inadvertent puncture of abdominal organs when entering the peritoneal cavity. A scalpel blade is used to penetrate the linea alba and enter the peritoneal cavity. The incision is extended the desired length with scissors or scalpel blade and forceps. Moistened laparotomy pads (sponges) are placed along the incision edges for protection during exploratory surgery. This is usually not necessary during ovariohysterectomy since the incision is small and manipulation is minimal. A Balfour self-retaining abdominal retractor can be introduced, if necessary, into the incision to facilitate visualization of abdominal structures (exploratory celiotomy). Surgical lights and air exposure of abdominal organs will quickly dry out abdominal structures. It is very important for the surgical assistant to keep exposed tissues moist to prevent damage and decrease adhesion formation. The technician should pay special attention to viscera moved external to the abdominal cavity. Viscera temporarily moved outside of the abdominal cavity should be covered with warm moist laparotomy pads. Abdominal viscera should be handled carefully and as little as possible. Whenever retraction or manipulation of structures is necessary, atraumatic technique is mandatory. Retract viscera with moistened laparotomy pads, manipulate viscera with moistened gloves, blot any excess hemorrhage with moistened sponges (do not wipe surfaces with sponges), and when using suction, be careful not to suck the walls of visceral structures against the suction orifice. A postoperative sponge count should be made before closing the abdomen to ensure all sponges are accounted for.

The abdomen is sutured closed in three layers. The linea alba is the layer of strength and must be securely closed. The subcutaneous tissues are then sutured to decrease the amount of dead space. This helps reduce the frequency of postoperative hematoma or seroma formation. The skin is then sutured to complete the celiotomy closure.

POSTOPERATIVE CONSIDERATIONS

During the first 24 hours, the skin incision should be examined carefully for swelling, drainage, excessive redness, dehiscence, and evidence of self-trauma. An Elizabethan collar should be considered if the animal appears to lick or chew the incision. Incision problems should be brought to the attention of the veterinarian. Incision monitoring should be continued for 2 weeks after surgery or until suture removal. Animals should be exercise restricted until the abdominal wound is healed. If there is evidence of dehiscence, the veterinary technician should notify the veterinarian immediately. Emergency closure may be necessary.

Some animals may be inappetent or vomit after celiotomy. Intestinal and pancreatic manipulation can lead to intestinal ileus (temporary loss of intestinal motility), nausea, and/or pancreatitis. One or two episodes of vomiting or lack of appetite for the first 24 to 48 hours after celiotomy is usually not concerning in and of itself. However, if the animal appears ill or vomiting and inappetence continues, further evaluation should be performed. Animals not eating or drinking after surgery should be supported with intravenous fluid therapy until oral alimentation is resumed.

GASTROINTESTINAL SURGERY

DEFINITION

Gastrotomy is incision (opening) into the stomach. *Enterotomy* is incision into the intestine. These are often done to obtain biopsies or to retrieve foreign material. Anastomosis is suturing portions of the gastrointestinal tract together to allow confluent ingesta flow. Anastomosis is performed after damaged tissue or tumor requires a segment of the gastrointestinal tract to be removed.

INDICATIONS

Gastrointestinal surgery has many indications. Gastrointestinal foreign body lodgment, neoplasia, biopsy for vomiting or diarrhea of unknown origin, gastric dilation and volvulus, gastrointestinal trauma, and gastrointestinal obstruction of unknown cause can all be reasons for abdominal exploration and gastrointestinal surgery.

PREOPERATIVE CONSIDERATIONS

Many animals undergoing gastrointestinal surgery have usually been recently vomiting or not eating for several days. The veterinary technician should stabilize the patient with appropriate fluid management to correct dehydration prior to surgery. The animal should be intubated as soon as possible with a cuffed endotracheal tube to help ward

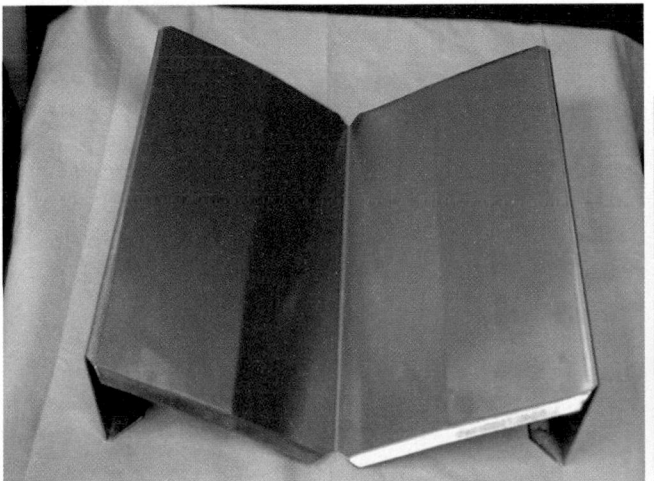
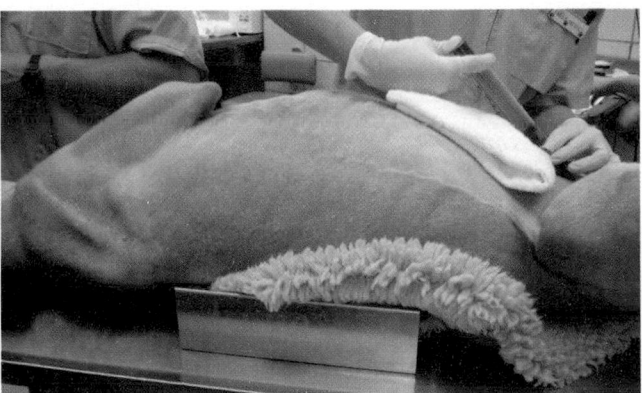

Figure 24-19 V-trough is used to stabilize large animals in dorsal recumbency for surgical preparation. **A,** Trough. **B,** Proper positioning.

off aspiration of stomach contents should the animal vomit during induction. The veterinary technician should make sure extra instruments are available in case the primary pack is contaminated with intestinal contents during the procedure. Prophylactic antibiotics are used if the gastrointestinal tract is to be entered.

TECHNIQUE AND INTRAOPERATIVE CONSIDERATIONS

The patient is prepared for a full midline celiotomy (Figure 24-18). An abdominal exploration is performed. Abnormalities are noted. Gastrointestinal masses are removed or a biopsy was performed. Foreign bodies leading to gastrointestinal obstruction are removed via gastrotomy or enterotomy. The normal gastrointestinal tract is pink, has visible vasculature on the surface, and has active motility. In some instances, devitalized tissue must be removed via resection and anastomosis. Devitalized intestine is discolored and lacks blood supply. Purple and red discoloration does not necessarily imply devitalization; blood supply must be evaluated by direct visualization of cut sections, Doppler, or injection of vital stains. If the tissue is questionable, it should be resected (Figure 24-20).

Characteristics of intestinal devitalization are:

- Lack of motility
- Black discoloration
- Green discoloration
- Gray discoloration
- Severe thinning of the visceral wall
- Lack of bleeding on cut section
- Lack of fluorescein dye uptake
- Lack of Doppler blood flow

For biopsy or foreign body removal, the affected portion of the gastrointestinal track is isolated with laparotomy pads (Figure 24-21). Laparotomy pads are placed to prevent intestinal contents from leaking into the abdomen if accidental spillage occurs. Stay sutures are placed to steady the tissue on either side of the incision. Biopsy is performed by making a stab incision into the stomach or intestine between the stay sutures and removing a full thickness portion of the tissue with a blade or scissors. If the incision is made simply to remove intraluminal material, the stab incision is extended enough to remove the material, and no tissue is removed for biopsy. The incision is closed in an interrupted pattern with absorbable, monofilament suture.

If a resection and anastomosis is to be performed, the vasculature to the portion of the intestine to be removed is ligated, the intestines are clamped with Doyen forceps or the surgical assistant supports the intestines with fingers to prevent ingesta from leaking onto the surgical field (Figure 24-21), the portion of the intestines to be removed is excised, and the viable intestinal ends are sutured together in an interrupted pattern similar to a biopsy site. After completion of the anastomosis, the intestine is evaluated for leakage. This is accomplished by occluding the intestine on either side of the anastomosis site and filling the enclosed space with sterile saline using a syringe and small-gauge needle. The surgeon and assistant check for leaks along

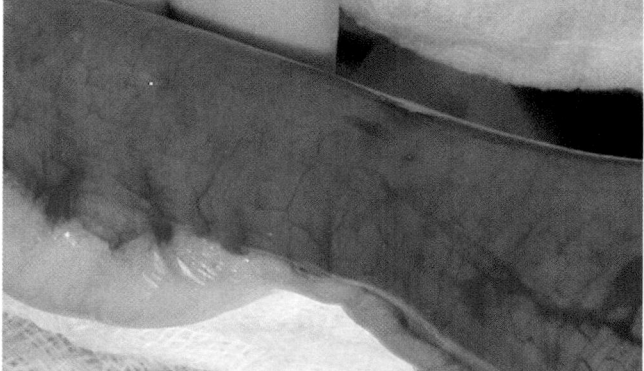

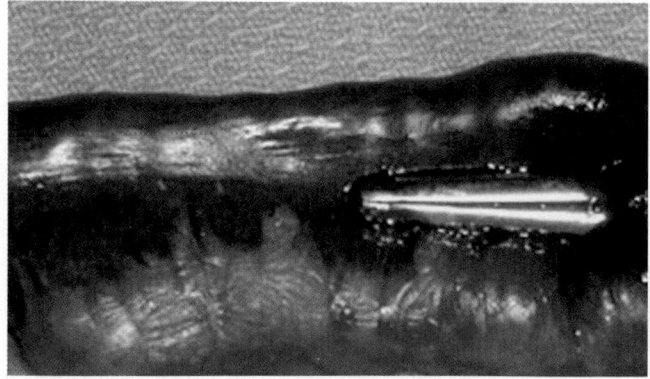

Figure 24-20 The normal intestine is pink with visible vessels and motility. Note the difference in color of the normal intestine (**A**) with the devitalized segment of bowel (**B**).

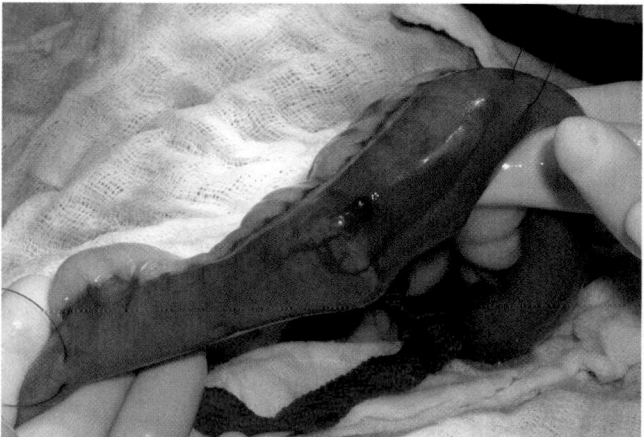

Figure 24-21 If a biopsy is to be performed on the gastrointestinal tract, the segment is packed off with laparotomy pads to prevent leaking ingesta from contaminating the abdominal cavity. Note the white pads surrounding the intestine. Ingesta is prevented from leaking from the cut surface of the intestine by placement of intestinal clamps or having an assistant gently pinch off the intestinal lumen on either side of the incision with fingers.

the incision. Leaks are sealed with additional suture (Figure 24-22). The intestine is flushed and the laparotomy pads are removed from the abdomen and surgical field being careful not to contaminate the rest of the abdomen or the surgical field with ingesta that might have leaked onto the pads. Omentum is placed over the incision and the abdomen is flushed. The celiotomy is closed routinely. Many surgeons will ask for a clean surgical pack, gloves, and drape to perform the celiotomy closure to prevent contamination of the celiotomy wound with ingesta from instruments used during the intestinal procedure.

TECHNICIAN NOTE

It is important to remember that gastrointestinal contents are not sterile. Materials that touch intestinal contents are considered contaminated and are removed from or kept in a separate place on the surgical field.

POSTOPERATIVE CONSIDERATIONS

Careful patient monitoring is important following intestinal surgery. The main consideration is evaluation for intestinal leakage. If intestinal dehiscence or leakage occurs, septic peritonitis is likely to follow. Animals should be monitored for inappetence, vomiting, fever, painful abdomen, abdominal enlargement, incision drainage, and shock, which are all potential indicators of peritonitis. Most animals are willing to eat within 24 hours of intestinal surgery. Minor vomiting (1 to 2 times) might be expected. However, protracted vomiting and inappetence should alert the technician to a potential impending problem with the intestinal surgery site. If intestinal leakage is suspected, an abdominal tap is performed. Material collected is evaluated for cell population and bacteria. If enough material is not obtained for evaluation on a simple abdominal tap, but leakage is still suspected, then a diagnostic peritoneal lavage should be performed. A septic abdominal tap warrants abdominal exploration and correction of the problem.

Feeding animals after intestinal surgery is also a consideration. The gastrointestinal tract requires food for cellular health and proper function. Intestinal surgery can result in ileus and may cause inappetence, nausea, and vomiting. However, animals without complications are most often willing to eat within 24 hours. Unless the animal is vomiting, oral alimentation should be initiated as soon as the animal has an appetite. Animals should be introduced to water first. If no vomiting occurs after water intake, then food is introduced. A small amount of highly digestible, bland food should be fed initially (1 to 2 tablespoons of Hill's Science Diet I/D, for example). If no vomiting occurs over 2 to 4 hours, another small amount can be fed. If vomiting does not occur, the amount fed can be gradually increased and frequency decreased. Animals are reintroduced to their normal or another maintenance diet gradually after recovery.

Monitoring as discussed for routine celiotomy should also be done.

GASTRIC DILATATION AND VOLVULUS

DEFINITION

Gastric dilatation-volvulus (GDV) is dilation of the stomach with ingesta and gas with rotation of the stomach into an abnormal position. This is a life-threatening condition that typically occurs in deep-chested, large, and giant breed dogs. The cause is not specifically known, but genetics and chest/abdomen configuration play a role. Some animals have often eaten a large meal, drunk a large portion of water, and/or engaged in heavy exercise following either; however, others have not. Some animals develop the condition during times of stress such as hospitalization or boarding. Vomiting, retching, and bloating (severe distension of the stomach) are classic clinical signs. Gastropexy is attachment of the stomach to the body wall. The goal is to have a permanent

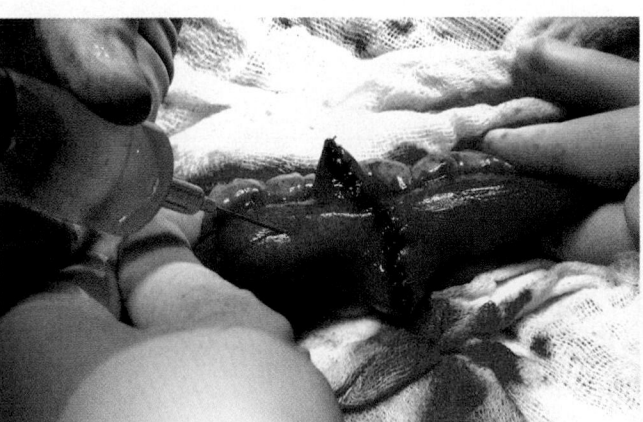
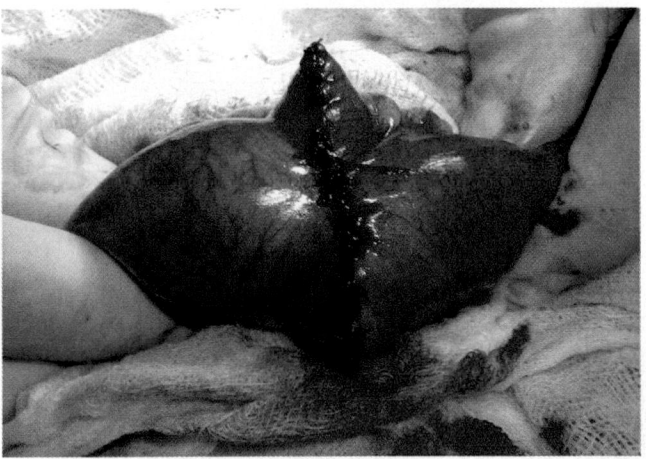

Figure 24-22 **A,** To check for leaks after intestinal anastomosis, the intestine is occluded on either side of the incision and the occluded segment of intestine is filled with sterile saline. **B,** The incision is checked for leakage while the segment is filled with saline.

adhesion form between the stomach and body wall. It is performed to substantially decrease the chance of stomach rotation, but it does not prevent bloating. Partial *gastrectomy* is removal of part of the stomach. *Splenectomy* is removal of the spleen.

PREOPERATIVE CONSIDERATIONS

Animals suffering from GDV usually present in shock. If left untreated, these animals will die from cardiovascular collapse. The enlarged stomach compresses the caudal vena cava and affects venous return to the heart. Hypovolemic shock results. Large-bore catheters should be placed immediately. It is important to place the catheters in the front legs or jugular vein since venous return from the caudal half of the body is impaired by the dilated stomach. These dogs are often very large and require a substantial amount of fluids. It is best to place at least two catheters. Baseline blood work, electrocardiogram (ECG), and blood gas should be obtained. The veterinary technician should review treatment of hypovolemic shock (see Chapter 26).

> ### ✎ TECHNICIAN NOTE
> Intravenous catheters should be placed in the front half of an animal suffering from GDV. Venous return is compromised from the back half of the dog due to compression of the vena cava from the dilated stomach.

After fluids are started, the stomach must be decompressed to help stabilize the animal and decrease the chance of gastric wall necrosis secondary to vascular compromise from the severe distention. A stomach tube is measured from the nose to the last rib (Figure 24-23). Stomach tubes are large bore and thick. The mouth is held open with a roll of tape or a gag with a hole big enough to pass the tube. An assistant should hold the mouth closed with the gag in place while another person passes the tube (Figure 24-24). The tube is lubricated and then gently passed down the esophagus to the stomach up to the premeasured mark. It is very difficult to impossible to pass a tube of that size into the trachea, but if the animal begins to cough, the tube should be removed and repassed. It would not be possible to pass the entire measured length of the tube down the trachea without causing severe destruction of the trachea and lungs. Over insertion of the tube may result in gastric rupture if the gastric wall is compromised due to vascular impairment. Gas is emptied from the stomach as the tube enters the stomach. Water can be pumped into the stomach to help break up ingesta. If the tube can not be passed, the animal can be sedated with an opioid and benzodiazepam and another attempt made. The veterinary technician must always remember to pinch off the gastric tube prior to removing it from the stomach (Figure 24-25). If the tube is not pinched, material from the tube can leak down the trachea as the tube is removed, causing aspiration pneumonia.

> ### ✎ TECHNICIAN NOTE
> While removing a gastric tube from a dog, the tube lumen should be pinched or clamped off to prevent leakage of tube contents down the trachea during removal.

If the tube cannot be passed after sedation, then the stomach should be decompressed by trocarization. The disadvantage of trocarization is the potential leakage of gastric contents into the abdominal cavity at the stomach puncture site or stomach rupture. For trocarization, the right side of the stomach is aseptically prepared behind the last rib. A large bore needle attached to a 60-cc syringe and three-way stopcock is gently passed into the dilated stomach

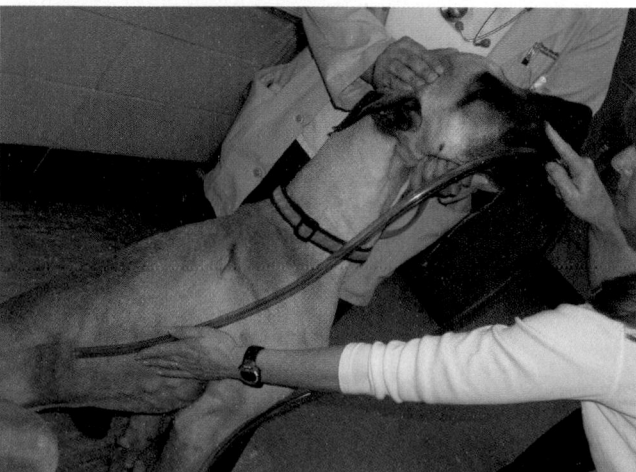

Figure 24-23 Before passing a stomach tube, the length of tube to be passed is marked by measuring from the nose to the last rib.

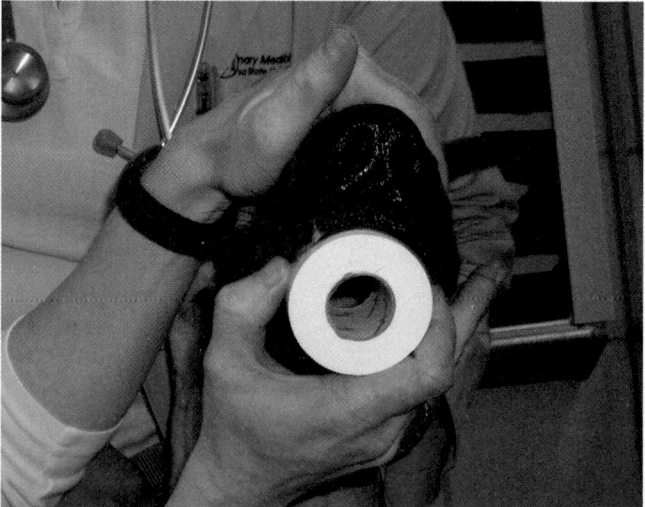

Figure 24-24 A roll of tape (pictured) or a mouth gag can be used to hold the mouth open while passing a stomach tube. The assistant should hold the mouth gag in place by holding the mouth shut around the gag.

percutaneously and air is aspirated until the stomach is decompressed enough to stabilize the dog.

After stabilization is under way and vital signs are improving, right lateral abdominal radiographs are obtained. This view is best for evaluating whether rotation of the stomach or simple bloat without rotation is present. Thoracic radiographs should also be performed since aspiration is a possibility. Due to vascular compromise to the stomach wall, the patient should also be started on broad spectrum antibiotics to help prevent septicemia should intestinal compromise lead to bacterial translocation from

the gastrointestinal tract to the blood stream. The animal is stabilized and then prepared for emergency surgery.

Anesthesia can be challenging in these cases. Respiratory compromise is often present due to the gas-distended stomach compressing the diaphragm. Blood pressure is often low and difficult to maintain. If possible, an arterial access port should be established for continuous pressure and blood gas monitoring. Additionally, cardiac arrhythmias may also occur and may need to be treated. The veterinary technician should review Chapter 19 for specific anesthetic techniques and monitoring.

TECHNIQUE AND INTRAOPERATIVE CONSIDERATIONS

The dog is prepared for a full ventral midline celiotomy. The abdomen is opened carefully to avoid puncture of the stomach since gas distention pushes the stomach against the ventral aspect of the abdomen (Figure 24-26). If the stomach is substantially distended at the time of surgery, further decompression should be performed to make manipulation easier. The veterinary technician should make sure that a stomach tube, bucket, and pump are available in the operating room. The tube should be gently passed down the esophagus after lubrication while veterinarian manipulates the tube into position within the stomach. The veterinarian can often gently express gas and fluid from the stomach through the tube. If decompression cannot be achieved in this manner, decompression can be performed with a syringe, three-way stopcock, and needle. The stomach must be handled with care. The tissue is often friable due to compromise of the tissues. Additionally, the ingesta and fluid that accumulates in the stomach following GDV is heavy and can contribute to tissue tearing during

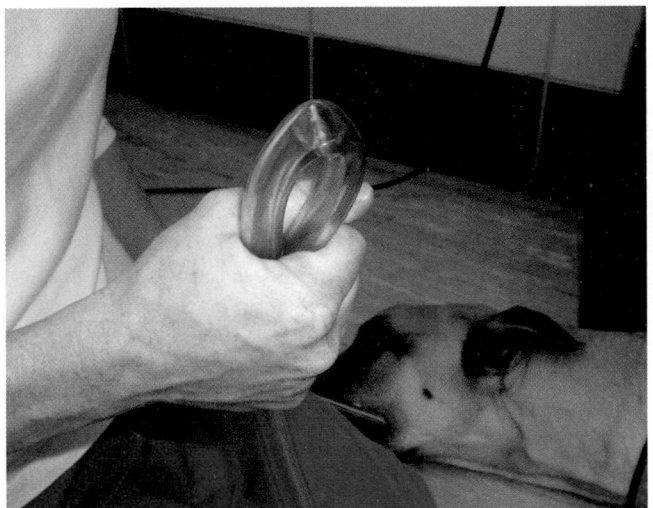

Figure 24-25 The assistant passing a stomach tube should pinch the tube off before removing the tube from the animal's stomach. This helps prevent aspiration of stomach contents into the lungs.

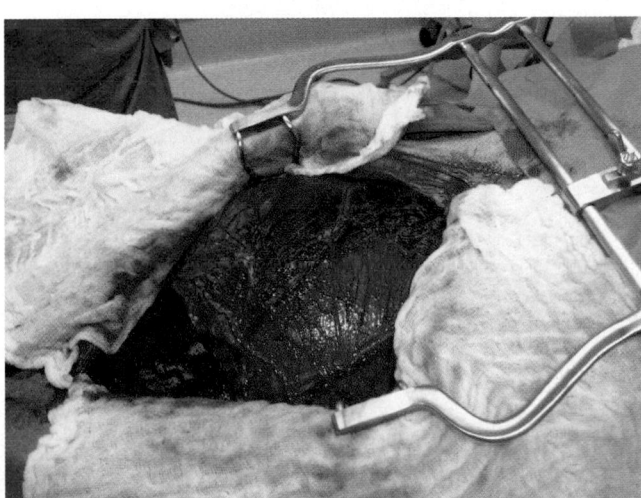

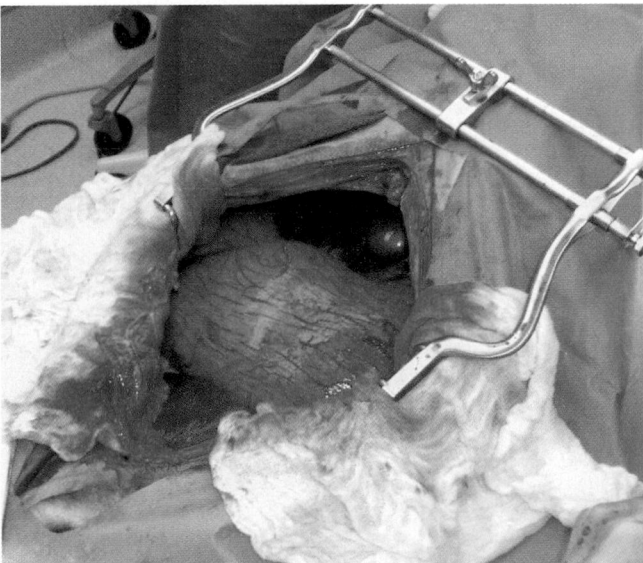

A   B

Figure 24-26 **A,** Note how the dilated, rotated stomach is pressed against the ventral abdominal wall and protrudes out of the abdomen. Inadvertent stomach puncture can occur if the abdomen is not entered carefully. **B,** The normally positioned stomach is still dilated, but recesses back away from the ventral incision and lies completely within the abdomen.

manipulation of the stomach back into the normal position. Extreme care must be taken to avoid inadvertent damage. Once the stomach is in its normal position, it is evaluated for viability. The stomach is often discolored at the start of the procedure, but may improve as blood supply and venous drainage returns. A complete abdominal exploratory is performed while circulation is allowed to return to the stomach. The spleen is carefully evaluated as well. Vascular compromise to the spleen can occur with dilation and rotation of the stomach, or the spleen may rotate as well. If the spleen is discolored, the vascular pedicle is relieved of compromise, and then the spleen is gently placed out of the abdomen and covered with moistened laparotomy pads while a gastropexy is performed. In most instances, the spleen will return to its normal character once blood supply is reestablished to it. After abdominal exploration, the stomach is reevaluated for viability. Partial resection is performed if needed.

A gastropexy is then performed on the right ventrolateral aspect of the body wall near the last rib. There are many different techniques for performing gastropexy, and the discussion of each technique is beyond the scope of this chapter. Which technique is used depends on the comfort level and skill of the surgeon performing the procedure. Pexy of the stomach into the celiotomy incision at the time of closure is not recommended since future abdominal surgery can result in accidental perforation of the stomach when the abdominal cavity is entered. The surgical assistant is responsible for retraction of tissues and suture manipulation to keep the procedure running smoothly. It will often help the veterinary surgeon if the assistant stands on the right side of the dog and holds the body wall up with towel clamps during the gastropexy. This will often expose the entire surgical field for the surgeon (Figure 24-27). After gastropexy, the spleen is reevaluated. If all or a portion of the spleen does not appear viable, all or part of the spleen is removed, respectively. The abdomen is flushed and the celiotomy incision is closed routinely.

POSTOPERATIVE CONSIDERATIONS

Dogs suffering from GDV can have many postoperative complications. Arrhythmias can continue for 2 to 3 days postoperative. Treatment for the arrhythmias should be initiated if vascular compromise is present or are expected based on the abnormality. The veterinarian should be alerted as to the type of arrhythmia present. Hypotension and hypovolemia can continue postoperative and should be treated as needed. Urination should be monitored since prolonged hypotension under anesthesia can affect renal function. A urinary catheter should be placed if urine production is questionable. Some dogs will require a blood transfusion due to hemorrhage associated with tearing of blood vessels during bloating and rotation of the stomach and/or spleen. If a partial gastrectomy was performed, the dogs should be monitored for evidence of gastric wall dehiscence. Some of these dogs continue to develop gastric wall compromise after decompression and surgery. Fever, persistent inappetence, and vomiting may be an indication that this is occurring. Signs are similar to intestinal incision dehiscence as previously discussed. Antibiotics should be continued for at least 7 days postoperative. Immediately after surgery antibiotics should be given intravenously to avoid oral administration. Gastrointestinal protectants such as H_2 blockers should also be administered for 3 to 5 days postoperative. Finally, gastric dilation can again occur in the postoperative period necessitating decompression. However, gastropexy should prevent rotation of the stomach.

Oral alimentation should be initiated slowly. Water is given in small amounts to start. If no vomiting occurs, food is gradually introduced. Feeding can start as soon as the animal is willing to eat, this is often within 24 hours of surgery. Some animals may require antiemetics in the perioperative period to help control nausea and vomiting. Long-term dietary management should be considered. When home, these dogs should be on a three- to four-times-a-day feeding schedule. If possible, a three-times-a-day

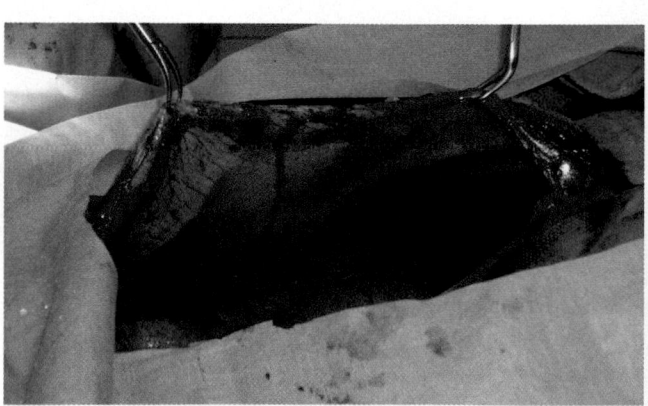
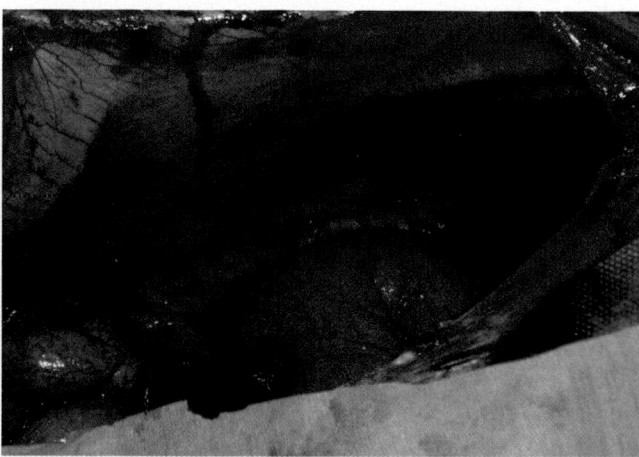

Figure 24-27 **A,** The surgical assistant can increase exposure for the surgeon during gastropexy by holding the abdominal wall up on the right side with towel clamps. **B,** Note how well this exposes the abdominal wall and the pylorus of the stomach.

feeding schedule should be continued the rest of the dog's life. Water should always be available, but gulping of water should be avoided. Heavy activity should be avoided after feeding. Owners should be warned that bloating can still occur even though gastropexy was performed, but surgery is likely to prevent gastric rotation which is more life threatening. Stomach decompression may be needed if bloat is severe.

OVARIOHYSTERECTOMY IN THE DOG AND CAT

DEFINITION

Ovariohysterectomy (spay) is surgical removal of the uterus and ovaries.

INDICATIONS

The primary indication for ovariohysterectomy is prevention of pregnancy and subsequent production of unwanted puppies and kittens. Other indications for ovariohysterectomy include endocrine imbalances, infections, injuries, cysts, tumors, prevention of unwanted behavior, and congenital abnormalities. Endocrine disturbances are associated with varied clinical manifestations, such as sterility, skin lesions, mammary tumors, pseudocyesis (false pregnancy), and nymphomania. Ovariohysterectomy before the first estrus will greatly decrease the chance of mammary neoplasia in dogs. Uterine diseases that may require ovariohysterectomy include metritis, pyometra, endometrial hyperplasia, neoplasia, injury, neglected dystocia, and congenital abnormalities.

PREOPERATIVE CONSIDERATIONS

Ovariohysterectomy is usually performed between 5 and 6 months of age, but it can be performed at almost any age and during any phase of the reproductive cycle. Performing ovariohysterectomy around 6 months of age decreases anesthetic risk in younger animals and usually allows the procedure to be performed before the first estrus. If performed during estrus or pregnancy, increased vasculature may be encountered with potential for increased hemorrhage. This is more important for dogs than cats. The most favorable time to spay a mature dog is 3 to 4 months after estrus. After whelping, the operation should be done as soon as the puppies or kittens have been weaned and lactation has ceased, about 6 to 8 weeks following parturition.

TECHNIQUE AND INTRAOPERATIVE CONSIDERATIONS

The patient is clipped and aseptically prepared for a ventral midline celiotomy. The skin incision extends caudally 3 to 6 cm from the umbilicus in the dog and from 2 cm caudad

to the umbilicus caudally 3 to 4 cm in the cat. When the abdominal cavity is entered, the uterine horns are located and exteriorized from the abdomen using a spay hook or digital manipulation. The ovarian arteries and veins (pedicles) are ligated with the appropriate-size absorbable suture material. The veterinarian or surgical assistant should check to ensure that both ovaries are completely removed after ligation and division of the ovarian pedicles. The uterine body is then exteriorized and ligated. The abdominal cavity is carefully examined for hemorrhage. The celiotomy incision is closed routinely.

Intraoperative complications include hemorrhage and anesthetic problems. If excessive intraabdominal blood is seen during surgery, both ovarian pedicles and the uterine stump should be evaluated before celiotomy closure. The abdominal incision will likely have to be extended. The left ovarian pedicle is evaluated by retraction of the descending colon to the right and viewing the pedicle just caudal to the left kidney. The right pedicle is evaluated by retraction of the descending duodenum to the left and viewing the pedicle just caudal to the right kidney. The uterine stump is visualized between the urinary bladder ventrally and the colon dorsally. Bleeding stumps are religated before abdominal closure.

Postoperative, intraabdominal hemorrhage can also occur and can be fatal if not treated appropriately (see the section on monitoring blood loss on p. 742). After ovariohysterectomy, the technician should monitor the animal carefully for the first 24 hours. Abnormalities should be promptly reported to the veterinarian in charge.

Incision complications can also occur after ovariohysterectomy. These include irritation, premature suture removal by the patient, seroma formation, infection, suture reaction, and dehiscence. Only rarely are these complications serious. The veterinarian should be alerted to impending incision complications.

Some animals experience renal dysfunction secondary to accidental ureteral ligation during surgery. Ligation typically occurs when overzealous attempts are made to alleviate hemorrhage from a bleeding stump with mass ligation of tissues and poor visualization. It is important to ensure that the ureters are visualized and are not in the mass of tissue to be ligated when controlling hemorrhage from bleeding ovarian or uterine stumps. Animals are unlikely to show signs of renal failure if only one ureter is ligated, but they may present for abdominal enlargement, abdominal pain, or signs consistent with renal infection at a later date. If both ureters are inadvertently ligated, the animal will begin to show signs within 24 hours and will die if steps are not taken to alleviate the obstruction of urine flow.

Body weight gain may occur as a late sequel to ovariohysterectomy. The reasons for this excessive weight gain are poorly understood but may be partially caused by ovarian endocrine deficiency. In actuality, obesity can be controlled by proper diet and exercise. Other late complications include loss of stamina in working dogs (eunuchoid syndrome) and urinary incontinence. Although incompletely understood, urinary incontinence may be related to endocrine alteration following ovariohysterectomy or scar tissue formation around the urinary bladder and proximal urethra. These appear to be rare complications.

PYOMETRA

DEFINITION

Pyometra is a condition of the uterus in which endometrial hyperplasia has resulted in increased uterine secretions and accumulation of fluid in the uterus with secondary infection. Progesterone production from the ovaries during diestrus contributes to uterine gland hyperplasia and the disease process. The process typically occurs in middle-aged to older dogs 4 to 8 weeks following estrus. *Muco metra* or *hydrometra* is enlargement of the uterus with a sterile mucoid or serous fluid, respectively.

INDICATIONS

Ovariohysterectomy is the recommended treatment for pyometra. This is especially true for closed (nondraining) pyometras. Some owners will elect conservative management for open (draining) pyometras in valuable breeding dogs, but this should be discouraged since septicemia and/or endotoxemia is possible and the incidence of recurrence is high. Conservative management of closed pyometras is not recommended due to the risk of uterine rupture, septicemia/endotoxemia, and possible death.

PREOPERATIVE CONSIDERATIONS

Intact female dog presenting with fever, lethargy, polyuria, polydipsia, vaginal discharge, abdominal pain, abdominal enlargement, inappetence, vomiting, and/or diarrhea should be evaluated carefully for pyometra. Animals with closed pyometras are more likely to have severe clinical signs. Baseline biochemical values and blood cell counts should be obtained. Many of these animals are dehydrated, inappetent, and have metabolic and/or electrolyte abnormalities at the time of presentation (renal or hepatic dysfunction, glucose imbalances, etc.). They should be started on intravenous fluids and their metabolic/electrolyte abnormalities corrected, if possible, prior to surgery. If left untreated, pyometra can result in septicemia/endotoxemia and possible death. Additionally, uterine rupture and peritonitis is also possible. Palpation of the abdomen should be done with extreme care and cystocentesis to collect urine should be avoided in animals suspected of having pyometra. Broad-spectrum intravenous antibiotic therapy is initiated prior to surgery.

TECHNIQUE AND INTRAOPERATIVE CONSIDERATIONS

The animal is prepped for a ventral midline celiotomy. A routine ovariohysterectomy is performed with some exceptions. The uterus is usually large, heavy, and friable (Figure 24-28). It should be manipulated with extreme care during the procedure to avoid rupture and contamination of the abdomen. This means that the celiotomy incision should extend from the xiphoid to the pubis so that excessive tension is not placed on the uterus during manipulation. Vessels are usually prominent and may be increased in number, so care must be taken to ligate and separate vessels appropriately to avoid hemorrhage. The uterine contents should be cultured for aerobic, and anaerobic bacteria and a bacterial sensitivity performed after the uterus is removed from the surgical field. This is performed via aseptic aspiration of the fluid with a needle and syringe before the uterus is contaminated. The abdomen should be flushed before closure. The abdominal closure is routine.

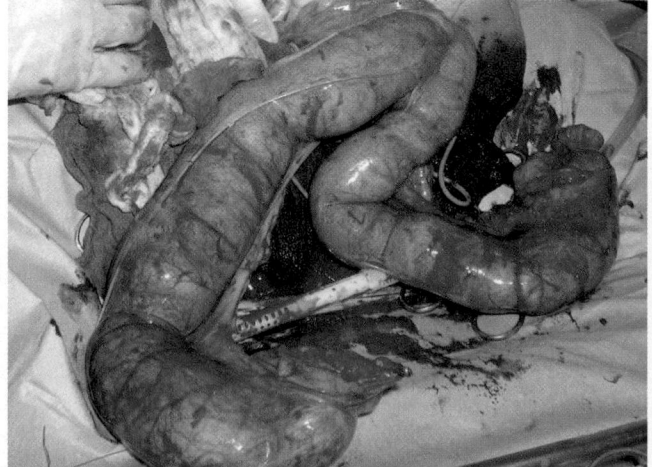
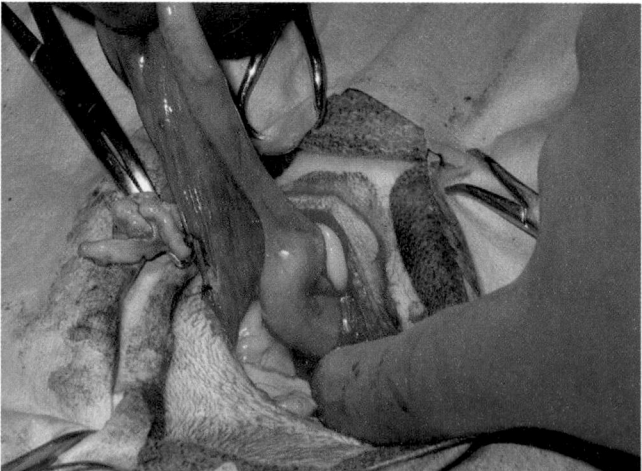

A   B

Figure 24-28 The uterus must be carefully handled in cases of pyometra since it is often large, friable, and heavy. Compare the pyometra uterus (**A**) with the normal uterus (**B**).

POSTOPERATIVE CONSIDERATIONS

Animals should be monitored as for ovariohysterectomy. Special considerations include continued antibiotic therapy in the postoperative period. Antibiotics are given intravenously until the animal is stable and eating. Antibiotic therapy is continued for 7 to 10 days after surgery based on culture and sensitivity results. Electrolyte and metabolic abnormalities can continue postoperative and monitoring for this is important. Abnormalities should be corrected. Intravenous fluids should be given until the animal is stable, eating, and drinking.

CANINE CASTRATION

DEFINITION

Canine *castration* (neuter) is the removal of both testicles. *Scrotal ablation* is removal of the scrotum with the testicles at the time of castration.

INDICATIONS

There are numerous indications for canine castration, the most common being an elective procedure in the young male dog to help prevent roaming, aggressiveness, unwanted breeding, or a combination of these. Several medical problems may also be treated by castration, including prostate disorders, anal and perianal tumors, perineal hernias, and testicular tumors. Older dogs with a well-developed scrotum or animals with scrotal abnormalities should undergo scrotal ablation to prevent severe scrotal swelling, improve postoperative aesthetics, and/or treat disease.

PREOPERATIVE CONSIDERATIONS

There is not an optimal age for canine castration, but the procedure is often performed around 6 months of age. Performing castration prior to the development of unwanted male behavior, before sexual maturity, may help prevent this behavior from occurring. Castration after development of this behavior will often improve behavior but may not eliminate it in all male dogs. Prior to surgery, a careful examination should be performed to ensure that both testicles lie within the scrotum.

TECHNIQUE AND INTRAOPERATIVE CONSIDERATIONS

The abdomen is clipped from the tip of the prepuce to the margin of abdominal skin and scrotal skin (Figure 24-29). The clipped area should extend widely into the inguinal region. The scrotum is typically not draped into the surgical field and is not normally clipped during surgical preparation. The scrotum has very delicate, thin skin that is easily subject to clipper burn and laceration. If, however, there are long scrotal hairs protruding into the surgical field, they can and should be trimmed without touching the clippers to the scrotal skin. If scrotal ablation is to be performed, the scrotum is clipped and prepared aseptically along with the rest of the surgical field.

For simple castration, the dog is secured in dorsal recumbency, and a standard surgical preparation of the prescrotal skin (craniad to the scrotum) is performed. A midline incision is made in the prescrotal skin. With gentle pressure, one of the testicles is pushed craniad into the incision. The testicle is then exteriorized through the incision by carefully incising over the common tunic (tissue that encases the testicle). The major vessels are then easily identified and ligated with two absorbable sutures. The remaining scrotal ligament is gently dissected from the testicle. The opposite testicle is handled in a similar fashion. The incision is closed with a continuous subcuticular suture pattern.

For scrotal ablation, the incision is made circumferentially around the base of the scrotum. The subcutaneous tissue is bluntly dissected to expose the testicles and associated structures. Castration is carried out via ligation of these structures as for simple castration. The testicles and scrotum are removed and the incision closed. Care must be taken to avoid removal of too much skin around the scrotum to prevent excessive tension on the closure.

POSTOPERATIVE CONSIDERATIONS

Several postoperative complications can occur. If the presurgical preparation is not done carefully so as to preclude

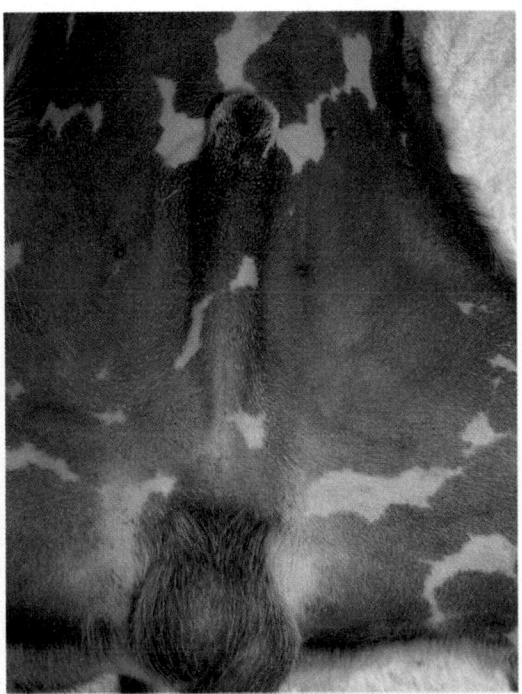

Figure 24-29 Proper positioning and preparation for canine castration.

scrotal dermatitis (clipper burn, excessive scrubbing), the dog will lick aggressively at the scrotum and the incision. This often results in severe inflammation and swelling of the scrotal and prescrotal skin. If this problem is not detected early, the results can be premature suture removal and wound dehiscence. The best treatment is prevention. If scrotal dermatitis does occur, the dog should be placed in an Elizabethan collar.

Another less common complication is hemorrhage. When the testicles are removed from the scrotal sac, free space remains in the scrotum. If there is any hemorrhage, either from the subcutaneous tissue or common tunic, the space will fill with a considerable amount of blood before there is enough pressure to create hemostasis, resulting in a large hematoma within the scrotum. If a hematoma is detected early, before the scrotum is full, cold compresses can be applied with slight pressure to the scrotal area to encourage hemostasis. If the scrotum becomes excessively large, not only is it unsightly but tremendous trauma and skin sloughing may also occur. At this point, removal of the scrotum may be necessary.

A scrotal seroma is more likely to occur than hemorrhage and can also result in tremendous scrotal swelling. In older dogs with a well-developed scrotal tissue, fluid accumulation after castration can be tremendous. Some advocate performing a scrotal ablation at the time of castration to help prevent this complication in older animals. Treatment is the same as for hematoma. It is very important to restrict activity in these dogs to decrease the amount of fluid accumulation.

FELINE CASTRATION

DEFINITION

Feline castration (neuter) is the removal of both testicles.

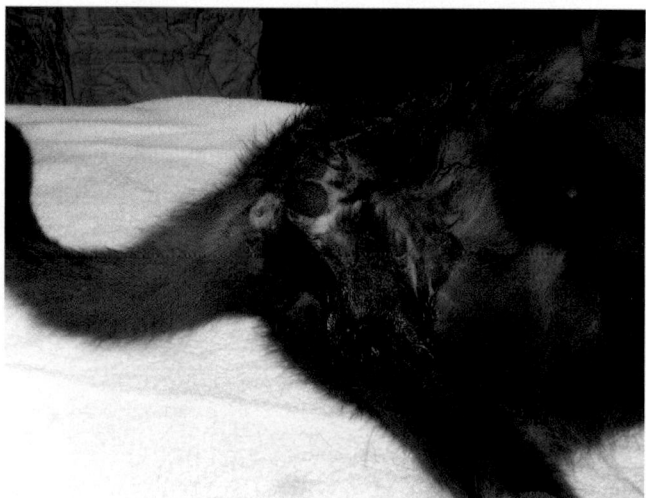

Figure 24-30 Proper positioning for feline castration. The legs are pulled forward and the cat is in dorsal recumbency.

INDICATIONS

The major indications for feline castration are to prevent fighting, roaming, and urine spraying and to decrease urine odor. Castration in the cat may provide a rapid response (2 to 4 weeks) to these objectionable characteristics, although complete resolution may not occur.

PREOPERATIVE CONSIDERATIONS

The cat is usually castrated while around 6 months of age. Preanesthetic evaluation should include palpation of both testicles to confirm the gender of the cat and to detect retained testicles before surgery.

TECHNIQUE AND INTRAOPERATIVE CONSIDERATIONS

There are several acceptable techniques for feline castration. The patient is generally placed in dorsal recumbency with the legs tied craniad (Figure 24-30). Unlike the dog, the scrotum is the site of the primary incision and should be aseptically prepared for surgery. Scrotal dermatitis is not a major concern in the cat, although you should avoid putting alcohol on the scrotum during surgical preparation. Warmed sterile saline is a good substitute for alcohol. The scrotal hairs are gently plucked from the scrotum with the thumb and finger. This is easily accomplished by grasping the base of the scrotum by the thumb and index finger of one hand and gently pushing the testicles into the scrotum (Figure 24-31). With the other hand, the thumb and finger are used to gently strip the hair from the scrotal skin. The scrotum is then scrubbed and draped in an aseptic manner.

An incision is made directly through the scrotum. The testicle is protruded through the incision by gentle pressure with the thumb and index finger. The testicle and its spermatic cord (vessels) are exteriorized and then may be ligated with suture, ligated with metal clips, or tied in a

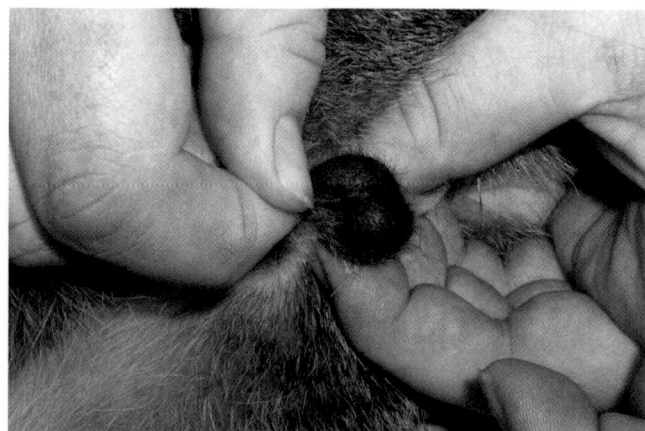

Figure 24-31 Technique for scrotal plucking to remove hair in preparation for surgery.

knot on itself, or the vessels can be separated from the vas deferens and tied in a square knot. The scrotum is left unsutured.

POSTOPERATIVE CONSIDERATIONS

Scrotal swelling and bleeding are the two most common complications of feline castration. Scrotal swelling is due primarily to traumatic surgical preparation and hair plucking. An Elizabethan collar may be necessary to control licking. If scrotal hemorrhage is noted after surgery, cold compresses on the scrotum for 5 to 7 minutes will help to encourage hemostasis. Severe hemorrhage can also occur and may actually occur intraabdominally. The veterinary technician should monitor these animals carefully (see discussion on blood loss) and bring clinical abnormalities to the attention of the veterinarian. Scrotal infection occurs rarely and should be treated with drainage (if not already draining), scrotal flushing/abscess drainage, Elizabethan collar, and appropriate antibiotics.

When the patient is sent home, the owner should be informed to change the litter from gravel type to shredded or pelleted type for the first 5 to 7 days. This will prevent pieces of litter from contaminating the surgical site.

CESAREAN DELIVERY

DEFINITION

Cesarean delivery derived its name from Caesar, allegedly the first to be born by such a technique. The procedure involves making an incision into the abdominal cavity and then into the uterus to deliver a neonate. It is usually performed on animals experiencing dystocia. *Dystocia* (Greek: *dys,* difficult + *tokos,* birth) literally translated means "difficult birth."

INDICATIONS

Cesarean delivery is indicated when a bitch or queen cannot deliver the pups or kits through the birth canal by normal uterine contractions, because of either maternal or fetal abnormalities. Some breeders schedule planned cesarean deliveries in dog breeds that might typically have birthing problems, such as bull dogs. Some of the common causes of dystocia are seen in Figure 24-32. Normal stages of parturition are discussed in Chapter 17.

PREOPERATIVE CONSIDERATIONS

The aim of treatment should be the successful delivery of live and undamaged puppies or kittens without harm to the dam. Medical therapy to increase uterine contracture or to treat metabolic abnormalities in the dam should be considered prior to surgery, however, a diagnosis of the cause of dystocia must be made first. Medical therapy may do more harm than good when used in the wrong type of dystocia. An example would be giving a drug (oxytocin) that would increase uterine muscular contraction in a dam that has a uterine obstruction due to malpositioned fetus or uterine torsion. When proper diagnosis of the type of dystocia is made, and medical therapy is either contra-indicated or not effective, the dam should be prepared for surgery. Metabolic alterations should be treated prior to or during anesthesia if possible.

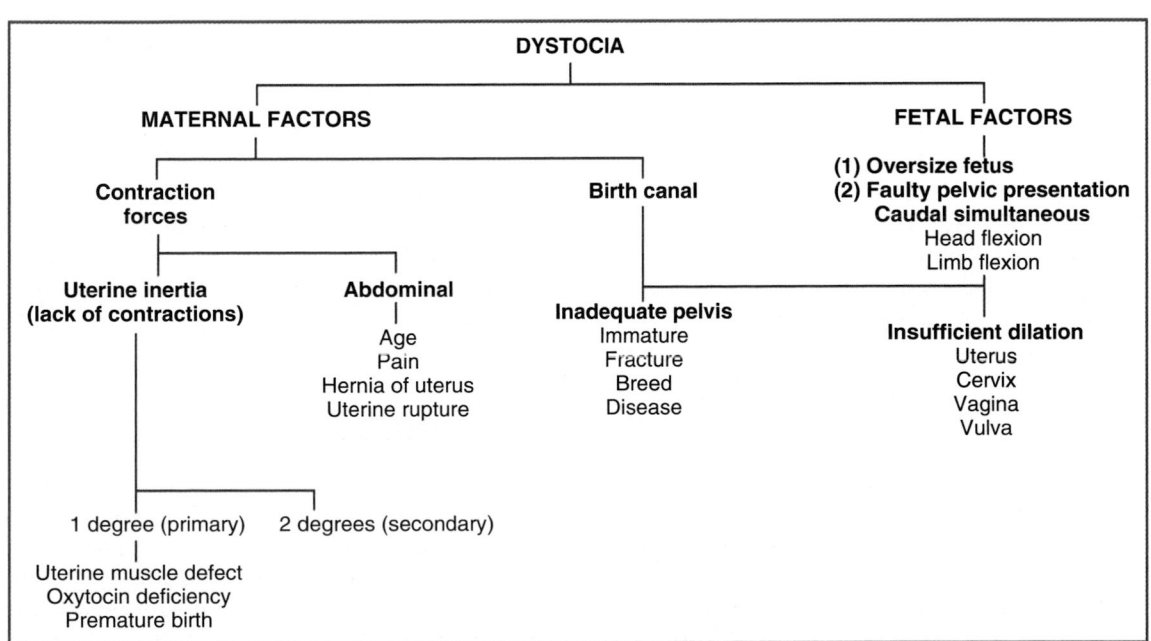

Figure 24-32 Common causes of dystocia.

The anesthetic regimen is of prime importance when considering cesarean delivery. The dam that is dehydrated and exhausted with potential metabolic abnormalities from a prolonged attempted delivery is a poor anesthetic candidate. Anesthetic complications may be encountered. The selected agents should have minimal effects on the newborn. A detailed discussion of anesthetic regimens for the dystocia patient is given in Chapter 19.

TECHNIQUE AND INTRAOPERATIVE CONSIDERATIONS

The patient is clipped *before* anesthesia. After anesthetic induction and maintenance, the dam is placed in dorsal recumbency. It is important to remember that the increased weight of the gravid uterus on the diaphragm may compromise the normal breathing capacity of the dam and intermittent manual respiration or a respirator should be considered.

✎ TECHNICIAN NOTE

It is important to do as much preoperative preparation in lateral recumbency as possible and then place the patient in dorsal recumbency just before the surgical preparation.

A ventral midline celiotomy is performed (Figure 24-18). The uterus is exteriorized and isolated with moistened surgical towels. Uterine isolation helps prevent the uterine contents from entering the abdominal cavity. An incision is made into the ventral aspect of the uterine body. Care is taken not to cut a fetus. A neonate and its associated fetal membranes are advanced through the uterine incision by applying gentle traction and pressure on the uterine wall. On presentation, the fetal membranes are removed, the umbilicus is clamped or ligated, and the neonate is handed to the assistant. The fetal membranes can be firmly attached to the uterus if the fetus was not to full term. Severe hemorrhage can result if the membranes are pulled from the uterus under those circumstances. Each successive neonate is handled in a similar fashion until all are delivered. The birth canal is checked carefully before closure to ensure that a fetus is not wedged there. The uterine incision is closed in two layers. The abdominal cavity is flushed to remove any debris that might have leaked into it from the gravid uterus. The celiotomy incision is closed in a routine fashion. The skin should be closed internally with an absorbable suture to prevent premature removal by the puppies or kittens during nursing.

Some owners prefer that the dam be spayed at the time of cesarean delivery. This can be accomplished in two ways. An en bloc removal of the gravid uterus can be performed. This entails clamping both ovarian pedicles and the uterine body, cutting the gravid uterus out of the dam, then going back and ligating all the vasculature in the dam. The gravid uterus is given to an assistant and the assistant cuts each neonate carefully from the uterus using sterile instruments and ligates or clamps the umbilicus. The neonates are then treated as previously described. The second method allows a formal cesarean delivery as already described followed by a routine ovariohysterectomy after uterine body closure. The technique chosen by the surgeon depends and preference and assistance available to care for the neonates. There is not a proven benefit or downfall to either technique if performed appropriately. Removal of the uterus and ovaries at the time of neonate delivery does not affect milk production or motherly instincts. Alternatively, the dam can be returned for ovariohysterectomy after the neonates are weaned.

POSTOPERATIVE CONSIDERATIONS FOR THE NEONATE

The assistant should be ready to grasp the neonate from the surgeon and immediately place it in a dry towel. The assistant can then massage the animal gently to stimulate respiration, dry any secretions around the mouth and nose, and dry the remainder of the body to decrease the chance of hypothermia. The mouth should be inspected for evidence of mucus that may be plugging the airway. Gentle suction of the nostrils or mouth may be necessary to remove debris. If the mouth and nostrils are clogged with mucus and suction does not remove the debris, the neonate can be cradled in the palm of the right hand while the left hand stabilizes the animal; it is then swung smartly downward in an arc, which removes any fluid by centrifugal force. The head should be firmly supported during this maneuver to prevent excess motion and cervical damage. Weak neonates or those with faint respirations may be stimulated by placing doxapram (a respiratory stimulant) under the tongue. A thorough examination for congenital defects is made, and the neonate is placed in an incubator or warm, padded area. Neonates stressed from the prolonged attempted delivery may not survive or may already be dead by the time cesarean is attempted.

The neonates should be returned to the dam as soon as she has recovered from anesthesia. Care should be taken not to return them so early that the dam may unknowingly harm them by stepping or lying on them. The dam should be returned to her home environment as soon as possible so that she can begin caring for the neonates and to prevent transmission of hospital organisms to the immune-challenged neonates.

POSTOPERATIVE CONSIDERATIONS FOR THE DAM

The dam should be awakened from anesthesia as soon as possible so that the neonates can begin nursing. The mother and neonates should be monitored carefully as the two are introduced. Most dams will accept the young readily, but some may be aggressive. If the dam appears painful, pain medication should be considered. It must be remembered that all systemically administered pain medications will be delivered to the neonates through the milk; therefore dosing should be low. Epidural drug administration prior to surgery will minimize the need for pain medication and transmission of these drugs to the neonate (see anesthetic management of cesarean delivery under the anesthesia section). Other considerations include the development of metritis secondary to retained fetal membranes or infection, excessive uterine hemorrhage from overzealous fetal membrane removal, and all the potential complications discussed for routine celiotomy or ovariohysterectomy, if that was performed at the same time. Some dogs may experience infertility after cesarean delivery due to scar tissue formation.

CYSTOTOMY

DEFINITION

Cystotomy means incision into the urinary bladder to expose the lumen or interior of the urinary bladder.

INDICATIONS

The most common indication for cystotomy in small animals is for removal of cystic calculi (bladder stones). A cystotomy is also indicated to remove tumors, to correct congenital defects, or to repair traumatic rupture of the urinary bladder. A final indication for cystotomy is placement of a cystostomy tube (a tube exiting the urinary bladder and abdominal wall) to provide an alternate outlet of urine in the case of tumor, calculi, or scar tissue causing obstruction of urine flow through the urethra.

PREOPERATIVE CONSIDERATIONS

Animals undergo cystotomy for various reasons. If urinary flow was obstructed, then stabilization of the patient prior to anesthesia and surgery should be performed. Severe metabolic and/or electrolyte abnormalities might exist. Imaging studies may be necessary to identify the extent of disease and its exact location.

TECHNIQUE AND INTRAOPERATIVE CONSIDERATIONS

The abdomen is widely clipped from the xiphoid to the pubis. In male dogs, care is taken to clip the hair from the prepuce. The preputial orifice and penis are then gently flushed with a 1% povidone-iodine (Betadine) solution (Figure 24-33).

The animal is placed in dorsal recumbency and prepared for surgery with a standard skin preparation. In male patients, the abdominal skin incision will curve laterally to avoid the prepuce (Figure 24-18, *D*). Care should be taken to thoroughly prepare this area aseptically. The prepuce is draped into the surgical field in the case of urinary calculi removal. This allows placement of a urinary catheter

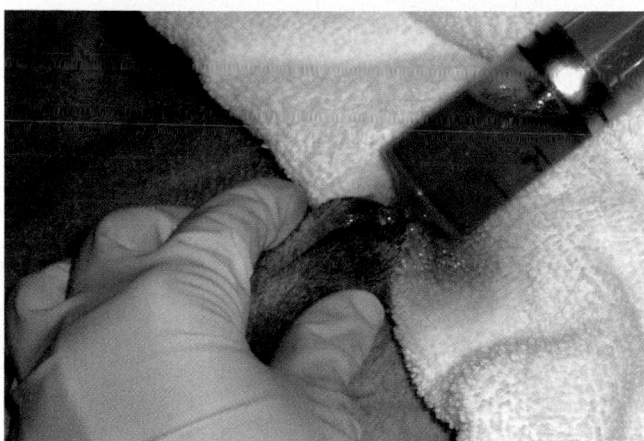

Figure 24-33 Proper technique for flushing the prepuce.

through the urethra for urethra flushing to aid in calculi removal. Although it is more common for urinary stones to lodge in the urethra of the male, a urethral catheter should also be passed in the female, because urethral calculi have been reported. The urinary catheter in the female dog should be placed aseptically prior to surgery. Care should be taken if bladder expression is attempted prior to celiotomy since an outflow obstruction due to tumor, calculi, or scar tissue may result in inadvertent bladder rupture. Bladder expression should be avoided in those cases or when urinary bladder wall fragility is expected, urinary flow obstruction or tumor, for example.

In the female, a standard caudal midline celiotomy is performed (Figure 24-18, *A*). In the male, a caudal midline skin incision is made from the umbilicus to the sheath of the penis and is then extended lateral to the sheath. The caudal superficial epigastric artery and vein lateral to the prepuce are encountered. These are ligated and transected. The sheath is retracted laterally, and a ventral midline celiotomy is performed. The bladder is exteriorized and packed off with laparotomy pads to preclude urine spillage into the abdominal cavity. If a urinalysis and urine culture were not obtained prior to surgery, a syringe and needle are used to obtain a urine sample prior to cystotomy. An avascular area on the ventral aspect of the bladder is visualized and two stay sutures placed along the intended incision line. An incision is made along the proposed incision line between preplaced stay sutures. If cystic calculi are present, they are removed and submitted for stone analysis. If biopsies are taken for a suspected tumor, samples are placed in formalin and submitted for histological analysis. Since calculi can lodge in the urethra, after removal, the entire lower urinary tract (bladder to urethra) is flushed with sterile physiologic saline solution until all calculi have been removed. The bladder wall is inspected for abnormalities and is then closed with a simple interrupted or inverting suture pattern. The laparotomy pads are removed, the abdomen is lavaged with sterile physiologic saline solution, and the incision is closed in a routine fashion.

In the case of calculi, a postoperative imaging study may be necessary to determine if all the calculi were actually removed.

POSTOPERATIVE CONSIDERATIONS

The animal should be placed on intravenous fluids after cystotomy to help dilute blood clots and flush the urinary bladder. Urine production should be carefully monitored. If the incision was close to or involved the proximal urethra, postoperative swelling can obstruct urine flow. The veterinarian in charge should be alerted if the animal is straining to urinate and does not produce a urine stream or has not produced urine in 12 hours. Some straining to urinate can be expected following cystotomy due to swelling and bladder irritation, but a urine stream should accompany the straining, and the bladder should be nearly empty afterwards. During the first 48 to 72 hours postoperative, a mild hematuria (bloody urine) with or without blood clots and frequent urination can be expected. Owners should be informed of this if the patient is released during this time.

✐ TECHNICIAN NOTE

During the first 48 to 72 hours following a cystotomy, a mild hematuria with or without blood clots and frequent urination can be expected.

Treatment ultimately depends on urinalysis, urine culture and the type of disease present (type of calculi, type of tumor, type of congenital defect). If cystic calculi were removed, stone analysis must be performed before an appropriate treatment regimen can be initiated. Therapy will likely involve dietary alterations and/or antibiotics. The owners should be informed that calculi recurrence is a possibility and that dietary recommendations should be followed strictly to help decrease that chance.

Postoperative complications are rare following cystotomy. They include urinary outflow obstruction due to swelling, celiotomy incision complications, uroabdomen secondary to urine leakage through the cystotomy incision, and recurrence of the primary problem. If the animal is unable to urinate following cystotomy, a temporary urinary catheter may have to be placed to keep the bladder decompressed until the surgical swelling decreases. This is not done routinely since catheter placement can cause further irritation to the healing cystotomy incision and increases chance of infection. If the animal is not producing urine or is producing minimal urine and abdominal distention is detected, a complete biochemistry panel, complete blood count, and paracentesis should be performed. Fluid taken from the abdomen should be spun for packed cell volume determination and should undergo creatinine and blood urea nitrogen determination. Values higher than serum values indicate a problem and should be reported to the veterinarian in charge. Urine leakage through a cystotomy incision is treated with an indwelling urinary catheter or reoperation and appropriate urinary bladder incision closure.

URETHROSTOMY

DEFINITION

Perineal urethrostomy is the process of making an external opening in the urethra in the area of the perineum that is large enough for passage of urine, mucus, crystals, and small calculi without obstruction. It bypasses the narrow penile urethra where obstruction often occurs. The procedure is performed in male cats with recurrent urethral obstruction secondary to feline urologic syndrome. Urethrostomy are also performed in other locations and are named by their location (scrotal urethrostomy, prescrotal urethrostomy, antepubic urethrostomy, etc.). *Scrotal urethrostomy* rather than perineal urethrostomy is performed in male dogs prone to calculi obstruction or with penile scar tissue preventing normal urination since this location provides the best functional outcome. The general technique is the same.

INDICATIONS

The primary indication for a perineal urethrostomy is multiple episodes of obstruction in association with feline urologic syndrome. Other less common indications include rupture of the penile urethra secondary to traumatic catheterization or blunt trauma (e.g., hit by car, abdominal kick), stricture of the penile urethra, or obstruction secondary to cancer.

PREOPERATIVE CONSIDERATIONS

A cat with feline urologic syndrome can present for examination with an array of clinical findings, as can dogs with urethral obstruction. The presentation often depends on the duration and completeness of the urinary obstruction. A common factor is straining to urinate. If the patient is brought for examination early, there is little chance that other organ systems are affected. If the patient is presented 12 to 24 hours after a complete obstruction, severe electrolyte abnormalities, cardiac arrhythmias, kidney dysfunction, and shock can be present. These patients must have the obstruction removed and be stabilized with establishment of normal renal function before surgery. Obstruction of urine flow is a *true* emergency situation in both cats and dogs.

Depending on the suspected cause and location of the obstruction, preoperative imaging studies will be necessary to determine the exact location and extent of the problem.

TECHNIQUE AND INTRAOPERATIVE CONSIDERATIONS

The hair on the perineum and external genitalia is clipped. For perineal urethrostomy, the cat is placed in ventral recumbency with the perineum elevated approximately 30

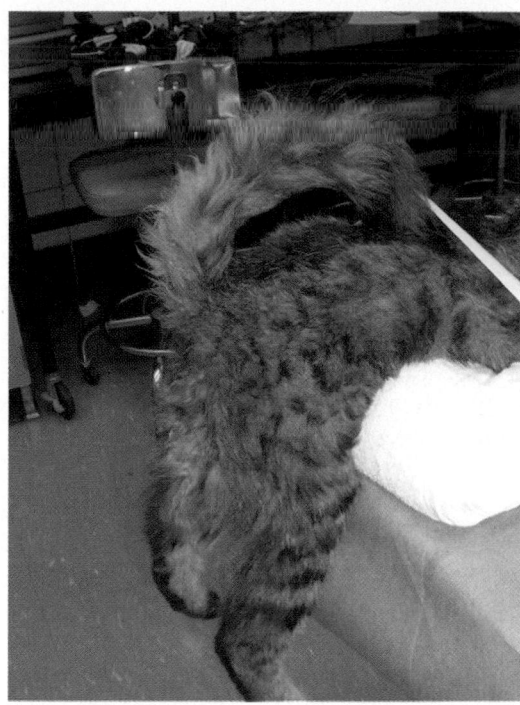

Figure 24-34 The perineal position can be used in the dog or cat.

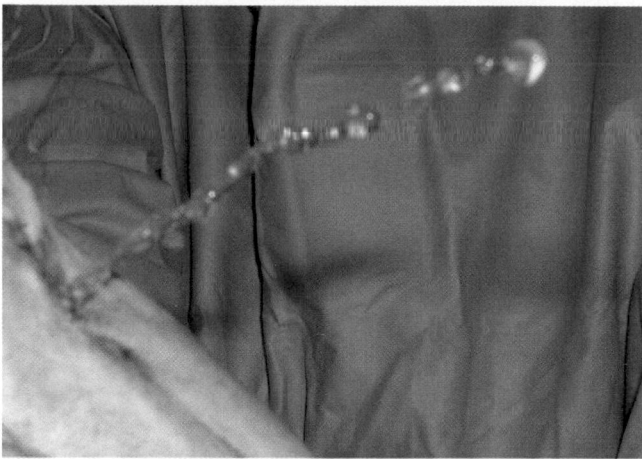

Figure 24-35 After urethrostomy in cats, the bladder should be gently expressed to ensure easy urine passage.

degrees (Figure 24-34). The tail is extended directly over the dorsal midline and immobilized with tape. A purse-string suture is placed in the anus to eliminate fecal contamination of the surgical field. Standard skin preparation is performed. For scrotal urethrostomy in male dogs, the animal is placed in dorsal recumbency, and the area is prepped as for castration and scrotal ablation.

For perineal urethrostomy, an elliptical skin incision is made around the scrotum and prepuce. The testicles are removed if the cat is intact. The penis is dissected free from its pelvic attachments. A catheter is placed in the urethra, and a longitudinal incision is made through the penile urethra extending craniad to the level of the pelvic urethra. The diameter of the pelvic urethra is approximately two times that of the penile urethra. This allows normal urination in the face of crystalluria (sandlike material in the urine) and mucous plugs. The urethral mucosa is sutured to the skin. The remaining portion of the penis is amputated during urethra suturing, and the urinary catheter is removed. This results in a new, permanent opening that will accommodate the excess mucus and crystals. The bladder should be expressed at completion of the procedure to ensure that a good urine stream is obtained (Figure 24-35). Scrotal urethrostomy in male dogs is performed the same way except that the penis is not removed. A skin incision is made in the area of the scrotum (castration with scrotal ablation is performed in intact dogs), followed by a urethral incision over a presurgically placed urethral catheter, and then suturing of the urethral mucosa to the skin as for perineal urethrostomy.

POSTOPERATIVE CONSIDERATIONS

The purse-string suture is removed. Immediate postoperative care includes placement of an Elizabethan collar and examination of the surgical site for evidence of hemorrhage. The Elizabethan collar is essential to keep the animal from licking the sutures. Mild hemorrhage during urination is expected for the first 24 to 72 hours after surgery (this may even continue for a couple weeks postoperative, especially in intact animals undergoing urethrostomy). This is usually of no consequence and will resolve on its own. Rarely is the bleeding severe enough to require additional surgery or transfusion. Animals should be placed on intravenous fluids for at least 24 hours after surgery, especially if urinary outflow obstruction was encountered, to maintain normal renal function and flush the urinary bladder and urethra.

The animal should be monitored carefully for normal urination in the early postoperative period. If no urine is produced for 12 hours after surgery, the bladder should be manually expressed until normal urination is seen. Postoperative catheters are *discouraged* because of the increased incidence of strictures at the surgery site. The urethrostomy site should be manipulated as little as possible. Ointments and warm cleansings are also discouraged. This may delay healing or aggravate hemorrhage. For cats, the use of shredded paper or pellets in the litter box is recommended for the first 7 to 10 days. Dietary alterations will likely be necessary depending on the composition of the mucous plug, grit, or calculi causing the obstruction and the presence or absence of a urinary tract infection. Owners will have to be counseled on the importance of dietary modification.

The most common late postoperative complication is stricture. This is generally manifested by chronic stranguria (straining to urinate). Complete obstruction of urine flow may also be noted. Stricture requires reoperation.

HERNIAS

The strict definition of *hernia* is protrusion of tissue from its normal cavity (generally the abdominal cavity) through a congenital or acquired defect in the wall of that cavity. Some common hernias in the dog and cat are umbilical hernias, inguinal hernias, and diaphragmatic hernias.

UMBILICAL HERNIA

DEFINITION

An *umbilical hernia* is one in which bowel or, more commonly, omentum and intraabdominal fat protrudes through a defect in the abdominal wall under the skin at the umbilicus. This hernia is most commonly congenital, and it is recognized on physical examination by the presence of a swelling at the umbilicus (Figure 24-36).

PREOPERATIVE CONSIDERATIONS

Most umbilical hernias are not life threatening and are surgically repaired at the time of ovariohysterectomy or castration. Very small hernias in young dogs (2 to 4 months of age) may be self-limiting. Larger hernias or those in older dogs (6 to 9 months of age) generally require surgical repair. Large umbilical hernias can result in intestinal entrapment within the confines of the hernia with resultant strangulation (loss of intestinal blood supply with devitalization and possible intestinal perforation). If intestinal strangulation occurs, surgical repair becomes an emergency.

TECHNIQUE AND INTRAOPERATIVE CONSIDERATIONS

The abdomen is widely clipped from xiphoid to pubis. The patient is placed in dorsal recumbency, and a standard skin

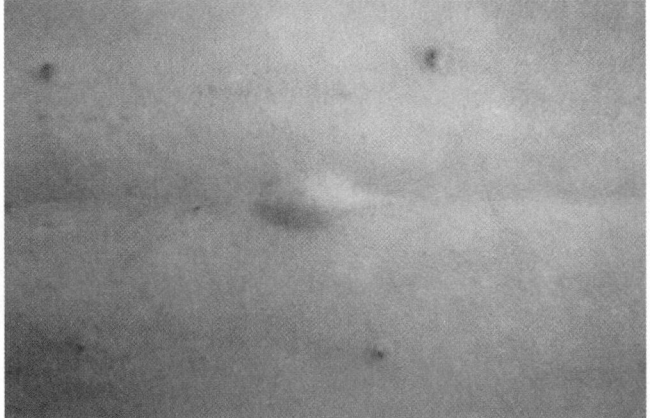

Figure 24-36 Note the raised lesion in the region of the umbilicus (umbilical hernia) on the ventral abdomen.

preparation is performed. A ventral midline incision is made directly over the hernia being careful not to perforate hernia contents. The skin is dissected away from the hernial sac; the contents are then exposed and are either replaced into the abdominal cavity (intestine) or excised (falciform or omental fat). The edges of the hernial ring are trimmed to ensure healing of the defect. The abdomen is closed in a routine fashion as for the celiotomy incision.

POSTOPERATIVE CONSIDERATIONS

Postoperative care is similar to that for any celiotomy incision. Recurrence is a rare complication of repair and reoperation is necessary for correction.

INGUINAL HERNIA

DEFINITION

An *inguinal hernia* is one in which intestine, uterus, broad ligament, intraabdominal fat, and/or another abdominal organ protrudes through the inguinal canal due to a defect in the constraints of the canal. This is more common in the bitch than in the male dog. An inguinal hernia is diagnosed on physical examination by the presence of a soft, doughy, nonpainful mass in the inguinal region. Inguinal hernias can develop early or late in life. It does not spontaneously regress, and surgical correction is necessary.

PREOPERATIVE CONSIDERATIONS

The opposite inguinal ring should be carefully palpated for weakness. Owners should be told that hernias can develop bilaterally even if a hernia is not present on the opposite side at the time of presentation. Owners should also be told that recurrence is rare, but possible.

TECHNIQUE AND INTRAOPERATIVE CONSIDERATIONS

The abdomen is widely clipped from the umbilicus to and including the inguinal area. The patient is placed in dorsal recumbency, and a standard skin preparation is performed. A midline skin incision is made in the caudal abdomen between the inguinal folds. The abdominal cavity is not entered. Lateral dissection is performed carefully to expose the affected inguinal ring with its hernial sac and external pudendal vessels. The hernial sac is emptied of its contents with gentle manipulation and pressure toward the abdominal cavity. The empty sac is then excised and sutured along with the margin of the inguinal ring. Care is taken during closure to avoid the external pudendal vessels that exit from the caudal medial aspect of the ring. The skin incision is closed as for celiotomy.

POSTOPERATIVE CONSIDERATIONS

The incision is monitored as any abdominal incision. The owner should monitor for recurrence or occurrence on the opposite side.

DIAPHRAGMATIC HERNIA

DEFINITION

A *diaphragmatic hernia* exists when abdominal contents protrude through an opening in the diaphragm into the thoracic cavity. Diaphragmatic hernias may be congenital or traumatic.

PREOPERATIVE CONSIDERATIONS

Any animal with a history of trauma or suspected trauma should be examined for presence of a diaphragmatic hernia. Diaphragmatic hernias can be life threatening or insidious and difficult to identify. Signs can also be masked by other problems. Presumptive diagnosis is based on a thorough physical examination. The classic signs of diaphragmatic hernia are a "tucked-up" abdomen (thin/empty abdomen), intestinal sounds in the chest, muffled heart and lung sounds, and dyspnea. However, some animals only have decreased lung sounds over the area of the hernia and mild exercise intolerance, if that. The diagnosis is confirmed by a thoracic radiograph.

An animal with a massive hernia will have a diminished intrathoracic space due to presence of abdominal contents within the thoracic cavity. The resultant space occupying mass does not allow the lungs to expand normally and compromises oxygen delivery to the blood. These animals can have life-threatening respiratory compromise and should be treated appropriately. Once the diagnosis of diaphragmatic hernia has been made, the animal should be stabilized. This includes *minimal* stress, oxygen cage or nasal oxygen insufflation, confinement, and constant monitoring for respiratory insufficiency or arrest. Sometimes holding the animal gently and with the head up and the rear legs hanging down will allow some abdominal contents to shift back into the abdomen. Along the same lines, the animal can be propped up such that the front half of the chest and shoulders are higher than the hindquarters. Intravenous access should be established in case of an emergency so long as the stress of catheter placement does not cause further respiratory embarrassment. Rarely is diaphragmatic hernia

---

TECHNICIAN NOTE

Diaphragmatic hernia patients should have oxygen and cage confinement to allow maximal oxygenation, minimal stress, and constant monitoring for respiratory insufficiency before surgery.

---

repair an emergency. Mortality is actually higher in those animals operated acutely for the problem. Only in cases of massive hernia with severe respiratory distress or severe gas distention of a herniated viscous (stomach) is immediate operation necessary.

TECHNIQUE AND INTRAOPERATIVE CONSIDERATIONS

One of the most critical time periods for an animal with a diaphragmatic hernia is anesthetic induction. It is very important to be thoroughly familiar with induction procedures as well as resuscitative techniques in the event of respiratory or cardiac arrest. The animal is placed in dorsal recumbency on an incline, with the head slightly higher than the hindquarters. It is important to remember that severe respiratory compromise may result when the animal is placed in dorsal recumbency and the technician should be prepared to breathe for the animal. Mechanical ventilation or intermittent manual respiration will be necessary throughout the procedure.

The skin is widely clipped from about 3 inches cranial to the xiphoid to the pubis. The lateral thoracic wall on at least one side, preferably the side of the hernia, should be clipped and aseptically prepared for potential chest tube placement. A ventral midline celiotomy from xiphoid to umbilicus is performed. The edges of the incision are protected with laparotomy pads, and a Balfour self-retaining abdominal retractor is placed to enhance visualization. The diaphragmatic defect is inspected, and any herniated contents are gently reduced into the abdominal cavity. If the herniated contents do not reduce easy, then the diaphragmatic defect is enlarged slightly to allow easy reduction. A thorough inspection of abdominal and thoracic viscera is made to rule out organ rupture or vascular compromise.

Diaphragmatic hernia repair requires working in a deep cavity. Gentle retraction of viscera to expose the defect during repair is necessary to preclude damage to abdominal organs to allow adequate visualization by the surgeon. The diaphragmatic defect is sutured with a nonabsorbable suture material in a simple continuous suture pattern. This will affect an air-tight and watertight seal. Air is evacuated from the chest by thoracocentesis through the diaphragm or with chest tube placement. The celiotomy is closed in a routine fashion. After celiotomy closure the chest cavity is once again aspirated from the lateral thoracic wall. If a chest tube was placed, evacuation of the thoracic cavity occurs through the chest tube.

POSTOPERATIVE CONSIDERATIONS

The patient should be monitored carefully for signs of respiratory distress. It is best to waken these animals with oxygen supplementation either through placement in an oxygen cage or through nasal insufflation. If a pulse oximeter is available, oxygen saturation should be checked frequently, especially as an attempt is made to wean the animal off oxygen. If dyspnea occurs or the animal cannot maintain normal oxygen saturation, the chest should be evacuated with a hypodermic needle, three-way stopcock, and a large syringe or through the chest tube. A rapid return to normal negative thoracic pressure and normal lung capacity should occur with evacuation of air and fluid.

If an indwelling chest tube was placed, periodic aspiration using positional changes (right lateral recumbency, left lateral recumbency, standing on hind legs, standing on front legs) will afford maximal removal of air and fluid. It is of utmost importance to keep the patient from chewing a hole in the drain or removing it from the chest cavity, and those involved in tube management should be informed on how the tube should be handled. An Elizabethan collar may be necessary and the chest tube should be covered with a bandage. It is also imperative to keep all connections on the chest drain air tight. A security clamp should be placed on the tube to keep air from leaking into the chest if the free end of the tube is inadvertently opened. Premature removal, puncture, or inappropriate management (leaving the three-way stopcock open to the atmosphere) can result in acute animal death secondary to pneumothorax and resultant pulmonary dysfunction. Proper management of a chest tube requires full-time patient monitoring. A chart quantitating the amount of air and fluid removed during a given period of time (12 to 24 hours) will help to determine when the tube should be removed. Most chest tubes are removed immediately following surgery once negative intrathoracic pressure is obtained or within 12 hours of hernia repair. Otherwise, the tube can safely be removed as the amount of air and fluid decreases toward zero.

LUMPECTOMY

DEFINITION

Lumpectomy refers to local surgical resection of a mass. The term often refers to cutaneous or subcutaneous masses.

INDICATIONS

Indications for lumpectomy include masses of cancerous origin, rapidly growing masses or masses that appear to be changing, ulcerative masses, nonhealing wounds, or masses that are impairing function.

PREOPERATIVE CONSIDERATIONS

Some masses are related to biochemical or blood cell alterations. Blood work should be performed to evaluate for these abnormalities. Abnormalities should be corrected prior to anesthesia if possible. Additionally, many animals undergoing surgery for mass resection are older and may have organ system failure, which should be evaluated before anesthesia. After a mass is diagnosed, fine needle aspirate of the mass is performed. If the mass is considered benign (i.e., lipoma), then resection can proceed or the owner can monitor the mass. If changes in the mass are noted, resection should be considered. If the mass appears cancerous, further workup for detection of metastasis should be considered and resection is strongly recommended. All surgically resected masses should be submitted for histologic evaluation. Removed masses are placed in formalin at a 1:10 ratio of mass to fluid.

TECHNIQUE AND INTRAOPERATIVE CONSIDERATIONS

The skin around the area to be resected is prepared for surgery. It should be remembered that a generous clip needs to be performed since normal margins will need to be removed with the mass. Additionally, large mass resections will require that normal skin around the mass be pulled into the surgical field during closure. If this skin was not prepared aseptically prior to surgery, it will contaminate the surgical field. Masses should be manipulated as little as possible prior to surgery. A sterile marker is used to draw an elliptical pattern around the mass to be removed. One to 3 cm of normal tissue is included in the resection plane with large margins being reserved for cancerous lesions. The mass is removed and the wound closed in three layers with absorbable suture placed internally. The mass is marked with ink or suture to note cranial and lateral margins. This will help future surgical planning if the mass was found to be incompletely resected according to histologic evaluation.

POSTOPERATIVE CONSIDERATIONS

The surgical wound should be monitored as any other surgical procedure. Large resections will result in tension on the incision line making dehiscence more likely. Animals should be exercise restricted until the wound is healed and sutures are removed. Owners should be told that further steps for treatment may need to be taken once a diagnosis is obtained (future surgery if complete resection was not obtained, chemotherapy, radiation therapy, etc.).

REMOVAL OF MAMMARY NEOPLASIA

DEFINITION

Mammary neoplasia is cancer of the mammary gland. It is the most frequently occurring neoplasm in the female dog and the third most frequently found tumors in the female cat. *Mastectomy* is removal of a mammary gland. *Radical mastectomy* is removal of a chain of mammary glands on one or both sides of the animal. *Lumpectomy* is removal of a mammary tumor with approximately 1 cm of normal marginal tissue, not the entire mammary gland.

GENERAL INFORMATION AND INDICATIONS

In dogs there is a significantly higher incidence of mammary gland tumors in nonspayed females or females that are spayed after their first estrus. Spaying before the first estrus cycle provides a definite protective factor against mammary tumor development.

In the initial stages, the tumor will usually appear as a small, pea-shaped, firm mass in one or more of the glands of the mammary chain. Long-standing or fast-growing tumors may present a sizeable mass with ulceration and drainage. Early diagnosis and therapy is best when dealing with mammary neoplasia.

Before surgery is considered, an examination for possible metastasis of the tumor is done. Malignant tumors will generally metastasize to the lymph nodes and lungs. Chest radiographs may detect pulmonary metastases, and abdominal radiographs may show iliac lymph node enlargement suggestive of metastasis. About 50% of mammary tumors in dogs are malignant, and about 80% to 90% of mammary tumors in cats are malignant. Surgical resection of tumors that have already metastasized does not improve prognosis. At the time of surgery, biopsy of regional lymph nodes should always be performed.

Surgery is currently considered the most effective therapy. The primary objective of surgical treatment is to remove completely the tumor tissue for potential cure and to obtain a histologic diagnosis of tumor type and behavior.

TECHNIQUE AND INTRAOPERATIVE CONSIDERATIONS

Two techniques are available for tumor resection. In dogs there appears to be no advantage to radical gland resection verses lumpectomy unless the tumor is incompletely excised. Lumpectomy affords the same long-term outcome as varying forms of mastectomy as long as the tumor is freely movable, small, and on the periphery of the gland. If the tumor is centralized within a gland, multiple tumors are present within a gland or a chain of glands, or the tumor is large and/or fixed, a more radical excision is warranted. Unlike in dogs, in cats recurrence is decreased if unilateral mastectomy is performed rather than local excision of the mass. If bilateral radical mastectomy is necessary, the procedure must be staged (removal of one side at a time) to allow less tension on the skin closure. The skin is clipped widely to include all affected mammary glands. The patient is placed in dorsal recumbency, and a standard skin preparation is performed. An elliptical incision is made, attempting to include a 1-cm margin around the tumor. The skin and tumor, with or without the mammary gland, are gently undermined and removed. The skin incision is often gaping after tumor excision if an entire gland is removed, requiring a meticulous subcutaneous closure. Subcutaneous tissues are closed with a simple interrupted pattern using absorbable suture material. An active drain may be placed if a large

amount of tissue is removed to help prevent fluid accumulation under the skin. The skin is closed in a routine fashion. The excised mammary masses are placed in formalin and sent to a laboratory for histopathologic evaluation.

POSTOPERATIVE CONSIDERATIONS

Major complications that can occur postoperatively are generally related to the tension placed on the skin to adequately close the wound when large amounts of tissue are removed. Seroma formation is common, especially if a drain was not placed at the time of surgery. It is best to bandage these patients for 48 to 72 hours postoperative to help prevent large amounts of fluid from accumulating under the incision and to make the animal more comfortable. Warm compresses may be needed after seroma development. Dehiscence is not common, but the incision should be examined daily for evidence of separation, especially if a large amount of tissue is removed. Bruising along the incision edges is common and should be expected. Immediate postoperative hemorrhage can occur. In the event of oozing blood, an abdominal bandage should be applied with gentle pressure. If a drain was placed, then a bandage should be placed over the drain. The drain is emptied several times a day and is removed when minimal drainage is noted. If the animal irritates the incision by licking, an Elizabethan collar should be applied until suture removal. An Elizabethan collar should be applied as long as a drain is in place to prevent self-inflicted pulling or breaking of the drain. The animal should be exercise restricted, especially if a large incision under tension is present, to help prevent dehiscence and seroma formation. Radical mastectomy is a painful procedure, and pain management should be continued for at least 5 days postoperative.

AMPUTATION

DEFINITION

Amputation refers to partial or complete removal of a body part such as a limb or a toe. This section covers limb amputation.

INDICATIONS

Indications for amputation include appendicular cancer not amendable to local excision or other treatment modality (amputation may be curative or may be done as palliative therapy in some instances), severe neurologic dysfunction resulting in repeated trauma of a limb, nonunion fractures that will not result in limb function with orthopedic repair, irresolvable osteomyelitis, vascular disease of the limb such as thrombosis or arteriovenous fistulas, and congenital deformity resulting in a nonfunctional limb not amendable to orthopedic repair. Simple limb fracture is not an indication for amputation, although some veterinarians may perform the procedure for that problem.

PREOPERATIVE CONSIDERATIONS

Amputation can involve considerable blood loss. It is important to perform presurgical blood work to determine PCV and TP. Transfusion should be given or anticipated depending on the animal's preoperative values. Additionally, coagulation times should be assessed. A thorough orthopedic examination should be done to evaluate the dog for any concurrent orthopedic problems. The owner needs to be aware of other orthopedic conditions that are diagnosed and how they may affect function following amputation. Orthopedic problems in other limbs can make ambulation after amputation difficult depending on the severity and type of problem. The owner should also be made aware of neurologic problems affecting other limbs. This too can lead to difficult ambulation after amputation. When amputation is done because of neoplasia, the animal should be screened appropriately for metastasis. The amputation must be planned such that adequate margins of normal tissue are obtained if cancer is involved. Amputation is a very painful procedure and analgesics are best initiated before surgery and continued without interruption in the postoperative period.

For rear limb amputations with disarticulation of the coxofemoral joint in intact male dogs, scrotal swelling is a major concern. Seroma formation after amputation is common and fluid tends to accumulate in the scrotum. Scrotal swelling can become so severe that ablation is necessary. Additionally, the scrotum is more visible after amputation and may not be aesthetically pleasing to some owners. It is best to perform a scrotal ablation and castration at the time of amputation in these dogs.

TECHNIQUE AND PERIOPERATIVE CONSIDERATIONS

The limb is suspended from an intravenous (IV) stand as for an orthopedic procedure. The limb is clipped and aseptically prepared for surgery. The clip should be generous and include the skin around the base of the limb to prevent contamination during closure. In general, a skin incision is made around the limb in the area to be amputated. Subcutaneous and muscle tissue are dissected and transected to remove the limb. Vessels are ligated and transected and nerves are blocked with local anesthetic and then transected. Depending on the site of amputation, the limb may need to be disarticulated or the bone severed in order to remove the limb. The remaining muscle and subcutaneous tissue are closed over the bone and/or wound bed. The skin is closed in three layers. If a large amount of dead space is present at the time of closure, a closed, active drain can be placed.

Thoracic limb amputation can be done by removing the scapula and the entire forelimb (forequarter amputation), disarticulation of the scapulohumeral joint, or by ostectomy (cutting of the bone) at the level of the proximal humerus. Forequarter amputation offers the advantages that the major vessels and nerves are well visualized, sectioning the bone is not required, and the prominent scapular spine will not be present as the scapular muscle mass atrophies. It is also indicated in neoplastic diseases of the humerus (especially proximal) or of the scapula. Disarticulation leaves a more full appearance to the thorax and requires less extensive dissection, but muscle atrophy over the scapula can be unsightly in some cases. If disarticulation is performed, the acromion process should be excised to improve appearance. Proximal humeral amputation may be faster for some.

Pelvic limb amputation can be accomplished by disarticulation of the coxofemoral joint or proximal femoral osteotomy. Proximal femoral osteotomy yields a more cosmetic result particularly in an intact male dog. It is also faster and easier than disarticulation. However, the remaining stump will move as the animal ambulates, and the owners must be made aware of this. Neoplastic diseases of the femur will require disarticulation to obtain a normal margin of tissue.

POSTOPERATIVE CONSIDERATIONS

Postoperative complications are not a major concern but should not be ignored. Animals undergoing amputation are painful and analgesics must be given. It is best to give analgesics as schedule doses rather than on an "as needed" basis. Analgesics will likely be required for 4 to 5 days after surgery.

Seroma formation is common. The area can be cold compressed for the first 24 hours after surgery, and then if a seroma forms, warm compresses can be initiated. The limb should be bandaged for the first 24 to 48 hours if possible. This will provide some comfort for the animal and help minimize seroma formation. The animal should be exercise restricted since motion will increase seroma size. Hematoma is also a possibility.

Seroma or hematoma formation after surgery can increase the chance of infection. If infection develops, the incision site will have to be opened, drained, and a culture and sensitivity obtained. Anemia can occur in the postoperative period due to blood loss at the time of surgery. Transfusion may be necessary. Intravenous fluids should be administered postoperative until eating and drinking resumes. Additionally, the animals should be kept in a well-padded area and be supported when being taken out for a walk. Tension on the incision line, seroma formation, or infection may lead to dehiscence. Depending on the cause and degree of dehiscence, this is managed conservatively or with surgical closure. Animals with neoplasia may develop metastatic disease or have tumor recurrence at the surgery site.

Amputation is generally more traumatic to the owner than their pet. Three-legged dogs and cats are excellent pets, and it is important to help the owner understand that. Most animals are ambulating within 24 hours of surgery, but some may take another day. Almost all are ambulatory within 2 days of surgery. Animals should be kept in the hospital until they are ambulating and their pain seems well controlled. Amputees have an excellent prognosis unless the limb was amputated for neoplastic disease. For neoplasia, the prognosis depends on the tumor type. Most owners are satisfied regardless of the reason for amputation, the age, breed, or weight of the animals, or the animal's survival time after surgery.

NEUROLOGIC PATIENT CARE

The most common neurologic disorder in the dog is spontaneous intervertebral disk disease. Disks are normally found between vertebral bodies in the spine and act as shock absorbers during spinal movements. With time, the disks can undergo degeneration and calcification. When this occurs, the normal shock-absorber-like effect is impaired, and extrusion (rupture) of the disk material into the spinal canal can occur. This puts pressure on the spinal cord and can cause an array of neurologic deficits or pain. Other neurologic disorders that may be encountered include atlantoaxial subluxation in toy breeds (abnormal articulation between the first and second cervical vertebra), acute spinal trauma (fracture, luxation), cauda equina (compression of the lumbosacral nerve roots), and cervical spinal cord malformation. Many animals with neurological problems are referred to specialty hospitals for surgery. However, the veterinary technician should be familiar with some of the procedures that might be performed and understand how to manage neurologic patients in general so that when they return to the veterinary hospital for care after surgery, the technician understands what to do.

One neurosurgical procedure occasionally performed in small animal practice is *intervertebral disk fenestration*. In this procedure each disk that is calcified or that may become calcified is removed (scraped) from the intervertebral space. This procedure is performed under some circumstances to help deter rupture of the disk material into the spinal canal, although its benefit is unproven. Dogs may develop spontaneous intervertebral disk extrusions in the cervical spine (neck) or the thoracolumbar spine (lower back). If the disk has already ruptured, a *decompressive* procedure must be performed to alleviate compression on the spinal cord. The most common decompressive procedures are the ventral slot (for cervical disk rupture) and hemilaminectomy or dorsal laminectomy (for thoracolumbar disk rupture). For acute disk herniation, the most commonly affected breed is the dachshund, but the beagle, Pekinese, poodle, and terrier breeds also frequently experience disk herniation.

SURGICAL TECHNIQUE AND PERIOPERATIVE CONSIDERATIONS

When an animal with substantial spinal column instability is anesthetized, the normal protective abilities of muscle support and conscious perception of pain are removed. Conditions that can result in substantial instability include spinal fracture/luxation and atlantoaxial instability. Animals with simple disk herniation or spinal malformation can also be worsened by excessive manipulation while under anesthesia. It is the responsibility of the veterinary technician, anesthesiologist, and surgeon to protect the animal from further neurologic damage by handling the spine with care while under anesthesia. It is important to keep the neck and back as straight as possible when moving the patient from one location to another. To accomplish this, the patient can be taped to a rigid, flat surface, can be carefully cradled in the arm, or placed in a stiff blanket sling supported on all sides. No matter how they are carried, one should be careful to avoid manipulation of the affected area. The means of transportation is often dictated by the size of the patient, but a rigid, flat surface is the preferred method for transporting patients with severe instability.

Patients undergoing cervical disk surgery are placed in dorsal recumbency with the head and neck in slight extension (Figure 24-37). The ventral aspect of the neck is widely clipped from the manubrium sterni to the cranial aspect of the larynx. A standard skin preparation is performed. A ventral midline incision is made through the skin and muscles to expose the intervertebral spaces. For fenestration, a dental tartar scraper, curved needle, fenestration hook, or curette can be used to remove the disk material from the interspace. Fenestration is carried out from the C2-3 to the C6-7 disk space. If decompression is needed, an oblong slot is made through the vertebral bodies into the spinal canal using a pneumatic or electric-powered burr. The disk material is then carefully removed from the spinal canal. A fat graft is placed over the spinal cord in the defect to prevent restrictive scar formation. The surgical wound is

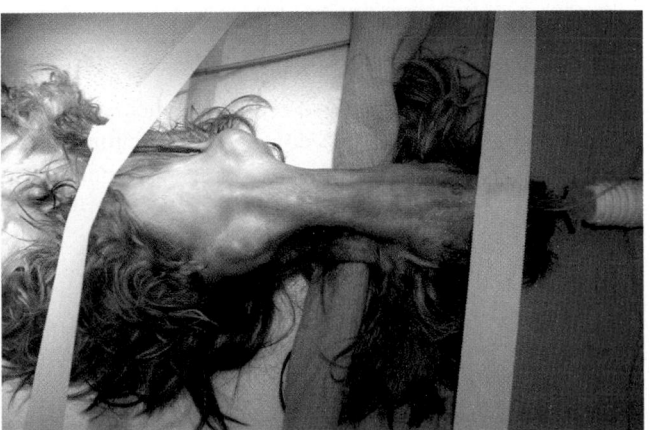

Figure 24-37 Proper positioning for cervical disk surgery.

closed in layers with a continuous suture pattern using an absorbable suture. The skin is closed in a routine fashion.

Animals undergoing thoracolumbar disk surgery are placed in ventral recumbency. For fenestration, the dorsum over the back is widely clipped from the midthoracic region to the pelvis. A standard skin preparation is performed. A skin incision is made from T11 to L6. Careful dissection between epaxial muscles (muscles of the back) allows palpation and limited visualization of the disk spaces. For fenestration, each space between T10 and L5 is curetted with a technique similar to that described for cervical disk fenestration. If decompression is needed, a portion of the bony lamina covering the spinal cord is removed with a pneumatic or electric-powered burr or bone rongeurs. The ruptured disk material is then carefully removed from the spinal canal. A fat graft is placed in the defect over the spinal cord. The muscles, subcutaneous tissue, and skin are closed in a routine fashion.

POSTOPERATIVE CONSIDERATIONS

The preoperative and postoperative care of neurologic patients depends on their neurologic status and the type of neurologic disease they have. Management for the non-ambulatory animal is demanding. These patients are subject to decubital ulcers (bed sores or pressure sores), urinary bladder infections, joint stiffness, muscle atrophy (muscle wasting), pneumonia, and gastrointestinal ulceration. Preventing these conditions from occurring is the main objective of proper postoperative management and should include the following:

- Passive range-of-motion exercises, muscle massages, and whirlpool baths encourage joint motion and muscular activity and help decrease chance of pressure sore formation. Passive range of motion should be performed at least three times a day until the animal is able to ambulate normally.
- Urinary bladder expression four or five times per day to keep the urinary bladder empty. This might lower the incidence of infection due to urine retention, help keep the animal clean, and prevent detrusor muscle atony secondary to bladder overdistention.
- Turn the patient frequently to reduce the incidence of pneumonia and to help prevent pressure sore formation. Slings and wheel chairs can be used to get the animals up and off pressure points for a period of time if their spinal injury is stable.
- Keep the patient well padded to prevent the formation of sores. A waterbed mattress works well for large dogs.
- Keep the animal clean and dry. Soiling will increase the chance of pressure-sore formation. This can be challenging when incontinence and immobility play a role.
- Observe of the stool for evidence of fresh blood (bright red on feces) or digested blood (dark, tarry feces), which

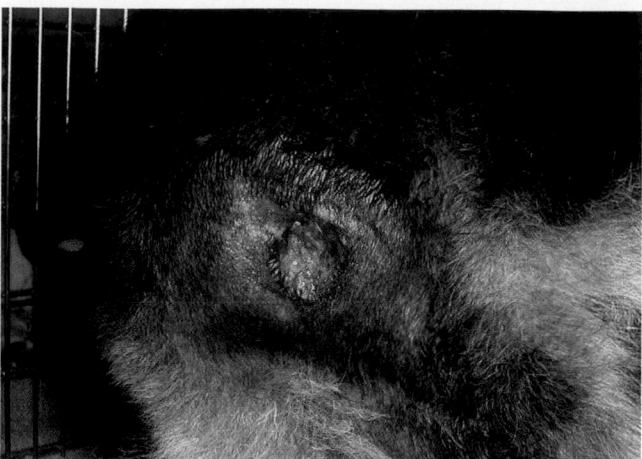

Figure 24-38 Decubital ulcer (pressure sore). The ulcer developed over the greater trochanter of this dog due to improper care during recovery from spinal surgery.

may be an indicator of colonic or gastric ulceration, respectively, following spinal cord injury, hospital stress, and/or steroid therapy
- Observe vomiting. If the vomitus contains coffee-ground-like material, it is indicative of gastric bleeding secondary to ulcer formation.
- Observe these animals daily for evidence of pressure sores. Sores tend to form over bone prominences, especially in large dogs (Figure 24-38). Pressure-sore formation can lead to sepsis and death if severe, and their presence should not be taken lightly. Prompt treatment should be initiated to prevent severe complications. Treatment consists of frequent flipping, whirlpool baths, massages, antibiotics, clipping and cleaning of the area, surgical debridement, and bandages to alleviate pressure over a prominence depending on the severity of the lesion. Prevention is the best form of therapy.

✎ TECHNICIAN NOTE

It is better to prevent pressure-sore formation than to have to treat a pressure sore once it occurs.

- Animals that have lost pain sensation to one or more limbs should be monitored carefully. These animals may begin to lick or chew the asensory portion of their limbs, especially if the area becomes traumatized. Some will even chew off toes or whole limbs. If an animal without sensation to a limb beings to lick the limb, an Elizabethan collar should be placed immediately.
- An animal that cannot walk should never be allowed to roam free. They will traumatize their skin as they drag themselves around and can develop serious abrasions and ulcers.

Animals with some motor function to the limbs and a stable spinal injury should be gotten up at least three times a day and encouraged to use their limbs. Ambulatory but ataxic animals should be supported when ambulating to help prevent falls that might lead to further spinal damage. All animals with neurologic injuries require cage rest and controlled activity to allow the spinal column to heal. They should all be leashed when outdoors (animals with cervical problems should always be placed in a harness rather than in a neck collar to prevent further cervical damage), crated when indoors, and restricted according to the surgeon's protocol. Owners should be carefully counseled on the importance of confinement for prevention of further spinal injury.

> **✎ TECHNICIAN NOTE**
>
> Animals with injuries to the cervical spine should always be placed in a harness rather than in a collar to prevent further cervical damage.
>
> All animals with a spinal injury will require cage rest whether surgery is done or not. It is important to emphasize to owners that cage rest is important for proper healing even if their pet is walking and feeling normal.

As can be seen from the preceding list, the veterinary technician and veterinarian must work diligently and continually to properly manage animals with neurologic dysfunction.

ORTHOPEDIC SURGERY

LONG-BONE FRACTURES

Preoperative Considerations
When an animal is brought to the veterinary hospital with a fracture, several steps must be taken to ready the animal for a permanent repair. First, the patient must be stabilized with respect to all other body systems (treated for shock, chest injuries, and abdominal injuries). Second, any open wounds associated with the fracture should be managed Third, the fracture must be immobilized by means of a bandage, cast, or sling if the fracture is in a location amendable to bandaging (review Chapter 4). Once these three things have been achieved, fracture repair can be safely considered. Most long-bone fractures are not life threatening and do not require emergency surgery. Stability of the animal determines when the fracture is repaired.

> **✎ TECHNICIAN NOTE**
>
> Most long-bone fractures are not life threatening and do not require emergency surgery.

Intraoperative Considerations
The limb is usually suspended from the foot (Figure 24-39). An extensive hair clip is required on all limb preparations. The limb will usually undergo extensive manipulation during reduction and repair. For this reason, the limb is

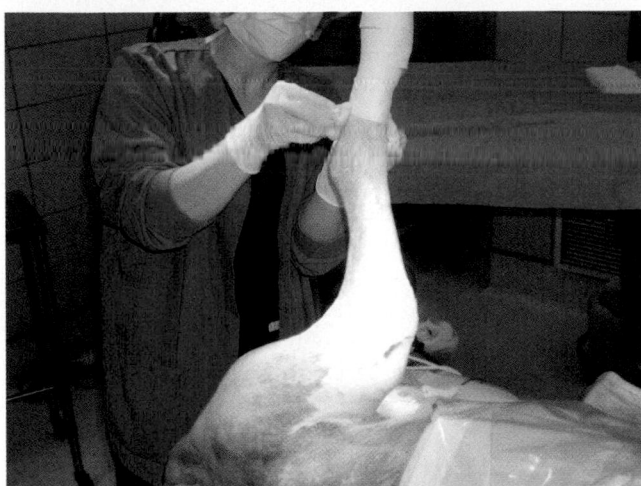

Figure 24-39 Proper limb positioning for limb preparation for orthopedic surgery.

clipped from the level of the metacarpus or metatarsus to the scapula or pelvis, respectively, including the medial and lateral aspects of the extremity. This may vary slightly, depending on the particular bone that is fractured, but the general rule should be a wide and thorough clip. The remaining hair at the tip of the paw is covered with a rubber glove or plastic wrap that is taped to the clipped skin.

Positioning
Animal positioning depends on the specific bone that is fractured. Generally, the following positions are recommended for each fracture:

- Femur: lateral recumbency, affected side up
- Tibia-fibula: lateral recumbency, affected leg down
- Humerus: lateral recumbency, affected leg up
- Radius-ulna: dorsal recumbency, affected leg craniad; or lateral recumbency, affected leg up
- Pelvis: lateral recumbency, affected leg up

With so much skin exposed, skin preparation is time-consuming, but it must be meticulous. The surgeon eventually covers the extremity with a sterile stockinette, but this should not preclude an adequate skin preparation.

Surgical Assistance
Orthopedic procedures are often very difficult and time-consuming and may demand the help of an assistant. Often, the veterinary technician is called on to participate as a surgical assistant and therefore should have a general understanding of orthopedic tissue handling (specifics of intraoperative assistance is covered in Chapter 23).

Several basic maneuvers commonly needed by the surgeon are often performed by the veterinary technician. They include retraction, muscle fatigue, alignment and reduction, and suction of the field. Proper techniques for each are discussed separately.

Retraction

Care should be taken to preserve the soft tissues in the operative field. It will be necessary to have functional muscle groups remaining when the bone is repaired. Retraction should be firm but not so traumatic as to bruise or tear the muscle. The tissues should also be kept moist. Tissue desiccation can cause tissue death and loss of function.

Muscle Fatigue

Large-breed dogs or fractures that are 3 to 5 days old may be difficult to reduce because of heavy muscle mass or severe muscle contraction, respectively. In such cases, constant steady traction on the muscle groups will cause them to fatigue and relax, thus facilitating reduction. Epidural anesthetics and/or paralytics can be used to aid in muscle reduction (review Chapter 19).

Alignment and Reduction

In order to repair fractured bones, the ends must be reduced and aligned. It is often necessary for an assistant to hold reduction during the fixation of the fracture. Pins, wires, screws, and plates of stainless steel may be used to achieve the necessary fixation.

Suction

Whenever a fracture occurs, bleeding into the fracture site can be massive. Some continuous oozing occurs during fixation. A clean surgical field is of the utmost importance in facilitating early and accurate reduction and fixation.

Postoperative Considerations

Some postoperative orthopedic patients may require external coaptation. Applied bandages should be managed as previously discussed. Animals undergoing orthopedic surgery will likely require passive range-of-motion exercises, but activity is limited otherwise. Animals should be encouraged to use the operated limb to increase blood supply to the fracture site, maintain joint and muscle health, and speed fracture healing. However, limb use should be slow, deliberate, and very well controlled. No off-leash activity, running, jumping, or playing with other animals should be allowed. A crate is the best place for these animals when the veterinarian, veterinary technician, or owner is not strictly controlling the animal. The only orthopedic procedure in which activity is strongly encouraged is femoral head and neck excision where rehabilitation, building of muscle mass, and encouragement of weight bearing is extremely important for optimal limb function. Animals are restricted to light activity for the first 2 weeks following femoral head and neck excision, but thay are then allowed to use the limb fully thereafter. It is also important to realize the relatively unsure gait of a three-legged dog or cat, and when exercising the animal, one must be certain to avoid slippery surfaces (vinyl or wet floors). Cement, grass, gravel, or dirt provides a much more sure-footed environment.

Rehabilitation is an important part of recovery in every orthopedic patient. Flexing and extending the affected limb along with muscle massage will improve blood flow and muscle tone as well as reduce muscle contraction. Therapy should be done for a period of 5 to 7 minutes each time and be repeated two to three times per day. A demonstration by the technician of the proper technique will aid the client in understanding the therapy. Slow leash walking is also performed to encourage limb use.

JOINTS

Preoperative Considerations

Most orthopedic procedures involving a joint are elective and rarely need emergency care. Traumatic fractures and luxations, however, do require urgent treatment. Preoperative management should include limiting the animal's activity. External coaptation is rarely necessary for nonurgent cases but will make the traumatically injured animal (animals with luxations or fractures) more comfortable. Indications for joint surgery include dislocations, ligament ruptures, infections, fractures, synovial biopsy, arthrodesis (surgical fusion of a joint) and treatment of osteochondrosis (abnormally thickened portion of the articular cartilage).

Intraoperative Considerations

An extensive clip, as for fractures, should also be done for joint surgery. Positions will vary depending on the joint involved. Generally, the following positions are recommended for each joint:

- Hip: lateral recumbency, affected leg up
- Stifle: lateral recumbency, affected leg up; or dorsal recumbency, leg hanging off the end of the table
- Shoulder: lateral recumbency, affected leg up
- Tarsus: lateral recumbency, affected leg up
- Elbow: lateral recumbency, affected leg up
- Carpus: lateral recumbency, affected leg up, or dorsal recumbency

Intraoperative assistance in joint surgery is similar to that necessary in fracture repair. Some special precautions should be taken while joints are exposed.

Retraction

Care should be taken *not* to place retractors in direct contact with the articular cartilage. This will damage the cartilage, and cartilage has a relatively poor response to trauma. When exposure of the joint is necessary, sharp retraction of the joint capsule will decrease trauma but increase exposure.

✏️ **TECHNICIAN NOTE**

Care should be taken *not* to place retractors in direct contact with the articular cartilage, and the cartilage should be kept moist to prevent permanent cartilage damage.

Flush

The cartilage should be frequently flushed with saline to keep it from drying out during the procedure. This is true of all tissues, but especially the articular cartilage because of its poor regenerative ability.

Postoperative Considerations

Postoperative care of patients undergoing joint surgery is variable, depending on the surgical procedure, the joint involved, and the surgeon's preference. Early passive range-of-motion activity with light joint usage is recommended for most animals undergoing joint surgery. Heavy joint use is discouraged in the early postoperative period. Joint use is increased gradually over the course of recovery, which is variable depending on the procedures performed. Joint immobilization is necessary in some cases, such as luxation, but can result in severe limitations in joint range of motion after recovery if care is not taken to rehabilitate the joint carefully.

CLIENT EDUCATION

When a patient is discharged from the professional care available in a veterinary hospital, it becomes the responsibility of the hospital staff to instruct the client to provide the same type of care at home. This requires that time be spent with the client and the pet to educate the client on appropriate treatment techniques. There are several methods of client education in surgical cases, the degree of difficulty of which is often associated with the type of surgical procedure performed (e.g., ovariohysterectomy versus fracture repair).

Whenever a patient is sent home with a sutured skin incision, the client must be instructed to observe the incision daily for evidence of swelling, redness, or drainage. The client should also watch the animal for aggressive licking,

removal of skin sutures, or both. The owner must be told to inform the veterinarian of problems.

If a patient is sent home with a bandage, a written discharge form should be given to the client describing in detail the proper management necessary to prevent complications.

In orthopedic cases, as well as in many elective soft-tissue surgery cases, the owner should be instructed specifically on what kind of limited activity should be enforced. If passive range-of-motion exercises are expected, the client should be given both oral and written instruction in providing the correct care. A demonstration by the technician of the correct method of therapy is helpful.

In many instances, such as complicated orthopedic and neurologic discharges, a handout explaining in detail the care necessary is very informative and provides a handy reference for the client if a problem arises.

The use of visual aids, such as a skeleton or overlay books that illustrate anatomy, can be effective in helping the client understand the scope of the problem. Clients are generally willing and very capable of handling postoperative care for their pets if instructed appropriately.

RECOMMENDED READING

Dunning D: Surgical wound infection and the use of antimicrobials. In Slatter D, editor: *Textbook of small animal surgery,* ed 3, Philadelphia, 2002, WB Saunders.

Shmon C: Assessment and preparation of the surgical patient and the operating team. In Slatter D, editor: *Textbook of small animal surgery,* ed 3, Philadelphia, 2002, WB Saunders.

Licroy MD, Bartels KE: Surgical lasers. In Slatter D, editor: Textbook of small animal surgery, ed 3, Philadelphia, 2002, WB Saunders.

Quandt JE: Postoperative patient care. In Slatter D, editor: *Textbook of small animal surgery,* ed 3, Philadelphia, 2002, WB Saunders.

Seim HB III, Creed JF: Restraint techniques for prevention of self-trauma. In Bojrab MJ, editor: *Current techniques in small animal surgery,* ed 4, Philadelphia, 1998, Lea & Febiger.

25

Small Animal Medical Nursing

SUSAN M. EDDLESTONE

INTRODUCTION

Small animal nursing has changed over the last few decades from attending to the basic needs of the patient such as feeding, walking, and cleaning to a more proactive role in the total needs of the medical patient. Problem solving is the basic skill needed to work with medical patients. This learned skill can be applied to almost every situation the medical nurse will encounter. Problem solving can be divided into several components: data collection, data interpretation, implementation of a plan, and evaluation of the response to the plan.

Data collection for the technician begins with *observation*. This is the single most important tool needed to successfully manage a medical patient. If change in a patient's condition is to be recognized, careful, detailed, and systemic observation is required. Also, needed is an understanding that clinical problems are dynamic and can change at any time for better or for worse. The technician will usually notice these changes more so than the veterinarian due to the longer period of time he or she will spend with the patient. In order to monitor a patient there needs to be an established baseline for the parameters being serially monitored. The precise system and nature of patient monitoring will vary depending on the specific clinical situation; however, the evaluation of all patients should take place according to a regular and reliable schedule. ■

Data interpretation by the veterinary technician consists of recognizing and correctly interpreting the observations that have been made. Stated differently, the technician must recognize and define the clinical problems. A clinical problem is anything that interferes with the well-being of the patient or anything that requires treatment or further diagnostic evaluation. Examples of clinical problems that might be recognized by the technician include diarrhea, vomiting, anorexia, and respiratory distress.

Once a problem is documented, a diagnostic or therapeutic plan is made. This may consist of repeating a clinical parameter such as a blood pressure reading or the patient's temperature before a more extensive plan is made. Once a clinical problem is positively identified, the attending veterinarian is consulted, and a diagnostic or therapeutic plan is implemented. For nursing to be optimally effective, a mechanism should exist for the ready exchange of information between technician and veterinarian. A team approach to animal health care is the ultimate goal, with veterinarian and technician each contributing their unique skills and abilities to the task of returning the patient to health. After a change of plan or treatment, continued observation of the patient is needed. The new plan or treatment may need to be altered again because of a changing clinical situation.

When implementing any diagnostic or therapeutic plan, it is important to remember that the quantity and nature of nursing care should always be individualized. One patient may readily accept a specific procedure, whereas another will resist to the point that the intended benefit is lost. Although excessive intervention may be detrimental to certain animals, this should not be construed as an excuse for medical neglect. The fundamental principle is that if a patient is not meeting a requirement for survival, the technician must promptly intervene. Certain animals require tremendous amounts of attention and affection from the

---

✎ TECHNICIAN NOTE

An integral aspect of any method of observation is the technician's ability to establish an accurate baseline for the parameter to be serially monitored.

technician simply to maintain the will to live during periods of separation from the owner.

Each technician and the head of every animal hospital should establish and maintain consistent standards of nursing care. Veterinary technicians have a professional and moral obligation to every patient to provide the following basic necessities:

- Clean, comfortable environment, as free of stress as possible
- Fresh food and clean water at all times unless restricted for medical reasons
- Adequate exercise and grooming care unless restricted for medical reasons
- Prompt and humane relief of suffering/pain
- Humane treatment of every patient with dignity at all times

GENERAL CARE

Grooming and bathing are aspects of the general care of the animal patient that are important for several reasons. First, a clean and well-groomed animal has an enhanced sense of well-being and potentially will recover from an illness more rapidly. Second, a clean animal is much less likely to develop severe contact dermatitis from urine scalding and fecal soiling of the skin, which, if it does occur, becomes another clinical problem to manage. Third, grooming and medicated baths are recommended for the prevention or treatment of many dermatologic problems. Bathing with shampoo that contains an insecticide is a useful adjunct in the control of ectoparasites. Finally, the cleanliness of the patient at the time of discharge is an indication to the owner of the overall quality of the health care provided.

Every animal hospital should have an adequate collection of grooming and bathing equipment and supplies, that is, combs, brushes, scissors, towels for drying, electrical dryers, and a selection of shampoos appropriate for different situations. Care must be taken to prevent the spread of infections, such as dermatomycosis, from one animal to another via grooming instruments. These instruments should be thoroughly cleansed in an appropriate disinfectant solution after each use.

When clipping or removing hair from an animal for medical reasons, it is important to obtain the owner's permission, whenever possible. This is particularly important in animals used for show purposes. In certain breeds, such as the Afghan hound, regrowth of hair is extremely slow.

BATHING

The basic technique for bathing dogs and cats is to thoroughly wet the coat and then apply small amounts of shampoo starting at the head and working back to the tail. Rubbing the shampoo into the coat until a lather is produced, again starting from the head and working back to the tail is a generally accepted bathing method. The eyes should be protected from chemical injury by instilling a drop of mineral oil or a small amount of boric acid ophthalmic ointment in each eye before the bath. Care should be taken to prevent water from entering the external ear canal; this can be accomplished by placing a small piece of cotton in each ear. Remember to remove the cotton when the bath has been completed. Thermal injury from excessively hot water can be prevented by constantly monitoring the water temperature. Thorough rinsing with clean water prevents irritation of the skin from residual shampoo. The axillary and scrotal regions of long-haired dogs are particularly vulnerable to residual shampoo irritation. If a cage dryer is used, caution must be exercised to prevent overheating (hyperthermia). Shampoos containing insecticides should be used only with the approval of the attending veterinarian because of the possibility of cumulative toxicity or drug interactions with medications or other topically applied insecticides. If insecticidal dips are used, correct dilutions are necessary to avoid toxic reactions. If a complete immersion bath is contraindicated, localized soiling of the animal may be handled with a sponge bath. Orthopedic or neurological patients may not be able to stand steady in the bath tub, and therefore a rubber mat should be placed in the tub to help reduce the risk of injury.

EXERCISE

Moderate exercise is beneficial for the general care of the animal patient. Exercise should take place in a secure, controlled, and safe environment so that injury or loss of the animal does not occur. Contraindications to exercise include many, but not all, respiratory, cardiovascular, and musculoskeletal problems. The decision whether to restrict exercise should be made after consultation with the attending veterinarian. Moderate exercise consists of taking the patient for a walk and can be considered the simplest and most basic form of physical therapy. It can be a useful means of reducing peripheral edema and improving muscle tone and strength.

> **TECHNICIAN NOTE**
> Moderate exercise consists of taking the patient for a walk and can be considered the simplest and most basic form of physical therapy.

FEEDING

The animal health technician plays a particularly pivotal role in ensuring that each patient remains in a positive energy balance, in which caloric intake exceeds metabolic requirements. The technician is in an excellent position to observe complete or partial anorexia and to take appropriate action to correct the situation. As long as the patient is not vomiting or the suppressed appetite is not due to a gastro-intestinal problem such as an ulcer or pancreatitis, there are a few things that should be tried to encourage the patient to eat. Substituting a more palatable food or texture such as canned food may solve the problem. Familiarity with the home feeding regimen will aid in the selection of palatable alternative diets. In certain instances, it may be advisable for the owner to prepare food at home and bring it to the hospital such as chicken or hamburger and rice. It is helpful to stock a variety of types of food, such as canned, semimoist, and dry, in a variety of flavors to satisfy even the most discriminating patient. Personal attention at feeding time such as talking to the patient and hand feeding the patient may work in some animals. Cats particularly may have an aversion to eating because they have lost the taste of food due to prolonged anorexia. Putting a small amount of canned food on the tongue or letting them lick it off the finger usually stimulates taste and interest in eating again. Force feeding, although not highly recommended, can be done in selected cases. This is done by mixing canned food with water for a slurry consistency and then administering the food with a syringe applied to the back of the animals mouth to stimulate the swallowing reflex. Care must be taken to avoid giving too much food at one time and to be sure that the animal is swallowing after each food bolus to prevent the patient from choking and/or aspirating food into the lungs causing life-threatening aspiration pneumonia. High-calorie density supplements, such as Nutrical (Evsco), may help to meet the caloric needs of the patient but by no means will meet the animal's daily require-ment by themselves. Gastric gavage (stomach tubing) can be done in patients requiring force feedings for an extended period of time because it is less stressful to the patient and the technician. (The technique is discussed in Chapter 15.) More commonly, other methods of enteral feeding are being used with increasing frequency and include placement of nasoesophageal, esophagostomy, gastrostomy, and jejun-ostomy tubes. Specially tailored complete diets may be administered through these enteral tubes. All but the nasoesophageal tubes have large enough diameters to allow the use of commercially prepared prescription canned diets blended with water and strained to be easily administered through the tube. Only liquids (CliniCare diet, Abbott Laboratories) can pass through the nasoesophageal tube. Being able to use these complete diets ensures adequate nutritional requirements are being met in a variety of disease states such as hepatic lipidosis in cats and renal failure. Total or partial parenteral nutrition (TPN/PPN) may also be chosen and consists of administering a sterile liquid that contains a complete or partial nutritionally balanced diet and is given intravenously through a fresh and aseptically placed jugular catheter. Aseptic technique is needed for every feeding. This feeding option is very labor intensive and introduces the risk of sepsis to the patient if not adminis-tered properly. It is usually chosen for the most critically ill patients when other feeding options are not possible. Giving

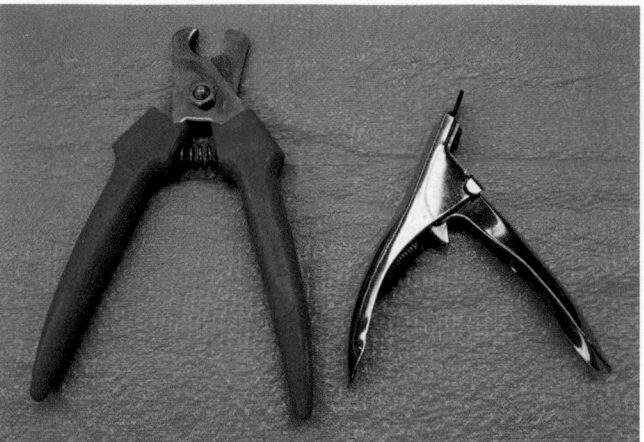

Figure 25-1 The two common types of nail trimmers, Whites *(top)* and Resco *(bottom)*. The Whites nail trimmer is useful for very long nails that have curled back toward the footpad.

appetite stimulants to cats (does not work in the dog) is usually done when trying to get a cat to eat that has been off feed for quite a while and has no current illness such as GI disease or nausea from a metabolic disease to prevent them from eating. These drugs will increase interest in eating but will not assure adequate calorie intake by the patient.

NAIL TRIMMING

Nail trimming (pedicure) is an important general care tech-nique. Excessive nail length results in altered gait and the potential accentuation of lameness problems. Excessively long nails are more likely to split or to be traumatically avulsed. Finally, untrimmed nails can become ingrown (usually into the footpads), resulting in cellulites or abscess formation.

There are two common types of nail trimmers available (Resco and Whites; Figure 25-1). To avoid cutting pigmented (black) nails too short in the dog, the cutting surface of the nail trimmer should be held parallel to the palmar or plantar surface of the digital footpads, and the nail cut in this plane. In cats, the nails can be exposed by grasping the paw between the thumb and index finger and sliding the skin on the dorsum of the paw away from the nails (Figure 25-2). Once exposed, the nails can be trimmed as described for the dog. It should be noted that nails that have not been trimmed regularly have a "quick" or nail vein that extends further out into the claw than that of regularly trimmed nails. In this situation, one should be conservative with regard to how much nail is trimmed. The center of the nail takes on a fleshy, shining appearance in the region next to the quick (Figure 25-3). This is an indicator to trim no further. Because some animals vehemently resent handling of their feet for nail trimming, it is a good practice to routinely give a pedicure to any animal anesthetized or tranquilized for any procedure. If the blood vessel in the nail is inadvertently severed (the "quick" is cut), silver nitrate

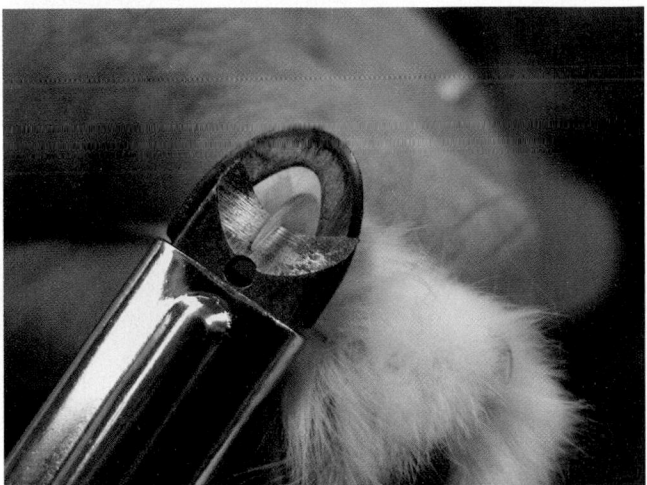

Figure 25-2 To trim the nails in cats, extend the claw by compressing the caudal part of the nail just in front of the footpad with the thumb and forefinger. At this point, one can visualize the vein or "quick" (pink area in claw), and the nail trimmer can be placed in front of the vein for trimming.

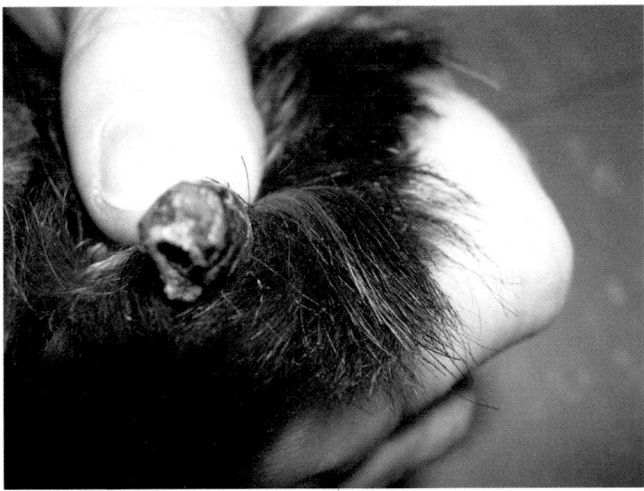

Figure 25-3 When trimming black nails, always trim a small amount at a time. Once you get close to the quick, you will note that the center of the nail begins to have a shiny, fleshy appearance. Once you see this, no further trimming is necessary.

sticks can be used to stop the hemorrhage by means of chemical cautery. Other products available for chemical cautery include styptic powder and blood-stop powder, which are available from numerous companies. Owners can be instructed on the proper technique of nail trimming so that this routine task can be performed at home.

EAR CLEANING

The external ear canal may accumulate cerumen, exudate, or cellular debris as a sequela to otitis externa or a foreign body (e.g., grass awn), which then requires cleaning. Certain breeds, notably poodles and terriers, may also accumulate

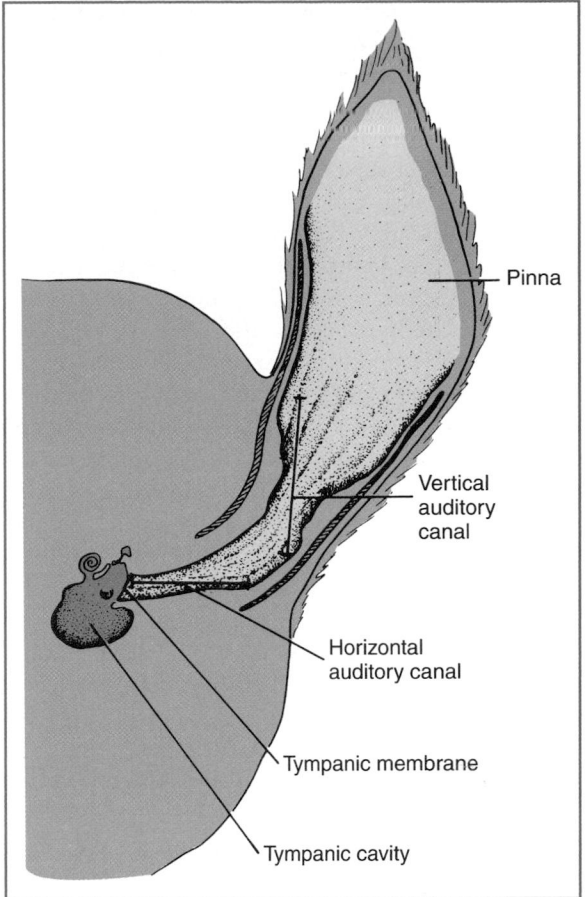

Figure 25-4 Schematic diagram of the anatomy of the canine ear.

excessive hair in the external ear canal. The initial and essential step in the treatment of any external ear problem is complete and thorough cleaning of the entire ear canal (Figure 25-4). Frequently, it is necessary to administer a short-acting general anesthetic or tranquilizer to properly clean the ears of patients that have painful ears and for patients that strongly resist ear cleanings. In some patients it may be necessary to remove hair from the ear canals, whereas in others it may be left alone. This will depend on the severity of the ear infection with the more severe inflamed ears responding to hair removal. A hemostat can be used to pull the hairs out, grabbing a small amount at a time. Excessive wax can be removed more easily if a ceruminolytic agent, i.e., dioctyl sodium succinate (Cerusol, Burns-Biotech labs), is instilled first to soften the wax. Caution should be used before instilling ceruminolytics and certain ear cleaners that contain chlorhexidine when the integrity of the tympanum is not known. Normal saline can be used for the initial cleaning agent until a proper ear canal exam can be performed to assess the tympanum. Using a soft rubber bulb syringe or a Luer-tipped catheter, excessive wax and debris can then be removed from the ear canals by gentle lavage with the chosen cleaning solution. Some practitioners advocate the use of pulsating streams of water from a dental hygiene apparatus (Water Pik, Teledyne Inc.) to clean the external ear canal. Approximately 5 ml of povidone-iodine (Betadine, Purdue-Frederick) or chlorhexidine solution (Nolvasan, Fort Dodge Laboratories) is added to approximately 236 to 384 ml of warm water. The stream of water should be applied in a rotating motion and directed parallel to the external ear canal. The excess water and debris can be collected in an ear irrigation basin or similar vessel. Avoid use of this method if the tympanum is not intact. Regardless of the irrigation system used, balls of cotton and cotton applicator sticks can then be used to gently wipe the wax from the external ear canal. It is important to remove only debris that is visible in the vertical canal so that debris is not pushed deep into the horizontal canal (Figure 25-4). Cleaning of the horizontal ear canal should be done only in the well-restrained patient and with caution to prevent damage to the tympanic membrane or the packing of debris deep into the horizontal canal (Figure 25-4). A second otoscopic examination should be performed after the ear canals are cleaned to evaluate the completeness of the ear cleaning. Once the ear canal is sufficiently clean, the canal should be carefully dried with clean cotton swabs, and the initial dose of prescribed otic preparation instilled into each canal.

Before cleaning, some of the debris should be mixed in mineral oil and smeared on a microscope slide to be examined under low-power magnification for the presence of *Otodectes* (ear mites). A small amount of the debris should also be smeared on a dry microscope slide and stained with Diff-Quik solution for examination under high-power magnification for overgrowth of bacteria and yeast. If the ear canal contains purulent debris, a sample should be obtained for cytological evaluation (smear), bacterial culture, and antibiotic sensitivity testing (sterile Culturette) before inserting instruments or cleaning solutions. Based on the cytology (yeast, bacteria) and mineral oil slides (mites), appropriate therapy can be initiated and then adjusted if necessary based on bacterial culture and sensitivity results when available in a few days.

> ✎ **TECHNICIAN NOTE**
>
> Ceruminolytics and disinfecting solutions containing chlorhexidine should be used with caution if the integrity of the tympanic membrane is not known. Cleansing with warm normal saline should be attempted first.

ANAL SACS

The anal sacs are reservoirs for the secretions produced by the anal glands. The anal glands line the walls of the anal sacs and produce a foul-smelling fluid that varies from serous to pasty in consistency and is brown to off-white. The anal sacs are paired structures, approximately 1 cm in diameter, that lie between the internal and external anal sphincter muscles on either side of the anal canal. Each sac opens into the lateral margin of the anus by a single duct, at

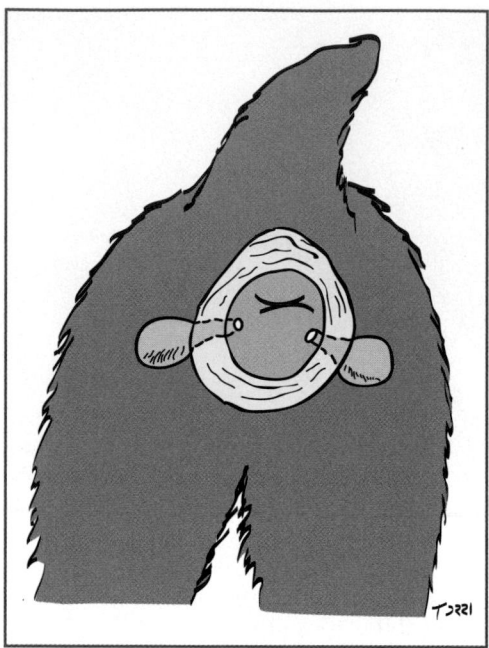

Figure 25-5 Schematic diagram of the anatomy of the canine anal sacs located approximately at the 4 o'clock and 8 o'clock positions.

approximately the 4 and 8 o'clock positions of the anus (Figure 25-5).

Clinical signs associated with impacted anal sacs include excessive licking of the perineum; "scooting" or dragging the perineum on the floor; abnormal carriage of the tail; and vague indications of pain or discomfort in the perineal region.

The anal sacs are best emptied, or "expressed," using the internal technique of inserting a lubricated, gloved forefinger into the rectum. The distended sacs are immobilized between the forefinger and thumb, which remains external to the anus. The sacs are generally found in a ventrolateral location. Gentle pressure is applied until the secretions are forced through the ducts. Because the ducts as well as the sac are occasionally compressed with this technique, if the sac cannot be expressed with gentle pressure, the finger and thumb are repositioned and pressure is reapplied. Paper towels, gauze, or cotton balls can be placed over the anus to collect the extremely unpleasant liquid from soiling the patient, environment, and the technician. External expression of the anal sacs is a technique that requires squeezing of the anal glands from the external anal sphincter. This technique is not recommended due to frequent occluding of the ducts, inability to completely empty the sacs, and excessive pain it may cause the patient.

BEDDING

The optimal means of keeping an ambulatory dog clean is by the appropriate use of bedding and exercise runs. Several types of bedding are routinely used in small animal practice; they include newspaper, other types of paper products, blankets, towels, and lamb's wool products. It is important that the bedding material selected be either disposable or readily and effectively cleaned between uses. Because occasionally dogs will ingest their bedding, it is also important that the material be safe and nontoxic. Most dogs are extremely reluctant to urinate or defecate in their cage; therefore keeping the cage and patient clean is facilitated by the regular use of walks outside or use of an exercise run to allow them to urinate and defecate. Specifically, dogs should be walked or placed in the runs several times daily for an adequate period of time.

Generally, cats are easier to keep clean than dogs during periods of hospitalization. Cats will use litter pans and groom and clean themselves unless they are seriously ill. Litter should be changed daily, and pans or trays should be either disposable or constructed of materials that will allow thorough cleaning and disinfection between uses. To avoid litter from getting into open wounds or surgical incisions, newspaper shredded into long strips can be used in the litter pan in place of gravel litter. It is unnecessary to walk or place cats in exercise runs unless the hospital stay is unusually long.

DECUBITAL SORES

Prevention and management of *decubital sores* (bedsores) and urine scald are extremely important aspects of the care of recumbent patients. Animals with various neurologic or orthopedic problems can be recumbent for prolonged periods and require special care. Urine and fecal soiling can cause serious problems that can complicate recovery from the underlying condition. Scalding from urine or diarrhea can be prevented by a light topical application of a protective compound, such as Aquaphor (Beiersdorf, Inc.) or petrolatum (e.g., Vaseline) to susceptible perineal or inguinal areas.

Decubital sores not only complicate recovery but can also be a source of sepsis, which can lead to the demise of the patient. The best treatment for decubital sores is *prevention*. Decubital sores develop over bony prominences as the result of continuous pressure and damage to the overlying skin. Various types of bedding have been advocated to reduce the frequency and severity of decubital sores; they include the use of air or water mattresses, foam padding, synthetic fleece, grids or grates, and straw. The material should either be disposable or have an impermeable surface that does not retain moisture or microorganisms and can be thoroughly cleaned. A potential problem with impermeable surfaces is that urine and moisture tend to remain in contact with the skin and can exacerbate the problem. Therefore care should be taken to keep the skin surface as dry as possible. This is why, for long-term management, straw is beneficial since adequate cushioning is available for the animal and urine drains through the straw and away from the patient.

TECHNICIAN NOTE

The best treatment for decubital sores is *prevention*.

Other routine measure that help to prevent decubital sores include frequent turning of the patient from side to side, intermittent use of slings or carts to prevent continuous pressure over the bony prominences, and frequent baths to keep the skin clean.

Once decubital sores have developed, they should be thoroughly cleaned with a surgical scrub. Surgical debridement of necrotic tissue may be necessary. After cleaning, the area should be completely dried. Soaking the affected area two to four times daily with a mild astringent will aid in keeping the decubital sore dry. A 1:40 astringent solution of aluminum acetate (Burow solution) may be made by dissolving one packet (Domeboro solution, Dome Laboratories) per pint of warm water. Ideally, the area of the decubital sore should be padded to prevent further pressure injury; however, the sore itself should remain exposed to the air to prevent retention of moisture. One way of accomplishing this is to fashion a "donut" from foam rubber and to fix this to the skin by means of adhesive tape. Unfortunately, it is difficult to maintain these pads in the proper location for long periods of time. Topical antimicrobials agents should be applied judiciously because many contain ointment or cream bases that form an occlusive dressing that will retain moisture. Further, it is questionable how beneficial they are in controlling an infected decubital sore.

GERIATRIC NURSING

With improved veterinary care, pets are enjoying an increased life span; consequently, the number of geriatric patients seen in small animal practices is increasing. The geriatric patient can be presented with a number of problems that directly influence the nursing process. These problems are generally related to or are secondary to degenerative diseases and other geriatric changes, such as arthritis, deafness, and blindness (see Chapter 13).

Dogs with arthritis or other degenerative diseases of the musculoskeletal system may be suffering from chronic pain. These animals are likely to react aggressively when an affected body part is touched or manipulated. Gentle handling when lifting or moving these patients and taking care to walk them at a slower pace than younger dogs is needed to avoid pain and fear in these patients. Dogs suffering from central nervous system disorders (e.g., a brain tumor or cerebral infarction) may also display aggressive behavior.

Deafness is another disorder that frequently accompanies old age. It is easy to surprise or startle a deaf, older dog, and certain dogs will instinctively respond by biting. When approaching a deaf dog, it is important that the patient is able to see you before you attempt to handle it or perform a procedure.

Blindness can occur in older dogs from cataracts, retinal degeneration, glaucoma, and other diseases. As is the case with deaf dogs, blind dogs should be approached cautiously. It is best to move slowly and speak while approaching the dog. Generally, elderly dogs and cats show less response to external stimuli. They appear to be less interested in their surroundings and frequently remain inactive for prolonged periods. In fact, they tend to resent any interference and react aggressively when disturbed. Some dogs forget previous training and may fail to respond to basic commands. Finally, the geriatric dog or cat is resistant to changes in daily routine. The stress of hospitalization alone can sometimes cause rapid deterioration. Obviously, it is impossible to correct or reverse many of the changes associated with aging; however, a willingness to provide gentle, compassionate nursing care is of paramount importance.

PEDIATRIC NURSING

The clinical situation that best illustrates the skills required in pediatric nursing is the hand rearing of orphaned puppies or kittens (see Chapter 12). The first step is to determine the caloric requirements of the puppy or kitten. During the first week of life, these requirements are approximately 27 cal/kg/day, 32 to 36 cal/kg/day during the second week, 36 to 41 cal/kg/day during the third week, and 41 to 45 cal/kg/day during the fourth week. A number of artificial milk replacers (Esbilac, Pet-Ag; Just Burn, Farnham) are available for use in puppies. KMR (Pet-Ag) is an artificial replacement for queen's milk. (See Table 25-1 for formula dosage.) The following formula can be used as a short-term emergency supplement in puppies: 8 oz of cow's milk mixed with two egg yolks and 1 tsp of corn oil. For an emergency formula in kittens, 4 oz of cow's milk can be mixed with two egg yolks and one drop of multivitamins. Once the total daily requirement has been calculated, this amount can be divided into four equal feedings. Frequent feedings are necessary to prevent overdistention of the stomach and subsequent emesis and aspiration pneumonia. Generally, it is faster and easier to use gavage via an orogastric tube than to bottle feed.

The technique for gavage is to use a soft rubber feeding tube (Fr 8 to 16). The tube is marked with a marking pen

or tape at a point equal to the distance between the tip of the nose and the eighth rib. The tube is advanced into the pharynx and down the esophagus to the level of the midthorax. A syringe can be used to inject the artificial milk replacer slowly. The stomach capacity of puppies and kittens can be calculated by using the following formula: body weight in grams times 5% equals the capacity of the stomach in milliliters. This milliliter amount should not be in a single feeding.

If the puppies or kittens are vigorous nursers, an alternative technique would be to use Pet Nursettes (Peg-Ag) or human premature baby bottle nipples. This technique is slower but may satisfy the pups and kittens more, so the incidence of litter mates nursing on each other will be reduced.

The neonatal puppy is essentially poikilothermic (body temperature varies with ambient temperature); therefore it is imperative that the ambient temperature of the whelping box be maintained between 30° C and 33° C. If hypothermia occurs, it will reduce feeding by the neonate and may enhance the pathogenicity of certain viruses, such as canine herpes. To detect hypothermia in neonates, it is desirable to use a low-reading clinical rectal thermometer.

A highly effective monitoring technique during the neonatal period is to weigh the neonates frequently. Newborn puppies and kittens should be weighed daily. Puppies should gain approximately 10% to 20% of their birth weight daily for the first week of life. Postage or food scales should be used to weigh each animal two or three times daily, especially during the first 2 weeks of life. Weight loss or failure to gain weight each day may be the first sign of illness. Puppies and kittens less than 2 weeks of age often do not defecate or urinate on their own. The mother stimulates these functions by gently licking the genitals and anus. This can be simulated by using a warm wet cloth to gently wipe the genital and anal area a few times daily.

> **✎ TECHNICIAN NOTE**
>
> A highly effective monitoring technique during the neonatal period is to weigh the neonates frequently.

PRACTICAL NURSING PROCEDURES

In many veterinary practices, it is the responsibility of the veterinary technician to monitor the patient's vital signs (i.e., temperature, pulse, respirations).

TEMPERATURE

One routine method for determining the body temperature of a small animal is to use a standard mercury-in-glass clinical rectal thermometer. Veterinary thermometers differ from those used in humans in that the storage reservoir for

Table 25-1 ORPHAN FORMULA DOSAGE FOR PUPPIES AND KITTENS

Age (wk)	Dosage* (ml/100 g body wt/day)
1	13
2	17
3[†]	20
4	22

*Divide and feed four times daily.
[†]Begin to feed solid food.

the mercury is short and spherical rather than elongated. Human thermometers can be used in dogs and cats without difficulty. Thermometers can be calibrated in Fahrenheit or Celsius degrees. A Fahrenheit reading can be converted to Celsius by using the following formula: degrees $C = (\text{degrees } F - 32) \times {}^5/_9$.

When taking the patient's temperature, one should first shake the thermometer so that the mercury is below the constriction in the glass tube. The thermometer is well lubricated with petrolatum, mineral oil, or a mild soap and inserted into the rectum with a gentle twisting motion. The thermometer is advanced into the rectum beyond the bulb and is held in place for the minimum period of time stated on the thermometer. The patient is restrained to prevent the thermometer from being broken. The thermometer is withdrawn, and the bulb and stem are wiped clean with an alcohol-soaked cotton swab. The thermometer is held horizontally and rotated until the magnified scale is clearly visible. Because of the constriction in the glass tube, the level of the mercury does not fall until it is shaken down. Finally, the thermometer should be stored in an antiseptic solution (e.g., benzalkonium chloride). Hot water should not be used for cleaning thermometers.

The more common and quicker method of obtaining a body temperature is with the use of digital thermometers (Figure 25-6). There are many brands available, and with most an auditory beep alerts the technicians when the reading is final.

Certain diseases that produce fever display a diurnal pattern (i.e., the temperature fluctuates) during the day. If the patient's temperature is taken just once per day, the periods of fever may not be recognized. If this situation is suspected, a temperature chart may be kept by taking and recording the temperature at regular intervals, for example, every 4 hours.

The normal rectal temperature in the dog is 101.0° F to 102.5° F. The normal rectal temperature in the cat is 100.5° F to 102.5° F. Excitement or activity can elevate the temperature above these limits. In rare clinical situations (i.e., rectal laceration, rectal prolapse), it may not be possible to measure the rectal temperature. In these situations, the temperature may be taken in either the axilla or the external ear canal. The temperature recorded in these sites will be significantly lower than the simultaneous rectal temperature. In general, 1° F can be added to an axillary or ear canal temperature to approximate rectal temperature. These alternative techniques for determining the body temperature are useful when the same site is used serially in an individual patient, and the results are compared. The temperature is taken by placing the bulb of the thermometer deep in the axilla or ear canal for several minutes.

Recently, infrared thermometers have been developed that record accurate body core temperatures by focusing the infrared beam on the tympanic membrane. This thermometer is helpful in those patients with very low rectal temperatures or in those for which taking a rectal temperature is contraindicated (Ototemp Veterinary, Exergen Corp.).

PULSE

The rate and character of the pulse are valuable means of assessing the cardiovascular status of the patient. The pulse can be palpated in any artery located close to the body surface. Using an index finger to palpate the pulse is best for sensitivity with the thumb being the least sensitive. The pulse is most commonly felt in the femoral artery. The femoral artery is palpated on the medial aspect of the thigh, proximal to the stifle. Palpation of the femoral pulse requires practice and can be difficult in a trembling patient or in a patient with short, heavily muscled legs. Alternative sites for taking the pulse are the palmar aspect of the carpus and the ventral aspect of the base of the tail. The *normal pulse rate* in adult dogs is 60 to 160 beats/min, up to 180 beats/min in toy breeds, and 220 beats/min for puppies. The maximum rate in cats is 240 beats/min.

The heart rate can be counted by palpation or auscultation at the point of maximal intensity of the heartbeat. The point of maximal intensity is located at the costochondral junction between the left fourth and sixth intercostal spaces. If the pulse rate is taken at the same time as the heart rate and the pulse rate is less, this is called a *pulse deficit*. A pulse deficit generally indicates an abnormal heart rhythm.

The dog can have heart and pulse rates that are "regularly irregular." Characteristically, the heart and pulse rates increase with inspiration and decrease with expiration. This normal variation is called *sinus* arrhythmia.

In addition to taking the pulse rate, it is beneficial to evaluate the pulse pressure and character of the pulse.

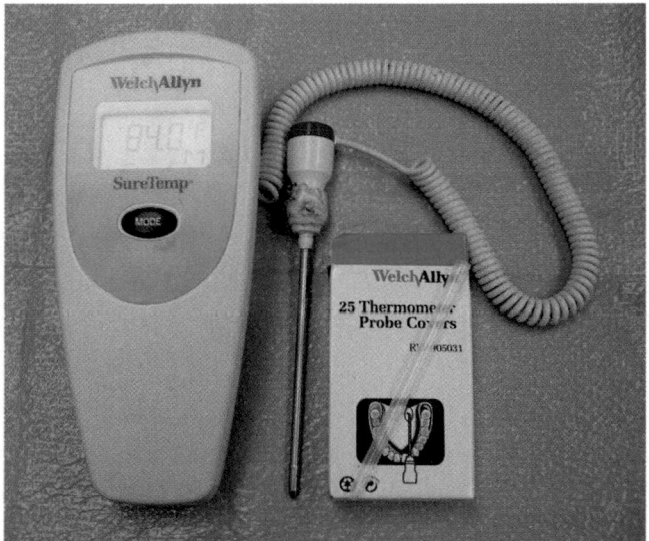

Figure 25-6 Digital electronic thermometer by Welch Allyn with removable and disposable plastic sheaths. These are very accurate and quick for the measurement of rectal temperature.

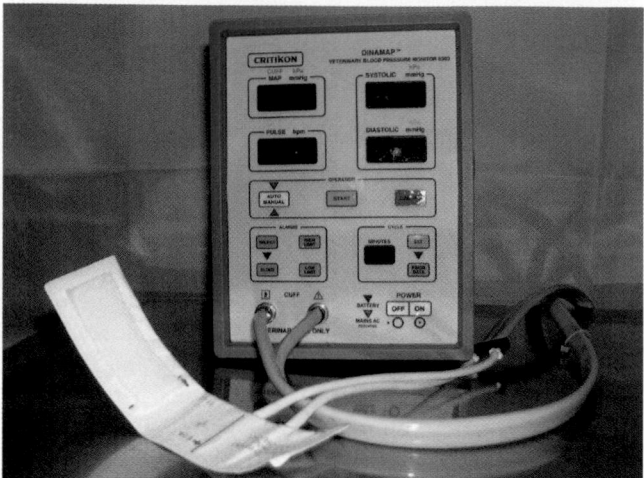

Figure 25-7 Dinamap 8300 (Citricon) instrument for noninvasive measurement of blood pressure.

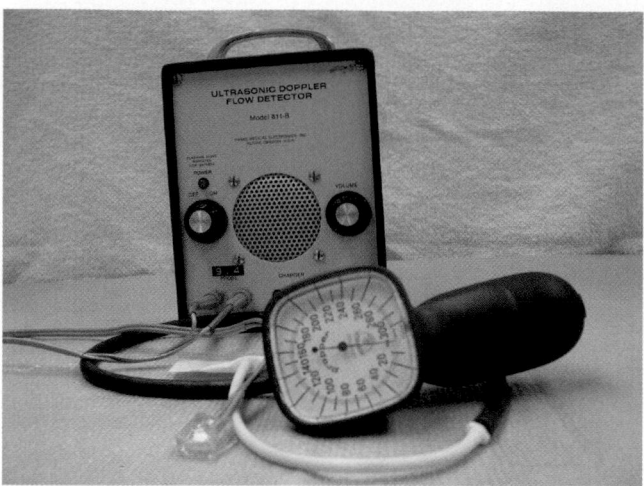

Figure 25-8 Parks 811-B (Parks Medical Electronics, Inc.) instrument for noninvasive measurement of blood pressure.

Decreased pulse pressure may indicate systemic hypotension (drop in blood pressure) secondary to a process such as hypovolemic shock. Instrumentation has been developed for the noninvasive measurement of blood pressure in the dog and cat using the ultrasound Doppler method (Dinamap 8300, Critikon [Figure 25-7], Parks 811-B, Parks Medical Electronics, Inc. [Figure 25-8]. Blood pressure readings are taken when the dog or cat has acclimated to the hospital environment to avoid falsely high readings. A neonatal cuff that has a width that is 40% the size of the limb circumference is placed over the medial tibial artery, which is found midway between the carpus and elbow or in the tibial area on a back leg. A small area is clipped free of hair distal to the cuff and transducer gel applied. The transducer is placed on top of the gel. Seven readings are taken for systolic and diastolic blood pressures. The highest and lowest values are omitted, and the remaining 5 values are averaged for the final value. The systolic readings are much more reliable than the diastolic readings with the Dinamap. The Parks ultrasound Doppler gives a more reliable reading in the cat. In the dog and cat the *normal systolic blood pressure* is less than 170 mm Hg and *normal diastolic blood pressure* is less than 120 mm Hg.

> ### ✐ TECHNICIAN NOTE
>
> In the dog and cat the *normal systolic blood pressure* is less than 170 mm Hg and *normal diastolic blood pressure* is less than 120 mm Hg.

RESPIRATION

The respiratory rate should be counted when the animal is at rest but not sleeping. Respiration involves both an inspiratory and expiratory phase. When counting the respiratory rate, it is necessary to count either inspirations or expirations but not both. The normal rate in the dog is between 15 and 30 breaths/min. Smaller breeds tend to have a more rapid rate of respiration than larger breeds. The rate in cats is between 20 and 30 breaths/min. In addition to determining the rate, it is important to characterize the respiratory status of the patient by inspection.

Several terms are used to describe respiratory function. *Tachypnea* refers to very rapid breathing. *Hyperpnea* indicates a condition in which the respiration is deeper and more rapid than normal. *Depth of respiration* indicates the volume of air inspired with each breath. Increased depth of respiration indicates a greater demand for oxygen. Shallow respiration can be caused by either metabolic derangement (e.g., acidosis) or mechanical injuries (e.g., fractured ribs). *Dyspnea* is a term used to indicate the subjective impression of increased difficulty or distress in breathing. *Labored breathing* is also used to describe difficulty in breathing and may include abdominal movements that occur simultaneously indicating the degree of increased effort to breath by using abdominal muscles. *Hyperventilation* is seen as shallow, rapid breathing and occurs in severe metabolic acidosis and sometimes in severe respiratory disease.

All hospitalized patients should have their vital signs monitored at least once per day. Depending on the underlying problem and the status of the patient, it may be necessary to monitor the patient more frequently. The temperature, pulse, and respiration rate should be recorded in the medical record every time they are taken. This will facilitate recognition of abnormalities as early as possible. Further, serial observations will permit recognition of clinical trends.

ADMINISTRATION OF MEDICATIONS

It is important for the animal health technician to be familiar with several basic principles of clinical pharmacology. These principles are important when considering the route of administration of various drugs. Drugs can be administered parenterally (e.g., by injection), orally, or topically. The parenteral techniques routinely used in veterinary medicine include the intravenous, intramuscular, and subcutaneous routes. The specific techniques used to administer drugs by these various routes are discussed in Chapter 3. The discussion in this chapter is concerned with the selection of an appropriate route in various clinical situations.

In choosing the route of administration, a variety of factors must be considered. First, the pharmacologic properties of the drug should be considered. Certain drugs are not adequately absorbed when given by a certain route (e.g., gentamicin is poorly absorbed from the gastrointestinal tract). Similarly, insulin must be given by injection because it is destroyed in the gastrointestinal tract. Other drugs cannot be given by a certain route because they produce severe tissue reactions (e.g., thiamylal sodium causes sloughing of the skin if it is given subcutaneously). Another pharmacologic factor to consider is the rate of absorption. If an animal is critically ill, the route of administration that will provide the earliest onset of action is preferred. For example, an animal with a severe, overwhelming infection should receive an antibiotic intravenously rather than orally.

It is also important to consider the patient when considering the route of administration. For example, it is generally inadvisable to administer oral medications to a vomiting patient or to an animal with severe respiratory compromise or distress. The temperament of the patient should also be considered. In a fractious animal, it may be impossible to administer drugs topically, orally, or intravenously. Subcutaneous or intramuscular injections may be the only feasible routes of administration. Finally, convenience and compliance of the client will influence therapeutic decision. Obviously, the topical and oral routes are preferred for treatment at home.

The principal advantages of the oral route are convenience and reduced risk of infection or abscess caused by faulty injection technique. Disadvantages of the oral route include the potential for aspiration of liquid medications and the potential for animals to spit out the medication, so the prescribed dose is not absorbed.

> **✎ TECHNICIAN NOTE**
>
> The principal advantages of the oral route are convenience and reduced risk of infection or abscess caused by faulty injection technique.

Advantages of parenteral injections include, in general, more rapid absorption and greater assurance that the prescribed dose is accurately delivered.

The major advantage to topical medication is that systemic effects are reduced and safety is thus increased. The major disadvantage is that most systemic illnesses do not respond to topical medication alone.

Whenever any drug is administered, it is essential to record the treatment (drug, dose, time) and route of administration completely and accurately in the medical record. The notation should be made immediately after administering the medication. If this procedure is consistently followed, patient care will improve because it is less likely that treatments will be omitted or inadvertently repeated. In addition to improving the level of patient care, it should be remembered that this policy is important because the medical record is a legal document, and every treatment should be recorded in case of subsequent litigation.

It is also of utmost importance that all medications, either those used in the hospital or those dispensed for use at home, be labeled correctly (see Chapter 21). The dispensing label information should include the complete name of the drug, size or concentration of the drug, number of tablets or capsules or milliliters of drug dispensed, dose and frequency of administration, name of the client, and name of the hospital. If potentially toxic drugs are dispensed, childproof containers should be used, as determined by state and federal regulations.

FLUID THERAPY

The veterinary technician generally will not be called on to formulate a fluid order in a hospitalized patient without supervision of the attending veterinarian. However, familiarity with certain fundamental points will allow the technician to participate actively in this essential process.

The total volume of fluid required to treat an animal can be approximated by considering the volume of fluid needed to rehydrate the patient, volume of fluid needed for maintenance requirements, and volume of fluid needed to correct ongoing losses.

Sensible losses are roughly equivalent to urine output. *Insensible losses* represent the fluid lost in the feces and during respiration. These losses are considered as part of the daily maintenance requirements. *Contemporary losses* are due to ongoing problems (i.e., vomiting, diarrhea).

The hydration status, and thus the rehydration requirement, can be assessed by the following physical examination criteria: skin turgor, dryness of the mucous membranes, capillary refill time, and degree of sinkage of the eyes into the bony orbit. Several laboratory criteria are beneficial, particularly if they are followed serially; these include the hematocrit, total protein determination, and urine specific gravity (SG). Finally, serial body weights can be valuable in determining changes in hydration status. One pound of body weight is equivalent to 1 pt or 480 ml of fluid.

By using the physical examination findings mentioned, the degree of dehydration is estimated as a percentage of body weight (Table 25-2). Thus an animal that shows only a slight alteration in skin turgor is approximately 5% to 6% dehydrated. Skin turgor is evaluated by pinching a fold of the skin and subjectively assessing the rate at which it returns to its normal position. This is not a valid test in older animals or animals that have recently lost weight due to the increased skin turgor that develops due to decreased

Table 25-2	DIAGNOSIS OF DEHYDRATION: PHYSICAL EXAMINATION FINDINGS

Dehydration (%)	Clinical Signs
<5	Undetectable
5-6	Skin slightly doughy, inelastic consistency
6-8	Skin definitely inelastic; eyes very slightly sunken in orbits
10-12	Increased skin turgor; eyes sunken in orbits, prolonged refill time, dry mucous membranes
12-15	Shock and imminent death

Box 25-1 CALCULATION OF FLUID REQUIREMENTS

Body weight (kg) × % dehydration × 1000 = ml fluid deficit*
(60 to 80 ml/kg) × Body weight (kg) = ml of daily fluid requirement*
Estimation of ongoing losses × 2 = ml of ongoing losses*

Example: 20 kg dog, 8% dehydrated, 100 ml vomitus
20 kg × 0.08 1000 = 1600 ml
(20 kg) × (60 mg/kg) = 1200 ml
100 ml × 2 = 200 ml
Total volume = 3000 ml/24 = 125 ml/hr

*Add together for total volume to be replaced in millileters over 24 hours. Divide total volume by 24 hours to get hourly fluid rate needed for digital pump administration of continuous fluids.

fat in the subcutaneous space. An animal that is 10% to 12% dehydrated will display pronounced changes in skin turgor; dry, tacky mucous membranes; prolonged capillary refill time; and eyes that are sunken into the orbits. The physical alterations associated with dehydration are a continuum, so an animal that is 8% dehydrated should have abnormalities midway between the end points described. It should be stressed that physical examination findings are at best very crude indicators of the degree of dehydration. The quantitative value of these parameters is improved if they are carefully and critically assessed over time.

The laboratory criteria used to assess the degree of dehydration evaluate the extent of hemoconcentration. Thus the higher the hematocrit and the total protein determination, the more hemoconcentrated and thus dehydrated is the patient. These laboratory tests are useful in detecting relative changes and do not necessarily measure the absolute hydration status of the patient. If the concentrating ability of the kidneys is normal, a urine SG of more than 1.035 in the dog and 1.040 in the cat provides further evidence that the patient may be dehydrated.

Because changes in body weight over short periods are caused by changes in fluid balance rather than by the loss or gain of body mass, an accurate daily weight can also be helpful in assessing changes in the hydration status of the patient.

Once the degree of dehydration has been estimated, it can be used in calculating the volume of fluids needed to rehydrate the patient. The percent dehydration is multiplied by the body weight in kilograms and then by 1000. This is the number of milliliters needed to rehydrate the patient.

In addition to the volume required for rehydration, the maintenance requirement must be incorporated in the calculation of the daily fluid order. The maintenance requirement consists of estimates of both sensible and insensible losses.

As mentioned, sensible losses refer to the urine output. Insensible losses represent the fluid lost from the body via the gastrointestinal and respiratory tracts. Although sensible and insensible losses will vary somewhat depending

on the clinical setting, a useful clinical approximation is 60 ml/kg/day (30 ml/lb/day). If the animal is not taking any liquids by mouth, a volume equivalent to the sensible and insensible losses (e.g., the maintenance requirement) should be included in the daily fluid order.

Most animals with problems that require fluid therapy do not have these problems resolve immediately on initiation of fluid therapy. Therefore contemporary or ongoing losses must also be considered in determining the daily fluid order. For example, if a patient has gastroenteritis, the volume of fluid lost with each episode of vomiting and diarrhea should be estimated and added to the rehydration and maintenance volumes. The volume of diarrhea and vomitus is frequently underestimated; therefore it has been recommended that the visual estimate be *doubled* to more accurately reflect the actual volume lost. Generally, the volume required to rehydrate the animal is not replaced immediately. Usually, the total volume is administered over the first 24 hours. Once rehydrated, maintenance requirement and ongoing losses are combined to calculate the fluid requirement for the next 24 hours and given over 24 hours (Box 25-1).

ROUTES OF FLUID ADMINISTRATION

Oral fluid administration is the preferred method because of reduced expense, ease of administration, and safety. Contraindications to oral fluid administration include vomiting and severe, life-threatening fluid imbalances that require immediate correction.

Many conditions respond well to subcutaneous administration of fluids. Fluids given subcutaneously should be warmed to body temperature and must be isotonic with extracellular fluid. Isotonic fluids have an osmotic pressure approximately equal to that of extracellular fluid. Never give subcutaneously dextrose solutions with a concentration of more than 2.5%; sloughing of skin and abscess formation are common sequelae. The volume and rate of subcutaneous

Table 25-3 FREE DRIP CALCULATIONS

$$\text{Drops per minute} = \frac{\text{total infusion volume} \times \text{drops/ml}}{\text{total infusion time (min)}}$$

For example, to administer 3000 ml over 24 hours using a 10 drop/ml drip set:

$$\frac{3000 \times 10 \text{ drops/ml}}{1440 \text{ min}} = 20 \text{ drops/min}$$

---

fluids that can be given will vary from patient to patient. A rough guideline for total daily volume is approximately 60 ml/kg (30 ml/lb). Absorption of subcutaneous fluids will occur over 6 to 8 hours; therefore this total daily dose can be divided and given every 6 to 8 hours. It is necessary and desirable to administer this divided dose in as many sites as possible. Subcutaneous fluid administration is safe and easy; however, it is not the recommended route of administration when prompt correction of severe deficits is required. Intravenous fluid administration is indicated when a patient is severely compromised with dehydration, hypovolemia, electrolyte imbalances, hypoglycemia, and so forth. The intravenous route is the most common way to give fluids in the hospital and is indicated particularly for serious, life-threatening illness and vomiting patients. Aseptic technique is required to place an intravenous catheter into the cephalic vein, saphenous vein, or jugular vein. The catheter and the fluid drip set must be kept sterile and free of blood clots to allow long-term use (3 to 5 days maximum) of the intravenous line. Heparinized saline or sterile saline may be used to periodically flush the catheter to prevent blood clots from forming in the catheter. Intravenous fluids can be given at a continuous rate using a digital fluid pump, or they can be given intermittently using the free-flowing drip method (Table 25-3).

The intraperitoneal route is not a routine method of fluid administration because peritonitis and intraabdominal abscess formation may result from this form of fluid therapy. The rate of absorption of intraperitoneal fluids is roughly equivalent to the rate of absorption of subcutaneous fluids and therefore the intraperitoneal route is not adequate when prompt correction is needed. The exception to this is the use of intraperitoneal fluid administration in the neonate and wildlife neonate, where this route may be very effective.

Signs of volume overload include restlessness, hyperpnea (increased respiratory rate), serous (watery) nasal discharge, chemosis (edema of the ocular conjunctiva), and pitting edema. Volume overload can be caused by either an excessive total volume or an excessive rate of fluid administration. Decreased cardiac function or decreased plasma protein can predispose to a volume overload state. If volume overload is suspected, the lungs should be auscultated for evidence of pulmonary edema, and the central venous pressure should be determined. Before the development of pulmonary edema or elevated central venous pressure, weight gain may be seen. Therefore it is advisable to weigh the animal three times daily while intravenous fluid therapy is being used, especially in those patients who are less able to handle a fluid load (e.g., patients with cardiac or renal disease). The placement of an indwelling urinary catheter (Foley) and urinary outflow collection system will allow quantitation of urine production. This will allow a more accurate assessment of how much fluid is coming out and how much intravenous fluids the patient actually needs to prevent overzealous fluid therapy.

Fluid therapy is a dynamic process that must be reassessed at frequent intervals and adjusted to obtain the maximum results. The technician's role in clinically assessing the patient is important in making appropriate adjustments. The chance of inadvertent fluid overload can be reduced by using indwelling intravenous catheters and administering fluids over prolonged periods of time rather than using rapid bolus techniques. In addition, Minidrip (Travenol Laboratories, Inc.) and Buretrol (Travenol Laboratories, Inc.) administration sets can be used in cats and small dogs. Also, syringe pumps are useful in administering fluids to cats and very small dogs (Medfusion 2010 [Medex, Inc.] Syringe Pump; Figure 25-9).

Several basic types of fluid are routinely used in small animal practice. They include physiologic (0.9%) saline, 5% dextrose in water, and extracellular fluid replacement solutions such as lactated Ringer's solution or Ringer's solution. Combinations of these basic fluid types are also used. These basic parenteral fluid types can be supplemented with concentrated solutions of electrolytes and dextrose to produce the desired fluid composition appropriate for the specific clinical situation (Table 25-4).

Frequently, antimicrobials are added to intravenous fluids for administration. A number of the commonly used antimicrobials are incompatible with certain fluids (Table 25-5). The physical incompatibilities include precipitation of the drug out of solution and chemical inactivation. In addition to these incompatibilities, it has been noted that when certain drugs are mixed in infusion solutions, inactivation occurs. For example, when carbenicillin is added to a solution containing gentamicin, the gentamicin is inactivated. As a general rule, it is undesirable to mix multiple drugs in a syringe or intravenous fluids. Frequently, the interaction is visible on mixing, but other times it will not be observed before administration.

CENTRAL VENOUS PRESSURE

The measurement of central venous pressure is a useful aid in evaluating the fluid status of a patient. When used and interpreted properly, it can substantially reduce the likelihood of excessive fluid administration. Measurement of the central venous pressure is a simple technique that can be performed in all veterinary practices.

Table 25-4 BASIC FLUIDS

	Fluid Composition per Liter					
Fluid Type	Na⁺	Cl⁻	K⁺	Ca²⁺	Lactate	kcal
Lactated Ringer's solution	130	109	4	3	28	9
Ringer's solution	147	156	4	5	0	0
0.9% Saline	154	154	0	0	0	0
2.5% Dextrose in ½ normal saline	77	77	0	0	0	85
5% Dextrose in lactated Ringer's solution	130	109	4	3	28	179
5% Dextrose in water	0	0	0	0	0	179
Normosol-R	140	98	5	0	0	18
Normosol-M in 5% dextrose Glucose 50	40	40	13	0	0	175

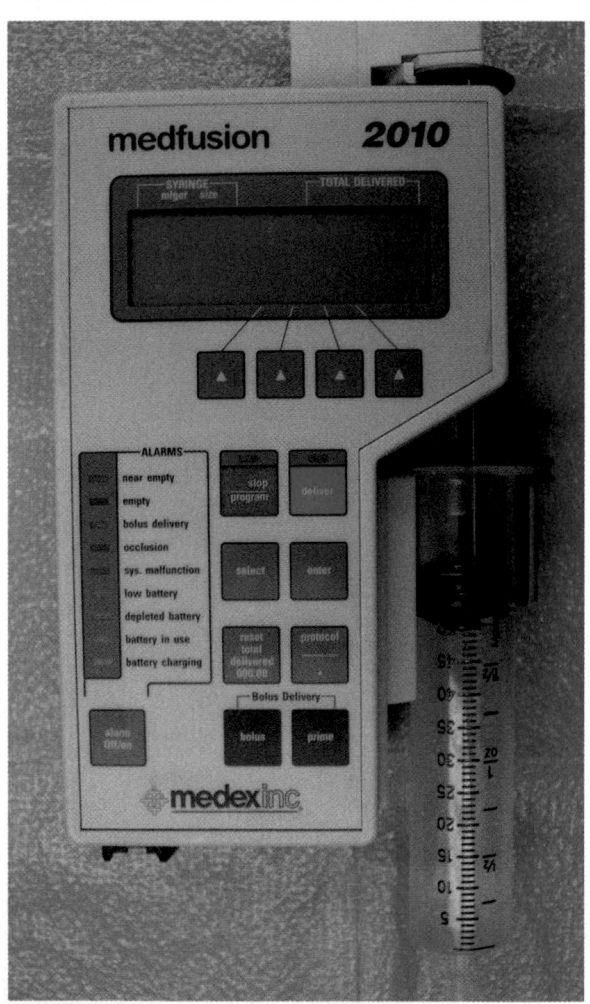

Figure 25-9 Medfusion 2010 (Medex, Inc.) Syringe Pump used for the administration of small volumes and slow rates of fluid to the cat and small dog.

Table 25-5 PHYSICAL INCOMPATIBILITIES OF ANTIMICROBIALS IN INTRAVENOUS SOLUTIONS

Antimicrobial	Incompatible With
Amphotericin B	Normal saline
Cephalothin sodium	Lactated Ringer's solution, calcium gluconate, calcium chloride
Chloramphenicol sodium succinate	Vitamin B complex with vitamin C
Chlortetracycline hydrochloride, oxytetracycline hydrochloride, tetracycline hydrochloride	Lactated Ringer's solution, sodium bicarbonate, calcium chloride
Penicillins	Dextrose-containing solutions with pH >8 (i.e., added sodium bicarbonate)
Penicillin G potassium	Vitamin B complex with vitamin C

To measure the central venous pressure, an indwelling intravenous catheter is placed in the cranial vena cava via the external jugular vein. It is very important that the catheter tip be located in the cranial vena cava. If the intravenous catheter is properly placed, a 2- to 5-mm fluctuation in central venous pressure will be noted with each respiration.

Next, a sterile three-way stopcock is attached to the intravenous catheter. The open line of the three-way stopcock is connected to the intravenous fluid source. The intravenous fluids are used to prime the manometer; that is, the manometer is filled to overflowing with the intravenous fluids. With the patient in lateral recumbency, the zero point of the manometer is positioned at the level of the sternum (Figure 25-10). The central venous pressure is equal to the level of intravenous fluid in the manometer once equilibrium has been established. To improve accuracy, this determination should be repeated a total of three times. If the pressure is high, prevent blood from entering the manometer because a blood clot may alter the measurements.

The following points are important considerations when measuring and interpreting central venous pressure measurements. Serial measurements should be performed with the same zero point and the patient in the same position. If the catheter is obstructed because of blood clots

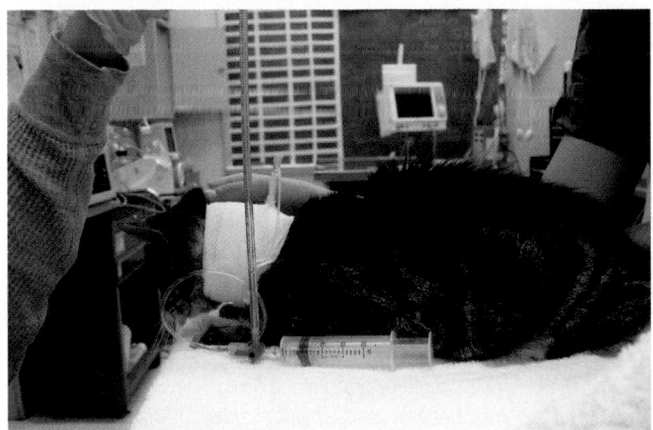

Figure 25-10 Use of a manometer to measure central venous pressure in a dog.

or kinking, the central venous pressure will be falsely elevated. Obstruction should be suspected if the level of the manometer does not fluctuate with respiration. Because continuous recording is not possible, pressure measurements are made intermittently. If intravenous fluids are not being administered between central venous pressure measurements, the catheter should be flushed with heparinized saline. Heparinized saline is prepared by adding 5 U of heparin per milliliter of saline. When evaluating the central venous pressure, it is better to evaluate trends rather than single measurements. Usually, changes of less than 3 cm of water are not significant. Using the sternum as the zero point, normal central venous pressure in the dog and cat varies between 0 and 5 cm of intravenous fluid. If the central venous pressure is consistently more than 8 to 10 cm of intravenous fluid, volume overload is suspected and fluid administration should be slowed or stopped.

✐ TECHNICIAN NOTE

Heparinized saline can be prepared by adding 5 U of heparin per milliliter of saline. For example, add 500 U of heparin to a 100-ml bag of saline.

BLOOD TRANSFUSION

Blood transfusion is an effective method of fluid replacement but a potentially hazardous form of treatment. Clear indications for its use must be present. The effectiveness of transfusion is temporary. Consequently, every effort must be made to identify and correct underlying problems.

Severe blood loss is an indication for transfusion therapy. Massive hemorrhage can occur after trauma, surgery or with defects of coagulation. Measurement of the packed cell volume (PCV) can be misleading immediately after acute blood loss because of compensatory vasoconstriction and splenic contraction. The PCV may remain normal for as long as 6 hours after an acute bleeding episode, but the total

protein will decrease soon after the bleeding episode and therefore can be used as an early indicator of blood loss. As the intravascular volume is restored by the redistribution of body fluids, the PCV will drop. Collectively, the following clinical parameters are better indicators of acute hemorrhage than the PCV: total protein, pulse pressure, depth and rate of respiration, mucous membrane color, capillary refill time, urine production, central venous pressure, and arterial blood gases.

In the treatment of chronic anemia, blood is used primarily for its oxygen-carrying capabilities and should not be considered definitive therapy. The decision to transfuse should be based on clinical signs (e.g., respiratory distress, weakness) rather than an arbitrarily determined PCV or hemoglobin concentration. Some animals with chronic anemia have been shown to be able to increase oxygen delivery at the tissue level by means of biochemical changes within the red cells. Thus one dog with a PCV of 12 may be well compensated, whereas another with the same PCV will be severely compromised and will require a transfusion.

Transfusions may be indicated to stop or prevent bleeding resulting from decreased number of platelets or abnormal platelet function, but large quantities of blood are needed to significantly raise the platelet count; therefore platelet-rich plasma is the preferred method to replace platelets. Because platelets survive for less than 12 hours in stored blood, freshly drawn blood should be used. Transfusion therapy is also useful in the treatment of hereditary or acquired bleeding disorders, such as hemophilia, Von Willebrand disease (vWD), or disseminated intravascular coagulation (DIC). As with platelets, some coagulation factors are labile, so transfused blood should be less than 12 hours old. The basis for this use is to provide adequate concentrations of the deficient coagulation factor at the bleeding site.

Transfusion of blood is indicated in autoimmune hemolytic anemia only in life-threatening situations. The transfused red blood cells (rbcs) may be hemolyzed by the patient's immune system due to antibodies attacking the cell membrane. Transfusions should never be withheld from a patient if needed, in fact, many patients with the refractory form of the disease may need several transfusions before the disease is under medical control. Giving rbcs to these patients may increase the risk of pulmonary thromboembolism due to the rapid destruction of rbcs. If transfusion is necessary as a life-saving measure, only the absolute minimum number of rbcs should be administered. An initial replacement volume of not more than 12 ml/kg of body weight would be acceptable in this situation.

Transfusions to correct leukopenia [low white blood cell (WBC) count] or hypoproteinemia (low serum protein) are of equivocal long-term benefit and require such large volumes to affect a significant rise in these parameters that they are impractical for this use.

There are 19 or more known blood groups in dogs. Canine blood groups are designated by the presence of specific *dog erythrocyte antigens* (e.g., DEA-1.1, DEA-1.2,

DEA-3, DEA-4). Any of these erythrocyte antigens can stimulate antibody production if it is transfused into a recipient that is negative for that particular antigen. DEA-1.1 is the most powerful stimulus for such antibody production. Reactions to DEA-1.2 are less pronounced; however, they can still be of clinical significance. Dogs positive for DEA 1.1 and 1.2 are referred to as blood group *A positive* (+) and dogs negative to these antigens are referred to as blood group *A negative* (−). Reactions to the other canine erythrocyte antigens are generally clinically insignificant. Antibodies directed against DEA-1.1 and DEA-1.2 do not occur naturally; consequently, clinically significant adverse reactions do not occur on first transfusion.

Because 60% of dogs have either DEA-1.1 or DEA-1.2 antigens, transfusion with blood from a random donor (i.e., untyped donor) has a good chance of stimulating DEA-1.1 or DEA-1.2 antibody production. On subsequent repeated random transfusions, the incidence of transfusion reactions may increase due to the patient being "sensitized" to that antigen. Besides the possibility of transfusion reactions, other problems associated with the transfusion of untyped blood include decreased survival of transfused cells in the recipient and hemolytic disease of newborn pups born to dams sensitized by transfusion.

Unfortunately, blood typing sera are not readily available. The availability of in-house blood typing cards for DEA 1.1 has become common use in many hospitals. Once the blood type is known, the donor's rbcs and serum should be cross-matched with the patient's rbcs and serum for incompatibility. If multiple blood transfusions are required, cross-matching should be performed to detect donor-recipient incompatibility for each transfusion. A major crossmatch is performed by combining two drops of a 4% suspension of the donor's rbcs suspended in the donor's serum with two drops of the recipient's serum and incubated in a test tube at room temperature for 15 minutes. The tube is centrifuged at 1000 revolutions per minute (rpm) for 1 minute, and the contents are examined for hemolysis. If hemolysis is present, the transfusion is incompatible, and that donor blood should not be used. A minor crossmatch is performed as above but tests the donor's serum against the patient's rbcs. In the dog, a major crossmatch is all that is necessary to detect incompatibility. In the cat, a major and minor crossmatch are needed.

Cats belong to either blood group A or B. Most cats in the United States belong to blood group A with only a small percentage having blood group B. European cats have a higher percentage of blood group B, but the majority have blood group A. Cats can have a life-threatening reaction to the first transfusion due to the inheritance of preformed antibodies to the opposite blood group. Therefore, in cats, blood typing and cross-matching should always be performed on the first and subsequent transfusions.

Blood Donors
Canine blood donors should not have DEA-1.1 or DEA-1.2 and should be negative for heartworms, *Ehrlichia canis,*

Babesia canis, and *Haemobartonella canis (Mycoplasma hemocanis).* Donor cats should be blood group A. One or two blood group B cats should be available for the occasional patient that needs this blood type. Donor cats should be negative for feline leukemia virus, feline immunodeficiency virus, and *Haemobartonella felis (Mycoplasma hemofelis).* In large blood donor programs, each animal should be permanently identified and have a permanent medical record.

> **✎ TECHNICIAN NOTE**
>
> Canine blood donors should be blood group A negative and also be negative for heartworms, *Babesia canis, Ehrlichia canis,* and *Haemobartonella canis (Mycoplasma hemocanis)* with serologic testing.

Routine periodic laboratory evaluation, that is, a complete blood count (CBC), biochemistry panel, urinalysis, fecal flotation, and heartworm testing, will help to assess the health status of donors. Routine immunizations should be performed as required. The donors should be fed a good commercial diet and receive a hematinic (vitamin and iron supplement).

The ideal canine donor is greater than 23 kg (50 lb), medium-build dog in good health and of good temperament. Approximately 10 to 20 ml of blood per kilogram of body weight may be drawn every 3 weeks without excessively stressing the canine donor. The ideal cat donor is greater than 3.6 kg (8 lb), not overweight, in good health and of good temperament. In the cat, approximately 60 ml can be drawn every 3 weeks without excessive stress to the donor.

Blood Collection
The donor may be sedated if necessary but in most dogs this is not necessary once they are use to the routine. A surgical aseptic preparation of the collection site is performed. The collection site in the dog and cat is the jugular vein. Blood collection should be performed rapidly and without interruption, using a single venipuncture of the vein to avoid excessive activation of the clotting cascade and damage to the rbcs. If acid citrate dextrose (ACD Evacuated Blood Collection Bottle, Diamond Laboratories, Inc.) is being used, a separate collection set should be used. If citrate phosphate dextrose (CPD) plastic blood pack units (with Integral Donor Tube, Fenwall Laboratories, Inc.) are used, the attached needle should be used. If vacuum bottles are used, care should be taken not to lose the vacuum at the time of venipuncture. Use of glass bottle blood collection systems should be avoided since they are not closed systems and allow the blood to be exposed to room air. Glass bottles also cause platelet inactivation and clumping on contact with the glass surface.

In the cat, a 19-gauge butterfly needle (Travenol Laboratories) and a large syringe containing the desired anticoagulant can be used.

Several anticoagulants are available for routine collection of blood. Blood drawn in heparin or sodium citrate must be used within 24 to 48 hours because of the lack of an rbc preservative, which results in marked increase in pH and the subsequent decrease in red cell adenosine triphosphate. These chemical changes result in rigid red cells that do not deform and thus are rapidly removed from the recipient's circulation.

If blood is to be stored for longer than 48 hours, either acid citrate dextrose (ACD Evacuated Blood Collection Bottle) or citrate phosphate dextrose (CPD Blood Pack Units with Integral Donor Tube) must be used as the anticoagulant and the blood stored at 1° C to 6° C. The temperature cannot vary by more than 2° C, and if the blood is out of refrigeration long enough to warm to 10° C (approximately 30 minutes), it must be used immediately. During storage, the blood should be gently mixed periodically. When collected and stored as described, blood drawn in ACD has an effective storage life of approximately 14 days, and blood drawn in CPD has an effective storage life of approximately 21 days. Blood stored in CPDA-1, with the added rbc preservative adenosine has an effective storage life of approximately 35 to 45 days.

Blood should be gradually warmed to approximately 37° C or room temperature before administration. Refrigerated blood can be warmed by placing the bag in a 40° C water bath. Care should be exercised to prevent excessive warming (more than 50° C). Excessive warming will cause hemolysis.

It is essential that strict asepsis be maintained during collection, storage, and administration of blood and blood products. Once a blood storage container has been entered, the stored blood should be used within 24 hours. Blood should be administered through a sterile blood administration kit (Blood Administration Set, Diamond Laboratories, Inc.). A micropore filter is suggested to reduce the transfusion of microemboli found in stored blood. Administration of blood and blood products can be given by the intravenous (the most common route), intraperitoneal, or interosseous routes (into the bone marrow). The intraperitoneal and intraosseous routes are used more in the neonate.

If the practice has a frequent demand for transfusion therapy, it is desirable to make optimal use of the available donors by separating blood into its components and administering only the needed component. Packed red cells can be produced by either centrifugation or by sedimentation of whole blood. Sedimented packed red cells are separated from plasma by gravity. The recovery of plasma is less efficient by this method; however, a centrifuge is not necessary. If collected in glass vacuum bottles, approximately 25% to 30% of the blood volume separates into plasma by 7 to 9 days, and 45% of the blood volume is available as plasma after 14 to 16 days. Plasma is harvested from the glass collection bottles with a sterile 17.5-cm needle and a sterile syringe. Blood in plastic packs separates more rapidly than blood in glass bottles. Plasma can be collected from plastic packs by means of either a sterile needle and syringe or a plasma transfer pack (Plasma Transfer Sets,

Fenwall Laboratories) and a plasma extractor (Plasma Extractor, Fenwall Laboratories). The plasma transfer packs have attached tubing and adaptors as well as sealable entry ports. Thus the plasma can be collected in a closed, sterile system. If the plasma is to be stored at refrigerator temperatures (1° C to 6° C) for longer than 24 hours, a closed system is essential. Plasma frozen at less than –20° C has a storage life of longer than 1 year. If frozen plasma is to be used to treat bleeding disorders, it should be frozen within a few hours of collection.

If the major indication for transfusion is decreased oxygen-carrying capability, the patient should receive packed red cells. Packed red cells can be administered rapidly with less risk of creating volume overload in a patient with compromised cardiovascular function. The use of packed red cells will also reduce the frequency of transfusion reactions caused by plasma protein incompatibility.

Plasma transfusions are used primarily to expand the extracellular fluid volume. Plasma is also used for its transient benefit in the management of hypoproteinemia. Fresh frozen plasma is a source of coagulation factors for the treatment of warfarin toxicity, DIC, and inherited coagulation factor deficiencies.

An alternative to packed rbcs is bovine hemoglobin solution (Oxyglobin, Biopure, Inc.) also referred to as an *acellular oxygen-carrying replacement fluid*. The advantages of bovine hemoglobin are no need for blood typing and cross-matching, no transfusion reactions and the convenience of having the product stored on the shelf up to 3 years. Caution is necessary in the cat due to possible pulmonary edema when given rapidly. Bovine plasma is an active colloid solution and can cause volume overload if given to a patient with heart failure or renal failure or to any patient if given rapidly or in large amount. Discoloration of serum, urine, and mucous membranes to a yellowish-brown is seen with bovine hemoglobin. Also, certain laboratory tests are affected by bovine hemoglobin in the serum.

Transfusion Reactions

Complications of blood transfusion can be both immunologic and nonimmunologic in origin. Immunologic reactions can result from the transfusion of incompatible blood. Incompatible rbcs in a previously unsensitized recipient will be destroyed 7 to 10 days after transfusion. If the recipient is subsequently exposed to incompatible blood, a more acute hemolytic reaction may occur. Clinical consequences of hemolytic transfusion reactions include the rapid development of tachycardia, hypotension, vomiting, salivation, and muscle tremors. Laboratory changes associated with significant acute hemolysis include hemoglobinemia, hemoglobinuria, and possible acquired coagulation disorders.

Delayed hemolytic reactions will sometimes occur following multiple transfusions. Delayed hemolysis should be suspected if the PCV drops unexpectedly 2 to 21 days after transfusion. The clinical and laboratory signs of acute hemolysis mentioned may not be detected in delayed hemolytic reactions. Transfusion reactions may also be caused by immunologic reactions caused by leukocyte, platelet, or plasma protein incompatibilities. Reactions between antigens and antibodies may activate the complement system and thus release vasoactive substances that may be responsible for trembling, vomiting, and urticaria (hives). Prior transfusion is not required for these reactions to occur. The use of antihistamines (diphenhydramine hydrochloride) approximately 30 minutes before transfusion may reduce these reactions.

Transfusion-induced fever is due to the response of the donor to foreign proteins. The initial step in controlling transfusion-induced fever is to slow the rate of transfusion. If no response is noted when the rate is reduced, the transfusion should be discontinued, and the patient observed closely for more severe signs of reaction. Bacterial contamination of the transfused blood will also produce fever and should be considered. Starting another transfusion after a period of time may eliminate the problem.

Nonimmunologic transfusion reactions are principally due to vascular overload. Signs of vascular overload include coughing, increased respiratory rate, respiratory distress, and vomiting. If there is evidence of preexisting cardiac dysfunction, the rate of administration of blood should be reduced to approximately 1 ml/kg/hr. Because vomiting is a potential adverse reaction to transfusion, food and water should be withheld from the patient during the transfusion as well as any medications scheduled to be given during this time.

✎ TECHNICIAN NOTE

Since vomiting is a potential adverse reaction to transfusions, if the situation allows, the patient should have food and water withheld and avoid the administration of medications during the transfusion.

PHYSICAL THERAPY

Physical therapy can be defined as the use of cold, heat, water, electrical impulses, and therapeutic exercise to treat an injury or disease. When used appropriately, these techniques can either prevent permanent dysfunction or hasten the return of normal function. Physical therapy is especially useful in treating diseases of the musculoskeletal and neuromuscular systems.

Physical therapy can be of tremendous value in reducing muscle spasm, relieving pain, resolving peripheral edema, improving blood supply to a specific site, improving muscle tone, and increasing the range of motion of a joint.

In veterinary practice basically five treatment modalities are employed: superficial heat, cold, massage, active exercise, and electrical stimulation. All these forms of treatment will influence blood supply and edema.

Superficial heat increases the temperature of local tissues, which results in increased metabolism, improved blood supply, and mild analgesia. In contrast, deep heat (e.g., *diathermy*) can potentially increase peripheral edema by increasing capillary hydrostatic pressure. Superficial heat can be applied by means of whirlpool baths, hot packs, or infrared radiation. Moist heat is preferred to dry heat because of its greater action in reducing pain and muscle spasms. Use of a whirlpool bath provides superficial heat as well as buoyancy to support the affected body part. The jet streams of warm water can also stimulate peripheral nerves and cleanse soiled areas. The technique for applying hot packs is to soak a towel or cloth in water as hot as the technician can comfortably stand, wring lightly, and apply to the affected part. As the temperature of the towel decreases, the towel can be rinsed with hot water and reapplied. Twenty minutes is an adequate period of time for this form of heat treatment.

In most traumatic injuries, *early* application of cold will reduce swelling and muscle spasm. Towels or cloths soaked in either cold water or ice water and wrung lightly are a means of applying cold to an animal patient. Alternatively, commercial cold packs or ice packs can be used; however, they should be used with caution in order to prevent cold-induced injury. The required time for treatment is usually 15 to 20 minutes.

If peripheral edema is present, massage may be beneficial. The technique for therapeutic massage consists of gentle stroking and light kneading of the involved area. An attempt should be made to direct the peripheral edema from the involved area toward the heart. This will enhance venous return of the edematous fluid.

Active movement should be encouraged as soon as it can be accomplished safely and without pain. Active movement can be accomplished by swimming the patient in a whirlpool or bathtub. Water treadmills are becoming more common in larger hospitals due to the benefit of exercise with minimal impact on joints. Most animals will swim with encouragement and then actively exercise a body part that otherwise would not be exercised. A towel or sling can be used for support and to keep the animal upright. When appropriate, therapeutic exercise can occur on any nonslippery surface. If the patient is not able to ambulate without assistance, a towel or sling can provide the necessary support. Active therapeutic exercise is of greater benefit than passive exercise.

Although not widely used in veterinary practice, electrical stimulation is beneficial in the treatment of some neuromuscular diseases and neurogenic atrophy.

Owners of animals that would benefit from physical therapy are usually willing to perform physical therapy at home. However, the owner must be carefully instructed on how to perform the treatment and why it will be beneficial to the patient. The technician is usually the best person in the practice to demonstrate the proper technique.

OXYGEN THERAPY

The primary indication for oxygen therapy is *hypoxia*, which refers to a deficiency of oxygen at the tissue level. Tissue hypoxia may be caused by a reduction in perfusion (reduced blood flow) or a reduction in oxygen content of the blood. Hypoxia is probably more common than is recognized in veterinary medicine since a caged animal at rest will not show signs until the oxygen content of the blood is severely reduced.

Hypoxia can be manifested in a variety of ways, and the veterinary technician must be alert to identify these changes. Abnormalities that may be noted in the cardiovascular system include tachycardia or arrhythmias. An increased respiratory rate, open-mouthed breathing, and dyspnea may also be noted. *Dyspnea* is the term used to indicate subjective difficulty or distress in breathing. With severe hypoxia, central nervous system changes may be noted and include drowsiness, altered motor abilities, or increased excitability. Finally, cold extremities may indicate an inadequate supply of oxygen at the tissue level. Cyanosis is not a reliable indicator of hypoxia, especially if the animal is anemic. *Cyanosis* refers to dark bluish or purplish discoloration of the skin and mucous membranes.

Although the basic defect in hypoxia is decreased oxygen availability at the tissue level, it can occur by a variety of mechanisms. For example, it can result from lung disease, decreased cardiac output, or severe anemia.

In small animal practice, oxygen therapy is used primarily in the following clinical situations: pulmonary edema, severe bronchopneumonia, upper airway disease in brachycephalic breeds such as English bulldog and Boston terrier, pulmonary trauma, collapse of lung lobes, and shock. Measurement of hemoglobin saturation is performed with pulse oximetry (Figure 25-11). A pulse oximeter is used by applying a clip to nonpigmented skin or mucous membrane such as the lip, tongue, pinnae, vulva or prepuce to allow reading of hemoglobin saturation in the peripheral blood vessels. Hemoglobin saturation is an indirect way to monitor whether a patient has adequate peripheral arterial blood circulation. It is also a good indicator of hypoxemia due to decreased ventilation of air to the lungs. Direct measurement of oxygenation of arterial blood is monitored with the more invasive arterial blood gas. Arterial blood gas analysis determines the partial pressure of oxygen available in the bloodstream, which is a direct indicator of whether a patient can oxygenate blood in the lungs normally. An arterial blood gas blood sample is taken from the femoral artery. Be careful not to incorporate air bubbles into the sample, and an immediate reading of the sample by a blood gas analyzer is imperative. A pulse oximeter reading less than 70% is considered decreased and an arterial blood gas P_{O_2} less than 95 mm Hg is considered decreased.

Methods of oxygen therapy include oxygen cages, human pediatric incubators, masks, nasal catheters, endotracheal tubes, and intratracheal catheters.

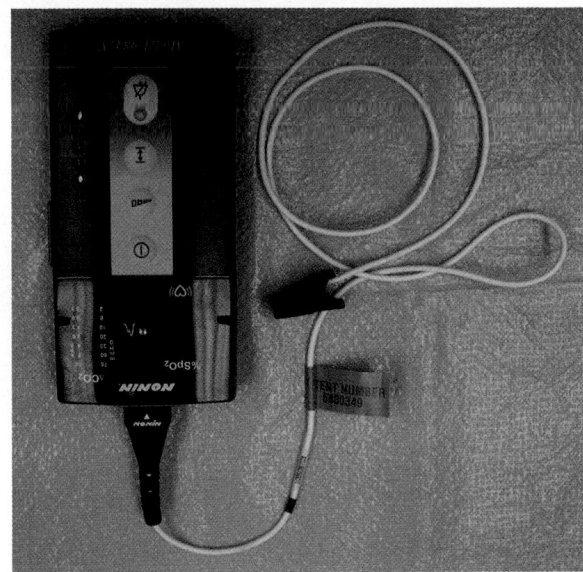

Figure 25-11 Pulse oximeter (Nonin 9847V) measures oxygen saturation.

Oxygen Cage

Oxygen cages for veterinary use are sold commercially. These cages permit control of not only the oxygen concentration but also temperature and humidity (Figure 25-12). These cages are useful in animals able to ventilate without assistance. However, they are expensive and consume large amounts of oxygen. Surplus human pediatric incubators are a less expensive means of providing similar therapy to small dogs, cats, or exotic animals. Oxygen cages and incubators should be flushed (filled) with oxygen after they have been opened. Some units are equipped with entry ports that allow access to the patient without excessive loss of oxygen.

An inspired oxygen concentration of 30% to 40% is adequate for animals requiring oxygen therapy. Excessively high oxygen concentrations can result in oxygen toxicity. Neonatal kittens appear to be particularly susceptible to retinal changes induced by oxygen toxicity.

Mask Induction

In certain circumstances, masks can be used to administer oxygen. Masks are available in a variety of sizes and shapes suitable for use in dogs and cats. If an oxygen mask is used, it is important to provide a high oxygen flow rate to prevent excessive accumulation of carbon dioxide. Administration of oxygen via a mask is suitable for short periods of time only and only in selected patients. Some patients will resist the use of an oxygen mask, and the resultant stress will negate any beneficial effect of the oxygen.

Intratracheal Catheter Induction

An alternative means of oxygen administration that is both inexpensive and effective is the intratracheal catheter. This technique is reserved for critically ill patients. The skin

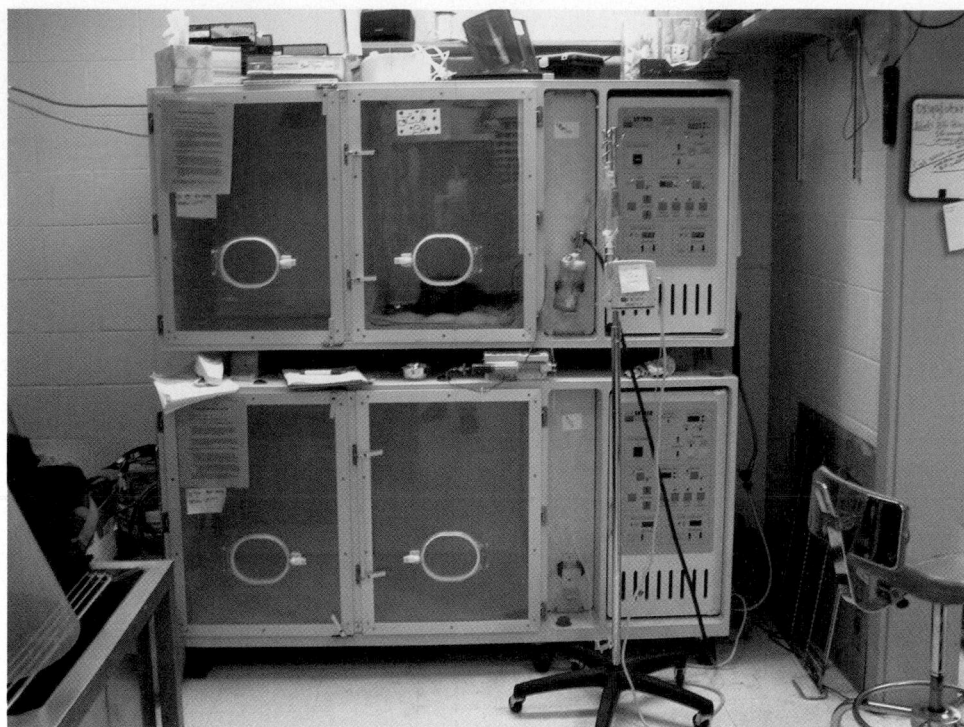

Figure 25-12 Small animal oxygen cage.

is aseptically prepared, and a local anesthetic is administered over the trachea in the midcervical area. An intravenous catheter (14, 16, or 18 gauge) is introduced into the trachea and advanced to a point craniad to the bifurcation of the trachea. The delivered oxygen should be humidified and administered at a flow rate of 0.5 to 4 L/min. The flow rate should be adjusted, depending on the size of the animal.

Nasal Catheter Induction

Nasal catheters can also be used to administer oxygen for brief periods to severely depressed animals. In this technique, a small (5 to 8 Fr) soft rubber feeding tube or urinary catheter is inserted through the external nares to the level of the caudal nasopharynx. The catheter can be coated with a topical anesthetic cream, or topical anesthetic drops can be instilled in the nostril to facilitate passage. Adhesive tape is attached to the catheter, and the tape is sutured to the forehead. An Elizabethan collar is used to prevent the patient from dislodging the catheter.

RESPIRATORY PHYSICAL THERAPY

Physical therapy of the respiratory system is a valuable adjunct to other forms of therapy for diseases of the lungs and airways. Appropriate physical therapy is also useful as a preventive measure in patients at high risk for the development of pulmonary disease. Secondary bronchopneumonia is a common complication in patients with lung lobe collapse. Stimulation of the cough reflex by

compressing the trachea will expand the lungs maximally and help prevent lung collapse. Regular turning of recumbent patients will enhance drainage and circulation and thus prevent hypostatic congestion.

Percussion (coupage), also known as *tapping* or *clapping,* is a technique of striking the animal's chest to loosen bronchial secretion and thus facilitate drainage. The chest is struck with the hand held slightly cupped with fingers and thumb closed so that a cushion of air is trapped between the technician's hand and the chest wall. Best results come from using both hands alternately in rapid sequence for several seconds, moving from ventral to dorsal on the lung fields. When done properly, this is a noisy procedure; however, it is not painful to the patient. If the animal is ambulatory, a brief walk after coupage will aid in mobilization of respiratory secretions.

Whenever possible, animals with pulmonary problems should be maintained in an upright position (i.e., sternal recumbency). If necessary, slings or supports should be used to maintain this posture. When this is not practical, alternating sides of recumbency by turning the patient from one side to the other, every 2 hours, can prevent hypostatic congestion from developing.

TOPICAL THERAPY

Topical therapy plays an important role in the treatment of dermatologic disease. It can be used to treat a specific disease, such as sarcoptic mange. More frequently, however, topical therapy is used either in conjunction with systemic medications or as a form of symptomatic therapy when the diagnosis is unknown.

Plain tap water is one of the most effective topical agents. Depending on how water is used, it can either hydrate or dehydrate the skin. Frequent wetting of the skin will stimulate evaporation from the skin and thus cause dehydration. This approach can be useful in managing any acute moist dermatitis ("hot spot"). In contrast, if a film of oil (e.g., Alpha Keri, Westwood Pharmaceuticals, Inc.) is applied immediately after soaking with water, evaporation is slowed or stopped, and the skin remains moist.

Soaks

Soaks are an effective means of handling localized acute eruptions. Soaks can be applied with moist towels or by placing the animal in a water-filled basin or tub. Soaks for local acute dermatosis should be applied for 10 to 15 minutes three or more times daily. The involved area should be kept constantly moist, and the warm temperature of the soak should be maintained by adding hot water as needed. Some of the solutions commonly used for soaks in veterinary medicine include water, aluminum acetate (Burow solution, Domeboro solution, Dome Laboratories), and magnesium sulfate or Epsom salts (1:65 solution in water, 1 tablespoonful per 1000 ml of water).

Astringents

Astringents precipitate proteins on the surface of an area of acute damage and form a beneficial covering. These agents do not penetrate deeply. Aluminum acetate is an excellent mild astringent. Another effective astringent is tannic acid. Tannic acid is combined with salicylic acid and alcohol in several products to form a potent astringent. These combination products are especially useful as part of the management of localized acute moist dermatitis; however, astringents should be applied only once to an involved area.

Baths

Cleansing baths are an important part of topical dermatologic therapy. Baths aid in the removal of dirt, debris, and scale. A variety of effective mild cleansing soaps or detergents are available. Mild dishwashing detergents or soaps (e.g., Joy, Palmolive Liquid) are effective and inexpensive. If a milder, less irritating product is desired, a balanced pH soap, such as Johnson's Baby Shampoo (Johnson & Johnson), can be used. If an even milder product is needed, vegetable oil soaps (coconut oil) are the most bland. Regardless of how mild the soap or detergent, it should always be thoroughly rinsed out of the coat with copious volumes of clean water.

A medicated bath can be applied as a shampoo or as a rinse applied to the animal after a routine cleansing bath. Medicated baths contain ingredients that enhance the actions of routine cleansing shampoos. Medicated shampoos should be lathered into the coat for 10 to 15 minutes. This allows the medicated component of the shampoo time for effect or limited absorption. Types of medicated baths used in small animal practice include colloidal oatmeal, tar-sulfur, sulfur-salicylic, and benzoyl peroxide products. Colloidal oatmeal (Aveeno, Cooper Care, Inc.; Epi-Soothe cream rinse, Allerderm, Inc.) baths are used for their soothing and antipruritic properties. Tar-sulfur shampoos (Lytar, Dermatologics for Veterinary Medicine, Inc.; Allerseb-T, Allerderm, Inc.) are used in the management of oily, flaky seborrheic conditions. Sulfur and salicylic shampoos (Sebalyte, Dermatologics for Veterinary Medicine, Inc.; Sebolux, Allerderm, Inc.) are used in the management of dry, flaky seborrheic conditions, and benzoyl peroxide shampoos (Oxydex, Dermatologics for Veterinary Medicine, Inc.; Pyoben, Allerderm, Inc.) are useful in the treatment of superficial pyoderma (bacterial skin infection), excessive crusting and debris problems, and oily seborrheic conditions. The underlying condition and the individual response to the medicated bath determine the required frequency of application.

Dips and Rinses

Dips or rinses use water as a means of delivering various antifungal or antiparasitic agents to the skin. Although applied to the skin, some of these agents have the potential to cause systemic toxicities. Clipping the hair and using cleansing baths help to obtain greater penetration in animals with excessive scale or crust. Dips that are useful in the treatment of dermatophytosis (ringworm) include dilute sodium hypochlorite solution, dilute Nolvasan solution (Fort Dodge Laboratories), dilute iodine solutions, or lime-sulfur solutions. Antiparasitic products used as dips or rinses include chlorpyrifos (Dursban), pyrethrins, pyrethroids, organophosphates (malathion), and carbamates. Amitraz (Mitaban, Upjohn Co.) is useful in the treatment of generalized demodectic mange.

Before using any topical agent the label should be checked to be sure it is safe to use in dogs, cats, puppies, and kittens. The age of young animals should be noted because some products are not recommended in the very young.

Powders

Powders are occasionally used in veterinary medicine as drying agents and vehicles for parasiticides and to reduce friction and irritation. When used as a drying agent, powders may be in the form of true powders, shake lotions, or pastes. Components that improve the drying action of various powdered products include talc, zinc oxide, cornstarch, and tannic acid. Carbaryl powders are a valuable part of flea control programs in the dog and cat. Labels should be checked carefully to be certain that the specific product is safe for dogs and cats. The powder must be worked down into the hair coat to increase the parasiticidal effect. This can be accomplished by rubbing the hair coat against the grain as the powder is applied. The powder should be applied to the entire body, excluding the face. Fractious or frightened cats can be treated by wrapping them in a thick bath towel and medicating small sections until the entire animal has been covered. Flea sprays can be used similarly.

Creams and Ointments

Creams and ointments are also used in the topical treatment of dermatologic problems. The area of treatment should be clipped, if not hairless, and protected from immediate removal by licking. For practical and economic reasons, the area to be treated should be relatively small. Ointments are thicker than creams and leave a greasy feeling when applied to the skin. Ointments and creams soften, lubricate, and protect the skin and aid in the removal of scale and crusts. Ointments and creams form an occlusive covering and therefore are not indicated for moist or oozing skin lesions.

Topical creams and ointments can be used to treat localized dermatophytosis (ringworm). They can be used as the sole type of therapy or as an adjunct to oral therapy or topical rinses. Creams and ointments must be restricted to small lesions because of expense and convenience. Effective topical fungicidal products used in veterinary medicine contain miconazole and thiabendazole. Because the use of ointments and creams alone is often insufficient to clear the infection or prevent reinfection, rinses or dips are important.

Otic Preparations

Most topical otic preparations contain various combinations of antibiotic, antiinflammatory, fungicidal, and parasiticidal agents. Topical antimicrobial agents are indicated whenever infection is present. Chloramphenicol, neomycin, polymyxin, and gentamicin are the commonly used antibiotics in these combination otic preparations. Neomycin and gentamicin have been reported to cause ototoxicity when used for prolonged periods in dogs with ruptured eardrums. (Gentamicin is inactivated by purulent exudate; therefore the ears must be thoroughly cleaned before use.)

Corticosteroids are used in these combination products because they decrease inflammation and the buildup of discharge and, consequently, decrease self-trauma by the animal. The antifungals are useful in treating dermatophytes and yeast organisms such as *Malassezia pachydermatis (Pityrosporon)*. Thiabendazole and miconazole are effective topical antifungal agents.

Certain drugs owe their efficacy to their ability to alter the pH in the ear canal. Acetic acid (dilute vinegar solution) and Domeboro Otic (Dome Laboratories) are specific examples.

Products that contain rotenone in oil or thiabendazole are used to treat ear mites. It is essential that treatment for ear mites be continued for at least 3 weeks and that all animals in the household be treated. Otic instillation of ivermectin, as a one-time application (on occasion, two to four treatments may be needed), has also been shown to be effective in the treatment of ear mites.

INFECTIOUS DISEASES

This section will discuss a number of common medical problems of dogs and cats. It is not intended to be a comprehensive review of internal medicine; rather, several specific problems have been selected that illustrate or emphasize important aspects of medical nursing.

CANINE RESPIRATORY DISEASE COMPLEX

Synonyms for canine upper respiratory disease complex include kennel cough and infectious tracheobronchitis. This complex is composed of a number of different disease processes. Causative factors include viral and bacterial agents as well as predisposing environmental factors. These factors may occur singly or in combination. Fever, coughing, ocular and nasal discharge, vomiting, diarrhea, lethargy, and depressed appetite may occur for 24 to 48 hours. The clinical signs are usually gone after 48 hours except for a dry, hacking cough, which can linger up to 2 weeks. The diagnosis of this complex is usually based on historical and physical examination findings rather than on laboratory tests. This problem is most often self-limiting, and the duration of signs generally is no more than 2 weeks.

Treatment involves nursing care and the correction of any environmental factors that may have predisposed to the illness. The dog should be kept in a warm space that is well ventilated and free of drafts and should be fed a highly palatable diet. Appetite will be enhanced if eyes and nose are kept free of accumulated discharge. If appetite is suppressed, the patient should be encouraged to eat canned dog food or even selected table food such as chicken and rice for increased palatability. Intravenous or subcutaneous fluid therapy is occasionally necessary. Steam or vaporizer therapy may provide symptomatic relief of the dry cough. Steam therapy can be performed by placing the dog in a steam-filled bathroom several times per day. Alternatively, cold-mist vaporizers can be used several times daily.

The decision to use antitussive (cough suppressant) therapy should be based on the frequency of coughing and how prolonged the episodes are. If codeine-derivative cough suppressants are used to excess, depression and anorexia will result.

Treatment with antibiotics usually is not indicated unless there is evidence of lower respiratory or systemic involvement, for example, fever. The presence of a green or yellow colored nasal discharge may also warrant antibiotic therapy. If antibiotic therapy is instituted, a complete regimen of 10 to 14 days at full therapeutic doses should be completed. The selection of an antibiotic would ideally be based on the results of culture and sensitivity testing of a transtracheal wash. If these are not available, chloramphenicol, beta-lactam penicillins, first-generation cephalosporins, or fluorinated quinolones are usually effective. The use of systemic products containing both antibiotics and corticosteroids is not indicated. Likewise, the intratracheal injection of any product is inappropriate therapy.

Because of the highly contagious nature of the causative organisms, an infected dog should be isolated from other hospitalized patients. If possible, hospitalization should be avoided. Once an outbreak occurs in a kennel or veterinary hospital, control is difficult. Ideally, the area should be kept vacant for approximately 2 weeks, and appropriate preventive measures should be instituted, consisting of the implementation of an effective vaccination protocol for every hospitalized patient. All dogs should preferably be vaccinated at least 10 days before exposure. At least every 3 years revaccination for the respiratory viruses of all patients over 1 year of age should be a consistent hospital policy. Vaccination with the intranasal vaccine for *Bordetella bronchiseptica* every 6 months is recommended for animals at high risk of exposure to the causative agents of infectious tracheobronchitis (e.g., frequent boarding or dog shows). The commonly used disinfectants, such as chlorhexidine (Novalsan) and benzalkonium (Roccal), effectively kill the causative bacteria and viruses.

FELINE RESPIRATORY DISEASE COMPLEX

The principal components of the feline respiratory disease complex are feline viral rhinotracheitis and feline calicivirus. Less frequently incriminated agents include feline reovirus, feline pneumonitis (*Chlamydia psittaci*), *Mycoplasma*, and *Bordetella* bronchiseptica.

Clinical signs of this complex include fever, cough, paroxysms of sneezing, and hypersalivation. As the infection progresses, mucopurulent ocular and nasal discharge, lacrimation, and open-mouthed breathing can be seen. Ulceration of the tongue, hard palate, and nasal pad has been reported with feline calicivirus. The severity of signs and the mortality are greatest in young (less than 1 year of age), nonvaccinated cats and kittens. The severity of the clinical signs will vary widely from patient to patient. The variability results from a number of interacting factors, which include the virulence of the virus, infecting dose of virus, and general health and immune status of the infected cat.

Diagnosis is based primarily on history and clinical signs rather than on laboratory findings. Occasionally, laboratory confirmation of the diagnosis by means of virus isolation or the demonstration of serum antibodies is indicated. The additional expense of laboratory confirmation is justified only when dealing with groups of cats having a chronic history of feline respiratory disease complex.

Treatment will vary, depending on the severity of signs. Some cats will show only mild, transient signs, and they require no treatment. Secondary bacterial infection will occasionally be a sequelae to the feline respiratory disease complex, and therefore a broad-spectrum antibiotic may be indicated in the very young kitten (<12 weeks of age).

General nursing care is of much greater importance than antibiotics in typical cases. Whenever possible, infected cats should be treated at home rather than in the hospital.

A vital part of nursing care is to gently clean away accumulated ocular and nasal discharge. If the nostrils are kept patent, the cat is more likely to continue eating due to the cat's reliance on smell to encourage appetite. To ensure that this happens, the owner should indulge the pet and provide highly palatable foods. Strongly flavored or odorous foods (fish flavored) are more likely to stimulate the appetite of an anorectic cat. Steam therapy is frequently useful and can be achieved by placing the cat in a steam-filled bathroom or by using a vaporizer.

In cats that become completely anorectic, subcutaneous or intravenous fluids may be required until the appetite returns to normal. Repeated syringe feedings may be attempted; however, in certain cats, the associated stress may negate any beneficial effect. Alternatives that appear to be better tolerated include nasoesophageal or pharyngostomy tubes. These procedures should be reserved for severely cachectic cats.

The virus is usually transmitted through direct contact with an infected cat. Sneezing with subsequent aerosolization of the virus will spread the virus a distance of approximately 15 to 20 cm. Fomite transmission via hands, clothing, letterboxes, and food and water dishes is a more significant means of transmission than aerosolization in veterinary hospitals. The agents responsible for the feline respiratory disease complex are sensitive to hypochlorite disinfection.

The best way to prevent outbreaks of feline respiratory disease complex in hospitalized cats is to have an effective immunization protocol that requires vaccination of the respiratory viruses at least every 3 years in cats over 1 year of age. Adequate ventilation will reduce the likelihood that infection will spread within the hospital. The humidity should be maintained between 30% and 50%. Disposable food trays and litter pans and autoclavable water dishes should be used. Cats should not be moved from one cage to another unless absolutely necessary during an outbreak. Cages should be thoroughly cleansed with a dilute hypochlorite solution. Finally, because the infection can be spread via hands and clothing, meticulous hygiene on the part of all hospital personnel is essential. It is important to understand that up to 80% of the cats that develop this respiratory complex remain lifelong carriers of the organism or organisms. They can pose a risk to other cats or can experience a recrudescence of the complex in stressful situations.

CANINE DISTEMPER

Canine distemper is an important viral disease of dogs because of the ubiquitous nature of the virus and the mortality associated with infection. The severity of signs will vary from a transient, subclinical infection to a severe fatal disease that involves several different organ systems. This variability is due to the differing virulence of various virus strains and differences in host immunity.

The initial phase of the infection is associated with fever, transient anorexia, lethargy, and a mild serous ocular discharge after an approximate 9- to 14-day incubation period. Obviously, these signs are not specific for canine distemper. Later, as the virus spreads to the respiratory and gastrointestinal systems, mucopurulent ocular and nasal discharge, coughing, diarrhea, and, occasionally, vomiting are noted. Many dogs are anorectic at this point and become severely dehydrated. Involvement of the central nervous system may occur and can be the only signs manifested by some dogs. These dogs may develop seizures or other evidence of neurologic disease. Some dogs will seemingly recover from the severe respiratory and gastrointestinal signs, but weeks or months later they develop neurologic signs that either are fatal or require euthanasia because of their severity.

Although the virus may survive in the environment for weeks at near-freezing temperatures (0° C to 4° C), it is susceptible to heat, drying, and ultraviolet light. Routine disinfection is usually effective in destroying the virus in a hospital or kennel. Patients suspected to have distemper should be housed separate from the rest of the hospital patients. An isolation ward or cat ward would be acceptable to prevent the spread of the virus to susceptible canine patients. Diligent washing of hands and avoiding fomite transmission after handling distemper suspects is also necessary to avoid spread of the virus.

FELINE PANLEUKOPENIA

Feline panleukopenia is a potentially severe, highly contagious parvoviral disease of cats. Synonyms are feline distemper and infectious enteritis.

The typical clinical signs associated with feline panleukopenia include lethargy, anorexia, vomiting, and diarrhea after a 7-day incubation period. Characteristically, the feces are yellowish and semiformed to fluid in consistency; they may be blood tinged. Severe dehydration may be present. The temperature may be elevated or subnormal. Feline panleukopenia can be an acute disease. Rarely, development of signs is so rapid that the owner may suspect malicious poisoning. Kittens and young cats appear to be more severely affected.

Diagnosis of feline panleukopenia is based on the presence of the clinical signs described above in the presence of a low total leukocyte count (less than 2000 WBCs/mm³). The low total count is primarily due to low numbers of neutrophils. The diagnosis of feline panleukopenia can be confirmed by virus isolation and serologic and histopathologic characteristics.

Treatment is primarily supportive because specific antiviral drugs are not available. The cornerstone of successful therapy is the correction of fluid and electrolyte imbalances and prevention of sepsis by the use of broad-spectrum antibiotics. Symptomatic control of vomiting and diarrhea is usually indicated. Another complication the technician should be aware of is the development of hypoglycemia. This may be manifested by the development of extreme weakness, seizure activity, or both.

The prognosis for recovery is good if the cat survives the initial 3 to 6 days of severe clinical signs. The prognosis for kittens and young cats is guarded. A rising WBC count indicates a more favorable prognosis. During the recovery phase, the WBC count may exceed 50,000/mm³ and reveal a significant leftward shift. This should not be confused with the development of another infection, because this can be a normal response.

If the queen is infected during pregnancy, fetal death or congenital defects in the kitten may result. The fetus is susceptible to the virus because most tissues have high cell-proliferation rates. If the fetus is infected just before or immediately after birth, the development of the cerebellum may be affected and hypocerebellum can occur. These kittens show balance and coordination problems beginning at about 3 to 4 weeks of age.

Fortunately, because of the availability of excellent vaccines, feline panleukopenia is currently an infrequent clinical problem.

FELINE LEUKEMIA VIRUS AND FELINE IMMUNODEFICIENCY VIRUS INFECTION

These two distinct retroviral infections in cats may cause similar clinical signs. Feline leukemia virus (FeLV) has been recognized for many years and may cause immunosuppression, neoplasia, or both. Lymphosarcoma and bone marrow disorders are the more common disorders associated with FeLV. The virus is transmitted between cats by direct contact through grooming, sharing food dishes, and fighting. The virus is easily killed in the environment, and isolation of an infected cat is adequate to prevent transmission to susceptible cats. Although most cats that are exposed to the virus successfully eliminate the infection, 1% to 3% of cats in single-cat households and up to 30% of cats in multiple-cat households will become persistently infected with the virus. These infected cats are then at risk for the development of the plethora of FeLV-related diseases. FeLV infection can be identified by an in-hospital test that detects viral antigen. There are many such in-hospital tests on the market and available to the practicing veterinarian. There are several vaccines available for the prevention of FeLV. These vaccines are not completely protective but do protect up to 70% of the vaccinated cat population.

Feline immunodeficiency virus (FIV), also called T-lymphotrophic T cell lentivirus (FTLV), is another virus that causes immunosuppression in the cat. Common clinical signs of infection with this virus include gingivitis, chronic diarrhea, generalized lymphadenopathy, fever, conjunctivitis, rhinitis, and dermatitis. It is notable that all these signs may be seen in cats infected with FeLV. FIV is found nationwide and, indeed, worldwide. Most cats infected with this virus will not become immune, which differs from FeLV infection. The disease is spread by inoculation of the virus through cat bites which allow blood transmission. Transmission of the virus by direct contact through grooming, sharing of food dishes, and close contact is less than that seen with FeLV. No treatment is available for this disease. Commercial kits detecting antibodies to this virus are available for in-hospital testing. A vaccine is currently available, however the efficacy has not been established. Also, this vaccine will cause a positive FIV antibody test, complicating the ability to clearly document FIV infection in vaccinated cats.

✐ TECHNICIAN NOTE

FeLV infection is spread by direct and repeated close contact such as grooming or sharing of food and water dishes, whereas FIV infection is transmitted by inoculation of the virus through cat bites.

ROUTINE IMMUNIZATION PROGRAM FOR DOGS AND CATS

One of the greatest areas of advancement in veterinary medicine in the past 50 years is in the prevention of infectious diseases. The purpose of any vaccination program is to prevent clinical disease by preventing or limiting infection. The vaccination program can also be the foundation of a complete well-animal health maintenance program. At the time of vaccination, owners should be counseled regarding nutrition, parasite control, and matters regarding reproduction. Chapter 11 provides a complete overview of canine and feline preventive health programs and vaccination recommendations.

A physical examination by the veterinarian at the time of vaccination is extremely important because a number of conditions will potentially influence the immunization procedure, such as pregnancy, debilitation, and fever.

Numerous factors influence the patient's ability to respond to vaccination. Factors that are of practical significance include colostral (maternal) antibodies, vaccine type, route of administration, age of the patient, nutritional status of the patient, and concurrent infection or drug therapy.

Colostral Antibodies

In puppies and kittens, approximately 95% of the circulating immunoglobulins come from absorption of *colostrum* (first milk) shortly after birth. These circulating immunoglobulins provide essential temporary protection, but they also have the ability to interfere with more permanent protection. Interference occurs because the vaccine does not reach the appropriate cells to stimulate the active immunity process. Consequently, it is necessary for the level of circulating immunoglobulins derived from the colostrum to be reduced before successful vaccination is possible. In

puppies born to bitches that have received vaccinations against canine distemper and infectious canine hepatitis, this period of uncertain response to vaccination may extend to 14 weeks of age. Thus the last dose of vaccine should be administered at 14 to 16 weeks of age to optimize the success of the vaccination program. Colostral immunoglobulins to canine parvovirus may persist for at least 16 weeks in puppies; therefore the last dose of vaccine for parvovirus should be given no earlier than 16 weeks of age. In the rottweiler and Doberman breeds, it is suggested that the last dose of parvovirus vaccine be given at 18 weeks of age.

An alternative technique to prevent or reduce the blocking effect of colostral antibodies on canine distemper vaccination is to use measles virus vaccine. Approximately 50% of puppies at 6 weeks of age will not respond to canine distemper virus vaccination, whereas the vast majority will respond to measles virus vaccine. The measles virus stimulates resistance against canine distemper in puppies regardless of circulating antibodies that the pup has acquired from the colostrum. Measles virus vaccine prevents clinical disease but does not prevent infection. Measles virus vaccine should be considered a temporary method of preventing canine distemper until the dog can respond to the canine distemper vaccine. There is no reason to use vaccines containing measles virus in dogs older than 16 weeks of age. There are no known public health dangers associated with the use of measles virus-containing vaccines. Measles virus vaccine does not provide protection against infectious canine hepatitis.

Methods of overcoming the effects of colostral (maternal) antibodies are not absolute. Therefore research is continuing in this area. Although colostral antibodies interfere with the immunization process, colostrum is extremely important for the protection of the neonate against a number of potentially harmful microorganisms. Puppies and kittens should never be deliberately deprived of colostrum.

Type of Vaccine

The type of vaccine is very important in formulating a successful vaccination program. Viral vaccines can be either *inactivated* or *modified live* virus vaccines. Because live virus vaccines depend on viral replication in the recipient animal to provide protection, the vaccine must be handled strictly according to the instructions supplied by the manufacturer. Inactivated vaccines are less labile; however, in general they must be administered several times to get an adequate protective response. It is impossible to state that one type of vaccine is categorically better than another; in the future, both inactivated and modified live virus types of vaccine will continue to be used.

To achieve the optimal response, the entire dose of vaccine should be given as recommended; the dose should not be split and given to more than one animal. Different vaccine products should not be mixed in the same syringe before administration. Frequently, vaccines contain preservatives that will interfere with another vaccine.

Route of Administration

The route of administration specified in the manufacturer's instructions should be followed. With certain viruses, significant differences in response occur, depending on the route of administration. For example, with measles virus and some rabies virus vaccines, the intramuscular route is much more effective than the subcutaneous route. The manufacturer's recommendations must be understood and followed for all vaccines.

With certain viruses (e.g., feline viral rhinotracheitis, calicivirus, feline infectious peritonitis) vaccines that produce local immunity have been developed. These vaccines are given by the intranasal and intraocular routes. An example of a bacterial disease for which an intranasal vaccine has been developed is *Bordetella bronchiseptica*. The basis for this approach is the concept that if the vaccine is administered by the same route that natural infection takes, greater local protection will be achieved. Unfortunately, these vaccines can produce mild clinical disease.

Because of the concern of development of feline sarcomas secondary to vaccination procedures, specific guidelines have been developed for vaccinating cats. Sarcomas have been associated more with rabies and feline leukemia virus vaccines than others. The suspected incidence of vaccine-induced sarcomas is approximately 1 in 1000 to 10,000 cases per year.

The suggested route of administration of rabies and feline leukemia vaccines is to give the rabies in the right rear leg (over the tibia) and the feline leukemia vaccine over the left tibia by the subcutaneous route. In this way, if a sarcoma does develop, amputation of the limb can be done to save the cat's life.

Age of Patient

The age of the animal is important, not only because of the persistence of colostral antibodies but also because of the relative immaturity of the immune response in the puppy and kitten during the first 2 weeks of life. This phenomenon is at least partially due to the hypothermia that exists during this period. Optimal functioning of the cells of the immune system depends on a normal body temperature. A puppy given vaccination at 8, 12, and 16 weeks and a kitten given vaccination 9 and 12 weeks should be revaccinated at 1 year of age to assure adequate response of the immune system to the vaccine.

Nutritional Status

An animal in poor nutritional condition may not respond adequately to vaccination. Generally, caution should be exercised in giving modified live virus vaccines to debilitated animals. However, a debilitated animal should be vaccinated if it is to be hospitalized. Although there is a chance the animal may not respond to the vaccination, it is also possi-ble that the animal will be protected from infection with a virulent organism. If a debilitated dog or cat is vaccinated, vaccination should be repeated when the patient's nutritional status has improved so that immunity is more certain.

Concurrent Disease or Therapy

Occasionally, dogs and cats presented for vaccination are incubating an infectious disease. A detailed history of possible exposure to infected animals as well as a complete physical examination may suggest this situation. However, it is impossible to definitively diagnose most infections in the incubation stage. If there is a history of exposure to an infected animal, the owner should be informed that there is a risk of their animal developing disease despite vaccination.

Certain infections and diseases may be associated with alteration of the immune system and may interfere with successful response to vaccination; examples include dogs infected with demodectic mange and cats infected with feline leukemia virus or feline immunodeficiency virus.

It has been suggested that certain virus vaccines may increase the susceptibility of the recipient animal to the development of the disease for which one is vaccinating against, if the animal is incubating or infected with another virus simultaneously. For example, dogs infected with the canine parvovirus that are subsequently vaccinated with a modified live distemper vaccine may be prone to develop distemper encephalitis because of infection with the parvovirus.

Modified live virus vaccines are not recommended in dogs and cats receiving immunosuppressive agents. Drugs that suppress the immune system are frequently given to animals with cancer or autoimmune diseases, such as immune-mediated hemolytic anemia. Commonly used immunosuppressive agents include cyclophosphamide, azathioprine, methotrexate, and corticosteroids. When corticosteroids are used at antiinflammatory dose levels (less than 2 mg/kg of body weight), the response to virus vaccines is not altered.

> ### ✏ TECHNICIAN NOTE
> Modified live virus vaccines are not recommended in dogs and cats receiving immunosuppressive agents.

Program Guidelines

When all the clinical factors discussed are considered, along with economic factors, it is safe to conclude that there is no single perfect vaccination program. Nonetheless, certain general guidelines are possible. Every veterinary hospital should establish a specific vaccination policy and protocol and adhere to it at all times. This will prevent errors of omission that could result if the vaccination policy is not clearly defined. Usually, the first vaccination should be administered when the animal is between 6 and 8 weeks of age. Animals should be revaccinated at 10 to 12 and 16 to 18 weeks of age. New vaccine guidelines recommend that revaccination should occur at 1 year of age or 1 year after the last puppy or kitten vaccine. Annual revaccination is unnecessary for most viral diseases, but for others it is of critical importance. Every 3 years vaccination is recommended for dogs and cats over 1 year of age that were properly vaccinated as puppies and kittens. Rabies vaccination could be given every 3 years as well but must be given based on the local county regulations, which can be as often as yearly.

Vaccine Reactions

Anaphylactic reactions to vaccines can occur after vaccinations are given. Typically it will occur on the second or third vaccination in the puppy or kitten series. Severe anaphylactic reactions occur immediately and up to 30 minutes after the injection. Severe reactions cause cardiovascular shock and respiratory arrest that can lead to death if not treated immediately with intravenous (IV) corticosteroids, epinephrine, and fluids. Vomiting, diarrhea, and urticaria are early signs of a reaction and should be treated immediately with IV fluids and corticosteroids. Milder reactions of vomiting and diarrhea should be noted in the medical record as a possible vaccine reaction. In severe life-threatening reactions, the animal should never be vaccinated again. In milder cases, the animal should be premedicated with an antihistamine (diphenhydramine hydrochloride) 20 minutes before the vaccination and monitored for at least 30 minutes after the vaccination before leaving the clinic. Many puppies and kittens will be lethargic or sleep more than usual the day after their vaccinations, and this is normal. Neurological signs such as seizure may occur in dogs within a few weeks after vaccinations and may be due to the distemper vaccine. This form of vaccine-related distemper is rarely fatal and usually resolves with treatment. Polyarthritis in cats may occur within weeks after vaccination and may be due to the calicivirus vaccine. Owners may notice a lump or hard nodule at the vaccination site, which may last for a few weeks. If it is present longer than 3 weeks, a biopsy should be taken to identify whether it is neoplasia or just a tissue inflammatory reaction.

PET-ASSOCIATED ZOONOSES

A zoonosis is a disease of animals that is transmissible to humans under natural conditions. The technician is frequently questioned by clients about the public health significance of animal diseases. Hospitalized animals may represent potential sources of zoonotic infection; thus these infections may be considered occupational diseases. (See Chapter 35.)

It is beyond the scope of this section to discuss all the pet-associated zoonoses, but several of the more important infections are described. It is important to stress that when

questions about human medical care arise, a physician should be consulted.

Canine brucellosis rarely occurs in humans. Transmission from an infected dog to a human can occur by contact with blood, urine, semen, milk, and infected tissues. Vaginal discharges, aborted fetuses, and placental material after abortion contain large numbers of bacteria. Infection in humans can be an insidious, chronic disease that resembles infection with other strains of *Brucella,* or it can result in relatively mild flulike symptoms.

Toxoplasmosis can be acquired by human exposure to cat feces containing infective oocysts. Cats are an obligate host in the life cycle of *Toxoplasma. Toxoplasma* oocysts can remain viable in the environment for as long as 6 months under ideal conditions. The following recommendations to reduce the exposure hazard from toxoplasmosis-infected cats should be followed.

Plastic gloves should be worn when cleaning litter pans or handling potentially contaminated soil.
Children's sandboxes should be covered, and basic principles of sanitation should be followed.
Immunodeficient people and women of child-bearing age should exercise extreme caution to reduce the risk of exposure.
Women contemplating pregnancy should have their antibody status determined by a physician.

Those with a significant titer against toxoplasmosis are probably protected from reinfection. Antibody titers in cats are of little value because they indicate exposure to the organism and do not indicate that the cat is currently infected or is actively shedding infective oocysts. An enzyme-linked immunosorbent assay (ELISA), currently available through the University of Georgia and Colorado State University veterinary schools, identifies immunoglobulin M (IgM) and immunoglobulin G (IgG) antibodies in a cat's serum and may provide evidence for an acute or a recent infection in a cat. It should be stressed to the concerned client that eating raw or improperly cooked meat probably is the most common source of human toxoplasmosis.

Campylobacter and *Salmonella* are bacteria that can produce pet-associated zoonoses. Pets appear to be relatively infrequent sources of *Campylobacter.* When pets are incriminated, it is usually a stray or recently adopted puppy or kitten that has had recent diarrhea. The incidence of *Salmonella* infection acquired from pets is unknown. Animals can be asymptomatic shedders of this organism for an average of 6 weeks. Because the route of transmission is the fecal-oral route, good sanitation is important.

Reports of human leptospirosis attributed to vaccinated pets have appeared in medical literature. The *Leptospira* bacteria that are used for routine immunization may not protect against subclinical infection and shedding of the organisms in the urine. Because transmission is via infected urine, good sanitation is essential.

Visceral larva migrans and cutaneous larva migrans are caused by the migration of animal parasite larvae in human hosts. The technician plays an important role in prevention by educating clients about the risks posed by pets infected with intestinal parasites. Treatment of infected animals and reducing environmental contamination will reduce the incidence of these problems.

Plague *(Yersinia pestis)* is an infectious disease of animals that is transmitted to humans by the bite of an infected ectoparasite, usually the flea. Although the majority of cases in humans result from exposure to infected wild rodents, domestic cats have been associated with a number of infections in humans. Infections have been reported in persons employed in veterinary hospitals. Cats with suppurative lymphadenitis (infected draining lymph nodes) should be considered plague suspects, and caution should be exercised by the veterinary technician when handling exudates or treating draining wounds.

Cat-scratch disease is a disease of humans that usually is associated with cat scratches or close contact with cats. Rarely, exposure to cats has not occurred, and other injuries are incriminated, such as splinters, thorns, or dog scratches. The causative agent is *Bartonella henselae*. It is presumed that cats simply act as vectors for the disease because they are not ill. Multiple cases in the same household have occurred over a period of months or even years. In immunocompromised patients (e.g., humans infected with the human immunodeficiency virus), the disease can cause severe problems and therefore may pose a significant risk to these individuals. Usually, the disease in humans is a mild, self-limited problem.

Rabies is an acute, fatal viral disease of the central nervous system that affects all mammals. Rabies is transmitted by infected secretions, usually saliva. In the United States, the skunk and bat are the most important sources of human exposure. However, raccoons, foxes, and unimmunized dogs and cats may also represent a hazard. In most areas of the world, the dog is the most important vector of rabies.

If human exposure to rabies is suspected, a physician or public health official should be consulted immediately. Technicians should be familiar with local laws governing the handling of animals who have bitten humans. Veterinarians and technicians that have a high exposure to rabid animals should be vaccinated for rabies virus with the human vaccine and have their serum titers checked periodically to assure adequate protection.

Animal bites can cause serious infectious complications, including cellulitis, lymphangitis, soft tissue abscesses, osteomyelitis, meningitis, and bacteremia. Humans who have undergone splenectomy are at particular risk of bacteremia and possibly death if the organism known as DF-2, isolated from the nasal and oral secretions of healthy dogs, is inoculated into tissues by a bite. Animal bites in the veterinary hospital should be washed thoroughly with a disinfectant solution (chlorhexidine) and examined by a physician for a prescription of antibiotics.

Box 25-2 BREEDS PREDISPOSED TO DEVELOPMENT OF GLAUCOMA

- Afghan
- American cocker spaniel
- Basset hound
- Beagle
- Bedlington terrier
- Brittany spaniel
- Dachshund
- Dalmatian
- English cocker spaniel
- English springer spaniel
- Fox terriers
- Great Dane
- Malamute
- Norwegian elkhound
- Saluki
- Samoyed
- Sealyham terrier
- Siberian husky
- Toy and miniature poodles

OPHTHALMOLOGY

GLAUCOMA

Glaucoma is defined as an increase in intraocular pressure. Glaucoma may cause blindness, and there are certain breeds predisposed to primary glaucoma (Box 25-2).

The signs in early glaucoma are often subtle and can be variable. Acute glaucoma is a painful process; signs include tearing, sensitivity to bright light, and pawing at the eye. Inspection of the eye may reveal congested episcleral blood vessels, a dilated nonresponsive pupil, and a cloudy cornea. In chronic glaucoma, the major finding is an enlarged globe.

The diagnosis is made by documenting an increased intraocular pressure. Several methods are used to measure intraocular pressure. Tonometers are the most accurate, but some are expensive. The Schiøtz tonometer is useful and costs approximately $300 to $400, which is well within the means of most veterinary practices (Figure 25-13). Tonopens are less cumbersome to use but can be cost prohibitive in smaller practices, costing approximately $1200.00 each (Figure 25-14).

Glaucoma is considered a medical emergency because delay in treatment may result in permanent damage to the eye. Several drugs are available to treat glaucoma, all of which work by either reducing aqueous production or increasing the opening at the drainage angle.

TECHNICIAN NOTE

Glaucoma is considered a medical emergency because delay in treatment may result in permanent damage to the eye.

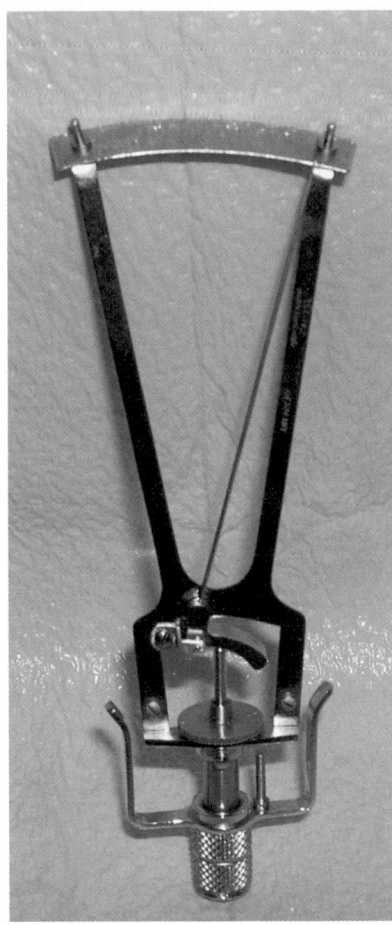

Figure 25-13 Tonometer (Schiøtz Tonometer) used for measurement of intraocular pressure. The tonometer is placed on the cornea to obtain the pressure reading.

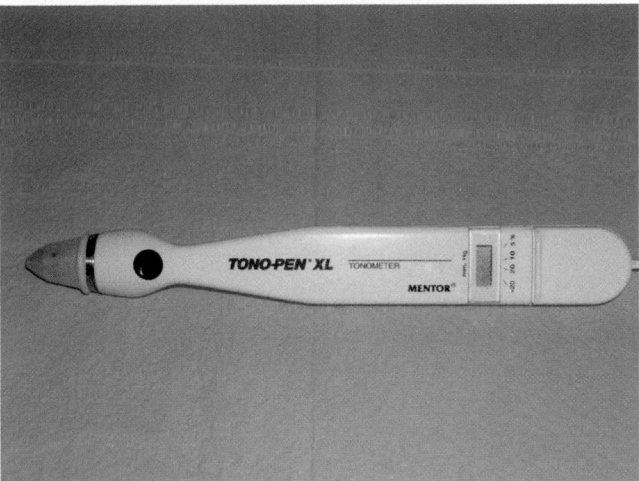

Figure 25-14 Tono-pen XL (Mentor) used for measure of intraocular pressure. Improved tonometer that is less cumbersome to use.

CATARACTS

A cataract is a focal or diffuse opacity within the lens and its capsule. Cataracts may be hereditary or nonhereditary. They should be differentiated from nuclear sclerosis, which is a normal aging change that decreases the clarity of the nucleus of the lens.

Inherited cataracts occur in many breeds and may be associated with other eye abnormalities. Different modes of inheritance have been reported in different breeds. Breeds reported to have inherited cataracts include the beagle, German shepherd, golden retriever, Labrador retriever, Afghan hound, American cocker spaniel, Boston terrier, poodle, and miniature schnauzer. Inherited cataracts have not been reported in the cat.

Cataracts can be the result of metabolic abnormalities, such as diabetes mellitus, inflammation, or trauma. Inflammatory diseases associated with cataracts include feline infectious peritonitis, feline leukemia virus, leptospirosis, and systemic mycoses.

There is no successful medical treatment for cataracts, but any associated inflammation should be treated.

Medications that dilate the pupil may be helpful in improving vision in cases of immature or hypermature cataracts. Currently, the only effective therapy for cataracts is surgical removal of the lens.

CORNEAL ULCERS

Superficial corneal ulcers may result from trauma, decreased tear production (keratoconjunctivitis sicca), aberrant eyelashes (distichiasis, districhiasis), inward rolling of the eyelid (entropion), and inability to blink. Animals with superficial corneal ulcers experience a significant amount of pain. This pain is manifested as excessive tearing, sensitivity to bright light, and squinting (blepharospasm). Corneal ulcers are diagnosed by using fluorescein dye. Fluorescein is a water-soluble dye that will not stain the epithelial layer but stains the underlying layers if the superficial epithelial layer is damaged.

Treatment should be directed first toward correcting the underlying cause. Once this has been accomplished, epithelialization of the ulcerated area is rapid and usually uncomplicated. Broad-spectrum antibiotics are generally used to eliminate infection. Antibiotic solutions and ointments that contain a corticosteroid should never be used with a corneal ulcer. Corticosteroids cause decreased healing with resultant deepening of the ulcer and possible corneal rupture. It has been shown that ointments may retard healing more than solutions; however, the difference in healing may not be clinically significant. One advantage to solutions is that the dose can be more easily controlled. Ophthalmic drops are applied by opening the upper and lower eyelid with one hand, tilting the patient's head slightly back, and then squeezing 1 to 2 drops of the solution into the eye with the other hand. Ophthalmic ointments are applied by the same restraint technique and then squeezing 1/8 inch of the ointment onto the cornea of the eye and then closing the eyelids shut for a moment to spread the medication. Systemic medications usually are not necessary with corneal ulcers. Occasionally, a surgical flap over the cornea or a special contact lens is necessary until epithelialization is complete.

DERMATOLOGY

Veterinary dermatology is an important part of small animal practice. Veterinary dermatology is a challenging discipline; although there are many causes of skin disease, there are only a limited number of ways in which the skin can react. Consequently, in many cases a specific etiologic diagnosis can be difficult to make.

It is beyond the scope of this chapter to consider all the common dermatologic diseases of dogs and cats. Instead, emphasis is placed on several diagnostic procedures that are commonly performed by veterinary technicians.

SKIN SCRAPING

Skin scraping is one of the most frequently used tests in veterinary dermatology. It should be part of the minimum data base whenever the diagnosis has not been established. The skin scraping is used to identify microscopic ecto-parasites such as *Demodex* and *Sarcoptes* as well as dermatophytes. The material and equipment needed to identify ectoparasites include mineral oil, scalpel blade, microscope slide, coverslip, and microscope. The material and equipment used to identify a dermatophyte include saline, scalpel blade, microscope slide, coverslip, potassium hydroxide solution, a heat source (e.g., Bunsen burner), and a microscope.

A representative area should be selected for the skin scraping. In general, an area that has not been disturbed or medicated should be selected. If a dermatophyte is suspected, an area near the margin of the lesion should be selected. If *Demodex* is suspected, a fold of skin should be gently pinched and the skin scraped until there is a slight ooze of blood. When scraping for ectoparasites, a drop of mineral oil should be placed on the scalpel blade so that it is possible to transfer the material to a microscope slide. When scraping for dermatophytes, saline or water is used to wet the blade to facilitate the transfer of the specimen to the microscope slide.

Once the accumulated material and mineral oil have been transferred, one or two drops of mineral oil are added, and the mixture is spread evenly with an application stick. A coverslip is added, and the specimen is carefully examined under the microscope. If parasites are not found, demo-dectic mange is generally eliminated as a diagnostic possibility; however, as many as eight to ten sites should be evaluated and found to be negative before eliminating sarcoptic mange as a possibility.

If a dermatophyte is suspected, a potassium hydroxide preparation should be examined. The material is collected, using the technique described, and placed on a microscope slide. Several drops of 10% potassium hydroxide are placed on the sample, a coverslip is added, and the slide is gently heated for 15 to 20 seconds. Alternatively, the preparation can be placed on the microscope stage and heated by the microscope light source for 15 to 20 minutes. Interpretation of the specimens obtained requires patience and experience. Identification of dermatophytosis can be made by finding branching mycelia. The mycelial filaments are uniform in diameter (2 to 6 μm), are divided into compartments, and vary in length and degree of branching. Hair shafts should be carefully examined for spores. The dermatophytes that infect animals generally have ectothrix spores, which form a prominent sheath on the outside of the hair shaft, in addition to growing inside the hair shaft.

If there is any doubt about the interpretation of the potassium hydroxide digestion, a fungal culture should be performed. A culture is considered the most reliable means of identifying dermatophytes.

The equipment needed for culture includes culture media, a sterile scalpel blade, sterile forceps, and alcohol swab. Appropriate culture media include Sabouraud media and dermatophyte test media (DTM).

Before a specimen is obtained, the area is cleansed with 70% alcohol to reduce bacterial contamination. A small scraping of superficial debris and hair should be obtained, using the sterile scalpel blade and forceps. Alternatively, a small tuft of hair can be plucked from the margin of a lesion, using mosquito hemostats. The hair sample should be deposited partially beneath the surface of the culture medium. The culture medium bottle cap should be left open one-fourth turn to provide aerobic conditions, and the specimen should be incubated at room temperature. Care should be taken not to inoculate the medium with too large a specimen because this may confuse interpretation of the results. A number of commercial media containing agents that inhibit the growth of bacteria and indicator dyes that help to differentiate pathogens from saprophytes are available (e.g., Fungassay, Pitman-Moore).

Another commonly used diagnostic technique in veterinary dermatology is bacterial culture of suspected pyodermal lesions. The technique used to obtain the specimen is extremely important because skin contaminants are usually present. A representative site should be selected, and an unopened lesion should be gently prepared with a surgical scrub. The lesion should be opened with sterile instruments, and a sterile swab should be inserted deep into the cavity or tract. Alternatively, after the area has been scrubbed, a sterile needle is introduced into the unopened lesion, and the purulent material is aspirated into a syringe. Inoculation of the culture medium should be made immediately. Direct smears should also be made immediately and stained with Gram stain.

CARDIOLOGY

CONGESTIVE HEART FAILURE

Congestive heart failure is a clinical term used to describe the state when the heart is unable to maintain adequate cardiac output. Because of decreased cardiac output, the body's tissues do not receive sufficient blood supply for normal function. The decreased cardiac output and the resultant increase in pressures within the vessels entering the heart stimulate complex compensatory mechanisms that contribute to the clinical signs of congestive heart failure. The term *congestive heart failure* does not indicate a specific etiology.

Tachycardia and cardiomegaly (heart enlargement) are general signs associated with congestive heart failure. However, depending on the principal site of involvement, signs of left-sided or right-sided heart failure will predominate.

Left-sided heart failure results from dysfunction of the left atrioventricular valve (mitral valve), ventricle, or both. Clinical signs associated with left-sided heart failure include cough, exertional dyspnea, orthopnea, and, at times, syncope. Characteristically, early in left-sided heart failure the cough occurs in paroxysms and at night or in the early morning. The cough in left-sided heart failure is usually secondary to the development of pulmonary edema or occurs because the left atrium has enlarged and compressed the left main-stem bronchus. *Exertional dyspnea* refers to labored breathing associated with increased activity. This may be manifested as decreased exercise tolerance or reluctance to exercise. *Orthopnea* means difficult or labored breathing in the recumbent position. *Pulmonary edema* refers to the accumulation of abnormal fluid in the interstitial spaces and alveoli of the lungs. It can be detected by auscultating rales (crackles) in the lungs or by observing the characteristic pattern on chest radiographs. Syncope, or fainting, results from decreased cardiac output to the brain.

Right-sided heart failure results from a pathologic condition of the right atrioventricular valve (tricuspid valve), right ventricle, or both. Clinical signs associated with right-sided heart failure include hepatic enlargement, ascites, pleural effusion, and subcutaneous edema. Increased pressure in the abdominal veins results in congestion and enlargement of the liver. Increased hydrostatic pressure in capillaries results in leakage of fluid and the subsequent development of ascites, pleural effusion, and subcutaneous edema. Subcutaneous edema is a relatively rare sign in the dog and is seen late in the course of the condition. (Box 25-3 provides a list of signs seen with left- and right-sided heart failure.)

Certain cardiovascular problems result in both left-sided and right-sided heart failure. Obviously, the signs described are not specific for heart disease. Consequently, when evaluating a patient for cough or ascites, the conditions to rule out should include noncardiac problems.

> **Box 25-3** CLINICAL SIGNS OF LEFT- AND RIGHT-SIDED HEART FAILURE
>
> **LEFT CONGESTIVE SIGNS**
> Pulmonary congestion and edema resulting in cough, tachypnea, dyspnea, orthopnea, pulmonary crackles, tiring, hemoptysis, cyanosis
> Secondary right-sided heart failure
> Cardiac arrhythmias
>
> **RIGHT CONGESTIVE SIGNS**
> Systemic venous congestion: high central venous pressure (CVP), jugular vein distension
> Liver and spleen enlargement
> Fluid in chest cavity (pleural effusion) causing dyspnea, orthopnea, and cyanosis
> Fluid in abdominal cavity (ascites)
> Subcutaneous edema
> Fluid in pericardial sac (pericardial effusion)

MITRAL INSUFFICIENCY

Mitral insufficiency resulting from chronic mitral (left atrioventricular) valvular fibrosis is the most frequently diagnosed form of heart disease in the dog. It is followed in prevalence by chronic tricuspid (right atrioventricular) valvular fibrosis, which causes tricuspid insufficiency. *Valvular insufficiency* is a term used to indicate functional incompetence (leakage) of the valve with subsequent regurgitation (backward flow) of blood from the ventricle into the atrium during ventricular systole.

The signs associated with chronic mitral insufficiency are those of left-sided heart failure (e.g., cough, exertional dyspnea, pulmonary edema). The specific cause of mitral valvular fibrosis is unknown; however, it appears to be associated with aging. Certain breeds appear to be predisposed, the majority of these being small breeds of dogs (e.g., miniature poodles). Mitral insufficiency as a cause of left-sided heart failure is much less common in the cat. The diagnosis of chronic mitral insufficiency is based on the clinical history, auscultation of the heart and lungs, thoracic radiography, and electrocardiography. Although the traditional treatment for this condition has included the use of cardiac glycosides (e.g., digoxin), recent evidence indicates that cardiac contractility is normal to increased in the majority of these dogs, and therefore digoxin is not indicated until late in the course of the failure state.

Initially, the use of diuretics such as furosemide (Lasix), a sodium-restricted diet, and exercise restriction are the primary mode of therapy. Treatment with vasodilators such as hydralazine (Apresoline), captopril (Capoten), and enalapril (Enacard) is also beneficial. These drugs work by decreasing the resistance against which the heart has to pump.

HEARTWORM DISEASE

Canine heartworm disease, caused by *Dirofilaria immitis,* is characterized principally by the presence of right-sided heart failure. The adult parasites lodge in the right atrium, right ventricle, right ventricular outflow tract, pulmonary arteries, and vena cava. The major effect of heartworm disease is to produce pulmonary hypertension (increased resistance in pulmonary arteries), which results in right-sided heart failure.

✐ TECHNICIAN NOTE

Canine heartworm disease, caused by *Dirofilaria immitis,* is characterized principally by the presence of right-sided heart failure.

Heartworm disease has a geographic distribution. The highest incidences of infection occur along the southeastern Atlantic and Gulf coasts. Gradually, heartworm disease has spread to most of the eastern and midwestern United States. Small endemic areas have also been reported in the western United States. With the increased travel of dogs from one region to another, heartworm disease is possible anywhere.

Mosquitoes are an intermediate host for the parasite. The disease is spread by mosquitoes ingesting microfilariae (immature parasites, the L_1 larvae) from the blood of an infected dog. The microfilariae undergo maturation within the mosquito to become an infective larva. Infective larvae (L_3 stage) enter the dog through the skin puncture wound produced by the mosquito and migrate to subcutaneous tissue, muscle, or fat. Two more molts occur within the dog's body, and the young adult heartworm arrives in the heart approximately 110 days after infection. The adult female heartworms begin producing circulating microfilariae 6 to 7 months after infection.

The most practical method to detect heartworm disease is to observe the presence of circulating microfilariae in the peripheral blood. The microfilariae of a nonpathogenic filarial worm, *Dipetalonema reconditum,* must be differentiated from those of *Dirofilaria immitis.* The most useful diagnostic characteristics of the microfilariae of *D. reconditum* are the blunt shape of the head and the serpentine progressive movement demonstrated in direct blood smears. There are three basic tests used to detect microfilariae. They include the direct smear, modified Knott's test, and filter tests. Each test has its advantages and disadvantages; however, if cost, sensitivity, and ease of species identification are considered, the modified Knott's test is preferred. During the past few years, serologic testing for heartworm disease has become the preferred method of documenting heartworm infection. There are multiple in-house kits available to detect heartworm antigens in dog serum, and these can be easily performed in practice.

It has been estimated that as many as 25% to 65% of dogs with heartworm disease have no circulating microfilariae.

This is referred to as *occult heartworm disease.* If heartworm disease is suspected based on history, physical examination, radiography, and electrocardiography, yet circulating microfilariae are not present, a serologic test for detection of adult heartworm antigens should be performed.

The treatment of heartworm disease can be divided into three phases. The first phase is to kill the adult heartworms (adulticidal therapy) that are present in the heart and blood vessels. The next phase is to eradicate the circulating microfilariae (microfilaricidal therapy). Finally, preventive medication (prophylactic therapy) is administered to those dogs at risk of developing heartworm disease. This would include any dog residing in or traveling to an endemic area.

Adulticide therapy consists of administering melarsomine dihydrochloride (Immiticide, Merial). It is an arsenical compound given by intramuscular injection into the epaxial muscles in the lumbar region. Two treatments are given 24 hours apart. If needed, a second treatment can be given 4 months later. In the clinically ill dogs, treatment to stabilize the disease is given, and then at a later date, the patient is treated with adulticide in two stages. One injection is given and then 1 month later two injections are given 24 hours apart. This allows a slower kill of heartworms with less chance of pulmonary reaction to dying worms.

The adult heartworms will die slowly over a 2- to 3-week period. Fever, coughing, and, in more severe cases, dyspnea and hemoptysis (coughing up blood) are the signs observed as the worms die and pass to the lungs (pulmonary thromboembolism). Prednisone therapy (1 mg/kg) is the accepted therapy for pulmonary thromboembolism. Administration of aspirin therapy (5 mg/kg once daily) is recommended in dogs with moderate to severe heartworm disease to reduce thromboembolism. It may be started 1 week before treatment and continued for 4 to 6 weeks after treatment.

To minimize the development of clinical pulmonary thromboembolism, it is important to restrict exercise for 3 to 4 weeks after completion of adulticide therapy. If the signs associated with pulmonary thromboembolism are severe, hospitalization and the administration of bronchodilators, antiinflammatory drugs, and antibiotics are recommended. DIC may occur in dogs with severe clinical signs. Treatment of advanced DIC is usually unsuccessful.

Microfilaricidal therapy is begun 3 weeks after adulticide therapy. Ivermectin (Ivomec), 50 µg/kg orally once, is the current accepted method of treatment for microfilaria, even though it is not approved by the U.S. Food and Drug Administration (FDA) for this function.

Heartworm disease may be prevented with the use of one of several products. Some of these also have protective activity against some endoparasites. Table 25-6 lists the products currently available for heartworm prevention in the dog.

Feline heartworm disease is far less common than canine heartworm disease due to dogs being the natural host for

Table 25-6 CURRENTLY AVAILABLE HEARTWORM PREVENTIVES

Trade Name	Ingredients	Company	Antiparasitic Activity
Multiples	Diethylcarbamazinc	Multiple	Roundworms Heartworm prevention
Filaribits	Diethylcarbamazine	Pfizer	Roundworms Heartworm prevention
Filaribits-Plus	Diethylcarbamazine Oxibendazole	Pfizer	Hookworms Roundworms Whipworms Heartworm prevention
Heartgard	Ivermectin	Merial	Heartworm prevention
Heartgard-30 Plus	Ivermectin Pyrantel pamoate	Merial	Heartworm prevention Roundworms Hookworms
Heartgard for cats	Ivermectin	Merial	Heartworm prevention Hookworms
Interceptor	Milbemycin oxime	Novartis	Heartworm prevention Hookworms Whipworms Roundworms
Sentinel	Milbemycin oxime Lufenuron	Novartis	Heartworms Fleas Whipworms Roundworms Hookworms
Revolution	Selamectin (topical)	Pfizer	Fleas Heartworms *Otodectes cynotis* Ticks Hookworms Roundworms
Proheart oral (once a month)	Moxidectin	Fort Dodge	No other antiparasitic activity
Proheart 6 injectible (once every 6 months)	Moxidectin	Fort Dodge	Hookworms

heartworms. In endemic areas, occasionally cats are infected with heartworms. Clinical signs differ from the dog with mild reactions causing occasional vomiting. Severe reactions cause severe respiratory distress due to pulmonary thromboembolism. Most cats presenting with the severe form do not survive. If they do survive, they are treated with corticosteroids for pulmonary thromboembolism and oxygen and then put on feline heartworm prevention to avoid further infections in the future (Table 25-6). Currently there are no safe and effective treatments to eliminate heartworms in the cat. Because the cat is not the natural host, the worms die over a 2- to 3-year period as compared to a 5- to 7-year period in the dog. Preventing further infection during this time may allow the cat to become heartworm free. Diagnosing heartworm infections in the cat is much more difficult than in the dog due to the lower number of worms infecting the cat. In-house antigen tests used in the dog are usually not sensitive enough to pick up antigen in the cat. Thoracic radiographs, angiography, positive antibody titer and clinical signs are used to diagnose feline heartworm disease.

CARDIOMYOPATHY

Cardiomyopathy is a general term that merely indicates that the basic pathologic lesion involves the heart muscle. Cardiomyopathies can be primary or secondary. Primary cardiomyopathies indicate that the myocardial disease is not due to any recurrent or preexisting cardiovascular or systemic disease. Primary cardiomyopathies in cats are further subdivided into hypertrophic, dilated, and restrictive forms. Secondary cardiomyopathies in dogs and cats are less frequent and are the result of diseases such as infection, metabolic disorders (e.g., uremia), endocrine problems (e.g., hyperthyroidism), and infiltrative processes (e.g., neoplasia).

Feline Cardiomyopathy

Hypertrophic cardiomyopathy is characterized by increased thickness of the myocardium and a small left ventricular lumen. Clinical signs are seen in middle-aged cats of all breeds. The most prominent sign is the sudden development of respiratory distress secondary to pulmonary edema. Hind-limb paresis (weakness) and severe pain may also be present. These hind-limb signs are caused by aortic thromboembolism (blood clots) disrupting the blood supply to the hind limbs. This problem can usually be diagnosed easily if femoral pulses are found to be poor or absent. Diagnosis of cardiomyopathy is based on history, physical examination, radiography, electrocardiography, and echocardiography. If echocardiography is not available, nonselective angiocardiography may be necessary for diagnosis. The basic initial therapeutic approach may include diuretics (e.g., Lasix, Hoeschst-Roussel Pharmaceuticals), cage rest, oxygen therapy, beta-adrenergic blockers such as propranolol (Inderal, Ayerst Laboratories), and calcium channel blockers such as diltiazem hydrochloride (Cardizem, Marion Merrell Dow). Long-term management consists of diuretics, beta blockers, calcium channel blockers, a sodium-restricted diet (feline H/D, Hill's), aspirin, and restricted activity. Aspirin is used to reduce the likelihood of aortic thromboembolism.

> ### ✎ TECHNICIAN NOTE
> Hypertrophic cardiomyopathy is characterized by increased thickness of the myocardium and a small left ventricular lumen.

Dilated cardiomyopathy is characterized by extreme ventricular dilation and moderate atrial enlargement. This results in impaired pump function of the ventricle. This type of cardiomyopathy is also known as *congestive cardiomyopathy*. Signs of right-sided heart failure usually predominate. In addition, cats may show a gradual onset of lethargy and anorexia and at times may be brought in dehydrated, hypothermic, and in cardiovascular shock. Respiratory distress secondary to pleural effusion and aortic thromboembolism resulting in hind-limb paresis is also occasionally seen. The basic therapeutic approach is to mechanically remove as much fluid as possible from the pleural cavity (thoracocentesis), administer digitalis (digoxin therapy), and administer diuretics. Aspirin is used as a preventive measure against aortic thromboembolism. Vasodilators, such as nitroglycerin ointment (Nitrol ointment, Kremers-Urban Co.), may have a role in the management of dilated cardiomyopathy.

Some cats with dilated cardiomyopathy have low plasma taurine levels, and cardiac function will increase with oral taurine supplementation of 250 to 500 mg daily. Cardiac function usually improves over a period of months, and if cats are placed on a diet containing ample taurine, cardiac drugs and taurine supplementation may eventually be discontinued. It should be stated that because this association of low taurine levels and cardiomyopathy in the cat has been made, almost all commercial and prescription diets have adequate levels of taurine, so low-taurine dilated cardiomyopathy is much less common than it used to be.

Restrictive cardiomyopathy is the least common form of primary feline cardiomyopathy. A synonym is *endomyocardial fibrosis*. Respiratory distress is the most common clinical sign. Diagnosis is similar to the other forms of primary cardiomyopathy. Response to therapy is generally poor.

Canine Cardiomyopathy

Primary cardiomyopathies in the dog are categorized as dilated (congestive), boxer cardiomyopathy, Doberman pinscher cardiomyopathy, and hypertrophic cardiomyopathy.

Dilated cardiomyopathy is most common in large and giant breed male dogs aged 4 to 6 years; however, English and American cocker spaniels are smaller-breed dogs that may be affected. Presenting signs often include weakness, lethargy, respiratory distress, cough, anorexia, weight loss and possibly ascites, and syncope. The left ventricle and atrium are dilated with decreased contractility. Diagnosis is confirmed by physical examination, radiography, electrocardiography, and echocardiography. Treatment consists of diuretics, a low sodium diet, arteriolar dilators, and positive inotropes, such as cardiac glycosides (digitalis, digoxin). The long-term prognosis is guarded in that most dogs with the dilated form of cardiomyopathy have an average life span of 6 to 8 months after the diagnosis has been made.

> ### ✎ TECHNICIAN NOTE
> Dilated cardiomyopathy is primarily a disease of large and giant purebred dogs, although medium-sized breeds, such as English and American cocker spaniels, are being diagnosed with increasing frequency with this acquired heart disease.

A specific cardiomyopathy occurs in boxers. These dogs may be asymptomatic or present with syncope and episodic weakness. Arrhythmias are common and may cause sudden death. Diagnosis is confirmed by the same methods as those used in dogs with dilated cardiomyopathy. Treatment with diuretics and antiarrhythmics, such as propranolol, may be useful; however, prognosis is still poor.

Doberman pinschers may present with a primary cardiomyopathy that is similar to congestive or dilated cardiomyopathy. Ventricular contractility is often severely compromised, and atrial arrhythmias are common. These dogs are often in fulminant congestive heart failure and require supportive care with oxygen, diuretics, positive inotropes, and vasodilators. Prognosis is poor.

Hypertrophic cardiomyopathy is the most uncommon primary cardiomyopathy in the dog. It is most often seen in German shepherd dogs and other large breeds. Presenting signs are referable to cardiac disease, and sudden death may occur. Treatment with diuretics and propranolol may improve cardiac output and clinical signs.

ENDOCRINOLOGY

Canine hyperadrenocorticism (Cushing syndrome) is a disorder that results from the excessive production of cortisol by the adrenal cortex. The clinical signs of canine hyperadrenocorticism include polyuria, polydipsia, abdominal distention, polyphagia, muscular weakness, dermatologic changes, and reproductive problems (anestrus, testicular atrophy). Cushing syndrome can result from excessive production of adrenocorticotropic hormone (ACTH) by the pituitary gland (pituitary-dependent hyperadrenocorticism) or from a functional tumor of the adrenal cortex. Pituitary-dependent hyperadrenocorticism is by far the most common, comprising approximately 80% of the cases. Diagnosis is based on measurements of the plasma cortisol levels after stimulation with ACTH or suppression with dexamethasone. Treatment is different for these two conditions. If a functional adrenal tumor is present, the recommended treatment is surgical removal. The drug used to treat Cushing syndrome caused by excessive ACTH production is mitotane (Lysodren, Bristol Laboratories). Side effects associated with the use of mitotane include anorexia, lethargy, vomiting, and depression. Hyperadrenocorticism is rare in the cat and usually is suspected due to the secondary consequences of the disease such as insulin resistance in a cat being treated for diabetes mellitus. Although there is much less known about this disease in the cat, diagnosis is similar to the dog. Treatment at this time is surgical removal of the adrenal glands. Medical therapy has not been as effective in the cat.

Canine hypoadrenocorticism (Addison disease) is caused by a lack of glucocorticoid and/or mineralocorticoid levels and activity. It is generally seen in the middle-aged female, and the most common signs are gastrointestinal (vomiting, anorexia), weakness, depression, and collapse. These signs may have a waxing-waning course.

In an acute crisis these patients may present in acute collapse and in hypovolemic shock. The classic laboratory abnormalities are a low serum sodium (Na^+) level and a high serum potassium (K^+) level, resulting in a low Na^+/K^+ ratio (usually less than 25:1). These patients may also be azotemic and have a low urine specific gravity, which could be confused with renal failure.

The most accurate means of diagnosis is to perform an ACTH stimulation test and show that the patient has a very poor response to this drug, because cortisol levels will not increase following ACTH administration.

The treatment consists of aggressive isotonic saline fluid therapy and supplementation with glucocorticoid and mineralocorticoid therapy. Prednisolone sodium succinate and desoxycorticosterone are the glucocorticoid and mineralocorticoid used to treat this disease. Addison disease in the cat has not been reported.

HYPOGLYCEMIA

Canine hypoglycemia is a clinical problem associated with a variety of diseases rather than a specific diagnosis itself. The signs associated with hypoglycemia include weakness of the rear legs, generalized weakness, focal or diffuse muscle twitching, incoordination, blindness, generalized seizures, and behavioral changes. These behavioral changes include aggressive behavior and anxiety as evidenced by incessant running, barking, and loss of bowel and bladder control. These signs tend to be episodic, regardless of the cause of hypoglycemia. Hypoglycemia should be considered a differential diagnosis in any dog that is having seizures or is comatose.

The first step in evaluating a patient with suspected hypoglycemia is to verify or document that hypoglycemia exists. Improper handling of blood samples may result in falsely low blood glucose levels. The blood glucose level can be lowered if the serum is not removed from the clot or if the specimen is stored at room temperature for a prolonged period. It is preferable to remove serum from the clot within 10 to 15 minutes of drawing the blood sample. If this cannot be done, use of sodium fluoride tubes may be helpful.

Once hypoglycemia has been verified, the signalment, history, clinical findings, and further laboratory tests may be needed to reduce the long and rather diverse list of conditions that may cause hypoglycemia. Functional beta-cell tumors (insulinomas of the pancreas), nonpancreatic tumors, hypoglycemia-ketonemia in pregnant bitches, glycogen storage diseases, septic shock, liver failure, juvenile and neonatal hypoglycemia, canine parvoviral diarrhea, and excessive insulin administration in diabetic patients are all examples of diseases that can cause hypoglycemia.

HYPOTHYROIDISM AND HYPERTHYROIDISM

Hypothyroidism is one of the most common endocrine disorders in the dog, but it is rare in the cat. Some of the common clinical signs include oily seborrhea, alopecia, thickened skin, weight gain, constipation, lethargy, and cold intolerance. There are some breeds with an apparent increased incidence of hypothyroidism (Box 25-4). The thyroid-stimulating hormone (TSH) stimulation test used to be the most accurate diagnostic test. TSH is no longer readily available; therefore a combination of three tests (total T_4, free T_4, and TSH levels) is used to diagnose the routine hypothyroid patient. Treatment of hypothyroidism consists of supplementation with thyroxine (T_4).

Box 25-4 BREEDS WITH AN APPARENT INCREASED INCIDENCE OF HYPOTHYROIDISM

- Afghan hound
- Airedale
- Beagle
- Boxer
- Brittany spaniel
- Chow chow
- Cocker spaniel
- Dachshund
- Doberman pinscher
- English bulldog
- Golden retriever
- Great Dane
- Irish setter
- Irish wolfhound
- Malamute
- Miniature schnauzer
- Newfoundland
- Pomeranian
- Poodle
- Shetland sheepdog

Hyperthyroidism is the most common endocrinopathy affecting cats older than 5 years of age, but it is rare in the dog. The most common clinical signs of hyperthyroidism are weight loss despite a good appetite, restlessness, hyperactivity, and diarrhea. In many cases, a thyroid nodule can be palpated in the ventrocervical region of the neck. The diagnosis can usually be confirmed by documenting an elevated serum T_4 level. Treatment may consist of medical therapy with methimazole (Tapazole, Eli Lilly and Co.), surgical removal of the thyroid nodule, and/or radioactive iodine (^{131}I).

✎ TECHNICIAN NOTE

Hyperthyroidism is the most common endocrinopathy affecting cats older than 5 years of age, but it is rare in the dog.

DIABETES MELLITUS

Diabetes mellitus is seen in the older dog and cat, and it is more common in the female dog and the male cat. Common clinical signs include excessive water intake (polydipsia), large volumes of urine (polyuria), weight loss in spite of a good appetite, and rapidly developing lens opacities (cataracts) in the dog. If the dog or cat is ketoacidotic, then weakness, vomiting, depression, and, possibly, coma may develop. The diagnosis of diabetes mellitus is made by documenting hyperglycemia, glucosuria, and, if the animal is ketoacidotic, ketonuria or ketonemia.

The technician's role in the treatment of patients with this endocrinopathy is twofold: (1) management of the ill ketoacidotic diabetic animal in the hospital and (2) education of clients concerning home management and treatment of their pets.

The ketoacidotic diabetic patient represents a true challenge for the veterinarian and technician alike, and it is important that they work in unison so that optimal patient care is achieved. The technician's role involves close monitoring of vital signs, ensuring fluids are given at the proper rate, frequent blood glucose determinations, and administering short-acting (regular/crystalline) insulin (see Table 25-7 for types of insulin). Because the ketoacidotic patient requires such close monitoring, the technician plays

a major role in the minute-to-minute and hour-to-hour evaluation of the patient, so minor changes in the patient's condition can be recognized early and the veterinarian be informed. Because of the complexity of the ketoacidotic diabetic patient, all these functions should be done under the direct supervision of a veterinarian.

The second aspect of diabetic management involves the instruction of the client concerning home management of the pet. This can be a time-consuming function, and the technician who has a good understanding of diabetes management can be a tremendous asset to the veterinarian. Examples of areas in which the client should be instructed and/or shown include how to mix the insulin, read the syringes, draw up the insulin into the syringe, give the subcutaneous injection, and read urine test strips for urine glucose measurement. Having the owner practice giving injections to the pet by drawing up sterile saline in the syringe and giving saline injections is extremely helpful to the hesitant owner. In addition, the client needs to be instructed (1) about the type of diet to be fed and how much and when to feed, (2) *not* to give the insulin if the pet does not eat in the morning, and (3) to give the animal Karo syrup orally and call the hospital immediately if the pet has a seizure. All these items can be compiled into a handout that the technician can develop with the aid of the veterinarian. This handout can then be given to the client, who can refer to it as needed at home.

THERIOGENOLOGY

POSTPARTUM DISORDERS IN THE BITCH

The postpartum bitch may be brought to an animal hospital for a variety of serious problems after whelping. These problems include mastitis, metritis, and eclampsia. *Mastitis* refers to inflammation of one or more mammary glands. In severe cases, affected glands are hot and painful, and the patient is systemically ill. Bitches with septic mastitis are depressed, anorectic, and reluctant to care for the puppies. In less severe cases, the bitch may not be symptomatic; however, the puppies may fail to gain weight or may show signs of septicemia. Systemic antibiotics are used to treat

---

Table 25-7 TYPES OF INSULIN USED IN DOGS AND CATS

Type of Insulin	Route of Administration	Onset of Effect	Duration of Effect
Regular crystalline	IV	Immediate	1-4 hr (d&c)
	IM	10-30 min	3-8 hr (d&c)
	SC	10-30 min	4-10 hr (d&c)
NPH	SC	30 min–2 hr	6-18 hr (d); 4-12 hr (c)
Lente	SC	30 min–2 hr	8-20 hr (d); 6-18 hr (c)
Ultralente	SC	30 min–8 hr	6-24 hr (d&c)
PZI	SC	1-4 hr	12-24 hr (d&c)

mastitis. Because the affected glands produce abnormal milk, and the antibiotics excreted in the milk may be harmful to the puppies, it is recommended that the puppies be hand fed.

Severe mastitis may progress to abscess formation or gangrenous mastitis. Surgical drainage and treatment may be required in these cases.

Stasis of milk in the mammary glands can occasionally result in enlarged, painful mammary glands. Galactostasis may be observed during pseudopregnancy or at the time of weaning when the body is attempting to resorb milk. Unlike mastitis, dogs with galactostasis are not systemically ill. Treatment consists of application of cool towels and compresses to decrease inflammation. Care should be taken not to massage the glands because this can stimulate additional milk letdown.

Metritis is a uterine disease of the immediate postpartum period. Signs usually develop within the first week of whelping. Metritis is associated with retained placentae, retained fetuses, and dystocia. Clinical signs suggestive of metritis include fever, depression, and reduced interest in the puppies. A foul-smelling, brown or reddish-brown vaginal discharge may be present; the normal discharge after whelping is nonodorous and greenish. The diagnosis is based on history, clinical findings, and laboratory results. Laboratory tests that are useful include vaginal cytologic studies, CBCs, and bacterial cultures.

Initial therapy consists of replacing fluid deficits, treating shock, if present, and initiating antibiotic therapy after cultures have been obtained. Medical drainage of the uterus can be attempted in valuable breeding bitches. In severe cases, ovariohysterectomy may be indicated to save the bitch's life.

Hypocalcemia (eclampsia) usually occurs 2 to 3 weeks postpartum in small bitches with large litters but occasionally can occur before birth. Presenting signs include weakness and trembling and may proceed to tonic convulsions. The temperature is usually elevated during convulsions.

Diagnosis is based on clinical signs in a lactating female and low serum calcium levels. Treatment includes preventing the puppies from nursing on the dam, giving the dam intravenous 10% calcium gluconate, and ensuring the dam receives oral calcium lactate or calcium gluconate and vitamin D at home. The puppies are hand fed with nursing bottles and milk replacer until 4 weeks old. It is highly recommended that the dam have an ovariohysterectomy due to the high recurrence rate of eclampsia. See Chapter 17 for additional information on animal reproduction.

CANINE BRUCELLOSIS

Canine brucellosis is primarily an infection of the reproductive tract, although other organ systems may be involved. *Brucella canis* also has been isolated from dogs with discospondylitis and chronic recurrent fever. Brucellosis is a frequent cause of infertility and other reproductive problems in both males and females.

Definitive diagnosis requires demonstration of the organism by a culture of blood or body fluids. Serologic tests can be diagnostic as well. The rapid slide agglutination test is an easy, readily available test; however, false-positive results occur. The rapid slide agglutination can be used as a screen, with positive tests being confirmed using an alternative technique (e.g., agar gel immunodiffusion).

The mode of transmission is venereal. However, infection can also result from the ingestion of infected material, for example, aborted fetuses, placentae, and vaginal discharge. Because of these means of spread, brucellosis can quickly become a kennel-wide problem.

Although a variety of antibiotic combinations have been recommended, therapeutic success cannot be guaranteed. After antibiotic therapy, some dogs will continue to harbor the organism and represent a risk to other dogs. Canine brucellosis is considered a possible zoonotic disease. For these reasons, some experts advocate removal of all infected dogs from the premises. Other experts feel that this position is extreme and instead recommend castration or ovariohysterectomy and antibiotic therapy for infected pet dogs.

Because treatment is not always successful, prevention is emphasized. All dogs should be tested before breeding or before introduction into a kennel.

PYOMETRITIS (PYOMETRA)

Pyometritis is a uterine disease that occurs during the luteal (approximately 1 to 2 months after estrus) phase of the reproductive cycle. It occurs in both bitches and queens. Pyometritis may be part of a complex that initially starts with cystic changes in the endometrium and endometrial hyperplasia. Prior estrogen therapy may predispose to pyometritis (see also Chapter 17).

Clinical signs are variable. A vaginal discharge may or may not be present, but, if present, the color of the discharge can be green, yellow, or reddish brown. Bitches with pyometritis frequently will be polydipsic and polyuric. Affected animals can be severely depressed and septic or clinically normal.

An enlarged uterus on radiographs and leukocytosis with a left shift are considered diagnostic. Fluid therapy to correct fluid and electrolyte deficits followed by emergency ovariohysterectomy is the treatment of choice in nonbreeding animals. In valuable breeding bitches, medical treatment with prostaglandin $F_{2\alpha}$ has been advocated to preserve the breeding life of the patient. Treatment with prostaglandin $F_{2\alpha}$ is expensive and potentially dangerous; therefore it should be strictly reserved for dogs of significant breeding value.

CANINE PROSTATIC DISEASE

Prostatic disease is occasionally seen in older intact male dogs. Clinical signs include straining to urinate (stranguria), painful urination (dysuria), blood in the urine (hematuria), and/or difficulty in defecation. The conditions that affect the prostate include benign prostatic hyperplasia, bacterial prostatitis, prostatic abscess, prostatic cyst, and prostatic neoplasia.

The following noninvasive techniques are used to evaluate the prostate: rectal palpation, routine radiology, sonography (ultrasound), urethrography, cytologic studies, and bacterial cultures of prostatic washes or the prostatic fraction of the ejaculate. Frequently it is difficult to differentiate neoplasia, infection, and hyperplasia with these noninvasive techniques. Consequently, surgical exploration and biopsy may be required to establish a definitive diagnosis.

Treatment varies, depending on the specific process. Dogs with benign prostatic hyperplasia respond to castration. Although estrogen therapy reduces the size of the prostate in benign prostatic hyperplasia, it is not recommended because of possible adverse reactions. Finasteride (Proscar, Merck & Co., Inc., West Point, Pa) has been shown to be an effective medical treatment for reduction of prostatomegaly secondary to benign prostatic hyperplasia. Prostatic abscesses and cysts require surgical drainage. Bacterial prostatitis and prostatic abscesses are treated with antibiotics. Prostatic neoplasia is generally highly malignant, and treatment is directed toward palliation rather than cure. Some dogs with prostatic cancer may benefit from castration because the tumors possess testosterone receptors.

GASTROENTEROLOGY

ACUTE GASTROENTERITIS

Acute gastroenteritis is one of the more common problems seen in canine practice. Some examples of conditions that may cause this problem include dietary indiscretion, viral gastroenteritis, bacterial gastroenteritis, gastrointestinal foreign bodies, gastrointestinal parasites, intussusception, ingestion of toxins, acute pancreatitis, and hypoadrenocorticism. The clinical history, signalment, and physical examination may suggest the diagnosis. Frequently, response to symptomatic therapy is used to assess whether further diagnostic study is warranted. The intensity and degree of symptomatic and supportive care are determined by the severity of clinical signs.

✎ TECHNICIAN NOTE

Acute gastroenteritis is one of the more common problems seen in canine practice.

The fundamental decision of whether to hospitalize the patient is based on a number of factors; they include the hydration status of the dog, severity and frequency of vomiting and diarrhea, presence or absence of blood in the vomitus or stool, and presence of fever or profound lethargy.

Non–patient-related factors to be considered include the client's ability to provide adequate care for the patient at home and ability of the client to pay for hospitalized care.

Clinical management of outpatients consists primarily of dietary restriction, administration of locally acting gastrointestinal medications, and use of fluid therapy when indicated. Dietary restriction is the most important aspect of the symptomatic care of acute gastroenteritis. The objective is to rest the gastrointestinal tract. This is accomplished by withholding all food for 12 to 24 hours, depending on the details of the case. If vomiting is severe, water is also withheld. If diarrhea is present and vomiting has not occurred, warm electrolyte-containing solutions can be given by mouth. During this period of symptomatic therapy, it is imperative that the patient be observed closely to prevent ingestion of foreign material and detect any worsening of clinical signs.

After food has been withheld for the prescribed period, small, frequent, bland meals should be offered. These meals should be low in fat, low in fiber, and easily digested and absorbed. These criteria are met by prescription diets, such as Prescription Diet I-D (Hill's), and by homemade diets, such as cottage cheese and boiled rice. These diets should be warmed before feeding. These frequent, small, bland meals should be continued for 2 to 3 days. If the patient is doing well, the regular diet and feeding schedule can be gradually reintroduced over the next 3 to 5 days. If clinical signs recur during this process, the dog should be reevaluated. Further diagnosis, evaluation, and more intensive supportive therapy may be warranted.

Although a vast number of locally acting preparations are available for the treatment of acute gastroenteritis, most have not been proved effective in controlled clinical trials. An over-the-counter preparation containing bismuth subsalicylate (Pepto-Bismol) has been shown to shorten the duration of symptoms in humans with experimental viral enteritis. It is theorized that the beneficial response is not due to the coating action of the product but rather to the salicylate inhibiting prostaglandin synthesis. Prostaglandins play a role in diarrhea by affecting both motility and secretory activity of the gastrointestinal tract. The technician should be aware that Pepto-Bismol may cause the stool to be dark to black, giving the false impression that melena is present when it is not.

✎ TECHNICIAN NOTE

Pepto-Bismol causes the stool to be colored black and therefore should not be confused with melena.

In animals that are slightly to mildly dehydrated, some form of fluid therapy is appropriate. Fluids can be administered by mouth if the patient is not vomiting. Commercial water and electrolyte solutions, such as Gatorade, can be used to restore hydration and correct electrolyte imbalances. Alternatively, a homemade solution can be prepared inexpensively. One formula that has been recommended consists of 3.5 g of sodium chloride, 2.5 g of sodium bicarbonate, 1.5 g of potassium chloride, and 20 g of glucose added to 1 L of water. Approximately 13.6 ml/kg/day of this solution will meet the maintenance requirements of the patient.

If the dog is mildly to moderately dehydrated or is vomiting, subcutaneous fluids are indicated. Lactated Ringer's solution or Normosol are the fluid of choice. If signs have been prolonged, the lactated Ringer's solution can be supplemented with potassium chloride. Generally, the dose of subcutaneous fluids is 4.5 to 9.0 ml/kg of body weight administered at multiple sites. This can be repeated if necessary.

Client education is an essential part of the symptomatic care for acute gastroenteritis. The client should be informed that a definitive diagnosis has not been established and that merely the symptoms are being treated. If the animal is getting worse or if the signs persist longer than 36 to 48 hours, the animal should be reevaluated. The technician should have a concerned, caring attitude during the outpatient visit so that if signs persist, the client will not hesitate to return or call for additional help. In many practices, it is standard procedure to telephone the client to receive follow-up progress reports. This ensures close client contact and thus improves the chances of successful management of the problem.

If initial clinical signs are severe or there is no response to symptomatic therapy, hospitalization is necessary. A major indication for hospitalization is the need for intravenous fluid therapy. Details about intravenous fluid therapy have been discussed.

Medications that alter the motility of the gastrointestinal tract may be indicated in cases of severe gastroenteritis. Improved understanding of the pathophysiology of intestinal motility has resulted in the more rational use of medications that are used to symptomatically treat vomiting and diarrhea. Anticholinergics decrease the resistance to intestinal flow and thus are of questionable efficacy in treating diarrhea. Antispasmodics are of minimal benefit as well.

Narcotics and narcotic-like drugs increase the rhythmic segmental contractions of the bowel, slow the passage of ingesta, and thus help to control diarrhea. These drugs should be used cautiously because of potential problems. Generally, they are reserved for more chronic or severe cases that are unresponsive to conservative therapy. A major disadvantage of the narcotic derivatives is that they can cause central nervous system depression. The decreased ingesta flow rate may result in increased absorption of toxins and altered bacterial flora in the gut. These compounds are contraindicated in the presence of intestinal obstruction.

Drugs used for the treatment of acute vomiting can be divided into several categories (Box 25-5).

Drugs used to decrease gastric acidity include antihistamines or H$_2$ blockers such as cimetidine (Tagamet,

Box 25-5 DRUGS USED FOR ACUTE VOMITING

DOPAMINE ANTAGONISTS
Metoclopramide (Reglan)
Domperidone

PHENOTHIAZINES
Chlorpromazine (Thorazine)
Prochlorperazine
Darbazine (prochlorperazine, isopropamide)
Tigan (trimethobenzamide)

ANTIHISTAMINES
Cyclizine hydrochloride
Diphenhydramine hydrochloride (Benadryl)
Dimenhydrinate (Dramamine)
Meclizine hydrochloride (Bonine)
Trifluoperazine

SK&F Lab Co.), ranitidine (Zantac,) and famotidine (Pepcid AC). Antacids do not decrease the secretion of acid; however, they neutralize the acid that is produced. Antacids must be given frequently because their duration of action is brief. Paradoxically, if antacids are not given frequently, total daily acid secretion increases. Antacids administered according to a schedule of two or three times per day are probably of no value and may, in fact, be harmful. In most practices, more frequent administration is not practical. Antidopaminergic drugs such as metoclopramide (Reglan) inhibit vomiting at the vomiting center in the central nervous system. Metoclopramide is contraindicated in intestinal obstruction due to its prokinetic or motility-stimulating activity. Phenothiazine-derivative tranquilizers, such as chlorpromazine, also work on the vomiting center of the central nervous system. These drugs are effective at controlling vomiting at much lower doses than the usual tranquilizer doses. These agents should be used with caution in dehydrated patients because of their blood pressure—lowering effects. Other antihistamines such as (Dramamine) act by inhibiting a neural center involved in vomiting called the *chemoreceptor trigger zone*. Vomiting induced by certain drugs, such as digoxin, is mediated by this center. Vomiting caused by motion sickness or vertigo may also respond to drugs in this group. Box 25-6 lists drugs used commonly for acute gastrointestinal disease.

When the patient has improved, oral fluids and frequent, small, bland meals can be instituted. After discharge from the hospital, the dog can be treated as already described under outpatient management.

CANINE VIRAL ENTERITIS

The two most important causes of viral enteritis in the dog are canine coronavirus and canine parvovirus. Other

Box 25-6 COMMONLY USED DRUGS FOR ACUTE GASTROENTERITIS

NARCOTICS
Diphenoxylate and atropine (Lomotil)
Loperamide (Imodium)
Parepectolin (paregoric, pectin, kaolin)

ANTICHOLINERGICS
Atropine
Scopolamine
Methscopolamine
Glycopyrrolate (Robinul-V)
Aminopentamide hydrogen sulfate (Centrine)
Prochlorperazine, isopropamide (Darbazine)
Amoforal (kanamycin, aminopeptamide hydrogen sulfate, pectin)

LOCALLY ACTIVE AGENTS
Kaopectate (kaolin, pectin)
Kao-forte (kaolin, pectin)
Pepto-Bismol (bismuth subsalicylate)

ANTIHISTAMINES
H_2 Blockers: Tagamet (cimetidine), Zantac (ranitidine), Pepcid AC (famotidine)

viral agents can occasionally produce gastroenteritis; they include canine distemper and canine rotavirus.

Clinical signs vary from subtle lethargy and anorexia to severe, rapidly fatal hemorrhagic gastroenteritis. Dogs of any age can be affected; however, the more severe cases typically occur between 6 and 20 weeks of age. On physical examination, the pups are usually febrile, depressed, and dehydrated. Vomiting or diarrhea may be observed. The stool may be watery, watery with flecks of blood, or severely hemorrhagic. Occasionally, infected dogs will display abdominal tenderness or pain. The presence of fever is more commonly associated with parvovirus than with coronavirus. A history of vaccination does not rule out viral enteritis because maternal antibodies may have prevented a protective immune response to the vaccination. It should be noted that the gastroenteritis and clinical disease secondary to coronavirus infection are much less severe than those seen with parvovirus infection.

Hemograms are usually normal with coronavirus enteritis but may be abnormal with parvovirus enteritis. Transient leukopenia is present in roughly one third to one half of dogs with parvovirus infections. Severely leukopenic patients may develop secondary infections because of a compromised immune system.

Plain abdominal radiographs do not reveal specific changes. Gastrointestinal contrast study changes may mimic small bowel obstruction. Abnormalities include dilated loops of bowel, tremendously prolonged passage time, and gas-capped fluid lines.

Definitive diagnosis is possible by several techniques. The viruses may be detected in the stool by electron microscopy. An ELISA performed on the feces can detect parvoviral antigen and can be used to demonstrate the virus in the feces during the period of active viral shedding. This period corresponds to the clinical illness. An easy-to-perform in-house test is available to check for parvovirus antigen in the stool (Probe-Canine Parvovirus Antigen test kit, Idexx Labs).

It should be stressed that the treatment of canine viral gastroenteritis is supportive because there are no effective antiviral agents. Treatment includes aggressive intravenous fluid therapy, antibiotics, injectable antiemetics, and keeping the animal clean and comfortable. One other complication seen with parvovirus infection, to which the technician should be alert, is the development of hypoglycemia. If profound weakness and/or seizures develop, a blood glucose level should be determined.

A myocardial form of canine parvovirus has been described in young pups. This form of the disease is characterized by sudden death in otherwise healthy pups; however, it is becoming less common. This may be because most pups have maternal antibodies at the critical period when they are susceptible to the myocardial form.

Both canine parvovirus and coronavirus are highly contagious. The major route of the infection is fecal-oral. Dogs showing clinical signs will shed large numbers of viral particles for 1 to 2 weeks. The canine parvovirus is hardy; therefore once the environment is contaminated, infective virus will survive for prolonged periods. The virus has been shown to remain infectious in dog feces held at room temperature for longer than 6 months.

Good sanitation will reduce the numbers of infective virus in the hospital environment. Keeping infected patients isolated from other patients and wearing disposable gloves, gowns, and shoe covers every time the patient is handled will prevent spread of the virus within the hospital. Dilute hypochlorite (chlorine bleach and water, diluted to a ratio of 1:32) solutions have significant viricidal properties. However, because the virus is ubiquitous the best means of prevention is an appropriate immunization program.

TECHNICIAN NOTE
Dilute hypochlorite (chlorine bleach and water, diluted to a ratio of 1:32) solutions have significant viricidal properties.

NEPHROLOGY AND UROLOGY

CANINE UROLITHS

A *urolith* is a pathologic stone formed from mineral salts found in the urinary tract. Clinical signs depend on location, number, size, shape, and whether there is concurrent urinary tract infection. Urolith classification is generally based on the predominant mineral component, such as phosphate or urate. In the dog, more than 90% of uroliths are located in the bladder and urethra and fewer than 10% are located in the kidneys. Although uroliths can occur in any breed, some breeds suspected to be at greater risk include the miniature schnauzer, Dalmatian, dachshund, pug, English bulldog, Welsh corgi, basset hound, Pekinese, and Scottish terrier.

If the urolith is located in the bladder, there may be no clinical signs, but more commonly stranguria, increased frequency of urination (pollakiuria), and hematuria will be seen. If the urolith is in the urethra, there may be frequent attempts to urinate and dribbling of urine. If the urethra is completely obstructed by the stone or stones, abdominal distention, pain, anorexia, depression, and vomiting will be observed.

Laboratory findings generally are not specific for uroliths. Radiology, including contrast studies such as cystograms and pneumocystograms or ultrasound, may be necessary to establish the diagnosis. Generally speaking, uroliths are managed surgically. A prescription diet (S/D, Hill's) has been advocated as a means of medically treating phosphate uroliths. The diet is high in sodium and low in protein and phosphorus and has an acidifying effect on urine. Dissolution of the uroliths occurs over a period of weeks. Unfortunately, this medical approach has several important limitations. A prescription S/D diet is effective in the dissolution of only phosphate calculi and is not recommended as a long-term maintenance diet.

The overall recurrence rate for bladder stones is high, approximately 25%. Therefore efforts to reduce the chance of recurrence are very important. The first step is to analyze the mineral composition of the stone because different stone types are managed differently. It is also important to determine whether infection is present and, if so, which antibiotics are most likely to be effective.

Several preventive measures are appropriate regardless of the stone type. These include elimination of any infection and stimulation of increased urine output. The urine output can be increased by salting the diet and thereby increasing water intake.

Depending on the specific stone type, it may also be desirable to initiate dietary therapy and modify the urine pH. Ammonium chloride is commonly used to acidify the urine, and sodium bicarbonate is used to alkalinize it.

Because the recurrence rate for uroliths is high, client education is extremely important. First, long-term therapeutic compliance will be achieved only if the importance of these measures is stressed to the client. Second, the owner should be aware of signs that indicate recurrence of the problem.

FELINE LOWER URINARY TRACT DISEASE

Feline lower urinary tract disease (FLUTD) is the term used to describe a condition of unknown etiology in cats characterized by dysuria, hematuria, pollakiuria, urinating in uncommon places, and occasionally urethral obstruction. Urethral obstruction, if it occurs, is potentially fatal because of the associated severe metabolic derangements. The emergency treatment of feline urethral obstruction is covered in Chapter 26.

Because recurrence of the urethral obstruction is frequent, some clinicians prefer to routinely use indwelling urethral catheters for a brief period of time after relief of the obstruction. The justification for the use of indwelling catheters is to maintain urine flow without the trauma associated with recatheterization and manual compression of the bladder. Indwelling urethral catheters should be used judiciously because of the risk of ascending urinary tract infection and catheter-induced injury to the bladder or urethra. Complications associated with the use of indwelling catheters can be minimized if an appropriate catheter is selected. Commercially manufactured polypropylene catheters (Sovereign tomcat catheters and open-end tomcat catheters, Sherwood Medical Industries) can be either too short or too long. Therefore care should be taken to select a catheter with an appropriate length. Soft, flexible polyvinyl catheters, such as the Sovereign sterile disposable feeding tube and urethral catheter, are preferred because of decreased damage to the urethral and bladder mucosa. To pass these catheters, they are kept frozen until immediately before use. This will make the catheter sufficiently rigid to allow passage in a male cat. The catheter should be well lubricated before passage.

Indwelling urethral catheters are generally secured by suturing the catheter to the prepuce. Adhesive tape is attached longitudinally and transversely to the end of the catheter. If the catheter is wet when the tape is applied, it may not stick. Two simple interrupted sutures on either side of the prepuce penetrate the tape and thus prevent movement of the catheter. If analgesia is required to place the sutures, the prepuce can be numbed by applying an ice cube for 1 or 2 minutes. When the catheter is sutured in place, it should be done in such a way that there is no chance of kinking. An Elizabethan collar should be used to prevent the cat from removing the indwelling catheter.

To prevent ascending urinary tract infection, sterile technique is required when placing and maintaining the indwelling catheter. The collection apparatus should be a closed, sterile system. The entire system—catheter, plastic tubing, and collection bottle—must be sterile initially and must be kept sealed to prevent bacterial contamination. Povidone-iodine ointment should be applied several times daily at the point at which the catheter exits the urethra.

Indwelling urethral catheters should be used for as brief a time as possible. The prophylactic use of antimicrobials does not reduce infection. If infection does develop, it is frequently caused by an organism resistant to the prophylactic antimicrobial.

Because the recurrence rate for feline urologic syndrome is high, preventive measures are an important aspect of its medical management. Unfortunately, because the etiology of feline urologic syndrome is unknown, preventive measures are largely empirical. The most frequently recommended preventive measures include providing an ample supply of fresh, potable water, cleaning the litter pan frequently, and lightly salting the food to increase water intake and thus urine volume. Exclusive feeding of diets that contain 20 mg of magnesium per 100 kcal or less and that maintain a urine pH of 6.4 or less is the most important preventive measure. Certain diets, such as C/D or Feline Maintenance (Hill's), meet this requirement. Although urinary acidification with ammonium chloride has been recommended, it should be emphasized that some diets, such as the ones mentioned above, cause urinary acidification, and additional acidifiers are contraindicated. The basis of acidifying the urine is to increase the solubility of this crystalline material, which is incriminated as the cause of feline urologic syndrome.

If ammonium chloride is used with a nonacidifying diet, it should be thoroughly mixed with the food to improve palatability. It should also be administered with every meal. Any change in diet or introduction of a food additive, such as ammonium chloride or salt, should be done gradually over several days. This will reduce the chances of the cat rejecting the new or altered food. Enteric-coated ammonium chloride tablets are not effective in the cat.

In recent years, calcium oxalate bladder stones have become recognized in the cat as a new cause of FLUTD. Calcium oxalate stores are more likely to form in an acid urine, and therefore cats that eat an acidifying diet may be at risk for the formation of calcium oxalate stones.

In addition, some cats with FLUTD have no definable cause but may benefit from drugs such as amitriptyline (Elavil) or glycosaminoglycans (Adequan).

CHRONIC RENAL FAILURE

Animals in renal failure should be fed diets containing reduced quantities of high-quality protein and adequate nonprotein calories. This can be accomplished by using prescription diets such as K/D (Hill's). K/D is a moderate protein-restricted diet available for dogs in canned, semimoist, and dry forms. Feline K/D is a canned product suitable for use in uremic cats.

If desired, homemade diets can be used. The following is a recipe for a moderately low protein diet for dogs:

$^{1}/_{4}$ lb regular ground beef
1 hard-boiled egg, finely chopped
2 cups cooked rice without salt
3 slices white bread, crumbled
1 tsp calcium carbonate
Balanced vitamin and mineral supplement

The meat should be braised, retaining the fat, and thoroughly mixed with the other ingredients. This recipe will meet the daily requirements of a 13.5-kg dog.

The following is an example of a homemade protein-restricted diet for cats:

$^{1}/_{4}$ lb liver
2 large hard-boiled eggs
2 cups cooked rice without salt
1 tbsp vegetable oil
1 tsp calcium carbonate
Balanced vitamin and mineral supplement

Dice and braise the liver, retaining fat. This recipe provides a total of 635 kcal/lb.

Many animals with renal failure are anorectic because of nausea and vomiting. Small, frequent meals are recommended to reduce the nausea. If the animal can tolerate food orally but is not eating, feeding by means of an orogastric tube is recommended. The diets described can be administered through a stomach tube if the ingredients are thoroughly mixed with water in a kitchen blender.

Supportive therapy for chronic renal failure includes the use of phosphorous binders, anabolic steroids, sodium bicarbonate, sodium chloride, calcium, and vitamin D metabolites. The use of these treatments should be based on documented abnormalities because the inappropriate or incorrect use of these agents can do more harm than good. Administration of subcutaneous fluids as a form of diuresis can be taught to the owner for use every other day or daily in advanced kidney failure. Surgically implanted subcutaneous catheters that do not require needle puncture for administration of fluids are a newer option for owners. Cats generally tolerate these catheters very well, and the owners can safely administer the fluids in a much shorter period of time due to the multiple fenestrations of the catheter allowing rapid fluid distribution without pocketing under the skin. This is also a less painful procedure for the patient.

ORTHOPEDICS

CANINE HIP DYSPLASIA

Hip dysplasia refers to a developmental problem of the canine coxofemoral joint. Subluxation of the femoral head leads to abnormal wear and eventual degenerative joint disease. The acetabulum is more shallow than normal, and the femoral head is flattened.

The etiology of hip dysplasia is multifactorial. Genetics and environmental factors such as nutrition appear to be important. Hip dysplasia is seen in most large breeds and is inherited by a polygenic mode of inheritance. This means that many genes are responsible for its development. It is also quantitative in its expression. In other words, affected dogs can show slight or severe changes. As is characteristic for traits with a polygenic mode of inheritance, hip dysplasia is modified by environmental factors. For example, it has been suggested that dogs fed a high-calorie diet during growth have an increased incidence, whereas dogs fed a low-calorie diet have a decreased incidence.

The Orthopedic Foundation of America in Columbia, Mo., is an organization established to evaluate the hip radiographs of potential breeding dogs. Radiologists identify those dogs with radiographically normal hip joints. Unfortunately, because of the factors mentioned, breeding two radiographically normal dogs does not ensure normal progeny. It is better to evaluate entire families (siblings and progeny) when selecting dogs to be included in a breeding program to decrease the incidence of hip dysplasia. It is also important to recognize that good hip joints should not be the sole criterion for selection. Other traits, such as disposition, working ability, and conformation, should also be considered.

The clinical signs of hip dysplasia vary tremendously from occasional slight discomfort to a severe disabling disease. It should be remembered that the clinical signs of hip dysplasia do not always correlate with the severity of hip dysplasia detected radiographically.

Dogs with hip dysplasia will respond differently to varying levels of exercise. Some dogs are most comfortable with minimal activity, yet others do best with a regular regimen of moderate exercise. Swimming is an excellent form of exercise, since muscle tone is increased with the hip joints in a non–weight-bearing position. Any exercise program should be instituted gradually. Forced sudden activity such as ball playing or rough play should be discouraged. Severely affected dogs should be treated symptomatically with analgesics and antiinflammatory drugs.

Several surgical procedures have been advocated for the treatment of hip dysplasia. They include procedures such as pectineal myotomy, pelvic osteotomy, excision arthroplasty, and total hip prosthesis. A discussion of these surgical procedures is beyond the scope of this chapter.

INTERVERTEBRAL DISK DISEASE

Intervertebral disk disease is a relatively common problem affecting the spinal cord of chondrodystrophoid and other breeds. Breeds commonly affected include dachshunds, Pekingese, cocker spaniels, poodles, pugs, and beagles. The chondrodystrophoid breeds tend to develop signs at an earlier age than the nonchondrodystrophoid breeds.

The intervertebral disks are structures located between the vertebrae and function as a shock-absorbing system. The disk itself is composed of two parts: the firm fibrous outer annulus and the softer inner nucleus. In intervertebral disk disease, the annulus undergoes degeneration, and the nuclear material protrudes or is completely extruded. The result is compression of the spinal cord with the subsequent development of neurologic signs. These signs vary from simple pain to complete paralysis.

Intervertebral disk disease can be managed either conservatively with strict cage confinement and antiinflammatory drugs or more aggressively with neurosurgery. Management decisions are based on the history, neurologic signs, and wishes of the owner.

If conservative therapy is elected, the technician plays a vital role. Extreme care should be taken in handling the patient because movement may result in the extrusion of additional disk material and worsening of signs. To reduce handling, these patients should be placed in lower cages whenever possible. Because these patients are frequently in severe pain, gentle, compassionate care is essential. Many cases will benefit from some of the physical therapy techniques described earlier.

Dogs with intervertebral disk disease receiving antiinflammatory drugs, such as dexamethasone, may develop secondary problems, such as gastrointestinal hemorrhage or acute pancreatitis. Consequently, these patients should be observed closely for fever, anorexia, abdominal pain, hemorrhagic vomiting, and diarrhea.

Additional information regarding orthopedics is found in Chapter 24.

Recommended Reading

Nelson and Couto: *Small animal internal medicine,* ed 3, St Louis, 2003, Mosby.

Greene C: *Infectious diseases of the dog and cat,* ed 2, Philadelphia, 1998, WB Saunders.

Feldman EC, Nelson RW: *Canine and feline endocrinology and reproduction,* ed 3, Philadelphia, 2003, WB Saunders.

Ford RB, Schultz RD: In Bonagura JD: *Kirk's current veterinary therapy XIII,* Philadelphia, 2000, WB Saunders.

Hand MS et al: *Small animal clinical nutrition,* ed 4, Marceline, Mo, 2000, Walsworth Publishing.

26

Emergency Nursing

Lee Ann Eddleman • Kirk Ryan • Steven Marks

INTRODUCTION

As the family pet has become a true family member, a greater awareness of treatment availability and the demands of pet owners for more advanced treatment options have spurred specialization within the veterinary profession. Since its inception, the field of veterinary emergency and critical care has grown exponentially and continues to respond to the needs of animals, pet owners, and the veterinary profession. Steady improvements have occurred in emergency and critical care techniques and in equipment and staff training. Likewise, the technician's role in the emergency room and the intensive care unit has grown. Technicians are the team members most directly involved with patient care (monitoring vital signs, administering medications appropriately, providing positive touch, and keeping patients clean and dry) and in maintaining accurate patient records (recording current status and therapies). This role is important in documenting patient response to treatment, in providing continuity of care, and in recognizing the onset of clinical problems. The field of emergency and critical care is incredibly dynamic. Team members are challenged by rapid changes within the profession (new methods, pharmaceuticals, and diets) and by rapid changes in each patient (new and evolving clinical problems in each case). Animals are frequently presented to the veterinarian with emergent and often life threatening injuries or illnesses. Such demands require that the veterinary facility be set up in a manner in which quick assessment, screening diagnostics, and immediate therapies are possible. ■

THE EMERGENCY CARE STATION AND RESUSCITATION AREA

Every veterinary clinic should contain a centrally located emergency care station and resuscitation area devoted to crisis management. This area should be designed to facilitate rapid triage and treatment. It should be easy to access and have adequate space to accommodate multiple staff members responding to a patient emergency. Emergency drugs and equipment should be stored within easy reach and in designated areas. Equipment and drug inventory of the emergency care station should be checked at each shift change and following each use to ensure all items are in working order and in adequate supply. As a minimum, this area should have a source of oxygen, a suction unit, adequate electrical capability, and sufficient lighting. In many veterinary practices, oxygen is supplied via anesthetic equipment. The ideal equipment is an oxygen source with a flowmeter and Ambu bag (Figure 26-1). While an anesthetic machine provides a familiar means of ventilation and access to sedation (if needed), it can also be a source of catastrophe when errors of anesthetic depth or pop-off valve closure occur. If an anesthetic machine is used, waste anesthetic gas scavenging systems should also be available. Ambu bags are especially useful because they are easily transported and inexpensive for providing artificial ventilation. The emergency care station should have a sufficient number of electrical outlets to supply monitoring equipment without the use of excessive extension cords, which can be clumsy, unsafe, and impede the movements of staff. Suction is often used in the emergency area to clear the airway or endotracheal tube of fluid (mucus, blood, exudates, vomitus, etc.)

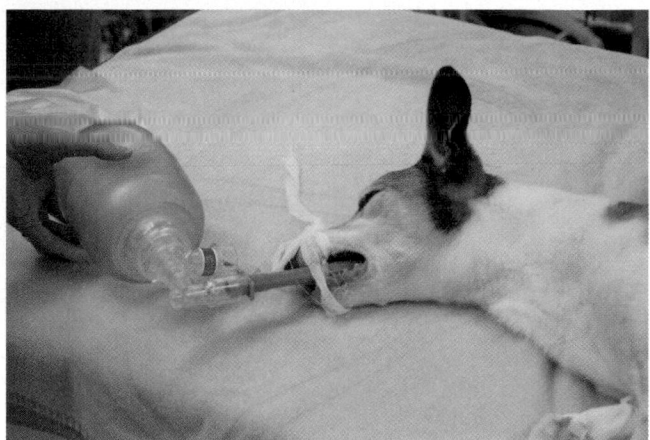

Figure 26-1 An endotracheal tube connected to an Ambu bag and oxygen source provides an ideal means to supply 100% oxygen and manually assisted ventilations.

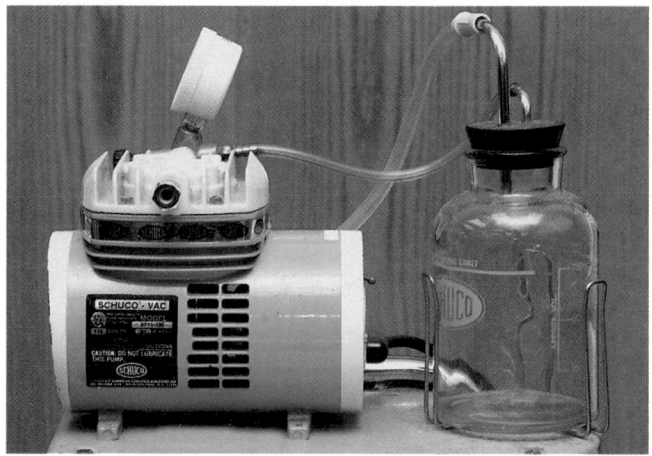

Figure 26-2 A suction unit similar to those used in a surgery suite should be centrally located and used in emergencies to clear airways of fluid and debris.

and facilitate endotracheal intubation. Many small practices have suction units with adjustable suction pressure, which are also used in surgery (Figure 26-2). The emergency area should have its own suction unit available. Standard fluorescent lighting can be augmented by well-positioned surgery lights.

> ### 🖉 TECHNICIAN NOTE
> An Ambu bag or anesthetic machine should be located close to the crash cart so that assisted ventilation can be started immediately after the animal is intubated.

CRASH CART

An integral part of being prepared for an emergency is a "crash cart" (Figure 26-3). This can be a fishing tackle box

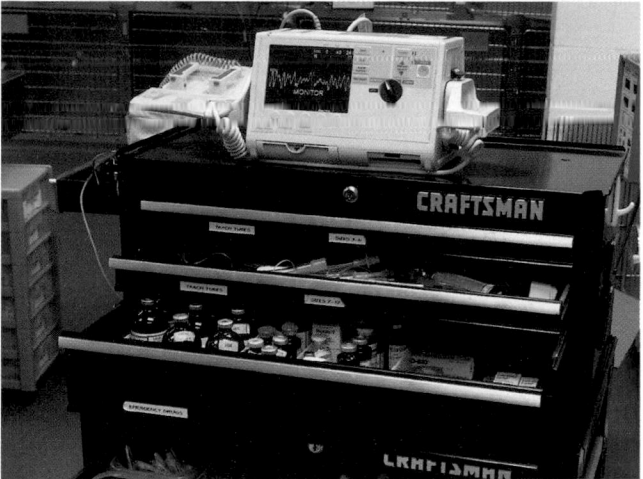

Figure 26-3 An effective "crash cart" is easily accessible and spacious enough to contain a vast array of emergency supplies.

with necessary items or a large cart on wheels with multiple drawers. A tool storage cart available at hardware stores can work quite well. The crash cart should be located at the emergency station and contain necessary items for treating the patient that is medically unstable. Additional crash carts may be placed in select locations throughout the hospital (i.e., operating room or dental suite). Basic supplies contained in the crash cart should include items necessary to establish an airway, venous access, emergency drugs, and a dose chart.

Airway supplies should include at least one laryngoscope with a small- and large-size blade. The laryngoscope battery and bulb light should be checked at each shift to make sure the equipment is in working order. Various sizes of clean endotracheal tubes and stylets should be placed in well-marked and organized places so that the appropriate tube can be located rapidly during an emergency. It is also helpful to maintain supplies needed to secure the tube in place once the animal has been intubated. Such supplies include tie gauze, or other tube securing material, and a clean empty syringe to inflate the cuff. Endotracheal tube cuffs should be checked at least once a week to ensure that they are functional and that no leak is present. Additional equipment to assist with airway control may be located in larger crash carts. This equipment should include a pair of sponge forceps, which may be used to clear the airway with gauze or to remove a foreign body without getting bitten. Normal per oral intubation is not always possible due to facial trauma or upper airway obstruction (tumor, foreign body, or severe trauma). In such cases, a transtracheal cannula or needle tracheostomy may be useful until a surgical tracheostomy can be performed or until airway obstruction can be otherwise resolved. Tracheal cannulae are attached to an oxygen source and inserted into the trachea between cartilage rings. Some items utilized for tracheal cannulae include large-gauge through-the-needle catheters, large-gauge

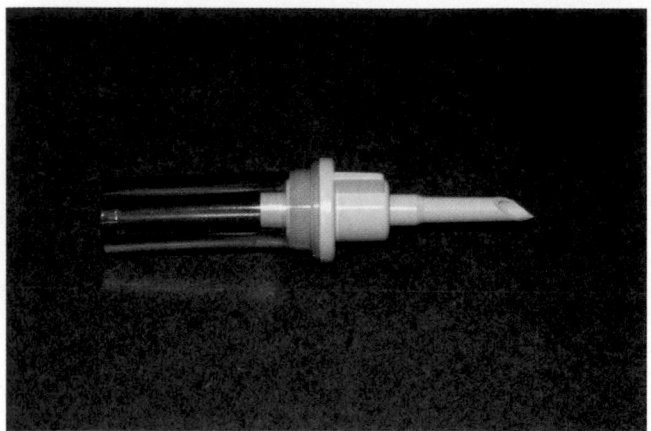

Figure 26-4 A macrodrip intravenous fluid set can be used as an emergency tracheal cannulae until more appropriate equipment can be readied.

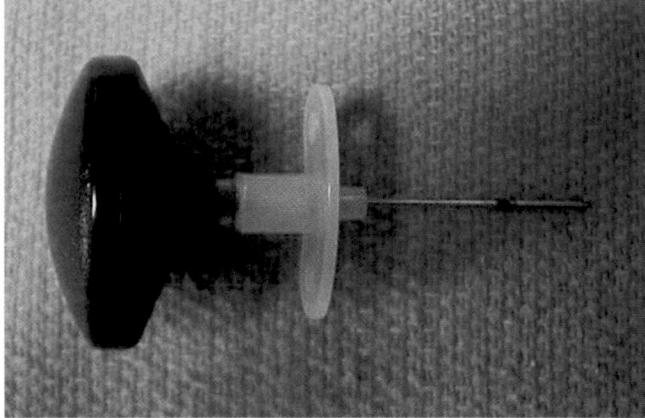

Figure 26-5 Commercially available bone marrow catheters are helpful when venous access is limited.

needles (attached to an extension set and 6-cc syringe adapter), or macrodrip intravenous (IV) fluid sets (Figure 26-4). In some situations, a small-diameter polypropylene catheter may be passed through the mouth into the trachea and used as a cannula to administer oxygen or as a guide (stylet) to direct an endotracheal tube. As previously noted, an Ambu bag or anesthetic machine should be located close to the crash cart so that assisted ventilation can be started immediately after the animal is intubated.

> ### ✏ TECHNICIAN NOTE
> Ambu bags are especially useful because they are easily transported and inexpensive for providing artificial ventilation.

Items to establish venous access should be kept in the crash cart for use in crisis patients who do not already have an intravenous (IV) catheter or who need additional venous access. A selection of various sizes of IV catheters should be well stocked and organized. In addition, bone marrow needles or intramedullary catheters are desirable for small patients (Figures 26-5 and 26-6). Bone marrow catheters are ideal for puppies, kittens, and exotic pets because the bone marrow cavity connects to the vascular system and small patients often have fragile or inaccessible veins. Commercially available bone marrow catheters, spinal needles, or 18- to 20-gauge hypodermic needles can be used for this purpose. Porous tape and gauze bandage material for stabilization of any vascular line will also be necessary and should be included in the crash cart inventory. Hair clippers and solutions for aseptic skin preparation should be within easy reach. Commonly used intravenous fluid solutions (i.e., lactated Ringer's, 0.9% saline solution), synthetic colloids (i.e., Hetastarch, Oxyglobin), hypertonic saline, and a pressure infusion bag should be kept close at hand for emergency fluid resuscitation.

A selection of emergency drugs, especially those used in the treatment of cardiopulmonary arrest should be kept

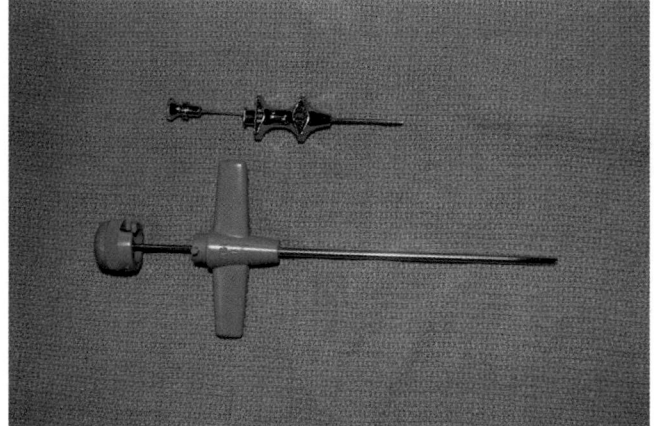

Figure 26-6 Examples of bone marrow catheters are shown.

in an area of the cart. Drug bottles should be well-labeled and kept in specific and consistent locations within the cart to facilitate their use during an emergency. Later in this chapter, cardiopulmonary resuscitation (CPR) is discussed in detail. Commonly used emergency drugs include atropine, epinephrine, lidocaine, and naloxone (Table 26-1). Drug dose and administration errors may be avoided if the veterinary staff is familiar with the location of the drugs and with the drug concentrations. If space allows, it may be helpful to have various sizes of sterile syringes with the needles already attached to facilitate rapid drug administration. During cardiopulmonary resuscitation attempts, some drugs may be administered via the endotracheal tube (see administration routes under the discussion of CPR). This requires utilizing a catheter of some sort (i.e., red rubber catheter cut to an appropriate length with a syringe adapter for syringe attachment or a similar size polypropylene urinary catheter). Two such catheters should be on hand (one for larger sized animals and one for small animals). Emergency situations rarely allow time for individual dose

Table 26-1 DRUGS FOR CARDIOPULMONARY RESUSCITATION

Drug	Formulation	Dosage	Indications
Atropine	0.54 mg/ml	0.04 mg/kg IV	Bradycardia AV block Asystole
Dobutamine	12.5 mg/ml	5-20 mg/kg/min CRI	Myocardial failure
Dopamine	40 mg/ml	5-10 mg/kg/min CRI	Low cardiac output
Epinephrine	1:1000 solution	0.2 mg/kg IV	V-fibrillation Asystole EMD
Lidocaine	20 mg/ml	2 mg/kg IV 50-100 mg/kg/min CRI	Ventricular arrhythmias
Magnesium chloride	200 mg/ml	2 g over 2 minutes IV	V-fibrillation V-tachycardia
Naloxone	0.4 mg/ml	0.03 mg/kg IV	EMD

calculations for each patient. During a crash scenario remembering and calculating doses can take time and introduce errors. At the same time estimated doses may be dangerously inadequate or over zealous. Therefore, some sort of centrally located drug dose chart should be posted at the emergency care station with a smaller version kept with drugs in the crash cart. A chart or drug card allows for simply reading the appropriate drug volume based on the species and body weight. Drug calculation programs are available that generate an emergency drug card that can be printed for all high-risk patients. Following each use, and at every shift change, the contents of the crash cart should be checked and re-stocked. The function of all battery or electrical items should be checked and replaced or recharged as necessary.

✎ TECHNICIAN NOTE

Drug bottles should be well-labeled and kept in specific and consistent locations within the cart to facilitate their use during an emergency.

A centrally located drug dosing chart should be posted at the emergency care station with a smaller version kept with drugs in the crash cart.

Following each use, and at every shift change, the contents of the crash cart should be checked and restocked.

Electrical defibrillation is indicated in the treatment of some cardiac arrhythmias (primarily ventricular fibrillation). Electrical defibrillators are available through many medical equipment distributors and may be combined with an electrocardiogram (ECG) monitor. This equipment should be located at the central emergency care station and used by experienced staff and doctors. Special training is required for the safe use of electrical defibrillators.

Depending on space, other items such as surgical packs for emergency procedures may also be stored in the crash cart. Common procedures performed in the emergency

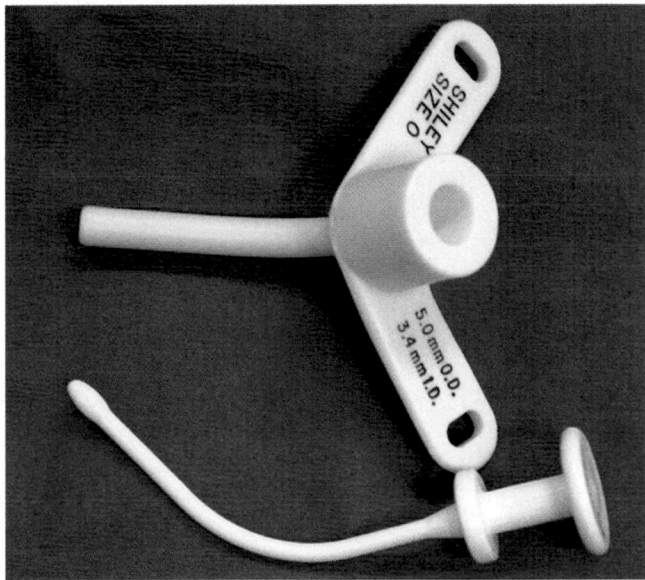

Figure 26-7 A temporary tracheostomy tube (with stylet) can be surgically placed to establish an airway when upper airway obstruction is present.

station include venous cut down, thoracotomy for open chest CPR, thoracic drain placement, and tracheostomy (Figure 26-7). Sterile instruments and drapes for these procedures should be available in the emergency area (if not in the crash cart). Basic bandaging and splinting supplies, irrigation fluids and sterile water-soluble lube (for clipping around and lavaging open wounds) should also be available.

LABORATORY

Next to the emergency care station, equipment should be close at hand to obtain baseline exam and laboratory parameters as determined by the doctors. Often these

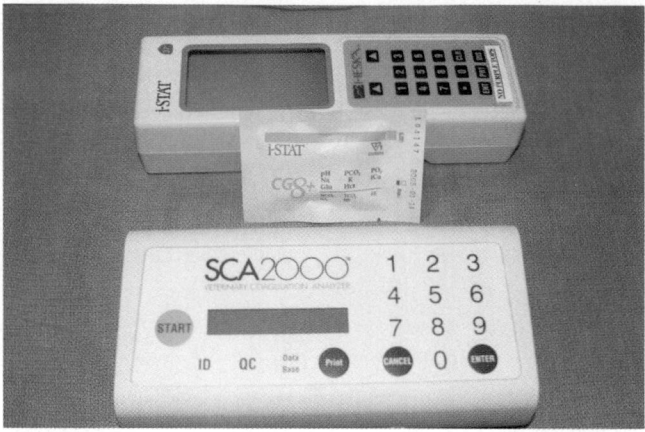

Figure 26-8 Automated blood analyzers are available for assessment of biochemical, arterial blood gas, and coagulation parameters (I-Stat, Symbiotics 3000).

parameters include but are not limited to temperature, pulse, respiration, mucus membrane color, capillary refill time, blood pressure, electrocardiogram (ECG) and oxygen saturation via a pulse oximeter. Basic laboratory data often includes packed cell volume, total plasma solids, blood glucose, blood lactate, blood urea nitrogen, and urine specific gravity. A rapid assessment of laboratory data can be obtained at the emergency station using "dip stick" test strips, glucometers, or point-of-care analyzers. Point-of-care testing equipment is available for coagulation assessments [prothrombin time (PT), partial thromboplastin time (PTT), activated clotting time (ACT) tubes, buccal mucosal bleeding time equipment], arterial blood gas analysis, and basic serum biochemistries. Automated blood analyzers (Figure 26-8) allow for multiple blood parameters to be assessed quickly and repeated later for comparison.

All veterinary hospitals should also have a basic laboratory area with a microscope set up to view blood smears or cytology samples. Blood smear examination can provide important diagnostic clues that may aid the emergency clinician (including red cell morphology, relative white blood cell numbers, and platelet count estimates).

Commercial test kits can also be kept at hand for rapid detection of toxin exposure (i.e., ethylene glycol) and infectious disease status (i.e., canine parvovirus, feline retroviruses, and heartworm disease). A card test and kits are available for rapid blood typing and for cross-matching. These supplies should be kept with a quick reference for the kit instructions and for interpretation of results. Other useful equipment may be kept in this area as determined necessary, such as an ultrasound unit.

FLUID THERAPY

Fluid therapy is a valuable asset in the treatment of critically ill animals. Although fluid therapy is commonly used in veterinary hospitals, there are often questions concerning which fluids are appropriate and what volumes should be delivered.

It is helpful to think of fluid therapy as expanding the animal's blood or plasma volume. This volume expansion lasts for a variable period of time depending upon the fluid administered and the animal's condition. Common reasons for providing fluid support in critically ill pets include

1. Maintaining hydration
2. Replacing fluid losses
3. Maintaining intravenous access and delivering other medications
4. Treatment of shock or hypoproteinemia
5. Increasing urine output
6. Correcting acid-base or electrolyte disturbances
7. Providing nutritional support

Crystalloid fluids are isotonic fluids consisting primarily of water with sodium or glucose. They are used for volume expansion and rapidly distribute into the extracellular space. However, only approximately 25% of crystalloid fluids remain in the vascular space after 1 hour. Crystalloids fluids are inexpensive and readily available in most practices. Examples of commonly used crystalloid solutions include 0.9% saline, lactated Ringer's solution (LRS), Normosol-R, and Plasma-Lyte. Colloid solutions are also used to expand vascular volume. They contain high-molecular-weight particles, which remain intravascular for longer periods of time. The hemodynamic effects of most colloids are similar to plasma and last longer than crystalloid fluids. Colloids can be used as single agent therapy or in conjunction with crystalloid fluids. Use of colloids can reduce the volume of crystalloid solution required in some animals. These agents are used in a variety of critical care cases. One disadvantage of using colloids is the additional expense incurred. Examples of synthetic colloids include hydroxyethyl starch (Hetastarch), Dextran 70, Dextran 40, and Oxyglobin.

The route of fluid administration is an important aspect of fluid therapy. Subcutaneous fluid administration is popular because it is quick and easy and can be used during home management or outpatient management of some animals. However, fluid absorption via this route may be slow and unpredictable. For this reason, overreliance on subcutaneous fluid therapy should be avoided. The intravenous route is often the best route to administer fluids in critical animals. Multiple large-bore catheters can be placed in peripheral or central veins to increase the veterinarian's ability to administer fluid and medications to sick animals. In some critically ill animals (especially puppies and kittens), venous access may be difficult to obtain. If venous access is limited, the intraosseous route can be utilized by using purpose made intramedullary catheters, stylet needles, or bone marrow needles. Once the animal is volume expanded, peripheral veins may be more accessible for intravenous catheterization.

The intravenous route is often the best route to administer fluids in critical animals

Appropriate fluid therapy is administered in phases as part of a complete treatment plan. This fluid therapy plan should be adapted to the needs of each individual case and based on solid patient monitoring. In planning fluid therapy, veterinarians often consider an emergency phase, a replacement phase, and a maintenance phase. Emergency fluid therapy in the treatment of shock is outlined elsewhere in this chapter. Replacement fluid therapy is intended to restore fluid balance to dehydrated animals. The volume of fluid to be replaced is calculated by estimating the percent dehydration and multiplying this number by the body weight in kilograms. The product of these numbers equals the replacement fluid volume in liters. For example, a 20-kg dog estimated to be 7% dehydrated would need 1.4 L of fluid (0.07 20 kg = 1.4 L). The rate of fluid replacement is dependent on clinical signs and the rate of loss. If the animal has become acutely dehydrated, then the volume may be replaced over 6 to 8 hours. If the loss has been chronic, it can be administered over 24 hours. Maintenance fluid requirements are calculated by well-established formulas. Most formulas are based on body weight (i.e., maintenance fluid dose = 60 ml/kg/day), although some believe that fluid requirements are best approximated by the basal energy requirement (30 kg body weight + 70 = fluid dose in ml/day). Ongoing fluid losses may continue in the hospitalized patient from fluid loss associated with vomiting, diarrhea, hemorrhage, or fluid effusion. Staff members should record and estimate the volume of such losses so that the veterinarian can devise an appropriate maintenance fluid therapy plan which takes such losses into consideration.

Staff members should record and estimate the volume of fluid losses due to vomiting or diarrhea.

Animals receiving fluid therapy must be closely monitored for both dehydration and fluid overload. Relying solely on calculated fluid rates places the animal at risk for either inadequate fluid therapy or "overhydration." Clinical signs and subjective parameters associated with overhydration include coughing, tachypnea, respiratory distress, nasal discharge, conjunctival edema (chemosis), and peripheral edema. Abnormal lung sounds may be due to pulmonary edema caused by over hydration. Objective parameters used to evaluate fluid therapy include hematocrit (or packed cell volume)/total protein (PCV/TP), body weight, central venous pressure, urine specific gravity, and urine output. The PCV/TP should be monitored frequently as shock and replacement fluid therapy is administered. If the hematocrit should decrease to less than 20% or the TP decreases by 50% or more of the initial value, veterinarians may consider

changes in fluid type or rate of administration. In addition, catheters and catheter sites should be routinely evaluated to check for catheter patency and guard against catheter-associated inflammation.

STANDARDS OF CARE AND EMERGENCY PROTOCOLS

The development of standardized procedures and patient care protocols is helpful in dealing with common clinical presentations and emergency situations. A standardized approach helps maintain an expected standard of care, allows the veterinary team to respond rapidly to a crisis, and minimizes confusion among staff members during an emergency. In addition, written procedure manuals can aid in the training of new staff members and serve as a reference for review by experienced team members. In developing a procedures manual, minimum standards of care should be agreed upon. If a group of clinics have shared staff or clientele (i.e., an emergency clinic that serves a community of veterinary practices), then agreed-upon procedures or protocols (between hospitals) can compound the benefits of smooth operation and consistent patient care with the benefits of better communication. In the same way, veterinarian and technician associations may play a role in advocating standards of care, in providing continuing education, and in creating a forum for professionals with common interests to share their experiences. Certain situations (trauma, shock, cardiopulmonary resuscitation) are common scenarios in all veterinary facilities and merit individual discussion in this chapter.

TRIAGE OF THE TRAUMA PATIENT

Animals presenting with a history of traumatic injury require rapid, accurate assessment and special monitoring to ensure good care and guard against secondary complications. The patient with multiple-body-system trauma is at a greater risk of complications due to the additive effects of each injury. "Triage" is the process of determining the priority of need and the proper order of treatment when evaluating a clinical situation. A standard protocol is used to identify which problems and which body systems should be evaluated first. In emergency cases, priority is given to treating respiratory, cardiac and vascular problems. Other body systems are subsequently evaluated in a systematic manner. Secondary complications of trauma include but are not limited to disseminated intravascular coagulation, sepsis, multiorgan failure, and distress due to pain.

Most veterinarians are familiar with mnemonics dictating the principles of triage. These mnemonics are useful in managing cases and in instructing staff members in a standardized approach to emergency situations and cardiopulmonary arrest. Initially, the ABC's of cardiopulmonary

Box 26-1   A CRASH PLAN: TREATMENT PRIORITIES
OVER A SPECTRUM OF BODY SYSTEMS

Airway	Cardiovascular	Pelvis
	Respiratory	Limbs
	Abdomen	Arteries/veins
	Spine	Nerves
	Head	

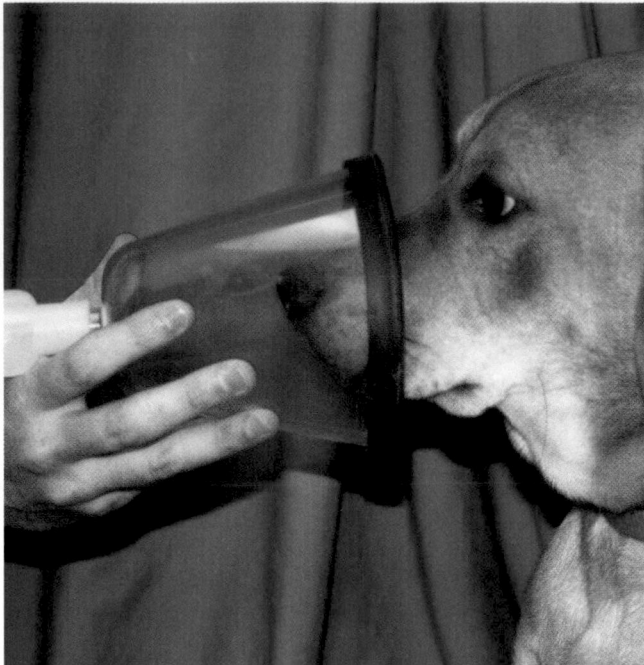

Figure 26-10   Supplemental oxygen may be supplied via a face mask.

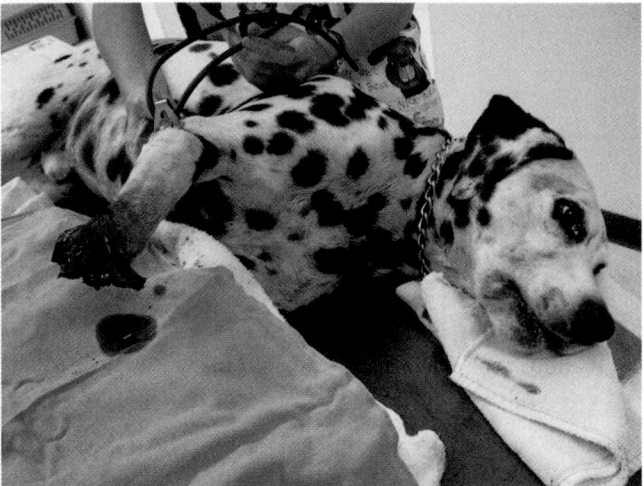

Figure 26-9   Tourniquet placement can control arterial bleeding from the extremities when the distal limb is not salvageable.

resuscitation illustrate a good assessment strategy for victims of cardiopulmonary arrest and also the acute trauma patient. Control of **a**rterial bleeding and rapid establishment of an **a**irway, followed by **b**reathing assistance and evaluation of **c**ardiac and **c**irculatory problems, ensures support of the vital life systems. Box 26-1 describes an alternative mnemonic, A CRASH PLAN, which refers to treatment priorities over an extended spectrum of body systems.

The great diversity of individual patient needs leaves room for debating the exact priorities in any given case. The real value of these schematic plans lies in their ability to standardize treatment and encourage rational stepwise thought during otherwise chaotic emergency situations.

Arterial bleeding is a serious priority for animals presented as an emergency. In part, this problem is uncommon, because animals with significant arterial hemorrhage may not survive long enough to reach a veterinary hospital. If arterial hemorrhage is present, direct pressure should be applied to the wound immediately. If the vessel is easily visualized, the vessel can be clamped. Placement of ligatures is time-consuming and is not an immediate priority during the initial emergency assessment. A tourniquet may be applied to a limb to control hemorrhage if the distal limb cannot be salvaged (Figure 26-9).

The respiratory system is the next priority. Evaluation can be done quickly and efficiently by observation and auscultation. Visual assessment of respiratory pattern and mucous membrane color can be combined with thorough auscultation. Oxygen supplementation should be provided if the patient is in respiratory distress or is not hemodynamically stable (as judged by pale or cyanotic mucous membranes, weak pulses, rapid heart rate, or presence of an irregular heart beat). Techniques for supplementation of oxygen include face mask (Figure 26-10) or blow-by technique (Figure 26-11), nasal cannula (Figure 26-12), placement in an oxygen cage (Figure 26-13) or oxygen canopy (Figure 26-14), and intubation with manual or mechanical ventilation with 100% oxygen.

Veterinarians and technicians should be alert to common and severe respiratory problems associated with trauma, including upper airway trauma/rupture, pneumothorax, hemothorax, pulmonary contusions, diaphragmatic hernia, and flail chest. Signs of upper airway trauma may include bloody respiratory discharge, increased respiratory effort, subcutaneous emphysema, and increased upper airway noise. In animals with pneumothorax and hemothorax, air or blood becomes trapped between the body wall and lung, resulting in pressure changes within the chest and collapse or compression of the lung. Clinical signs of hemothorax or pneumothorax include rapid shallow breathing (a restrictive breathing pattern) and respiratory distress. Flail chest results from two or more consecutive ribs that are broken in two places, which results in respiratory pain and paradoxical motion of the chest wall (i.e., a segment of the chest wall

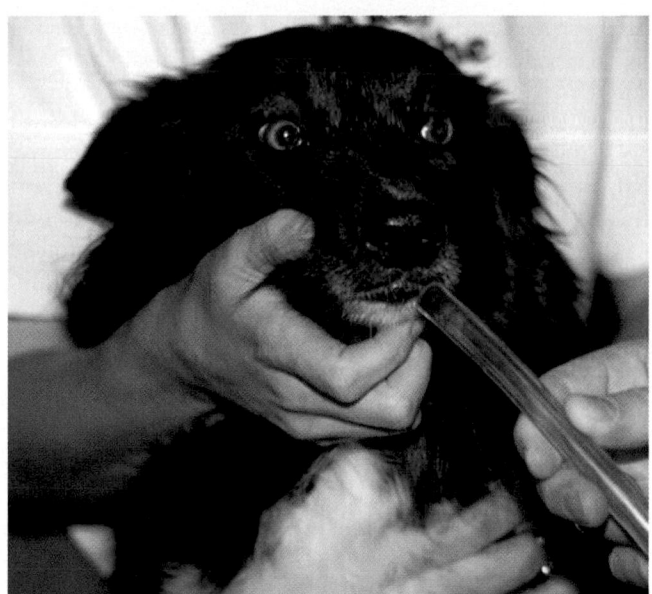

Figure 26-11 A high rate of oxygen flow from an oxygen source can be administered by the "blow-by" technique to provide temporary noninvasive oxygen supplementation.

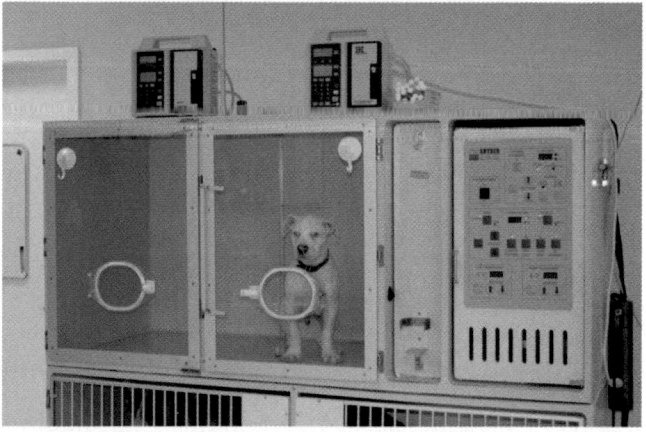

Figure 26-13 An oxygen cage offers a high-tech but noninvasive means of providing oxygen therapy.

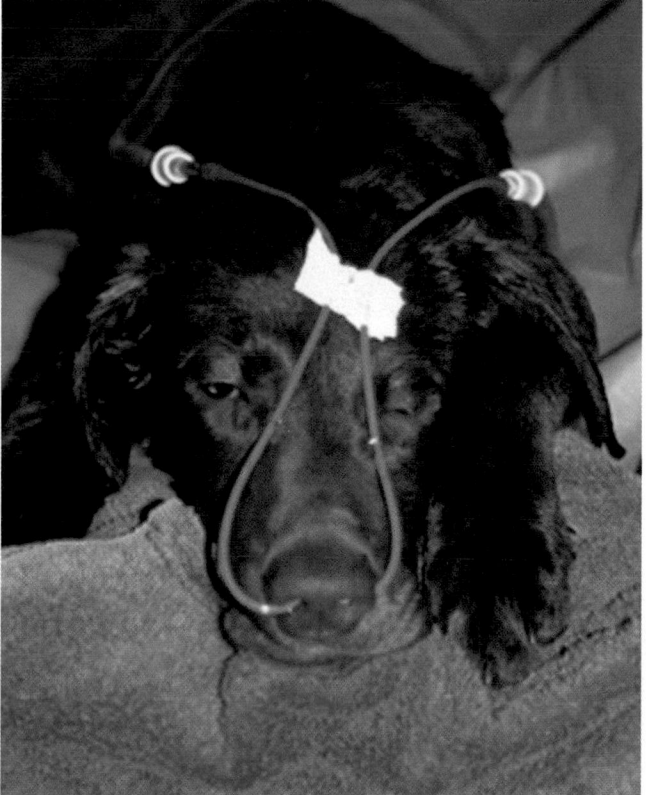

Figure 26-12 Bilateral nasal canulae can be attached to an oxygen source for comfortable and durable oxygen supplementation.

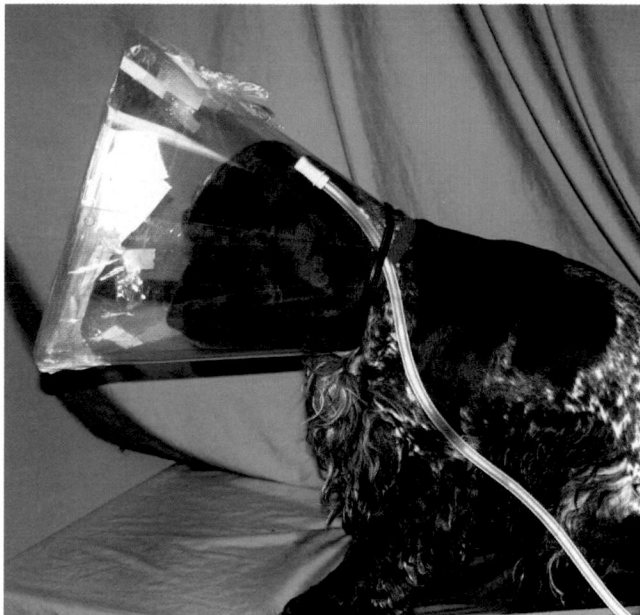

Figure 26-14 An oxygen canopy can be constructed from an Elizabethan collar and used in most veterinary hospitals.

collapses during inhalation and expands during exhalation). Rapid recognition of these problems is imperative because additional emergency procedures including thoracocentesis and thoracic drain placement may be required for animals with these conditions. Thoracocentesis is a diagnostic, as well as therapeutic, procedure and can be the difference between life and death until a thoracic drain can be placed. Additional diagnostics may include thoracic radiographs, pulse oximetry, and arterial blood gas analysis. Respiratory injuries often benefit from oxygen supplementation, but severe injuries may require mechanical ventilation.

🖉 TECHNICIAN NOTE

Thoracocentesis is a diagnostic, as well as therapeutic, procedure and can be the difference between life and death until a thoracic drain can be placed.

The cardiovascular system is clearly a priority system and is often assessed in combination with the respiratory system. Thoracic auscultation combined with mucous membrane color (capillary refill time) assessment and femoral artery pulse palpation will provide quick evaluation of the cardiovascular system. An ECG will assess cardiac electrical activity and detect the presence of heart rhythm disturbances. Often, monitoring equipment can be set up during the animal's initial assessment so that the ECG can be performed as an extension of the physical exam.

Blood loss must be evaluated and addressed immediately. Mucous membrane color, capillary refill time, and hematocrit with total plasma solids should be evaluated as soon as possible. If outward hemorrhage is apparent, this must be addressed and replacement with fluid therapy and/or blood products should be considered. Remember that internal hemorrhage may be occurring, which is not easily observed in sites such as the pleural space and peritoneal cavity. An abdominal pressure bandage may be placed if abdominal or pelvic injuries (i.e., femur or pelvic fractures, road rash) are outwardly evident. Application of such a bandage may help preempt a worsening hemoabdomen and prevent further cardiovascular decompensation. Proper application of abdominal pressure bandages is important. First, a folded gauze pad or a rolled towel is placed on midline (Figures 26-15 and 26-16) and secured with gauze cling (Figure 26-17). Further tension may be applied with cohesive bandage material (Figure 26-18). Care is taken not to secure the bandage so tightly that the animal has discomfort or impaired respiration. Thoracocentesis and abdominocentesis may be considered if patient monitoring suggests the presence of ongoing unrecognized hemorrhage. If ongoing

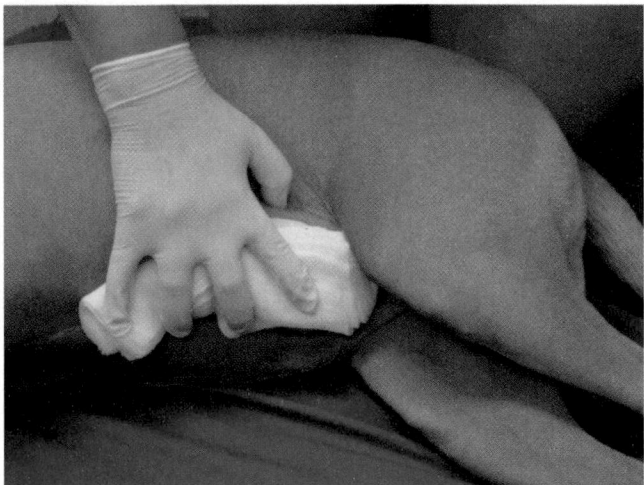

Figure 26-15 In the initial step of applying an abdominal pressure bandage, folded gauze is placed on midline to provide a padded site of pressure.

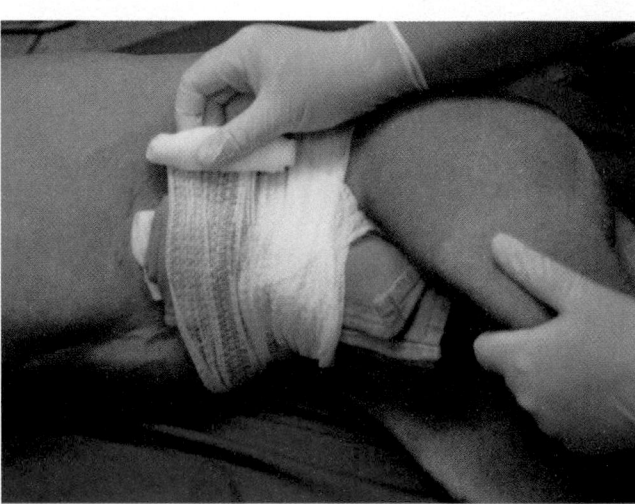

Figure 26-17 Gauze cling is used to secure the bandage material on midline and apply appropriate tension.

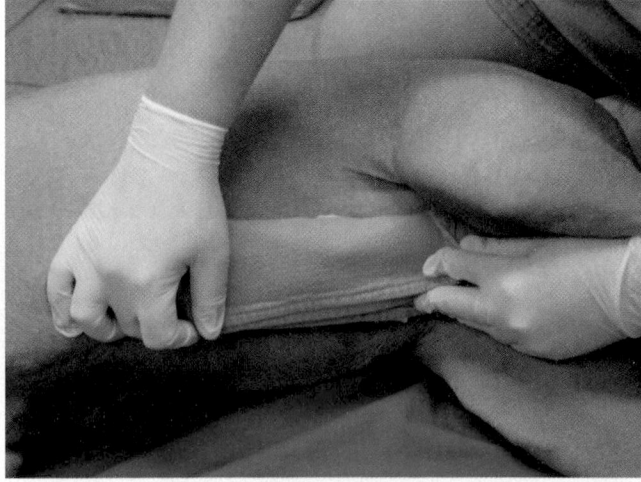

Figure 26-16 A rolled towel may be placed on top of the gauze pad to add to the cushion and further focus the bandage pressure.

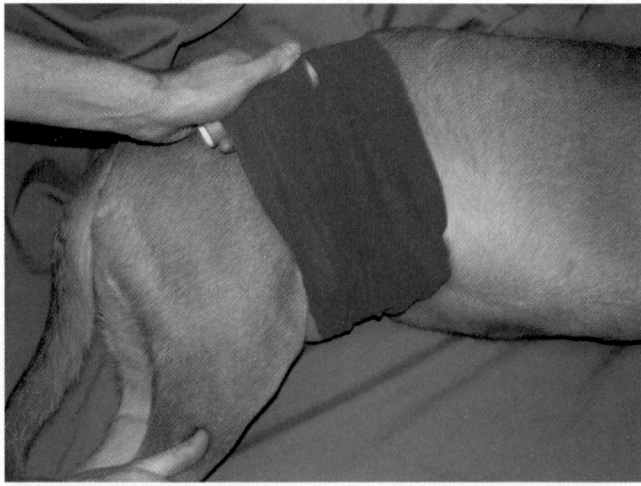

Figure 26-18 Additional layers of bandage material are applied to secure the bandage.

abdominal hemorrhage is detected, surgery may be considered once appropriate attempts have been made to ensure the animal is hemodynamically stable.

Neurological evaluation of the trauma patient is difficult. Recognizing severe head trauma with changes in intracranial pressure should be a priority. Changes in mentation and level of consciousness along with changes in pupillary light response and pupillary size may be an indication of increased intracranial pressure. Increased intracranial pressure results from hemorrhage, edema, and inflammation that occur secondary to trauma. Although decompressive surgeries are sometimes used in people with increased intracranial pressure, most veterinary cases of head trauma are medically managed with drugs that reduce intracranial pressure (mannitol, furosemide). This difference may in part be due to the ability of people to have brain imaging without general anesthesia. The specific uses of drugs in the treatment of head trauma are controversial. Corticosteroids reduce intracranial inflammation but may have other harmful side effects. Veterinarians often disagree on the use of steroids for head trauma. Mannitol and furosemide are diuretics that can reduce cerebral edema. However, mannitol is contraindicated in animals with active intracranial bleeding. In systemically unstable animals with head trauma, treating hypotension is a priority. Restriction of fluid to prevent cerebral edema in the face of hypotension should be avoided. In these cases, volume expansion with colloids may be more beneficial than the use of crystalloids because smaller volumes can be used.

Thorough palpation of the spine followed by assessment of extremity sensation and tendon reflexes should be part of a complete neurologic examination after other triage priorities have been assessed. A syndrome of "spinal shock" may interfere with interpretation of the neurologic exam for up to 24 hours. Abnormal postures such as Schiff-Sherrington, decerebellation, and decerebrate rigidity may provide clues to severe neurologic injury.

> **TECHNICIAN NOTE**
>
> A syndrome of spinal shock may interfere with interpretation of the neurologic exam for up to 24 hours.

Orthopedic injuries should be stabilized whenever possible. A splint placed on bone fractures must incorporate the joint above and the joint below the fracture site to provide adequate stabilization of the injury. Early closure of contaminated soft tissue injuries is not a priority in animals with concurrent internal injury and circulatory compromise. Instead, sterile bandages may be applied to keep the wounds clean and moist, until they can be dealt with safely.

> **TECHNICIAN NOTE**
>
> A splint placed on bone fractures must incorporate the joint above and the joint below the fracture site to provide adequate stabilization of the injury.

Although the emergency trauma case can be a very stressful and hectic event for the veterinary team, it is important to follow a systematic approach to the patient. It is imperative that the patient be thoroughly examined and triaged on initial presentation as well as closely monitored during hospitalization.

TRIAGE OF THE CRITICAL CARE PATIENT

Outside the realms of trauma and cardiac arrest, the principles of triage can be applied to many cases. Management of treatment priorities in a similar stepwise fashion is the basis for providing quality medical care. The complex and lethal nature of illness in emergency and critical care medicine makes a priority-based approach imperative. Such cases often demand a critical response from a team of staff members, similar to those responding to acute trauma. Consequently, the above triage decisions are readily, and even necessarily, adapted to a variety of cases during the treatment of critically ill pets.

Severely ill animals are often hospitalized with a limited or vague clinical history. In such patients, a systematic body systems review (including a triagelike review of basic life support systems) will document a stoic animal's true clinical condition and may help determine the nature and extent of disease. Appropriate triage of body systems during daily interactions with the patient (including serial physical exams), facilitates the recognition of new problems and important clinical changes. Abnormalities in the respiratory, cardiac, and circulatory systems often require common supportive therapies, regardless of cause. For instance, a recumbent animal with gray mucous membranes, tachycardia, weak pulses, a poor capillary refill time, and hypothermia will benefit from oxygen supplementation, intravenous fluid therapy, and external warming irrespective of the final diagnosis.

The value of a team approach cannot be overstated. Nursing and technical staff often have a unique insight into the health of hospitalized animals by virtue of the time spent providing nursing care and administering treatments. Veterinarians can take advantage of this insight by listening to their staff and requesting additional clinical information. It may be beneficial to review the principles of triage with staff members in the context of critical care. In this way, an appropriate and standardized response to serious illness will ensure good practice even when a "red flag" (like polytrauma) is absent.

SECONDARY COMPLICATIONS

Secondary complications of trauma and critical illness are common in veterinary medicine. Although technicians are not called upon to make a diagnosis or formulate treatment plans, a detailed understanding of such complications can be beneficial. For example, well-trained staff members can prepare for and anticipate complications by knowing appropriate clinical signs and monitoring techniques. This knowledge can enable experienced staff members, who are familiar with commonly performed diagnostic and treatment strategies, to better assist the veterinarian with the recognition and treatment of these problems. A proactive approach is appropriate in order to provide the best defense against these complications.

PAIN

Staff members trained in the recognition and treatment of pain can help ensure that appropriate analgesia is provided in a compassionate and preemptive manner as part of sound medical care. Many analgesic drugs (i.e., opioids) have cardiac and respiratory depressant effects, which can be dangerous in systemically unstable animals. Nonsteroidal antiinflammatory drugs (NSAIDS) have little effect on the cardiopulmonary system but may have side effects that affect the gastrointestinal and renal systems. However, if the patient is stable with regards to the cardiopulmonary system and central nervous system, systemic administration of analgesics may be safely considered. In less stable animals the use of regional or local analgesia techniques may be considered. Local anesthetic block of flail chest segments can be a primary treatment of this condition.

Detection and assessment of pain is often a challenge in veterinary patients because animals can not directly communicate their physical condition and there are no pathognomonic signs of pain. Common signs frequently associated with pain include vocalization, depression, anorexia, tachypnea, tachycardia, hypertension, hypotension, pale mucous membranes, aggression, abnormal postures, excess salivation, and dilated pupils. Abdominal pain in particular may be expressed by a classic "praying" or "play bowing" position in which the forequarters are crouched with the abdomen and hindquarters elevated from the ground. It is important to note that animals who do not exhibit any of these signs are not necessarily pain free. All trauma victims should be assumed to experience some degree of pain. Victims of polytrauma, by extension, experience severe pain. Many critical illnesses, such as pancreatitis, meningitis, and cancer, are clearly painful problems. Obtunded animals, such as those with severe head trauma, may be unaware of or unable to express their pain. Pain management is an important component of treating these diseases. Regardless of the underlying conditions, untreated pain causes further stress and harmful physiologic changes.

DISSEMINATED INTRAVASCULAR COAGULATION

Trauma causes intense severe inflammation, poor blood perfusion, and widespread tissue/vessel injury that act as normal triggers for coagulation (blood clot formation). In most cases, the body's natural homeostatic mechanisms prevent widespread abnormal clotting by balancing clot formation with clot resolution. However, in animals with massive injuries, severe inflammation and tissue damage, the natural balance between clot formation and clot prevention/resolution may be disrupted. When this happens, massive activation of coagulation overwhelms the body's clot prevention and clot dissolution functions. Instead of controlled clot formation confined to sites of injury, systemic clot formation begins on a widespread basis. This phenomenon is referred to as disseminated intravascular coagulation (DIC).

In DIC, microclots form throughout the body's capillary network disrupting blood flow to vital organs (especially in the kidneys, brain, heart, and lungs). Blood pools in the capillaries behind the clots, causing stagnant flow, increased blood viscosity, and further tissue damage from ischemia and necrosis. Ongoing clot formation results in consumption of platelets and depletion of clotting factors and regulatory proteins, which causes a paradoxical inability to clot and bleeding tendency. Once the normal balance is disrupted, a vicious downward spiral is initiated, and a rapid, frequently fatal self-propagating cycle begins.

Clinical signs of DIC are often masked by those of the primary disease or trauma. In the early stages of DIC, the body is clotting excessively (hypercoagulable), and signs of thrombosis predominate. Signs of thrombosis include unexplained edema, cold extremities, tachypnea, pale mucous membranes, hypotension, and neurologic signs. In later stages of DIC (i.e., once clotting factors have been consumed), bleeding tendencies predominate. Progressive signs associated with the hypocoagulable state include unexplained hemorrhage or bruising (hematoma, intraocular bleeding, hemoabdomen or thorax, and excessive bleeding from venipuncture sites). Tiny pinpoint bruises known as *petechiae* commonly appear on the skin (especially along the ventrum and inguinal areas, Figure 26-19) and mucous

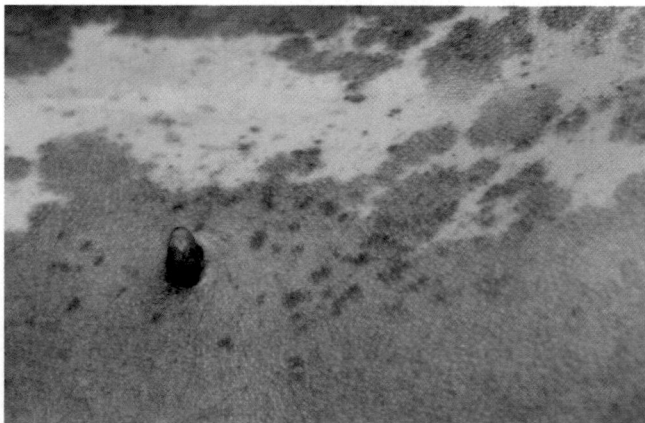

Figure 26-19 The bleeding tendency associated with DIC often results in small hemorrhages called *petechiae*, which are often seen on the thinly haired skin of the ventrum.

membranes (especially the gums and sclera, Figure 26-20). Large petechial hemorrhages, known as *ecchymoses*, form in similar areas (Figure 26-21).

DIC is always a secondary complication of some other severe disease. Common veterinary causes of DIC include polytrauma, pancreatitis, heatstroke, cancer, liver disease, immune-mediated hemolytic anemia, and snake envenomation. Unfortunately, there is no single specific sign or test for the diagnosis of DIC. Diagnosis of DIC is based on supportive lab findings and clinical signs in animals with severe underlying disease. Decreased platelet count (due to platelet consumption) is a consistent and early finding. Another reliable indicator of DIC is red blood cell morphology. Schistocytes or fragmented red cells are often seen in cases of DIC due to the effects of fibrin strands and microclot formation. Fibrin strands span small blood vessels and "rough up" the red cells resulting in distorted borders and red cell fragments that may be seen on the blood smear. Standard tests of clotting function are used to detect clotting factor deficiency. These tests include the PT, PTT, and the ACT. The advent of in-house coagulation time analyzers increases the ability of practitioners to monitor trends in all bleeding times (PT, PTT, ACT). The ACT has the benefit of being performed in-house without expensive equipment, but it requires special tubes containing sterile diatomaceous earth (Figure 26-22). Trends in ACT can be very helpful in cases where DIC is anticipated. Without sequential data, only the acute or end-stage patient may be diagnosed. Measurement of anticoagulant proteins (i.e., antithrombin levels) and by-products of clot breakdown (i.e., fibrin degradation products and D-dimers) have also been used in the diagnosis of DIC. Serum levels of fibrin degradation products (FDP) and D-dimers increase in DIC because fibrin clots are being formed and dissolved in a massive unregulated manner. Antithrombin is a natural anticoagulant regulatory protein that gets consumed in fulminant DIC.

TECHNICIAN NOTE
Schistocytes or fragmented red cells are often seen in cases of DIC.

Successful treatment of DIC lies in resolution of the primary disease whenever possible. Blood product therapy and anticoagulants are used to interrupt the self-propagating cycle of coagulation in DIC and to help the animal compensate for coagulation imbalance. Plasma products and fresh whole blood transfusions help replenish depleted clotting factors, provide anticoagulant regulatory proteins, and manage anemia caused by blood loss. Whole blood may also provide some fresh platelets, but it should be noted that these platelets are generally few in number and survive only a very short time. Heparin is an anticoagulant commonly used in conjunction with plasma. If heparin is used at moderate to high doses, it should be tapered prior to discontinuing therapy. Supportive care with fluid therapy and oxygen supplementation should not be overlooked. Unfortunately, treatment of DIC is often unsuccessful

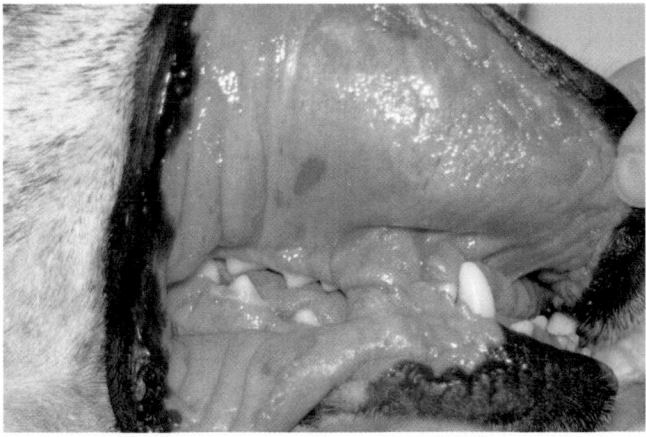

Figure 26-20 This dog suffered from DIC as a complication of heatstroke, and petechial hemorrhages are noted on the gums.

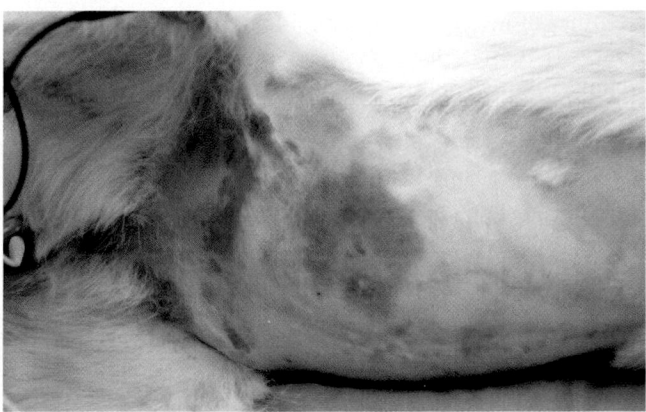

Figure 26-21 Larger hemorrhages, known as *ecchymoses*, are visible on the ventrum.

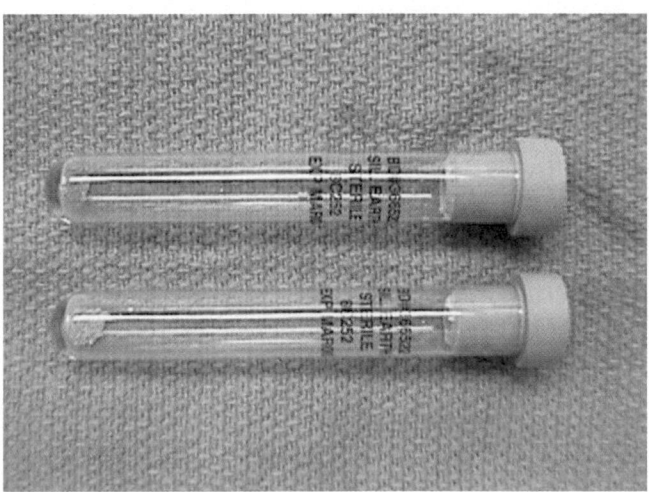

Figure 26-22 The activated clotting time (ACT) is a convenient countertop coagulation test requiring special tubes.

because many underlying conditions cannot be rapidly resolved and continue to propagate coagulation imbalance. In addition, once compensatory mechanisms are overwhelmed, it is exceedingly difficult to restore the body to a state of healthy equilibrium.

SHOCK AND THE SYSTEMIC INFLAMMATORY RESPONSE SYNDROME

The clinical syndrome known as *shock* is defined as perfusion failure and impaired delivery of oxygen to tissues. The imbalance between tissue oxygen demand and oxygen delivery is a key to understanding the causes and treatments of shock. When the fluid and oxygen demands of the tissues are not met (due to increased tissue demands, impaired fluid/oxygen delivery, or both), then ischemia, necrosis, organ failure, and death can occur rapidly.

In the early stages of shock, impaired perfusion triggers natural compensatory mechanisms (vasoconstriction, increased heart rate, increased cardiac contractility) that maintain blood pressure and increase cardiac output. This early or compensated phase of shock is known as the *hyperdynamic phase*. Clinical signs during this phase relate more to signs of the compensatory response than to perfusion failure and include increased heart rate and respiratory rate, rapid capillary refill time, injected mucous membranes, and increased pulse pressure. These findings can be subjective and easily missed, as the weakness, depression, and altered consciousness associated with later stages of shock are either absent or mild. Unless close monitoring has been performed by alert staff members, clinical signs in the early stages of shock may go unrecognized. The most recognizable clinical signs of hyperdynamic shock include brick red (injected) mucous membranes and bounding pulses. Early recognition and treatment may prevent further progression of shock.

TECHNICIAN NOTE

The most recognizable clinical signs of hyperdynamic shock include brick red (injected) mucous membranes and bounding pulses.

Uncompensated or hypodynamic shock ensues if there is progressive underlying disease or if compensatory mechanisms and treatment fail to restore normal blood flow and oxygen delivery. During uncompensated shock, cardiac output and systemic blood pressure are inadequate and blood flow is preferentially distributed to vital organs (brain, heart) at the expense of other tissues. This shunting of blood exacerbates the oxygen deficit and fluid imbalance in other tissues and can lead to organ failure. The commonly recognized clinical signs of uncompensated shock are associated with circulatory failure and include rapid heart rate, weak pulses, prolonged capillary refill time, pale mucous membranes, hypothermia, overt weakness, depression, and loss of consciousness. Eventually, prolonged hypoxia results in vascular paralysis, systemic vasodilation, and fulminant

cardiovascular collapse. This terminal phase of shock is irreversible and rapidly fatal.

Shock is a state of emergency that is associated with many causes. When subdivided according to underlying cause, general categories of shock are hypovolemic shock, distributive shock, cardiogenic shock (including obstructive shock), and septic shock. Hypovolemic shock is the most common form of shock in small animals. In this form of shock, perfusion failure results from a reduction in circulating blood volume caused by bleeding, dehydration (vomiting, diarrhea, increased urine output), or effusive fluid loss (i.e., abdominal fluid accumulation). Distributive shock is associated with maldistribution of blood flow associated with pathologic vasodilation. In this syndrome, pooling of blood in capillaries and veins results in a decrease in effective blood volume (regardless of intravascular volume or cardiac output). Common causes of distributive shock include trauma, heatstroke, envenomation, and anaphylaxis. As its name implies, cardiogenic shock is associated with decreased cardiac output. Cardiogenic shock can occur from many primary heart diseases such as cardiomyopathy, valvular disease, and cardiac arrhythmias. A subset of cardiogenic shock known as *obstructive shock* is associated with obstruction of blood flow. Common causes of obstructive shock include pericardial disease, heartworm disease, pulmonary hypertension, and pulmonary thromboembolism.

Septic shock can be triggered by primary infectious diseases, but it can also occur due to secondary infections. Extensive tissue damage is the hallmark of many diseases. For example, trauma, heatstroke, envenomations, and pancreatitis all result in significant tissue injury, disruption of blood flow, and severe inflammation. In these diseases areas of poorly perfused, devitalized tissue provide a good setting for bacterial growth. Infection in such areas is difficult to combat because disruptions in blood flow prevent systemically administered antibiotics from reaching the site of infection. In addition, poor perfusion results in ischemia, hypoxia, and continued tissue damage, which support bacterial growth. Bacterial toxins escalate the inflammatory response and exacerbate tissue damage. In small localized areas of infection, a heightened immune response aids in the clearance of infection. However, in animals with widespread injury or tissue damage, the exaggerated inflammatory response is maladaptive, leading to uncontrolled systemic inflammation. Systemic inflammatory mediators result in widespread vasodilation, vascular permeability changes, impaired myocardial function and activation of the coagulation cascade, which results in perfusion failure, impaired oxygen delivery to tissues, and spread of infection. This syndrome is referred to as septic shock. Hyperglycemia may occur in the early phase of septic shock due to the effects of stress hormones on metabolism. In later stages, hypoglycemia predominates as glucose is consumed by both bacteria and body demands.

A systemic inflammatory response syndrome (SIRS), which parallels septic shock, can be triggered by inflammatory mediators and products of tissue damage associated with critical illness even in the absence of infection. As is the case with other forms of shock, SIRS patients may go through an early hyperdynamic phase followed by an uncompensated or hypodynamic phase. In the hyperdynamic phase, circulatory collapse is temporarily held at bay by compensatory mechanisms that increase cardiac output and maintain vascular tone and volume. During this phase, bounding pulses and brick red mucous membranes may be noted. Clinical manifestations of SIRS include circulatory changes, thermoregulatory dysfunction (fever or hypothermia), depression, tachypnea, and DIC. Recognition of septic shock and SIRS in individual patients is based on clinical findings, supportive history, and laboratory data. Fulminant septic shock and SIRS are associated with a syndrome of multiple-organ dysfunction (MODS). Kidney failure is particularly common, and therefore urine production should be monitored. Hypoproteinemia is commonly noted in advanced stages of septic shock and SIRS due to impaired protein synthesis associated with liver dysfunction and protein loss caused by vascular permeability changes and inflammatory exudates.

TREATMENT OF SHOCK

Treatment of underlying diseases is important in the management of animals in shock. For instance, steps should be taken to control active hemorrhage in bleeding animals and transfusion should be considered. Animals with septic shock should receive appropriate antibiotics and animals with heart disease should be treated with appropriate medications. Unfortunately, management of underlying conditions takes time and often is only partially effective. Therefore, animals diagnosed with SIRS or other states of shock should receive treatment based on triage priorities similar to those animals in cardiac arrest.

Restoring oxygen delivery and perfusion to the tissues is a priority. Oxygen supplementation should be provided immediately via face mask during initial resuscitation efforts. This allows a staff member to continually monitor the patient during treatment. Nasal oxygen catheters or an oxygen cage (or canopy) may also be used. Preventing circulatory collapse is the number one treatment priority during management of these syndromes. This is accomplished primarily with aggressive fluid therapy to restore effective vascular volume. Fluid therapy is often administered "to effect," which means that shock fluids are administered until monitoring parameters indicate that treatment has had the desired effect. Shock dosages of crystalloid solutions are 90 ml/kg/hr in the dog and 45 to 60 ml/kg/hr in the cat. When using crystalloid therapy in the dog, shock dosages of fluid can be administered in quarter dose increments. A quick formula for this administration is to take the body weight in pounds and multiply by 10. For example, for a 40-lb dog, 400 ml will be approximately a quarter shock dose. This can be given over 15 minutes and the animal reevaluated. A pressure bag may be helpful

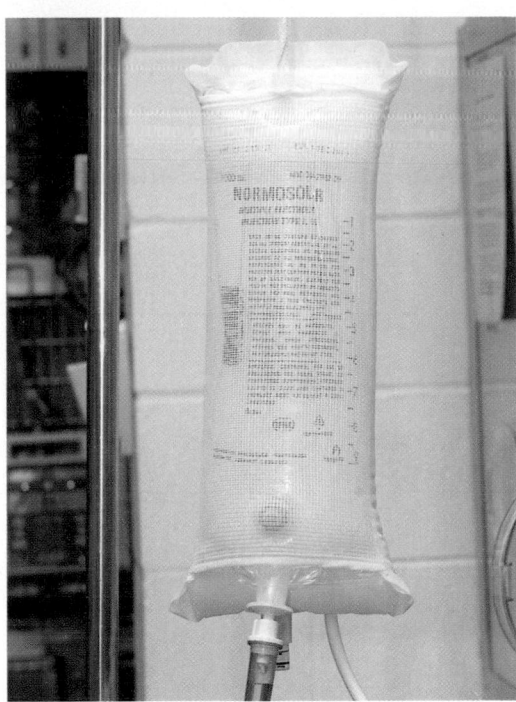

Figure 26-23 Intravenous fluid bags can be placed within a pressure bag to increase the rate of fluid administration.

for administering large fluid volumes over a short period of time (Figures 26-23). For cats the same formula can be used; however, you must divide the dose in half (or use the body weight in kilograms and "add" a zero, i.e., multiply by 10). Colloid fluids are also used to restore vascular volume. Colloid doses depend on the type of colloid used. Blood products such as whole blood and plasma may also be used in some cases during resuscitation efforts. Oxyglobin is a hemoglobin-based oxygen-carrying solution made from polymerized bovine hemoglobin. When administered intravenously, Oxyglobin acts like a colloid but also has oxygen carrying capacity, which has made it a popular resuscitation fluid for some clinicians. These fluid doses are a guideline, but higher doses may be necessary. Appropriate fluid therapy often results in normalization of heart rate, blood pressure, and mucous membrane color. Additional monitoring parameters include central venous pressure, urine output, blood lactate levels, hematocrit, and total protein. It should be noted that unusually large crystalloid and colloid fluid volumes may be necessary to maintain vascular volume in unstable animals, and intensive patient monitoring is critical. Animals with refractory hypotension, despite appropriate fluid therapy, may be candidates for use of vasopressor drugs (dopamine, dobutamine). Veterinarians generally give these drugs as a constant rate infusion to increase vascular tone and cardiac output. At low dose levels in dogs, dopamine selectively increases renal perfusion, which can be helpful in restoring urine output. At moderate doses, beneficial effects on systemic blood pressure predominate. However, at high doses, dopamine has an adverse effect on renal perfusion and may worsen kidney failure. Dobutamine primarily increases blood pressure by enhancing cardiac contractility and cardiac output. Both drugs can be associated with cardiac arrhythmias and ECG monitoring and careful auscultation may be helpful.

> ### ✎ TECHNICIAN NOTE
>
> A quick formula for quarter-dose shock fluid calculation is to take the body weight in pounds and multiply by 10 ("add" a zero). For cats the same formula can be used; however, you must divide the dose in half (or use the body weight in kilograms and multiply by 10).

PERFUSION FAILURE AND REPERFUSION INJURY

Reperfusion injury is a cellular injury that develops as blood flow returns to a previously ischemic area. During cardiopulmonary arrest and shock, oxygen-starved tissues develop an anaerobic metabolism and become depleted of the cellular energy stores known as *adenosine triphosphate* (ATP). These conditions alter certain enzyme systems responsible for adenine (an ATP precursor) metabolism and also destabilize white blood cell membranes. Upon reestablishment of oxygenation and perfusion (as occurs with successful resuscitation and fluid therapy), the altered enzyme systems (in the presence of oxygen) generate harmful molecules called *oxygen free radicals*. In addition, the membrane-damaged white blood cells release inflammatory mediators (including oxygen free radicals) that contribute to the reactive environment. Further activation and extension of inflammation and vascular damage ensues, resulting in thrombosis and edema. Widespread injury may result in systemic disorders such as DIC, SIRS, and multiorgan dysfunction. All vital organ systems can be affected by reperfusion injury, increased oxygen demands, and inflammation. For this reason, all systems must be monitored closely and supported, with special attention paid to basic life support systems.

CARDIOPULMONARY ARREST

Cardiopulmonary arrest is defined as the cessation of breathing and effective blood circulation. In most veterinary patients, cardiopulmonary arrest occurs as the terminal stage of an advanced disease. However, arrest can occur as a complication of any critical illness and even in healthy patients undergoing anesthesia. Resuscitation efforts attempting to reverse the state of arrest is commonly known as *CPR*, or more properly, cardiopulmonary cerebrovascular resuscitation (CPCR). The acronym CPCR emphasizes the importance of maintaining perfusion and oxygen delivery to the central nervous system during and after an arrest. Attention to nervous system needs is important so that resuscitation offers a chance to return an animal to full

function rather than simply returning cardiopulmonary function to a brain dead animal.

In an arrest, time is crucial if resuscitation is going to be successful. Therefore, being prepared and having trained personnel is essential to management of arrest situations. Specific equipment and facility recommendations have been addressed previously in this chapter. One of the most important aspects of emergency preparedness involves knowing which patients are likely to arrest. These patients include those with heart disease, respiratory disease, hypothermia, multisystem failure, trauma, and shock. Contributing factors include hypoxia, heightened vagus nerve stimulation (vagal tone), acid-base disturbances, electrolyte abnormalities, and anesthesia. Common diseases associated with heightened vagal tone include gastrointestinal disease, respiratory disease, neurologic disease, and ophthalmic disease. The most commonly recognized source of vagus-mediated arrest occurs in weak and vomiting animals. Vomiting is accompanied by a reflex slowing of the heart rate (bradycardia), which is mediated through the vagus nerve. In susceptible animals, this slowing of the heart rate can be extreme and lead to cardiac arrest. Other stimuli for vagus-mediated arrest include urination and defecation. However, there are many factors involved in an arrest scenario, because each individual animal deals with disease, traumatic insult, or stress differently. Sudden changes in the animal's physical status can alert you to impending arrest. In all high risk patients, it is important to frequently monitor respirations, pulse rate/character, mucous membranes color (for pallor or cyanosis), and body temperature. Anesthetized patients should also be monitored for unexplained changes in anesthetic depth. Recognizing an impending arrest and alerting other team members are the first steps in resuscitation.

CARDIOPULMONARY CEREBROVASCULAR RESUSCITATION

Resuscitation efforts (CPCR) may be divided into two phases: basic life support and advanced life support. As noted in the preceding discussion of triage, the steps of resuscitation may be correlated with letters of the alphabet to assist with training and remembering the order of steps. Basic life support involves the important first steps or ABC's of resuscitation. If these steps are not successful, subsequent efforts at resuscitation are futile.

BASIC LIFE SUPPORT

In basic life support, *A* is for airway. Staff members responding to a potentially arrested animal should note if the animal is breathing. If respirations are absent or weak, the mouth should be opened, and the oropharynx examined for possible obstruction. Common sources of airway obstruction include respiratory secretions, aspirated vomitus, blood, ingested foreign material, and mass lesions (hematomas, neoplasia, etc). If obstruction is noted, the airway should be cleared with suction or manual removal of foreign material. Caution is indicated to avoid being bitten, although most animals in partial or full states of arrest have limited or no capacity to bite. A sponge forceps and gauze may be helpful in clearing some exudates. Once the airway is cleared, staff members should note whether these steps have stimulated the animal to breathe.

If the animal does not begin to breathe, then the patient must receive ventilation assistance. *B is for breathing.* Mouth-to-nose resuscitation may be performed by sealing the lip margins and blowing into the animal's nose. This method requires no special equipment and will deliver about 16% oxygen. This level of oxygenation is inadequate and should only be done temporarily until a higher supply of oxygen can be provided. Mouth-to-nose resuscitation efforts carry some risk to caregivers treating animals with potentially zoonotic diseases. Endotracheal intubation and ventilation with an Ambu bag in room air provides 21% oxygen. The best method of assisted ventilation is endotracheal intubation and delivery of 100% oxygen from an oxygen source. Ideally, animals should be intubated in lateral recumbency to prevent elevation of the head and positional changes that impair cerebral blood flow. Many times, however, intubation is performed more rapidly and accurately using a laryngoscope with the animal in sternal recumbency. Rapid intubation is imperative, and delays or failure can be catastrophic to further resuscitation. Following intubation, the tube should be secured with a gauze tie. If intubation is not possible, a narrow orotracheal catheter or transtracheal cannulae is sometimes useful. However, a large-bore airway is preferred and may require a surgical tracheostomy. During assisted ventilation, the first two breaths administered should be long breaths lasting a full 2 seconds, followed by patient assessment. In some instances, restoring an open airway will lead to recovery of spontaneous respirations by the patient. If not, the animal should be manually ventilated at a rate slightly higher than the expected normal. Assisted ventilation should expand the chest by 30%, with a slightly longer expiration than inspiration. If the breathing circuit contains a manometer (i.e., most anesthetic machines), a pressure of 10 to 20 cm of water should be obtained with each breath.

Acupuncture is a method that can be attempted to treat respiratory arrest when other efforts have failed. The acupuncture point is Governor Vessel 26 (VG 26) of Jen Chung. This point is located at the nasal philtrum at the level of the ventral edge of the nares. A 25-gauge needle is applied to the bone at this point, and then twirled to induce breathing.

C is for circulation. Once the airway is established and ventilation provided, circulation must be assessed by palpation of pulses (or apex heart beat) and auscultation of the heart. Peripheral pulses are nonpalpable when the mean blood pressure is less than 60 mm Hg. An apex heart beat may be indistinguishable when the pressure is less

than 40 mm Hg. It is important to note that some animals suffer respiratory arrest without cardiac arrest. Improper chest compressions can increase stress to the patient and precipitate cardiac arrest in some cases. Once cardiac arrest has been confirmed, chest compressions should be started immediately.

Positioning of the animal during compressions depends on the animal's size, the shape of the chest (barrel chest versus deep and narrow chest), and the ability to deliver adequate compressions. There are two theoretical models to explain forward motion of blood during CPCR. In small animals and/or those with a narrow chest conformation chest compressions (during closed-chest CPCR) and direct cardiac massage (during open-chest CPCR) apply forces to the heart that mimic the normal heart mechanics. This is known as the *cardiac pump.* In large animals and those with barrel chests, changes in chest conformation limit the direct effect of chest compressions on the heart. In these cases increased intrathoracic pressure during compression results in forward blood flow from the heart, which serves as a passive blood reservoir. This is referred to as the *thoracic pump* model, which is thought to play a significant role in medium- to large-size animals during CPCR. To optimize the cardiac and thoracic pumps, animals less than 15 lb (7 kg) should be placed in lateral recumbency. Animals greater than 15 lb may be placed in either lateral or dorsal recumbency. The point of compression (hand placement) for the cardiac pump is located directly over the heart (Figure 26-24). For the thoracic pump, the point of compression is located at the widest part of the chest (Figure 26-25).

Effectiveness of CPCR should be assessed by palpating for a pulse and evaluating the mucous membrane color. If available, an ECG can be extremely beneficial at this point to assess the heart and also to evaluate the effectiveness of resuscitation efforts. Traditionally, a pulse and/or an electrical waveform on ECG should be generated with each compression. If available, end-tidal CO_2 (capnography) is a reliable indicator of perfusion. Other monitoring equipment

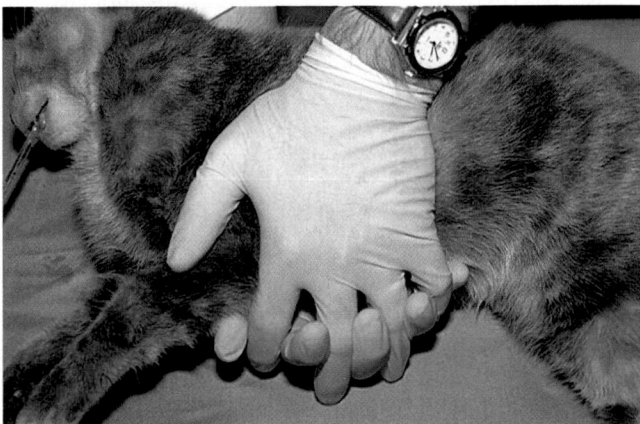

Figure 26-24 Correct placement of hands in an animal less than 15 lb for the administration of chest compression, which simulates cardiac contractions (the cardiac pump).

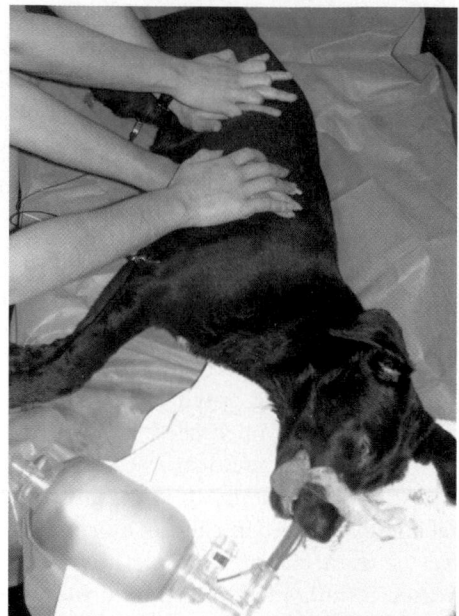

Figure 26-25 Appropriate hand placement for chest compressions utilizing the thoracic pump theory. Also, note placement of the hands for abdominal compressions.

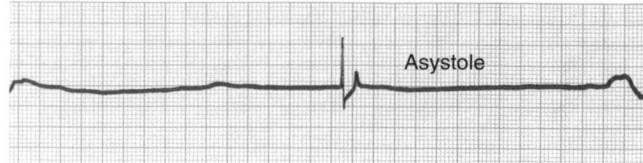

Figure 26-26 This ECG is from an arrested animal in asystole (flat line). A single "escape beat" is also present.

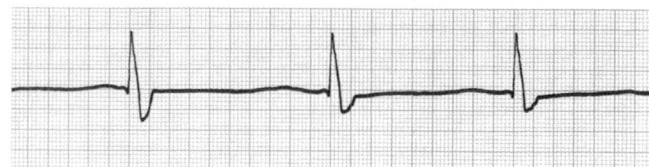

Figure 26-27 This ECG is characteristic of electrical mechanical dissociation (EMD).

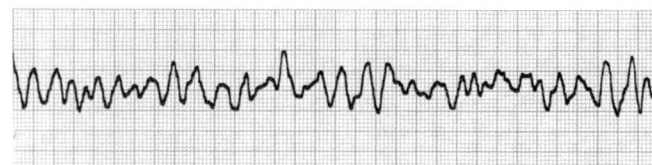

Figure 26-28 This ECG demonstrates ventricular fibrillation.

(ECG, pulse oximeter, venous blood gas analysis, and lactate levels) also provides useful quantitative information. A change in technique may be required to improve effectiveness, such as changing places with another team member, changing the animal's position, and/or altering your compression technique. Ventilation and chest compressions may be interposed or administered simultaneously. Administering ventilations and compressions simultaneously enhances the thoracic pump by increasing intrathoracic pressure during the compression (systole) and increasing venous return and atrial filling during relaxation (diastole). This is thought to assist in a forward flow of blood, which favors cerebral circulation over myocardial blood flow. Once compressions have begun, a solid rhythm can develop if the breaths are administered simultaneous to the compressions. This rate should be 120/min for animals less than 15 lb and 80 to 100/min for animals greater than 15 lb. Interposed abdominal compressions assist in directing blood in the lower half of the body back toward the heart (via increased intraabdominal pressure) and may be administered by another team member (see Figure 26-25).

> ### ✎ TECHNICIAN NOTE
> Effectiveness of CPCR should be assessed by palpating for a pulse and evaluating the mucous membrane color.

Open-chest CPCR is mostly indicated in animals with chest trauma (flail chest, pneumothorax, and diaphragmatic hernias) due to the interference of such injuries on closed-chest compressions. In this method of CPCR, the chest is surgically opened on the left side at the fifth intercostal space, and compressions are applied to the heart from the apex to the base. Care should be taken not to twist the heart, which can occlude major vessels. Nontraumatic occlusion of the descending aorta during open-chest CPCR may improve coronary and cerebral blood flow. Open-chest CPCR is only beneficial if initiated early in the resuscitation effort. The decision to perform an emergency thoracotomy for open-chest CPCR should be made within 2 minutes of cardiopulmonary arrest.

ADVANCED LIFE SUPPORT

Advanced life support requires interpretation of an ECG and administration of drugs based on cardiac output, blood pressure, and the presence of arrhythmias. These steps in resuscitation are important only after basic life support has been established (i.e., the animal is being ventilated and adequate circulation is provided). If the animal has responded to resuscitation efforts and has a perfusing rhythm, advanced life support may not be necessary. Unfortunately, in many cases, life-threatening arrhythmias and hypotension are common and require treatment.

Common drugs used in CPCR include atropine, epinephrine, naloxone, lidocaine, and magnesium chloride or sulfate. Proper use of an ECG allows recognition of specific arrhythmias so that appropriate drugs may be administered and patient response to therapy can be gauged. There are three basic arrhythmias seen during an arrest. These include asystole ("flat-line") (Figure 26-26), nonperfusing rhythms (electromechanical dissociation or pulseless electrical activity) (Figure 26-27), and ventricular fibrillation (Figure 26-28). Intravenous drug doses are listed in Table 26-1.

In many cases, asystole and nonperfusing rhythms are preceded by progressive bradycardia. Bradycardia can be a sign of imminent arrest and should prompt notification of other staff members. Sinus bradycardia may be treated with atropine as the animal is monitored. During asystole, both electrical and mechanical cardiac activity has stopped. Asystole is treated with atropine and/or epinephrine with repeated doses administered if no response is observed. Electrical mechanical dissociation (EMD) is a common terminal arrhythmia in cats and dogs. The hallmark of this arrhythmia is the presence of ECG complexes with no cardiac contractions to generate a pulse [hence the synonym, *pulseless electrical activity* (PEA)]. This rhythm can have a diverse appearance, but often mimics a ventricular arrhythmia with wide bizarre QRS complexes occurring at a slow rate. EMD is treated with naloxone, megadose atropine, or epinephrine.

Ventricular fibrillation is a common arrhythmia in people suffering myocardial infarction. It also occurs in cats and dogs during cardiopulmonary arrest. In dogs, ventricular fibrillation may be preceded by rapid ventricular tachycardia (especially when multifocal ventricular beats or R-on-T phenomenon are present). When ventricular fibrillation is diagnosed, it must be converted as soon as possible for resuscitation to be successful. Conversion of this arrhythmia may be attempted prior to initiation of basic life support. Treatment of choice for this arrhythmia is electrical defibrillation. This necessitates the availability of an electrical defibrillator. If this is not available chemical defibrillation may be attempted using drugs such as magnesium chloride. A strong precordial thump is potentially effective as a last resort.

Electrical defibrillators should only be used by specially trained personnel (Figure 26-29). Tips for appropriate use of an electrical defibrillator include:

1. Apply adequate pressure to the chest with the paddles.
2. Use the largest paddle surface area.
3. Use a proper conducting gel or saline solution-soaked gauze.

Alcohol should never be used near defibrillator paddles due to the risk of fire. The recommended dose is 2 to 4 joules/kg. Initially, use a setting at the lower end of the dose range, and repeat or double the dose if no response is seen. Open-chest defibrillation requires specific paddles and a modified dose (usually one tenth of the transthoracic dose).

Drugs administered during CPCR may be ineffective due to poor perfusion and failure of the drugs to reach their target tissues (primarily the heart). A central vein catheter (i.e., jugular catheter, Figure 26-30) is the CPCR drug administration route of preference during closed-chest

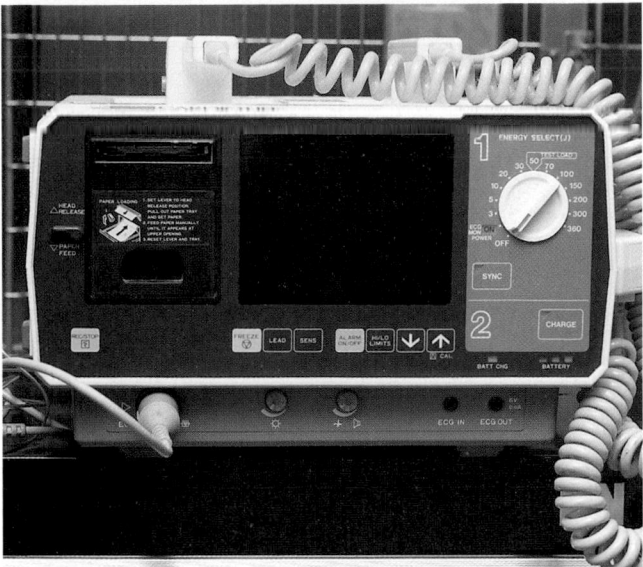

Figure 26-29 An electrical defibrillator and ECG are located on top of the crash cart for treatment of ventricular fibrillation during cardiac arrest.

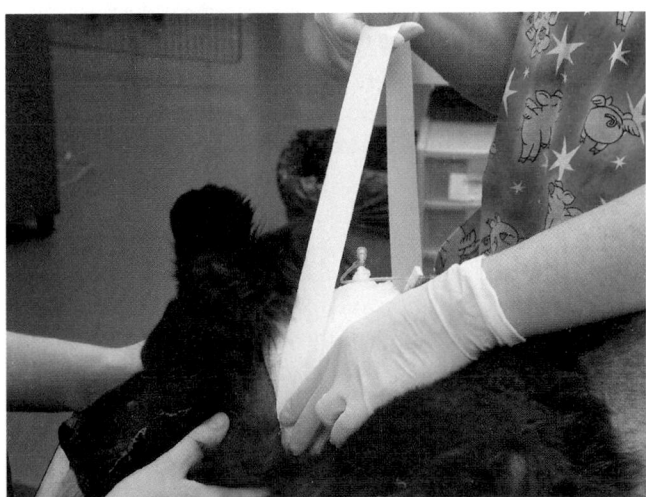

Figure 26-30 Placing jugular catheter in a critically ill dog.

CPCR. These catheters facilitate delivery of the drug(s) directly to the heart or its close proximity. The next best route is intratracheal administration. This route of administration takes advantage of alveolar membranes, which have a large surface area and receive a high blood flow separated by a narrow diffusion barrier. An acronym to remember which drugs can be administered by the intratracheal route is LEAN (lidocaine, epinephrine, atropine, and naloxone). Intratracheal drugs are administered via a catheter passed through the endotracheal tube (Figure 26-31). Insertion of drug into the catheter must be followed by a flush of air or saline to ensure drug deposition in the airways. A deep breath administered via manual ventilation helps to further distribute the drug. Drug doses administered by this

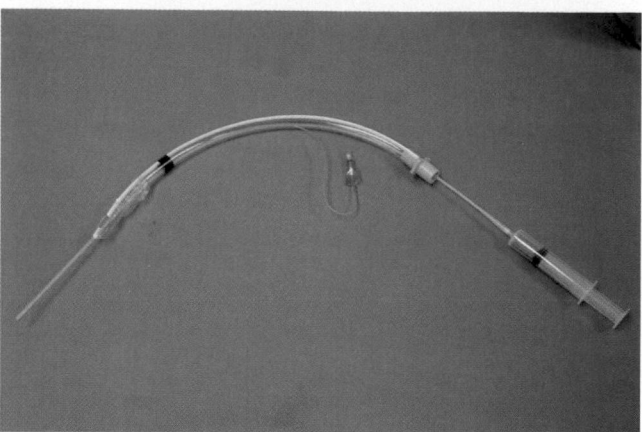

Figure 26-31 A polypropylene catheter passed through an endotracheal tube can be used for the intratracheal administration of some drugs during CPCR.

route are rapidly estimated by doubling the intravenous dose. Small drug volumes may require dilution for effective administration. Drug uptake by the pulmonary circulation is impaired by conditions such as pulmonary edema, which negates this as a suitable route. Good communication between team members performing CPCR is imperative because a vigorous chest compression delivered at an inopportune moment may result in exhalation of medications administered intratracheally.

Drugs may be administered via a peripheral intravenous catheter (i.e., cephalic or saphenous vein catheters) if a central line or intratracheal access is unavailable or contraindicated. All drugs administered peripherally must be followed with a good flush of saline solution to ensure delivery into the circulation and toward the heart. Intraosseous catheters and intralingual injection are another means of peripheral administration. Placement of an intraosseous catheter (or intralingual injection) in the arrested patient can be rapid and does not need to interrupt the CPCR attempt. Intralingual drug doses are usually double the standard intravenous drug dose. The last route for drug administration is intracardiac. This is chosen last because of the challenge of hitting a flaccid heart, the need to stop CPCR to administer drugs, and the risk of damaging the heart. However, in open-chest CPCR, intracardiac drug administration is preferred. Usually, one tenth of the intravenous dose is injected directly into the left ventricle.

Crystalloid fluids or colloids may be beneficial if hypovolemia was a predisposing factor of the arrest or to compete with peripheral vasodilation. However, fluid support of peripheral circulation is not a high priority during CPCR. Fluids may be contraindicated during CPCR due to the risk of overhydration associated with a failed cardiac pump. Overhydration may elevate right atrial pressures, which impedes coronary blood flow and further compromises the myocardium.

The decision to initiate CPCR is made on a case-by-case basis according to the wishes of an informed pet owner.

Many critically ill animals face an already grave prognosis. Following an arrest and successful resuscitation, the risk of re-arrest and subsequent death is high. "Do not attempt resuscitation" orders may be indicated after discussion with the clinician and pet owner. Consequently, assessing the patient's risk of arrest and addressing the desires of the client are important early on. If the patient does not respond to CPCR within 20 minutes, continuation of the resuscitation effort is unlikely to succeed. Successful resuscitation rates in veterinary medicine are approximately 10%. Fortunately, certain patients do respond to basic and advanced life support. Many of these cases have a reversible disease process and/or a treatable cause of arrest. A written record of everything done during the CPCR should be made for the team to learn from and for the client record. Regardless, the real work begins following successful resuscitation.

✐ TECHNICIAN NOTE

A written record of everything done during the CPCR should be made for the team to learn from and for the client record.

PROLONGED LIFE SUPPORT

Proper postresuscitation management has two primary focuses. First, primary factors leading up to the arrest should be identified and treated. Second, problems associated with both the acute loss of cardiopulmonary function and the trauma of the resuscitation effort should be recognized and managed.

The central nervous system is particularly sensitive to injury during states of shock or cardiopulmonary arrest. In health, cerebral blood flow is locally controlled and maintained by baroreceptor reflexes that maintain blood flow and protect the brain from hypertension and volume overload. This autoregulation of cerebral blood flow is lost during ischemia, leaving the central nervous system susceptible to further injury during and after resuscitation. Cerebral ischemia and reperfusion injury results in neuron cell death, and it is a serious complication of cardiopulmonary arrest and resuscitation. Initially, neurologic exams should be done hourly. Pupillary light response, responsiveness to stimulation, respiratory pattern, motor responses, and motor postures should be noted. Normal pupil size and pupillary light responses (PLR) are positive signs. Slow PLRs, anisocoria, and pinpoint pupils that are nonresponsive to light are progressively guarded neurologic indicators. Nonresponsive bilaterally dilated pupils indicate severe neuronal damage and a poor prognosis. Recent administration of atropine during the arrest should be ruled out as a cause of dilated nonresponsive pupils. Brainstem damage should be suspected in patients lacking a corneal reflex or swallow/gag reflex. Breathing patterns also reflect brainstem function, and erratic breathing patterns and periods of apnea (breathlessness) are poor prognostic indicators. A posture in which the animal demonstrates opisthotonus with rigidity in all four limbs defines the *decerebrate posture*. This indicates severe brainstem injury with a grave prognosis.

> ### ✏ TECHNICIAN NOTE
> Recent administration of atropine during the arrest should be ruled out as a cause of dilated nonresponsive pupils.

The cardiovascular system is clearly "ground zero" during cardiac arrest. In addition, abnormalities associated with other organ failure may further impact heart rhythm and blood pressure. Changes in heart rhythm, vascular tone, and cardiac output predispose to systemic hypotension and re-arrest. Consequently, it is imperative to continuously monitor the ECG and blood pressure in the postresuscitation period. Accurate blood pressure measurements may be obtained using direct and indirect methods. Direct blood pressure measurement is ideal but requires an arterial catheter and specialized equipment. Indirect blood pressure measurements may be obtained with Doppler or oscillometric methods. Arrhythmias causing clinical signs or hemodynamic compromise should be treated. Oxygen therapy has relatively few complications in the short term, and it is a useful treatment because of increased myocardial oxygen demand and when pulmonary disease is present.

Acute kidney failure is a common problem associated with states of shock and cardiac arrest. Following resuscitation, the kidneys are particularly susceptible to ongoing damage caused by unrecognized or untreated hypovolemia and hypotension. Consequently, monitoring of kidney and electrolyte parameters should be performed frequently in the postresuscitation period. Decreased urine production is associated with severe kidney failure and carries a poor prognosis. Urine output should be monitored hourly for at least 24 hours after an arrest. Veterinarians sometimes use an "ins and outs" fluid therapy plan to maintain fluid balance when kidney function is in question. In such cases, fluid doses are balanced with calculated fluid losses. Strict attention should be paid to maintaining adequate hydration and blood pressure. Although hypertension should be avoided, hypotension is common, and the mean arterial blood pressure should be maintained within normal limits to guarantee adequate kidney blood flow. Appropriate fluid therapy will maintain hydration without causing volume overload. Central venous pressure, repeated PCV/TP, and body weight measurements may be useful indicators of volume status. Hemodialysis and peritoneal dialysis are available at certain specialized treatment centers.

Primary respiratory disease is a common factor leading up to cardiopulmonary arrest. Respiratory complications of arrest/resuscitation include pulmonary edema due to congestive heart failure, noncardiogenic edema associated with hypoxia, and pulmonary thromboembolism. Vigorous chest compressions during resuscitation efforts may result in pulmonary contusions, rib fractures, atelectasis, and/or edema, and these injuries must be addressed in the post resuscitation treatment plan. Optimal respiratory therapy may require ventilation support and monitoring of arterial blood gas analysis. If blood gas analysis is not available, monitoring should include pulse oximetry and/or capnography.

Blood glucose concentrations should be monitored frequently, because many patients which arrest develop hypoglycemia. Normal blood glucose concentrations should be maintained by adequate supplementation when indicated. Hyperglycemia should be avoided.

MEDICAL TREATMENTS IN THE POSTARREST PERIOD

Many variables affect the outcome and management of an arrested patient. These variables include the animal's underlying diseases and reason for arrest, in addition to the experience and equipment available to the resuscitation team. There is a general consensus regarding the difficulties facing the team and the syndromes associated with the postarrest period, but disagreement exists regarding treatment methods, treatment priorities, and which therapies result in the best outcome. All therapies of postarrest patients are somewhat controversial due to an inability to create a standardized model. Many drugs may be useful in the postresuscitation patient and the list continues to grow. The following is a brief review of medical therapies and the rationale behind their use.

Mannitol is an osmotic diuretic sometimes used in the management of acute renal failure and cerebral edema. The mannitol molecule resides in the vascular space and draws water from the interstitial spaces between cells, thereby decreasing edema and expanding the vascular volume. As mannitol is excreted by the kidneys, its osmotic effects "pull" water with it into the urine. It is also an oxygen-free-radical scavenger. As such, it may aid in the treatment of reperfusion injury. Some caution is advised in the use of mannitol, because it can exacerbate volume overload. At high doses, mannitol may be nephrotoxic and is contraindicated in hypovolemic animals.

Furosemide (Lasix) is a potent diuretic that is commonly used in the treatment of pulmonary edema and kidney failure (with decreased urine production). The diuretic effects of furosemide increase urine output and may enhance the effects of mannitol. In addition, furosemide may also improve renal blood flow. In cases of pulmonary edema, furosemide causes volume contraction, which decreases edema formation and hastens resolution of edema.

Glucocorticosteroids (i.e., dexamethasone sodium phosphate, prednisolone sodium succinate, and methylprednisolone sodium succinate) are extremely controversial as to appropriate usage. They may be beneficial in stabilizing cellular membranes, thereby decreasing the release of membrane arachidonic acid (a precursor to many inflammatory mediators). Methylprednisolone sodium succinate is also a free-radical scavenger. As such, it is one of few drugs capable of rapid action against the oxygen free radicals created during reperfusion injury.

Dobutamine, a synthetic catecholamine, is a positive inotrope and may be administered to maintain mean arterial blood pressure. These effects increase cardiac output and perfusion, which along with other obvious benefits may reduce pulmonary edema. The related drug, dopamine, can be used to increase renal perfusion in canine patients at low doses and to increase systemic blood pressure at higher dosages. The use of dopamine in feline patients is controversial and limited to the systemic blood pressure effects of the drug.

Sodium bicarbonate is utilized in the treatment of severe life-threatening acidosis. However, caution is warranted because overzealous therapy is both harmful and easy to accomplish. Severe alkalosis, unpredictable acid-base disturbance between tissue compartments, and shifts in the oxygen-dissociation curve can be attributed to overdoses. Blood pH must be monitored via serial venous or arterial blood gas analyses.

Lidocaine is an antiarrhythmic drug used to treat ventricular tachycardia. Care should be taken to accurately interpret the ECG tracing, because this drug may be contraindicated in ventricular escape and isolated premature ventricular complexes. The latter are common arrhythmias observed in the immediate postresuscitation period. Although abnormal, these rhythms do provide functional blood perfusion in many cases. Abolishing a perfusing ventricular rhythm with lidocaine may result in development of a nonperfusing rhythm and death.

Because all body systems are affected by cardiopulmonary arrest, a whole body approach to monitoring and therapy is required. For this reason, successfully resuscitated arrest victims are among the most critical and labor-intensive patients and the prognosis is often poor. Those patients successfully resuscitated will require constant monitoring, therapy, and support for several days. The postresuscitation patient requires tremendous nursing care and 24-hour monitoring.

PATIENT MONITORING

For veterinary technicians, the majority of time in the clinic is spent providing patient care of which a large portion, especially in critical care, is devoted to monitoring. The primary objectives of critical care monitoring include (1) evaluation of current status, (2) evaluating the response to therapy, and (3) detecting new problems. Continuous 24-hour monitoring should be provided to patients who are very critical or unstable, whereas 8-hour monitoring intervals may be acceptable in improved or stable patients.

Both subjective parameters and objective parameters are combined to provide the most complete evaluation of patient progress so that sound treatment decisions can be made. Subjective parameters include hydration status and mentation (attitude, alertness, appetite). Objective parameters include body weight, urine production, vital signs (i.e., temperature, pulse, respirations), and lab results. Special techniques are often utilized to enhance our ability to monitor, diagnose, and treat critically ill veterinary patients. The most important tool in monitoring any patient is serial physical exams and assessment by a trained and attentive caregiver. Expensive equipment may be helpful in some situations but will never replace a hands-on nursing approach. Likewise, continuity of care is important so that dedicated caregivers can recognize patient trends, alert the veterinary team, and respond appropriately. A rational approach to patient monitoring can be loosely organized around the principles of triage and body system anatomy.

> ✎ **TECHNICIAN NOTE**
>
> The most important tool in monitoring any patient is serial physical exams and assessment by a trained and attentive caregiver.

RESPIRATORY SYSTEM

Care should be taken to minimize stress in animals with respiratory difficulty (dyspnea). Oxygen supplementation is an important treatment in some animals and can be provided via blowby, nasal cannulae, face mask, oxygen canopy, or oxygen cage/incubator. In all patients (especially those with known respiratory disease), it is important to note the rate, pattern, and effort of breathing. Obstructive airway disease (i.e., laryngeal paralysis or tracheal foreign material) is often characterized by a slow and deep respiratory pattern with harsh or whistling upper airway noise. Restrictive respiratory disease (i.e., pleural effusion, chest wall injuries) often manifests as a rapid and shallow breathing. Respiratory distress can be detected by frequent monitoring of respiratory rate, mucous membrane color, and respiratory effort. A significant abdominal component or effort during inspiration is abnormal. All lung fields and the upper airways should be ausculted. Additional sounds with inspiration or expiration should be noted and significant changes recorded in the medical record and reported to the doctor. Fluid and air in the pleural space often results in muffled heart and lung sounds. Percussing the thoracic wall during auscultation may aid in determining air or fluid in the pleural space. Certain lower airway disorders, such as pneumonia and pulmonary edema, are characterized by crackles during each phase of respiration.

Monitoring equipment such as a pulse oximeter (Figure 26-32) and capnograph can provide additional information to the veterinary team. These monitors are frequently used

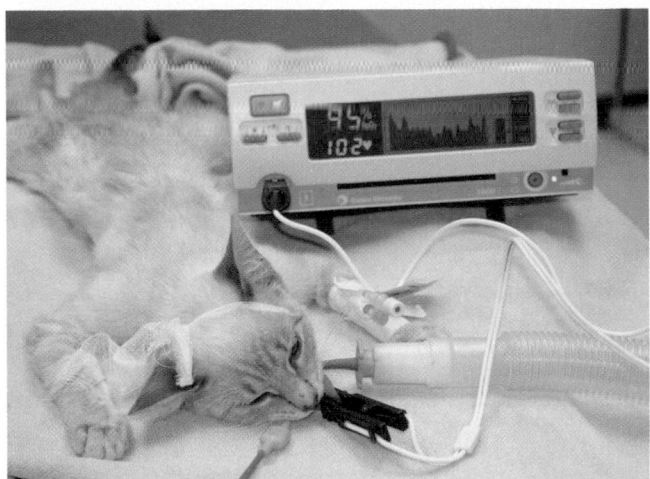

Figure 26-32 A pulse oximeter provides a convenient and reliable means to monitor oxygenation in critical or anesthetized animals.

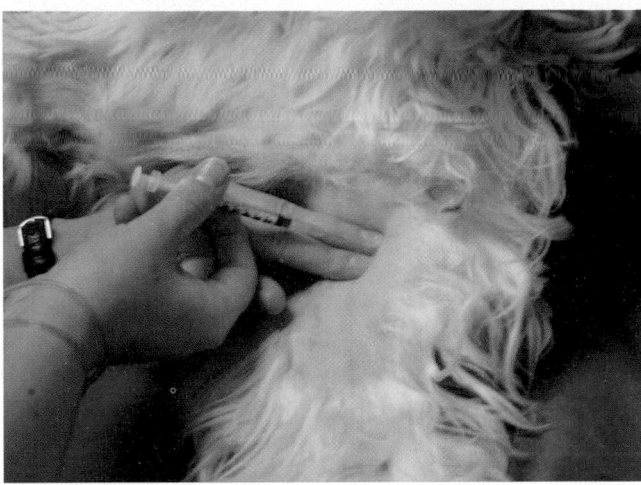

Figure 26-33 The femoral pulse is palpated prior to arterial blood sample collection from the femoral artery of a dog.

for anesthesia monitoring but can also be used for continuous monitoring of critically ill patients. Pulse oximetry uses an infrared sensor to count the pulse rate and provide a noninvasive measure of arterial hemoglobin-oxygen saturation (usually in per cent). Infrared sensors are made to clip onto the tongue, lip margin, or flank. Rectal probes (with sanitary covers) for recumbent patients are also available. It is important to note that the pulse oximeter reading is an oxygen saturation value and is not identical to the blood oxygen content or arterial oxygen partial pressure (PaO_2). The structure and biochemistry of hemoglobin allows saturation to remain high despite some significant changes in blood oxygen content. Thus, the pulse oximeter is a good crisis prevention tool, but does not provide fine details about the oxygenation and ventilation status of the patient. If the pulse oximeter detects a problem with oxygen saturation, a blood gas analysis and oxygen supplementation may be ordered. In normal patients the oxygen saturation should remain above 95%. Poor perfusion at the probe site, hypothermia, and movement will impede the sensor's ability to obtain an accurate reading. If the pulse oximeter sensor triggers an alarm, manual palpation of the pulse, auscultation of the heart, and check of the mucous membranes should be performed immediately before adjusting the equipment.

TECHNICIAN NOTE

The pulse oximeter is a good crisis-prevention tool, but it does not provide fine details about the oxygenation and ventilation status of the patient.

Capnography also uses infrared technology to estimate the carbon dioxide concentration of expired air. By incorporating a capnometer into the breathing circuit of intubated animals, the end-tidal CO_2 (CO_2 concentration at the end

of expiration) can be measured. The end-tidal CO_2 is an estimate of $PaCO_2$, which can be useful in monitoring the efficiency of mechanical ventilation. Capnometry can also be used to confirm endotracheal intubation and to detect airway occlusion. If an endotracheal tube is misplaced into the esophagus or occluded by exudates, end-tidal CO_2 will be negligible. Additionally, capnographs have been used to assess the efficacy of resuscitation efforts during CPR. Successful resuscitation is expected to result in progressively increased end-tidal CO_2 values as forward blood flow returns CO_2 from the tissues.

Arterial blood gas analysis provides specific data on the oxygenation, ventilation, and acid/base status of the pet. Normal ranges for arterial blood gas values are published elsewhere. Values for oxygen (O_2) and carbon dioxide (CO_2) are expressed as a pressure in units of millimeters of mercury (mm Hg). Arterial blood samples may be drawn from the femoral artery, dorsal pedal artery, or lingual artery by palpating the pulse and guiding the needle into the artery by tactile sensation (Figure 26-33). The femoral artery and dorsal pedal arteries are the most common sites of arterial blood sampling. Lingual artery samples may be obtained in anesthetized or comatose animals, but they should be avoided due to the risk of inducing a large oral hematoma, which can obstruct the airway and interfere with swallowing. Acquiring arterial blood samples may be too stressful for some patients. By definition ventilation is determined by the carbon dioxide level (PCO_2) as determined by arterial blood gas analysis. Hypoventilation (decreased ventilation) results in increased blood carbon dioxide, which can cause neurologic signs and acidosis. Hyperventilation ("blowing off CO_2") results in decreased carbon dioxide and may occur with respiratory disease or as a compensatory response to metabolic acidosis. Oxygenation is indicated by the PaO_2, and a low value indicates hypoxemia. Signs of hypoxemia include cyanotic (blue) mucous membranes, weakness, rapid heart rate, increased respiratory rate, and increased respiratory effort.

By calculating the difference between alveolar oxygenation and arterial oxygenation, arterial blood gas data can be used to assess the efficiency of oxygen transfer to the blood by the lung. In patients that are hypoxemic, this *alveolar-arterial gradient (A-a gradient)* calculation can provide a single value to assess and monitor the animal's oxygen exchange. The alveolar oxygen content (A) is calculated by the alveolar gas equation: $A = (BP - 47) 0.21 - P_{CO_2}/0.8$, where BP is the barometric pressure (760 mm Hg at sea level), 47 is the vaporization pressure of water (a constant physical property of water), and 0.21 is the oxygen percent of room air. This formula is only used when the patient is breathing room air. In the formula above, P_{CO_2} is obtained from the arterial blood gas analysis and 0.8 is the respiratory exchange quotient (a mathematical constant). At elevations near sea level, the formula simplifies to $A = 150 - P_{CO_2}/0.8$. The arterial oxygen content (a) is the P_{aO_2} obtained from the arterial blood gas analysis (in mm Hg). In animals with normal oxygen exchange, the *A-a* gradient is less than 10 mm Hg. As a general rule, an *A-a* gradient over 30 mm Hg is an indication for oxygen therapy.

In order to determine how responsive the patient is to oxygen therapy, an arterial sample is collected while the patient is on supplemental oxygen, and a second arterial blood gas analysis is performed. The original *A-a* calculation is invalid for patients receiving oxygen therapy. Instead, oxygenation is assessed by evaluating the ratio of arterial oxygen to inspired oxygen (P_{aO_2}/F_{IO_2}). P_{aO_2} is obtained from the blood gas analysis. F_{IO_2} is the fraction (percent) of oxygen being supplemented in decimal form. For example, a dog receiving 100% oxygen would have an F_{IO_2} of 1.0. Most of the time, animals receiving oxygen therapy by mask or nasal catheters have an F_{IO_2} of close to 40% ($F_{IO_2} = 0.4$). By definition an animal's disease is responsive to oxygen if the P_{aO_2}/F_{IO_2} value is greater than 250. As a general rule of thumb, the P_{aO_2} should be approximately five times the F_{IO_2}.

CARDIOVASCULAR SYSTEM AND PERFUSION/HYDRATION

Monitoring of common physical exam findings can be key to detecting serious health problems. Technicians should be comfortable using a stethoscope and familiar with the basic principles of cardiac auscultation and pulse palpation. The detection of a new heart murmur, irregular heart beats (arrhythmia), and/or changes in heart or lung sounds can be signs of an impending crisis. For example, animals that are "overhydrated" may develop crackles characteristic of pulmonary edema. Factors that decrease sound intensity include obesity, pleural or pericardial effusion, and hypovolemia. Likewise, pulse character and quality are important clues to the hydration status and stability of the critically

ill pet. Pulse strength will be diminished and it will be difficult to palpate pulses if the mean arterial blood pressure is less than 60 mm Hg. Common sites to palpate a pulse are the femoral, dorsal pedal, or lingual arteries. Pulse rates should parallel the heart rate, rhythm, and quality. Comparing the pulse rate and heart rate during auscultation can aid in detecting "pulse deficits" that may be produced by irregular heartbeats.

✎ TECHNICIAN NOTE

Comparing the pulse rate and heart rate during auscultation can aid in detecting "pulse deficits" that may be produced by irregular heartbeats.

Monitoring of hydration status and peripheral perfusion is very crucial in the critically ill or injured patient. Helpful monitoring parameters include texture and color of mucous membranes, capillary refill time, quantitation or close estimation of urine output compared with fluid intake, thoracic auscultation, pulse rate and character, serial body weights, and temperature (both core body temperature and peripheral limb temperature). Physical signs of overhydration include serous nasal discharge, chemosis (conjunctival edema), peripheral edema, body cavity effusion, and weight gain. Noninvasive monitoring equipment such as an ECG and indirect blood pressure equipment can provide additional information regarding the pet's cardiovascular status. Evaluation of the ECG complexes may provide clues to electrolyte abnormalities and other diseases (heart blocks, pericardial effusion). Patients at greater risk of decompensation may require more invasive monitoring techniques. Examples of at-risk patients include animals with heart disease, pneumonia, and renal disease. Invasive monitoring techniques include PCV, TP, direct blood pressure, and central venous pressure (CVP) measurement. Trends in observations will provide the most information and allow for early problem detection and intervention. Diligent record keeping and consistency in monitoring techniques are imperative.

BLOOD PRESSURE

In humans blood pressure is often expressed as a fraction, with systolic pressure as the numerator and diastolic pressure as the denominator. Mean arterial pressure is calculated from the systolic and diastolic values. A similar fraction can be used in cats and dogs. Normal systolic blood pressure varies between species, but generally ranges from 100 to 150 mm Hg. An ideal mean blood pressure ranges from 75 to 90 mm Hg. Arterial blood pressure can be monitored directly or indirectly and provides more information than simple subjective assessments of pulse character. Systolic values more than 90 mm Hg and diastolic values greater than 60 mm Hg are required to maintain adequate perfusion of vital organs (namely, the kidneys and brain).

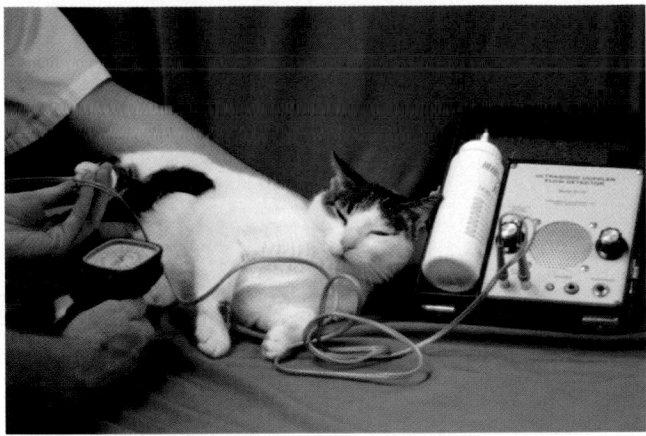

Figure 26-34 Indirect blood pressure measurement using ultrasound Doppler equipment provides an accurate reading of the systolic blood pressure.

A systolic blood pressure over 175 mm Hg indicates hypertension. However, stress of illness and anxiety associated with hospital visits can increase the blood pressure significantly in nervous animals. In cats and dogs, pulses should be palpable if the mean arterial blood pressure is greater than 60 mm Hg.

Indirect blood pressure is obtained using either oscillometric or Doppler equipment. Oscillometric blood pressure monitors often come in combination with an ECG and pulse oximeter and are popularly used in monitoring anesthetized or sedentary animals. These monitors use a blood pressure cuff to determine systolic, diastolic, and mean arterial pressures and can be programmed to take readings at regular intervals. To ensure an accurate measurement, cuff size should be proportionate to the size of the animal. As a general rule, the diameter of the cuff should approximate 40% of the circumference of the limb at the site of cuff placement. Common sites of cuff placement include the metacarpus, metatarsus, and tail. Doppler blood pressure equipment uses an ultrasound crystal and monitor to audibly locate the arterial pulse (Figure 26-34). Hair is clipped over an artery (usually the ventral digital artery or tail artery). The ultrasound crystal with ultrasound gel is positioned over the palpable pulse so that the Doppler elicits a clear sound with each pulse. Subsequently, a blood pressure cuff is applied to the patient as described above and a sphygmomanometer is used to inflate the cuff until the audible pulse can no longer be heard. Finally, pressure is released in the cuff until the pulse can be heard again. The pressure at which the pulse is again detected is equivalent to the systolic blood pressure. This technique is more labor intensive for monitoring, because this procedure must be manually performed. In addition, mean and diastolic blood pressures are not reliably obtained by this technique. However, many prefer Doppler equipment because the audible pulse is reassuring and allows a subjective assessment of the accuracy of data.

Direct blood pressure measurement is more invasive because it requires catheterization of an artery and specialized equipment. This method is considered the most accurate method of blood pressure measurement. Since most arteries can not be directly visualized at the time of arterial puncture, arterial catheters are placed using digital palpation of the pulse as a guide. Common arteries for catheterization include the dorsal pedal artery and femoral artery. Once in place, the arterial catheter is connected to a monitor via commercially available transducer equipment. The monitor displays a pulse waveform and reads out a systolic, diastolic, and mean blood pressure. Comparing the waveform deflection with an ECG allows staff members to note pulse pressure created by each cardiac contraction. This can be helpful in determining the effects of transient arrhythmias. Staff members should be trained in the use and care of arterial catheters. No medications should be administered via intraarterial injection, and arterial catheters must be appropriately labeled to prevent confusion. Arterial catheters are flushed slowly and regularly to prevent clot formation. Arterial catheters must be properly secured to prevent animal movement from disconnecting equipment. If equipment becomes detached from the catheter hub, an open arterial catheter can result in rapid severe blood loss, which is particularly dangerous in small animals.

CENTRAL VENOUS PRESSURE

In the healthy body, venous pressures are maintained lower than arterial pressures to facilitate forward blood flow. Blood flows from arteries to veins and back to the heart, in part, by following this natural pressure gradient. Most discussions of blood pressure refer to systemic arterial blood pressure. However, venous blood pressures are also important. CVP refers to the blood pressure of the thoracic vena cava, which is used to monitor fluid balance and the efficacy of fluid therapy. A normal central venous pressure is 0 to 5 cm H_2O. Values less than zero indicate hypovolemia or dehydration or inadequate fluid therapy. Values trending upward to 8 or 10 indicate an increase in vascular volume and adequate fluid therapy. Sudden increases in CVP or values above 10 may indicate venous congestion, increased thoracic pressure, and volume overload. Patient status should be closely reviewed. CVP values are usually used in

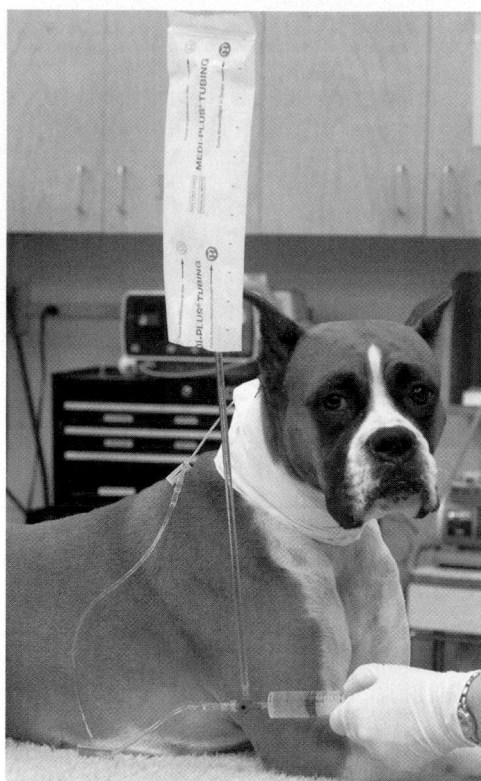

Figure 26-35 Central venous pressure measurement (using manometer equipment connected to a central catheter) can be used to monitor hydration and fluid therapy requirements.

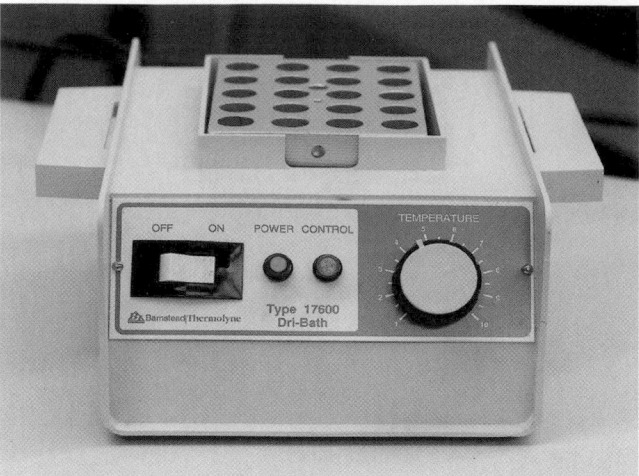

Figure 26-36 Purpose-made heating blocks are available to warm ACT tubes to body temperature before and during the test.

conjunction with subjective measures of hydration status (heart rate, mucous membrane appearance, skin turgor).

Measurement of central venous pressure requires placement of a long catheter in a central vein. Most commonly, jugular vein catheters are placed that reach into the thoracic vena cava (Figure 26-35). Equipment for measuring CVP can be constructed from a three-way stopcock that separates a manometer (in cm H_2O) and a saline-filled syringe from an extension set. The extension set and manometer are flushed with normal saline and the extension set is connected to the patient's central line catheter. The animal is placed in sternal or lateral recumbency and the apparatus is held so that the zero mark of the manometer is in the approximate position of the distal catheter tip. In most small animals this position is approximated by the location of the heart (i.e., the sternum in laterally recumbent animals and the point of the elbow during sternal recumbency). After flushing the catheter to ensure smooth flow of blood, the stopcock is opened between the patient and the manometer. After several seconds, the saline column of the manometer will equilibrate with the pressure at the end of the catheter, reflecting the central venous pressure.

COAGULATION STATUS

Assessment of an animal's coagulation status may be helpful in assessing unexplained bleeding and detecting DIC.

Evaluation of a blood smear may detect red blood cell morphology changes and allow an estimation of platelet numbers. The presence of schistocytes or fragmented red blood cells along with a decrease in platelet numbers may be seen with DIC, splenic tumors, and severe heartworm disease. A high percentage of echinocytes can be seen in animals suffering from snake envenomation. A normal platelet count is between 200,000 and 500,000 platelets per microliter in most species. Although a complete platelet count is advised, rapid assessment or confirmation of platelet numbers may be obtained by estimating the platelet numbers on a blood smear. This can be done by counting the number of platelets per high-power field and multiplying by 15,000. A better estimate is obtained if several high-power fields are assessed and averaged. Platelet clumping, which is common at the edge of blood smears, can make platelet estimates invalid.

✎ TECHNICIAN NOTE

A high percentage of echinocytes can be seen in animals suffering from snake envenomation.

The ACT test is used as a quick and inexpensive method of screening clotting factor status. Commercially available tubes containing sterile diatomaceous earth (see Figure 26-22) are post-warmed to body temperature (Figure 26-36). Two milliliters of patient blood is placed in the tube and gently rocked a few times to mix with the contents. The tube temperature should be maintained at body temperature. After 60 seconds, the tube is tilted every 5 seconds to evaluate for any sign of clot formation. The activated clotting time is the time from introduction of blood to the tube until the first evidence of detectable clot is noted. Normal values are 90 to 120 seconds for the dog and 70 to 90 seconds for the cat.

The buccal mucosal bleeding time (BMBT) evaluates platelet function and is used most often as an in-house screening test for von Willebrand disease (an inherited disease effecting platelet adhesion). A commercially available

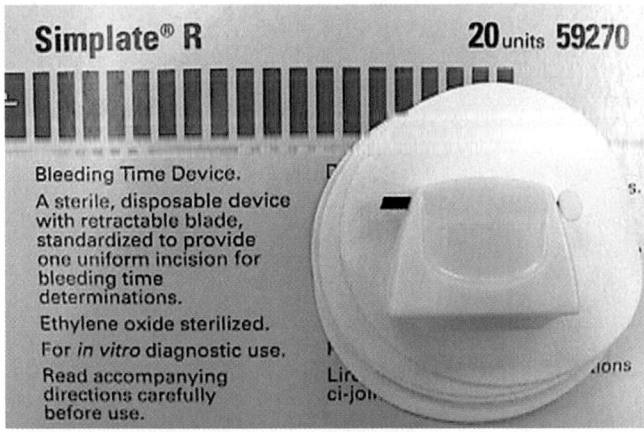

Figure 26-37 Commercially available lancet devices and filter paper are used in the buccal mucosal bleeding time test.

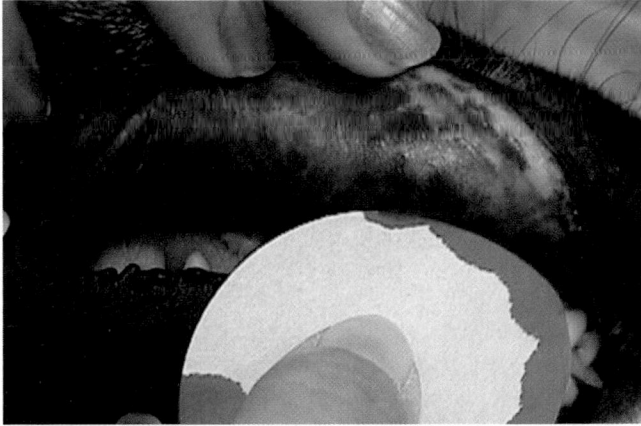

Figure 26-39 Blood flowing from the cut is blotted away with filter or absorbent paper to permit visualization of the site without disturbing the incision.

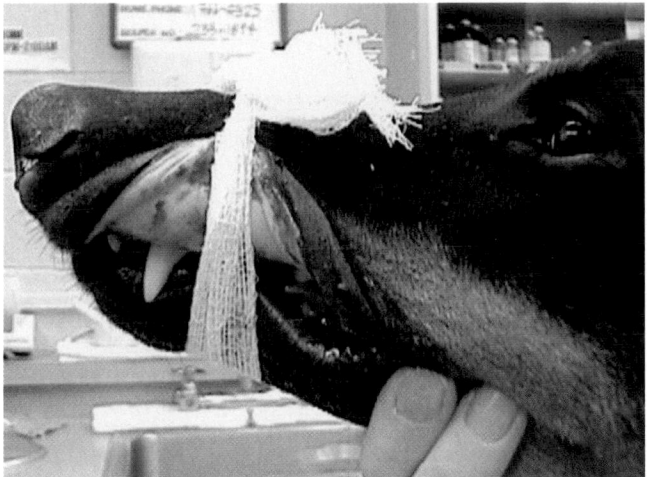

Figure 26-38 The lip is positioned appropriately, and a standardized incision is made in the buccal (check) mucosa.

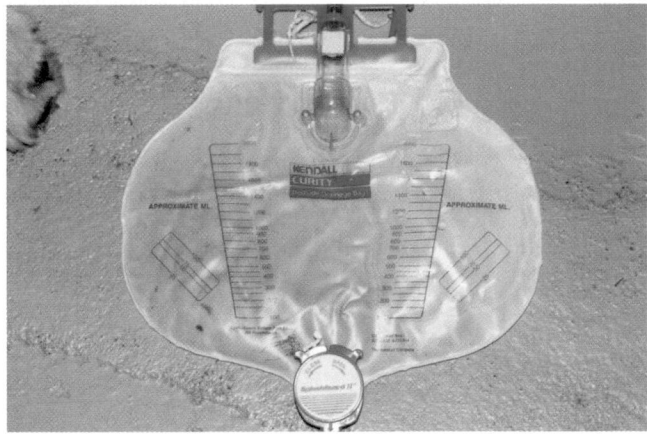

Figure 26-40 Sterile urine collection bags connected to an indwelling urinary catheter can be used to monitor urine production and maintain cleanliness.

lancet device (Figure 26-37) is used to make a standardized incision (specific size and depth) into the buccal mucosa on inside of the cheek (Figure 26-38). The blood flowing from the cut is blotted away with filter or absorbent paper to permit visualization of the site without disturbing the incision (Figure 26-39). The time required until bleeding stops is the buccal mucosal bleeding time, which represents the time for formation of an initial platelet plug. Normal time for the dog is less than 4 minutes. Following completion of the test, renewed bleeding at the site can occur if the incision is disturbed or if the animal has other coagulation problems, but such bleeding does not effect the reported time.

RENAL/URINARY SYSTEM

Ideally, all hospitalized animals should have a urine sample obtained for urinalysis. Urine specific gravity is important information in determining urinary tract health and in interpreting changes in kidney parameters and the urine

sediment. Because urine specific gravity and blood values for blood urine nitrogen (BUN) and creatinine can be affected by fluid therapy and medications (such as diuretics like furosemide and mannitol), posttreatment blood and urine samples should be obtained. However, if such samples cannot be readily obtained, fluid therapy should not be delayed, particularly if the animal is in shock or otherwise unstable.

Urine output should be estimated in all animals and recorded in the medical record. In critical cases, close monitoring of urine production may be performed via urine collection through indwelling urinary catheters or specifically designed cages that allow urine to drain through a grate to be collected. Indwelling urinary catheters attached to sterile collection sets and bags are an excellent and accurate way to monitor urine output as well as maintain patient comfort (Figure 26-40). Because catheters may clog, kink, or change position so that urine collection is impaired, urine collection equipment should be regularly inspected and replaced if faulty. Minimum urine production is 2 to

4 ml/kg/hr. Inadequate urine production may be an indication for changes in fluid therapy and should be interpreted with other patient data (i.e., body weight, CVP, etc.) and reported to the veterinarian.

CENTRAL NERVOUS SYSTEM

Unfortunately, few objective parameters are available to monitor the central nervous system. Serial physical and neurologic exams are perhaps the best means of detecting new or ongoing problems. Changes in mentation, responsiveness, level of consciousness, and respiratory patterns may indicate changes in neurologic status and should be reported. Likewise, pupillary size and responsiveness to light are important signs to monitor. Increased intracranial pressure results in a syndrome of brainstem and cerebral herniation whereby pressure shifts compress the brain against solid connective tissue and bone. Early signs of increased intracranial pressure include mental dullness, tachypnea, tachycardia and dilated pupils. Later, signs include bradycardia, fixed pinpoint pupils, seizures, coma, and death. Early recognition and intervention are key to the management of this syndrome. Animals at risk for brain herniation include those with head trauma, hydrocephalus, brain tumors, and encephalitis. Herniation can also be a complication of some diagnostic procedures, such as spinal fluid collection and myelogram.

ABDOMINAL CAVITY

Each patient should receive a daily physical examination and repeat exam as indicated by monitoring parameters. Palpation of the abdomen may detect abdominal distension due to fluid accumulation, organ enlargement, and intestinal gas (or free abdominal gas). Abdominal pain can be detected by the presence of discomfort, splinting, or vocalization. Animals with unexplained abdominal pain or distension warrant further investigation.

Abdominocentesis is a procedure to confirm the presence of abdominal fluid and to collect samples for fluid analysis. During this procedure, the abdomen is clipped of hair and aseptically cleaned with surgical scrub. A needle attached to syringe is inserted into the abdomen near the umbilicus, and gentle suction is applied to withdraw fluid (Figure 26-41). Care is taken not to redirect the needle blindly within the abdomen, as this may result in unnecessary pain and potential injury to abdominal organs. Fluid collected in this manner may be submitted for culture and cytology. Abdominocentesis is commonly performed to detect active hemorrhage, infection (peritonitis) ascites, uroabdomen, and neoplastic effusions. If a minute amount of fluid is suspected, a four-quadrant tap may be performed in which the four areas of the abdomen centered around the umbilicus are sampled. If no sample is obtained, a diagnostic

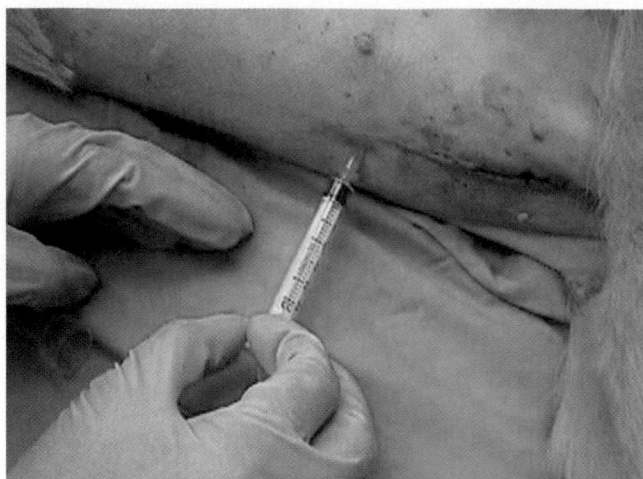

Figure 26-41 During abdominocentesis, a needle attached to syringe is inserted into the abdomen near the umbilicus, and gentle suction is applied to withdraw fluid.

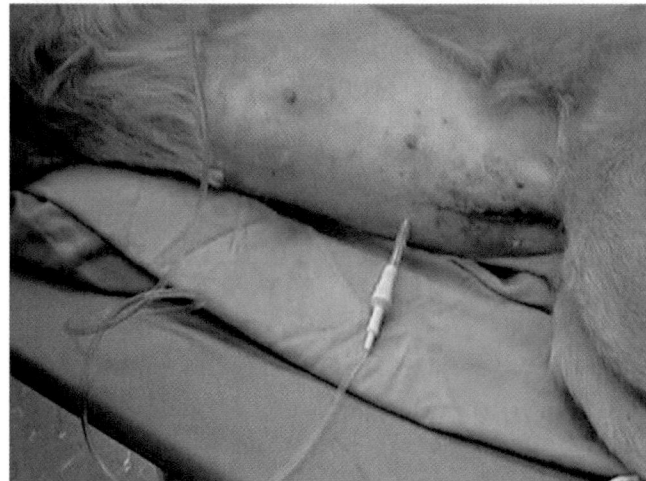

Figure 26-42 During diagnostic peritoneal lavage, sterile saline is injected into the abdomen via a catheter or needle and allowed to mix with abdominal contents prior to abdominocentesis.

peritoneal lavage (DPL) may be performed. DPL is a modified procedure for collecting small amounts of abdominal fluid. In this procedure, the animal is prepared as described above. Prior to fluid withdrawal, a volume of 10 to 20 ml/kg of sterile warm isotonic saline is instilled into the abdomen (Figure 26-42). After a brief moment to adjust the animal's position and allow the instilled fluid to mix with abdominal contents, standard abdominocentesis is performed. The added fluid may dislodge adherent debris and mix with isolated fluid pockets that can then be collected during abdominocentesis for fluid analysis.

TECHNICIAN NOTE

Abdominocentesis is commonly performed to detect active hemorrhage, infection (peritonitis) ascites, uroabdomen, and neoplastic effusions.

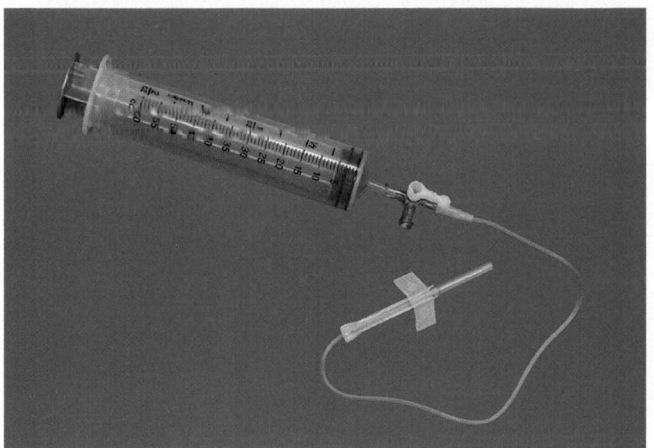

Figure 26-43 Thoracocentesis may be performed with a butterfly catheter connected to a three-way stopcock and syringe.

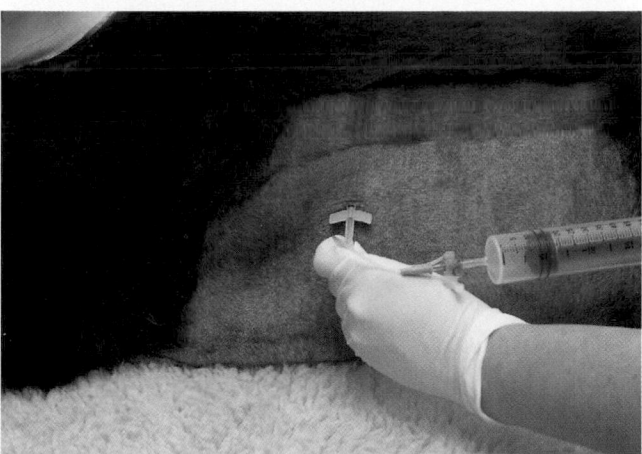

Figure 26-44 Thoracocentesis is often performed with the animal in sternal recumbency.

THORACIC CAVITY

Animals with cardiac and respiratory disease often have similar clinical signs (namely, coughing, labored breathing, exercise intolerance, and collapse). Unfortunately, these signs can occur with many different causes, including upper airway congestion, pulmonary edema, pleural effusion, pneumonia, primary heart disease, and thoracic neoplasia. A thorough physical exam often directs diagnostics tests to differentiate respiratory from cardiac problems. Muffled heart and respiratory sounds often indicate fluid or air in the pleural space (between the lungs and chest wall). Mild to moderate amounts of pleural fluid may result in severe respiratory compromise due to inhibition of normal lung expansion. Crackles heard during the different phases of breathing usually indicate pulmonary disease such as pneumonia or pulmonary edema. In general, crackles indicate relatively severe pulmonary disease. Chest x-rays are commonly used to confirm, classify, and document the presence of cardiorespiratory disease.

If thoracic fluid is documented on x-rays or clinically suspected, thoracocentesis to remove the fluid is indicated as therapy and to obtain diagnostic samples. Thoracocentesis is usually performed with the animal comfortably restrained in sternal recumbency. During this procedure, one or both sides of the chest are clipped of hair (in the area of rib spaces 7 through 9) and cleaned with surgical scrub. A butterfly catheter (or needle with extension set) is attached to a three-way stopcock and syringe (Figure 26-43). The needle is advanced into the chest along the cranial aspect of a rib to avoid discomfort and bleeding associated with nerve and vessel bundles located behind each rib (Figure 26-44). As the needle is inserted into the chest, an assistant controls the syringe and maintains the stopcock in the closed position to prevent environmental air from entering the chest during inspiration. Once the needle is positioned in the pleural space, the stopcock is opened to allow the

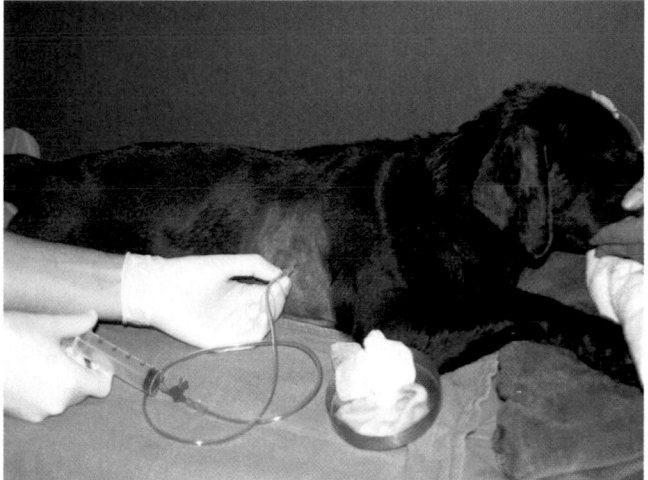

Figure 26-45 A thoracic drain is shown immediately following placement.

assistant to suction fluid from the pleural space into the syringe. If a large amount of fluid must be removed, the stopcock is closed to the patient as the syringe is repeatedly emptied. Samples for culture, cytology, and fluid analysis are often obtained early during the procedure. Thoracocentesis may be performed as an emergency diagnostic procedure in animals with severe respiratory distress and suspected pleural fluid. Air can also accumulate in the pleural space. This condition is referred to as a *pneumothorax* and often results from traumatic rupture of airways or severe pulmonary disease. In such cases, air leaks outside of the lung and is contained inside the chest, resulting in increased intrathoracic pressure and collapse of the lung. Thoracocentesis (as described above) may also be used to remove air from the pleural space. If fluid or air continues to accumulate in the chest, "chest drains," or thoracostomy tubes, may be placed that allow repetitive or continuous drainage of air/fluid from the pleural space (Figures 26-45 and 26-46).

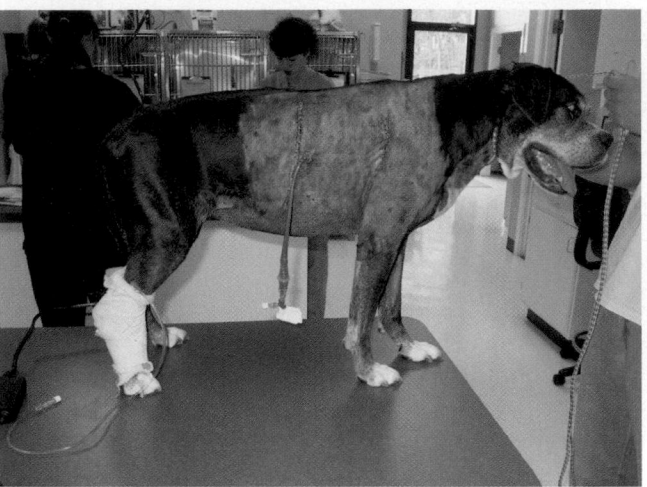

Figure 26-46   A thoracic drain is shown in a standing dog.

CONCLUSION

The best monitoring plan uses multiple parameters and a standardized approach to interpreting and responding to problems during triage, cardiopulmonary resuscitation, and standard patient care. Emergency and critical care veterinary hospitals treat the sickest and often the most unpredictable animals. These unique challenges emphasize the importance of basic patient care and advanced monitoring techniques. Providing comfort and basic needs should be a nursing priority. In addition, technicians must be aware of common clinical problems and anticipate the needs of the patient and alert the veterinarian to new problems and impending crises.

Familiarity with a variety of monitoring techniques and diagnostic procedures will allow for the best possible care.

Continuing education is an important component of providing the best possible care. The Association of Veterinary Emergency and Critical Care Technicians (AVECCT) is a technician association created under the auspices of the Veterinary Emergency and Critical Care Society (VECCS). This association, which was recognized by the North American Veterinary Technician Association (NAVTA) in 1996, is devoted to recognizing, educating, and networking technicians with specialty interest and training in emergency and critical care.

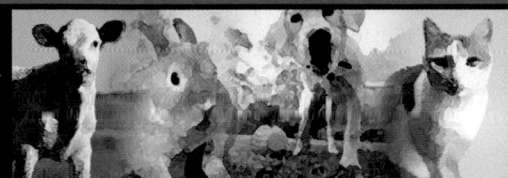

Toxicology

JILL A. RICHARDSON

INTRODUCTION

Animals have a natural curiosity and many are adept at accessing areas where baits, cleaners, chemicals, and medications are stored. Some pets can pry caps from child-resistant bottles or chew through heavy plastic containers. Products such as flavored medications or pest control baits may be attracting to animals, and in some cases, even small amounts can be dangerous. Therefore, proper and prompt treatment of poisonings, including stabilization and decontamination, is essential. The purpose of this chapter is to discuss management of poisoning in pets.

Toxicants may be of biologic origin, manufactured chemicals, or naturally occurring chemicals. A toxicant is any substance that when introduced into or applied to the body can interfere with the life processes of cells of the organism. A toxin (biotoxin) is a noxious or poisonous substance that is formed or elaborated during the metabolism and growth of certain microorganisms and some higher plant and animal species. Decontamination is the process of removing or neutralizing injurious agents. Additional definitions of terms that are pertinent to this chapter are located in Box 27-5. ■

TECHNICIAN NOTE

Toxicants may be of biologic origin, manufactured chemicals, or naturally occurring chemicals.

MANAGING POISON EMERGENCIES

Make sure to keep your clinic organized with a dedicated area in the clinic for emergency management of poisoned patients. The designated area should be centralized and stocked with key emergency supplies and drugs commonly used in toxicology (Box 27-1). Maintain a library of related references in your clinic such as a current veterinary drug formulary, a current *Physician's Desk Reference* (PDR), and clinical toxicology textbooks. Be wary of using the Internet as a sole source of information as there are thousands of sites with erroneous information.

Often, the first instinct of an animal owner whose animal has been exposed to a poison is to call a veterinary clinic. The technician should be able to recognize what constitutes a toxicological emergency and what does not, give basic first aid advice, and provide clear directions to the hospital, if needed. The following questions should be asked to evaluate the situation:

1. What is the current clinical status of the animal? Severe clinical signs necessitate immediate veterinary assistance.
2. What was the animal exposed to and through what route (oral, ocular, dermal)?
3. Has the owner taken any steps to treat the animal?
4. How old is the animal and how much does it weigh?
5. How much was ingested (milligram or quantity)?
6. When was the exposure?
7. Is the animal a male or female? If female, is she lactating or pregnant?
8. Does the animal have any history of health problems?
9. Is the animal currently on medication?
10. Has the animal had any recent surgeries?

This information can be helpful to prepare for the office visit. After reviewing this information with your staff veterinarian, basic first aid advice or at-home decontamination recommendations may be given and/or the client told to bring the animal into the hospital. While waiting for the client's arrival, the technician can prepare the necessary equipment and medication (Box 27-1). In addition, the technician can help investigate the toxicant by scanning a reference in the clinic library or by consulting with veterinary

Box 27-1 DRUGS COMMONLY USED IN TOXICOLOGY

DRUGS USED IN DECONTAMINATION
Hydrogen peroxide
Syrup of ipecac
Apomorphine
Xylazine
Activated charcoal
Cathartics (Sorbitol, magnesium sulfate, sodium sulfate, psyllium)
Drugs used to control tremors or seizures
Diazepam
Barbiturates
Methocarbamol inhalant anesthetics
Miscellaneous drugs
Yohimbine hydrochloride
Pyridoxine
Flumazenil
N-Acetylcysteine
Naloxone
Digibind
Propranolol
Metoprolol
Atropine
2-PAM, pralidoxime chloride

Phenothiazines (chlorpromazine/acepromazine)
Methylene blue
Vitamin K_1
4 MP, fomepizole
Ethanol
Pamidronate
Calcitonin
Sodium bicarbonate
Cholestyramine
Gastrointestinal protectants (misoprostol, Carafate, H_2 blockers)
Physostigmine
Vitamin C
Calcium gluconate
Furosemide
Ammonium chloride
Chelators
Succimer: lead, arsenic, mercury
Deferoxamine mesylate-Iron
Calcium EDTA lead
D-penicillamine: mercury and lead
BAL (British Anti-Lewisite or dimercaprol): lead, arsenic, mercury

The information above is a partial list of drugs used in veterinary toxicology. Please note this list is not all-inclusive.

toxicology specialists at the American Society for the Prevention of Cruelty to Animals (ASPCA) Animal Poison Control Center (888-426-4435.)

TECHNICIAN NOTE

While waiting for the poisoned patient to arrive, the veterinary technician can help investigate the toxicant by consulting a veterinary toxicology specialist at the ASPCA Animal Poison Control Center at 888-426-4435.

ASSESSMENT OF THE ANIMAL'S CONDITION

Initial management of a potential toxicoses starts with assessing the condition of the pet. The assessment should be performed quickly and include the following: an examination of the respiratory rate, capillary refill time, mucous membrane color, heart rate, and core body temperature. Examination of a pet that is unconscious, in shock, seizing, or in cardiovascular or respiratory distress must be conducted simultaneously with stabilization measures. With stable animals, the technician should obtain a comprehensive history of the pet and the exposure, and perform a thorough physical examination.

STABILIZATION OF VITAL FUNCTIONS

As a general rule, treat the patient not the poison (Box 27-2)! Establishing stabilization of the patient is essential before

Box 27-2 STEPS: MANAGING POISON EMERGENCIES

Assess the following: What clinical signs is the animal exhibiting? Is the animal seizing? Is the animal breathing? What is the animal's heart rate? What color are the animal's mucous membranes? Is the animal in shock? What is the core body temperature? Is there any evidence of hemorrhaging?

Stabilize the animal. Administer oxygen if necessary. Control seizures. Correct any cardiovascular abnormality. Perform a systematic exam once the animal is stabilized and obtain a comprehensive history of the animal and the exposure.

Decontamination. Perform the appropriate method(s) of decontamination.

Control clinical signs. Administer the specific antidote, if applicable. Preventive measures such as gastric protection or antibiotics may be needed. Correct acid-base balance, hydration, and electrolytes, if needed.

Good nursing care until full recovery. Monitor the systems most likely to be affected by the toxin. Chemistry panels, coagulation panels, or diagnostic tests may be needed. Appropriate supportive care should be given until the animal completely recovers.

attempting any type of decontamination. A patent airway should be established and artificial respiration given if the animal is dyspneic or cyanotic. Artificial respiration may be required. The cardiovascular system should be monitored closely, preferably with a constant electrocardiogram (ECG) monitor, and any cardiovascular abnormality should be corrected. The placement of an indwelling intravenous catheter may be necessary for the administration of medications and intravenous fluids.

DECONTAMINATION

Signalment and history are crucial when dealing with a toxicosis and often affects the manner in which the animal is treated. Always get complete and accurate data about the animal.

There is no doubt that appropriate decontamination procedures have saved many animal lives. However, depending on the particular situation, certain methods of decontamination are more beneficial than others. Patient's age, weight, and previous medical history can affect the method of decontamination.

EXTERNAL EXPOSURES

OCULAR IRRIGATION

With any ocular exposure, the eyes should be flushed repeatedly with water or saline solutions for a minimum of 20 to 30 minutes. Eye flushing should begin as soon as possible and often requires treatment at the pet's home by the pet owner. Ocular exposure to corrosive agents should be considered an emergency. The eyes should be examined for corneal damage and monitored closely for excessive redness, lacrimation, or pain. Follow-up examinations or ophthalmic consultation may be needed to establish level of corneal damage.

BATHING

For dermal exposures, the animal should be bathed in a mild liquid dishwashing detergent. Baths may need to be repeated to completely remove sticky or oily toxicants. Afterward the animal should be rinsed well with warm water and towel dried to prevent chilling.

ORAL INGESTION

DILUTION

Dilution with milk or water is recommended in cases of corrosive ingestion. A dosage of 1 to 3 ml/lb is suggested.

EMESIS

Emesis is the technical term for inducing vomiting. The patient's species, length of time since ingestion, the animal's previous and current medical condition, and the type of poison can effect the decision to induce emesis.

Dogs, cats, pigs, and ferrets are able to vomit. Emesis is contraindicated in rodents, rabbits, birds, horses, and ruminants. Emesis is usually only productive within 3 hours of ingestion and is more likely to be productive if the animal is fed a small moist meal before inducing vomiting.

Any animal who has a previous history of cardiovascular abnormalities, epilepsy, or recent abdominal surgery or is severely debilitated is not a candidate for emesis induction. Emesis should not be induced in any animal that (1) is severely depressed or in a coma (as it could lead to aspiration), (2) is hyperactive (as this could trigger a seizure), (3) has already vomited.

Another factor affecting the decision to induce emesis is the nature of the substance ingested. Emesis is contraindicated for corrosive materials such as cationic detergents, acids, and alkali. Induction of vomiting is not recommended with corrosives because of reexposure of the esophageal tissues to the corrosive material. Dilution with milk or water in combination with demulcents and gastrointestinal protectants is recommended in cases of corrosive ingestion.

Emesis is also contraindicated with hydrocarbon ingestion with the main concern being possible aspiration. Examples of hydrocarbon containing products include lubrication oils, fuel oil, butane, propane, kerosene, mineral spirits, and gasoline.

EMETIC AGENTS

A 3% hydrogen peroxide solution has been shown to be an effective emetic for dogs, cats, ferrets and pigs. The mechanism of action of hydrogen peroxide is to cause a mild irritation to the gastric mucosa. The dosage for hydrogen peroxide is 1 teaspoon per 5 lb and should not exceed 3 tablespoons. Typically, vomiting occurs within 15 or 20 minutes as long as there is food in the stomach and the peroxide is fresh. If not, peroxide can be repeated one additional time.

Syrup of ipecac (never use the fluid of ipecac) is another product that owners may have in their homes. It acts both through gastric irritation and also stimulates chemoreceptor trigger zone, but it should be used cautiously as overdosing or repeated doses may cause cardiovascular problems.

Apomorphine hydrochloride is considered to be the preferred emetic agent by most small animal clinicians. Apomorphine is available in an injectable solution and as a capsule for conjunctival use.

Salt should never be used as an emetic. Salt is not an effective agent and there have been cases of sodium toxicities reported as a result of its use as an emetic agent.

✐ TECHNICIAN NOTE

Owners can be advised to give the emetic hydrogen peroxide at a dose of 1 teaspoon per 5 lb of body weight (not to exceed 3 tablespoons).

ACTIVATED CHARCOAL

Activated charcoal adsorbs a chemical or toxicant and facilitates its excretion via the feces. It is administered when an animal ingests organic poisons, chemicals, or bacterial toxins or if enterohepatic circulation of metabolized toxicants can occur. The recommended dose of activated charcoal for most species of animals is 1 to 3 g/kg body weight. Repeated doses of activated charcoal every 4 to 8 hours at half the original dose may be indicated when enterohepatic recirculation occurs.

Activated charcoal can be given orally with a large syringe or with a stomach tube. In symptomatic or uncooperative animals, anesthesia may be needed. A cuffed endotracheal tube should always be used in the sedated or clinically depressed animal to prevent aspiration.

Activated charcoal is contraindicated in animals that have ingested caustic materials. These materials are not absorbed systemically, and the charcoal may make it more difficult to see oral and esophageal burns. Other chemicals that are not effectively absorbed by activated charcoal include ethanol, methanol, fertilizer, fluoride, petroleum distillates, most heavy metals, iodides, nitrate, nitrites, sodium chloride, and chlorate.

CATHARTICS

Cathartics increase the clearing of intestinal contents. Cathartics are used to enhance the elimination of activated charcoal and adsorbed toxicant. Cathartics can be added to solutions of activated charcoal, or a combination of activated charcoal and cathartic can be purchased. Contraindications for using cathartics include patients with diarrhea or dehydration.

ENEMAS

Enemas are helpful when elimination of toxicants from the lower gastrointestinal tract is desired. The general technique is to use plain warm water or soapy warm water. Premixed enema solutions for humans are contraindicated in small animals due to potential electrolyte/acid-base imbalance.

GASTRIC LAVAGE

Gastric lavage is a method of gently pumping the stomach contents out of the animal. Gastric lavage should not be performed in cases of caustic or petroleum distillate ingestion and should always be performed under general anesthesia using a cuffed endotracheal tube to protect the airway and prevent aspiration. The procedure involves inserting a fenestrated lavage tube two to three times the diameter of the endotracheal tube; it should be placed to the level of the xiphoid cartilage. The stomach should be lavaged repeatedly with physiological temperature water until the fluid drawn out of the stomach is clear in color.

ENTEROGASTRIC LAVAGE

Enterogastric lavage, also known as the *through and through* lavage, may be necessary when potentially lethal oral exposures have occurred. Following a gastric lavage, the stomach tube is left in place. An enema is performed to eliminate large pieces of fecal matter from the colon and upper large intestines. The distal end of the enema tube is attached to a water faucet and body temperature water is slowly allowed to fill the tube and enter the intestinal tract in a retrograde manner. Water is allowed to flow until the water flows from the stomach tube. This process is continued until the color of the fluid passing out of the stomach tube is clear.

SUPPORTIVE CARE

The technician plays a critical role by routinely evaluating vital signs and any parameters likely to be affected by the toxicants. Hydration can be assessed in the pet by checking skin turgor, capillary refill time, and the moisture of the oral mucous membranes. The animal's body temperature should also be monitored closely.

Blood samples may be needed to perform complete blood count, chemistry panels, or clotting profiles to monitor the effects of the poison. Some toxicants, such as iron, copper, acetaminophen, and arsenic, can cause liver damage, while others, such as estrogen, lead, and antineoplastic medications, can cause anemia.

Daily fluid requirements should be maintained with compensation made for excessive fluid loss or to correct dehydration. Debilitated animals may require additional supplementation. An infusion pump should be used to prevent overhydration. The animal should be monitored for wet lung sounds or the development of a heart murmur, which could indicate overhydration. Pets with cardiovascular disease are at a higher risk for overhydration. Closely monitor pets with indwelling catheters to prevent entanglement in the line or chewing.

Diuresis may be beneficial for exposures to toxicants that can cause kidney damage or to enhance elimination of the toxicant. Examples of toxicants that can cause kidney damage include ethylene glycol antifreeze, zinc, mercury, oxalic acids, nonsteroidal antiinflammatory drugs, diquat herbicide, and aminoglycoside antibiotics. Adverse effects associated with diuresis include pulmonary edema, cerebral edema, metabolic acidosis or alkalosis, or water intoxication. Close monitoring is therefore necessary.

Ancillary measures, such as nutritional support, are key components for complete recovery for the pet. Anorectic cats and ferrets are at risk of developing hepatic lipidosis and hypoglycemia; therefore, it is extremely important to maintain nutritional requirements. A pharyngostomy tube may be necessary to provide adequate nutrition to the animal. Good nursing care should be continued until the pet completely recovers.

Box 27-3 QUICK REFERENCE CHART OF TREATMENT PROTOCOLS

OCULAR IRRIGATION

Flush exposed eyes repeatedly with water or saline solutions.

Minimum of 20 to 30 minutes of irrigation is recommended.

After flushing, eyes, should be treated with lubricant ointments.

Follow-up examinations should also be performed to establish level of corneal damage.

BATHING

Animal should be bathed in a mild liquid dishwashing detergent.

Baths may need to be repeated to completely remove the toxicant.

The animal should be rinsed well with warm water.

The animal should be towel dried to prevent chilling.

EMESIS

Emesis has best results within 2 to 3 hours postexposure.

Feeding the animal a small moist meal before inducing vomiting increases chances of an adequate emesis.

Dogs, cats, ferrets, and potbelly pigs are examples of animals that can vomit.

ACTIVATED CHARCOAL

Adsorbs a chemical or toxicant and facilitates its excretion via the feces.

The recommended dose of activated charcoal for most species of animals is 1 to 3 g/kg

Activated charcoal should not be given to animals that have ingested caustic materials.

CATHARTICS

Enhance elimination of the activated charcoal.

Cathartics are not to be used if the animal has diarrhea or is dehydrated.

ENEMAS

Useful when elimination of toxicants from the lower gastrointestinal tract is desired.

Premixed enema solutions for humans are contraindicated in small animals due to potential electrolyte/acid-base imbalance.

Some of the guidelines discussed in this chapter can be used to aid in the management of toxicoses in pets. Assessing the condition of the pet, stabilizing the animal, preventing absorption of the toxicant, controlling the signs, and instituting ancillary measures are critical areas in which the technician plays a key role. The best way to avoid serious problems due to toxicosis is poison prevention. Being cautious with harmful substances by "pet proofing" the home environment is the only safe choice. The technician can educate pet owners on ways to make their homes poison safe. However, if a pet is exposed to a toxicant, prompt action will be needed to avoid a potentially life-threatening problems. Refer to Box 27-3 for a quick reference chart of treatment protocols.

> **TECHNICIAN NOTE**
>
> Assessing the condition of the pet, stabilizing the animal, preventing absorption of the toxicant, controlling the signs, and instituting ancillary measures are critical areas in which the technician plays a key role. The best way to avoid serious problems due to toxicosis is poison prevention.

HOUSEHOLD HAZARDS

HOUSEHOLD CLEANING AGENTS

Acids

Hydrochloric, sulfuric, nitric, phosphoric acids, oxalic acid, and sodium bisulfate are examples of acids. Common sources of acids include toilet bowl cleaners, drain openers, metal cleaners, antirust compounds, gun barrel cleaners, automobile battery fluid, and pool sanitizers. Acids are corrosives and can produce severe burns on contact with tissue. Acids produce tissue damage at the site of contact. Severity of tissue damage produced is directly related to the concentration. Concentrated acids may produce severe burns on contact with any part of the body, as well as the gastrointestinal tract, if ingested. When acids are diluted or have higher pH, they do not cause corrosion, only irritation. Most cases of exposure to acids that are irritants usually result in mild self-limiting signs of nausea, vomiting, or diarrhea. Oxalic acids include ethanedioic and dicarboxylic acid and can also cause kidney damage.

Alkali

Alkali are used as drain openers, oven cleaners, bleaches, industrial cleaners, denture cleaners, bathroom and household cleaners, radiator cleaning agents, and hair relaxers and in alkaline batteries, electric dishwasher soaps, some oven-cleaner pads, and cement.

Lesions from alkalis are typically deeper and more penetrating than those from acidic compounds. The ability of alkalis to generate corrosive injury depends on the concentration, pH, viscosity, amount ingested, and the duration of contact with tissue. Serious corrosive injury is unlikely to occur from substances with a pH less than 11. Alkali with a pH of 12.5 can cause esophageal ulcers, while those with a pH of 14 or more can cause esophageal perforation.

Bleaches

Household bleaches are used as a bleaching or oxidizing agent, a deodorant, or disinfectants. Household bleaches mainly contain less than 5% sodium hypochlorite, while household mildew removers contain up to 5% calcium hypochlorite. Nonchlorine bleach or colorfast bleaches may contain sodium peroxide, sodium perborates, or enzymatic detergents. Commercial bleaches may also contain other bleaching agents such as sodium peroxide, sodium perborate, sodium carbonate, or oxalic acid.

Household bleaches contain low concentrations of bleach and are mild to moderate mucosal irritants. Commercial forms of alkaline bleach contain higher concentrations, and if the pH is 11 to 12 or greater, it can produce partial-thickness chemical burns. At higher concentration, corrosive effects could be seen.

DETERGENTS

Detergents are nonsoap surfactants in combination with inorganic ingredients such as phosphates, silicates, or carbonates. Detergents are classified according to their charge in solution: nonionic, anionic, and cationic surfactants.

Anionic and nonionic detergents are found in shampoos, dishwashing detergents, laundry detergents, and electric dishwashing detergents. Anionic and ionic detergents are irritants, and their toxicity is generally limited to cutaneous, ocular, oral, or gastrointestinal irritation. They are considered to be low in toxicity. However, when used in coordination with caustic substances such as sodium tripolyphosphate and various carbonates they can be corrosive.

Cationic detergents can be found in fabric softeners, some potpourri oils, hair mousse, conditioners, germicides, disinfectants, and sanitizers. Cationic detergents are rapidly absorbed and may produce severe local and systemic toxicity. Oral ulcerations, stomatitis, and pharyngitis can be seen in the cat at concentrations of 1% or less.

FIRST AID TREATMENT OF EXPOSURES TO CORROSIVE AGENTS

For recent ocular exposure to corrosive acids or alkali a minimum of 20 to 30 minutes irrigation with tepid tap water or physiological saline is recommended. Afterward the eye should be examined by a veterinarian and closely monitored for evidence of corneal ulceration.

Following dermal exposure to corrosives, the animal should be bathed immediately with a mild liquid hand dish detergent or a noninsecticidal shampoo. The animal should be monitored and treated as needed by a veterinarian for burns, erythema, swelling, pain, or pruritus. Veterinary treatment for skin damage and may include pain medication, antiinflammatory agents, and antibiotics.

In cases of ingestion of corrosive agents, do not induce vomiting, because of potential corrosive effects. Preferred initial treatment should be oral dilution with a few laps of milk or water. Following, the patient should be monitored and treated by a veterinarian for oral or esophageal burns. With ingestion of oxalic acid products, additional care with intravenous fluids is necessary to prevent kidney problems.

MISCELLANEOUS HOUSEHOLD ITEMS

ANT BAITS

Ant and roach baits are common objects found in households. The product names may vary, and they may be referred to as *hotels*, *discs*, *stations*, *systems*, *traps*, *baits*, or *trays*. The baits usually contain inert ingredients such as peanut butter, breadcrumbs, sugar, and vegetable or animal oils. Insecticides used most commonly in these baits are sulfluramid, fipronil, avermectin, boric acid, and hydramethylnon. These insecticides have a very wide safety range and are present in very small quantities within the baits, making them a hazard of low toxicity to dogs and cats.

SILICA GEL PACKETS

Silica gel is used as a desiccant and often comes in paper packets or plastic cylinders. They are used to absorb moisture in leather, medication, some food packaging, and some types of cat litter. Silica is considered "chemically and biologically inert" upon ingestion. However, with ingestion, it is possible to see signs of GI upset, such as nausea, vomiting, and inappetence, although signs are expected to be mild or not present with small ingestion. Additional problems could occur if the silica gel was used as a desiccant in medication, since silica could possibly absorb qualities of the medication.

TOILET WATER WITH TANK CLEANING DROP-IN TABLETS

Toilet tank "drop-in" tablets typically contain corrosive agents (alkali or cationic detergents). Corrosive effects could be seen if the actual tablet was chewed. But, when a tank "drop-in" cleaning product is used in a toilet, the actual concentration of the cleaner is very low in the toilet bowl of water. With dilution by the bowl water, the cleaning agent is just a gastric irritant. Common signs seen with ingestion include mild vomiting and nausea.

GLOW NECKLACES

Dibutyl phthalate, also known as *n*-butyl phthalate, is a liquid found in various glow-in-the-dark products. Jewelry containing dibutyl phthalate is commonly sold at fairs, carnivals, and novelty stores. Pets are often attracted to the glowing jewelry. Almost all pets that bite into glow-in-the-dark jewelry drool or foam at the mouth excessively in response to the bitter taste. Some pets will also exhibit hyperactivity and aggressive behavior most likely due to being uncomfortable with the unpleasant taste.

LIQUID POTPOURRI

Liquid potpourri may contain essential oils and cationic detergents, both of which can be harmful. Because product labels may not list ingredients, it is wise to assume any liquid potpourri contains both ingredients. Essential oils can cause mucous membrane and gastrointestinal irritation, central nervous system (CNS) depression, and dermal hypersensitivity and irritation. Severe clinical signs can be seen with potpourri products that contain cationic detergents (see discussion under Detergents). Dermal exposure to cationic detergents can result in redness of the skin, tissue swelling, intense pain, and ulceration. Ingestion of cationic detergents can lead to tissue necrosis and inflammation of the mouth, esophagus, and stomach.

BATTERIES

Flashlights, remote controls, battery-operated toys, watches, calculators, hearing aids, etc., all provide the opportunity for animals to be exposed to batteries. The alkaline material within a battery can cause burns that can penetrate deeply into the local tissue. In addition, battery casings may result in gastrointestinal obstruction if swallowed. When batteries are chewed and the contents released, alkaline burns can result. Signs of foreign body obstruction may occur when casings are swallowed. Treatment of battery exposures is as for exposure to any alkaline product and includes observation and treatment by a veterinarian (see discussion under Alkali). Radiographs are often used to determine the location of the battery when the casing is missing.

CIGARETTES AND OTHER NICOTINE PRODUCTS

Tobacco products contain varying amounts of nicotine with cigarettes containing 13 to 30 mg and cigars containing 15 to 40 mg. Butts contain about 25% of the total nicotine content. Signs often develop quickly (usually within 15 to 45 minutes) and include excitation, tachypnea, salivation, emesis, and diarrhea. Muscle weakness, twitching, depression, tachycardia, shallow respiration, collapse, coma, and cardiac arrest can follow the period of excitation. Death occurs secondary to respiratory paralysis.

PENNIES

Ingestion of coins by pets, especially dogs, is not uncommon. Of the existing U.S. coins currently in circulation, only pennies pose a significant toxicity hazard. Pennies minted since 1983 contain 99.2% zinc and 0.8% copper, making ingested pennies a rich source of zinc; one penny can cause a zinc toxicosis. Other potential sources of zinc include hardware such as screws, bolts, or nuts, all of which may contain varying amounts of zinc. In the stomach, gastric acids leach the zinc from its source, and the ionized zinc is readily absorbed into the circulation, where it causes intravascular hemolysis (breaks apart the red blood cell.)

Veterinary treatment is always required for ingested pennies. Treatment may include inducing vomiting or removal of zinc-containing objects using an endoscope or through surgery. Often treatment includes blood replacement therapy, as needed, intravenous fluids, and other supportive care.

MOTHBALLS

Veterinary treatment of mothball ingestion is always required. Mothballs may be composed of either 100% naphthalene or 99% paradichlorobenzene. Naphthalene-based mothballs are approximately twice as toxic as paradichlorobenzene, and cats are especially sensitive to naphthalene. One 2.7-g mothball contains 2700 mg of naphthalene. Naphthalene causes Heinz bodies, hemolysis, and, occasionally, methemoglobinemia. Paradichlorobenzene primarily affects the liver and central nervous system, although methemoglobinemia and hemolysis have been reported in humans.

MOLDY FOOD (TREMORGENIC MYCOTOXINS)

Tremorgenic mycotoxins produced by molds on foods are a relatively common, and possibly underdiagnosed, cause of tremors and seizures in animals. Because of their relatively indiscriminate appetites, dogs tend to be most commonly exposed to tremorgens than cats. These toxins are produced from a variety of fungi; however, tremorgens produced by *Penicillium* spp. are the most commonly encountered. These molds grow on practically any food, including dairy products, grains, nuts, and legumes; compost piles may also provide a source of tremorgens. Tremorgens have several different mechanisms of action: some alter nerve action potentials, some alter neurotransmitter action, and others alter neurotransmitter levels. The overall effect is the development of muscle tremors and seizures.

> **✐ TECHNICIAN NOTE**
>
> Tremorgenic mycotoxins produced by molds on foods are a relatively common and possibly underdiagnosed as cause of tremors and seizures in animals.

Box 27-4 QUICK POISONOUS PLANT REFERENCE

CARDIOTOXIC PLANTS

Convallaria majalis	Lily of the valley
Nerium oleander	Oleander
Rhododendron	Rhododendron, azalea, rosebay
Taxus species	American, Japanese, English, and Western yew
Digitalis purpurea	Foxglove
Kalanchoe spp.	Kalanchoe

PLANTS THAT COULD CAUSE KIDNEY FAILURE

Certain species of lilies, in cats only
Rhubarb (*Rheum* species), leaves only
Grapes, raisins

PLANTS THAT COULD CAUSE LIVER FAILURE

Cycads (*Cycad* species)
Amanita phalloides, mushroom

PLANTS THAT CAN CAUSE MULTIPLE EFFECTS

Autumn crocus (*Colchicum* species): Can cause bloody vomiting and diarrhea, shock, kidney failure, liver failure, bone marrow suppression.
Castor bean (*Ricinus* species): Usually a lag period of 48 hours before signs appear. Beans are highly toxic! Two to four beans can be lethal to adult humans!
Mushrooms: Always assume that any ingested mushroom is highly toxic until a mycologist identifies that mushroom. Toxic and nontoxic mushrooms can grow in the same area.

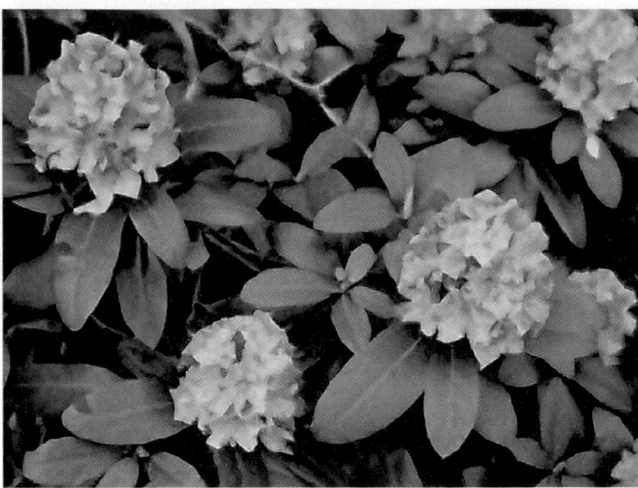

Figure 27-1 Members of the *Rhododendron* species, including azaleas and rhododendrons, contain grayanotoxins that can lead to cardiovascular dysfunction.

RHODODENDRON SPECIES

Members of the *Rhododendron* species, including azalea and rhododendrons, contain grayanotoxins, which can lead to cardiovascular dysfunction (Figure 27-1).

Clinical signs in dogs and cats include vomiting, diarrhea, abdominal pain, weakness, depression, cardiac arrhythmias, hypotension, shock, cardiopulmonary arrest, pulmonary edema, dyspnea, CNS depression, and seizures. Signs generally occur within 4 to 12 hours of ingestion and may persist for several days. Poisonings have also been reported in ruminants and horses. Veterinary treatment and observation is always recommended.

ICE OR SNOW MELTS

The most common ingredients in ice melts are sodium chloride, potassium chloride, magnesium chloride, calcium carbonate, and calcium magnesium acetate. A few ice melts contain urea. Sodium ion toxicosis is possible after large ingestion of ice melts, salt, or rock salt. Signs reported in one dog with fatal hypernatremia (increased sodium level in blood) from salt ingestion included vomiting, increased thirst, increased urination, fine muscular fasciculation, sinus tachycardia, metabolic acidosis (acidic blood pH), and seizures.

DANGEROUS PLANTS

These are a wide variety of common plants that can be poisons to animals, if consumed. Refer to Box 27-4 for a list of some of these plants.

CARDIAC GLYCOSIDE–CONTAINING PLANTS

Hundreds of cardiac glycosides have been identified in various plants, including oleander *(Nerium oleander)* (Figure 27-2), lily-of-the-valley *(Convallaria majalis)*, and foxglove *(Digitalis purpurea)* (Figure 27-3). In most cases, all parts of the plant are toxic, and even small amounts can cause significant clinical signs.

Clinical signs generally develop within several hours of ingestion, and signs may persist for several days after removal of plant material from gastrointestinal tract. Clinical signs seen most commonly involve the gastrointestinal tract and cardiovascular system. Veterinary treatment and observation is always recommended.

CASTOR BEANS

Castor beans *(Ricinus communis)* are often used in jewelry, and the oil extracted from the seeds is used medicinally

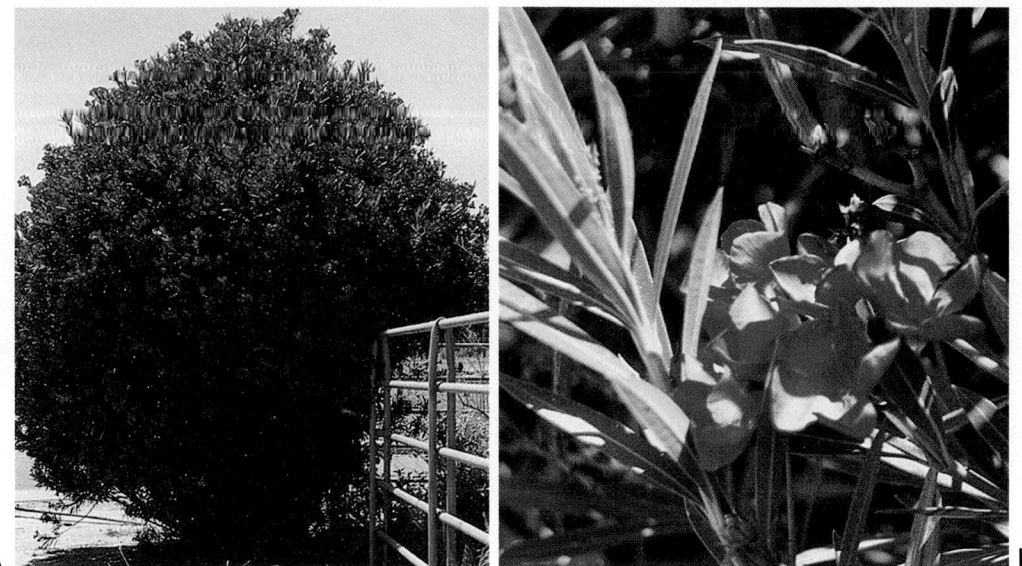

Figure 27-2 **A** and **B,** *Nerium oleander.* There are hundreds of cardiac glycosides identified in various plants, including oleander, lily-of-the-valley, and foxglove.

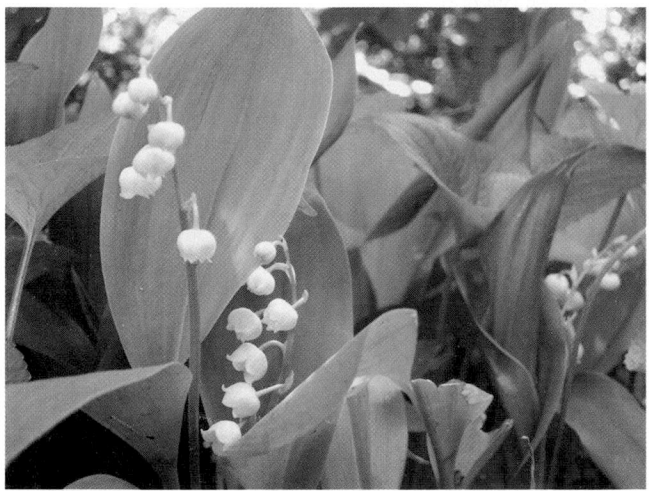

Figure 27-3 *Convallaria majalis,* or lily-of-the-valley. (Courtesy Rachel Hayes.)

(castor oil) Ricin is the toxic principle of castor beans and is considered to be one of the most potent plant toxins known. All parts of the castor bean plant are toxic, but the seeds contain the highest concentration of ricin. In humans, ingestion of one seed is potentially lethal. Veterinary treatment and observation is always recommended.

CYCAD PALMS

Cycad palms (Cycas, Zamia) are found naturally in the sandy soils of tropical to subtropical climates but may also be grown as houseplants in more temperate climates (Figure 27-4). Cycasin is considered to be the toxic principle that is responsible for the hepatic and gastrointestinal signs generally seen with toxicosis. Most parts of the plant are toxic, but the seeds contain a higher concentration of cycasin and are more often associated with toxicosis in small animals. Ingestion of one or more seeds has resulted in liver failure and death in dogs.

LILIES

Easter lilies *(Lilium longiflorum)* (Figure 27-5), tiger lilies *(Lilium tigrinum),* Rubrum or Japanese showy lilies *(Lilium speciosum* and *Lilium lancifolium),* and various day lilies *(Hemerocallis* species) can cause acute renal failure and death in cats. (Figure 27-6 and 27-7). The toxic principle is unknown. Even minor exposures (a few bites on a leaf, ingestion of pollen, etc.) may result in toxicosis. All feline exposures to lilies should be considered potentially life threatening.

Affected cats often vomit within a few hours of exposure to lilies, but the vomiting usually subsides after a few hours, during which time the cats may appear normal or may be mildly depressed and anorexic. Within 24 to 72 hours of ingestion, oliguric to anuric renal failure develops, accompanied by vomiting, depression, anorexia, and dehydration.

Elevations kidney blood values can occur as early as 12 to 18 hours after ingestion. Death due to acute kidney failure generally occurs within 3 to 6 days of ingestion.

Veterinary treatment and observation is always recommended with lily ingestion in cats. Early decontamination by a veterinarian (emesis, oral activated charcoal, and cathartic) in combination with intravenous fluid therapy has been

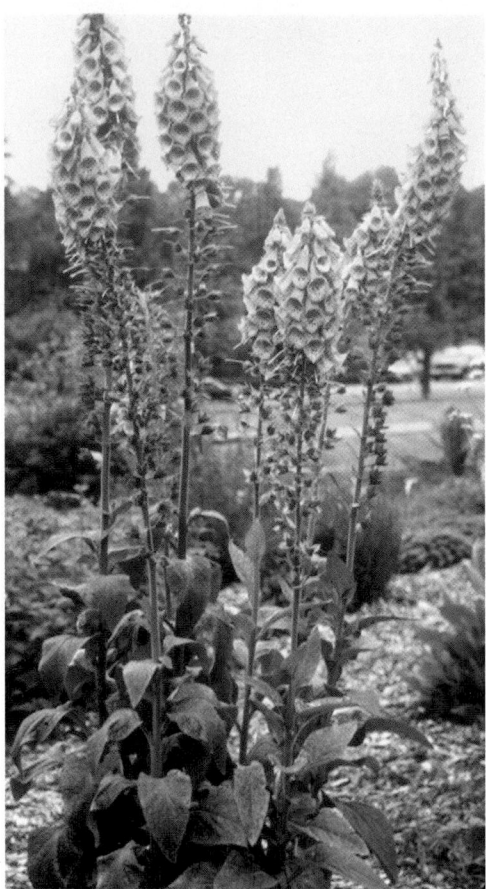

Figure 27-4 *Digitalis purpurea*, or foxglove.

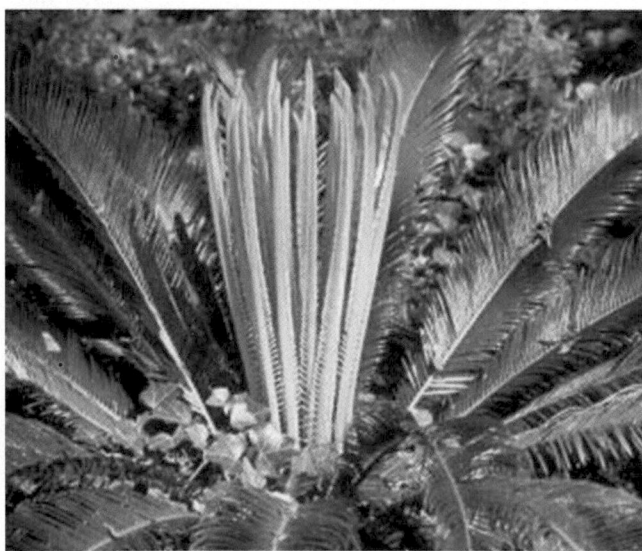

Figure 27-5 Cycad palms are found naturally in the sandy soils of tropical to subtropical climates but may be used as houseplants in more temperate climates.

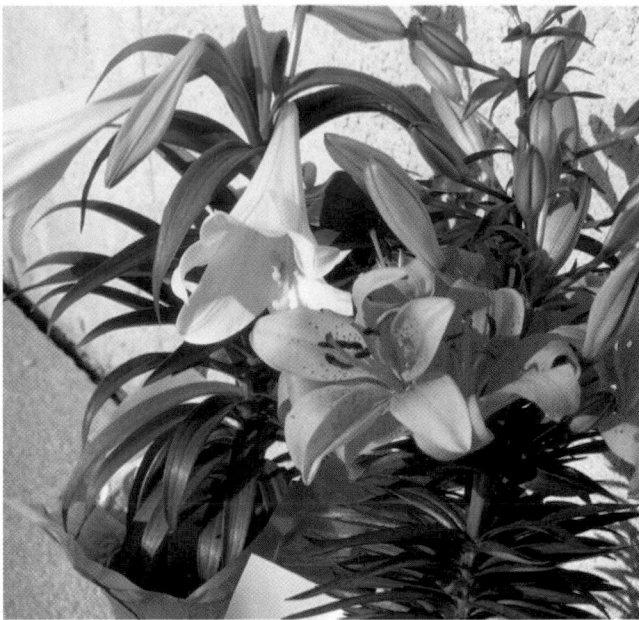

Figure 27-6 *Lilium longiflorum*, or Easter lily. Acute renal failure and death can occur in cats that consume various lilies. These include the Easter lily, tiger lily, day lily, and the Rubrum or Japanese showy lily.

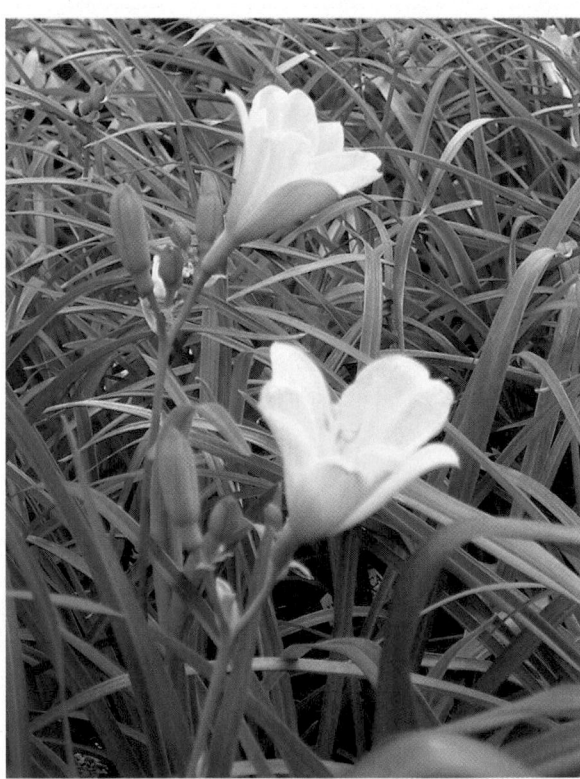

Figure 27-7 *Day lily.* (Courtesy Rachel Hayes.)

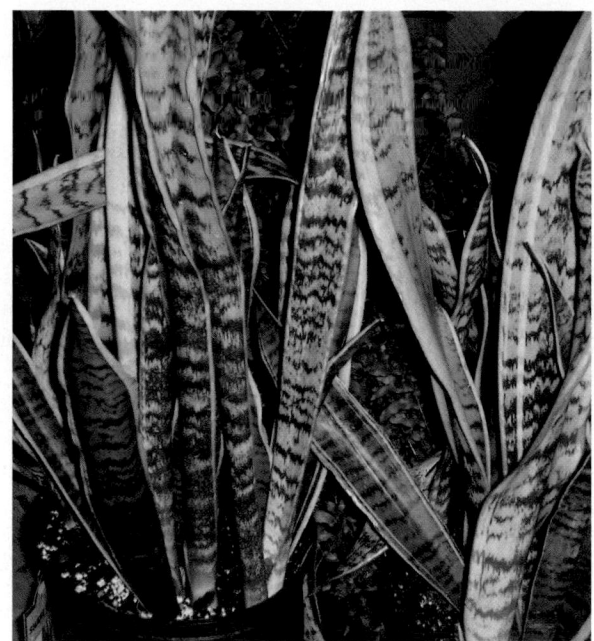

Figure 27-8 *Mother-in-law tongue.* (Courtesy Rachel Hayes.)

shown to effectively prevent lily-induced kidney failure. Conversely, delaying treatment beyond 18 hours frequently results in death or euthanasia due to severe kidney failure. Dialysis can be of help with severely affected animals, but it is not commonly available.

GRAPES AND RAISINS

Some types of grapes and raisins have been shown to cause kidney failure in dogs when eaten in quantity. The basis for kidney failure following consumption of grapes or raisins is unclear, but this is being studied closely in the veterinary community.

ONIONS AND GARLIC

Onion and garlic (*Allium* spp.) are members of the genus Allium. The primary toxic principle is *n*-propyl disulfide, which is thought to cause oxidative damage to erythrocytes, resulting in hemolysis. Toxicosis from fresh, dried, or, powdered plant material has been reported in dogs and cats. Feeding commercial baby food containing onion powder caused toxicity in cats.

CALCIUM OXALATE–CONTAINING PLANTS

Philodendron species, calla lily (*Zantedeschia* sp.), elephant ears (*Caladium* sp.), dumb cane (*Dieffenbachia* sp.) mother-in-law's tongue (*Monstera* sp.) (Figure 27-8), peace lily (*Spathiphyllum* sp.), pathos (*Epipremnum* sp.), and certain other varieties of plants contain insoluble calcium oxalate crystals in their plant material. Chewing of the plant

material can cause the crystals to be expelled into the oral cavity and can result in painful oropharyngeal edema. Clinical signs associated with these plants include oral irritation, intense burning and irritation of the mouth, lips, tongue, excessive drooling, vomiting, and difficulty in swallowing. Airway compromise from tissue swelling could be life-threatening, although severe effects are a rare occurrence.

> ### TECHNICIAN NOTE
> The most dangerous forms of pesticides include: snail bait containing metaldehyde, fly bait containing methomyl, systemic insecticides containing disyston or disulfoton, and zinc phosphide.

PESTICIDES

The most dangerous forms of pesticides include snail bait containing metaldehyde, fly bait containing methomyl, systemic insecticides containing disyston or disulfoton, and zinc phosphide.

FLY BAIT

Methomyl is a highly toxic carbamate insecticide that can be found in fly baits. Carbamate insecticides competitively inhibit both acetylcholinesterases and pseudocholinesterases. Acetylcholinesterase inhibitors cause muscarinic, nicotinic, and CNS system effects. Exposure to methomyl may lead to cholinergic crisis with increased salivation, lacrimation, urinary incontinence, diarrhea, gastrointestinal cramping, and emesis (SLUDGE) syndrome, but the most obvious sign is severe seizures. Hypertension and slow heart rate or cardiorespiratory depression may occur. Immediate veterinary treatment and observation is always required as signs can occur within minutes of methomyl ingestion.

SNAIL OR SLUG BAIT

Metaldehyde is a polymer of acetaldehyde and is commonly found in snail or slug bait and is very toxic. Onset of clinical signs is typically within 30 minutes to 3 hours. Common clinical signs seen with metaldehyde ingestion include increased heart rate, nervousness, panting, drooling, incoordination, hyperthermia, tremors, and seizures. In some cases, liver failure may occur within 2 to 3 days after exposure. Veterinary treatment and observation is always required.

GOPHER OR MOLE BAIT

Zinc phosphide is used in mole and gopher baits and is considered to be highly toxic. Following ingestion, phosphide is converted to phosphine gas by stomach acid (the conversion is enhanced with presence of food and water.)

Released phosphine gas causes severe respiratory distress. Clinical signs are seen soon after ingestion, typically within 15 minutes to 4 hours. Death occurs secondary to respiratory failure. Veterinary treatment and observation is always required.

SYSTEMIC INSECTICIDES: DISULFOTON, OR DISYSTON

Disulfoton (also known as *disyston*) is a selective, systemic organophosphate insecticide and is very highly toxic. Systemic insecticides are applied to the soil and then are actively taken up by plant roots and translocated to all parts of the plant. Onset of clinical signs is 2 to 8 hours postingestion and signs can last for several days. Clinical signs seen with a toxicosis include typical cholinesterase inhibitor SLUDGE signs, but they can also have hemorrhagic diarrhea and liver and pancreatic enzyme elevations. Veterinary treatment and observation is always required. Good nursing care is essential. Prognosis is good to guarded depending on the severity of the signs. Complete recovery from acute effects may take several days or weeks.

RAT OR MOUSE BAIT

There are three main types of rat or mouse baits available commercially: anticoagulants, bromethalin, and chole-calciferol. Other pesticides, such as strychnine, aldicarb, and zinc phosphide may be used to control wild rat and mouse populations.

Anticoagulants (Table 27-1) include:

Short acting: warfarin
Long acting: pindone, diphacenone, difethialone,
    chlorophacinone, brodifacoum, and bromadiolone

The anticoagulant rodenticides act by competitive inhibition of vitamin K epoxide reductase, thus halting the recycling of vitamin K. In early cases of toxicoses, the prothrombin time (PT) when checked between 36 and 72 hours will be elevated, but the animal will still appear clinically normal. Beyond 72 hours, hemorrhage is a possible effect. The presence of circulating clotting factors in normal animals is the reason for the delay in the development of signs.

Clinical signs of anticoagulant poisoning may not be observed for 5 to 10 days postingestion and include hemorrhage, pale mucous membranes, weakness, exercise intolerance, lameness, dyspnea, coughing, and swollen joints. Often the animal is not presented to the veterinarian until signs are severe.

Animals with clinical signs should be stabilized immediately. Transfusions with whole blood or plasma may be necessary to replace clotting factors. Decontamination is only effective early; remember, clinical signs are usually delayed 5 to 10 days postingestion. Any elevation in the prothrombin time (PT) warrants full treatment with vitamin K_1. No treatment is indicated if PT remains normal; however, recent vitamin K_1 administration could result in misleading PT values because new clotting factor synthesis only requires 6 to 12 hours. Oral vitamin K_1 is an antidote for anticoagulants. Vitamin K_1 should be given with a fatty meal to enhance absorption.

> **✎ TECHNICIAN NOTE**
>
> Oral vitamin K_1 is an antidotal for anticoagulants. Vitamin K_1 should be given with a fatty meal to enhance absorption.

BROMETHALIN

Bromethalin is an uncoupler of oxidative phosphorylation. Bromethalin causes a reduction of adenosine triphosphate (ATP). ATP is necessary to sustain the sodium/potassium ion channel pumps. When the pump mechanism is inhibited, fluid buildup occurs, which results in fluid-filled vacuoles between myelin sheaths. This leads to decreased nerve impulse conduction.

Clinical signs of bromethalin toxicosis could occur within 24 hours up to 2 weeks and include muscle tremors, seizures, hyperexcitability, forelimb extensor rigidity, ataxia, CNS depression, loss of vocalization, paresis, paralysis, and death.

Aggressive decontamination is most important with bromethalin ingestion. Repeated doses of activated charcoal (every 8 to 12 hours) is recommended. Supportive care should be given, as needed, for clinical signs. The prognosis is poor for animals showing severe signs. Animals exposed at lower doses exhibiting paralysis may recover. Agents such as mannitol, furosemide, and corticosteroids may reduce the cerebral edema. Unfortunately, these drugs were of little benefit in reducing the severity of signs in experimental animals. Ginkgo biloba has been used experimentally in rats with bromethalin poisoning, although true benefit is not known.

CHOLECALCIFEROL

Cholecalciferol (vitamin D_3) increases intestinal absorption of calcium, stimulates bone resorption, and enhances kidney reabsorption of calcium. This results in a serum calcium increase. This can lead to kidney failure, cardiovascular abnormalities, and tissue mineralization.

Table 27-1 ANTICOAGULANT RODENTICIDES

Type of Anticoagulant	Minimum Duration of Therapy
Warfarin	14 days
Bromadiolone	21 days
Brodifacoum and others	30 days

Clinical signs usually have a delay in onset and usually occur 18 to 36 hours postingestion. The most common signs seen with cholecalciferol toxicosis include vomiting, diarrhea, inappetence, depression, polyuria, polydipsia, and cardiac arrhythmia. Kidney failure arises from the deposition of calcium in the kidney.

Aggressive decontamination is most important with cholecalciferol ingestion. Repeated doses of activated charcoal (every 8 to 12 hours for 1 to 2 days) is recommended.

Close monitoring of the serum calcium, phosphorus, creatinine, and blood urea nitrogen (BUN) is recommended.

Renal effects are treated with fluid diuresis. Prednisone and furosemide are often used with treatment. Pamidronate inhibits osteoclastic bone resorption and has been used successfully to treat cholecalciferol poisoning. Alternatively, salmon calcitonin has been used to decrease calcium levels.

ANTIFREEZE PRODUCTS

METHANOL

Methanol (also known as *methyl alcohol* or *wood alcohol*) is found most commonly in "antifreeze" windshield washer fluid and varies in concentration from 20% to 100% (with 20% to 30% being the most common form.) Methanol's metabolite, formaldehyde, is rapidly oxidized by aldehyde dehydrogenase to formic acid, which can cause metabolic acidosis if significant quantities are ingested and retinal toxicity in humans and nonhuman primates. In general, alcohols are rapidly absorbed from the gastrointestinal tract. The minimum toxic dose in dogs is 8.0 g/kg (or 3 oz of 100% methanol). The most common exposures occur with dogs and usually involve chewing on containers or lapping up spills. With small exposures in dogs and cats, only mild gastric upset is seen. Recent small ingestion is treated with dilution (milk and water) that may help minimize gastric upset. Large exposure would be expected to only occur when there is no other water source available. In the case of a large ingestion, the animal should be monitored and treated for acidosis.

PROPYLENE GLYCOL

Propylene glycol is the main ingredient in "safer" forms of engine antifreeze/coolants. Propylene glycol is approximately three times less toxic in dogs than ethylene glycol. According to a study, no clinical signs were seen when a dog was given an acute dose of 20 ml/kg.

In toxic quantities, acidosis, liver damage, and renal insufficiency are possible from propylene glycol. Clinical signs of propylene glycol toxicosis include CNS depression, weakness, ataxia, and seizures. With large ingestion, diuresis and supportive care, such as treatment for acidosis, should be given.

ETHYLENE GLYCOL

Ethylene glycol (EG) is the most dangerous form of antifreeze. Most commercial antifreeze products contain between 95% and 97% ethylene glycol. The minimum lethal dose of undiluted EG antifreeze is 4.4 to 6.6 ml/kg in dogs and 1.4 ml/kg in cats. EG can cause metabolic acidosis and acute renal tubular necrosis. In most cases of EG poisonings, vomiting is seen within the first few hours, and then within 1 to 6 hours signs of depression, ataxia, weakness, tachypnea, polyuria, and polydipsia occur. By 18 to 36 hours acute renal failure occurs.

TECHNICIAN NOTE

Ethylene glycol is the most dangerous form of antifreeze. Most commercial antifreeze products contain between 95% and 97% EG.

Diagnosis

Peak levels of EG are reached within 1 to 4 hours postingestion. There is one commercial EG kit available for veterinary use (EGT Kit PRN Pharmacal, 800-874-9764). EG tests can be run as early as 30 minutes postingestion up to 12 hours. The EGT Kit is labeled for dogs and detects a level greater than 50 mg/dl. Since cats are more sensitive than dogs, the kit may not be sensitive enough to diagnose a toxicosis in the cat. Some human labs may run a quantitative EG analysis to detect levels and could be considered with feline exposures. False-positive test results can occur from propylene glycol (in some types of activated charcoal solutions and also from some injection solutions such as pentobarbital and diazepam) or from formaldehyde.

Treatment

Induction of emesis is only helpful with recent exposures (<1 hour.) To prevent false-positive EG tests, it is recommended to take a blood sample before administering activated charcoal since many products contain propylene glycol as inactive ingredients. Although its effectiveness is controversial, activated charcoal can be given within 1 to 3 hours of ingestion. Gastric lavage with activated charcoal could be considered but would only be effective early.

EG is metabolized via alcohol dehydrogenase to glycoaldehyde, which is then metabolized to glycolic acid, which is then metabolized to glyoxylic acid. Glycoaldehyde is more toxic than EG. The formation of glycolic acid is thought to be responsible for causing metabolic acidosis. The goal of treatment of EG toxicoses is to slow down the metabolism.

Fomepizole (Antizole Vet by Orphan Medical, 888-8-ORPHAN) is used to inhibit alcohol dehydrogenase and is considered the preferred treatment for treating EG toxicoses in dogs but is not effective in cats.

Ethanol can be used in cats and dogs. Ethanol also competes with EG as a substrate for alcohol dehydrogenase; however, it does have several unfavorable side effects, which include CNS depression, hyperosmolality, and metabolic acidosis. Fluid diuresis and correction of acidosis with sodium bicarbonate is also an important part of therapy. Peritoneal dialysis should be considered with anuric animals. Prognosis is good with early aggressive treatment (<8 hours of ingestion.)

DANGEROUS HUMAN MEDICATIONS

Please note, any medication can be dangerous to an animal, depending on the dose and frequency. The following is a list of potentially dangerous medications. All require veterinary consultation, treatment, and monitoring.

ACETAMINOPHEN

Acetaminophen is a synthetic nonopiate derivative of p-aminophenol. Acetaminophen toxicity can result from a single toxic dose or repeated cumulative dosages, which lead to methemoglobinemia and liver damage. In dogs, acetaminophen is used therapeutically for analgesia at a dose of 10 mg/kg q12h. Clinical signs of toxicity are not typically observed in dogs unless the dose exceeds 100 mg/kg, at which dose hepatotoxicity is possible. At 200 mg/kg, methemoglobinemia is a possibility. In cats, 10 mg/kg has produced signs of toxicity.

Clinical signs of acetaminophen toxicity are related to methemoglobinemia and hepatotoxicity. Clinical signs include depression, weakness, tachypnea, dyspnea, cyanosis, icterus, vomiting, methemoglobinemia, hypothermia, facial or paw edema, hepatic necrosis, and death.

> ### ✎ TECHNICIAN NOTE
> Clinical signs of acetaminophen toxicity include depression, weakness, tachypnea, dyspnea, cyanosis, icterus, vomiting, methemoglobinemia, hypothermia, facial or paw edema, hepatic necrosis, and death.

IBUPROFEN

Ibuprofen is a substituted phenylalkanoic acid with nonsteroidal antiinflammatory, antipyretic, and analgesic properties. Ibuprofen has been used therapeutically in dogs at 5 mg/kg, but because it can cause gastric ulcers and perforations, it is generally not recommended.

According to studies of acute ingestion of ibuprofen in dogs, vomiting, diarrhea, nausea, anorexia, gastric ulceration, and abdominal pain can be seen with doses of 50 to 125 mg/kg; these signs in combination with renal damage can be seen at doses at or above 175 mg/kg; and at doses at or above 400 mg/kg CNS effects such as seizure, ataxia, and coma may occur. Cats are considered to be twice as sensitive as dogs because they have a limited glucuronyl-conjugating capacity.

Most common signs of ibuprofen toxicoses include anorexia, nausea, vomiting, lethargy, diarrhea, bloody diarrhea, ataxia, increased urination, and increased thirst. Postmortem lesions associated with ibuprofen toxicoses include perforations, erosion, ulceration, and hemorrhage of the gastrointestinal tract.

The primary goal of treatment is to prevent or treat gastric ulceration, renal failure, CNS effects, and possibly hepatic effects. Prognosis is good if the animal is treated promptly and appropriately. Delay in treatment can decrease survival potential with large exposures.

ASPIRIN

Aspirin is used therapeutically in dogs and cats [acceptable daily doses (ADDs)]. Aspirin must be used cautiously in cats because of their inability to rapidly metabolize and excrete salicylates. Symptoms of toxicity may occur if given doses frequently or without stringent monitoring. Aspirin should be used cautiously in neonatal animals; adult doses may lead to poisoning. Symptoms of acute aspirin overdosage in dogs and cats include depression, vomiting (may be blood tinged), anorexia, hyperthermia, and increased respiratory rate. If treatment is not provided, muscular weakness, pulmonary and cerebral edema, hypernatremia, hypokalemia, ataxia, and seizures may all develop with eventual coma and death.

MA HUANG, PSEUDOEPHEDRINE, AND EPHEDRINE: SYMPATHOMIMETIC ALKALOIDS

Ma huang is used as an herbal weight loss aid aid contains the sympathomimetic alkaloids ephedrine and pseudoephedrine. Ephedrine and pseudoephedrine act as stimulants and are also found in cold and flu medications as nasal decongestants and are similar in structure to amphetamines. They can cause increased blood pressure, tachycardia, ataxia, mydriasis, hyperactivity, tremors, and seizures. Ephedrine and pseudoephedrine are eliminated by the kidneys. The half-life varies with urine pH. With an overdose, it is common to see clinical signs last for over 24 hours.

ISONIAZID

Isoniazid (INH) is a medication used to treat tuberculosis and has a very narrow margin of safety. Isoniazid is available as an elixir, injectable, syrup, and tablets in strengths of 50, 100, and 300 mg. Overdoses produce life-threatening signs: seizures, acidosis, and coma. Pyridoxine (vitamin B_6) is a direct agonist of INH.

CALCIPOTRIENE: VITAMIN D DERIVATIVES

Calcipotriene is a synthetic derivative of vitamin D_3. It is used as a topical ointment to treat psoriasis in humans. An overdose of calcipotriene can cause hypercalcemia that

Box 27-5 GLOSSARY

ACIDS
Compounds whose water-based solutions have a sour taste, turn blue litmus paper red and can combine with metals to form salts and yield hydrogen ions or protons when dissolved in water.

ADSORBENT
Solid substance that attracts and holds a substance to its surface.

ALKALI
Alkaline substances produce hydroxide ions on contact with water.

AMINOGLYCOSIDE ANTIBIOTICS
Group of broad spectrum antibiotics. Common examples are streptomycin, gentamicin, amikacin, kanamycin, tobramycin, and neomycin.

BIOTOXIN OR TOXIN
Noxious or poisonous substance that is formed or elaborated during the metabolism and growth of certain microorganisms and some higher plant and animal species.

CATHARTICS
Medications, through their chemical effects, that serve to increase the clearing of intestinal contents.

CATIONIC DETERGENTS
Nonsoap surfactants that are in a positive state.

CORROSIVE
Highly reactive substance that causes obvious damage to living tissue.

DECONTAMINATION
Removal or neutralization of injurious agents.

EMESIS
Act of vomiting.

ENTEROHEPATIC RECIRCULATION
Occurs with some compounds that are metabolized in the liver. The metabolites are emptied in the bile and are reabsorbed in the small intestines.

HEPATOTOXIC
Compound that is toxic to liver cells.

HYDROCARBONS
Any of a large class of organic compounds containing only carbon and hydrogen. Examples would be natural gas, propane, butane, kerosene, gasoline, and motor oil.

METABOLIC ACIDOSIS
Metabolic derangement of acid-base balance where the blood pH is abnormally low.

NEPHROTOXIC
Toxic or destructive to kidney cells.

NONSTEROIDAL ANTIINFLAMMATORY DRUGS
Large group of antiinflammatory agents that work by inhibiting the production of prostaglandins. Examples include ibuprofen, ketoprofen, naproxen, and aspirin.

TOXICANT
Any substance that when introduced into or applied to the body can interfere with the life processes of cells of the organism. Toxicants may be of biologic origin, manufactured chemicals, or naturally occurring chemicals.

TOXICOSIS (PLURAL FORM, TOXICOSES)
Any disease of toxic origin.

TOXIN (OR BIOTOXIN)
Noxious or poisonous substance that is formed or elaborated during the metabolism and growth of certain microorganisms and some higher plant and animal species.

---

can result in kidney failure, cardiac failure, and possibly death. In most cases, dogs that have ingested toxic levels of calcipotriene start showing signs of lethargy, weakness, and inappetence within 1 to 2 days postexposure. Serum calcium levels would be expected to increase within 12 to 72 hours. Hypercalcemia, hyperphosphatemia, azotemia, proteinuria, and tissue mineralization can occur with overdoses. Bradycardia and cardiac arrhythmia are also expected.

5-FLUOROURACIL: ANTIMETABOLITES

5-Fluorouracil (5-FU) is an anticancer topical cream. It is used in human patients to treat solar and actinic keratoses and some superficial skin tumors. Topical fluorouracil is available as 1% or 5% cream [5-FU can inhibit ribonucleic acid (RNA) processing and functioning as well as deoxyribonucleic acid (DNA) synthesis and repair]. The toxicity effects of 5-FU, as with other anticancer agents, is mainly through its destruction of rapidly dividing cell lines such as bone marrow stem cells and epithelial layer of the intestinal crypts.

Early effects seen with 5-FU, in the dog, include generalized grand mal seizures, tremors, vomiting, and ataxia. Cardiac arrhythmia, respiratory distress, and hemorrhagic gastroenteritis are also seen. Clinical signs develop within 1 hour and are usually life threatening. Often death occurs within 6 to 16 hours after exposure. In those that survive initial effects, it is possible to see bone marrow suppression with evidence of neutropenia 4 to 20 days after exposure.

Recommended Reading

Konnie P, editor: *Clinical veterinary toxicology*, St Louis, 2004, Mosby.

Roger WG, Shawn M: *Handbook of small animal toxicology and poisonings*, St Louis, 2004, Mosby.

Peterson ME, Talcott PA: *Small animal toxicology*, Moscow, ID, 2001, University of Idaho.

Mindy GB: Dermal decontamination: dealing with sticky situations, *Vet Technician** 24(8):538-540, 2003.

Moorman M: Bromethalin: it's not what you think, *Vet Technician* 24(7):484-486, 2003.

---

*Toxicology Brief is a column written by ASPCA Animal Poison Control Center veterinary technicians for *Veterinary Technician*, a peer-reviewed journal published monthly by Veterinary Learning Systems.

Steenbergen VM: Acetaminophen and cats, *Vet Technician* 24(1):43-45, 2003.

Foss T: Liquid potpourri and cats, *Vet Technician* 23(11):686-689, 2002.

Bough MG: Castor bean toxicosis: one mean bean, *Vet Technician* 23(8):498, 2002.

Steenbergen VM: Beautiful lilies: a potential cat-astrophe, *Vet Technician* 23(4):236-237, 2002.

Richardson JA:·Poison prevention and management primer, *Vet Technician* 23(3):150-156, 2002.

Tamara F: The hazards of ice melts to dogs and cats, *Vet Technician* 23(2):94-104, 2002.

Moorman M: Anticoagulant rodenticides now more toxic to pests and pets, *Vet Technician* 23(1):34-36, 2002.

Simmons DM: Onion breath, *Vet Technician* 22(8):424-427, 2001.

Hull W: Ethylene glycol testing, *Vet Technician* 22(4):201-206, 2001.

Farbman D: Death by chocolate? Methylxanthine toxicosis, *Vet Technician* 22(3):146-147, 2001.

Farbman D: 'Tis the season to be informed: toxic potential of holiday plants, *Vet Technician* 21(11):630-631, 2000.

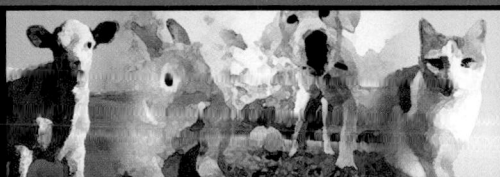

28

Veterinary Dentistry

ASHLEY B. OAKES

INTRODUCTION

Every pet with teeth will need dental care at some point in its lifetime. Whether the pet mouse, snake, or horse will receive the quality of dental care dogs and cats now receive remains to be seen. As dental home care products continue to improve, clients have more options available to provide dental care for their pets. It is not uncommon to find photographs in veterinary and dental literature of exotic animals such as killer whales, dolphins, and sea lions opening wide for dental care. Preventive dentistry (tooth brushing, dental cleanings) is important to maintain good health and quality of life in pets just as it is for humans. Most family veterinary offices provide routine professional dental cleanings for their patients. Some practices also provide advanced dental care, such as endodontics, exodontia, and periodontal treatments. Dental radiography has a place in every veterinary practice that examines and cleans teeth. Veterinary technicians play an important role in providing these dental services to the client's pets. It is important that the dental technician or veterinary dental assistant have a good understanding of the different dental problems and treatment options available for these problems.

This chapter provides a detailed discussion of periodontal disease and its prevention with proper diet, routine professional dental cleanings, and dental home care. Because veterinary technicians often perform dental scaling and polishing procedures, it is important to have a good understanding of the necessary equipment and its proper use and care. Dental radiology is extremely beneficial in veterinary medicine because patients often do not show obvious signs of dental pain. Veterinary personnel must examine the teeth closely and radiograph teeth with abnormalities and/or use periodic survey films. The procedures for taking diagnostic dental radiographs

are covered. The remainder of the chapter addresses the specialty branches endodontics, exodontia, orthodontics, and restorative dentistry. ■

ETHICAL AND LEGAL ASPECTS

The level of dental care a veterinary technician may provide varies from state to state, and the rules for the particular state in which a person is working need to be reviewed before providing dental care. The American Veterinary Dental College (AVDC) published a position statement (American Veterinary Dental College, 1998) regarding veterinary dental heath care providers. The purpose of this statement was to develop a means to safeguard veterinary dental patients and ensure the qualifications of persons performing veterinary dental procedures. The AVDC considers it appropriate for the veterinarian to delegate maintenance dental care and certain dental tasks to veterinary technicians.

Tasks appropriately performed by veterinary technicians include dental prophylaxis and certain procedures that do not result in alterations in the shape, structure, or positional location of teeth in the dental arch. A veterinarian may direct a technician to perform these tasks providing the veterinarian is physically present and supervising the treatment and providing the technician has received appropriate training.

The AVDC supports advanced training of veterinary technicians to perform additional ancillary dental services (e.g., taking impressions, making models, charting veterinary dental lesions, taking and developing dental radiographs, performing nonsurgical subgingival root scaling and debridement) providing that they do not alter the structure of the tooth.

The AVDC supports appropriate training of veterinary assistants (not registered, certified, or licensed) to perform

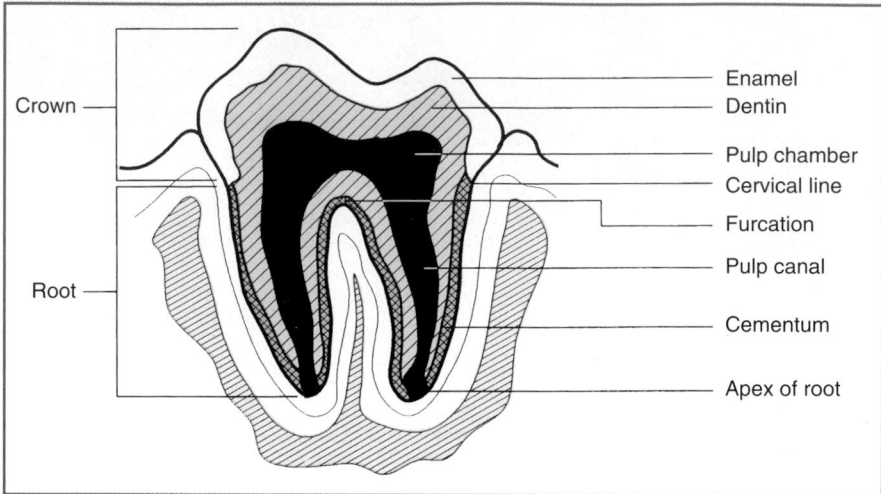

Figure 28-1 Typical external and internal gross anatomy of a tooth. The model is a premolar. (From Bojrab MJ, Tholen M: *Small animal oral medicine and surgery,* Philadelphia, 1990, Lea & Febiger.)

the following dental services: supragingival scaling and polishing, taking and developing dental radiographs, taking impressions, and making models.

VETERINARY DENTAL ORGANIZATIONS

Many of the veterinary specialty fields are opening up opportunities for veterinary technicians to achieve advanced training and recognition in a particular field. The Academy of Veterinary Dental Technicians (AVDT) received provisional recognition by the National Association of Veterinary Technicians of America (NAVTA) in 2002. Individuals interested in achieving this specialty training need to be a credentialed veterinary technician with at least 1 year of experience prior to applying to the AVDT. The AVDT requires a 2-year training program under the supervision of a mentor. The applicants will have to complete several requirements during this time. Once the requirements have been successfully completed, the applicant is then invited to sit for the examination. Technicians that pass the exam will be given the title of Veterinary Technician Specialist in Dentistry, which is written as VTS (Dentistry). Information is available on their Web site (www.avdt.us) or by contacting the secretary Ms. Sara Sharp at 303-753-6961 or email address DBLTRBSLS@aol.com.

The American Society for Veterinary Dental Technicians (ASVDT) was established in 1994. This organization currently has over 6000 members who have taken and passed a self-taught home study video and workbook course. All veterinary staff personnel are eligible to take the examination (i.e., veterinary technicians, veterinary assistants, veterinarians, receptionists, kennel workers). The purpose of the course is to improve the individual's dental knowledge to better serve clients and their pets. To find out more about the ASVDT, contact Mr. Gerry Selin at 800-613-3647.

Membership to The American Veterinary Dental Society (AVDS) is open to veterinarians, veterinary technicians, and dental hygienists who wish to join, and membership includes a subscription to the quarterly *Journal of Veterinary Dentistry.* The AVDS can be contacted c/o Walker Management Group at 800-332-AVDS.

DENTAL MORPHOLOGY AND OCCLUSION

Dogs and cats have four types of brachyodont teeth: incisors, canines, premolars, and molars. The incisor teeth are positioned in the front of the mouth and are used for gnawing and grooming. The canine teeth are distal to the incisors. They are very long and are used for grasping and tearing. The premolars and molars (often referred to as *cheek teeth* based on their location) are used for shearing and grinding. Brachyodont teeth have a short crown height and do not continue to grow once they have erupted (Figure 28-1). Humans, carnivores, and pigs have brachyodont teeth. The teeth of horses and the cheek teeth of ruminants are hypsodont teeth. Hypsodont teeth have a long crown height and continue to erupt through most of the animal's life span.

Mammals are diphyodonts, meaning that they have two sets of teeth. The first set is called the *deciduous teeth* (baby teeth), and these are replaced with permanent teeth as the animal matures. Mammals show great variety in the number and types of teeth each species has. Dental formulas are used to classify the types and numbers of teeth that a species should have. The dental formulas for the deciduous and permanent dentition of the dog and cat are listed in Box 28-1. The dental formula lists the dentition on one side of the jaw (maxilla or mandible) preceded by the number 2 to compensate for the duplicate set of teeth on the opposite side of that jaw. The maxillary formula is placed on top of the mandibular

Box 28-1 DENTAL FORMULAS FOR THE DOG AND CAT

Dog deciduous 2 × (3i/3i, 1c/1c, 3p/3p) = 28
Dog permanent 2 × (3I/3I, 1C/1C, 4P/4P, 2M/3M) = 42
Cat deciduous 2 × (3i/3i, 1c/1c, 3p/2p) = 26
Cat permanent 2 × (3I/3I, 1C/1C, 3P/2P, 1M/1M) = 30

Table 28-1 DOG AND CAT PERMANENT DENTITION

DOG PERMANENT DENTITION

MANDIBLE	TOOTH	ROOTS
Incisors	1st, 2nd, 3rd	1
Canines	1	1
Premolars	1st	1
Premolars	2nd, 3rd, 4th	2
Molars	1st, 2nd	2
Molars	3rd*	1 (or 2)

MAXILLA	TOOTH	ROOTS
Incisors	1st, 2nd, 3rd	1
Canines	1	1
Premolars	1st	1
Premolars	2nd, 3rd*	2
Premolars	(3rd*), 4th	3
Molars	1st, 2nd	3

CAT PERMANENT DENTITION

MANDIBLE	TOOTH	ROOTS
Incisors	1st, 2nd, 3rd	1
Canines	1	1
Premolars	1st, 2nd	Not present
Premolars	3rd, 4th	2
Molars	1st	2

MAXILLA	TOOTH	ROOTS
Incisors	1st, 2nd, 3rd	1
Canines	1	1
Premolars	1st	Not present
Premolars	2nd	1
Premolars	3rd*	2 (or 3)
Premolars	4th	3
Molars	1st*	1 (or 2)

*Anatomical variation in root numbers is common. There may be an extra root, or it may be partially fused to the normal root(s).

formula, and the tooth type is abbreviated with a letter *I* for incisor, *C* for canine, *P* for premolar, and *M* for molar. Deciduous teeth are abbreviated with lowercase letters and permanent teeth with uppercase letters. The total number of teeth in the mouth is on the right side of the equation.

The number of tooth roots each tooth has is also very important to know. This number will vary among species. For instance, it is important to know that the maxillary fourth premolar (carnassial tooth) of dogs and cats has three roots because these teeth are often treated for dental problems. Anatomical variation does occur, so careful examination and dental radiographs are helpful to determine when an animal has an additional or missing tooth root. The maxillary third premolar is a two-rooted tooth in most dogs and cats, but it is not uncommon to find a third palatal root on some dogs and cats. The number of roots commonly found on the teeth of dogs and cats is listed in Table 28-1 along with the location where we find anatomical variation.

The majority of dogs and cats have a scissors bite (Figure 28-2, *A*). When the teeth are properly aligned in scissors occlusion, there is maximal function of all teeth with no occlusal trauma (irritation to soft tissues or other teeth). We do see variations of dental occlusion in dogs and cats depending on the breed of animal and skull type as well as malaligned teeth from numerous other causes (genetics, retained deciduous teeth, idiopathic). The teeth in normal occlusion (scissors bite) have the following relationships.

INCISORS

The mandibular incisors should be palatal to the maxillary incisors and the incisal one third of the mandibular incisors should rest on the cingulum of the maxillary incisors. The cingulum (Figure 28-3, *A*) is a ledge located on the palatal side in the gingival third of the incisor tooth.

CANINES

The mandibular canine should rest distal to the maxillary third incisor and mesial to the maxillary canine, and it should be centered in between these two maxillary teeth.

PREMOLARS

The premolar cusp tips point to the interdental space of the opposing premolar teeth. The mandibular fourth premolar cusp tip points in the interdental space between the maxillary third and fourth premolars. The mandibular first premolar is mesial to the maxillary first premolar. The premolars are not in occlusion with the opposing premolar teeth, but when the mouth is closed, the cusp tips should intersect a dorsal plane drawn midway between the mandibular and maxillary occlusal planes (Figure 28-2, *B*).

CARNASSIAL TEETH

The maxillary fourth premolar tooth should occlude buccal to the mandibular first molar tooth.

MOLARS

The occlusal surface of the maxillary molars should occlude with the occlusal surface of the mandibular molars.

There are four classes of malocclusions that are utilized. For the purpose of this chapter the discussion will be limited to the three main types. A class I malocclusion (Figure 28-4) is when the maxillary and mandibular jaw lengths are of proper proportion but one or more teeth are tipped or rotated out of the normal line of occlusion. *Neutroclusion* is a descriptive term used to describe this malocclusion. Class I malocclusions (neutroclusion) are the most common type of malocclusion that receive orthodontic correction in pets. Common examples of class I malocclusions are lingually displaced mandibular canines (base narrow canines) and anterior cross bite. When the mandibular canines are displaced lingually, they usually cause occlusal trauma with the palatal tissue and/or maxillary gingiva because of their long crown height. Severe cases can result in complete

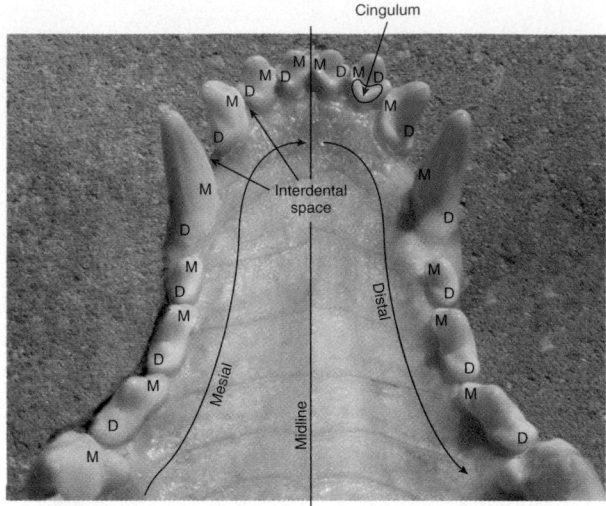

M = Mesial surface
D = Distal surface

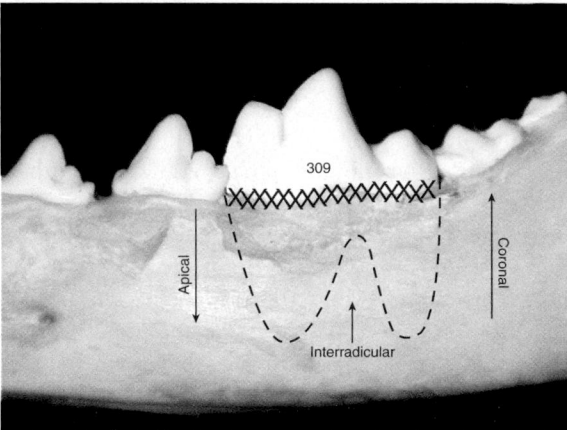

$\diagdown\!\!\times\!\!\times\!\!\times$ = Gingival or cervical area

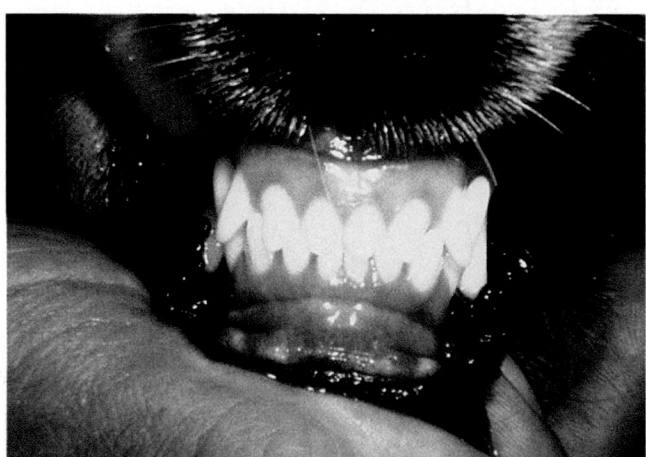

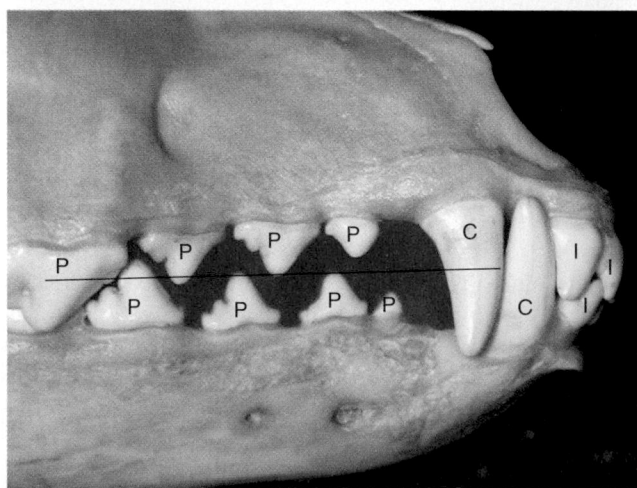

Figure 28-2 Normal scissors occlusion in a dog: *I*, incisors, *C*, canines, *P*, premolars, *M*, molars. **A,** Anterior view of a dog. **B,** Lateral view of a dog skull. Note how the premolar cusp tips (with the exception of the short first premolar teeth) contact the line midway between the maxillary and mandibular occlusal planes.

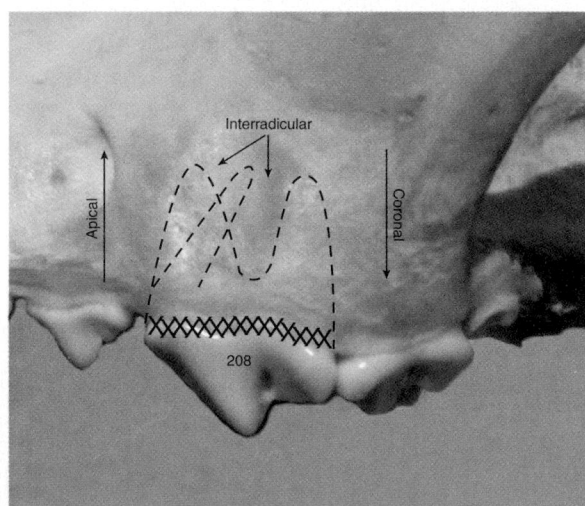

$\diagdown\!\!\times\!\!\times\!\!\times$ = Gingival or cervical area

Figure 28-3 Positional terminology commonly used in dentistry. **A,** is a palatal view of the dog maxilla. The midline is marked with a line, and the mesial and distal tooth surfaces are marked with an M or D, respectively. The cingulum is visible on the maxillary incisors. **B,** The mandibular first molar and **C,** the maxillary fourth premolar in a dog skull. The *X*'s indicates the cervical or gingival area of the teeth.

penetration of the palatal bone resulting in an oronasal fistula.

An anterior cross bite is when one or more maxillary incisors are displaced palatally so that they are lingual to the mandibular incisor(s). A posterior cross bite is when one or more premolar or molar teeth are displaced palatally (maxillary) or buccally (mandibular) from their normal relationship. These three malocclusions can exist in a class II or III malocclusion as well, so the entire dentition must be examined to make the proper classification.

A class II malocclusion (distoclusion) (Figure 28-5) is when the mandibular dentition is positioned distal to its normal maxillary counterpart. A class II malocclusion can be a result of an abnormally long maxilla or an abnormally short mandible.

A class III malocclusion (mesioclusion) (Figure 28-6) is when the mandibular teeth occlude mesial to their normal maxillary counterpart. This condition can be a result of an abnormally short maxilla or an abnormally long mandible.

The terms *brachygnathic* and *prognathic* refer to the length of the mandible in relation to the maxilla. Less informed individuals will commonly use terms such as *parrot mouth* or *brachygnathic* to describe a class II malocclusion and *undershot* or *prognathic* to describe a class III malocclusion. This terminology is not ideal because it does not always correctly identify the abnormal jaw. For instance, bulldogs might be described as having a prognathic malocclusion (long mandible), but the abnormality causing the malocclusion is actually a chondrodysplastic maxilla (failure of the maxillary bone to grow properly). It is important to have a general understanding of these terms so that veterinary professionals and personnel can understand and communicate with breeders and pet owners that use these terms. A detailed study of occlusion is necessary before considering orthodontic treatment for pets or counseling breeders on malocclusions.

The shape of a dog or cat's skull must also be evaluated when performing a dental occlusion evaluation. We recognize three types of skulls: brachycephalic, mesaticephalic (or mesocephalic), and dolichocephalic. Brachycephalic breeds have a wide skull with a short maxilla. Examples of these breeds are boxers, bulldogs, and Persian cats. Mesaticephalic breeds have a well-proportioned skull width and maxillary length. Examples are Dalmatians, Labrador retrievers, and German shepards. The dolichocephalic breeds have a narrow skull and long maxilla, and some examples are the sight hounds (greyhound, whippet) and Siamese cats. It is better to classify the brachycephalic breeds occlusion as a normal class III occlusion (breed normal) because we know that they do not have a scissors occlusion and we expect to see a mesioclusion relationship of the teeth in these breeds.

A wry bite is a condition where one segment of the jaw is disproportionate to the other segment. For instance the left mandible is longer than the right mandible. The disproportionate jaw length can occur in either quadrant of the maxilla or mandible.

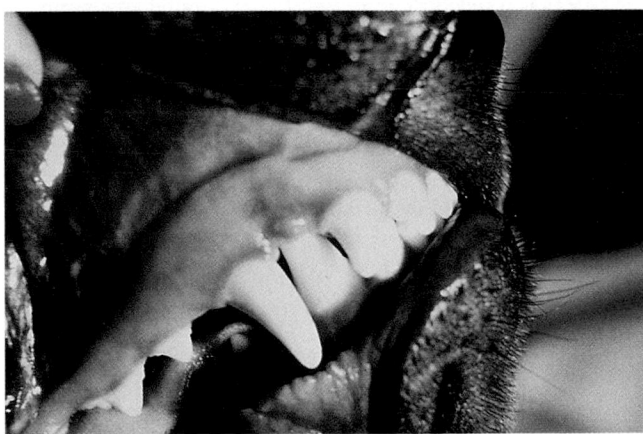

Figure 28-4 Class I malocclusion (neutroclusion) in a dog. The right mandibular canine is tipped lingually and occludes into the maxillary gingival tissue.

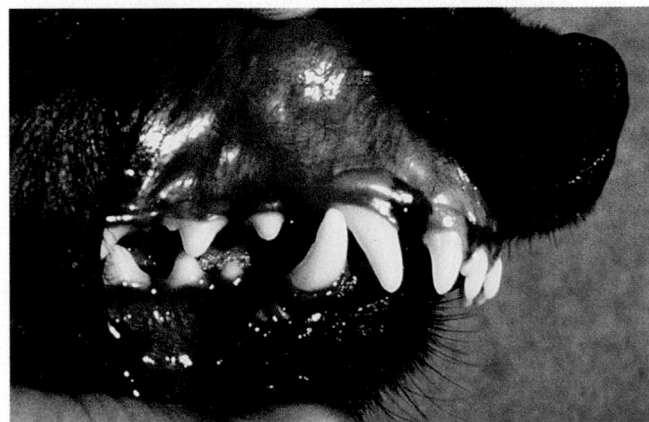

Figure 28-5 Class II malocclusion (distoclusion) in a dog.

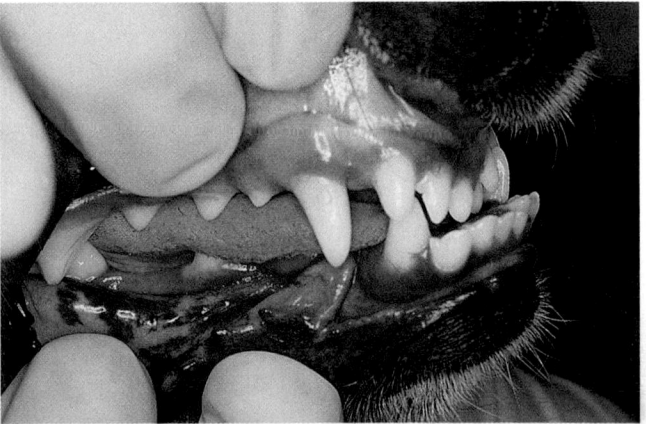

Figure 28-6 Class III malocclusion (mesioclusion) in a dog.

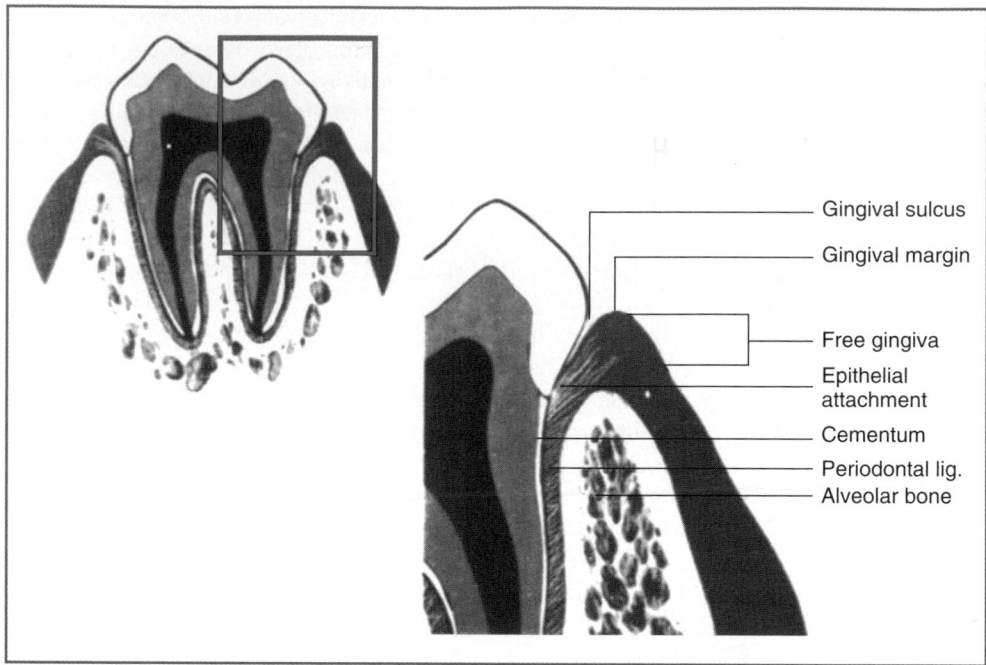

Figure 28-7 Structures collectively referred to as the *periodontium*. The tooth is suspended in the socket by the periodontal ligament. (From Bojrab MJ, Tholen M: *Small animal oral medicine and surgery,* Philadelphia, 1990, Lea & Febiger.)

PERIODONTICS AND PERIODONTAL DISEASE

Periodontics is the branch of dentistry concerned with the study and treatment of the periodontium. The periodontium is composed of the supporting structures of the tooth. These supporting structures are the gingiva, periodontal ligament, alveolar and supporting bone (tooth socket), and the cementum of the tooth root (Figure 28-7). Healthy gingiva has a sharp, tapered edge (margin) that lies closely against the crown of the tooth. The free gingiva forms a moat around the tooth called the *gingival sulcus.* The epithelial attachment of the gingiva to the cementum of the tooth root forms the bottom extent of the gingival sulcus. The depth of this sulcus ranges from 1 to 3 mm in a healthy mouth of a dog and is up to 1 mm deep in the cat.

Periodontitis means inflammation of the structures around the tooth (Greek *peri,* around + *odous,* tooth + *itis,* inflammation). It is the most common disease of animals and humans and is caused by plaque. Approximately 80% of dogs and 70% of cats have some form of periodontal disease by 3 years of age.

Plaque is a white, slippery film that collects around the gingival sulcus of the tooth. It is composed of bacteria, food debris, exfoliated cells, and salivary glycoproteins. Over time, plaque will mineralize on the teeth to form dental calculus, a brown or yellow deposit (Figure 28-8). As the plaque collects around the tooth, it damages the gingival tissues by releasing bacterial endotoxins. The animal's immune system further damages these tissues through the release of harmful by-products from white blood cells as they attempt to

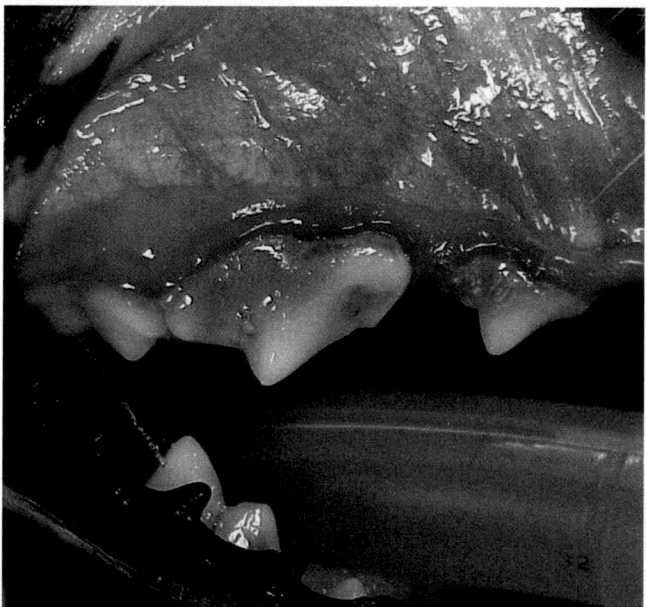

Figure 28-8 The calculus and plaque deposits on these teeth have caused the gingiva to become inflamed (gingivitis). (Courtesy Dr. Alfred G. Stevens, Sherwood South Animal Hospital, Baton Rouge, La.)

destroy the bacteria. In the early stages, the gingiva becomes inflamed and bleeds easily. This stage is called *gingivitis* (Figure 28-8). As the disease progresses and destruction of the periodontium begins to occur (e.g., loss of alveolar bone, periodontal ligament, and gingiva), an irreversible stage of disease begins that is termed *periodontitis* (Figure 28-9).

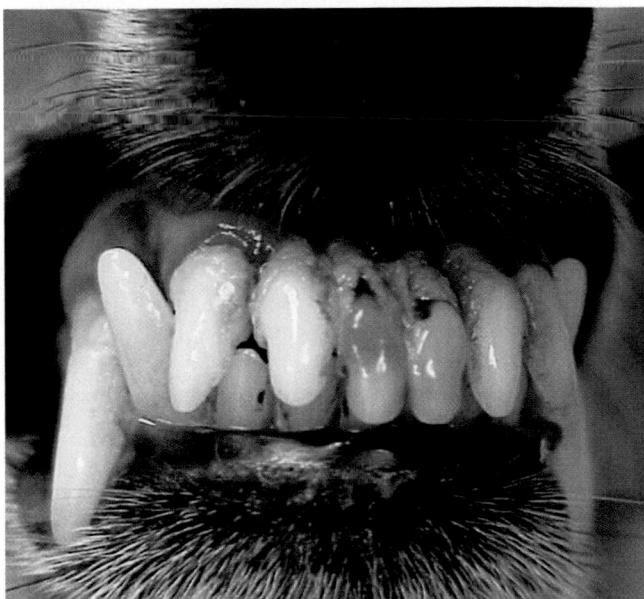

Figure 28-9 Periodontal disease has destroyed a significant portion of the alveolar bone and periodontal ligament of these incisor teeth. The gingiva has receded from the crowns of these teeth, and the tooth roots are now exposed. (Courtesy Dr. Alfred G. Stevens, Sherwood South Animal Hospital, Baton Rouge, La.)

TECHNICIAN NOTE

The key to prevention of periodontal disease is to minimize plaque accumulation by means of proper diet, routine professional dental scaling and polishing, and daily teeth brushing or mouth rinsing.

Periodontal disease is difficult to control once it has developed. For this reason, great emphasis must be placed on its prevention. Many diseases can contribute to the severity of periodontal disease, but the bacteria in plaque are believed to be the primary cause.

When periodontitis is already present, destruction of the periodontal tissues has begun and will continue if not treated. Once the periodontal ligament is destroyed, it is extremely difficult to replace. As the tooth begins to lose its periodontal tissue, it becomes more susceptible to plaque accumulation in the deep periodontal pockets that form around the tooth root or roots. When the tooth loses a significant portion of its periodontium, it becomes mobile (loose) and will eventually fall out. This is nature's way of clearing the infection from the body. The infection, however, is usually present for months to years before the tooth is eventually lost. During this time, the bacteria can gain entrance to the animal's bloodstream and become systemic, spreading to numerous organs such as the liver, kidney, heart, and lungs.

For patients with periodontal disease, the treatment goal is to remove the plaque and calculus from the teeth and to minimize plaque reattachment. Treatments to minimize plaque accumulation include those listed for prevention of

Box 28-2 PERIODONTAL DISEASE

Grade 1: Reversible gingivitis.
Grade 2: Advanced gingivitis/early periodontitis—some attachment loss present (1 to 2 mm).
Grade 3: Moderate periodontitis—moderate attachment loss (3 to 6 mm). These teeth have a fair to guarded prognosis.
Grade 4: Advanced periodontitis—advanced attachment loss (>6 mm). These teeth usually have a poor prognosis.

periodontal disease, as well as periodontal surgery when deep periodontal pockets have formed around tooth roots.

Root debridement and subgingival curettage are important procedures in periodontal treatment. *Root debridement is* the removal of calculus from the diseased tooth roots. Curettes are used to clean the root surface using multiple overlapping strokes in vertical, horizontal, and oblique directions as necessary to clean the root surface. Pressure created with each stroke ranges from firm to light as the tooth root is cleaned. Care must be taken not to gouge the root surface. It was once felt that the tooth root cementum under the calculus was diseased and needed to be removed along with the calculus. This approach was called *root planing*. Present-day research seems to favor a less aggressive approach to cleaning the exposed tooth root surface. This approach is called *root debridement,* and the goal is to remove the root calculus while preserving the tooth root cementum.

The gingiva covering these roots must be cleaned of foreign debris and granulation tissue as well. This procedure is called *subgingival curettage,* and curettes are used for this procedure too. The blade of the curette is directed toward the pocket lining, and digital pressure is placed on the gingival tissue to support it while the tissue is debrided.

Ultrasonic instruments can be very beneficial for subgingival cleaning, but precautions must be taken. The ultrasonic frequency can actually lyse bacteria in the periodontal pocket. The instruments are efficient at calculus removal and help prevent hand fatigue. They do generate heat and a continuous water supply must be present to strike the instrument tip to keep it cool. Special ultrasonic instrument tips must be used to work in the narrow confines of the periodontal pocket space. These tips are smaller than the supragingival tips.

Subgingival curettage and root debridement can be done without incising and elevating the gingival tissue as long as there is sufficient access to the roots and gingival pocket epithelium to thoroughly debride the area. This process is called *closed root debridement.* If the gingiva impedes proper cleaning of the tooth roots, the gingiva should be incised and reflected to allow visualization and instrumentation of the roots for proper debridement. This technique is termed *open root debridement* and must be performed by a veterinarian or dentist under the direct supervision of a veterinarian.

A grading system is helpful to categorize periodontal disease and determine appropriate treatment (Box 28-2). Grade I periodontal disease is a reversible gingivitis and requires routine dental cleaning. Grade II periodontal disease is an early form of periodontitis. There is some attachment loss (approximately 1 to 2 mm), and root debridement or subgingival curettage may be required. Grade III periodontal disease is considered a moderate degree of periodontitis; attachment loss is in the range of 3 to 6 mm and root debridement, subgingival curettage, and periodontal surgery are often required. These teeth have a fair to guarded prognosis. Grade IV periodontal disease is severe periodontitis; attachment loss is greater than 6 mm, and the tooth has a poor prognosis. Many of these teeth are extracted. Efforts to save these teeth require root debridement, subgingival curettage, periodontal surgery, and possibly periodontal splinting. (The attachment losses mentioned above apply to dogs, not cats.)

ADVANCED PERIODONTAL PROCEDURES

Several types of gingival flap procedures are used to expose the diseased tooth roots when deep periodontal pockets are present. The instruments required to create the gingival flaps are a scalpel blade (no. 11 or 15) and handle as well as a periosteal elevator. Small elevators, such as the Cislak EX-9, are commonly used for single teeth or small surgery sites. Larger periosteal elevators, such as the Molt 9, are used for larger teeth and/or surgery sites (Figure 28-10). Once the roots and pocket lining are exposed and debrided with an ultrasonic scaler and curette, the surgery site is lavaged with 0.2% chlorhexidine followed by sterile saline. The tissue is reapposed with 4-0 absorbable suture material placed interdentally in a simple interrupted pattern, and digital pressure is applied to the gingiva for 60 seconds. The patient should be placed on a soft food diet for 1 week and have the mouth rinsed daily with a 0.2% chlorhexidine solution for 2 weeks. The owner should start brushing the teeth 1 week postoperatively and be very gentle around the surgery site.

Loose teeth can be stabilized by splinting them to adjacent teeth. This helps prevent tooth loss while the periodontium is healing. A thorough dental cleaning with radiographs, root debridement, and subgingival curettage must be performed before splinting the loose teeth. Splinting is

performed only if the pet owner is willing to provide dental home care and have the teeth professionally cleaned as needed. If the owner does not properly clean the splints and teeth, the splints will retain foreign debris and worsen the condition. Pets with advanced periodontal disease may require professional dental cleaning every 3 to 4 months.

PROPER DIET

The semimoist and canned pet foods are tacky and tend to stick to the teeth. This accelerates plaque accumulation.

> **✎ TECHNICIAN NOTE**
>
> Dry pet food is the diet of choice for minimizing the rate of plaque accumulation on the dentition. Several dry pet food manufacturers have diets designed to minimize plaque and calculus formation.

Tartar control pet products have entered the marketplace. The active ingredients are sodium hexametaphosphate (HMP) and sodium tripolyphosphate. The tartar control products work by sequestering the calcium in plaque fluids to reduce calculus formation. Research studies on dogs and cats have shown that these products can reduce calculus up to 46% in dogs and 30% in cats.

Hill's Pet Nutrition has produced a pet food called t/d that is nutritionally balanced and designed to help minimize calculus buildup. The t/d biscuit fibers are longer than traditional fibers and are primarily oriented in one direction to keep the biscuit from crumbling readily when the dog or cat bites into it. This design allows the biscuit to mechanically scrape the sides of the teeth clean as the teeth penetrate the biscuit.

Proper chew toys should be encouraged. Rawhide bones and chews are excellent for exercising the teeth and periodontium to help maintain a healthy mouth. Some pets have a desire to chew on hard objects such as rocks. Hard objects can damage the teeth and should be removed from the pet's environment when possible. Any chew toy has the potential to cause damage, so the owner should monitor the pet while using these items.

The Veterinary Oral Health Council (VOHC) is a committee of veterinary dentists and dental scientists with experience in scientific protocols and study design. The council members review research submitted by pet food manufacturers that wish to state on their packaging that their product has the VOHC seal of approval. If the product merits the VOHC seal, the consumer can be reassured that regular use of the product has been shown to reduce the severity of periodontal disease in pets.

DENTAL SCALING AND POLISHING

Most pets are admitted to the veterinary clinic in the morning for a dental cleaning. The veterinarian or veterinary technician should admit the pet for the dental procedure.

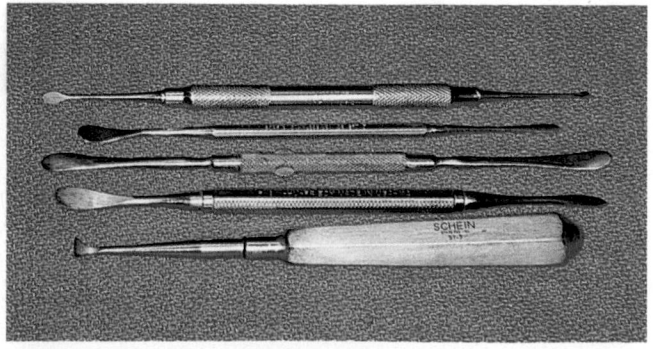

Figure 28-10 Periosteal elevators. *Top to bottom:* Cislak Ex-9, Schein no. 7, Freer, Molt no. 9, Schein ST 7.

Ideally the pet has been examined prior to the dental appointment to identify any serious dental problems and have preanesthetic blood work submitted when necessary. If this has not been done prior, it should be done at this time. It is important to confirm that the pet has been fasted and have the owner sign the anesthesia and dental procedure consent form. The owner should write the phone numbers where they can be reached in case unforeseen dental problems are detected. Many veterinary clinics have the owners state on the procedure release whether they give permission for tooth extraction. It is also a good idea to specifically ask the owner what they wish to have done if attempts to contact them fail and the pet needs dental treatment beyond a cleaning. An example of such a dental procedure consent form is show in Figure 28-11.

Before beginning the dental cleaning procedure, the dental treatment area should be prepared. The proper instruments should be out for easy access, and they should be clean and sharp (Figure 28-12). The veterinarian should give the patient a preanesthetic examination and evaluate the oral cavity and periodontium for signs of bacterial infection. When oral infection is present, preoperative antibiotics should be given to help prevent the systemic spread of oral bacteria to internal organs. Patients with moderate or advanced periodontal disease should begin antibiotic treatment at least 3 days before the dental cleaning procedure.

The patient is anesthetized, and a cuffed endotracheal tube is used to prevent water and foreign debris from entering the trachea. Care should be taken not to over inflate the endotracheal tube cuff, which could damage the trachea. In 1994 the American Veterinary Medical Association Professional Liability Insurance Trust received 18 claims on pets (all cats) diagnosed with subcutaneous emphysema following an anesthetic procedure. All cases were intubated, and 16 patients were under anesthesia for dentistry procedures. The cause of the subcutaneous emphysema was not confirmed in every case, but tracheal tears were found in some of the cases. To avoid injury to the trachea, disconnect the animals from the anesthesia circuit when repositioning them, minimize movement of the endotracheal tube, and inflate the cuff just enough to stop the leak of anesthetic gases.

> ### ✎ TECHNICIAN NOTE
> To avoid injury to the trachea, disconnect the patient from the anesthesia circuit when repositioning is needed, minimize movement of the endotracheal tube, and inflate the cuff just enough to stop the leak of anesthetic gases.

The patient's head should be placed on a slight incline (nose downward) if possible. This can be done by tilting a surgery table or placing a rolled towel under the animal's neck to ensure that the pharynx is higher than the nose (Figure 28-13). This allows water and debris to run out of the mouth while mechanical scalers are being used.

Once the anesthetized patient is prepared, the technician should don the proper attire and begin the dental cleaning. Proper attire consists of a mask, gloves, eye protection (glasses or a shield), cap, and laboratory coat. It is important to wear these protective coverings because large numbers of bacteria are aerosolized during the mechanical scaling procedure, and these could be inhaled or could saturate clothing, leading to contamination of other areas in the hospital.

The dental cleaning begins with a thorough examination of the oral cavity. The mouth is propped open, and the cheeks and tongue are lifted to evaluate all areas of the mouth thoroughly. Do not forget to examine the tongue, tonsils, and pharynx as well. Just before beginning the oral examination a chlorhexidine rinse can be given to the oral cavity to decrease the bacterial load substantially. This increases safety for the pet and dental care provider. Clinical findings should be recorded at either the beginning or the end of the procedure. Important findings to include are areas of ulceration, missing teeth, mobile teeth (loose teeth), periodontal pockets, receded gingiva, furcation exposure, degree of periodontal disease, and fractured teeth (Figure 28-14). Box 28-3 and Figure 28-3 defines and illustrates dental terminology that is useful for describing specific locations in the mouth.

Missing teeth are often the result of tooth exfoliation from advanced periodontal disease but they can be missing because of other causes. If there is a space present where the tooth should be and the pet has a history to periodontal disease, there is a good chance it lost the tooth or the tooth was extracted previously. *Hypodontia* or *oligodontia* are terms used to describe animals with a reduced number of teeth. Anodontia is when an animal does not have any teeth. If the history of a missing tooth is not known, it is important to take a radiograph of the area to make sure the tooth is not impacted or that there are no diseased root fragments remaining.

Mouth gags for veterinary patients are available through supply companies. Most dog and cat mouth gags work well for the intended species, but care should be taken not to put excessive tension on the jaws with a powerful mouth gag. If the resistance of the springs is to great, it will create a lot of pressure on the temporomandibular joint (TMJ) that may result in postoperative problems for the pet. If the mouth gags appear to open the pets mouth too wide, you can avoid this by customizing a mouth gag with a tuberculin syringe or a 3-cc syringe case. Remove the plunger if using the syringe and cut the ends to the appropriate length. This creates a hole large enough for the canine teeth to fit in and opens the mouth without excessive force.

Tooth mobility can be recorded on a scale of 1 to 3 (Box 28-4). Multirooted teeth can develop furcation exposure as periodontal disease progresses. A furcation is the area between adjacent tooth roots on a multirooted tooth. The maxillary fourth premolar has two furcations. One is the mesial furcation created by the mesiobuccal and palatal

Veterinary Clinic   *Dr(s). Name & Credentials*
Street Address
City, State, Zip Code
Office Telephone Number
Office Fax Number

Anesthesia and Dental Treatment Consent Form

Owner's Name: _____

Pet's Name: _____ Breed: _____ Sex: _____

Our goal is to provide your pet with as healthy a mouth as possible. Your commitment to this goal is important to our long-term success.

DENTAL PROCEDURES CAN RUN FROM $ TO $ OR HIGHER.

I, the undersigned, certify that I am the owner/agent of the animal described above. I give (Veterinary Clinic Name) permission to perform the following procedures:

_____

Estimates of complications (based on information available at this time) for my animal from the procedure(s) listed above are:

_____% may have reoccurrence of the same problem after treatment (or surgery)
_____% may develop infection at the surgery site
_____% may have persistent infection of the treated tooth root(s)
_____% may fracture the treated tooth or dislodge the filling
_____% may have complications or death from anesthesia and/or surgery
_____% _____
_____% _____

Please check one of the following below:

[ ] Perform any extractions, x-rays, or periodontal surgery necessary to avoid another anesthetic later.

[ ] Call me first, but if you cannot reach me by telephone, you may proceed with any procedure(s) deemed necessary.

[ ] Do nothing else unless you reach me by telephone. I understand that you will wake my pet up without doing even the simplest of any additional procedure(s). I also understand that should I agree to the recommended procedure(s) at a later date, there will be additional charges for the anesthetic and procedure(s).

The estimated cost of the procedure(s) described to me will be in the range of $_____ to $_____.
I understand this is just an estimate and the final bill may be more or less than this estimate.

Signature: _____ Date: _____

Between 9:00 AM and 4:00 PM I can be reached at _(_____)_____

Figure 28-11 Anesthesia and dental consent form. The appropriate dollar amounts and percentages are filled in for the particular case.

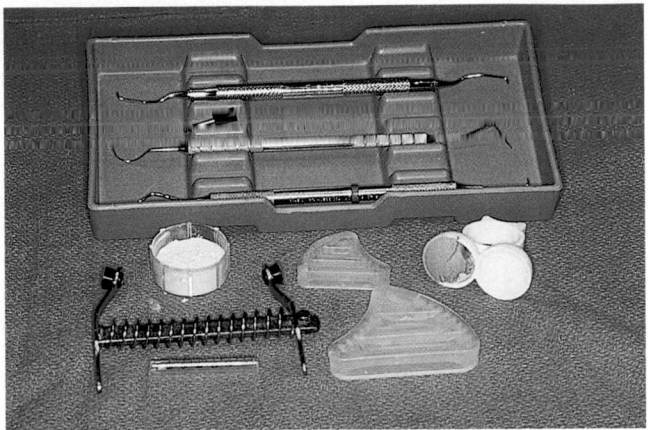

Figure 28-12 Dental cleaning tray (subgingival curette, explorer and periodontal probe, supragingival curette, Prophy cup), Prophy paste in ring, variety of mouth gags, flour pumice.

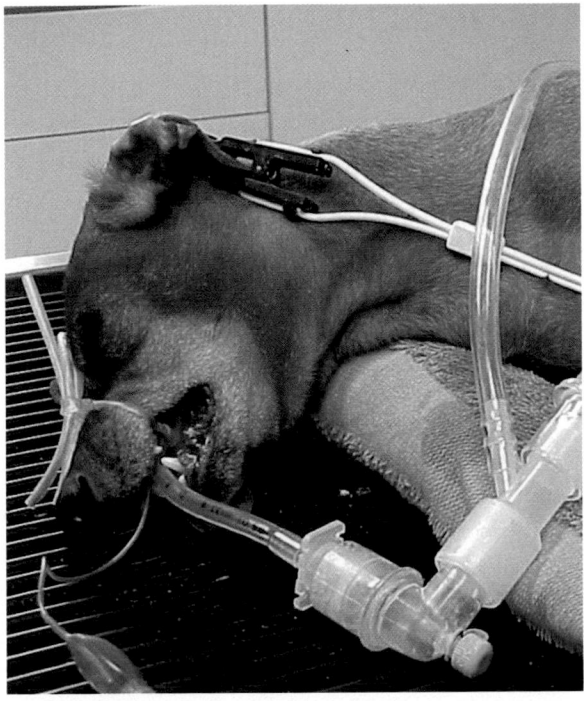

Figure 28-13 Proper patient positioning for dental scaling and polishing. Note that the head is placed in a downward position. (Courtesy Dr. Alfred G. Stevens, Sherwood South Animal Hospital, Baton Rouge, La.)

Box 28-3 DENTAL TERMINOLOGY FOR DIRECTION AND LOCATION

apical: Toward the apex of the tooth root
buccal: Side of the tooth that faces the cheek (posterior teeth)
cervical: Toward or at the cementoenamel junction (neck) of the tooth
coronal: Toward the crown of the tooth
distal: Side of the tooth that is farthest from the midline of the maxillary or mandibular dental arch
gingival: Area of the tooth toward or at the gingival tissue
incisal: Biting surface of the anterior teeth
interdental: Area between two adjacent teeth in the same arch
interradicular: Area between roots of multirooted teeth
labial: Surface of the tooth nearest the lips; term used to describe the front surface of incisor teeth as opposed to the distal surface that faces the tongue
lingual: Side of the tooth that faces the tongue (applied to mandibular teeth)
mesial: Surface of the tooth that is closest to the midline of the maxillary or mandibular dental arch
occlusal: The chewing surfaces of the caudal teeth
palatal: The side of the tooth that faces the palate (applied to maxillary teeth)

Box 28-4 TOOTH MOBILITY

Grade I: Slight tooth movement
Grade II: Moderate tooth movement of 1 mm
Grade III: Marked tooth movement of more than 1 mm

Box 28-5 CLASSIFICATION OF TOOTH FURCATION EXPOSURE

Class I: The furcation can just be detected with a dental probe with very minimal bone involvement.
Class II: The periodontal probe can be placed into the furcation but not all the way through to the other side
Class III: The periodontal probe can be passed all the way through the furcation to the other side of the tooth.

---

roots. The second is the buccal furcation created by the mesiobuccal and distal roots. As periodontal disease progresses and bone is lost around the tooth roots, the furcations become exposed to the oral cavity. These spots should be identified and recorded. There is a classification system for furcation exposure that should be noted on the pet's dental chart (Box 28-5). Sites of furcation exposure can be difficult to clean and periodontal disease can rapidly accelerate in these areas. Keeping good records on these areas is helpful so that they are not missed on future dental

treatments and the owner can be shown where the problem areas are for diligent home care.

It is preferable to refer to the teeth by number rather than having to use the laborious descriptive terminology (e.g., 208 as opposed to "the left upper fourth premolar"). Most people who do a large volume of dentistry will adapt a numbering system. Unfortunately there are several numbering systems in existence, which can cause confusion. The most commonly used system is the Modified Triadan System. Teeth in the maxillary right quadrant are assigned

Veterinary Clinic Name
Street Address
City, State Zip Code
Phone Number
Fax Number

Dr(s). Name & Credentials

Canine Dental Record

Patient: *Patch Smith*

Date: *4/1/04*

Reason for Visit: _____

History: *Eats dry food only; chews on bones* _____

NPO ✓

Right Upper Quadrant   Left Upper Quadrant

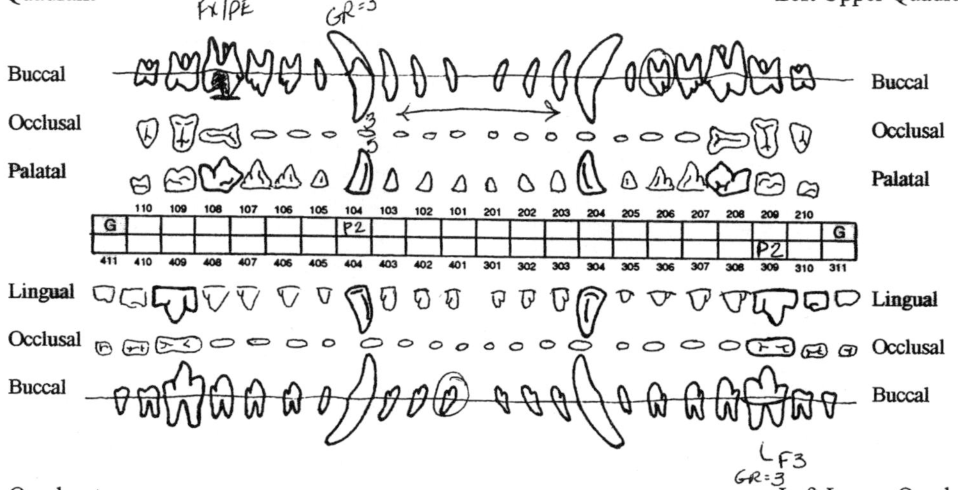

Buccal   Buccal
Occlusal   Occlusal
Palatal   Palatal

Lingual   Lingual
Occlusal   Occlusal
Buccal   Buccal

Right Lower Quadrant   Left Lower Quadrant

KEY

CE - Cervical Erosion	F1 - Grade 1 Furcation	GH - Ging. Hyperplasia	M1 - Grade 1 Mobility	ONF - Oronasal Fistula
D - Discolored Tooth	F2 - Grade 2 Furcation	GR - Gingival Recession	M2 - Grade 2 Mobility	PE - Pulp Exposure
E - Enamel Defect	F3 - Grade 3 Furcation	HX - Hemisection	M3 - Grade 3 Mobility	PH - Pulp Hemorrhage
FX - Fractured Tooth			M4 - Grade 4 Mobility	PN - Pulp Necrosis
			O - Missing Tooth	RD - Retained Deciduous Tooth

RR - Retained Root   ↻ - Rotated Tooth
SN - Supernumerary Tooth
T - Twinning   ↔ - Crowding
W - Worn Tooth
                            ↓ or ↑ - Super-erupted Tooth

Calculus
None
Slight (s
Moderate (m)
Heavy (h)

Gingivitis
None
Mild (1)
Moderate (2)
Severe (3)

Periodontitis
None
Early (P1)
Moderate (P2)
Advanced (P3)

Diagnosis: *Fractured 108 with pulp exposure; crowding of maxillary incisors; grade II periodontal disease of 104 with 5mm pocket on palatal aspect and 3 mm pocket on buccal side. Also 3mm of gingival recession for total attachment loss on buccal side of 8mm (5mm pocket + 3mm recession = 8mm total attachment loss). Missing teeth 206 & 401; grade II periodontal disease of 309 with grade III furcation exposure + 3mm gingival recession on buccal aspect; Moderate calculus & gingivitis.*

Figure 28-14 **A,** Canine dental record: note each tooth has a three-digit number.

Veterinary Clinic Name
Street Address
City, State Zip Code
Phone Number
Fax Number

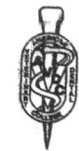

Dr(s). Name & Credentials

Feline Dental Record

Patient:_____   Date:_____

Reason for Visit:_____

History:_____
_____
_____NPO_____

Right Upper Quadrant   Left Upper Quadrant

Buccal

Occlusal

Palatal

| 109 | 108 | 107 | 106 | | 104 | 103 | 102 | 101 | 201 | 202 | 203 | 204 | | 206 | 207 | 208 | 209 |

G   G

| 409 | 408 | 407 | | 404 | 403 | 402 | 401 | 301 | 302 | 303 | 304 | | 307 | 308 | 309 |

Lingual

Occlusal

Buccal

Right Lower Quadrant   Left Lower Quadrant

KEY

D - Discolored Tooth	F1 - Grade 1 Furcation	GH - Ging. Hyperplasia	M1 - Grade 1 Mobility	ONF - Oronasal Fistula
E - Enamel Defect	F2 - Grade 2 Furcation	GR - Gingival Recession	M2 - Grade 2 Mobility	PE - Pulp Exposure
ERR – External Root Resorption	F3 - Grade 3 Furcation	HX - Hemisection	M3 - Grade 3 Mobility	PH - Pulp Hemorrhage
FORL – Feline odontoclastic	F4 - Grade 4 Furcation	IRR – Internal Root Resorption	M4 - Grade 4 Mobility	PN - Pulp Necrosis
Resorptive Lesion	FX - Fractured Tooth		O - Missing Tooth	RD - Retained Deciduous Tooth

RR - Retained Root   ⟳ - Rotated Tooth
RSP – Root Resorption
SN - Supernumerary Tooth ⟷ - Crowding
T - Twinning
W - Worn Tooth   ↑ or ↓ - Super-erupted Tooth

Calculus	**Gingivitis**	**Periodontitis**
None	None	None
Slight (s	Mild (1)	Early (P1)
Moderate (m)	Moderate (2)	Moderate (P2)
Heavy (h)	Severe (3)	Advanced (P3)

Diagnosis:_____
_____
_____
_____
_____
_____
_____
_____
_____
_____
_____

B

Figure 28-14 B, Feline dental record.

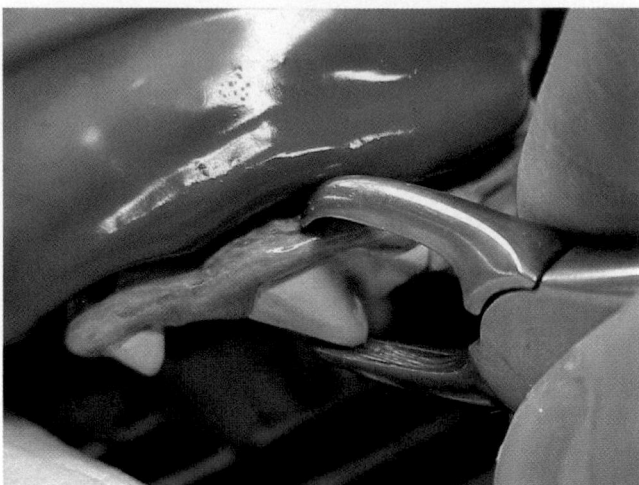

Figure 28-15 Large pieces of calculus can be quickly removed with forceps. Care should be taken not to place excessive pressure on the tooth, especially cusp tips, to avoid fracturing the tooth. (Courtesy Dr. Alfred G. Stevens, Sherwood South Animal Hospital, Baton Rouge, La.)

the 100 series, left maxillary quadrant 200 series, left mandibular quadrant 300 series, and right mandibular quadrant 400 series. Each tooth within the quadrant has a two-digit number starting at the anterior midline and moving along the dental arch in a caudal direction. The right maxillary first incisor is 101, right maxillary second incisor is 102, right maxillary third incisor 103, right maxillary canine 104, and so on. The left maxillary canine is 204, left mandibular canine is 304, and right mandibular canine is 404 (Figure 28-14). Deciduous teeth are assigned the 500 series for right maxillary quadrant, 600 series for left maxillary quadrant, 700 series for left mandibular quadrant, and 800 series for right mandibular quadrant.

Felids have fewer teeth than canids, so the system is modified in felids to keep numbers consistent. In other words, no. 108 should refer to the right upper fourth premolar whether discussing a dog, hyena, cat, or lion. Since the cat has three maxillary premolars instead of four like the dog, the 105 number is skipped and the first tooth behind 104 (maxillary right canine) is 106 (Figure 28-14). The feline mandible has only two premolars, so 305, 306, 405, and 406 are skipped, and the numbering starts with 307 and 407. Keeping these numbers consistent among species allows veterinary personnel to quickly learn the tooth by one specific number. When someone says tooth 208 is fractured, one should think of the left maxillary fourth premolar (carnassial tooth) since its anatomic shape is very similar for all mammalian carnivores.

Large pieces of calculus can often be easily removed with calculus-removing forceps (Figure 28-15). If the patient has minimal amounts of calculus present, the calculus can be removed with hand scaling instruments alone. Electric and air-driven mechanical scalers can be used on patients with significant amounts of calculus present (most patients!)

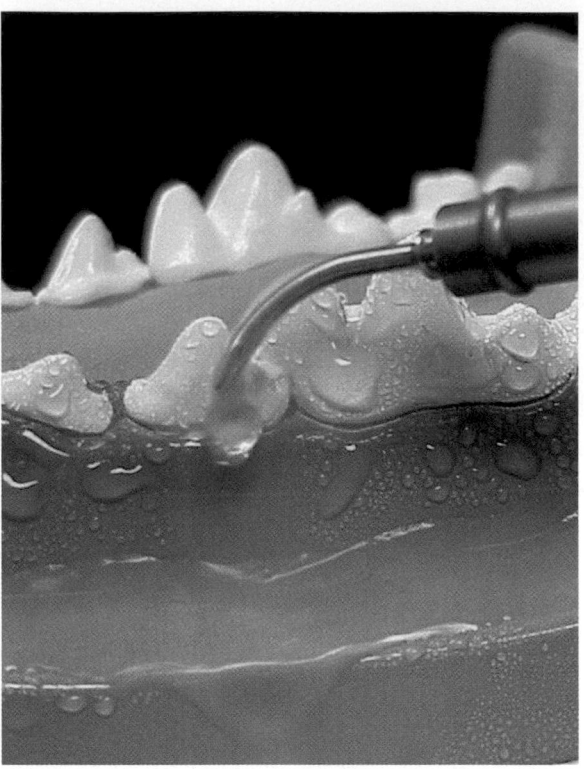

Figure 28-16 An ultrasonic scaler is used to clean the tooth of calculus and plaque deposits. The water helps cool the instrument tip and flush debris off the tooth and gingiva. (Courtesy Dr. Alfred G. Stevens, Sherwood South Animal Hospital, Baton Rouge, La.)

because they remove calculus rapidly (Figure 28-16). Since the mechanical vibrations of the tips of these scalers dislodge the calculus, minimal pressure is used when operating these instruments. Most of these instruments generate heat owing to the rapid vibrations, so it is imperative to use irrigation to cool the working tips of these instruments so that the pulp tissue does not receive thermal damage.

> **✎ TECHNICIAN NOTE**
>
> When using mechanical scalers, the instrument must be kept moving on the tooth surface and should not be on the tooth for more than 10 to 15 seconds to avoid heat buildup.

If the scaling of a tooth is not completed in 10 to 15 seconds, the adjacent tooth can be scaled while the first tooth cools. Once cool, the first tooth can be scaled again.

Most dental cleaning procedures require the use of mechanical and hand scalers. Hand scalers can be used to reach those areas that are inaccessible to the mechanical scaler.

There are a large number of different types of dental scalers and curettes on the market. It is important to understand the different components of these instruments so that they can be used properly and aid the technician's decision on which instruments to purchase. Scalers and curettes

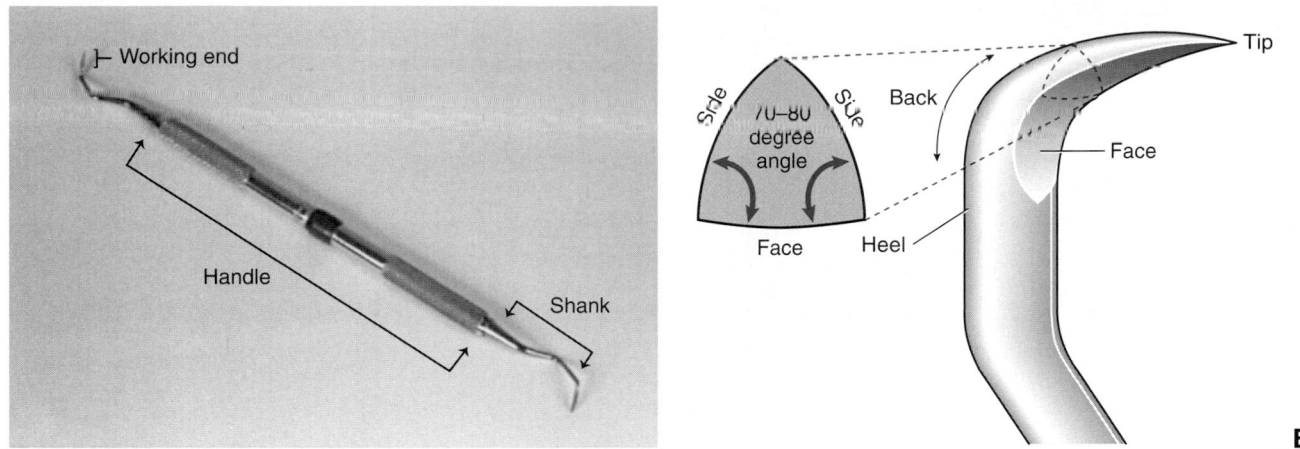

Figure 28-17 **A,** Supragingival scalers are used to scale the crowns of the teeth. Jacquette scaler is shown here. **B,** Drawing of the working end. The face of the instrument joins the sides to create a blade edge of 70 to 80 degrees.

are designed with three main components: the handle, shank, and working end (Figure 28-17). The handles can be purchased in slim to wide diameters and be hollow or solid, based on personal preference. The shank attaches the handle to the working end and allows adaptation of the working end to the tooth surfaces. The shank is the most variable part of the curette. A relatively straight shank is good for working in the anterior segment of the mouth and in deep periodontal pockets. An angled shank improves instrumentation in the distal segment of the mouth where space is minimal.

The working end of the instrument has several components: the blade or cutting edge, back, face, heel, and toe or tip. The blade is the portion that cleans the tooth and gingival pocket epithelium. The face of the working end is the flat surface, which creates one of the edges of each blade. The back is the rounded bottom of the working end. These instruments can be purchased as single or double ended depending on whether they have a working end at one or both ends of the handle. Double-ended scalers are designed so that one end adapts to the anterior surface of the tooth and the other end adapts to the distal surface. The term *scaler* includes supragingival (above the gingival margin) and subgingival (below the gingival margin) scalers. All curettes can be used subgingivally because they have a round toe and back to help prevent damage to the gingival tissue (Figure 28-18). They may be used supragingivally as well. Supragingival scalers are not to be used subgingivally because they have a pointed tip that could damage the gingival sulcus (Figure 28-17, *B).* Supragingival scalers are often referred to as *scalers* and subgingival scalers as *curettes.*

Dental scalers should be held in a modified pen grasp (Figure 28-19). The thumb and index finger hold the handle close to the shank. The middle finger is placed just in front of the index finger to further support the instrument. The ring finger is placed on a stable surface (e.g., the tooth or gingiva) to act as a fulcrum and support the hand. The strokes of the scaler should be made through the wrist and not the fingers to avoid operator hand fatigue.

To remove subgingival calculus from the gingival sulcus, the curette is placed to the bottom of the gingival sulcus with its curved smooth back toward the gingival epithelium. Once it is seated at the bottom of the sulcus, the cutting edge is turned to engage the calculus on the tooth root. The curette is then pulled toward the crown to dislodge the calculus and remove it from the sulcus. This pull stroke is repeated until all the calculus has been removed from the tooth. Proper instrument positioning takes practice and concentration. It is important to master this technique to ensure that the instruments do not damage the gingival tissue and the subgingival calculus is completely removed.

After the teeth have been properly scaled, they must be polished. This step is performed to smooth the microscopic pits and scratches on the tooth surface created by the scaling procedure and routine chewing. If this step is skipped, the plaque will rapidly return because of increased surface area created by the scratches. Polishing is achieved using a slow-speed handpiece with a Prophy cup attached and filled with Prophy paste. Enough pressure should be applied to just flare the edge of the Prophy cup. Flaring the edge will allow it to be gently inserted into the gingival sulcus to polish subgingivally (Figure 28-20).

All surfaces of the tooth crown should be polished. The rotational speed should be kept slow (4000 rpm or less), and the polisher should be constantly moved on the tooth surface to prevent thermal damage to the tooth and gingiva. The tooth should not be polished for more than 5 seconds, or thermal damage could result. If the polishing is not

TECHNICIAN NOTE

All surfaces of the tooth crown should be polished. The rotational speed should be kept slow, and the polisher should be constantly moved on the tooth surface to prevent thermal damage to the tooth and gingiva.

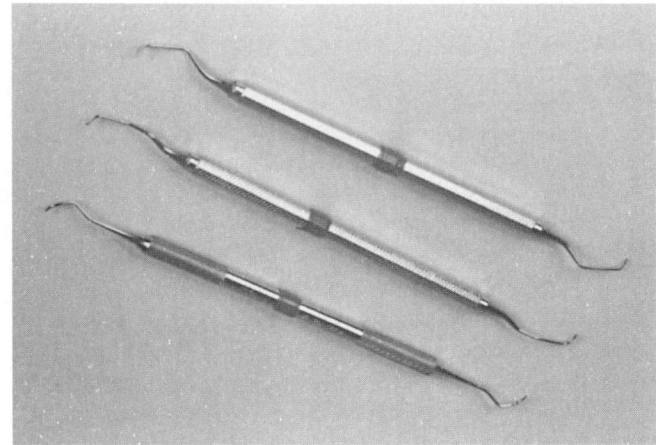

A

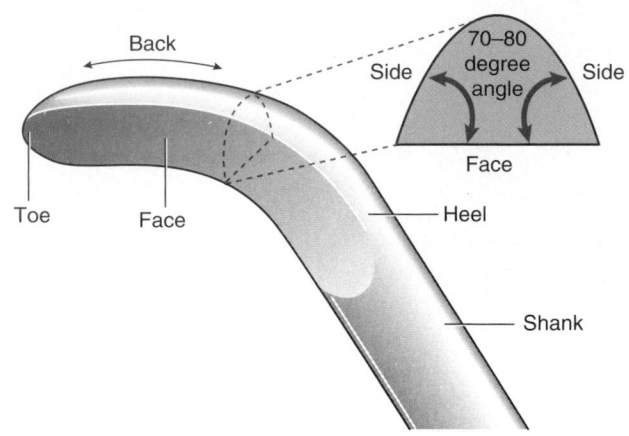

B

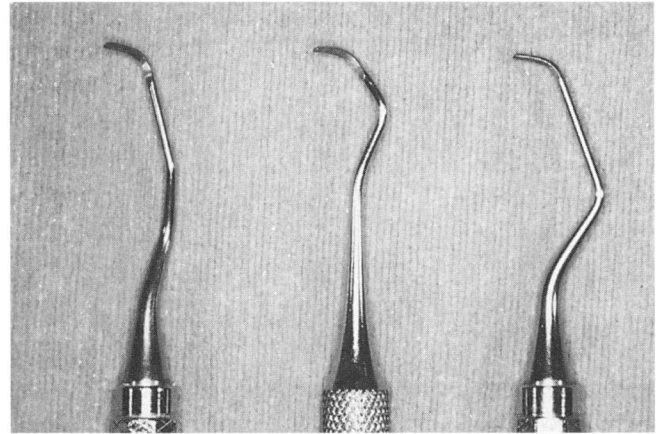

C

Figure 28-18 Curettes can be used subgingivally (below the gingival margin) to scale tooth roots and debride the gingival sulcus. Note the rounded toe and curvature of the instrument. Curettes are available with different angles to the shank to improve access to the tooth roots. **A,** Double-ended curettes. **B,** Drawing of the working end. **C,** Shank and working end of curettes.

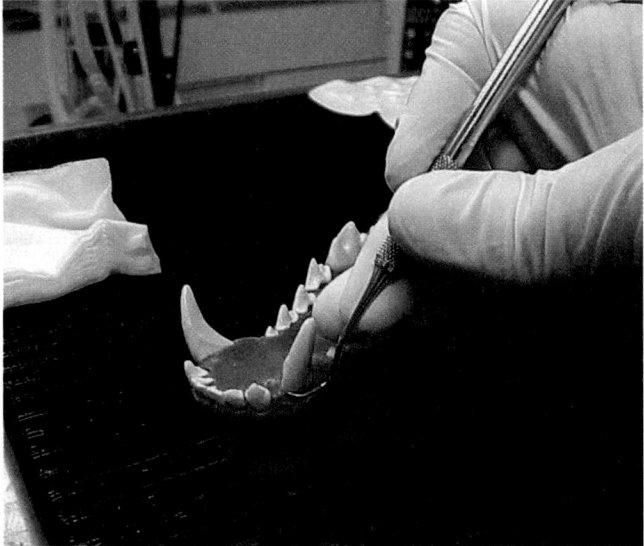

Figure 28-19 The scaler is held in a modified pen grasp. (Courtesy Dr. Alfred G. Stevens, Sherwood South Animal Hospital, Baton Rouge, La.)

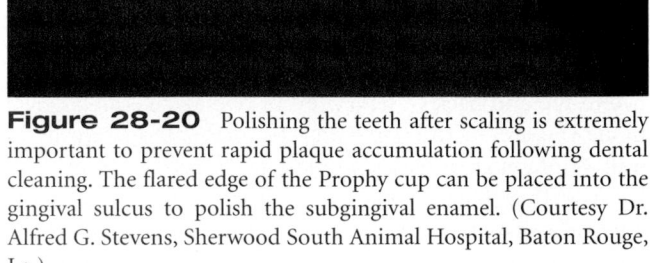

Figure 28-20 Polishing the teeth after scaling is extremely important to prevent rapid plaque accumulation following dental cleaning. The flared edge of the Prophy cup can be placed into the gingival sulcus to polish the subgingival enamel. (Courtesy Dr. Alfred G. Stevens, Sherwood South Animal Hospital, Baton Rouge, La.)

completed in 5 seconds, another tooth should be polished, and the unfinished tooth can be polished once it has been given time to cool.

Ample Prophy paste should be kept in the Prophy cup to help prevent excessive heat generation and to smooth

the tooth surface. Several polishing pastes are available. For routine dental cleanings, the fluoride-containing pastes are preferred. Fluoride strengthens enamel, decreases tooth sensitivity, has antimicrobial properties, and decreases the rate of plaque reattachment. The zirconium silicate pastes

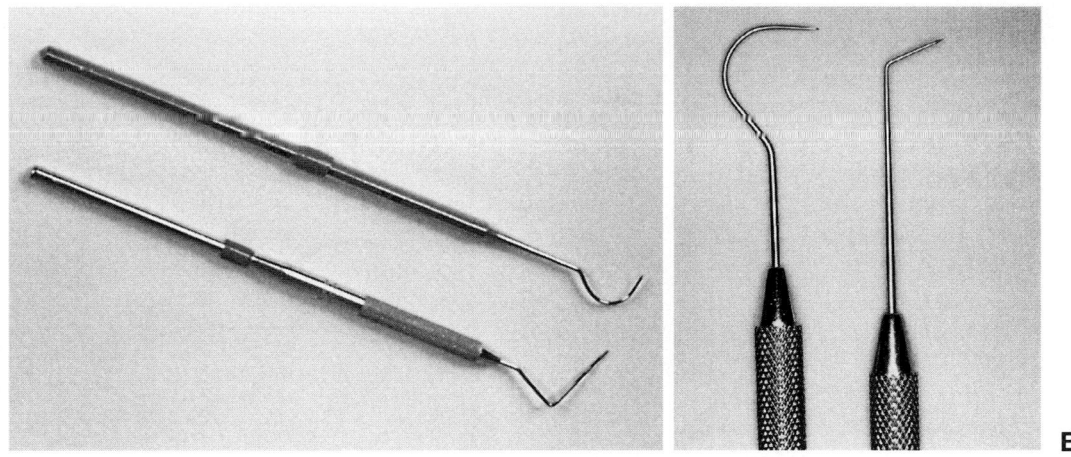

A   B

Figure 28-21 **A,** Dental explorer *(top)* and periodontal probe *(bottom).* The periodontal probe is marked in millimeter increments to measure periodontal pocket depth. The dental explorer has a fine tip and is used to detect subgingival calculus and tooth abnormalities. **B,** Shepherd's hook explorer *(left)* and no. 6 explorer *(right).*

(sodium or potassium aluminum silicates) are very effective polishing pastes and will not abrade the tooth enamel.

The oral cavity is rinsed of Prophy paste and calculus after all surfaces of the teeth have been polished. The gingival sulcus should be irrigated to remove debris if present. Irrigating systems or syringes can be purchased, or a blunt needle on a syringe can be used. A dilute 0.1% chlorhexidine solution is an excellent irrigation agent because of its antibacterial property, but other solutions can be used, such as physiologic saline, 3% hydrogen peroxide, or zinc ascorbate.

The teeth are checked for any abnormalities and remaining plaque after they have been scaled and polished. Plaque disclosing solutions, such as Reveal (Henry Schein Inc.), are available to enhance visualization of areas of plaque retention. Drying the teeth with air will further enhance visualization of any remaining plaque and calculus.

A dental explorer is used to check for subgingival pathologic changes, such as root caries or erosion, calculus, and tooth root furcation exposure. Explorers come in a variety of shapes to aid exploration of the periodontal pockets in the different areas of the mouth (Figures 28-7 and 28-21). Commonly used explorers are the shepherd's hook for dogs and the no. 6 for cats. The tip of the explorer has a sharp delicate point that gives good tactile sensation to the operator's hand when exploring the subgingival area.

A common problem of feline dentition is the development of idiopathic feline odontoclastic resorptive lesions (FORLs) (Figure 28-22). It is estimated that 20% of cats are affected by this problem. The lesions are usually found at the neck of the tooth (the junction of the enamel of the crown and the cementum of the tooth root), which is often hidden by the gingiva. Cats must be examined closely for these lesions. Often the gingival tissue over these lesions is inflamed. A dental explorer must be used to check for irregularities below the gingiva. Early detection and restora-

tion of these lesions may prevent the continued resorption of the tooth. Unfortunately most teeth with FORLs are identified in the advanced stages of the disease when pulp exposure and root resorption is present. When the resorption has progressed this far, the tooth cannot be saved and should be extracted (see exodontics for further discussion). Dental radiographs of these teeth are necessary to evaluate the severity of resorption.

A periodontal probe (Figure 28-21, *A)* must be used to check the level of epithelial attachment in the gingival sulcus of each tooth. The probe is placed parallel to the long axis of the tooth root, and multiple sites along each tooth should be checked (Figure 28-23). The clinical probing depth of any periodontal pocket should be recorded on the pet's dental chart and is a measurement taken from the gingival margin to the epithelial attachment level (base of the pocket). These instruments are extremely beneficial in detecting occult oronasal or oroantral fistulas. These fistulas originate along the palatal aspect of the maxillary teeth when periodontal disease has destroyed the palatal bone along the root of the tooth. Oronasal fistulas are a common problem on the palatal aspect of maxillary canines of small breed dogs like dachshunds and Chihuahuas. Oroantral fistulas communicate with the sinus cavity and usually occur around the maxillary fourth premolars.

Oronasal and oroantral fistulas are classified as occult when the tooth is still present because it hides the pathology. If the tooth has been lost the fistula is easily visualized. These fistulas subject the pet to chronic infection, so it is important that they are identified during the oral examination. Treatment for oronasal or oroantral fistulas requires tooth extraction (if still present) and oral surgery to create a tissue flap to close the lesion. They can be difficult to resolve due to the nature of the lesion and the owner must be forewarned of the possibility of dehiscence. Client education is very important because they are often unaware of the problem since the

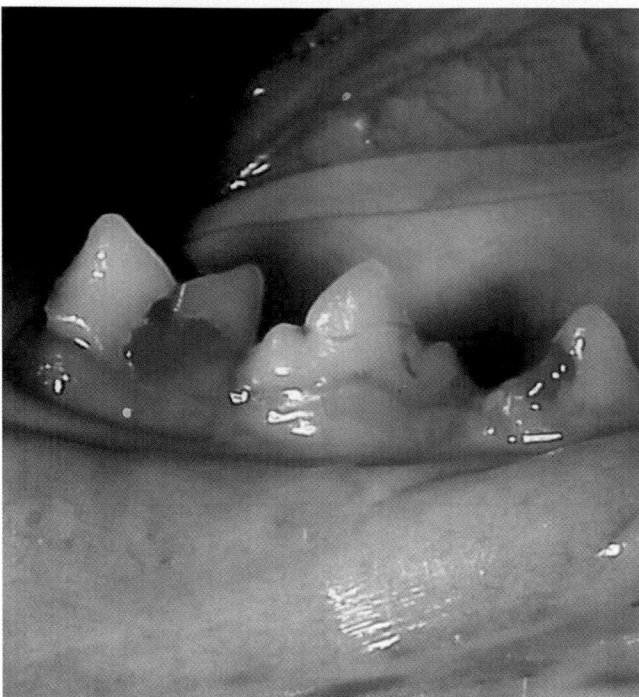

Figure 28-22 Feline odontoclastic resorptive lesion. A dental radiograph is necessary to evaluate the tooth roots. (Courtesy Dr. Alfred G. Stevens, Sherwood South Animal Hospital, Baton Rouge, La.)

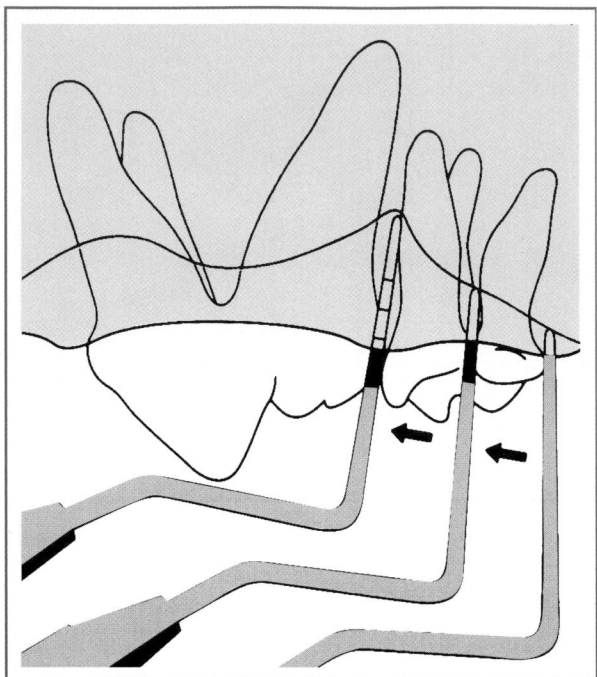

Figure 28-23 Multiple sites on a tooth should be probed to detect any deep pockets present. (From Emily P, Penman S: *Handbook of small animal dentistry,* ed 2, Oxford, England, 1994, Pergamon Press.)

tooth has hid the pathology. These patients will often have a history of chronic halitosis, sneezing, and/or nasal discharge.

Periodontal probes come in a wide variety of calibrations, which are either color coded or notched and measure pocket depths up to 10, 11, or 12 mm. The probes are either round or flat. It is useful to have a variety of probes, but the most popular probe is a color-coded probe that measures 3-, 6-, 9-, and 12-mm increments. Factors that affect the probing depth of a periodontal pocket are epithelial attachment level, alveolar bone loss, gingival margin swelling (reversible), and gingival recession. Gingival recession should be measured with the periodontal probe from the level of the cementoenamel junction (CEJ) of the tooth to the gingival margin and recorded on the dental record. This value plus the clinical probing depth will equal the amount of attachment loss for that particular tooth (attachment loss = clinical probing depth + gingival recession). Any problems noted during the dental cleaning should be brought to the attention of the veterinarian, and dental radiographs should be taken if indicated. After scaling, polishing, and sulcus irrigation have been performed and all problems have been addressed, the animal can recover from anesthesia. Box 28-6 lists the seven steps to a complete dental cleaning.

DENTAL HOME CARE

The final stage of dental cleaning is client education on dental home care treatment along with the dispensing of

---

Box 28-6 STEPS FOR DENTAL CLEANING

1. Preanesthetic examination/anesthesia and dental procedure consent form signed by owner and phone numbers verified.
2. Anesthetize patient; don protective clothing; rinse pet's mouth with 0.12% chlorhexidine solution.
3. Perform oral examination and dental charting.
4. a. Remove calculus from crowns and roots.
   b. Take dental radiographs if needed.
5. Polish teeth.
6. Rinse oral cavity and pharynx of all foreign debris.
7. Perform medicated oral rinse and/or fluoride gel treatment.
8. Recover pet from anesthesia.

---

dental home care products. Many products are available to encourage good compliance and meet individual needs.

When the owner comes to pick up the pet, he or she should be taken into an examination room, where the technician can demonstrate the proper brushing technique on a dental model. The owner should be instructed to start slowly with the pet and to use ample praise. The owner should then be asked to repeat the brushing procedure on a dental model to ensure correct technique. The pet can then be brought in to the owner. The owner should be shown how to properly grasp the muzzle so that the pet is not injured when brushing the teeth. Daily dental home care is the best way to prevent the accumulation of plaque. For owners with

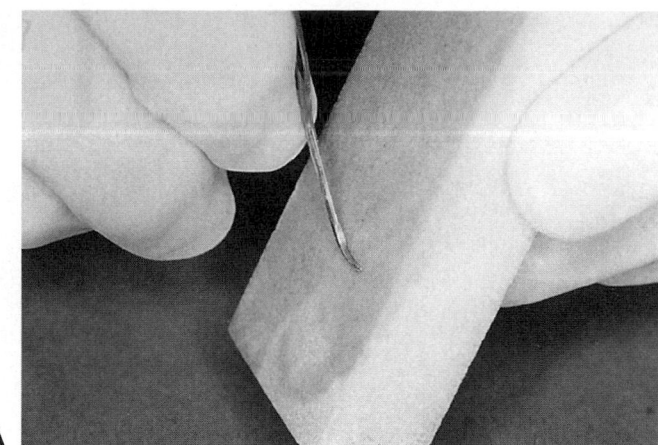
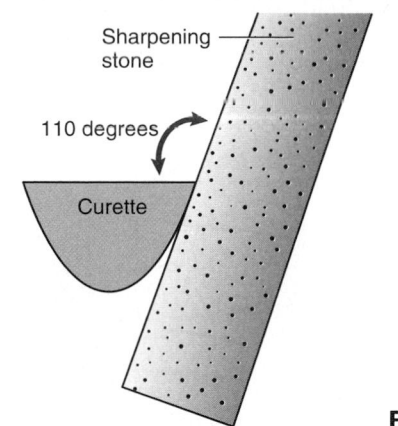

Figure 28-24 **A,** The sharpening stone should be kept at an angle of 100 to 110 degrees to the scaler face to maintain the proper shape of the instrument. **B,** Curette face in cross section to sharpening stone showing the 100- to 110-degree angle.

busy schedules, however, a home care session on alternate days or three times per week will still provide benefits to the pet.

> ### 🖊 TECHNICIAN NOTE
>
> The key to success with dental home care is finding a product that works well for the owner and is acceptable to the pet. With patience, praise, and guidance, the owner should be able to find a dental home care treatment that will work for his or her pet.

The owner should be informed of any dental problems the pet might have as well as the date on which the pet's next dental cleaning will be due. As a general rule, pets with healthy mouths or mild to moderate gingivitis will benefit from annual dental cleanings. Those with early periodontitis will probably require a dental cleaning every 6 to 8 months, and those with moderate to severe periodontitis may require a dental cleaning every 3 to 4 months.

The key to success with dental home care is finding a product that works well for the owner and is acceptable to the pet. There are many different types of toothbrushes available. Dog and cat toothbrushes can be purchased, or the owner can buy a child's soft-bristled toothbrush. Some pets will not tolerate a toothbrush and may respond better if the owner uses a sponge-type swab or a gauze pad wrapped around the owner's finger. If this is unacceptable to the pet, or if the owner risks being bitten, a mouth rinse or spray can be used.

Pet toothpaste formulas are well tolerated by most pets because they like the malt, poultry, or beef flavoring that has been added. Human toothpaste should not be used on pets. The flavors of the veterinary chlorhexidine and zinc ascorbate oral rinses and spray products are not as well liked by pets. However, they are excellent for keeping oral bacterial levels under control and for healing damaged gingival tissue. They can be applied more quickly than pastes and are easier to use on animals that will not tolerate much handling.

With patience, praise, and guidance, the owner should be able to find a dental home care treatment that will work for his or her pet.

SHARPENING DENTAL SCALERS

Dental scalers must be kept sharp to work properly. Dull instruments burnish calculus into the tooth rather than remove it and can cause operator hand fatigue. There are several different methods to sharpen scalers. A helpful instructional textbook is *It's About Time to Get on the Cutting Edge* by Hu-Friedy, which is available through most dental supply companies. An oiled sharpening stone should be used to sharpen dental scalers. The finer grades of sharpening stones (e.g., the Arkansas stone) maintain a smoother cutting edge, remove less metal, and as long as instruments are sharpened frequently the sharp edge is rapidly restored. A thin layer of oil should be placed on the surface of the stone before sharpening. The instruments should be cleaned before sharpening, and sharpening should be performed in a well-lit area.

A simple sharpening method is the moving flat stone, stationary instrument technique. The flat stone is held at an angle of 100 to 110 degrees to the face of the curette or sickle scaler (Figure 28-24). This angle will maintain the 70- to 80-degree bevel of the cutting edge (Figures 28-17, *B*, and 28-18, *B*). Begin sharpening with short up and down strokes starting at the heel of the instrument and working toward the toe or tip of the instrument. The technician's dominant hand should hold the stone, and the other hand should hold the instrument with the face up and parallel to the floor. The instrument hand should be braced on a stable surface, such as a counter or tabletop. Sharpening always finishes on a down stroke, and greater pressure is placed on the down strokes than on the up strokes. Once the stone reaches the tip of the supragingival scaler the stone is removed on completion of the down stroke. The rounded

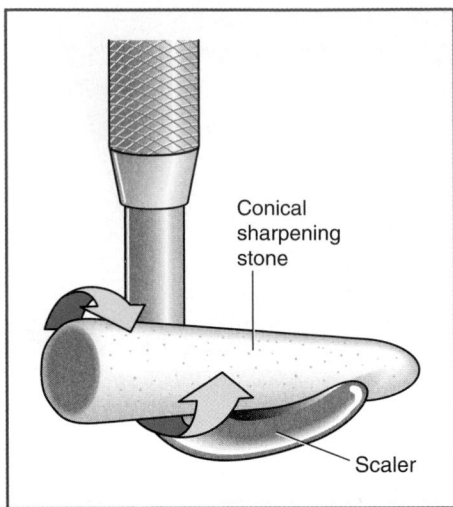

Figure 28-25 The conical sharpening stone is rolled across the face of the scaler to remove wire edges.

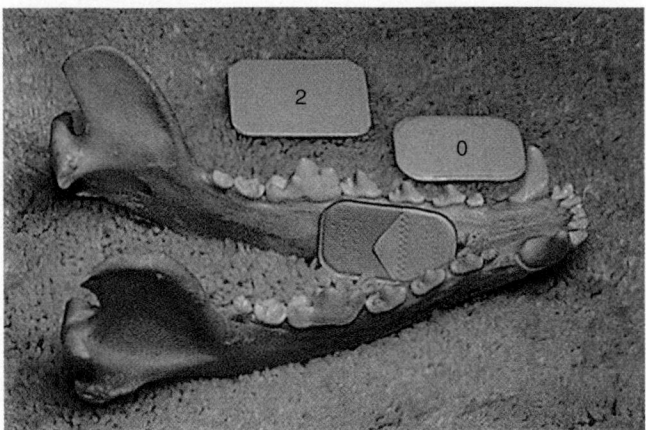

Figure 28-26 Intraoral dental film size 2 and size 0.

toe must be maintained on curettes to avoid soft tissue trauma. As the stone approaches the toe, the sharpening is continued, maintaining the same angle around the toe to finish on the down stroke.

The instruments should be checked for sharpness on an acrylic stick. A sharp instrument easily engages the acrylic and shaves thin strips off with little effort. The sharpening procedure is repeated until the instrument is properly sharpened. The wire edges are then removed from the face of the instrument by rolling a round stone over the face a few times (Figure 28-25). Finally, the instrument is cleaned of oil and metal debris and sterilized.

Instruments need to be sharpened based on use. If a scaler is used very little, it may be able to go through three or four procedures without dulling. If a dental case requires extensive hand scaling, the scaler may require sharpening after that case. A good rule of thumb is to check scalers frequently with an acrylic stick to identify the dull instruments.

DENTAL RADIOGRAPHY

Dental radiography is an important tool in the diagnostic and prognostic evaluation of oral disorders in veterinary medicine. As advances have been made in veterinary dentistry, there has been a demand for high-quality dental radiographs to evaluate teeth and oral structures more accurately. The use of dental radiograph machines and intraoral dental film in veterinary medicine has increased dramatically during this time.

Traditionally, radiographs of the teeth, mandible, and maxilla were taken to evaluate disorders such as oral masses, fractured jaws and teeth, and facial pain and swelling. Many veterinarians are now using this diagnostic aid to assess problems such as discolored teeth, feline odontoclastic resorptive lesions, and periodontal disease and to aid in the treatment of endodontically compromised teeth, dental restorations, and difficult extractions.

Dental radiographs can be taken with the film placed in the mouth (intraoral technique) or outside the mouth (extraoral technique). Intraoral dental film is a nonscreened flexible film (Figure 28-26). Regular screened or non-screened x-ray film can be used for extraoral radiographic views (see Chapter 9) and a limited number of intraoral views. Nonscreened x-ray films provide greater detail than the screened films but require increased exposure times.

There are several advantages of the intraoral radiographic technique over the extraoral technique. Perhaps the greatest advantage of the intraoral technique is the ability to minimize the superimposition of teeth and surrounding structures on the area of study. Intraoral dental film can be purchased in sizes small enough to fit in the mouth next to the tooth or teeth to be studied. The closer the x-ray film is to the subject of interest (the tooth), the better the detail. The aiming cylinder of the dental radiograph machine can be moved and angled to radiograph the tooth of interest and be placed close enough to the tooth to eliminate the opposite dental arch.

When using the extraoral technique, there is usually some degree of superimposition of teeth from the contralateral arches that are in the path of the primary beam (Figure 28-27). The teeth in the opposite arch may obstruct the view of the teeth of interest, and dental abnormalities could be missed.

The film focal distance (FFD) for the dental radiograph machine is 16 inches or less, in contrast to the standard radiograph machines for which an FFD of 36 to 40 inches is commonly used. The shorter FFD of the dental radiograph machine allows closer placement of the anode to the tooth, eliminating the opposite dental arch, surrounding soft tissue, and/or bone from the path of the primary beam. The shorter FFD also minimizes harmful scatter radiation, as does the small cone size and lead lining, which many of the dental radiograph cones contain.

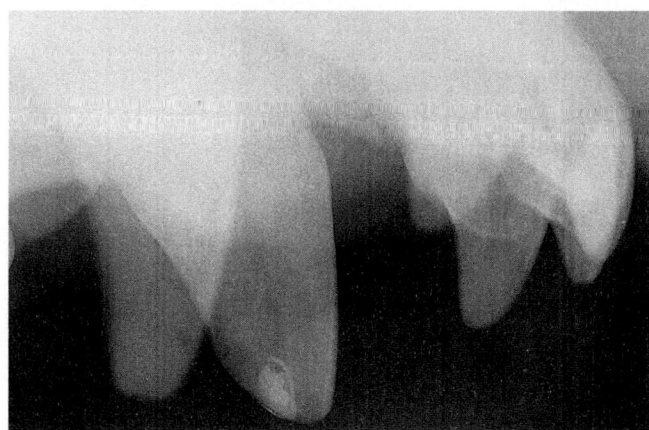

Figure 28-27 Superimposition caused by placing the film extraorally. The teeth in the contralateral arch are interfering with the image of the area of interest.

The extraoral views require the patient to be placed in many different positions so that the skull is angled in order for the primary beam to avoid the surrounding oral structures. This proper positioning takes time and skill. Intraoral dental film can be placed in the mouth, and the tube head of the x-ray machine can be moved instead of the patient. The patient is placed in dorsal recumbency to radiograph the mandible and in ventral recumbency to radiograph the maxilla. A complete evaluation of all four oral quadrants requires at least six to eight views.

Intraoral dental film can be processed by hand or piggybacked to a regular film with electrical tape and automatically processed. Extraoral nonscreened x-ray film may not be compatible with the automatic processor's developer and might require hand developing. The extraoral nonscreened x-ray film is considerably more expensive than the smaller intraoral dental film. If rapid developer and fixative are used, intraoral dental film can be hand developed in approximately 2 minutes, which is helpful in minimizing anesthesia time. Many veterinary clinics are switching to digital radiography, which uses a sensor instead of dental film and does not require developer or fixer. The sensor sends the image to the computer, which shows the image in 10 to 15 seconds. Images can be enhanced with the programs software as well. Digital radiography requires less radiation exposure than traditional radiographic films. Digital radiography will most likely be the standard technique in the years ahead.

To use the intraoral radiographic technique, one must master the bisecting angle technique. The bisecting angle technique was developed to minimize image distortion caused by the inability to place the dental film parallel to the central axis of the tooth. Placing the film parallel to the teeth in the maxillary arch and anterior mandible is particularly difficult because of the flat palate and impeding soft tissue structures of the mandibular symphysis. To utilize the bisecting angle technique, the film is placed as close to

the tooth as possible. The primary x-ray beam is then aimed perpendicular to the plane that bisects the angle created by the plane of the central axis of the tooth to the plane of the dental film. The bisecting angle (or bisector angle) is the imaginary plane that divides this angle created between the tooth and film into two equal parts (Figure 28-28). Distortion of the tooth is minimized but is still present because the film is closer to the crown of the tooth than it is to the root apex.

> ### ✎ TECHNICIAN NOTE
>
> To use the intraoral radiographic technique, one must master the bisecting angle technique. The bisecting angle technique was developed to minimize image distortion caused by the inability to place the dental film parallel to the central axis of the tooth.

The buccal object rule (tube shift technique or Clark's rule) is useful for object localization as well as isolating structures for better visualization. Objects that are lingual to a reference point will move in the same direction as the change in position of the tube head (either rostrally or distally), and objects buccal to the reference point move opposite the direction of the tube head. For example, the left upper fourth premolar tooth (208) of the dog or cat has two mesial roots (mesiobuccal and palatal roots) and one distal root. When we radiograph this tooth, we may need to distinguish the mesiobuccal root from the palatal root on the radiograph. If the tube head is positioned rostral to the upper fourth premolar and the radiograph taken in a rostrocaudal oblique projection, the most mesial root on the radiograph of 208 will be the palatal root followed by the mesiobuccal and finally the distal root in that order (Figure 28-29, *A*). An acronym to help remember this rule is SLOB, which stands for same lingual, opposite buccal. The tube head was placed mesial (or rostral) to 208, so the root that moved with it was the palatal (lingual) root. If we were to take a caudorostral oblique (shift the tube head distal to 208 and project toward the nose), the palatal root would also shift distally (same lingual) and the mesiobuccal root would shift mesially (opposite buccal) so that it appears as the first root on the radiographic image of 208 (Figure 28-29, *C*).

To change the position of the tube head for a rostrocaudal or caudorostral oblique projection, the position-indicating device (PID) remains perpendicular to the bisecting angle but the tube head is simply angled obliquely at the object. The PID is either in a slightly more anterior oblique projection or posterior oblique projection as compared with the lateral projection (Figure 28-29, *B*).

INTRAORAL RADIOGRAPHY IN THE DOG AND CAT

Intraoral radiographs of the mandibular premolars and molars are obtained by using standard radiographic technique. The film is placed on the lingual side of the teeth and parallel to the central axis of the teeth. The dental x-ray

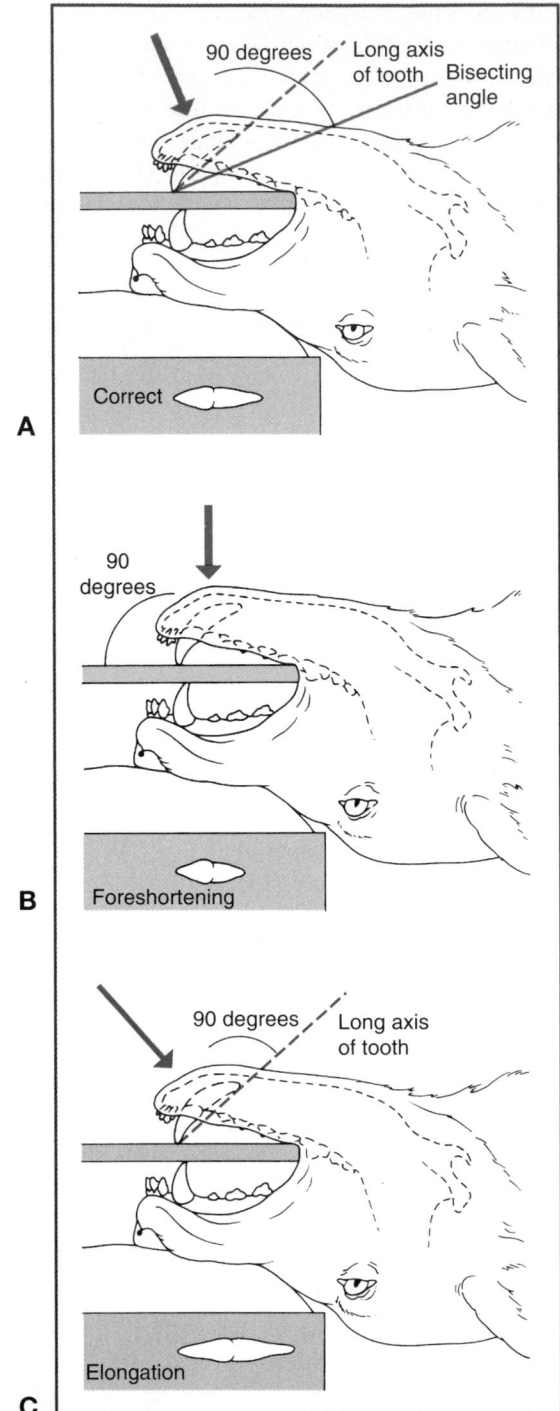

Figure 28-28 **A,** Bisection angle technique produces an accurate image of the tooth. **B,** Direction of the x-ray beam at right angles to the film shortens the tooth's image. **C,** Direction of the x-ray beam at right angles to the long axis of the tooth elongates the tooth's image. (From Emily P, Penman S: *Handbook of small animal dentistry,* ed 2, Oxford, England, 1994, Pergamon Press.)

beam is then aimed perpendicular to the film (Figure 28-30). This is the only area in the oral cavity of the dog and cat where the standard technique can be used.

The mandibular incisors can usually be radiographed on one dental film. The animal is placed in dorsal or lateral recumbency with the dental film as close to the incisors as possible on the lingual side. The PID is then centered over the first incisors pointing in a caudal direction with the x-ray beam aimed perpendicular to the bisecting angle. The apices of both mandibular canines can be obtained in this view if the dental film extends far enough caudally (Figure 28-31). The frenulum of the tongue may prevent proper placement of the intraoral film in some pets, particularly cats. If this becomes a problem, the tongue can be placed between the teeth and the film.

To obtain a radiograph of the mandibular first, second, and third premolars in a dog and third premolars in the cat where the symphysis prevents proper parallel placement of the film, place the animal in dorsal recumbency. Position the film on the lingual side of the teeth as close to the teeth and ventral border of the mandible as possible. Direct the PID at the teeth from a lateral position, and aim the x-ray beam at the bisecting angle (Figure 28-32).

Radiographs of the maxillary dentition are commonly taken with the bisecting angle because the flat palate makes it difficult to place the film parallel and in close apposition to the tooth roots. The maxillary incisors are radiographed with the same technique as is used for the mandibular incisors except the animal is placed in sternal or lateral recumbency (Figure 28-33). The apices of the maxillary canines are usually superimposed over the first and second premolars in this view. The maxillary canines should be radiographed from a lateral or rostrocaudal oblique view using the bisecting angle technique (Figures 28-29, *B,* and 28-34).

To radiograph the maxillary premolars and molars the animal is placed in sternal or lateral recumbency. The film is placed as close to the tooth as possible on the lingual side of the dentition. Maxillary premolars one through three can be viewed with the tube head placed lateral to the teeth (Figure 28-34). If the animal has crowding or rotation of these teeth, additional views in a rostrocaudal oblique position may be required to improve visualization of tooth roots.

Rostrocaudal or caudorostral oblique views are needed to isolate the different tooth roots of the maxillary fourth premolar and first and second molar teeth. A rostrocaudal view of premolar four provides an isolated view of the anterior tooth roots, but the distal root may be superimposed over the first molar. An additional view of the tooth from the caudorostral oblique projection will isolate the distal root, but the anterior roots may now be superimposed over the third premolar. The crowns of the molar teeth will superimpose their roots, so the technique may need to be adjusted to penetrate the additional structures.

In cats and in brachycephalic dogs, the zygomatic arch may be superimposed over the maxillary premolar tooth

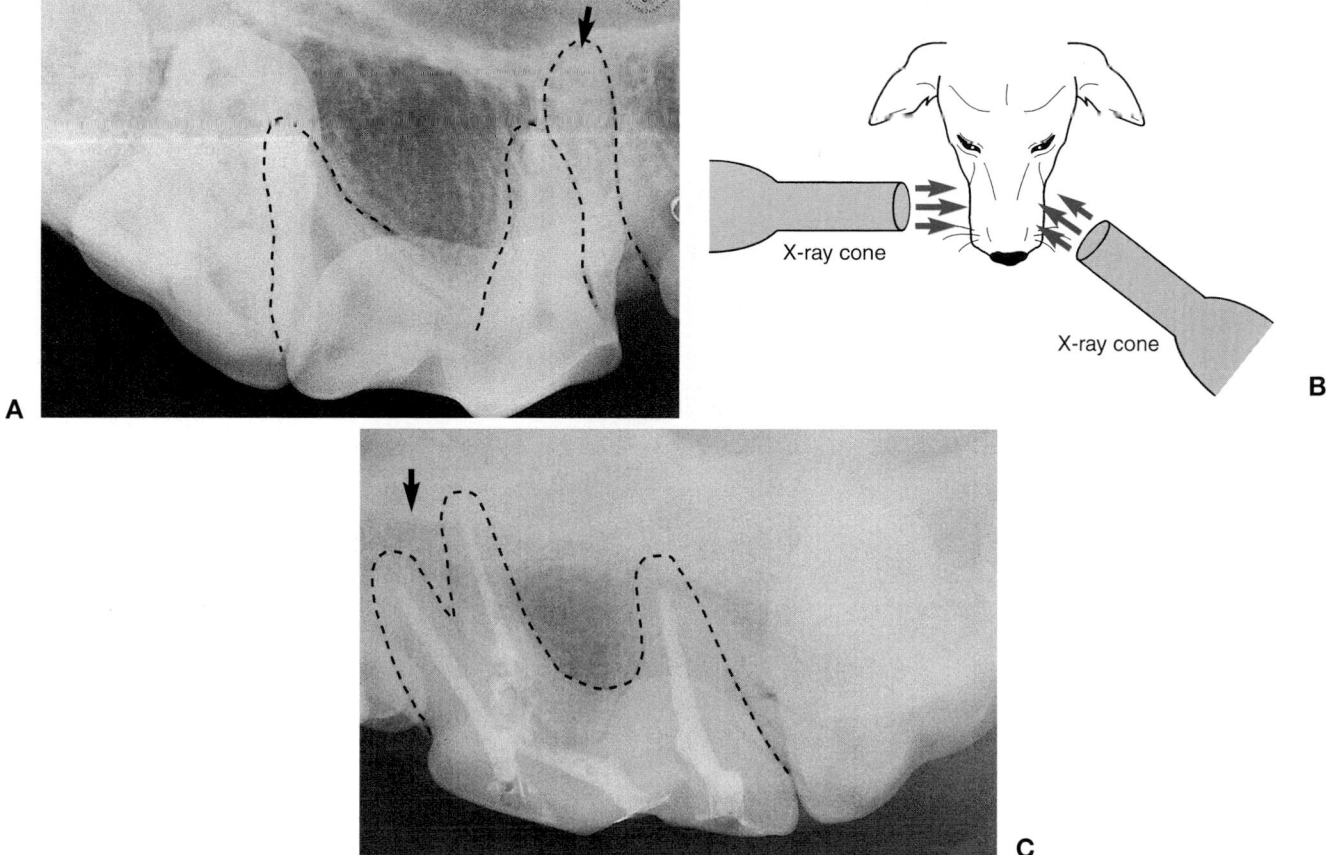

Figure 28-29 **A,** Rostrocaudal oblique view of the upper fourth premolar tooth *(arrow)* of the anterior roots. The most mesial root is the palatal root. **B,** This diagram illustrates how the position-indicating device (PID) is positioned to take an oblique view. **C,** Caudorostral oblique view of the upper fourth premolar. The most mesial root is the buccal root *(arrow).* Note the nice separation.

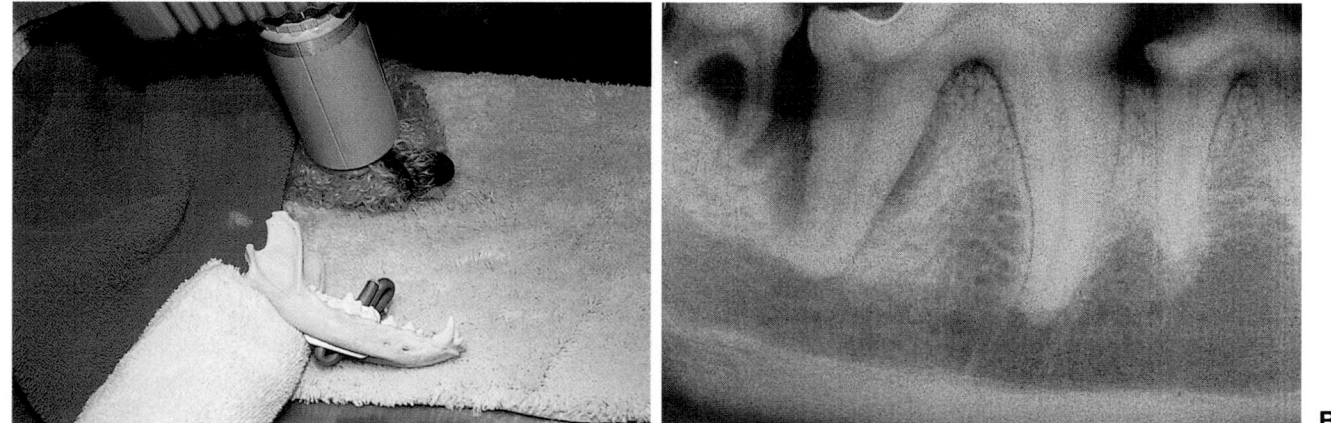

Figure 28-30 **A,** Proper positioning for a radiograph of the mandibular premolars and molars. **B,** Radiograph of teeth 408, 409, and 410. The area of interest in this study was 409.

roots. If the PID is placed in a rostrocaudal oblique position, the zygomatic arch can be shifted off the area of interest.

When one is learning the positioning techniques for intraoral dental radiographs, it is easiest to place the dog or cat in sternal recumbency for views of the maxillary dentition, in dorsal recumbency for views of the anterior mandible, and in lateral recumbency for views of the mandibular premolars and molars. As one masters the technique, the animal can be left in lateral recumbency (since many veterinarians perform dental procedures with

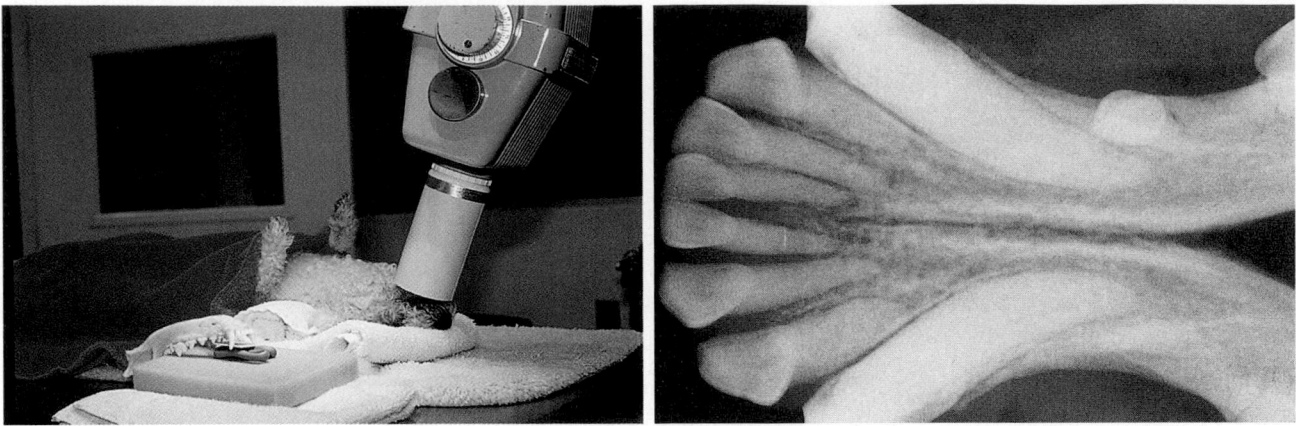

Figure 28-31 **A,** Positioning for a study of the mandibular incisors and canines. **B,** Radiograph of the mandibular incisors and canines.

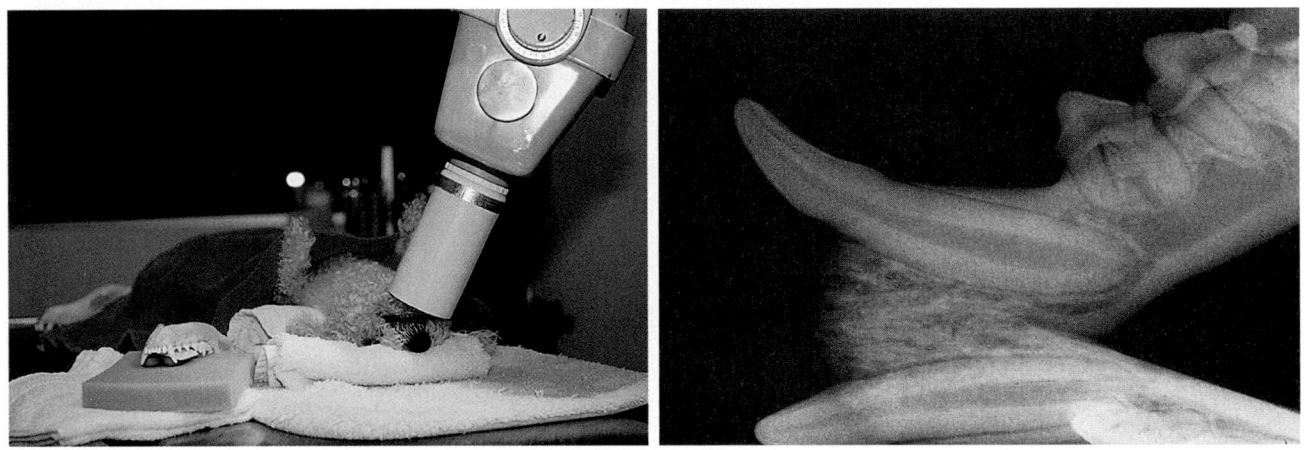

Figure 28-32 **A,** Positioning for a study of the rostral mandibular premolars. This can also be used to obtain a lateral view of the incisors and canine tooth. **B,** Radiograph of 304, 307, and most of 308 in a cat. Note the incisor teeth are missing.

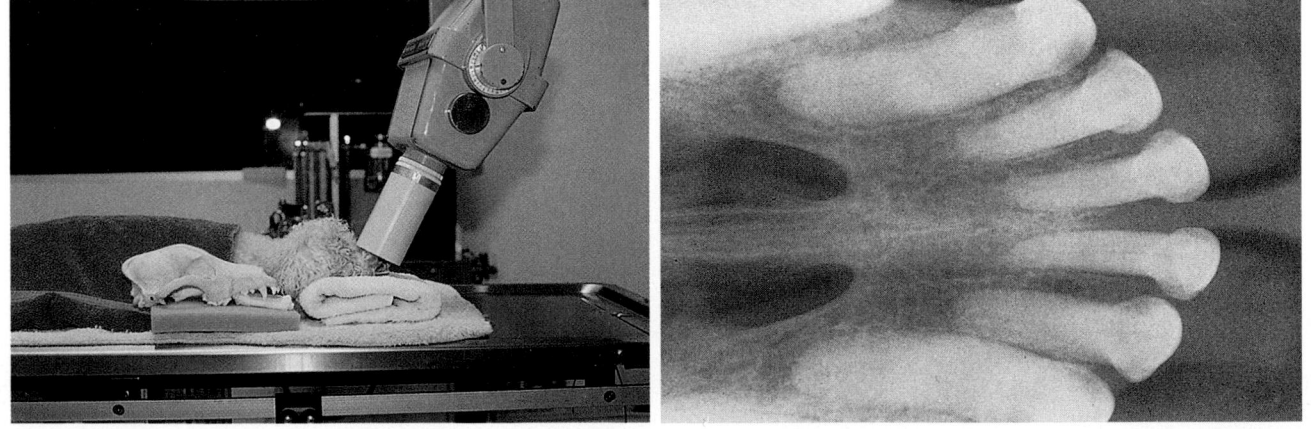

Figure 28-33 **A,** Positioning for a study of the maxillary incisors. **B,** Radiograph of the maxillary incisors.

the animal in this position) and the views taken following the same principles. Film holders are often needed for many of these views to keep the film from moving once it is placed in proper position. Gauze squares and Flexi-film holders (Dr. Shipp's Laboratories) are useful for this purpose (see

Figures 28-30, *A,* and 28-31, *A*). Box 28-7 is a technique chart to serve as a reference for taking intraoral radiographs with a dental x-ray machine and intraoral film.

An intraoral dental film packet has four main components (Figure 28-35). The film itself is wrapped in black

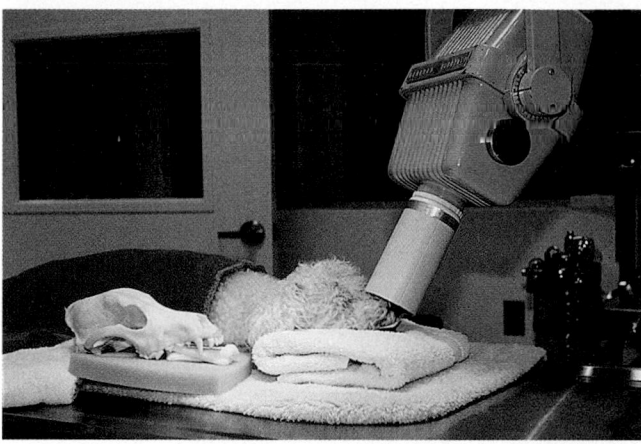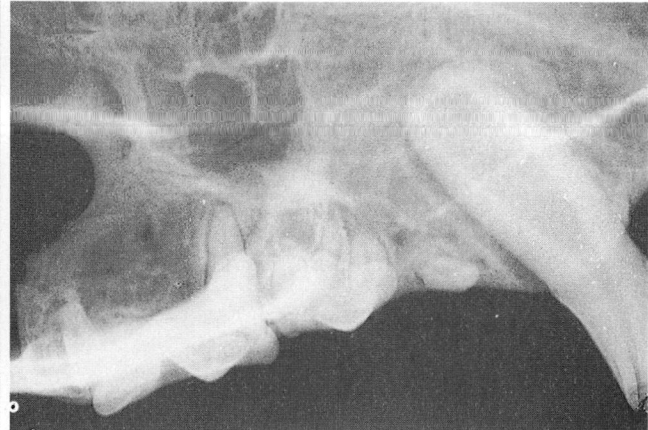

A **B**

Figure 28-34 **A,** Positioning for a study of the maxillary premolars. This can also be used to obtain a lateral view of the maxillary incisors and canine tooth. **B,** Radiograph of 204, 206, 207, 208, and 209 in a cat.

Box 28-7 EXPOSURE TIME USING D SPEED INTRAORAL DENTAL FILM

- Cats: 0.1 to 0.3 sec
- Dogs: 0.2 to 0.5 sec
- Dental machine: 70 kVp, 15 mA, FFD 12 inches

FFD, Focal-film distance; kVp, kilovolts peak; mA, milliamperes.

✎ TECHNICIAN NOTE

When one is learning the positioning techniques for intraoral dental radiographs, it is easiest to place the dog or cat in sternal recumbency for views of the maxillary dentition, in dorsal recumbency for views of the anterior mandible, and in lateral recumbency for views of the mandibular premolars and molars.

---

paper to protect it from light exposure. The back of the film contains lead foil to shield the film from backscatter radiation that could cause film fog. These components are then wrapped in a paper or plastic outer wrap that is moisture resistant. Intraoral dental film is available in D, E, and most recently F speeds. The exposure time of E speed film is 50% less than D speed, but there is less sharpness and more film fogging with E speed film. F speed film requires about 50% to 60% less exposure time than D speed and has image quality comparable to D speed film.

Intraoral dental film comes in three styles: periapical, bitewing, and occlusal. The composition of the film does not vary in the different film sizes. In veterinary medicine the periapical and occlusal sizes are used primarily. Periapical films are used to evaluate the crown, root, and periapical region and come in the following three sizes: size 0 ($^7/_8 \times 1^3/_8$ inch), size 1 ($^{15}/_{16} \times 1^9/_{16}$ inch), and size 2 ($1^1/_4 \times 1^5/_8$ inch). Size 0 is used commonly in cats and small breed dogs. Size 2 is used for medium to large breed dogs and for single tooth studies, such as an endodontic case.

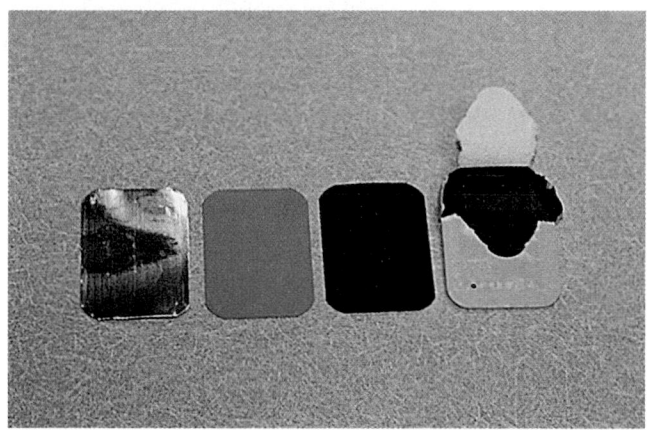

Figure 28-35 Components of intraoral dental film. *Left to right,* Outer water-resistant wrapper, black paper, dental film, lead foil.

Occlusal film is size no. 4 film and is used to evaluate a larger area of the mandible or maxilla than would be seen on a single periapical film. It is commonly used for full mouth dental radiographic studies in medium to large breed dogs to get more teeth per film with each radiation exposure. The dimensions of no. 4 film are $2^1/_4 \times 3$ inches.

Digital radiograph systems use sensors or phosphor storage plates (PSP) to record the image that is then transfered to a computer. The image is stored in the computer and viewed on the computer monitor. The software allows the image to be enhanced if desired. There is no need for developing the image, and the image is viewed on the computer within seconds after the exposure is taken.

Digital radiograph sensors can be cumbersome as they are rigid and have a cord that connects to the computer. The sensor sizes are similar to intraoral dental films but the actual active area that records the image is slightly smaller than this. These sensors are several thousand dollars each so great care must be taken not to damage them. The

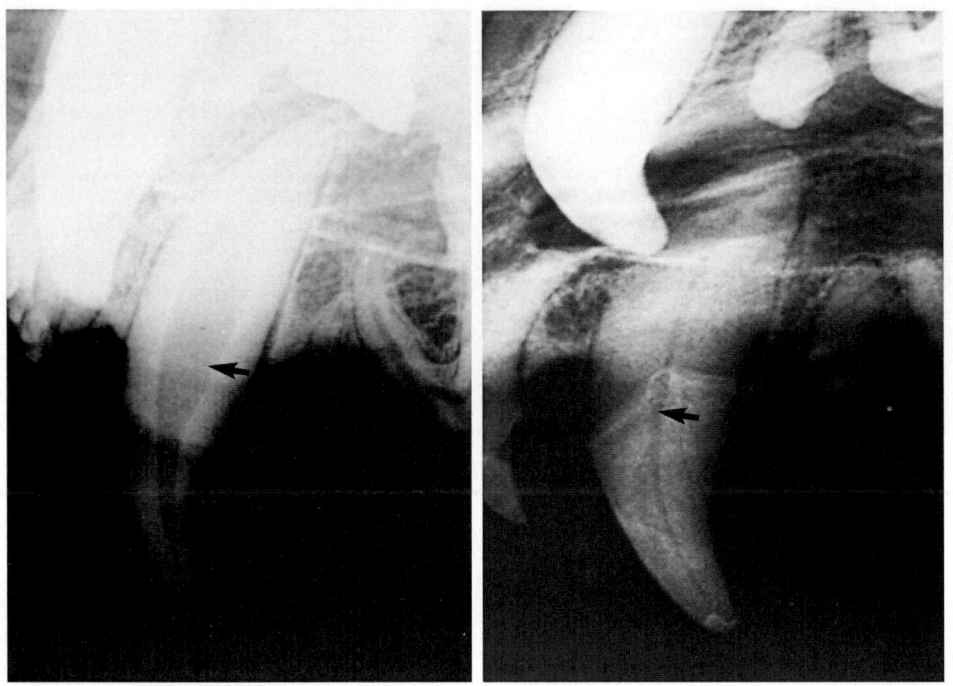

A   B

Figure 28-36   **A,** Large pulp chamber and canal in a young cougar's canine tooth *(arrow).* **B,** As animals age, dentin is deposited, and the pulp chambers and canals narrow *(arrow).*

PSPs, on the other hand, are similar to an intraoral dental film in size and flexibility. The PSP is placed in a thin plastic protective sleeve to record the image in the patient's mouth. It is then removed from the sleeve and placed in a scanner to record the image in the computer. The image is then removed from the film with an eraser plate (or other source of bright light) so that it can be used again. The PSPs can be used up to 1000 times and are relatively inexpensive.

ENDODONTICS

Endodontics deals with the study and treatment of the inside of the tooth (pulp) and periapical tissues. The periapical tissue is located around the tip (apex) of the tooth root. The tooth pulp consists of nerves, blood vessels, lymphatics, and connective tissue. The pulp tissue is found in the pulp chamber (crown) and pulp canal (root) of the tooth and enters the tooth through numerous small openings in the apex of the tooth root called the *apical delta.*

The dental pulp is important to the development of the tooth in a young animal. It supplies the nutrients needed by the odontoblasts to deposit dentin. This makes the walls of the root and crown thicker, so the tooth is stronger. Once the dog or cat is past 10 to 18 months of age, the majority of the dentin has been deposited, the tooth walls are fairly thick, and the root apex should be closed. As the animal continues to age, the pulp chamber and canal will become smaller because the odontoblasts will continue to deposit dentin (Figure 28-36).

The treatment options for teeth with endodontic disease will depend on the age of the animal, duration of endodontic disease, and anatomy of the tooth. Conventional root canal therapy is usually performed on dogs and cats 12 months of age and older with endodontic disease. Treatment involves removing the dead or dying pulp tissue from the tooth with small files or reamers, disinfecting and shaping the root canal, and filling the canal (obturation) with an appropriate material to seal the apex from the periapical tissues. Radiographs are necessary to ensure that a proper apical seal has been achieved. A detailed discussion of this procedure will follow below.

Among the most common causes of endodontic disease in dogs and cats are pulp exposures from fractured teeth as well as dental abrasion (wear from a foreign object) and attrition (wear from tooth on tooth). Many dogs will cause severe abrasion of their teeth by chewing on hard objects such as rocks or fences. The teeth most commonly fractured are the canines and the maxillary fourth premolars (carnassial) (Figure 28-37). Attrition and abrasion usually occur on the incisors and canines but can be seen on the premolars and molars as well. If the dental wear occurs slowly, the odontoblasts will deposit tertiary dentin over the pulp tissue to prevent pulp exposure as enamel and dentin are lost. The pulp tissue may be visualized through the tertiary dentin as a brown or red dot (Figure 28-38). A dental explorer should be run over the tooth surface to make sure the pulp tissue is not exposed. When the pulp tissue is exposed, the tip of the dental explorer will drop down into the pulp chamber as it crosses the surface of the tooth.

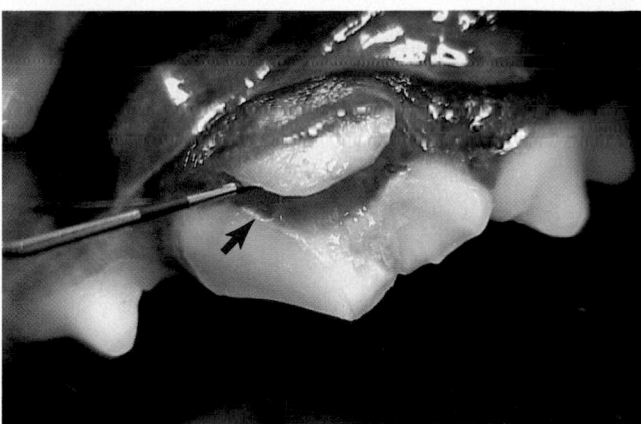

Figure 28-37 Slab fractures of the maxillary fourth premolar teeth are a common problem in dogs. This fracture extends subgingivally, and can expose the pulp *(arrow)*. (Courtesy Dr. Alfred G. Stevens, Sherwood South Animal Hospital, Baton Rouge, La.)

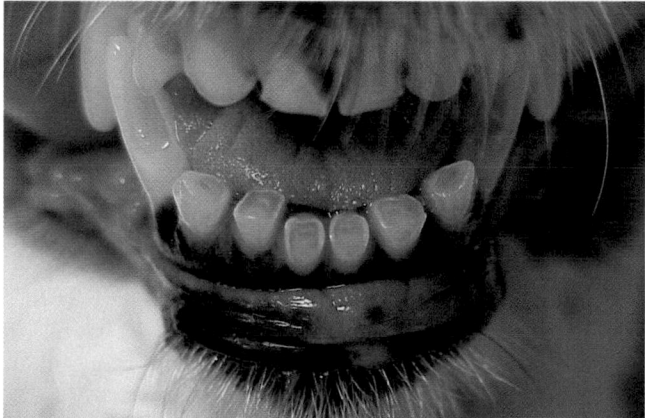

Figure 28-38 Severe abrasion of the incisors and canine teeth. The brown or red dots *(arrow)* in the center of these teeth are the pulp tissues below the less opaque tertiary dentin. (Courtesy Dr. Alfred G. Stevens, Sherwood South Animal Hospital, Baton Rouge, La.)

In fresh fractures the tooth may bleed from the center. If the tooth is treated within the first 48 hours, a vital pulpotomy procedure may be successful. This procedure involves removing the coronal pulp tissue (the pulp tissue in the tooth root remains), covering the pulp tissue with calcium hydroxide, and sealing the coronal exposure site with appropriate dental restorative materials.

All teeth with exposed pulp tissue should be treated either by endodontic treatment (conventional root canal, pulpotomy) or by extraction. If left untreated, infection from the exposure site will spread to the periapical tissues, and a periapical abscess may develop. This condition is seen fairly frequently in dogs with maxillary carnassial tooth abscesses. The owner will notice swelling or a draining tract just below the dog's eye, and treatment is usually sought (Figure 28-39). Surprisingly, only about 20% of periapical abscesses will form a fistula to the skin, which means that

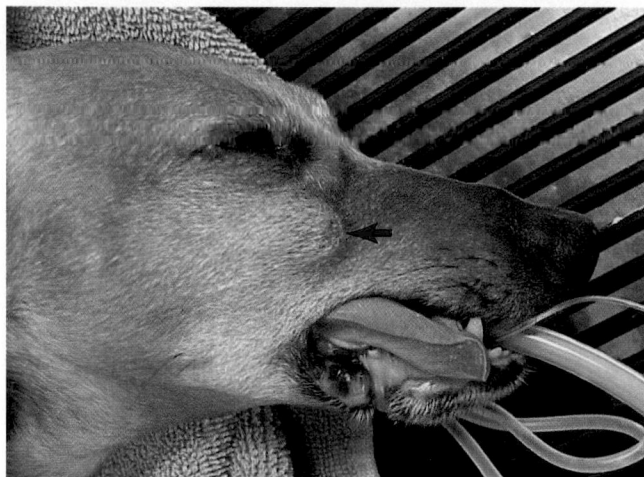

Figure 28-39 Infraorbital swelling and draining tract *(arrow)* from an abscessed upper fourth premolar. (Courtesy Dr. Alfred G. Stevens, Sherwood South Animal Hospital, Baton Rouge, La.)

unless the teeth of these pets are being examined for endodontic disease, many abscesses go untreated. These abscesses can be very painful and are a source of infection, which can spread to other teeth and the bloodstream.

✎ TECHNICIAN NOTE

All teeth with exposed pulp tissue should be treated either by endodontic treatment (conventional root canal, pulpotomy) or by extraction.

Other signs of endodontic disease include discolored teeth and painful teeth. Diagnosing a painful tooth in an animal can be difficult, but when there is a question, a dental radiograph can be taken to assess the periapical area for signs of disease.

CONVENTIONAL ROOT CANAL THERAPY

Box 28-8 lists equipment and supplies needed for conventional root canal therapy. These items should be ready for use before the root canal treatment is started.

A preoperative radiograph is taken to evaluate the tooth root and periapical region. The veterinarian will make the appropriate access to the root canal through the crown of the tooth with a dental bur of proper size determined by the size of the tooth being treated. The canal may have pulp present that will require removal with a barbed broach (Figure 28-40). The broach is placed in the canal and rotated to ensnare the pulp. The broach and pulp tissue are removed from the canal. This step is repeated until all pulp has been removed. Many teeth will not have any visible pulp tissue remaining (necrotic pulp), and the barbed broaches will not be needed.

The next step is to begin filing the root canal in order to clean and shape the canal for proper obturation. *Obturation* means to fill the canal. There are several types and sizes of

Box 28-8 ROOT CANAL INSTRUMENTS AND MATERIALS

- A dental cleaning tray with supragingival scaler and small blade subgingival curette, dental explorer and probe, new Prophy cup, flour pumice (See Figure 28-12.)
- Several dental films, dental film positioner, dental machine turned on and set to the proper technique for the patient
- Barbed broaches, endodontic files with endodontic stops, measuring gauges
- Canal irrigants, endodontic irrigation needles, canal lubricant, dental dam
- Engine-driven endodontic files (rotary files) and corresponding handpiece
- Tongue depressors, gauze squares
- Round ($\frac{1}{2}$, 1, or 2) or pear-shaped (330) carbide or diamond burs
- Gutta-percha cones, cannulas, and syringes; machinery used to heat gutta-percha should be turned on and filled with gutta-percha if extended heating times are required (i.e., Ultrafil and SuccessFil products)
- Glass bead sterilizer should be turned on
- Endodontic cement and mixing pack, spreaders and pluggers, sterile paper points
- Restorative materials and dentinal bonding agent

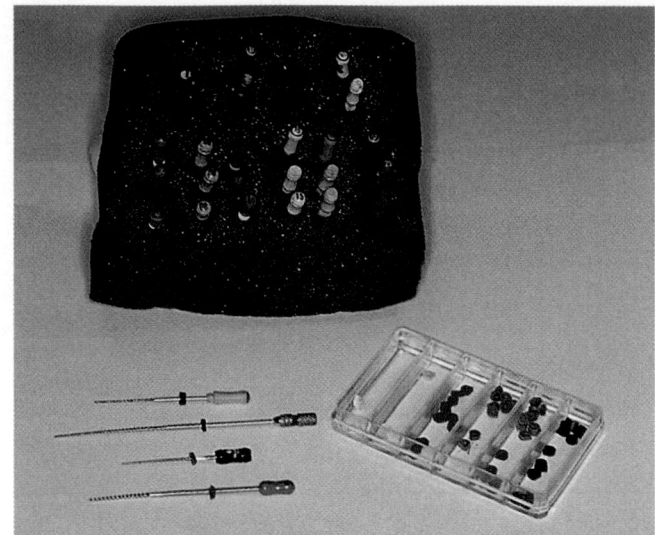

Figure 28-41 A sterile sponge and sterile endodontic files are organized and ready for use. Endodontic stops are in the container on the right. Different file lengths and types are displayed below the sponge. *Top to bottom,* 30-mm size 20 H file, 60-mm size 25 H file, 25-mm size 40 K file, and 40-mm size 35 K file.

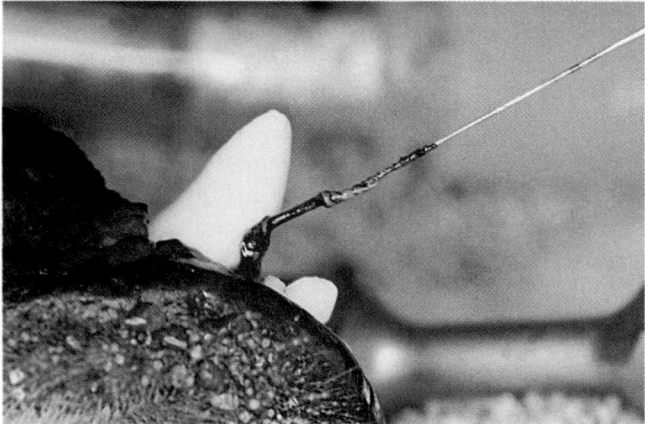

Figure 28-40 A barbed broach is used to remove pulp tissue from the tooth.

files. Hedström and K files are the most commonly used files (Figure 28-41). Hedström files have a sharper edge and can remove dentin faster than K files. They are used in a push-pull motion. They are more susceptible to file fracture than K files, however. K files are used in a push quarter clockwise turn-pull motion. Their edges are not as sharp, so dentin removal is less efficient than with Hedström files, but they are structurally sounder and less likely to fracture in the canal. The files are available in a number of different lengths and diameters. The smallest diameter file is a no. 6. They increase in diameter by even number increments from 6 to 10 and then they increase by increments of 5. For

instance, the following diameters exist: 6, 8, 10, 15, 20, 25, 30, 35, 40, and so on until file 60, at which point the diameter increases by 10. The largest diameter file is a 140. The length is 21 mm, 25 mm, 30 mm, or 31 mm. Special veterinary files are available for canine teeth that are 40 mm, 60 mm, or, most recently, 120 mm (Figure 28-41). This variation in length is necessary so that the tip of the tooth root can be reached in very long teeth (canines). The variation in diameter is necessary so that the narrow canals of old and/or small animals as well as the large canals of young or big animals (lions, horses) can be properly filed.

Files should be removed from the package and placed in an organized manner. In our practice we place the files in a piece of foam in increasing diameter from 6 to 40 or 45, and all the files in this group should be a standard length (e.g., 21 mm). The files in the foam can be autoclaved, and when the veterinarian is ready to perform the root canal, the foam of files will be sterile and in an organized manner. Several files of each diameter should be included. For instance, we put three of each size from 6 to 25. Two of these three files are K files, and the other one is a Hedström file. The files are organized with the two K files in front and the Hedström file in back (Figure 28-41). This attention to detail is helpful in minimizing anesthesia time because root canals can take 1 to 2 hours depending on the tooth and degree of skill.

Endodontic stops are small pieces of rubber that go around the file to mark a specific length (Figure 28-41). The file is placed in the root canal, and a radiograph is taken to make sure the file goes all the way to the apical extent of the root canal system (Figure 28-42). The distance from

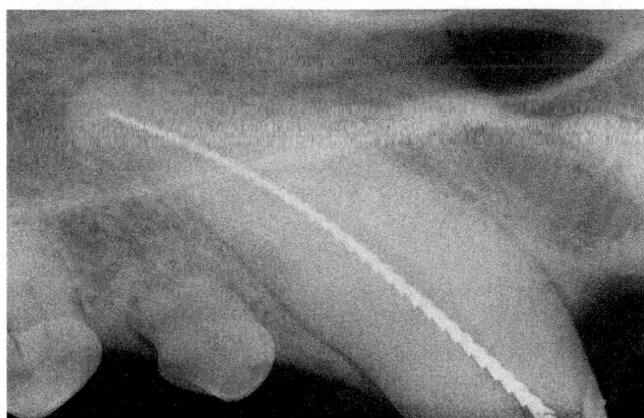

Figure 28-42 This radiograph verifies that the file is at the proper working length because the file tip goes all the way to the apical extent of the root canal.

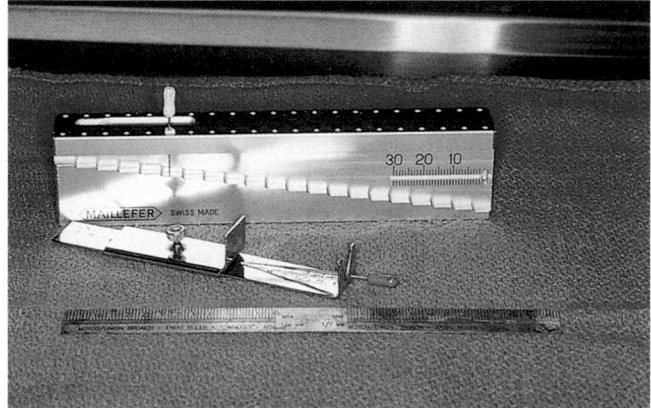

Figure 28-43 Measuring gauges used to measure the working length of the root canal. The two gauges at the top are used to quickly slide the endodontic stop to the correct length.

the endodontic stop (placed at a convenient location on the crown of the tooth) to the file tip is called the *working length*. The rest of the files are set to this length to ensure the root canal is filed to the proper depth. Measuring gauges are available that allow quick adjustment of the endodontic stop to the proper working length (Figure 28-43).

If rotary files are used they can be placed in a sterile sponge in order from smallest diameter to largest as well. The handpiece that attaches to these files should be set up. It will either be attached to the low-speed handpiece of the air-driven dental unit or have an electrical connection. The rotary engine-driven files may have two different file types available. The first type is a shorter file with a greater diameter increase along the taper. These files are referred to as *orifice shapers,* and they are used to open the coronal third of the root canal. The other set of files will be longer and should reach the apex of the tooth. The diameter of these files does not increase as rapidly along the taper.

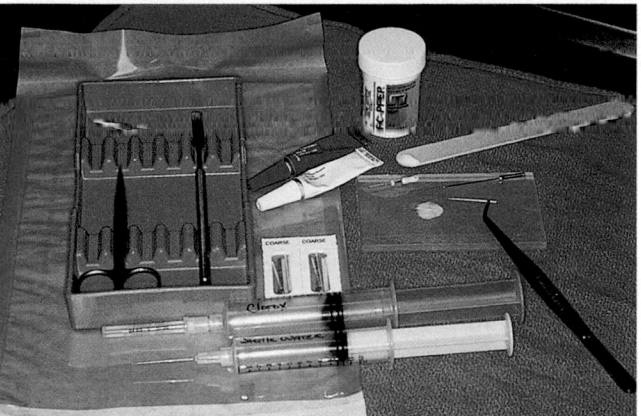

Figure 28-44 Root canal irrigants *(bottom),* paper points, and sterile glass slab with endodontic cement. The small jar contains a canal lubricant. Some of the lubricant has been placed on a tongue depressor. The files can be coated with lubricant without contaminating the stock bottle. The pink tray is autoclaved with the glass slab, cotton forceps, spatula, and iris scissors. The cement is mixed with the spatula on the glass slab.

Canal lubricants are sold that are used to soften the dentinal walls to ease filing and help prevent file breakage. One of these lubricants should be on hand. An irrigant is used in between file sizes to rinse the canal of dentinal shavings and other debris. The most common irrigant is sodium hypochlorite (i.e., Clorox bleach) because of its excellent disinfecting properties and ability to break down organic debris (pulp). Endodontic irrigation needles are placed on the syringe that contains the irrigant. These needles have a blunt end with a side opening to prevent forcing noxious irrigant periapically (Figure 28-44).

After the canal has been properly cleaned and shaped by the files, it is then ready for obturation. This simply means filling the canal with a material that will seal it from the periapical area. The canal should have a final rinse of sterile water, then it is dried with sterile paper points. Successive paper points are inserted and removed until the points come out of the canal dry. An endodontic sealer is then applied to the canal walls. Sealer application can be done with a sterile paper point, K file, or spiral paste filler on a slow-speed handpiece (Figure 28-44).

Gutta-percha is used to provide the bulk of the filling agent. It is a radiopaque viscoelastic material that can be vertically and laterally condensed to adapt to the shape of the root canal. The material can be heated to allow it to flow into the canal and adapt to the canal shape easier. Ultrafil cannulas are heated in a specially designed heater. When the heater indicates that the cannula is ready (flashing light), it is attached to a syringe and injected into the canal. The Thermafil system has gutta-percha coated on a file. The appropriate size gutta-percha coated files are selected based on the size of the canal and with the aid of a size verifier file. The correct size verifier file will fit passively in the root canal to the appropriate working length. The

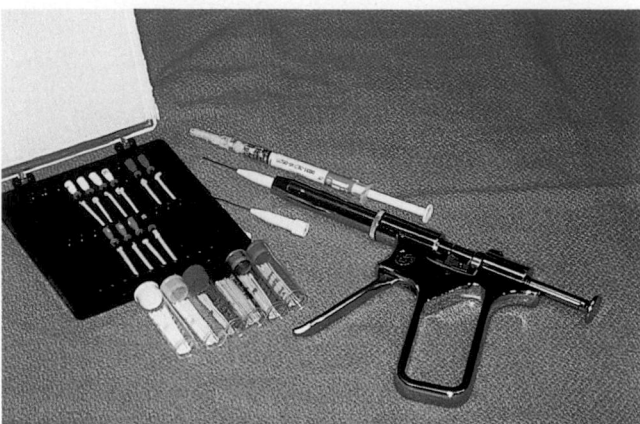

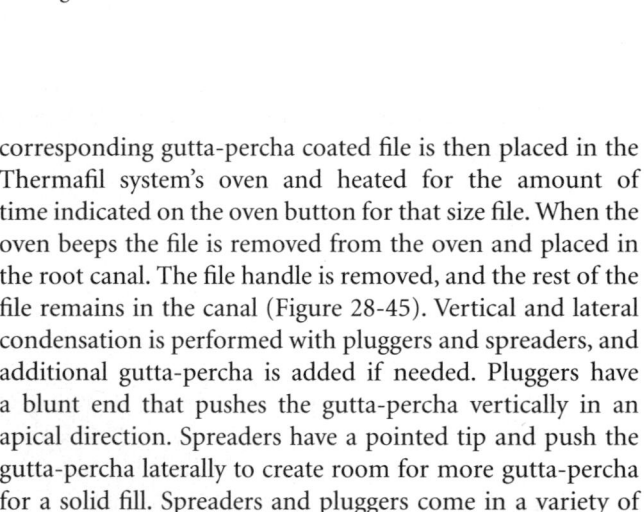

Figure 28-45 Gutta-percha products. The TB syringe contains gutta-percha (SuccessFil), the white cannulas go in the silver gun to inject gutta-percha (Ultrafil), and the gutta-percha–coated files in the black box are inserted into the canals and the handle is removed. These three techniques require heating of the gutta-percha before placement. The gutta-percha points in the vials are color coded to indicate size. These are placed in the canal without heating but can be heated once in the canal if desired.

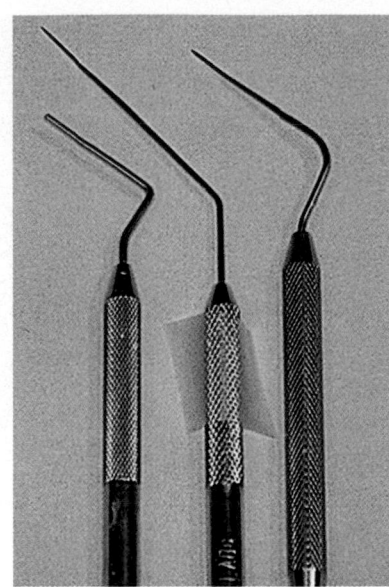

Figure 28-46 An endodontic plugger (*left*) and endodontic spreaders (*middle* and *right*). The spreaders have a pointed end, and the pluggers have a flat end.

corresponding gutta-percha coated file is then placed in the Thermafil system's oven and heated for the amount of time indicated on the oven button for that size file. When the oven beeps the file is removed from the oven and placed in the root canal. The file handle is removed, and the rest of the file remains in the canal (Figure 28-45). Vertical and lateral condensation is performed with pluggers and spreaders, and additional gutta-percha is added if needed. Pluggers have a blunt end that pushes the gutta-percha vertically in an apical direction. Spreaders have a pointed tip and push the gutta-percha laterally to create room for more gutta-percha for a solid fill. Spreaders and pluggers come in a variety of lengths and sizes (Figure 28-46). Extra long veterinary length spreaders and pluggers are available as well.

Once obturation of the canal has been accomplished, the restorative filling material is placed. This can be done with a single filling material or in two layers with an intermediate and final filling material used. Composite fillings cannot be placed next to eugenol because eugenol can interfere with the set of the composite. Gutta-percha does contain a large amount of eugenol. Glass ionomers are a commonly used intermediate or final filling material. If used as an intermediate filling material, a composite final filling material is then used for optimal esthetics.

Teeth that have undergone pulp death do become more brittle over time because of the lack of hydration that was originally provided by the pulp tissue. A good history should always be taken to try to determine how the pet fractured the tooth. If inappropriate chew toys are in the environment, these should be removed when possible. A metal cap may be desired to help prevent fracture of the tooth in the future.

EXODONTICS

Some people feel that tooth extraction is equivalent to failure for a dentist. Although it is fantastic to be able to save teeth for pets, it is not always in the pet's best interest to save a very diseased tooth. A good history from the owner is necessary to determine his or her level of commitment to the pet's oral health. If owners do not feel they can brush their pet's teeth daily or at least 3 times per week and are not likely to bring the pet back for professional dental care as necessary, then tooth extraction may be the best option for the pet. It can be very disheartening to have a pet go through advanced periodontal therapy only to see that the owner is not following through with the dental care at home and the pet returns to the office with an infected mouth and oral pain. The veterinary practice's ultimate goal is to provide the pet with a healthy and comfortable mouth.

Sometimes owners are willing to provide all the treatment necessary, but the tooth is too damaged to have successful results. In either scenario tooth extraction will be necessary. Very loose teeth can be easy to extract and sometimes fall out on their own when the technician is cleaning the teeth. These teeth should be set aside for the veterinarian to examine to make sure no portion of the root remains in the mouth, and they should be recorded on the dental record. Teeth with a healthy periodontium can be very difficult to extract, especially if they are multirooted. Tooth extraction techniques will be discussed so that the technician can have the appropriate equipment on hand for the veterinarian. In many instances a preoperative radiograph of the

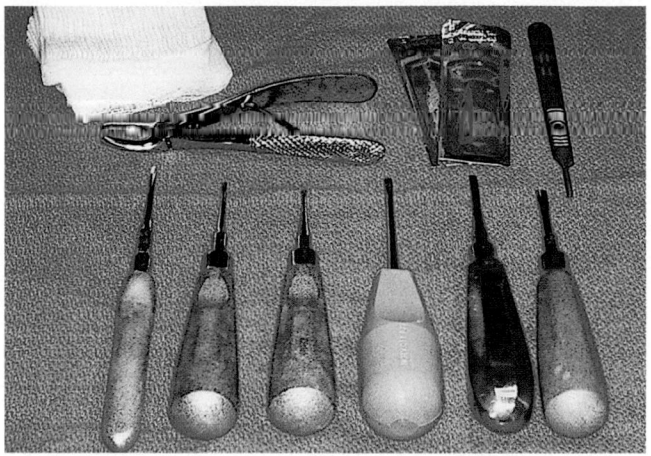

Figure 28-47 An assortment of dental elevators is necessary. Elevators with a small narrow blade are used initially, and as the periodontal ligament breaks down, larger-bladed elevators can be used. Small breed extraction forceps, scalpel blades and handle, and gauze sponges are on hand as well. Dental elevators *(left to right):* Cislak 100c, Cislak EX5, Cislak 301MX, luxator, Cryer 34S, E34.

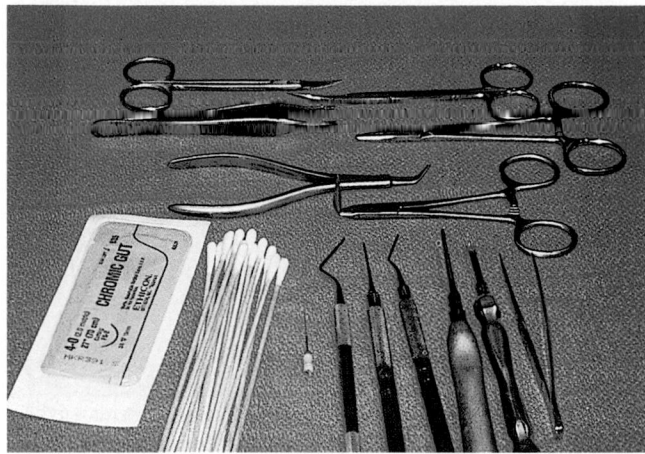

Figure 28-48 Small root-tip picks are necessary to retrieve broken roots or to extract teeth in very small animals. Dental elevators *(left to right):* Schein ST11, Cislak WA1, Cislak WA2, Cislak 100C, and a Farenkrug. A small tip tissue forceps or an endodontic file can also work well to retrieve loose root tips. Small root-tip forceps and suturing instruments should be on hand.

tooth will be taken to evaluate the roots and surrounding bone so that risk factors are minimized.

A no. 11 or 15 scalpel blade is used to sever the epithelial attachment of the gingiva around the cervical region of the tooth (neck). If the tooth is multirooted a periosteal elevator (Cislak Ex-9, Schein ST 7, Molt 9) (see Figure 28-10) can be used to lift the gingiva off the buccal or lingual bone to visualize the furcation. Vertical releasing incisions may be needed to allow further elevation of the gingiva to expose alveolar bone for removal over the tooth roots or to create a mucogingival flap to close the extraction site. Next, a small dental elevator is placed in the periodontal ligament space and rotated to put pressure on the tooth root (Figure 28-47). Pressure is held for 5 to 10 seconds, and then the elevator is advanced apically and rotated against the root in the opposite direction to create pressure and hold again. The goal is to fatigue the periodontal ligament and avoid tooth root fracture. Larger elevators are used as the periodontal ligament breaks down and allows more room to place a larger instrument (Figure 28-47). The veterinarian will therefore need a surgery pack of small to large dental elevators, a periosteal elevator, scalpel handle and blade, gauze squares, extraction forceps, suture, needle holders, thumb forceps, and scissors (dissection and suture).

Sometimes a root will fracture, and additional instruments will be needed to retrieve the retained tooth root. Small dental elevators called *root tip picks* are helpful for root tip retrieval as are very small tipped extraction forceps called *root tip forceps* (Figure 28-48). Cotton tip applicators are helpful to bloat hemorrhage in the alveolar socket to visualize the root tip. Once all tooth root material has been extracted, the socket should be debrided of any calculus

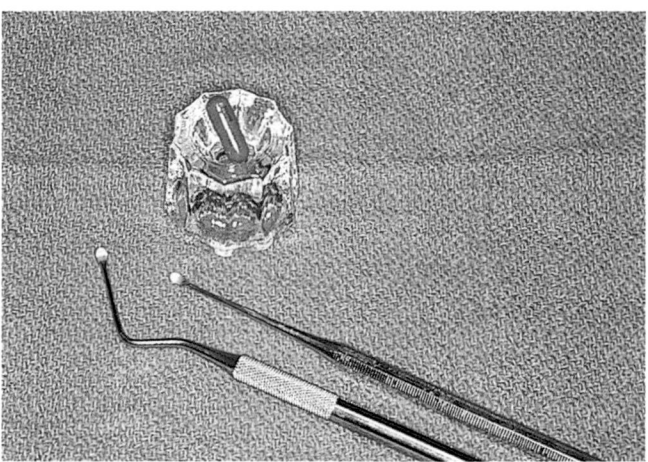

Figure 28-49 Bone curettes (Lucas 75, Schein ST10) and a tetracycline capsule in a dental dappen dish. The tetracycline powder can be poured into the dappen dish and placed into the alveolar socket with the bone curette.

and excessive granulation tissue with a spoon curette (Figure 28-49). If the site is to be closed with a mucogingival flap, tetracycline powder can be placed in the socket before closing the site if the animal is mature. The pet should be given soft food for 7 to 14 days following treatment and be given antibiotics and pain medications as deemed necessary by the veterinarian. Regional nerve blocks are very helpful with pain management and can be given at the time of surgery. The owner can resume tooth brushing in 3 to 14 days but may wish to avoid the extraction site until the pet no longer seems tender.

Tooth extraction is considered a surgical procedure in most instances, and serious complications can arise that the owner should be made aware of before admitting the pet for the procedure. Complications to address with the owner are those associated with anesthesia as well as the possibility of hemorrhage, eye trauma if working on teeth in the mid- to caudal maxilla, and jaw fracture. Iatrogenic jaw fracture can easily occur when extracting diseased mandibular first molars or canine teeth in cats or small breed dogs if care is not taken.

> ### ✐ TECHNICIAN NOTE
> Tooth extraction is considered a surgical procedure in most instances, and serious complications can arise that the owner should be made aware of before admitting the pet for the procedure.

Sometimes it is not possible to perform a complete tooth extraction because of tooth root ankylosis or resorption. When this occurs, the tooth root is fused to the adjacent alveolar bone. This is a common problem in cats with FORLs. It is possible to remove the crown and coronal one third to one fourth of the tooth root(s) and intentionally leave the remainder of the tooth root(s). This procedure is called *crown amputation* and it has been shown to cause less post-operative discomfort and minimal complications for cats with FORLs or ankylosed tooth roots provided there is no sign of an endodontic abscess or periodontal disease involving the remaining root fragment(s). The tooth crown and coronal root segment are removed with a dental bur and high-speed hand piece with water irrigation. The crestal alveolar bone is smoothed with the dental bur, and the gingiva is closed with absorbable suture over the crown amputation site. Postoperative care for these patients is the same as for traditional extraction cases.

ORTHODONTICS

Orthodontics is concerned with the correction and prevention of irregularities and malocclusion of the teeth. The primary reason for performing orthodontic correction of malaligned teeth in veterinary medicine is to alleviate a painful malocclusion or a malocclusion that will lead to endodontic or periodontal disease. When genetic malocclusions are suspected, the owner should be counseled on the problem in order to prevent breeding of these animals and the propagation of inferior genes.

Interceptive orthodontics involves the extraction of retained deciduous teeth that will usually cause displacement of the permanent dentition (Figure 28-50). This treatment can be extremely beneficial, and many abnormally erupting permanent teeth will correct spontaneously after extraction of the retained deciduous teeth. The most important factor determining success with this treatment is early detection of the problem. Many puppies and kittens have completed

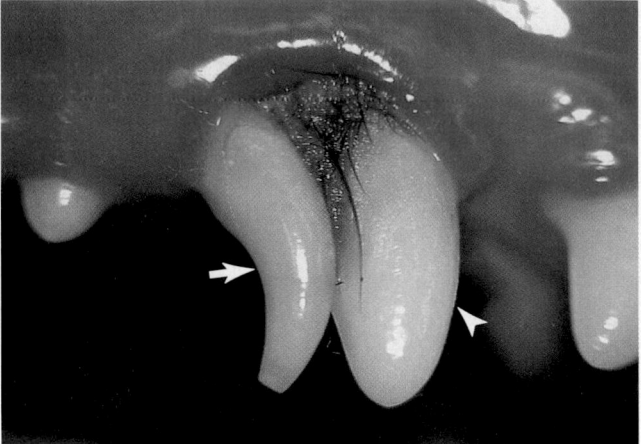

Figure 28-50   A retained deciduous maxillary canine tooth *(arrow)* has displaced the permanent canine tooth mesially (toward the nose) *(arrowhead)*. The abnormal tooth alignment can lead to periodontal disease and interfere with other teeth or oral soft tissues. (Courtesy Dr. Alfred G. Stevens, Sherwood South Animal Hospital, Baton Rouge, La.)

their vaccination series by the time they reach this mixed dentition stage and will not be seen again until 6 months of age if the owner has elected to neuter the pet. To prevent this condition from going undetected, the owner should be instructed to monitor the dentition closely to ensure that the deciduous tooth is shed before the emergence of the permanent tooth. Dental models can be used to show the owner the difference between deciduous teeth and permanent teeth. Dental examinations can be scheduled to ensure that a dental problem does not go undetected.

Retained deciduous teeth can occur in any breed of dog or cat, but it is most often seen in small breed dogs such as Yorkshire terriers, poodles, and dachshunds. Deciduous teeth should be shed prior to eruption of their permanent counterpart. When retained deciduous teeth are identified they should be extracted before they cause malalignment of their permanent counterparts. Retained deciduous teeth cause a predictable displacement of the permanent tooth. Most all permanent teeth will erupt lingual or palatal to the retained deciduous teeth with one exception. Maxillary canine teeth erupt mesial to the retained deciduous teeth. This is noteworthy because this malalignment will decrease the space between the maxillary canine and third incisor where the mandibular canine occludes. When this space is too narrow, the mandibular canine tooth will have interference with either one or both maxillary teeth and severe tooth wear (attrition) can occur. The pet will also have difficulty closing the mouth properly.

Extraction of retained deciduous teeth is a very rewarding procedure, but care must be taken. Deciduous teeth have long hollow roots that are thin walled and can fracture easily. The goal is to remove the entire tooth root to create a space for the permanent tooth to move into. The immature jaw contains numerous developing permanent tooth buds

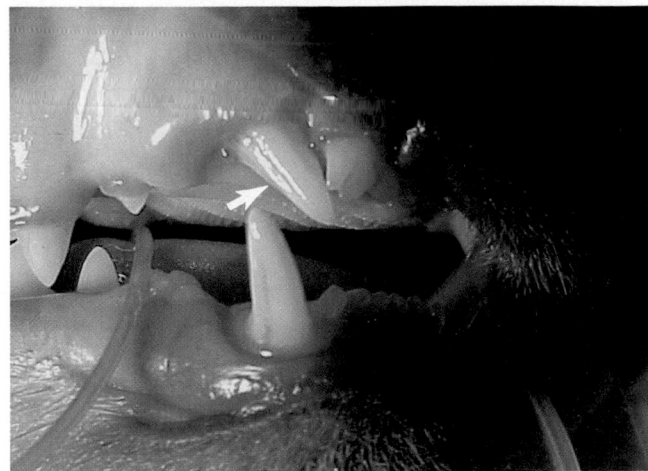

Figure 28-51 Mesially displaced maxillary canine tooth. The maxillary canine tooth is displaced mesially *(arrow)* and is striking the mandibular canine tooth when the mouth is closed. (Courtesy Dr. Alfred G. Stevens, Sherwood South Animal Hospital, Baton Rouge, La.)

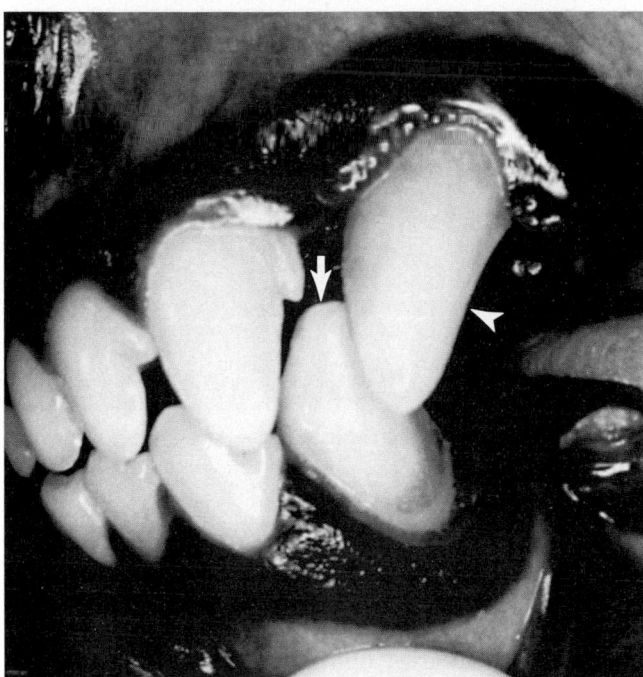

Figure 28-52 The mandibular canine tooth *(arrow)* has been shortened to prevent it from impinging on the palate. The maxillary canine tooth *(arrowhead)* is displaced mesially, preventing the mandibular canine tooth from returning to its normal position.

that can be damaged by dental elevators and stained by hemorrhage. The owner needs to be cautioned of the possibility of permanent tooth damage or discoloration. A skilled veterinary dental surgeon can significantly minimize these complications.

Some of the most common dental malocclusions seen are lingually displaced mandibular canine teeth (see Figure 28-4), mesially displaced maxillary canine teeth (Figures 28-51 and 28-52), and even or level bites. These malocclusions can be corrected by orthodontics in most cases, but the owner must be willing to invest the time to clean the oral appliance and return for rechecks as needed. Orthodontic treatment generally costs more than tooth extraction and involves more anesthetic procedures, but it is less invasive than extraction. Orthodontics can be an important treatment option when considering alternatives to extraction of large teeth such as the canines, or multiple teeth, such as the six incisors in a dog with an even bite. Many cases that present with the malocclusions listed above can be corrected rapidly with orthodontic treatment.

Crown height reduction with or without a vital pulpotomy is another option for animals with malocclusions, particularly severe malocclusions. This procedure entails shortening the tooth to remove the interference it is causing with another tooth or surrounding soft tissue. This method is less invasive than extraction, removes the animal's source of discomfort, and achieves results more quickly than does orthodontics. However, it does permanently alter the appearance of the tooth (see Figure 28-52). The pulp chamber is often exposed when the crown is reduced sufficiently. When this occurs, a vital pulpotomy will be necessary to protect the pulp tissue.

IMPRESSIONS AND MODELS

Veterinary technicians and dental assistants can be given the task of taking an impression and pouring a stone model if an orthodontic study model is needed. These stone dental models will aid treatment and serve as a record for treatment progress. The orthodontic appliances are often constructed from these models as well.

Alginate is the material that records the imprint of the teeth. The teeth should be cleaned before the impression is made. The appropriate size dental impression tray is selected for the patient. The area of interest must fit into the tray without touching the sides, and the tray must completely cover these teeth. Impression trays made for dogs and cats can be purchased. These trays are designed for the anterior portion of the mouth from about the level of the third premolar forward. This is where most of the treated orthodontic problems occur in dogs. Cats are rarely treated by orthodontic means because of poor patient acceptance.

The jar of alginate should be agitated (fluffed) with the top on before use and should be allowed to sit for at least 5 minutes after agitation so that the dust will settle. Level scoops of alginate are placed in a rubber mixing bowl. The scoop comes in the jar of alginate. A proper scoop of alginate will be level on the surface and will not contain filling voids. Gently tap the scoop of alginate to eliminate any voids, and then level the surface with the blade of the alginate spatula (Figure 28-53).

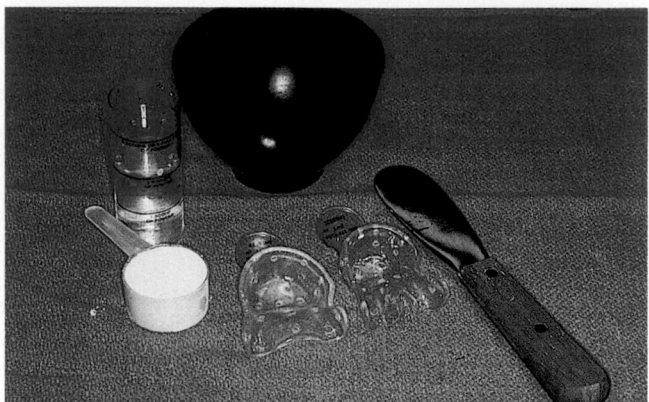

Figure 28-53 Materials used to take an alginate impression: rubber mixing bowl, alginate spatula, impression trays (mandibular and maxillary), alginate scoop, and water measuring cylinder.

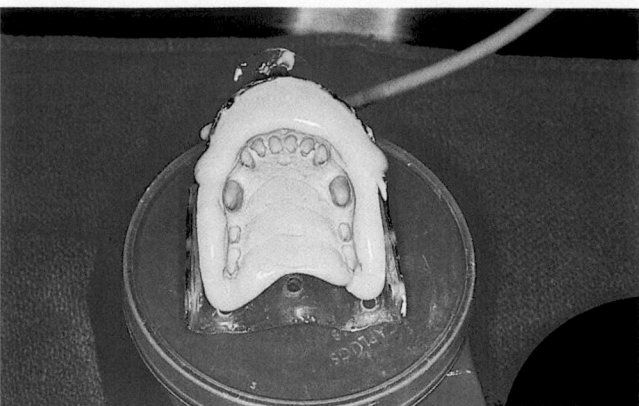

Figure 28-54 Alginate impression of the rostral maxillary dentition.

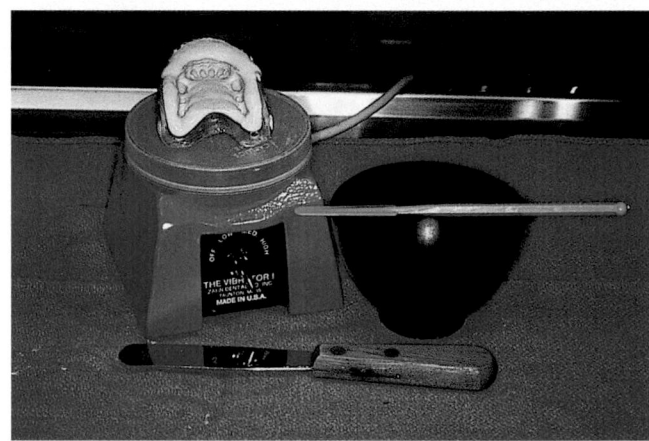

Figure 28-55 Materials used to pour a stone dental model: rubber mixing bowl, small blade spatula, narrow blade spatula, laboratory vibrator, and alginate impression.

Alginate spatulas have a wide blade that is used to blend the alginate powder with the water. A cylinder comes with the alginate to measure out the proper amount of water. The cylinder is clear plastic with three lines on it. Water is filled to the first line if one scoop of alginate is used, the second line if two scoops of alginate are used, and so on. The amount of alginate used is based on the size of the impression tray. The water is added to the alginate all at once, and the spatula is used in a stirring action to wet the powder. Once the powder is wet, the wide blade is used to start spatulating. The term *spatulate* means to spread and smear the alginate from one side of the bowl to the other in a back and forth motion. The bowl is held in the palm of the hand while the dominant hand works the spatula. Once the alginate is mixed, it is loaded into the impression tray with the spatula. The lips of the animal are held away from the teeth, and the tray is placed over the teeth. The tray should be held steady while the material sets. This takes about 5 minutes from the start of the mix. Cold water and room temperature will increase the set time, and warm water and room temperature will shorten the set time. The extra alginate around the rim of the impression tray can be touched periodically to determine when it is set. Once the material sets, it is similar to rubber and will not stick to the finger when touched. The impression tray and alginate are then removed from the teeth in one quick pulling motion in the direction of the long axis of the teeth.

Once removed from the teeth, the impression should be inspected to be sure the area of interest was adequately recorded (Figure 28-54). The material should then be rinsed off and a moist paper towel placed on it until the stone can be poured into it. The sooner the stone is poured, the more accurate the impression will be since alginate is susceptible to desiccation and overhydration. Most technicians pour the stone as soon as the animal is recovered from anesthesia or sooner when safely possible.

Dental stone is used to make the positive image of the mouth. The stone comes in a powder form and is mixed with water. The powder can be weighed out and mixed with a specified volume of water. Experienced technicians can determine the approximate amount of water and stone powder by the thickness of the mix. A good mix will slowly run off the mixing blade when held above the bowl. The rubber mixing bowls and a narrow blade spatula are used for the stone (Figure 28-55).

Once the stone is mixed, the alginate impression should be cleared of excess water by gently tapping or shaking it. The impression is then held on a laboratory vibrator while small amounts of stone are placed on the impression and allowed to run into the teeth. This step is critical because if an air bubble gets trapped in the teeth, the stone model will be missing part of the tooth. The vibrator serves two purposes. First, it helps to remove bubbles from the stone, and second, it causes the stone to flow into the teeth. Once the teeth have been filled with stone, the rest of the stone can be added at a faster rate since this step is less critical. The stone mix can then be made thicker by adding more powder.

This portion can be placed on the top of the model to give it a strong base. The vibrator is not used for this step. Optimal working time for the stone is about 10 minutes. Complete set of the stone takes about 1 to 2 hours.

The model should be removed from the alginate impression after the stone has had at least 45 minutes to set. Do not wait several hours because the alginate will dry and stick to the stone model. The model should be carefully pulled from the alginate and inspected to make sure all teeth are adequately recorded. If a portion of a tooth is missing, this could be a result of an air bubble or the tooth could have broken off and still remain in the impression. The canine teeth are particularly susceptible to fracture because of their long curved anatomy. If the stone tooth breaks, it can be glued back on the model. The model should then be labeled with the pet's name and the date.

RESTORATIVE DENTISTRY

The goal of restorative dentistry is to restore a tooth as closely as possible to its natural structure and function. No restorative material is as strong as the original tooth structure, so an attempt is always made to preserve as much of the original tooth as possible. Indications for restorative dentistry include teeth with dental caries (cavities), fractured teeth, and endodontically treated teeth.

Dental caries rarely occurs in the dog and cat. When present, the carious tooth structure must be completely removed and the defect restored. If left untreated, the caries will dissolve the enamel and dentin and gain access to the pulp tissue. The tooth will eventually be destroyed.

Fractured teeth are frequently restored to return function and maintain periodontal health. The cheek teeth (premolars and molars) have a natural design called the *cervical bulge* that deflects food away from the gingival sulcus. When the teeth lose this proper contour they can become predisposed to periodontal disease. Fractured teeth can be restored with restorative materials alone or in combination with retention pins or posts or both. Pins and posts do not add strength to the restoration but aid in retaining the restoration. Restoration of the bulge on the upper fourth premolar is usually best achieved with a metal crown because of the powerful shearing forces this area receives.

Caps or prosthetic crowns are placed on teeth with fractured crowns to protect the tooth, to improve function, and sometimes to improve esthetics. The silver-colored

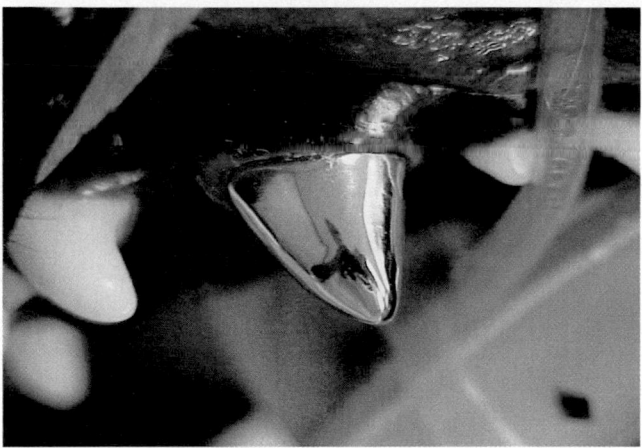

Figure 28-56 A non–precious metal crown has been cemented to the maxillary canine tooth after the tooth was traumatically fractured and received endodontic treatment. (Courtesy Dr. Alfred G. Stevens, Sherwood South Animal Hospital, Baton Rouge, La.)

metal caps, which are made of non–precious metals, are the most common type used because of their greater strength and lower cost when compared with gold or porcelain caps. The teeth most commonly capped in dogs are the canines and maxillary fourth premolars (Figure 28-56). In the cat, the canine is the most commonly capped tooth.

Veterinary dentistry is a specialty field in veterinary medicine. Advanced procedures require strong background knowledge of the materials used, the anatomy and physiology of the teeth and periodontium, and the principles applied to each procedure. It is important for the general practitioner and veterinary technician to be able to identify dental abnormalities and to be able to recommend treatment alternatives to the owner. The pet can then be referred for advanced dental procedures if the owner wishes to pursue treatment.

Recommended Reading

DeForge DH, Colmery BH: *An atlas of veterinary dental radiology,* Ames, 2000, Iowa State University Press.

Holmstrom SE, Frost P, Eisner ER: *Veterinary dental techniques,* ed 2, Philadelphia, 1998, WB Saunders.

Torres HO et al: *Modern dental assisting,* ed 5, Philadelphia, 1995, WB Saunders.

Wiggs RB, Lobprise HB: *Veterinary dentistry principles and practice,* Philadelphia, 1997, Lippincott-Raven.

29

Equine Medical and Surgical Nursing

LAIS R.R. COSTA • LESLIE TALLEY • RUSTIN M. MOORE

INTRODUCTION

The role of the veterinary technician in equine practice is to be a team member with a goal of providing efficient, quality health and nursing care for horses. A skilled, observant veterinary technician with equine-specific training is an invaluable resource in an equine hospital. Technicians are expected to provide patient monitoring, treatment, surgical assistance, nursing care, and client education. Providing veterinary care for horses is particularly cumbersome because they are large, fractious, and fragile animals. Skilled technical support with expertise in patient handling and restraint, specialized instrumentation, and equine-specific disease is crucial for the equine veterinarian to provide quality intensive care or perform advanced techniques. Familiarity with equine behavior will allow the veterinary technician to recognize abnormal behavior, permitting the early recognition of colic, pain, neurologic disease, and respiratory distress during patient monitoring, for example. The technician is often the first to identify a change in patient status and may save valuable time at a crucial turning point for therapeutic intervention. Familiarity with equine-specific surgical equipment will reduce surgical time and improve patient prognosis. Recognition of the unique layperson's language in equine medicine and surgery will help the technician recognize the significance of the patient's historical data and physical examination findings and improves client communication. Equine technical support imparts a tangible contribution to the quality and efficiency of patient care in a hospital setting. ▪

PHYSICAL EXAMINATION OF THE EQUINE PATIENT

A thorough physical examination is an integral part of the diagnostic assessment and monitoring of ill horses. Because

veterinary technicians play an important role in the day-to-day monitoring of hospitalized patients, learning to perform a thorough and complete physical examination is vital (see Chapter 2). A knowledgeable veterinary technician should ensure the safety of the handler, the examiner, and the patient when performing a physical examination. Handling the ill horse is inherently dangerous because most horses are more difficult to control when in pain or under stress. It is crucial to record all observations and findings of the physical examination in the medical record. The medical record provides the only record of the patient's progress or deterioration, and moreover it is a legal and scientific document (see Chapter 33).

> **✎ TECHNICIAN NOTE**
>
> The veterinary technician plays a pivotal role in the day-to-day monitoring of and caring for hospitalized patients; therefore the ability to be observant and to perform a thorough and complete physical examination is vital.

Physical examination should begin with observation of the equine patient from a distance and overall inspection of the animal and its surroundings, followed by a detailed assessment of each body system. The observation of the patient from a distance provides a more accurate assessment of the animal's mental status and attitude (the animal's interaction with its environment and other animals and response to external stimuli; thus the animal may appear bright and alert, depressed, obtunded, demented, responsive or unresponsive, excitable, etc.). Observation from a distance also allows assessment of the horse's breathing pattern and respiratory effort. Young horses and foals are likely to have increased respiratory rate and shallow breathing when approached. The horse's general body condition should be noted. The ribs should not be visible but should be easily palpated in a horse in ideal body condition. The horse's use and the physiologic demands, such as intense training, pregnancy, and lactation, should be considered when assessing body condition. Moreover, horses with mild depression or mild abdominal pain are more likely to demonstrate their true behavior when observed from a distance, whereas they may appear relatively normal when approached and examined. Several signs can indicate the horse is experiencing mild abdominal discomfort or pain. Those signs include pawing the ground with the front feet; kicking at the abdomen with the rear feet; looking at the flank or abdomen; curling the lip; posturing or straining to urinate or defecate; playing in the water bucket; lying down in sternal, lateral, or dorsal recumbency; and rolling on the ground.

Inspection of the horse's environment can also provide important information. Evidence of disrupted stall bedding could be an indicator of the horse being cast (unable to stand because the horse lies down too close to the wall) or could be an indication that the horse has experienced discomfort such as colic (abdominal pain). Exposed bare stall floor often indicates pawing of bedding. The amount of hay, feed, and water in the stall can be an important indicator of the horse's appetite and water intake. The amount, character, and quantity of feces in the stall and observation of the horse's drinking, urination, and defecation can also yield important information.

Close inspection of the horse should include evaluation of the head for swelling, wounds, and asymmetries; the nostrils for the presence and character of nasal discharge and for flared nostrils; and the eyes for ocular discharge (epiphora), the character of ocular discharge, and "squinting" (blepharospasm). Serous nasal discharge is often present in horses with viral respiratory disease, whereas horses with an infection of the frontal or maxillary sinuses or guttural pouches or horses with pneumonia often have a mucopurulent nasal discharge. Horses may have evidence of blood at the nostrils (epistaxis) as a result of guttural pouch mycosis, ethmoid hematomas, or exercise-induced pulmonary hemorrhage. Epiphora may be associated with a primary ocular disease or occlusion of the nasolacrimal duct system, or it may manifest secondary to a viral respiratory disease. Blepharospasm is usually a sign of ocular pain and is commonly observed in horses with corneal ulceration and uveitis. Coughing is generally a sign of lower respiratory tract disease [such as pneumonia, recurrent airway obstruction (RAO)] and can be productive or nonproductive. The presence of inspiratory or expiratory noise usually reflects an obstructive disease of the upper respiratory tract (nostrils to trachea). Dyspnea (difficult breathing) is characterized by flared nostrils, rapid and shallow thoracic excursions, and, if very severe, cyanotic mucous membranes; this should be brought to the attention of the attending veterinary clinician immediately. Flared nostrils (Figure 29-1) combined with the presence of prominent external abdominal oblique musculature ("heave line") extending anywhere from the tuber coxae toward the elbow (Figure 29-2) and a forced expiration usually indicate hat the horse has obstructive airway disease.

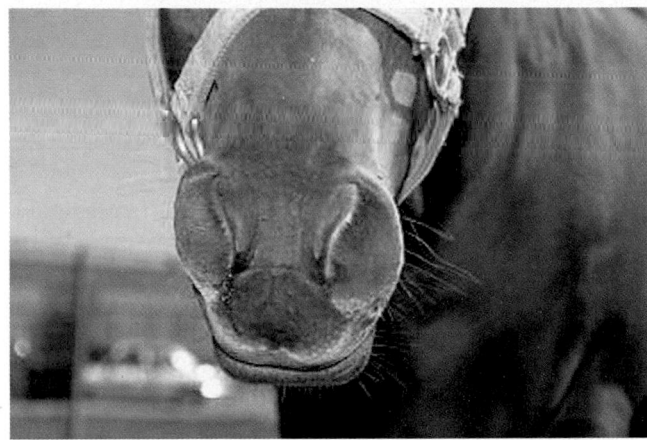

Figure 29-1 Flared nostrils on a horse with recurrent airway obstructive disease.

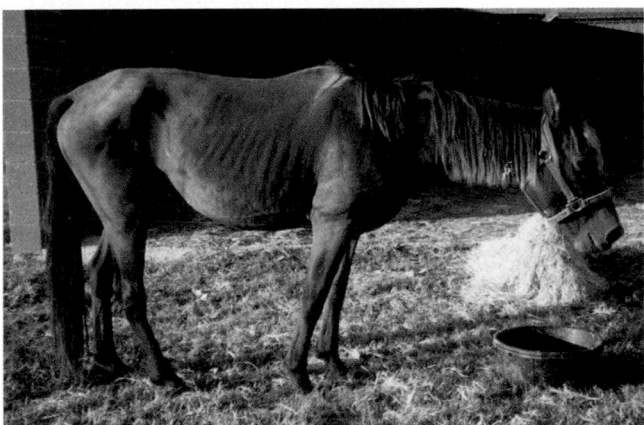

Figure 29-2 Horse with increased expiratory effort and heave line caused by obstructive airway disease.

Evaluation of the manner in which the horse ambulates in the stall can provide important information regarding the musculoskeletal and neurologic systems. Horses with laminitis (founder) often stand with their rear limbs camped underneath their torso and their front limbs extended in front of their torso in order to take weight off the toe and have an arched and tense back (Figure 29-3). These horses may ambulate in the stall, but it is particularly painful when they are forced to turn. Horses with navicular disease may stand with the heels of the front feet elevated. Horses with severe unilateral limb lameness may stand with all their weight on the unaffected limb and may hold the affected limb in a slightly flexed position. Evidence of ataxia (incoordination), generalized weakness, head tilted to one side, involuntary muscle tremors, and circling are suggestive of neurologic disease. Horses spending long periods in sternal or lateral recumbency because of painful musculoskeletal ailments (e.g., laminitis, rhabdomyolysis or "tying up," botulism) or neurologic diseases (hepatic encephalopathy, severe spinal cord disease) may often develop decubital ulcers (Figure 29-4).

Monitoring of vital signs, including rectal temperature, respiratory rate, heart rate, and character of the pulse, is very important. One must be careful when taking a horse's rectal temperature and take appropriate safety precautions to prevent self-injury. Some horses resent having their rectal temperature taken and will kick. The horse should be approached from the left side, standing as close to its body as possible. The handler should also be located on the left side of the horse. One should slowly work toward the rear of the horse, carefully raise the tail, and slowly insert a

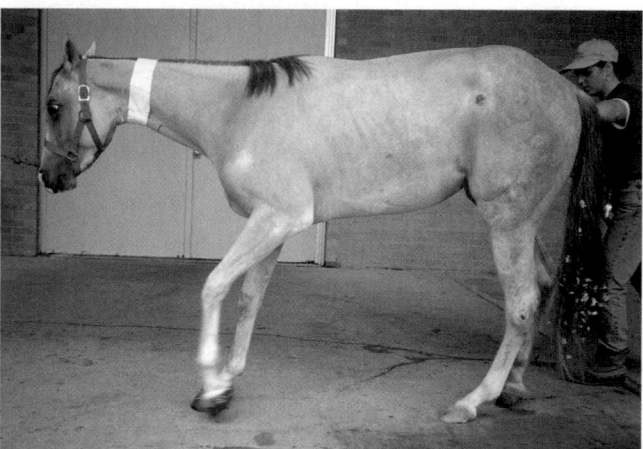

Figure 29-3 Typical posture of a horse with laminitis walking or turning on a hard surface.

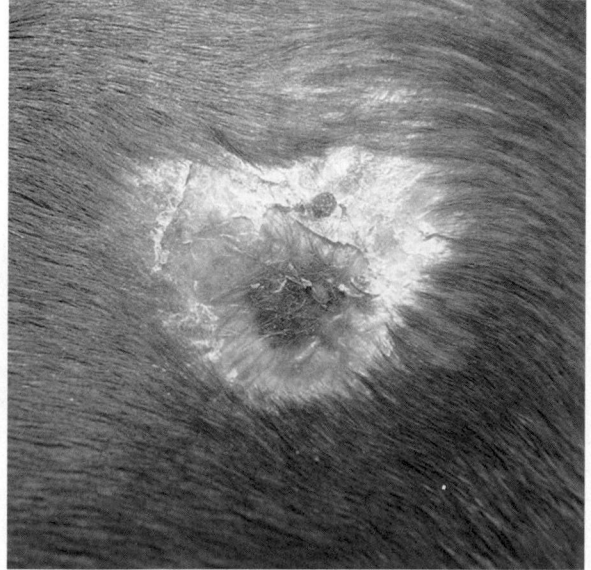

Figure 29-4 Pressure sores (or decubital ulcers) on a horse secondary to prolonged recumbency.

lubricated thermometer into the rectum. Some horses will clamp down their tail. Do not stand directly behind the horse when taking the temperature because a kick could cause serious injury or death. The thermometer should be attached to a string or piece of rubber tubing and an alligator clip so that it can be attached to the tail hairs, which will prevent it from dropping to the floor during defecation. The normal rectal temperature of adult horses is approximately 37° C to 38.5° C (99° F to 101.5° F). An increased rectal temperature usually indicates an inflammatory or an infectious process somewhere in the body, but hyperthermia can occur after exercise and secondary to environmental conditions (hot, humid, poor ventilation), especially in anhidrotic (unable to sweat) horses. Hypothermia can occur regardless of the environmental temperature, particularly in foals and also in old and debilitated horses. The heart rate of adult horses should range from 25 to 50 beats/min and is generally 30 to 40 beats/min. The respiratory rate is generally 8 to 20 breaths/min. The heart rate can be determined by auscultating the heart or by obtaining the pulse from the linguofacial or transverse facial arteries (Figure 29-5).

The heart rhythm should also be assessed during auscultation of the heart; second-degree atrioventricular block is a common arrhythmia in adult horses and usually is alleviated by exercise. Atrial fibrillation is characterized by an irregular cardiac rhythm and can be confirmed on an electrocardiogram by a rapid and irregular rate and absent P waves. Auscultation and percussion of the thoracic cavity are important to assess the status of the lower respiratory tract and thoracic cavity. Both lung fields should be auscultated carefully (Figure 29-6). Frequently a rebreathing bag is used during auscultation of the lungs in adult horses to increase the depth of breathing by increasing the inspiratory and expiratory volumes and thus exacerbating adventitious sounds (Figure 29-7). A muzzle secured to the halter will aid in the prevention of the bag occluding the nostrils. Abnormal lung sounds, such as crackles and wheezes, can be auscultated in horses with pneumonia. End-expiratory wheezes can often be heard in horses with

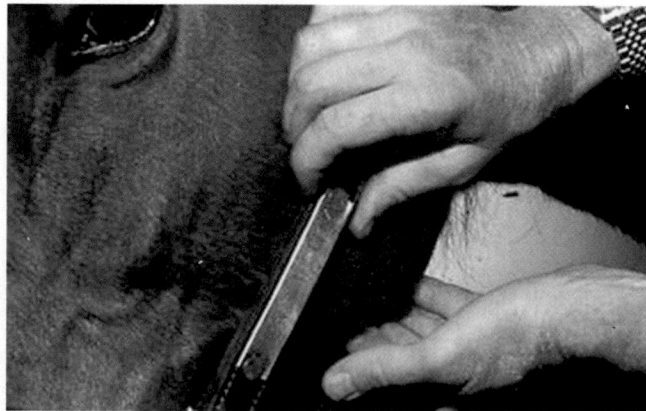

Figure 29-5 Determination of pulse rate and arterial pulse pressure through palpation of the facial artery.

RAO. In horses with pleural effusion, the heart and lungs sounds can be muffled, and a fluid line can be frequently identified by auscultation and percussion of the thorax.

Oral mucous membranes should be assessed for color, moistness, capillary refill time after blanching, icterus, and petechiae. The oral mucous membranes should typically be light pink in color and moist to the touch. The capillary refill time should be less than 2 seconds. Cyanotic (whitish blue) mucous membranes often indicate severe hypoxemia (insufficient quantity of oxygen present in the blood) and are often observed in horses with respiratory disease. Dark pink to bright red mucous membranes are often observed in horses with endotoxemia. Dry, tacky mucous membranes often reflect volume depletion and are frequently observed in horses that are dehydrated or in shock. The sclera should

also be examined for injection and icterus; this is particularly important in neonatal foals (Figure 29-8).

The veterinary technician is also expected to be able to collect venous blood samples. Venous samples can be taken from the jugular veins using a vacutainer and a vacutainer cuff attached to the needle. Alternative sites for venous blood collection include the cephalic veins and the transverse facial vein, but only in debilitated or nonfractious horses. The transverse facial vein is most generally used for collection of small volumes of blood (e.g., 2 to 5 ml for routine monitoring of packed cell volume and total plasma protein, although larger volumes may be drawn from this site. Using a small gauge (21- to 25-) needle and a 1-, 3-, or 5-ml syringe, insert the needle parallel and approximately 2 cm ventral to the facial crest. Aspirate gently and adjust the depth of the needle until blood fills the syringe (Figure 29-9).

Auscultation and percussion of the abdominal cavity (Figure 29-10) should be performed carefully and thoroughly, especially in horses with gastrointestinal tract diseases (colic, diarrhea). The abdominal cavity is generally arbitrarily divided into right and left dorsal and ventral quadrants for purposes of auscultation and percussion. In addition, the degree of abdominal distention should be assessed and monitored. This can be performed by subjective visual observation or can be assessed more objectively by measuring abdominal circumference at a consistent site. Monitoring of abdominal distention is especially useful in colicky foals.

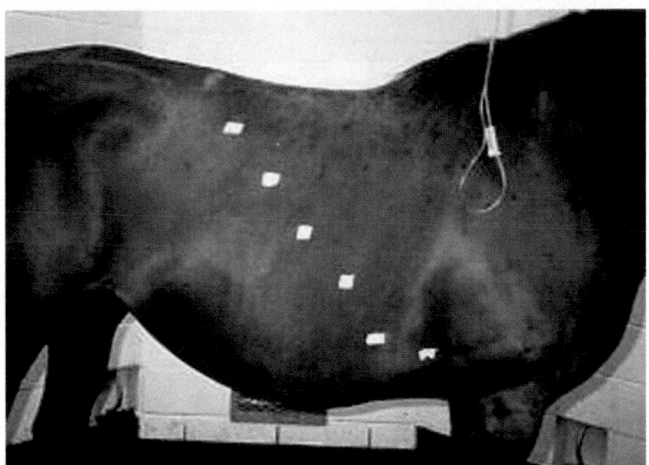

Figure 29-6 Outline of the lung fields in the horse.

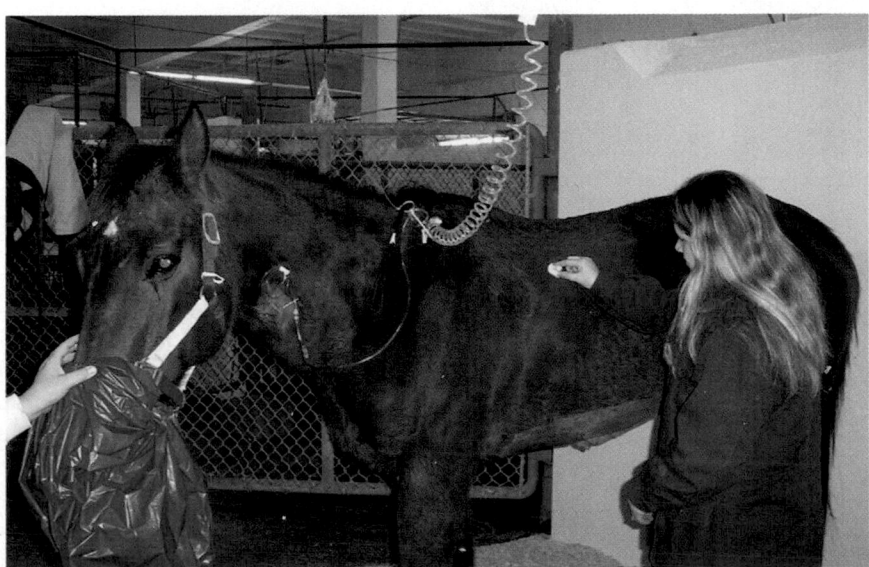

Figure 29-7 Use of a rebreathing bag to stimulate the horse to breathe more deeply to accentuate both normal and abnormal lung sounds during thoracic auscultation.

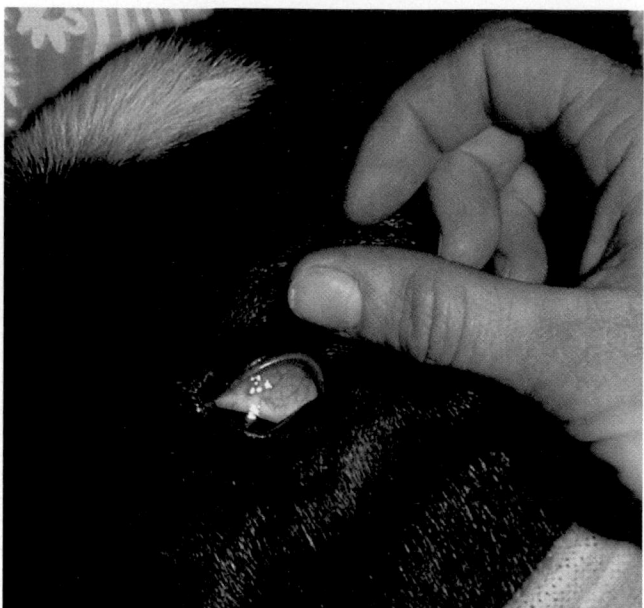

Figure 29-8 Scleral injection in a neonatal foal is suggestive of sepsis.

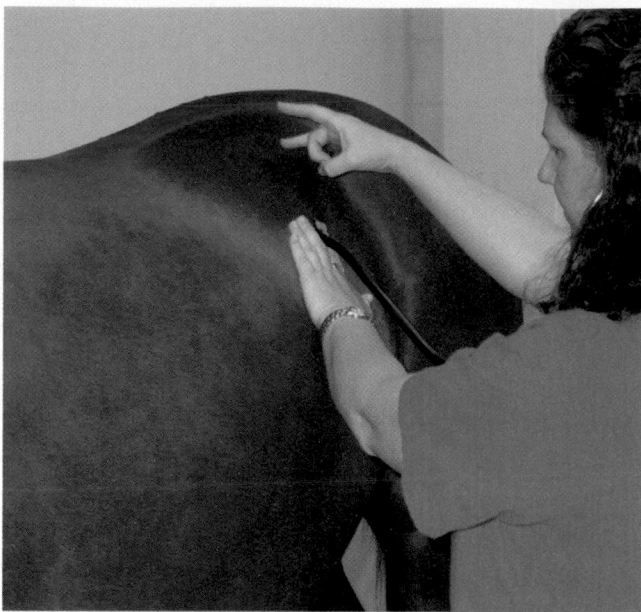

Figure 29-10 Auscultation and percussion of the abdominal cavity.

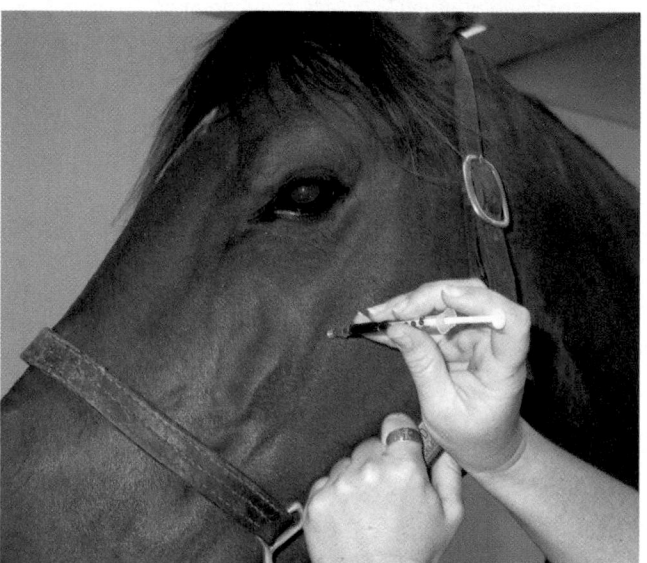

Figure 29-9 Blood collection at the dilation of the transverse facial vein.

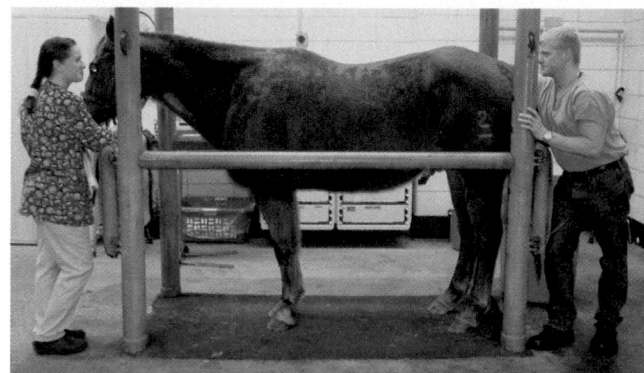

Figure 29-11 Rectal examination of a horse that is physically restrained with the use of stocks.

> ### TECHNICIAN NOTE
>
> Horses are unable to evacuate their stomach by vomiting; therefore it is important that the veterinary technician become knowledgeable and proficient in nasogastric intubation to prevent a catastrophic rupture of the stomach.

Last, rectal examination is important in the evaluation of adult horses with conditions involving the abdominal cavity, and it is often considered an extension of the physical examination of horses with colic, diarrhea, or weight loss. A rectal examination should only be performed by a veterinarian in horses that are properly restrained (Figure 29-11). Rectal trauma can be sustained during a rectal examination and can lead to a tear or perforation that is fatal. Likewise, digital rectal palpation of a young foal suspected to have a meconium impaction should be carefully performed by a veterinarian.

Because ill horses are predisposed to develop laminitis, the digital pulse and hoof heat should be evaluated often. The digital pulse can be palpated at the level of the fetlock over the abaxial surface of the sesamoid bones (Figure 29-12). Normally the pulse can be palpated, but it should not be bounding. Although subjective, evaluation of hoof heat can be useful, particularly if there is a unilateral disease process. Hoof heat increases secondary to laminitis, sole abscess formation, and other infectious or inflammatory conditions of the foot. The digital pulse can increase subsequent to

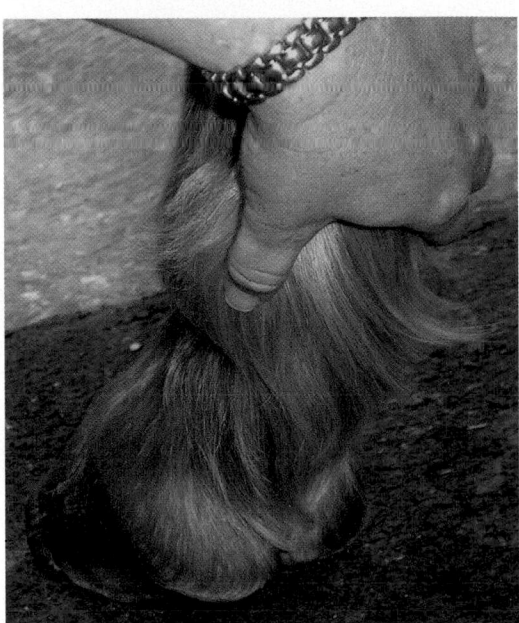

Figure 29-12 Location for palpation of digital pulse in a horse.

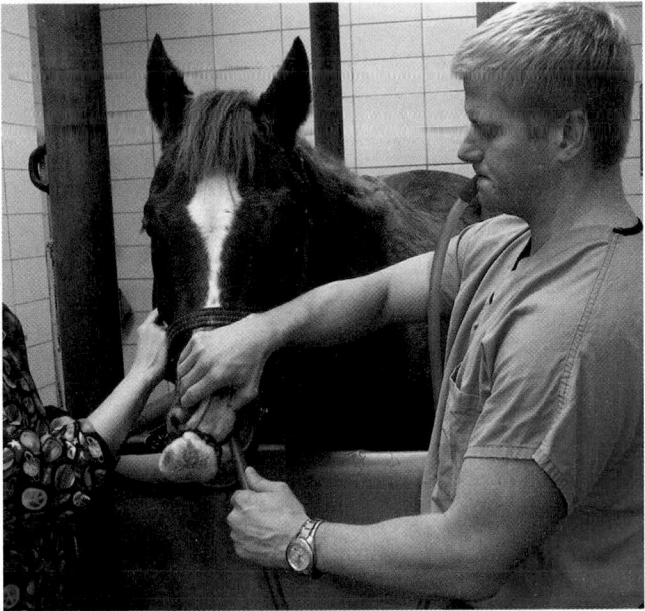

Figure 29-13 Nasogastric intubation in an adult horse.

any disorder of the foot, but an increase occurs commonly with laminitis, sole abscess, and third phalanx fractures. Laminitic horses are reluctant to move, particularly when turning or stepping on a hard surface. Proper management measures and therapy for acute laminitis should be instituted as soon as possible.

Passage of a nasogastric tube is an essential part of the examination and treatment of horses with colic. Because horses are unable to evacuate their stomach by vomiting, it is important that the technician becomes knowledgeable and proficient in nasogastric intubation to prevent a catastrophic rupture of the stomach. The nasogastric tube can be passed by standing on the horse's left side and placing the right hand on the bridge of the nose to control movement of the horse's head (Figure 29-13). The end of the nasogastric tube to be passed into the stomach should be held in the left hand, and the opposite end of the tube should either be held in the mouth or draped around the neck of the person passing the tube. Lubrication of the end of the tube with warm water or a water-soluble jelly may facilitate the passage through the nasal canal. The thumb of the right hand is used to push the tube into the ventral meatus of the nasal passages. The tube should be advanced slowly through the nasal passages because if the tube briskly contacts the ethmoid turbinates, profuse bleeding can occur. As the nasogastric tube is advanced through the nasopharynx the neck should be flexed to facilitate swallowing of the tube and to avoid placing the tube into the trachea. Once the horse swallows the tube, the nasogastric tube should be advanced. The person passing the nasogastric tube should confirm that the tube is within the esophagus by obtaining negative pressure when sucking back on the tube or by visually observing or manually palpating the tube within the

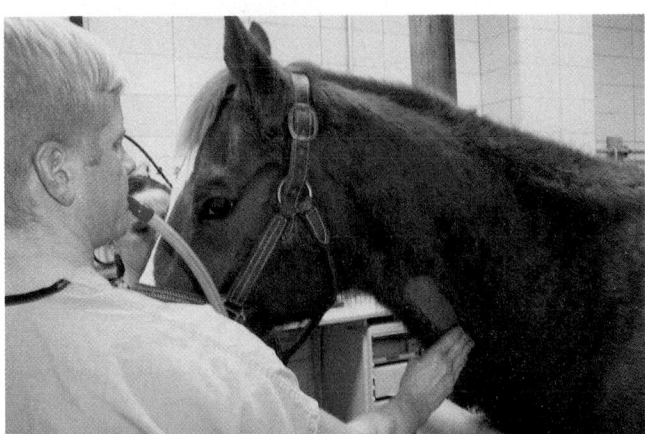

Figure 29-14 Confirmation that the nasogastric tube is within the esophagus.

esophagus on the left side of the neck above the jugular groove (Figure 29-14). Adult horses often cough vigorously when the nasogastric tube is accidentally passed into the trachea; however, severely depressed and sedated horses may not cough at all. After it has been confirmed that the tube is within the esophagus, air can be blown through the tube to dilate the esophagus as the tube is being advanced into the stomach.

TECHNICIAN NOTE

Special care should be taken when intubating the stomach of a neonatal foal. Neonatal foals often do not have a normal swallow reflex, and they rarely cough when the tube is located in the trachea. Avoid blowing into the nasogastric tube because accidental rupture of the foal's stomach can occur.

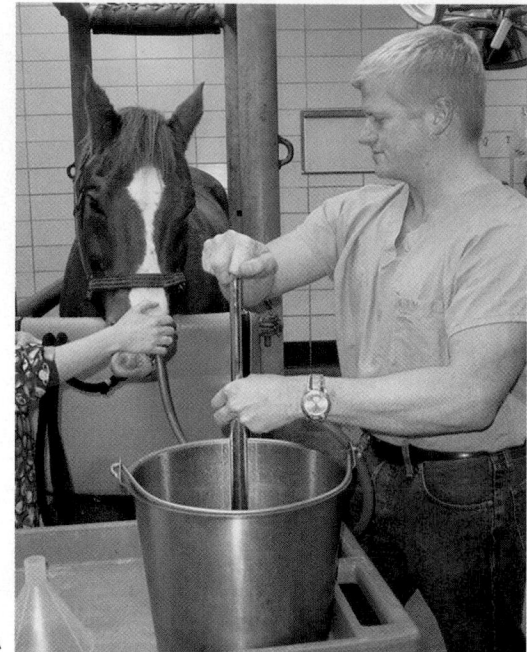

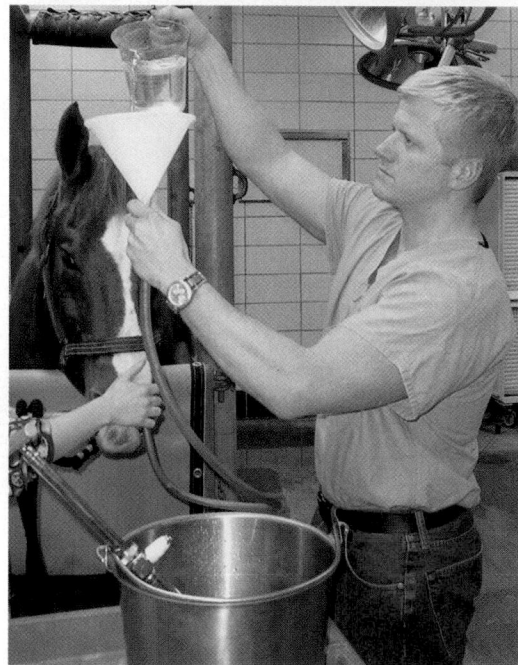

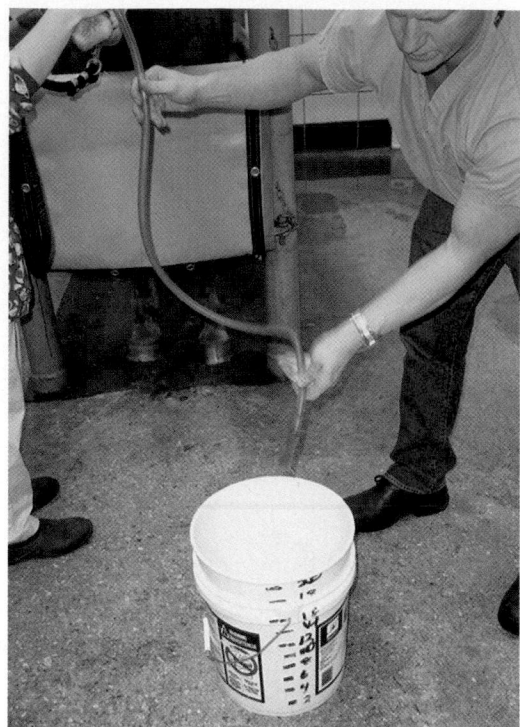

Figure 29-16 Evacuation of fluid from the stomach of a horse through a nasogastric tube.

Figure 29-15 Once in the stomach, the nasogastric tube should be primed with water to initiate a siphon effect. This can be achieved by filling the tube with water through the use of either a pump (**A**) or gravity flow with a funnel (**B**).

Once the tube is within the stomach it should be primed with water to obtain a siphon effect. The nasogastric tube can be primed by pumping water or allowing water to flow by gravity through a funnel (Figure 29-15, *A* and *B*). Once the tube is primed, the end of the tube should be lowered to allow stomach contents to flow (Figure 29-16); sometimes it is helpful to pull the tube out in small movements until flow becomes steady. It is helpful to use a tube of as large a diameter as possible to facilitate removal of feed material from the stomach. It is also helpful to have several fenestrations along the end of the tube to encourage drainage, as some fenestrations become occluded with feed material. The quantity of fluid that is placed within the tube and stomach for priming should be subtracted from the total amount of fluid obtained to determine the net amount of reflux, which should be recorded in the medical record. This provides a monitoring tool for determining the magnitude of the intestinal obstruction, determining whether ileus (abnormal intestinal motility) is improving, and monitoring fluid therapy. Moreover, the character of the gastric fluid (e.g., hemorrhagic, yellow, fermented grain, putrid smell) and the pH of the fluid will provide important information.

If no net reflux is obtained, then fluids or medications such as mineral oil (intestinal lubricant), magnesium sulfate (osmotic cathartic), dioctyl sodium succinate (surface-acting agent), psyllium hydrophilic mucilloid (bulk laxative), and bismuth subsalicylate (intestinal protectant) may be administered through the nasogastric tube. The total capacity of the stomach of adult horses is not very large, and no more than 6 to 8 L should be administered at one time. In horses being administered oral fluids, 6 to 8 L can be administered every 2 to 4 hours. In situations where net reflux is obtained

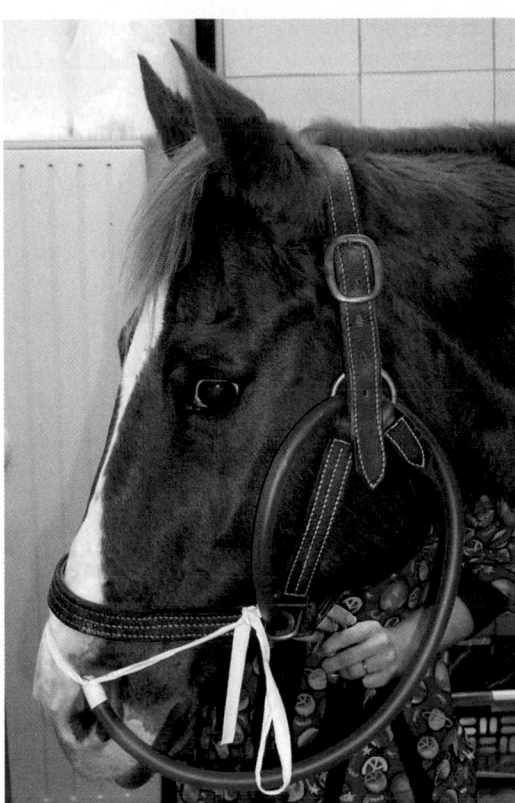

Figure 29-17 Technique for securing a nasogastric tube in the proper position. Adhesive tape can be applied to the tube and then tied to a securely fitting halter. This will help prevent dislodgment of the tube.

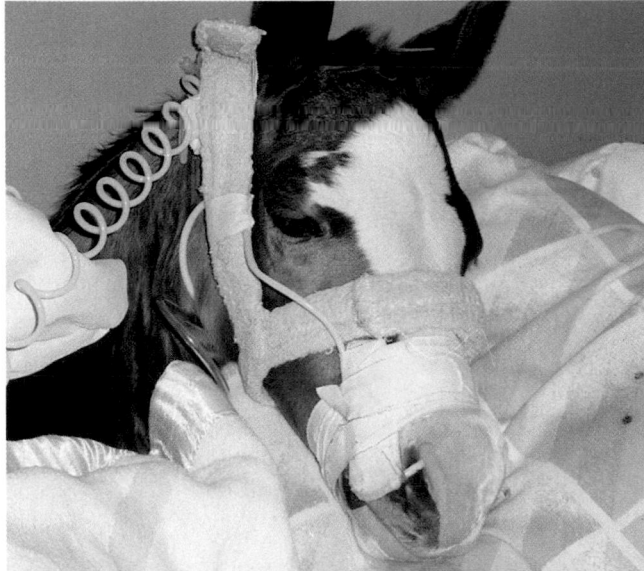

A

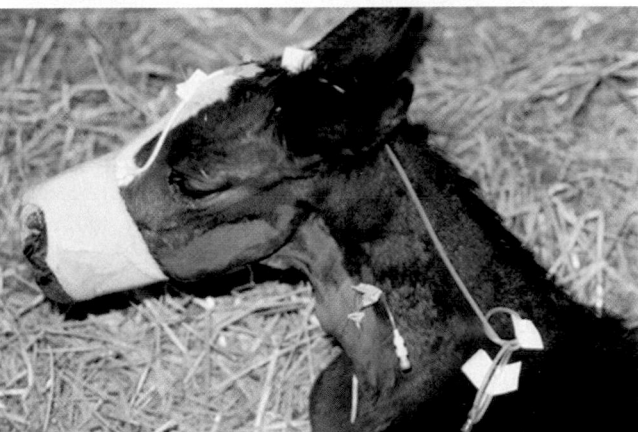

B

Figure 29-18 **A,** Nontraumatic technique for securing a nasogastric feeding tube in a foal (by using a tongue depressor taped to the nasogastric tube and then taped to the foal's maxilla with adhesive tape placed circumferentially around the foal's muzzle. (Courtesy Dr. J. Palmer.) **B,** Alternative technique for securing a nasogastric feeding tube in a foal (by suturing the tube to the nostril and securing to the maxilla with Elasticon adhesive tape placed circumferentially around the foal's muzzle).

or when fluids are being administered via nasogastric tube, the tube can be secured in place with adhesive tape and tied to the halter (Figure 29-17). If the tube is kept in place because the horse is continuously refluxing, the external end of the tube may be left unplugged to allow spontaneous drainage. Alternatively, the horse with voluminous continuous reflux may be checked hourly, and the amount of reflux quantified. Indwelling nasogastric tubes are not benign; horses with tubes that are kept in place for long periods can develop inflammation and ulceration of the pharynx and esophagus. Therefore, horses that salivate or chew excessively should be closely monitored because these horses are prone to develop esophageal ulceration or perforation. Nasogastric tubes can become fragmented, and the tube fragments could potentially cause gastrointestinal tract obstruction.

A similar method is used for nasogastric intubation in foals, but a smaller diameter, more pliable tube should be used. Indwelling tubes are often used for feeding sick foals; the end of the tube should be placed in the middle or distal esophagus rather than the stomach. When priming the tube with water or administering medication via a nasogastric

tube in foals, the fluid should be administered with a funnel via gravity flow. It is often helpful to secure the tube to the foal's nostril with a tongue depressor attached to the tube and taped to the foal's head (Figure 29-18, *A*). Alternatively, the tube can be secured with a tape butterfly and suture to an elastic tape around the foal's head (Elasticon, Johnson & Johnson) placed over the bridge of the nose (Figure 29-18, *B*).

The technician should be familiar with the normal range of vital signs in foals and the differences among adult horses. Temperature should range from 37.3° C to 38.8° C (99° F to 101.8° F). The heart rate varies considerably in foals

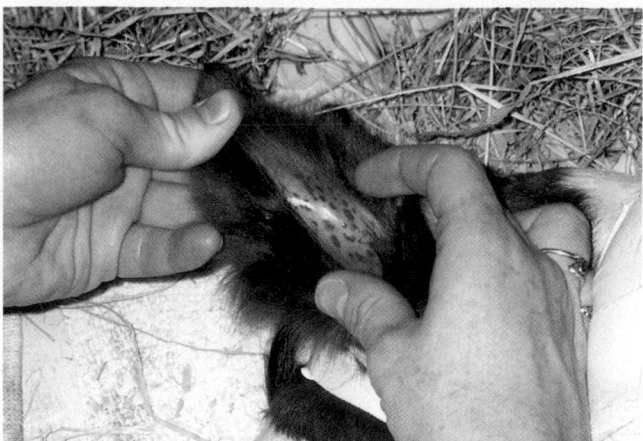

Figure 29-19 Presence of petechial hemorrhages in the pinna of newborn foal is suggestive of sepsis.

within the first week of life; it is usually 40 to 80 beats/min in the immediate postpartum period, increases to 120 to 150 beats per minute during the next several hours, and then stabilizes at approximately 80 to 100 beats/min during the first week of life. The respiratory rate in the neonatal foal is approximately 60 to 80 breaths/min in the immediate neonatal period and decreases to approximately 30 breaths/min within 1 hour of birth. Thoracic auscultation is not a reliable indicator of lower respiratory disease in the foal; often only subtle abnormalities are detectable on auscultation, even in the presence of severe pulmonary disease.

Physical examination of foals is similar to that of adult horses; however, there are several areas that need to be more closely evaluated in foals than in adult horses. The sclera, mucous membranes, and pinna should be evaluated for the presence of icterus and petechiae (Figure 29-19). Icterus and petechiae are often associated with neonatal sepsis and hemolysis. The umbilicus should be observed and palpated for heat, pain, swelling and moisture, which are indicators of umbilical remnant disease; ultrasonography may help in further evaluation of umbilical remnant disease. All joints of foals should be evaluated and palpated on a daily basis; effusion (joint swelling) or periarticular swelling and heat are indicators of joint infection. See Neonatal Care for more information.

RESTRAINT OF THE EQUINE PATIENT

Proper restraint of the equine patient is important to protect the handler, examiner, and patient from injury or death (see Chapter 1). Both physical and chemical methods can be used to achieve proper restraint (see Chapter 1). The handler should always stand on the same side of the horse as the examiner. This is important because if the horse is anxious or fractious and is moving, the handler can turn the horse's front end toward the examiner so that the rear limbs of the

horse go away from the examiner. This will prevent injury from occurring secondary to the horse kicking the examiner. The handler should always lead the horse from its left side. The snap of the lead shank should be attached to the ring of the halter on the chin strap. A cotton or nylon lead shank can be used with or without a chain attached. The chain is useful when handling fractious or difficult horses. The chain portion of the shank can be placed over the bridge of the nose, under the chin, or over the gums to provide more secure control of some horses. This may be particularly necessary in stallions. The chain should be placed through the rings of the halter on the chin strap and on both sides of the halter, and then the snap should be attached to the ring on the chin strap. Care must be taken when using the chain in this manner because many horses are not accustomed to this and may rear or resist handling.

> **TECHNICIAN NOTE**
> Horses can be dangerous; therefore proper handling and restraint of the equine patient are critical to protect the handler, examiner, and patient from injury or death.

Technicians are often involved in conducting lameness or neurologic examinations of equine patients. When walking or jogging a horse, the handler should walk or jog along on the horse's left side and allow approximately 1 foot of shank between the right hand and the horse's head. This allows the horse to have some movement of its head, which can be important when conducting a lameness examination. This also enables the handler to stay far enough away from the horse to prevent getting stepped on. The handler should not look back at the horse when walking or jogging because this often causes the horse to resist forward movement. The surface where the horse is being walked or jogged is important. A hard surface, such as concrete or asphalt, allows one to better hear and sometimes better observe a subtle lameness, but this kind of surface can cause damage to unshod hooves and can be slippery, particularly if wet. Therefore caution must be taken when handling horses on this type of surface.

In a hospital setting, horses can be placed in stocks for performing many necessary procedures. Although this helps control the horse's movement, it is not the best method of restraining some horses. Some very anxious or fractious horses can actually cause more injury to themselves if placed in stocks. Therefore the horse's temperament and level of training should be taken into consideration when contemplating the use of stocks for restraint. When placing a horse in stocks, both the front and rear gates should be opened and the handler should walk through from rear to front and allow the horse to follow. An assistant should close the gate behind the horse and secure it before the handler closes the gate at the front of the stocks. This will prevent the horse from suddenly backing out of the stocks before the rear gate can be closed. Many stocks have a set

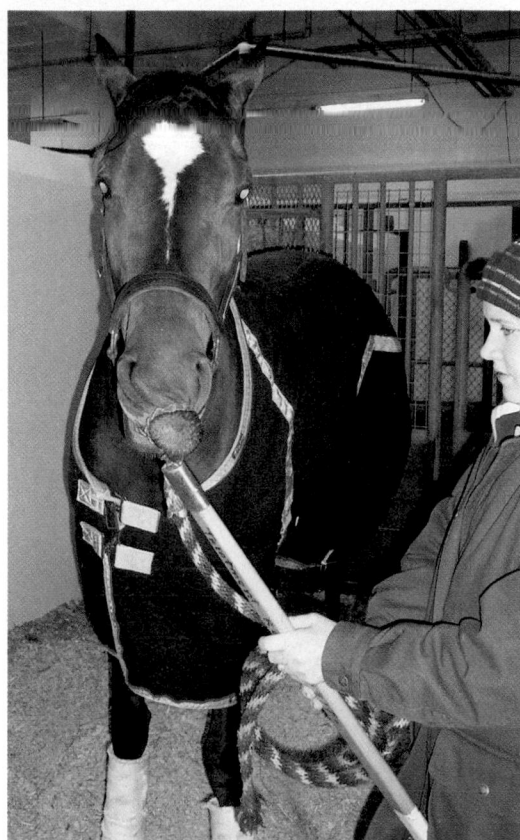

Figure 29-20 Technique for restraining a horse with a nose twitch.

of cross ties at the front. Many horses can be secured with cross ties, but they should not be used on fractious horses. Rather, the handler should remain at the horse's head. Horses should always be untied or released from the cross ties before the rear gate is opened to avoid the animal panicking and potentially injuring itself. Horses should never be left unattended in stocks because they can easily become frightened or anxious and attempt escape. This can lead to severe injury, sometimes necessitating humane destruction.

A twitch can be used as the sole method of physical restraint or can be used in combination with other forms of physical or chemical restraint (Figure 29-20). A chain or rope twitch can be placed over the horse's upper lip and tightened by rolling it toward the horse's poll. This should help prevent it from coming off the lip. The twitch should be placed on the nose from the side where the handler is standing. The restraining effects of a twitch have a limited period of effectiveness; therefore the twitch should not be placed on the lip until immediately before it is needed. Some horses resist twitching, particularly if they have had it performed several times in the past. Other horses will tolerate it at first but then start resisting it. If the procedure is lengthy, then taking the twitch off for a period may prevent the horse from becoming very anxious. It may be

better to use chemical restraint in certain horses in which lengthy procedures are being performed. Other forms of physical restraint, such as twitching an ear or the skin in front of the scapula, will provide variable degrees of restraint and are not widely accepted by many people. When restraining horses for certain procedures, such as nerve blocks during a lameness evaluation, one of the horse's limbs can be picked up and held off the ground by an assistant. This often helps prevent the horse from lifting the limb that is being worked on.

Chemical restraint (sedation or tranquilization) is probably the most effective and safest form of restraint, but it can sometimes interfere with certain procedures. For example, sedation can alter the gait of horses and interfere with interpretation of a lameness or neurologic examination. Some sedatives also have analgesic properties that could possibly alleviate or alter lameness. Sedation can also interfere with interpretation of an upper airway endoscopic examination. Because some sedatives have muscle-relaxing properties, they can alter abduction and adduction of the arytenoid cartilages and can alter function of the epiglottis and soft palate. Therefore, if sedation is required during an endoscopic examination of the upper airway, this should be taken into consideration when interpreting the endoscopic findings.

> **✎ TECHNICIAN NOTE**
>
> Chemical restraint (sedation or tranquilization) is probably the most effective and safest form of restraint, but it can sometimes interfere with certain procedures.

The most commonly used drugs for chemical restraint include alpha$_2$ agonists (e.g., xylazine, detomidine), narcotic agonist/antagonists (e.g., butorphanol), and phenothiazines (e.g., acepromazine). These can be administered alone or in different combinations; they can be administered intravenously or intramuscularly. Xylazine and detomidine are potent sedatives that have muscle-relaxing and analgesic properties. They provide marked visceral analgesia, which makes them effective in controlling pain associated with colic. The duration of effect depends on the dose and the route of administration; xylazine lasts 20 to 30 minutes when administered intravenously. Detomidine is more potent and has a greater duration of effect; this can be beneficial in some instances but can also cause problems because it can mask pain for an extended period. Moreover, detomidine has more cardiovascular side effects than xylazine. Butorphanol is a narcotic, and it is best used in combination with one of the alpha$_2$ agonists or acepromazine. Acepromazine provides tranquilization but no muscle relaxation or analgesia. It is frequently used in combination with other drugs. It can lead to marked hypotension and therefore should not be used in horses that are dehydrated or in shock. It can also cause permanent penile paralysis (paraphimosis) in stallions.

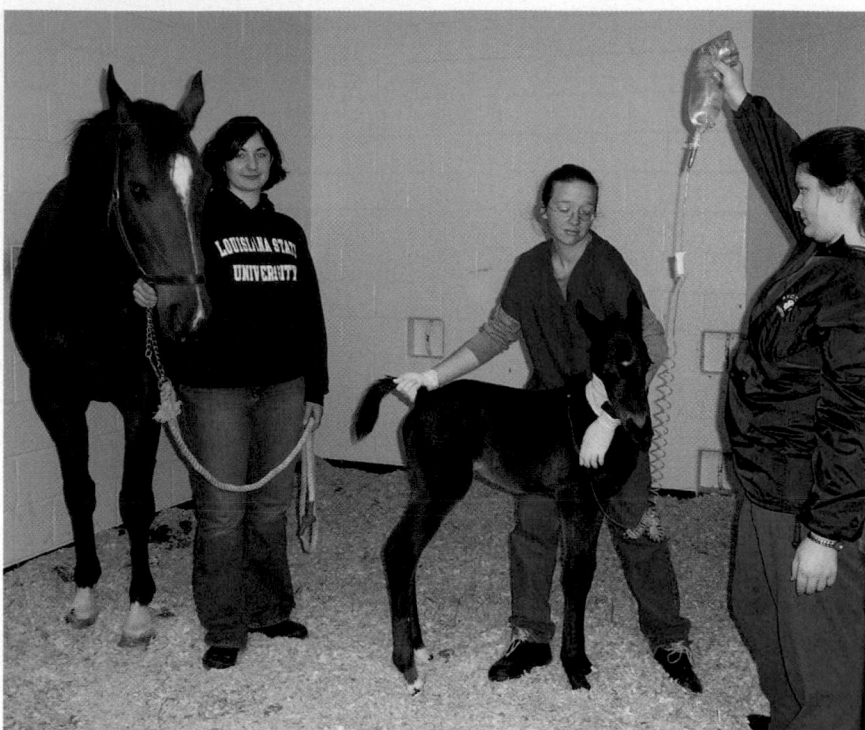

Figure 29-21 Technique requiring three people for restraining both the mare and her young foal in order to treat the foal.

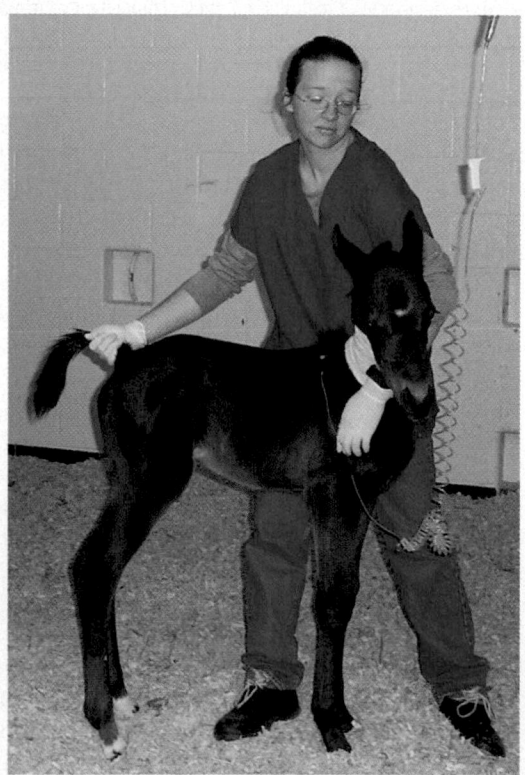

Figure 29-22 Technique for restraining a young foal.

Foals are restrained differently from adult horses. Because most foals have not usually been trained to be led by a halter, attempts at leading foals with a halter can lead to injury. Some older foals may be lead by a halter and a rope looped around the hindquarters; this method should only be used by experienced handlers. Many times the foal can be moved by walking the mare to the desired location and allowing the foal to follow. This also works well when attempting to evaluate the foal's gait. When the foal needs to be restrained, it is probably best to have at least two and preferably three people; one person should handle the mare, one should restrain the foal, and the other should examine or treat the foal (Figure 29-21). Foals are probably best restrained by holding one arm around the lower portion of the foal's neck and grasping the tail at its base with the opposite hand (Figure 29-22). Some foals tend to sink in the rear end if the handler tries to support them by holding too much tension on their tail. Therefore the tail should be used as a handle to help control the foal's movement rather than as a method to support the foal's hindquarters. Foals should not be placed in stocks because the stocks are too large for their body size and foals are generally not trained to stand. Horse trainers have many other effective methods of walking and restraining foals. Foals can be chemically restrained with tranquilizers or sedatives as with adult horses; the dose must be adjusted to body weight.

CARE OF HOSPITALIZED PATIENTS

In the equine hospital setting, veterinary technicians are often responsible for primary patient monitoring, administration of medications, general daily care of horses, and supervision of lay technical support. This section provides an overview of daily management of equine patients in the hospital setting.

PATIENT MONITORING

The level of patient monitoring required for a hospitalized horse will depend on the severity and nature of its disease. Horses hospitalized for elective surgery (castration, bone chip removal) require a thorough physical examination at presentation to ensure they are healthy surgical candidates. During hospitalization, elective patients usually require twice daily monitoring of heart rate, temperature, respiratory rate, appetite, and fecal output. Horses with infectious disease or extensive traumatic injuries require antibiotic administration and patient monitoring every 6 hours. Neonates; horses with colic (medical or surgical), diarrhea, renal failure, or respiratory distress; and any critically ill patients need constant intravenous fluid administration and intensive care monitoring. Most will be monitored continuously or hourly for signs of discomfort, abdominal pain, respiratory distress, shock, laminitis, gastrointestinal motility, heart rate, respiratory rate, hydration, and capillary refill time. Recumbent foals are particularly fragile and labile (Figure 29-23). A 24-hour attendant is required to maintain an esophageal feeding tube, intravenous fluids, oxygen therapy, and sternal recumbent positioning. In addition, the attendant will administer medications and monitor heart rate, temperature, character and rate of respiration, mental status, abdominal distention, and urinary output.

Patient monitoring forms are designed to identify trends in physical signs, and patient treatment forms are designed to coordinate treatment periods when several individuals may be responsible for administering medications. Treatment sheets and monitoring forms may be combined for low-maintenance, elective patients (Figure 29-24). However, for intensive care patients, monitoring should be more detailed and indicated appropriately in a flow sheet. Considering the diversity of conditions of intensive care patients, the flow sheet should outline the parameters to be evaluated, such that the evaluation of a horse with colic (Figure 29-25) or a horse with diarrhea (Figure 29-26) would differ from the evaluation of a neonate (Figure 29-27) or any other intensive care patient (Figure 29-28).

A separate treatment sheet should be used to outline the detailed medication schedule, the route, the dose of the drug per unit body weight, the strength, and the total amount given to the patient (Figure 29-29). The intensive care unit (ICU) flow sheets for all patients in the hospital

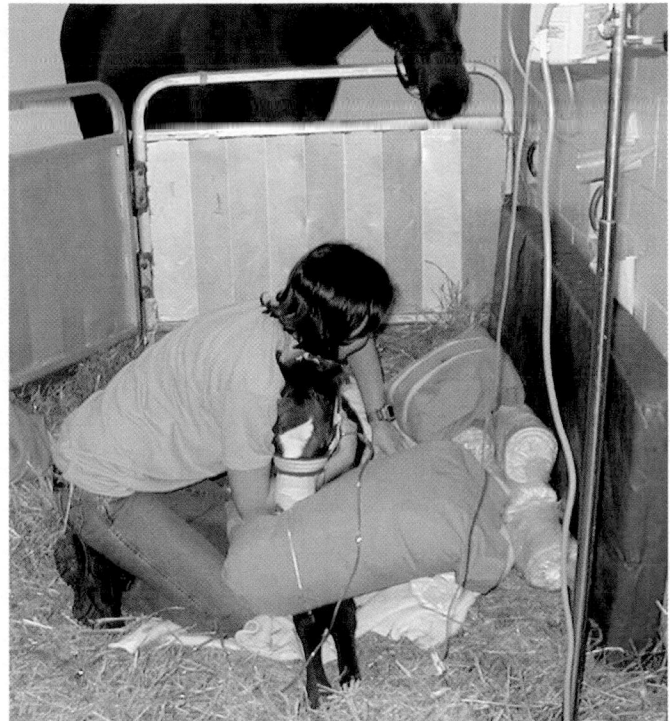

A

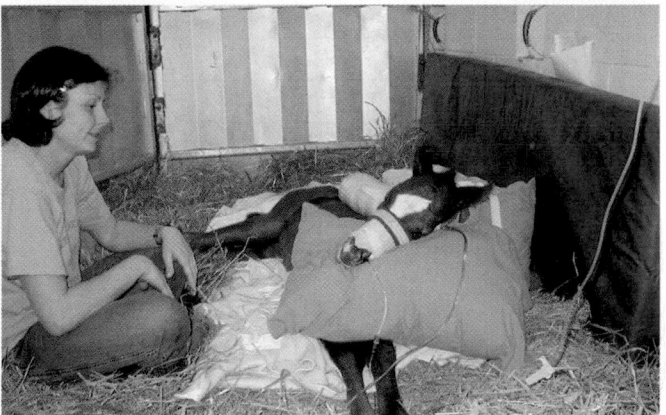

B

Figure 29-23 A, Technique positioning and assisting a recumbent foal. B, Veterinary technician monitoring and providing nursing care to the recumbent foal.

may be assembled in a central area to allow one technician to easily identify treatment periods and thus coordinate efforts. It is important to recognize that monitoring and treatment forms are a permanent part of the medical record, which represents a legal document to record all events during hospitalization.

Horses with infectious, contagious diseases should be hospitalized in isolation facilities. The most common infectious diseases that require an isolation protocol are colitis (salmonellosis) and strangles (*Streptococcus equi*). Personnel should be supplied with disposable gloves, boots, and body suits to wear while attending to isolation cases; a disinfectant foot dip should be used when entering and exiting each

Text continued on p. 920

EQUINE TREATMENT SHEET
SID, BID, TID, and QID

Date	T	P	R	Treatment	7AM	1PM	3PM	7PM	11PM	1AM

Person Administering Treatment Should Initial Box Under the Appropriate Time

Figure 29-24 Elective patient flow sheet for monitoring of patient's progress and treatments.

COLIC FLOW SHEET

Clinician: _____
Student: _____
Date: _____
Page: _____ of _____

Date: _____	AM/PM	AM/PM	AM/PM	AM/PM	AM/PM	AM/PM	AM/PM	AM/PM	AM/PM	AM/PM	AM/PM	AM/PM
Attitude												
Temperature												
Heart rate												
Resp. rate												
Refill/color												
Est hydration												
GI sounds RD/RV												
LD/LV												
Feces												
Urine												
Digital pulse												
PCV _____ % TP _____ g/dl												
N-G reflux vol												
Rectal exam												
Abdominal centesis												
Lab submitted												
Fluid type												
Fluid rate												
Drugs (record doses, routes, rates on the treatment sheet)												
Signature:												

Instructions: _____
_____
_____

Heart rate more than _____
PCV more than _____ less than _____
TP more than _____ less than _____
Respiratory rate _____ __ temp _____
Signs of colic

COLIC FLOW SHEET

Figure 29-25 Colic flow sheet for intensive care unit patients to identify monitoring, treatments, and administration schedule.

DIARRHEA/ISOLATION FLOW SHEET

Clinician: _____
Student: _____
Date: _____
Page: _____ of _____

Date: _____	AM/PM	AM/PM	AM/PM	AM/PM	AM/PM	AM/PM	AM/PM	AM/PM	AM/PM	AM/PM	AM/PM	AM/PM
Attitude												
Temperature												
Heart rate												
Resp. rate												
CRT/MM color												
Est hydration												
GI sounds RD/RV												
LD/LV												
Feces output consistency												
Fecal culture												
Urine vol./ua												
PCV _____ % TP _____ g/dl												
Digital pulse												
Water consumption electrolyte water*												
Feeding/appetite												
Evaluate catheter site												
Fluid therapy rate Fluid therapy vol												
Lab submitted												
TX: drugs/dose												
Initials:												

Instructions: _____
_____
_____

- **Measure and refill water buckets (plain and electrolyte water)**

DIARRHEA/ISOLATION FLOW SHEET

Figure 29-26 Diarrhea flow sheet for quarantine intensive care unit patients to identify monitoring, treatments, and administration schedule.

NEONATOLOGY/ICU FLOW SHEET

Clinician:
Student: _____
Date: _____
Page: _____ of _____

Date: _____	AM/PM	AM/PM	AM/PM	AM/PM	AM/PM	AM/PM	AM/PM	AM/PM	AM/PM	AM/PM	AM/PM	AM/PM
Attitude												
Temperature												
Heart rate												
Resp. rate												
CRT/MM color												
Est hydration												
GI sounds RD/RV LD/LV												
O2 suppl.												
Feces output consistency												
Urine vol./ua												
Blood glucose												
PCV _____ % TP _____ g/dl												
DIP/CK umbilicus												
Feeding nursing												
Milk from mare												
Fluid therapy rate Fluid therapy vol												
Lab submitted												
TX: drugs/dose												
Initials:												

Instructions: _____
_____
_____

If recumbent, turn foal q2 hours

NEONATOLOGY/ICU FLOW SHEET

Figure 29-27 Neonatal flow sheet to identify monitoring, treatments, and administration schedule for critically ill newborn foals.

ICU FLOW SHEET

Clinician: _____

Student: _____

Date: _____

Page: _____ of _____

Date: _____	AM/PM	AM/PM	AM/PM	AM/PM	AM/PM	AM/PM	AM/PM	AM/PM	AM/PM	AM/PM	AM/PM
Attitude											
Temperature											
Heart rate											
Resp. rate											
Refill/color											
Est hydration											
GI sounds RD											
RV											
LD											
LV											
Feces output consistency											
Urine vol./ua											
Digital pulse											
PCV _____ % TP _____ g/dl											

Drugs (record doses, routes, rates on the treatment sheet)

Signature:											

Instructions: _____

_____

_____

Heart rate more than _____
PCV more than _____ less than _____
TP more than _____ less than _____
Respiratory rate _____ __ temp _____
Signs of colic

ICU FLOW SHEET

Figure 29-28 Intensive care unit flow sheet to identify monitoring, treatments, and administration schedule for critically ill patients. This helps readily identify trends that may indicate a deterioration in the patient's condition.

MEDICATION RECORD			

Clinician: _____
Student: _____
Admission date: _____

Please initial and date all entries

Time given:

Medication																
Date	Drug	Dosage	Route													

MEDICATION RECORD

Figure 29-29 A medication record should list all the medications, the drugs' concentration, the dose per body weight, the total amount, the appropriate route, and the times to be administered. Following administration, the medication must be recorded promptly.

stall, and the protective boots, gloves, and suits should be discarded when exiting the isolation area. Horses in isolation should not be walked in areas where other horses are grazing, and waste from the stall should be disposed of in an inaccessible area. If possible, personnel attending to isolation cases should not attend to foals or immunocompromised patients.

📝 TECHNICIAN NOTE

Horses with infectious, contagious diseases should be hospitalized in isolation facilities. The most common infectious diseases that require an isolation protocol are colitis (salmonellosis) and strangles (*Streptococcus equi*).

Recumbent horses are a particular challenge to manage effectively in a hospital setting. Neurologic and musculoskeletal diseases are the most common problems resulting in recumbency in horses. Horses and foals that are recumbent will quickly develop pressure sores over the point of their hip (tuber coxae), elbows and head. Manure and urine soaked bedding must be removed frequently. The hair coat and skin integrity will degrade in a wet and dirty environment. Pressure sores rapidly become deep and may infect underlying bony structures. In addition, recumbent horses may have decreased intestinal motility and failure to void urine, and they are predisposed to developing colic, urinary bladder distention, and even rupture. Therefore laxatives and soft laxative feeds, such as fresh grass and bran mash, should be offered to recumbent horses to facilitate evacuation and prevent impaction. Horses unable to defecate should have feces manually removed twice daily. Placement of an indwelling urinary catheter or periodic catheterization of the urinary bladder is necessary when managing recumbent patients. Recumbent horses should be deeply bedded on straw, placed on a padded mat, or placed on a waterbed to prevent development of pressure sores. Creating a "bowl" by layering sand or peat as a base and covering the surface with straw will aid in wicking the urine away from the horse. Banking the edges will help the horse to position its head and neck above the level of the stomach. Their position should be changed every 4 hours; multiple attendants are required to move an adult recumbent horse. A sling can only be used in horses that can support their own weight but are too uncoordinated to remain standing (Figure 29-30). The sling acts as a safety net to catch them when they stumble. Horses cannot be supported solely by the sling because of the constriction of breathing and development of sling-induced pressure sores. Rarely can recumbent adult horses be managed for more than 1 or 2 weeks without development of life-threatening complications (pneumonia, urinary tract infection, colic, pressure sores).

FEEDING

Whenever possible, hospitalized patients should be offered feed similar to what they are fed at home. Sudden changes in diet can predispose horses to colic or diarrhea. In some instances, feeding must be specialized to accommodate the patient's disease. Horses with diarrhea should not be offered rich, calorie-dense feeds, such as corn, barley, or alfalfa, that may exacerbate colitis. Grass hay, bran mash, and oats are the most appropriate feeds for horses with diarrhea. After colic surgery or medical resolution of colic, horses should be offered soft, laxative feeds, such as bran mash,

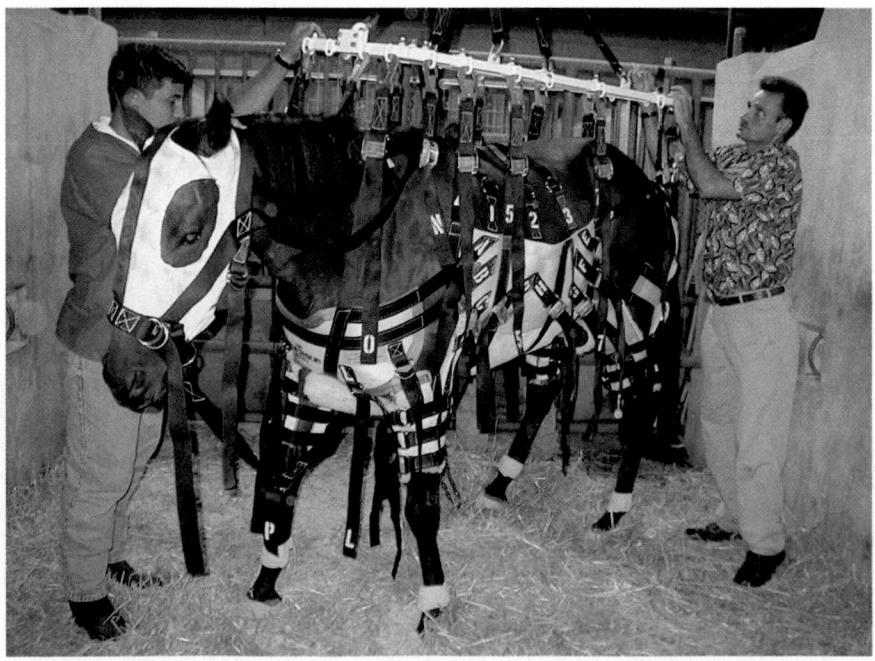

Figure 29-30 Use of a sling and hoist to provide some balance and support to an ataxic or weak horse.

fresh grass, and small amounts of good-quality hay. Feed should be offered frequently in small quantities to horses with gastrointestinal tract disease rather than offering two large daily meals. Horses with allergic airway disease (heaves, RAO) should be offered water-soaked hay and dust-free complete pelleted diet (i.e., the fiber content greater than 25%). Horses with inappetence owing to infectious disease should be offered highly palatable, calorie-dense feeds to increase energy intake (see Chapter 15).

THERAPEUTICS

Medication in tablet form is best administered to horses by crushing the pills with a mortar and pestle and mixing the powder with corn syrup, molasses, or applesauce. The resultant solution is sticky and palatable and can be placed directly in the horse's mouth with a syringe. Alternatively, the prepared medication may be placed over feed, but the attendant must observe closely to ensure medication placed over feed is completely ingested.

Oral medications may also be administered via nasogastric intubation. The nasogastric tube is passed through the nasal passages into the esophagus and stomach. Proper placement of the nasogastric tube should be confirmed before administration of medications. The tube should be visualized as it passes through the cervical portion of the esophagus (Figure 29-14), negative pressure should be obtained when the examiner aspirates on the tube, and the aroma of stomach contents may be noted as gas escapes from the tube. Inadvertent administration of medication into the lung using an improperly placed nasogastric tube (in the trachea) can result in death of the horse.

Nonirritating, sterile solutions can be administered intramuscularly in horses. Intramuscular injections should be administered using an 18- to 20-gauge, 1.5-inch needle. The needle should be placed independent of the syringe. Attach the syringe and aspirate to ensure the needle is not in a vein. The volume of medication to be injected at a single intramuscular site should not exceed 20 ml. Sites for intramuscular injection include the semimembranosus or semitendinosus muscle and the musculature of the neck. The appropriate region for injection in the neck is above the cervical spine, cranial to the scapula, and below the nuchal ligament (Figure 29-31, *A*). Before intramuscular injection, the site should be properly cleaned and wiped with alcohol (Figure 29-31, *B*). Because of excessive postinjection swelling, the pectoral muscles are not recommended for intramuscular injection. The gluteal muscles are not recommended for intramuscular injection, because this region cannot effectively drain if an abscess forms at the injection site. In rare instances, postinjection abscesses in the gluteal muscles may drain into the abdominal cavity. Irritating medications, such as phenylbutazone, tetracycline, and thiamylal, should never be administered intramuscularly.

> ### ✎ TECHNICIAN NOTE
>
> Sites for intramuscular injection include the semimembranosus or semitendinosus muscle and the musculature of the neck.
>
> Because of excessive postinjection swelling, the pectoral muscles are not recommended for intramuscular injection. The gluteal muscles are not recommended for intramuscular injection, because this region cannot effectively drain if an abscess forms at the injection site. In rare instances, postinjection abscesses in the gluteal muscles may drain into the abdominal cavity.

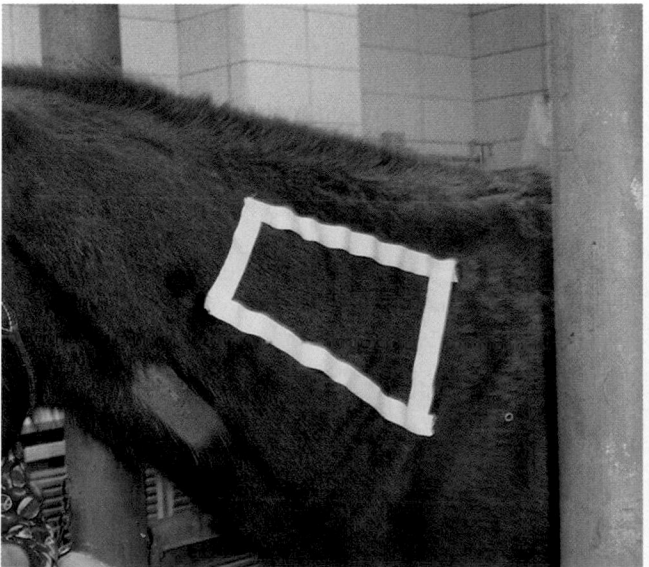 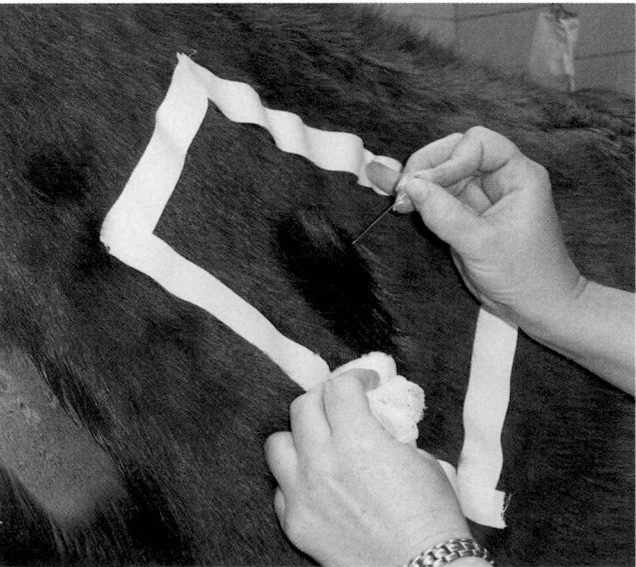

Figure 29-31 **A,** Location considered safe in the cervical region of horses for the administration of intramuscular injections. **B,** Technique for administering intramuscular injections: the skin should be cleansed and then swabbed with an alcohol-soaked gauze pad before insertion of the needle, and the needle (1.5 inch) should be inserted intramuscularly to its hub to deposit the medication deep within the muscle.

Intravenous medications may be administered directly into the jugular vein, using an 18-gauge, 1.5-inch needle. The jugular vein is most superficial and most distant from the carotid artery in the proximal one third of the neck. The needle should be seated in the jugular vein to the hub without the syringe attached to ensure the needle has not been accidentally placed in the carotid artery. Blood flows continuously and slowly from an 18-gauge needle in the jugular vein, whereas blood spurts in a pulsatile manner from a needle placed in the carotid artery. Inadvertent intracarotid injection may result in seizure, coma, permanent neurologic deficits, or death.

An intravenous catheter can be placed for repeated administration of medications or continuous fluid infusion. Intravenous catheters may be placed in the jugular, cephalic, and lateral thoracic (spur) veins in horses. Catheters should be placed aseptically and secured appropriately to prevent their dislodgment (Figure 29-32). Teflon catheters are relatively irritating and should be replaced every 3 days. Silastic catheters can remain in the vein as long they are patent and show no signs of infection. Central venous catheterization using a wire-guided polyurethane catheter is often used in critically ill patients. Polyurethane catheter are less traumatic and less thrombogenic, and therefore they are especially ideal in peripheral veins such as lateral thoracic and cephalic veins. Intravenous catheters should be flushed with heparinized saline flush (2 to 10 U/ml) every 4 to 8 hours, and monitored twice daily for heat, swelling, pain, and positioning. Infection at the catheter site may occur in the subcutaneous tissue or within the vein (septic thrombophlebitis). Septic thrombophlebitis can be life threatening in horses.

The ideal antibiotic is effective against a wide range of bacterial organisms (broad spectrum), easy to administer, and nontoxic (see Chapter 21). Penicillin has good efficacy against common gram-positive pathogens in the horse (*Streptococcus zooepidemicus, S. equi*) and is relatively safe. It is frequently administered intramuscularly (procaine

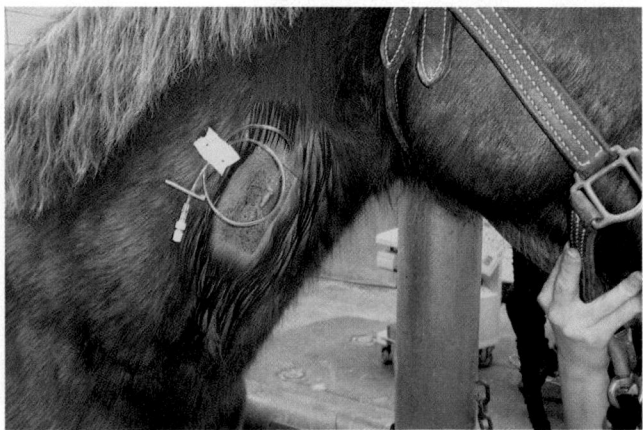

Figure 29-32 Technique for securing a catheter in the jugular vein of a horse.

penicillin) and intravenously (potassium penicillin). Procaine penicillin should never be administered intravenously. Life-threatening anaphylactoid reactions are reported with procaine penicillin administration and should be treated with epinephrine. Aminoglycoside antibiotics (gentamicin, amikacin sulfate) are efficacious against gram-negative pathogens and can be administered intramuscularly or intravenously. These antibiotics are nephrotoxic, and renal function should be monitored during the period of administration. Trimethoprim-sulfa antimicrobials have a moderate gram-positive and gram-negative spectrum, are administered orally, and are used for treatment of mild to moderate infection. Ceftiofur sodium has a good gram-positive and gram-negative spectrum, may be administered intramuscularly or intravenously, and is used for moderate to severe infection. Metronidazole is administered orally or per rectum to treat anaerobic bacterial infections. There are specific indications for administration of tetracycline, erythromycin, and rifampin in horses, but these antibiotics are not widely used because of the risk of antibiotic-induced colitis. Chloramphenicol is used sparingly in horses because of the human health risk of idiosyncratic, fatal aplastic anemia after exposure during administration.

There are many analgesic medications available for horses. Phenylbutazone, ketoprofen, and flunixin meglumine are nonsteroidal antiinflammatory drugs (NSAIDs) that provide mild to moderate pain relief without sedation or immunosuppression. The NSAIDs also reduce fever (antipyretic) and inflammation. Phenylbutazone is the most widely administered analgesic of horses and is most effective for treatment of musculoskeletal pain. Ketoprofen, meclofenamic acid, and naproxen are less commonly used drugs that provide mild to moderate analgesia for musculoskeletal pain. Flunixin meglumine is more effective for soft-tissue and visceral pain. In addition, flunixin meglumine may combat the effects of endotoxemia in horses with gastrointestinal tract disease. Xylazine and detomidine are alpha$_2$-agonist sedative analgesic medications that provide immediate relief of moderate to marked pain with moderate to profound sedation. Xylazine provides 20 to 30 minutes of sedation and analgesia, whereas detomidine provides up to 1 hour of sedation and analgesia. Butorphanol is a narcotic agonist/antagonist that provides up to 1 hour of sedation and analgesia for moderate to severe pain. Acepromazine has no analgesic properties, and it only provides moderate tranquilization. Acepromazine causes hypotension, and it can lead to the development of persistent paraphimosis in stallions.

Corticosteroids have potent antiinflammatory properties and are administered for allergic airway disease, allergic skin conditions, immune-mediated disease, and joint inflammation. Corticosteroids are administered topically, orally, parenterally (intravenously or intramuscularly), and intraarticularly. Adverse effects of corticosteroid administration include immunosuppression, polyuria or polydipsia, poor hair coat, muscle wasting, poor wound healing, laminitis, and progression of degenerative joint disease. Therefore corticosteroids are administered with caution in instances with specific indications for their use.

Dimethyl sulfoxide (DMSO) is a common antiinflammatory drug used in horses to relieve swelling and edema associated with central nervous system trauma, traumatic musculoskeletal injuries, laminitis, and myositis. DMSO may be administered topically, orally, or intravenously (diluted in crystalloid fluids as a 10% to 20% solution). The technician should wear gloves while handling the product. Rapid intravenous administration may result in hemolysis, hematuria, and sweating in horses.

ENDOSCOPY

Fiber-optic endoscopes of different lengths allow evaluation of the upper respiratory tract (nasal passages, sinuses, ethmoid turbinates, nasopharynx, guttural pouches, trachea, bronchi), proximal gastrointestinal tract (esophagus, stomach, duodenum), distal gastrointestinal tract (rectum), and urogenital tract (uterus, urethra, urinary bladder). The endoscope is frequently used for evaluating athletic horses with poor performance and those making respiratory noise. The endoscope can be used with horses standing (Figure 29-33) or with horses exercising on a high-speed treadmill (Figure 29-34). The latter enables the upper respiratory tract to be evaluated dynamically as the horse exercises. The most common abnormalities detected in the upper respiratory tract include left laryngeal hemiplegia, dorsal displacement of the soft palate, epiglottic entrapment, arytenoid chondritis, and subepiglottic cysts. The endoscope can also be used to determine the source of mucopurulent nasal discharge or epistaxis. The most common source of mucopurulent nasal discharge is the lower airway;

endoscopy would enable observation of this material in the trachea and bronchi. Other possible sources of discharge could be guttural pouch empyema or sinusitis. Horses with maxillary sinusitis often have mucopurulent discharge exiting the nasomaxillary opening into the nasal passages. Potential sources of epistaxis include ethmoid hematoma, guttural pouch mycosis, and exercise-induced pulmonary hemorrhage. The endoscope is also used to obtain a tracheal wash or bronchoalveolar lavage sample in horses with inflammatory or allergic lung disease.

TECHNICIAN NOTE
The endoscope is frequently used for evaluating athletic horses with poor performance and those making respiratory noise.

The endoscope is useful for evaluating horses with esophageal obstruction (choke) to determine the location and cause of the obstruction. It is also useful for evaluating the integrity of the esophagus after resolution of the choke to determine if the mucosa is ulcerated, which could predispose the esophagus to form a diverticulum or stricture. Development of the long endoscope (3 m) has allowed examination of the stomach and duodenum in foals and adult horses for gastric and duodenal ulceration. Endoscopy has revealed that the incidence of gastric ulceration in adult performance horses is greater than previously suspected. This enables the clinician to document the presence and severity of ulceration and monitor the response to treatment.

The endoscope is often used to assess the integrity of the urethra and urinary bladder in horses with hematuria (blood in the urine), stranguria (slow and difficult urination), and pollakiuria (frequent urination in small amounts). It may reveal erosive or neoplastic lesions in the urethra.

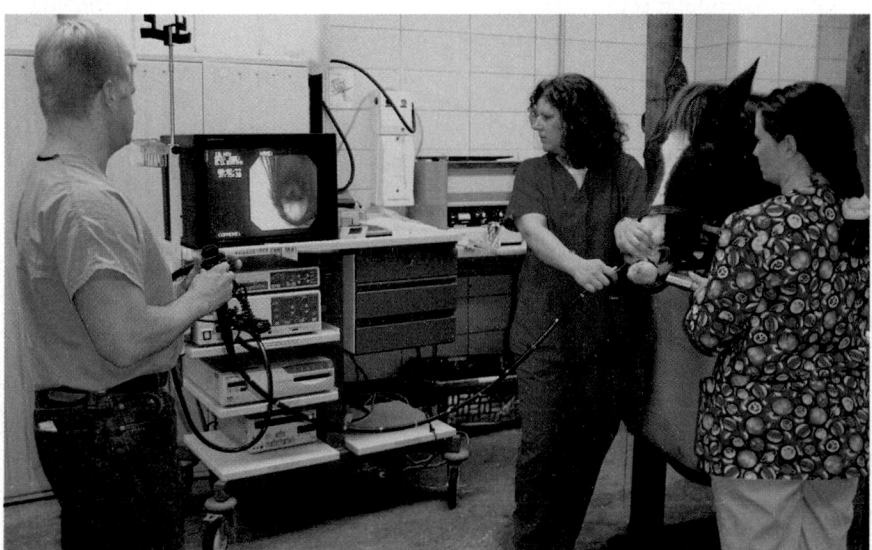

Figure 29-33 Use of endoscopy at rest to evaluate the upper airway and esophagus and stomach of a horse.

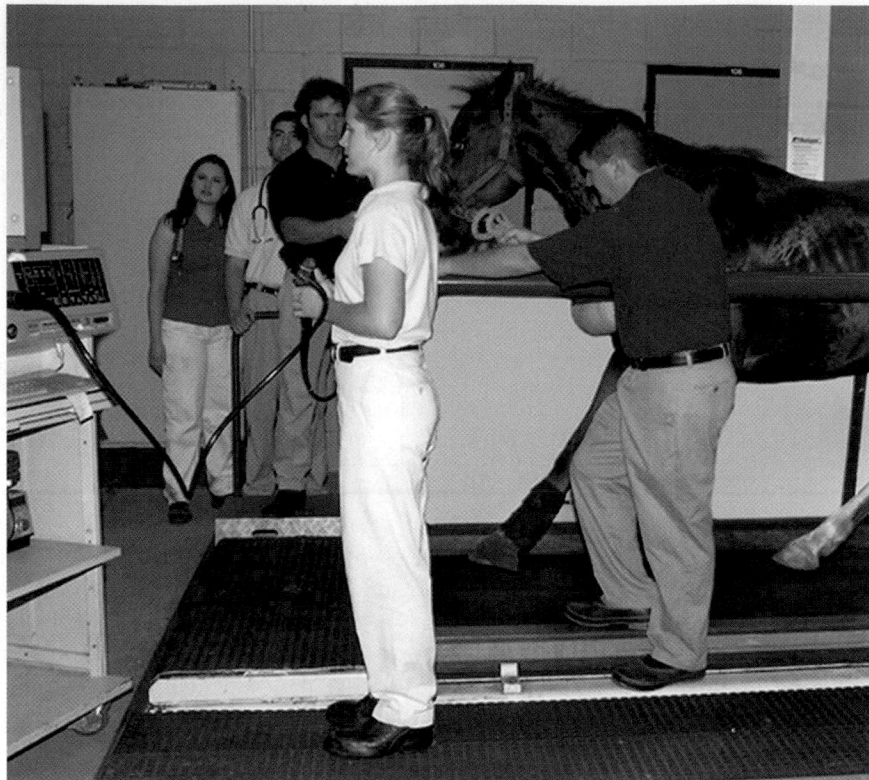

Figure 29-34 Use of dynamic endoscopy to evaluate the upper airway of a horse during exercise.

Urinary bladder abnormalities that can be identified endoscopically include inflammatory and neoplastic diseases and cystic calculi. The endoscope has been used to assess the uterine lining for cysts and other pathologic conditions.

The technician is integrally involved in the care, use, and maintenance of the endoscope and associated equipment. There are specific instructions on the proper methods for cleaning and disinfecting the endoscope. It is important that the proper methods be followed to ensure that infectious agents are not transmitted from one patient to another and to prevent damage to the endoscope.

IMAGING TECHNIQUES

The veterinary technician in equine practice often participates in diagnostic imaging techniques. In some instances, the technician may be solely responsible for obtaining radiographic or scintigraphic images for interpretation by the veterinarian. The technician must recognize good-quality images on the basis of technique and positioning and understand indications for special radiographic studies. The technician must have adequate knowledge of anatomy to ensure proper execution of diagnostic studies. Additional information on imaging techniques may be found in Chapter 9.

PLAIN FILM RADIOGRAPHY

Plain film radiography is used to identify disruption of bony structures, such as fracture, osteochondrosis, osteomyelitis (bone infection), malalignment (luxation, subluxation), or degenerative joint disease (arthritis). If it is necessary to be near the horse when the x-ray examination is performed, lead aprons and gloves should be worn. Long-scale [low milliamperage (mAs), high kilovolt peak (kVp)] techniques are used for plain film radiographic technique to preserve resolution of soft tissues and bone. Portable radiograph machines are typically used to image the carpus, hock, skull, and distal limbs in adult horses. The standard focal spot-to-film distance using portable radiographic units is 85 cm. To obtain detailed radiographs of the coffin and navicular bone, the horse's shoes should be removed and the frog should be packed with Play-Doh. Portable radiograph units may also be used to image the thorax, abdomen, and cervical spine in neonatal and weanling foals. Large overhead radiograph units (1000 mA, 150 kV) are required to image the spine, thorax, elbow, shoulder, stifle, and hip in adult horses. The standard focal spot-to-film distance using overhead radiographic units is 100 cm. Radiographs of the thorax, cervical and thoracic spine, elbow, and stifle may be obtained in standing, sedated horses. However, high-quality radiographic imaging of the lumbar spine, shoulder, and hip usually requires general anesthesia. It is important to label the radiographs correctly with the name of the patient, the date of examination, the affected limb, and the radiographic marker used for orientation. Radiographic markers are generally used when performing radiographs of the limbs; the markers are placed externally on the radiographic cassette in a location that will either be lateral or dorsal to the limb.

> ### TECHNICIAN NOTE
>
> In some instances, the technician may be solely responsible for obtaining radiographic or scintigraphic images for interpretation by the veterinarian.

CONTRAST RADIOGRAPHY

Special radiographic techniques use a contrast agent to better define or outline lesions suspected clinically or radiographically but not visualized on survey (plain film) radiographs. Positive-contrast agents are most commonly used in equine radiography for investigation of puncture wounds or draining tracts (fistulogram), joints (arthrogram), bladder (cystogram), spinal cord (myelogram), and esophagus (barium swallow). Short-scale (high mAs, low kVp) techniques are used to highlight visualization of the contrast agent. Triiodinated, water-soluble contrast materials are used for the fistulogram, arthrogram, and cystogram. Nonionic, water-soluble benzoic acid derivatives are used for myelographic examination, and oil-based barium solutions are used for evaluation of the gastrointestinal tract. The fistulogram is most commonly used to outline foreign bodies or a sequestrum (dead bone) or to define the extent of a penetrating wound. A fistulogram can easily outline involvement or penetration of a synovial structure, such as a joint or tendon sheath. Arthrograms allow a complete evaluation of articular cartilage integrity, synovial membrane proliferation, and joint capsule integrity. A surgical skin preparation is required before injection of sterile contrast agent into a joint. Positive-contrast cystography can only be performed in foals and is used to identify a tear in the bladder wall or persistent urachal remnants. Myelography is used to diagnose cervical stenotic myelopathy (wobbler's syndrome) wherein the cervical spine is malformed and narrowed, which compresses the spinal cord. Attenuation or obliteration of the contrast column is identified at vertebral sites where the cervical vertebrae are compressing the spinal cord. A barium swallow may be useful for investigating dysphagia, esophageal motility, esophageal integrity, gastric emptying, and duodenal structures (foals only).

ULTRASOUND

Ultrasound examination is useful for investigating soft-tissue structures and body cavities. The ultrasonic image is formed by ultrasound waves reflecting from tissue interfaces. The reflection of ultrasound waves is caused by the

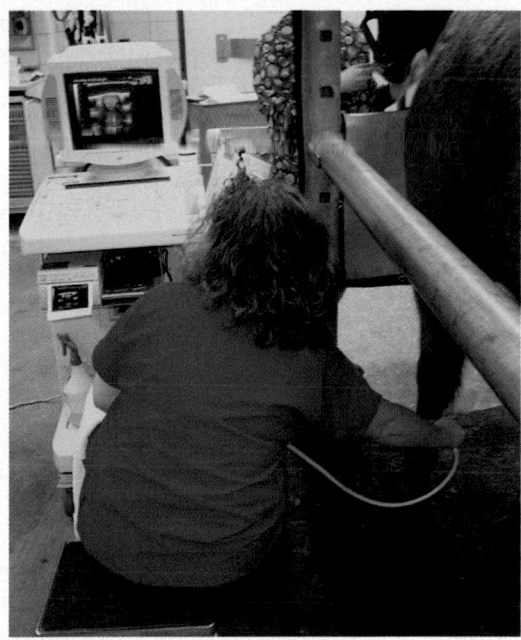

Figure 29-35 Use of ultrasonography to evaluate soft-tissue structures, such as a tendon injury in a horse with suspected flexor tendinitis.

difference in acoustic impedance between tissues. The knowledge of anatomy is necessary for execution of ultrasonographic studies. Ultrasound can be used to investigate any soft-tissue structure, solid organ, or swelling but is most commonly used in horses to examine tendon, lung, heart, pleural space, abdominal organs, and reproductive tract. It is important to recognize that air impedes ultrasound penetration; therefore investigation of gas-filled intestines and air-filled lung is unrewarding. Tendon ultrasound allows the examiner to identify and monitor core lesions, tears, and fibrosis of the tendons during the healing process (Figure 29-35). Ultrasound examination of the heart is termed *echocardiography* and is used to identify congenital defects, valvular disease, and abnormalities of myocardial contractility. Ultrasound examination of the thorax is particularly useful in horses with pleuropneumonia to identify the location, depth, and character of pleural fluid. Identification of free gas, fibrin, or highly cellular fluid within the pleural space using ultrasound examination is a poor prognostic indicator in horses with pleuropneumonia. Pulmonary abscesses can only be identified if they communicate with the pleural space; deep pulmonary abscesses cannot be visualized because air in the lungs impedes ultrasound penetration. Abdominal ultrasound in foals is used to identify peritoneal effusion resulting from ruptured bladder, enlarged umbilical structures, and gastrointestinal dilatation and intestinal intussusception (telescoping of the bowel). In adult horses, abdominal ultrasound is used predominately to investigate solid visceral organs, such as the liver, kidney, and spleen. Reproductive ultrasound examination is used to identify the appropriate time for breeding, follicular development, early pregnancy diagnosis (15 days), twins, and metritis (dense fluid accumulation in the uterus) and evaluation of the fetus and placenta.

Therefore, ultrasonography is a useful noninvasive diagnostic technique that provides immediate diagnostic information. Moreover, ultrasonography can be utilized to guide a number of invasive procedures such as the biopsy of organs (e.g., liver, lung, and kidney) or abnormal masses and the aspiration of structures (lymph nodes, masses) and cavities (e.g., abdominocentesis, thoracocentesis, and amniocentesis).

NUCLEAR SCINTIGRAPHY

Nuclear scintigraphy is performed by injecting a radioactive isotope intravenously and monitoring its distribution in the soft tissues and bones. Technetium-99m is the most commonly used radioactive isotope. For bone scan, technetium is combined with phosphate compounds that eventually localize within bones after intravenous administration. Localization of phosphate-labeled technetium is identified using a gamma camera. Bony uptake of phosphate-labeled technetium is greater in regions of high bone turnover or increased blood flow. Areas of increased uptake are termed *hot spots* and usually indicate an abnormality or disease process. Nuclear scintigraphy is indicated in horses with obscure, unlocalized lameness (using local anesthesia) and localized lameness with normal radiographic examination. Hot spots may identify nondisplaced fractures or stressed or damaged bone. In the soft-tissue phase, usually done 30 minutes postinjection of the isotope, images of support structures of distal limbs are captured. Nuclear scintigraphic examination is quickly performed on an entire limb or multiple limbs, whereas radiographic examination of an entire limb is cost and time prohibitive. In instances of unlocalized lameness, a plain film radiographic examination should be performed after nuclear scintigraphy to identify bony abnormalities. Serial nuclear scintigraphic imaging should be performed in horses with normal plain film radiographic examination to monitor progression and healing of the injury.

A white blood cell scan can be performed to identify occult infection. In this procedure, the patient's white blood cells are isolated from a blood sample (60 ml) and labeled with technetium-99m. These technetium-labeled white blood cells are injected back into the patient, and the patient is scanned with a gamma camera. The white blood cells travel to a focus of infection and create a hot spot detectable with the gamma camera. This technique may be used to identify a tooth root abscess, osteomyelitis (infected bone), and intraabdominal or intrathoracic abscesses.

CLINICAL PATHOLOGY

Clinicopathologic testing provides important information for the veterinarian to identify functional impairment of an organ system, confirm a clinical diagnosis, assess response to therapy, and formulate a prognosis. The normal values of many clinicopathologic tests vary among species. In addition, there are species-specific characteristics associated with diseases and significance of abnormal findings. This section concentrates solely on equine-specific alterations in clinicopathologic values in health and disease (also see Chapter 6).

SERUM CHEMISTRY

A serum chemistry panel provides specific information pertaining to the liver, kidney, muscle, and serum electrolyte concentrations. The serum sample should be drawn into a tube without anticoagulant (red-top tube) and submitted to the laboratory. Some laboratories can perform chemistry profiles in heparinized blood samples (green top). If there will be more than a 1-hour delay in submission, the tube should be centrifuged, serum or plasma removed, and stored in the refrigerator. Delayed sample submission without centrifuging produces artificially low serum glucose and high serum potassium concentrations. Horses normally have yellow serum due to high serum bilirubin compared to other species. Serum bilirubin concentrations will increase dramatically if feed is withheld for more than 24 hours. Fasting hyperbilirubinemia in horses is a normal physiologic response and is not indicative of liver disease. Most species develop low serum albumin with chronic liver disease because of decreased production; however, horses maintain production of albumin even with marked impairment of liver function. Reliable indicators of liver dysfunction in horses are high serum gamma glutamyltransferase (GGT) activity, high serum sorbitol dehydrogenase (SDH) activity, high serum bile acid concentrations, and low blood urea nitrogen (BUN) concentrations.

✒ TECHNICIAN NOTE

Horses normally have yellow serum due to high serum bilirubin compared to other species. Serum bilirubin concentrations will increase dramatically if feed is withheld for more than 24 hours. Fasting hyperbilirubinemia in horses is a normal physiologic response and is not indicative of liver disease.

In most species, renal failure produces low serum calcium and high serum phosphorus concentrations. Horses are obligate calcium excreters, and chronic renal failure often produces a marked increase in serum calcium concentration. Reliable indicators of renal failure in horses include high serum creatinine and BUN and electrolyte abnormalities, including low sodium and chloride and high potassium and calcium. The large colon of horses exchanges a vast amount of electrolytes and fluids on a daily basis. Horses with colonic inflammation may develop marked electrolyte abnormalities before development of diarrhea. Low serum sodium, chloride, and potassium in horses with abdominal pain or depression often indicate loss of electrolytes into the lumen of the colon and impending diarrhea.

Serum creatine phosphokinase (CK) is an indicator of muscle damage in all species. Horses have large muscle masses in comparison to ruminants and small animals. Moderate increases in serum CK (two to four times normal) readily occur in horses following prolonged transport, prolonged recumbency, exercise in an unconditioned horse, or rolling owing to abdominal pain. Moderate increases do not usually indicate primary muscle disease. Horses with primary muscle disease, such as exertional rhabdomyolysis (tying up, azoturia, Monday morning sickness), have increases in serum CK activity of up to 200 times normal values.

HEMATOLOGY

A complete blood count (CBC) provides information pertaining to the red blood cell (RBC) count, RBC morphology, total white blood cell (WBC) count, differential WBC (including neutrophils, lymphocytes, eosinophils, monocytes), WBC morphology, and fibrinogen concentration. Samples for CBC should be submitted in a tube with ethylenediamine tetraacetic acid (EDTA) anticoagulant (purple-top tube). The RBCs are most easily estimated, using the packed cell volume (PCV); low PCV is indicative of anemia. Horses have a large muscular spleen that normally contains up to one third of the circulating RBC volume. With excitement and exercise, PCV in horses can increase by as much as 50% secondary to splenic contraction. Therefore the resting PCV is highly variable and must be serially evaluated in excitable patients. In addition, the response of the spleen to massive hemorrhage precludes use of the PCV to estimate the magnitude of blood loss for at least 24 hours. The normal range of PCV depends on the breed. Hot-blooded breeds (thoroughbreds, Arabians, quarter horses) have higher resting RBC counts, compared with cold-blooded breeds (ponies, draft horses).

Evaluation of the total and differential WBC count is important to identify the presence of infection. In most instances, bacterial infection will manifest as an increase in WBC count (leukocytosis) characterized by an increase in the number of mature neutrophils (mature neutrophilia). Fibrinogen is a coagulation factor and an acute-phase reactant in horses. The liver produces fibrinogen in response to bacterial infection and inflammation within 72 hours, and fibrinogen concentrations remain increased until the infection is resolved.

Horses are particularly sensitive to circulating endotoxin released from the cell wall of gram-negative bacteria. Endotoxin causes margination and sequestration of WBCs. Therefore a profoundly low WBC count (leukopenia) characterized by low neutrophil count (neutropenia) and immature band neutrophils (left shift) is indicative of either gram-negative septicemia or gastrointestinal disease with mucosal absorption of gram-negative bacteria. High eosinophil counts (eosinophilia) are indicative of massive parasite infestation or possibly allergic diseases, and low lymphocyte counts (lymphopenia) are observed in horses with early viral infections.

URINALYSIS

Urinalysis is essential for evaluation of primary renal disease. Urine can be collected as a voided sample or after catheterization of the bladder. Urinary catheterization is performed in the standing horse. Females should have the perineum washed with mild soap and water. A sterile gloved hand is inserted into the vagina approximately 10 cm, feeling for the urethral orifice on the floor of the vagina. Using one finger to guide a sterile lubricated catheter, the catheter is inserted into the urethra and advanced. Males need to be sedated, and the penis is then grasped, gently extruded, and washed thoroughly with mild soap and water. While wearing sterile gloves, a sterile flexible stallion catheter is inserted into the urethral orifice, advanced until urine flows from the catheter. If no urine is spontaneously voided, slight negative pressure from a syringe attached to the catheter may produce a sample.

Normal horse urine is usually alkaline (pH 7 to 9) and contains many calcium carbonate crystals. Alkaline urine usually produces a false-positive reaction for protein on urine dipsticks. Horses have a large number of mucous glands located within the renal pelvis; therefore normal horse urine may appear very thick and mucoid. Normal horse urine may appear red or bloody in the snow, which often alarms novice horse owners. Truly red urine is abnormal and results from the presence of frank blood (primary urinary tract disease), hemoglobin (hemolytic anemia), or myoglobin (myositis). Differentiation of these sources of red urine requires special testing of urine and serum samples. Urine specific gravity and urinary electrolyte excretion ratios should be obtained to investigate primary renal function. Urine specific gravity indicates the ability of the kidney to concentrate urine, and normal values in resting horses should be 1.020 to 1.035. Urinary electrolyte excretion ratios indicate the ability of the kidney to conserve electrolytes. Identification of WBCs and bacteria indicates a urinary tract infection.

EVALUATION OF BODY FLUIDS

Evaluation of cerebrospinal, synovial (joint), and abdominal cavity fluid provides important information pertaining to inflammation, infection, or neoplasia within that particular body cavity. These body fluids are analyzed for total protein, total cell count, differential cell count, and bacterial culture.

Any form of neurologic disease in horses constitutes an indication for cerebrospinal fluid (CSF) analysis. Because some of neurologic diseases have zoonotic potential, such as rabies, the CSF must be collected and handled with caution (e.g., protective eyewear or face shields, lab coats and gloves) in order to avoid or minimize exposure to the infectious agent. CSF is collected in standing, sedated horses with spinal cord disease from the lumbosacral space using a 6-inch, 18-gauge spinal needle. In horses with brain and brainstem disease, CSF is collected in anesthetized horses from the atlantooccipital space using a 3-inch, 18-gauge spinal needle. Normal nucleated cell counts are less than five cells per microliter (predominately lymphocytes), and normal total protein concentration is variable depending on the laboratory but is usually less than 80 mg/dl (higher than in other species). Abnormalities in protein and cell counts can identify an inflammatory, infectious, or neoplastic process, but results of CSF analysis are often nonspecific. Antibody to the causative agents of several equine neurologic diseases (rabies, protozoal myelitis, herpes myeloencephalopathy, equine encephalomyelitis) can be detected in CSF, which provides specific information regarding the cause of neurologic signs. Complications associated with CSF tap include iatrogenic (operator-induced) spinal cord trauma and introduction of bacteria into the central nervous system.

Joint effusion, pain, or heat is an indication for arthrocentesis (joint tap) in horses. Synovial fluid is obtained by needle aspiration of almost any joint on the limbs of horses. Before needle aspiration, the hair must be clipped and a sterile preparation must be performed over the joint. Normal synovial fluid is highly viscous and will string 2 to 3 cm between your fingers before breaking. Normal synovial fluid is clear yellow in color and does not clot. Normal total protein is less than 2 g/dl and the normal cell count is less than 300/μl (less than 10% neutrophils). Analysis of synovial fluid can differentiate between synovial inflammation and infection. Bacterial culture of synovial fluid can identify the offending bacteria in horses with septic arthritis. Complications associated with arthrocentesis include iatrogenic septic arthritis and trauma to joint structures.

Abdominal pain, abnormal rectal examination, abdominal distension, and fever of unknown origin are indications for abdominocentesis in horses. Abdominal fluid is obtained by placing an 18-gauge, 1.5-inch needle into the peritoneal space of the ventral abdomen (Figure 29-36). The needle should be placed one hand's breadth behind the sternum, off the midline to the right of the horse (to avoid the spleen). If a 1.5-inch needle is insufficient to reach the peritoneal cavity, a teat cannula or female dog urinary catheter may be used. The use of a teat cannula is more invasive and increases the risk of traumatic bowel rupture. Normal abdominal fluid total protein is less than 2.5 mg/dl, and normal total nucleated cell count is less than 5000/μl (50% neutrophils). Analysis of abdominal fluid can identify devitalized bowel in horses with acute abdominal pain (colic), abdominal abscess, tumor in horses with a mass in the abdomen identified via rectal palpation, and ruptured bladder in foals with abdominal distention. Complications of abdominocentesis include traumatic bowel rupture, intraabdominal hemorrhage from trauma to the spleen, and iatrogenic septic peritonitis.

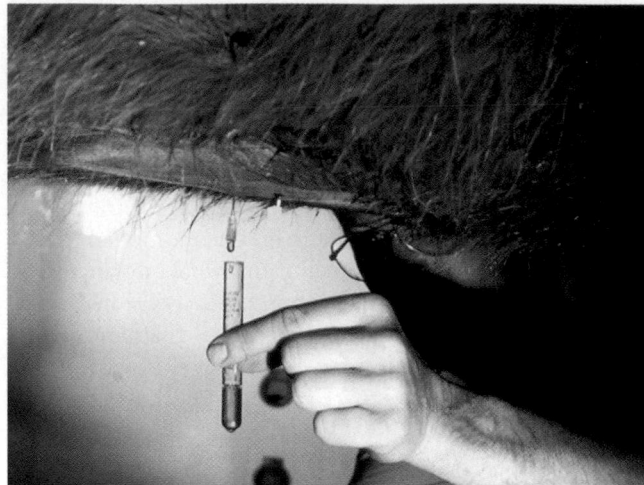

Figure 29-36 Technique for performing abdominocentesis in a horse.

BACTERIAL CULTURE AND SUSCEPTIBILITY TESTING

The veterinary technician often plays an important role in bacteriologic testing of specimens collected from patients with infectious diseases (see Chapter 8). Specimens (blood, joint fluid, abdominal fluid, urine, wound exudate, infected bone, etc.) are frequently collected from horses with infectious diseases for culture. Following the proper procedures during collection and transport of these specimens to the laboratory for culture and susceptibility testing improves the chances of growing the causative organism. There are specific guidelines that should be followed for collection and transport of different types of specimens. For example, blood is usually placed in a special enhancement medium immediately after collection for transport to the laboratory. Likewise, there are special methods for collection and transport of samples submitted for aerobic and anaerobic culture. Identifying the causative agent in an infectious process and determining its in vitro susceptibility pattern to antibiotics are often critical in choosing the appropriate antibiotic regimen. Therefore the technician contributes greatly to the successful outcome of equine patients with infectious diseases. Fecal samples are often submitted for *Salmonella* spp. or *Clostridium* spp. cultures from horses with diarrhea. Fecal samples for *Salmonella* culture should be submitted daily for 5 consecutive days. If no salmonellae are isolated from these five samples, then one can be reasonably confident that the horses are not shedding *Salmonella* organisms. Fecal samples may be tested for *Clostridium* toxins instead or in conjunction with samples for *Clostridium* culture; samples should be submitted daily for 3 consecutive days. Fecal samples may be submitted to other diagnostic tests as enzyme-linked immunosorbent assay (ELISA) for rotavirus.

PREVENTIVE HEALTH CARE

The equine veterinary technician may be a valuable resource for client education in areas of general horse care, vaccination programs, deworming protocols, and interstate shipment guidelines. Specific information in these areas will depend on geographic location. The technician and veterinarian should prepare standard recommendations that are appropriate for their region and clientele.

VACCINATION

Vaccination plays a crucial role in equine management programs in preventing and controlling infectious disease within a herd. Appropriate vaccination protocols will differ among horses depending on geographic location, age, use, and reproductive status. All horses must be vaccinated against tetanus and Eastern, Western, and West Nile encephalitis; and vaccinations against influenza, rhinopneumonitis, and rabies are highly recommended (see Chapter 11). The frequency of vaccination for these five diseases depends on age and reproductive status. Geographic and epidemiologic circumstances dictate indications for administering vaccines to protect horses from botulism, strangles, equine viral arteritis, rotavirus, and Potomac horse fever. Initial vaccination schedules for naive horses should be administered according to manufacturer recommendations.

TECHNICIAN NOTE

All horses must be vaccinated against tetanus and Eastern, Western, and West Nile encephalitis; and vaccinations against influenza, rhinopneumonitis, and rabies are highly recommended.

The equine veterinary technician may be a valuable resource for client education in areas of general horse care, vaccination programs, deworming protocols, and interstate shipment guidelines.

When a vaccine is administered to a patient, it must be recorded in the patient's medical record. The information about the vaccine's manufacturer, the location of the injection, and the date and time of vaccination should be noted. Vaccinations are administered either subcutaneously or intramuscularly, depending on manufacturer instructions. Vaccinations are frequently given in the neck musculature; however, local inflammatory reactions may make the horse reluctant to lower or raise its head. The impact of local reactions can be diminished by administering vaccines deep within the semimembranous or semitendinosus muscles. Administration of vaccines into the pectoral or gluteal muscles is not recommended in horses.

Tetanus is a highly fatal neurologic disease in horses. It is characterized by a stiff, stilted gait, hyperexcitability, seizure, and coma. The causative organism is ubiquitous in the environment. The most common portals of entry for disease in horses include a subsolar abscess, penetrating wound, and infected intramuscular injection site. Tetanus toxoid (inactivated) is a safe and efficacious vaccine for preventing clinical disease. Healthy horses without risk factors should be vaccinated for tetanus annually. Horses that acquire penetrating wounds or subsolar abscesses or require surgery (colic, castration) should receive a booster vaccine if the most recent vaccination was administered more than 3 months before this incident. Unvaccinated horses at high risk of development of tetanus (wounds, subsolar abscess, surgery) should receive tetanus antitoxin in addition to tetanus toxoid to provide immediate protection against disease. Tetanus antitoxin is associated with fatal serum hepatitis, and administration should be limited to cases at high risk of disease.

There are four main types of viral equine encephalitis: Eastern, Western, Venezuelan, and West Nile. The viral equine encephalitides produce rapidly progressive, highly fatal neurologic disease in horses. Mosquitoes transmit the infection to horses; therefore disease incidence is seasonal in most geographic regions. Vaccines for Eastern and Western equine encephalitis are highly efficacious, and clinical disease in vaccinated horses is rare. Vaccine for West Nile has been available since 2001, and it also appears to be very efficacious. All horses in the United States should be vaccinated against Eastern and Western equine and West Nile encephalomyelitis virus before the mosquito season, which is generally in the spring. Horses that live in southern states with a year-round mosquito season should be vaccinated in the fall and summer in addition to the spring vaccination. Brood mares should receive a booster of their vaccination in the tenth month of gestation (use only killed vaccines in pregnant animals) to ensure adequate colostral antibody protection for the foal. Vaccination against Venezuelan equine encephalomyelitis is not routinely recommended because the disease has not been reported recently in the United States and does not currently pose a threat to the U.S. horse population except those near the Mexican border.

Influenza is a highly contagious respiratory disease in horses and is characterized by fever, cough, and depression. The intramuscular influenza vaccines do not provide consistent protection from influenza virus challenge, but vaccination programs do reduce the incidence of disease within the herd and the severity and duration of disease in individual horses. On the other hand, intranasal influenza vaccine closely resembles the protective immunity achieved with natural infection. Sedentary adult horses, not exposed to other horses, are at low risk of contracting influenza and may be vaccinated only once or twice per year. Young horses and horses engaged in performance activities (racing, showing, training) are at high risk of contracting influenza because of their exposure to other horses and should be vaccinated every 4 months or 3 to 4 weeks before exposure to other horses. Brood mares should be vaccinated with the injectable vaccine against influenza in the tenth month of pregnancy to ensure adequate colostral transfer of antibody against influenza for the foal. Some horses may suffer a transient systemic reaction characterized by fever, inappetence, and depression several days after influenza vaccination.

Equine herpesvirus (the causative agent of rhinopneumonitis) is a highly contagious virus that produces respiratory disease, abortion, and neonatal and neurologic disease in horses. Protection against respiratory disease following equine herpesvirus vaccination is inconsistent and relatively short lived. Sedentary adult horses, not exposed to other horses, may not be vaccinated or vaccinated only once or twice per year, whereas young horses and horses engaged in performance activities should be vaccinated every 4 months. Inactivated univalent vaccines should be administered to brood mares during the third, fifth, seventh, and ninth months of pregnancy to prevent abortion. Although 100% protection against abortion is not achieved, the incidence of abortion caused by equine herpesvirus is significantly decreased by adherence to a proper vaccination program. None of the current vaccines claim to provide protection against the neurologic form of herpesvirus in horses.

Rabies is a rapidly progressive, fatal neurologic disease in horses. Although the incidence of rabies is low, equine infection does represent a human health hazard. The most likely source of infection in horses is the bite of a rabid wild animal. Skunks, foxes, raccoons, and bats are the most common reservoirs in North America. Horses should be vaccinated against rabies on an annual basis. Vaccinated horses that have been exposed to a rabid animal should be revaccinated promptly and observed for 90 days. Unvaccinated horses with a known rabies exposure should be observed for 6 months and should not be vaccinated.

Botulism is a rapidly progressive, fatal neurologic disease in horses characterized by profound weakness, muscle fasciculations, and dysphagia (inability to swallow). The causal organism produces a neurotoxin that may gain entry to the body by colonizing the intestinal tract (foals), infected wounds, or contaminating feedstuffs. Colonization of the intestinal tract in foals occurs in particular geographic regions of the United States, especially Pennsylvania, Ohio, and Kentucky. Foals in endemic regions may be protected by vaccination of mares with botulism toxoid before foaling.

Strangles is a highly contagious respiratory disease of horses caused by *Streptococcus equi*. Although strangles is common in young horses, vaccination is not routinely recommended. The injectable vaccine induces incomplete, short-term immunity against infection, whereas natural disease provides protection against infection for up to 10 years. In addition, injectable vaccines are commonly associated with swelling and abscess formation at the injection site and immune-mediated reactions (purpura hemorrhagica). Therefore routine vaccination should be limited to herds with endemic clinical disease and rapid turnover of horses. The recently developed modified live intranasal vaccine induces mucosal immunity, providing better

protection and fewer side effects, but it should not be given to pregnant mares and young foals.

Equine viral arteritis is a contagious viral disease that produces limb swelling, abortion, and respiratory disease in horses. Stallions can develop a persistent infection in their reproductive tract, which they readily transmit to mares during breeding. The vaccine for equine viral arteritis is approved for use in stallions and nonpregnant mares under the supervision of the U.S. Department of Agriculture (USDA). Pregnant mares should not be vaccinated for equine viral arteritis. Vaccination induces seropositivity and may interfere with testing requirements for export.

Potomac horse fever is caused by *Ehrlichia risticii* and produces diarrhea, fever, abortion, and laminitis. The mode of transmission is not completely elucidated, but it is suspected to involve an arthropod vector. Geographically, clinical disease is observed predominantly in states east of the Mississippi. Two inactivated bacterins are commercially available and should be administered to horses living in or traveling to endemic regions of the United States. Vaccination should precede the months of peak disease incidence (March through October).

Systemic reactions may occasionally occur after vaccine administration. Anaphylaxis is a systemic reaction characterized by angioedema (wheals) throughout the entire body (Figure 29-37, *A* and *B*). Anaphylaxis may be life threatening, manifested as rapid increase in respiratory and heart rate, hyperexcitability and excessive sweating over the entire body, culminating with cardiovascular shock and respiratory distress. Anaphylaxis should be treated immediately with epinephrine; fluid therapy may be administered in severe cases. Local reactions characterized by swelling, heat and pain are more common and are generally self-limiting. Administration of NSAIDs may speed recovery of local swellings, fever, and pain associated with vaccination. Fatal local reactions are rare and are associated with infection of the injection site with clostridial organisms (malignant edema or clostridial myonecrosis).

DEWORMING

Internal parasite control is an essential part of an effective preventive medicine program for all horses and is especially beneficial in young horses (see Chapter 7). Effective internal parasite control will allow young horses to grow to their full potential and will reduce the incidence of colic in horses of any age. An effective internal parasite control program should be directed at control of ascarids (large roundworms), small strongyles, large strongyles, and bots. Adult ascarids predominately affect young horses, live within the lumen of the intestinal tract, and may produce colic. Ascarid larvae migrate through the lungs and may produce parasitic pneumonia. The larvae of large strongyles migrate through the vascular system of the intestinal tract and may reduce blood flow and cause colic. Bot larvae attach to the stomach wall, creating inflammation, irritation, and potentially

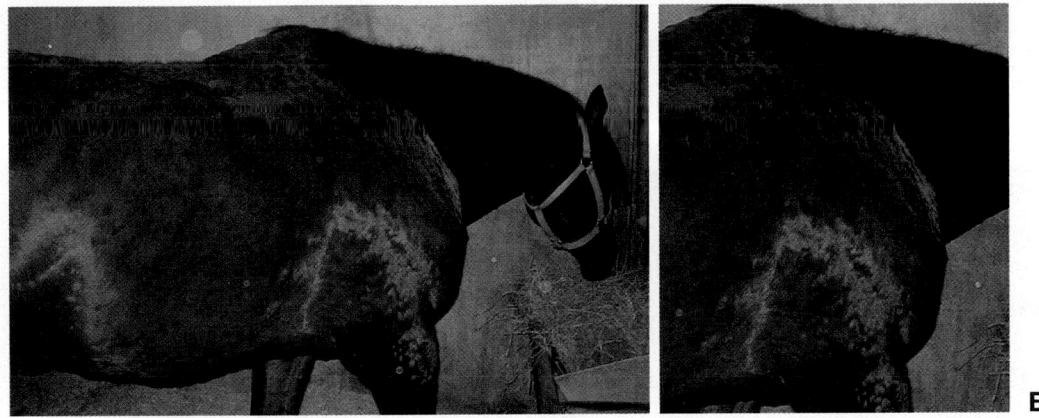

Figure 29-37 **A,** Horse with wheals throughout the body indicating an anaphylactic reaction. **B,** Closer view of the wheals (raised areas of pitting edema).

obstruction. Small strongyles encyst into the intestinal wall, which impairs nutrient absorption and creates inflammation. Small strongyles are particularly difficult to control because they have developed resistance to many of the commercially available anthelmintics.

The frequency of anthelmintic administration depends on geographic location. In the northern United States, a seasonal deworming program can be used wherein dewormer is administered from March through November at 8- to 12-week intervals. A boticide should be administered after the first frost in the northern United States and Canada. In the southern United States, dewormer should be administered year-round at 8- to 12-week intervals. Foals should be dewormed beginning at 8 weeks of age. Properly administered paste dewormers have an efficacy equal to tube deworming. Daily administration of pyrantel tartrate is effective in controlling small strongyles, large strongyles, and ascarids. This product is added to the feed daily and kills larvae before their migration. A boticide (ivermectin) must be administered in the fall of the year in addition to daily administration of pyrantel tartrate. Daily deworming is more expensive than interval deworming. Larvicidal deworming effective against encysted small strongyles includes single-dose moxidectin and 5 consecutive days of fenbendazole at twice the regular dose. The effective anthelmintic commonly used against equine tapeworms is a double dose of pyrantel pamoate; however, a new commercially available combination of ivermectin and praziquantel is also effective against tapeworms.

DENTAL CARE

Dental care is an important but frequently neglected part of health maintenance programs for horses. Regardless of age, the teeth of all horses should be examined annually. Dental problems may interfere with mastication, contribute to systemic infection, and cause chronic weight loss. Abnormal eating habits, such as dropping grain, excessive

salivation, dropping feed boluses (quidding), or tilting of the head during mastication, are indications of dental problems. Thorough examination of the oral cavity often requires sedation, a flashlight, and a mouth speculum (gag). The frequency of routine dental care depends on the age and occlusal anatomy of the individual horse. Normal horses have three pairs of incisors, three pairs of premolars (second, third, and, fourth premolars), and three pairs of molars on each arcade. Males usually have canine teeth, whereas females usually do not. Some horses will have "wolf teeth," which are remnants of the upper first premolar. Wolf teeth are small, round teeth adjacent to the second premolar (first cheek tooth). They often interfere with the bit and require removal between 12 and 18 months of age. Wolf teeth can be removed in standing, sedated horses.

Horses have a hypsodontic dentition, meaning their teeth continue to elongate and wear throughout their lives. Therefore dental surfaces that are not opposed by the adjacent arcade because of abnormal anatomy, malalignment, or malocclusion develop sharp, protruding enamel surfaces called *points* and *hooks*. The upper arcade of normal horses is wider than the lower arcade; therefore points develop on the buccal (cheek) surface of the upper arcade and the lingual (tongue) surface of the lower arcade. Often the upper arcade is shifted rostrally (with respect to the lower arcade), and hooks will develop on the rostral surface of the first cheek tooth on the upper arcade and the caudal surface of the last molar on the lower arcade. Dental hooks and points can cause erosion and ulceration of the tongue and cheek, dropping feed, and weight loss. Most hooks and points can be removed by floating (rasping) the teeth with dental floats (Figure 29-38, *A* and *B*). Large hooks may be removed using molar cutters. Many of the severe, often untreatable malocclusions and wear abnormalities seen in older horses can be prevented by regular dental care.

The most common malocclusive disorder in horses is parrot mouth, or prognathism, and there is likely a heritable component to this disorder. Prognathism is characterized as

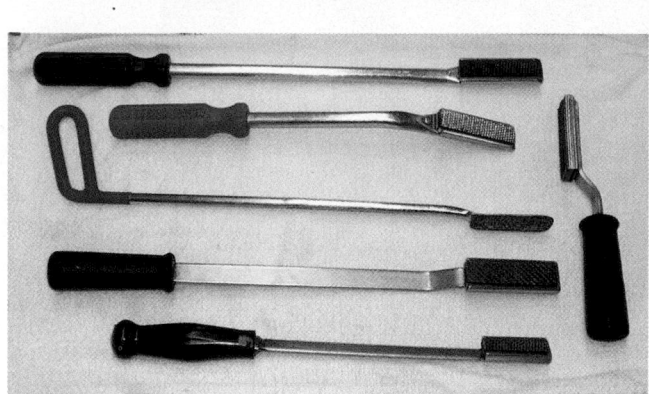

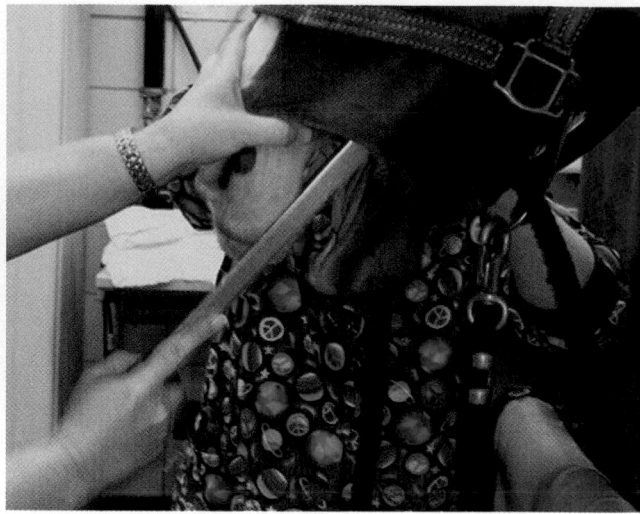

A   **B**

Figure 29-38 **A,** Tooth floats used to file off the enamel points of the upper and lower cheek teeth of horses. **B,** Technique for floating teeth in a horse.

an unsoundness in horses and results in difficult prehension of food and dental hooks on the first cheek tooth (upper) and last molar (lower). Dental examination should be performed every 6 months in horses with prognathism.

> ### ✐ TECHNICIAN NOTE
> The most common malocclusive disorder in horses is parrot mouth, or prognathism, and there is likely a heritable component to this disorder.

Horses affected with a tooth root infection typically present with malodorous nasal discharge. The tooth roots of the last four teeth on the upper arcade are located within the maxillary sinus; therefore infected tooth roots result in secondary sinusitis. Although the most commonly involved teeth are the first molar and fourth premolar, skull radiographs are necessary to identify the affected tooth. Removal of the affected tooth is the only effective treatment approach. Teeth generally cannot be removed from the oral cavity. Rather, teeth are repelled from their roots via an incision into the maxillary sinus or trephination in the maxilla or mandible (with the horse under general anesthesia) and driven into the oral cavity for removal.

Young horses (2 to 3 years) may retain deciduous caps after eruption of the permanent teeth. Retained caps can produce ulcerations on the cheeks, inadequate mastication, and dropping of feed and should be removed if retained for more than a few months. Retained caps can be removed in standing, sedated horses.

EQUINE INFECTIOUS ANEMIA

Equine infectious anemia (EIA) is a persistent viral disease of horses that results in anemia, fever, and weight loss; however some horses may be inapparent carriers. The virus

is transmitted from infected horses by large biting flies, tabanids. Once infected, horses become permanently infected and therefore are carriers of the virus for the rest of their lives. Infected horses produce antibodies to the virus, so they will test positive in the agar gel immunodiffusion test (Coggin's test) or the ELISA for EIA virus. Horses must have a negative (Coggin's) test for EIA within 6 months for issuance of health certificates for interstate travel, international travel, show, and sale. A USDA-accredited veterinarian must draw blood for testing and provide a detailed description of the horse on specified forms. The health certificate for interstate travel cannot be issued until the negative test is returned from a state or federally recognized laboratory. Horses that are not traveling or sold should still be tested on a yearly basis. If a positive test is obtained, the entire herd is quarantined until all horses on the premises are tested (usually 60 days). Only the state veterinarian can release the quarantine. Because horses that test positive for EIA are persistent carriers, they serve as a reservoir of the virus. Therefore, infected horses must be quarantined for life (within a distance greater than 200 yards from other horses) or euthanized. The veterinary technician may be involved in collection of blood, completing submission forms, and sending samples for EIA testing under the direct supervision of the attending veterinarian.

SELECTED MEDICAL DISEASES

EQUINE RESPIRATORY DISEASE

Strangles is a common, highly contagious respiratory disease of horses caused by the bacterial pathogen *Streptococcus equi.* Strangles typically produces swelling and abscesses of the submandibular and retropharyngeal lymph nodes.

Affected horses have fever, depression, poor appetite, and painful swellings under the mandible. The abscesses under the mandible enlarge, rupture, and drain a large volume of purulent exudate. Horses may develop abscesses within the guttural pouch, thorax, abdomen, and central nervous system. Development of abscess in abnormal locations is termed *bastard strangles*. These cases are particularly difficult to treat successfully. Horses with complicated cases of strangles should be treated with antibiotics, and *S. equi* is typically sensitive to penicillin. Horses with strangles should be maintained under strict isolation protocol. Recovered horses remain contagious and represent a threat to susceptible horses for approximately 6 weeks after recovering from clinical disease. Immunization against *S. equi* is controversial (see Vaccination).

Influenza is a highly contagious viral respiratory disease in horses characterized by an increased body temperature of 40° C (104° F), cough, and depression. The incubation period is short (2 to 3 days), and horses remain ill for 3 to 4 days. Equine influenza virus is transmitted through a herd via aerosolization of virus during coughing. The virus damages the clearance mechanisms in the lung and predisposes horses to bacterial pneumonia. Horses should be rested for a minimum of 3 weeks after recovery from viral respiratory disease. Immunization against influenza is recommended (see Vaccination).

Equine herpesvirus is a very contagious virus that produces respiratory disease, abortion, and neonatal and neurologic disease (ascending paralysis) in horses. The clinical signs of respiratory disease caused by equine herpesvirus are milder but hardly distinguishable from equine influenza. The incubation period is longer (2 to 10 days), and horses may remain ill for 4 to 5 days. Equine herpesvirus is transmitted through the herd by aerosol transmission, respiratory secretions, and fomite transmission. Protection against respiratory disease following equine herpesvirus vaccination is inconsistent and relatively short lived. Abortion secondary to equine herpesvirus occurs in the seventh to eleventh month of gestation, and the mare does not appear sick at the time of abortion. Vaccination is recommended for performance horses and brood mares. Neurologic disease caused by equine herpesvirus is not common. Affected horses demonstrate signs of incoordination, inability to urinate, and poor tail tone. Recovery from neurologic diseases is prolonged (2 to 3 months), and horses may not return to completely normal neurologic function. None of the currently available vaccines claims to provide protection against the neurologic form of herpesvirus in horses.

Equine viral arteritis is a contagious viral disease that produces limb swelling, conjunctivitis, abortion, and respiratory disease in horses. Limb swelling is painful and results from vasculitis (inflammation of blood vessels). Stallions infected after puberty develop a persistent infection in their accessory sex glands (ampullae) and transmit the viral infection to mares during breeding. Abortion can occur at any point during gestation and results from viral damage to the blood vessels of the placenta. The vaccine for equine viral arteritis is approved for use in stallions and nonpregnant mares under the supervision of the USDA. Pregnant mares should not be vaccinated against equine viral arteritis.

Recurrent airway obstruction (RAO) or heaves, formerly known as chronic obstructive pulmonary disease (COPD), is an allergic airway disease that causes narrowing of small airways (bronchoconstriction) and excessive mucous production. The clinical signs of COPD are cough, nasal discharge, flared nostrils, increased respiratory rate, increased expiratory effort, and wheezing. The severity of clinical signs may range from exercise intolerance to severe respiratory distress (dyspnea) at rest. Most affected horses are allergic to the molds present in hay and straw. Ideally, horses should be maintained at pasture, and hay should be removed as the source of roughage in the diet. A similar form of this disease is observed in horses during the summer months in the southern United States. Summer pasture–associated obstructive pulmonary disease (SPAOPD), or summer heaves, usually occurs from May to November, and it is believed to result from exposure to mold spores present on the pasture. Horses cannot be "cured" of heaves , but the disease can often be controlled with appropriate management practices. Changing the environment to remove offending allergens is the single most important principle in the treatment of COPD and SPAOPD. Medical therapy of horses with heaves may be intermittently necessary in moderate to severely affected horses and consists of corticosteroids to reduce inflammation and bronchodilator therapy to relax small airways.

The guttural pouches are two large symmetric dilations of the eustachian tube that are present in all Equidae. They are located just above the pharynx and larynx and can be accessed during endoscopic examination through small openings in the dorsal lateral nasopharynx. The internal and external carotid arteries and several cranial nerves travel superficially under the surface of the guttural pouch lining and are vulnerable to damage from pathologic conditions. The purpose of the guttural pouches may be to lower the temperature of the blood that is traveling to the brain (internal and external carotid arteries) during exercise. Bacterial infection of the guttural pouch is termed *guttural pouch empyema* and is often associated with strangles. Fungal infection of the guttural pouch is termed *guttural pouch mycosis*, and the causative agent is often *Aspergillus* sp. The fungal plaque usually forms over the internal carotid artery, adjacent to nerves that control swallowing. Horses may have life-threatening blood loss from rupture of the internal carotid artery or dysphagia from damage to the nerves. Accumulation of air in the guttural pouches (guttural pouch tympany) occurs in foals and weanlings and is usually associated with an abnormality of the opening to the pouches. It can occur unilaterally or bilaterally and is characterized by a fluctuant, nonpainful swelling in the throat-latch region. Guttural pouch empyema is characterized by accumulation of mucopurulent material in the pouches, which is often secondary to retropharyngeal lymph node abscess formation from a streptococcal infection.

GASTROINTESTINAL DISEASE

Choke refers to obstruction of the esophagus. Chronic dental disease and retained deciduous caps are common predisposing conditions for development of choke. Horses that are in overcrowded environments may bolt their feed and become choked. Removing the competition usually alleviates this behavior. The esophagus is usually obstructed by grain or hay, and most horses will continue to attempt to eat despite their inability to swallow. Clinical signs include anxiety, gagging, excessive salivation, and feed and saliva coming from the nostrils. The obstruction can be visualized via endoscopic examination and in most instances can be relieved by manipulation and hydropulsion using a nasogastric tube. Horses must be heavily sedated to lower their head during manipulation of the nasogastric tube to prevent water and feed from entering the trachea. Aspiration pneumonia is a significant complication and must be addressed in all cases. Esophageal stricture or rupture is a less common complication and occurs in horses with circumferential damage to the esophageal mucosa.

✎ TECHNICIAN NOTE

Choke refers to obstruction of the esophagus.

Young horses are particularly prone to development of gastric ulceration. Stress, a high-grain diet, musculoskeletal pain, and administration of NSAIDs are common predisposing factors. Clinical signs of gastric ulceration are bruxism (grinding teeth), hypersalivation, and abdominal pain after eating. Foals with gastric ulceration will often lie still in dorsal recumbency with their forelimbs over their head or extended out straight. Human antiulcer medications, such as histamine H_2 blockers, intestinal protectants, and hydrogen ion pump blockers, are used to treat gastric ulceration in horses. Most equine facilities administer prophylactic antiulcer therapy to hospitalized foals because of the stressful environment.

Colitis in horses can result in rapid, life-threatening fluid loss (hypovolemia), shock, endotoxemia, electrolyte loss, and acid-base imbalance as a result of diarrhea. Some horses may develop hypovolemic shock and electrolyte imbalance before the appearance of diarrhea. In addition to diarrhea, clinical signs of colitis include depression, inappetence, abdominal pain, tachycardia (increased heart rate), injected (brick red) mucous membranes, and prolonged capillary refill time. Etiologic agents that produce life-threatening diarrhea in horses include *Salmonella*, *Clostridium*, and *Ehrlichia risticii*. Horses with diarrhea should be considered contagious and maintained under isolation protocol. Intravenous fluid therapy is crucial to support the cardiovascular

system, replace fluid losses, and correct electrolyte and acid-base imbalance. Complications of colitis include laminitis (founder), cardiovascular collapse, cardiac arrhythmias, and thrombophlebitis.

Phenylbutazone toxicosis in horses can produce renal insufficiency and oral, gastric, and colonic ulceration in horses. The colonic ulcers occur in the right dorsal colon and are the most difficult aspect of phenylbutazone toxicity to treat. Colonic ulcers secondary to phenylbutazone toxicity can produce abdominal pain, marked protein loss, melena (blood in manure), peritonitis, colonic stricture, or colonic rupture. Dehydration and excessive dosages are the most important predisposing factors for development of phenylbutazone toxicosis.

NEUROLOGIC DISEASE

The five most common disorders of the spinal cord are cervical vertebral myelopathy caused by stenotic or dynamic compression of the spinal cord (wobblers), equine protozoal myelitis, equine herpesvirus myeloencephalopathy (rhinopneumonitis), equine degenerative myeloencephalopathy, and vertebral fracture. Damage to the spinal cord causes spinal ataxia (incoordination of the limbs without abnormalities of the brain and brainstem), which may progress to dog-sitting and recumbency (Figure 29-39). Diagnostic aids to differentiate these diseases include neurologic examination, cervical radiographic examination, myelographic examination, and CSF analysis. CSF can be obtained at the lumbosacral space in standing, sedated horses, and at the atlantooccipital space in anesthetized horses. The CSF travels from the cranial area in a caudal direction. Therefore CSF should be obtained at the lumbosacral space in horses with spinal cord disease and at the atlantooccipital space in horses with brain and brainstem disease. Because some

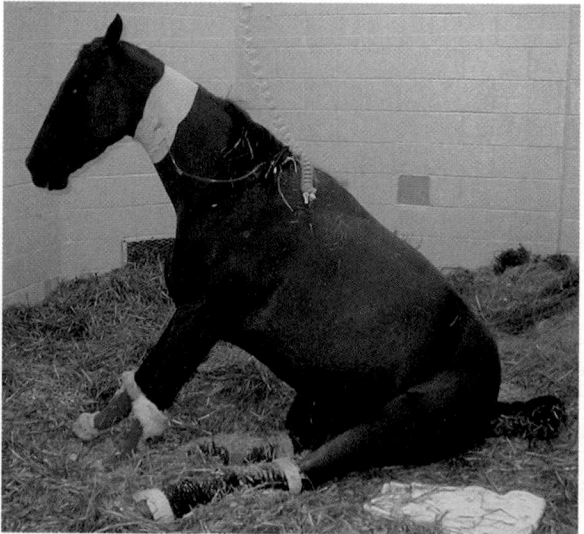

Figure 29-39 Horse in dog-sitting position due to a spinal cord dysfunction.

neurologic infectious diseases have zoonotic potential, most notably rabies, precaution must be taken when collecting and handling CSF samples from horses with neurologic signs in order to minimize exposure to the infectious agent.

Cervical vertebral myelopathy is a manifestation of developmental orthopedic disease characterized by compression of the cervical spinal cord by malformed or unstable cervical vertebrae. Males are affected four times more frequently than females, and thoroughbreds appear to be predisposed. Clinical signs of symmetric incoordination usually begin between 6 months and 3 years of age. The hind limbs are usually more severely affected than the forelimbs. The likelihood of disease is determined by evaluation of plain film of cervical radiographs, and the diagnosis is confirmed by myelographic examination. Surgical stabilization improves the neurologic status of some patients.

Equine protozoal myelitis (EPM) is the most common cause of spinal ataxia in the United States. Horses are dead-end, aberrant hosts of the protozoan parasites. *Sarcocystis neurona* is the most common of the protozoan parasites that cause spinal cord disease in horses; opossums are the primary hosts of this parasite, and horses are likely infected via fecal-oral transmission. Birds are the secondary hosts and do not appear to be infectious for horses. The clinical signs of EPM are directly referable to the location of the organism in the central nervous system. Therefore, EPM should be considered in any horse demonstrating neurologic signs. Most horses with EPM (85%) demonstrate signs referable to spinal cord damage, such as ataxia, weakness, and muscle atrophy, generally asymmetrical (Figure 29-40). Other signs such as cranial nerve deficits may occur. The diagnosis is confirmed by identification of antibody to the organism in CSF. Treatment of EPM consists of administration of antiprotozoal drugs; the most used treatment for EPM is a combination of two antibiotics that inhibit folic

acid metabolism: sulfadiazine and pyrimethamine, for an average period of approximately 120 days. Folic acid supplementation should be administered to prevent development of anemia during treatment. Another antiprotozoal treatment for EPM is ponazuril.

Equine herpesvirus can produce respiratory disease, abortion, and neonatal and neurologic disease in horses. The neurologic form is characterized by ascending paralysis with the hind limbs more severely affected than the forelimbs. Horses often demonstrate urinary incontinence, poor tail tone, and penile prolapse. Diagnosis is confirmed by cytologic analysis of CSF. Administration of corticosteroids may improve recovery if administered early in the disease process. Prognosis for return to normal neurologic function is approximately 80%.

Equine degenerative myelopathy results in symmetric spinal ataxia with both the forelimbs and hind limbs equally affected. Clinical signs appear between 6 months and 2 years of age, and the disease appears to be familial in some breeds. There is no definitive antemortem diagnostic test, and diagnosis is usually made on the basis of the neurologic examination, CSF analysis, cervical radiographs, and myelographic examination. Dietary supplementation with vitamin E may prevent progression of disease and may result in improvement in clinical signs in some instances. The prognosis for return to normal neurologic function is poor.

The most consistent clinical sign associated with vertebral fracture is pain. The cervical vertebrae, caudal thoracic vertebrae, and thoracolumbar junction are the most common sites of vertebral fracture. Cervical vertebral fracture results in tetraparesis (weakness of all four limbs), whereas fracture of the thoracic and lumbar vertebrae produces paraparesis (weakness of hind limbs) or paraplegia (paralysis of hind limbs). Diagnosis is confirmed by plain film radiography. If the fracture is nondisplaced, nuclear scintigraphy may aid in identification of the fracture site. Surgical correction may be attempted for fractures of the cervical vertebrae, but repair of thoracic or lumbar vertebrae is not attempted.

The four most common disorders of the brain and brainstem in horses are rabies, equine viral encephalitis (Alphaviruses: Eastern, Western, Venezuelan; Flavivirus: West Nile), leukoencephalomalacia (moldy corn toxicity), and head trauma. Damage to the cerebrum may produce altered mentation, altered states of consciousness, head pressing, and seizure (Figure 29-41). Damage to the brainstem may potentially damage the cranial nerves, which control the muscles of facial expression, facial sensation, mastication, swallowing, balance, vision, taste, and ocular position (Figure 29-42). Brainstem lesions also lead to

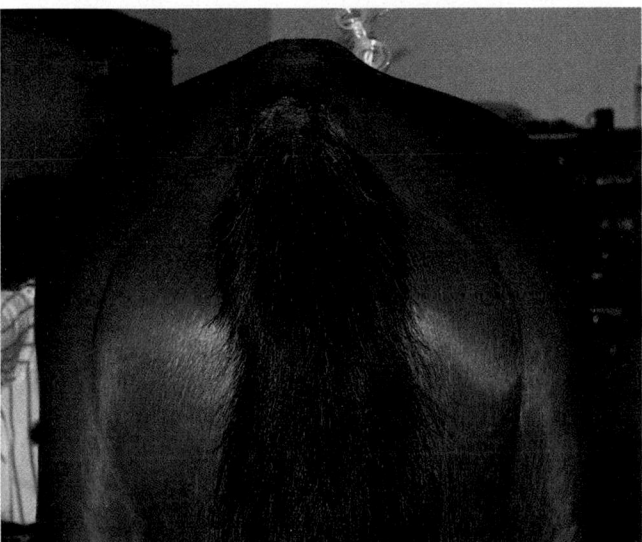

Figure 29-40 Asymmetrical gluteal muscle atrophy in a horse with spinal cord dysfunction involving a lower motor neuron.

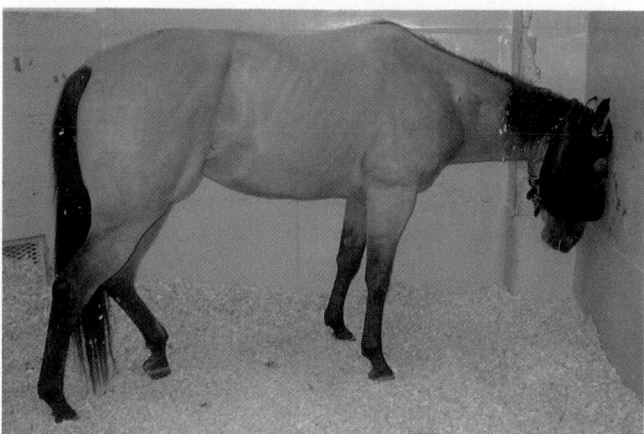

Figure 29-41 Horse head pressing as a sign of cerebral dysfunction.

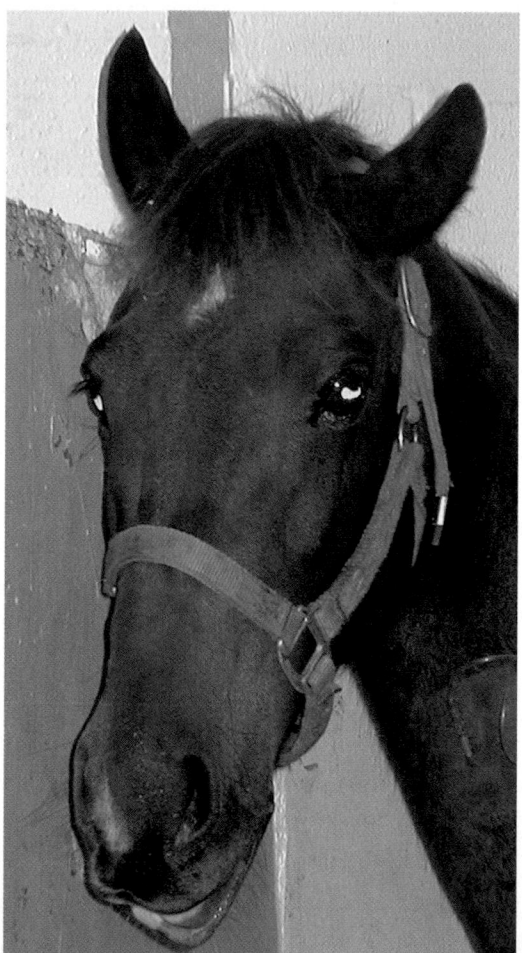

Figure 29-42 Horse with facial nerve paralysis (flaccid facial musculature, droopy ear and eyelid on the affected side) as signs of brainstem dysfunction.

incoordination of the limbs and altered breathing patterns. Diagnostic aids for evaluation of horses with cerebral or brainstem dysfunction include CSF analysis and skull radiographs.

Rabies is a zoonotic infection (infectious to humans) and is universally fatal. Horses usually acquire the infection by a bite wound from a rabid skunk, fox, or bat. Clinical signs are highly variable but often begin as fever, hind limb ataxia, and hyperesthesia (hyperresponsiveness to touch). Neurologic signs rapidly progress to involve the brain and brainstem. The duration of neurologic signs before death is relatively short, varying from 3 to 10 days. There is no accurate antemortem test for rabies; therefore it is very important to be cautious when handling horses with suspected rabies. The diagnosis of rabies is confirmed by fluorescent antibody stain of brain tissue. People handling potentially rabid horses should avoid contact with saliva, wear gloves, protective eyewear, disposable outerwear, wash hands thoroughly, and avoid contact with CSF. A list of individuals that had contact with the potentially rabid horse must be kept, and these individuals must be informed of the result of the test (generally 24 to 48 hours). Postexposure rabies vaccination should be administered to humans in contact with rabid animals. Individuals with occupational exposure to livestock and wildlife should undergo a prophylactic rabies vaccination series.

> **TECHNICIAN NOTE**
>
> Rabies is a zoonotic infection (infectious to humans) and is universally fatal.

The equine viral encephalitides (Eastern, Western, Venezuelan, West Nile) are transmitted to horses by mosquitoes. Clinical signs of Eastern, Western, and Venezuelan encephalitis are practically indistinguishable and include profound depression, fever, ataxia, head pressing, dementia, and multiple cranial nerve abnormalities. The clinical signs of West Nile encephalitis include weakness and ataxia, which are often asymmetrical, involving the hind limbs or both forelimbs and hind limbs, muscle fasciculations, and cranial nerve deficits (such as droopy lip). The mortality rate is extremely high with Eastern equine encephalitis (75% to 100%), moderate with Venezuelan (40% to 80%), and lower with Western (30% to 50%) and West Nile (36% to 44%). Treatment consists of supportive care to provide hydration, nutrition, and a clean, dry environment. The prognosis is poor with Eastern equine encephalitis and guarded with Western, Venezuelan, and West Nile encephalitides. Diagnosis is confirmed by serologic test (a high titer or a fourfold increase in antibodies to Eastern, Western, and Venezuelan viruses identified by complement-fixation, neutralization or hemagglutination-inhibition assays, or a positive IgM capture ELISA for West Nile and Venezuelan) or, in case of postmortem samples, fluorescent antibody or virus isolation in brain tissue. The viral encephalitides can be prevented by vaccination 1 month before mosquito season. In southern regions of the United States, vaccinations should be administered two or three times per year.

Equine leukoencephalomalacia (moldy corn toxicity) is caused by ingestion of a fungal toxin produced by *Fusarium moniliform.* This mold has a predilection for corn, and affected kernels are usually pink to brown. The fungal toxin produces liquefactive necrosis of the cerebral cortex, and clinical signs include profound depression, head pressing, altered states of consciousness, incoordination, and aimless wandering. Treatment consists of supportive care, and the prognosis for recovery is poor. Horses often die within 24 hours of manifesting neurologic signs.

Horses acquire two types of skull fractures depending on the nature of their traumatic injury. Horses that suffer frontal impact with a solid object develop depression fractures of the frontal and parietal bones. The common neurologic signs observed in horses with this type of fracture are referable to cerebral damage and include depression, seizure, stupor, and aimless wandering. Horses that flip over backward develop fractures of the petrous temporal bone and the junction of the basisphenoid and basioccipital bone. Neurologic signs associated with these fractures include abnormalities of balance, incoordination of limbs, nystagmus (rhythmic eye movement), abnormal respiratory patterns, and coma. Diagnosis is confirmed by radiographic examination of the skull. Treatment consists of supportive care and antiinflammatory therapy (corticosteroids, DMSO). Surgical decompression of frontal and parietal fractures may improve the neurologic status of some horses.

Occasionally, the neurologic disease may progress to the point that the horses become dangerous to themselves and the personnel handling them, for instance, in cases of violent seizures unresponsive to therapy, dementia, aggressiveness, and mania. These horses must be handled as rabies suspects and exposure of personnel must be minimized. In some cases the veterinarian may elect to euthanize the animal, and that must be done by the safest means possible, and with limited exposure to people. The use of ropes and tranquilizer guns may facilitate securing the animal before entering the enclosure. The animal is secured usually in lateral position, with a head rope, fore and rear legs tied or held with ropes. The veterinarian should approach the horse from the top of the neck to avoid a kick or strike. This should give adequate venous access with limited exposure.

DERMATOLOGIC DISEASE

Equine dermatophytosis (ringworm) is a fungal infection of the superficial layer of skin. The fungi commonly involved are *Trichophyton* and *Microsporum* spp. Transmission of the fungal infection is by direct contact between affected animals, and younger animals (less than 4 years old) are more likely to be affected. Infected areas of skin have a bull's-eye appearance with circular patches of hair loss with a circle of inflammation at the periphery of the lesion. Diagnosis is confirmed by fungal culture on commercially available dermatophyte culture medium. Although the infection is usually self-limiting, application of topical antifungal drugs will speed recovery.

Dermatophilosis (rain scald, rain rot) is a common bacterial infection caused by *Dermatophilus congolense* that produces crusting lesions. The crusts can be pulled out with a tuft of hair, and the remaining lesion is a glistening yellow crater. The organisms readily colonize wet, macerated skin, and therefore the disease is common in the winter and spring. An impression smear of the tuft should be stained with Wright's stain, and organisms are identified as a double chain of cocci with a "railroad track" appearance. The organisms are usually easily cultured and form an applesauce-like colony on specialized growth medium. Affected horses should be bathed with an iodine-based or chlorhexidine shampoo and placed in a dry environment. Administration of penicillin will speed recovery in severely affected horses.

Culicoides hypersensitivity is a syndrome characterized by mane and tail rubbing whereby affected horses develop an allergic pruritic skin condition secondary to the bite of *Culicoides* flies. The classic body regions affected include face, ears, mane, withers, rump, base of the tail, and ventral abdomen. The dermatitis usually begins as a seasonal condition, but its severity and duration increase as the horse ages. Pruritus usually is noted during the fly season but will vary in length depending on geographic location. The condition is diagnosed by correlating the historical findings of seasonal pruritus with physical evidence of self-mutilation, especially in the mane and tail areas. Intradermal skin testing can be useful in confirming the diagnosis. Treatment involves reducing insect exposure and concomitant use of antiinflammatory medication. Because *Culicoides* breeds in stagnant waters, affected horses should be moved from proximity to ponds, lakes, or irrigation canals. Water troughs and barrels should be cleaned frequently and the water kept fresh to prevent use as breeding sites by the flies. Because *Culicoides* feeds primarily at dusk, night, and dawn, horses should be kept stabled during these times. Stabling is most effective if the doors and windows can be closed and if the stall is lined with a fine-mesh screen. Frequent application of insecticide to the screen may also be useful. Ceiling fans help reduce exposure because *Culicoides* cannot fly well in brisk breezes. Application of insecticides and repellents is a necessary part of disease control. The most effective products are those containing pyrethrins with synergists and repellents. Frequent bathing not only decreases scale and crust but also seems to decrease pruritus. Corticosteroid therapy may be required in some horses to control the pruritus.

Equine sarcoid is a benign, locally invasive tumor of skin and is the most common tumor in horses. These tumors produce either raised, hairless lesions with a corrugated surface that often bleed when traumatized, known as *fibroblastic sarcoids,* or a flattened form known as *verrucous sarcoids.* The cause of sarcoid is unknown, but a viral agent is suspected. Surgical resection, cryotherapy (freezing), laser therapy, immunotherapy (intralesional mycobacterial cell wall extract), radiotherapy (iridium 191), and chemotherapy (intralesional cisplatin) are accepted treatment modalities with variable success. It is difficult to predict response to a given treatment modality, and combination therapy is often necessary.

Melanomas are relatively common skin tumors that develop particularly in gray horses. They occur most commonly in the perineal region but can occur on other areas of the body. Melanomas appear as darkly pigmented nodules in the skin. They are usually benign but tend to progress and can cause mechanical problems, such as interfering with defecation. Most clinicians believe it is better not to attempt surgical removal unless they are located in an area that interferes with tack or they are so large that they interfere with normal body functions. These tumors often become more aggressive following unsuccessful attempts at complete surgical removal. Administration of cimetidine has been reported to be effective in some horses in causing reduction in size or resolution of melanomas, but it does not seem to be effective in all horses. Once the cimetidine is discontinued, the tumors usually enlarge.

OPHTHALMOLOGIC DISEASE

Recurrent uveitis (moon blindness, periodic ophthalmia) is the most common cause of blindness in horses. Affected horses experience episodes of intraocular inflammation characterized by blepharospasm, corneal edema, and hypopyon (inflammatory cellular exudate in the anterior chamber). Over time, the episodes become more frequent and severe and produce permanent ocular lesions, including retinal degeneration, cataracts, synechiae (adhesions of the iris to either the lens or the anterior chamber), and low ocular pressure. The disease may be unilateral or bilateral. Recurrent uveitis is classified as an unsoundness in horses, which constitutes failure during prepurchase and insurance examinations. Recurrent uveitis cannot be cured but can be controlled in some instances with long-term anti-inflammatory therapy (aspirin). Acute episodes are treated with ophthalmic preparations containing atropine and corticosteroids; systemic antiinflammatory therapy may be beneficial, including flunixin meglumine, phenylbutazone, or aspirin. It is an immune-mediated condition, and many factors have been implicated (heredity, parasites, leptospirosis); the inciting cause of uveitis is unknown. Horses with end-stage uveitis are blind and have very small, collapsed, ocular globes (phthisis bulbi).

> ### TECHNICIAN NOTE
> Recurrent uveitis (moon blindness, periodic ophthalmia) is the most common cause of blindness in horses.

Corneal ulceration commonly results from ocular trauma. Corneal ulceration can be detected by application of fluorescein dye to the surface of the eye. Defects in the corneal surface will stain an apple-green color. Corneal ulceration in most horses responds readily without

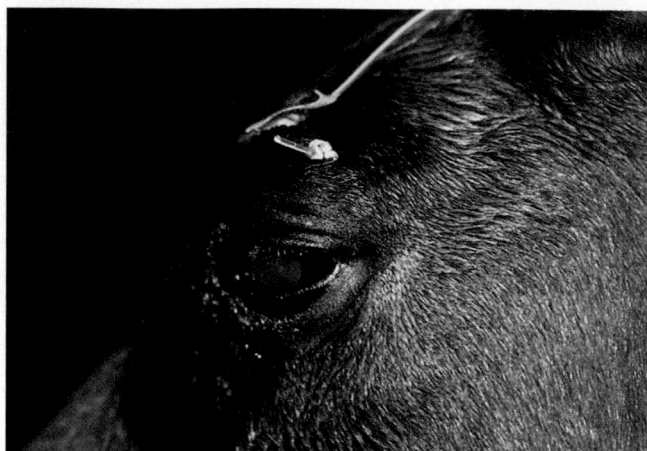

Figure 29-43 Subpalpebral eye lavage system for administration of ophthalmic medication without touching the affected eye.

complications to administration of ophthalmic antibacterial ointment (bacitracin, neomycin, polymyxin B). In some instances, the ulcer will be colonized by *Pseudomonas* or *Aspergillus* spp. These organisms produce collagenase, which destroys the cornea and creates a "melting" corneal ulcer. These ulcers are rapidly progressive and prone to uveal prolapse or ocular rupture. Frequent antibiotic dosage regimens may require placement of a subpalpebral lavage system, wherein polyethylene tubing is placed into the eyelid and exits the conjunctiva dorsal to the globe (Figure 29-43). The port of the tubing can be braided into the horse's mane, which facilitates frequent dosing for a painful eye. Aggressive topical antibacterial therapy may be successful, but suturing a conjunctival pedicle flap to provide blood supply to the affected area may be necessary to save the globe in some instances. Deep, melting corneal ulcers often heal with a fibrous scar that may impair vision in the future.

NEONATAL CARE

The normal gestation period of mares varies considerably, ranging from 320 to 360 days. As a mare approaches parturition, the udder begins to enlarge ("bagging up") and may leak small amounts of colostrum that dry over the ends of the teats ("waxing"). Increasing calcium and magnesium concentrations in milk correspond to impending (less than 24 hours) parturition and can be detected using commercially available foal predictor kits. In mares with placentitis, parturition can not be predicted by the increase in milk calcium. Parturition occurs in three stages. Stage 1 is under voluntary control of the mare and is characterized by repositioning of the fetus to a dorsosacral position and initial uterine contractions; it generally lasts a few hours, although it can be interrupted for hours to days. External signs of stage 1 labor include restlessness, sweating, pacing, inappetence, and raising the tail. The onset of stage 2 labor is signaled by rupture of the chorioallantoic membrane and release of allantoic fluid (breaking water). Delivery of the foal should be complete within 20 to 40 minutes of the onset of stage 2 of labor. The third stage of labor begins after expulsion of the foal and is defined by expulsion of the fetoplacental membranes. Fetoplacental membranes should be passed within 1 hour of expulsion of the foal. Retained placenta (failure to pass fetal membranes within 3 hours of delivery) is an emergency in mares and may result in toxic metritis and laminitis. After parturition, the umbilicus is dipped in a chlorhexidine or an iodine solution, foals are examined for developmental anomalies and traumatic injury, the mare's reproductive tract is examined for traumatic injury, and the placenta is inspected for completeness and evidence of thickening or infection. (See Chapter 17 for additional information on reproduction.)

Premature foals are born before 320 days of gestation, whereas foals that present with prematurity but have a normal (320 to 360 days) or abnormally long (>360 days) gestational length are referred to as *dysmature*. Signs of prematurity include small body size, silky and fine hair coat, domed head, floppy ears, tendon and ligament laxity, weakness, and incomplete ossification of the cuboidal bones (carpi and tarsi). If the latter is suspected, then weight bearing should be limited, and radiographs of at least one carpus and one tarsus should be taken as soon as possible to evaluate the degree of cuboidal bone ossification. Appropriate treatment must be instituted to minimize the risk of compressing the cartilaginous cuboidal bones, which will result bone deformity.

> ✎ **TECHNICIAN NOTE**
>
> Premature foals are born before 320 days of gestation, whereas foals that present with prematurity but have a normal (320 to 360 days) or abnormally long (>360 days) gestational length are referred to as *dysmature*.

Normal foals should stand within 1 hour, suckle within 2 hours, and pass meconium within 3 hours of parturition. It is important for the foal to ingest the colostrum ("first milk") produced by the mare. Colostrum contains immunoglobulins and other factors and provides protection against infection. Foals are born without immunoglobulin in their blood, and the immunoglobulin in colostrum represents the only form of immune protection (passive transfer of immunity). The immunoglobulins in colostrum are absorbed intact by the foal's intestinal tract for the first 18 hours of life. After that time, the intestinal tract will no longer absorb the large immunoglobulin proteins (gut closure). Foals that do not receive adequate colostral maternal immunoglobulins shortly after birth are said to experience *failure of passive transfer*. Failure of passive transfer can occur with failure or delay to suckle, premature gut closure, failure of the dam to produce good-quality colostrum, and leakage of colostrum before parturition and is the single most important predisposing factor for development of life-threatening neonatal infections.

Adequate transfer of immunity should be assessed at 18 to 24 hours of life, using one of the several commercially available immunoglobulin G (IgG) test kits that provide a semiquantitative measurement of IgG concentration in serum, plasma, or whole blood. The test to measure the foal's IgG is often performed by the veterinary technician. Early assessment of passive transfer is often indicated in high-risk pregnancies and can be performed at 12 hours of age; although blood IgG levels may increase some, most of the absorption occurs in the first 8 to 12 hours. If the foal has not received adequate colostrum, it should be supplemented by intravenous plasma transfusion, using either commercial hyperimmune plasma or plasma collected from an appropriate donor as soon as possible. Moreover, if signs of sepsis are present blood cultures should be collected using sterile technique and broad-spectrum antibiotic therapy instituted immediately. The antibiotic therapy should be modified appropriately in accordance with the organism cultured. Bactericidal antibiotics with a broad spectrum, particularly activity against gram-negative organisms, may also be recommended to prevent bacterial infection in neonatal foals.

Normal foals suckle every 30 to 40 minutes and are very active. Foals are particularly fragile, and failure to suckle is the first sign of disease. Neonatal septicemia is the most common life-threatening disease of foals and results from entry of bacteria via the gastrointestinal tract, respiratory tract, and umbilicus (navel ill). Clinical signs include depression, fever, tachycardia, injected mucous membranes, icterus and petechiae seen on the mucous membranes and pinna (see Figures 29-8 and 29-19), recumbency, respiratory distress, shock, hypothermia, and coma. If untreated, neonatal septicemia usually results in death of the foal. Septic arthritis (joint ill) and osteomyelitis are common sequelae to neonatal septicemia that are difficult to cure and may produce permanent damage.

Hypoxic-ischemic (HI) syndrome is a result of prolonged birth asphyxia associated with insufficient placentation, difficult labor (dystocia), premature placental separation (known as *red bag*, Figure 29-44), and premature umbilical cord rupture and failure to rupture placental membranes. The organs most susceptible to the HI injury include the central nervous system, the gastrointestinal tract, kidneys, and liver, respectively. Neonatal maladjustment syndrome (dummy foal) is a manifestation of HI encephalopathy. Foals may show neurologic abnormalities since birth or may develop those abnormalities within 24 hours after birth. The range of neurologic abnormalities includes failure to suckle, hyperresponsiveness, depression, bizarre vocalization (barkers), failure to recognize the dam, stupor, seizures, and coma. The neurologic signs result from neuronal damage associated with the hypoxia and ischemia in the brain and brainstem; edema and hemorrhage are commonly seen. Less commonly, the HI injury affects the other organs mentioned above, resulting in necrotizing enterocolitis and renal and liver insufficiencies.

Other causes of neonatal distress include constipation (meconium impaction), abnormal intestinal distention associated with enterocolitis, uroperitoneum associated with ruptured urinary bladder, all of which manifest as signs of abdominal discomfort, distention, and straining (Figure 29-45, *A* and *B*). Additionally, the newborn may present with respiratory difficulty due to profound anemia because of neonatal hemolysis resulting from incompatible blood type with mare (referred to as *neonatal iso-erythrolysis*), congenital cardiac abnormalities, fractured ribs, and neonatal respiratory distress syndrome (resulting from pulmonary immaturity and primary or secondary surfactant dysfunction).

Foals readily develop gastric ulceration under conditions of stress. Signs of abdominal discomfort, bruxism, and salivation are indicative of gastrointestinal ulceration, and therefore prophylactic antiulcer medication may be administered to all foals under intensive care.

> ### ✎ TECHNICIAN NOTE
>
> Regardless of the primary disease process, neonatal intensive care is a daunting task. The veterinary technician attending to the recumbent foal must be diligent, thorough, aseptic, and observant.

Normal foals suckle approximately 30 times per day, ingest 15% to 20% of their body weight in milk, and gain 1.0 to 2.5 kg (2.2 to 5.5 lb) per day. Adequate nutritional support is of paramount importance in neonatal care. Nutritional support can be provided to the foal by feeding the mare's milk using a small nasoesophageal feeding tube. The mare should be hand milked every 2 hours, but if the mare does not produce sufficient milk to meet the nutritional requirements of the foal, equine milk replacers may be used. Nonevaporated goat's milk may be used as a substitute; cow's milk should only be used as a last option, and it should be modified by the addition of lime water; calf milk replacers should be avoided. Total parenteral nutrition (TPN) is an intravenous nutritional support that may be necessary in foals with poor gastrointestinal motility and primary gastrointestinal disease. Parenteral nutrition requires a dedicated intravenous catheter and a constant infusion pump. Moreover, TPN may predispose or exacerbate septicemia; therefore appropriate handling and strict sterile technique are required when giving parenteral nutrition. Intravenous fluid therapy is often necessary to support the cardiovascular system, correct electrolyte abnormalities, and maintain acid-base balance.

Recumbent neonatal foals require intensive supportive care consisting of a 24-hour attendant, constant intravenous infusion system, nutritional supplementation, oxygen supplementation, and accessible blood gas and electrolyte analyzers. Recumbent foals are sometimes placed on a foal bed, which is designed to allow the attendant to care for the foal from one side and the mare to access the foal from

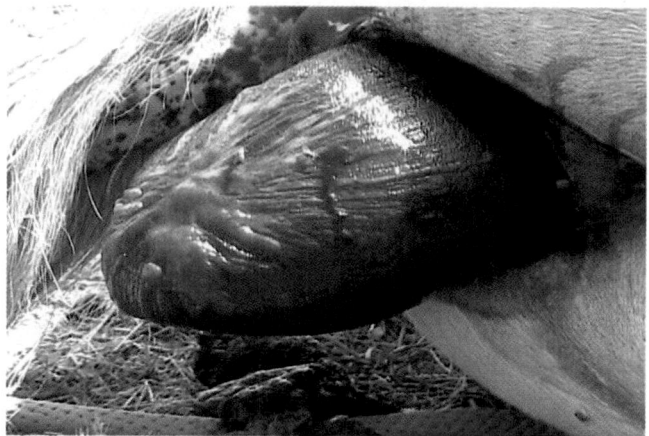

Figure 29-44 Mare with premature placental separation (red bag), which is often associated with prolonged birth asphyxia.

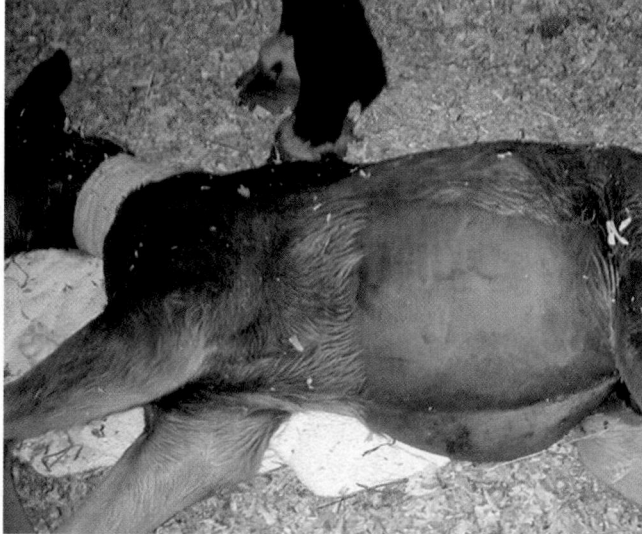

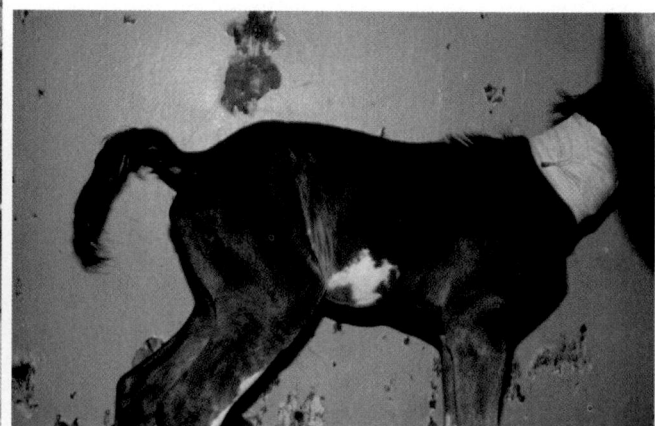

Figure 29-45 **A,** Foal with abdominal distention showing signs of discomfort. **B,** Foal straining as a sign of abdominal discomfort.

A   B

the other. Foals should be maintained in sternal recumbency to prevent collapse of the down lung, allowing maximal ventilation. Foals must be kept clean and dry, and their position should be changed every 2 hours. Recumbent foals are prone to corneal ulceration, therefore, triple antibiotic ointment or artificial tears should be placed in their eyes every 4 hours. Additional protection can be maintained by placing padded head protection on the foal. Commercially available soft helmets work well (Figure 29-46); an inexpensive alternative is gauze placed in a ring around the eyes and secured with tape (Figure 29-47). Heart rate, respiratory rate and character, temperature, mucous membrane character, capillary refill time, abdominal distention, and gastrointestinal motility should be monitored every 2 hours. Urinary and fecal output should be recorded. Observe the umbilicus during urination to note any urine leakage from the umbilical stump. This is commonly referred to as a *patent urachus*. Arterial blood gas, PCV, total protein, serum electrolyte, and serum glucose concentrations should be determined every 4 to 12 hours depending on the severity of the disease. Palpation of the umbilicus and joints should be performed at least daily.

Most recumbent foals demonstrate some degree of respiratory insufficiency. Oxygen can be supplemented to the foal using nasal insufflation with humidified 100% oxygen at 4 to 8 L/min. If nasal insufflation is inadequate, the foal may require mechanical ventilation to ensure adequate oxygenation. Mechanical ventilation requires nasotracheal or endotracheal intubation and positive pressure ventilation. Pulmonary function can be monitored using serial arterial blood gas evaluation obtained from the greater metatarsal artery, the median artery (in the medial aspect of the antebrachial region), or the brachial artery (as it crosses the medial aspect of the proximal forearm). Pulse oximetry is a noninvasive alternative for monitoring arterial oxygen saturation.

Regardless of the primary disease process, neonatal intensive care is a daunting task. The veterinary technician attending to the recumbent foal must be diligent, thorough, aseptic, and observant. Deterioration in patient status occurs rapidly and without warning. Meticulous patient care and monitoring will allow rapid correction of the therapeutic plan, which often determines the final outcome for neonatal foals. Additional information on neonatal care of the foal is found in Chapter 12.

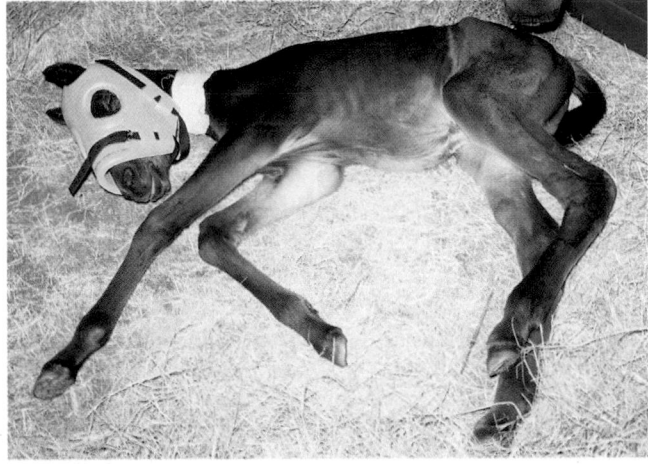

Figure 29-46 Helmet for protection of the head and eyes of newborns.

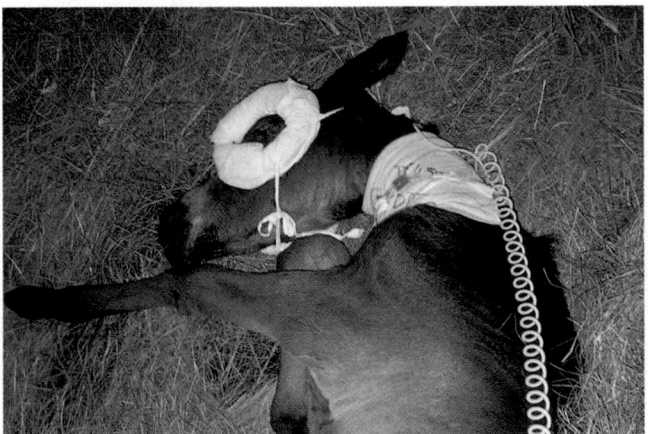

Figure 29-47 Protection of the eyes in recumbent foals, made with rolled gauze and white tape.

DYSTOCIA

Dystocia means "difficult birth" and is relatively uncommon in horses compared with cattle. However, when dystocia occurs in mares, it is usually a serious problem. Because parturition is rapid in horses and the expulsive efforts of the mare are violent, veterinary obstetric manipulations are difficult and exhausting. Care must be taken at all times to avoid injuring the reproductive tract of the mare. There are many causes of dystocia in the mare; the most frequent ones include premature placental separation and abnormal presentation of the fetus, especially when either the head or limbs or both are deviated. Because the neck of the foal is relatively long, it can easily become twisted. Sometimes the foal may come hind feet first (rare), or if the hind feet are retained, the tail comes first. This latter situation is true breech position. Transverse presentation is also rare in mares. Other occasional causes of dystocia include an excessively large fetus or fetal monsters (e.g., hydrocephalus). An anatomic or physiologic abnormality in the mare herself may cause dystocia. For example, a mare that has sustained a pelvic fracture can develop callus formation, which impairs the shape and size of the birth canal. Another cause of dystocia is torsion of the uterus. This may occur during gestation, particularly during the last trimester.

Dystocia in mares is corrected using a variety of methods, depending on the cause of the dystocia, the status of the foal, and the condition of the mare. Sometimes the dystocia can be corrected by manipulating fetal position or presentation with the mare standing, with or without the use of sedation or an epidural anesthetic. Placement of a nasotracheal tube will prevent the mare from exerting an abdominal press and will relieve straining. Sometimes a short-acting anesthetic protocol combined with rolling the mare on her back or hoisting her hind limbs is enough to relieve the dystocia and provide the veterinarian with sufficient relaxation in the mare to deliver the fetus. Fetotomy is sometimes performed to relieve dystocia, particularly if the fetus is dead. Fetotomy is a process in which a dead foal is cut into pieces while within the uterus and removed. Caution must be taken while performing a fetotomy to prevent serious injury to the reproductive tract of the mare.

✏ TECHNICIAN NOTE

Most cesarean deliveries are performed in the mare with general anesthesia. Generally, time is critical for saving the foal and for the overall health and well-being of the mare. The technician must be prepared for the surgery and have the necessary equipment, personnel, and drugs ready for reviving the foal if necessary.

Most cesarean deliveries are performed in the mare with general anesthesia. Generally a cesarean delivery is performed though a caudal ventral midline or flank incision in mares. Time is usually critical for saving the foal and for the overall health and well-being of the mare. The technician must be prepared for the surgery and have necessary equipment, personnel, and drugs ready for reviving the foal if necessary. The same instruments that are used for colic surgery are often used for cesarean delivery, but additional instruments may be necessary. If the foal is alive, the technician or other personnel need to be prepared and equipped to revive it. The foal will usually be depressed from the effects of general anesthesia and may need vigorous rubbing and drying. Oxygen should be available, as well as heat lamps and a nasotracheal tube and Ambu bag to ventilate the foal. Forceps to clamp the umbilicus should be readily available if excessive bleeding occurs. A suction device to remove mucus and stomach contents from the airway should be attended to by the technician or other personnel. The technician should be cognizant and attentive to the needs of the surgeon during this time even though the foal is requiring assistance.

A piece of straw inserted in the nostril is one of the most practical methods of initiating respiratory movements in a newborn foal. The foal's neck should be extended to help ensure a patent airway. The foal should be vigorously dried because fluid will conduct heat away from the animal, resulting in hypothermia and a weak foal. The foal can be resuscitated with the self-inflating nonrebreathing Ambu bag. Air can be delivered through a cone-shaped face mask similar to the one used to induce anesthesia in small animals. The mask must fit tightly over the nostrils and mouth. Mouth-to-nose ventilation may be performed and is done by covering one nostril, closing the mouth, and blowing in the opposite nostril. A few short breaths are all that is usually required. Overinflation can obviously cause perma-nent damage to the lungs. Frequently the veterinarian may order intravenous fluids, respiratory stimulants, and drugs to support the cardiovascular system. The foal should be kept warm (not hot) with heat lamps, circulating warm water pads, and blankets. The next important thing is to ensure that the foal consumes or is administered an adequate amount of colostrum to provide passive immunity to infectious agents during the first few weeks of life (see Neonatal Care). Enteral feeding of foal that underwent severe asphyxia may be contraindicated, as it may contribute to the development of neonatal necrotizing enterocolitis.

SURGERY OF THE FEMALE CAUDAL REPRODUCTIVE TRACT

Perineal surgery is relatively common in equine practice. Primiparous mares develop rectovaginal and cervical lacerations during foaling. Abnormal perineal conformation can lead to reproductive unsoundness. Mares with abnormal conformation can develop pneumovagina or pneumouterus secondary to aspirating air into the reproductive tract. They also can develop vesicovaginal reflux in which urine pools in the cranial vaginal cavity; this can drain into the uterus during estrus when the cervix is opened, leading to endometrial inflammation. Most surgical procedures to correct these caudal reproductive tract abnormalities are performed in standing mares that have been sedated, and a caudal epidural anesthesia is used.

A caudal epidural anesthesia is performed after clipping the hair over the tail head and aseptically preparing the skin. An 18-gauge, 1.5-inch needle is inserted through the skin between the last sacral and first coccygeal vertebrae or between the first and second coccygeal vertebrae and advanced (Figure 29-48). The correct location can be confirmed by checking to see if local anesthetic placed in the hub of the needle is drawn into the epidural space. Once the correct location has been identified, the local anesthetic is injected. The most commonly used agents for horses are lidocaine, mepivacaine, or xylazine. A caudal epidural anesthetic will desensitize the perineal region. Because horses will also develop incoordination in their rear limbs following the procedure, care should be taken when moving them until the effects of the anesthetic dissipate.

There are several surgical procedures for correcting caudal reproductive tract abnormalities. The most important factor in the eventual success of repairing a rectovaginal tear is that the mare's feces be made soft (cow patty consistency) and kept soft for at least 30 days after surgery. This decreases the straining and tension placed on the repaired rectal shelf. The most effective method for getting the feces soft is to remove hay and other coarse roughage from the diet and feed the mare on lush pasture or a complete pelleted feed. Administration of mineral oil or magnesium sulfate to the diet also helps soften the feces.

The most commonly preformed perineal surgery is Caslick's operation. This is performed in many fillies on

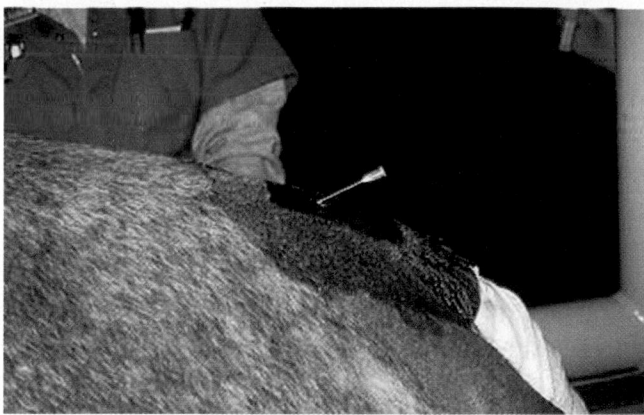

Figure 29-48 Technique for injecting a caudal epidural anesthetic between the first and second coccygeal vertebrae in a horse using an 18-gauge, 1.5-inch needle.

the racetrack and in mares with poor vulvar conformation to prevent pneumovagina and fecal contamination of the vagina, respectively. This procedure is usually performed with sedation and local anesthetic infiltration of the edge of the vulva. The edges of the dorsal vulvar labia are incised and then sutured using a continuous suture pattern. The closure is extended down to the level of the pelvic floor. The suture should not be any lower than this because it may interfere with urination and contribute to urine pooling.

UROGENITAL TRACT SURGERY

Urinary calculi occur infrequently in horses. Urinary calculi in horses are usually composed of calcium carbonate and have a spicular appearance. These calculi may develop in the kidney or urinary bladder. Small-diameter calculi can be passed during normal urination and go unnoticed. Clinical signs of urinary calculi include stranguria (slow and difficult urination or straining to urinate), pollakiuria (frequent urination), and hematuria (bloody urine). Horses that develop renal calculi will develop signs of abdominal discomfort when the stones become lodged in the ureter. In addition, cystic (urinary bladder) calculi that become lodged in the urethra in male horses cause an inability to urinate and subsequent abdominal pain. Urinary calculi can be diagnosed based on clinical signs, urinalysis, palpation of the urinary bladder per rectum, and endoscopic evaluation of the urethra and urinary bladder. Occasionally a calculus can be palpated in the proximal urethra of male horses at the level of the ischial arch. There are several techniques and certain instruments available for removing urinary tract calculi.

TECHNICIAN NOTE

Urinary calculi occur infrequently in horses. Urinary calculi in horses are usually composed of calcium carbonate and have a spicular appearance. These calculi may develop in the kidney or urinary bladder.

Foals commonly develop diseases of the umbilical remnants, including infection (navel ill) in the umbilical arteries, veins, and urachus. These foals often become depressed, inappetent, and febrile. Many foals also develop secondary septicemia and septic arthritis. Umbilical remnant infection may be diagnosed based on clinical signs of swelling, heat, or drainage in the umbilical area. However, foals can have infection within these structures and be normal on palpation. Transabdominal ultrasonography is also helpful in diagnosing diseases of the umbilical structures. Foals with umbilical remnant infection require treatment with broad-spectrum antibiotics; many of these foals require surgical removal of the affected structures. Surgery for umbilical remnant disease involves a similar approach and instrumentation as for repairing an umbilical hernia. It is necessary to proceed with caution and have suction available and ready while dissecting the umbilical structures to prevent contamination of the abdominal cavity.

Patent urachus is a condition wherein foals dribble urine from the umbilicus because a patent canal between the urachus and urinary bladder is present at birth or develops in the postnatal period. Because those that develop in the postnatal period often occur secondary to an infectious process, it is imperative to rule out umbilical remnant infection and systemic infectious disease. Foals with a patent urachus may be treated nonsurgically by applying an irritant, such as iodine solution, or using silver nitrate sticks on the external surface of the urachus to promote scarification and closure. This is probably most effective in those foals that have a patent urachus at birth. Foals that do not respond to this treatment or those that have an infectious process occurring in the umbilical remnants should have an umbilical remnant resection.

Castration is one of the most commonly performed surgeries in horses. It is usually performed in the field and does not require extensive surgical facilities or instrumentation. Although under most circumstances castration is performed under short-acting intravenous general anesthesia, it can be performed in the standing horse with heavy sedation and infiltration of a local anesthetic into the scrotum and spermatic cord. The most common drugs for castration with the horse under intravenous anesthesia include xylazine/ketamine or xylazine/thiobarbiturate; both combinations can be used with or without guaifenesin. It is important to document that both testicles have descended into the scrotum before commencing with castration in the field. One needs to be prepared for a more extensive surgery requiring entrance into the abdominal cavity (as in a retained testicle); this needs to be planned for because it often takes more time than a routine castration. If both testicles cannot be palpated in the scrotum, then the testicle may be located intraabdominally, in the inguinal canal, or immediately outside the external inguinal ring. A horse with a testicle located outside the abdominal cavity, but not within the scrotum, is referred to as a *high flanker*. If the testicle cannot be palpated in the scrotum, then sedation may relax the horse and the cremaster muscle and allow the examiner to palpate the testicle or a portion of it. If the testicle still cannot be palpated after sedation, then a rectal examination with or without ultrasonography may help confirm the location of the testicle. Involvement of the veterinary technician for castration includes general restraint, handling, administering and monitoring anesthesia, preparation of the surgical site, and preparation of instruments.

Castration is usually performed with the horse in lateral recumbency with the upper rear limb pulled forward and tied around the horse's neck. Castration involves making an incision over each testicle parallel to the median raphe through the skin and subcutaneous tissue. The testicles are removed by crushing then cutting the spermatic cord proximal to the testicle and epididymis, using emasculators (Figure 29-49, A). The emasculators should be placed on the spermatic cord so that the cord is crushed on the side toward the body wall and cut on the side toward the scrotum (Figure 29-49, B). There are numerous types of emasculators, and each surgeon may have an individual preference. The entire spermatic cord may be crushed and cut simultaneously within the tunic (closed castration) or the tunica albuginea may be opened and the emasculators can be applied to the vascular structures separately (open castration); this is often done in aged stallions that have an excessively large-diameter spermatic cord. The spermatic cord should be examined after the emasculator is removed to make sure there is no bleeding. The skin incisions are stretched manually to promote drainage.

Postoperative care usually includes strict stall confinement for 24 hours and then controlled exercise (hand walking) once or twice daily for 1 to 2 weeks to promote drainage, prevent excessive swelling, and prevent or reduce stiffness and soreness. The horse should be monitored closely during the first day after surgery for signs of excessive hemorrhage, evisceration of intestine or omentum (herniation), or excessive swelling.

If the testicle has not descended (cryptorchidism), then surgery is more involved and requires anesthesia of longer duration. Cryptorchidectomy (removal of a cryptorchid testicle) also requires the surgeon to use a different surgical technique than for routine castration. The testicle can be approached through various incisions, but an approach through the inguinal ring is most often used. A sponge forceps is used to grasp the structures that lead to the scrotum (gubernaculum), and the testicle is extracted from the inguinal canal. In some horses the testicle cannot be retrieved in this manner, and the surgeon must manually

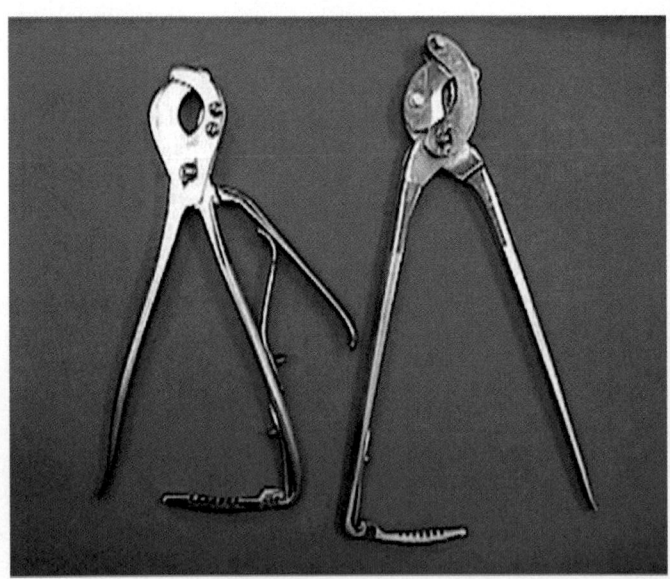

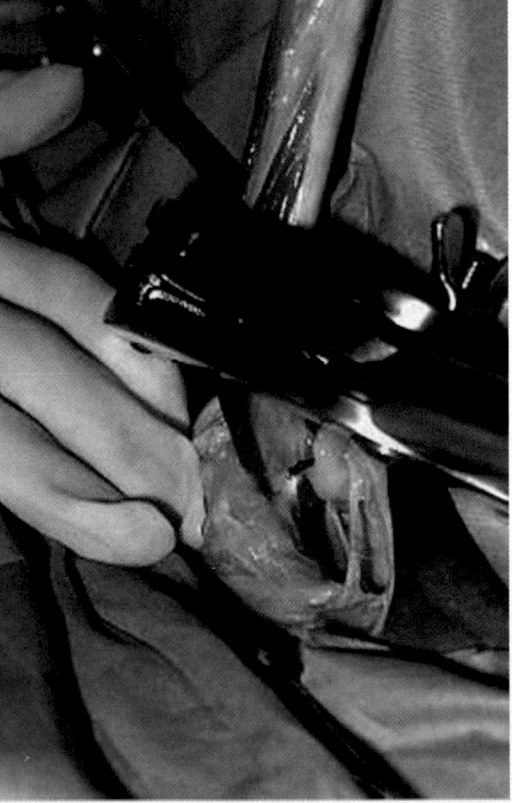

A   B

Figure 29-49 **A,** Emasculators used to crush and cut the spermatic cord of horses during castration. **B,** Use of emasculators during castration of a horse: the emasculators are placed around the spermatic cord so that the nut on the emasculators is located toward the testicle, ensuring that the spermatic cord is crushed toward the body side and the cord is cut toward the testicle side.

explore the inguinal canal or caudal abdominal cavity. Once the testicle is retrieved, it is removed using a similar technique as described for routine castration. Following removal of the retained testicle, the other one is removed in a routine manner. Occasionally horses have both testicles retained.

It is believed that cryptorchid horses are more at risk for evisceration after surgery. To prevent this, some surgeons may elect to temporarily pack a length of gauze soaked in sterile saline or an antiseptic into the subcutaneous areas of the inguinal canal. The gauze packing is held in place with large sutures in the skin and is usually removed in 24 to 72 hours. Other surgeons place interrupted absorbable sutures in the external inguinal ring.

Ovariectomy is performed in mares with diseased ovaries, in mares with normal reproductive tracts for use as teaser mares, and in some mares used as performance horses that have unacceptable behavior associated with estrus. An ovariectomy can be performed unilaterally or bilaterally depending on the reason for the procedure. Diseased ovaries are usually enlarged and require removal through an incision in the ventral body wall (caudal midline or diagonal paramedian) or the flank. The most common cause of ovarian disease necessitating removal is neoplasia; the most common types of ovarian neoplasia include granulosa theca cell tumors and teratomas. Mares with granulosa theca cell tumors often display abnormal behavior, such as anestrus, persistent estrus or nymphomania, or stallion-like behavior. Ovarian tumors and other ovarian diseases are diagnosed based on clinical signs, rectal examination, and transrectal ultrasonography. Nondiseased ovaries of normal size can usually be removed through a flank incision or via an incision in the vaginal wall (colpotomy) in standing sedated mares with either local anesthetic infiltration in the body wall or a caudal epidural anesthetic. Hemostasis of the ovarian pedicle is provided either by transfixing with multiple sutures, application of an automatic stapling device, or crushing with a chain écraseur. Complications include hemorrhage, abdominal pain, myositis, and other problems related to anesthesia and abdominal surgery.

HERNIA REPAIR

Herniation of omentum or abdominal viscera through the abdominal wall can occur with an umbilical hernia, inguinal (scrotal) hernia, or incisional hernia. Umbilical hernias are usually congenital and are relatively common in foals. Small hernias may close spontaneously as the foal grows, whereas others require surgical intervention. Umbilical hernias can be repaired using several different methods. Generally the body wall is closed with either interrupted or continuous absorbable suture. Some surgeons open the peritoneum (open herniorrhaphy) and others leave the peritoneum intact (closed herniorrhaphy). If an umbilical hernia is large or it has not closed by several months of age,

then it should probably be surgically repaired. The owner should be instructed to manually reduce hernial contents at least daily; if at any time the hernia cannot be reduced, the horse should be examined by a veterinarian immediately. If intestine becomes incarcerated in the hernia, then vascular compromise can occur leading to ischemic injury.

Inguinal or scrotal hernias can occur in horses of any age, but newborn foals and adult breeding stallions are probably the most commonly affected. Frequently the herniated contents do not become incarcerated and can be easily reduced. The hernia should be reduced at least daily in foals because intestine could become incarcerated, which would necessitate emergency surgery. Sometimes, these hernias will spontaneously resolve in foals, but many foals require surgical repair. Because the tissues are friable in foals, successful surgical repair can be difficult. Scrotal hernias in adult horses most commonly occur in stallions shortly after breeding. In most instances, the herniated structure or structures become incarcerated (not reducible), which necessitates immediate surgery. Incarceration of intestine within the scrotum will result in a large, firm, and cold scrotum on the affected side secondary to compromised testicular blood flow. The blood supply to the intestine also becomes compromised, resulting in ischemic injury. Generally the testicle on the affected side is removed and the affected segment of intestine often requires resection. This necessitates preparation of the horse for inguinal and ventral midline surgery.

Acquired body wall herniation occurs in horses subsequent to trauma and following surgery. Blunt trauma such as a kick can lead to disruption of the body wall musculature. Body wall hernias occur secondary to abdominal incisions; these occur more frequently in horses that develop incisional infection or other complicating factors. Small body wall hernias can be repaired primarily by suturing the defect. Larger body wall defects require the use of mesh implants. It is critical that there be no residual incisional infection present at the time of mesh herniorrhaphy and that aseptic technique be followed during placement of the mesh.

MUSCULOSKELETAL DISEASE

Laminitis (founder) is a serious, often life-threatening disease of horses. It involves ischemic necrosis and inflammation of the sensitive laminae of the feet. It often involves both front feet or all four feet. However, it can occur in only one fore or rear foot if there is a severe lameness in the opposite limb. The cause of laminitis is unknown, but horses with serious infectious or inflammatory diseases resulting in endotoxemia, such as ischemic or inflammatory bowel disease, pleuropneumonia, septic metritis, and grain overload, are predisposed. Certain medications, such as corticosteroids, have also been incriminated as a potential cause of laminitis. Laminitis occurs almost exclusively in adult horses; it rarely occurs in horses less than 1 year of age.

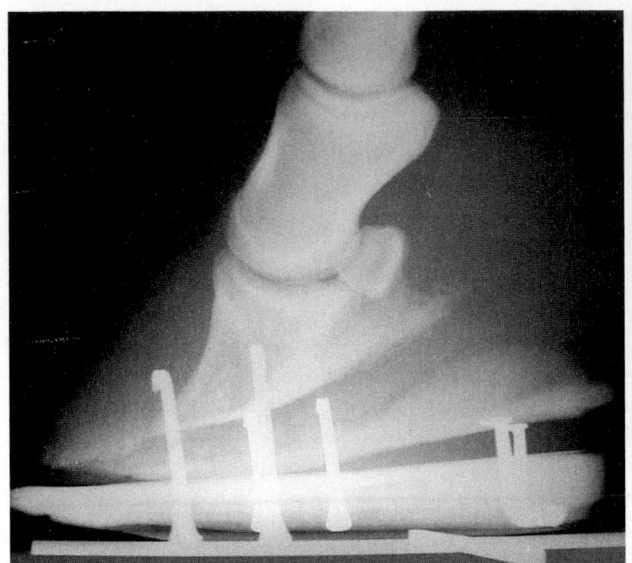

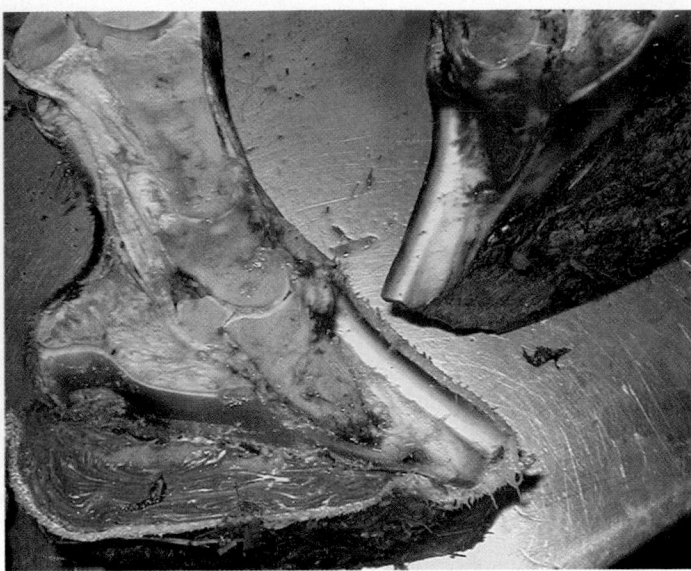

A   B

Figure 29-50 **A,** Lateral radiograph of the front foot of a horse with laminitis that has evidence of coffin bone rotation. **B,** Gross pathologic photograph of sagittal section of both front feet of a horse with bilateral laminitis that has undergone coffin bone rotation.

> ✎ **TECHNICIAN NOTE**
>
> Laminitis (founder) is a serious, often life-threatening disease of horses. It involves ischemic necrosis and inflammation of the sensitive laminae of the feet. It often involves both front feet or all four feet.

Acute laminitis occurs in the initial stages of the disease, resulting in extreme pain and reluctance to move. Horses often have increased heat in the hooves and have a pronounced or bounding digital pulse. They are reluctant to walk, turn, or allow their feet to be picked up. They stand with a characteristic stance with their rear legs camped underneath their torso and their front feet camped out in front (Figure 29-3). Chronic laminitis occurs when, because of degeneration of the sensitive laminae on the coffin bone (distal phalanx), the dorsal laminar attachments to the insensitive laminae of the hoof detach and the coffin bone rotates. In severe chronic laminitis, the rotated coffin bone may protrude through the sole of the foot. A lateral radiograph of the foot is usually required to determine whether coffin bone rotation has occurred (Figure 29-50). In more severe cases, all laminar attachments may become detached, and the coffin bone is displaced distally within the hoof wall. Horses that have distal displacement of the coffin bone develop a characteristic depression at the coronary band and are termed *sinkers*. Horses with chronic laminitis develop characteristic concentric rings on the hooves as well as an abnormal shape of the hooves (Figure 29-51).

The main focus of treatment of horses with laminitis involves reducing inflammation and providing analgesia with antiinflammatory drugs (phenylbutazone), promoting digital blood flow with vasodilator drugs (acepromazine, isoxsuprine, topical glyceryl trinitrate), and mechanically supporting the distal phalanx by providing frog support

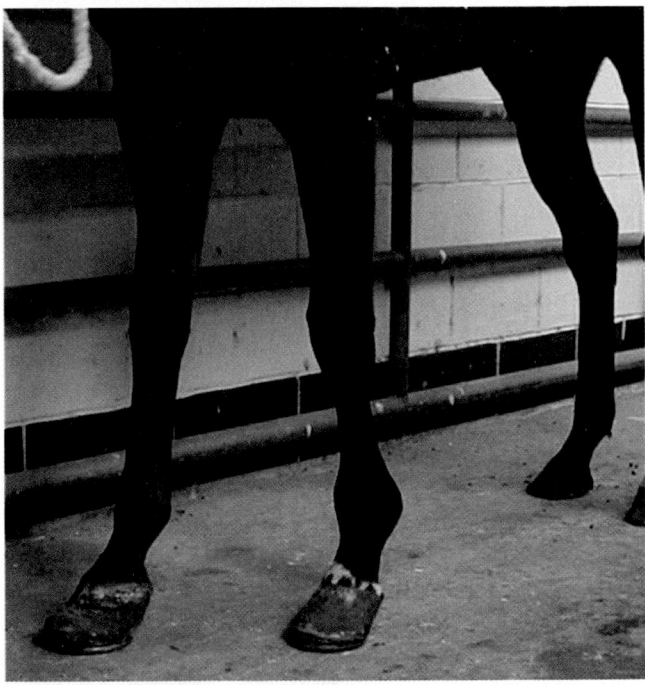

Figure 29-51 Abnormal hoof growth in a horse with chronic laminitis in both front feet.

(frog pads or heart bar shoes). Nursing care is also an important component of the therapeutic regimen, particularly in chronic laminitis. Because laminitis is extremely painful, horses often spend long periods of time lying down. This necessitates care of decubital ulcers. Preparing the stall bedding as described in the section Care of Hospitalized Patients in this chapter will aid in the prevention of pressure sores. In addition, they often develop subsolar abscesses that require daily soaking and bandaging. The prognosis for return of the horse to athletic competition depends on the occurrence and severity of rotation or sinkage of the coffin bone. Most horses that have appreciable rotation do not return to athletic function. The prognosis for horses that develop distal displacement of the coffin bone is poor.

Rhabdomyolysis (myositis, tying up, azoturia, Monday morning sickness) is an acute inflammatory disease of muscle. It can be initiated by exertion or by a change in either the diet or the amount of exercise. It is characterized by a stiff, stilted gait with firm or hard muscles. The most commonly affected muscles are those of the hind limb and back. Severely affected horses may be reluctant to move, and some may become recumbent and be unable to rise. Affected horses are often anxious, sweat excessively, and have elevated heart and respiratory rates and body temperature. Horses often have dark, discolored urine secondary to myoglobinuria. Confirmation of this disease is often based on increased serum muscle enzyme (creatine phosphokinase, aspartate aminotransferase) concentrations. Treatment involves exercise restriction, diet modification, intravenous fluid therapy, NSAIDs (phenylbutazone, flunixin meglumine), muscle relaxants, and tranquilization.

Bog spavin is a term used to describe the accumulation of synovial fluid (effusion) in the tarsocrural joint of the hock. Fluid can accumulate secondary to osteochondrosis, synovitis, and arthritis. Degenerative joint disease (arthritis) is a common performance-limiting condition of horses and can affect numerous joints. *Bone spavin* refers to arthritis in the distal intertarsal and tarsometatarsal joints of the hock. *High ring-bone* and *low ring-bone* refer to arthritis in the proximal interphalangeal (pastern) and distal interphalangeal (coffin) joints, respectively. *Osselet* is a term to describe arthritis in the metacarpophalangeal or metatarsophalangeal (fetlock) joint.

Tendinitis (bowed tendons) is an injury involving primarily the superficial digital flexor tendon and occasionally the deep digital flexor tendon of the front limbs. This injury is usually sustained secondary to racing or other strenuous activity. There are different degrees of tendinitis ranging from mild edema and inflammation to tendon fiber separation to tendon fiber tearing or disruption. When tendon fibers tear the result is hemorrhage and inflammatory debris accumulating in a cavity within the tendon, which is known as a *core lesion*. Treatment of tendinitis includes hydrotherapy, NSAIDs, support bandages, topical antiinflammatory agents (sweats, poultices), and exercise restriction or controlled exercise. Several surgical procedures have been used to either treat tendinitis or prevent its recurrence. The most commonly performed surgery is tendon splitting, which evacuates the core lesion and allows more rapid vascularization and healing of the area. The prognosis for return to athletic function depends on the severity of the injury; some horses with severe core lesions can return to athletic function if given appropriate treatment and time for convalescence.

Osteochondrosis is a form of developmental orthopedic disease in which the articular cartilage and underlying subchondral bone do not develop appropriately. This can result in the formation of osteochondritis dissecans (cartilage flaps), osteochondral fragments, cartilage erosion, and subchondral bone cysts. These abnormalities often manifest as joint effusion and lameness when young horses are first put into strenuous exercise. Many of these lesions are amenable to treatment via arthroscopy, resulting in the horse returning to athletic function.

Subsolar abscess is a common cause of severe lameness. Horses usually will not bear weight on the limb. There is palpable heat in the hoof and a bounding digital pulse similar to that in a horse with laminitis. However, the difference is that subsolar abscesses usually occur only in one foot. Pain can be localized by applying focal pressure to the sole of the foot with hoof testers. Occasionally, purulent debris will accumulate and migrate, and an area breaks open at the coronary band and drains (gravel). Treatment involves paring out the sole until the abscess is located to provide drainage. The foot should be kept bandaged to keep it dry and clean. The affected foot can be soaked daily in a solution of povidone-iodine (Betadine) and magnesium sulfate (Epsom salts) and then rebandaged. The horse should be given analgesics (phenylbutazone) for a few days. Appropriate tetanus prophylaxis should be administered. The foot needs to be protected from dirt and debris until the area fills in with granulation tissue and is covered with cornified tissue.

Septic arthritis is a common occurrence in adult horses secondary to iatrogenic inoculation of joints during arthrocentesis or joint surgery or subsequent to traumatic joint injuries. It occurs commonly in foals subsequent to hematogenous spread from a focus of infection, such as the umbilicus (navel ill), lungs (pneumonia), or intestinal tract (enteritis). The cornerstone of treatment of septic arthritis includes broad-spectrum antibiotics administered systemically, intraarticular antibiotics, NSAIDs, and joint drainage and lavage.

Horses frequently sustain severe musculoskeletal injuries, such as long-bone fractures or disruption of tendons or ligaments. These injuries often require stabilization with the use of bandages, splints, or casts before transport to a referral hospital. Successful stabilization of these injuries and safety of transport are important considerations in the outcome of these cases. Most severe injuries should be bandaged and splinted or casted to a level at least one joint above the injury. A heavy Robert Jones bandage should be applied and then rigid splints placed on the lateral and either the dorsal or palmar aspects of the limb to provide appropriate support. Splints can be made out of rigid materials, such as wood, steel, or aluminum. The splints should not be excessively heavy or bulky but must provide appropriate support. Horses with phalangeal fractures can be casted with their distal limb in flexion or can be placed in a commercially available device such as a Kimsey splint (Figure 29-52).

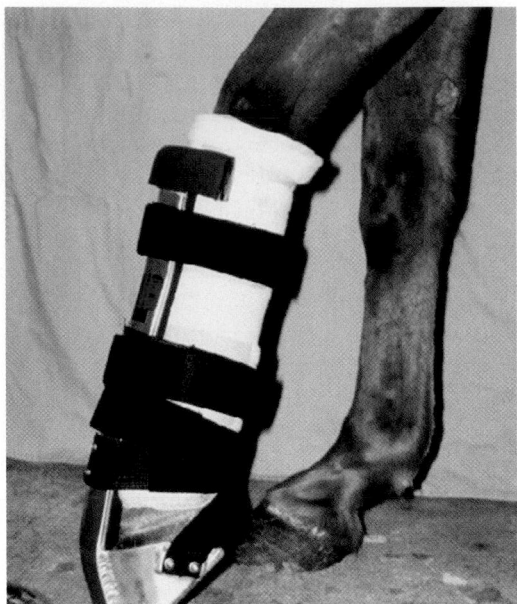

Figure 29-52 Use of Kimsey splint to stabilize fractures or joint subluxations in the lower limb of horses.

Horses with limb injuries should be hauled in a trailer with partitions to provide some support for them to balance themselves. The head should be tied loosely enough to enable the horse to use the head and neck for balance. Horses with front limb injuries should be transported with their head toward the rear of the trailer, and those with rear limb injuries should be transported with their head toward the front of the trailer.

SURGERY OF THE EQUINE PATIENT

PREOPERATIVE PREPARATION OF THE EQUINE PATIENT

Numerous procedures are required in preparation of the equine patient for anesthesia and surgery. Many if not all of these procedures involve the veterinary technician. It is probably wise that a checklist be developed that the technician can use to make sure all procedures are performed. This is particularly helpful in a hospital where more than one technician is working on the same case. Because of the dense hair coat of horses, thorough grooming is necessary. This may include simply brushing or currying the horse's coat, or it may require that the horse be bathed. The aim of grooming is to remove as much loose hair, dander, and dirt from the horse's body as possible, thereby keeping such material out of the operating room. If the horse is shod, the shoes are generally removed before surgery to prevent injury to the horse during recovery from anesthesia or damaging the recovery stall flooring. Some therapeutic shoes may not be removed to avoid damage to the hooves.

If the shoes must be left on, wrapping them with gauze and elastic tape will provide some protection from injury from the shoes during recovery. The horse's feet need to be picked out and cleaned. One of the main responsibilities of the technician will be to clip a wide area of hair in the vicinity of the surgery site before anesthetic induction. If the surgery will be performed on a limb, then the hair can be clipped the day before surgery and the limb can be cleaned and a bandage placed to keep the site clean. The final aseptic preparation is performed once the horse is under anesthesia. Clipping the hair and cleaning the surgery site before anesthetic induction will reduce anesthesia time.

> **✏ TECHNICIAN NOTE**
> A checklist should be developed to ensure that the technician performs all procedures required for preparation of the equine patient for anesthesia and surgery.

It is important that the technician consult the clinician as to the exact site that should be clipped. Areas of the mane and tail should be clipped only under special circumstances. Most owners are adamant that these areas should not be clipped for cosmetic purposes. The hair of the mane and tail takes months to years to grow out, and unnecessarily clipping these areas may cause needless delay in a show horse's convalescence. The location of the skin incision and the appropriate part of the horse to clip before surgery can usually be found in equine surgical textbooks. However, because of variation among surgeons, the technician should always consult the surgeon before clipping the patient.

Unlike ruminants and small animals, horses do not regurgitate or vomit. Adult horses are generally held off feed for approximately 12 hours to allow time for emptying of the stomach, which may allow the horse to ventilate more easily. Horses are generally provided water during this time. Young foals that are still nursing are generally not held off feed before anesthesia, but, if they are, it is usually only for 1 to 2 hours. A complete physical examination should be performed, including auscultation of the heart and lungs. In adult horses, a rebreathing bag may need to be used to increase the respiratory effort sufficiently to hear air moving through the lung fields. An electrocardiogram should be performed if there is any evidence of an abnormal heart rhythm detected during auscultation. Preoperative blood work usually includes a complete blood count (CBC) and fibrinogen determination. Some clinicians also perform a chemistry profile depending on the age and health of the horse.

Before general anesthesia, an intravenous catheter is placed in one of the jugular veins. The location of the catheter is important to provide access without compromise to the surgical site. The anesthetic agents for induction are administered through the catheter. Some anesthetic agents (thiobarbiturates) and perioperative medications (phenylbutazone) are irritating if injected perivascularly. Therefore it is imperative that the catheter be placed into the vein and appropriately secured. Catheter placement can be performed by the clinician or by the technician under the supervision of the clinician. Perioperative medications such as antibiotics and NSAIDs are usually administered before anesthetic induction. However, if an infectious process is suspected, then the surgeon may opt to start antibiotics after a sample has been obtained at surgery for culture and susceptibility testing. In this case, the medication can be administered during anesthesia or after recovery; this will depend on the medication and the condition of the patient while under anesthesia. Because horses are generally intubated with an endotracheal tube through the oral cavity, it is important that the mouth be thoroughly washed out before anesthetic induction; this will reduce the chance that feed material will be carried into the airway during intubation. Once the horse is intubated, the cuff should be inflated to prevent saliva and other materials from draining into the lower airway and leading to aspiration pneumonia.

INTRAOPERATIVE NURSING

The technician should consult the surgeon regarding which instruments will be required. In a hospital where there is more than one technician and several surgeons, a card system that has the necessary instruments listed for each surgical procedure should be used. This will allow the technician to know the different requirements of individual surgeons. One common difference among surgeons is the type of suture material chosen to close wounds. The technician must learn to adapt to these individual preferences. It is recommended that the technician have all the available instruments close to the surgery. Even if the instrument is used infrequently, it is better to have it nearby rather than waste time looking for it once it is needed. Time-wasting activities lead to prolonged anesthetic time, which could lead to increased morbidity or mortality. Correctly labeled radiographs are essential for most limb surgery. The radiographs should be placed on a radiographic view box in the operating room. The technician should have available gloves, gowns, and drapes and all other supplies that are anticipated to be used. In some lower limb surgeries, an Esmarch bandage (Latex Rubber Bandage/Tourner Wrap, Smiths & Nephew Richards) and tourniquet are used to assist with hemostasis during surgery. An Esmarch bandage is a flat, gum-rubber elastic bandage that is wrapped around the limb in a spiral fashion from distal to proximal to a point above the surgical site. At this point, an inflatable tourniquet is applied and secured. The aim of the Esmarch bandage is to force blood out of the limb, while the tourniquet prevents blood from entering into the site. The Esmarch bandage is removed after the tourniquet is fully inflated. The use of an Esmarch bandage and tourniquet enables the surgeon to operate in a bloodless field and results in a shorter surgery time. Following surgery, a pressure bandage is applied and the tourniquet is released.

TECHNICIAN NOTE

In a hospital where there is more than one technician and several surgeons, a card system that has the necessary instruments listed for each surgical procedure should be used.

The technician must help ensure that the patient is properly padded. Because of their body weight, horses are prone to myositis (muscle damage) that can be life threatening. The pressure of the horse's body and the hypotension that can occur during anesthesia can result in hypoperfusion of the muscles. If this condition is prolonged, the muscles can undergo metabolic change, resulting in extreme soreness and pain. In severe cases, muscle pigment (myoglobin) is released into the bloodstream and excreted in the urine (coffee-colored urine); the pigment can lead to kidney damage. The first sign that muscle damage has occurred during anesthesia is manifested during recovery. Usually the front or rear limb, or both, on the side the horse is lying on will be affected. However, the uppermost limb or any limb in a horse in dorsal recumbency can be involved. The horse may be unable to bear weight on the limb. If a forelimb is involved, the horse will drag the limb in a flexed position and will be unable to bear weight; this is associated with triceps damage. If the hind limb is involved, the horse may knuckle in the lower joints and walk on the dorsal aspect of the fetlock, and the limb will collapse as the horse tries to bear weight. Most horses show some improvement over the first few days, but some horses are unable to rise. Management of a postoperative recumbent patient presents a number of problems to clinicians and technicians. Appropriate padding materials are an inflatable waterbed, semi-inflated tire inner tubes under the shoulder and hip, dunnage bags, or foam rubber pads.

The patient and the surgery site must be positioned so that it is comfortable to the surgeon and safe for the patient. This will help ensure that the surgeon does not become fatigued or frustrated and a subsequent compromise in technique does not occur. It is not wise to overextend, overflex, abduct, or adduct the limbs because of potential complications of myopathy and neuropathy.

Aseptic preparation of the surgery site, surgical instruments, and the surgeon is imperative to a successful and uncomplicated surgery. It is the responsibility of all personnel involved to maintain asepsis, but the technician or technicians should assume primary responsibility for ensuring that the surgical site is properly prepared and the instruments are properly sterilized and packaged. The technician must be cognizant of all activities in preparation for surgery and during the surgical procedure. If a technician observes a break in aseptic technique it should be brought to the attention of the surgeon so that the problem can be remedied. The techniques involved in sterilization of surgical instruments and supplies and aseptic preparation of the surgery site are covered in Chapter 24.

POSTOPERATIVE NURSING

Technicians play a vital role in the postoperative care of the equine patient. Although veterinarians are responsible for the patients' care, technicians are often primarily involved with postoperative monitoring, administering medications, changing bandages, grooming, and other tasks required on postoperative patients. Monitoring the postoperative patient is similar to previously discussed patient monitoring. Although all body systems should be evaluated, the important things to consider in the postoperative patient are the presence and magnitude of postoperative pain, whether the patient is febrile, and whether there are any signs of infection (swelling, erythema, heat, pain) at the incision site. The postoperative patient should be examined for any complications such as pneumonia, diarrhea, jugular vein thrombophlebitis, or laminitis.

> ### ✎ TECHNICIAN NOTE
> Although veterinarians are responsible for the patients' care, technicians are often primarily involved with postoperative monitoring, administering medications, changing bandages, grooming, and other tasks required on postoperative patients.

Technicians are generally responsible for administering medications postoperatively. This may involve giving antibiotics or NSAIDs orally, intravenously, or intramuscularly. Many horses that undergo surgery have an intravenous catheter that is used in the postoperative period to administer perioperative antibiotics. The duration of antibiotic therapy depends on clinician preference and the type and severity of the underlying disease process. Many horses are administered NSAIDs in the postoperative period for their antiinflammatory and analgesic properties.

Horses undergoing limb surgery generally have a bandage placed on the limb at the conclusion of surgery before recovery from anesthesia. The limbs are often kept bandaged until the skin sutures are removed 10 to 14 days postoperatively. The bandages should probably be changed every 2 to 3 days initially or more frequently if they become wet or soiled from the outside or if wound drainage soaks through from the inside. There are several types of materials used for limb bandages in horses and several methods of application (see Chapter 4). In general, a sterile nonadherent material is usually placed directly against the incision and held in place with sterile, soft roll gauze (Kling, Johnson & Johnson). The next layer of the bandage is usually a sterile, soft combine that covers the circumference of the limb for the entire distance of the bandage, which is also held in place with soft roll gauze. This layer can be skipped if the outer bandage that is placed is a thick, sterile combine material. Next, a thick layer of rolled cotton, sheet cottons, or combine material is placed on the limb and secured with soft roll gauze. An Ace bandage, Elasticon (Johnson & Johnson), or Vetwrap (Animal Care Products/3M) can be used as the final layer of the bandage. Elasticon is useful for securing the top of the bandage to the skin above it and the bottom of the bandage to the foot below. This helps seal the bandage and prevent debris from getting between the skin and the bandage. All layers of the bandage should be applied in the same direction (dorsal to palmar or plantar) and with even tension; this should help prevent constriction of the tendons in the metacarpal or metatarsal area and subsequent tendinitis (bandage bow). When the bandages are changed postoperatively the incision should be examined for swelling, heat, exudate, and pain on palpation. The limb should be monitored for excessive swelling above and below the bandage. The exudate should be removed, the wound gently cleaned, and the bandage reapplied. If there has been an appreciable change in the horse's gait or in the incision from the last bandage change, this should be brought to the immediate attention of the veterinarian.

COLIC

Colic is a general term used to describe abdominal pain; many diseases can result in abdominal pain or signs that mimic abdominal pain. Diseases of the gastrointestinal tract are the most common causes of abdominal pain in horses. Because of the anatomy and physiology of the gastrointestinal tract and the fact that horses experience varying degrees of parasitic infestations (e.g., *Strongylus vulgaris*), they are more predisposed to colic than are most other animals. It is one of the most common and important diseases of horses and is one in which the veterinary technician plays a vital role in assisting in the diagnosis and both medical and surgical treatment. The technician is also intimately involved in the daily monitoring and treatment of horses with colic.

> ### ✎ TECHNICIAN NOTE
> *Colic* is a general term used to describe abdominal pain; many diseases can result in abdominal pain or signs that mimic abdominal pain.

The typical cause of colic in horses is an obstruction to flow of ingesta and gas in the gastrointestinal tract, causing intestinal distention, stretching of the intestinal wall, and tension on the mesentery, all of which lead to pain that is manifested in a variety of behavioral signs. Not all signs of abdominal pain are attributable to intestinal obstruction. For example, a mare that is near parturition will show similar signs owing to uterine contractions. A horse with an obstruction of the urinary tract (urethral calculus) may also show signs of abdominal pain. Although it is important that the veterinary technician recognize signs of colic, the diagnosis of the actual cause of colic is the responsibility of the veterinarian. Various signs of abdominal pain are often displayed by horses with different types and magnitudes of colic; however, certain signs are common to most. Mild signs of colic include inappetence, stretching more frequently than normal, yawning, and looking at the flank. Other signs include playing with water or frequent urination. More obvious signs of colic include pawing the ground, stamping the feet, walking the stall, kicking the abdomen, and violent rolling. Some horses will actually sit like a dog or roll into dorsal recumbency to relieve the pain. Horses with colic often sweat profusely, have increased heart and respiratory rates, and have congested mucous membranes.

The causes of gastrointestinal tract–related colic include volvulus (twisting of the intestine), intestinal incarceration, impactions of feed material or foreign bodies, obstruction caused by enteroliths (stones that form in the intestinal tract), parasitic infections, displacement of the intestine, tympany (primary gas distention), and inflammatory bowel disease (anterior enteritis, enterocolitis). Volvulus can occur in numerous portions of the intestinal tract, but it most commonly occurs in the small intestine and large colon. The small intestine frequently becomes incarcerated (entrapped) in numerous sites, such as the inguinal ring, epiploic foramen, mesenteric rent, and a diaphragmatic hernia. Intestinal incarceration and volvulus result in obstruction of the intestinal lumen and occlusion of the intestinal blood vessels resulting in intestinal distention and ischemic necrosis of the bowel wall. Therefore these horses display severe abdominal pain and usually develop signs of shock owing to absorption of endotoxin through devitalized bowel. These horses require emergency abdominal exploration with correction of the volvulus or reduction of the incarceration; depending on the duration and magnitude of the disease, the affected segment of intestine often requires resection. Because of the anatomy of the gastrointestinal tract, horses are predisposed to large intestinal displacement. Large colon displacement results in luminal obstruction but no vascular occlusion. Therefore these horses develop mild to severe abdominal pain depending on the magnitude of the luminal distention but do not develop intestinal ischemia. Treatment usually involves surgical correction. However, one particular type of large colon displacement (entrapment of the large colon in the nephrosplenic space) is sometimes correctable by rolling the horse under general anesthesia.

Horses develop impactions in the ileum, cecum, and large and small colon. Many of these horses can be treated medically with intravenous or oral fluids, lubricants (mineral oil), cathartics (magnesium sulfate), and analgesics. Other horses with intestinal impactions require surgery to evacuate the intestinal contents to prevent rupture. Intestinal contents are usually evacuated through an incision in the bowel wall (enterotomy), and the lumen is lavaged to remove as much of the contents as possible. The enterotomy incision is then sutured. Intestinal obstruction can occur secondary to an enterolith (stone) lodging in a segment of the large intestine that has a reduced diameter (pelvic flexure, transverse colon, small colon). Enterolithiasis results from mineral deposition that forms around a nidus within the intestinal tract. Sometimes horses pass numerous small-diameter stones

in the feces, whereas large-diameter stones may develop and obstruct the lumen; these large-diameter stones frequently cause abdominal pain secondary to luminal distention and require removal through an enterotomy. Horses can develop intestinal obstruction secondary to ingestion of foreign bodies; young curious horses are most commonly affected, and the most common type of foreign bodies is fibrous (nylon rope or string, hay netting, feed sacks, rubber fencing, hair). Occasionally a horse will be able to pass these fibrous foreign bodies, but often surgery is required to remove the foreign body and relieve the intestinal obstruction.

Although parasite-related causes of colic are less common now than in the past because of the development of effective anthelmintic drugs and management strategies, they still represent a possible cause of colic, especially on farms with poor preventive medicine programs. Larvae of *Strongylus vulgaris* (blood-sucking worms) migrate through the mesenteric arteries causing arteritis; this can lead to thromboembolic colic wherein segments of the intestine become infarcted. Ascarids (*Parascaris equorum*) usually cause a problem in young horses. The problem usually arises after deworming a heavily infested foal when a large number of adult ascarids die and obstruct the intestinal lumen (ascarid impaction). The best way to prevent this is to begin effective deworming programs early in the foal's life or to use a dewormer that is not especially effective in a heavily infested foal. Once the ascarid impaction occurs, the most effective treatment is evacuation of the worms via an enterotomy. Tapeworm (*Anoplocephala perfoliata*) infestation has been anecdotally related to cecocolic and ileocecal intussusception and to development of cecal impactions. These parasites are frequently identified in the cecal lumen in horses with these conditions, but no cause-and-effect relationship has been confirmed. The most effective treatment regimen for tapeworms is twice the recommended dose of pyrantel pamoate. Small strongyles are probably the most important intestinal parasite in horses because of their resistance to benzimidazole anthelmintics. Infestation with small strongyles can cause poor doeing, weight loss, diarrhea, and colic (see Chapter 7).

Horses with inflammatory bowel disease often have signs of abdominal pain, fever, increased heart and respiratory rates, congested mucous membranes, diarrhea, and nasogastric reflux. These horses are usually best treated with intravenous fluids, gastric decompression, and administration of intestinal protectants, antibiotics, analgesics, and antiinflammatory drugs.

The prognosis for horses with colic depends on the type of abnormality and its magnitude and duration. In general, horses with simple obstruction (no compromise in blood flow) of the intestinal tract (impaction, enterolith, displacement, tympany) have a good prognosis for survival with appropriate medical or surgical treatment. Horses with strangulating obstruction (compromised blood flow) of the intestinal tract (volvulus, incarceration, intussusception) have a more guarded prognosis, but some of these horses will survive and be functional if treated early and appropriately. The prognosis for horses with parasitic and inflammatory bowel diseases depends on the severity and duration before treatment and the development of life-threatening complications, such as laminitis.

The veterinarian will conduct a thorough examination and perform several diagnostic procedures in an attempt to arrive at an accurate diagnosis of the cause of colic. Most of these procedures will either directly or indirectly involve the veterinary technician. Such procedures include a rectal examination, nasogastric intubation, abdominocentesis and abdominal fluid analysis, collection of blood for CBC and chemistry profile, transabdominal ultrasonography, urinalysis, fecal flotation for intestinal parasites, and fecal cultures for *Salmonella*. The technician may be involved in organizing the instruments and supplies for performing these procedures or actually participate in the procedures.

The veterinary technician will be intricately involved in both medical and surgical treatment of horses with colic. Medical treatment is usually appropriate for impactions, tympany, and spasmodic colic, whereas surgical treatment is necessary for intestinal volvulus and incarceration, enterolithiasis, fibrous foreign body obstruction, and intestinal displacements. Fortunately, most horses with colic respond to conservative treatment, such as analgesic, anti-inflammatory, or antispasmodic drugs; intestinal lubricants or cathartics; intravenous or oral fluids; restriction of feed; and controlled exercise. Only a small percentage of horses with colic require surgery. Sometimes surgery is necessary to arrive at an accurate diagnosis. Abdominal surgery is a major undertaking and requires a full team to perform it in an effective and efficient manner.

ABDOMINAL SURGERY

Adult horses and foals frequently undergo abdominal surgery for gastrointestinal and urogenital tract disease. Although a flank incision in a standing, sedated horse is sometimes used for horses with colic or other abdominal disease, the most common approach to the abdominal cavity is through a ventral midline incision with the horse under general anesthesia and positioned in dorsal recumbency (Figure 29-53). Because most horses with colic requiring surgery will be operated on with the patient under general anesthesia, the veterinary technician will be involved in the preparation of the horse for surgery. This will include placing a catheter, administering perioperative medications, passing a nasogastric tube, washing out the mouth, clipping the hair, preparing the anesthetics, aseptically preparing the incision site, and opening surgical packs at the time of surgery. Most colic patients can be clipped before anesthesia, but if the horse is in severe pain, it may be done after anesthetic induction for the safety of the horse and personnel. The hair should be clipped from rostral to the xiphoid area to the udder or preputial area and to the flank folds on either side; clipped hair and other debris can be removed

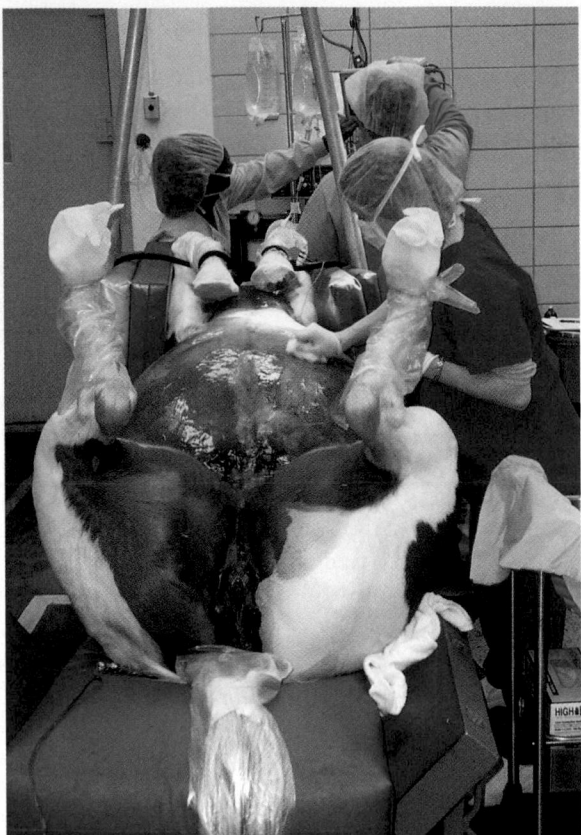

Figure 29-53 Preparation of the ventral abdominal area for abdominal surgery in a horse with colic that is under general anesthesia and positioned in dorsal recumbency.

with a vacuum. The incision site (ventral midline) may be shaved to remove the hair remaining after clipping, and the clipped area is then aseptically prepared. The incision is draped with four small drapes or towels, and then a large, water-impermeable drape is placed that covers the entire horse. The incision is usually made from the umbilicus rostrally toward the xiphoid until the necessary exposure is achieved, but the incision can be extended caudal to the umbilicus. This is particularly necessary for urogenital tract surgery, such as a cystotomy for removal of cystic calculi. Once the incision is made, a thorough exploration is usually performed depending on the reason for surgery. Once the abnormality is identified it is corrected. Suction is often necessary to decompress gas from the gastrointestinal tract or aspirate fluid such as urine from the bladder during a cystotomy.

✐ TECHNICIAN NOTE

The most common approach to the abdominal cavity is through a ventral midline incision with the horse under general anesthesia and positioned in dorsal recumbency.

There are numerous surgical techniques and manipulations that the veterinarian may perform at the time of abdominal surgery. They are too numerous to describe here, and the veterinary technician will become familiar with them through instruction and experience. Many specialized instruments are required for abdominal surgery (see Chapter 24). One group of instruments that has become increasingly popular with veterinary surgeons for use in equine abdominal surgery is gastrointestinal stapling equipment. The technician must become familiar with the different instruments and cartridges. Intestinal resection and anastomosis often require specialized instruments and supplies.

Once the cause of colic or other abdominal problem has been corrected and the horse has recovered from anesthesia, the veterinary technician becomes even more closely involved with patient management. Horses usually require administration of intravenous fluids, antibiotics, antiinflammatory drugs, and other medications in the postoperative period. The veterinary technician usually administers or oversees administration of these medications. The technician may also be involved in nasogastric intubation, blood collection, intravenous catheterization, and changing bandages. In addition, the technician will often be responsible for feeding and watering, exercising, grooming, and monitoring the horse.

ARTHROSCOPIC SURGERY

Arthroscopy is commonly performed for the diagnosis and treatment of joint disease. It is commonly performed for removing osteochondral chip fractures, treating cartilaginous and bony abnormalities associated with osteochondrosis, treating septic arthritis, and evaluating causes of joint lameness that have no definitive radiographic abnormalities. Depending on the joint being evaluated and the type and location of the lesion, the horse may be positioned in dorsal or lateral recumbency. It is necessary to have the radiographs on a view box in the operating room so that the surgeon can evaluate them intraoperatively. During arthroscopy the technique of triangulation is used whereby the lesion forms one corner of the triangle and the arthroscope and surgical instruments serve as the other two corners of the triangle. Generally the arthroscope is placed in the joint on the side opposite the lesion, and the surgical instrument is placed in the joint on the same side as the lesion. The portal for placement of the arthroscope is usually made by making a small (1-cm) incision in the skin and subcutaneous tissue and then using a sharp trocar to advance the arthroscopic cannula through the fibrous joint capsule and synovial lining. Once the cannula has penetrated the joint cavity, the sharp trocar is replaced with a blunt obturator to pass the cannula across the joint; this prevents iatrogenic damage to the cartilage. The skin incisions are usually made before joint distention in the carpus but after joint distention in other joints. The joint is distended with sterile polyionic fluid to facilitate placement of the arthroscope. Once the arthroscope is in place, the joint is evaluated; once the lesion is identified, the most appropriate location for the instru-

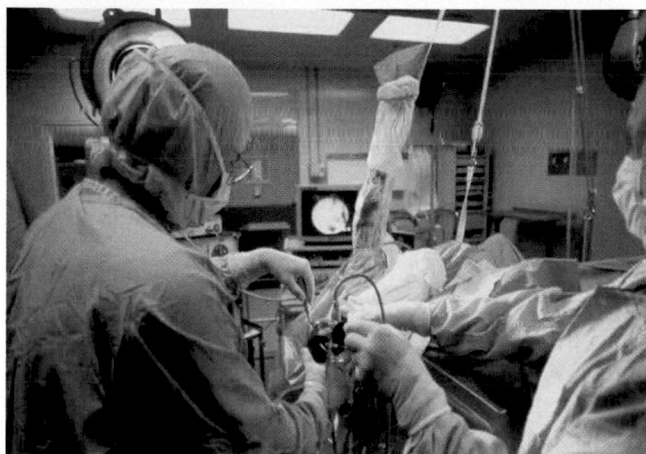

Figure 29-54 Use of arthroscopy for evaluating joint disease in horses. The arthroscope is inserted into the joint and attached to a camera that projects the image on a television screen for easy viewing by the surgeon and other personnel.

ment portal is determined by using a needle to triangulate the lesion with the arthroscope. Once the appropriate location for the instrument portal is identified, the instrument portal is made with a scalpel blade (no. 11 or 15). The appropriate instrument is placed into the joint. The instruments commonly used in arthroscopy include a blunt probe for palpating intraarticular structures, rongeurs for removing osteochondral fragments, and curettes for debriding diseased cartilage and bone. A fenestrated cannula is often used at the end of surgery to facilitate removal of cartilage and bone debris via lavage. Motorized equipment is available and is sometimes necessary for debridement of large areas of diseased bone.

The surgeon uses specific instruments for arthroscopy, and these may vary depending on the joint involved and the individual surgeon's preference. Generally there will be a standardized set of arthroscopy instruments that are packaged together. Instruments are steam sterilized, but if they are to be used on more than one case per day, they are sterilized with a cold sterilization solution before each use. Following sterilization, the instruments are packed in a sterile stainless steel pan that is later used to rinse disinfecting solution off the arthroscopy instruments. One of the most important and most expensive instruments is the arthroscope; it should be handled carefully to prevent damage. Additional items necessary are a sterile needle (usually 18-gauge) and syringe, which are used for distending the joint. During arthroscopic surgery, the joint is kept distended with sterile physiologic solution; this solution is usually delivered with a pump through a sterile intravenous set.

Many hospitals perform arthroscopy using a video camera so that the entire procedure can be viewed on a television screen (Figure 29-54). This causes less strain on the surgeon's eye, makes the procedure more educational for surgery assistants and technical staff, provides an opportunity to videotape the procedure, and probably allows the procedure to be performed with fewer breaks in aseptic technique. To provide the intense light required to illuminate the inside of the joint, a fiber-optic light source and light cable are required. It is essential that the technician be familiar with the assembly and function of the arthroscopic equipment and the proper care, cleaning, and disinfecting of the instruments. The arthroscopy instruments are disinfected using a cold sterilization solution such as activated dialdehyde (Cidex, Surgikos); the instruments, arthroscope, and light cables are soaked for a minimum of 10 minutes. One should read the manufacturer's recommendations regarding the time required for disinfecting. To avoid delays, the instruments can be placed in the sterilizing solution at the start of anesthesia. This will also ensure adequate sterilization time. Before using the instruments, they are transferred sterilely into an empty sterile tray. The instruments are then rinsed with sterile saline to remove the sterilization solution.

After the surgical site has been aseptically prepared and draped and the instruments removed from the sterilizing solution, the technician will be responsible for attaching the fiber-optic cable to its light source. The system that delivers the fluid to distend the joint must also be connected to the appropriate fluid source. Once the system is connected to the fluid source, the surgeon must run fluid through the system to flush all air bubbles out of the tubing so that they do not enter the joint. Electric fluid pumps are generally used to maintain joint distention; these may be manually or pressure controlled.

Following surgery, all specialized arthroscopy equipment and instruments need to be cleaned. The arthroscope lens should be examined for scratches, and the video camera should be dried carefully. If several arthroscopy surgeries are scheduled for the day, then the instruments are placed in the cold sterilization solution in preparation for the next surgery.

ORTHOPEDIC SURGERY

Orthopedic surgery has become more common in horses. Athletic horses develop numerous orthopedic conditions that are amenable to surgical correction. Historically, fractures of long bones in adult horses were considered irreparable. However, with advanced techniques and more rigid surgical implants many of these injuries are potentially correctable. Certain bony fractures are amenable to surgical correction using bone screws that are placed in lag fashion to stabilize the fracture by creating compression of the bone fragments (Figure 29-55). Although developing an understanding of the principles of lag screw fixation and the instrumentation involved will help the equine technician in preparing instruments and assisting with surgery, this area is beyond the scope of this book. Major fractures of long bones in horses are best repaired with screws and bone plates to prevent movement at the fracture site while the

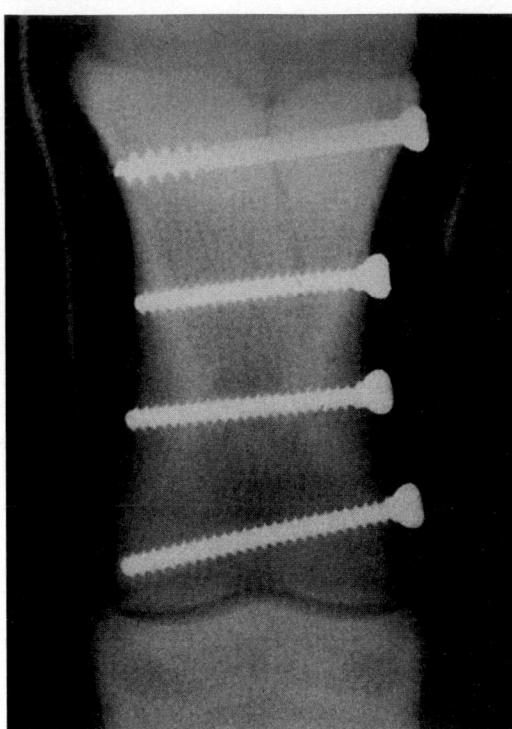

Figure 29-55 A proximal phalanx fracture in a horse repaired with cortical bone screws placed in lag fashion to compress the fracture line.

bone heals under rigid fixation. Although aseptic technique is imperative for all surgical procedures, it is especially crucial to the overall success of orthopedic surgery in horses. If bony infection develops, it can lead to instability of the implants and fixation failure, which often necessitates euthanasia. It is the responsibility of all personnel to follow aseptic protocol. The technician should strive to maintain asepsis by monitoring the activities of all personnel involved in surgery. Orthopedic surgery requires the use of several specialized instruments and implants; because many of these surgeries are performed on an emergency basis, it is imperative that the technician make sure instruments are available and ready for use. Many orthopedic injuries that are surgically repaired require the use of external coaptation (cast) for anesthetic recovery or for longer periods postoperatively (see Chapter 4). Therefore the technician should anticipate this need and have the appropriate materials available at the conclusion of surgery. The technician may also be needed to assist with anesthetic recovery of the orthopedic equine patient.

Postoperative monitoring of the orthopedic patient is vital for early detection of potential problems. It is particularly important to observe how the horse is using the affected limb in the stall; any dramatic change in use of the limb may signal an impending problem (infection or cast sores). The cast should also be monitored for heat, odor, or exudate, which would indicate the development of cast sores. The most common locations for sores to develop in association with a half-limb cast are at the proximal, dorsal aspect of the metacarpus or metatarsus, at the palmar or plantar aspect of the fetlock over the sesamoid bones, and over the heel bulbs. Bandages need to be changed frequently, and the incision sites should be monitored for swelling, erythema, and discharge. Drains are commonly used in orthopedic surgery following repair of a long bone. Drains can be useful in preventing seroma formation, but they can serve as potential routes for inoculation of the surgery site. Therefore it is important to maintain these drains sterile by keeping a clean, sterile bandage on the leg. This may require changing the bandage more frequently than once daily.

> ✎ **TECHNICIAN NOTE**
>
> Postoperative monitoring of the orthopedic patient is vital for early detection of potential problems. It is particularly important to observe how the horse is using the affected limb in the stall; any dramatic change in use of the limb may signal an impending problem (infection or cast sores).

UPPER RESPIRATORY TRACT SURGERY

Abnormalities of the upper respiratory tract can be performance limiting to athletic horses and, if severe, can also be life threatening. Many obstructive diseases of the upper respiratory tract are amenable to surgical correction. The most common of these are left laryngeal hemiplegia, epiglottic entrapment, dorsal displacement of the soft palate, and arytenoid chondritis. Others are subepiglottic cysts, guttural pouch empyema, guttural pouch tympany, and guttural pouch mycosis.

Left laryngeal hemiplegia ("roarer") is a condition resulting in paralysis of the left arytenoid cartilage, which prevents it from being abducted during inspiration. This results in the arytenoid collapsing and being pulled into the airway secondary to the negative pressure that is generated during inspiration. The cause of this condition is unknown, but it results in a recurrent laryngeal neuropathy. Because this nerve normally provides innervation to the major abductor muscle of the arytenoid cartilage, the cricoarytaenoideus dorsalis, a neuropathy results in muscle atrophy and an inability to abduct the arytenoid. As the name implies, this condition occurs almost exclusively on the left side (95%); it is believed that this is related to the longer length of the nerve on the left side and the fact that it may become damaged from the vibrations as it courses around the aortic arch. This condition is diagnosed using endoscopy at rest or during exercise on a high-speed treadmill; the left arytenoid cartilage is not fully abducted during inspiration and in severe cases actually collapses into the airway. Horses with this condition make a characteristic inspiratory noise (roaring) and develop exercise intolerance. Surgical treatment is a prosthetic laryngoplasty, which involves placing a suture between the cricoid cartilage and the muscular process of the arytenoid cartilage to mimic the action of

the cricoarytaenoideus dorsalis and abduct the arytenoid cartilage (tieback). The laryngeal ventricles (saccules) are also everted and resected (ventriculectomy or sacculectomy) through either a ventral laryngotomy or by use of an endoscopically guided laser. Approximately 70% of horses treated with a prosthetic laryngoplasty and sacculectomy return to athletic function. Most horses will continue to make some noise, and in some the noise may not improve. The laryngotomy incision is usually left open to heal by second intention. This requires daily cleaning with gauze sponges with saline or water followed by application of petrolatum to the skin around the incision and on the mandible and neck to prevent skin scald from the drainage. It usually takes approximately 3 weeks for the incision to heal. Some clinicians partially close the incision, which reportedly shortens the time required to heal.

> ✎ **TECHNICIAN NOTE**
>
> Left laryngeal hemiplegia ("roarer") is a condition resulting in paralysis of the left arytenoid cartilage, which prevents it from being abducted during inspiration.

Epiglottic entrapment is a condition where the aryepiglottic membrane that extends from the arytenoid cartilage to the ventral surface of the epiglottis hypertrophies and rolls upward to envelope the rostral and abaxial portions of the epiglottis. Normally the epiglottis should have a serrated edge and a distinct vascular pattern present on the dorsal surface. When the epiglottis becomes entrapped, the serrated edge and vascular pattern can no longer be seen. The shape or outline of the epiglottis can still be observed (unlike that seen with a dorsal displacement of the soft palate), but the tip appears more rounded and the abaxial surface is smooth rather than serrated. In more chronic cases, the tip of the epiglottis may become ulcerated. The cause of epiglottic entrapment is unknown, but it is believed these horses have an instability between the caudal edge of the soft palate and the epiglottis and that the aryepiglottic membrane hypertrophies and makes the epiglottis more rigid. Epiglottic entrapment can be intermittent or permanent. Some horses can continue to perform athletically with an entrapped epiglottis, but it does appear to affect performance in most horses. Treatment of epiglottic entrapment includes transecting the aryepiglottic membrane to release the epiglottis. This can be done using several techniques. First, it can be performed with a hooked bistoury placed through the nasal passages in a standing sedated horse with or without endoscopic guidance; care must be taken to prevent trauma to other structures and to prevent laceration of the soft palate. Second, it can be performed in an anesthetized horse with a mouth speculum by manually guiding a hooked bistoury and transecting the membrane on midline. Third, it can be performed using an endoscopically guided laser in a standing sedated horse. Finally, in more severe or chronic recurring cases the aryepiglottic membrane can be resected through a ventral laryngotomy. The prognosis for return to athletic performance is good, but entrapment can recur. Some of these horses may develop dorsal displacement of the soft palate after the entrapment is released. Horses that have the entrapment released using the hooked bistoury or laser can generally resume training in a few days, whereas those treated via resection through a laryngotomy require approximately 3 weeks before resuming training.

Dorsal displacement of the soft palate (DDSP) is generally a dynamic obstructive disease of the upper respiratory tract that occurs during exercise. Normally the soft palate remains ventral to the epiglottis. However, if the epiglottis is small or flaccid or the caudal edge of the soft palate is flaccid, the soft palate can become displaced dorsal to the epiglottis during strenuous exercise. The cause of this condition is unknown, but it is believed the factors listed above predispose the palate to become displaced during inspiration when negative pressure is generated in the upper airway. This condition usually is intermittent, occurring during strenuous exercise and dissipating once exercise has stopped and the horse swallows. Because horses are obligate nasal breathers, dorsal displacement of the soft palate interferes with the horse's breathing. Horses with DDSP usually make a characteristic gurgling or snoring type of noise, which will dissipate as soon as they swallow and replace the palate into its normal position.

Treatment options for a horse with DDSP include placing a cloth or leather tie on the horse's tongue and pulling the tongue rostrad and tying the tongue to the mandible in the interdental space. The epiglottis, tongue, and sternothyrohyoideus muscles are attached to the hyoid apparatus. Because the tongue is attached at the rostral aspect of the hyoid apparatus and the sternothyrohyoideus muscles are attached at its caudal aspect, a tongue tie prevents caudal retraction of the hyoid apparatus, including the epiglottis. This seems to help approximately 50% of horses with DDSP because it prevents caudal retraction of the epiglottis and maintains normal epiglottic-palate alignment. Because of its noninvasive nature, the tongue tie is generally the first thing attempted in horses with DDSP. If this does not work, a section of the sternothyrohyoideus muscles can be resected in the midcervical region; this also prevents caudal retraction of the hyoid apparatus. This myectomy procedure helps in approximately 50% of horses with DDSP that fail to respond to a tongue tie. If this procedure does not work, then the caudal margin of the soft palate can be resected (staphylectomy). There are two theories as to why this may help prevent DDSP. First, it is believed the caudal edge of the palate becomes more fibrous as it heals with scar tissue; this makes the caudal edge more rigid and therefore more resistant to displacement. The other theory is that, if the palate does displace, then it enables the palate to be replaced more easily. Regardless of the mechanism it seems that it helps prevent DDSP in approximately half of the horses that do not respond to the tongue tie or myectomy.

Arytenoid chondritis is an inflammatory, degenerative condition of the arytenoid cartilages resulting in a proliferative mass on one or both arytenoids. This usually results in an obstructive disease of the upper airway with signs similar to the conditions described earlier. These cartilages are usually enlarged and more fibrous than normal, which prevents them from being effectively treated with a tieback. The treatment of choice is to remove the affected arytenoid cartilage through a ventral laryngotomy. Because of the time required for dissection in the laryngeal region during an arytenoidectomy, a tracheotomy is usually performed in the middle or proximal trachea to provide a mechanism for ventilation during anesthesia. The tracheotomy can be performed either before anesthetic induction or once the horse is anesthetized. These horses are prone to upper airway obstruction postoperatively and need to be closely monitored. The tracheotomy tube is usually left in place, at least for a couple of days, until it is believed the horse has an airway of adequate diameter for breathing. It is imperative that these horses be monitored closely while the tracheotomy tube is in place to make sure it does not become dislodged or obstructed with mucus or other discharge. The laryngotomy and tracheotomy sites require daily cleaning and application of petrolatum on the skin around the incisions. Both these incisions will heal by second intention in approximately 3 weeks.

Bacterial infection of the guttural pouch (empyema) usually is a sequela to strangles or retropharyngeal lymph node abscesses. Clinical signs include swelling in the throatlatch region and a bilateral mucopurulent nasal discharge. Horses with guttural pouch empyema can be treated conservatively with antibiotics and guttural pouch lavage; this may be effective in many horses that are treated early in the course of the disease. However, in more chronic cases the mucopurulent material becomes inspissated and forms gelatinous concretions (chondroids) that lie in the floor of the guttural pouches. Resolution of empyema requires removal of the chondroids, and long-term effective drainage can usually only be achieved with surgical drainage. Several approaches are reported for surgical drainage of the guttural pouches, but the most common surgical approach for guttural pouch empyema is the modified Whitehouse technique; the incision is made in the skin on the ventrum of the throat region just axial to the linguofacial vein and is followed by blunt dissection into the pouch. The guttural pouch is lavaged intraoperatively. Indwelling catheters can be placed into the guttural pouches in standing sedated horses under endoscopic guidance; these catheters enable frequent lavage of the pouches. The guttural pouches should not be lavaged with irritating solutions because of the proximity of blood vessels and nerves coursing through the area. The incision is managed similarly to a laryngotomy or tracheotomy incision.

Guttural pouch tympany is an accumulation of air in the guttural pouches; this occurs in foals and weanlings and is usually associated with an abnormality of the opening to the pouches. It can occur on one or both sides and is characterized by a fluctuant nonpainful swelling in the throat-latch region. If unilateral guttural pouch tympany is present, then it is usually treated by surgically creating an opening in the septum between the left and right pouches; this is usually approached through an incision in Viborg's triangle on the affected side. If bilateral tympany is present, then creating an opening in the septum will not effectively drain the two sides. Therefore the opening to one or both of the guttural pouches is surgically revised through a Viborg's triangle approach. Surgical revision of the guttural pouch opening may be performed on only one side with creation of an opening in the septum to enable both pouches to evacuate the air through one opening.

Guttural pouch mycosis can be life threatening. Fungal plaques form in the lining of the guttural pouches; if the plaques involve vascular structures such as the internal carotid artery, then severe fatal hemorrhage can occur. Fatal hemorrhage is often preceded by several episodes of substantial epistaxis. However, once the diagnosis is made, surgery should not be delayed. The most accepted method of surgical treatment involves either direct ligation or use of a balloon-tipped catheter to occlude either the internal carotid artery, external carotid artery, or both depending on which vessels are affected. Both the internal and external carotid arteries can be ligated unilaterally with no untoward effects. The major potential complication of external carotid artery occlusion is blindness. Once the affected vessels are ligated, the fungal infection is treated by lavage of the guttural pouches and instillation of antifungal medication into the pouch via indwelling catheters or via the endoscope.

SURGICAL MUSCULOSKELETAL DISEASES

Flexural and angular limb deformities (crooked legs) are abnormalities of the limbs that arise from abnormal development of bones and musculotendinous structures in the limbs. Flexural limb deformities result in overflexion of certain joints. There are three main manifestations of flexural limb deformities in horses. These can be present at birth or develop during the first few months or years of life. Carpal flexural deformities result in the front limbs being flexed or buckled forward at the carpus. This may range from mild deformity to a severe deformity that prevents the foal from standing. Mild to moderate cases are often amenable to treatment with controlled exercise combined with application of bandages and splints that extend from the ground to the elbow or tube casts that extend from just above the fetlock to the middle portion of the antebrachium. Intravenous administration of oxytetracycline may be beneficial to help relax the musculotendinous structures.

The second type involves flexural deformity of the distal interphalangeal (coffin) joint, which results in a characteristic clubfoot-shaped hoof (Figure 29-56). This often is first noticed when the foal is a few months of age and can progress to the point that the foal walks on the toe or the

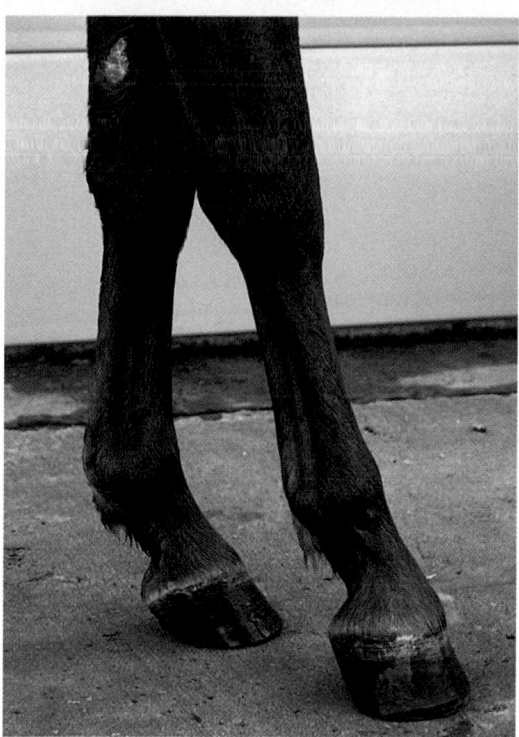

Figure 29-56 Flexural deformity of the distal interphalangeal (coffin) joint of the right front limb in a horse.

dorsum of the hoof wall. Mild to moderate cases (those in which the foot has not passed the vertical plane) often respond to corrective trimming (lower heel) and application of an extended toe shoe, which helps to stretch out the deep digital flexor tendon. More advanced cases usually require surgical transection of the inferior check ligament, which lengthens the deep digital flexor musculotendinous unit.

The third type of flexural deformity involves the metacarpophalangeal joint and is characterized by an increased steepness to the pastern and fetlock (Figure 29-57). This usually begins to develop around 1 year of age but may occur as late as 2 years. It can progress until the horse knuckles over at the fetlock. This condition commonly occurs in rapidly growing heavily muscled horses such as 1- to 2-year-old quarter horses. Conservative treatment involves controlled exercise, dietary management (balanced minerals, low energy and protein), management of pain (arising from osteochondrosis or physitis) with NSAIDs, and application of bandages and splints that extend from the ground to the elbow. More severely affected horses or those that do not respond to conservative treatment may be successfully treated surgically by performing a superior check or inferior check ligament desmotomy or both, depending on whether the superficial digital flexor or deep digital flexor tendons or both are involved.

Angular limb deformities are deformities that develop in the appendicular skeleton in a medial-to-lateral direction. These deviations can be present at birth or develop during the first few months of life. Mild deformities may self-correct,

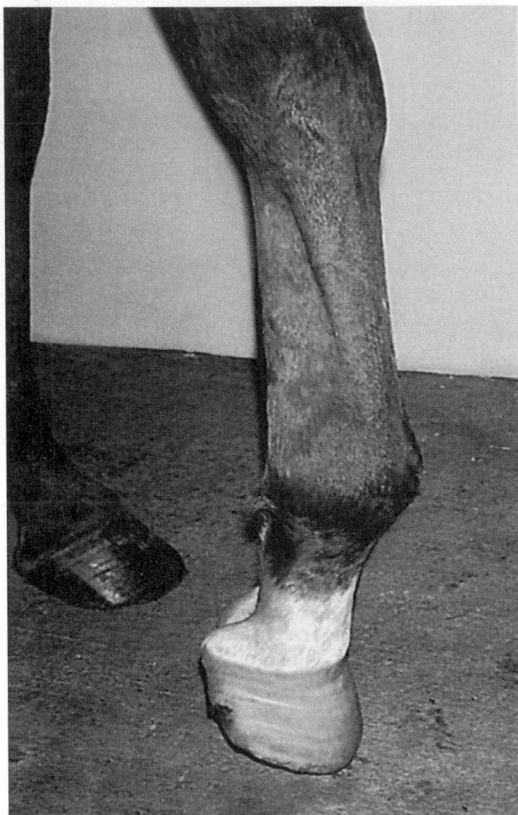

Figure 29-57 A flexural deformity of the metacarpophalangeal (fetlock) and the carpal (knee) joints in a yearling horse.

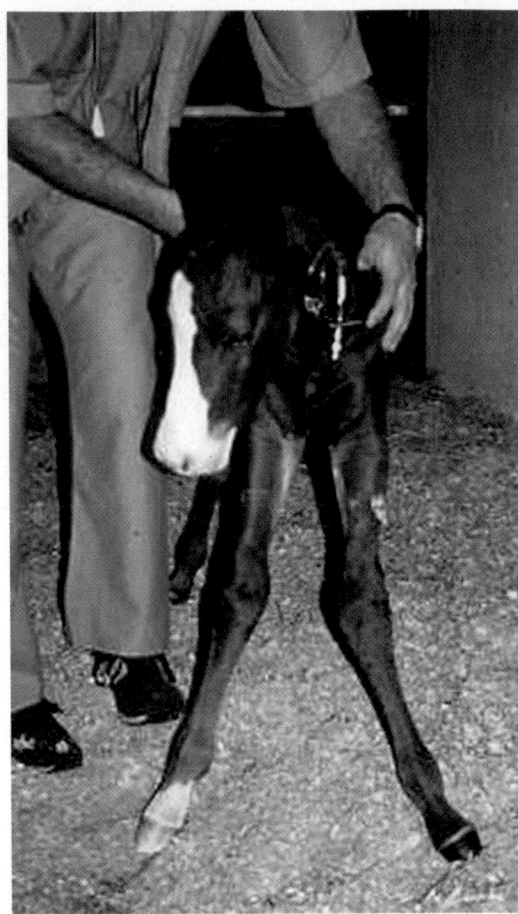

Figure 29-58 Bilateral carpal valgus deformity in a foal. It is more severe in the left front leg.

others may persist but not worsen, and still others may become more severe with time. These deformities are named in reference to the joint involved and the direction of the deviation. The most common deviation is carpal valgus, where the limb distal to the carpus deviates laterally (Figure 29-58). Other common deviations include fetlock varus, where the limb distal to the fetlock deviates medially (Figures 29-57 and 29-59), and tarsal valgus. These deviations can occur because of disproportionate growth of bone on either side of the growth plate, incompletely ossified cuboidal bones in the carpus and tarsus, or ligamentous laxity. The deviations in foals with incompletely ossified cuboidal bones or ligamentous laxity can usually be manually straightened, whereas those with disproportionate growth at the physis cannot.

Treatment of mild to moderate angular deviations may include stall rest with controlled exercise, depending on the age of the foal. Successful surgical procedures have been developed to treat moderate to severe deformities. Transection and elevation of the periosteum near the affected growth plate on the concave (short) side of the limb will stimulate more rapid bone growth, which usually leads to correction of the disproportionate growth. Periosteal transection and elevation can be repeated in 4 to 6 weeks if the deformity has not been completely corrected. The deformities do not overcorrect with this procedure. In more

severe deformities or in older foals with less growth potential, the growth on the convex (or long) side of the bone can be slowed by performing transphyseal bridging. This is usually performed by placing a screw on either side of the growth plate and then tightening a figure-of-eight wire around the screw-heads to provide compression of the growth plate. Use of transphyseal bridging can lead to correction of more severe deformities, but it is imperative that these implants be removed at the correct time to prevent overcorrection leading to the opposite type of deformity. Foals with deviations of the carpus or tarsus subsequent to ligamentous laxity or incompletely ossified cuboidal bones are best treated with stall rest with controlled exercise combined with application of full-limb bandages and splints or tube casts extending from the distal cannon bone to the proximal radius or tibia.

EMERGENCY SITUATIONS AND PROCEDURES

Several emergency situations can arise that necessitate immediate action on the part of a technician or clinician to

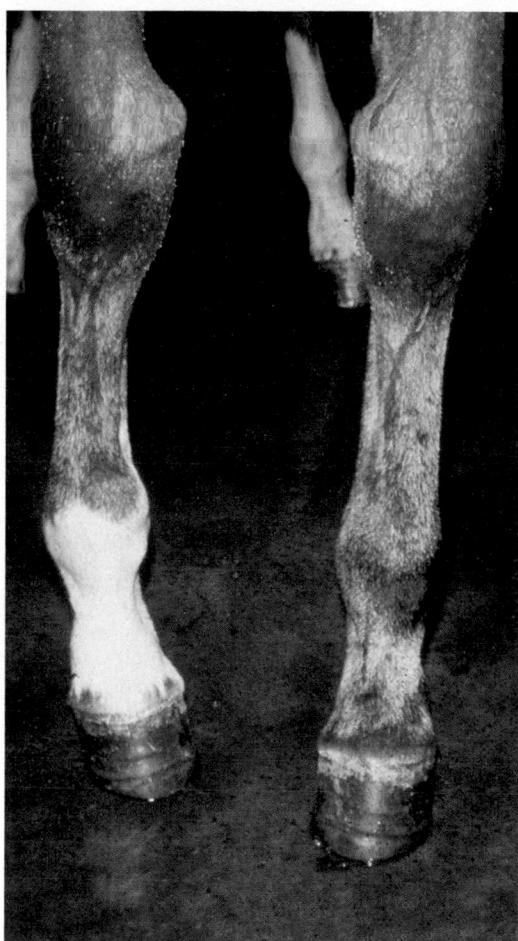

Figure 29-59 A valgus deformity of the right carpus and a varus deformity of the left carpus in a foal.

prevent death of a horse. One of the most common emergency situations is the development of upper airway obstruction leading to dyspnea. Obstructive diseases involving the nasal passages, nasopharynx, and larynx can be alleviated by a tracheotomy. A tracheotomy is generally performed at the junction of the middle and proximal thirds of the neck on the ventral midline. An incision is made on the ventral cervical midline through the skin, subcutaneous tissue, and cutaneous colli muscle parallel to the trachea. The paired sternothyrohyoideus muscles are then split on midline to expose the tracheal rings. The membrane between two adjacent rings is then cut with a scalpel on the ventral surface for a distance of approximately one half the circumference of the tracheal rings. Care should be taken not to cut the tracheal rings and not to cut vital structures adjacent to the trachea (carotid artery, recurrent laryngeal nerve, jugular vein). Many times the tracheotomy must be performed on an extremely anxious horse or after the horse has collapsed from insufficient oxygen. Therefore one should be careful not to get into a situation where injury occurs.

Veterinary technicians should become familiar and comfortable with the dosages and indications for drugs commonly used in emergency situations. A list of drugs and doses along with the drugs and syringes should be kept readily available in several locations throughout the hospital. These can be prepared in small emergency packs.

Occasionally horses develop reactions to certain drugs. These may be anaphylactic reactions resulting in shock or death or allergic-type reactions resulting in skin wheals. Horses may develop a reaction to procaine penicillin, which usually results in an anaphylactoid reaction. These horses usually require treatment with corticosteroids and epinephrine. They may recover or die subsequent to pulmonary edema. Horses often develop skin wheals in response to drugs or environmental allergens (Figure 29-37, *A* and *B*). The drugs that most commonly cause these wheals in horses are NSAIDs and trimethoprim-sulfa antibiotics.

Intracarotid injection of drugs can cause seizurelike activity. This can be life threatening to the horse and is potentially injurious to the handler and other personnel in the vicinity. The chance for this can be minimized by using an 18-gauge needle that is unattached from the syringe and directed down the jugular vein. Normally, if the needle is in the jugular vein, blood will slowly ooze out of the needle hub only if the jugular vein is occluded. If the carotid artery is inadvertently entered with the needle, then blood will exit in a pulsatile manner. If this occurs, do not inject the medication. The needle should be removed, and compression should be applied to decrease hematoma formation. The needle should be reinserted into a different location using the same technique.

ANESTHESIA FOR THE EQUINE PATIENT

The veterinary technician may be directly or indirectly involved in anesthesia of horses. Frequently the technician is primarily responsible for all aspects of anesthesia, including selection of induction and maintenance anesthetic agents, instrumentation, monitoring, and recovery of patients. It is important that the technician be familiar with the properties and recommended doses of the anesthetic agents being administered and the equipment (ventilator, blood pressure monitor, anesthetic machine, etc.) being used (see Chapter 19). Numerous complications can arise, and it is important that the technician be familiar with the methods of treating these complications, including the correct drugs and doses for treating hypotension and cardiac arrhythmias. Because it is important to maintain mean arterial blood pressure at 70 mm Hg or greater to help prevent myopathies and neuropathies, blood pressure should be monitored via an indirect or direct method. Hypotension is usually treated by decreasing the depth of anesthesia, increasing the rate of administration of intravenous fluids, and administration of vasoactive drugs, such as dobutamine, dopamine, or phenylephrine. It is important to monitor how well the horse is being oxygenated and ventilated during anesthesia; this can be done most effectively by monitoring arterial blood gases. The technician should monitor recovery from anesthesia and be prepared for any potential complications.

TECHNICIAN NOTE

Frequently the technician is primarily responsible for all aspects of anesthesia, including selection of induction and maintenance anesthetic agents, instrumentation, monitoring, and recovery of patients.

Recommended Reading

Auer JA, Stick JA, editors: *Equine surgery,* Philadelphia, 1999, WB Saunders.

Koterba AM, Drummond WH, Kosch PC, editors: *Equine clinical neonatology,* Philadelphia, 1990, Lea & Febiger.

Orsini JA, Divers TJ: *Manual of equine emergencies,* ed 2, Philadelphia, 2003, WB Saunders.

Reed S, Bailey W, Sellon D, editors: *Equine internal medicine,* ed 2, Philadelphia, 2003, WB Saunders.

Robinson NE, editor: *Current therapy in equine medicine,* ed 2, Philadelphia, 1987, WB Saunders.

Robinson NE, editor: *Current therapy in equine medicine,* ed 3, Philadelphia, 1991, WB Saunders.

White NA, Moore JN, editors: *Current practice of equine surgery,* Philadelphia, 1990, Lippincott.

White NA, Moore JN, editors: *Current techniques in equine surgery and lameness,* Philadelphia, 1998, WB Saunders.

30

Food Animal Medical and Surgical Nursing

Marjorie S. Gill

INTRODUCTION

With fewer veterinarians choosing food animal practice, practice owners have been finding it increasingly difficult to hire an associate. For these individuals optimizing the use of veterinary technicians is of great importance. Capitalization of technician skills can help meet client needs and improve practice productivity and efficiency. As a part of the professional team, the veterinary technician can assist in the restraint and handling of animals for examination, sample collection, diagnosis, and treatment. Technicians can also prepare equipment, supplies, and animals for surgery as well as assist during the surgical procedure.

Additional tasks performed by veterinary technicians in food animal practice may include performing laboratory procedures and diagnostic tests, patient care, diagnostic imaging, anesthesia, preparation of pharmacological and biological agents, administration of injections and other treatments, ration balancing, body condition scoring in cattle and small ruminants, metabolic profiling of herds/flocks, monitoring records of postparturient cows, and planning herd consultation visits. Technicians are also very helpful in client education, for example, instructing producers about the proper technique for placement of growth implants in feedlot cattle and explanation of proper injection techniques based on meat quality assurance guidelines.

Veterinary technicians can also be trained to perform necropsies and collect tissue specimens. They could then describe their findings to the veterinarian or take digital pictures of the necropsy for review later by the veterinarian. Technicians may also possess special talents or training such as expertise in artificial insemination or corrective foot work that could be offered as a service to clients. A cognizant, well-trained, and knowledgeable technician can anticipate the needs of the veterinarian and producer thereby enhancing the productivity of the professional team.

Finally, with current concerns of bioterrorism and foreign animal diseases in the United States (currently bovine spongiform encephalopathy), the food animal veterinary technician will play a key role in dissemination of accurate information when handling public questions and concerns.

This chapter serves as an overview of the common medical and surgical conditions encountered in all food animal species and includes information on diagnostic sampling and testing. Common diagnostic sampling techniques are outlined such that the veterinary technician can prepare the animal for sampling by the veterinarian or even obtain samples themselves for use by the attending veterinarian. ∎

TECHNICIAN NOTE

Capitalization of veterinary technician skills in food animal practice can help meet client needs and improve practice productivity and efficiency.

COMMON DISEASES AND CONDITIONS OF CATTLE

CARE OF THE NEONATE AND NEONATAL DISEASES

Food animal veterinarians are often asked to assist cows and heifers having difficulty calving. Oftentimes the calves born via forced fetal extraction or cesarean section (C-section) are compromised. While the veterinarian attends the mother, especially in the case of a cesarean, the veterinary technician can provide intensive care to the neonate if necessary. The most important step is to make sure the calf is breathing. All mucus should be cleared from the nose, mouth, and upper airway. There are several ways to achieve this. The calf may be hung upside down with the head off the ground to allow drainage of these fluids. A bulb syringe also works well to remove mucus from the nose and mouth, and it also provides nasal stimulus to breathe. A piece of straw or hay can also be used to tickle the nose and stimulate respiration. If all else fails, a technique known as *gin chung*, placing a small-gauge needle in the nasal septum, is often a successful respiratory stimulus. If these techniques fail, artificial respiration can be provided by mouth-to-nose resuscitation or by raising and lowering the uppermost forelimb while simultaneously pressing and releasing the rib cage. For difficult cases a small amount of doxapram hydrochloride, a respiratory stimulant, may be injected under the tongue to induce respiration. Once the calf is breathing, it should be vigorously rubbed dry with a towel and the umbilical cord dipped in strong (7%) iodine.

Colostrum ingestion soon after birth is an important part of neonatal survival and prevention of infectious disease. Cattle and other ruminants (including sheep and goats) have a thick syndesmochorial placentation that prevents the in utero transfer of large molecular weight immunoglobulins. These species are essentially agammaglobulinemic at birth and rely on ingestion and absorption of colostrum rich antibodies and nonantibody immune factors.

Transfer of immunity can be compromised by colostrum deficiencies, ingestion failure, or absorption failure. Immunoglobulins are absorbed by pinocytosis by specialized epithelial cells in the jejunum and ileum. These cells are replaced soon after birth by normal intestinal epithelium and absorption terminates Therefore, it is important that the neonate receives colostrum within the first 6 to 8 hours of life. The calf should receive colostrum at the rate of 10% of its body weight within the first 12 hours (4.5 L/45 kg of body weight in 12 hours).

Several tests are available for detection of failure of passive transfer (FPT) including single radial immunodiffusion (SRID), sodium sulfite precipitation, zinc sulfate turbidity, and serum protein analysis. Serum concentration of IgG using the SRID should be greater than 1600 mg/dl. Serum protein can be measured using a refractometer. A serum protein greater than 5 mg/dl in the absence of dehydration is indicative of successful passive transfer; values less than 4.5 mg/dl are consistent with FPT. For valuable calves treatment may be achieved by plasma transfusion at the rate of 20 to 40 ml/kg body weight.

Partial or total failure of passive transfer can make a calf susceptible to a variety of disease conditions. Compromised calves are more likely to develop umbilical infections (omphalophlebitis), which may lead to any combination of the following problems: septicemia, septic arthritis, anterior uveitis, meningitis, vegetative endocarditis, pneumonia, and diarrhea. Calves experiencing these problems should immediately be given broad-spectrum antimicrobial agents, supportive therapy such as fluids with dextrose and electrolytes, and other treatments specific to the problems encountered. If omphalophlebitis is present and does not respond to antimicrobial therapy, surgical removal of infected umbilical remnants should be considered if the patient is a good surgical candidate. Anterior uveitis and hypopion often respond to application of ophthalmic preparations of antibiotics and atropine. Septic arthritis may be treated with IV regional antibiotic perfusion or implantation of antibiotic impregnated polymethylmethacrylate (PMMA) beads near affected joints.

✐ TECHNICIAN NOTE

Colostrum ingestion soon after birth is an important part of prevention of infectious diseases in neonates.

Diarrhea, a common problem in young dairy and beef calves, has multiple infectious and noninfectious causes. Viral etiologies include rotavirus, coronavirus, and bovine viral diarrhea virus (BVD). Bacterial enteritis may result if the calf is infected with *Escherichia coli*, *Salmonella* spp., or clostridia and protozoal diseases such as cryptosporidia and coccidiosis may also cause calf diarrhea. In addition, a variety of management conditions including stress, poor nutrition, and improper sanitation may cause or contribute to development of diarrhea. Regardless of cause, affected calves often develop watery diarrhea, rapidly leading to severe dehydration, metabolic acidosis, hypoglycemia, shock, and hypothermia. Treatment is aimed at quick replacement of lost fluids and correction of acidosis and electrolyte abnormalities. Sick calves should be started on warm intravenous (IV) fluids such as Normosol (Abbott Laboratories) supplemented with dextrose and bicarbonate as indicated. Milk and milk products should be withheld during treatment of diarrhea but for no longer than 48 hours total. In herds in which calf diarrhea is a persistent problem, it may be necessary to vaccinate cows and heifers prior to calving. Many polyvalent vaccines are available, and the product(s) used can be tailored to the needs of the individual herd (see Chapter 11).

Calves should be fed whole milk or quality calf milk replacer. Although milk replacers are never as complete as whole milk, the product chosen should be of good quality and meet the following standards: protein level 20% to 22% and all protein must be milk derived (dried skimmed milk, dried whey, whey protein, casein, etc.), crude fat 18% to 20%, and fiber less than 10%. In general, calves are fed 10% of their body weight divided twice daily. This amount may need to be adjusted based on individual needs. It is important to carefully follow label directions when mixing milk replacers since a solution that is too concentrated or too dilute can cause problems such as nutritional diarrhea.

Well-informed veterinary technicians can question clients concerning the quality of their milk replacers, the method of mixing the milk replacer, and the technique of calf feeding and can then make appropriate recommendations to owners.

CONDITIONS OF THE DIGESTIVE SYSTEM

ACTINOMYCOSIS AND ACTINOBACILLOSIS

Two common conditions of the head in cattle include actinobacillosis (woody tongue) and actinomycosis (lumpy jaw). Woody tongue is caused by a gram-negative bacterium, *Actinobacillus lignieresii*, which is a normal inhabitant of the mouth of cattle. The organism may gain entry into the soft tissues of the mouth through wounds caused by weed or plant awns resulting in a granulomatous abscess usually of the tongue. The tongue becomes hard with a diffuse nodular swelling. Clinical signs include excessive salivation and inability of the animal to prehend food normally causing anorexia and weight loss. The tongue may become so swollen that it protrudes from the mouth (Figure 30-1). Diagnosis is usually based on clinical signs and examination of the tongue; however, biopsy and culture of the organism confirms the diagnosis. Successful treatment of this disease involves using sodium iodide and antibiotics. Sodium iodide is administered intravenously, and care must be taken during administration as perivascular injection may result in tissue sloughing. Woody tongue typically responds to treatment within a few days, but occasionally, repeated doses of sodium iodide may be necessary until signs of iodism occur (lacrimation, anorexia, dandruff, coughing). Prevention includes reduced exposure of the cattle to scabrous feeds and plant awns (foxtails, horse nettles, pigweed) by keeping pastures as clean as possible.

Lumpy jaw is the common name for the disease caused by *Actinomyces bovis*. This organism is gram positive and also a normal inhabitant of the mouth of ruminants. This bacteria gains entry through wounds in the mouth and infection results in osteomyelitis of the mandible and less commonly the maxilla. Affected cattle present with a hard, immovable, nonpainful bony mass of the mandible or maxilla (Figure 30-2). If the mass becomes large enough or involves tooth roots, it may result in pain, inability to masticate, and subsequent anorexia with weight loss. Treatment of lumpy jaw is the same as described for woody tongue; however, this disease is much less responsive to treatment. Repeated doses of sodium iodide are often necessary just to arrest the growth of the lesion. A more radical treatment involves surgical debridement and curettage of fibrous tissue and infected bone. The surgery is not without risk as these patients often lose significant amounts of blood and may require blood transfusions during the surgical procedure. Still, surgical treatment followed by medical treatment offers the best long-term prognosis for valuable animals.

PHARYNGEAL TRAUMA AND ABSCESSATION

Pharyngeal trauma occurs relatively frequently in cattle and may result in cellulitis, abscess, or hematoma formation. It is almost always caused by trauma associated with the improper use of a balling gun, long dose syringe, speculum, paste dewormer gun, or a rigid stomach tube. Less commonly, a foreign body (sharp stick or wire) may penetrate the pharynx.

Clinical signs include anorexia, salivation, malodorous breath, extension of the head and neck, feed coming from the nares, and mild bloat. In more severe cases, fever, obvious pharyngeal swelling, dysphagia, coughing, and

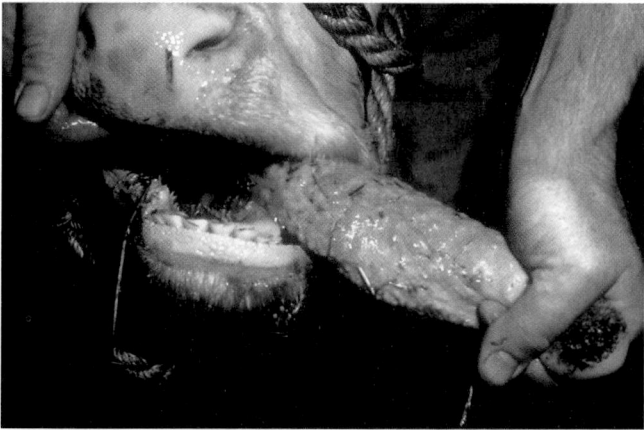

Figure 30-1 Bull with actinobacillosis (woody tongue). The tongue is enlarged and nodular in appearance.

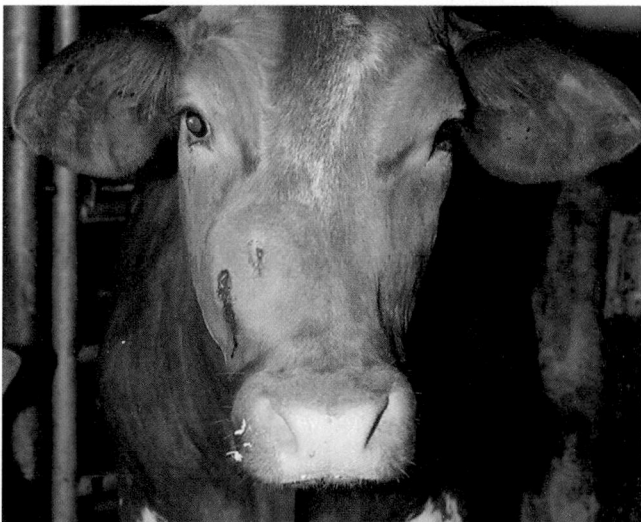

Figure 30-2 A bony mass on the maxilla of a cow with actinomycosis (lumpy jaw).

aspiration pneumonia may occur. Careful digital palpation of the pharynx per os is often diagnostic. Always wear gloves during palpation of the mouth or pharynx in cattle because of the concern of rabies. Endoscopy and radiography may be of great benefit in diagnosing the site of the lesion, extent of the cellulitis, and the presence of a foreign body.

Treatment requires aggressive use of antimicrobial drugs for 10 to 14 days. Nonsteroidal antiinflammatory drugs (NSAIDs) may help reduce the inflammation in the early stages of the disease. Supportive therapy is also very important especially if the animal cannot eat or drink. Feed and water may be forced with the use of a soft stomach tube or via a temporary rumenostomy. If a retropharyngeal abscess develops, it is best to drain the abscess into the pharynx by manually enlarging the original laceration.

The best way to prevent this condition is to exercise caution when using balling guns, dose syringes, and stomach tubes and make sure restraint is adequate to prevent excessive movement of the animal and subsequent injury. The veterinary technician can play an important role in educating the client/producer concerning proper use of this equipment.

> ✎ **TECHNICIAN NOTE**
>
> Pharyngeal trauma in cattle can be prevented by careful use of oral dosing equipment.

GRAIN OVERLOAD (CARBOHYDRATE ENGORGEMENT, LACTIC ACIDOSIS)

Grain overload in ruminants results from consumption of excessive amounts of highly fermentable carbohydrate feeds with production of large quantities of lactic acid in the rumen. Cattle with grain overload rapidly develop clinical signs of depression, anorexia, bloat, diarrhea with large amounts of grain, dehydration, incoordination, and recumbency leading to death.

Excess carbohydrate ingestion leads to increased production of volatile fatty acids in the rumen, which lowers rumen pH and decreases rumen motility. *Streptococcus bovis* organisms then multiply producing lactic acid, which further lowers rumen pH (4.0 to 5.0). The acid-resistant *Lactobacillus* spp. then proliferate, producing more lactic acid. With the increased osmolarity of the rumen fluid, body water is drawn into the rumen creating a "splashy rumen" and leading to loss of body water with severe dehydration and metabolic acidosis. Thus, affected animals, if not treated early, may develop severe metabolic acidosis leading to shock and acute death. Animals that do not die from the acute acidosis may subsequently develop secondary problems such as rumenitis with liver abscesses, laminitis (founder), and/or polioencephalomalacia.

Diagnosis is based on history of sudden exposure to large amounts of grain, typical clinical signs, and a rumen pH of

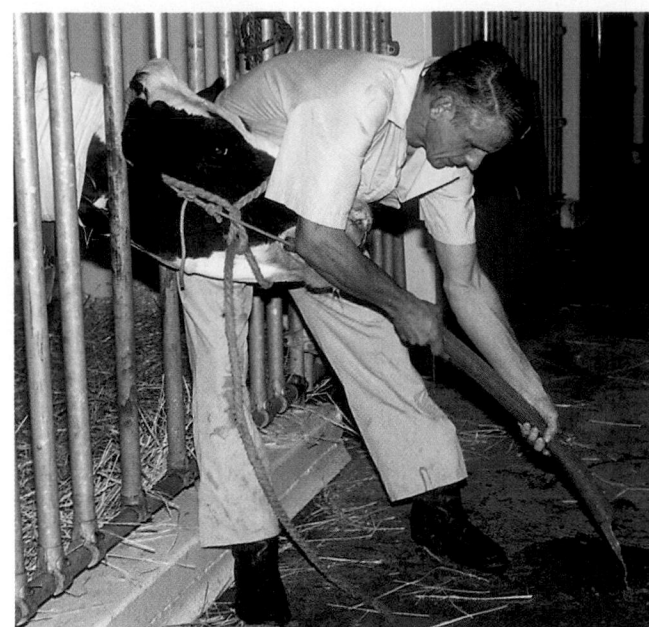

Figure 30-3 Rumen lavage or flushing using a large-bore stomach tube (Kingman tube).

less than 5.0. Ruminal fluid analysis can be a valuable tool in diagnosis of this and other rumen abnormalities.

Medical treatment involves removal the rumen contents with a large-bore stomach tube (Kingman tube), which is accomplished by repeated flushing of water into the rumen followed by outflow of rumen contents (lavage) (Figure 30-3). In addition, animals are given oral antacids, antibiotics (usually penicillin), NSAIDs when rehydrated, and thiamine, which all help prevent liver abscesses, polioencephalomalacia, and laminitis. In more severe cases, IV fluids with sodium bicarbonate should be administered to correct dehydration and acidosis. It may be necessary in some cases to perform a rumenotomy to remove all rumen contents. Whether an animal is treated medically or surgically, rumen transfaunation is often helpful to reestablish normal rumen microflora and improve appetite during the convalescent period. Prevention of grain overload involves making dietary changes very gradually. Rumen adaptation to dietary changes may take as long as 6 weeks. The veterinary technician can be instrumental in helping owners understand nutrition and the importance of making slow dietary adjustments in ruminants.

Analysis of rumen fluid is useful to establish the etiology of indigestions due to abnormal fermentation such as occurs with previously described grain overload. These are diagnostic tests that can be performed relatively quickly by a veterinary technician, providing the veterinarian with diagnostic information as to the cause of the indigestion and treatment appropriate to the condition. Samples may be collected by using a 2- to 3-m-long × 1-cm-inner-diameter (ID) stomach tube. Nasogastric passage of the tube prevents continuous struggling during sample collection and reduces the amount of saliva (no mouth device) that can contaminate the sample and falsely elevate its pH. Samples may also be obtained via centesis of the left paralumbar area using an 18-gauge, 12- to 15-cm needle.

Evaluation of the fluid sample includes assessment of color, consistency, odor, pH, sedimentation velocity, microscopic examination, rumen chloride, and redox potential. Normal color of rumen fluid is olive or brownish-green. Grain overload results in fluid that is milky gray, while prolonged stasis or decomposition in the rumen changes the color to dark green or black. Consistency of normal rumen fluid is slightly viscous, and salivary contamination increases viscosity. The odor of normal rumen fluid is aromatic and strong, but it develops an acid smell with grain overload, a putrid odor with stasis and decomposition, and an ammonia scent with urea toxicity.

The pH of rumen fluid is normally 6.5 to 6.8 (5.5 to 6.5 high grain diets). In general, anorexia will usually result in elevation of rumen pH. Values below 5.5 and above 7.0 can cause anorexia because of an alteration in the normal microbial population. A pH <5.5 is suggestive of grain overload, while a pH >7.5 may indicate overzealous use of antacids or urea toxicity.

Evaluation of sedimentation velocity should be performed soon after sampling and serves as a crude evaluation of microbial activity. The sample is placed in a tube and observed for the time it takes for sedimentation to occur. Fine particles sink and coarse particles float, being buoyed by gas bubbles of fermentation. Normal sedimentation takes 4 to 8 minutes. Grossly inactive fluid shows very rapid sedimentation, and frothy ingesta may show no sedimentation.

Microscopic exam is performed to assess type of bacteria present as well protozoal activity. Observation of protozoa requires no stain and they can be easily seen at ×40 to ×100 magnification. Normally, ciliate and flagellate forms of various sizes, and shapes are present and very active. The importance of protozoa is their sensitivity to abnormalities in rumen fluid; the larger species are more sensitive to change, and all protozoa die at a pH <5. In the normal animal, gram-negative bacteria predominate in the rumen. Grain overload results in mostly gram-positive bacteria (*Streptococcus* spp. and *Lactobacillus* spp.).

Rumen chloride is normally less than 25 mEq/L and may be elevated in cases of vagus indigestion (failure of pyloric outflow and reflux of chloride back into the rumen). The redox potential tests uses new methylene blue (NMB) test to evaluate anaerobic fermentative. To perform the test 1 ml of 0.03% NMB is mixed with 20 ml rumen fluid (control sample is untreated rumen fluid). The microflora, if active, reduce NMB and it loses its color, and this usually takes about 3 minutes (1 to 3 minutes if on a grain diet, 3 to 6 minutes if on a hay diet). Animals with prolonged anorexia, postgrain overload, or those receiving indigestible roughage may have a redox potential >15 minutes.

RUMEN TYMPANY (BLOAT)

Gas production is a normal occurrence during rumen fermentation and healthy animals are capable of eructating far more gas than the rumen produces. However, in some cases, abnormal distention of the rumen with gas may occur resulting in bloat. Bloat is classified as either primary where eructation is normal but the gas cannot be expelled or secondary which is due to a failure of eructation. Primary bloat occurs when large amounts of legumes or grain are ingested resulting in development of froth in the rumen. Failure of eructation or secondary bloat may be associated with esophageal foreign bodies (choke), motor function abnormalities of the rumen such as vagus indigestion, body position (lateral recumbency), hypocalcemia, or pharyngitis. Bloat is also described as free gas bloat or frothy bloat depending on the cause.

Clinical signs include distention of the left paralumbar fossa, discomfort (grunting, colic), dyspnea with openmouth breathing, anorexia, salivation, anxiety, depression terminally, and sudden death.

Treatment of free gas bloat involves passing a stomach tube either via the nasogastric or orogastric route. If bloat is due to the animal's position, the animal should be helped into sternal recumbency or a standing position. If hypocalcemia is the underlying problem, administration of calcium is therapeutic. Forced exercise also stimulates rumen motility and eructation. In addition, rumen stimulants improve motility and normal belching. If an animal is critically bloated and passing a stomach tube is too stressful, an emergency procedure called *rumen trocarization* should be performed using a large bore trocar to enter the rumen through the left paralumbar fossa.

Frothy bloat requires different treatment in that the froth must first be consolidated into larger pockets of gas before it can be expelled. In order to reduce surface tension, several products may be used including poloxalene, household detergent (Tide, 2 to 3 oz.), mineral oil, or dioctyl sodium sulfosuccinate (DSS). Once the frothy bloat becomes a free gas bloat it can be eructated or relieved via tube. Nutritional management such as preventing excessive exposure to grain or legumes is important to prevent bloat in ruminants.

TRAUMATIC RETICULOPERITONITIS

Traumatic reticuloperitonitis (TRP), or hardware disease, which results from penetration of the reticulum by a foreign body, is one of the most common gastrointestinal problems affecting the forestomach compartments of mature dairy cattle. The indiscriminate eating habits of cattle, in contrast to small ruminants, can lead to accidental ingestion of foreign materials that settle in the reticulum (Figure 30-4).

✍ TECHNICIAN NOTE

To prevent grain overload and other indigestions in cattle, dietary changes should be made gradually over at least a 6-week period.

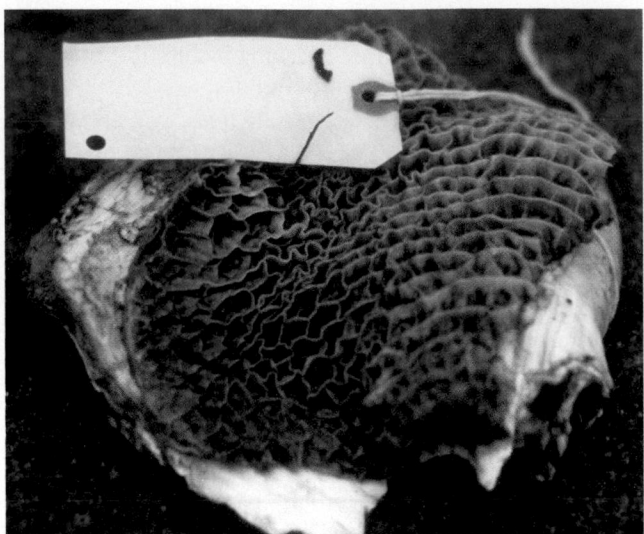

Figure 30-4 Metallic foreign body (wire) found in the reticulum of a cow with traumatic reticuloperitonitis (hardware disease).

The foreign bodies ingested by cattle are most often wires and nails but also include steel objects. Most foreign bodies are ferromagnetic. Subsequent to ingestion of a foreign body, four outcomes are possible:

Attachment of the object to a magnet without further disease problems

Penetration of the reticular wall with acute inflammation and mild clinical disease if there is not penetration into the peritoneal cavity

Perforation of the reticular wall into the peritoneal cavity with acute localized TRP

Migration of the foreign body with penetration into the peritoneal or thoracic cavity and resulting abscessation (thoracic, reticular, hepatic), vagal indigestion, pericarditis, myocarditis, or other secondary problems.

Acute cases of TRP result in anorexia, a sharp decrease in milk production, reluctance to rise or move, cranial abdominal pain, and kyphosis. Uncomplicated cases may improve in 3 to 5 days, but progression of the severity of signs may indicate either a failure to contain a localized peritonitis or extension of infection to other organs. A heart rate >90 beats/min or a fever >40° C generally indicates more severe disease such as diffuse peritonitis or pericarditis. A heart rate <64 beats/min is suggestive of vagus indigestion syndrome.

A differential white blood cell count (WBC) is a more reliable indicator of inflammation than is a total WBC. A neutrophilia (>4000 cells/μl) with a left shift can be expected in acute cases, but in chronic cases these changes are less consistent. A high plasma fibrinogen concentration (>1000 mg/dl) usually occurs in both acute and chronic cases of TRP.

Peritoneal fluid analysis may be helpful in diagnosis of TRP, especially in chronic cases when WBC changes are infrequently observed. It may be necessary to sample multiple sites due to the size of the rumen and the fact that cattle are capable of localizing infection by formation of a large amount of fibrin. Failure to obtain a fluid sample does not rule out TRP. A relatively accurate diagnosis of peritonitis can be made if the nucleated cell count >6000 cells/μl and the total protein >3 g/dl (a more accurate diagnosis can be made if a differential is performed and neutrophils account for >40% of the cells and eosinophils for <10%).

Reticular or cranioventral abdominal radiography or ultrasonography can offer valuable assistance in diagnosis and treatment of TRP.

Medical treatment of TRP is often successful. Even if a foreign body has perforated the reticular wall, in approximately half of the cases, it will return to the lumen. Medical treatment is geared toward treating reticulitis/peritonitis and preventing further perforation of the reticulum by the use of broad-spectrum antimicrobials and oral administration of a magnet.

Surgical intervention may be necessary if TRP fails to respond to conservative treatment, if a foreign body is observed outside the reticulum on radiography, or if an intraabdominal or thoracic abscess is suspected. The approach of choice is a left flank exploratory laparotomy and rumenotomy using transruminal exploration. The rumenotomy site is the dorsal sac of the rumen using one of two recommended rumenotomy procedures: use of a rumen board (Weingarth apparatus) or suturing the rumen wall to the skin. Most abscesses that form secondary to TRP are located on the medial wall of the reticulum and are usually tightly adhered. These abscesses are the most common causes of vagal indigestion associated with TRP. These tightly adhered abscesses can be lanced and drained into the reticulum or omasum and then explored for the presence of a foreign body.

TECHNICIAN NOTE

Traumatic reticuloperitonitis (hardware disease) may lead to peritonitis, liver or reticular abscesses, pericarditis, vagal indigestion, or other secondary problems.

Indications for performing paracentesis or abdominocentesis include evaluation of accumulated abdominal fluid and diagnosis of abdominal diseases such as traumatic reticuloperitonitis, peritonitis, abomasal ulcers (perforating), abomasal rupture, ruptured bladder or ureters, abdominal neoplasia (lymphosarcoma, mesothelioma), or intestinal obstruction/rupture. In monogastrics, the most ventral aspect of the abdomen on the midline is the usual site for abdominocentesis; however, in cattle, centesis on the midline usually results in puncture of the rumen. Also, because bovine abdominal disorders are often localized (or effectively walled off), centesis of a single site might not reflect disease elsewhere in the abdomen. Centesis of four sites on the ventrolateral abdomen may be most productive. These areas represent four abdominal quadrants; left cranial, left caudal, right cranial, right caudal.

Sampling should begin where the problem is suspected, such as start with the left cranial quadrant if hardware disease is likely. The animal should be standing and properly restrained. The area of centesis is surgically clipped and prepared. To approach the left cranial quadrant, palpate the foramen of the subcutaneous abdominal vein. The site to tap is one hand's breadth cranial and one hand's breadth (6 cm) medial to the foramen, or half way between the xyphoid and umbilicus and half way between the midline and milk vein. The right cranial quadrant has the same landmarks as the left cranial quadrant only on the right side. This site would be most useful if abomasal disease is suspected. The left caudal quadrant can be located directly anterior to the attachment of the udder to the body (comparable location in the male) in the paramedian area. The right caudal quadrant has the same landmarks as the left caudal quadrant only on the right side. These sites are sampled using an 18-gauge, 3.8-cm needle and collecting any fluid in ethylenediaminetetraacetic acid (EDTA) and serum tubes. Each quadrant sample should be individually analyzed if several sites are tapped unless it is necessary to combine samples because of small volumes. A sterile teat cannula may be used instead of a needle, but this requires some local analgesia and a small skin incision.

The sample is evaluated and classified as a transudate, which is a serous fluid accumulation due to alteration in pressure, or an exudate, which may be a result of abdominal infection. Transudates are clear, colorless, odorless, have a protein <2.5 g/dl and cell counts <5000/μl, and may be due to hypoproteinemia or hypoalbuminemia. Exudates are usually turbid and have a protein >3 g/dl and cell counts >10,000 cells/μl. Evaluation of peritoneal fluid in cattle includes assessment of volume, color, turbidity, total protein, chemical analysis (urea nitrogen, creatinine), cell count, and cytology. In clinically normal animals, the ratio of neutrophils to mononuclear cells (eosinophils) is 1:1 with the exception of normal cows less than 2 weeks postpartum that may have total nucleated cell counts >10,000 cells/μl and neutrophils or eosinophils predominate.

To evaluate cytology, a direct smear may be prepared or the sample may need to be centrifuged if cellularity is low. Hematologic stains such as Wright's stain, NMB, or Diff-Quik (Baxter S/P) can be utilized to examine neutrophil morphology (degenerative changes, bacteria). Classification of inflammatory fluids (exudates) are as follows:

1. Acute inflammation with 80% to 85% neutrophils (the rest of the cells are lymphocytes, eosinophils, macrophages), which may be nondegenerate as with a noninfectious irritant or degenerate as may occur with sepsis

2. Chronic active (subacute) inflammation with 50% to 70% nondegenerate neutrophils and 20% to 50% monocytes or macrophages

3. Chronic inflammation with >50% monocytes and macrophages

✎ TECHNICIAN NOTE

Abdominocentesis with evaluation of accumulated abdominal fluid may aid in the diagnosis of abdominal diseases such as traumatic reticuloperitonitis, peritonitis, abomasal ulcers (perforating), abomasal rupture, ruptured bladder or ureters, abdominal neoplasia (lymphosarcoma, mesothelioma), or intestinal obstruction/rupture.

ABOMASAL DISPLACEMENTS AND VOLVULUS

Abomasal displacement is a common problem of high-producing dairy cows fed high concentrate, low roughage diets. Displacements are most likely to occur in the first 6 weeks after calving. Predisposing factors include high grain diets with increased amount of volatile fatty acids in the abomasum, hypocalcemia, concurrent diseases such as mastitis, metritis, and ketosis, and lack of exercise. Increased volatile fatty acids, histamine release with concurrent diseases, and hypocalcemia may lead to abomasal dilatation and atony and subsequent displacement of the abomasum from its normal right paramedian position to the left or right paralumbar area. Left abomasal displacement (LDA) is much more common than right abomasal displacement (RDA). Abomasal volvulus may occur after displacement to the right and carries a poorer prognosis than LDA or RDA because of compromise of the innervation and blood supply that occurs when the abomasum twists. AV can quickly lead to development of shock and toxemia if not diagnosed and treated early.

LDA, RDA, or abomasal volvulus can be diagnosed by auscultation of a distinct "ping" in the left or right paralumbar fossa area since the gas trapped in the abomasum produces a characteristic "metallic pinging" sound when thumping the area over the gas cap while simultaneously ausculting with a stethoscope.

The Liptak test can also be used as an aid in diagnosing LDA. After percussion of the abomasum on left side under the last few ribs, an area just below the gas ping, which corresponds to the fluid level in the abomasum, is clipped and surgically prepared. Centesis is performed using an 18-gauge, 10- to 12-cm needle. Fluid with a pH <4.5 confirms the presence of an LDA. Also, aspiration of gas with a characteristic "burnt almond" odor is indicative of an LDA.

Surgery is usually necessary to correct abomasal displacements, and abomasal volvulus requires immediate surgical intervention. The choices of surgical approach and technique depend on the direction of the displacement, the presence of volvulus, the condition of the animal, and the surgeon's preference. Postsurgically, the diet should be restricted to roughage only and grain should be introduced very gradually into the diet once recovery is complete.

DIARRHEA IN THE ADULT

Common causes of acute diarrhea in adults include coccidiosis, dietary gastroenteritis, acute salmonellosis, acute BVD, and winter dysentery. Chronic diarrhea in the adult may be due to gastrointestinal (GI) parasites, Johne's disease, chronic BVD, chronic salmonellosis, BLV, chronic renal disease, or chronic liver disease.

Winter dysentery, believed to be caused by a coronavirus, is an acute, contagious diarrheal disease of adult cattle. It is seen more commonly in dairy herds in the winter, and it is considered an epizootic disease since it spreads rapidly through infected herds. Morbidity is high but mortality rare. The disease presents as a rapid onset of explosive diarrhea, mild depression, partial anorexia, and decreased milk production in affected animals. The disease can spread through an entire herd in 2 weeks and those individuals affected first usually recover within 1 week. The greatest economic loss to the producer is loss of milk production due to body water loss secondary to severe diarrhea. No treatment is available, and most animals recover spontaneously; however, sick cows can be treated symptomatically with intestinal astringents, protectants, and absorbents. Provision of fresh drinking water and free-choice salt is also beneficial.

The most frequent cause of chronic diarrhea in cattle is parasitic infection, especially by *Ostertagia ostertagi* and *Nematodirus*. In adult cattle, the most common clinical parasitic disease is type II or pre-type II ostertagiasis.

In pre-type II disease, the fourth-stage *Ostertagia* larvae burrow into the abomasal wall and encyst instead of maturing into adults. This occurs in the fall in the northern United States and in the spring in the south. During encystment, the acid-secreting parietal cells of the abomasum are destroyed causing an increase in the pH of the abomasum. With the pH above 5, pepsinogen is no longer converted to pepsin, resulting in impaired protein digestion.

Type II ostertagiasis occurs in the spring in the northern United States and in the late summer, early fall in the south when large numbers of encysted larvae emerge into the lumen of the abomasum and mature. Much more damage occurs to the abomasal glands during emergence than during dormancy. Because of the extensive damage, clinical signs often persist long after the parasites are removed by effective anthelmintics.

Clinical signs include unthriftiness, weight loss, pale mucous membranes, diarrhea, and dependent edema in severe cases. Severe parasitism and associated clinical cases are more likely to occur when conditions are crowded, nutrition is marginal, and deworming programs are inadequate.

Parasite eggs may be absent in some cases of type II ostertagiasis. Increased serum pepsinogen concentration may be helpful in diagnosis in cases of type II ostertagiasis (excessive amounts of pepsinogen are in the GI tract as a result of mucosal damage or decreased conversion to pepsin; the pepsinogen leaks into the bloodstream). For treatment of these parasitic conditions, please refer to Chapter 7.

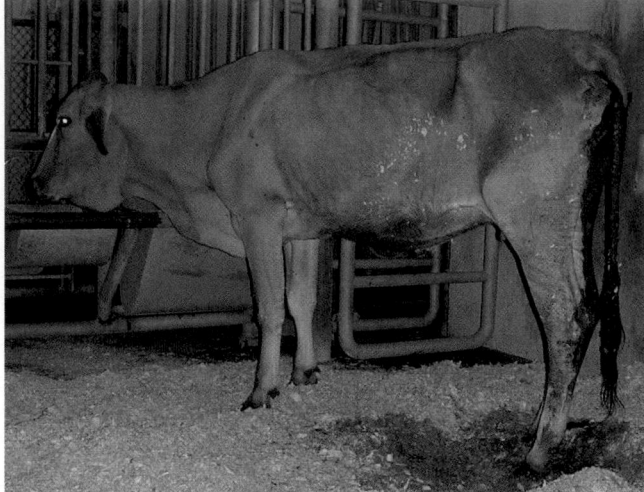

Figure 30-5 Severe emaciation, intermandibular edema, and chronic diarrhea in a cow with Johne's disease.

✎ TECHNICIAN NOTE

The most frequent cause of chronic diarrhea in cattle is parasitic infection.

Johne's disease, characterized by chronic diarrhea and weight loss, is caused by *Mycobacterium paratuberculosis*, a slow-growing, acid-fast organism. The bacterium is transmitted from infected cows to their calves via the fecal-oral route with calves less than 6 months being the most susceptible to infection. Once the organisms have been ingested by the calf, they are taken up from the intestinal lumen by cells covering the Peyer's patches, particularly in the distal ileum, and are phagocytized by macrophages. The organisms reside and grow within macrophages eventually causing a severe granulomatous reaction with thickening of the intestinal wall. This leads to protein malabsorption and a protein-losing enteropathy so that even though these animals have good appetites, they continue to experience diarrhea and weight loss (Figure 30-5). Although infection occurs early in life, clinical signs do not usually develop until the animal is at least 2 years of age.

Johne's is a terminal disease with no effective treatment. It can be very difficult to diagnose due to a lack of reliable tests. There are several serological tests available that may help diagnose this disease; however, most tests are clouded by false-positive and false-negative reactions. A deoxyribonucleic acid (DNA) test has recently become available, but it is relatively expensive and not 100% reliable. Once clinical signs are advanced, a rectal mucosal biopsy may be beneficial to achieve a quick diagnosis. Often the diagnosis is made based on history, clinical signs, and lack of response to conventional treatments such as antimicrobial and anthelmintic therapy (for both nematodes and trematodes).

Control programs have been outlined for producers who wish to eliminate the disease from their herd. These programs involve the use of repeated serologic testing, fecal cultures, culling of positive animals as well as clinically ill animals, and maintenance of separate disease-free and infected herds. These programs are costly and labor intensive, so most producers choose to live with the disease, culling clinically affected cows and their exposed offspring. A vaccine, the use of which is state controlled, is available and is used to control the development of clinical disease in herds with a high incidence of Johne's disease.

Salmonellosis typically manifests as an acute diarrhea, but in rare cases individuals become chronically infected and have recurring bouts of diarrhea with or without fever, anorexia, and dehydration. Chronically infected cattle usually lose weight and become unthrifty. Salmonellosis is often associated with leukopenia, hyponatremia, hypokalemia, and hypoproteinemia. Submission of multiple fecal samples of adequate volume (up to 60 ml) for culture is necessary to establish a diagnosis. Culture of a rectal biopsy may enhance recovery of the organism.

Salmonellosis should be suspected when chronic diarrhea is preceded by an outbreak of acute diarrhea in a herd, especially if the outbreak was associated with the introduction of new livestock, a feed change, a water change, or a flood.

Other clinical diseases caused by Salmonella include septicemia, especially in the neonate, and abortion in adults. Severe cases may progress to endotoxemia, shock, and subsequent death. Animals that survive may continue to carry and shed the organism, posing a threat to other animals. Treatment includes antimicrobial drugs, nonsteroidal antiinflammatory drugs, and fluid therapy particularly in young calves with septicemia and/or endotoxemia.

BVD is a common virus-induced gastroenteritis affecting all ages of cattle. BVD manifests as sudden onset of fever, depression, anorexia, oral and gastrointestinal ulcers and erosions, and diarrhea (sometimes with blood and mucus). The disease may progress rapidly through a group of animals. BVD also plays an important role in respiratory tract diseases in cattle by causing immunosuppression and susceptibility to secondary bacterial pathogens causing pneumonia. The virus is also responsible for abortions, in utero infection, and birth defects. Exposure of pregnant cattle to the noncytopathic strain of BVD between days 80 and 125 of gestation may result in an infected fetus, which becomes immunotolerant to the virus. Later in life, the calf may be exposed to cytopathic strains of BVD, which results in acute mucosal disease(MD) or chronic diarrhea (chronic BVD or BVD-MD), which has a nearly 100% mortality rate; affected calves rarely live to a year of age. Clinical signs of BVD-MD include intermittent or persistent diarrhea, weight loss, anorexia, unthriftiness, crusty eyes or muzzle, blunting of oral papilla (Figure 30-6), and chronic coronary band lesions. These cattle are also leukopenic and anemic and have no titer to BVD when serology is performed.

Diagnosis of BVD is made on physical exam, characteristic necropsy findings including linear erosions in the esophagus, necrosis of the Peyer's patches, blunted papillae in the buccal mucosa and epithelial erosions on the tongue

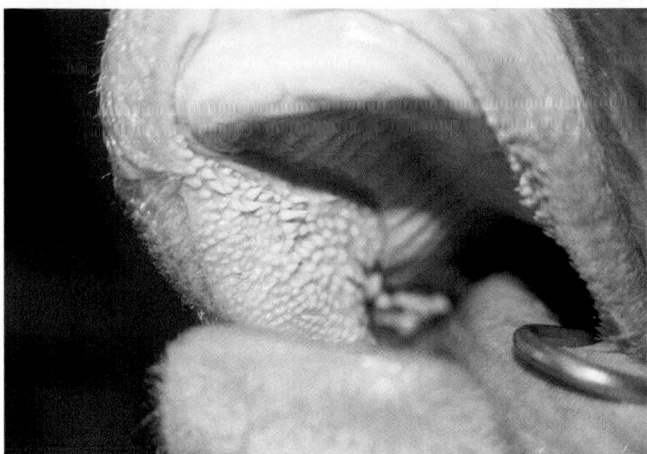

Figure 30-6 Blunted oral papilla seen in a calf with chronic BVD (BVD-MD).

and ruminal pillars, virus isolation from tissues or the buffy coat of whole blood samples, and serology (paired samples 2 to 4 weeks apart are most helpful).

There is no treatment for BVD, but antimicrobials are often used to prevent secondary bacterial infections. Vaccination of dairy and beef animals is important to help prevent the disease. Both killed and modified live vaccines are available (see Chapter 11). Use of the modified live vaccines should be avoided in pregnant cows, calves nursing pregnant cows, and immunosuppressed animals. Vaccination of calves experiencing chronic BVD using the modified live vaccine may result in death of the animal.

> ✎ **TECHNICIAN NOTE**
>
> Bovine virus diarrhea (BVD) may cause gastroenteritis, respiratory tract diseases, immunosuppression, abortions, in utero infection, and birth defects in cattle.

DISEASES OF THE RESPIRATORY SYSTEM

BOVINE RESPIRATORY DISEASE SYNDROME

Bovine respiratory disease syndrome (BRDS) affects all ages of cattle but particularly beef calves during the first 45 days in the feedlot and dairy calves younger than 6 months of age. The syndrome is caused by a complex interaction of respiratory viruses, bacteria, and stress. Transportation, cold weather, close confinement, stress with immunosuppression, and exposure to viral and bacterial pathogens predispose to the development of respiratory disease.

A number of viruses including infectious bovine rhinotracheitis (IBR), BVD, parainfluenza virus (PI_3), bovine respiratory syncytial virus (BRSV), and respiratory coronavirus as well as bacteria such as *Mannheimia haemolytica* and *Haemophilus somnus* produce respiratory disease in susceptible, immunocompromised animals. Generally,

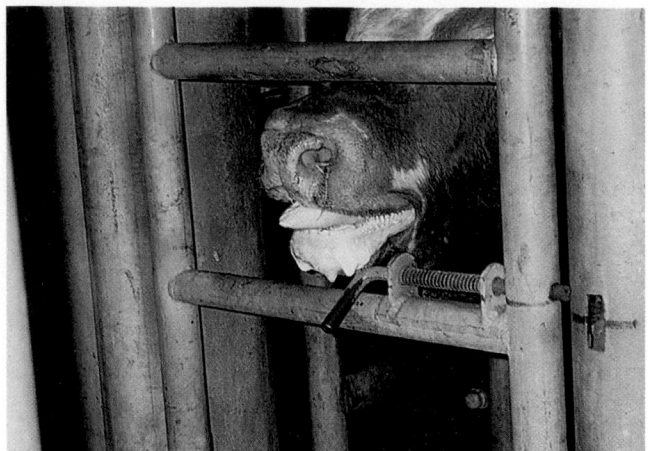

Figure 30-7 Severe dyspnea and open mouth breathing in a calf with shipping fever.

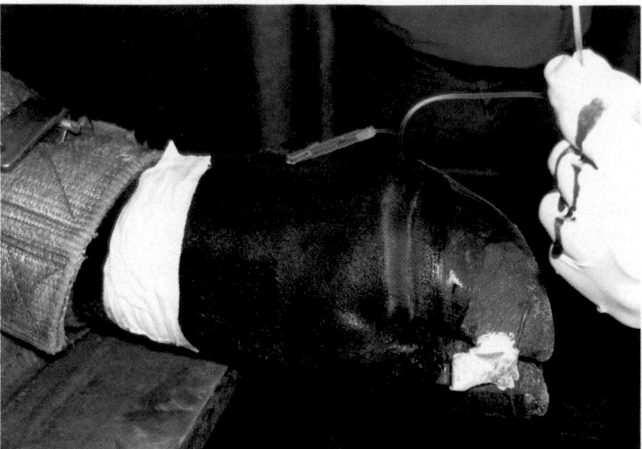

Figure 30-8 Injection of lidocaine for intravenous retrograde analgesia of the bovine foot after placement of a tourniquet above the fetlock.

infection with one or more of the respiratory viruses occurs first, followed by bacterial infection of the lower respiratory tract or bronchopneumonia. BRDS in feedlot cattle is often referred to as *shipping fever*.

Cattle with BRDS experience depression, standing with their heads lowered, anorexia, fever 40° to 41.5° C (104° F to 107° F), mucopurulent ocular and nasal discharge, cough, and dyspnea (Figure 30-7). Morbidity and mortality within a group may be quite high.

Diagnosis of BRDS is based on a history of calves undergoing stress, typical clinical signs of pneumonia, and presence of bronchopneumonia on necropsy. Samples from a transtracheal aspirate can be submitted for cytology, bacterial isolation, and antimicrobial sensitivity as well as virus isolation in cases of respiratory disease in cattle. Successful treatment of the disease hinges on early diagnosis and institution of appropriate antimicrobial therapy. Individual sick animals should be isolated from the rest of the group and treated with broad-spectrum antimicrobial therapy for at least 5 days. Antimicrobial agents typically used for treatment of shipping fever include ceftiofur sodium or hydrochloride (Naxcel or Excenel, both produced by Pharmacia & Upjohn, Kalamazoo, Mich.), florfenicol (Nuflor, Schering-Plough, Union, N.J.), tilmicosin (Micotil, Elanco, Indianapolis, Ind.), tetracycline (LA200, Liquamycin, Pfizer Animal Health, New York, N.Y.), and fluoroquinolone (Baytril, Bayer, Shawnee Mission, Kan.). When large numbers of animals are ill, antimicrobial agents may be added to the water to simplify treatment. In addition, fresh water, hay, and adequate shelter should be provided. A procedure known as *metaphylaxsis* is now commonly employed by feedlots and involves treatment of cattle with long-acting antimicrobial agents such as Micotil upon arrival to the feedlot. Preconditioning (castration, dehorning, implanting, acclimation to feed and water, deworming, and vaccination) of calves prior to weaning and vaccination before transport from stocker to feeder operations decreases

stress on the cattle during these transitions and may prevent development or lessen the severity of disease. Vaccines typically used to prevent respiratory disease outbreaks include IBR, PI_3, BVD, BRSV, *Mannheimia haemolytica*, and *Haemophilus somnus*. For more information refer to Chapter 11.

> **✐ TECHNICIAN NOTE**
>
> BRDS, which affects primarily feedlot calves and dairy calves younger than 6 months of age, is caused by a complex interaction of respiratory viruses, bacteria, and stress.

DISEASES OF THE MUSCULOSKELETAL SYSTEM

REGIONAL ANALGESIA AND REGIONAL ANTIBIOTIC PERFUSION TECHNIQUES AND PMMA IMPLANTS

Regional analgesia (IV retrograde analgesia) of the foot/distal limb is commonly performed prior to claw amputation or corn removal, although the regional block can also be used for other surgeries or painful techniques of the foot or distal limb, or as a diagnostic aid in lameness exams. A tourniquet is applied distal to the hock or carpus in the midmetatarsal or midmetacarpal area. A superficial vein is located, either the common dorsal metacarpal (metatarsal) vein or the palmar/plantar metacarpal (metatarsal) vein, and surgically prepared. An intravenous injection of 15 to 30 ml of 2% lidocaine will provide analgesia in 5 minutes, which will persist until the tourniquet is released (the tourniquet should not be left in place more than an hour) (Figure 30-8). An alternative to this technique involves placing the tourniquet above the tarsus or carpus to achieve analgesia more proximally. Accordingly, more lidocaine should be used to block this larger area. This same technique can be

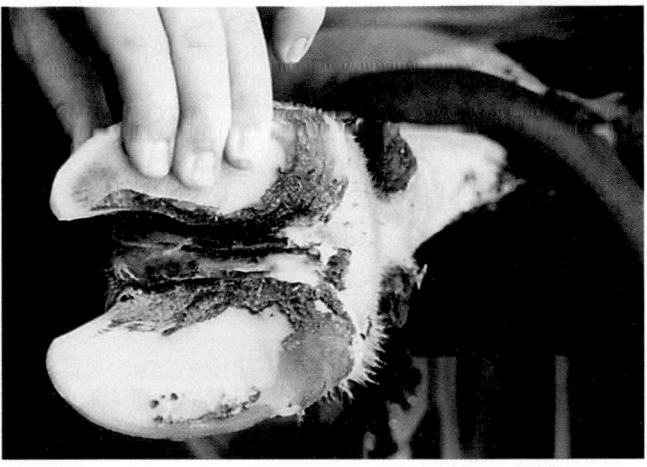

Figure 30-9 Interdigital necrobacillosis or foot rot in a cow.

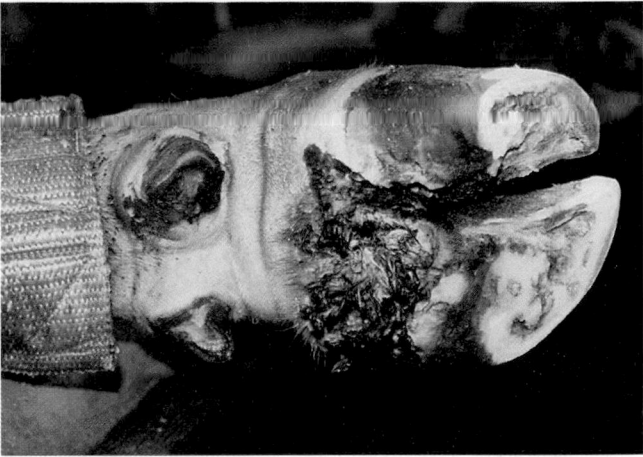

Figure 30-10 Papillomatous digital dermatitis or hairy heel warts of the hind feet cause severe lameness in affected dairy cattle.

used to perform regional perfusion of antibiotics to the distal limb for the purpose of treating localized infections such as foot rot with cellulitis. A cephalosporin is injected through the catheter and allowed to perfuse the limb distal to the tourniquet for approximately 45 minutes. Both of these techniques are primarily used in cattle but can be applied to all food animal species. Recently, a technique involving the implantation of antibiotic-impregnated PMMA beads subcutaneously near infected joints has shown promise for treatment of septic arthritis in calves. The beads slowly release antibiotics into the joint and appear to be more effective than systemic antibiotic treatment or joint flushing alone. Techniques such as joint flushing, PMMA bead implants, regional perfusion, and systemic antibiotics used in combination work well to resolve septic arthritis.

LAMENESS

Lameness is commonly encountered in cattle and is most often (88%) caused by lesions or problems in the foot. Upper leg problems such as anterior cruciate ligament rupture, coxofemoral (hip) luxation, fractures, and arthritis account for the remaining 12% of lameness seen. When foot problems occur, they are most often seen in the claws that bear the most weight, front medial and hind lateral claws.

Common foot conditions especially in dairy cattle include foot rot, laminitis, white-line abscess ("gravel"), sole ulcer, underrun heel and sole, and hairy heel warts. It is important to examine all foot problems early since many conditions can quickly lead to osteomyelitis and/or septic arthritis if not properly treated. Regardless of the cause of lameness, it can lead to loss of production due to decreased milk production, weight loss, delayed breeding or anestrus,

---

TECHNICIAN NOTE

Lameness is commonly encountered in cattle and is most often (88%) caused by lesions or problems in the foot.

---

and culling. Intensive housing and feeding of large groups of animals has lead to an increased incidence of lameness.

INTERDIGITAL NECROBACILLOSIS

Interdigital necrobacillosis, or foot rot, in cattle is an infection of the interdigital skin and underlying tissues caused by the synergistic effects of *Fusobacterium necrophorum* and other anaerobic bacteria. Infection results in an ulcerated, foul-smelling area between the claws with resultant lameness (Figure 30-9). There may be swelling apparent above the coronary band and in severe cases cellulitis up to the carpus or hock may occur. The disease is particularly prevalent when cattle are kept in wet, muddy conditions. If left untreated, foot rot can invade the deeper tissues of the foot causing septic arthritis, osteomyelitis, and chronic lameness.

Treatment of foot rot in cattle can be successfully accomplished with aggressive topical treatment. In some cases it may be necessary to debride necrotic tissue and even bandage the foot with antimicrobial agents to promote healing. In cases where cellulitis has occurred it may be necessary to use parenteral antibiotics or the regional antibiotic perfusion technique previously described. Foot rot usually has a low morbidity in any given herd, but in cases where there is a high incidence of foot rot it may be necessary to initiate the use of a footbath containing zinc sulfate for prevention or treatment of foot rot.

PAPILLOMATOUS DIGITAL DERMATITIS

Papillomatous digital dermatitis (PDD), or hairy heel wart, has become an important cause of lameness in dairy cattle worldwide. Initially, PDD appears as a superficial inflammation of the skin of the bovine digit but progresses to the typical mature lesions that are circumscribed, erosive, or proliferative and are usually located on the hind feet, adjacent to the interdigital ridge and heel bulbs (Figure 30-10). Granulation tissue develops with outgrowths of

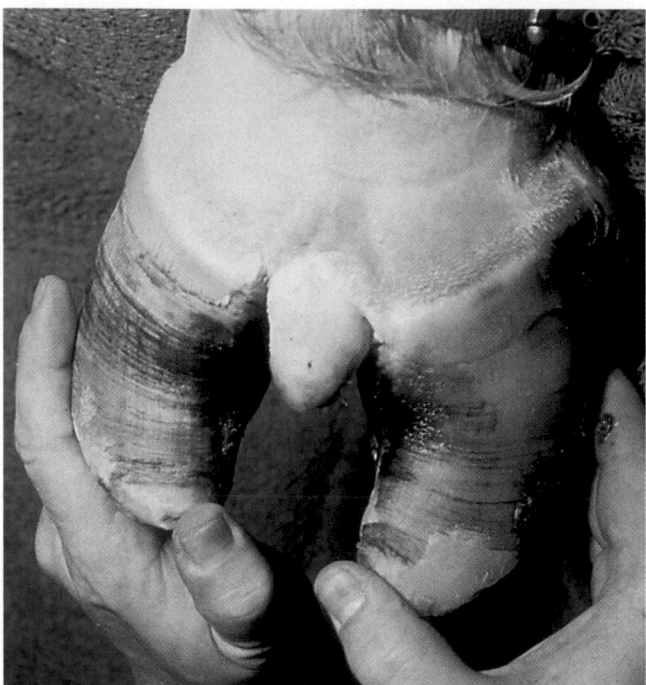

Figure 30-11 Interdigital hyperplasia (fibroma or corn) between the toes of a bull's foot.

dermal tissue that grossly resembles hair, thus the common name, *hairy heel wart*. The disease seems to be contagious with a fairly high morbidity within any given herd.

At this time the etiology of PDD is still controversial; it is believed to be a multifactorial disease in which infectious agents are primarily involved. Economic impact includes decreased milk production, impaired reproductive performance, an increased number of cows culled, and cost of treatment and control. Antibiotics such as oxytetracycline, lincomycin, or lincomycin/spectinomycin have been used as well as nonantibiotic products such as triplex (solubilized copper, a peroxy compound, and a cationic agent). Treatment is beneficial but does not appear to be curative as disease outbreaks are common once a herd is infected.

LAMINITIS

Laminitis, or founder, is a diffuse, aseptic inflammation of the corium (sensitive lamina) of the feet. Acute laminitis occurs sporadically and may be due to sudden excess grain ingestion (see Grain Overload), or it may occur secondary to other diseases that occur during the postparturient period such as retained placenta, metritis, mastitis, ketosis, or abomasal displacement. Chronic laminitis is more often associated with constant feeding of high-grain diets as occurs commonly in high-producing dairy cows, feedlot cattle, or show cattle.

Clinical signs include stiffness, pain, reluctance to walk and difficulty in rising. Affected animals spend a lot of time lying down, and when they do stand, they may stand with their backs arched, front legs crossed, or kneeling on the front legs in an attempt to redistribute body weight because of the pain. Acute cases of laminitis are treated by correcting any existing underlying problem and administration of NSAIDs. Laminitis often leads to serious sequela including sole ulcers, white-line disease, abnormal hoof growth with horizontal or vertical hoof wall cracks (normal hoof growth is about 0.5 cm per month), underrun heel and sole, and even osteomyelitis or septic arthritis. Frequent foot trimming helps prevent development of these problems.

> ### ✒ TECHNICIAN NOTE
> Acute laminitis may be due to sudden excess grain ingestion or may occur secondary to other diseases that occur during the postparturient period such as retained placenta, metritis, mastitis, ketosis, or abomasal displacement.

INTERDIGITAL HYPERPLASIA

Interdigital hyperplasia (interdigital fibroma, corn) is a thickening of the interdigital skin, which causes a mass to protrude between the claws (Figure 30-11). One or more feet may be involved, but the hind feet are more commonly affected. Beef breeds, especially bulls, have a higher incidence of corns. Fibromas develop in response to chronic irritation between the claws. Hereditary predisposition is suspected. Spreading of the toes and other conformational problems probably contribute to irritation of the interdigital skin.

The size of the mass varies from a noticeable thickening of the skin to a size of 3 cm or more. A large mass can cause pain and the fibroma may become eroded, ulcerated, and even infected leading to more swelling and pain. Lameness varies, depending on the size of the mass, from absent to severe. Size of the corn and degree of lameness are guides in determining whether removal is necessary. Surgical excision is accomplished using IV retrograde analgesia as described above.

SOLE (RUSTERHOLZ) ULCERS

A sole ulcer is a circumscribed loss of sole that exposes the corium (sensitive lamina or "quick"). The typical location of the lesion is near the axial (inside) aspect of the hind lateral claws near the heel-sole junction. Lesions are usually bilateral involving both hind lateral claws. In some cases sole loss is not evident, but there is a circular area of hemorrhage beneath the sole or the sole is yellow and soft; the ulcer becomes apparent when the undermined sole is trimmed away. Lameness usually isn't severe until granulation tissue develops from the exposed corium and protrudes from the defect in the sole. This granulation tissue retards development of new sole. These ulcers may become infected with extension of infection into the deeper tissues (navicular bursa, coffin joint and flexor tendons).

Sole ulcers are probably the direct result of laminitis. It is not certain but the higher incidence of ulcers in the lateral hind claws versus medial hind claws suggests anatomical or mechanical difference. Pressure on impact is greater at the heel-sole junction of the lateral claw. Localized ischemia from laminitis can lead to erosion of the sole.

Lameness can be severe and is worse when the granulation tissue protrudes or if deeper tissues are involved. The animal may abduct its leg slightly (an attempt to put more weight on the medial claw) or stand with the heel extending beyond the gutter. Since the condition is often bilateral, both hind feet should be checked even though lameness may be apparent in only one leg (usually the lesion is more advanced in one foot than the other). Treatment is aimed at controlling granulation tissue and preventing extension of infection into the deeper tissues. Treatment involves excision of excessive granulation tissue, placement of a wooden block on the medial claw to take weight bearing off the lateral claw, and use of a caustic substance such as copper sulfate or phenol-formalin with a bandage to control the granulation tissue. Prognosis is good if there is no deep infection; however, treatment requires time and money.

WHITE-LINE DISEASE

The white line is the area of fibrous connective tissue that joins the rigid hoof wall to the more resilient sole. Since the white line is soft, it is more vulnerable to penetration by foreign material. Dirt-filled cracks and fissures in the white line are not uncommon in normal feet, but when abscesses develop under the sole, lameness follows. Factors predisposing to white-line disease are continuously wet feet and animals with previous bouts of laminitis, which result in poor horn quality and decreased white-line strength.

A serious sequela to white-line disease is infection of the navicular bursa. Although the bursa is protected from direct penetration or infection by the flexor tendon, it is still vulnerable at the edges of the tendon. Occasionally, infection extends up along the wall, abscesses in the navicular bursa, and drains above the abaxial coronet (called *gravel*).

White-line abscesses cause lameness. The animal may walk or stand with the heel slightly raised or the limb abducted (again, an attempt to shift weight to the medial claw). Hoof testers help localize the lesions that are not obvious. Black lines, cracks and fissures should be followed and pared out. Opening of an abscess will often result in release of watery black exudate and gas. If the navicular bursa is involved, the heel will be swollen, hot, and painful. The sole should be pared to allow adequate opening and drainage of the abscess, and the lateral wall should be trimmed to prevent packing of dirt and manure back into the abscess hole.

UNDERRUN HEEL AND SOLE

This condition is also referred to as *stable foot rot* and occurs primarily in the hind feet. The erosive process begins at the heel bulb initially as pits or pockmarks, and then parallel

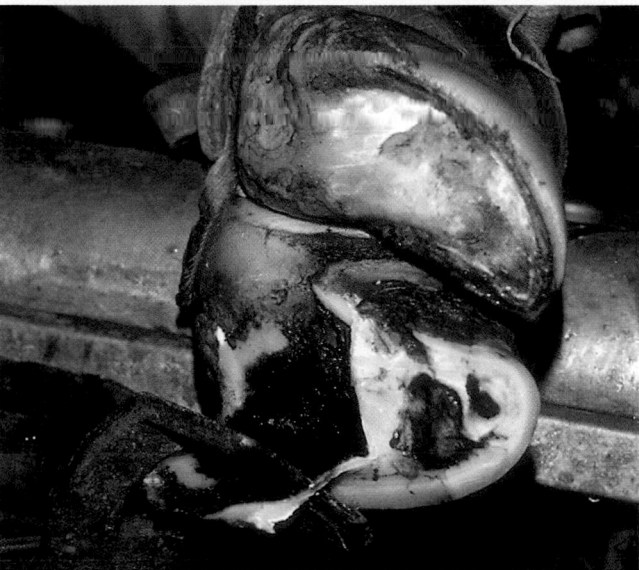

Figure 30-12 Debris packed between layers of sole causing lameness in a bull with underrun heel and sole.

horizontal grooves develop and fill with black necrotic material. The anaerobic bacteria *Fusobacterium necrophorum* and *Bacteroides nodosus* have both been isolated from these cases. The sole can separate to form a flap that may extend to the toe with a new sole developing underneath (Figure 30-12). Debris can become packed between the sole layers causing lameness. Underrun heels may not cause lameness unless there is infection of deeper structures or a lot of debris gets pack between the sole layers.

This condition may result from chronic laminitis, which causes hoof overgrowth (especially at the toe) and shifting of the animal's weight to the area of the heel. The abnormal and underrun sole should be removed to treat this condition. If sensitive lamina is exposed, the foot may need to be topically treated with antimicrobials and bandaged until the area becomes tough enough to bear weight. A wooden block on the opposite claw may be helpful during the healing process. Prevention includes regular hoof trimming to keep the animal from walking on its heels and the use of footbaths or regular topical treatment to control anaerobic bacterial infection in the area.

CLAW AMPUTATION

Diseases of the foot may become so severe that they cannot be treated, thus necessitating amputation of the affected digit. Any of the previously discussed conditions of the foot as well as other diseases may lead to infection of deeper tissues with resulting osteomyelitis of first phalanx (P1), second phalanx (P2), or third phalanx (P3) and/or septic arthritis of the proximal or distal interphalangeal joints (pastern or coffin joint). In cases of advanced infection, removal of the infected claw may be the only treatment option. This procedure is performed using the previously described IV retrograde block. The affected claw is then removed at a level necessary to remove all infected tissue using OB wire (it should be noted that amputation can only be performed distal to the fetlock joint). The claw should be removed at a cosmetic angle and through bone rather than through a joint. The foot is then bandaged snugly after topical antibiotic application. Bandage changes should be done every 3 days until any exposed bone is covered with granulation tissue. The entire healing process takes about 6 weeks. Cattle can support weight on one claw but will eventually experience breakdown of supporting structures of the remaining claw. The time it takes for breakdown depends on the claw removed, the weight and use of the animal, and the surface on which the animal must stand. It is undesirable to remove any claw in a bull, except for salvage purposes, and it is not generally a good choice to remove a weight-bearing claw (front medial or hind lateral) in cows, although sometimes there is no choice.

> ### ✎ TECHNICIAN NOTE
> Diseases of the foot may become so severe that they *cannot* be treated, thus necessitating amputation of the affected digit.

WOODEN BLOCK APPLICATION

Wooden blocks or commercial rubber shoes may be glued to the bottom of healthy claws in order to reduce or eliminate weight bearing on a diseased or painful claw. These devices are adhered to the claw using an acrylic material (Technovit, Jorgensen Laboratories, Inc.). Wooden blocks may last as long as 6 weeks and may be allowed to wear off naturally unless they are wearing abnormally, in which case they may be manually removed earlier. Blocks or shoes help promote healing of affected claws as well as making the animal more comfortable when standing or moving.

BLACKLEG AND MALIGNANT EDEMA

Infections by *Clostridium chauvoei* (blackleg) and *Clostridium septicum* (malignant edema) are two important causes of lameness and sudden death in young cattle. These bacteria produce spores that enter the animal through either the digestive tract or skin wounds, producing a severe necrotizing myositis and cellulitis. Affected animals develop high fever and lameness due to severe muscle damage. The swollen muscle mass often contains gas pockets that are palpable subcutaneously as crepitus.

Animals with these infections are usually found dead. Those animals caught in the early stages of infection may be treated with high doses of penicillin along with debridement and topical treatment of the wounds; however, prognosis for recovery is poor. The best way to prevent these clostridial diseases, as well as others, is to vaccinate calves with a multivalent bacterin at 2 months of age followed by a booster 4 to 6 weeks later (see Chapter 11). Cows should be vaccinated prior to calving to provide colostric protection to their calves.

HEMOLYMPHATIC SYSTEM

LYMPHOSARCOMA

The adult form of lymphosarcoma (LSA) is associated with BLV and is the most common neoplastic disease of cattle. Lymphosarcoma is mostly likely to affect cattle between the ages of 2 and 6 years. Although many cattle are exposed to BLV and any given herd may have a high incidence of cattle with titers to BLV, the actual number of cattle that develop neoplastic disease is small (<5%). Malignant tumors may develop in peripheral or deep lymph nodes, lymph tissue behind the eye or around the spinal cord, abomasum, heart, kidney, uterus, or other organs; therefore, clinical signs may vary greatly depending on the organ(s) or system(s) involved. Occasionally a lymphocytosis with the presence of neoplastic lymphocytes is apparent when a complete blood cell count (CBC) is performed. Diagnostic tests to help confirm lymphosarcoma may include a CBC, lymph node biopsy, paracentesis, thoracocentesis, a cerebral spinal fluid (CSF) centesis, or a BLV titer. A positive titer to BLV only suggests exposure to the virus but does not confirm neoplastic disease. There is no treatment or vaccine available, and the disease is always fatal. Since BLV titers are so prevalent in cattle herds, it is unlikely that a test and cull program would ever be initiated. Because the virus is spread by infected lymphocytes, every effort should be made to prevent transfer of blood between infected and noninfected animals (e.g., by changing needles and disinfecting surgery instruments between animals).

> ### ✎ TECHNICIAN NOTE
> Malignant tumors associated with adult lymphosarcoma due to BLV may develop in peripheral or deep lymph nodes, lymph tissue behind the eye, or around the spinal cord, abomasum, heart, kidney, uterus, or other organs; therefore, clinical signs may vary greatly depending on the organ(s) or system(s) involved.

ANAPLASMOSIS

Anaplasmosis, caused by the intraerythrocytic organism, *Anaplasma marginale*, is primarily a disease of adult cattle. Red blood cells infected with the organism are removed from the circulation by the liver and spleen and are subsequently destroyed resulting in a severe anemia. Resulting clinical signs from the development of acute anemia include pale mucous membranes, icterus, weakness, and depression or aggressive behavior due to anoxia to the brain. Anaplasmosis often causes sudden death without obvious clinical signs, and it must be differentiated from other causes of sudden death such as anthrax, clostridial diseases, bloat, and lightning. The organism is sensitive to tetracycline, so this drug is used for treatment as well as prevention of the disease. There is currently no commercial vaccine available for prevention of anaplasmosis.

ANTHRAX

Bacillus anthracis is the etiologic agent of this acute disease causing sudden death in animals and humans. Anthrax is endemic in many areas of the southern United States. Since people can easily contract the disease, it is important not to perform a necropsy on any animal suspected of having anthrax. Exposure of anthrax bacilli to the air, as in the case of necropsy, results in spore formation by the organism and permanent contamination of the surrounding environment. If anthrax is strongly suspected as the cause of death, the area federal veterinarian should be notified immediately. Anthrax-contaminated carcasses should be buried in lime or incinerated. A live vaccine is available, and its use should be considered in high-risk areas. The organism is sensitive to penicillin, but in most cases treatment cannot be initiated quickly enough. In recent years anthrax has become an important issue in cases of bioterrorism.

✏ TECHNICIAN NOTE

Anaplasmosis, anthrax, clostridial diseases, lightning, and bloat are causes of sudden death in cattle.

REPRODUCTIVE SYSTEM/ MAMMARY GLAND

MASTITIS

Mastitis is inflammation of the mammary gland due to invasion of the streak canal of the teat by a variety of bacterial pathogens. Economically, mastitis is one of the most important diseases in the dairy industry, and it is the single most common disease syndrome in adult dairy cows. Anatomically, the mammary gland is relatively resistant to infection, but severe environmental contamination of the teats, injury to the streak canal, or improperly functioning milking machine equipment may predispose the udder to infection.

Clinical signs of mastitis vary considerably based on the etiologic agent and may present as an asymptomatic subclinical infection to one in which the gland is markedly swollen and the milk is grossly abnormal. In general, mastitis can be subdivided into two broad but overlapping categories based on source of infection: contagious and environmental. Contagious mastitis is spread from an infected mammary gland to a healthy one via contaminated milking equipment, nursing calves, or by the milker's hands. *Streptococcus agalactiae* and *Staphylococcus aureus* are examples of bacteria causing contagious mastitis. Environmental mastitis results when bacteria within reservoirs in the environment gain access to the mammary gland and cause infection. Those organisms characteristically associated with environmental mastitis include the coliform bacteria. Other mastitis-causing organisms that fall between these two broad categories, maintaining alternate niches either in the host or in the environment include *Streptococcus dysgalactia* and *Streptococcus uberis*. Mastitis, depending on the etiology, causes various abnormal secretions ranging from the presence of milk with flakes or clots to purulent material. The degree of inflammatory response varies also depending on cause. Other classifications of mastitis include acute or toxic mastitis usually caused by coliforms or *Staphylococcus aureus*, chronic mastitis caused by *Staphylococcus aureus*, or acute gangrenous mastitis, the cause of which may be *Staphylococcus aureus* or *Clostridium perfringens*. Cows with toxic mastitis are usually very ill, have watery or serous secretion from the affected gland(s), and have low serum calcium such that they may resemble a case of milk fever. Gangrenous mastitis causes gangrene of the gland with a distinct blue line of demarcation separating normal and affected tissues. Secretions from affected glands are watery and serosanguineous, the gangrenous portions will be cold to the touch, and these portions of the gland will eventually slough. Toxic and gangrenous mastitis may cause death of the cow.

Mastitis is best diagnosed by clinical examination of the udder and milk and the use of the California Mastitis Test (CMT). The CMT is performed by mixing equal parts of CMT reagent and milk. A plastic paddle with four separate compartments is provided with the test kit so that each quarter can be individually evaluated. The reagent reacts with leukocytes that are usually present in large numbers when mastitis is present. When this reaction occurs, the reagent-milk mixture thickens or gels in proportion to the number of white cells present and indicates the severity of the inflammation. The greater the reaction, the higher the CMT score. CMT scores are designated as negative, trace, 1, 2, and 3 with corresponding cell counts of 100,000, 300,000, 900,000, 2,700,000, and 8,100,000. Aseptic collection of a milk sample for culture and antimicrobial sensitivity often provides information on etiology and appropriate drug therapy.

Depending on the etiologic agent, mastitis can be successfully treated if recognized early. Treatment of mastitis involves the use of appropriate antimicrobial therapy, systemic and/or intramammary. Frequent stripping of affected quarter(s) helps remove infected secretions and promotes quicker recovery. Cows with toxic mastitis may need intensive treatment with NSAIDs, IV fluid therapy, and calcium in those cows with hypocalcemia. Only antibiotics approved for use in dairy cows should be administered for the treatment of mastitis. In addition, antibiotic milk witdrawal times should be closely monitored. The veterinary technician should be familiar with these approved drugs and their withdrawal times and can serve as an important resource for education of the dairy farmer.

Prevention of mastitis is of paramount importance in the dairy industry. Control may be achieved by implementation of the Five-Point Plan for Mastitis Control, which includes

1. Hygiene: pre- and postmilking teat dipping and efforts to keep cows clean and dry between milkings.
2. Use proper milking procedures with well-functioning equipment when milking.
3. Practice dry cow treatment of every quarter of every cow and develop a veterinary-prescribed therapeutic plan for clinical cases.
4. Cull cows as necessary based on economics.
5. Maintain good records on each cow concerning production, reproduction, milk quality, and clinical mastitis.

> ✏️ **TECHNICIAN NOTE**
>
> Control of mastitis in cattle may be achieved by implementation of the Five-Point Plan for Mastitis Control.

DYSTOCIA

Dystocia or difficult calving in cattle is relatively common, especially in first-calf heifers, and frequently requires veterinary assistance. Dystocia may result from fetal oversize, maternal undersize, or fetal malposition. In order to recognize if a problem exists, the veterinary technician should be familiar with the normal signs of impending parturition as well as the stages of parturition. When a cow or heifer is nearing parturition, relaxation of the pelvic ligaments, swelling of the vulva, and udder development occur. During stage I of labor, the cervix dilates and the chorioallantoic membrane ruptures, releasing a large volume of clear, yellow fluid. Stage II is marked by the appearance of fetal extremities at the vulva along with the amniotic membrane. Normally the cow or heifer will deliver the calf within 2 hours of this observation. If delivery takes longer than 2 hours or if the cow stops straining, the cow should be examined and veterinary assistance may be indicated. Stage III involves passage of the placenta.

When dystocia is suspected, the cow should be quickly and thoroughly examined to rule out hypocalcemia as a cause of uterine inertia. Prior to vaginal examination, the vulva and perineal area should be thoroughly cleaned with a mild disinfectant. A sterile, nonirritating lubricant such as carboxymethylcellulose can be used to perform the vaginal exam, and it may be pumped into the uterus to facilitate manipulation, repositioning, and delivery of the calf. Once any malposition is corrected, obstetrical chains can be placed on the legs of the calf to apply traction for delivery. The chains should be looped above the fetlocks and half-hitched below the fetlocks to more evenly distribute the pulling forces on the legs. A single loop of the chain on each leg is much more likely to result in physeal fractures. If the calf's head is in normal position, a snare may be placed around the head to aid delivery. Excessive force should be avoided during forced fetal extraction in order to prevent nerve injury to the cow and fractures of the calf's legs. A mechanical calf extractor can be used carefully when manual traction is unavailable. If the calf cannot safely be delivered by this technique, then fetotomy or cesarean section should be considered.

Fetotomies are usually reserved for removal of calves that are dead or emphysematous. It involves the use of specialized instruments to dissect the dead calf in utero in order to deliver it more easily.

Cesarean section is indicated when there is a chance of delivering a live calf. Several approaches are available for cesarean section including flank approaches (right or left), paramedian approaches (right or left), or the ventral midline approach. The technique used is determined by the size, temperament, and physical condition of the cow as well as the veterinary surgeon's preference.

> ✏️ **TECHNICIAN NOTE**
>
> During forced fetal extraction, obstetrical chains should be looped above the calf's fetlocks and half-hitched below the fetlocks to more evenly distribute the pulling forces on the legs to prevent physeal fractures.

VAGINAL AND UTERINE PROLAPSE

Vaginal prolapse is a fairly common occurrence in cattle (Figure 30-13). It usually occurs in pluripara cows during

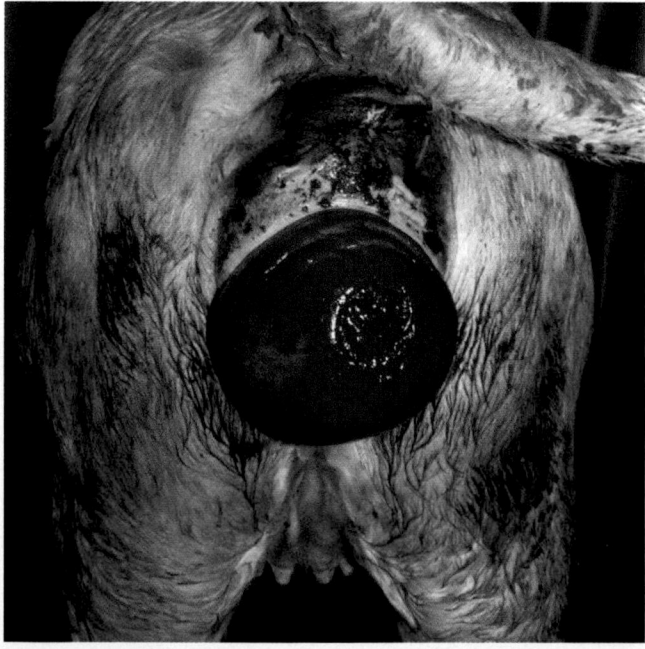

Figure 30-13 Vaginal prolapse in a prepartum cow. Recurrence during subsequent pregnancies is common.

the last 2 months of gestation and tends to recur during subsequent pregnancies. Hereford, Santa Gertrudis, and Holstein breeds seem to be more commonly affected. Factors that influence the development of vaginal prolapses include increased estrogen levels in late pregnancy, increased fetal size with increased intraabdominal pressure in late pregnancy, bulky diets causing increased intraabdominal pressure, recumbency that forces the urinary bladder and other organs into the pelvic cavity and places pressure on the constrictor vestibuli muscle, and obesity with proliferation of pelvic fat (vaginal prolapse can occur in overconditioned, nonpregnant heifers). A new population of vaginal prolapse cows is emerging in embryo donor cows that are super-ovulated. Hormonal extremes are a suggested cause of vaginal prolapse in these cows.

Initially the vaginal prolapse may be intermittent, only protruding when the animal is lying down, but eventually it progresses to the point that it remains prolapsed at all times. Although vaginal prolapses are not emergencies, they should be repaired soon after noticed by the owner. The most common method of repair is the Buhner technique (see below). Since this condition usually occurs prior to calving, the cow will need to be observed closely for signs of impending parturition. Owners should be advised to cull these cows since this is likely to recur with subsequent pregnancies.

Uterine prolapse is very common in the cow due to the anatomic suspension of the uterus (Figure 30-14) It occurs at parturition or shortly thereafter while the cervix is fully dilated. The uterus invaginates and the uterine mucosa

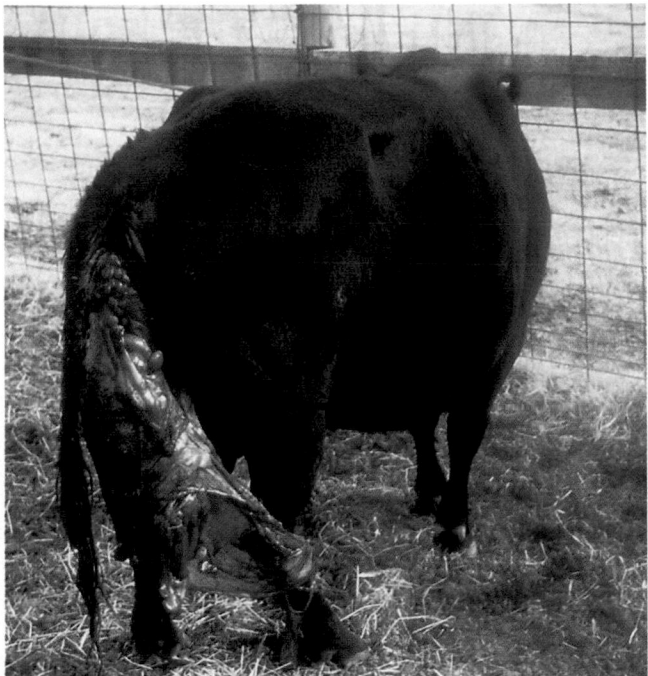

Figure 30-14 Uterine eversion with exposure of the caruncles in a postpartum cow.

protrudes through the vulvar lips. Uterine prolapse is more likely to occur in first-calf heifers and is not likely to recur at subsequent calvings. Factors playing a role in the development of uterine prolapses include concurrent hypocalcemia, recumbency such as that due to obturator nerve paralysis, dystocias with excessive straining, excessive force used during fetal extraction, and unnecessary traction on retained placentas.

Uterine prolapses are considered emergencies due to the possibility of shock from exposure of uterine mucosa, fatal hemorrhage due to rupture of the middle uterine arteries, and concurrent hypocalcemia. In addition, the urinary bladder and/or intestines may also be involved within the prolapse.

To prevent uterine prolapse, it is wise to force the animal to stand as soon as possible after calving and administer oxytocin to begin uterine involution.

Treatment consists of replacement of the prolapsed portion and application of a retention suture (Buhner) to prevent recurrence. This is best accomplished with the animal in a standing position with the aid of a caudal epidural (as previously described under urolithiasis). If the cow is already down and cannot get up, attempt to elevate the hindquarters or pull the cow's hind legs straight out behind her as she lies in sternal recumbency; an epidural helps maintain this position. Prior to replacement of the uterus, placenta is removed atraumatically if possible, the uterus is cleansed with warm water and a mild disinfectant, and the uterus is lubricated to facilitate replacement. Elevation of the uterus makes it easier to replace. The uterus is inserted a little at a time, making certain the apical end of each horn has been completely returned to its normal position. Oxytocin (40 IU), calcium if necessary, intrauterine antibiotics, and systemic antibiotics should be administered. The vulva is then sutured using the Buhner suture technique.

The Buhner suture technique is useful for retention of both vaginal and uterine prolapses. It is a buried pursestring suture that simulates the action of the constrictor vestibula muscle. To begin the suture pattern, a 1-cm horizontal skin incision is made midway between the dorsal commissure of the vulva and the anus. Another horizontal incision is made at the ventral commissure of the vulva. The Buhner needle is inserted into the ventral incision, driven deeply (5 to 8 cm) and directed out of the dorsal skin incision. The eye of the needle is threaded with Buhner suture tape, and the needle is pulled out through the ventral incision. The procedure is repeated on the opposite side resulting in two free ends of tape from the ventral incision. The suture is tightened so that only two to three fingers can be inserted into the vagina. This allows for normal urination but prevents reprolapse of the vagina or uterus. This suture may be completely buried and left in place indefinitely. The Buhner suture tape is particularly strong, will not disintegrate, and is well tolerated by the tissues. The tape may be tied such that it can be untied as the cow begins to calve as in the case of prepartum vaginal prolapse.

RETAINED PLACENTA (FETAL MEMBRANES)

After calving, the placenta is usually passed within 2 to 4 hours and is considered retained if it has not been expelled by 8 to 12 hours. Retained placenta is more common in dairy cows than beef cows. The cause is unknown, but it is more likely to occur following the birth of twins, following abortion during the last half of pregnancy, and in cases of dystocia. Selenium and vitamin A and E deficiencies have been suggested to cause an increased incidence of retained placentas.

Manual removal of the placenta should be avoided since this may result in endometrial damage and infection with prolonged uterine involution and delayed breeding. Retained placenta and endometritis may be treated with intrauterine infusions of appropriate antibiotics. Although uterine infusion is controversial, most veterinarians agree that cows with signs of systemic illness due to retained placenta should receive parenteral antibiotic therapy.

If abortion is the cause of retained fetal membranes, vaccination of cows and heifers for diseases causing abortion should be considered (see Chapter 11). If nutrition is suspected as a predisposing factor, the ration should be evaluated making certain that it contains recommended levels and ratios of calcium, phosphorus, vitamins A and E, and selenium. An injection of vitamin E/selenium 1 month prior to calving may reduce the incidence of retained placenta in problem herds.

FIBROPAPILLOMAS OF THE PENIS

Fibropapillomas of the penis in bulls are caused by the bovine papilloma virus (Figure 30-15). They tend to occur in young bulls housed together and are contracted from warts on other parts of the body when the bulls display homosexual behavior by "riding" each other. The warts may result in hesitancy or refusal to breed and may become large enough that they prevent extension (phimosis) or retraction (paraphimosis) of the penis. Surgical removal of the wart(s) is one treatment option and may be performed in conjunction with vaccination with either a commercial or autogenous wart vaccine. Recurrence is not uncommon.

PREPUTIAL PROLAPSE

Preputial prolapse tends to occur in bulls of *Bos indicus* influence (i.e., Brahman, Zebu) due to several predisposing breed, related factors including a pendulous sheath, long prepuce, large preputial orifice, and the absence of retractor prepuce muscles. The prepuce may become traumatized due to environmental exposure because of the inability of the bull to keep the prepuce within the preputial cavity, or trauma may occur as an accident during breeding. Once traumatized, the prepuce begins to swell and prolapses further, making it susceptible to further injury (Figure 30-16). The affected prepuce is treated initially by soak in warm water with Betadine and Epsom salts to reduce swelling and control infection. The prepuce is returned to the preputial cavity and wrapped with a tube in place to prevent further trauma. Once the inflammation and infection are under control, surgery (reefing) to remove scar tissue and shorten the prepuce may be considered if the bull is valuable. Without surgery, recurrence rate for preputial trauma and reprolapse is high.

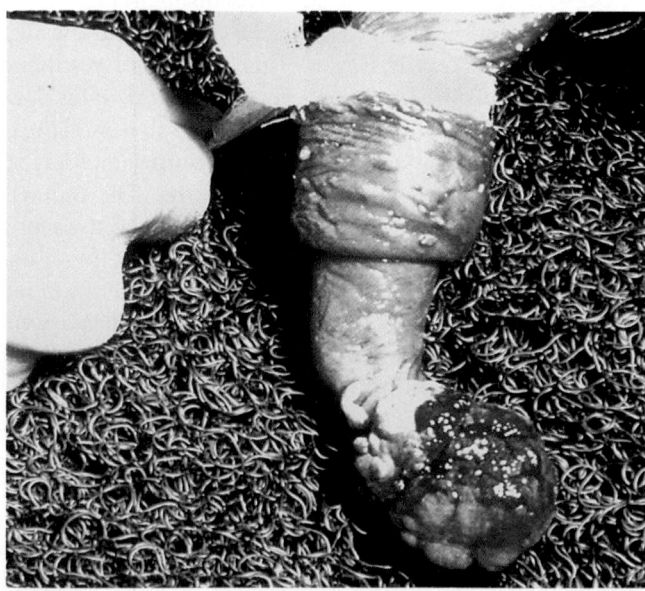

Figure 30-15 Fibropapillomas (warts) of the glans penis in a bull.

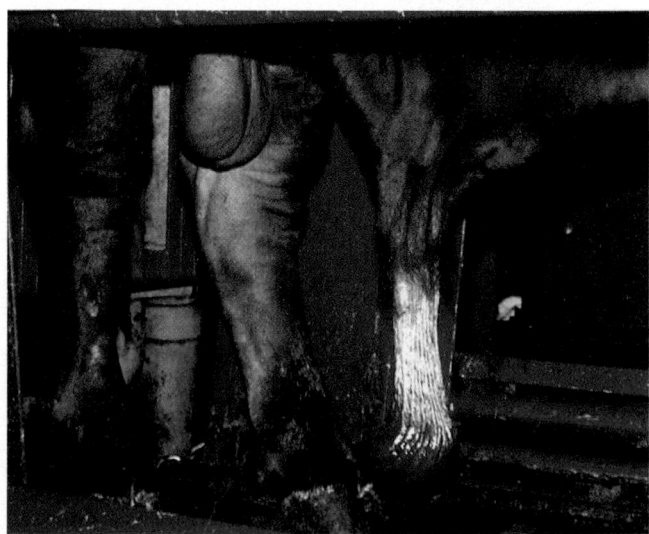

Figure 30-16 Prolapse of the prepuce of a *Bos indicus* bull with a pendulous sheath.

METABOLIC DISORDERS

PERIPARTURIENT HYPOCALCEMIA (MILK FEVER)

Milk fever is a common metabolic problem in periparturient dairy cows usually occurring within 48 hours of calving. It is unlikely to occur in first calf heifers, but the incidence of the condition increases with the age of the cow. It reportedly is more likely to occur in the Jersey breed. Milk fever is the result of a severe decline in serum calcium level (normal, 10 mg/dl). Hypocalcemia results from feeding of diets high in calcium during the late dry period (the last 2 months of gestation), which causes a lack of response by the parathyroid gland and a decrease in vitamin D levels. As a result, the cow is slow to mobilize calcium reserves from the bone when there is a sudden demand for calcium at the beginning of lactation.

Cows with hypocalcemia develop muscle tremors, weakness, and a staggering gait eventually leading to recumbency. Cows with milk fever often lie in sternal recumbency with their head turned into their flank. Affected cows have a dry nose, rumen atony with bloat, and no urine or feces production. Some cows with milk fever may be found in lateral recumbency. The heart rate is increased and pupils dilated. Unless the cow is treated quickly, she may die of the effects of low serum calcium. It is important to get a down cow up as soon as possible since recumbency leads to development of severe myositis of the muscles of the limbs and subsequent nerve damage resulting in a permanent "downer" cow.

Slow administration of calcium gluconate IV is the treatment of choice. Cows often respond rapidly to calcium therapy and will begin to lacrimate, eructate, urinate, and defecate. If the initial treatment helps but the cow does not stand, it may be necessary to administer additional calcium subcutaneously. If the cow does not respond to treatment, she should be reevaluated for persistent hypocalcemia or concurrent problems such as mastitis, metritis, or musculoskeletal or nerve damage. Cows in the very early stages of milk fever (prior to recumbency) often respond to administration of oral calcium gel.

Prevention of milk fever is achieved by providing a well-balanced, low-calcium diet during the dry period. The total dietary intake of calcium should not exceed 20 g per head per day. It is important to keep dry cows separate from the rest of the herd so that they can be fed properly not only to prevent milk fever but also to prevent overconditioning and fat liver syndrome.

KETOSIS (ACETONEMIA)

Ketosis occurs in high-producing dairy cows during the first few months of lactation if they are unable to meet the energy demands of lactation. In order to provide energy for milk production, the cow begins to mobilize fat, the breakdown of which results in the formation of ketone bodies that accumulate in the blood. Ketosis in dairy cows may result from a primary deficiency in energy intake, or it may occur secondary to a disease process such as abomasal displacement, mastitis, or metritis, which can cause anorexia.

Ketones have a characteristic odor that can be detected in the breath, milk, and urine of affected cows. Excessive amounts of ketones as well as low blood glucose may cause the cow to display nervous symptoms known as *nervous ketosis*.

Ketosis responds to administration of energy sources such as glucose IV, propylene glycol per os, or where appropriate, systemic corticosteroids. It is important to determine the cause of ketosis and to correct the underlying problem. The cow's ration should be examined to make certain it contains adequate digestible energy to meet requirements for maintenance and lactation.

CARDIOVASCULAR SYSTEM

VEGETATIVE OR VALVULAR ENDOCARDITIS

Vegetative or ulcerative lesions may develop on the heart valves, in particular the right atrioventricular (AV) valve, as a result of septic emboli from other sites such as omphalophlebitis or navel infection in calves. These lesions, if severe, may interfere with blood flow leading to congestive heart failure (CHF). The etiology is bacterial, usually *Arcanobacterium pyogenes* or α-hemolytic streptococcus in cattle. Vegetative endocarditis in pigs is usually due to streptococcus or *Erysipelothrix*. If fragments detach from the heart valve, embolic endoarteritis and abscesses in showered organs may follow. Clinical signs in cattle include history of a poor doing animal, presence of a murmur or thrill, exercise intolerance, CHF with jugular vein distention and dependent edema in advanced cases, and fluctuating fever (Figure 30-17). Clinical pathology in acute cases may show leukocytosis (>100,000 WBC) with a left shift, while chronic cases may have a normal CBC. Three serial blood cultures performed as the body temperature rises may yield bacterial growth. On necropsy the valve lesions may be large and cauliflower-like or small and wartlike. In chronic cases

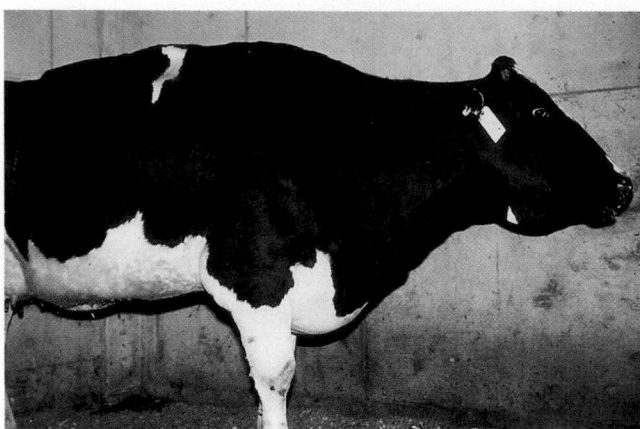

Figure 30-17 Ventral midline edema and jugular pulse in a cow with congestive heart failure.

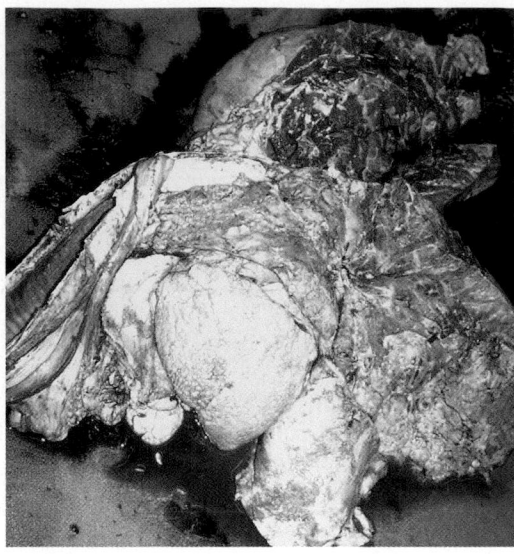

Figure 30-18 Severe fibrin formation with purulent exudate on the heart of a cow that died of pericarditis.

valves may be shrunken and distorted or scarred. Treatment is not very successful due to inadequate penetration of the lesions with antibiotics and the presence of irreversible damage to the valves. Penicillin at high levels (44,000 IU/kg bid) for long periods of time (2 to 3 weeks) has given the best results, although cephalosporins may also prove beneficial and are commonly used to treat young calves. Echocardiography, when available, is quite useful for visualizing valve lesions.

PERICARDITIS

Pericarditis causes inflammation of both the parietal and visceral surfaces of the pericardial cavity. True pericarditis is always infectious and nearly always exudative. It may be due to a blood-borne infection but is usually due to traumatic pericarditis, an extension of traumatic reticuloperitonitis. Pericarditis develops after penetration of the pericardial sac by a metallic foreign body (often occurs close to parturition). It results in a mixed bacterial infection that causes severe local inflammation. Inflammation causes deposition of fibrinous exudate leading to a friction rub (Figure 30-18). Effusion then develops creating splashing sounds around the heart especially if the fluid is mixed with gas, or it may cause muffled heart sounds. Fluid accumulation compromises heart function and can lead to CHF. Clinical signs include pain as evidenced by kyphosis, abduction of the elbows and shallow abdominal respirations. The temperature is slightly elevated, 103° F to 106° F. Pericardial friction sounds, fluid splashing sounds, or muffled heart sounds may be auscultated. Signs of CHF occur late in the course of the disease, and death is usually due to toxemia or CHF. Most cows die within 1 to 3 weeks, but a few persist with chronic pericarditis. These cows often have a leukocytosis (16,000 to 30,000 WBC). Pericardiocentesis can be performed at the four or fifth intercostal space at the level of the elbow on the left side to confirm the presence of pericarditis. Necropsy findings vary from hyperemia

and fibrin deposition to accumulation of purulent exudates, fibrin, and thickened pericardium/epicardium to adhesion of the pericardium to the epicardium as the condition progresses from acute to chronic. A metallic foreign body may also be present. Treatment is not very successful and requires long-term use of antibiotics. Pericardiocentesis provides only temporary relief and pericardiotomy (fifth or sixth rib resection) for drainage and flushing purposes can be attempted but is not highly successful.

> **◢ TECHNICIAN NOTE**
>
> Pericarditis in cattle is usually due to penetration of the pericardial sac by a metallic foreign body.

URINARY SYSTEM

UROLITHIAISIS

Urolithiasis is the result of formation of calculi (uroliths) within the urinary tract. The result of these uroliths varies from minor urinary tract irritation to complete obstruction of urine flow. The nonclinical manifestation of this condition is referred to as *urolithiasis*, while the clinical form is termed *obstructive urolithiasis*. When complete obstruction occurs, there is marked distention of the urinary bladder with eventual rupture of the bladder, the urethra, or both. Depending on the site of rupture, urine accumulates in the ventral subcutaneous tissues (urethra) or in the abdomen (bladder) resulting in swelling commonly referred to as *water belly*.

Although there is no sex predilection for development of calculi, males are much more likely to become obstructed

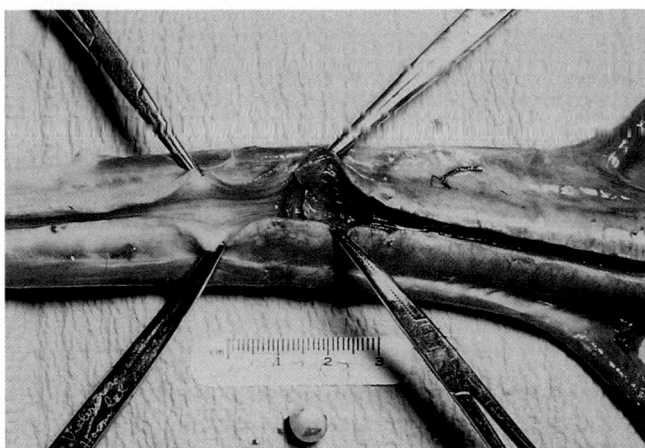

Figure 30-19 Identification of a calculus causing obstructive urolithiasis at the distal sigmoid flexure in a bull. Note urethral necrosis at the site where the calculus was lodged.

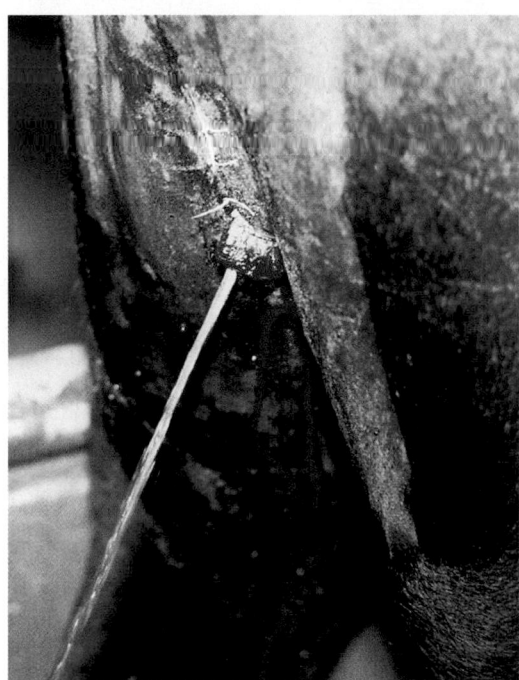

Figure 30-20 Perineal urethrostomy performed as a salvage procedure for treatment of obstructive urolithiasis in a steer.

due to the length, shape, and size of their urethra. The most common site of obstruction in cattle is the distal sigmoid flexure of the penis (Figure 30-19). Feedlot animals receiving grain rations with high phosphorus levels are predisposed to developing phosphate calculi.

Clinical signs of acute urethral obstruction are attributable to trauma to the urinary tract epithelium and bladder distention. Early in the course, the animal repeatedly assumes a posture for urination but little or no urination results from these attempts to void. As bladder distention progresses, the animal may tread, stretch, tail swish, and kick at its abdomen. Blood and/or crystals may be present on the preputial hairs. Nonspecific signs such as anorexia, mild bloat, and lethargy are also common. Owners often misinterpret these signs as evidence of acute gastrointestinal disorders especially since affected animals may show signs similar to colic. After the bladder or urethra ruptures, straining ceases and the animal may go through a brief phase of euphoria; however, azotemia [increased blood urea nitrogen (BUN) and creatinine] and dehydration quickly develop. If urethral obstruction is diagnosed early, before azotemia develops or before the bladder or urethra rupture, the animal may be immediately slaughtered. If not, medical and/or surgical treatment should be initiated quickly.

Medical management involves the use of muscle relaxants to facilitate passage of the calculi, antimicrobial therapy for urinary tract infection, and the use of a urinary acidifier such as ammonium chloride. Medical therapy alone is rarely successful, so it may be necessary to consider surgery in some cases. Perineal urethrostomy may be chosen as a salvage procedure particularly for feedlot steers or bulls of low economic value (Figure 30-20). This surgical approach allows for relief of obstruction and resolution of the uremia before slaughter. Long-term, urethral stricture has been a problem with this technique. The procedure is performed with the animal standing and analgesia provided by an epidural block. A caudal or low epidural provides loss of sensation to the anus, vulva, perineum, and caudal aspects of the thighs. It is used for relief of tenesmus and obstetric straining and vaginal, rectal and uterine prolapse repair, and surgical procedures of the perineal area. Injection is made between the first and second coccygeal (Cy1 to Cy2) vertebrae or in the sacrococcygeal space. The space is located by moving the tail up and down and while palpating for the first obvious articulation caudal to the sacrum. Using aseptic technique, an 18-gauge, 3.8-cm needle is inserted through the space on the midline at a 10-degree angle (tip of needle directed cranially) until a drop of lidocaine placed in the hub of the needle is sucked into the space. An alternative approach involves insertion of the needle until it hits the floor of the spinal canal at which time the needle is backed out slightly to enter the epidural space. There should be no resistance to injection. The dose of lidocaine used is 0.5 to 1 ml of 2% lidocaine per 45 kg body weight with which the animal should have adequate analgesia but remain standing.

The low approach is often preferred for perineal urethrostomy. This allows the penis to be diverted caudally at such an angle as to prevent urine scald to the hind legs. It also makes it possible to perform repeated procedures higher if necessary. The skin incision is made beginning at the dorsal aspect of the scrotum or scrotal remnant and extending dorsally on the midline for 10 to 15 cm. The incision is continued until the penis is encountered. The retractor penis muscles may be the first structures seen and are frequently mistaken for the penis. These muscles are superficial to the penis, pink, soft, and easily separated into two structures. The penis is a relatively firm, single structure covered by the white tunica albuginea. Once the penis has been located, it is bluntly dissected from the surrounding tough fascia and pulled caudally out of the incision. The penis is transected at a length adequate to allow the transected end to exit the perineal incision without tension leaving a 2- to 3-cm stump exposed. The stump is sutured to the skin of the lower part of the incision using a mattress suture that surrounds the corpus cavernosum penis (CCP) and passes under the urethra. This suture limits hemorrhage from the CCP. In addition, the urethra can be split for several centimeters and spatulated by suturing the urethral mucosa and tunica albuginea to the skin using 2-0 or 3-0 absorbable suture material. This optional technique is intended to limit stricture of the urethral opening. The remaining skin incision is closed with simple interrupted sutures of nonabsorbable suture material. Urethral obstruction may recur due to additional calculi or because of stricture of the urethrostomy site.

An alternative surgical procedure that can be used for valuable breeding bulls or "pets" is the ischial urethrostomy, a temporary urethrostomy with catheter placement. This technique allows for urine egress through a Foley catheter placed in the urethra at the level of the ischium, just below the anus, and antegrade or retrograde flushing of the distal urethra to remove calculi. When the tube is pulled, the urethrostomy usually heals by second intention without stricture formation. This procedure can be useful for preservation of fertility in valuable breeding bulls.

Dietary management is the key to control and prevention of obstructive urolithiasis. The calcium to phosphorus ratio of the overall diet should be in the range of 2:1 to 2.5:1. A continuous supply of fresh, clean water should be available at all times, and salt may be added to the ration up to 4% to promote water intake and diuresis. In addition, vitamin A may be added to the ration to help prevent desquamation of epithelial cells in the bladder. Prophylactic use of urinary acidifiers is advocated; administration of ammonium chloride at 1% to 1.5% of the ration is recommended.

> ✐ **TECHNICIAN NOTE**
> Perineal urethrostomy may be chosen as a salvage procedure for feedlot steers with obstructive urolithiasis.

CONTAGIOUS BOVINE PYELONEPHRITIS

Contagious bovine pyelonephritis, caused by *Corynebacterium renale*, is an ascending urinary tract infection often affecting females due to their short, wide urethra. Infection occurs more often in the periparturient period when cows are more stressed and the urogenital tract is more susceptible to entry of bacteria.

Clinical findings include hematuria, pyuria, straining (stranguria) and discomfort during urination, and frequent urination (pollakiuria). Affected cows may have a fluctuating fever, variable appetite, and decreased milk production. If the left kidney is affected, rectal palpation may reveal an enlarged, fluctuant, painful kidney.

Treatment is often unrewarding but may be attempted using high doses of penicillin (44,000 U/kg b.i.d.) for long periods of time. In valuable animals in which only one kidney is affected, nephrectomy may be indicated.

NERVOUS SYSTEM

RABIES

Rabies is a fatal, viral, neurological disease of warm-blooded animals. Rabies is most often transmitted by the bite of an infected wild animal with skunks, raccoons, and foxes being the greatest threat to domestic livestock. Two forms of rabies may occur: the furious form in which the affected animal demonstrates hyperexcitability, fear, or rage or the dumb form in which extreme depression, paresis, or paralysis manifest.

Clinical signs of rabies may include bloat, tenesmus, bellowing, aggressiveness, and increased sexual activity. *Hydrophobia*, the common name for rabies, stems from the inability of the animal to drink due to pharyngeal/laryngeal paralysis. Death occurs within 10 days of the onset of clinical signs. Definitive diagnosis is made by fluorescent antibody testing of the brain, the presence of Negri bodies (cytoplasmic inclusions in neurons) on histopathology, and mouse inoculation.

Several vaccines are available for use in cattle and sheep (see Chapter 11). Rabies poses a serious human health concern; therefore care should be taken when handling animals suspected of having rabies (i.e., gloves should be worn during oral examination). A veterinary technician who practices in areas where rabies incidence is high should strongly consider being vaccinated for rabies.

> ✐ **TECHNICIAN NOTE**
> Rabies poses a serious human health concern; therefore gloves should always be worn during oral examination of animals suspected of having rabies.

POLIOENCEPHALOMALACIA (POLIO)

Polioencephalomalacia is a central nervous system (CNS) disease that results from an underlying defect in thiamine metabolism. The disease may occur secondary to grain overload as previously discussed, or other sudden ration changes may precipitate its development. The coccidiostat amprolium administered at high doses or for long periods of time has induced polioencephalomalacia.

Affected animals show neurological signs including blindness, ataxia, depression, opisthotonus, dorsomedial strabismus, convulsions, coma, and death. Polioencephalomalacia, if treated early, responds well to treatment with thiamine; however, the longer the animal has been affected, the longer it takes for recovery, and recovery may not be complete (i.e., blindness may persist). Addition of thiamine or brewer's yeast to the ration in high-risk situations may be beneficial in preventing disease.

LISTERIOSIS

Listeria monocytogenes is responsible for three different clinical syndromes in ruminants: septicemia, abortion, and neurological disease. Neurological involvement produces fever, anorexia, depression, proprioceptive deficits, head tilt, and circling. Cranial nerve dysfunction causes unilateral drooping of the ear, eyelid, nose, and lips with excessive salivation. While ingestion of contaminated corn silage is blamed, consumption of any rotting contaminated vegetation can serve as the source of infection.

The organism is sensitive to tetracycline or penicillin, but treatment of listeriosis is often unrewarding. No vaccine is available for protection against this disease. The organism has zoonotic potential and poses a serious human health risk when contaminated milk, milk products, or meat have entered the food chain.

THROMBOEMBOLIC MENINGOENCEPHALITIS

Thromboembolic meningoencephalitis (TEME) is the result of septic emboli in the brain secondary to septicemia caused by *Haemophilus somnus*. Animals affected with TEME show neurological signs that are consistent with the areas of brain that are damage by the emboli. The organism is found primarily in the respiratory tract and usually causes pneumonia. It is not unusual for some individuals to develop neurological disease after an outbreak of pneumonia in a group of feedlot cattle.

Diagnosis is made by finding the characteristic hemorrhagic lesions scattered throughout the brain. With confirmation of the disease, treatment of the herd with tetracycline may be beneficial in preventing more cases and vaccination with *Haemophilus bacterin* may be indicated.

OBTURATOR AND SCIATIC NERVE PARESIS AND PARALYSIS

The obturator and/or sciatic nerves may sustain damage during dystocia or forced fetal extraction resulting in "calving paralysis." Treatment consists of the use of NSAIDs early, good nursing care, housing the animal on a soft surface with good footing, lifting the cow or heifer for short periods

of time at least a couple of times a day, rolling the cow from side to side several times daily to prevent severe muscle compression, and hobbling cows or heifers that can stand but cannot adduct their hind legs.

> **⬥ TECHNICIAN NOTE**
>
> During dystocia or forced fetal extraction, the obturator and/or sciatic nerves may sustain damage resulting in "calving paralysis."

DISEASES OF THE EYE

INFECTIOUS BOVINE KERATOCONJUNCTIVITIS

Infectious bovine keratoconjunctivitis (IBK), or pinkeye, is an infectious and contagious ocular disease of cattle characterized by conjunctivitis and keratitis with ulceration (Figure 30-21). Ultraviolet light and mechanical irritants such as dust and weeds may disrupt the corneal epithelium, allowing entry of *Moraxella bovis*, the etiologic agent of pinkeye. Flies have been shown to act as vectors for the bacteria.

Initial clinical signs include lacrimation, blepharospasm, and photophobia. Corneal inflammation followed by ulceration eventually develops. If ulceration becomes deep, the cornea may rupture and vision will be lost.

Individual treatment of pinkeye involves subconjunctival injection of antibiotics, usually procaine penicillin G (Figure 30-22). Eye patches may be applied to affected eyes to decrease photophobia and protect the eye from flies. More severe cases may require surgery such as a third eyelid flap or tarsorrhaphy (suturing the lids closed) to protect deeper ulcers as they heal. In the case of herd outbreaks

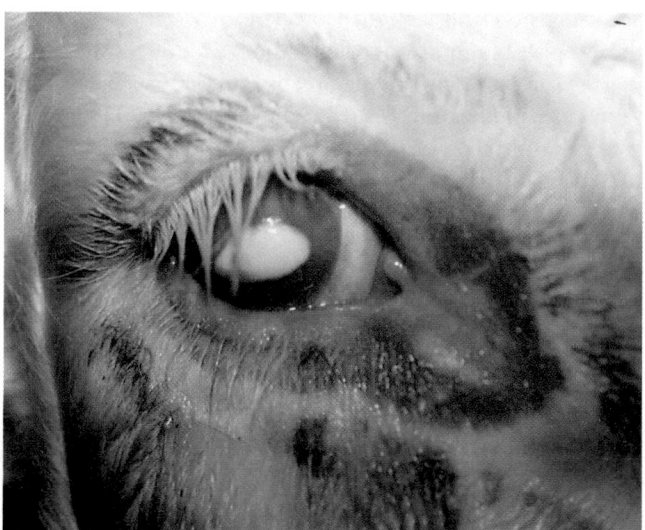

Figure 30-21 A large central corneal ulcer with abscess in a bull with infectious bovine keratoconjunctivitis (IBK, pinkeye).

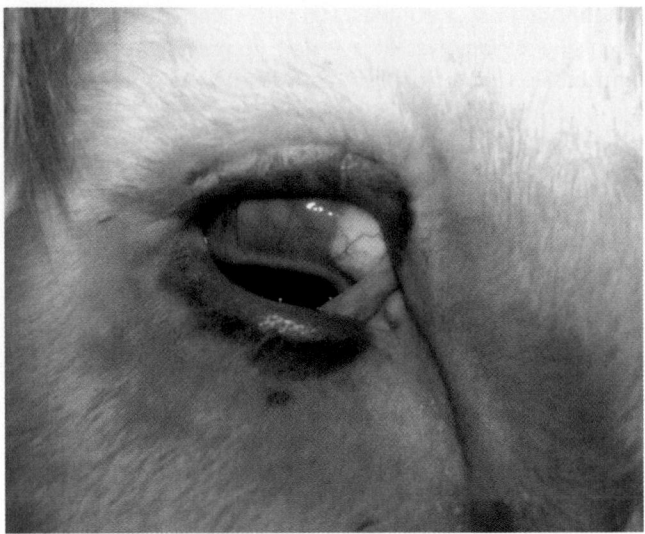

Figure 30-22 Procaine penicillin G injected subconjunctivally for treatment of IBK (pinkeye).

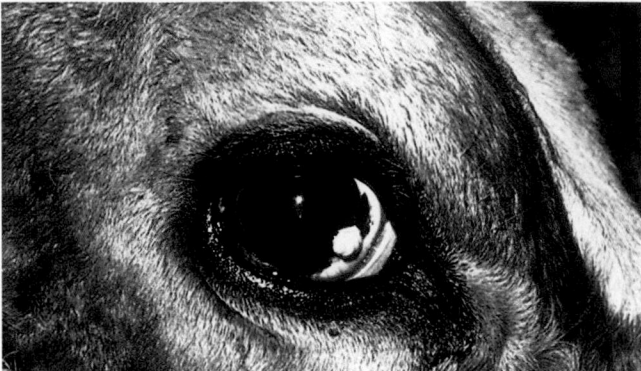

Figure 30-23 OSCC (cancer eye) lesion of the medial canthus of the eye of a cow.

it may be impractical to treat each animal with local therapy, so systemic antibiotics, such as long-acting tetracycline, can be administered to the group.

OCULAR SQUAMOUS CELL CARCINOMA (CANCER EYE)

Ocular squamous cell carcinoma (OSCC), the most common tumor of cattle, is estimated to cause annual losses of $20 million in beef cattle in the United States. Losses result from condemnation of affected carcasses and loss of prime breeding stock.

The etiology is multifactorial; there appears to be a genetic predisposition for development of ocular squamous cell tumors, and exposure to ultraviolet radiation (amount and intensity) and lack of protective pigmentation around the eye play an important role. Tumors occur predominantly in Herefords but also other breeds with similar patterns of periocular pigmentation such as Simmentals and Holsteins. It is seldom seen in animals less than 4 years of age and peak age of occurrence is 8 years. The tumors begin as benign plaques or papillomas that often progress quickly to squamous cell carcinoma. Common sites for development of malignancy in decreasing order of prevalence are the lateral and medial limbus (Figure 30-23), eyelids (especially lower), third eyelid, and medial canthus.

Treatment modalities include cryotherapy, radiofrequency hyperthermia, immunotherapy, chemotherapy, radiation therapy, and surgery (keratectomy, lid resection, or extirpation). Although commonly referred to as *enucleation*, the term *extirpation* is more accurate. Extirpation is removal of all the contents of the bony orbit. Since this procedure is commonly performed for advanced cases of OSCC where removal of all ocular tissue is crucial and because cosmetic appearance is not as important in cattle, we are more likely to perform extirpation rather than evisceration or enucleation of the eye.

Extirpation is performed with the aid of a retrobulbar or Peterson eye block. To perform the Peterson block an 18-gauge, 12-cm needle bent to a slight curve is used to block cranial nerves II, IV, V, and VI as they emerge from the round foramen. The needle enters the skin at the angle produced by the supraorbital process and the zygomatic arch and is directed medially. The concavity of the needle is directed caudally so that the point of the needle will pass around the cranial border of the coronoid process of the mandible and to the pterygopalatine fossa of the skull. A reliable indication of proper position is a severe twitching of the eyelids. Once the proper position is located, 5 cc of local anesthetic is injected. The needle is repositioned slightly two more times with injection of 5 cc of local anesthetic each time. Aspiration is essential prior to injection to avoid depositing lidocaine in the CSF, possibly resulting in sudden death. Before withdrawing the needle completely, it is redirected caudally just beneath the skin along the zygomatic arch to block the auriculopalpebral nerve. The four-point retrobulbar block is performed by injecting through the eyelids, both dorsally and ventrally, and at the medial and lateral canthi using a slightly curved, 18-gauge, 12-cm needle that is directed to the apex of the orbit. Five to 10 ml of local anesthetic are injected at each site. Exophthalmos, corneal anesthesia, and mydriasis indicate a satisfactory retrobulbar block.

The eye is surgically prepared, and the lids are sutured or clamped together. A transpalpebral incision is made approximately 1 cm from the lid margins (unless the disease extends beyond this margin). The skin incision is full thickness but does not penetrate the palpebral conjunctiva; the conjunctival sac helps contain contaminated ocular structures during surgery. Sharp dissection is continued 360 degrees around the bony orbit. The orbital ligament is incised at the medial canthus, and the muscles, adipose, lacrimal glands, and fascia are removed. The optic artery can be ligated, significantly reducing hemorrhage, or the lids can be tightly closed and a gauze stent placed over the incision to provide pressure and hemostasis. The lids are closed with appositional or everting interrupted sutures using non-absorbable no. 3 suture material. If excessive skin must be removed such that the incision cannot be closed, the orbit can be packed with gauze that is removed in 48 to 72 hours. The incision is left to heal by second intention. NSAIDs and antibiotics may be administered prior to surgery.

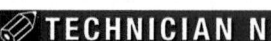

> **TECHNICIAN NOTE**
>
> OSCC, the most common tumor of cattle, results in large economic losses to cattle producers.

DISEASES OF THE SKIN

CUTANEOUS PAPILLOMAS (WARTS)

Warts, a benign neoplasia caused by the papilloma virus, are very common in young cattle. They appear as tan, white, or gray protruding masses with a dry, horny surface. They vary greatly in size and shape and can persist for 3 to 12 months at which time they often spontaneously regress.

Small warts may be crushed or surgically removed to help stimulate development of natural immunity and hasten healing. Cryosurgical treatment has also been successful. Use of autogenous and commercial vaccines has met with variable success. Since warts are usually self-limiting, no treatment may be necessary; however, in long-standing, severe, or nonresponsive cases, the immune status of the patient must be considered, and slaughter or euthanasia may be necessary.

DERMATOPHYTOSIS (RINGWORM)

Trichophyton verrucosum is the fungus responsible for ringworm in cattle. Ringworm is most likely to occur in calves housed in crowded conditions in the winter. Multiple circular lesions develop particularly around the head and neck. The lesions, which are several centimeters in diameter, consist of an area of alopecia surrounding a slightly raised, whitish accumulation of dry, scaly skin. If left untreated, most lesions heal on their own in 2 to 3 months especially if calves are turned out to pasture and exposed to the sunlight in the spring.

If treatment is desired especially in the case of show animals, topical agents such as iodine, bleach (1:10 in water), chlorhexidine, Captan, 5% lime sulfur, and thiabendazole may be useful. Immunocompetency of the animal should be questioned in cases that do not respond spontaneously or with treatment.

DERMATOPHILUS (STREPTOTRICHOSIS, RAIN SCALD)

Dermatophilus is caused by the bacterium *Dermatophilus congolensis*. The bacteria invade the skin and produce crusts, which cause matting of the hair giving it a typical "paintbrush" appearance. The disease is more prevalent during periods of heavy rainfall or high humidity. Trauma, abrasions, concurrent disease, and poor nutrition make the skin more susceptible to infection. The disease may be transmitted by insect vector or direct contact with infected animals.

Treatment is accomplished by removal of crusts by grooming followed by repeated iodine- or chlorhexidine-based shampoos. More severe cases may require systemic antimicrobials such as penicillin or long-acting tetracycline. Exposure to the sunlight and disinfection of grooming equipment and housing helps control reinfection and spread of the bacteria.

> **TECHNICIAN NOTE**
>
> Dermatophilus or rain scald, a common bacterial skin disease of cattle, is more prevalent during periods of heavy rainfall or high humidity.

BEHAVIOR

Since veterinary technicians are often responsible for the handling and restraint of cattle, it is important that they have a basic understanding of cattle behavior (see Chapter 1). Handling cattle can result in less stress to the cattle and increased safety for the handler if one has an understanding of the behavioral characteristics of the species. Minimizing excitement and stress is important since isolation, handling, and transportation stresses can lower conception rate and suppress immune function. Nearly half of all bruises on livestock are due to rough handling with a cost of $46 million annually to the U.S. livestock industry.

Cattle have excellent wide-angle vision (>300 degrees) but have difficulty with depth perception at ground level while moving along with their heads elevated. In order to see depth at ground level, the animal must lower its head, which may be one reason cattle stall when they see shadows. It is important to know that approaching an animal directly from the rear in its blind spot may result in the handler getting kicked if the animal is startled. Cattle are more sensitive to high-frequency noises than are people, and loud noises can cause distress in livestock.

When moving cattle in an open area or pasture, it is important to know they will tend to follow fences. Shadows that fall across an alley or chute can cause cattle to stop moving; handlers should be careful about projecting moving shadows across the animal's line of vision. Cattle movement is facilitated by eliminating harsh contrasts of light and dark in loading ramps, chutes, and handling areas and sudden changes in floor level or texture. Cattle may also stop moving at puddles, drain grates, and bright spots of sunlight. Cattle have a tendency to move toward a more brightly illuminated area provided the light is not glaring in their eyes or causing a reflection off standing water on the ground. Care should be taken if leading halter broken cattle from dim to bright light as they may unexpectedly run toward the light. It is sometimes difficult to move cattle under a roof or into a building for handling, but they will enter more readily if moved single file.

Cattle will tend to balk at the sound of clanking metal in chutes; rubber stops will help reduce the noise level. Moving or flapping objects (i.e., a coat hanging on a fence or a refection from a truck bumper) will also cause cattle to stall. If cattle see people standing in front of the squeeze chute, they will frequently refuse to approach. However, a person in front of a squeeze chute containing an aggressive cow/bull may actually be advantageous to catching the head as the animal charges.

Movement of cattle in large pens is sometimes facilitated by a piece of cloth or plastic tied to a stick (commercial slap sticks are available). The noise and movement of these instruments causes the cattle to move away from the stimulus. Herding dogs should only be used in open areas where there is sufficient space for the cattle to move away. Electric prods should be used as sparingly as possible on cattle. Cattle quickly learn to associate the sound of the buzzer with receiving an electric shock and can often be moved by the noise alone. Cattle movement is more efficient if the working parts of the handling facility (squeeze chute) are oriented toward the "home" pasture or pen.

The flight zone of cattle is that space surrounding the animal that will elicit avoidance or escape when encroached upon. When a person enters an animal's flight zone, it will move away. If the handler penetrates the flight zone too deeply (gets too close to the animal), the animal will either bolt and run away or, if cornered, turn back and run past the person or charge the person. The best place for a handler to work animals is on the edge or perimeter of the flight zone. In this position the animal will move away from the handler in an orderly manner (i.e., not show extreme flight behavior). The cattle will generally stop moving when the handler retreats from the flight zone.

The size of the flight zone depends on their relative degree of tameness. The flight zone of cattle raised on range may be many times greater than the flight zone of feedlot cattle. The "flight distance" can be roughly estimated by slowly walking toward the animal and noting how close the animal can be approached before it starts to move away. Flight distance can also be influenced by previous experience. Animals that have been handled gently and those that have been reared in close contact with people will have shorter flight distances than those handled roughly or with minimal human contact.

It is important not to invade the flight zone too deeply when moving cattle down an alley; if the animals attempt to turn back, the handler should retreat from the flight zone, which should terminate their escape behavior. Cattle sometimes rear up in a single-file chute or alley when the handler approaches too closely; backing up will allow the animal to settle down.

Cattle exhibit a strong tendency to follow and are highly motivated to maintain visual contact with each other. A single-file chute or alley should be long enough to take advantage of the animal's tendency to follow the leader. Cattle show visible signs of distress when isolated. This is especially true of Brahman-type cattle. An animal left alone in a crowding pen after the other animals have entered the alley or single-file chute may attempt to jump the fence to rejoin its herd mates. A lone steer or cow may become highly aroused and charge the handler. Many serious handler injuries have occurred when a steer or cow, separated from its herd mates, refuses to enter the single-file area. In this case, the handler should release the animal from the crowding pen and bring it back with another group of cattle.

Cattle should only be able to see one pathway of escape in the direction you want them to go and will move into a squeeze chute more easily if they can see other cattle ahead of them. Cattle can be driven most efficiently if the handler is situated at a 45- to 60-degree angle to the animal's shoulder. If the handler is behind the animal's shoulder ("point of balance"), the animal will move forward. If the handler is ahead of the animal's shoulder, forward movement will cease and the animal will back up, if possible.

> ✎ **TECHNICIAN NOTE**
>
> Handling and restraining cattle can result in less stress to the cattle and increased safety for the handler if one has an understanding of the behavioral characteristics of the species.

COMMON SURGICAL PROCEDURES PERFORMED ON CATTLE

DEHORNING

If possible, calves should be dehorned within the first month of life (or when the horn buds are first palpable) using a dehorning iron. The electrothermal dehorning technique is easy to perform when the calf is young, produces desirable, cosmetic results, and is much less stressful to the young calf. Dehorning of beef calves is commonly performed at the time of weaning in conjunction with castration, vaccination, and other management procedures. This age group is usually dehorned using a Barnes dehorner or scoop to remove the horn (Figure 30-24). Hemostasis, which is crucial, is provided by pulling or twisting the cornual artery. Calves older than 6 months may have exposed frontal sinuses after dehorning and may be at greater risk for development of sinusitis. Dehorning mature cattle often requires analgesia via a cornual nerve block. The block is performed by injecting 10 ml of 2% lidocaine under the frontal crest halfway between the lateral canthus of the eye and the base of the horn. Large horns are removed with a dehorning saw or Gigli wire. Another method of dehorning cattle is

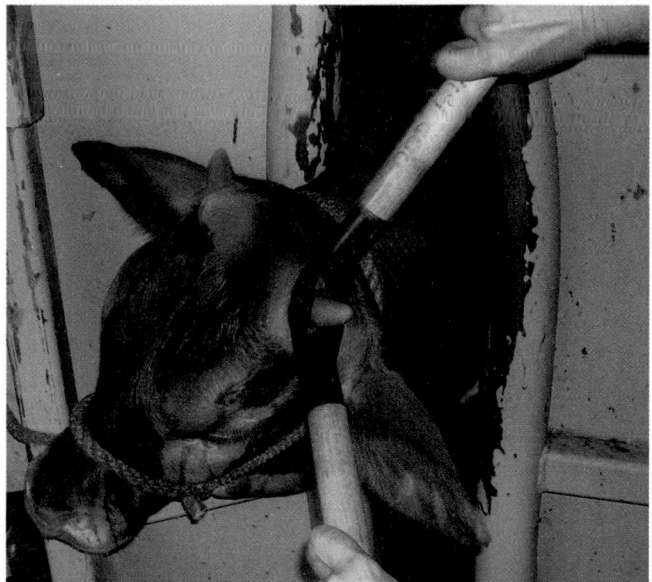

Figure 30-24 Use of a Barnes dehorner or scoop for removal of the horns in a young calf.

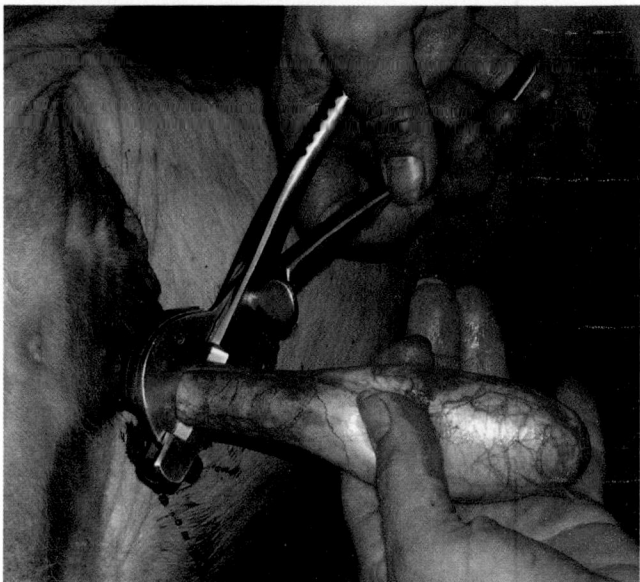

Figure 30-25 Castration of a calf by emasculation after removing the bottom half of the scrotum.

surgical or cosmetic dehorning, which is usually performed on show cattle. This method requires local or regional analgesia. An elliptical incision is made around the base of the horn, the horn is removed, and the skin incision is closed. This surgical technique allows for a more cosmetic appearance to the poll and reduces the chances of postoperative hemorrhage or infection.

CASTRATION

Several techniques are available for castration of calves. As with dehorning, castration is best performed when the calf is young as it is easier and less stressful to the calf at that time. Castration of young calves is often done without analgesia. Small calves can be adequately restrained on the ground, while larger calves are restrained in a chute with the tail pushed tightly up over the back. A technique commonly employed is the "open" method in which the bottom one third to one half of the scrotum is excised exposing the testicles. In very young calves the testicles are pulled until the cords break. In older calves the cord can be sharply transected or an emasculator that crushes and cuts can be used to separate the cord (Figure 30-25). Another less commonly utilized technique is a "closed" castration using an emasculotome, which crushes the cord within the scrotum without cutting the scrotal skin. This technique is also referred to as *bloodless castration* or *pinching*. Castration in young calves has also been performed by application of an elastrator band. It is important to make certain that both testicles are below the band when the procedure is completed. It takes 2 to 3 weeks for the scrotum and testicles to slough. This technique has been associated with development of tetanus; therefore vaccination for tetanus may be advisable.

LAPAROTOMY

Laparotomy or celiotomy is performed for the purpose of diagnosis and/or treatment of abdominal disease. The site chosen for laparotomy is dictated by the procedure being performed and the preference of the surgeon. A left flank laparotomy is typically performed for rumenotomy, correction of left abomasal displacement, and cesarean section, while a right flank laparotomy may be indicated for abdominal exploration, correction of left or right abomasal displacement, abomasal volvulus, and intestinal obstruction (such as intussusception or cecal volvulus) (Figure 30-26). A paramedian or ventral midline laparotomy may be preferred for cesarean section, correction of abomasal displacement, or approach to surgical treatment of abomasal ulcers. Left or right flank laparotomies are performed with the animal standing and restrained in a chute or stocks. After clipping and scrubbing the flank for a laparotomy procedure, a line block, inverted L block, or paravertebral block can be administered to provide analgesia for the surgical procedure.

✎ TECHNICIAN NOTE

Laparotomy or celiotomy is performed for the purpose of diagnosis and/or treatment of abdominal disease.

SUPERNUMERARY TEAT REMOVAL

Removal of extra teats is of most value in young dairy heifers, but it is also performed in beef heifers intended for show. Often this procedure is performed at the time of brucellosis vaccination. The extra teats are removed flush with the skin and parallel to the normal folds of the udder

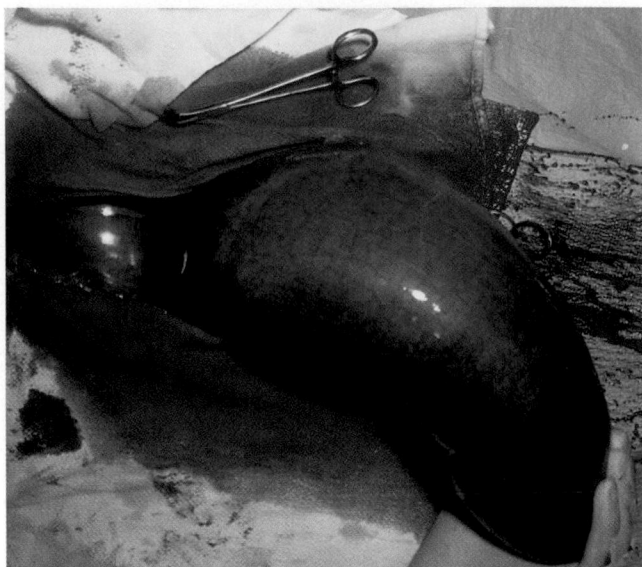

Figure 30-26 A right flank laparotomy approach for correction of an intestinal obstruction (cecal volvulus) in a cow.

using curved scissors. In young calves, suturing the skin is not usually necessary. Care must be taken not to remove any of the four normal teats.

COMMON DISEASES AND CONDITIONS OF SMALL RUMINANTS

CARE OF THE NEONATE

One of the most important components of successful rearing of lambs is establishment of a strong ewe-lamb bond. Factors that may interfere with the bonding process include

1. Lambing in a group housing situation
2. Conditions that prevent the ewe from licking the lamb immediately after birth
3. Separation of the lamb from the ewe during the first 24 hours for any reason

Sheep are gregarious and stay together as a group even during lambing, which may result in lamb "stealing" by late pregnant ewes due to their maternal instinct. Lambing in individual pens (lambing jugs, 4 feet square and 30 inches high) helps prevent this from happening. Licking of amniotic fluid from the lamb by the ewe clears the airway and stimulates breathing as well as allowing the ewe to identify that lamb as her own. Intervention during or right after parturition by the owner or veterinarian might confuse

the ewe as to whether or not the lamb is hers. Ewes are capable of identifying their own lamb(s) after only a few hours of contact, whereas lambs require several days to identify their mothers. This is another reason for utilizing individual lambing pens. Treatment of the lamb for hypoglycemia, chilling, or illness should be performed in the lambing pen if at all possible since separation of the lamb for more than 1 hour may result in rejection of the lamb by the ewe.

The first week of life is the most critical for the lamb; as much as 50% of lamb and kid mortality occurs during this time, the first 48 hours being most critical. Two major problems that may occur are hypothermia and hypoglycemia. The relatively large body surface of a lamb (versus body mass) can serve as a significant drain of body heat and energy. A 55° F environmental temperature with a 12 mph breeze has an evaporative cooling effect equivalent of –25° F to a newborn; thus it is important to protect newborns from direct wind. Lambs and kids are born with minimal body fat stores; therefore hypoglycemia can develop if the newborns do not ingest colostrum (high in fat) within the first 12 to 24 hours. The dam's udder should be checked immediately postpartum to make sure it is functional. Ewes tend to have a thick wax plug that blocks the end of the teat prior to initial nursing. Occasionally the lamb is unable to remove the plug when it begins to nurse, which results in unsuccessful nursing. Another reason to examine the ewe's udder is for presence of ovine progressive pneumonia (OPP) mastitis. The ewe's udder and milk will appear normal; however, the udder will feel firm when palpated due to the presence of fibrous connective tissue that occurs with OPP. Fibrous tissue development in the udder results in markedly decreased milk production. Lambs should be examined for congenital problems that might affect nursing such as cleft palate, brachygnathous, prognathism, and tongue myopathies associated with vitamin E/selenium deficiency.

Hypothermia and hypoglycemia can usually be prevented with good management practices. Individual lambing pens work well to allow for bonding of the ewe and lamb, help keep the lamb warm, and allow the owner or veterinarian to check the ewe's milk supply and intervene if problems should arise. Pens should be built to prevent drafts and may even be designed with a supplemental heat source (heat lamp) for the lamb(s). It is helpful to have frozen sheep or goat colostrum available in case it is needed. Cow colostrum can be utilized, however, a small percentage of lambs have developed neonatal isoerythrolysis-type syndrome around 10 days after ingesting cow colostrum. Commercial lamb and kid milk replacers are available for orphan rearing or to supplement lambs/kids from poor producing mothers. Lambs/kids need to be fed 10% to 15% of their body weight divided into 3 to 4 feedings during the first few days after birth. Later, twice-a-day feeding is adequate. They should be offered hay and starter rations early, but milk should be their major energy source until they are 5 to 6 weeks old. If a lamb or kid is hypoglycemic and hypothermic, it is best to rewarm the animal prior to any oral therapy. During a hypothermic crisis the lower esophageal sphincter relaxes, and milk or oral supplements may be regurgitated and aspirated unless the animal is alert and sternal. Rewarming when core body temperature is low is best achieved by immersing the neonate in warm water (100° to 105° F) while supporting the head.

Sometimes lambs sustain "mama trauma" in the maternity pens, so it is important that the pens be of adequate size for large ewes. Lambs are sound sleepers, and it is instinctive for the ewe to roust the lamb(s) by pawing. Vigorous pawing in a small pen may result in fractured limbs, fractured ribs, and/or pneumothorax in the lamb. Signs of trauma include lethargy, lameness, inability to rise, dyspnea, or sudden death in the lamb(s). Securing a corner of the pen and providing a heat source in that area attracts the lamb(s) away form the ewe to rest and provides safety from the ewe's feet.

> ### TECHNICIAN NOTE
> The key to successful rearing of lambs is establishment of a strong ewe-lamb bond; lambing in individual pens (lambing jugs) helps establish this bond.

GASTROINTESTINAL SYSTEM

JOHNE'S DISEASE

Johne's disease in small ruminants has several unique features as compared to the disease in cattle. The most important difference is that Johne's in small ruminants is not characterized by diarrhea. Secondly, although Johne's is more infective to younger animals, exposed adults can develop clinical signs of the disease. Fecal culture, which is the "gold standard" in cattle, is unreliable and of no practical use in small ruminants because ovine strains, in particular, are difficult to grow. Agar gel immunodiffusion on a serum sample is fairly accurate and a good screening test to run.

ENTEROTOXEMIA

Enterotoxemia, caused by *Clostridium perfringens*, is recognized worldwide as a common, frequently fatal disease of goats. Aspects of enterotoxemia peculiar to goats include a propensity for diarrhea to occur, severe enterocolitis at necropsy, and frequent failure of vaccination to protect from development of clinical disease. The main cause of caprine enterotoxemia is *C. perfringens* type D, a gram-positive anaerobic rod that produces two main toxins the most significant of which is epsilon toxin. Many outbreaks of caprine enterotoxemia involve dairy goats raised under intensive or semiintensive management conditions, whereas the greatest losses in sheep occur in lambs in feedlots receiving concentrate rations. Sudden feed changes have been associated with outbreaks of enterotoxemia, although outbreaks have occurred in situations where feeding practices were consistent. Specific feed changes include sudden accidental exposure to grain, turnout to lush pasture, feeding of bran/molasses mash to recently fresh does, feeding of bread or other bakery goods to goats, and feeding of garden greens to goats unaccustomed to green feed. Intestinal tapeworms are thought to predispose feedlot lambs to enterotoxemia by slowing GI transit time of grain rations allowing for more extensive proliferation of clostridia. In ruminant species it is believed that commensal *C. perfringens* type D organisms reside in the gut without much damage, but sudden ingestion of readily fermentable carbohydrate-rich feeds serves as a nutrient substrate for rapid proliferation of the organism. Excess carbohydrate intake may also reduce gut motility enhancing proliferation of *C. perfringens*, which increases the concentration and pathologic potential of the epsilon toxin. The toxin is necrotizing and neurotoxic. Death is due to damage of vital neurons, generalized toxemia, and shock. Clinically lambs show lethargy, overt neurological signs, minimal diarrhea, and death as opposed to kids, which show more prominent diarrhea and colic and fewer neurological signs, followed by death.

Glucosuria often occurs in goats affected with enterotoxemia, and soft or pulpy kidneys found on necropsy soon after death helps support the diagnosis. The most convincing evidence of enterotoxemia is detection of epsilon toxin in diarrheic feces or intestinal contents (samples should be immediately refrigerated or frozen and sent to the lab). An enzyme-linked immunosorbent assay (ELISA) test is available to identify the toxin.

Treatment includes balanced fluids with bicarbonate, NSAIDs, type C and D antitoxin (as much as 15 to 20 ml IV every 4 hours until stabilized), and antibiotics. In addition, cathartics and absorbents such as activated charcoal, $MgSO_4$, and/or kaolin-pectin have been used. In the face of an outbreak, previously vaccinated goats should be boostered and unvaccinated animals should be vaccinated (to be repeated in 2 to 3 weeks) and given antitoxin. Any feeding of excessive carbohydrates should be immediately discontinued. Goats are considered highly susceptible to enterotoxemia and should be vaccinated at a maximum 6-month interval. In herds with a history of disease, 4-month vaccination intervals may be more appropriate. Initial vaccinations should be followed by booster vaccination 3 to 4 weeks later, then semi- or triannual vaccinations should followed by booster vaccination 3 weeks prior to parturition for maximum benefit for the newborns. Kids should be vaccinated at 4 to 6 weeks of age and again at weaning. Vaccines with *C. perfringens* type C and D with or without tetanus are preferable to polyvalent clostridial vaccines available for cattle.

> ### TECHNICIAN NOTE
> Goats are considered highly susceptible to enterotoxemia and should be vaccinated at a maximum interval of *6 months*.

RESPIRATORY SYSTEM

PASTEURELLA PNEUMONIA

Pasteurella multocida and *Mannheimia haemolytica* are both inhabitants of the pharynx of healthy animals but may cause pneumonia in sheep and goats. Risk factors for development of pulmonary infection include initial infection with viral or mycoplasmal respiratory diseases, temperature extremes, overcrowding, respiratory tract irritants, transport, and other handling stresses. Clinical signs include bilateral nasal discharge, coughing, anorexia, and high fever. *Mannheimia haemolytica* causes an enzootic pneumonia with hemorrhagic bronchopneumonia as the primary lesion. Treatment includes the use of an antimicrobial to which the organism is sensitive. Drugs similar to those used for respiratory disease in cattle (i.e., ceftiofur) may be effective, but there use is extralabel. Vaccines for pneumonic pasteurellosis are available but are of questionable efficacy.

OVINE PROGRESSIVE PNEUMONIA

OPP manifests as progressive respiratory failure but also causes mastitis ("hard bag"), neurological signs, and arthritis. The pulmonary form predominates in the United States, and clinical signs include exercise intolerance, open mouth breathing, exaggerated expiratory effort, and an occasional dry cough. In the later stages of the disease weight loss occurs despite good appetite. The disease causes an interstitial pneumonia, and affected animals usually die within 3 to 8 months of the onset of clinical signs. Diagnosis is based on clinical signs, necropsy, and serology using either AGID or enzyme-linked immunosorbent assay (ELISA) (specificity of both is comparable, but ELISA is slightly more sensitive).

MUSCULOSKELETAL SYSTEM

FOOT ROT

Lameness in multiple animals is usually due to contagious foot rot caused by *Dichelobacter nodosus* and *Fusobacterium necrophorum*. Initial signs occur 10 to 20 days after exposure and include inflammation of the interdigital skin, followed by slight undermining of the sole at the heels. The undermining eventually progresses to the sole and wall. Some sheep are resistant to infection, some improve and clear the infection spontaneously, and others become chronic carriers of the disease. The usual source of bacteria is chronic carrier sheep or surfaces contaminated within the last 2 weeks by an infected animal. Infected feet have a characteristic foul odor.

Successful treatment involves thorough inspection of all animals and trimming and treatment of all affected animals. Animals should be divided into affected and unaffected groups and placed on clean pastures after treatment. As new cases develop in the unaffected group, they should be moved to the affected group. As cases in the affected group heal and respond to treatment, they should be placed in a third clean pasture. Footbaths are very useful for treatment after trimming and may contain copper sulfate, zinc sulfate, or formalin. Zinc sulfate (10% to 20%) may be the best choice since it is less irritating than the other two. Copper sulfate poses a threat if sheep can drink the bath water, and formalin is a carcinogen and an environmental hazard. Once a treatment program has been initiated, all sheep should be checked weekly, trimmed if needed, and placed in the footbath. After 4 weeks of treatment, any animals with obvious hoof abnormalities or any that are still lame should be culled. Segregation of infected sheep and goats and culling of chronic carriers are essential for successful foot rot control. Vaccination can increase an animal's resistance to the organism, but it has little value in treating an active infection.

> **TECHNICIAN NOTE**
>
> The most common cause of lameness in sheep and goats is contagious foot rot caused by *Dichelobacter nodosus*.

TETANUS

Spores of the bacterium *Clostridium tetani* may infect wounds resulting in tetanus. In an anaerobic environment, such as a wound, the organism produces several potent neurotoxins that are responsible for the typical clinical signs.

The disease commonly occurs following puncture wounds or surgical procedures such as castration, tail docking, and dehorning. Animals with tetanus develop progressive muscle tetany characterized by stiff, erect ears, rigid extension of the limbs ("saw horse" stance), and prolapse of the third eyelid (Figure 30-27). Affected animals are hyperresponsive to external stimuli such as loud noises. Ultimately death is due to respiratory failure.

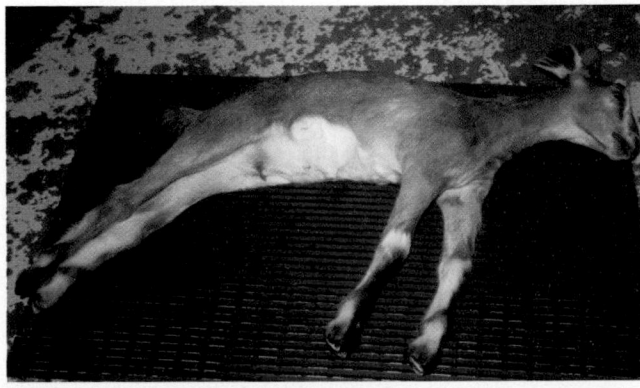

Figure 30-27 Severe extensor rigidity ("saw-horse" position) in a kid with tetanus.

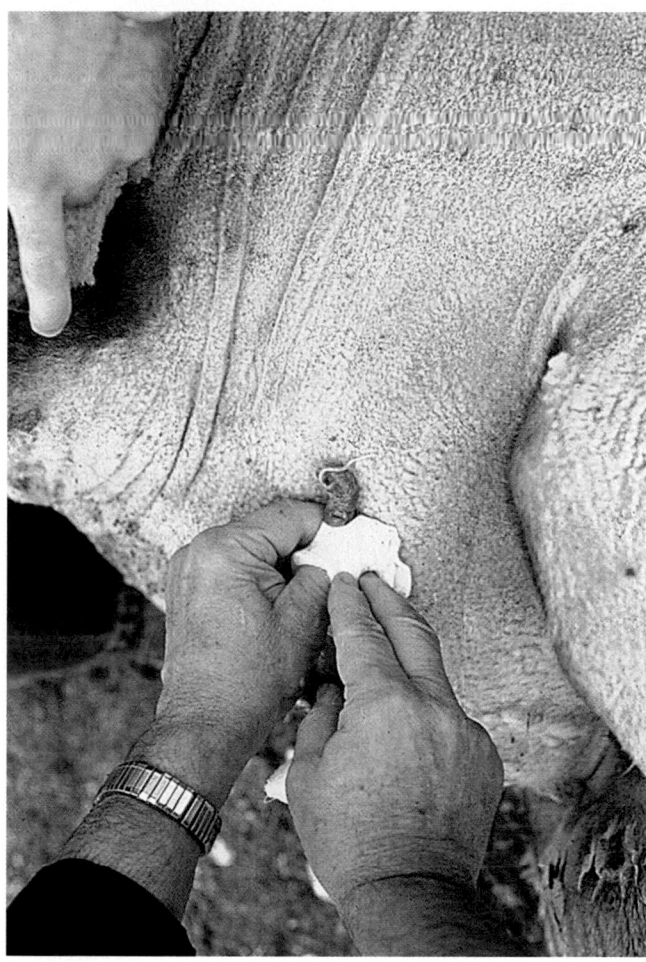

Figure 30-28 Examination of the urethral process in a wether for the presence of calculi (urolithiasis).

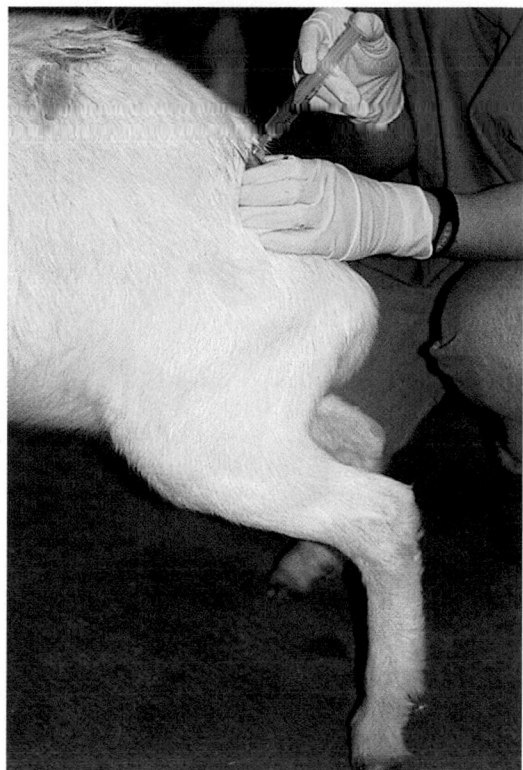

Figure 30-29 Administration of a lumbosacral epidural in a goat results in loss of motor control to the hind legs.

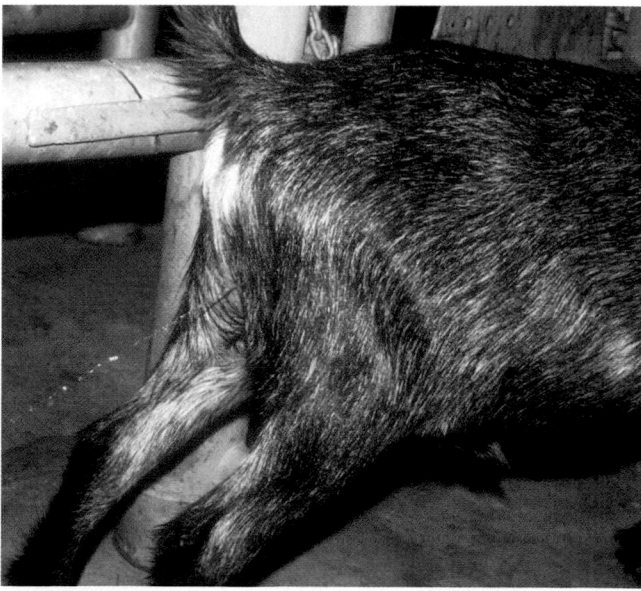

Figure 30-30 Perineal urethrostomy, a surgical treatment for obstructive urolithiasis, is prone to stricture formation in small ruminants.

sloughed by itself during a previous episode of obstruction. Immediate urethral patency may occur after urethral process amputation; however, reobstruction is common. Consequently, it appears that urethral process amputation alone rarely results in a long-term cure.

Urethral catheterization with saline flushing may be attempted to relieve obstruction; however, the bladder is difficult to catheterize due to the presence of the suburethral diverticulum in ruminants and complications associated with catheterization include urethritis, urethral rupture, and urethral damage leading to stricture.

Perineal urethrostomy may be suitable in cattle as a salvage procedure (Figure 30-30). Urethrostomy frequently results in stricture formation in the urethra and is probably not a good choice for pets due to shortened life span.

Cystotomy and/or tube cystostomy have become the procedures of choice for treatment of obstructive urolithiasis and often result in prolonged life and preservation of breeding capability in breeding males. Using this procedure, calculi can be removed from the bladder, and normograde and retrograde urethral flushing can be attempted. In addition, a Foley catheter placed in the bladder allows urine

egress while the urethra and bladder heal (Figure 30-31). The catheter is then removed when it is determined the animal can urinate a normal stream consistently from the urethra.

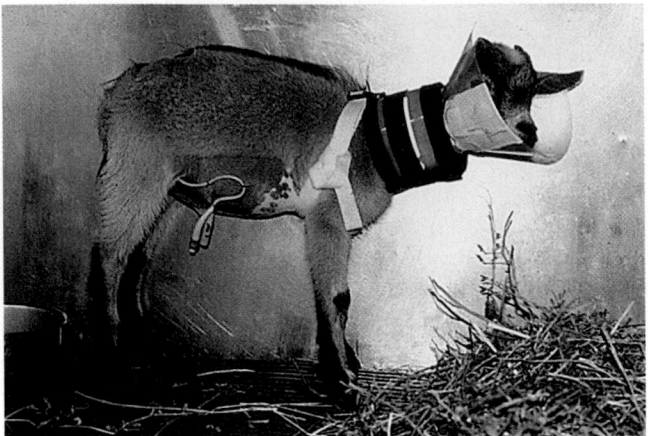

Figure 30-31 Temporary tube cystostomy allows urine egress while the urethra and bladder heal postobstruction.

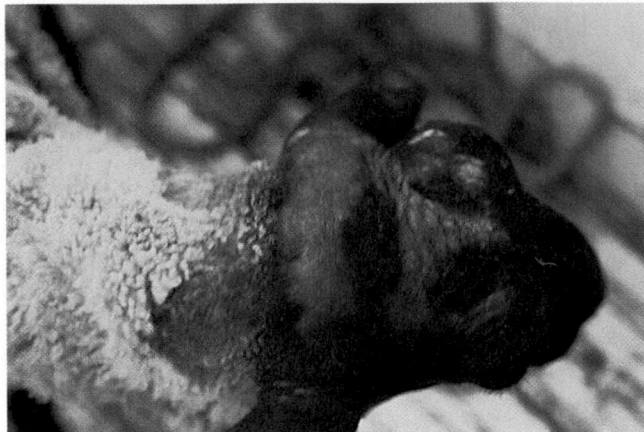

Figure 30-32 A ewe with scrapie exhibiting pruritus and wool loss over the poll.

> ✎ **TECHNICIAN NOTE**
>
> Male small ruminants are at high risk for development of obstructive urolithiasis due to the feeding of excessive grain in the diet.

NERVOUS SYSTEM

CAPRINE ARTHRITIS-ENCEPHALITIS

Caprine arthritis encephalitis most often affects dairy goats and causes a nonresponsive arthritis (usually carpi) in adults and an acute leukoencephalomyelitis in young goats. It may also cause chronic pneumonia (interstitial), chronic encephalomyelitis, chronic weight loss, and "hard udder." Clinical disease is less common than infection, and only about 15% of seropositive goats ever develop clinical disease. The primary mode of transmission is through infected colostrum and milk of infected dams. Lactating goats housed together can seroconvert, but there is no evidence of nonlactating goats spreading the disease. There is also no evidence that the disease is spread during breeding. The arthritic form is seldom seen prior to 1 to 2 years of age. In general, the ELISA test developed for detecting caprine arthritis-encephalitis (CAE) virus infection is more sensitive than are the available AGID tests. Positive tests in kids <90 days old may reflect colostric transfer of antibody; likewise, a negative serological test result cannot be used to exclude a diagnosis of CAE because the time required for seroconversion is variable (some goats take months to years to seroconvert). A PCR test for CAE is available and will detect positive goats sooner, but the test is labor intensive and expensive. Therefore, serology will probably continue to be used more widely for eradication of CAE in individual herds.

SCRAPIE

Scrapie is a transmissible spongiform encephalopathy (prion protein) that manifests primarily as weight loss—generally takes years to develop the disease, so weight loss is seen primarily in adults. Other clinical signs include pruritus with wool loss (Figure 30-32), ataxia, fine muscle tremors of the face, head pressing, abnormal gait, and disorientation. Scratching of the sheep's back will usually elicit nibbling or licking of the lips. Confirmation can only be achieved by histopathologic exam of the brain. Scrapie is a reportable disease, and there is no known treatment. Genetic testing can be performed to predict the susceptibility of individual sheep to the scrapie prion. A scrapie eradication program is currently in place, and veterinary technicians will play an important role in this regulatory work.

PREGNANCY TOXEMIA

Pregnancy toxemia is a metabolic disease that commonly affects pregnant ewes and does during late gestation. Clinical signs can occur in pregnant animals that are over-conditioned, thin, or in normal body condition. Affected animals are generally pregnant with multiple fetuses and in their last month of gestation. The condition is typically limited to ewes or does in their second or subsequent pregnancies; it is uncommon in dams carrying a single fetus or yearlings bred for their first pregnancy. Clinical cases usually follow a period of negative energy balance resulting in hypoglycemia, increased fat catabolism, ketonemia, and ketonuria in susceptible animals. Traditionally, annual feed costs for the ewe flock account for 50% of yearly out-of-pocket expenses for producers; therefore, this area of expenditure may be targeted for cost reduction to improve profitability resulting in an increased incidence of pregnancy toxemia in a flock.

A diagnosis of pregnancy toxemia should be considered whenever late pregnant ewes or does exhibit neurologic signs or motor weakness leading to death within 3 to 10 days. Clinical signs include anorexia, hypoglycemia, ketonemia, ketonuria, weakness, depression, incoordination, mental dullness, and impaired vision, followed by recumbency and death. Urine can easily be checked for ketones using commercially available urine test strips. Recumbency is generally indicative of a poor prognosis. Characteristically, affected animals linger for several days to a week before dying. Differential diagnoses include hypocalcemia, listeriosis, polioencephalomalacia, hypomagnesemia, trauma, parasitism, and meningeal worm migration. While treatment of the individual animal is often necessary, the owner should be reminded that prevention in the rest of the flock/herd is usually more important and cost effective than is treatment of the individual animal. Treatment often includes propylene glycol (100 ml twice daily PO), IV dextrose or glucose at 5 to 7 g every 4 hours (100 ml of 5% dextrose every 4 hours, for example), 20 to 40 units of protamine zinc insulin every other day for 3 days, B vitamins and calcium borogluconate if hypocalcemia is a problem. In addition, corticosteroids may be used to promote gluconeogenesis, increase appetite and induce parturition or abortion, and assist lung maturation in the fetuses. A recent report suggests that a single subcutaneous injection of 160 mg of a slow-release formulation of recombinant bovine somatotropin in combination with glucose and electrolyte treatments may show promise for increasing both ewe and lamb survival.

Body condition scoring of ewes or does 4 to 6 weeks prior to the expected date of parturition allows detection and adequate time for correction of problems. Late gestation body condition scores should increase to a 3 to 3.5 level at parturition. Palpation of the lumbar epaxial musculature is a rapid and relatively simple means of evaluating the body condition score (BCS) in sheep (Box 30-1).

OPHTHALMIC SYSTEM

PINKEYE

Pinkeye, or infectious keratoconjunctivitis, is usually caused by *Chlamydia psittaci* in sheep and *Mycoplasma conjunctivae* in goats, although either organism can cause pinkeye in both species. Carrier animals and apparently uninfected animals in a herd or flock serve as an important source of infection. Both organisms may persist for months in ocular tissue and is spread by contact with infected ocular secretions. Clinical signs, regardless of the cause, include conjunctival hyperemia, epiphora, photophobia, blepharospasm, corneal edema, vascularization of the cornea, and ocular discharge. Severe cases may result in corneal ulceration or corneal abscessation. Both infections are self-limiting and recovery can be expected in a few weeks; however, treatment with tetracycline systemically and/or topically is recommended

Box 30-1 BODY CONDITION SCORE FOR SHEEP

0. Absence of lumbar musculature and subcutaneous fat, leaving a profound depression between the tips of the dorsal and transverse spinous processes
1. Moderate concavity between the dorsal and transverse spinous processes
2. Mild concavity between the dorsal and transverse spinous processes
3. No depression (straight line) between the dorsal and transverse spinous processes
4. Slight bulging (convexity) between dorsal and transverse spinous processes
5. Profound convexity between the dorsal and transverse spinous processes (cannot palpate spinous processes)

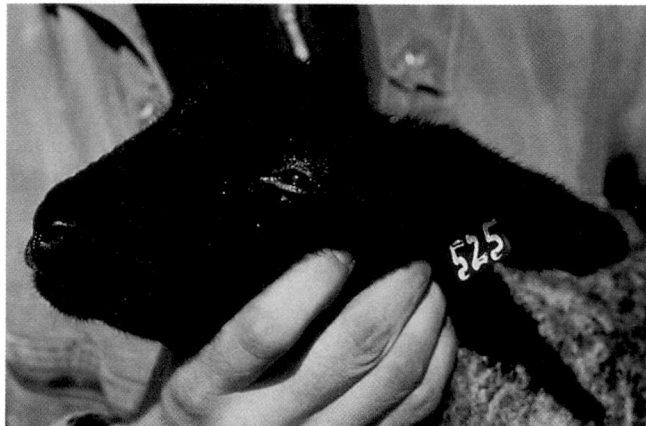

Figure 30-33 A lamb with corneal irritation due to congenital entropion or inward rolling of the lower eyelid.

to prevent spread of infection and development of severe eye lesions with loss of sight.

TECHNICIAN NOTE

Pinkeye or infectious keratoconjunctivitis, usually caused by *Chlamydia psittaci* in sheep and *Mycoplasma conjunctivae* in goats, is often treated with tetracycline in both species.

ENTROPION

Entropion, or inward rolling of the eyelid, has been reported to be the most common ocular disease of neonatal lambs (Figure 30-33). The congenital or primary form involves only the lower lid but is usually bilateral. Clinical signs of blepharospasm, photophobia, eye rubbing, and keratoconjunctivitis are ordinarily observed in lambs during the first few days to weeks of life. Initial treatment is conservative and involves administration of ophthalmic antibiotics and manually rolling the lower lid outward. If this is

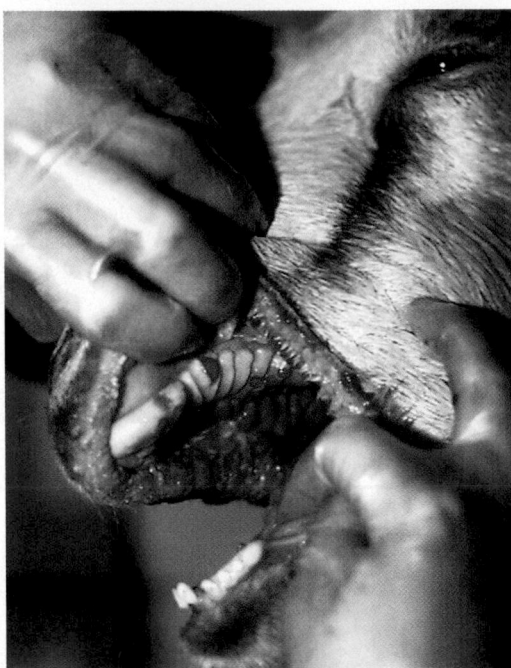

Figure 30-34 Ulcerative and proliferative lesions in and around the mouth of this doe are due to contagious ecthyma, or orf.

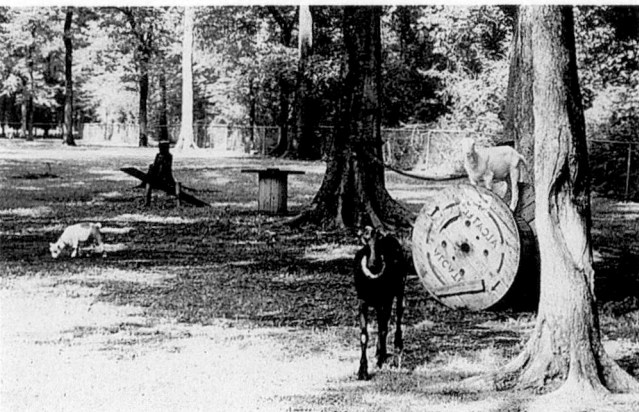

Figure 30-35 Goats are excellent climbers and should be provided with safe areas to climb and play for recreation.

unsuccessful, other treatment options include injection of penicillin or tetracycline in a linear fashion parallel to the lower lid or clamping of the skin of the lower lid below and parallel to the lid margin with mosquito forceps for 30 seconds. Both techniques should create sufficient inflammation and fibrosis to keep the lower lid rolled out. Another technique involves placement of two or three vertical mattress sutures in the lower lid to roll out the lid margin. Congenital entropion is considered to be a heritable trait, so affected animals should not be kept for breeding.

INTEGUMENTARY SYSTEM

Contagious ecthyma (soremouth, orf), a common viral disease of small ruminants, causes crusty, proliferative lesions around the mouth and nose of lambs and kids and similar lesions on the teats and udder of the ewes and does (Figure 30-34). Infection is self-limiting, taking 4 to 6 weeks to run its course. Since it is a viral disease, there is no treatment; however, antimicrobials may be given to prevent secondary bacterial infection. Supportive therapy may also be administered to those lambs and kids too painful to nurse. A live virus vaccine is available, but its use should be limited to those flocks/herds already experiencing a problem. The virus is zoonotic (transmissible to humans), so care should be taken when handling infected animals or administering the live vaccine (wear gloves).

BEHAVIOR

Goats tend to flock together in extended family groups and have strong hierarchical structure in the herd. Both males and females will establish social dominance in their respective groups through head-to-head combat. Since goats use their horns to advantage during fighting, it is best if all goats in a group either be horned or dehorned to avoid excessive bullying by horned goats.

When goats are threatened or upset, they will turn to face an intruder or stranger and make a characteristic sneezing noise (sheep have a similar response). Goats will orally investigate everything in their environment, so destructible items should be kept out of their reach. They are agile and are excellent climbers often found in trees, on rafters, or on top of vehicles (Figure 30-35). A rock pile or other elevated area within their pen or pasture will provide recreation and help control hoof overgrowth. Goats are notorious for learning to open gates and thus may escape their enclosure or may get into excessive amounts of stored feed (grain overload). Since goats can climb and get caught in fencing, electric fencing is recommended for their safety.

Goats are adaptable worldwide due to their efficient browsing ability and effective utilization of relatively poor quality roughages. Goats and sheep are seasonally polyestrous in temperate climates, breeding primarily in the fall. Bucks develop a stronger odor during breeding (rut) and may become quite aggressive during this time.

Sheep have wide-angle vision and can see behind themselves without turning their heads. Solid fencing should be utilized when moving sheep as they respect solid barriers and are less apt to be distracted or spooked. When moving sheep, it is important to know that they move toward light and will follow other sheep due to their flocking instinct.

COMMON SURGICAL PROCEDURES PERFORMED ON SMALL RUMINANTS

Lumbosacral epidurals are useful for alleviating pain during procedures performed caudal to the umbilicus. The animal will lose motor control to the hind legs and should be confined to a small, well-bedded area to prevent injury. A lumbosacral epidural is performed at the lumbosacral junction that can easily be palpated in small ruminants. A 20-gauge, 3.8-cm needle is utilized for this technique. The needle is inserted perpendicular to the dorsal midline until a slight popping sensation is encountered. If the epidural space has been entered, injection should be very easy. An alternative is to advance the needle until bone is felt, then back the needle out slightly and attempt injection. If cerebrospinal fluid (CSF) is encountered, the subarachnoid space rather than the epidural space has been entered. It is acceptable to inject lidocaine into this area if aseptic technique has been used during the procedure, but the lidocaine dose should be reduced to half of that used for epidural injection. Analgesia will take several minutes if in the epidural space and will be almost immediate if injected into the subarachnoid space. The dose of lidocaine used for this procedure is 5 to 8 ml/45 kg body weight.

The optimal time for disbudding/dehorning kids is 3 to 5 days in buck kids and 5 to 7 days in doe kids. At this age the procedure is less invasive as the horn buds have not yet attached to the underlying bone and there is less chance of regrowth if dehorned properly at this age. Many owners perform this procedure with restraint only; however, the kid may be sedated with xylazine and butorphanol. In addition, a ring block of 1% lidocaine around the base of the horn will provide local analgesia. The horn bud is removed by first burning with the dehorning iron and either allowing the bud to slough or by excising the bud after burning around its base. Care should be taken not to leave the iron on too long (5 to 10 seconds per side) to avoid thermal meningitis. The burning procedure may be repeated, allowing the area to cool between burns, until a uniform ring of copper-colored skin is apparent around the entire horn bud bases (Figure 30-36).

Factors causing rectal prolapse in sheep include short tail docking, overconditioning of lambs (increased pelvic fat), straining due to urolithiasis, diarrhea, dystocia, or conditions that increase abdominal pressure such as coughing. Short tail docks are performed strictly for cosmetic reasons in show lambs and may result in loss of innervation to the rectum and anal sphincter, which comes from S3 to Cy5. A resolution to the American Veterinary Medical Association (AVMA) suggests that lamb tails not be docked shorter than the distal end of the caudal tail fold. Methods for rectal prolapse repair include pursestring suture after replacement (strictly a salvage procedure), injection of irritating solutions (tetracycline, strong iodine in oil) at 3 to 4 points perirectally, and rectal amputation.

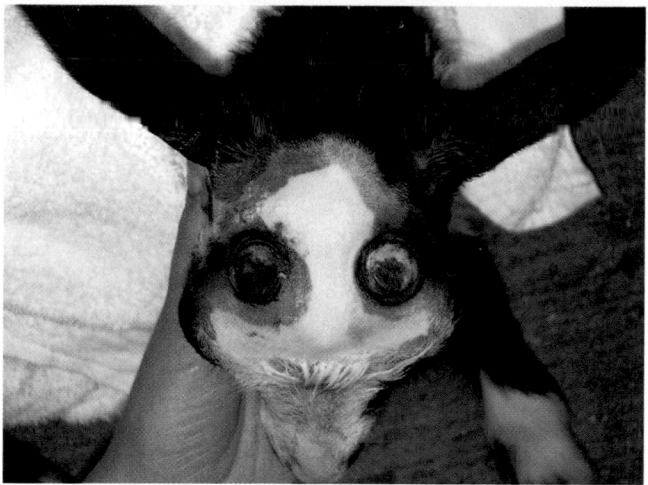

Figure 30-36 Disbudding kids is performed by burning the horn buds with an electric dehorning iron prior to 2 weeks of age.

TECHNICIAN NOTE

The optimal time for disbudding/dehorning kids is 3 to 5 days in buck kids and 5 to 7 days in doe kids.

COMMON DISEASES AND CONDITIONS OF SWINE

CARE OF THE NEONATE

Neonatal pigs have little fat store and therefore require supplemental heat during the first few weeks of life. During the first week the temperature of their sleeping area should be 92° F to 95° F, the second week 89° F to 92° F, and the third week 86° F to 89° F. Colostrum intake soon after birth is important in this species. Adequate nutrition is also very important since hypoglycemia can quickly develop in the undernourished piglet. Hypoglycemia may then lead to a weakened piglet that is susceptible to a variety of diseases or crushing by the dam when she lies down. Frequent observation of the sow/gilt and the pigs will help determine if nursing behavior is normal. Piglets that are hungry will circle the dam and squeal weakly. In this case the sow/gilt should be examined to determine if she has mastitis or some other disease that requires immediate treatment. Baby pigs raised in confinement need iron dextran injections at 3 days of age (Figure 30-37). Needle teeth should also be clipped at this time to prevent injury to the dam's udder and to other piglets in the litter (Figure 30-38). Tails may also be docked at the same time to help prevent tail biting later, and castration may also be performed (Figure 30-39). These are common pig processing techniques that are much less

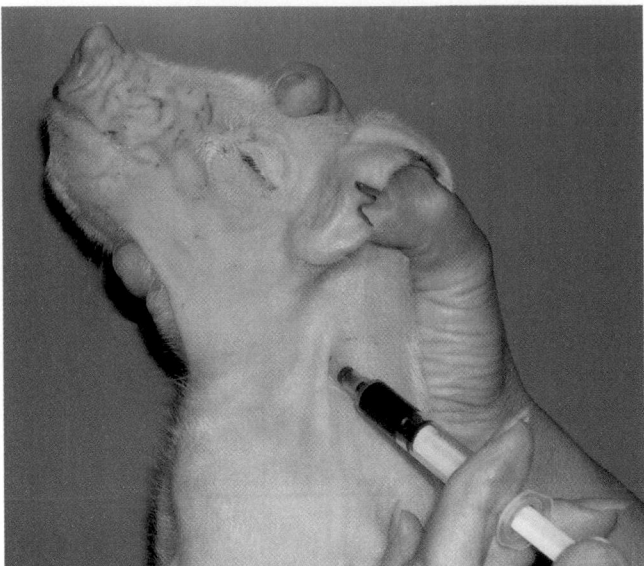

Figure 30-37 Baby pigs raised in confinement require iron dextran supplementation by 3 days of age.

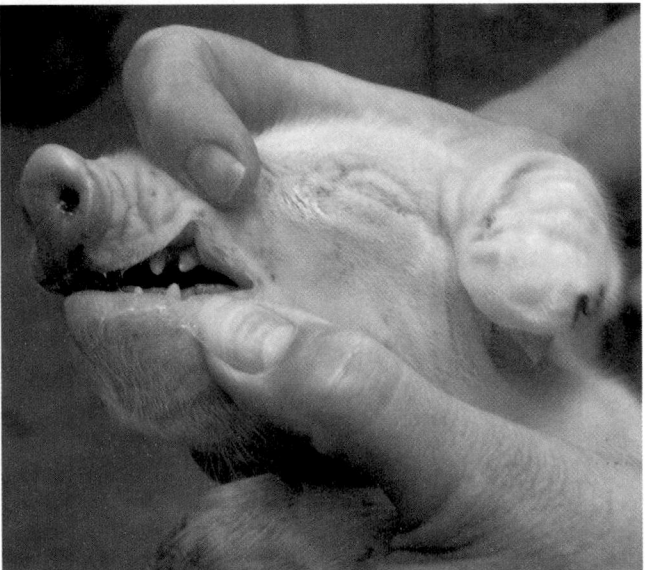

Figure 30-38 Needle teeth in neonatal pigs should be clipped to prevent bite injuries to the dam and littermates.

stressful to the pig if performed at a few days of age. If hypoglycemia develops, the piglet(s) may be treated with 5 to 10 cc of 5% dextrose injected by aseptic technique intraperitoneally. Pigs that are rejected, orphaned, or not receiving adequate nutrition by the mother may be supplemented with a milk replacer designed for pigs. Young pigs quickly learned to drink from shallow pans and therefore do not usually require bottle feeding, which can be labor intensive. These piglets can also be offered prestarter feeds at a very early age. Being nosey by nature and exploring their environment, they learn to eat solid feed quickly. A homemade milk replacer that can be used to raise piglets

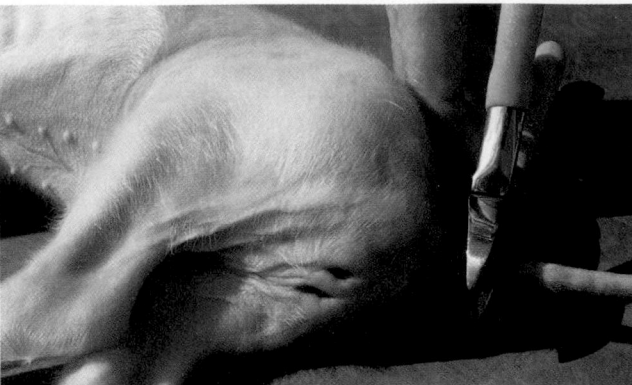

Figure 30-39 Tail docking is often performed at several days of age to prevent tail biting in pigs kept in confinement. Also note recent castration incisions.

(more appropriate for potbellied pigs) consists of 1 qt of whole cow's milk, 1 oz of white corn syrup *or* honey, and 1 oz of cream *or* corn oil.

> **TECHNICIAN NOTE**
>
> Prevention of hypothermia and hypoglycemia in the neonatal period is important to successful pig rearing.

MULTISYSTEMIC DISEASES

ERYSIPELAS

Erysipelas is caused by a bacterium that enters the body through lymphoid tissue such as tonsil or intestinal lymph tissue or via breaks in the skin. Up to 50% of healthy swine may carry and shed the organism. Septicemia quickly develops after infection, and the organisms tend to localize in the skin, heart, and joints. Infection causes a high fever and may produce characteristic diamond skin lesions. This form often results in death if not recognized early. The chronic form of the disease is more likely to result in vegetative endocarditis or chronic, nonsuppurative polyarthritis with lameness. The treatment of choice for the acute form is penicillin, but nothing is effective for treatment of the chronic form. Immunization against erysipelas is very effective and inexpensive and should be provided at weaning and repeated every 6 months.

PSEUDORABIES VIRUS (AUJESZKY DISEASE, MAD ITCH)

Swine are considered the natural host of pseudorabies virus (PRV), and although many other species are affected by this virus, most are dead-end hosts. Infection in baby pigs results in development of neurological signs and in some cases vomiting and diarrhea. Mortality in this age group is very high. Weaning and growing pigs exhibit fever, pneumonia, a dry nonproductive cough, and flulike signs. Death loss can be high in nursery age pigs but fairly low in finishers. Infection in adults may cause reproductive problems including early embryonic death, abortion, or stillbirths in pregnant sows or gilts. Serologic tests (ELISA) are used for screening herds for PRV. There is no treatment for PRV, and vaccination for the disease is closely regulated by state officials. There is currently a pseudorabies eradication program in place in the United States.

TECHNICIAN NOTE

Pseudorabies virus is responsible for development of neurological signs in baby pigs, flulike signs in growing pigs, and embryonic death, abortion, or stillbirths in pregnant sows or gilts.

PORCINE REPRODUCTIVE AND RESPIRATORY SYNDROME

Infection with the viral disease porcine reproductive and respiratory syndrome (PRRS) is prevalent in U.S. swine herds. The virus enters the body through the respiratory tract replicating in the pulmonary alveolar macrophage resulting in interstitial pneumonia. A viremia follows and the virus may cross the placenta infecting embryos or fetuses. General clinical signs include fever, lethargy, inappetence, and cyanosis of the ears, vulva, tail, abdomen, and snout ("blue ear disease"). The respiratory syndrome is manifest by labored breathing, increased secondary respiratory infections, increased postweaning mortality and decreased rate of gain and feed efficiency. The reproductive syndrome includes abortion, stillbirths, fetal mummies, and birth of weak piglets. Diagnosis is based on clinical findings, histopathology, virus isolation, immunofluorescence, and/or polymerase chain reaction (PCR). Serology is also available, but since seroprevalence is high in U.S. swine herds, presence of antibodies does not necessarily mean the herd is experiencing clinical disease due to PRRS. There is no treatment for PRRS, but antimicrobials may be administered in the event of secondary bacterial infections. A modified live vaccine is available. Control measures are variable and dependent upon the current herd status and the goals of the producer.

GASTROINTESTINAL SYSTEM

DIARRHEA IN YOUNG PIGS

Differentials for baby pig diarrhea include enterotoxigenic *Escherichia coli* (ETEC) or colibacillosis, rotavirus, coronavirus or transmissible gastroenteritis (TGE), clostridial enteritis, coccidiosis, and parasites (*Strongyloides ransomi* or threadworms).

ETEC is the most important primary cause of diarrhea in piglets less than 5 days of age. Pathogenic strains are spread to susceptible pigs via the fecal-oral route. These strains of bacteria adhere to the lining of the small intestine via pili or fimbriae and produce enterotoxins. Dehydration and electrolyte abnormalities often result in death. Fecal pH is usually high (>8) in pigs experiencing colibacillosis due to secretion of bicarbonate into the intestinal lumen. In contrast, malabsorptive diarrheas such as those caused by viruses and protozoa usually have a fecal pH of 7 or lower. Diarrheic stools are watery or pasty and yellowish. Definitive diagnosis is based on the isolation of large numbers of *E. coli* with appropriate virulence factors from the small intestine of affected pigs at necropsy. No villous atrophy occurs in the small intestine with colibacillosis. Treatment involves the use of antimicrobials to which the bacteria show sensitivity as well as supportive care such as fluid and electrolyte therapy. Prefarrowing vaccination of the sow with a Kohler milk culture (oral vaccination of the sow with a live culture of the farm-specific strain of ETEC) or a commercial bacterin or subunit vaccine may be beneficial in preventing disease in the neonate.

TGE, caused by a coronavirus, occurs in an epizootic and enzootic form. The epizootic or acute form affects pigs of all ages. It causes vomiting, diarrhea, high morbidity, and high mortality in pigs less than 2 weeks of age and anorexia, vomiting, and diarrhea with low mortality in growers, finishers, and adults and usually occurs in the winter months. The enzootic or chronic form of TGE primarily affects pigs from 1 to 8 weeks of age and may occur year round. With this form diarrhea is usually not seen before 6 to 7 days and not after 2 weeks after weaning. Morbidity and mortality are much lower than with the epizootic form. Diagnosis is based on clinical signs, particularly in the epizootic form, presence of villous atrophy in the jejunum seen on histopathology, detection of viral antigen (ELISA, immunofluorescence, or electron microscopy), and a fecal pH of less than 7. Supportive care with fluid and electrolyte therapy and antimicrobials for prevention of secondary bacterial infections may reduce death losses. Vaccines, both injectable and oral, are available for sows and pigs for prevention of TGE.

Rotavirus is similar to enzootic TGE though usually less severe. Diarrhea almost always occurs 3 to 4 days after pigs are weaned. Histopathology reveals villous atrophy in the small intestine and the duodenum is *not* spared as in TGE. Treatment of rotavirus is as described for TGE. Vaccines are available for oral vaccination of pigs at 7 and 21 days of age.

Coccidiosis (*Isospora suis*) is responsible for diarrhea in 7- to 10-day-old piglets. Coccidiosis is more of a problem in production units with continuous farrowing operations and poor sanitation. Mixed infections, especially with *E. coli*, are common. Affected piglets have yellow to green watery feces without blood. The fecal pH in these cases is usually acidic. Diagnosis is based on clinical findings, fecal floatation, and necropsy with histopathology and impression smears from the small intestine demonstrating merozoites. No coccidiostats are available for use in swine, so extralabel recommendations for treating baby pigs are oral amprolium or oral trimethoprim/sulfa. To reduce the chances of coccidiosis, all-in, all-out farrowing with cleaning and disinfection of premises is recommended.

Clostridium perfringens type C causes enterotoxemia in 3- to 4-day-old pigs. Piglets consume the organism from carrier sows and the bacteria attach to and invade the jejunal villi producing toxins that cause intestinal necrosis. Death results from secondary bacteremia, hypoglycemia, and toxemia. The peracute form may cause sudden death without prior clinical signs. The acute form has a 2- to 3-day course and causes a bloody diarrhea with shreds of necrotic mucosa. The subacute form had a longer duration with pigs that gradually waste away, while those pigs that have the chronic form become chronically stunted. Hemorrhagic diarrhea in nursing pigs is highly suggestive of clostridial enteritis. Characteristic gross lesions include bloody fluid and necrotic membranes in the jejunum and large gram-positive rods may be apparent on histopathology. Treatment is usually ineffective once clinical signs are obvious. Administration of type C antitoxin may benefit some cases. Vaccination of the sow prefarrowing with *Clostridium perfringens* type C toxoid and improved sanitation are effective in prevention of this disease.

Despite the cause of diarrhea in young pigs, good nursing care is important to survival. Free-choice oral electrolyte solutions should be provided in shallow pans. Antimicrobials may be used if there is a risk of secondary bacterial infection. Finally, it is important to keep the piglets warm, at least 32.2° C (90° F), to prevent energy loss and rapid wasting.

> ### 🖋 TECHNICIAN NOTE
>
> Baby pig diarrhea may be caused by ETEC or colibacillosis, rotavirus, coronavirus or TGE, clostridial enteritis, coccidiosis, and parasites (*Strongyloides ransomi* or threadworms).

DIARRHEA IN GROWER AND FINISHER PIGS

Swine dysentery, salmonellosis, proliferative enteropathy (ileitis), and whipworms are all differential diagnoses for diarrhea in growing and finishing swine.

Swine dysentery is caused by a spirochete, *Brachyspira hyodysenteriae*. Morbidity with this disease in untreated herds may reach 90%. The disease is spread from pig to pig by the fecal-oral route. Once the bacteria are ingested, they attach to the colonic mucosa and produce virulence factors that cause a catarrhal colitis. The colon loses its re-absorptive capacity, leading to diarrhea and dehydration. Diarrhea begins with soft yellow feces that progresses to diarrhea with large amounts of mucus and flecks of blood, then to a watery mixture of blood, mucus, and shreds of

mucofibrinous exudate. Affected pigs become thin, weak, emaciated, and dehydrated. Most pigs recover in 2 weeks and may become chronic poor doers but up to a third may die. Diagnosis is based on clinical findings, gross lesions in the colon, observation of the organism by darkfield microscopy, examination of silver-stained histological sections, culture, or PCR. Several drugs including carbadox, lincomycin, tiamulin, and bacitracin methylene disalicylate have helped in the treatment of swine dysentery. Prevention of this disease requires maintenance of a closed herd. Vaccination is not very useful in control. Eradication of swine dysentery from an infected herd is possible and probably advisable from an economic standpoint. It may be accomplished without depopulation and involves culling, meticulous sanitation, and segregated early weaning.

Proliferative enteropathy (porcine proliferative enteritis, "garden-hose gut"), also transmitted through the feces, is caused by *Lawsonia intracellularis*. Clinical findings include intermittent diarrhea (hemorrhagic in older pigs), anorexia, weight loss, melena, and anemia. Gross lesions of thickened intestinal mucosa, or garden-hose gut, are usually limited to the distal third of the small intestine. Treatment is aimed at prevention by segregated early weaning, all-in, all-out pig production, stress reduction, and good sanitation.

RESPIRATORY SYSTEM

ATROPHIC RHINITIS

Atrophic rhinitis (AR) is a chronic, progressive disease of swine that results in atrophy of the nasal turbinates. Although AR is a multifactorial disease, *Bordetella bronchiseptica* and *Pasteurella multocida* are the primary infectious agents involved. The two pathogens together produce a more severe and persistent nasal atrophy than either agent alone. Environmental factors such as high ammonia levels, stress, concurrent disease, and suboptimal nutrition also play a role in development of AR. Piglets acquire the infectious agents from nose-to-nose contact with a chronically infected dam, and transmission may also occur among young pigs. Nationwide, probably 80% of swine herds are affected to some degree by turbinate atrophy. Early clinical signs include sneezing and mucopurulent nasal discharge in young pigs. Later, twisted or shortened snouts, excessive lacrimation, epistaxis, decreased growth rate and decreased feed efficiency are apparent in grower/finisher pigs. Necropsy and slaughter checks can be utilized to assess the degree of turbinate atrophy and the prevalence of disease in a herd. At least 20 pigs should be evaluated by cross-sectioning the snout at the level of the second premolar. The severity of the lesion is then evaluated by measuring in millimeters the space between the ventral turbinate and the floor of the nasal cavity and comparing it to an existing scoring scale. Treatment and control involves use of antimicrobial agents in the feed to maintain rate of gain in pigs in the presence of

AR. Vaccines are also available and are of greatest benefit when used in the dam prefarrowing. All-in, all-out farrowing, improved ventilation, control of concurrent diseases, farrowing older sows, and provision of adequate nutrition all help control incidence of AR. Eradication may be achieved by depopulation and repopulation with AR-free swine. Other options for eradication include specific pathogen-free (SPF) programs and segregated early weaning.

Bordetella bronchiseptica can also cause pneumonia in very young pigs. Clinical signs include fever, anorexia, and coughing in nursing or recently weaned pigs. The disease causes an anteroventral hemorrhagic consolidation in the lung. Antimicrobials based on sensitivity should be administered to affected pigs and vaccination of pigs with *Bordetella* bacterins aids in prevention.

> ### TECHNICIAN NOTE
>
> Atrophic rhinitis (AR), a chronic, progressive disease of swine, results in atrophy of the nasal turbinates, twisted or shortened snouts, excessive lacrimation, epistaxis, and decreased growth rate and feed efficiency in growing/finishing swine.

SWINE INFLUENZA

Swine influenza is a viral disease of swine that produces high fever, up to 108° F (42° C), anorexia and a deep, dry "barking" cough. The disease is characterized by a high morbidity (nearly 100%) and low mortality. The clinical signs of the epizootic form of swine influenza are dramatic, distinctive, and highly suggestive of the disease although diagnostic tests such as FA, IHC, ELISA, PCR, serology, and virus isolation are available for definitive diagnosis. There is no specific treatment for swine influenza but good nursing care and antimicrobial administration for prevention of secondary bacterial respiratory infections is suggested. Vaccines are available for protection against swine influenza. Though rare, swine influenza may be zoonotic and cause serious illness and even death in humans; therefore, it is the veterinarian's responsibility to prevent infected animals from appearing at public exhibitions.

MYCOPLASMA PNEUMONIA

Mycoplasma hyopneumoniae is the most common cause of chronic pneumonia in swine with most herds being affected to some degree. The organism is spread by contact and aerosol and disease may be mild but other bacterial infections such as *Pasteurella multocida, Streptococcus suis, Actinobacillus pleuropneumoniae,* and *Salmonella choleraesuis* may occur due to compromised pulmonary defenses caused by *Mycoplasma.* The disease is usually not apparent until pigs are 3 to 6 months old when a chronic, nonproductive cough induced by exercise develops. The primary economic significance of the disease is the decreased growth rate experienced by affected pigs. Characteristic lung lesions

are a purple to gray consolidation of the anteroventral lung. Several feed and water additives such as lincomycin, tylosin, tetracycline and tiamulin have been shown to reduce the severity of pneumonia and improve feed efficiency. All in, all-out rearing throughout the growing/finishing period is probably the most important management technique for control of pneumonia. Vaccines are also available and may reduce lesions and improve weight gain.

> ### TECHNICIAN NOTE
>
> *Mycoplasma hyopneumoniae,* the most common cause of chronic pneumonia in swine, results in significant economic losses due to decreased growth rate in affected pigs.

PLEUROPNEUMONIA

Actinobacillus pleuropneumoniae, the etiology of pleuropneumonia in swine, most frequently causes clinical disease in pigs from 12 to 16 weeks of age. The disease is spread among pigs by direct contact and aerosol transmission. Pigs may become susceptible when passive immunity from the sow wears off and a high level of exposure can cause serious and often fatal disease. Recovered swine become carriers and can expose other susceptible animals to the disease. The peracute form causes sudden death without clinical signs. The acute form results in fever of up to 107° F (41.7° C), labored breathing, coughing, and often death within 36 hours. Pigs with the chronic form may display intermittent coughing, reduced appetite, and decreased weight gains. Lung lesions include pulmonary hemorrhage, edema and/or necrosis, usually more severe in the caudal lung lobes, with a fibrinous pleuritis. Chronic cases may develop abscesslike nodules and fibrinous pleuritis with adhesions. Acute cases may be treated with parenteral ceftiofur or high doses (10 times label dose) of procaine penicillin G. Administration of commercially available vaccines to pigs after weaning (twice, 2 to 4 weeks apart) can reduce the severity of the disease. Antimicrobials added to the feed or water may be effective in prophylaxis.

PASTEURELLA PNEUMONIA

Pasteurella multocida is the most common bacterial isolate from pneumonic swine lungs. The organism is a common inhabitant of the upper respiratory tract of swine and is an opportunistic pathogen. Other infections that impair pulmonary defense mechanisms (mycoplasma, ascarid migration, influenza) render the lung susceptible to *P. multocida* infection. Clinically affected pigs have dyspnea, pyrexia, up to 107° F (41.7° C), moist productive cough, and anorexia. The organism causes a purulent bronchopneumonia with an anteroventral distribution. Severe cases may develop fibrinous pleuritis and pericarditis. Affected animals should be treated parenterally with antimicrobial agents based on sensitivity. Since pasteurellosis is almost always a secondary infection, prevention of primary problems is important. Vaccination with *P. multocida* bacterins may offer some protection.

MUSCULOSKELETAL SYSTEM

Porcine stress syndrome (PSS) is also known as *malignant hyperthermia* (MH) or *pale soft exudative pork* (PSE). Susceptibility to PSS is caused by a single autosomal recessive gene, and disease is manifest only in pigs that are homozygous recessive for this gene. This defective gene is closely associated with desirable characteristics such as good feed conversion and high percent lean. The gene for PSS has been identified in almost every breed of swine but is especially prevalent in the Pietrain breed. Stress, halothane, and other anesthetics may precipitate the development of PSS. The severity of clinical signs is related to the degree of stress, and signs include muscle and tail tremors, dyspnea, alternating blanched and reddened areas of skin, elevated body temperature (hyperthermia), cyanosis, muscle rigidity, and death. At slaughter or on postmortem the musculature is pale, soft, and watery. Susceptibility to stress can be diagnosed with a DNA probe test, which will identify both homozygous and heterozygous carriers. Once clinical signs develop, the affected animal may be treated by removing the stress, applying external cooling, and administration of dantrolene sodium, if available. It is more important to prevent this condition by genetic selection of breeding stock that is not stress susceptible.

REPRODUCTIVE SYSTEM

Agents responsible for abortion and reproductive failure in swine include pseudorabies virus, brucellosis, porcine reproductive and respiratory syndrome, porcine parvovirus, and leptospirosis.

Porcine parvovirus (PPV) is present in nearly 100% of swine herds worldwide. If the virus infects a male or nonpregnant female, the pig seroconverts and eliminates the virus with no clinical signs. If a pregnant female becomes infected, the virus crosses the placenta and infects rapidly dividing fetal cells. If the pregnancy is less than 30 days, the embryo is killed and resorbed by the dam. Between 30 and 70 days of gestation, the fetus is killed and mummified, and >70 days of gestation, the fetus mounts an immune response and survives to term, although it may be born weak or dead. The only clinical signs of PPV are those of reproductive problems in pregnant sows/gilts. Mummies of different sizes, stillbirths, and live pigs may be present in the same litter. Abortions are not typical of parvovirus infection in swine. Since the virus is ubiquitous, a single positive titer is not very useful in confirming a diagnosis of reproductive failure due to PPV. Prevention may be achieved by natural exposure of gilts to sows prior to breeding. Natural infection usually results in lifelong immunity. Vaccines are available but immunity only lasts 4 to 6 months, so vaccination must be repeated prior to each breeding. Vaccination may interfere with development of natural immunity.

Leptospira pomona and *Bratislava* are the primary serovars that are adapted to swine, although other serovars may incidentally infect pigs. The bacteria are shed through the urine and reproductive discharges of infected animals and enter susceptible animals through mucous membranes or broken skin. Once infected, a bacteremia develops and the organism localizes and multiples in the kidney and in pregnant females may cross the placenta and infect and kill the fetuses. Aborted, weak, and stillborn pigs may be the only obvious clinical signs. Diagnostic tests include demonstration of high antibody titers in the dam (interpret in light of vaccination status) or in fetal fluids, culture of the organism, darkfield microscopy of urine or fetal fluids, fluorescent antibody of fresh tissue, and PCR techniques. Treatment may be accomplished with the use of tetracycline in the feed or administration of parenteral tetracycline. Many monovalent and multivalent vaccines are available for protection of breeding stock; however, the immunity is short-lived, so animals should be vaccinated every 6 months at breeding.

> ✎ **TECHNICIAN NOTE**
>
> Pathogens responsible for abortion and reproductive failure in swine include pseudorabies virus, brucellosis, PRRS, porcine parvovirus, and leptospirosis.

NERVOUS SYSTEM

Salt poisoning, also known as *sodium ion toxicosis* or *water deprivation*, occurs in commercial as well as pet swine due to overconsumption of excess sodium (direct salt poisoning) or inadequate water intake (indirect salt poisoning) or possibly both. Water deprivation causes a hyperosmolarity of the CNS so that when water is consumed, the osmotic pressure draws water into the CNS causing cerebral edema. Affected pigs show signs of restlessness, pruritus, constipation, and thirst followed by depression, blindness, convulsions, and death. Salt toxicity is a well-recognized entity in commercial swine, but descriptions of medical treatment of affected animals is limited as it is usually not economically feasible to treat individual commercial pigs. Successful treatment of pet pigs has been reported. Treatment consists of slow rehydration with fluids that will gradually return sodium to a normal level. In one report, successful treatment of two potbellied pigs with salt toxicity was achieved using $^1/_2$ strength lactated Ringer's in 2.5% dextrose.

BEHAVIOR

The pig's normal response to fear is vocalization and attempts to escape. They are naturally curious and spend a great deal of time exploring their environment. The prehensile organ of the pig is the snout, and in general they have a keen sense of smell. Pigs have poor eyesight, so with poor eyesight and a reliance on smell, pigs are reluctant to venture into areas with unusual odors and changes in light intensity. Once familiar with their surroundings, they begin to investigate by rooting with their snout, which may lead to destructive behavior. Co-mingling pigs, such as occurs at weaning, results in reestablishment of hierarchy in newly mixed pigs. This reordering usually occurs within 12 to 24 hours with the dominant pig establishing itself first, followed by number two, three, and so on. Some changes of rank may occur within the middle members, but the top and bottom of the order remains fairly stable. The dominance hierarchy of swine is referred to as *bidirectional*, a subordinate pig sometimes directing antagonistic behavior toward a higher ranking pig; however, this does not affect the social status between individuals. In established hierarchies, the dominant pig assumes a recumbent position, and its belly is nuzzled by subordinates, possibly an allogrooming ritual. The best group size for socialization is not known for sure, but the order seems to become more complex when a group size is over 20.

Abnormal behavior is more likely to develop because of stressful living conditions. An abnormal behavior may either be a new behavior or a normal behavior that has become misdirected or exaggerated. Abnormal behavior can be a valuable indicator of environmental (physical, climatic, or social) or managerial deficiencies. Tail biting begins as misdirected investigative behavior (harmless nibbling) at weaning that can escalate to vicious biting, an expression of predatory aggression and appetite for blood. Tail biting can cause an ascending infection of the spinal cord or spinal abscesses and even hind limb paralysis and death. Contributing factors include stress of weaning (often begins at weaning), climatic stress, overcrowding, or an imbalanced diet. The behavior can be controlled by providing diversions like toys (bowling balls, inner tubes) for pigs to play with in their pens. Commercial pigs in confinement have their tails docked to prevent this problem; however, tail docking may then lead to ear biting if the underlying problem is not corrected. Also, removing the "biter" often controls the problem within a group.

Ear biting and flank biting are different expressions of the same problem(s) that result in tail biting. In addition to the aforementioned reasons, ear biting may be initiated by fighting for social rank. Flank biting may begin by flank sucking that is misdirected nursing behavior (more likely to occur when piglets are weaned younger than 20 days) that escalates to varying levels of destructive behavior to the victim.

Aggression in the extreme may be an abnormal behavior. Some aggression in pigs is normal. In a group situation, such as within a litter, a pecking order is established by fighting. This begins as early as birth when a teat order is established. Since more milk is produced in the cranial mammary glands, the stronger, more assertive piglets will fight to claim these teats. This is the reason for trimming needle teeth shortly after birth to prevent serious injury to the piglets and to the sow's udder. Once teat preference is established, that order remains until weaning. In older groups of pigs, if groups are mixed or a pig is added or removed, the pecking order must be reestablished usually by fighting. Mature boars have well-developed tusks for slashing and will bite each other as a part of their normal aggressive behavior. If strange boars are mixed, they will fight and may seriously injure each other. Boars raised together undergo a dominance procedure but typically do not violently fight each other. Sows and weaned pigs will also fight, and even though they do not have tusks, they will bite. Sows and young pigs will also ram their heads against an opponent's head or torso. Baby pigs are often observed play fighting in preparation for normal pecking order establishment later in life.

Pigs normally keep their sleeping and feeding areas clean from an early age. Poor manure habits or pen fouling may be indicative of environmental or management problems such as overcrowding, high ambient temperature, or inappropriate airflow pattern (resting area should be draft-free). Lameness and diarrhea may contribute to the problem.

Dam aggression toward piglets (hysteria) or savaging of baby pigs is usually exhibited by gilts. These same gilts may be normal during subsequent farrowings. Possible causes of hysteria include stress due to inability of the gilt to make a "nest," human interference during farrowing, and perhaps genetic predisposition. Management of the condition includes removal of pigs as they are born and reintroducing the entire litter once parturition is complete as initiation of nursing often calms the gilt.

POTBELLIED PIGS NUTRITION AND HUSBANDRY

Without proper knowledge of the potbellied pig's husbandry and nutritional needs, health and behavior problems are inevitable. According to one report, approximately 50% of potbellied pigs are abandoned or rehomed before they are 1 year of age. This occurs because of unrealistic expectations of the owners and their unwillingness or inability to provide for the pig's environmental needs. The most common misconception held by pet pig owners is that their potbellied pig will only weigh 40 to 50 lb when fully grown. Although a few pigs remain small, most of them will weigh closer to 120 pounds when mature, and they do not reach full size until they are 2 to 3 years old. Breed standards set by the North American Potbellied Pig Association describe a pig weighing no more than 95 lb and having a maximum height of 18 inches at the shoulder, at 1 year of age. The most common nutritional disease of potbellied pigs is obesity; however, many stunted and malnourished pigs are also seen owing to their owner's misguided attempt to keep them small. A number of companies have developed diets specifically for miniature pigs. Miniature pigs should never be fed commercial swine feeds; feeds for miniature swine are lower in protein and fat and have a higher fiber content than commercial swine rations. Miniature pig feeds are generally classified as starter, grower, breeder, or maintenance. Starter rations are intended for newly weaned pigs. The most appropriate ration for the average potbellied pig is the maintenance ration, which contains 12% protein, 2% fat, and 12% to 15% fiber. Most potbellied pigs are adopted by owners at 6 to 8 weeks of age and are spayed or neutered in the first few months. They begin to lead sedentary lifestyles early, so maintenance rations are probably the best choice for these pigs. If the pig is not spayed or neutered and/or it leads a very active life, grower rations may be a better choice. Some commercially available potbellied pig feeds have urinary acidifiers to help prevent cystitis, so if this seems to be a problem, this specialty ration may be considered. Recommendations concerning amount to feed potbellied pigs varies; some references suggest 2% to 2.5% of their body weight, others suggest 1 cup of feed per 50 to 80 lb. These are general guidelines, and owners must be advised to feed their pets according to body composition.

Although the potbellied pig should have a rotund potbelly, they should never have turgid, fat-filled jowls or rolls of fat hanging over their hocks. They should have ribs that can be felt but not seen (Figure 30-40). Appropriate treats for the pig include low-fat, low-salt (see salt poisoning under swine) snack foods such as popcorn (air popped without salt or butter), and small amounts of dried or fresh fruit. Requiring that the pig earn its treats is one way of continually reinforcing the pig's position as a subordinate member of the family. Obesity is likely to be the leading cause of health problems and decreased life span in pet pigs. Arthritis, heart disease, and kidney failure are just a few possible geriatric diseases that may be hastened by obesity. Sometimes entropion and corneal damage occur in morbidly obese pigs. Water intake in pigs is important for prevention of cystitis, urolithiasis, and salt poisoning. Pigs have a habit of alternating between eating and drinking and may make a mess at feeding time. Owners should be advised not to restrict water for this reason. Food and water should be provided in an easy to clean environment such as a shower stall or by placing the food and water in a large shallow try to make cleanup easier. Pigs are also particular about the temperature of their drinking water, so the water should not be allowed to get too cold in the winter or too hot in the summer as this may restrict intake and cause problems. Pigs are foraging animals that normally spend much of their day either in search of food or at rest. When kept as a pet, pigs are fed two to three small meals a day and

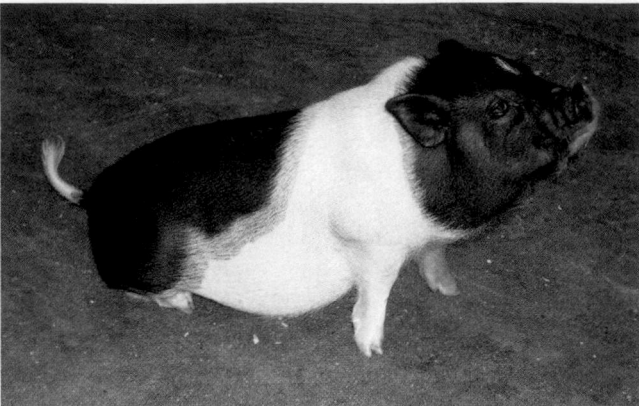

Figure 30-40 A healthy potbellied pig of appropriate size for its age.

spend little time looking for food or eating. There are a variety of ways to extend mealtime, which increases the pig's exercise and makes them a more active participant in the acquisition of their food. In good weather the pig's ration may be broadcast over the grass in the yard. A rooting box can also be constructed out of wood or by utilizing a plastic wading pool. The box is filled with large smooth stones and their food can be spread among the stones. This not only extends feeding time but also allows the pig to fulfill its rooting needs in an acceptable place. Other useful techniques include the use of a Manna Ball or Buster cube, which allows the pig to slowly acquire its food while exercising at the same time.

> ### ✎ TECHNICIAN NOTE
> Obesity is the most common nutritional disease of potbellied pigs and is likely to be the leading cause of health problems and decreased life span in pet pigs.

RECOMMENDED READING

Smith BP: *Large animal internal medicine*, ed 3, Philadelphia, 2002, Mosby.

Cowart RP: *An outline of swine diseases*, ed 2, Ames, 2001, Iowa State University, Blackwell Science.

Pugh DG: *Sheep and goat medicine*, ed 1, Philadelphia, 2002, WB Saunders.

Rebhun WC: *Diseases of dairy cattle*, ed 1, Philadelphia, 1995, Lippincott, Williams & Wilkins.

Cooper VL: Diagnosis of neonatal pig diarrhea. *Vet Clin North Am: Food Animal Prac* 16:117-133, 2000.

Wills RW: Diarrhea in growing-finishing swine. *Vet Clin North Am: Food Animal Prac* 16:135-161, 2000.

Tynes VV: Potbellied pig husbandry and nutrition. *Vet Clin North Am: Exotic Animal Prac* 2:193-207, 1999.

Tynes VV: Preventive health care for pet potbellied pigs. *Vet Clin North Am: Exotic Animal Prac* 2:495-510, 1999.

Fubini SL, Ducharme NC: *Farm animal surgery*, ed 1, St Louis, 2004, WB Saunders.

31

Nursing Concepts in Alternative Medicine

Laurie McCauley • Christine Jurek

INTRODUCTION

Complementary and alternative therapy can be a very exciting and rewarding part of veterinary medicine. Whether you work in a conventional or nonconventional practice, you will have clients who seek a more natural approach to their pet's care than standard veterinary medicine provides. In fact, quite often clients feel more comfortable speaking with a technician about less mainstream ideas than they do with a veterinarian.

The purpose of this chapter is to give you a basic knowledge and understanding of the most common complementary and alternative medicine modalities used in veterinary practice today. It is not meant to be a comprehensive explanation of each modality, nor is it intended as a "how to" guide. The following modalities will be discussed: acupuncture and traditional Chinese medicine, chiropractic, homeopathy, herbal medicine, physical therapy and rehabilitation, massage, and miscellaneous therapies. For those interested in more information about alternative medicine, we have included a list of recommended reading and resources at the end of the chapter.

On one end of the spectrum is perfect health, and on the other end is disease. Most patients fall somewhere in between. Holistic medicine seeks to bring the patient to an ever greater state of general health and well-being rather than the conventional approach of simply treating disease. ■

✐ TECHNICIAN NOTE

The term *holistic* refers to a "whole-animal" approach to health care. It focuses on wellness as an ongoing, dynamic process with great variability in the state of health.

An animal in perfect health has bright eyes and a shiny coat and is muscular and fit, energetic, and robust. This animal is not only in balance internally, but it is also able to adapt to its environment in a much greater capacity. It is able to rebalance and heal easily after it receives an external insult, such as exposure to an infectious agent or trauma. Anything less than perfect health leaves room for improvement. The technician has a tremendous opportunity to contribute to holistic health care of the veterinary patient, both as an assistant and as a therapist under the supervision or direction of the veterinarian.

MASSAGE

Massage is defined as a systematic and scientific manipulation of the soft tissues of the body for the purpose of obtaining or maintaining health. Massage has been performed for thousands of years. There are over 70 types of human massage philosophies, many of which can be applied to animals.

TYPES

Shiatsu is a Japanese form of massage that literally means "finger pressure." Shiatsu practitioners use finger pressure on specific points in the body (correlating to acupuncture points) to increase circulation and stimulate the nervous system.

In *trigger-point massage*, or myotherapy, the therapist feels for taut bands or knots that have a point of maximal tenderness. Pressure on this point can cause local pain, referred pain, and muscle spasms in humans as well as animals. The manual technique for deactivating a trigger point is *ischemic compression*. By applying direct pressure over the point, the tissue becomes ischemic (blood is pushed out of the tissue) and then, when the pressure is removed, hyperemic (blood quickly infiltrates the tissue). This will often relieve the tension, band, or knot, as well as the pain.

This pressure is usually held for 8 to 15 seconds, and if a spasm is felt during the pressure, it should be maintained until the muscle stops firing.

Sports massage can be broken into event massage and maintenance massage. Event massage (relating to a massage done on an athlete before, during, or after competing) can be broken down into preevent, interevent, and postevent. The goal of preevent massage is to leave the animal relaxed and ready for the event. Interevent massage keeps the patient tuned up and ready for the next event, while postevent massage flushes out metabolic waste and reduces muscle spasms and soreness. The goal of maintenance massage is to help prevent injury and expedite the healing of injured tissue.

TTEAM is a system of massage for teaching physical awareness of the body. Originally designed for horses, and based on the human work of Dr. Feldenkrais, TTEAM is a form of massage that is devoted to nonhabitual motion to reeducate the nervous and musculoskeletal systems. It has an impact on an emotional level as well as aiding focus, coordination, and balance. A major difference between TTEAM and other forms of massage is that while massage works on the deeper tissue, TTEAM manipulates only the skin. Although this was originally designed for horses, all species may benefit from this therapy.

Swedish massage is the most commonly used massage system in North America. These techniques began in the late 1700s and will be discussed for use on animals. Studies have shown that massage is beneficial in reducing stress, enhancing blood and lymph circulation, decreasing pain, promoting sleep, reducing swelling, enhancing relaxation, and increasing oxygen capacity of the blood.

TECHNIQUES

Effleurage is the most commonly used stroke in animals. It is a gliding stroke that follows the contour of the body. Hand over hand, thumb over thumb, or one hand on either side of the body are the most common variations. It is repeated several times at the beginning and end of the massage to evaluate the tissue and enhance blood flow (warm it up and then aid in flushing lactic acid). Animals usually prefer these strokes flowing with the hair. Although effleurage is often thought of as a light stroke, deeper strokes are used to lengthen muscles and aid in stretching.

Pétrissage, or kneading, consists of rhythmic lifting, squeezing, and releasing the tissue. It assists in removing metabolic waste and increasing circulation. The hands form a C shape and can be alternated in a circular motion, can "roll" the skin, or can spread up and out to help widen or broaden the muscle (Figure 31-1).

Friction is the manipulation of tissue to increase circulation. It is commonly used over tendons when tendonitis is present, over knots and trigger points, and over joint capsules with excessive fibrous tissue. It is also used to break up skin adhesions and scar tissue (wait 3 to 4 weeks after

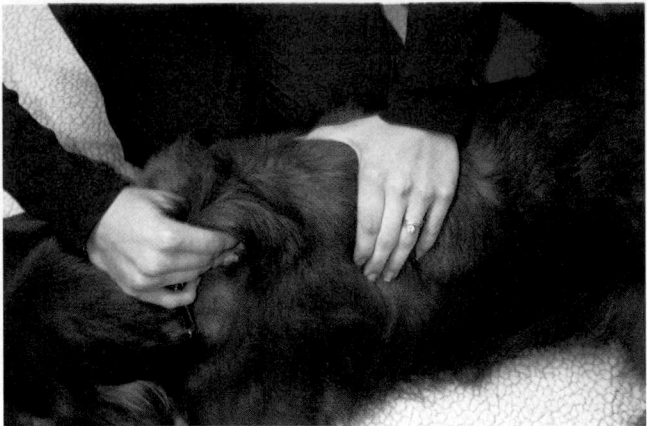

Figure 31-1 Pétrissage: dog receiving pétrissage; notice the C shape to the hands and the alternating pattern to the hands.

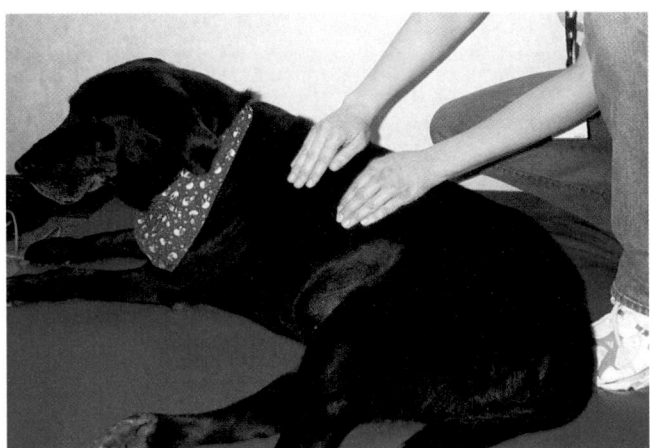

Figure 31-2 Tapotement: Coupage, a form of tapotement, is performed on a dog. Note the hands are cupped and alternating. The motion starts at the base of the ribs and moves forward.

injury or surgery before applying this technique). When applying this to deep tissue, one finger or thumb is placed on the skin and either rubs the skin or is attached to the skin and rubs the tissue underneath. This can be done longitudinally (with muscle fibers), across fiber (perpendicular to the muscle fibers), circularly, diagonally, or in a J pattern.

Tapotement is a tapping motion of the hands or fingers. When done for a short time, it stimulates nerve endings (preevent sports massage or to tone atrophied muscles). When done longer, it has a more sedative effect. Coupage, which is used to loosen phlegm congestion in the lungs, is a form of tapotement. The hands are cupped, and the strokes start at the caudal aspect of the ribs and move forward. Proper positioning using wedges or pillows can help maximize the effectiveness of coupage. This stroke may be continued for 5 to 10 minutes on each side (Figure 31-2).

Vibration is a rapid shaking or slower rocking of the tissue. Speed of vibration will affect outcome: faster vibration will be stimulatory while slower speeds will be inhibitory. It differs from tapotement in that the therapist's hands do not leave the patients skin. It can aid in relaxing muscles, reducing trigger point activity, and, when used over a joint capsule in the proper position, can act as a joint mobilization.

SWEDISH MASSAGE

Swedish massage breaks down the massage into several elements and movements. The elements include intention, touch, pressure and depth, excursion, speed, rhythm and continuity, duration, and sequence. The movements that we will discuss include effleurage, pétrissage, friction, tapotement, and vibration. *Intention* is the consciously sought out goal of the therapist. Therefore the massage outcome is different if the therapist wants to create relaxation versus invigoration. *Touch* is the vehicle of massage and conveys the intention. *Pressure* is the force applied to the surface, usually through the therapist's hands. *Depth* is the distance traveled into the patient's tissue. The therapist controls the force, but the patient has more control over the depth. Often, applying less pressure slowly will increase depth, whereas fast, higher pressure will cause splinting (muscle contracting in a protective reflex) to occur. *Excursion* is the length of one massage stroke. In a cross-friction massage, meant to relieve tendonitis, the excursion may be only 1 to 2 cm, but in a beginning effleurage stroke, the excursion may be from the head all the way to the tip of the tail. *Speed* refers to how fast the hand moves over the patient. In an invigorating preevent sports massage the speed will be much faster than if the therapists' goal is to achieve relaxation. The repetition or regularity of the stroke defines its rhythm, similar to music. The concept of *continuity* in massage refers to the uninterrupted flow of strokes and to the unbroken transition from one stroke to the next. It is hard for the patient to relax if the rhythm is not smooth or if the continuity is not fluid. *Duration* is the length of time devoted to one area. In humans, a relaxing massage does not usually last more than 1 hour without creating muscle soreness. Small animal massage duration is usually 30 minutes and large animal duration, like the human, is approximately 1 hour. A *sequence* is the arrangement of the massage strokes.

A typical example of a sequence would be

- Start with effleurage on the face and head.
- Continue down the back and sides.
- Use pétrissage over the paraspinal muscles (including kneading, circles, or strokes going with or perpendicular to the muscle fibers).
- Apply ischemic compression on trigger points if found.
- Move on to one side of the neck.
- Carry on down the forelimb.
- Perform effleurage, with strokes running from the toes to the heart to flush toxins.
- Continue by using skin rolls along the body wall.

- Apply the same techniques you used in the forelimb to treat the rear limb.
- Gently flip the patient over if a canine or walk around to the other side if an equine.
- Repeat your techniques on the other side.
- Finish up with a final effleurage.

Signs of relaxation include sighing, yawning, licking the lips, hanging the head (equine), burping, or flatulence. Signs that the pressure is too great include increased respiratory rate, opening the eyes (if previously closed), fidgeting, and incessant licking (canine), or swishing the tail (equine).

CONTRAINDICATIONS

There are several contraindications to massage, and there are also *endangerment sites.* Endangerment sites are areas of the body that are delicate and are relatively unprotected. Contraindications include massage over bacterially or virally infected lesions, over open wounds, over the area of an acute injury or inflammatory condition, over an area of hemorrhage, or following a recent high fever. Some endangerment sites include the throat, eyeballs, brachial plexus, abdomen (deep, near the aorta), and over the kidneys.

Precautions should be taken when massaging a patient with heart disease or over a neoplastic area.

The technician, if properly trained, can play the key role in massage therapy. Most massage certification courses are open to technicians, allowing them to be the primary massage therapist for the animal patients. Training schools will be listed at the end of this chapter.

TECHNICIAN NOTE

Effleurage is the most commonly used stroke in animals. It is a gliding stroke that follows the contour of the body.

The technician, if properly trained, can play the key role in massage therapy. Most massage certification courses are open to technicians, allowing them to be the primary massage therapist for the animal patients.

PHYSICAL THERAPY AND REHABILITATION

Physical therapy is a relatively new modality in both the human and animal realm. It has been used with horses and companion animals for just over 20 years, and although much has been learned, there is still much we do not know. *Physical therapy* or *rehabilitation* is defined as the use of many modalities to relieve pain, build strength, and reeducate patients to walk in a balanced manner after an injury or illness. Many conditions may benefit from physical rehabilitation (Box 31-1).

Tools we will discuss in this section include hydrotherapy, land treadmill, neuromuscular stimulation, therapeutic

Box 31-1 COMMON CONDITIONS SEEN AT
REHABILITATION FACILITIES

MUSCULOSKELETAL
Osteoarthritis
Rheumatoid arthritis
Hip dysplasia
Muscle contracture
Wobbler's disease
Discospondylosis
Soft-tissue injuries
Sprain, strain, muscle tears
Joint injuries
Tendonitis and bursitis
Postsurgical including but not limited to
Hip surgeries
Cranial cruciate ligament tear surgery
Fracture repair
Arthrodesis
Amputation
Osteochondrosis dissecans
Postsurgical complications including but not limited to
Non–weight bearing
Loss of range of motion

NEUROLOGICAL
Intervertebral disk disease
Fibrocartilaginous embolism
Neuropathy
Degenerative myelopathy
Wobbler's disease
Discospondylosis
Postsurgical complications including but not limited to
laminectomy
Postsurgical complications including but not limited to
decreased neurological function

OTHER
Circulatory deficiency
Wound healing

ultrasound, pulsed signal therapy, electromedical horizontal therapy, passive range of motion (PROM), therapeutic exercises, cryotherapy, and heat therapy. Other therapies used in rehabilitation that are discussed in this chapter but not in this section include massage, magnets, acupuncture, and chiropractic.

HYDROTHERAPY

Hydrotherapy was used in 400 BC by Hippocrates to treat rheumatism and paralysis. In the United States, in the 1970s, it was found that when racehorses swam after an injury, they were able to return to the track faster then their comrades who did not have access to water. Unfortunately, it was also found that they increased muscle mass without the benefit of strengthening the bone (which is done when there is a

compressive force), so they were also more likely to fracture a limb shortly after returning to the track. To get the best of both worlds, the underwater treadmill was invented. In 1998 the first underwater treadmill was designed for use specifically in companion animals. Walking on an underwater treadmill in a warm water environment has the benefits of increased joint range of motion, improved muscle flexibility and mobility, enhanced circulation, and facilitation of front-to-rear and side-to-side balance. Because it can relieve pain and increase muscle strength while putting decreased weight on the joints, it is extremely beneficial in the treatment of osteoarthritis. It is also an invaluable tool when working with patients with neurological deficits, as many patients can take steps in water before they have voluntary motion on land. Swimming, without an underwater treadmill, also has many of these benefits. However, dogs most commonly swim with stronger strokes in the forelimbs compared with the rear limbs. This may not be the best treatment if the goal is to strengthen the rear limbs. Also, paralyzed patients tend to improve more quickly with walking on the underwater treadmill. Massage, stretching, and exercises can also be done in the water before, during, or after swimming or walking on the underwater treadmill. Racehorses often use swimming or wading in water as a conditioning tool.

Dynamic variables in the aquatic environment include buoyancy, resistance, flexion and extension of the limbs, speed, and patterning. Buoyancy can be added if a life vest is worn; this makes swimming easier. Using jets or water wings can increase resistance, making swimming more of a workout. By changing the depth of the water, resistance, buoyancy, and flexion/extension are affected. The deeper the water, the more the buoyancy and the easier it is for the patient. Slightly above shoulder depth creates the most buoyancy without losing flexion of the limbs. If decreased flexion is warranted, then the water level should be above the shoulder as this is more of a gait with the animals walking on their toes. The most resistance with the least buoyancy occurs when the patient walks at about elbow depth. Resistance can be increased with the use of water wings or balloons. To maximize flexion, either balloons or water wings can be used (Figure 31-3), or the water level can be lowered to just above the joint you want to flex. Altering treadmill speed will affect the speed of the patient, and thereby change the intensity of the workout. Patterning can be defined as teaching the body to act in a certain way without conscious thought (an example for people would be riding a bicycle or skiing). With animals we can work on proper gait by moving their limbs or stimulating limbs to move in a certain pattern. An example would be to work on a walking gait, a trotting gait, or a pacing gait.

Although the doctor determines the variables associated with the hydrotherapy, the technician plays a very important role. The technician's role is to be in the pool with the canine patient, facilitate correct motion, monitor the patient, and provide the massage, stretching, or exercises. Before going

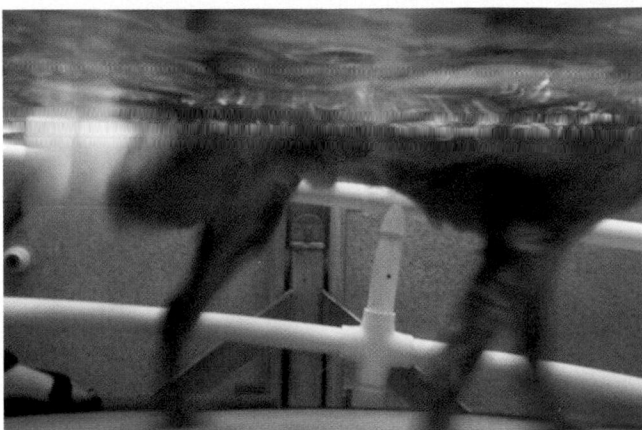

Figure 31-3 Dog in pool with water wings. Water wings are used to increase flexion at the stifle.

in the pool, if the patient is fecal incontinent, the technician can use a cotton swab to rectally stimulate the patient to defecate outside. When the patient is done with the pool, the technician may towel dry and/or blow them dry. The technician should also be responsible for pool care (testing the water and adding any chemicals that may be needed). The technician would be responsible for holding the lead attached to the horse's halter in an equine swim.

LAND TREADMILL

Land treadmills are used for increasing strength and endurance as well as reeducating front-to-back balance and normal foot placement. Front-to-back balance comes into play when an animal has made a habit of shifting their weight in one direction to favor a painful limb. When the pain is removed from the limb, the compensation remains. By walking either just uphill or just down hill, this habit can be altered. By walking uphill, a patient with nonclinical hip dysplasia can strengthen the muscles around the hip, decreasing laxity and delaying the onset of clinical signs. When a patient places a limb laterally after surgery, it will often place the limb back in normal position when walking on a treadmill, especially if the treadmill is at an angle that decreases the weight on that limb. Although treadmills recreate the same motion as walking on land, fewer muscles are utilized to do so. This is because the belt movement reduces the body's need for self-propulsion. As such, the benefits of the treadmill are maximized when the treadmill is used to go up or down hill.

The goal of teaching the canine patient to use the treadmill is to have them be comfortable getting on at one end, off at the other end when done, and to enjoy the workout in between. To make the transaction easier, have the patient walk across the treadmill three times (sitting and then standing on the third pass). On the fourth pass start the treadmill. Do not start too slowly, as this is awkward. Quickly go to a normal pace where there is no hesitation between steps. Keep them looking forward so that habits of side winding do not start. Many dogs will pace on a treadmill.

The technician's role is to teach the patient to use the treadmill without fear, to monitor the patient for gait changes and weariness while on the treadmill, and to record time, speed, angle, and progress of the patient.

ULTRASOUND

Ultrasound is the use of sound waves to treat tissue. It works by producing heat, but it also has some nonthermal effects that are not fully understood. The therapeutic value of ultrasound includes increased collagen extensibility, increased blood flow, increased range of motion due to changes in contractility of muscle, decreased pain and muscle spasm, increased enzyme activity, changes in nerve conduction velocity, accelerated wound healing due to facilitation of the inflammatory process, and enhanced transdermal delivery of medication (phonophoresis).

Variables that determine the amount of heat produced by the sound wave include frequency, intensity, duty cycle, duration of exposure, and the size and type of the tissue to be treated. At a frequency of 1 MHz the depth of penetration is 4 to 5 cm, whereas at a frequency of 3 MHz the penetration is only 1 cm. The proximity of the bone and the thickness of the tissue determine the frequency that is used. The intensity determines if there will be thermal or nonthermal effects. Intensities over 1.0 W/cm^2 produce thermal effects that increase circulation and help reduce joint contractures. Intensities under 1.0 W/cm^2 produce nonthermal effects that enhance wound healing. The duty cycle is the fraction of time that the sound wave is emitted during a pulse period. In a continuous mode the intensity is constant and may cause "unstable cavitations," which can be destructive to tissue but may be beneficial for stretching scar tissue. In a pulsed mode, most commonly 20% or 50%, the wave is interrupted in an on/off pattern. Pulsed ultrasound is used to enhance healing and remove swelling. Time is determined by the size of the area being treated. As sound increases the temperature in the tissue, it is very important to continuously move the sound head. If it is held stationary, burns of the skin, muscle, or periosteum may result (Boxes 31-2 and 31-3).

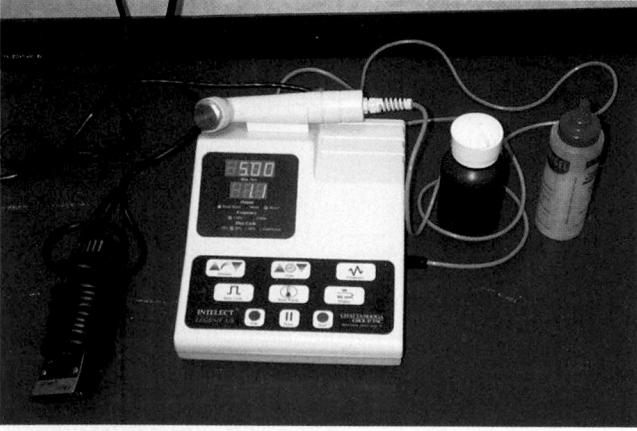

Figure 31-4 Ultrasound setup: Setting up the ultrasound is one of the technician's responsibilities.

The technician's role in ultrasound is to shave the area, clean the area with alcohol, and perhaps to administer ultrasound treatment under the doctor's supervision (Figure 31-4).

NEUROMUSCULAR STIMULATION

Neuromuscular electrical stimulation (NMES) is the application of electrical current to elicit a muscle contraction. The main purpose of NMES in rehabilitation is for muscle strengthening. Clinical uses include reducing disuse atrophy (after surgery or injury), reversing muscle atrophy (the patient that is not using a limb after surgery or injury), and strengthening selected muscles (neuromuscular reeducation).

> ### TECHNICIAN NOTE
> Neuromuscular electrical stimulation (NMES) is the application of electrical current to elicit a muscle contraction.

A voluntary muscle contraction recruits small-diameter, slow-twitch, type I, fatigue-resistant fibers first. Constant tension of the muscle is maintained by asynchronous recruitment of those fibers—some are relaxing as others are contracting. An electrically induced muscle contraction recruits large-diameter, fast-twitch, type II fibers first due to their low threshold to electrical excitation. These fibers tend to be recruited simultaneously, and as they fatigue, tension in the muscle will begin to decrease. With continued NMES therapy, studies have revealed that properties of the fast-twitch, type II muscle fibers began to resemble those of the slow-twitch, type I muscle fibers and decrease the fatigability of the muscle. Pads are placed over the motor point of the muscle (the area that the least amount of electricity is needed to produce a contraction, usually where a nerve enters the muscle) and a distal point on the muscle. If a solid contraction can not be created, the proximal pad should be rearranged to make sure it is truly over the motor point (Box 31-4).

The technician's role in NMES is to shave and clean the skin with alcohol, apply the gel and pads, and utilize the NMES machine to obtain a strong yet pain-free contraction (Figure 31-5). Knowledge of the anatomy is essential to performing this task. The muscles and muscle groups that are routinely stimulated include triceps muscles, paraspinal muscles, gluteal muscles, hamstring muscles, quadriceps muscles, and cranial tibial muscles. The forelimb flexor muscles, forelimb extensor muscles, deltoid muscles, and gastrocnemius muscles may also be stimulated.

BIOELECTRIC STIMULATION

Electricity is found naturally in all of us. In ancient Greece, physicians used electric eels in footbaths to relieve pain and enhance circulation. It is known that certain electrical

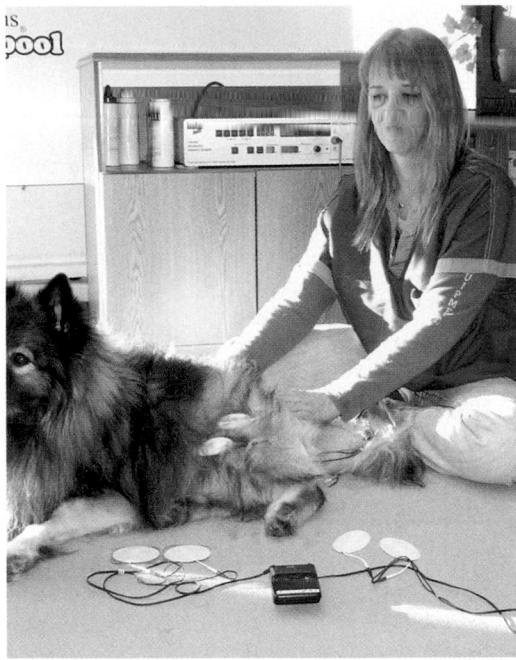

Figure 31-5 A dog receives NMES from the Hako-Med unit, which is visible in the background. A smaller, handheld NMES unit is visible on the floor in the foreground.

impulses help facilitate bodily functions including actions needed for healing. Bioelectric therapy can be classified as stimulatory, which includes therapies that operate within a range of 1 and 1000 pulses per second (Hz), and multifacility, which include therapies that operate within a range of 1000 to 100,000 Hz. Stimulatory therapies have the benefits of electroanalgesia, pain management, vasoconstriction, vasodilatation, edema reduction, reinnervation acceleration, and muscle stimulation. Multifacilitory therapy benefits include acute pain reduction, vasoconstriction and vasodilatation, muscle stimulation, and antiinflammation.

Several types of devices that can deliver electricity through the patient are transcutaneous electrical nerve stimulation (TENS) units, interferential units, and horizontal units. Most units have attached leads (Figure 31-5) that are placed on either side, or in the case of interferential units on all four sides of the area to be treated. With most units, patients need to be shaved and have their skin cleaned with alcohol to remove hair and dead skin. The exception would be the horizontal stimulation units (Hako-med). With this unit water and gel are used to increase conductivity, eliminating the need to shave. Reusable or carbon pads are attached to the unit's leads with gel to increase conductivity. The frequency is set and the amplitude is adjusted so that the patient feels a sensation but has no pain or muscle contraction.

TENS units most frequently use frequencies of 75 to 100 Hz and are mostly used for pain relief. The down side of TENS units are that the pain often returns relatively quickly.

Interferential therapy can be used with one frequency in one direction and another in a perpendicular direction so that where they are superimposed there is summation and then cancellation of the current. It can also be used with two pads on one side for topical treatment or muscle stimulation. This therapy is most effective in treating deep, aching, and chronic pain but can also be used for acute pain and electroanalgesia. The frequencies used are usually 4000 Hz in one direction and 4001 to 4100 Hz in the other direction. This puts the frequency in the periphery at the 4000-Hz range and between 1 and 100 Hz (often scaling up and down) where the frequencies cross.

Horizontal therapy uses changing and scanning of frequencies from 1 to 12,400 Hz to obtain effects within the tissue that is both stimulatory and multifacilitory in the same treatment. This therapy is effective in treating acute pain, chronic pain, pain associated with osteoarthritis, and edema. It can be used to relieve muscle tension in patients who have generalized excessive muscle tightening and spasms. It can also be used for electroanalgesia (short-term analgesia for use during uncomfortable procedures like debridement). Although this technology has been around for over 10 years, within the last few years a pool has been developed to connect to the electrical unit. This allows the small animal patient to be submerged in warm water with whirlpool jets while the electrical current flows through the water. The whirlpool aids in treatment as well as hides the current. This is very beneficial for patients with osteoarthritis in multiple joints.

The technician's role in bioelectric stimulation is to administer the treatment. This includes shaving if needed, applying gel and pads, and setting the machine to the proper frequency and intensity. Additional training with the individual units will be needed before this can be done effectively.

PASSIVE RANGE OF MOTION

Passive range of motion (PROM) is the use of stretching to prevent the loss of normal range of motion, to return normal range of motion if absent, to increase cartilage nutrition in the joint, and to stimulate cartilage regeneration. Most of the nutrition received by the chondrocytes (cartilage cells) comes from the capillary-rich synovial capsule, which then bathes the cartilage via the synovial fluid. If the joint is stationary, then the joint fluid is not circulated and there is less nutrition available to the chondrocytes. In studies done in rabbits, after stabilizing a joint for 7 days, microscopic degenerative changes had already started in the cartilage.

If PROM is to be done postsurgically or in a joint with restricted motion, each joint being stretched should be done separately. However, when PROM is performed on a patient with a neurological disorder where it will be used to prevent loss of motion and increase cartilage nutrition and regeneration, then each limb is done as a whole. The rules of PROM include:

1. It should never hurt.
2. If the patient is lying on their side, keep the limb being worked on parallel to the ground to prevent torque of the joints.
3. Flex the most proximal joint first and work distally.
4. Do not let the stifle go under the rib cage.
5. Hold the limb flexed for 10 seconds, hold it in extension for 10 seconds (to the front, then 10 seconds to the back), and repeat this 10 times.
6. Massage the muscles you are stretching.
7. Guide the limb, do not pull it.
8. Do not hyperextend the carpus or tarsus because permanent tendon or ligament damage may occur. These joints are flexed and relaxed, unless there is a contracture issue involving these joints.
9. If it is postsurgical PROM, set up your hands on either side of the joint on which you are working (one joint is worked on at a time), and then move your eyes too and keep them on the surgery joint to prevent inadvertent motion of this joint.
10. The hip and shoulder joint have rotation as well as flexion and extension. Start with small circles and gradually increase the motion performing 10 rotations. Stabilize the distal joints.

The technician can take a very active role in PROM, performing this modality under a veterinarian's direction. This can be used successfully in equine as well as canine patients.

EXERCISES

Exercises are used for strengthening specific muscles or muscle groups, building endurance, enhancing balance and proprioception, and reeducation of normal posture and gait. Examples of exercises and their purpose are listed in Table 31-1. Many of these exercises are custom made for the individual patient and condition (Figure 31-6).

It has been shown that a graded exercise program consisting of hand walking and utilizing ultrasound, returned horses to racing faster than either stall rest or being put out to pasture.

The technician's role in exercises is to lead the patient in doing the exercises or to teach the owner to perform the exercises at home.

CRYOTHERAPY AND HEAT THERAPY

Cryotherapy, or cold therapy, when applied to the body, removes heat. Some of the actions are vasoconstriction, which reduces postsurgical bleeding and bruising (when the cooling agent is removed, there is a rebound vasodilatation—red coloration may be seen in the skin), slowed

Table 31-1 Exercises

Exercises	Type	Use
Sit to stand	Strengthening	Rear limbs
Walking on a hill	Endurance	Whole body
Zig zag	Proprioception	Side closer to the top
Parallel to top	Strengthening	
Balance board	Balance	Limbs on the board
	Proprioception	Limb not on the board
	Strengthening	
Goosing (abdominal contractions)	Strengthening	Posture
Cavaletti poles	Proprioception	Gait training Flexing limbs
Flexing limbs*	"High five" or "wave"	Strengthening forelimb

*tc \l 4 Flexing limbs.

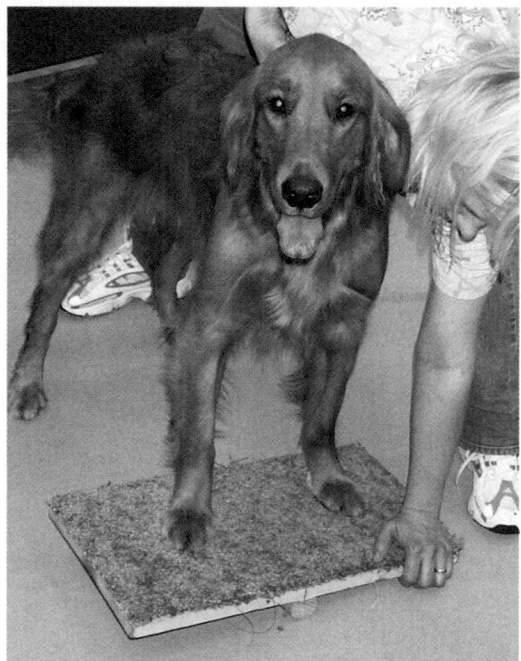

Figure 31-6 Exercises: A dog increases his forelimb balance and proprioception on the rocker board.

nerve conduction (thereby decreasing pain sensation), and decreased enzyme activity (decreasing inflammation). The first 72 hours after an injury is the destructive phase of inflammation in which only cold and not heat therapy should be used. After that period, heat may be applied between cryotherapy sessions. An example would be 10 to 15 minutes of cold, 10 to 15 minutes of heat, and 10 to 15 minutes of cold up to three times daily. Very small patients may require less time. Horses do not need more then 15 minutes of cryotherapy and heat therapy on their limbs. Postsurgically, cold can be applied by filling a Dixie cup ³/₄ full and freezing it. The paper is unraveled and gauze can be placed at the incision to prevent water from contaminating the incision. Commercial cool packs are easy to keep in the freezer. Frozen peas can also be used as they are moldable and hold the cold fairly well. A mixture of alcohol and water in a Ziploc freezer bag at a ratio of 2:1 stays cold and malleable. Double bagging is recommended. If the patient is shaved or short coated, wrapping the peas or alcohol bag in a towel may be required. In horses, running a cold hose over an injury is also very effective. Therapeutic ice boots are also available for equine extremities. Sweat wraps in horses commonly contain dimethyl sulfoxide (DMSO), Furosin, and dexamethasone surrounded by plastic wrap and a quilted wrap. This is thought to decrease inflammation.

The actions of heat include increasing enzyme activity (beneficial 72 hours after the insult), increasing circulation, increasing muscle contractility, increasing collagen's ability to stretch, and decreasing pain. The recommended method is wet heat. A hand towel, for small areas, or bath towel, for larger areas, may be folded into thirds and rolled (to be unrolled around a joint) or accordion folded to be placed over a flat surface. Run the towel under warm to hot water, and apply to the area. If you cannot keep your hand on the towel because it is too hot for you, then it is also too hot for the patient. A big thick towel or plastic wrap may be placed over the wet towel to keep the heat in. Heat can be applied for 10 to 15 minutes between cryotherapy sessions, preceding exercises to warm up the muscles and joints, or if an area is cold to the touch on exam (signifying a chronic condition with decreased blood perfusion). Heat can also be used over an area of infection once the patient is taking antibiotics to enhance the drugs penetration into the area.

CONTRAINDICATIONS

Do not use cryotherapy and heat therapy over areas that do not have sensory sensation as tissue damage may occur.

The technician's role in cryotherapy and heat therapy is to treat the patient and to instruct the clients on home care.

> ### ✎ TECHNICIAN NOTE
>
> *Physical rehabilitation* is defined as the use of many modalities to relieve pain, build strength, and reeducate patients to walk in a balanced manner after an injury or illness.

Walking on an underwater treadmill can relieve pain and increase muscle strength while putting decreased pressure on the joints. Therefore it is extremely beneficial in the treatment of osteoarthritis.

Ultrasound can be used to remove scar tissue, decrease pain and inflammation in muscles, accelerate wound healing, and treat tendonitis and bursitis. Passive range of motion (PROM) is used to prevent the loss of normal range of motion, return normal range of motion, increase cartilage nutrition, and to stimulate cartilage regeneration.

ACUPUNCTURE

The term *acupuncture* comes from the Latin words *acus*, meaning "needle," and *pungure*, meaning "to pierce." It is the technique of piercing the skin with a needle at specific, predetermined "acupuncture points." It is now known that these points can be stimulated by more than just needles, they can also be stimulated by injection of fluid, laser, ultrasound, surgically implanted material, and electrical stimulation.

Acupuncture has been used for over 4000 years in the East as one medical method within traditional Chinese medicine (TCM). TCM is a system of medicine that includes herbology, massage, and nutritional and lifestyle management. Early Chinese veterinary applications of acupuncture started with the domestication of animals. Veterinary acupuncture came to the United States in the early 1970s, and in 1974 the International Veterinary Acupuncture Society (IVAS) was organized with the aim of fully integrating acupuncture into Western veterinary science. Acupuncture is used to treat all species from ferrets and birds, to dogs and cattle, to elephants and killer whales.

In the United States, acupuncture is increasingly utilized as a modality in the treatment of musculoskeletal, neurological, cardiovascular, respiratory, gastrointestinal, reproductive, and dermatological disorders. Although it has the ability to help many areas of the body, pain management is probably the most common use of acupuncture today.

TERMINOLOGY AND RECORD KEEPING

Acupuncture points are connected through pathways that are called *meridians* or *channels*. In TCM it is believed that the body's vital energy or life force (bioelectricity) circulates in a cyclic predetermined course through the meridians. In most species, there are 14 classical meridians: 12 are associated with specific organ systems on which they have a primary influence, and two run on the midlines of the body. The paired organ-related meridians are named lung (LU), large intestine (LI), stomach (ST), spleen (SP), heart (HT), small intestine (SI), bladder (BL), kidney (KI), pericardium (PC), triple heater (TH), gallbladder (GB), and liver (LV). The unpaired channels are the conception vessel (CV) that runs on the ventral midline and the governing vessel (GV) that runs on the dorsal midline. Individual acupuncture points are named and recorded by pairing the meridian and a number (for example, LV3 is the third point on the liver meridian, and SP6 is the sixth point on the spleen meridian). In addition, there are "extra" points that do not lie on meridians, and trigger points, which are temporary tender areas that can move on and off the meridians in episodes of pathology.

ACUPUNCTURE THEORIES

According to TCM theory, energy circulates through each meridian every 24 hours. The meridians run on the surface of the body, where acupuncture points can be accessed and manipulated. A blockage of energy circulation manifests as dysfunction or disease. Medical conditions that can be helped by rehabilitation result from stagnant energy circulation or lack of sufficient energy to function optimally. Stagnant energy manifests as painful spasms or swelling, while deficient energy manifests as atrophy or weakness. To bring the body into balance and to facilitate healing, it is necessary to stimulate or sedate energy levels at acupuncture points. There are many theories about how acupuncture works. The most current acupuncture theories discussed in the human literature are as follows:

1. Gate theory
2. Endogenous opioid theory
3. Autonomic nervous system input theory
4. Humoral theory
5. Bioelectric theory

GATE THEORY

The gate theory explains the analgesic effects of acupuncture. It has been shown that different types of neurons transmit pain. When an acupuncture needle is inserted, thin myelinated nerve fibers carry a message to the spinal cord. The neurotransmitters are released and taken up by the interneurons. When the impulse from the unmyelinated pain nerve fibers cause the release of neurotransmitters, the receptors are full and the "gate" is closed to that signal with little to no message of pain reaching the brain.

ENDOGENOUS OPIOID THEORY

Opioids have been used for many years to combat pain (i.e., poppy, morphine, torbutrol). Depending on where the needles are placed, acupuncture has been shown to release beta-endorphins, met-enkephalins, and leu-enkephalins in both the blood and cerebral spinal fluid. These endogenous opioids can be reversed with naloxone (an injectable agent used in veterinary medicine to reverse the effects of morphine). Opiates are also known to have systemic effects that can be produced by acupuncture. For example, opiate receptors in the gut are responsible for decreasing peristalsis and increasing segmental contractions, thus effectively controlling diarrhea.

AUTONOMIC NERVOUS SYSTEM THEORY

This theory looks at how needles inserted into the skin can have an effect on the muscles and organs of the body. Numerous viscerosomatic (relating the organs to the muscles) relationships have been studied, and it has been found that visceral and somatic fibers have adjacent tracts in the spinal cord and distribution in the dorsal gray matter. Examples of this relationship include muscle cramping seen secondary to inflammation of the intestines and the phenomenon of

"referred pain," which is when there is pain felt in one part of the body but it is different from the part of the body that was stimulated.

HUMORAL THEORY

This theory was first postulated after studies showed that a transfer of blood, cerebrospinal fluid (CSF), or brain tissue from an animal under acupuncture analgesia to an animal not receiving acupuncture resulted in analgesia of the recipient. This analgesia was generalized and reversed by naloxone. Beta-endorphins are released by acupuncture and may contribute to analgesia, but it is not the only important component. Serotonin is also important and increases 30% to 40% in the systemic circulation after acupuncture. Acupuncture has also been shown to cause systemic increases in growth hormone, prolactin, oxytocin, luteinizing hormone, white blood cells, immunoglobulins, antibodies, and interferons, depending on which points are stimulated.

BIOELECTRIC THEORY

Becker and Reichmanis, in 1976, proposed a theory that the healing and analgesic properties of acupuncture are based on a direct current (DC) system. In this system, electric signals are generated and propagated by Schwann cells, satellite cells, and Glial cells. Acupuncture points, like amplifiers, would boost the DC signal along the nerve pathways. Insertion of a metal acupuncture needle would, in effect, short-circuit the system and block pain perception. In this system, acupuncture points boost the DC signal along the meridian, comparable to an amplifier boosting electricity along a high-power tension wire.

TECHNIQUES

Dry needling is performed using stainless steel acupuncture needles. These needles are 25 to 36 gauge, and range from $1/2$ to 2 inches long when used with companion animals or up to 4 inches long when used with large animals. Large animal practitioners will often use hypodermic needles in their patients (Figure 31-7).

Moxibustion is the burning of dried leaves of the *Artemisia vulgaris* or mugwort plant. The moxa stick can be moved slowly over an acupuncture point or placed on an inserted needle. This is often used for animals with degenerative changes who do better in warm dry climates than when it is cold or damp. In TCM this adds energy to a deficient area.

Aqua-puncture is the injection of a solution into an acupuncture point. The most commonly used substance is vitamin B_{12}, although electrolyte solutions, saline, DMSO, vitamin C, antibiotics, herbal extracts, homeopathics, and local anesthetics can be used. It is thought that either the pressure on the point or the solution itself will stimulate the nerve fibers.

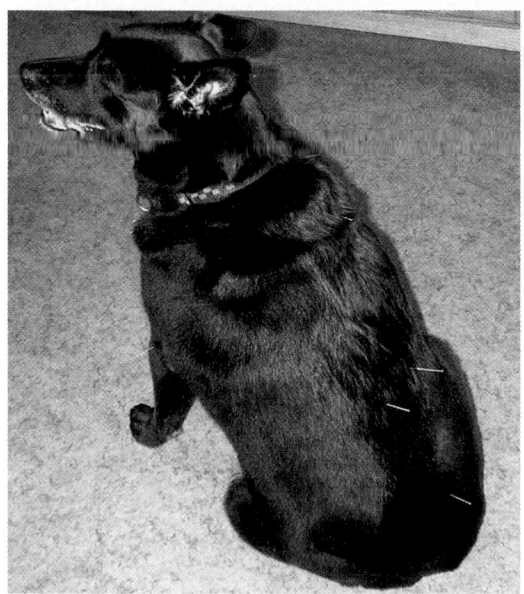

Figure 31-7 Acupuncture: A dog has acupuncture treatment for spondylosis.

Electro-acupuncture is the passing of electrical energy through acupuncture points. Stimulation is accomplished by connecting an electronic device to the inserted needles. Indications include paralysis or paresis, severe and chronic painful conditions, or conditions not responsive to dry needling.

To achieve a continuous stimulation of an acupuncture point, various materials may be surgically implanted at acupuncture points, called *implantation*. Though catgut, stainless steel, and silver can be used, the most common implant is gold in the form of solid beads or wires. This technique is most commonly used for young dogs with painful hip dysplasia, older dogs with coxa-femoral arthritis, or epilepsy. This is considered a surgical procedure.

Low-intensity or "cold" lasers have been used to stimulate acupuncture points. *Laser puncture* is a noninvasive form of intense light therapy using various frequencies and wavelengths that promote positive physiologic changes within cells. It is used to (1) stimulate acupuncture points, (2) enhance healing of wounds and burns, and (3) treat acutely inflamed joints.

Ultrasound can be used to stimulate an acupuncture point, but it is not commonly done, perhaps because of the cost and also the necessity of shaving at each acupuncture point.

Microcurrent therapy is the use of a machine that generates a microcurrent of electricity that can be used on acupuncture points or directly over areas of pain or muscle spasm.

Acupuncture needles can be placed in the tissue perpendicularly or at an angle. When removing the needles they should be gently pulled in the same direction that they went in. If there is resistance when removing the needle, tapping around the needle, rolling it back and forth, or

gently holding down the skin on either side of the needle while pulling the needle gently will ease it from the tissue. Occasionally the needles will come out crooked, which is not unusual because they bend very easily. All needles should be accounted for and placed into a sharps container.

The technician's role in acupuncture includes having a general understanding of how and why acupuncture works and to be able to discuss this with clients, charting the points in the record, aiding in patient restraint or diversion if needed, assisting in easing patient anxiety if present, and removing and counting the needles.

> ### 🖉 TECHNICIAN NOTE
>
> Acupuncture points are connected through pathways that are called *meridians* or *channels*.
>
> The humoral theory was first postulated after studies showed that a transfer of blood, CSF, or brain tissue from an animal under acupuncture analgesia to an animal not receiving acupuncture resulted in analgesia of the recipient.
>
> If there is resistance when removing the needle, tapping around the needle, rolling it back and forth, or gently holding down the skin on either side of the needle while pulling the needle gently will ease it from the tissue.

VETERINARY CHIROPRACTIC

Chiropractic is perhaps one of the most familiar and most utilized complementary therapies that are used to treat veterinary patients. The term is derived from the Greek *cheir* ("hand") and *praxis* ("practice"). The purpose of chiropractic is to manually restore reduced motion in the spine and limbs, thereby improving patient mobility, comfort, and in many cases nervous system function. A. E. Homewood defined *chiropractic* as "that science and art which uses the inherent recuperative powers of the body and deals with the relationship between the nervous system and the spinal column, including its immediate articulations, and the role of this relationship in the restoration and maintenance of health."

The technician is an important team member in a practice that utilizes chiropractic. The involvement may include writing down exam findings and treated areas as well as assisting with restraint and client communication. The technician should have a basic knowledge of the procedure as well as what abbreviations or chiropractic notations are used at the practice.

HISTORY

Manipulation of the spine is an ancient practice. References were made to this form of treatment as early as 2700 BC in China. Even Hippocrates noted the effects of this type of therapy, as he notes, "Look well to the spine for the cause of disease." Chiropractic began in the United States in 1895 with D. D. Palmer, who began to treat the spine as a primary method of healing his patients. His son, B. J. Palmer, followed in his father's footsteps and further developed chiropractic into a system of medicine. He founded the first school of chiropractic in Davenport, Iowa. He claimed to have treated animal patients as well as people in his hospital at the school.

Chiropractic is becoming a more accepted and mainstream treatment in humans. In fact, most major health insurance carriers now cover chiropractic care. This increased accessibility to people has contributed significantly to the increased demand for chiropractic care for veterinary patients. Also contributing to wider acceptance is the growing amount of research that has been done on chiropractic in humans. In fact, many of these same studies utilize animals as models for human disease, thus creating even more applicable research for veterinarians.

In most states veterinary chiropractic adjustments must be performed by a trained professional (either a veterinarian or a chiropractor). Training leading to certification in veterinary chiropractic is available to both groups of professionals through postgraduate courses, but it is not yet a part of standard or elective coursework in either profession. In the United States, certification is available to both veterinarians and chiropractors through the American Veterinary Chiropractic Association, which was founded in the 1980s. This involves approved course work (consisting of at least 200 hours of lecture and hands-on labs), a certification examination (written and practical), and the completion of several case reports. In order to remain certified, a doctor must complete 40 hours of continuing education every 2 years.

> ### ✎ TECHNICIAN NOTE
>
> Proper chiropractic technique requires a great deal of time and effort to learn. This is why chiropractors who administer to human patients go to school for 3 to 4 years before practicing. It is important that *only* a thoroughly trained professional adjust an animal patient. A weekend short course is a nice introduction, but it is not enough to prepare anyone to treat patients. Imagine a person taking a weekend course in veterinary nursing trying to take on the responsibilities that you have worked so hard to prepare for!

Chiropractic is much more than the stereotyped "bone out of place." A chiropractic problem, known as a *subluxation* or *vertebral subluxation complex* (VSC), involves an abnormal relationship between two adjacent vertebrae. This is an anatomically complex area known as the *motor unit* (Figure 31-8). It consists of muscles, ligaments, connective tissue, a spinal nerve and other smaller nerves, blood vessels, lymphatics, and cerebrospinal fluid. The hallmark, or "triad" of signs that occur with a subluxation, includes altered mobility, pain on palpation, and abnormal tension in the surrounding (paraspinal) muscles.

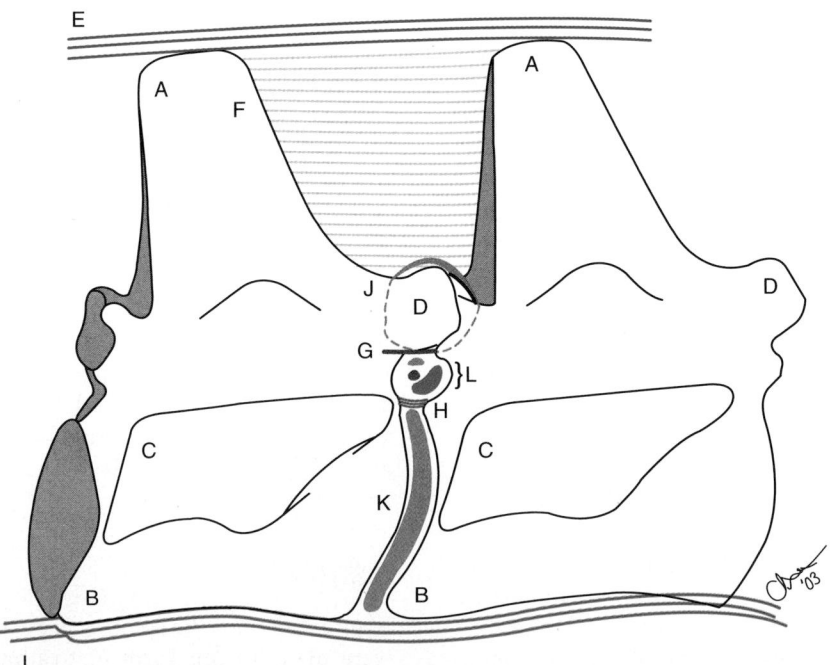

Figure 31-8 The motor unit is a complex anatomic and dynamic area that consists of two adjacent vertebrae and the tissues in between. *A*, Dorsal spinous process. *B*, Vertebral body. *C*, Transverse process. *D*, Articular facet joint. *E*, Supraspinous ligament. *F*, Interspinous ligament. *G*, Ligamentum flavum. *H*, Dorsal longitudinal ligament. *I*, Ventral longitudinal ligament. *J*, Joint capsule. *K*, Intervertebral disk. *L*, Intervertebral foramen.

There are many explanations about how subluxations occur that have been validated by scientific research. The causes of subluxation can vary from overt trauma to minute repetitive stress to the area, such as abnormal spinal movement secondary to left forelimb lameness. Clinical signs range from mild discomfort to reduced reflexes to serious organ dysfunction. By determining where abnormal motion exists and correcting reduced motion in the spine, we can restore normal biomechanics to the body as well as resetting normal neurologic pathways, thus aiding proper nervous system function.

The chiropractic appointment begins with a clear and detailed history. Typically, the patient has previously received a thorough "Western" medical workup prior to the chiropractic appointment, but this is not always the case. The examination proceeds with observation of posture and gait, palpation of the spinal column as well as the extremities (limbs and tail), neurological evaluation, and review of diagnostic images and lab work. It is as detailed (or more so) than a typical general physical examination. Problem areas are recorded, usually using American Veterinary Chiropractic Associations (AVCA) notations. This creates a uniform way of communicating with other doctors who use chiropractic (much as abbreviations for a CBC or blood chemistry are universally understood).

Once the problem areas are identified, the doctor determines whether a chiropractic adjustment is an appropriate therapy for the patient at that time. Sometimes more diagnostics may be required, either in the future or prior to any adjustment being performed. For example, a horse may present with neurologic deficits consistent with equine protozoal myelitis (EPM), and a spinal fluid analysis and EPM test may be indicated. A dog may present for lameness, and the doctor may find cranial drawer motion in the left stifle, indicating anterior cruciate ligament rupture. In both of these cases, chiropractic may help these patients and could be an appropriate therapy to perform at the initial visit, but other primary therapies are warranted. In some cases, such as when patients present with acute paralysis secondary to intervertebral disk disease, it may be more appropriate to obtain further diagnostics (such as radiographs and a myelogram) prior to adjusting the patient to be sure that any areas of active disk disease are avoided.

The next step is for the doctor to adjust the patient. Although treatment principles are similar, each doctor has a unique technique that he or she has developed. The AVCA certifies doctors who are able to perform the basic techniques, but advanced techniques and variations may be learned. Often it is easiest to treat patients in a standing position (Figure 31-9). However, sometimes a sitting or sternal recumbent position may work better for small animal patients. Cats, in particular, are easier to treat while lying on the treatment table rather than being forced to stand. The best position for a patient is one that is comfortable for the patient and allows the doctor to adjust properly. The adjustment should generally be painless for the patient, although sometimes a problem area may present some momentary mild discomfort. If a seriously painful area is found, the doctor will likely avoid treating that area altogether, at least until further diagnostics have been done. It is important to keep the patient relaxed and make the treatment a positive experience (both for the patient and the client), so all of the problem area may not be corrected in one visit. Following the treatment, the doctor will instruct the client on aftercare and follow-up visits, as well as any additional recommendations.

Restraint is particularly important for the first-time patient, because they are unsure about the process and may be nervous or frightened. Restraint can be very simple, such as gentle petting, kind words, or a food distraction (Figure 31-9). Often a patient may need to be repositioned so that the doctor is in the best position to perform the necessary adjustment. Most patients accept and in fact enjoy the treatment, so generally only gentle physical restraint is necessary. It may, however, be necessary to use more rigorous methods of restraint if the situation warrants. Some canine or feline patients may need to be muzzled (especially if they are regular patients at a general practice—they may be expecting a blood draw or a vaccine rather than a relaxing and comfortable treatment). Some horses will require twitching or hobbling, especially if they are not used to being routinely handled. In large animal practice, sometimes the technician may be required to stabilize nearby segments so that an adjustment may be more effective or specific. Proper technique is required in order to provide the most effective treatment, as well as for assistant safety. Occasionally, although most doctors avoid it, chemical restraint

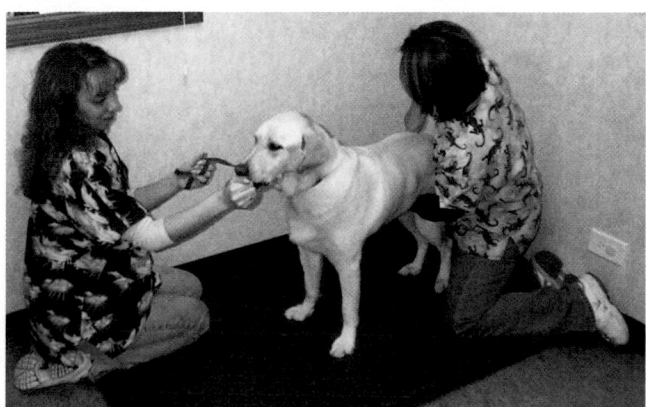

Figure 31-9 Chiropractic adjustment: A technician uses food to gently restrain a patient in a standing position while the doctor performs an adjustment.

is necessary for some patients to relax enough to receive a safe and effective treatment. This is much more likely to happen early in the treatment program, and most patients will not need to be sedated more than once or twice. The technician should become comfortable with all anticipated restraint techniques prior to their use because any unfamiliarity or nervousness may contribute to patient anxiety, and it is very important for the patient to be as relaxed as possible. Practicing on staff pets is often a very good method of developing proficiency in this important role.

Following the treatment, the technician may be asked to follow up with the client the following day, so it is important to be familiar with expected results as well as the doctor's recommendations for aftercare. It is also helpful to be able to answer commonly asked questions about the exam, treatment, or aftercare. If there is a situation which deviates from the normal response, the doctor can be alerted and the patient can be reevaluated in a timely fashion.

ALTERNATIVE CONCEPTS IN NUTRITION

One of the most commonly asked questions in veterinary practice is what should I feed my pet? Quite often, the technician is the staff member responsible for educating clients about nutrition. This is a very important way that you can influence the health of your patients and become an outstanding part of the veterinary health care team. Basic nutrition is essential knowledge for every technician in every practice type of veterinary with no exceptions. Counseling clients on proper nutrition to optimize the recovery of their pet is an important aspect of providing the best and most complete health care. This section is meant to expand upon basic knowledge of animal nutrition and introduce some novel concepts in companion animal nutrition.

Nutrition becomes an even more commonly discussed issue in holistic practice, because it is the foundation of achieving a state of ideal health. In fact, many clients who seek alternative care for their pets are already very educated about nutrition, sometimes even more than the staff. On the downside, misinformation and hype abounds, especially in the Internet age. It can be difficult to convince a client that a vegetarian diet is inappropriate for cats when the lady at the health food store swore it cured her Fluffy's cancer. It is therefore becoming a very important issue at any practice, because these clients need sound nutritional advice from an "expert" who is confident and well-informed. Whether you or your doctors advocate a holistic approach to nutrition, it is imperative that you understand it and can justify your recommendations to these well-informed but sometimes misinformed clients.

A good holistic diet is based on using whole, natural ingredients in a balanced ration. For small animals, the most wholesome healthy diet is a *balanced*, home-prepared diet. In the case of herbivores, the best diet is pasture provided on a soil with balanced minerals, supplemented with hay

and grain only when necessary. The term *balanced* is an important one because an improperly prepared or unbalanced diet can cause disease or at the very least be a hindrance to attaining ideal health. Balance can be achieved with each meal, as it is with commercial pet foods, or it may be achieved on a daily to weekly basis, as our own diets do. It is also important to note that a healthy water source, such as spring water, is as important to the patient's overall health.

✎ TECHNICIAN NOTE

Not every client is willing or able to provide a balanced, home-prepared diet for their pet. There are many excellent nutritious and wholesome commercially prepared pet foods that are easily accessible to the client.

Some recommendations may simply be unattainable for large animal patients, but we can do the best to optimize the resources that are available, such as proper pasture management and using sources of good quality hay and grain, along with supplementation to balance the mineral and vitamin component of the diet. Soil testing and hay analysis for nutrient content is fortunately fairly easily accessible and should be utilized regularly as food sources change.

HOME-PREPARED DIETS

Meat used in the home-prepared diet for carnivores may be raw or cooked, depending on the owner's preference and the pet's constitution. Raw diets are quite an area of controversy, and there is a great deal of information available on this topic. The theory behind raw diets is that a wild carnivore (feline or canine) catches prey and eats it, no cooking involved. Raw meat does contain more enzymes and is truly more "what nature intended." It is more highly digestible and contains more unspoiled nutrients than the cooked version (think about our vegetables). While this is certainly undeniable, most people are unable to provide a fresh catch for their domestic cat or dog. Our raw meat is processed and packaged. This brings about the problem of bacterial contamination, which the carnivore is generally (but not always) well equipped to handle because of the more acidic pH of their stomach and intestines. This is actually much more of a concern to the humans in the household who will be handling the food. Care must be taken to educate clients about the health risks posed to them and their families, especially when there are very young, elderly, or immunocompromised members of the household.

Where raw bones are concerned, it is true that they do not splinter or break teeth as cooked bones do, but they are not without their dangers.

On the subject of vegetables, these should be cooked (lightly steamed) and chopped or minced or grated because carnivores are less able to break down plant cell walls to obtain the nutritious substances inside. Generally, in the wild, the most substantial plant source is what is contained in the herbivorous prey's GI tract. This has already gone through part of the digestive process, and the nutrients

Many dogs, when introduced to raw bones, are too enthusiastic about their new diet and consume large pieces, which can cause gastrointestinal (GI) obstruction. This is not as common an occurrence in cats, but it is not inconceivable. Bones must be introduced very carefully, and if the pet is overzealous, the bones may be ground or a calcium powder must be substituted. This is not as ideal for dental health, but safety is more important.

are thus available for use by the carnivorous predator. The bottom line on raw diets is that they can be a wonderful way to enhance an animal's health if properly prepared and balanced, but they are not indicated for every pet, nor are they the cure for every disease or disorder.

Each patient must be assessed to find the best diet for him or her that is also feasible for their caretaker. An acceptable alternative to home-prepared meals may involve choosing several (3 to 4) commercial diets and rotating them in order to provide overall balance in nutrients. For example, one diet may give an animal less than an ideal (although meeting *minimum* requirements) amount of a certain micronutrient. By rotating diets, this will likely balance out in the long run, because another diet may have more of that nutrient.

Remember that holistic medicine is about treating each patient as an individual. With that in mind there is no best diet for every animal.

NUTRACEUTICALS

The use of *nutraceuticals* is quickly becoming more mainstream in both human and veterinary medicine. The term refers to nutritional supplements that are not herbs and not approved for use as drugs but are thought to convey therapeutic benefit to the patient. There are many types of neutraceuticals. They are used to *treat* many conditions as well as assist the general health and well-being of the patient. The following is a brief list of the more commonly used nutraceuticals (Table 31-2).

As the name implies, this type of supplement uses animal products to supply nutrients (steroids, enzymes, and raw materials of some organs such as liver) to the patient. The theory behind use of glandulares is that by providing sources of whole tissue to an subject with a dysfunctional or suboptimally functioning organ or gland, the patient will receive the necessary substances to improve function and hopefully heal his or her own diseased tissue. This comes about by providing

It is very important to have a reputable source for these products because they are made from animal products. There are a handful of companies in the United States that use human-grade ingredients in their products and have rigorously standardized and tested their products. These companies often provide guidelines for dosing and administration to animals. One company is now making products specifically for dogs and cats, using a powdered form that is quite palatable. This type of therapy is also sometimes a moral and ethical dilemma for holistic practitioners due to animal use, but the more reputable companies try to be as ethical and humane as possible in their formulations.

The technician should be familiar with the glandular-type and nutraceutical products used by the practice. In addition, he or she should be aware of the many types of diets that are appropriate and inappropriate for patients and able to explain to the client the recommendations of the veterinarian.

Table 31-2 COMMONLY USED NUTRACEUTICALS

Nutrient	Primary target area(s)	Function
Glucosamine chondroitin, Perna mussel	Joints	Promote joint lubrication. Reduce progression of or prevent arthritis. Reduce pain and improve mobility.
Shark and bovine cartilage	Joints	Reduce pain and improve mobility.
	Cancer	Anticancer function (shark cartilage is significantly more potent).
MSM	Muscle	Supports muscle function and metabolism.
SAM-E	Liver	Antioxidant.
Coenzyme Q 10	Heart, gingiva	Antioxidant: reduces free-radical damage.
Taurine	Heart, eye	Amino acids: used when deficiency occurs.
L-Carnitine	Heart	Antioxidants/free-radical scavengers.
Superoxide dismutase		
Vitamin E/selenium		
Vitamin C		
Vitamin A		
Essential fatty acids (EPA, glandulares, cell therapy, and glandulare-like products)	Skin	Inhibit inflammation.

HERBAL MEDICINE

Herbal, or *botanical*, *medicine* refers to the practice of using plant materials (including flowers, stems, leaves, bark, seeds, and roots) to treat patients. Herbal medicine is the most ancient known medicine and is the foundation of modern medicine. Using plants as medicine predated written communication, and evidence of its use is widespread in ancient cultures. It is still a large practice in the world today, with an estimated 80% of the world's population using this form of therapy as a primary means of health care. Even today, about 20% of our drugs are derived from some plant source. The technician should become familiar with the herbal pharmacy, just as he or she knows about the drugs on the shelf.

HERBS VERSUS DRUGS

Information about the medicinal use of herbs can be found in the Materia Medica, which is similar to a drug formulary. Many have not been proven safe in pregnancy, and some are very toxic to cats. This is very important to remember, because many clients equate herbs with complete safety and need to be educated on proper use as well as side effects, just as they should with any medication prescribed.

> ### 🖉 TECHNICIAN NOTE
>
> Herbs tend to be less toxic than drugs because the therapeutic substances are not as concentrated. Plants also contain other substances that can act synergistically with the active compound. Herbs are not, however, to be used carelessly. There are many herbs that are extremely safe at many times the therapeutic dose, but others, like some drugs, have a very low margin of safety.

In the United States, herbs are regulated as a food. The FDA requires a rigorous testing procedure in order to approve a substance as a drug, at a cost to the manufacturer of over $230 million. Because a natural substance cannot be patented, no pharmaceutical company would fund the research required for approval. Currently, we rely mainly on testing based in Europe and Asia to substantiate the effects of herbal therapy. Unfortunately, this does nothing to assure us of the quality or purity of the products because of the lack of FDA regulation. The herbal practitioner, therefore, must be cautious about the source of the prescribed herbs. This is another issue that must be emphasized to clients, who often do not understand the difference between the medication purchased at the practice versus the bottle they buy at the local supercenter.

If practicing with a veterinarian who uses therapeutic herbs, the technician should be familiar with commonly used preparations just as he or she has knowledge of the commonly used drugs in the pharmacy. The technician may also be asked to assist in preparation and dispensing herbal products, as well as explaining their proper use to the client.

WESTERN HERBS

Western herbal medicine is becoming a common practice in veterinary medicine. With the holistic movement in human medicine, most people are now familiar with products such as Echinacea, Ginseng, and St. John's wort. Proper dosage and administration for animals has not been scientifically proven, but doses for the more commonly used herbs have been fairly well established.

The herbs come in many different forms (Figure 31-10), and each has advantages and disadvantages when used in animal species. Bulk herbs are the most commonly used preparation for herbivores. The product is often dried and prepared (chopped or powdered). Some of the tastier herbs are also administered to carnivores in this form. Capsules and tablets are often used for carnivores because they are more easily disguised. Teas are prepared by straining the herbs into water. They are fairly easy to prepare, but not always readily accepted by animals (depending on the patient and the herb.) Extracts are made by concentrating the herb in alcohol or glycerin. A standardized extract is much like a drug, where a specific amount of active ingredient is measured rather than a measurement of the herb itself. Milk thistle, for example, is often sold as a standardized extract containing 70% silymarin. Poultices and compresses are used topically for short periods. They are made by soaking the herb or extract in hot water, then allowing it to cool. The product is then held in place manually or with gauze for a short period. Ointments are also used topically, and are generally left in place. Essential oils may be used topically, and some can also be taken internally in extremely dilute form. They are very concentrated and must be used cautiously.

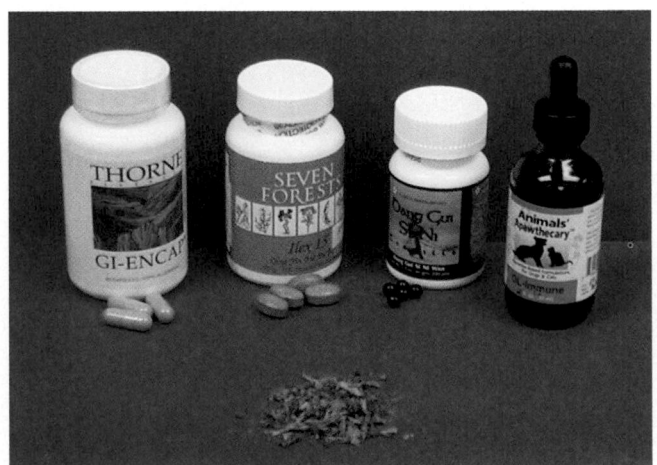

Figure 31-10 Commonly used herbal preparations *(clockwise, left to right)*: Capsules, tablets, tea pills, liquid, dried herbs.

Herbs may also be used to support the general health of the patient (known as *tonification*). When used in this way, the herbs are taken over a long period of time. Gingko is often used in this way to support mental function in geriatric patients. Herbs may also be used in detoxification, such as use of milk thistle to help protect and support the liver after steroid therapy.

Administration of most herbs is generally best done on an empty stomach. For herbivores, this may be impossible. The next best way to administer is with a small amount of water. Sometimes salt-free broth or clam juice works well for small animals. If food is the only way to get the herb to the patient, then try to avoid giving the herb with a full meal. It is also best to avoid any foods with strong flavor, such as peppermint, near the time of administration.

CHINESE HERBAL MEDICINE

Chinese herbs actually consist of many substances, including minerals, as well as animal tissue. Individual botanical herbs may be used in the same way that Western herbs are. In fact, there is some overlap between Chinese and Western herbs. The main difference between the two is the use of the TCM system in patient diagnosis and treatment with Chinese herbs.

TCM has previously been discussed in the section on acupuncture. The Chinese herbal practitioner must have a clear TCM diagnosis when prescribing an herbal therapy. This involves a TCM examination, including tongue and pulse diagnosis. Herbal medicine is considered "stronger" than acupuncture. Practitioners often use properties and taste of the herbs in order to choose the most appropriate herb or formula. In fact, most TCM practitioners in China use acupuncture only in acute cases, and prescribe herbs along with it in order to bring about a more thorough treatment. Often, for more chronic conditions or to help patients maintain health, herbs alone are used. For example, the herb Ma Huang, or Ephedra, is used to "disperse congestion in the lung" and "release the exterior." In terms of TCM, the patient may be diagnosed with an exterior cold excess pattern of disease. In terms of our knowledge of pharmacology, this substance dries mucous membranes, and derivatives are used to treat the common cold, which is an exterior pathogen.

The formulas are named for their function or their main ingredients. For example, for this reason the practitioner using Chinese herbs should undertake formal training. Forms are similar to Western preparation (Figure 31-10), including tablets and pills, powders, granules, liquid teas and extracts, and topical preparations (ointments, plasters, and liniments). Many of the formulas come in tiny tablets known as *tea pills*.

These are quite handy when treating cats, but large dogs may require 10 or more pills per dose!

As with Western herbs, and perhaps even more importantly, Chinese herbs must come from a reputable source with assurance of quality control. The use of animal products in many formulations makes this a more serious concern. There are several companies in the United States that distribute products of uniform quality that are produced under the most ethical circumstances possible. (For example, some animal products from endangered species are substituted with a similar product from a related domestic animal.) For some holistic practitioners, the use of animal products may result in a moral dilemma, and these doctors may choose to avoid these products in their pharmacy.

AYURVEDIC HERBS

Ayurvedic means the science of life. Similar to TCM, it emphasizes health and wellness, not just treatment of disease. It originated in India, and is believed to predate TCM, and even to have contributed to its foundation. It includes not only herbal prescriptions, but also diet, massage, exercise, and meditation as part of a patient's therapy. The goal of this system of medicine is to balance the three elements of nature, known as *Doshas*, which exist in every living organism.

Like Chinese herbs, ayurvedic herbs may be prescribed based on pharmacology (like Western herbs), according to the three Doshas (similar to yin, yang, and qi), or based on taste and temperature. For example, licorice is considered a sweet herb. Sweet herbs are considered to be cold and wet and are used to nourish and soothe. In terms of pharmacology, licorice reduces the breakdown of prostaglandin, which protects the stomach from excess acid. Thus it is a treatment for stomach ulcers, which cause a burning sensation.

The technician who works with a practitioner who treats patients using the above herbal therapies should be familiar with the more commonly used herbs: indications, contraindications, and precautions, as well as appropriate dosage. Awareness of common herb-drug interactions is also important. The technician may be asked to prepare the herbal formula, to administer, to dispense, and to explain a prescribed formula to the client. This requires a thorough knowledge of the herbal pharmacy.

VETERINARY HOMEOPATHY

Homeopathy is a system of medicine that is based on the principle that "like cures like." It involves treating each patient as an individual based on his or her group of symptoms. Practitioners use extremely diluted versions of herbs and other substances, which are called *remedies*, to treat patients. It is sometimes difficult to understand, but it can generate amazing results when used by a skillful practitioner. The technician should understand the basic principles of homeopathy and be able to properly administer and store remedies as well as explain these things to clients.

HISTORY AND PRINCIPLES

Samuel Hahnemann, a German physician, first used and developed homeopathy in the late 1700s. At the time, medications were given to patients without any assurance of safety. The scientific process as we know it did not exist, and trial and error determined which substances would be good medications and which would do more harm than good. One example of a commonly used medicine at that time is arsenic, which we know today as a poison. This astute doctor recognized that symptoms of disease were expressions of the body's attempt to restore homeostasis in response to imbalance or insult.

Hahnemann postulated that giving a patient a medication that would simulate the disease would stimulate the body's own defenses, and the patient would heal. This is similar to, though not completely the same as, the principle of vaccination. It is the reverse of allopathic (or Western/modern) medicine, which uses drugs to counteract symptoms, thereby suppressing them. For example, if you use cortisone to treat a rash, your symptoms will return if you do not repeat the dose for many days, sometimes even more severely than initially experienced. You may later show signs of a more serious disease, such as a stomach ulcer. Western medicine would consider the two conditions to be unrelated, but a homeopath considers them both to be signs of disorder in the body.

Hahnemann also determined that the more he diluted medicine, the stronger the beneficial effects became, while the harmful effects diminished or disappeared altogether. Although important, this was not his most profound discovery. Whereas most physicians were concerned with treating one symptom, the "chief complaint" as we know it, Hahnemann astutely observed that these medications had many multiple effects on the body (some beneficial, some harmful, and some neither beneficial or harmful). He decided to try his medications, which were then completely safe, on healthy patients. For example, if you were healthy and took cold medicine, you might experience a dry nose and throat as well as drowsiness or even inability to sleep, depending on the drug combination. He recorded everything his patients told him about the effects the medicine had on them, and he observed every detail that he could, from physical signs to emotions that his patients experienced. This practice is known today as a *proving*.

Hahnemann believed that the medication should match the symptoms more closely. He began collecting much more detailed information about his patients, and he was able to be more precise when choosing a medicine for each individual. A perfect example is the common cold: No two people exhibit the same exact symptoms, even though they may have the same exact virus that caused the disease. In fact, many people exhibit the same cold symptoms each time they are sick, regardless of the strain of the virus.

Because of the safety and efficacy of his medicine, others sought to learn how to treat patients in this manner. Hahnemann recorded his philosophy and findings in a book entitled *The Organon of Medicine*. Homeopathy is still widely practiced today in Europe, although less so in the United States. The earliest mention of veterinary homeopathy came from Hahnemann himself, when he stated in a lecture in the early 1800s that a similar approach was also applicable to animals. Today there are organizations and courses available worldwide for veterinarians who would like to practice homeopathic medicine.

PRACTICE

When a patient is seen by a homeopathic practitioner, a clear and detailed history is essential to a successful outcome. The owner is asked many questions, some of which may seem minute and unimportant. Any previous diagnostics and therapies (as well as responses) should be noted, even for minor problems. The patient is observed, and details about his or her physical status as well as personality and reactions to certain situations are noted and recorded. This should always include a thorough Western physical examination, because these findings may lead to symptoms not discovered by the owner (such as a fast heart rate). The doctor may also note something of a serious nature that may need a Western approach prior to using homeopathy. For example, an older patient in congestive heart failure that presents to the hospital dyspneic and cyanotic needs to be stabilized first. Once out of a life-threatening situation, then the patient can be evaluated, and a more long-term approach can be taken.

Minute details can be very important when treating patients homeopathically. Even the way the patient greets the doctor can be important in finding the correct remedy. All of the details are recorded, and a list of remedies that are appropriate for each sign or symptom is compiled. This is called *repertorizing*. From this list, the most appropriate remedy is prescribed. In modern times, much of this work can be done by computer, although some practitioners still do all of their research by hand.

The remedy is then dispensed to the owner with specific instructions on dosage and administration. Homeopathic remedies come in several strengths, called *potencies*. Potency is inversely proportional to dilution: the less actual substance present, the stronger the medicine. In general, it is best to use the lowest potency (or least most) necessary to bring about a cure. Sometimes the dose will be given only once, sometimes multiple times. The remedy should be discontinued when the symptoms cease or the patient shows improvement. Occasionally a patient will experience an exacerbation of symptoms, called an *aggravation*. This usually passes within a few hours and is not generally a concern. Usually it indicates that the correct remedy was

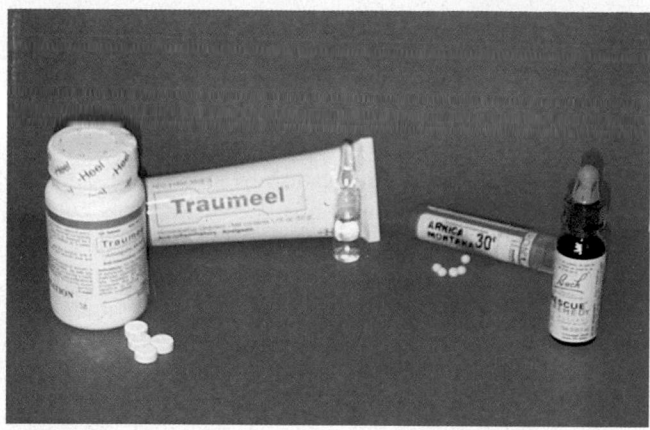

Figure 31-11 Homeopathic preparations *(clockwise, left to right):* Ointment, injectable (foreground), tablets, pellets, liquid (flower essence).

Table 31-3 HOMEOPATHIC PREPARATIONS

Form	Administration
Pellets (sugar) or tablets	Use whole (dispense from cap into the patient's mouth, avoiding contaminating the cap) or crush between a folded sheet of paper. Pour into patient's mouth or drop between the lips and gum. Can also be dissolved in distilled or spring water and administered by dropper.
Liquid	Use dropper and apply on tongue or between cheek and gums.
Topical	Apply to affected area.
Injections	May be used SQ, IM, intralesionally. Often used in acupuncture points.

chosen, but if the patient becomes weaker, an antidote (another remedy) to the prescribed remedy can be given. Antidotes to each remedy are listed in the Materia Medica.

> **TECHNICIAN NOTE**
>
> It is very important that the remedy be handled properly and that it be given exactly as directed.

The remedies are fragile compared to Western medications. There are several forms (Figure 31-11). They should not be touched and should be administered away from food whenever possible. The remedy is effective as soon as it gets into the mouth, so as long as it touches the lips, gums, or tongue, it does not need to be swallowed. Remedies should never be returned to the bottle. They should be stored at room temperature away from moisture (keep container sealed) in a dark place, preferably in a cabinet away from strong herbs, Western medication, and magnetic fields (microwaves, computers, stereo speakers) (Table 31-3).

Homeopaths believe things that suppress symptoms actually drive disease deeper into the body or create more imbalance. Depending on how "deep" or serious the disorder is, it may take a succession of several remedies to restore a patient to health. Changes in symptoms are noted, and a new remedy is chosen until the patient is healthy. Homeopathy can be used at many levels. The least complex is treatment of *acute disease*, which should quickly restore health to a vital, strong patient. An example of this is the use of Arnica montana to treat a patient with bruising due to trauma. Next is treatment on a *constitutional* level, which takes into account the very nature (physical traits, personality, emotions) of the patient as well as disease symptoms, past and present. The goal is to help the patient restore and maintain a state of health. The most complex is *miasmic* treatment, in which the ultimate goal of therapy is to prevent disease by addressing genetic weaknesses. This is quite challenging in the veterinary patient, and it is therefore not often undertaken.

> **TECHNICIAN NOTE**
>
> A disorder that may seem minor by traditional medicine may actually be quite serious from a homeopathic perspective. Similarly, a patient may be considered healthy by Western standards, but may still be imbalanced, and thus in need of further treatment when undergoing homeopathic treatment.

Homeopathy can be further divided into *classical homeopathy*, in which the patient is treated with one remedy at a time, and *modern homeopathy*, in which the patient is given a combination of remedies to match his or her given set of symptoms. The combination therapy can be used in a more Western approach. For example, a combination therapy called *Traumeel* (Figure 31-11) is a commonly used treatment for bruising, trauma, inflammation, and arthritis. It comes in several forms (oral tablets and liquid, injectable, and cream) and contains arnica, calendula, Echinacea, and several other individual remedies that work together to provide the desired effect.

From a scientific standpoint there has been much research on homeopathy. The individualized nature of the treatments can make it difficult to "prove" from a Western standpoint, but many double-blind, placebo-controlled studies exist. Research on the biphasic nature of medication has assisted our understanding of how diluted forms of medication can have the opposite effect of the therapeutic dose of the same medicine on the body. For example, a clinical dose of atropine causes drying of mucous membranes, but a tiny dose has been shown to increase secretions of mucous membranes. Both in vitro as well as clinical studies have shown homeopathic remedies to be effective, but thus far we do not understand exactly *how* they work.

BACH FLOWER REMEDIES

Flower essence therapy, developed by Edward Bach in the 1930s, uses an approach similar to homeopathy to treat patients. Bach believed that all substances used to treat patients be completely nontoxic. He developed 37 essences derived from plants (flowers, bushes, trees) and one from water (Rock Water) for a total of 38 remedies. They are not diluted to the extent that homeopathic remedies are.

The use of flower essences is based more on a psychological or emotional than physical level. Bach himself described 12 pathological emotional states that he believed would lead to physical disease if left untreated. For example, the remedy aspen is used to treat patients with fear of the unknown, and holly is used to treat patients exhibiting jealousy or suspiciousness. Of course, the emotional nature of animals can be difficult to determine, but it is not unreasonable and can be quite rewarding. Flower essences may, like homeopathy, be used in acute situations as well as treating patients on a constitutional basis.

The individual essences are all provided as a liquid. The most common remedy used is called *rescue remedy* (Figure 31-11), and it is a combination of five flower essences (Rock Rose, Cherry Plum, Star of Bethlehem, Clematis, and Impatiens). The preparation may also be found in a cream. It is used to treat animals in times of stress, anxiety, or trauma. For those interested in using flower essences, rescue remedy is an excellent starting point and can be used in such situations as trauma and surgery recovery or even for the frightened and panic-stricken boarding patient. The remedies are administered like homeopathic remedies, but they are generally sold in stock bottles. The stock flower remedy should be diluted in spring water or a combination of water and alcohol (increases shelf life) to make a treatment bottle. Generally two drops of each stock remedy (four if using rescue remedy) are placed in a 1-oz glass amber vial with a dropper. Up to five remedies may be combined in one treatment bottle (rescue remedy only counts as a single remedy). They are given by the dropper directly into the mouth. They may also be added to drinking water (from a few drops in a bowl for a cat to 15 drops per gallon for a horse). Another method is using the remedy in a spray bottle as a mist (usually into the environment), which is a very effective and stress-free means of treating birds and small mammals. It can also be used topically. Administration is generally repeated at various intervals. In an acute situation, it may be as often as every 30 seconds. For a less urgent situation, it may be daily for several days or weeks. They should be stored like homeopathic remedies.

These flower remedies, like their homeopathic counterparts, are very safe to use and can have a profound effect on a patient when the correct remedy is given. They are often used as an adjunct to other therapies that do not do as much to address the emotional aspect of healing. As you can well imagine, the technician can be of great value to the veterinarian who practices homeopathy. By assisting in observation of the patient as well as client education, the technician can have a substantial impact on the success of the treatment.

MISCELLANEOUS THERAPIES

LASER

Laser stands for light amplification by stimulated emission of radiation. Albert Einstein first introduced this concept in 1917. Low-level laser therapy (LLLT) is the stimulation of tissue with low-energy lasers to achieve a therapeutic effect. LLLT's most common indications include treating acupuncture points (Figure 31-12), trigger points, edema, wounds and ulcers, postoperative pain (seen commonly in human dentistry), stomatitis and gingivitis, and temporomandibular joint dysfunction. The lasers most commonly used in LLLT are the visible red helium-neon (HeNe) and the invisible infrared (IR) gallium-arsenide (GaAs) lasers and gallium-aluminum-arsenide (GaAlAs) lasers. Laser beams differ from conventional light by being monochromic (one color creates a narrow spectrum) and by being coherent (having the waves stay together and be consistent). Most lasers have polarized light (light waves oscillate in the same plane), have a small divergence (nearly parallel beam), and a high mean output power (MOP), indicating that many watts are put out. LLLT may be indicated for soft-tissue trauma, wounds, tendonitis, and pain relief. Some of the biologic effects seen with LLLT include accelerated cell division, increased leukocyte phagocytosis, stimulation of fibroblasts and collagen formation, degranulation of mast cells (which may explain why it can be used in acupuncture, as mast cell degranulation occurs when a needle is placed in an acupuncture point).

Precautions

Lasers may induce retinal lesions and are therefore classified by their irradiation properties. Some are utilized solely by the veterinarian.

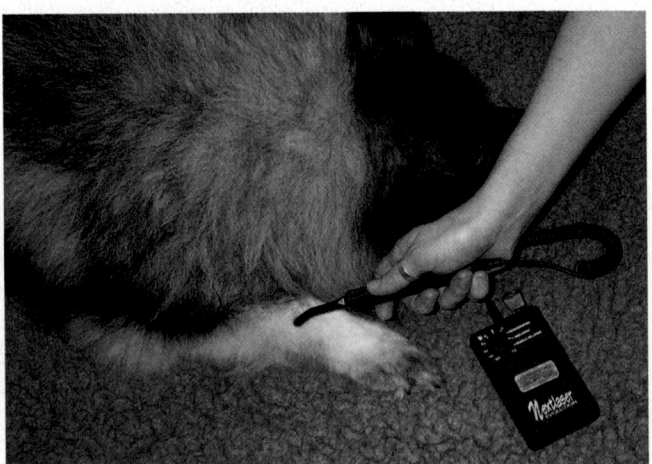

Figure 31-12 Laser acupuncture can be used for painful or swollen areas or with animals that are sensitive to needles.

The technician's role in LLLT is to document the veterinarian's treatment and be able to answer questions asked by clients regarding LLLT.

MAGNETS

Magnets have been used for centuries in medicine. Magnetism can be separated into stationary magnets, which have a north and south pole, and electromagnetic therapy, which utilizes electricity of different frequencies along with magnets to create an electromagnetic field. The units of measurement for magnetism are gauss (G) and tesla (T). Most therapeutic magnets range from 1000 to 3000 G. Below 500 G has been deemed ineffective. The north and south poles of a magnet are reported to have different effects. The effects of using the north pole end of the magnet include pain relief, stimulation of bone healing, the enhancement of vasoconstriction, decreased blood pressure, and, by decreasing mitosis, slowing the growth rate of cancer cells and bacterial cells. The effects of using the south pole end of the magnet include strengthening and promoting growth by stimulating cell multiplication (therefore should not be used with bacterial or viral infections or close to tumors), enhancement of vasodilatation, slowing bone healing, and increasing ascites, edema, and inflammation. Some therapeutic magnets have both north and south poles that may be held on given area or wrapped over an area. Products are available that place magnets in horse blankets or leg wraps and dog and cat beds and collars.

In electromagnetic therapy, pulsating electromagnetic waves are produced by electrical charges undergoing acceleration. These waves can be generated with different frequencies and can create different physiologic changes in the body. For instance, it is known that there is an electrical field around each joint that plays a part in the continual regeneration of cartilage and connective tissue. There is a disturbance in this field if osteoarthritis or inflammatory joint disorders are present. Pulsed signal therapy (PST) is one type of pulsed electromagnetic field therapy (PEMF). This allows reconstruction of the disturbed electrical field, which returns the natural regeneration capabilities and reactivates the chondrocytes (cartilage cells) and connective tissue to increase production of proteoglycan and collagen, which aids in repairing cartilage defects. Most of the research has been done in osteoarthritis, but there have also been significant improvements after treating many other conditions including tendon and ligament injuries (this should not be used in partial cranial cruciate tears because the scar tissue is important in joint stabilization, and this removes early scar tissue) and wound healing. PEMF has been used extensively in equine sports medicine for musculoskeletal and neurological conditions. It has been used successfully to treat navicular disease, tendon injuries, arthroses, spavins, delayed wound healing, and diseases of the thoracolumbar spine. Artificial insemination centers also use PEMF on bulls that suffer from degenerative lumbosacral diseases to extend their productive capacity.

The technician's role in magnet therapy is to answer question the clients may have, apply stationary magnets to the patients, and position and sit with patients during PEMF therapy (Figure 31-13).

AROMATHERAPY

Aromatherapy is the therapeutic use of volatile essential oils to obtain a physiologic or psychological effect. Oils are distilled or extracted from plants and are considered the "last possible and most sublime" parts of the plant. Flowers, buds, fruits, peel, leaves, bark, wood, roots, and seeds can be used. The oils can be applied topically by themselves or in a massage oil, ingested (not common), or administered by nebulization (the oil is made into a mist and inhaled). The effect of inhalation is most likely due to rapid absorption by both the nasal and lung mucosa. Plants or parts of the plants can also be burned and the smoke inhaled. Potential uses of aromatherapy include antibacterial and antifungal (tea tree oil and thyme oil), relaxation or sedation (lavender oil), behavior modification (positive or negative), conditioning (citronella bark collars), and medicinal.

The technician's role in aromatherapy is to apply the oils at the recommendation of the veterinarian and to have a basic knowledge of their treatment purpose, as well as be able to discuss their use and benefits.

> ### ✎ TECHNICIAN NOTE
>
> Some of the biologic effects seen with LLLT include accelerated cell division, increased leukocyte phagocytosis, stimulation of fibroblasts and collagen formation, and degranulation of mast cells.

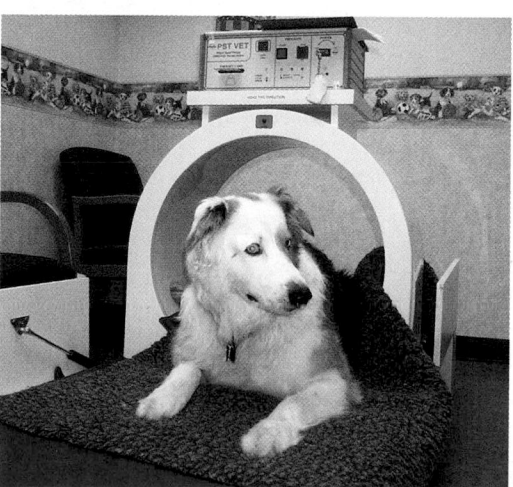

Figure 31-13 PST has an 80% to 85% success rate of treating osteoarthritis with good to excellent results. Since there is a 13-inch-diameter treatment area, often feet, hocks, stifles, hips, and lower back can be treated at the same time.

Most therapeutic magnets range from 1000 to 3000 G. Below 500 G has been deemed ineffective.

SUMMARY

Complementary and alternative veterinary medicine encompasses a vast amount of material. This chapter offers an overview of some of the more common modalities used today and is not a comprehensive guide to alternative medicine. Many of the individual subjects discussed in this chapter have their own texts written on the subject and are taught in courses lasting months to years. The technician may become the "clinic expert" in many of these modalities (i.e., massage, swim therapist, or Bach flower remedies) and can be a good source of client information in the other modalities (i.e., acupuncture and chiropractic therapy). As many clients are looking into alternative medicine for themselves, they are seeing the benefits and are looking into sharing the experience with their animals. There are numerous opportunities to be a part of the thrilling and gratifying fields of complementary and alternative medicine. Additionally, as more veterinarians are becoming certified in these areas, the employment opportunities will continue to grow.

RECOMMENDED READINGS

Books

Gersh MR: *Electrotherapy in rehabilitation*, Philadelphia, 1992, FA Davis.
Graham H, Gregory V: *Bach flower remedies for animals*, Scotland, 1999, Findhorn Press.
Michlovitz SL: *Thermal agents in rehabilitation*, ed 3, Philadelphia, 1996, FA Davis.
Pitcairn RH: *Dr. Pitcairn's complete guide to natural health for dogs and cats*, Emmaus, Pa, 1995, Rodale.
Pontinen PJ: *Low level laser therapy as a medical treatment modality*, Tampere, 1992, Art Urpo Ltd.
Salvo SG: *Massage therapy principles and practice*, St Louis, 2003, WB Saunders.
Schoen AM: *Veterinary acupuncture: ancient art to modern medicine*, St Louis, 1994, Mosby.
Schoen AM, Wynn SG: *Complementary and alternative veterinary medicine: principles and practice*, St Louis, 1998, Mosby.
Tisserand B, Balacs T, editors: *Essential oil safety: a guide for health care professionals*, New York, 1995. Churchill Livingstone.
Wynn SG, Marsden SM: *Manual of natural veterinary medicine: science and tradition*, St. Louis, 2002, Mosby.
PDR people's desk reference for essential oils, 1999, Essential Science Publishing.
Schwartz C: *Four paws five directions: a guide to Chinese medicine for cats and dogs*, Berkley, CA, 1996, Celestial Arts Publishing.
Wulff-Tilford M, Tilford G: *All you ever wanted to know about herbs for pets*, Irvine, CA, 1999, Bowtie Press.

Journals

Haussler KK: Chiropractic evaluation and management. *Vet Clin North Am, Equine Prac* 15(1): 195-207, 1999.

Videos

Schreiber M: *Sports massage for the equine athlete*, Middleburg, Va, 1990, Equissage Associates, 800-843-0224.
Vaughn L, Jones D: *Body works for dogs*, Pound Ridge, Clarksville, Md, 2000, Animals Healing, www.animalshealing.com. 877-929-1515.
Whalen-Shaw P: *Massage for your dog*, Circleville, Ohio, 1999, Integrated Touch Therapy, 800-251-0007.

Contacts

Bio-Magnetic Therapy Systems, Boca Raton, Fla, 561-362-4090 (call for CD with research), www.pstvet.com.
Ken Becker (contact person): Hako-med Systems, 1-800-562-0708, www.hakomed.com.

Professional Organizations

Academy of Veterinary Homeopathy, *www.theavh.org*.
American Holistic Veterinary Medical Association, 410-569-0795, www.ahvma.org.
American Veterinary Chiropractic Association, 918-784-2231, www.animalchiropractic.org.
International Veterinary Acupuncture Society, *www.ivas.org*.
Veterinary Botanical Medicine Association, www.vbma.org.

Massage Schools

Equissage: Round Lake, Va, 800-843-0224, www.equissage.com.
Healing Oasis: Sturtevant, Wis, 262-878-9549, www.thehealingoasis.com.
Integrated Touch Therapy, Circleville, Ohio, 800-251-0007, www.integratedtouchtherapy.com.
TTEAM Training USA, PO Box 3793, Santa Fe, NM, 800-854-TEAM.
TTEAM Training Canada, 5435 Rochdell, Vernon, BC, Canada, 604-545-2336.

Rehabilitation Training

Animal Rehab Institute, Loxahatchee, Fla, 561-792-6889, www.animalrehabinstitute.com.
North East Seminars, University of Tennessee, www.NESeminars.com.

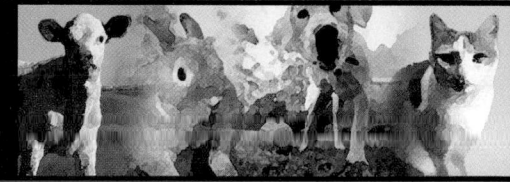

32

Veterinary Practice Management

DENNIS M. McCURNIN • ROGER L. LUKENS

INTRODUCTION

Each veterinary practice is a professional business that offers medical care to animals with their owners' consent. Only willing owners consent to pay a fee for professional services provided by the veterinary team. The total cost of operating a medical business providing these services is paid by the gross income of the practice. Therefore marketing efforts must effectively attract (and retain) sufficient clients to each practice or it will go bankrupt. No professional veterinary business will survive if it is not profitable.

The highest quality of care possible for the animals must be offered to their owners in a cost-effective (not cost-cutting) manner; this is extremely important to both patients and their owners. A high-quality practice requires keeping up with the latest medical knowledge and technologies. It also requires the most effective and caring communication possible with owners by the entire veterinary team. Quality communication is absolutely necessary to inform, educate, and obtain owner compliance for the veterinarian's recommendations to benefit the animal.

The profitability of the practice and the care of the client's animal are at risk if the veterinary team fails to deliver quality medical care for the animal coupled with caring effective communication with the owner. The services of the veterinary team are not successful unless the patient is helped and the client understands the service, the client is pleased with the caring attitude of the team, the client tells others of his or her enthusiasm for that practice, and the client wants to return for future veterinary care of pets. Veterinary technicians are very important to the success of the veterinary team in accomplishing these goals.

Effective management of the veterinary practice as a business is also necessary because of increased competition, growing malpractice threats, new technology, free Internet information, Internet pharmacies, shifting client expectations, and continuing inflation of medical equipment, supply, and personnel costs. All these risks and challenges must be well managed to enhance both productivity and quality of patient care.

It has been said, "What is good business may be bad medicine, and what is good medicine may be bad business." Veterinary practice represents the *art* of balancing both business and medicine to meet the needs of patients, clients, and the veterinary team. ■

VETERINARY PRACTICE MANAGEMENT AREAS

Veterinary students are naturally interested in managing nursing care of patients. They must realize the necessity of effective client communication to benefit the patient and begin to understand the business side of medicine. This develops only after gaining significant experience in a veterinary practice. Managing equipment, facility, staff, and marketing is not of much interest until the student has experienced problems or limitations in these areas that have a negative impact on patient care (or technician salary).

Each of these management areas (Box 32-1) must be coordinated with the other areas to meet the veterinary team's goals for the operation (mission statement and strategic plan). A successfully managed practice enjoys success and accomplishment with people, both internally and externally. Failure to properly manage patients, people, and the business ultimately leads to a reduction in the quality of service rendered, staff dissatisfaction, staff turnover, a disorganized practice, dissatisfied clients, and decreasing business.

Box 32-1 MANAGEMENT AREAS

- Facility design
- Patient care
- Client communications
- Human resources
- Finance
- Marketing
- Building
- Equipment
- Medical records
- Inventory control
- Computerization

VETERINARY FACILITIES

The type of practice facility will vary greatly according to the needs of the clients and the species of animals served by the practice staff. *Facility design* must accommodate the needs of the patients, the number of clients served, the interests of the veterinarians, the level of care to be provided, and the financing available for investing in the facility. Many facilities are simply expanded and remodeled. Occasionally the existing facility is totally replaced with one redesigned to meet the above goals.

The practice may limit veterinary service to a single species (feline, equine, swine, cattle), to small animals (dogs, cats, exotic pets), to large animals (any livestock, horses), to exotic animals, or to a mixed practice (all species). Each type of practice has unique requirements for a facility that is designed to accommodate their patients and clients. Large animal and mixed practices may provide all veterinary services on the owner's premises, have haul-in facilities for these species, or provide both options as a convenience to the client.

The majority of practicing veterinarians are general practitioners who offer *primary care* level of services. They increasingly refer problem cases to specialists at referral practices (*secondary care* providers) or veterinary schools (*tertiary care* providers). These specialists are board-certified in surgery, internal medicine, dermatology, ophthalmology, or other areas. Once treatment by the specialists is finished, the patient and client are transferred back to the primary care provider. Primary care providers are also able to use the skills of consultant specialists to read x-rays and ultrasound images as well as electrocardiograms (ECGs) or consult with specialists by telephone or via the Internet without referring the case.

Many diseases are not fully understood because diagnostic methods are unavailable, clinical treatments are inadequate, and prevention is not yet possible. Therefore this network of referring practitioners not only is providing the best quality of care possible, but it also is the foundation of supporting clinical research at the tertiary care centers at the veterinary schools. Both clinical and basic science research is absolutely necessary to discover the pathogenesis of unsolved diseases, new and effective diagnostics, effective treatments, and ultimately, the preventative steps necessary to avoid patient death and client despair.

Box 32-2 VETERINARY FACILITY NOMENCLATURE

OFFICE
Room where limited or consultative type of practice is conducted

MOBILE FACILITY
A vehicle for making house or farm calls *or* a vehicle equipped with special medical and/or surgical facilities; both must have a permanent base of operations (published address and telephone number)

CLINIC
Outpatient practice facility *not* offering overnight patient confinement

HOSPITAL
Inpatient practice facility offering overnight hospitalization of patients; sometimes called *primary care facility*

EMERGENCY FACILITY
Emergency practice facility that focuses primarily on treating and monitoring emergencies with veterinarian and staff who are always available (during specified hours of operation) and is equipped to provide timely and appropriate level of emergency care

ON-CALL EMERGENCY SERVICE
Veterinarians and staff who are not on premises all the time but are available via on-call basis to handle emergency calls

REFERRAL CENTER
Staff of board-certified specialist veterinarians who receive referrals from the primary care practitioners of the above facilities; sometimes called *secondary care facility*

ANIMAL MEDICAL CENTER
A large facility (veterinary teaching hospitals, large corporate practices) offering consultative, clinical, and hospital services to referred clients and their local veterinarian; also performs significant research on animal health problems and conducts advanced professional education programs; sometimes called *tertiary care facility*

FACILITY NOMENCLATURE

Numerous terms are applied to veterinary facilities. The American Veterinary Medical Association (AVMA) has developed guidelines (Box 32-2) for consistency in naming veterinary facilities to avoid confusion by the general public. In addition, many state practice acts and regulations not only have been updated to specify standards of practice and professional competency for both veterinarians and technicians but also have adopted facility and equipment requirements and hired inspectors to ensure that these standards are being met. The American Animal Hospital

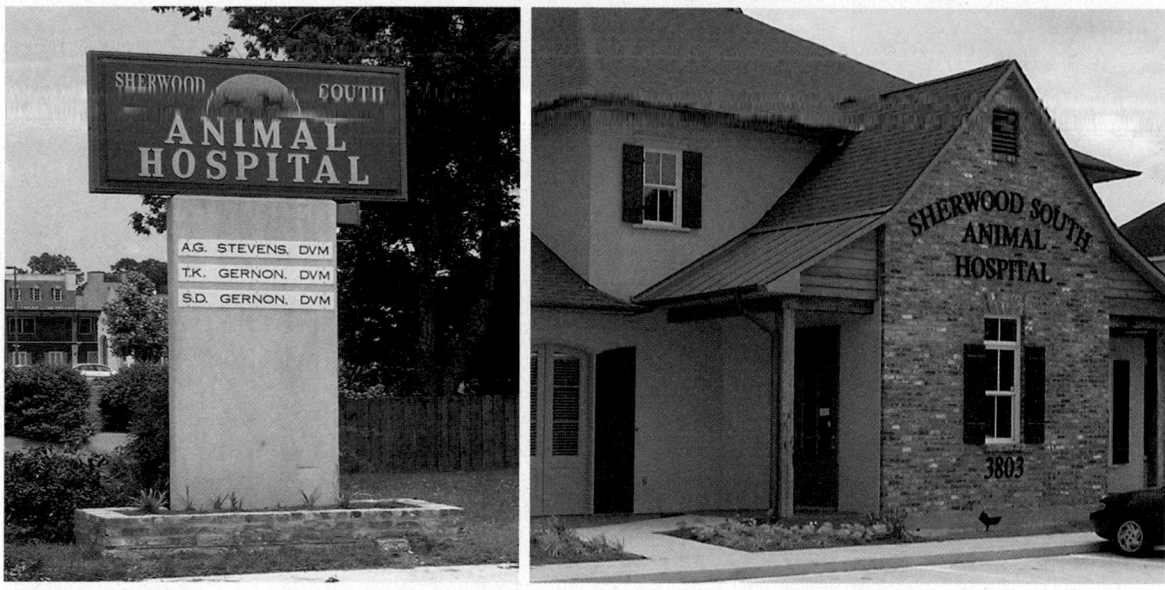

Figure 32-1 **A,** Hospital signs should be professional and clearly visible from the street. **B,** Signs directly on the building may also be used.

Association (AAHA) also has extensive standards of excellence that cover most of the management areas listed in Box 32-1. These must be met to have the hospital accredited by AAHA.

MANAGEMENT OF HOSPITAL AREAS

The small animal hospital (Box 32-2) is the most complete facility for primary care practice for small animals. It provides the best model for discussing location, function, and management of each of the facility areas in this chapter. Good management of hospital areas is the foundation to understanding the principles of improving the efficiency of any practice. Conversely, lack of attention to facility area management ultimately leads to inefficiencies, disorder of the practice, staff frustration, loss of income, and decrease of the quality of client service and patient care.

Small animal hospital facilities are designed to provide overnight hospitalization, complete surgical facilities, and sufficient examination rooms to provide outpatient services. They also must have ancillary support areas to provide reception, laboratory, pharmacy, imaging, diagnostic procedures, treatment, and inpatient ward space. The appropriate size and location of each area in the hospital are related to the number of veterinarians and support staff in the practice and the number of clients and patients served.

Patient management and possibly client management are obviously the most interesting and necessary management topics for entry-level veterinary technicians. It often takes more experience and a desire for advancement before veterinary technicians become very interested in the other areas of practice management (Box 32-1). Students need to develop a working knowledge of the principles of

management of hospital areas in order to be effective technicians and to prepare for future advancement in the veterinary technology profession. This understanding is also critical for assessing practice differences when searching for the best employment opportunity (see self-marketing section at end of this chapter).

Outside Areas

Location is the primary factor (other than referrals from satisfied clients) in attracting new clients. Location will often dictate slow or rapid practice growth. Location provides visibility for potential clients and allows existing clients to easily find the practice. Prime locations within shopping centers and on main streets are expensive during the initial investment period but will repay the investment by increasing practice growth and increasing real estate value. Location of the facility should also be considered by veterinary technicians when selecting a practice for employment.

Further, the *practice sign* must be evaluated for visibility and professional appearance. The optimum would be a well-placed, neat professional sign that allows the client clear visibility and direction (Figure 32-1). The sign becomes even more important during an emergency. Some form of lighting will allow clients to identify the building entrance after dark. A lit sign is also an excellent marketing tool.

Attention must be given to the *parking lot area.* Litter must be picked up, and plants and grass must be tended. The parking lot entrance and exit should be clearly marked by signs. Parking spaces should be reserved for clients only, with employee parking behind the building or in a remote area away from the building entrance (Figure 32-2).

The entrance to the veterinary facility should be in full view and well marked to allow easy access by clients. If

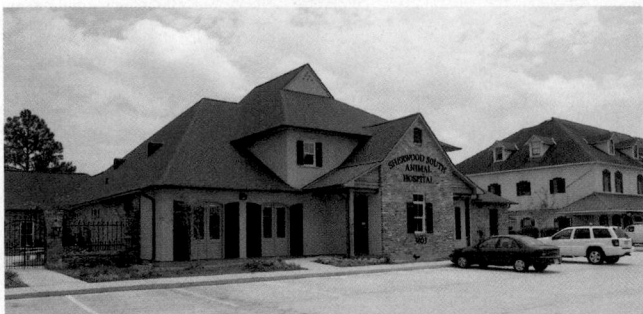

Figure 32-2 Client parking lot should be clearly designated and clean.

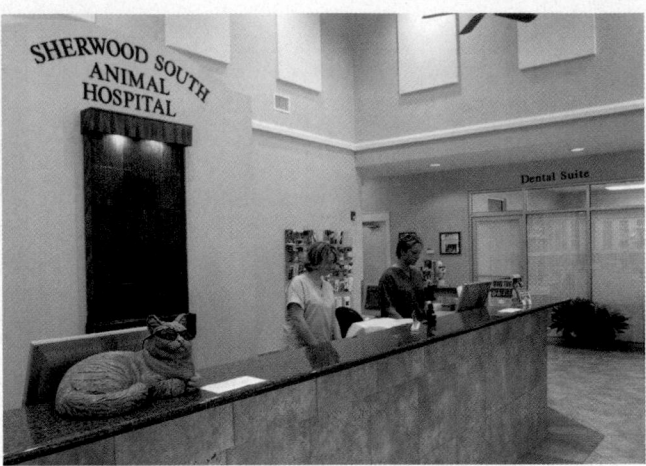

Figure 32-3 Reception area should give a warm, comfortable feeling to clients and staff.

more than one entrance is available (i.e., small animal and large animal or canine and feline), each entrance should be well marked. To prevent client congestion, the entrance and exit should be separate. Practice employees should not use the public entrance of the building. Further, routine deliveries and service activities should enter and exit the building away from client contact when possible.

Professional activities within a veterinary hospital can be grouped into four areas: outpatient, inpatient, surgical, and support. Depending on the practice size and type, the veterinarian, technician, or both may work in all four areas or focus on one or more areas. Effective management of each of these areas is needed to improve service and patient care.

> **TECHNICIAN NOTE**
>
> The four professional areas of activity within a hospital are outpatient, inpatient, surgical, and support service.

Outpatient Area

The first area to be discussed is the outpatient area. This area is composed of the *reception area, examination rooms, laboratory, pharmacy,* and *public restrooms.* Most commonly, clients will only have access to this area of the hospital. Special attention must be paid to maintain the outpatient area in a clean, organized, quiet, and odor-free condition. Because the client's first contact is with the outpatient area, lasting impressions are made that may raise or lower the overall client confidence in the quality of caring. A disorganized, dirty, smelly, noisy area will be remembered just that way. Veterinarians, technicians, and other staff must be well groomed, clean, and professionally attired. A professional appearance is mandatory for a professional image. All personnel in the outpatient area should also refrain from smoking, eating, and drinking when clients are present.

The *reception area* should always be considered by all hospital employees as a reception or client greeting area and not as a waiting room. The reception area should be comfortable and project a feeling of warmth, not a sterile feeling. Plants will help to create this warm feeling, but they must be well cared for. Dead or dying plants in the

reception area will not send a positive message to the client. Warm colors will also help to brighten the area. Reading material, if present, should be complete and not torn or half missing. A bright reception area with attractive wall hangings and plants will help relax clients (Figure 32-3).

The clients should spend only a short period of time in the reception room before being escorted to one of the *examination rooms.* This requires effective appointment scheduling and dedication to timely service. As a general rule, two examination rooms should be available in the outpatient area for each veterinarian. Therefore, in the typical two person practice, four examination rooms should be available. The examination areas should be decorated in warm tones, as should the reception area. Medications, examination equipment, records, and so forth should be secured or out of sight so that neither clients nor their children will be tempted. It is extremely important that the examination room be clean and in excellent repair because the client will spend the greatest amount of time there (Figure 32-4). A soiled floor or wall covering, dirty sink, and marred door will be noted and remembered by the client.

The *laboratory* and *pharmacy* should be well organized and clean. Clients will only occasionally visit these areas and should always be accompanied by a hospital employee. In some practices, the laboratory and pharmacy will be combined for more efficient use of floor space. They are usually located behind the examination rooms and accessible to the inpatient treatment areas (Figure 32-5). The pharmacy may also have Occupational Safety and Health Administration (OSHA) required material safety data sheet (MSDS) files and an eye wash station (Figure 32-6). The *public restrooms* should be cleaned and inspected regularly and should be conveniently located for client use.

Inpatient Area

The second work area is the inpatient area, consisting of a *treatment area, patient wards* and/or *large animal stalls,*

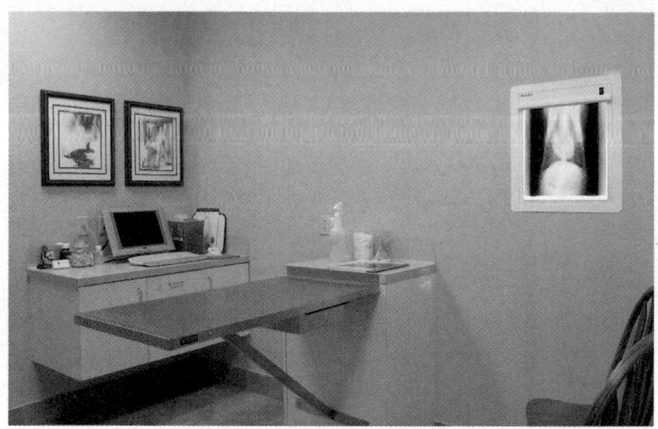

Figure 32-4 Examination rooms should be warmly decorated, clean, and in excellent condition.

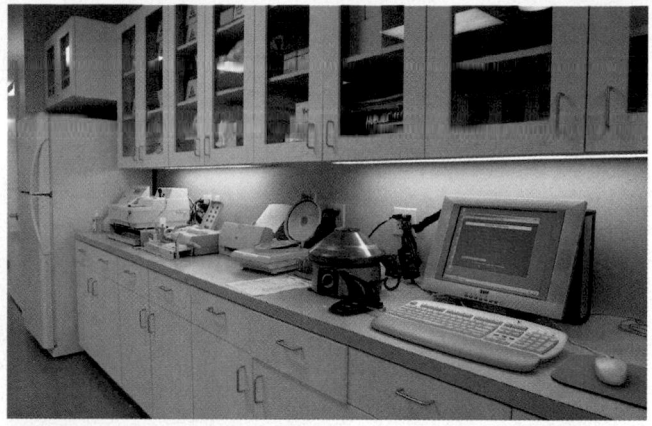

Figure 32-5 The laboratory is located just beyond the examination rooms.

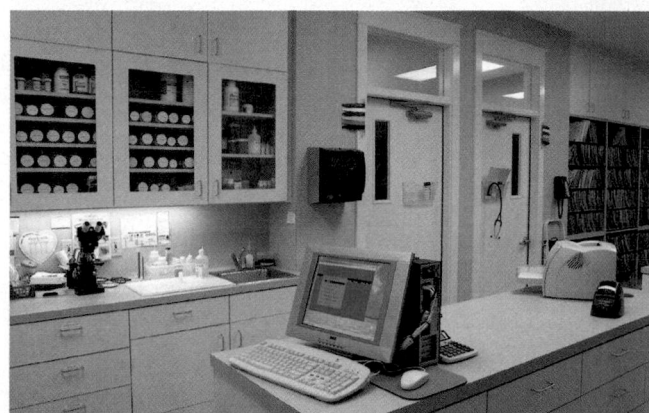

A

Figure 32-6 **A,** Pharmacy is located near examination rooms and inpatient treatment area. **B,** Drug shelf storage in pharmacy. **C,** Glass door refrigerator for storage of vaccines and biologicals.

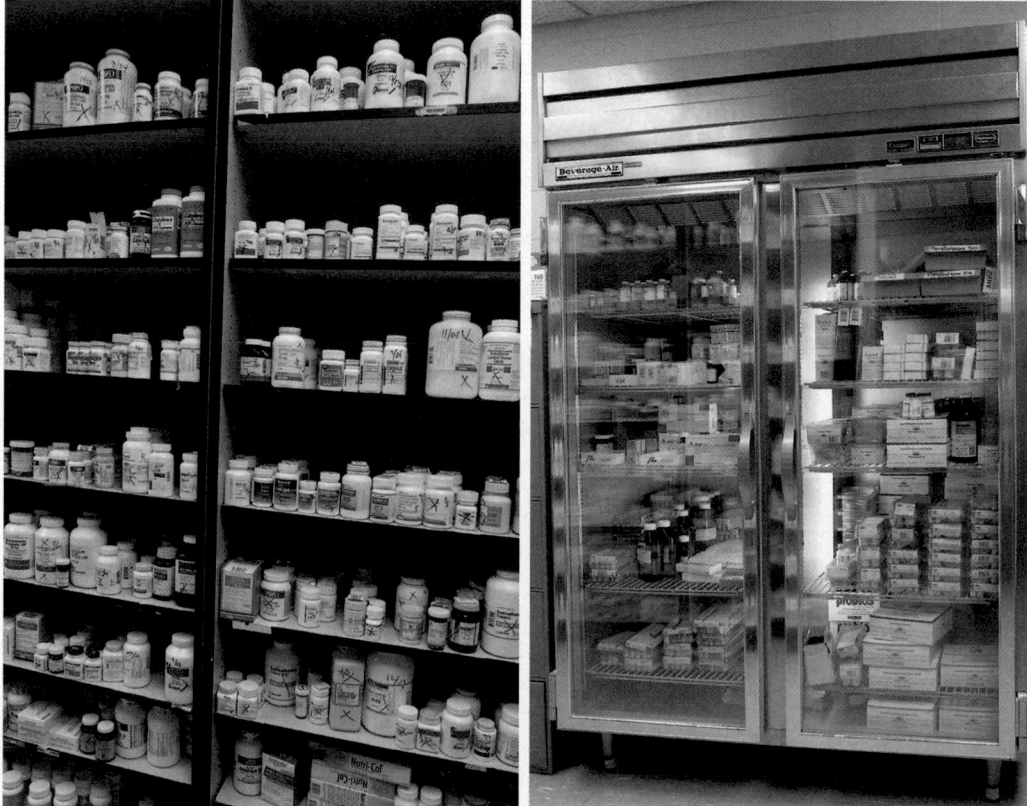

B

C

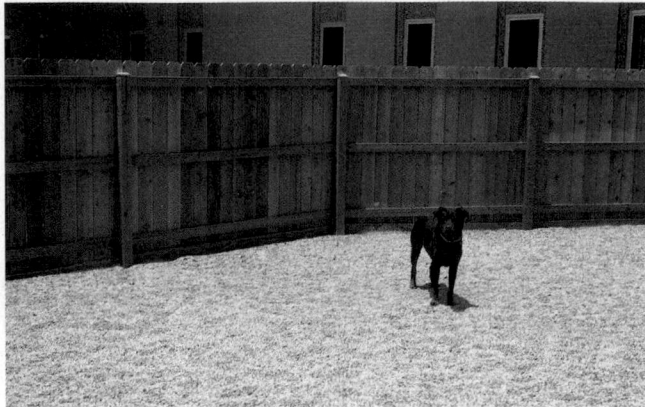

Figure 32-7   For security, fenced enclosures should always be used for outside exercise.

isolation area, exercise area, an area in which *necropsy* is performed, a *kitchen,* and a *bathing* and *grooming* area. The client has much less contact with this area than with the outpatient area, but constant attention must be given to maintain a clean, odor-free environment to prevent nosocomial infections of patients (Box 32-3).

Kennels, runs, and *stalls* must be cleaned several times during the day. Hospitalized patients must have closer attention than animals who are just boarding. Sick animals often cannot control urination and defecation; therefore more frequent attention to these areas will be required. Some pets are not used to eliminating indoors and will be reluctant to urinate and defecate unless they are in an exercise run. To maintain a quiet environment in public areas of the hospital, patient wards must be well insulated to reduce noise.

If large animals are hospitalized, adequate holding stalls will be necessary, with regular attention given to cleaning the stall and grooming and exercising the patient. When exercising either a large animal or a small animal patient, absolute security must be maintained at all times to prevent escape. Fenced areas should always be used to ensure that in the event of escape, the animal will still be contained (Figure 32-7). The veterinarian, hospital, or both assume all liability for an animal entrusted to them. Few experiences will match the helpless feeling of watching an escaped dog, cat, horse, or cow run off into the distance (especially if close to a busy street or highway).

Because of the security problem, the ward or stall area of the hospital should be adjacent to the *exercise area,* with an escape-proof fence or walls connecting the two. Exercise

areas for small animals ideally should be located within a well-insulated area of the hospital in which the temperature and humidity can be maintained at a constant level. Most city zoning laws will allow a small animal hospital to be located in proximity to residential areas because modern construction techniques use totally enclosed, attractive, and well-insulated designs.

> ✎ **TECHNICIAN NOTE**
>
> Animal security within the hospital must always be a high priority. Animals that escape are the legal responsibility of the hospital.

Large animal or mixed hospitals (caring for both large and small animals) will usually be required to locate in a less developed area of a city to allow exercise areas and odors to be properly addressed. Fewer veterinary hospitals now board animals on a regular basis. When boarding is offered, it should be explained to the client as "veterinary-supervised boarding." The recent trend has been away from construction of large boarding facilities as part of an animal hospital. Because of both the cost of construction and the cost of hospitalization, most veterinary practices work on an outpatient basis whenever possible. Construction and labor costs have made long-term hospitalization a financial burden to both client and veterinarian.

In certain instances, animals with infectious diseases must be hospitalized. Adequate *isolation facilities* must be available before a patient with an infectious disease is admitted. The isolation area should have only one entrance and exit, with proper disinfectant and clothing protection available. The air-handling system for the isolation area must be separate from the remainder of the building to prevent aerosol transmission of contagious disease organisms. In the event adequate isolation facilities are not available on the premises, the case should be referred to a veterinarian who has the proper facility. All treatments and handling of the infectious patient should be done by one or two persons only. The patient should be treated within the isolation

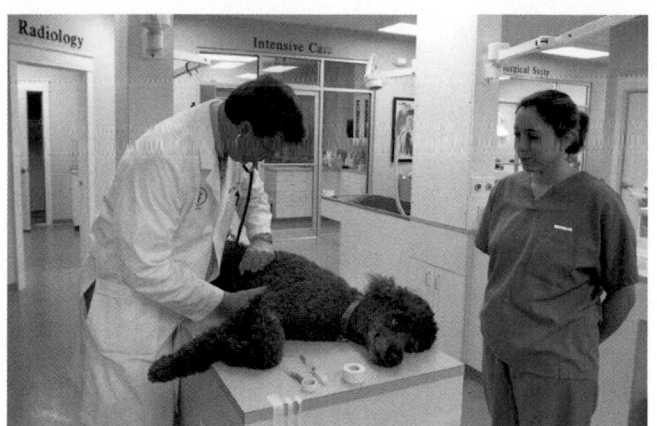

Figure 32-8 Centralized treatment area accommodates both outpatient and inpatient treatment.

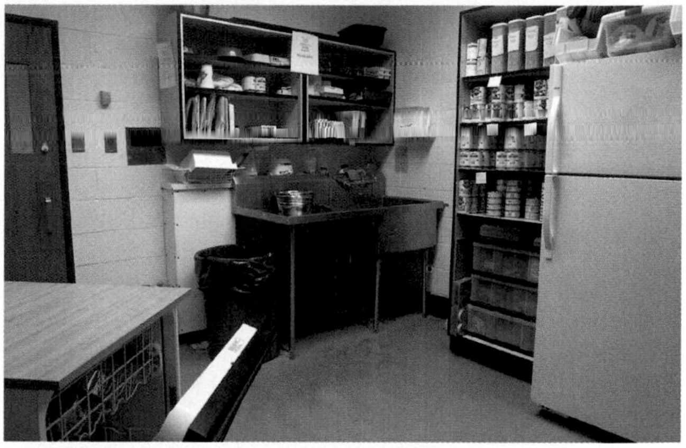

Figure 32-9 Hospital kitchen should contain diet materials, dishwasher, counter space, and refrigerator.

facility and should not be taken to the main treatment room. Staff must be trained to follow stringent isolation protocols to prevent nosocomial infections (Box 32-3).

The *treatment area* should be the central hub of the hospital (Figure 32-8). Patients from both the wards (inpatients) and examination rooms (outpatients) will be moved to this area for diagnostic procedures, medication administration, and recheck procedures (cast, bandage, or splint changes or removal). Certified veterinary technicians are increasingly performing the prescribed medical treatment and other nursing procedures while the veterinarian is performing surgery or seeing outpatients. One of the technical staff should have the primary responsibility for organization and cleanliness of the treatment room.

On occasion, clients may accompany the patient to the treatment area to assist with a bandage change or other minor procedure. The area therefore must be presentable at all times. In addition to the routine treatment functions carried out in the treatment room, many hospitals also use this room for preparation of the surgical patient. In the smaller practice, the treatment room may also contain x-ray facilities, laboratory equipment, or both. Because of the high traffic volume in the treatment area, hair and other debris will build up rapidly and should be removed with a vacuum cleaner on a regular basis to prevent nosocomial infections.

The *kitchen* in a small animal hospital should be an area in which animal food is stored and prepared. Usually, both canned and dry foods are available, and it should be stored in dry, rodent-proof containers. An automatic dishwasher is of great value if any quantity of dirty pans must be cleaned on a daily basis. It will also sanitize the pans with very hot water and remove soap and significant residues that cause digestive problems in sensitive patients. Hot and cold running water, a sink, countertop space, and a refrigerator should be available in the kitchen (Figure 32-9). Human food and drinks must not be stored in this refrigerator (OSHA regulations).

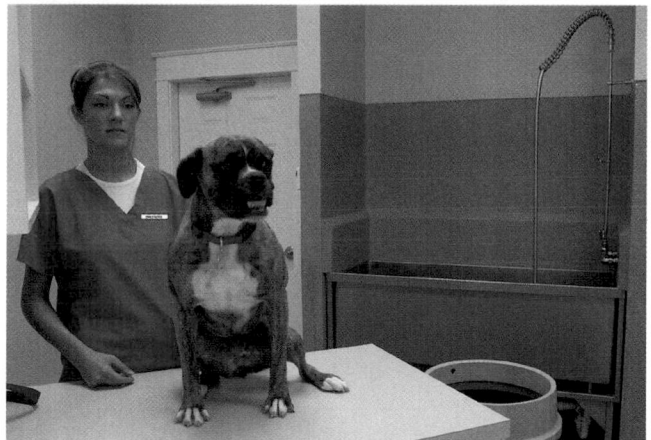

Figure 32-10 Custom pet bathing tub in background designed to aid in controlling animal during bath.

In the large animal hospital, the *feed room* will usually contain several grain mixtures and ration supplements. All materials must be stored in dry, rodent-proof containers. Grass hay, alfalfa, and bedding straw should be stored in a dry area protected from the weather to prevent mold and mildew. Moldy hay or alfalfa should never be fed to an animal because of possible toxicity and allergies.

The *bathing-grooming* area in the small animal hospital will usually consist of a raised bathroom tub [elevated about 60 to 90 cm (Figure 32-10)], a combing table, and a dryer cage. It is critically important that all patients dismissed from the hospital be clean and dry. Grooming services within the hospital may not be offered, but attention to daily grooming of all patients by all employees is necessary. Attention to grooming is also important for the equine patient and is usually done in the stall on a daily basis.

The final area to be discussed within the inpatient work area of the hospital is the *necropsy area*. The veterinary technician is able to perform a prosection (initial dissection) for the veterinarian to quickly inspect all organs for lesions and decide what specimens should be collected. The technician will collect, properly prepare, and ship the designated specimens to a diagnostic laboratory with the history (see Chapter 3). The necropsy area should be located in an isolated place in the building and be well lighted and well ventilated. Hot and cold running water and a drain should also be present. Necropsy tables or racks are used for small animals, whereas the necropsy floors usually are used for dissecting large animals. Gloves, boots, and aprons should be available in addition to specific necropsy instruments and specimen bottles. The availability of a 35-mm camera, digital camera, or video camera is helpful to record specific lesions.

Acceptable carcass disposal, preferably cremation, must be offered to owners. The body may also be released to the owner for owner burial.

In conclusion, the hospital inpatient area is the most labor-intensive section because of patient contact. Most hospitals expend the greatest amount of effort in maintaining this area. Most employees spend their greatest amount of time in this area performing direct animal care, diagnostic procedures, and nursing treatments. The outcome of most cases will also be determined here.

Surgical Area

The third work area in the hospital is the *surgical area*, which consists of the *preparation room, operating rooms, radiology section,* and *recovery room*. All four areas in the surgical section must be in close proximity to one another. Frequently the surgeon may need to obtain a postoperative radiograph of a fracture reduction to determine bone alignment or implant placement. When neurosurgery is to be performed, the surgeon may request a myelogram just before surgery; this requires that the patient be moved from the preparation room to the radiology area, back to the preparation room, and then into surgery.

As stated earlier, the *preparation room* may also be the treatment room. All presurgical preparation of the patient, surgeon, and technician should take place outside the operating room. Instrument preparation and sterilization usually will be completed in the preparation room. Clipping and scrubbing the patient and hand scrubbing of the surgeon and technician should be done before entering the operating room. A vacuum cleaner should be available in the preparation room to remove all loose hair from patient, table, and floor.

The *operating room* itself should be a "dead end" room with only one entrance-exit (Figure 32-11). Dust-carrying bacteria are easily stirred into the air when people walk through the room and will settle into the open surgical incision. No one should enter the operating room without proper clothing, shoes, cap, and mask. The operating room should be used only for surgical procedures and must not double as a treatment or examination room. Storage cabinets should be kept to a minimum and should contain only items that are used in surgery. Items used elsewhere

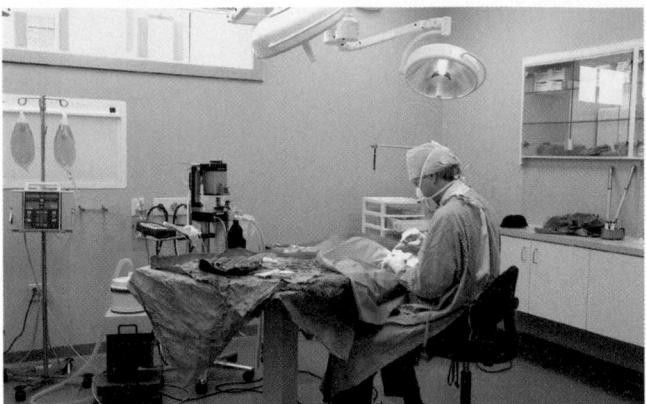

Figure 32-11 Surgical room with one door for both entrance and exit, ceiling-mounted lights, and minimal countertops.

in the hospital should not be stored in the operating room. Countertops should be kept to a minimum because flat surfaces collect dust and must be wiped down daily. Some flat surface is desirable to allow opening of packs and layout of instruments.

> **TECHNICIAN NOTE**
> The operating room (OR) must be used only for surgery and cannot be used as an examination or treatment room.

Wall-mounted radiographic viewers should be present to allow several views of a body part to be observed at once. Surgery lights, oxygen outlets, and patient monitors should be ceiling- or wall-mounted when possible. Floors, walls, and ceiling should be washable, smooth, and seam free to allow complete and easy cleaning. Cleaning under the surgery table base, the top of surgical lights, the floor, and flat surfaces (window ledges, countertop, etc.) should be performed daily. The air-handling system for the operating room should be separate and should create a slight positive pressure to prevent dust and other debris from entering the room from other rooms when the door is opened.

All cleaning materials and utensils used in the operating room should be restricted to use in this room. Mops and sponges that are used elsewhere in the building and are then used in the operating room will bring additional contamination into the room. The cleanliness of the operating room should be everyone's concern to prevent nosocomial infection of the surgical patient.

The *radiology area* should be located near the operating room, the preparation room, and the treatment area (for diagnostic workups). The radiology section should not be visited by clients during film exposure because of potential radiation exposure. Protective aprons, gloves, and film exposure badges should always be worn by all personnel in radiology. The technician will usually be responsible for equipment maintenance, exposure, developing, and filing radiographs (Figure 32-12). In most surgical orthopedic

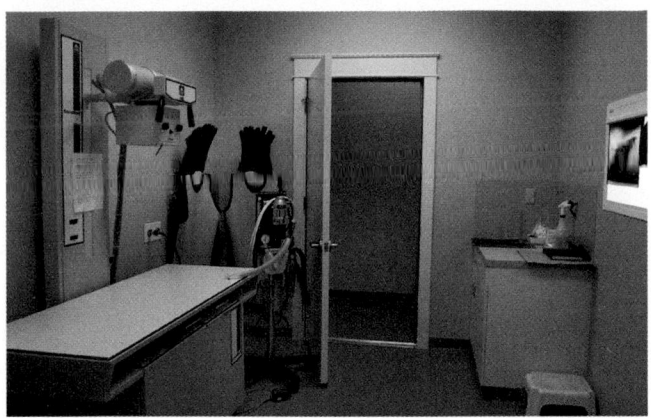

Figure 32-12 Radiology room with x-ray machine and protection equipment hanging on the wall. The automatic film processor is not visible through the open door.

cases, the radiology area will be visited after surgery to evaluate bone alignment or metal implant placement or both before placing the patient in the recovery room.

The surgical patient in the recovery area should be monitored at all times by a technician until the endotracheal tube has been removed. The recovery area may be in a room adjacent to the treatment room or behind a glass partition in the treatment room, or the recovery process may occur on a blanket on the treatment room floor. Whenever surgical recovery occurs, the patient should be closely monitored by the technical staff. *Under no circumstances* should any patient recovering from anesthesia be left unattended in the ward, in a stall, or elsewhere with an endotracheal tube in place.

In review, the surgical work area is a very technical and equipment-oriented area. Clients will not be permitted in this areas except in unusual circumstances. The skill level of technical support in this area must be very high, requiring familiarization with anesthesia (induction and administration), emergency procedures, radiology, surgical assisting, medical-surgical nursing, use of fiber-optic equipment, sterile technique, sterilization, monitoring equipment hookup, electrosurgical equipment, and necropsy techniques.

Support Area

The fourth work area of the hospital is the hospital support area. This area contains, somewhat by default, some of the "leftovers," but it also contains the planning and management areas of the hospital. The support area contains the *professional offices, business management office, library, employee lounge,* and *storage-inventory* areas.

TECHNICIAN NOTE

The support area of the hospital contains the professional offices, business management office, library, employee lounge, and storage areas.

In smaller practices, the *professional office, business management office,* and *library* will be in one room. In some multiperson practices, each veterinarian may have an office or large desk area in addition to the hospital manager's office. Larger practices may also have a library and conference room combination in which weekly staff meetings and conferences can be held.

The role of the hospital manager will vary according to practice size and management philosophy, but his or her office will usually be in proximity to the admissions-discharge functions of the hospital. Credit policy, accounts receivable, inventory control, purchasing, receiving orders, accounts payable, computer information management, management reports, personnel activities, and so forth will usually be handled by the hospital manager. In many practices, some of these functions are divided among the staff, and the veterinarian or veterinarians will assume the overall management role. For most veterinary technicians, some management skills will be required for advancement. Hospital management is now developing into a specialty area of veterinary medicine for nonveterinarians.

The *professional office* of the veterinarian functions as a client consultation area, a medical management area for discussing new products with drug company salespeople, and a professional management area for writing medical records, contacting clients, and discussing difficult or interesting cases with other veterinarians or staff. Many office hours are spent by the practicing veterinarian in studying and reading textbooks, journals, Internet articles, and reference materials and evaluating computer information. Veterinary technicians must also keep up with the latest advances in animal nursing, imaging, laboratory procedures, and management issues. Most states also require a minimal number of hours of approved continuing education for both certified veterinary technicians and licensed veterinarians.

The last portion of the support area is *storage*. From the management viewpoint, hospital storage space is the most expensive floor space in the building because this space produces the least income. Therefore the storage areas must be given close attention so that this valuable space will function as efficiently as possible. Supplies and equipment that are no longer used or usable should be removed to make room for the essential items. Inventory control (avoiding overstocking or understocking) and space organization will ensure maximal utilization. Items that can be hung on the wall or ceiling should be removed from the floor. Metal or wooden shelving will organize space for bulk drugs, food, and cleaning supplies. Flammable or toxic materials should be safely marked and stored away from foods or drugs.

In summary, the four major hospital work areas (outpatient, inpatient, surgery, support) are somewhat separate in function but are related in patient care and support. The smaller the practice, the less distinct will the areas be. Further, the smaller the practice, the fewer the number of technical staff and assistants, resulting in less opportunity for the veterinary technician to focus on one work area. This is not to imply that the smaller practice is less desirable. Sometimes, to the contrary, the small practice can provide more personal satisfaction because of closer contact with the entire operation and a diversification of job roles. Each technician and each veterinarian need to choose the type of practice with staffing utilization patterns that provide the greatest personal and professional satisfaction.

TRAFFIC FLOW

The four work areas that have been discussed are important from both client-patient and hospital organization viewpoints. The client wants personalized and professional service that is efficient, thorough, and cost effective. If each employee fully understands and enjoys his or her work area, the client and patient will usually experience satisfaction if all communicate effectively. However, the veterinary team must be efficient at handling the necessary number of patients to provide the needed cash flow required to stay in business. An efficient traffic flow (i.e., the movement of the client and patient from admission to dismissal) becomes very important to accommodate the required number of clients each day.

LARGE ANIMAL FACILITIES

Whereas about 75% of veterinarians practice in small animal facilities, about 4% of the practices in the United States are equine and 10% are primarily food animal (swine, dairy, and/or beef) practices. A decreasing number (less than 10%) are mixed practices in which veterinarians see both large animal and small animal patients. If the livestock population is high in an area, a group practice may have several large animal veterinarians each focusing on a specific species for providing diagnostic, treatment, and surgical services as well as preventive medicine consultation.

LARGE ANIMAL MOBILE UNITS

Veterinary diagnostic and preventive medicine services for a herd of animals require the veterinarian to visit the owner's facility on the farm or in the stable. The large animal practice often makes use of a mobile facility (Figure 32-13) for conducting these farm visits. These visits require stringent sanitary precautions to prevent transmitting disease among animal facilities. Washing hands, changing to clean coveralls, chemical disinfecting of boots, and cleaning of equipment between farm calls are paramount to prevent disease transmission among farms and to gain and keep the confidence of the livestock owner.

Mobile facilities used to serve large animal patients and clients may vary from a car with a few portable "grips" in the trunk, to a van with a set of drawers and containers, to a specially designed mobile truck unit. The truck units are usually fully equipped with refrigeration for biologicals plus hot water and a supply of disinfectants, drugs, vaccines, medical supplies, restraints, diagnostic and treatment

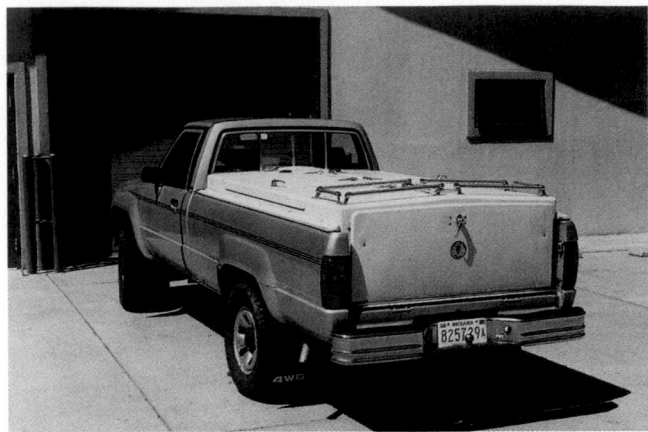

Figure 32-13 A veterinary mobile unit is equipped with hot water, a refrigerator, and many compartments for equipment and supplies.

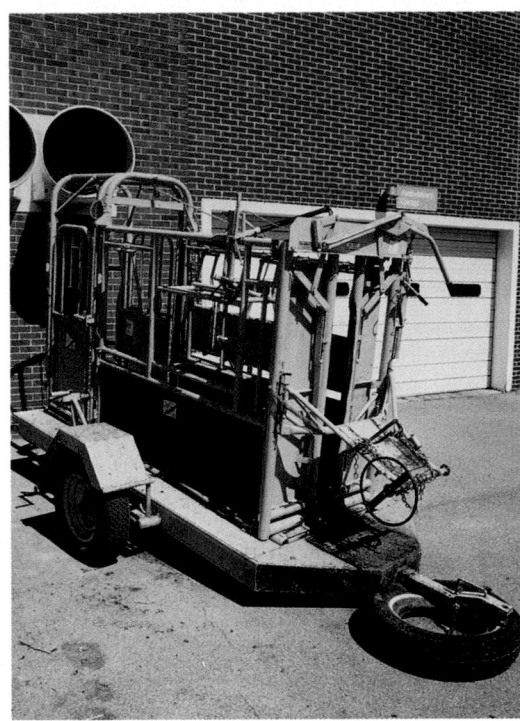

Figure 32-14 A portable cattle chute on wheels is pulled behind the ambulatory truck to the farm. It has a head table on front for head work and a palpation cage on back for reproductive examinations.

equipment, and sometimes even mobile x-ray units. Everything needed for a series of planned visits plus unexpected emergencies must be on board! The water supply and disinfectants are used to clean and disinfect hands, boots, and equipment after every farm call. A portable cattle chute may be also pulled behind the mobile unit to the farm to process herds of cattle (Figure 32-14).

A veterinary technician may be responsible for stocking, organizing, and maintaining the large animal mobile unit.

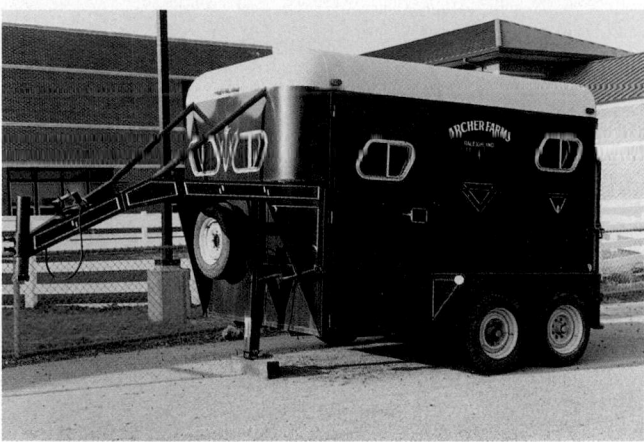

Figure 32-15 A stock trailer is used by animal owners to transport farm animals to the large animal hospital for treatment.

The mobile unit inventory will vary depending on the nature of the practice, the preferences of the veterinarian, and the species served. Preparing inventory lists and organizational charts for this daily activity ensures that the veterinarian will have what is needed on every call. Obviously, there is a wide range of specific supplies necessary for the routine practice of large animal veterinary medicine. This inventory must be replenished frequently, organized for easy and quick access, and cleaned and disinfected on a daily basis as well as after every farm call. Many technicians desire to assist veterinarians on farm calls and become efficient at maintaining and organizing the mobile unit.

LARGE ANIMAL HAUL-IN FACILITIES

Some veterinarians with mixed and large animal practices provide haul-in facilities for individual patients to be trucked or brought by trailer into the practice (Figure 32-15). Unloading chutes and gates for cattle trucks and stock trailers are provided at the large animal outpatient entrance. A few even provide holding corrals and squeeze chutes for processing a truckload of cattle or sheep. Unloading chutes for cattle, sheep, and swine must adjust to different heights to accommodate the trucks, pickups, and trailers used for transporting the animals. It is paramount that fencing and panel arrangements be constructed to prevent escape from the premises if the animal escapes from the head-catch or alleyway or when unloading.

When haul-in facilities for large animals are provided, each of the areas previously discussed for a small animal facility will be present for serving large animal patients. They may be in separate or combined rooms. In larger facilities they will often be separate from the small animal areas. Frequently, some areas will be used for both small animal and large animal service (e.g., the reception area, laboratory, conference rooms, pharmacy, public restrooms). Large mixed hospitals often have a separate pharmacy for large animal supplies, separate public restrooms, and possibly a

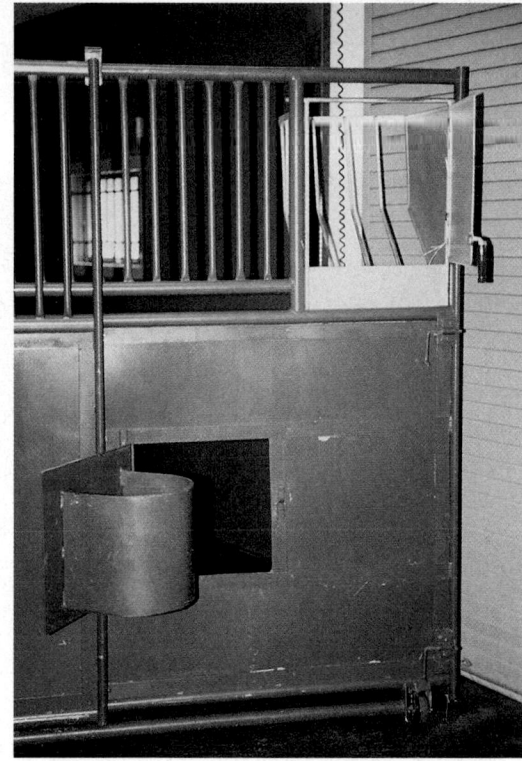

Figure 32-16 Large animal stall door has minidoors to feed and water large animal patients without having to enter the stall.

separate reception area. The nature of the large animal facilities of each practice is quite variable depending on the needs of the livestock population and owners served by the practice.

The *large animal inpatient treatment area* may be the same as the outpatient examination area for large animal patients. An alleyway with a head-catch or squeeze chute is used for bovine patients, a stock is used for equine patients, and pigs or sheep may be treated in their stall. When haul-in facilities are available for large animals, patient wards with a few stalls (Figure 32-16) are usually provided. These will often be indoors to protect the patients from bad weather, although outdoor pens may be used in good weather. Also, isolation areas in a different barn are sometimes necessary to prevent the spread of infectious disease.

Examination rooms are always separate because large animal examinations require stocks for horses (Figure 32-17), a squeeze chute and head-catch for cattle, and large special examination tables for restraining cattle on their side for hoof work or minor surgery. Cattle chutes (Figure 32-14) are manual or hydraulic squeeze chutes located at the end of an alleyway. A head-catch on the front of an alleyway will suffice for some cattle examinations and procedures. The alleyways leading to the chutes are sometimes arranged in a circular manner to facilitate easier cattle movement to the examination area. Because of the size of these species, staff should be well trained in restraint and safety procedures; this ensures protection for the both large animal

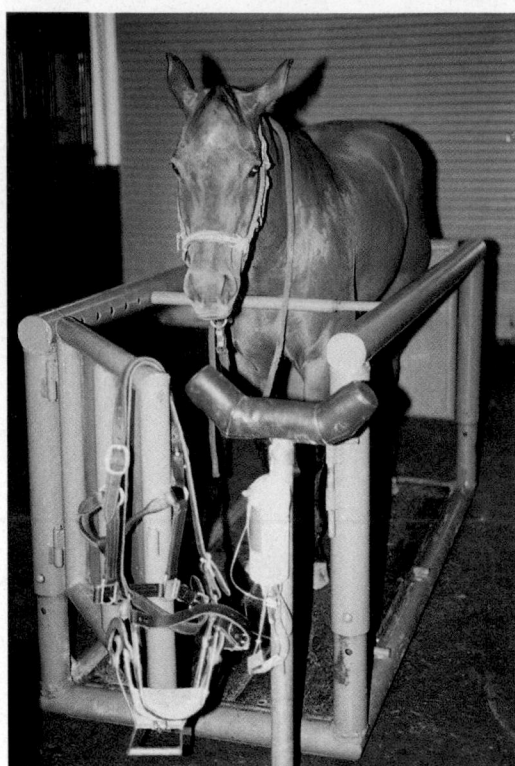

Figure 32-17 Horse in stocks with bar in front of chest to keep horse back against rear door. Mouth speculum is used to perform equine dental procedures.

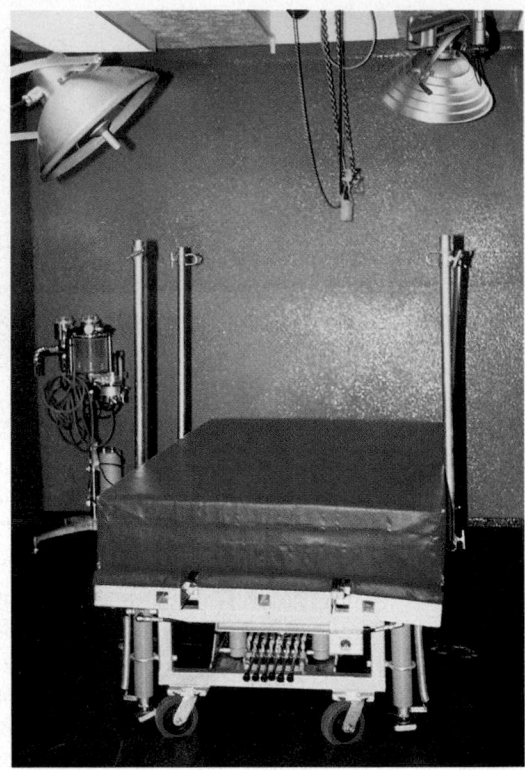

Figure 32-18 Large animal surgery table with anesthesia machine and padded walls of recovery room for recovering anesthetized horses.

patients, owners, and staff. A variety of restraint procedures are used (see Chapter 1).

Most food animal practices also use the treatment area as a minor, nonsterile surgical room. Because of the large patient size and the extensive amount of hair and excrement large animals bring to these areas, high-pressure hoses and disinfectant systems are necessary, along with removable floor drain traps. Most mixed practices use the same support areas for the small and large animal clients and patients with the exception of storage of cleaning equipment, lawn mowers, large animal hoof equipment, general supplies, and bulk pharmacy.

The *surgical room* in the equine practice facility is organized to provide the same stringent asepsis as provided in a small animal surgery. However, because the patient is much larger, mechanical or hydraulic equipment designed to lift the horse is provided. Larger equine practices have an induction room (may also be the treatment and minor surgery area), an operating room with a large animal radiology machine, and a padded recovery room. The surgical area is equipped with a surgical table on which the horse is placed after being induced with general anesthesia (Figure 32-18). Anesthesia is maintained with an equine gas anesthesia machine (Figure 32-19).

An area where a *necropsy* can be appropriately performed must also be available (see Chapter 5). Necropsies are more frequently performed when a *large* animal dies than for a

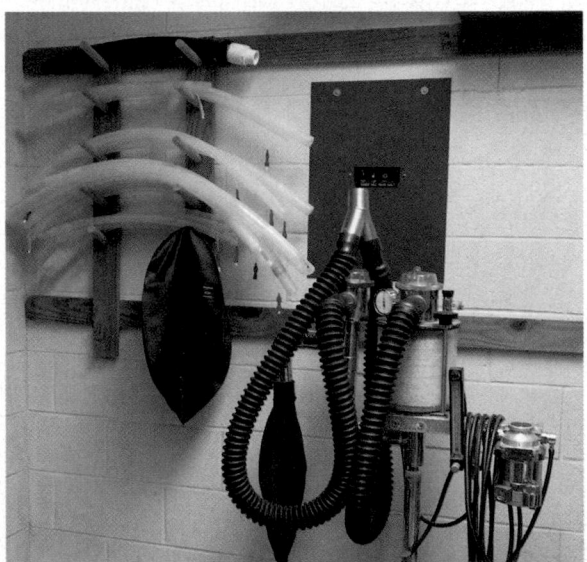

Figure 32-19 Large animal endotracheal tubes, rebreathing bags, and related anesthesia equipment stored on a rack for quick access.

small animal. Because of the economic value of large herds or flocks, necropsies of dead animals are often done to determine if the rest of the herd or flock is threatened. Confirmation of the diagnosis will often require submission of specimens to a state or university diagnostic laboratory

technicians. Therefore, although each of the members of the veterinary health care team has a different role, members must be hired and organized to work together efficiently as an effective team rather than as competing or isolated individuals.

The veterinary health care team is composed of the veterinarian(s), practice manager, veterinary technician(s), veterinary technologist(s), veterinary technician specialist(s), veterinary assistant(s), ward staff and receptionist(s). Refer to the introduction for a description of team members except for practice manager, ward staff, and receptionist which will be discussed here.

VETERINARY PRACTICE MANAGER

Veterinarians also managed their practices through most of the last century when one-person practices predominated. An increasing number of veterinarians (especially in group practices) are delegating the business management responsibilities to a practice manager. Medium-sized practices may divide these duties between several members of their veterinary team. In large practices a full-time, bachelor of science (BS) trained individual may serve as the veterinary practice manager (VPM).

Because veterinary practices are small businesses, the practice manager's role is to facilitate an efficiently operated and profitable medical business. The duties of the manager usually include hiring, supervising, and terminating personnel; managing inventory; handling client financial issues; facilitating accounting procedures needed for case control; analyzing progress toward goals; and developing and initiating new protocols for areas of hospital operation.

The owners, in concert with the hospital manager and other team members, must develop the mission statement and strategic plan for growth or change. The practice manager is delegated the responsibility for making day-to-day management decisions to meet theses goals for the business. The practice manager must also unite the team of veterinarians and support staff to work well together to meet the practice goals. Another management challenge necessary for business is the development of a marketing plan for the practice (discussed at the end of this chapter).

WARD STAFF

Ward staff members are individuals trained on the job to follow specific protocols for the cleaning and sanitation required to prevent nosocomial infections. They perform the basic husbandry required for keeping patients clean, groomed, fed, watered, and exercised with the safety and comfort of each patient taken into consideration. Ward staff must observe and record patient appetites, attitudes, bowel movements, and urinary output and alert the staff about observed abnormal behavior. They also move patients from the wards to the treatment area, to the reception for discharge, or to surgery. They may also be assigned basic janitorial duties in the rest of the hospital. Ward staff can also double as veterinary assistants.

RECEPTIONISTS

Receptionists facilitate client service, communicate a sense of friendliness and helpfulness, and organize appointments so that clients do not have to wait an unreasonable amount of time. The receptionist is a key position in any hospital operation. The "life blood" of the practice (clients) must filter through the receptionist via the telephone and one-on-one contact in the reception area. The old adages that "you don't have a second chance to make a first impression" and "the receptionist will make or break the practice" are key issues for selecting receptionists.

Receptionists have the critical role of handling the fee payments, billings, and daily cash records. These duties must be performed effectively to keep the business running smoothly, clients happy, and the rest of the veterinary team aware of what is happening with clients and their pets. Receptionists are often the last person communicating with the client at checkout and can assess the general client satisfaction level when clients leave the premises. The business needs satisfied clients who will return as continuing clients and refer their friends and associates. The receptionist's effectiveness is key to practice growth and happy clients!

PERSONNEL MANAGEMENT

Personnel management is important because the greatest percentage of overhead is in personnel. All personnel must work as a team to ensure productivity. Working *with* someone is always better than working *for* someone. All practice employees (including veterinarians) must be as productive as possible to provide a profitable and pleasant work environment. Veterinarians and technicians are usually not professionally trained to be managers. Both must work together to have a successfully managed practice, which will result in greater career satisfaction, not just a job.

Regardless of the size of the practice and how it is managed, each position within the practice should have a backup person who is cross trained in that area to take over when sickness, vacation, and emergencies arise. Without a cross-training plan, the practice may become crippled when one person is gone. This is especially true in smaller practices.

In most practices, the staff duties can be divided into the following job areas: (1) reception, (2) examination room or outpatient duties, (3) inpatient duties, and (4) building, kennel, and barn maintenance. The reception area is staffed and operated by one or more receptionists.

They must be friendly and caring people. The entire mood of the practice and, to a great extend, the attitude of the client will be determined by the communication skills and judgment of the receptionist. For example, the receptionist should screen patients and schedule undiagnosed medical problems or cases requiring radiography earlier in the day so that the client will have a diagnosis before the day's end. Emergencies obviously need immediate attention. The receptionist greets clients, starts the medical record by obtaining some history, answers questions by telephone, makes appointments, handles the records for patient dismissal, answers general medical questions, quotes certain fees, maintains a schedule of all veterinarians, handles money and bank deposits, and manages accounts receivable and other duties as assigned. In short, an effective receptionist in most practices is a super person.

A veterinary technician is usually assigned to *examination room* duties. In some practices, the receptionist and examination room duties will be performed by one person. The role of this individual may include backup or fill-in for the receptionist in addition to assisting in the examination rooms; obtaining medical histories; filling prescriptions; restraining patients; administering medications; demonstrating treatment techniques to clients; obtaining blood samples; performing laboratory work; escorting patients to the wards; dismissing patients; maintaining the examination, laboratory, and pharmacy areas in a clean and orderly manner; and other duties necessary for smooth patient flow in the public areas of the hospital. Efficiency is enhanced with multiple examination rooms and an assistant or orderly assigned to assist both technician and veterinarian. Every patient must be examined by a veterinarian to make the diagnosis to ensure existing problems are not overlooked (e.g., hernias, retained testicles, external parasites). Patients should not be admitted unless a veterinarian has had contact with the patient and client to establish a legal client-patient-veterinarian relationship.

The duties in the *inpatient area* are more isolated, and there is usually less client contact. Most of these duties are performed by a team of technicians and assistants. These duties include administering or monitoring anesthesia or both; preparing patients for surgery; monitoring surgical and postsurgical patients; surgical assisting; collecting laboratory samples; performing dental cleanings; administering and monitoring treatments; exposing and developing radiographs; performing laboratory tests; maintaining medical records; maintaining surgical and anesthesia logs; providing direct medical and surgical nursing care; and maintaining the surgery, treatment, and radiology areas.

Maintaining *building, barn,* and *wards* in a clean and orderly manner and other duties necessary for hospitalized patients to be well cared for are usually delegated to assistants and caretakers and supervised by a veterinary technician. Animal caretakers and ward staff clean, bed, and feed patients, allowing the veterinary technician to perform additional technical support functions. The role of the technician is determined by the staffing and delegation patterns as well as the size and type of practice.

A veterinary technician must be able to work in all areas of the hospital. The most common technical support utilization in veterinary practices involves the generalist type of veterinary technician. For a technician to function

---

Box 32-5 SOCIETIES WITH OR DEVELOPING SPECIALTY CERTIFICATION PROGRAMS

Academy of Veterinary Emergency and Critical Care Technicians (AVECCT) www.AVECCT.org: AVECCT members can be certified as veterinary technician specialists in emergency and critical care *and will use* VTS (Emergency/Critical Care) after their name and state certification [i.e., Jane Doe, RVT, VTS (Emergency/Critical Care)].
Academy of Veterinary Dental Technicians (AVDT) www.AVDT.US
Academy of Veterinary Technician Anesthetists (AVTA) www.AVTA_VTS.org
Veterinary Hospital Managers Association, Inc. (VHMA) www.VHMA.org: To be certified, a VHMA member must be actively employed as a veterinary practice manager (not necessarily a technician or DVM), achieve 18 college credit hours in business management, pass VHMA written and oral examinations, and participate in 6 days of management continuing education every 2 years. The designation of certified veterinary practice manager (CVPM) is conveyed to successful applicants (i.e., Jane Doe, CVPM; if a registered technician, Jane Doe, RVT, CVPM).

---

effectively as a generalist, a broad base of information and techniques must be mastered and maintained with cross training in all technical areas. Being a high-quality generalist is not an easy task.

Large private and institutional teaching hospital practices have the case load to allow the technical staff to become very skilled in one area. Examples of these areas would be surgery, intensive care, anesthesiology, cardiology, internal medicine, ophthalmology, dermatology, radiology, clinical pathology, and office management. Specialty societies and certifications for veterinary technicians are now available in critical care, dentistry, anesthesia, and management (Box 32-5).

DELEGATION PRINCIPLES

Personnel costs may be reduced by hiring the correct personnel for the job and delegating properly. Too many practices are still trying to hire a new veterinarian to perform veterinary technician duties. Many also hire veterinary technicians to perform non–income-producing duties of assistants and caretakers. Consequently, the practice spends more money than necessary on personnel and frustrates a new veterinarian or technician in the process as well as limiting income produced.

Both veterinarians and veterinary technicians should be paid according to gross income produced; therefore aides and assistants hired at near minimum-wage levels should be relied on as much as possible to perform most non–income-producing tasks, such as restraint, general cleaning, and animal husbandry. Veterinarians should focus on making diagnoses, prescribing treatments, and performing surgery while delegating billable treatments, such as anesthesia, dental prophylaxes, imaging, and laboratory procedures, to certified veterinary technicians.

JOB DESCRIPTIONS

Regardless of position in the hospital setting, all personnel should have a detailed job description. A job description will allow both employee and management to maintain a clear understanding of current and new areas of responsibility. Job descriptions are also very useful when hiring new employees or replacing employees.

Through the use of the job descriptions (expectations) and periodic performance evaluations, employees can be rewarded according to their performance, poor workers can be guided and encouraged to improve, and chronically poor workers can be discharged. One of the most common mistakes in personnel management is to put off regular employee evaluations. Personnel problems resulting from poor work performance do not just go away, they only become worse. Therefore a job evaluation system that is applied equally and fairly to all employees needs to be maintained. Employees cannot improve performance unless they are given an opportunity to identify shortcomings. If improvement is not observed within a reasonable period of time, both the practice and employee will probably be better off with employee dismissal.

HIRING PROCEDURES

When hiring a new employee, it is important that all employees have input into the decision if teamwork is to be expected. This is a very important decision. The cost of selection, training, and adaptation can equal 1 year's salary. A bad choice means disruption, turnover, and a loss of thousands of dollars to the practice.

A simple method of candidate evaluation that will satisfy most employees is to have two or three employees interview each candidate first and then make recommendations to the veterinarian. The screening committee should establish some specific questions for each interviewer to ask each candidate using the job description prepared for that specific job. The recommendations made to the veterinarian should include job suitability, personality, professionalism, knowledge, experience, dress, and other interview assessments. The veterinarian should have the final word on hiring and firing unless a practice manager has been hired for personnel management.

The major steps in the hiring process are as follows:

1. Analyze personnel requirements.
2. Develop a specific job description.
3. Develop a set of interview questions.
4. Announce and advertise the position.
5. Review the applications and resumes.
6. Rank the candidates for interview.
7. Check references.
8. Interview the top-ranked two to four candidates.
9. Make a final selection.
10. Offer the job to the best candidate and set salary.
11. Establish a starting date.

The analysis of personnel requirements will be done by the veterinarian or office manager based on the needs of the practice or business. Once the general need for the position or positions has been established (or replacement approved), a detailed job description must be prepared or the previous job description updated. The job description is usually developed on one page and consists of four or five job functions outlined in one or two sentences each. Each job function is then assigned a percentage of time. Once the job description is developed or updated, it can be used to write the advertisement to search for a specific individual. To prepare for the interview, a set of interview questions needs to be developed.

Some interview questions are unlawful or discriminatory and must not be asked (e.g., questions on race, religion, national origin, gender, handicaps, marital status). Questions should always be open ended (Box 32-6) and allow the candidates to express themselves. The following requests and questions could be considered when preparing interview questions:

1. Please review your previous position.
2. Describe your best boss.
3. Describe your worst boss.
4. What did you like best about your last position?
5. What did you like least about your last position?
6. What specific skills and abilities do you have that apply to this particular position?
7. What are your short-range and long-term employment goals?
8. What accomplishments have made you most proud?
9. What type of working relationships do you want to cultivate?
10. How do you feel about constructive criticism and formal performance evaluation?
11. How do you feel about being on call several times per month?
12. Do you have any questions you would like to ask?

During the interview, the evaluator should ask each candidate the same questions so the responses can be objectively compared. The interview period is the time to evaluate motivation, personal appearance, and personal hygiene. The job description, salary, and benefits should be reviewed. Each interviewer or interview team should limit their part of the interview to 30 minutes.

After the interview, personal references should be checked and past supervisors contacted. When all the above material has been collected and weighed, the individual who is the best person (and match) for the position should be offered the job.

Box 32-6   COMMUNICATION TECHNIQUES
FOR INTERVIEWING CLIENT

- Open-ended (or probing) questions
  Who?
  How?
  What?
  When?
  Where?
- Answers will be detailed descriptions.

- Leading (yes/no) questions
  Did? (this happen, you like it, etc.)
  Was it? (good, bad, etc)
- Answers will be yes or no even if client is not sure!

ONE-WORD ACKNOWLEDGMENT
Use one word (e.g., oh, OK, yes) with eye contact and voice inflection that imply you understand and want him or her to continue talking. This can be done with eye contact, nonverbal signs of active listening, and verbal silence with some clients.

ACCENT QUESTIONS
Restate one or two words used by the client in a questioning tone, which serves to request the client to elaborate on the description of events or signs.

PARAPHRASING
Restate client statements (in your own words) to check with the client whether you understand what the client is trying to say before going on in the interview. Use paraphrasing periodically in each segment of the interview to give the client an opportunity to clarify or confirm your understanding.

SUMMARIZING
Restate main points at the end (or at end of major segments) to emphasize key points and inform the client about what is going to happen next.

When the final selection has been made, the most common initial contact will be by telephone. During the telephone call, the job description should be reviewed, salary and benefits discussed, and starting date established. When the above steps are followed, the best candidate should be more easily identified and successfully hired. Other candidates should be notified that the position has been filled with the applicant who best matched the position.

A potential problem in personnel management is inadequate internal communication. To avoid internal disputes, weekly (or monthly) staff meetings should be held to update all employees on various aspects of hospital operation. Often, notes on a blackboard just do not do the job! These meetings can also be used to develop teamwork via group problem-solving techniques.

✎ TECHNICIAN NOTE
Practice staff meetings should be held at least once per month to ensure open communication.

ROLE OF VETERINARY TECHNICIANS AND VETERINARIANS IN MANAGEMENT

Technicians have an ever-increasing role in practice management. In most practice situations, technicians will be involved in management of the patient, client, equipment, and inventory. They may also be involved in staff, facility, and business management. To develop management skills, one must be willing to assume increasing levels of responsibility. As the practice changes in staffing, number of cases, facility, type of clients, new technologies, and so forth, the veterinary technician must adapt his or her management skills to these changes.

The role of the veterinary technician in management will vary depending on the type of practice and the previous experiences of the technician and the veterinarian. The technician who can (1) conceptualize the vision and goals set by the veterinarian for the practice, (2) efficiently organize each area in which he or she is given responsibility, (3) become a productive team player and a good communicator, and (4) develop the ability to solve problems constructively to enhance both patient care and the veterinary team will usually be given a greater role in practice management.

To be effective, the veterinarian-owner must act as overall hospital chief executive officer (CEO) and delegate appropriate areas of responsibility to the veterinary technician as well as to other members of the team. Effective delegation of responsibility to the technician must include billable (income producing) technical procedures of medical and surgical nursing. Ideally, veterinarians diagnose, prescribe, and perform surgery; and technicians perform venipunctures, laboratory tests, and prescribed treatments; expose and develop radiographs; and anesthetize, prepare, and manage recovery of surgical patients. The veterinary technician should also delegate most non–income-producing tasks to lesser paid aides, assistants, or animal caretakers. Clinic aides restrain, move, feed, and exercise the animals and assist both technicians and veterinarians when needed. Receptionists handle scheduling, receiving, discharging, billing, and related front office duties. There should be a direct relationship between the salary level paid and the income produced (productivity) for each veterinary technician and veterinarian in a practice if effective delegation is occurring.

✎ TECHNICIAN NOTE
The veterinary technician should delegate most non–income-producing tasks to assistants or aides.

Practice management efforts are necessary in all types of practice. To be effective the veterinarian and veterinary technician must be human resources managers. This requires both excellent communication skills and a policy and procedures manual for the practice team. It involves hiring, training, and scheduling performance appraisals and discharge of staff. The veterinarian and technician must work together with the rest of the staff as both a management team and a medical team.

Unfortunately, most colleges provide little training in hospital or people management for either technicians or veterinarians because it takes students so much time and effort to gain the medical expertise, technical skills, and confidence necessary to succeed medically. However, there are many new resources available to meet this need for management training after graduation, including continuing education short courses, books, journals, organizations, Internet courses (i.e., veterinary information network—www.VIN.com), and consultants.

✎ TECHNICIAN NOTE

Never argue with a dissatisfied client.

PATIENT MANAGEMENT

Patient management and client management go hand in hand. Both should be handled together, but for the sake of this discussion they are treated separately.

Patient management can best be described by outlining the typical case as it moves through the hospital. The first contact is with the receptionist. The receptionist should move the patient and client as quickly as possible into an examination room. A patient presented as an emergency should receive priority. An emergency case is always any case that the *owner* feels is an emergency. Most of these cases are not emergencies, but each should be managed as if it were to ensure client satisfaction with quality of service.

In many practices, the patient will be escorted into the examination room by a veterinary technician. The technician will continue to develop the medical record by obtaining the temperature, pulse, respiration, and weight of the patient. Additional informational questions are asked to establish a preliminary history, and a brief physical examination may also be helpful to the veterinarian (Box 32-6).

Once the veterinarian enters the examination room, the patient and owner should be introduced to the veterinarian by the technician. Name tags should be worn by all personnel to help clients remember whom they have met and who is the veterinarian. A veterinary assistant or technician should assist the veterinarian in the physical examination by restraining the patient as necessary. If blood, urine, or skin specimens are needed, the technician should usually take the patient to the treatment room and conduct these procedures away from the client with the help of an assistant while the veterinarian is seeing another client and patient. Once a diagnosis has been made by the veterinarian, the patient will either be treated and released or be hospitalized.

If the patient is to be treated and released, the technician will often administer treatment and will prepare prescriptions as needed. The technician will explain (or demonstrate) how to administer home medications or treatments and will then escort the client to the receptionist for dismissal and fee payment.

When the patient is to be hospitalized, the assistant or technician will escort the patient to the ward and ensure that the necessary items are present to make the patient comfortable. The veterinarian will establish each treatment regimen and evaluate its success. During hospitalization, the technician will maintain and manage most routine treatments, therapy, laboratory tests, and medical records while delegating exercise, feeding, restraint, and grooming to assistants or animal caretakers. Often the daily phone contact with the client will be through the technician. A blackboard or bulletin board in the treatment room can be used to remind personnel of the diagnostic, treatment, and surgery schedules for hospitalized patients. All patients should be evaluated several times each day, and these evaluations should be documented with appropriate entries into the medical record. Walking through ward rounds can be very helpful to all personnel to keep everyone updated on each case.

The dismissal of a hospitalized patient is similar to that of the outpatient except that dispensed medications and patient cleanup must be completed before the owner's arrival. When dismissing a hospitalized patient, the following points should be considered:

- An itemized fee statement should be ready at the time the owner is called to pick up the animal.
- All medications should be dispensed in child-proof containers with proper labels.
- The veterinarian should be available for consultation with the client.
- The technician should be available to demonstrate treatment and home care techniques with handout instructions for home reference.
- Fee collection should take place.
- The next appointment or recheck should be scheduled.
- The patient should be presented dry, clean, and odor free.

Some conditions dictate that the patient be presented before fee collection and the scheduling of the next appointment. When this occurs, someone should be available to hold or control the animal until the client has completed the dismissal process.

The technician can be extremely valuable during the dismissal process by explaining to the client what to do if specific possible events occur (through reinforcement of directions given by the veterinarian). Clients will often ask technicians questions that they forgot or were afraid to ask the veterinarian.

Most clients will judge the medical care an animal has received by the condition and appearance of the animal at dismissal. The patient should always be as clean or cleaner than when admitted. If an animal soils itself just before dismissal, always clean or bathe the animal before sending it home even if the client has to wait a few minutes longer.

The client should be informed that the animal has accidentally soiled itself and that you are cleaning it up: "We certainly do not want him to leave dirty." When dismissing surgical patients, in addition to the animal itself being clean, the surgical incision, bandages, splint, or cast must be clean and dry. The surgery technique will often be judged by the neatness of hair removal at the surgical site and the appearance of the incision.

✎ TECHNICIAN NOTE

Never send home a patient that has soiled itself or has an unpleasant odor.

INVENTORY MANAGEMENT

The purpose of inventory management and control is to always have every drug, vaccine, or supply item available when needed for use (or sale) yet not waste money acquiring and storing extra supplies that are not needed in the near future. This is a delicate balance because the amount and selected use of drugs and supplies can change rapidly. Close attention to inventory levels of surgical supplies, pet food, pharmaceuticals, vaccines, x-ray film, and other items will ensure that an adequate stock is maintained without oversupply if an effective inventory control system is being used to reorder and replenish items before they are gone.

If too much stock is on hand, extra money and storage space are committed and the stock will be paid for long before the last of it is used. If too little is kept on hand, needed items will sometimes not be available to provide the preferred treatment for the patient or an opportunity for profiting from the sale of a product will be missed. If the right amount is on hand, the doctors and staff always have what is needed, large amounts do not have to be ordered and stored, and much of it is used before the payment to the supplier is due creating the needed cash flow to pay the supplier.

Inventory is the second largest expense area of operating a veterinary practice. Drugs should be used and be replaced about every 45 to 60 days (a turnover rate of six to eight times per year). The formula that is used for computing turnover rate is listed in Box 32-7. Turnover can be computed for every item in the inventory, averaged for the total inventory, or focused on the 20% of the items that account for the majority (80%) of uses (Pareto's law). Some inventory items will naturally turn over every 2 to 3 weeks (12 to 18 times per year), such as pet food, and often much or all of the item will be sold, generating income before the supplier requires payment.

Practice managers, sometimes veterinary technicians or a veterinarian, and occasionally reception staff or an assistant will be assigned responsibility for inventory control. Sometimes the responsibilities are divided among several staff members. One person should be the primary person placing

---

Box 32-7 INVENTORY MANAGEMENT FORMULAS

Turnover rate* of an item = Yearly inventory expense for item ÷ Average cost of item on hand at any one time

Average cost of inventory on hand at one time = (Inventory at midyear + Inventory at year's end) ÷ 2

*Pareto's law, or the 80/20 rule, states that 20% of the items account for 80% of the annual inventory expenses; this suggests that the above formulas should be used to evaluate and adjust the turnover rate of the biggest expense items to attain the "ideal turnover rate." Modified from *Lukens and Landon's effective inventory control*, West Chester, Pa, 1993, SmithKline Beecham (Pfizer).

---

orders, making sure that what is received is what was ordered and/or billed, and authorizing payment for the shipments. It is also important to set up an inventory master list of all items in stock in the hospital; keep a pharmacy library of all company product inserts, catalogs, and ordering procedures; and keep a file of MSDSs for all products as required by OSHA.

Considerable money is involved in inventory purchases. Much can be lost through inadequate inventory control procedures. This loss may occur because the business was billed for materials that were never shipped or never received at the practice, or the business was double-billed for one shipment, billed for damaged goods, or billed for more or different items than were received. Back orders that are not canceled when the product is reordered elsewhere double the inventory! Losses also occur because of ordering too many months' supply of perishable vaccines, biologicals, antibiotics, and reagents that deteriorate beyond the printed expiration date on the container and are no longer effective or legally safe to use. Oversupply also crowds the shelf and storage space and leads to more misplacement and over-ordering or loss from not rotating new items to the back and oldest products forward to be used first. The best stock rotation system is "first in, first out" (FIFO).

The sales representative's responsibility is to sell their product and "deals" that may provide more product than can be used in 1 or 2 months. It makes little sense to buy and store a year's supply of an item, no matter how much the price has been reduced. On the other hand, during a seasonal increase of use of a product, it will make sense to buy a large supply instead of the normal 1-month supply, particularly if the price has been cut significantly.

There are many computerized and manual inventory systems available for upgrading a current practice's procedures on inventory control. Because computerized systems require the input of everything that is sold and used in order to be accurate, they are only moderately successful in providing all the inventory control information needed (see Chapter 34). Manual procedures, such as identifying minimum stock reorder points on the shelf, posting want lists or reorder bins for all staff to use, and taking frequent inventory count of all supplies, can go a long way to help the computerized inventory control process be a success.

An effective inventory control system should be easy to use, ensure that all medications and supplies are available when needed, and reduce expenses by achieving a turnover rate of 8 to 12 times per year. It should provide a signal when each item needs to be reordered, track seasonal variations, track past usage rates, and provide purchase cost information to keep the pricing and supply of products current. It should ensure ordered items are actually received and back-ordered items are tracked so that overordering does not occur. It should also be easy to account for when and where items are used so that cost can be allocated to various profit centers within the practice. It should ensure proper monitoring and handling of Drug Enforcement Agency (DEA) controlled substances, provide a procedure for checking invoices to make sure they are accurate for amounts ordered and prices quoted, and periodically assess the value of the inventory. It should also reduce the cost of ordering the supplies by taking advantage of minimum orders for prepaid shipments and discounts for early payments when available. The inventory control system should also allow the practice to obtain the best prices available, identify expired or outdated items for prompt removal and return to suppliers for credit if provided, and enable the manager to detect staff pilferage if it occurs. (Modified from *A Guide to Inventory Management for Veterinary Practices/Effective Inventory Control,* 1993, SmithKline Beecham.)

All these desirable results of managing inventory will not occur if someone is not put in charge of inventory control and given adequate time and support by all members of the veterinary team to accomplish the assignment!

CLIENT MANAGEMENT

The most important person in any practice is each client. The practice of veterinary medicine is truly a *people business.* Everyone in the practice must enjoy working with and problem solving for the clients served by the practice. Veterinarians and technicians who do not like working with clients and their animal problems should not be employed in practice because they are ineffective with client communication. Many other professional careers are now available for individuals who desire less public contact.

🖉 TECHNICIAN NOTE

The most important person in any practice is each client!

VALUE OF THE CLIENT

The availability of veterinary services in the United States appears to be at an all-time high. New schools of veterinary medicine and expanded enrollment at existing schools have resulted in this increased availability of graduate veterinarians. The net result of the increasing supply of veterinary practitioners is increased competition for clients among established and new practices.

The practices that will financially survive must offer expanded services that are competitive. Practices can become more cost effective by using both technicians and assistants effectively to leverage the veterinarians' productivity while expanding service.

How valuable is each client? The practice will collapse unless old clients are retained and new clients are continually entering the practice. Clients are the lifeblood of the practice. Everyone in the practice works for the client. Some practices would like to think that they control their clients, but client loyalty is seldom mandated. Loyalty is won with hard work and dedicated caring service to each client.

The only unique product that a veterinary practice has to offer is service. If everyone in the practice understands that his or her primary role is to provide the finest quality medical care possible to the patient with the end result being a pleased and informed client, the practice will grow. If the staff attitude becomes one of negative feelings toward clients (e.g., not another one of these!), the practice clientele will dwindle. A practice's facilities, equipment, and techniques may be the finest available, but they will remain unused until enough clients willingly authorize or request that practice's services.

CLIENT SELECTION OF A VETERINARIAN

How does a client select a veterinarian? Most clients with small animals will select a veterinarian because the practice location is convenient. Following closely after practice location, recommendations from friends are ranked next. Once a practice is selected, the individual veterinarian will be evaluated in the following areas: friendly and caring personality, gentleness in handling the animal, communication skills, and professional knowledge. In the selection process it becomes readily apparent that practice location, facility appearance, and recommendations from satisfied clients are extremely important to practice growth.

Once the client enters the hospital the ability of the veterinarian and staff to project a concerned, caring personality, the expertise used in carefully handling the animal, and the clarity of the communication are the most important determining factors. It is interesting to note that professional knowledge falls to the bottom of the list. The general public has a limited informational basis by which to judge the professional knowledge of a physician, dentist, attorney, or veterinarian.

🖉 TECHNICIAN NOTE

Practice location and personal referrals are the two most common methods by which new clients find a veterinarian.

When does the veterinary technician have an impact on the client selection process? Clients always view the hospital staff as an extension of the veterinarian. Therefore a friendly personality, gentle patient-handling techniques, and caring communication skills become critically important in this whole process.

Clients with large animals usually select a veterinarian based on recommendations from others. Once the veterinarian arrives at the farm or ranch, the retention and satisfaction issues are the same as the ones used by small animal owners, with the addition of economic return. In food animal practice the veterinarian must become an economic asset to the overall farm profitability or the client can not afford to seek veterinary services. Companion animal practice (i.e., small animal, horse) has some economic limits, but the sentimental and emotional attachment (human-animal bond) of the client to the animal is relied on to extend that economic limit, which the food animal client may not do.

EVALUATION OF THE CLIENT

The technician's attitude toward himself or herself will be reflected in how clients are handled. People who are happy and positive about themselves and what they are doing will find that this attitude dominates client relations. One of the most contagious attitudes is enthusiasm. Enthusiastic people turn other people on! Enthusiasm is caught, not taught. The client must be handled effectively so that staff members do not cause a positive client to become negative. Conversely, veterinary personnel should deal with a negative client in a friendly and positive manner, identifying his or her concerns and needs and trying to help find a solution.

Generally, after working with a client for a short period of time, a staff member will get enough feedback to make some judgments about the client's expectations. These expectations are in the form of client-pet relationships, client-hospital relationships, and one-on-one personal relationships. One should not judge clients by their outward appearances only. Clients who appear to have nothing materially may value their animal highly and spend their resources to support veterinary care. In contrast, clients who drive up in a luxury car and have expensive clothes may not have the animal's best interests in mind and may be financially overextended. You cannot always judge a book by its cover, and you cannot judge people by their appearance.

> ✎ **TECHNICIAN NOTE**
>
> Do not judge the client's ability to pay by his or her appearance.

In most instances the technician and veterinarian will have to discuss the perceived pet's value with the client and give the client the opportunity to express himself or herself. One of the most important roles in client communication is to establish the value of the animal within the client-pet relationship. Some clients will be difficult to really figure out, and veterinary personnel may never feel they understand the client's intent or interest level.

CLIENT TRAFFIC FLOW PATTERNS

When the client first enters the reception area, the admission process begins. The receptionist initiates the proper business and medical records for each case. The client is escorted into one of the examination rooms. A preliminary history and examination [including temperature, pulse, and respiration (TPR)] may be taken by the technician before the veterinarian arrives. After examination and consultation with the veterinarian, either the client will leave the animal (hospitalization for further diagnostic tests, treatment, surgery, or observation) or the patient will be treated and, if necessary, medication will be dispensed before the patient returns to the receptionist for dismissal. In the event the patient is dismissed (outpatient), the client settles the account and is scheduled to return for a reexamination or to call with a follow-up report. During the routine outpatient visit, the client usually only contacts the outpatient work area. The client traffic pattern for an outpatient visit is reception to admission to examination (to pharmacy to laboratory) to dismissal.

If the patient is hospitalized, the client may have some contact with the inpatient area in addition to the outpatient area. A typical client traffic pattern in the hospitalized case would be reception to admission to examination to treatment area or surgical area to hospitalization to admission (discussion of dismissal and payment-credit policy). The client would leave the hospital and return to the reception area on the day of dismissal.

On dismissal of hospitalized cases, the client enters the reception area and usually receives patient information from the receptionist or technician. The client then proceeds to the examination room for a brief consultation with the veterinarian followed by home care instructions and demonstrations from the technician (Figure 32-21). To reduce confusion at dismissal, it is advisable for the client to return to the dismissal area and settle the account before the patient is presented. Once the patient has been returned to the client, communication may be difficult during the reunion process.

In addition to the routine and outpatient client traffic pattern, a third type of contact exists when the client visits a hospitalized patient. In this event, the client usually makes an appointment with the receptionist to visit the animal at a specific time that is convenient to both client and the hospital operation. When the client arrives, he or she will proceed directly to the examination or treatment room. Visiting patients in the ward is usually discouraged because other patients in the ward are disturbed. During the visit with the animal, a technician (or veterinarian) should be present to answer questions concerning care and progress made by the patient. The client should always visit with

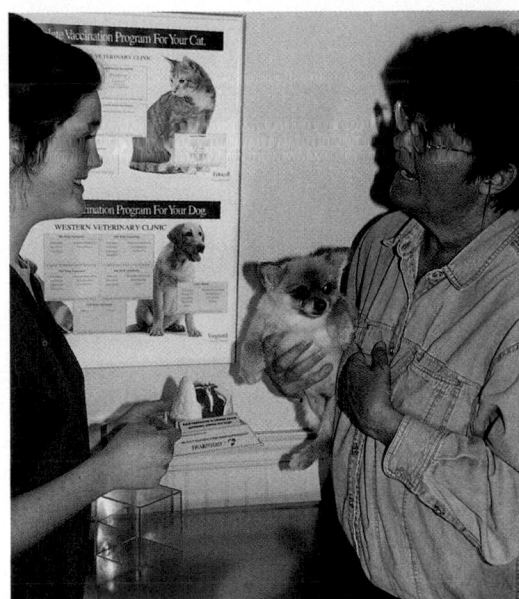

Figure 32-21 Veterinary technician uses a heartworm model to enhance client understanding of the impact of heartworm disease.

the veterinarian at some point in the examination room or the treatment room or in the veterinarian's private office.

Client visits are often beneficial for both the hospitalized patient and the client. The mental attitudes of client and patient can be strengthened, and communication can be improved between veterinarian and client. Client visits should be encouraged rather than discouraged.

OFFICE PROCEDURES

General office procedure knowledge is required of all staff in a veterinary practice. Staff (veterinarians, technicians, assistants, office managers) all need to have a working knowledge of how appointments are made, personnel staffed, fees developed and collected, inventory ordered and controlled, and pet insurance utilized. Most practices have a limited number of staff positions, and therefore everyone must have the ability to perform basic office procedures. The ability to perform other jobs is obtained through cross training.

The additional information needed to perform the work of others is acquired by being cross trained through working in different jobs while being trained in one's new job. This allows most jobs to be temporally performed by different people when a person is out sick or on vacation. In small businesses this ability to fill in with other staff is essential to maintain a smooth-running business.

APPOINTMENTS

Companion animal practices can operate either through the use of an appointment or a walk-in system. Each system has

advantages and disadvantages, but the appointment system is preferred by most veterinarians. Appointments allow the practice to control the flow of clients and patients into specific time periods that will improve the efficiency of the work schedule. When more clients are scheduled, most staff can be made available during the busier periods; on the other hand, when no appointments are scheduled, staff numbers can be reduced.

The appointment system usually functions around the scheduling of consultation times (office visits) in 15-, 20-, or 30-minute blocks. When 15-minute blocks are used, then four appointments per hour can be scheduled. Companion animal practices usually schedule 3 or 4 hours of appointment times in the morning and afternoon. A typical appointment period might be from 8:00 AM to 12:00 noon and 3:00 PM to 6:30 PM. Between noon and 3:00 PM, case workups, treatments, and surgery are performed.

Because of clients' work schedules, practices are now scheduling consultations in the evening to help meet the needs of the working family. Several evenings may be scheduled from 6:00 PM to 8:00 PM. Saturdays are also becoming more important to many clients, because Monday through Friday are filled with work and family activity. In many practices, Saturday is becoming the busiest day of the week.

The walk-in practice is the other method of scheduling. When using this work schedule, clients simply come in whenever they want and wait to be seen. The advantages to the client are not having to make an appointment and being able to drop in at the practice when it is convenient. The disadvantages are the length of wait time and the congestion when several clients come in at the same time. For the practice, the major disadvantage is not being able to plan and somewhat control and spread the workload to prevent several people coming at the same time.

To change from a walk-in practice to an appointment schedule requires planning and client communication. The first step is to set up 1 hour for appointments in the morning and 1 hour for appointments in the afternoon. Then as clients come into the practice for service or call the practice, explain that for the convenience of the client the practice has changed to an appointment schedule. Each client should be encouraged to use the appointment system the next time. As more and more clients are educated about the use and convenience of the appointment system the 1-hour periods are expanded. Eventually, only 30 minutes of unscheduled time is left in the morning and afternoon for walk-ins and semiemergencies.

Emergency cases are accepted at any time and are given priority over all appointments. However, if an appointment and a walk-in client come into the practice at the same time, the appointment is always given preference. Walk-in clients are always serviced, but they should not be given priority over an appointment unless it is a true emergency. Walk-in clients should never be turned away just because they do not have an appointment.

PRACTICE SCHEDULING

More and more people are now employed outside the home, so clients often have difficulty in visiting the practice between 8 AM and 5 PM, Monday through Friday. To help solve this problem, many practices now are expanding their consultation hours in the evening and on Saturdays. Some practices also offer early drop-off or late pickup service. This requires the veterinarian to communicate directly with the owner before the pickup or drop-off time.

The technician will also need to be able to discuss the case with the owner when he or she arrives at the practice during these extended hours, since the veterinarian may not always be available.

In addition to extending the hours, the staff must be scheduled to provide coverage during all practice hours. If the practice is open 6 days per week and operates 10 hours per day, support staff must be limited to a work schedule of 40 hours per week, so that overtime can be kept at a minimum. Veterinarians who are nonowners are usually scheduled between 38 and 48 hours per week.

The larger the number of employees in the practice, the more scheduling flexibility is available. Early morning, late evening, and Saturday periods are usually rotated so that everyone shares in these hours. If part-time employees are used, they could be scheduled into these extended hours and relieve full-time staff. The use of part-time employees greatly increases the flexibility to cover the expanded hours necessary to meet clients' needs. Part-time employees are more available now for both professional and support staff and can be readily used for coverage of extended hours.

PROFESSIONAL FEES

The only money available for funding a veterinary practice is collected from the clients as professional fees for professional medical services and products purchased. Loans from a bank will have to be obtained to cover deficits when there are more expenses than income. Therefore the veterinary business is vulnerable to failure if sufficient income is not received from enough clients to pay the operating costs of the business.

There are no government subsidies, few if any donations, and small amounts of money from pet insurance companies paid to veterinary practices. Therefore all employees must understand that their salary level is directly related to the health of the business and their productivity in generating income from billable tasks and product sales. Health care teams must be effectively organized with this principle in mind or the business will deteriorate.

Each veterinary practice should set fees based on what it costs to deliver services. However, the methods used for determining fees vary from practice to practice just like the cost of land and staffing of the facilities will vary. Methods used to set fees vary from accounting methods for establishing fees based on the cost of offering the service to a competitive guess of trying to match or undercut the price that other practices charge to just estimating what each client can afford. Only the accounting method is an acceptable business procedure. In 2002 another business method of evaluating fees was developed (National Commission of Veterinary Economic Issues (NCVEI). This on-line service can be accessed by any AVMA member at www. NCVEI.org. Specific fees can be observed based on national, regional, and state data.

Many veterinarians try to discount fees to a level they think the client can afford. However, it is impossible to accurately judge what a client can afford and is willing to spend. Only the client can freely decide what the animal means to him or her and what he or she is willing to pay. Discounting fees will eventually lead to reducing the quality of medical service, and that is unfair to the patient. It may also expose the team to charges of negligence and legal liabilities if the quality of care is below the accepted standard of care offered in similar practices in the area.

The practice manager or accountant must be able to identify the indirect costs and direct costs of operating the business via the financial reports to set or adjust the fees. Several steps are required to arrive at the appropriate fee for each procedure based on the cost of providing that service or product. First, direct costs are identified for each procedure related to the expendables used (drugs, bandages, film, etc.). Amortization of equipment costs over the equipment's expected useful life is also computed. For example, depreciating an x-ray machine over 7 years of useful life requires determining the number of x-rays taken per year from the radiology records. This will allow one to calculate the amount that must be included in the radiology fee for each x-ray taken. The machine will be paid for in the 7 years if the projected number of x-rays is taken (i.e., if the projected number of radiograph exposures is accurate).

The indirect costs (overhead) of operating a business must be computed. These include purchase or rental of the land, construction or rental of the building, the monthly cost of the utilities, facility upkeep, as well as taxes and interest on the debt. A new furnace, remodeling costs, and additions to the facility are either included as an annual cost or spread over several years. This cost of operation is added to each fee assessed as a percentage of overhead expense. It is spread over the number of expected client transactions in each fee to recover the indirect costs of overhead.

The biggest cost of running a professional business is the payroll for staff. Veterinarians' salaries, whether they are owners or employees, and the salaries of the rest of the veterinary team must all be prorated to each fee. The accountant does this for each procedure based on time input for each of the team members. Therefore an estimate of the normal time the receptionist, veterinarian, veterinary technician, and veterinary assistant spend to support each service must be computed. Time is valued per minute using each salary level and adding the payroll overhead costs (often 30% or more of salary). This is multiplied by the average time each person spends on the procedure and added to that fee. Once computed, all fees should be reviewed semiannually and adjusted as cost increases occur because of inflation. Obviously, fees must be refigured if anything major changes with staff time, the length of the procedure, or the purchase of new equipment.

The goal is to charge fair and equitable fees to cover the practice's cost of providing each service to clients. The fees should support using modern equipment, paying appropriate salaries to keep an effective team employed, and providing a fair return on the investment to the owners for taking business risks.

Fees fall into two groups: *shopped fees* or *nonshopped fees.* The shopped fees (examination fee, vaccination fee, and elective surgery fees: neuter, spay, declaw, etc.) should be competitive with other area practices. The level of shopped fees should be controlled by the going rate of other practices in the immediate practice area. Clients will judge the level of all practice fees by how competitive the shopped fees seem to them when they call and shop your practice.

The other group of fees are the nonshopped fees (clients do not call and shop these services), which include all other services in the practice. Examples of nonshopped fees are treatment for diarrhea or vomiting, fracture repair, chest x-ray, complete blood count, general anesthesia, cystotomy, angiogram, and cataract surgery. Most fees in practice are nonshopped. Therefore the practice can assess a fair fee for any of these services without concern about what other local practices are charging. The only fees that must be competitive are the shopped fees.

✏ TECHNICIAN NOTE

The only fees that must be competitive are the shopped fees.

The nonshopped fees should be increased by the inflation rate on at least an annual basis. If the annual inflation rate reaches 6%, then the nonshopped fees should be adjusted on a quarterly or monthly basis. The rate of medical inflation can be estimated by multiplying the consumer price index (CPI) by a factor of 2 to 3. Smaller, regular increases are not noticed by the client as much as one large annual increase. The major fees that attract client attention are the shopped fees, and these are only adjusted when local area practices adjust theirs. Computerization allows fee adjustments to be made easily and quickly even when done on a monthly basis.

Practice computerization (see Chapter 34) has allowed practices to have a much more detailed listing of fees for services and products. Fee codes can easily run into the thousands but are carefully adjusted and accounted for by the computer. This allows the client to receive a very detailed invoice at the conclusion of the practice visit. Computer software can also provide the client with a detailed fee estimate before service. This allows the client to make an informed decision about the level of service desired before the service is actually provided. This level of client communication is necessary to control collections and monthly billing.

Practice managers, owners, and the accountants that set up the accounting system of the practice will use monthly and yearly statistical summaries of incomes and expenses for evaluating changing trends for different procedures in all areas of the hospital, including profit centers. Trends of change from month to month and year to year are easy to track and recognize. The productivity of each veterinarian and veterinary technician can also be tracked with computerization software and salaries adjusted up or down based on productivity. In general the software should provide the business reports containing necessary information to make management decisions on what fees should be raised or lowered. This system enhances and rewards motivation and helps manage change. In summary, the accounting procedure for setting professional fees provides the basis for managing an effective business that will change as costs and demand for services change. The fees should be evaluated and adjusted at least twice yearly as appropriate to keep the fees in line with the costs and practice goals.

COLLECTIONS AND BILLINGS

Most practices have a standard payment policy of payment in full at the time service is provided. Cash payment is always the best method of payment. However, some services can be very expensive, and payment in full may not be possible at the time the service is rendered. Therefore alternative payment plans are usually required if the service is to be provided.

Alternative payment plans include the use of bank credit cards (Master Card, Visa, Discover, American Express, etc.), medical credit cards (Care Credit), and local bank credit and practice credit accounts. After all the above payment plans are discussed, the practice credit account should always be used as the last option. When internal credit is provided, specific controls must be in place. The usual controls for practice credit include approval of a credit application, a 50% deposit at the time the estimate is given, the balance to be paid in three or four monthly payments, 1.5% per month interest charge on the unpaid balance, and payment of a monthly billing fee (usually $3 to $8). The monthly billing fee covers the cost of billing each client (computer time, personnel time, stationery, envelopes, postage).

The collection of a 50% deposit based on the fee estimate at the time of admission is the standard way of determining how the client will pay the account. All hospitalized cases should have a written fee estimate prepared before service. Routine outpatient services usually do not receive a written fee estimate. True emergency cases are an exception. When a written fee estimate is prepared on a hospitalized case, the client will be informed by the business manager, technician, or veterinarian that it is hospital policy to collect a 50% deposit before performing the requested services and the balance of the account will be payable at dismissal. This allows the client and the practice the opportunity to discuss case finances before the service.

If the client determines the estimated services are too costly, then the veterinarian will have an opportunity to recommend another possible treatment or method that is less costly or discuss credit options. By making routine use of fee estimates and deposits the level of practice credit can be carefully controlled. The level of accounts receivable (practice credit) in a practice should not exceed 25% of the average of 1 month's gross income. As an example, the level of accounts receivable should not exceed $25,000 in a practice grossing $100,000 per month ($1,200,000 annual gross income). If the level of accounts receivable goes beyond 25%, a more strict credit policy needs to be put in place or enforced.

Effective communications related to collecting the fee from the client begin with confident receptionists, technicians, and veterinarians who understand how the fee is computed and are confident that it is deserved and fair and truly represents the quality of service provided. An educated staff is more confident, positive, and informed in discussing fees with clients, whether at the time of fee estimates or at the time of payment or billing.

Billings charged by clients for future payments are called *account receivables*. The more account receivables grow, the less cash is available to pay ongoing expenses that includes the payroll of the practice. Therefore the goal must be to collect (not charge) a fee according to a defined practice policy in a business manner that does not offend or alienate clients.

Most companion animal veterinarians attempt to collect all fees and not allow clients to charge. Increased credit card availability has allowed most clients to delay actual payments by transferring the charges to a credit card. This provides almost immediate payment to the business by the credit card company and prevents the practice from losing a significant amount of money from clients who will not or can not pay their bills in the future. Credit card payment allows money to be immediately available to pay inventory purchases, apply to payroll, or pay other bills.

If credit is to be provided, the practice manager should be involved before the services are provided to approve the client's credit application, establish down payment amounts, and develop a repayment schedule. Charging fees and sending monthly billings by mail are more common with large animal practices. Established clients with excellent credit who have a large number of animals may negotiate a monthly payment instead of payment for each service rendered.

CASH CONTROL

Cash control is best accomplished using some form of fee slips in triplicate that are numbered serially. One copy is kept in the examination room, one stays with the daybook ledger of income received, and one is given to the client. With this method, if someone's payment is unintentionally

(or intentionally) omitted from being recorded in the daybook ledger, the numbered fee slip can be traced back to determine who that client was and what happened. This system allows errors to be corrected, prevents embezzlement, and provides a way to track clients who may have forgotten to check out and pay for a service. Computerized systems should also have these and other cash control features.

Petty cash is often needed by staff to purchase stamps and incidental supplies from local businesses. A procedure must be set up to track petty cash to prevent embezzlement and meet U.S. Internal Revenue Service (IRS) business deductibility rules. Generally, a cash box accessible to approved staff for petty cash is set up with a set amount of cash, for example, $100. The petty cash box must always contain $100 made up of the total value of signed and dated purchase receipts, cash, and temporary IOUs made out by the person as he or she removes petty cash to get supplies. When the person returns, his or her receipt plus change must equal the IOU, which is removed and replaced by the change and signed receipt. When petty cash gets low, the receipts are taken out of the box, totaled, and entered into business records as petty cash expenses. A check for expenses is made out for that amount and cashed, and that amount of cash is returned to the petty cash box. This prevents suspicion of embezzlement if every person follows this procedure, preferably overseen by the practice manager. It also makes sure all expenses are accounted for when monthly and annual reporting is due.

All staff and veterinarians should record all supplies and products taken from the practice for personal use even when these are provided free as a staff benefit. This prevents embezzlement and pilferage, accounts for the level of benefit actually provided, and keeps everyone honest and above suspicion by management, co-workers, and the IRS. It encourages honesty, avoids destructive suspicions, and promotes trust if followed by all employees, including practice owners. Consulting accountants, owners, and the practice manager have resources to set up standard business procedures for the receptionist and staff to follow to develop a smooth operating veterinary business.

BUSINESS MANAGEMENT

Professionals as a whole would often like to abstain from the business side of practice and concentrate exclusively on professional (medical) activities. In reality, without the business side of any profession, there would be few opportunities to practice that profession. The business management aspects of practice can become as challenging as patient management. Lack of available time, lack of interest, and minimal experience are limiting factors.

Clinical signs of poor business management are lax credit policies, increasing accounts receivable (total dollars clients owe), reduced operating capital, lowered gross income, lowered net income, increasing personnel costs, increasing overhead, reduced client numbers, and reduced average transaction fee per patient. Tests used to identify problems of poor business management include complete review of monthly business information to establish trends, comparison of this month's data to the same month 1 year ago, review of the fee schedule, review of the credit policy, review and comparison of inventory levels, and turnover rates.

Prognosis is generally good once the diagnosis of poor business management has been supported by a review of the diagnostic tests. Treatment will usually need to continue for the life of the practice. Some recommended treatments for the poor business management syndrome follow:

Establish a firm written credit policy.
Make use of a written fee estimate sheet to itemize all patient charges.
Before admission, have the owner sign and retain one copy of the estimate sheet.
The credit policy should be clearly stated on the fee estimate sheet (see an example of a fee estimate form in chapter 33).
Make use of appointment systems to schedule clients for the most efficient use of time.

The practice fee schedule should be reviewed and updated at least every 3 to 6 months, and a current printed fee schedule should be available near each telephone. Accounts receivable need to be monitored monthly, with legally appropriate follow-up telephone calls and letters to stimulate payment in a timely manner.

Accounts payable should be handled in a way to obtain discounts for prompt payment. Accounts that do not provide discounts should be paid near the due date to conserve working capital. No account should be allowed to become past due. A poor credit image for the practice is difficult to remove.

One tool for analyzing and correcting poor business management is the office computer. The office computer can provide on-line storage and have information readily available at the push of a button. The computer can provide income analysis, accounts receivable information, inventory control, client information analysis, patient diagnosis analysis, on-line medical record, and so forth. Computerization is becoming increasingly cost effective, and well-designed programs are now available through several vendors. Additional information about computers in veterinary medicine is found in Chapter 34.

If these treatments are properly applied, the outcome from "poor business management syndrome" should be complete recovery. The result of improved management is a sound and stable veterinary practice that pays dividends to clients, patients, and employees.

PET INSURANCE

Health insurance has had a significant role in funding the costs of human medicine for several decades as a third-party payer insulating patients from most of the medical and surgical costs. Dental insurance also impacts dentistry practice. Pet insurance [veterinary pet insurance (VPI)] was introduced into veterinary medicine about 1982. Most pet insurance policies will cover specified services, have limits, co-payment levels, and deductibles, similar to human medicine policies. Some policies provide wellness benefits that include routine vaccinations, physical examinations, and dental services.

Recently, more companies have been encouraged to offer pet insurance because more pet owners value their pet as a member of the family and want some protection against catastrophic costs from unexpected accidents and disease. If these policies increase in number, they may help the business of veterinary practice. More patients will have major unexpected costs covered, wellness programs will be supported for saving money by preventing some costly treatments, and fewer owners will choose unnecessary euthanasia of their animals. Thus everyone benefits including the animal when the client has pet insurance.

CLIENT COMMUNICATION

Excellent interpersonal communication skills can serve to develop and expand veterinary service markets. Improved communication between client and veterinarian results in more personalized professional care. Reduction in spendable income of clients may reduce demand for elective procedures, but this can be offset by providing a more comprehensive preventive medicine program through improved communication skills. Clients are unable to make service selections until they fully understand all options.

Common courtesy and genuine concern affect all professions and businesses. It has been said, "I don't care how much you know until I know how much you care!" The world as a whole is becoming more depersonalized. When a veterinary practice loses sight of the individual client, the personal service feeling is lost to both the client and patient. Courtesy begins with acknowledging clients as soon as they enter the reception room, carefully explaining why an appointment is helpful, calling clients by name, asking about the clients' families—in short, treating clients as important guests in your hospital.

Courtesy also extends to telephone manners. All calls should be answered by the third ring; the caller should be greeted by "Good morning, this is ABC Animal Hospital, this is Kathy speaking. How may I help you?" The caller immediately knows he or she has reached the correct hospital and Kathy is there to help. Telephone courtesy is just as important as personal courtesy because most clients have their first contact with the hospital by telephone.

If the veterinary staff of a hospital treat each caller and each client with common courtesy, the impression the client will receive is genuine concern. A lack of concern for people and their pets' problems is a common complaint voiced by clients of many veterinary practices. If veterinary personnel treat each client as they would like to be treated when selecting or securing service, the result will be more happy clients who experience courtesy and concern.

Closely accompanying the issue of courtesy and concern is effective communication. The majority of complaints against veterinarians are the result of ineffective or misunderstood communication between veterinarian or staff and client. To communicate completely, staff members must have concern for *both* animal and client. In addition, they must learn to *listen* to the client and then communicate a caring attitude as well as information that is understandable and effective. Most people *hear* other people talking, but few people have developed the ability to *listen* effectively to what is communicated. The successful veterinary team must develop this ability.

To ensure effective communication consider these four rules:

1. Use terminology the client will understand; scientific terms can be confusing to the client.
2. Do not rush through the information just because you are hurried or because it appears to be "common knowledge" to you, or the client will feel "brushed off."
3. Do not assume a superior manner or tone to the extent the client feels "put down."
4. Use effective communication techniques for obtaining a history (Box 32-6).

In short, show concern and respect. Attempt to treat each client with respect, honesty, and as a very special person even if you do not agree with him or her. If the communication is open, honest, and caring, it will be effective and most problems can be prevented. One of the most common reasons for veterinarians to refer clients to other veterinarians is because of the failure to communicate effectively with the client.

Listening is an extremely important communication skill. The skill of listening must be practiced on a regular basis to become effective. Many people would rather talk than listen. Often, the client will assist in the diagnosis by providing important clues in the history if only someone will listen. Active listening involves listening to clients and then verbally rephrasing their messages back to them for verification. This technique ensures that the client was heard correctly and the technician or veterinarian received the entire message.

Listening requires understanding both the "music" and the "words." The correct words must be sent and received. In addition, the nonverbal music (facial expressions, hand gestures, body stance, etc.) must also be observed and understood to allow complete communication.

CLIENT EXPECTATIONS

Most clients expect the following five things during a consultation with a veterinarian: examination of the animal, diagnosis (cause if possible), prognosis (predicted outcome), treatment plan, and fee estimate. Communication of prognosis, treatment plan, and fee estimate is difficult for most veterinarians. Clients feel unprepared to make judgments without this information and often complain if complications occur. Malpractice (professional negligence) concerns can be virtually eliminated if these areas are effectively handled with the client. Again, the veterinary technician should be part of the communication team in these areas. Clear, effective communication is a team effort and absolutely necessary for client compliance and quality patient care.

COMMON COMPLAINTS FROM CLIENTS

When dealing with a cross section of the public, as most practices do, the goal of complete satisfaction for all clients can never be obtained. However, when clients do have complaints, careful attention must be given to them. To reduce the number of complaints from clients, several potential problem areas will be addressed. The more common areas of client complaints are fees, courtesy and concern, communication, appointment schedule, sanitation, and quality of patient care.

Every client deserves a complete explanation and breakdown of all anticipated costs of each service to be performed. Whenever communication is incomplete, client complaints will result. One of the most sensitive issues practitioners deal with is financial estimates. Quoted fees must be written down and honored unless revised with full consent of the owner. The most common client complaint will concern fees. The use of a fee estimate sheet and up-front, open communication will eliminate most fee complaints.

Another common client complaint area centers on the quality of care offered to the patient and client. Often, animal owners are hesitant to accept one veterinarian's opinion. As in human medicine, seeking multiple opinions on a case has become routine. Specialists have become more common in veterinary practice, and veterinary clients are requesting second and third opinions. Multiple opinions have been good for both the patient and client, but they require veterinarians to be thorough and up to date with their information and techniques.

THE DIFFICULT CLIENT

Some clients remain difficult to deal with regardless of the best efforts of everyone in the practice. Some of these difficult people actually enjoy being difficult. The attitude of the difficult client toward technical and reception staff may be different from the attitude toward the veterinarian. A very difficult, demanding person can suddenly become quite reasonable when the veterinarian enters the room. When this happens, the technician should not feel he or she has failed but rather should work a little harder to understand and win the client's trust.

In dealing with someone who is politely complaining, listen to their perceptions and feelings and attempt to convey that you understand the problem (you will appear to be agreeing; this will help to reduce the level of the confrontation). A good example would be the common complaint that fees are too high, which can be answered by, "Yes, fees are high. Everything is high these days!"

In situations in which the client appears to be unreasonable about the complaint, establish the specific problem (i.e., fees, unsatisfactory treatment result, poor communication) and then indicate to the client you would like for him or her to speak to the veterinarian. Once the unreasonable client has been identified, escort the client out of the reception room and into an examination room away from other clients; then the veterinarian can handle the problem as quickly as possible.

The most difficult people to reason with are people who have been drinking or are on drugs. Be careful how you handle these people. Do not argue or confront them because they could become violent and uncontrollable. In situations in which drugs or alcohol has been consumed to excess, law enforcement officials should be contacted to handle the situation.

Never argue with a dissatisfied client. The client is "always right, even when wrong." In other words, clients have a real concern that must be acknowledged and understood. If a client leaves angry, 10 other people are told how terrible you, your veterinarian, and your hospital are. When the client leaves the practice enthusiastically, he or she will only tell three other people. We cannot have clients leaving angry. Sometimes we must all "eat a little crow" to keep the client's good will. In the long run, this will benefit all concerned.

PROFESSIONAL MARKETING

Some professionals feel uncomfortable with the idea of marketing because the scope of marketing activity has been poorly understood. Often, the connotation of marketing is advertising. However, advertising is only a small portion of the total marketing picture for a professional business.

Professional marketing has numerous definitions, but the one that will be used here is "the communication of professional services and goods offered to existing and potential clients." The veterinary technician must understand marketing principles to be an effective communicator of professional services and goods offered by the practice.

Definition

Professional marketing consists of all activities that increase client awareness of professional services and goods. Marketing occurs through effective client relations; professional appearance of the hospital, clinic, or ambulatory vehicle; listening to owners' opinions; a convenient practice location; a polite support staff; offering full-service care; sending clients service reminders; being neat and clean; using business cards; sending clients educational newsletters or E-mail notes; providing nutritional counseling and dietary management; providing emergency service; offering pet and livestock supplies; giving career talks at high schools; leading 4-H, Future Farmers of America (FFA), or scouting groups; attending dog/cat/horse shows; having producer or client education nights; being involved in a community service club; setting up a Web site on the Internet; advertising in the yellow pages of the telephone book; providing handout material to clients; having an attractive and well-located building sign; sending thank-you and sympathy cards to appropriate clients; appearing as a guest on radio and television shows; writing a newspaper animal column; using attractive letterhead stationery; becoming active in professional associations; and group advertising in the newspaper about the annual rabies vaccination clinic.

Animals are totally dependent on owner awareness of health care needs. Professional marketing should be designed to help more animals by informing and serving more clients. If successful, it will result in increased practice income through increasing client numbers, increasing the revisit rate; or the amount of each client transaction. It requires balancing improved animal health and public health with the needs and goals of the practice. One of the most critical questions a veterinarian should ask is "What business am I in?" To be able to conduct a successful professional business, one must be clear about specific business objectives. Some practitioners believe as long as high-quality medical and surgical skill is delivered, the client will continue to use their service based on the quality of service alone. Fortunately, clients today are usually well-informed consumers and are looking for both quality *and* value. The average client lacks the professional background to accurately judge the quality of medical or surgical services performed. However, clients do have the ability to judge the quality of caring communication that *they* received personally, which influences their perception of the value of the professional service received. Therefore clients' perceived value of services is their reality of the practice's quality.

Veterinary medicine is in the *people service* business. The profession cares for animals but provides professional service to their owners. Patients cannot come to the practice without the owners! If each staff member understands that she or he is in the people service business, a completely different orientation will take place. When clients call on the telephone, for example, they are not interrupting the veterinarian's or technician's time in the examination room or surgery room; they are the reason for the existence of the examination room and surgery room. Veterinary practices do provide high-quality professional service to animals but only after the agreement and financial support of the owner. Also, only satisfied clients return and refer others.

✏ TECHNICIAN NOTE

Client phone calls are not an interruption because clients are the reason for the existence of the practice.

The professional success of most veterinarians and technicians is the result of *interpersonal skills* rather than strictly clinical skills. The ability to relate well to people and their problems will allow the practice the opportunity to provide high-quality veterinary medicine (Figure 32-22).

Once the practice is viewed as a people service business, marketing of those services becomes possible. The product to be marketed is *high-quality, people-oriented professional veterinary medical* service.

Marketing techniques must benefit the profession as a whole to achieve maximal success. The overall program must promote the *benefits* of veterinary services rather than the specific service.

If one were to compare the benefits of a program of immunization with one that sold a vaccination, the long-term effects are evident. A program that details the benefits of immunization can build a preventive medicine program through a physical examination, dental care, nutritional management, and so forth on an annual basis. The approach of selling a vaccination is just that—promoting a vaccine.

The program of promoting the benefits of a high-quality, people-oriented professional veterinary medical service must be the end goal.

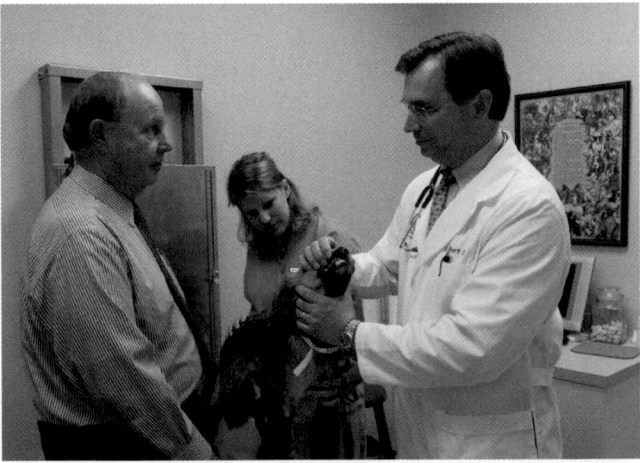

Figure 32-22 Client, technician, and veterinarian communicate as a team about patient care.

Marketing techniques will not overcome the effects of poor client relations within a practice. Unless effective client communication and client orientation are practiced on a client-by-client basis, marketing will be unsuccessful.

Practice Marketing

The first step in a marketing plan is to determine client needs. One must listen closely to services being requested by each client. Determine what service trends are going on within the practice in response to economic growth of the community. As an example, both spouses usually work today. This results in some people being unable to seek veterinary care during the traditional 8 AM to 5 PM period. The typical client also has less free time to devote to shopping around at several stores for items when all items could be purchased at one convenient location. By listening to clients and observing service needs, the practitioner may opt to extend the practice hours two evenings per week and open later in the mornings on those days. The practice may also expand services to include veterinary-supervised boarding and offer selected nonprofessional supplies, such as grooming aids.

The practice owner must determine the direction of the marketing plan by listening to client needs and gathering additional facts concerning community trends. The marketing process will then be guided by current facts and psychodemographic information.

Specific Marketing Techniques

Professional marketing can be divided into *internal* and *external* marketing. Internal marketing techniques are the day-to-day activities that occur within each practice, whereas external marketing involves techniques used outside the practice. The purpose of both internal and external techniques is to enlarge the number and size of the client transaction.

Internal Marketing

Internal marketing is aimed primarily at the existing client base. Internal marketing techniques attempt to educate and inform current clients about the various veterinary services and service programs available. They also should generate client enthusiasm for the practice. The following methods are meant to serve as an idea base and not as a complete listing of techniques for internal marketing.

Client Relationships. The most important technique to use in any marketing program is personalized, sincere client care. Most clients require as much attention and care as the patient. Clients today want both high technology and high touch. Personalized service that emphasizes each individual client will allow the opportunity for excellent communication to be established. Both veterinarian and technician must be skilled communicators as well as technically skilled professionals. All staff must support these efforts.

Practice Appearance. The visual appearance of the clinic, hospital, or ambulatory vehicle is the first outward signal to the client concerning the potential quality of service. One must consider the appearance of the building (repair, paint, cleanliness) and the grounds (Figure 32-23). Plants and grass must be neat and trimmed and the parking lot clean and well signed for parking. The interior of the building must also be clean, well cared for, and odor free. Silent marketing messages are sent to clients through the appearance of the facility.

A practice facility does not have to be new or have the latest equipment to project a positive professional image. The older facility that has been given proper care and maintenance will exhibit a strong marketing message of "we care" to people passing by each day.

Support Staff Utilization. Most internal marketing carried on within a practice will be through the veterinary team members. Support staff activities will augment the efforts of the veterinarian in client relations and personal appearance. Primarily, veterinary technicians and receptionists will be responsible for recommending services or goods and following up on hospital programs that require appointments or individual client contact. These team members are regarded as an extension of the veterinarian and must have a professional approach to client management.

Technical staff will usually deliver the majority of client education with the assistance of receptionists. Handout materials, visual aids, and video presentations will help the staff in their educational efforts. The staff will need detailed information concerning the various preventive health programs from the veterinarian. To be able to promote the product, everyone needs to be clear about the product. Therefore the veterinarian and the support staff must work together as a service team, all delivering the same high-quality service.

Professional sales point displays can add another level of service for clients. These displays need continuous monitoring by support staff to provide "on the spot" professional information. Areas in which support staff should have in-depth knowledge include nutrition, parasite control

(internal and external), grooming aids, dental care, immunization programs, obedience training, and rearing orphan animals. In addition, support staff must be on the constant lookout for new clients and additional services. Staff members who are active in dog clubs have continual access to new potential clients. New clients may not be aware of services offered, and so all staff members must be willing to provide program information at any time. When certain key support staff members are given a small percentage of income from all new services and new clients they provide the practice as an incentive, a new wave of enthusiasm may develop in everyone.

Full-Service Care. Listening to client needs will verify that clients want full-service care when possible. People are exposed to 1-hour photo processing, 1-hour eyeglasses, 7-Eleven, fast food restaurants, K-Mart, Wal-Mart, drive-through banking, and so forth. Convenient, fast, economic, one-stop shopping is the rule for single-parent families and families in which both husband and wife work. People are now asking for this same type of convenient service in their veterinary care. In small animal practice, full-service care would include prepurchased counseling concerning pets, human-animal bond and behavioral problem counseling, pediatric care, preventive medicine, nutritional counseling, nutritional management, veterinary-supervised boarding, geriatric care, dentistry, bereavement counseling, cremation service, and full routine veterinary care. The service would extend from birth to death.

In a full-service practice, various programs can be packaged for marketing. The goal of marketing is to sell a *program,* not an individual service. The emphasis of a quality practice is to provide preventive health care, not just disease treatment. A small animal practice must develop a complete health maintenance (wellness) program for new puppies and kittens as well as puppy training classes. This program carries into adulthood and on into the geriatric period. The wellness program could include annual physicals, periodic routine blood screens, nutritional counseling, dental care, and immunizations. Nutritional counseling would include pediatric, adult, and geriatric care as the patient matures. As clients continue their regular contact with the practice to purchase foods, the practice has a regular opportunity to market other health preventive care services.

Client Reminders. One of the more successful early attempts at practice marketing was through the use of a vaccination reminder system for small animals. During the early discussions on the use of a recall system, many practitioners felt it was unprofessional to send a reminder card to clients because it was advertising. No one was considering the service provided to the client and animal. Most veterinarians thought only of how it would appear to other veterinarians.

Charles, Charles and Associates discovered that sending vaccination reminders was even more important to clients than having boarding facilities or an attractive building. Clients want to be reminded when specific services are to

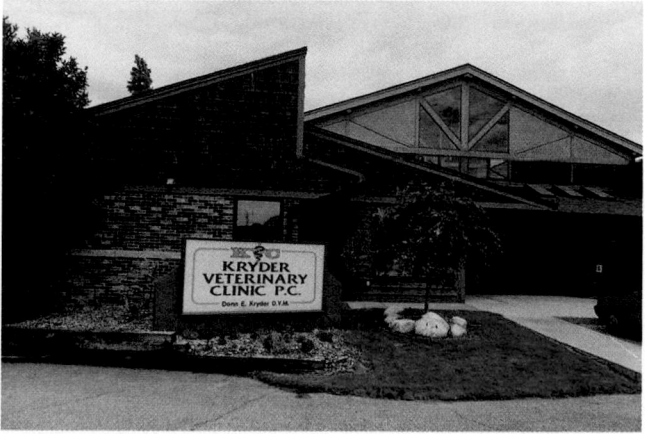

Figure 32-23 Exterior appearance of the hospital should provide a positive image.

be done. However, clients prefer to receive reminders by mail rather than by telephone.

A reminder system is a major marketing feature of most practice management computer software packages. A system that has the capacity to generate only one reminder is not nearly as valuable as a system that will produce a second and third reminder if the client does not respond. Using a system that will generate an additional second or third notice to be sent will greatly increase the service return rate.

Most practices now accept the use of a reminder system as a valuable marketing tool for routine immunizations. The reminder system must be expanded to include other routine services for clients. Additional use in small animal practice could be in the areas of dental hygiene (routine cleaning), annual physical examination, geriatric care, hip-dysplasia evaluations, follow-up laboratory testing, heartworm evaluation, and so forth. The suggestion of an annual physical examination may appear on the surface to be a poor recommendation in light of physicians now recommending fewer annual physicals. However, considering that the dog and cat age seven to nine times as rapidly as humans and that the diligent veterinarian and technician are able to find a potential problem on almost every physical examination, many clients will take advantage of the service when offered. When performing the examination, the veterinarian and technician must explain and demonstrate the findings to the client (i.e., potential problems with ears, eyes, teeth, anal sac, hair coat, obesity) (Figure 32-24).

Small animal geriatric care is another relatively untapped market area. When patients reach a specific age (i.e., 7 to 8 years of age), a reminder letter could be sent to the client providing information on specific conditions to be monitored. The letter could approach the client in the following way: "on the spot." This letter could be developed and recalled by the computer at a specific age.

Another area in which a reminder system could be used is to recall young animals that have been previously vaccinated but not yet neutered. The recall of unneutered animals is an opportunity to market ovariohysterectomy and castration services. This reminder may attract some clients who would otherwise go to a low-cost spay and neuter clinic. A personalized letter could detail the specific features of the service, which is not possible from the spay and neuter clinics.

The use of a recall system allows the market to be segmented (targeted). An example of market segmentation would be to send all feline owners a reminder about leukemia vaccination.

Personal Appearance. The personal appearance and hygiene of each staff member reflect the quality of the practice. Many clients relate personal appearance to the sanitation and level of quality of the practice. If someone does not care enough to change a dirty smock, coveralls, or boots, why should he or she care enough to provide the highest-quality service? Not only should hand washing occur between all patients, but also it should be practiced in front of the client. This enhances client awareness of disease prevention efforts. Personal appearance marketing works just as building appearance—an outward signal of internal quality (Figure 32-25). A professional image is perceived by the client when all hospital members have a professional appearance. Staff uniforms, shirt and tie, dress, and smocks for doctors are recommended.

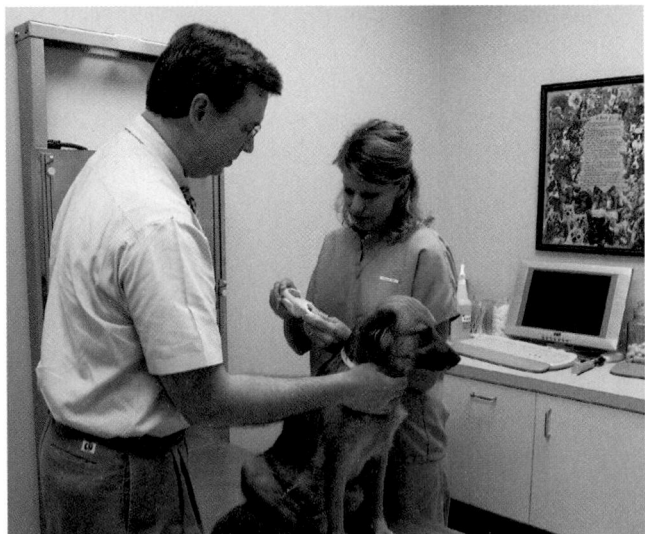

Figure 32-24 Technician explaining a diagnosis to client using visual aid.

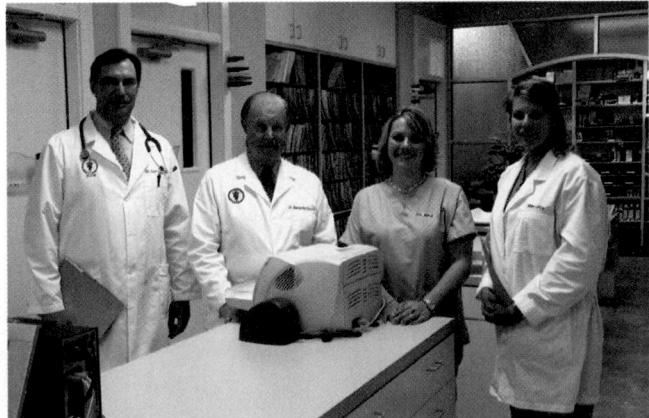

Figure 32-25 A professional appearance is a marketing tool.

Handout Materials. Marketing with handout materials has been used for a number of years. The quantity and quality of commercially available handouts are excellent. Most commercial companies realize the value of client-oriented professional literature. These pieces should be carefully reviewed by the practice so that only acceptable material is made available to clients. Once the material has been reviewed and useful pieces selected, all staff must be made familiar with how and when they should be used. A professional rubber stamp can be purchased with the practice name, location, and telephone number on it and used to personalize all commercial handout materials. A professional print shop may also be used to imprint the practice information on all brochures. Handout material must be handed directly to the client by the veterinarian or technician to be most effective (Figure 32-26). Handout materials displayed in the reception room for clients to pick up are often not well utilized. Clients will pick up material from a display rack and take it home, but few will ever read it.

In addition to commercial handouts, materials may be purchased from veterinary organizations. AVMA, the American Association of Equine Practitioners, and AAHA, among others, provide useful client handout materials.

Practices may also produce their own informational material. Quality handouts on whelping, ovariohysterectomy, cystic calculi, colic, mastitis, and so forth can be easily prepared on the computer. Discharge instruction handouts are very effective because clients often forget verbal explanations and instructions. Practice information brochures can also be produced to more fully explain practice hours, services, equipment, facilities, and staff function (Figure 32-27). Other forms of handout materials used on a regular basis are business cards and letterhead stationery. They

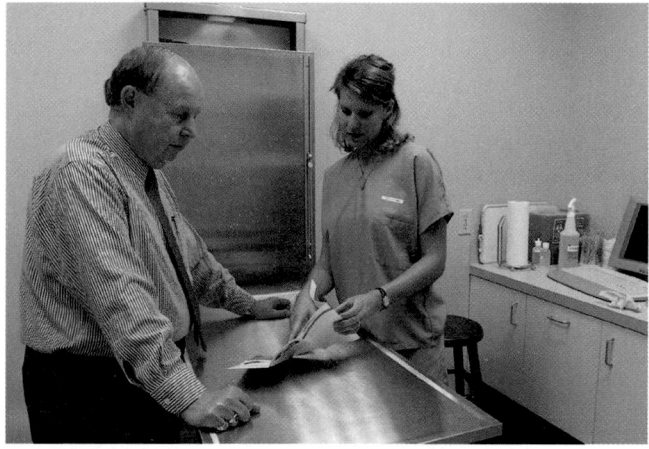

Figure 32-26 Technician explaining and providing a handout to client.

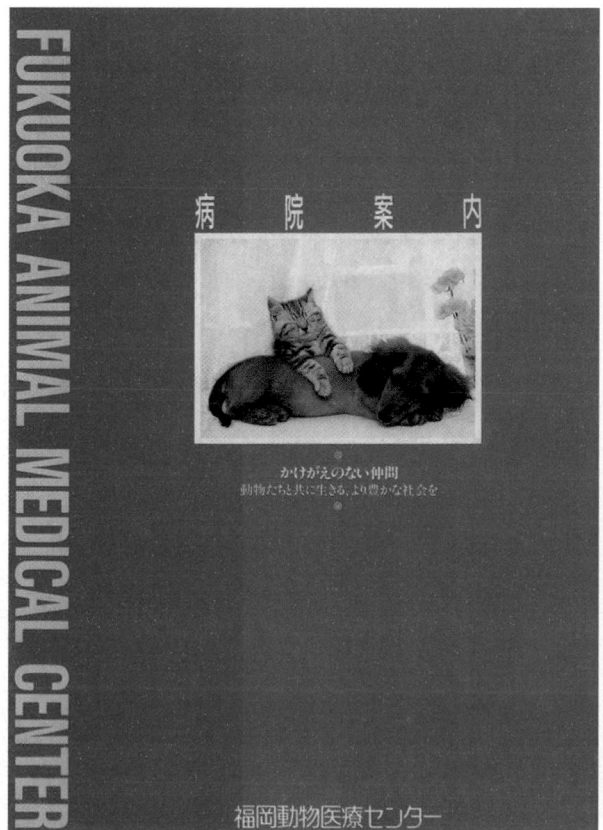
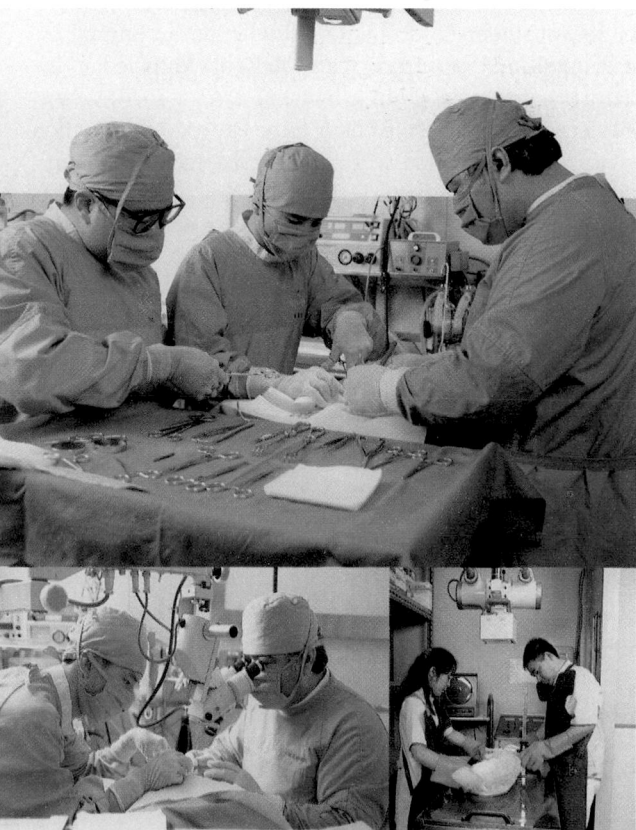

Figure 32-27 Practice information pamphlet. **A,** Cover. **B,** Inner page. (Courtesy Fukuoka Animal Medical Center, Fukuoka, Japan.)

are effective forms of marketing. Business cards should be made available to clients from *both* veterinarians and key support staff, especially certified veterinary technicians and receptionists.

Sympathy and Thank-You Communications. A very personal marketing approach is to appropriately use sympathy and thank-you types of communication. One may choose to use commercially prepared cards or develop a letter format on the computer that can be personalized. Regardless of the format used, the use of personal messages to specific clients for specific purposes has an everlasting positive effect. In the case of clients newly referred by current clients, a note or card to both the referring clients (thanking them for the referral) and the new clients (welcoming them to the practice) is appropriate. As the use of the Internet becomes more common, E-mail notes could also be used

The sympathy card or personal note is helpful when a pet dies to demonstrate open concern for the feelings of the client during his or her emotional loss. The expression helps the client deal with the loss and allows the client to understand the "I care" attitude of the practice for both the client and pet.

Newsletter or E-mail. The use of newsletters will increase client activity through improved understanding and education about veterinary services. Educational goals for newsletters should be to inform animal owners of the signs of illness, to make seasonal animal health care recommendations (i.e., heat stroke in summer), to review health care programs, and to introduce key staff members. Many clients do not understand how to tell whether an animal is ill or in serious condition. This lack of knowledge is especially true for cat and horse owners.

Newsletters will allow the client to be exposed to specific pieces of information that will help owners to know when to call a veterinarian for help. Total health care plans can also be explained to allow the owner to be aware of full-service health care that extends beyond vaccinations. The newsletter should help market the benefits of healthy animals.

Newsletters can be sent to specific segments of clients in the practice computer base; however, they can also be provided through a hand-generated list or passed out to all clients as they enter the practice. Most veterinarians do not have the experience or time to compose a complete newsletter three or four times per year. The practice manager, veterinary technicians, and receptionists may develop articles for a practice newsletter, or consideration can be given to purchasing a professionally edited newsletter service.

Each newsletter should be personalized by the practice to allow the reader easy access to the practice's location and telephone number. Another advantage newsletters have in overall marketing is the ability to reach the nonuser. If the client receiving the newsletter passes it on to a nonclient friend, the nonclient has an opportunity to be exposed to various veterinary services offered by the practice.

A spin-off use of the newsletter could be through the use of news notes or Internet letters. News notes are

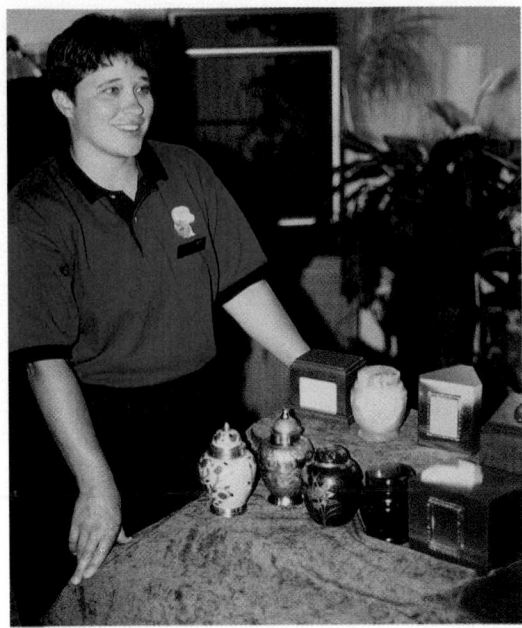

Figure 32-28 Veterinary technician shows a variety of urns for ashes of cremated patient. These services and compassion for the family's grief are greatly appreciated by clients.

postcard-size updates mailed to the client three or four times per year. As more clients become connected to the Internet, short E-mail letters can be used in place of newsletters sent by regular mail. Internet notes allow rapid and economical communication.

Special Services. Practices can either expand existing services or add new services to increase their market share. In a small animal practice, market expansion might be in the areas of birds and exotic service, bereavement counseling, prepurchased evaluation of pets to determine suitability for family, behavior counseling, nutritional counseling (i.e., puppy, adult, senior), dental care (i.e., endodontics, periodontics, orthodontics), geriatric care, cremation service (Figure 32-28), emergency care, and intensive care unit. Because most small animal clinics cater to dogs, many cat owners do not feel welcome or comfortable in an environment with dog pictures on the walls and barking dogs in the reception area. Practices that want to increase feline clients might be well rewarded by considering the needs of cats and cat owners when remodeling. Having a separate reception area for cats and keeping cats in a separate ward should be a starting point. Previous lack of recognition of these needs may be the primary reason for serving fewer cat owners than dog owners with professional veterinary care.

Sales Point Displays. When displays are being considered as an internal marketing technique, several important points must be contemplated if they are to be successful. First, the practice must define the clients' needs. The specific products must be carefully selected and priced. An appropriate location or locations must be established in the clinic or hospital that may be monitored at all times by the

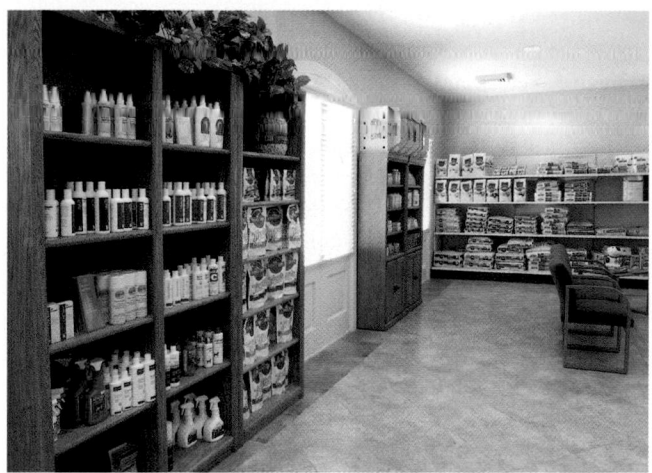

Figure 32-29 Professional display in reception area.

technical staff (Figure 32-29). The products must be attractively arranged and kept neat and clean. Prices must be clearly marked on all products.

The most important difference between a hospital or clinic display and a retail store display is the *professional* advice that is provided with each item sold. Professional counseling is not available at the feed store, grocery store, department store, Internet shops, or mail-order outlet. The technical staff will pay a key role in providing product information for the client.

Professional displays may include limited product lines confined to an examination room, a specific area of the reception room, or a special room adjacent to the reception room.

Animal Care Talks. Veterinary technicians and veterinarians can both become involved in providing veterinary medical care talks to grade school and high school students as well as to adult clients. The most effective and unique visual aid is a live animal. These presentations can provide information on routine animal health care, first aid activities, signs to look for when an animal is ill, and general information on educational requirements of veterinarians and technicians. These presentations also help to change the established norms about animal care.

When a presentation has become polished, service clubs in the community make excellent audiences. Talks to service clubs are helpful to enhance awareness of quality medical care provided by the individual practice and the profession. A slide or computer presentation that features both veterinarian and technician in their team roles is very effective.

The veterinary technician could present information on care of the new puppy or kitten, exotic pets and birds, first aid, feeding the pet, whelping and queening, hip dysplasia, parasite control, pet obedience training, and pet selection. Client education programs should be given on a regular basis and offered at convenient times. Attendees should be provided with handout material to take home for future reference.

When the education program is held at the practice, a complete tour of the facilities should be planned. Clients are interested in seeing hospital equipment and understanding more about hospital care. An annual hospital open house is an excellent image builder to clients. Having a "behind the scenes" tour is something most clients have not had an opportunity to experience. Many will be "amazed" to see x-ray, anesthesia, surgery, and laboratory equipment "just like in a human hospital." Children are especially impressed with show-and-tell demonstrations using live animals.

By providing client education opportunities, the client becomes more bonded to the practice. When veterinary problems arise, the client is more apt to contact the practice that has provided an inside look and veterinary medical information.

External Marketing

Most external marketing activities are aimed at expanding current client activity and identifying new nonclient activity. External marketing can be carried out by an individual practice, group practice, organized veterinary medicine, and commercial companies.

Some types of external marketing are currently being used in many practices. The use of an Internet Web site, newsletters (direct mail to nonclients), telephone yellow page advertising, building signs, client education nights, community service activities, and AVMA's National Pet Week materials expands the image of the practice to clients and nonclients. When a practice wants to penetrate into the nonclient base, one must make use of selected forms of advertising.

Professional Advertising. Professional advertising includes hospital signs, telephone book listings, practice newsletters, vaccination reminders, and professional business cards. However, the focus on advertising in this discussion will center more on the more hard-core forms of advertising: yellow pages of the telephone book, newspapers, magazines, radio, direct mail, and telephone. Attitudes concerning advertising differ between the professional and the consumer. A great majority of professionals (physicians, dentists, attorneys, veterinarians) are against advertising for a variety of reasons: it seems to be unprofessional and unethical, and it lowers status, credibility, and sense of dignity. Just as professionals feel strongly negative toward advertising, consumers feel strongly positive. Consumers generally believe advertising by a professional would not compromise that professional's credibility, status, image, or dignity as long as it is honest and not misleading. In fact, most consumers believe advertising by professionals would help them make a more intelligent choice.

Telephone Yellow Pages. When a yellow page advertisement is deemed appropriate for external marketing purposes, several guidelines should be followed. First, the advertisement should not be larger than one-fourth page; advertisements larger than one-fourth page are perceived as being more unprofessional by the consumer. Second, the advertisement should be set in one color (preferably black). The use of multiple colors (e.g., red, green) is again perceived by the consumer as being less professional. Finally, the advertisement should provide as much information as possible about the practice and its services.

Internet Web Page. Web pages are the newest form of marketing for veterinary practices and organizations. Many practices are using their own Web site to provide public access to information about the practice, its staff, pet care, and services provided, and they include pictures for a virtual tour of the medical facility and procedures. A Web page may also provide the practice clientele with the ability to make an appointment on-line, as well as provide quality information about pet selection, training, feeding, and selected medical conditions. The practice Web page can be updated frequently and may replace the need for practice newsletters and maybe practice brochures. Other quality sources for veterinary-related information on the Internet can be reviewed and approved and set up as a link to the practice Web page (see www.avma.org for initial links to the Virtual Library, PetVet, Care for Pets, and the ElectronicZoo on the Internet).

Newspapers. Newspaper advertising, like telephone yellow page advertising, is useful for initial impact when opening or expanding a practice. Many professionals will have a newspaper listing when opening a new practice, when relocating an existing practice, or when adding new associates to an existing practice. The continual use of newspaper advertising for veterinarians has been largely prohibited by cost.

Probably the best form of newspaper advertising for veterinarians is the "animal care information" format. Weekly animal care information columns are a public service, and newspapers are always seeking educational material. Pet columns have become popular reading as the public begins to acknowledge and understand the human-animal bond. To address the need for weekly newspaper columns, several private column services have sprung up that will provide the practitioner with 52 professionally written articles on animal care each year. This service can be purchased by individual veterinarians or through associations.

Radio and Television. Veterinary associations can obtain air time essentially free by participating in talk shows. The subject of animals, animal care, and animal behavior is a fascinating subject to most listening and viewing audiences. A number of the larger radio and television markets have regularly scheduled talk shows (some hosted by veterinarians) that have a question-and-answer format

devoted to animal care. The talk show format is an excellent opportunity for associations that have articulate and knowledgeable veterinarians and technicians to sell veterinary medicine for the profession as a whole.

Recently, popular television programs, such as Animal Planet and Emergency Vets, have had a large impact on marketing the veterinary profession. Likewise, the earlier James Herriot books and televised Public Broadcasting System (PBS) series attracted many animal lovers to the profession. All these media events help public awareness of the high level of medical care provided by the veterinary profession.

Community Activities. Veterinary practices that engage in community activities have a much wider client base.

Veterinarians and technicians should become involved in community service through Girl Scouts, Boy Scouts, 4-H Veterinary Science Leader, school boards, humane societies, country clubs, Rotary, Lions, and church activities. Potential client contacts are made in the course of being involved and contributing to these organizations. In addition, one becomes more knowledgeable about the species, breed, and show-circuit problems when participating in animal breed clubs.

One should not join a community activity only to make client contacts. Practice is too time consuming for both veterinarian and technician to become involved in too many activities or activities that are not personally rewarding. However, a reasonable involvement in some of these activities is an important marketing tool in addition to being necessary for supporting the community.

GRADUATE TECHNICIAN SELF-MARKETING

Veterinary technicians must learn to choose employment in practices in which veterinarians will delegate sufficient billable technical tasks to allow the technician to also generate income. This must be sufficient for adequate leveraging of the veterinarian's productivity to provide the technician an adequate salary sufficient to stay in the veterinary technology profession. The IAMS publication, *How to Market Yourself—A Veterinary Technician Placement Program,* is an excellent resource to plan this critical choice. Also see Recommended Reading at the end of this chapter.

✐ TECHNICIAN NOTE

Leveraging the veterinarian's productivity through delegation of billable tasks to the technician should provide adequate salary support for the technician.

The second phase of technician marketing occurs after the initial adjustment period of employment. Once a technician is a productive and trusted part of the veterinary team, strategies must be undertaken to improve and enhance the technician's productive role on the veterinary team. "I can do that" spoken at appropriate times is one of many ways to encourage greater delegation. Keeping a log of technical duties performed by the veterinarian and preparing an analysis of potential time (and money) that could be saved through delegation can also be effective. The same process can be applied to tasks performed by the technician that could be economically done by a minimum-wage assistant. Additional information concerning the financial rewards of the use of the veterinary technician is available at www.NCVEI.org.

Obviously, there must be some role delineation between technicians and assistants and between veterinarians and technicians while maintaining the most productive teamwork possible. In general, tasks should be delegated to the lowest paid person who can perform them correctly, especially when other income-producing tasks are available.

SUMMARY

Practices that will flourish in the twenty-first century will be those that integrate well-trained technicians with responsible client communication, deliver high-quality medicine and surgery, maintain excellent client-patient and personnel-business management, fully utilize current technology, practice in attractive facilities aided by a good location, and practice preventive maintenance on the facility, equipment, and grounds. These flourishing practices will be exciting and rewarding for clients, patients, and staff.

Recommended Reading

Ackerman L: *Business basics for veterinarians,* Lincoln, Neb, 2002, ASJA Press.

American Veterinary Medical Association: *Your professional image,* Schaumburg, Ill, 2000, The Association.

Finch L: *Telephone courtesy and client service,* Schaumburg, Ill, 1991, American Veterinary Medical Association.

Gerson RF: *Beyond customer service: keeping clients for life,* Schaumburg, Ill, 1993, American Veterinary Medical Association.

Haberer JB, Webb MW: *Teamwork: 50 ways to make it work in your practice,* Schaumburg, Ill, 1996, American Veterinary Medical Association.

Heinke ML, McCarthy JB: *Practice made perfect, a guide to veterinary practice management,* Lakewood, Colo, 2001, AAHA Press.

Lukens RI, Landon RM: *Effective inventory control,* West Chester, Pa, 1993, SmithKline Beecham (Pfizer).

Petit TH: *Hospital administration for veterinary staff,* Goleta, Calif, 1994, American Veterinary Publications.

Wise JK: *US pet ownership and demographics sourcebook,* Schaumburg, Ill, 2004, American Veterinary Medical Association.

MANUALS AND DIRECTORIES

AAHA hospital standards and accreditation manual, Denver, 2005, American Animal Hospital Association.

2005 AVMA membership directory and resource manual, Schaumburg, Ill, 2005, American Veterinary Medical Association.

How to market yourself: a veterinary technician placement program, Dayton, 2000, The IAMS Co.

Waltham veterinary hospital management, ed 3, Vernon, Calif, 1998, Waltham.

JOURNALS

DVM: The Newsmagazine of Veterinary Medicine, Cleveland, Advantstar Communications, monthly.

Trends, Denver, American Animal Hospital Association, monthly.

Veterinary Economics, Lenexa, Kan, Veterinary Medicine Publishing Group, monthly.

Veterinary Practice News, Mission Viejo, Calif, monthly.

MANAGEMENT SHORT COURSES

Veterinary Management Development School, Denver. Contact AAHA for details.

Veterinary Management Institute at Purdue University. Contact AAHA for details.

INTERNET SITES

www.avma.org (information on veterinary medicine and links to pet care sites)

www.avma.org/navta/ (veterinary technology profession information)

www.NCVEI.org (financial information for the veterinary profession)

33

Medical Records

JOANNA M. BASSERT

INTRODUCTION

The keeping of medical records in veterinary practices has become increasingly more sophisticated during the past several decades. Now with the use of computers, faxes, and E-mail, medical record keeping has taken on a new look and a greater level of complexity. Not surprisingly, even the term *medical record keeping* seems outdated as the phrase "veterinary medical health information management" more accurately describes the plethora of written and electronic records that are now routinely maintained by veterinary practices. Free from the confines of federal and state regulations that define medical record keeping in human hospitals, veterinary practices are able to apply a creative spectrum of approaches to record keeping. In this way, the individual needs of veterinary practices, in terms of business and medical information, may be effectively met by practice owners and managers.

Veterinary medical records include a wide range of forms and logs that document the treatment and care of animal patients. The results of physical examinations, laboratory tests, and diagnostic procedures, such as radiographic imaging, ultrasound, electrocardiograms, and endoscopy, are examples of information that is included in the record. In addition, medical records document treatment protocols, such as the administration of medication and intravenous fluids, surgery, wound care, and radiation or physical therapy. Medical records also describe the progress of patients, list daily observations, and chart vital signs and other monitoring data. Finally, medical records document euthanasia and postmortem examinations and include important authorization and consent forms.

The number and types of forms and logs that comprise medical records vary from practice to practice. Large

teaching hospitals, for example, such as those associated with schools of veterinary medicine, tend to have extensive medical records in which a separate form is used for each department, procedure, or study. Private companion animal practices, on the other hand, often employ shorter medical records that combine information into a concise chart or folder, which is easy to store and interpret. Finally, ambulatory food animal and equine practices often employ the most abbreviated form of medical record by using carbonized billing sheets as both medical record and invoice.

This chapter discusses the many approaches to medical record keeping that one sees in veterinary medicine. It offers a comprehensive "dissection" of the patient record, presents a variety of filing systems and clarifies the ethical and legal issues that accompany the record keeping process. ∎

FUNCTIONS OF THE MEDICAL RECORD

The Institute of Medicine has organized the functions of the medical record into two broad categories: *primary purposes* and *secondary purposes*. Primary purposes support the patient's medical care such as the documentation of diagnostic procedures, diagnoses, prognoses, and treatment. Secondary purposes are not clinically based but rather include evaluations of medical information for business, legal, and research purposes.

PRIMARY PURPOSES

Supports Excellent Medical Care
The medical record is a critical tool that enables and supports the effective treatment and care of animals, and it

does this in many ways. First, it assists the veterinary health care team in correctly identifying the patient and the owner. There are, after all, many black Laborador retrievers that look alike and many owners named Smith, Jones, or Brown. In this way, the medical record helps to prevent confusion of the identities of the patients and their owners. Second, it helps in the generation of an effective diagnostic and treatment plan. It documents the veterinarian's physical exam findings, lists the diagnostic procedures and tests to be performed, and records the veterinarian's ideas regarding differential diagnoses. The medical record also enables practitioners to document patient responses to treatment, so plans may be adjusted as needed. As time passes and members of the health care team change, the medical record supports continuity of care. It helps practitioners, who are not familiar with the patient, to understand the medical history and conditions of the animal. In this way, it provides an avenue for communication between each of the members of the veterinary health care team so that treatment can be accurately and effectively administered.

Documents Communication

The medical record also documents communication with the client, which is particularly important when there are many members of the veterinary health care team assisting the same client. Take-home instructions, for example, will be included in the medical record, so any confusion about home care by the client (owner) can be quickly clarified. In addition, the medical record assists in the generation of reminder cards that help pet owners to stay current in their pet's preventive medical plan. In these ways, good communication is critical for providing a logical, continued plan of patient care for both the health care providers and for the pet owner.

Interactions with clients and their pets are also aided by the use of medical records. Financial limitations, for example, and the behavioral idiosyncrasies of the pet may be recorded. In addition, the veterinarian-client relationship can be further enhanced when the names of other family members and important family activities are noted in the record as reminders for future topics of informal discussion.

SECONDARY PURPOSES

Supports Business and Legal Activities

The medical record lists all of the services rendered to the pet owner whether it is boarding a dog or spaying a cat. This documentation verifies billing and serves as legal evidence of services received by the owner. It can be used to assess the workloads of staff members, formulate income analysis, make budgetary plans, perform actuarial calculations, maintain inventory, and generate a marketing strategy. In addition, it plays an important role during hospital accreditations and helps assess compliance with standards of care.

The medical record is used as a legal document in a court of law and is valuable during litigation. It serves as evidence

of procedures performed and treatments administered and provides specific dates and times of events. In this way, the medical record is critical in defending against malpractice suits. Special care must be taken, therefore, to ensure that the record is complete and accurate. Keep in mind that in a court of law, the prevailing view is "not recorded, not done." In addition, insurance companies may require the medical record to assess whether a claim is to be paid.

Supports Research

The medical record is a key element in the preparation of case studies and presentations for conferences. Information from medical records is collected to develop registries and databases, which assist in the conduction of retrospective studies and in predicting clinical outcomes. It is used to teach veterinary medical and veterinary technician students. To maintain confidentiality, all patient markers are removed from the record before they are used for any purpose other than patient care (Box 33-1).

✐ TECHNICIAN NOTE

A comprehensive medical record supports excellent medical care, research, and good business practices. It also helps to protect practices during malpractice litigation.

Box 33-1 SUMMARY CHART: FUNCTIONS OF THE MEDICAL RECORD

I. PRIMARY PURPOSES
Supports Excellent Medical Care
A. Identifies correct patient and owner
B. Supports generation of diagnostic and treatment plans
C. Supports continuity of care
D. Supports communication
    1. Among health care team members
    2. With the owner
    3. Personalizes veterinarian-client relationship

II. SECONDARY PURPOSES
Supports Business and Legal Activities
A. Verifies billing.
B. Supports actuarial calculations.
    1. Income analysis
    2. Budgetary plans
    3. Staff workloads
C. Supports inventory maintenance.
D. Supports formulation of marketing strategy.
E. Supports hospital accreditation.
F. Acts as a legal document.

Supports Research
A. Case studies and presentations
B. Registries and databases
C. Education of veterinarians and veterinary technicians

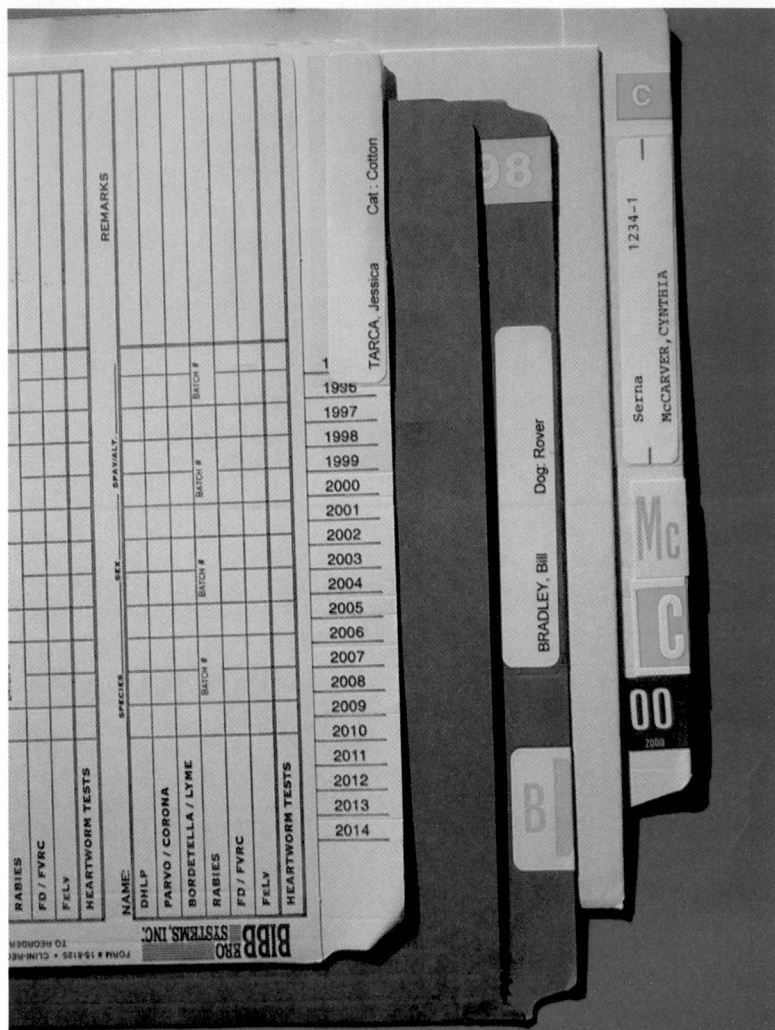

Figure 33-1 Shown are a variety of letter-size folders. The color and style of the folders can vary as well as whether charting is stamped on the cover. Color-coded decals are placed on the edge of the folders to facilitate filing.

TYPES OF PATIENT RECORDS

With use of computers and veterinary practice management software, veterinary hospitals are managing information better and more efficiently than ever before. Still, the vast majority of practices continue to employ hard copy, paper-based medical records, in addition to using computers. This chapter concentrates on the *written* record, while Chapter 34 concentrates on the *digital* record and the use of computers in information management.

Medical records come in a variety of shapes and sizes. They typically appear as letter-size folders that contain a variety of forms and charts held in place by fixed clips. However, they can also come in the form of large index-type cards on which the veterinarian makes handwritten notes. In addition, ambulatory food or equine practices often carry simple carbonized forms that serve as both a record of the services rendered and the charges assigned. Let's examine each type of medical record in greater detail.

LETTER-SIZE FOLDERS

The vast majority of veterinary practices today make use of 8 × 10 inch folders in which medical information is stored and organized (Figure 33-1). Each patient has its own folder. Tabs are located at the edge of one end of the folder to facilitate the placement of color-coded decals. Some folders have grids printed on the outside of the cover on which critical information, such as the animal's immunization history, can be written, In this way, the staff can quickly visualize key pieces of information. More commonly, however, veterinary practices use folders with a plain manila cover.

Letter-size folders are typically stored vertically on shelves, which are kept behind or near the receptionist's desk for easy retrieval. Some particularly large practices may have record rooms in which a mobile shelving system may be employed. In these systems, large shelves are mounted on tracks so that they can be moved easily from one location to another when pushed. Mobile shelving systems save space

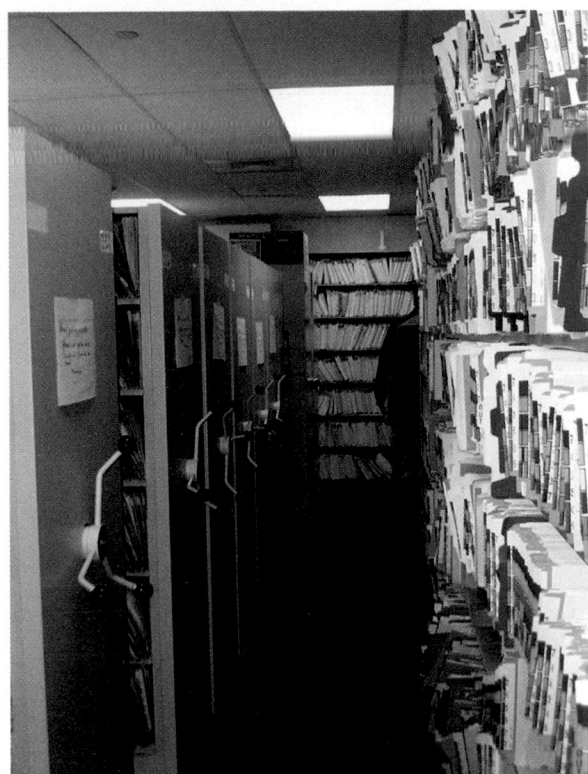

Figure 33-2 Mobile shelving creates more storage space for medical records. These shelves move on tracks that are fixed to the floor. Each shelf is moved by turning the wheel-crank located on the side of the shelf.

because shelves may be positioned up against one another when access to their records is not needed (Figure 33-2).

CARD FILES

To conserve space and cost, some veterinary practices use a card file system instead of maintaining letter-size folders. One type of card used is 5 × 8 inches, which is stored in a file pocket (Figure 33-3). Laboratory data and other reports can also be stored in the pocket with the animal record. As more and more writing space is needed, additional cards can be stapled to the original card. If a family has more than one animal, there is a separate card for each patient, but the cards are often clipped together and filed as one unit.

Another card system involves the use of a 10 × 16 inch card, which can accommodate more information per card than the 5 × 8 system. The 10 × 16 inch card can be folded in half to facilitate handling.

Card files are typically stored in file drawers rather than on shelves and are generally organized in alphabetical order according to the first letter of the last name of the client.

A plastic strip along the top of the folder contains a letter for each month and numbers that help receptionists to keep track of when reminder cards should be mailed. In addition, the strip contains hooks that enable the file to be suspended on a rack in the file drawer.

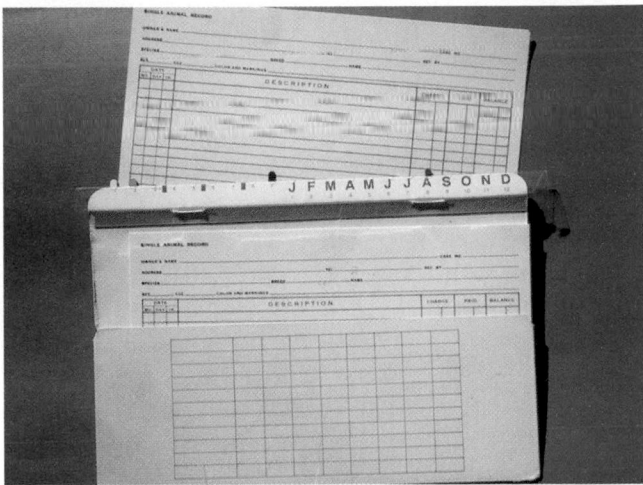

Figure 33-3 The card-style record with pocket folder, though once popular, are not as commonly used as the letter-sized folders.

Due to their small size and limited writing space, information contained on cards is brief. The patient information is usually entered in reverse chronological order. The date and information regarding each appointment is entered on a separate line. Each card file must contain owner and patient information along with sufficient data to allow the proper and adequate care of the animal. However, in our modern, litigious society, keeping thorough and complete records is increasingly more important as detailed medical information is often requested in a court of law. In addition, practices seeking accreditation by the American Animal Hospital Association (AAHA) are required to use letter-size folders. For these reasons, cards, though once popular, are not as commonly used today as letter-size folders can accommodate a more comprehensive animal health record.

CARBONIZED SHEETS (AMBULATORY LARGE ANIMAL PRACTICES)

Ambulatory food animal and equine practitioners work long hours and put many miles on their trucks as they travel from farm to farm. The use of lengthy medical records, therefore, is impractical in a situation where there is little storage space (in the truck) and where paper might blow out the window. Many ambulatory practitioners, therefore, make hand written notes on carbonized invoice sheets that are loaded into a sturdy metal dispenser. Once procedures are performed, diagnostic and treatment notes as well as billing information may all be included on the invoice pages. A copy is given to the owner. The original is kept on file at the practice's home base, where the sheets may be stored in 8 × 10 inch files along with the results from laboratory tests. A veterinarian who spends long days on the road might joke that this system is in keeping with the Veterinary Medicine Paperwork Reduction Act, but it is also cost effective and practical. Throughout the year, but particularly in the spring, during lambing and foaling season when practitioners receive remarkably little sleep, the carbonized sheets provide adequate documentation and communication in a time-efficient manner. This helps the veterinarian meet the heavy demands of ambulatory practice.

Although there has not been enough legal pressure to warrant changing the carbonized-invoice system that is used by the vast majority of ambulatory food and equine practitioners, a few veterinarians have begun to use laptop computers in the trucks to assist with record keeping. In this situation, the practitioner enters diagnostic, treatment, and billing information into a portable laptop computer that can be plugged into the cigarette lighter or run on batteries. The data can later be transferred to the practice's networked computer system when the veterinarian returns to the office to restock the truck. Some ambulatory practitioners use an index of bar codes, each one representing a different diagnosis, procedure, or medication. The veterinarian scans the appropriate bar codes to create an invoice and to document the diagnosis and treatments rendered. Instructions to the owner might also be generated. A small portable printer would enable the document to be printed on site and subsequently given to the owner. Wireless capabilities are also being explored by some progressive ambulatory practices.

It is impractical for food animal veterinarians, who are responsible for the health of entire herds of livestock, to maintain an individual record for every animal treated. In this situation, records are kept on the herd as a whole. Immunizations and reproductive histories are maintained for the group, although individual records may be generated for animals that have undergone special surgical or treatment procedures.

Large animal teaching hospitals and full-service equine clinics, commonly have hospitalized surgery, medicine, and neonatal patients, and often employ the standard 8×10 inch file record system. In this situation, each patient has its own medical record. In-house treatments and procedures are recorded in the record by hospital staff members. An invoice is generated separately and is typically given to the owner for payment before the animal is allowed to be discharged and loaded onto the trailer. Specific examples of hospital forms for equine patients can be found in Chapter 29.

FORMAT OF THE PATIENT RECORD

As mentioned, veterinary medical records are not subject to the federal and state regulations that one sees in the human medical field. Therefore, there is a wide range of approaches to record keeping, which vary from practice to practice. Most methods, however, fall into one of three categories:

1. Source-oriented medical record (SOMR)
2. Problem-oriented medical record (POMR)
3. Combination of source- and problem-oriented medical records

TECHNICIAN NOTE

Most companion animal practices use a combination of SOMR and POMR.

SOURCE-ORIENTED MEDICAL RECORD

The source-oriented method is typically used in records that have limited space such as in the card- or pocket-type records. Information comes from various sources and is entered chronologically by office visit or period of hospitalization. In this way, the most recent information is located last. Typically the date is entered in the far left-hand column of a line on the card, and the entry is made to the right of that. Physical exam findings, the database, diagnoses, and treatments are all listed. The veterinarian often makes entries in a "free form" that integrates information from various sources as it becomes available or comes to mind. The source-oriented method is easy to learn and takes little time to complete; however, it can lack detailed documentation, which may prove vital during litigation. Remember, "if it is not written down, it didn't happen."

PROBLEM-ORIENTED VETERINARY MEDICAL RECORD

The problem-oriented veterinary medical record (POVMR) is used in conjunction with the folder-type medical record and is used in teaching hospitals, AAHA-accredited hospitals, and many private companion animal practices including specialty and emergency centers. The format helps to provide a whole view of the patient and supports a logical and organized approach to clinical medicine. It fosters excellent communication, team-oriented medical care and rapid retrieval of information. Veterinary teaching hospitals find the POVMR particularly helpful when veterinary medical and veterinary technology students first learn to approach medical cases. The format provides a structured way to walk students through complicated cases, one problem at a time. In addition, a requirement for AAHA-accreditation is use of the problem-oriented format.

Though the components of the POVMR can vary somewhat, it most commonly includes the following:

1. Client and patient information
2. History
3. Physical examination
4. Master problem list and working problem list
5. Progress notes, assessment, and plan
6. Pertinent forms: surgery, anesthesia, radiography, special imaging, and laboratory reports
7. Case summary
8. Fee information

These components can be further subdivided into more specific units of information (Box 33-2).

Box 33-2 Standard Information for Veterinary Medical Records*

CLIENT INFORMATION
Name of owner
Address
Home phone number
Alternate phone number
If applicable, referring person
Additional information if co-owned

PATIENT INFORMATION
Name of animal
Signalment: species, breed, age, sex, and spayed or neutered.
Color and markings
If applicable, tattoo, microchip number, and identification (ID) number

PERTINENT HISTORY
Presenting complaint
Last normal
Frequency of episodes
Client observations and/or concerns
Current medications
Allergies
Current diet

PREVIOUS HISTORY
Previous problems
Previous treatments and responses (including transfusions)
Previous surgeries
Previous medications
Previous diagnostic tests
Immunization history
Environmental history
Travel history
Patient's weight history
Previous diet

PHYSICAL EXAMINATION FORM
Master problem list and working problem list
Progress notes:
Date
Physical examination findings

Problems
Tentative diagnoses
Definitive diagnoses
Prognoses
Therapeutic plans
Changes in therapy
Medications administered and dispensed
    Name of medication
    Expiration date
    Time
    Date
    Dosage and directions
    Fluid rate
    Route of administration
    Frequency
    Duration of treatment
    Identification of individuals
    Cautionary notes
    Slaughter withdraw and/or milk withholding dates (food animal)
Procedures performed in chronological order
Client communications

PERTINENT FORMS
Laboratory reports
Reports and assessments of diagnostic procedures (endoscopy, radiography, ultrasound, and special imaging)
Description of surgical and dental procedures, including duration of procedure and name of surgeon
Anesthesia record
Consultation reports with specialists or other referring veterinarians (dermatology, oncology, cardiology, ophthalmology, surgery, internal medicine, dentistry, and neurology)
Signed consent forms
Client waivers or deferrals of recommendations
Client phone log
Discharge instructions
Necropsy report

FINANCIAL RECORDS

Information compiled from Peden AH: *Comparative records for health information management*, AVMA Guidelines for Basic Information for Records and the American Animal Hospital Association Standards of Accreditation.

COMPONENTS OF THE POVMR

CLIENT AND PATIENT INFORMATION

Typically the receptionist first takes the name, address, and phone number of the client when the first appointment is made. This information is confirmed later when the owner arrives for the appointment. It is particularly important to record the correct spelling of the owner's first and last name. Even seemingly simple names such as *Megan Brown* may be spelled *Meaghan Brown* or *Meghan Browne*. Do not assume to know the correct spelling of the client's name; always confirm it. This will prevent subsequent filing and client-identity errors.

Cell phone numbers and E-mail addresses of the owner may also be important to obtain when the owner is in the office. In addition, the receptionist might want to have a general idea of the client's schedule for the day and where she or he can be reached at what time. This is particularly critical if the pet is undergoing surgery or a procedure that requires anesthesia. Unexpected events or findings can occur during clinical procedures, and the veterinarian may need to consult the owner immediately. Sometimes the owner must make important decisions over the phone, such as the extent of treatment to be performed, while the animal is on the surgery table and/or under anesthesia. In this situation, good communication and care for the patient is maximized if the client can be contacted.

In addition to the client information, the receptionist also records the age, breed, sex, and species of the patient. This information is collectively known as the *signalment*. In some veterinary practices it is imprinted, together with the client information, on the top of each medical record form using a plastic hospital card. When using a wide range of forms, as is done in many veterinary teaching hospitals, it is important to always remember to stamp each and every form. Refer to Figure 33-4 for an example of a client/patient information form.

The signalment of the patient is the first critical bit of information that helps the veterinarian in problem solving. Cancerous tumors, for example, are less likely to occur in puppies than in older dogs. Similarly congenital abnormalities, such as a cleft palate, are often first noticed in young animals, so it is rare to first diagnose them in older animals. Similarly there are certain conditions that are typically seen in large breeds of dogs and rarely seen in small breeds. Also, disorders may typically be seen in cats but not in dogs. In this way, the signalment immediately assists the veterinarian to hone in on certain disorders and rule out others.

HISTORY FORM

A comprehensive history includes both previous and recent history information. It is typically taken during each new-patient visit and during visits from those patients that have not been seen in several years. Some practices have two history forms: one in which the previous history information is recorded and the other for recent history information. Figure 33-5, *A* shows an example of a history form in which both the previous and recent history information is recorded together.

Previous history information includes the following:

1. Origin: animal's birth place and date
2. Preventive medicine program: immunizations, parasite control, dental care program, ear care program
3. Behavior: usual disposition and temperament, unusual behavioral events
4. Environment: kept in doors or out, presence of other pets in the home, level of exposure to non–family-owned pets, travel history
5. Known allergies and reactions: atopy, food, contact with substances, medications, blood transfusions

6. Reproduction: neutered, estrus cycles, when bred, number of litters
7. Previous conditions, trauma, or surgical operations
Recent history information includes
   1. Presenting complaint and circumstances
   2. Last normal
   3. Frequency of episodes
   4. Current medications
   5. Treatment efforts
   6. Comments and concerns of the owner
   7. Current diet
   8. Information from previous or referring veterinarian

PHYSICAL EXAMINATION FORM

The physical examination is one of the most important diagnostic procedures and, if performed carefully and systematically, can provide the clinician with the critical information that ultimately leads to a diagnosis. The physical examination form, therefore, is structured in such a way as to help the veterinarian and the veterinary technician to examine each anatomical system without overlooking anything. Notes are made directly on the form. "WLN," for example, may be written, which means "within normal limits," or "B & A" may be written, meaning "bright and alert." There is a wide variety of abbreviations that clinicians use when completing medical record forms. Refer to Figures 33-5, *B*, and 33-6 for examples of a physical examination form.

DATABASE

In the POVMR, the signalment, history, physical examination and diagnostic tests are collectively known as the *database*. The database forms the foundation of information on which veterinarians are able to make their diagnoses and therapeutic plans. Each veterinary hospital, however, may have its own variation on the standard database. Animals admitted for either a routine visit or a hospital stay may have, for example, a complete blood count, urinalysis, and fecal analysis. In this way, the database can vary depending on the needs of the patient. The tests done on the first visit will be considered the original database, and any subsequent visits should provide data for current problems.

In many emergency and critical care units the database is considered to include five or six important pieces of information that are key in treating the critical patient. These include the: pact cell volume, total solids, potassium, blood urea nitrogen, dextrose, and urinalysis. These data can be acquired quickly with a small amount of blood, a countertop centrifuge and analyzer, and dipsticks.

MASTER PROBLEM LIST

A defining part of the problem-oriented veterinary medical record is the problem list. The master problem list includes

Text continued on p. 1076

DATE _____

CASE NUMBER _____

COMPANION ANIMAL CLIENT/PATIENT INFORMATION FORM

Please provide the following information for our records: **PLEASE PRINT!**

OWNER INFORMATION

OWNER'S NAME	SOCIAL SECURITY NUMBER

STREET ADDRESS

CITY STATE	ZIP CODE	PARISH OR COUNTY

TELEPHONE NUMBER(S) (Area Code, if long distance) →	HOME	BUSINESS

DRIVER'S LICENSE NUMBER	PLACE OF EMPLOYMENT	HOW LONG?

ANIMAL INFORMATION

ANIMAL SPECIES (Dog, Cat, Other)	BREED

ANIMAL'S NAME	SEX	HAS ANIMAL BEEN SEXUALLY ALTERED? ☐ Yes ☐ No

COLOR	BIRTHDATE (Month/year, or approximate)	The undersigned owner or agent certifies that the herein described animal has a maximum value of approximately **$**

REFERRAL INFORMATION

WERE YOU REFERRED BY A VETERINARIAN? ☐ Yes ☐ No	IF YOU WERE REFERRED BY A VETERINARIAN, PLEASE COMPLETE THE FOLLOWING:

VETERINARIAN'S NAME	PHONE

STREET ADDRESS

CITY/STATE	ZIP CODE

You will be advised of estimated cost and anticipated procedures. Please feel free to discuss the proposed treatment and its cost with the veterinarian. A minimum deposit of 50% of the initial estimated charges will be required for hospitalization of an animal patient.

STATEMENT OF OWNERSHIP AND CONSENT: I am the owner of the above described animal, or have authorization from the owner to consent to its treatment.

I hereby authorize the performance of professionally accepted diagnostic, therapeutic, anesthetic, and surgical procedures necessary for its treatment.

I accept financial responsibility for these services.

I have read the above consent and understand why the above procedures may be necessary. I also have been told of the possible complications and alternatives to the listed procedures.

PAYMENT CHOICE: ☐ Cash   ☐ Check   ☐ Bank Card

SIGNATURE (Owner/Agent)	DATE

Figure 33-4 Client and patient information form.

VETERINARY HOSPITAL OF THE UNIVERSITY OF PENNSYLVANIA
3900 DELANCEY STREET
PHILADELPHIA, PA 19104

RABIES SUSPECT ? ___ YES ___ NO	CHANGES FROM LAST VISIT ___ NONE ___ AS NOTED
MANAGEMENT	**BEHAVIOR**
ORIGIN – GEOGRAPHIC LOCATION FROM WHOM – WHEN	USUAL DISPOSITION
	UNUSUAL BEHAVIOR PATTERN
STATES AND COUNTRIES KEPT IN	**ENVIRONMENT**
	OTHER ANIMALS
WHERE KEPT	WITH HEALTH PROBLEMS
ALLOWED TO RUN FREE?	
USUAL DIET	RELATED DISEASE (IN OWNER'S FAMILY)
PREVENTION	**ALLERGIES / REACTIONS**
	DIET
RABIES VACCINATION DATE GIVEN	
DATE DUE	MEDICATION / TREATMENT
COMBINATION VACC. DATE GIVEN	BLOOD COMPONENT THERAPY
_____ VACC. DATE GIVEN	X-MATCHED
HEARTWORM Seasonal Y N	**REPRODUCTIVE**
BRAND _____ Year 'round Y N	NEUTERED
FLEA/TICK Seasonal Y N	
BRAND _____ Year 'round Y N	LAST ESTRUS
	BRED
PREVIOUS CONDITIONS, PROBLEMS, OR OPERATIONS	(LIST, WITH DATE, IF KNOWN)

PRESENTING PROBLEM OR COMPLAINT   (INCLUDE TREATMENT BY OTHER VETERINARIANS)

HISTORY

B-1
FORM CONTROL NO.

A

Figure 33-5 **A,** Example of a comprehensive history form.

PHYSICAL EXAMINATION

Attitude at time of Exam (Circle one)
(Vicious, excited, alert, depressed,
comatose, other_____)
Nutritional state (Circle one)
(Obese, overweight, normal, underweight, cachectic)

Temp.	Pulse/min.	Resp./min

State of Hydration: good, fair, poor. (Circle one)   Weight (from scale)   kg.

SYSTEMATIC EXAMINATION (Use space below as needed)

Oro-Pharyngeal

Eyes

Ears

Respiratory

Cardiovascular

Gastrointestinal and Anus

Rectal

Uro-Genital

Integument

Lymph Nodes

Musculo-Skeletal

Nervous

Physical Exam Performed By:

(Student's signature)

PROBLEMS:
1.
2.
3.
4.

B

Figure 33-5—cont'd B, This physical examination form is printed on the back of the comprehensive history form shown in Figure 33-5, A.

TEACHING HOSPITAL AND CLINICS
School of Veterinary Medicine
Louisiana State University
Baton Rouge, Louisiana 70803

SMALL ANIMAL   NUMBER

Date: _6/20/06_

Temp _102.5_ °F   Attitude _BAR_

Fem. Pulse _100_   Charac. _normal_   Resp. _24_

Memb. Color _pink_   Cap. Refill Time _< 1.5 sec_

Hydration _normal_   Body Weight _70 #_

Color & Consistency of feces on Therm. _normal_

Body Condition — Underweight ☐   Overweight ☒   Normal ☐

NAME _____

CASE NO.
BERNARD DAVIS   66444
1087 TARA BLVD
BATON ROUGE, LA 70825   HOME _____

CAN LABCIES   BREED   SEX
BO BLK 11/30/96
ANIMAL'S NAME   DATE OF BIRTH

COLOR—IDENTIFYING MARKS

SYSTEM REVIEW

1. Integumentary	2. Otic	3. Ophthalmic	4. Musculoskeletal
☐ Normal	☐ Normal	☑ Normal	☑ Normal
☑ Abnormal	☑ Abnormal	☐ Abnormal	☐ Abnormal

5. Nervous	6. Cardiovascular	7. Respiratory	8. Digestive
☑ Normal	☑ Normal	☑ Normal	☑ Normal
☐ Abnormal	☐ Abnormal	☐ Abnormal	☐ Abnormal

9. Lymphatic	10. Reproductive	11. Urinary
☑ Normal	☑ Normal	☑ Normal
☐ Abnormal	☐ Abnormal	☐ Abnormal

DESCRIBE ABNORMAL:

2) Moderate otitis externa — erythema, waxy exudate, bilateral

1) multiple dermal, epidermal, and subcutaneous masses
— R lateral stifle, R cranial shoulder, L muzzle, L distal cranial antebrachium

EXAMINER _K. Ryan DVM_

PHYSICAL EXAMINATION   MEDICAL RECORDS   V-1

Figure 33-6 Another example of a physical examination form.

JONATHAN HART DVM
2441 TREASURE HILL BLVD
HOUSTON, TEXAS 70550

210 389 4726

BERNARD DAVIS   66444
1007 TARA BLVD
BATON ROUGE, LA 70825

CAN LAB F/S
BO BLK 11/30/96

IMMUNIZATION PREVENTATIVE RECORD

DATE	5/10/03	6/14/04								
RABIES	X	X								
DA2PL	X	X								
PARVO	X	X								
FVRCP										
FELV VACC.										
FELV/FIV										
FECAL	neg.	neg.								
HEARTWORM	neg.	neg.								

	PROBLEM LIST	DATE ENTERED	DATE RESOLVED
1.	Elective Ovariohysterectomy	8/10/95	8/10/95
2.	Malassezia-otitis externa	8/10/95	8/17/95
3.	Dental prophylaxis	11/3/98	11/3/98
4.	Gastroenteritis — small bowel diarrhea	3/15/99	3/18/99
5.	Uncomplicated UTI	2/3/05	2/16/05
6.	Recurrent UTI — E. Coli	3/14/05	3/28/05
7.	Recurrent UTI	6/10/05	6/20/05
8.	Right Renomegaly; Cystic kidney mass	6/20/05	
9.	Right unilateral nephrectomy	6/23/05	6/23/05
10.	Renal carcinoma	6/24/05	
11.	Lethargy, anorexia,	7/2/05	7/5/05
12.			
13.			

BREED=   SEX=

Figure 33-7 Immunization history record and master problem list.

the major medical disorders experienced by a patient during its lifetime. These medical problems are listed in chronological order, and a date is noted when and if they are resolved. In this way, the master problem list serves as a snapshot overview of the patient's medical history. At a glance, the clinician can determine what happened, when, and how long it lasted. Refer to Figure 33-7 for an example of a master problem list. A summary of the preventive medical history may accompany the master problem list, which includes the dates when immunizations were administered and the results of fecal analysis and feline leukemia and heartworm tests.

> **✎ TECHNICIAN NOTE**
>
> The working problem list helps the veterinarian to evaluate symptoms, think critically and arrive at a final diagnosis.

WORKING PROBLEM LIST

The working problem list (Figure 33-8 and Table 33-1) is often used in veterinary teaching hospitals and assists the clinician and student in working through problems that are relevant to the current hospital stay. For example, if the patient is hospitalized and is subsequently diagnosed with autoimmune hemolytic anemia, the working problem list may list symptomatic problems initially until the final diagnosis is made.

Compare the working problem list with the master problem list. Notice that the master problem list is essentially a list of final diagnoses rather than a list of symptoms. The working problem list helps the clinician to list clinical signs as they become apparent without offering a specific diagnosis. When a final diagnosis is reached, such as autoimmune hemolytic anemia in this case, the diagnosis can be added to the master problem list.

PROGRESS NOTES

The on-going management of veterinary patients is documented in the progress notes (Figure 33-9). Each time a patient visits the veterinary hospital, notes are made to summarize the visit. The date of the appointment, physical examination findings, and the reason for the visit are noted. If the animal is sick, problems are listed and a tentative diagnoses or list of differential diagnoses is generated. If diagnostic procedures are performed, the findings are entered and a definitive diagnosis may be noted together with therapeutic plans, the medication given, and the patient's prognosis. Communications with the client and any changes in therapy are also noted.

When the patient is hospitalized, progress notes are used to record the daily events. In many practices and in teaching hospitals, the patient is examined carefully at the beginning of each day. Therapeutic treatment and plans are evaluated

Table 33-1 WORKING PROBLEM LIST

Problem Number	Active Date	Problem
1	6/20/05	Depression/lethargy
2	6/20/05	Pale yellow mucous membrane
3	6/20/05	Mild tachycardia
4	6/21/05	Anemia
5	6/21/05	Icterus
6	6/22/05	Autoimmune hemolytic anemia

and adjusted according to the progress of the patient. This process is called a *morning SOAP*. SOAP is an acronym for subjective, objective, assessment, and plan. In teaching hospitals, the SOAPs are typically performed by the veterinary medical students and residents. In private practices, veterinary technicians often complete the first half (S and O) of the SOAP, while the latter half (A and P) may be completed by the veterinarian. The subjective portion of the SOAP refers to the way the patient appears from the point of view of the casual observer. The patient, for example, may be "standing, panting, and wagging its tail," or the patient may be "awake, but in left lateral recumbency." Vocalizations, body posture, attitude, and positions are all noted as "subjective."

> **✎ TECHNICIAN NOTE**
>
> *SOAP* stands for subjective, objective, assessment, and plan.

The objective portion of the SOAP includes physiological data such as temperature, pulse, and respiration. The examiner would also note any vomitus, urination, and defecation and would describe the color and consistency of these, if applicable. If the patient were on intravenous fluid therapy, a small sample of blood would be drawn and the pact cell volume, total solids, and results from the azo- and dextro-dipsticks would be recorded. Other easily accessible data such as sodium and potassium values might also be noted here. If the patient had surgery, notes regarding the surgical site, number of sutures present, and the level of swelling or drainage would also be made. If a urinary catheter and collection bag had been placed, urine output would be recorded.

Under the section assessment, the examiner would record the status of the patient. If the patient had undergone surgery, for example, the note might read "nonremarkable recovery postoperative" or "localized inflammatory response to suture material." An assessment for a medical case might read "polyuria and polydipsia noted with hyperglycemia. Diabetes mellitus likely."

Plan refers to the course of action that will be taken that day. Perhaps the patient will be discharged and given

VETERINARY TEACHING HOSPITAL
LOUISIANA STATE UNIVERSITY

WORKING PROBLEM LIST

BERNARD DAVIS   66444
1087 TARA BLVD
BATON ROUGE LA 70825

CAN LAB F/S
BO BLK 11/30/96

PROBLEM NUMBER	ACTIVE DATE	PROBLEM	DATE RESOLVED
①	6/20/05	Recurrent lower urinary tract signs (stranguria, pollakiuria)	6/24/05
②	6/20/05	Polyuria/polydipsia	
③	6/20/05	Right renomegaly; Cystic kidney mass	6/24/05
④	6/24/05	Renal carcinoma	

MEDICAL RECORD

Figure 33-8 Working problem list.

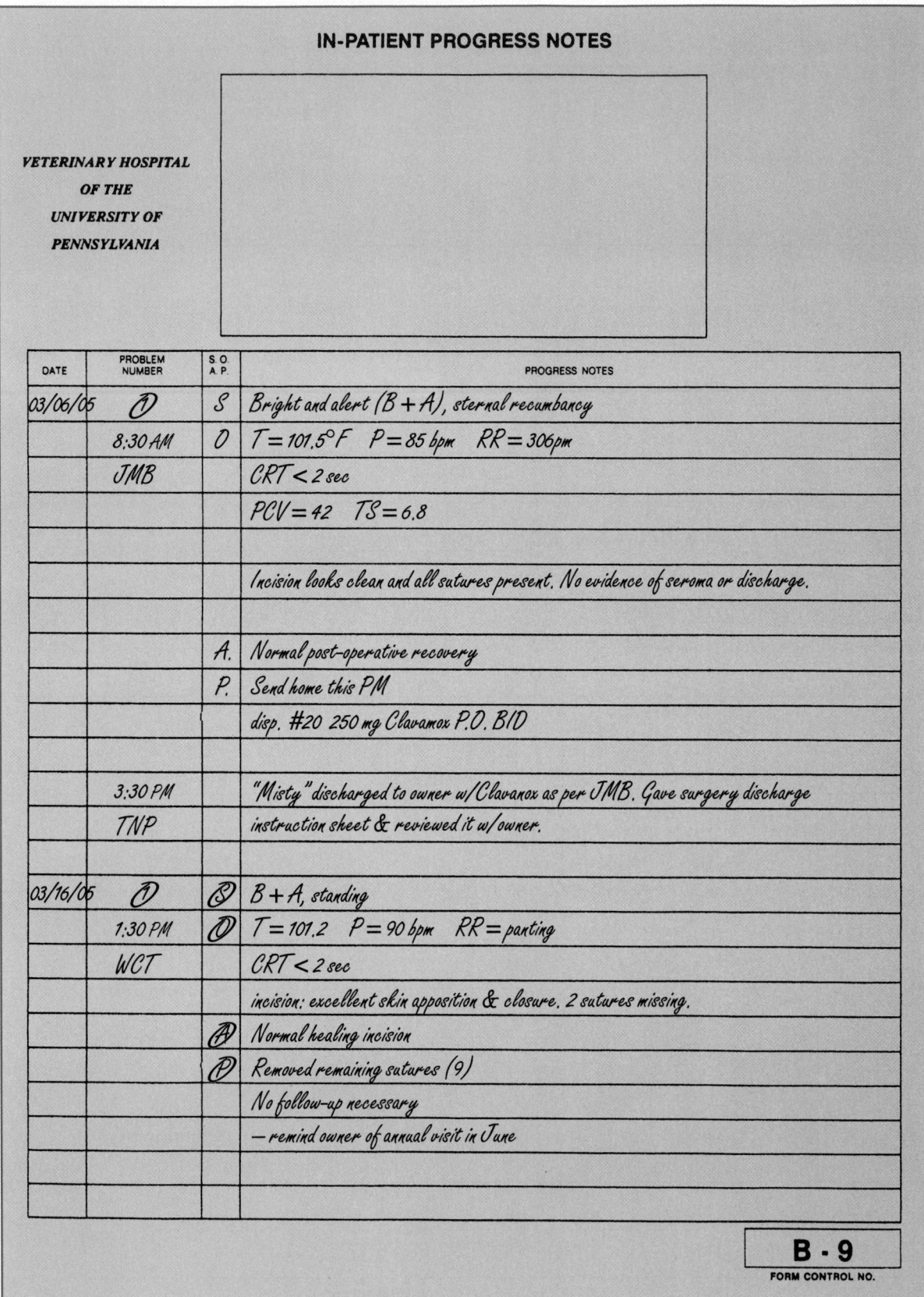

IN-PATIENT PROGRESS NOTES

VETERINARY HOSPITAL
OF THE
UNIVERSITY OF
PENNSYLVANIA

DATE	PROBLEM NUMBER	S.O. A.P.	PROGRESS NOTES
03/06/05	①	S	Bright and alert (B + A), sternal recumbancy
8:30 AM		O	T = 101.5°F P = 85 bpm RR = 30 6pm
JMB			CRT < 2 sec
			PCV = 42 TS = 6.8
			Incision looks clean and all sutures present. No evidence of seroma or discharge.
		A.	Normal post-operative recovery
		P.	Send home this PM
			disp. #20 250 mg Clavamox P.O. BID
3:30 PM			"Misty" discharged to owner w/Clavamox as per JMB. Gave surgery discharge
TNP			instruction sheet & reviewed it w/owner.
03/16/05	①	S	B + A, standing
1:30 PM		O	T = 101.2 P = 90 bpm RR = panting
WCT			CRT < 2 sec
			incision: excellent skin apposition & closure. 2 sutures missing.
		A	Normal healing incision
		P	Removed remaining sutures (9)
			No follow-up necessary
			— remind owner of annual visit in June

B - 9
FORM CONTROL NO.

Figure 33-9 Inpatient progress notes.

take-home medication, or perhaps the patient will undergo more diagnostic testing and observation. The medication to be given, procedures, and treatment plans to be performed are all described in this portion of the SOAP.

In teaching hospitals, an assessment and plan are sometimes written for each of the problems in the working problem list separately. Because this approach can lead to a lot of paperwork, an alternate method is to write an assessment and plan for the patient as a whole. Often the conditions and special circumstances of the case determines which approach is taken.

Any incoming information from a referring veterinarian or an animal's owner would also be placed in the progress notes section in chronologic order. Communication with the owner either in person, by telephone, or by E-mail is recorded in the progress notes in chronological order.

> ### 🖉 TECHNICIAN NOTE
> Be sure to initial the entries you make in the medical record. In a court of law, handwriting alone may be shown to be inadequate in identifying the author.

WARD TREATMENT SHEETS AND CAGE CARDS

Carrying out the treatments of hospitalized patients can be complicated, particularly in busy practices with heavy caseloads and in practices that treat emergency and critical care patients. To assist the veterinary health care team in carrying out the prescribed treatments efficiently, a treatment grid may be used. The grid may be part of a letter-size, ward treatment form that is kept in the patient's file (Figure 33-10), or it may be stamped on a card that is placed on the cage of the patient. The grid lists the treatments to be given and specifies the times throughout the day when each of the treatments should be completed. Specific doses, methods of administration, and cautionary notes should be noted. In most practices, the medications and supplies needed to complete the treatments are kept near the patient for convenience. Some practices store a patient's medications and treatment supplies in bins on a table or shelf along with the patient's medical record (Figure 33-11, *A*). Other practices prefer to use baskets that can be suspended from the patient's cage together with the ward treatment sheet (Figure 33-11, *B*). In either case, it is important to label the medications and supplies clearly with the patient's name, signalment, and owner information.

Cage cards are used to identify the patient and the reason for the hospitalization. The owner and patient information is stamped on the card. In some practices that do not use separate ward treatment sheets, the treatment grid is also stamped on the cage card and lists the procedures to be performed. In some specialty practices, the color of the card may be used to indicate the hospital division that is treating the patient. A red card, for example, might indicate surgery, while a blue card might indicate internal medicine or cardiology.

PERTINENT FORMS

Depending upon the size and caseload of the veterinary practice, there may be separate forms for different hospital departments, specialists, or diagnostic procedures. Anesthesia, surgery, recovery, and pain management forms, for example, may all be pertinent to a patient that has undergone a surgical procedure (Figures 33-12 to 33-14). Similarly, the results of diagnostic procedures, such as radiography and endoscopy, and laboratory tests may all be found in the medical record of an animal that presented with an esophageal foreign body (Figures 33-15 to 33-17).

LABORATORY DIAGNOSTIC SUMMARY AND FLOW SHEET

The laboratory diagnostic flow sheet is a compilation of laboratory data collected from an individual animal. It can be used for outpatients or inpatients. It shows at a glance the different laboratory values for the tests that have been performed on the patient. Specific values can be compared on the different dates for blood counts, chemistry panels, blood gases, urinalyses, and coagulation rates (Figure 33-18). This sheet is of particular value when evaluating internal medicine cases such as animals with diabetes, anemia, chronic renal failure, hepatic failure, Addison disease, and Cushing disease. Two spaces at the bottom of the left column are reserved for additional laboratory data that are not already listed in the grid.

CONSULTANTS

Teaching and referral hospitals are often divided into departments. Specialties such as behavior, dermatology, medicine, neurology, nutrition, oncology, ophthalmology, orthopedics, and surgery are examples of the departments that can make up a large teaching and referral center. As cases are worked up, specialists may be consulted to address specific problems that the patient is experiencing. Therefore a consultation form would be employed, and the consulting veterinarian's findings, diagnosis, and recommendations would be recorded. Refer to Figure 33-19. A copy of the consultation form is kept in the patient's record.

CASE SUMMARY AND DISCHARGE INSTRUCTIONS

When the patient is ready to be discharged, a summary of the case is written and discharge instructions are prescribed by the clinician. In some practices, the summary and home instructions are included on the same form. A copy of the form is given to the owner, and the veterinarian or veterinary technician reviews it with the owner before the animal leaves

Ward Treatment Sheet

ADDRESSOGRAPH:

Marjory Wyeth
431 Chadds Ford Drive
Chalfont, PA 18329
(610) 523-1896
"Misty" MC DSH
dob: 3-10-03

PROBLEM LIST

— weight loss

— anorexia

— vomition

— azotemia

Treatment Orders: Date: _9/4/06_ Appetite _poor_ Weight: _3.5_ kg.

22g. intracath. placed Ⓡ femoral vein. Continue maintenance fluids as below. Please monitor fluid input/urine output carefully. Note evidence of vomition/defication/eating. Call me if there is a change in status.

_____
Cindy Crown
(Student's Signature)

_____
David Mills, VMD
(Clinician's Signature)
cell (215) 943-2360

Treatments:	8	9	10	11	N	1	2	3	4	5	6	7	8	9	10	11	M	1	2	3	4	5	6	7	8
① Hep. cath	X						X						X					X							X
② Lact ringers IV, 10 ml/no. 3 rate/line	X		X			X			X		X		X		X			X		X					X
③ TPR/UO	X						X						X					X							X
④ PCV/TS/Azo/Dex	X						X						X					X							X

VASCULAR ACCESS

TIME	T	P	R	TIME	PCV	TS	AZO	DEX	UOP	Cath/Site	Comments
8 AM	100.2	150	33	8:15	53	7.5	30	100	3cc	Ⓡ femoral intracath.	

B - 8

FORM CONTROL NO.

Figure 33-10 Ward treatment sheet.

PROGRESS REPORT 9/3/04 10 AM	SIGNATURE
S) depressed & lethargic	D Mills
lateral recumbancy	
O) T = 99.2 P = 140 RR = 23	
CRT = 3-4 sec., dry, tacky mm.	
PCV = 30 TS = 5.5 AZO = 20 Dex. 95	
U/O: none pulses: thready, weak	
A) chronic renal failure w/anemia & hypothermia, CV shut down, condition grave	
P) continue fluids & meds as prescribed	
order repeat CBC/CS	

B - 8

Figure 33-10—cont'd

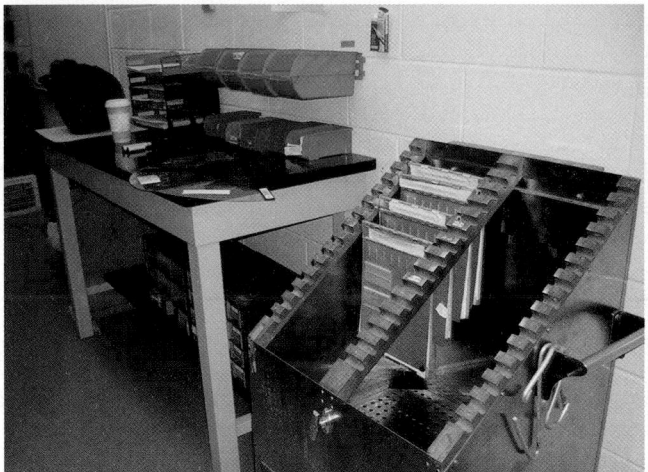
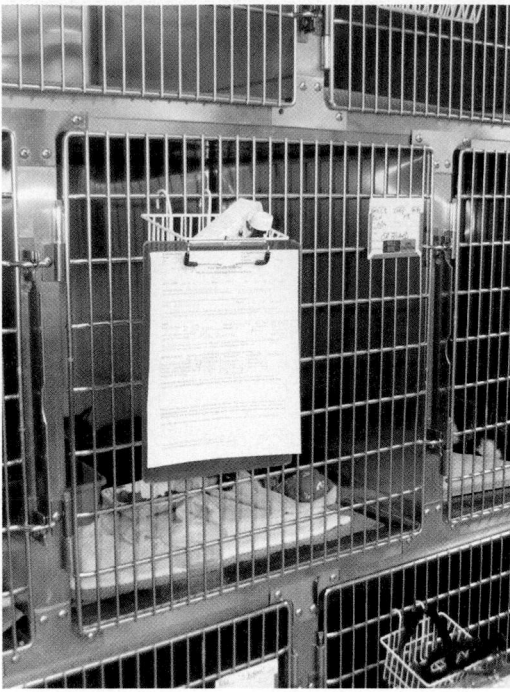

A   **B**

Figure 33-11   A, Some practices use individual bins to store the medications and supplies of each patient. These are kept near the medical record and are labeled with the patient's name. Notice that records kept on the wards are stored in protective metal holders. The record is removed from the holder before it is filed. **B,** Some practices store patient medications in wire baskets that can be attached directly to the door of the patient's cage. Medical records can also be attached to the cage as well. Both the record and the medications must be labeled clearly.

the hospital. In this way, the owner has a written account of the pet's diagnosis and treatment, which can be referred to frequently. Also, the discharge instructions are written out clearly and then reviewed directly with the owner (Figure 33-20). Often the clinician's name and contact information are included on the form so that the owner can call if questions or problems arise. If the animal was hospitalized at a specialty and referral center, the veterinarian often writes a formal letter to the referring veterinarian summarizing the case. In some veterinary practices, a copy of the case summary and discharge instructions form is mailed to the referring veterinarian in lieu of a formal letter.

Several days after a patient is discharged, the veterinarian often completes a follow-up call to the owner. This enables the clinician to assess the patient's progress at home and gives the owner an opportunity to ask questions. Pet owners are often grateful and appreciative of the special care that a follow-up call represents.

CONSENT AND AUTHORIZATION FORMS

Consent and authorization forms document in writing an understanding between the veterinary practice and the pet owner. The forms outline the specific conditions, risks of the procedure, and responsibilities of the two parties. In keeping with the doctrine of informed consent, completed authorization forms provide veterinary practices with legal evidence that the owner was informed of important information and that the owner agreed to pursue a particular course of action based on the circumstances and information given to them.

In many practices, consent forms are generated in those areas where there is the greatest potential for bad feelings due to poor communication. Obtaining authorizations to perform surgery, necropsy, and euthanasia are a few examples of situations where *written* owner permission, as well as verbal communication, is critical. During emergencies, for example, owners can be particularly emotional and may have difficulty making clear decisions. Owners who decide to euthanize their seriously injured pet may regret their decision later. They may blame the veterinary staff for feeling "pressured into it" or feel that they were not given all of the necessary information needed to make a sound choice. Authorization forms, such as the one in Figure 33-21, verifies the identity of the owner and frees the practice of liability in performing euthanasia. Signed consent forms are part of the medical record and should be stored and filed with the medical records.

A common source of consternation in veterinary practices is miscommunication regarding the cost of services. Many

Text continued on p. 1097

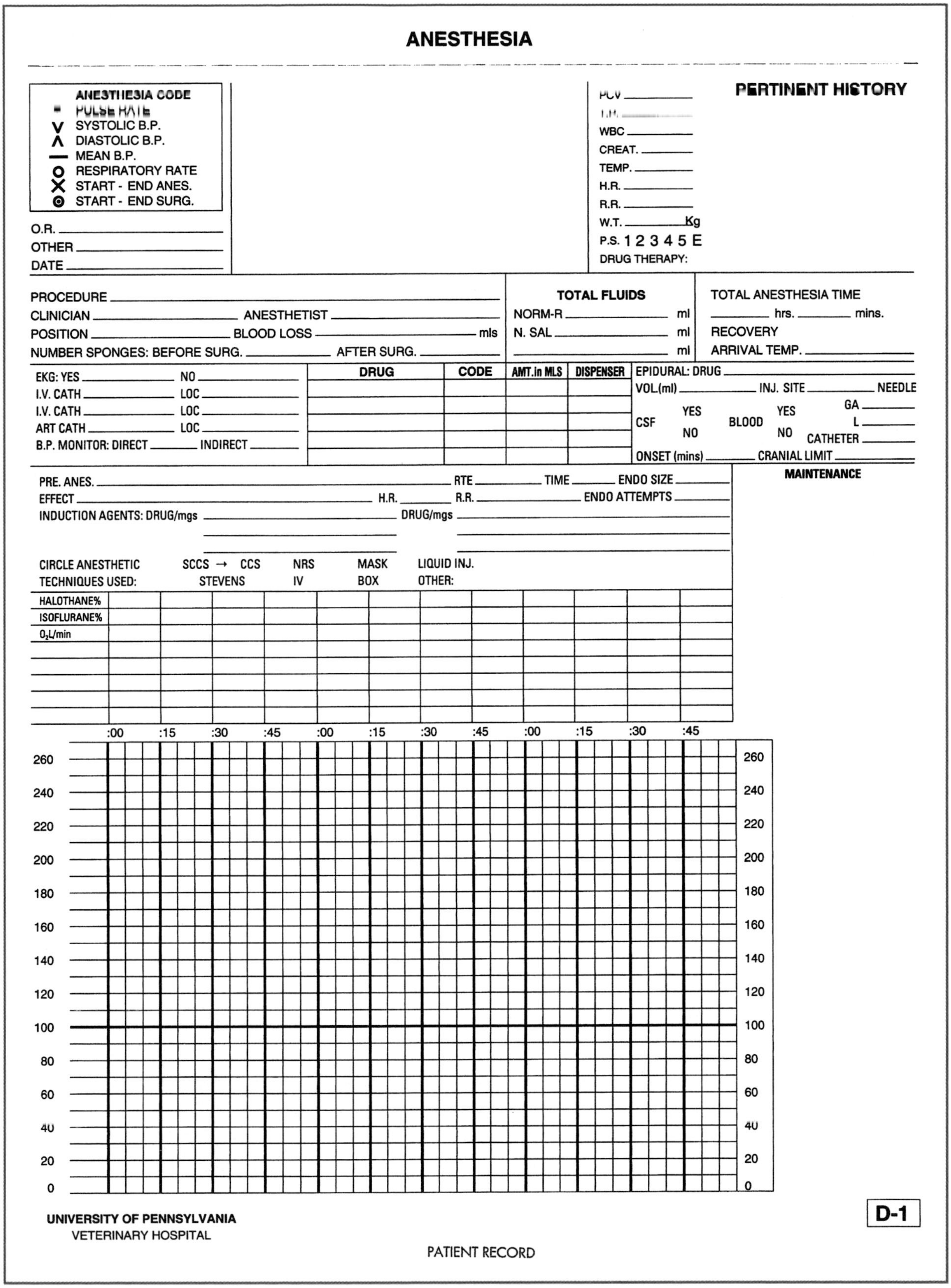

ANESTHESIA

ANESTHESIA CODE
- ▪ PULSE RATE
- V SYSTOLIC B.P.
- Λ DIASTOLIC B.P.
- — MEAN B.P.
- O RESPIRATORY RATE
- X START - END ANES.
- ⊙ START - END SURG.

O.R. ______
OTHER ______
DATE ______

PCV ______
T.P. ______
WBC ______
CREAT. ______
TEMP. ______
H.R. ______
R.R. ______
W.T. ______ Kg
P.S. 1 2 3 4 5 E
DRUG THERAPY:

PERTINENT HISTORY

PROCEDURE ______
CLINICIAN ______ ANESTHETIST ______
POSITION ______ BLOOD LOSS ______ mls
NUMBER SPONGES: BEFORE SURG. ______ AFTER SURG. ______

TOTAL FLUIDS
NORM-R ______ ml
N. SAL ______ ml
______ ml

TOTAL ANESTHESIA TIME
______ hrs. ______ mins.
RECOVERY
ARRIVAL TEMP. ______

EKG: YES ______ NO ______
I.V. CATH ______ LOC ______
I.V. CATH ______ LOC ______
ART CATH ______ LOC ______
B.P. MONITOR: DIRECT ______ INDIRECT ______

DRUG	CODE	AMT. in MLS	DISPENSER

EPIDURAL: DRUG ______
VOL.(ml) ______ INJ. SITE ______ NEEDLE
CSF YES / NO BLOOD YES / NO GA ______ L ______ CATHETER ______
ONSET (mins) ______ CRANIAL LIMIT ______

PRE. ANES. ______ RTE ______ TIME ______ ENDO SIZE ______
EFFECT ______ H.R. ______ R.R. ______ ENDO ATTEMPTS ______
INDUCTION AGENTS: DRUG/mgs ______ DRUG/mgs ______

MAINTENANCE

CIRCLE ANESTHETIC TECHNIQUES USED: SCCS → CCS STEVENS NRS IV MASK BOX LIQUID INJ. OTHER:

HALOTHANE%
ISOFLURANE%
O_2L/min

:00 :15 :30 :45 :00 :15 :30 :45 :00 :15 :30 :45

260 240 220 200 180 160 140 120 100 80 60 40 20 0

D-1

UNIVERSITY OF PENNSYLVANIA
VETERINARY HOSPITAL

PATIENT RECORD

Figure 33-12 Anesthesia record.

Continued

ANESTHESIA

DATE _____

PROCEDURE _____

CLINICIAN _____ ANESTHETIST _____

ANESTHESIA CHARGES

(Includes all Anesthesia Drugs,
1 500 ml. Fluid, 1 Administration Set, 1 Catheter)

TOTAL TIME   CHARGES

Anesthesia: _____ hrs. _____ mins. _____

Radiology: _____ hrs. _____ mins. _____

ADDITIONAL ANESTHESIA CHARGES: QUANTITY   CHARGES

EXTRA FLUIDS _____

_____

STERILE TUBE: _____

DATA BASE: _____

DRUGS _____

_____

_____

_____

OTHER _____

_____

_____

ISTAT _____

ARREST CHARGE _____

EMERGENCY FEE _____

               TOTAL ANESTHESIA _____ $ _____

SURGERY CHARGES:

PROFESSIONAL SERVICE FEE _____

OPERATING ROOM CHARGE _____

DISPOSABLE DRAPES _____

EMERGENCY FEE _____

OTHER _____

INITIAL _____

               TOTAL _____ $ _____

CHARGE SHEET

Figure 33-12—cont'd

ANESTHESIA

DATE ___ _____

PROCEDURE _____

CLINICIAN _____ ANESTHETIST _____

(TIME) (AM/PM)
ANESTHESIA STARTED _____

SURGERY STARTED (INCISION) _____

SURGERY FINISHED _____ / ANESTHESIA FINISHED _____

COMPLICATIONS: ARRESTED   YES _____   NO _____

RESUSCITATED   YES _____   NO _____
(Successfully)
EUTHANIZED   YES _____   NO _____

CALCULATIONS: WEIGHT x DOSE = AMOUNT;   AMOUNT ÷ CONCENTRATION = VOLUME   (pre-op, induction, oxygen, fluids)

Figure 33-12—cont'd

DATE _____

**TEACHING HOSPITAL AND CLINICS
SCHOOL OF VETERINARY MEDICINE**

SURGERY/PROCEDURE: _____

_____

CLINICIAN _____

ANESTHESIA STUDENT _____

STUDENT _____

SMALL ANIMAL RECOVERY ROOM

BODY WT. _____

❑ **WILL BITE**   ❑ **WILL NOT BITE**

POST OPERATIVE ANALGESIA

Drug	Time	Amount Drug mg	Route	Initials

INSTRUCTIONS: Patient vital signs should be monitored and recorded every 30 minutes until T° = 99.0° F or more and/or patient is ambulatory. IV catheters should remain in place until patient is completely recovered and is ready to return to the wards.

PATIENT VITAL SIGNS

Time	Temp	Pulse Rate	Resp. Rate	MM Color	Treatments/ Medications/Observations	Initials

SPECIAL INSTRUCTIONS: _____

_____

PRE-OPERATIVE ANESTHETICS: _____

ANESTHETICS/INTRA-OP MEDS: _____

RETURN TO WARDS? _____ **WARD/CAGE NO.** _____ **REMOVE CATHETER POST-RECOVERY?** _____

Figure 33-13 Postoperative recovery record.

Veterinary Hospital of University of Pennsylvania
PAIN MEDICATION FORM

Patient _____ Clinician _____

Case # _____ Breed _____ Weight _____ kg

Pertinent Information: _____

Date	Drugs Ordered	Route	How Often	Dose mg/kg	Total Amount	Comments	Init.

Date	Time	Drug Given	Amount	Route	Pre √List	Post √List	Effective? Comments:	Init.

	pre	post	pre	post	pre	post	pre	post	pre	post	pre	post	pre	post	pre	post
TIME																
Heart Rate																
Resp. Rate																
Temperature																
Blood Pressure																
Vocalization																
Restlessness/Agitation																
Resents Handling Area																
Depression/Inactivity																
Insomnia/Reluctant to Lie Down																
Other																
Other																
Other																

Figure 33-14 Pain medication form.

		RADIOGRAPHS	DATE:

IN	OUT		RADIOLOGY
			CLINICIAN
CLINICIAN:			MEDICAL INFORMATION
			PENN HIP
SERVICE:			TECH	# RADS

PRELMINARY REPORT: DATE: _____   RAD: _____

RAD. FINDINGS:

DIAGNOSIS:

FINAL REPORT: DATE: _____   RAD: _____

RAD. FINDINGS:

DIAGNOSIS:

UNIVERSITY OF PENNSYLVANIA
VETERINARY HOSPITAL

RADIOLOGY

Figure 33-15 Radiology record.

ABDOMINAL RADIOGRAPHS

DATE:

IN	OUT

CLINICIAN:

SERVICE:

RADIOLOGY
CLINICIAN
MEDICAL INFORMATION

TECH	# RADS

LEFT LATERAL

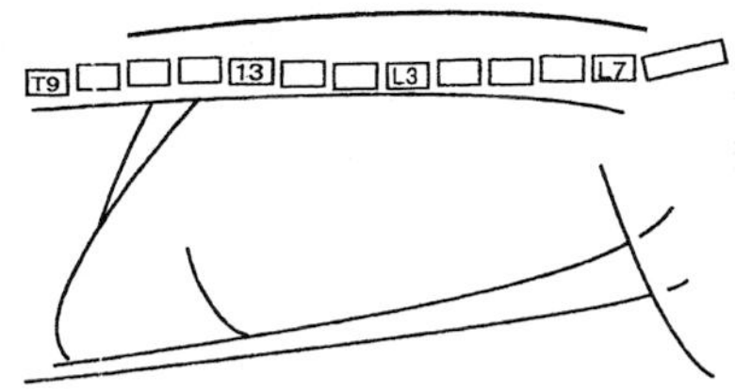

T9 13 L3 L7

RIGHT LATERAL

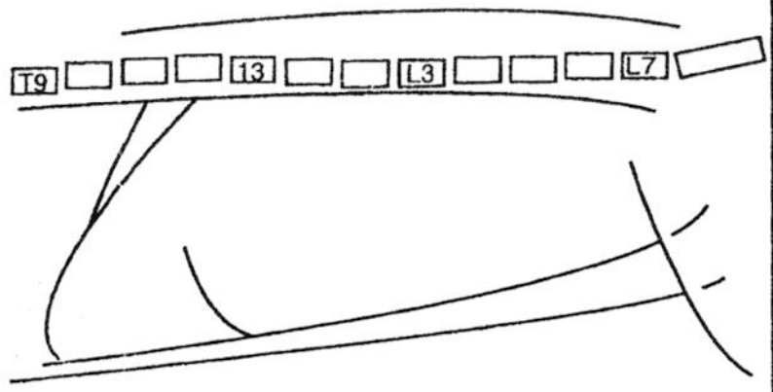

T9 13 L3 L7

LT / RT LATERAL

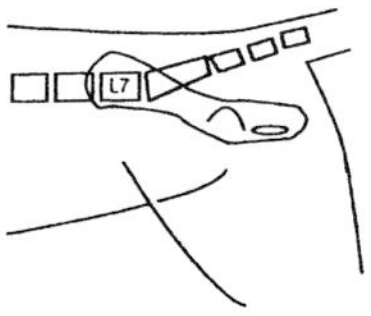

L7

VD / DV

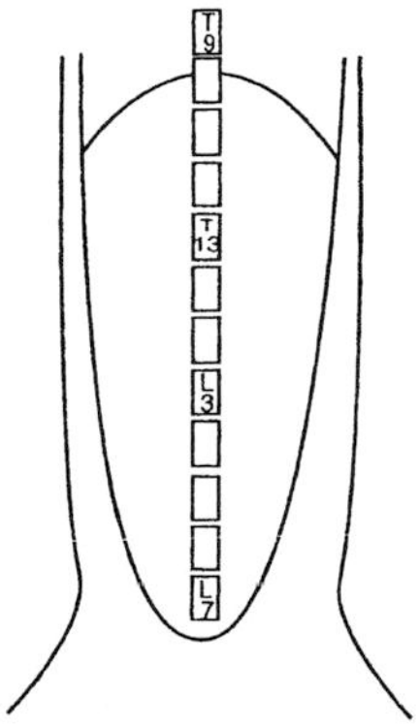

T9
T13
L3
L7

PRELIMINARY REPORT: DATE: _____ RAD: _____

RAD. FINDINGS:

DIAGNOSIS:

FINAL REPORT: DATE: _____ RAD: _____

RAD. FINDINGS:

DIAGNOSIS:

UNIVERSITY OF PENNSYLVANIA
VETERINARY HOSPITAL

RADIOLOGY

Figure 33-15—cont'd

AMHERST BUSINESS SOLUTIONS, INC.
(610) 584-1633
Fax (610) 277-5418

ENDOSCOPY

STUDENT _____

DOCTOR _____

DATE _____

TENTATIVE DIAGNOSIS

PROCEDURE

☐ 1305   Upper Gastrointestinal Endoscopy   _____ Video
☐ 1306   Lower Gastrointestinal Endoscopy   _____ Biopsy
☐ 1307   Rigid Proctoscopy
☐ 1308   Endoscopic Tube Gastrostomy
☐ 1309   Tracheobronchoscopy   _____ Urease
☐ 1310   Rhinoscopy
☐ 1311   Laparoscopy   _____ Culture
☐ 1312   Upper and Lower G.I. Endoscopy
☐ 1313   Emergency Foreign Body Retrieval   _____ Cytology
☐ 1314   Outpatient Endoscopy Clinic
☐ 1315   Cystoscopy
☐ 1316   Otoscopy

Description of Endoscopy

**VETERINARY HOSPITAL OF THE
UNIVERSITY OF PENNSYLVANIA**

Figure 33-16 Endoscopy record.

CLINICAL PATHOLOGY

VHUP

☐ ICU
☐ ES
☐ PRE-OP

DATE

TENTATIVE DIAGNOSIS

IN	STUDENT
OUT	DOCTOR

TIME OF SAMPLE COLLECTION

_____ AM/PM

HEMATOLOGY

☐ CBC
☐ Inst. counts only (ICO)
☐ Chemo. ICO

☐ PLT-inst. _____ $10^3/\mu l$
☐ PLT-manual _____ $10^3/\mu l$
☐ TP _____ gm/dl
☐ PCV _____ %
☐ WBC _____ $10^3/\mu l$
☐ Retic _____ %
    PCV _____ %
    corrected _____ %
    RBC _____ $10^6/\mu l$
    absolute _____ $10^3/\mu l$

☐ Retic with CBC _____ %
    corrected _____ %
    absolute _____ $10^3/\mu l$

☐ Extra blood smears (3)

☐ Smear Evaluation.

Technician _____

DIFFERENTIAL | **RELATIVE** | **ABSOLUTES** | **RBC MORPHOLOGY**

DIFFERENTIAL	RELATIVE	ABSOLUTES	RBC MORPHOLOGY
Neutrophils	____ %	____ $/\mu L$	Anisocytosis _____
Bands	____ %	____ $/\mu L$	Microcytosis _____
Lymphocytes	____ %	____ $/\mu L$	Macrocytosis _____
Monocytes	____ %	____ $/\mu L$	Polychromasia _____
Eosinophils	____ %	____ $/\mu L$	Hypochromasia _____
Basophils	____ %	____ $/\mu L$	Spherocytosis _____
Meta.	____ %	____ $/\mu L$	Poikilocytosis _____
Myelo.	____ %	____ $/\mu L$	Types
Promyelo.	____ %	____ $/\mu L$	
Unclassed	____ %	____ $/\mu L$	

nRBC _____ /100 WBC
corrected WBC count _____ $/\mu l$
Neutrophil toxic change
  + __ ++ __ +++ __ ++++ __

PLATELETS
Adequate ☐
Decreased ☐
Increased ☐

COMMENTS:

BLOOD CHEMISTRY
*requires **red top tube** 3 ml. min. req.*

Standard Profile ☐
Liver Profile ☐
Electrolyte Profile ☐
Pancreatic Profile ☐
Renal Profile ☐

INDIVIDUAL TEST

Glucose ☐ ____	ALT ☐ ____
BUN ☐ ____	AST ☐ ____
Creatinine ☐ ____	LDH ☐ ____
Phos. ☐ ____	SAP ☐ ____
Ca ☐ ____	GGT ☐ ____
Mg ☐ ____	Bili. T ☐ ____
Na ☐ ____	BILI. D ☐ ____
K ☐ ____	Chol. ☐ ____
Cl ☐ ____	Trig. ☐ ____
CO_2 enz ☐ ____	Lipase ☐ ____
Protein ☐ ____	Amylase ☐ ____
Albumin ☐ ____	CK ☐ ____

ROUTINE URINALYSIS

☐ COLLECTION METHOD:

COAGULATION SCREEN
*requires sodium citrate **blue top tube***

COMPLETE (PT, PTT, FDP, PLAT,
  RBC FRAGMENTS): ☐
INDIVIDUAL:

	CTRL	PAT.
PT		
PTT		

FDP ☐
D-DIMER ☐

BLOOD TYPE
*requires **purple top tube***

☐ FELINE _____
☐ CANINE _____

CROSS MATCH
*requires **purple top tube** or blood bag seg.*

DONOR	MAJOR	MINOR
_____	_____	_____
_____	_____	_____
_____	_____	_____

AMMONIAS
*requires **green top tube***

NH_3 RESTING ☐ ____
NH_3 TOL. (POST) ☐ ____

CLINICAL PATHOLOGY (6/96)

UNIVERSITY OF PENNSYLVANIA

VETERINARY HOSPITAL

MEDICAL RECORDS

C - 1
FORM CONTROL NO.

Figure 33-17 Clinical pathology report.

Hospital Name _____

Address _____

City _____ State _____ Zip Code _____

SIGNALMENT

LABORATORY DIAGNOSTICS FLOW SHEET

CHEMISTRY PANEL	DATES				HEMOGRAM	DATES			
GLUCOSE mg/dL					WBC ($\times 10^3$)/μL				
AST U/L					RBC ($\times 10^6$)/μL				
ALT U/L					HGB g/dL				
ALP U/L					HCT %				
CK U/L					MCV fl				
T. BILIRUBIN mg/dL					MCH pg				
T. PROTEIN g/dL					MCHC g/dL				
ALBUMIN g/dL					PLT ($\times 10^3$)/μL				
GLOBULIN mg/dL					PCV/TS %				
CHOLESTEROL mg/dL					SEGS ($\times 10^3$)/μL				
UREA NITROGEN mg/dL					BANDS ($\times 10^3$)/μL				
CREATININE mg/dL					LYMPHS ($\times 10^3$)/μL				
CALCIUM mg/dL					MONO ($\times 10^3$)/μL				
PHOSPHORUS mg/dL					EOS ($\times 10^3$)/μL				
SODIUM mmol/L					BASOS ($\times 10^3$)/μL				
POTASSIUM mmol/L					nRBC				
CHLORIDE mmol/L					RETIC %				
TCO$_2$ mmol/L					**URINALYSIS**				
ANION GAP mmol/L					COLOR				
BLOOD GAS					TURBIDITY				
pH					SPECIFIC GRAVITY				
PCO$_2$ mm Hg					pH				
PO$_2$ mm Hg					PROTEIN mg/dL				
HCO$_3$ mmol/L					GLUCOSE mg/dL				
TCO$_2$ mmol/L					KETONES				
BASE EXCESS					BILIRUBIN				
COAGULATION					HEMOGLOBIN				
ACT sec					VOLUME				
PT sec PATIENT/CONTROL					CASTS (+/–)				
PTT sec PATIENT/CONTROL					WBC				
FDP μg/mL					RBC				
BMBT (Sec)					EPITH CELLS (+/–)				
					CRYSTALS (+/–)				
					BACTERIA (+/–)				

Figure 33-18 Laboratory flow sheet with reference ranges.

CLINICAL PATHOLOGY REFERENCE RANGES

	units	CANINE	FELINE	EQUINE	BOVINE
Total leukocytes	($\times 10^3/\mu L$)	6-17	5.5-19.5	5.5-12.5	4-12
Neutrophils	($\times 10^3/\mu L$)	3-11.5	2.5-12.5	2.7-6.7	0.6-4
Bands	($\times 10^3/\mu L$)	0-0.3	0-0.3	0-0.1	0-0.1
Eosinophils	($\times 10^3/\mu L$)	0.1-1.2	0-1.5	0-0.9	0-2.4
Basophils	($\times 10^3/\mu L$)	rare	rare	0-0.2	0-0.2
Monocytes	($\times 10^3/\mu L$)	0.1-1.4	0-0.8	0-0.8	0-0.8
Lymphocytes	($\times 10^3/\mu L$)	1-4.8	1.5-7	1.5-5.5	2.5-7.5
Erythrocytes	($\times 10^6/\mu L$)	5-8.5	5-10	6.5-12.5	5-10
Hemoglobin	(g/dL)	12-18	9-16	11-19	8-15
Hematocrit	(%)	35-55	28-45	32-52	24-46
MCV	(fl)	60-77	39-55	34-58	40-60
MCH	(pg)	21-27	13-17	10-18	11-18
MCHC	(g/dL)	32-36	30-36	30-35	30-36
Platelets	($\times 10^3/\mu L$)	200-700	200-700	100-600	100-800
Plasma protein	(g/dL)	6-7.8	6-7.5	5.2-7.8	6-8
Fibrinogen (HPP)	(mg/dL)	–	–	100-500	100-700
Glucose	(mg/dL)	75-115	85-115	70-100	60-100
ALT	(IU/L)	<100	<90	–	–
AST	(IU/L)	<60	<40	<350	<150
CK	(IU/L)	<285	<300	<300	<300
ALP	(IU/L)	<135	<45	<300	<140
GGT	(IU/L)	–	–	<45	<45
T. Bilirubin	(mg/dL)	<0.4	<0.2	<2.0	<0.5
T. Protein	(g/dL)	5.7-7.4	6.0-8.1	6.0-8.0	6.4-8.2
Globulins	(g/dL)	2.1-4.1	2.8-4.9	2.0-4.4	2.7-4.5
Albumin	(g/dL)	2.9-4.0	2.9-3.5	3.0-4.1	3.1-4.0
BUN	(mg/dL)	6-22	15-30	14-27	10-24
Creatinine	(mg/dL)	0.4-1.5	0.6-2.2	1.2-2.5	0.7-1.8
Calcium	(mg/dL)	8.6-11.2	8.9-11.0	10-13	8.5-11.1
Phosphorus	(mg/dL)	2.5-5.5	3.1-5.8	1.9-4.7	4.0-7.2
Cholesterol	(mg/dL)	130-240	90-160	–	–
Magnesium	(mmol/L)	–	–	0.60-0.95	0.70-1.10
Amylase	(IU/L)	<900	<900	<20	–
Lipase	(IU/L)	<600	<400	<20	<50
Bile acids, fasting	(μmol/L)	<5	<2	–	–
Bile acids, post	(μmol/L)	<20	<20	–	–
Ammonia, fasting	(μmol/L)	<32	–	<55	–
SDH	(IU/L)	–	–	<7	<15
Sodium	(mmol/L)	140-155	140-155	130-145	135-150
Potassium	(mmol/L)	3.5-5.5	3.0-5.5	3.0-5.0	3.5-5.0
Chloride	(mmol/L)	105-120	110-125	95-110	95-110
Total CO_2	(mmol/L)	20-28	20-28	24-30	21-31
Anion gap	(mmol/L)	8-20	8-20	6-15	6-15
pH		7.31-7.50	7.24-7.40	7.30-7.43	7.35-7.50
PCO_2	(mm Hg)	29-42	29-42	36-50	35-44
HCO_3	(mmol/L)	17-24	17-24	21-30	20-30
TCO_2	(mmol/L)	18-25	18-25	22-31	21-31

Figure 33-18—cont'd

CONSULTATIONS

Date: _____

_____
IN/OUT
_____

Consultation Requested by

_____

Dr. / Service to be Consulted

_____

Location of Animal

		Usual Fee	Other Fee
Animal Behavior	1101 ☐		
Dermatology	1102 ☐		
Medicine	1103 ☐		
Neurology	1104 ☐		
Nutrition	1105 ☐	_____
Oncology	1106 ☐	1110
Ophthalmology	1107 ☐	
Orthopedics	1108 ☐	
Surgery	1109 ☐	

For completion by Attending Clinician	Consultation for: ☐ Diagnosis Only ☐ Recommended Treatment/Return Patient

Brief History: _____
_____

Clinical Signs and Duration:_____
_____

Tentative Diagnosis and Current Treatment: _____
_____
_____
_____

Consultant's Findings, Diagnosis & Recommendations

_____
_____
_____
_____
_____
_____
_____
_____
_____
_____
_____
_____
_____
_____
_____
_____
_____

_____   _____
Date   Consultant's Signature

B-4
FORM CONTROL NO.

UNIVERSITY OF PENNSYLVANIA
VETERINARY HOSPITAL

Figure 33-19 Consultation form.

Please use ballpoint pen.
(press firmly)

CASE NUMBER:

CLIENT'S NAME:

ANIMAL'S NAME:

VETERINARY HOSPITAL OF THE
UNIVERSITY OF PENNSYLVANIA

WARD

DISCHARGE DATE

DISCHARGE DIAGNOSES FOR RECORD CODING
(INDICATE "T" FOR TENTATIVE OR "C" FOR CONFIRMED)

_____

_____

_____

YOUR VETERINARIAN IS:_____ YOUR DOCTOR'S TELEPHONE # IS ____(215) 898-_____

RE-EXAMINATION

☐ AN APPOINTMENT HAS BEEN SCHEDULED FOR YOUR PET TO BE SEEN AGAIN ON _____ AT _____ a.m. / p.m.

☐ YOUR PET NEEDS A RE-EXAMINATION IN _____ DAYS / WEEKS / MONTHS

  IF AN APPOINTMENT NEEDS TO BE CHANGED OR ARRANGED, PLEASE CALL (215) 898-4680 (9:00 - 4:30, Mon. - Fri.)

☐ NO RE-EXAM NECESSARY AT THIS TIME

MEDICATIONS AND DIRECTIONS FOR USE:

_____

_____

_____

SPECIFIC INSTRUCTIONS: (If an emergency should develop in the evening or the weekend, please call (215) 898-4685.)

_____

_____

_____

_____

_____

_____

_____

_____

_____

_____

I have received the above animal and I have been given the opportunity to ask questions about these instructions.

_____   _____ _____   _____
Owner or Owner's Agent   Date   Time   Staff Nurse

DISCHARGE INSTRUCTIONS

OWNER'S COPY

B-1

FORM CONTROL NO.

Figure 33-20 Summary and discharge form.

UNIVERSITY OF PENNSYLVANIA
3850 SPRUCE STREET
PHILADELPHIA, PA 19104-6010

Veterinary Hospital　　　　　　　　　　　　**EUTHANASIA RECORD**

DATE _____ CASE # _____

OWNER'S NAME _____

ADDRESS _____

CITY, STATE _____ PHONE _____

DESCRIPTION OF ANIMAL _____ BREED _____ SEX _____

COLOR AND/OR MARKINGS _____ PATIENT'S NAME _____ AGE _____

　　　I, THE UNDERSIGNED, HEREBY CERTIFY THAT I AM THE OWNER OR AUTHORIZED AGENT FOR THE OWNER OF THE ANIMAL DESCRIBED ABOVE. I UNDERSTAND THAT BY SIGNING THIS AGREEMENT I AUTHORIZE THE VETERINARY HOSPITAL OF THE UNIVERSITY OF PENNSYLVANIA AND ITS' AGENTS OR REPRESENTATIVES TO HUMANELY EUTHANATIZE THIS PATIENT AND I AGREE TO RELEASE THE UNIVERSITY AND ITS' AGENTS OR REPRESENTATIVES FROM ANY AND ALL LIABILITY ASSOCIATED WITH THE PERFORMANCE OF THIS SERVICE.

SIGNATURE _____ DATE _____

ADDRESS (if different than above)_____

WITNESS _____ DATE _____

I CERTIFY THAT, TO THE BEST OF MY KNOWLEDGE, THIS PATIENT HAS NOT BITTEN ANY PERSON OR ANIMAL WITHIN THE PAST 10 DAYS.

SIGNATURE _____ DATE _____
　　　　　　　(IF PATIENT HAS BEEN INVOLVED IN A BITE INCIDENT SEE REVERSE SIDE OF FORM)

E - 5
FORM CONTROL NO.

Figure 33-21 Euthanasia record.

I, the undersigned, hereby certify that my animal named, _____
has bitten the following people or animals:

_____   _____
Name of person bitten or owner of animal bitten   Name of animal bitten

_____   _____

_____   _____

_____   _____

_____   _____

To the best of my knowledge, the bite(s) occurred on _____
                                                                   (date)

at the following address _____

I hereby give the Veterinary Hospital of the University of Pennsylvania and it's agents or representatives the authority to contact appropriate Public Health Authorities regarding this bite incident(s) and to proceed with procedures for the diagnosis of rabies as deemed necessary by VHUP personnel or Public Health Authorities.

Owner's
Signature _____ Date _____

E - 5
FORM CONTROL NO.

Figure 33-21—cont'd

veterinary hospitals, therefore, have developed fee-estimation and consent-for-treatment forms (Figures 33-22 and 33-23). These forms give owners a written estimate of the cost of the procedures, verify ownership, and establish an agreement in the event that the animal is abandoned by the owner. This empowers the practice to take action in the event that the owner cannot meet his responsibility to pay for services and/or retrieve their pet.

Obtaining consent from the owner is recommended whenever there is an indication that a client might end up being a problem. Often legal difficulties can be avoided by identifying potentially difficult clients in advance. Having

the owner's written consent to restrain their own pet during an examination, for example, may protect the practice later if the client is bitten. Sometimes an owner that normally insists on holding their own pet during an office visit may decide not to after reading and signing a consent form that lists the risks of restraining an animal.

LOGS

In addition to the documents contained within the patient record, medical information is maintained continuously in

VETERINARY HOSPITAL OF THE
UNIVERSITY OF PENNSYLVANIA

CONSENT FOR TREATMENT AND/OR ADMISSION

CLIENT PLATE

I, the undersigned owner, or owner's agent, of the pet identified above, certify that **I am/I am not** (circle one) over **eighteen** years of age, and hereby consent to the examination of my pet by staff veterinarians at VHUP. I also agree that after consultation with me, VHUP's doctors may prescribe medication for, treat, hospitalize, anesthetize, sedate, and/or perform surgery on my animal. I understand that some risks always exist with anesthesia, surgery, and/or certain diagnostic procedures and treatments and that I am encouraged to discuss any concerns I have about those risks with my attending veterinarian before the procedure is initiated. Should some unexpected life-saving emergency care be required and my attending veterinarian be unable to reach me, VHUP's staff has my permission to provide such treatment, and I agree to pay for such care.

I understand that an estimate of the costs of veterinary services will be provided to me and that I am encouraged to discuss all fees attendant to such care before services are rendered and during my pet's ongoing medical treatment. If my pet is hospitalized, I agree to pay a deposit of one half of the estimated fees and assume financial responsibility for the balance of all services rendered on a cash, credit card or check basis at the time my pet is discharged from the hospital. In the event my pet is hospitalized for more than 48 hours and my attending doctor is unable to reach me, I understand it is my responsibility to call the hospital at least every 48 hours to inquire as to the medical status of my pet and the fees incurred for medical services up to that day. In the event of an open balance, I agree to pay a monthly billing fee equal to 1.5% of the unpaid balance.

I understand that VHUP faculty and staff have teaching and research functions in addition to their clinical duties. In fulfilling their mission, they may generate photographs, x-rays or other images of patients and/or make use of blood or tissue samples in performing their studies. I consent to the taking of photographs and other images and the use of such images and blood or tissue samples for teaching and research purposes provided that 1) they are obtained as part of the normal diagnostic and therapeutic work-ups and 2) neither my animal nor I are identified in any publications, reports or presentations without permission. I understand that staff members will not obtain additional samples nor perform additional procedures beyond those necessary for the clinical care of my pet without additional oral or written consent.

I further agree that I, or an authorized agent of mine, will pick up my pet and pay for all accrued charges within 5 days after receiving written or oral notification that my pet is ready to be discharged from the hospital. Such notice will be given at the address maintained on the hospital's patient/client record or the address listed below. I agree that if I fail to comply with this policy, VHUP may handle the abandonment of my pet in the best interests of the animal and the hospital.

HAVE YOU TALKED WITH YOUR VETERINARIAN ABOUT THE FOLLOWING?

- **The reasonable medical and/or surgical treatment options for your pet?**
- **Sufficient details of the procedures for you to understand what will be performed?**
- **How fully your pet might respond or recover and how long it could take?**
- **The most common complications and how serious they might be?**
- **The length and type of follow-up care and restraint required?**
- **How much all of the care is expected to cost?**

_____   _____
Signature of Owner or Agent   Date

_____   _____
Signature of Parent or Legal Guardian   Date
if owner/agent less than 18 years of age

Figure 33-22 Consent for treatment and/or authorization for admission to hospital.

HOSPITAL NAME _____
ADDRESS_____
CITY_____STATE ___ ZIP CODE _____

DATE: | **TIME:**

CLINICIAN:

FEE ESTIMATE	
NAME _____ CASE NO. _____	
STREET _____	
CITY, STATE, ZIP _____	
PHONE BUS. _____ HOME_____	

SPECIES	BREED	SEX
ANIMAL'S NAME		DATE OF BIRTH
COLOR—IDENTIFYING MARKS		

					$
INITIAL EXAM	Routine Visit	Referral		Emergency	
HOSPITALIZATION NO. OF DAYS	Standard	ADDITIONAL FEES FOR : Isolation		ICU	
LABORATORY Data base	Clin Path Microbiology Parasitology	LASMDL Endocrinology Histopathology		Cytology Immunology Other	
RADIOLOGY Survey Exams	Ultrasound	Other			
DIAGNOSTIC PROCEDURES Consultations	ECG EEG EMG ERG	CSF Tap Endoscopy Skin Test Biopsy		Aspirate/Washes Ultrasound Special Exams Other	
ANESTHESIA Sedation	Local	General		Other	
SURGERY O.R. Fee	Materials Supplies	Professional Service		Implants Other	
THERAPEUTICS Vaccinations Medicated Bath/Dip	In–Hosp.Trmt Fluids Transfusions	Oxygen Therapy Physical Therapy		Deworming Dentistry Other	
PHARMACY Hospital Meds	Bandage Materials	Discharge Meds		Special Diets	
OTHER	Contingencies/Comments:				

You have been advised of estimated costs and procedures. Please feel free to discuss the proposed treatment and its cost with the veterinarian. A minimum deposit of 50% of the initial charges will be required for hospitalization of an animal patient.

Amt. of Deposit $ _____ Receipt # _____ TOTAL ESTIMATE $

STATEMENT OF OWNERSHIP AND CONSENT: I am the owner of the above described animal, or have authorization from the owner to consent to its treatment.

I hereby authorize the performance of professionally accepted diagnostic, therapeutic, anesthetic, and surgical procedures necessary for its treatment.

I accept financial responsibility for these services.

I have read the above consent and understand why the above procedures may be necessary. I also have been told of the possible complications and alternatives to the listed procedures.

I will not hold _____ or its agents liable in any manner regarding the care, treatment, or safekeeping of the animal described above.

I understand that if further services are required for this animal (even if for treatment of the same condition), additional expenses will occur. Do not allow the total bill to exceed $ _____without my authorization.

I have read and understand the above statement and have received a copy of this estimate.

_____ _____
Signature (Owner or agent) | Date

White: Client   Canary: Discharge Office   Pink: Medical records

Figure 33-23 Fee estimation form.

logs that are located throughout the veterinary hospital. In many practices, there are logs for radiology and special imaging, surgery, anesthesia, controlled substances, ultrasound, clinical laboratory, and euthanasia. In addition, some practices have unexpected death, drug reaction, and medical waste logs. Any division of the veterinary hospital or specific activity could conceivably have a log that records the daily activity in that particular aspect of the hospital. Some large practices, therefore, may have 8 to 12 different types of logs, while smaller practices may have two to four logs.

The logs serve two purposes:

1. They provide additional documentation for legal support.
2. They provide data for quick analysis and retrospective studies.

A practice that is interested in examining the average length of surgery, for example, can quickly calculate that figure based on data in the surgery log. In radiology, techniques could be evaluated by examining the recorded settings in the x-ray log. Typically, logs are kept in binders or bound composition books so that pages cannot be lost or discarded accidentally.

Some of the commonly used logs are listed below.

RADIOLOGY LOG

The radiology log records the technique used for every x-ray taken. It includes the following:
- Patients name and identification (ID) number
- Client's name
- Date
- Study type
- Measurement of body thickness
- Technique used: milliamperes (mAs), time, kilovolts peak (kVp)
- Radiographic findings or diagnosis

The radiology log is typically completed by the veterinary technician (Figure 33-24) and is particularly helpful when improved exposure technique is desired and repeat films are requested.

> **TECHNICIAN NOTE**
>
> The radiology log is especially helpful to technicians who wish to review and improve previous exposure techniques.

SURGERY LOG

Although there is much variation from practice to practice regarding the content and structure of the surgery log, most contain the following information:

- Date
- Animal and owner's name
- Case number
- Patient's weight
- Name of surgeon
- Surgical procedure
- Duration of surgery
- Complications

The surgery/anesthesia log is particularly helpful when completing retrospective studies regarding the cost of performing each surgical procedures and regarding surgical

Radiology Log													
Date	Case No.	Owner	Patient	Species	Study	Grid	Thickness (cm)	KVP	MA	Time Sec.	MAs	Tech. Initials
5/10/05	3246	Marshall	"Ed"	K-9	Abd.	Yes	21	90	300	1/30	10	cd
5/10/05	2671	Edward	"Wayne"	K-9	FR ext	No	6	60	100	1/20	5	df
5/10/05	6342	Kahn	"Nathanial"	Iguana	LF ext	No	1	50	100	1/20	5	cd
5/11/05	4563	Marshall	"Will"	Feline	Thorax	Yes	8	60	75	1/10	7.5	cd
5/12/05	4532	Pattison	"Hatchie"	Feline	Abd.	Yes	10	60	100	1/10	10	df
5/12/05	6543	Bassert	"Serena"	K-9	LH ext	No	6	60	100	1/20	5.0	cd
5/12/05	8964	Rose	"Suzie"	Feline	Thorax	Yes	8	60	75	1/10	7.5	df
5/12/05	8964	Rose	"Suzie"	Feline	Abd.	Yes	5	50	100	1/10	10	my
5/14/05	6751	Stern	"Gadget"	Snake	Skull	No	1	50	100	1/20	5.0	lb
5/14/05	7602	Berson	"Pete"	K-9	Adb.	Yes	14	76	300	1/40	7.5	cd
5/14/05	4398	Yates	"Mila"	K-9	Abd.	Yes	23	94	300	1/30	10	my
5/14/05	8743	Busch	"Abby"	K-9	Abd.	Yes	18	84	300	1/30	10	cd
5/14/05	4032	Brass	"Rose"	Feline	Thorax	Yes	8	60	75	1/10	7.5	lb
5/14/05	6302	Ash	"Sue"	K-9	Abd.	Yes	22	92	300	1/30	10	cd

Figure 33-24 Example of a radiology log.

complications (Figure 33-25). Some practices have separate surgery and anesthesia logs, while other practices combine the information to prevent redundancy.

ANESTHESIA LOG

The anesthesia log documents the anesthesia protocol used in surgical and nonsurgical procedures. Dental procedures, thorough ear examinations and bone marrow aspirates are all examples of procedures that would require anesthesia but that might not be entered into the surgery log. Information contained in the anesthesia log might include the following:

- Patient's and owner's name
- Patient's weight
- Relative risk category or result of physical exam

- Anesthetic protocol, including type and dosage of each anesthetic agent
- Anesthesia start and end time
- Number of intubation attempts
- Surgical procedure and name of surgeon
- Anesthetist's name
- Complications

The anesthesia log complements the information entered on the anesthesia form (Figure 33-12). Some of the information is repeated and is found in both the log and the form. However, the advantage of the log is that it is easily accessible (the notebook often sits out) and represents a summary of all of the anesthesia cases. The anesthesia form, on the other hand, although it contains more detailed information, is not as accessible and contains information about *one* anesthesia case.

SURGERY LOG

CASE NUMBER	CLIENT	PATIENT WEIGHT	SURGEON	ANESTHESIA	PROCEDURE	MAJOR	MINOR	TIME	FEE

Figure 33-25 Example of a surgery log.

NECROPSY LOG

The necropsy log is a compilation of data regarding the death of animals. It includes the date and cause of death and type of necropsy performed (Figure 33-26). It also contains the owner's name, case number, species, name of the veterinarian performing the evaluation, histopathology and gross findings, and special tissue submitted. The log is typically kept in the necropsy area.

CONTROLLED SUBSTANCES LOG

The Comprehensive Drug Abuse and Control Act (the Act) is federal law that was passed by Congress in 1970 and regulates the possession of drugs that have the potential to be abused. These drugs are called *controlled substances*. In the Act, the drugs are categorized according to their potential for addiction. The categories range from Schedule I drugs, which are the most addictive, to Schedule V drugs, which are the least addictive. Schedule I drugs include LSD, heroin, crack cocaine, and peyote and have no accepted medical use. All of the other scheduled drugs (Schedules II, III, IV, and V) must be securely stored in a locked cabinet and inventoried separately from noncontrolled drugs. An inventory of all controlled substances must be made every 2 years, though most practices do this annually. The inventory and should include the following:

1. Name, address, and DEA registration number
2. Date and time the inventory is performed
3. Contents of the inventory
4. Signature of the person taking the inventory

A separate inventory record must be kept for each Schedule II drug. The records for Schedule III, IV, and V drugs may be combined into one log, but must be kept separate from the other practice records. In addition, all drug-log information must be kept in a bound composition book or book in which the pages cannot be torn out without notice. Although specific requirements vary from state to state, a typical controlled-substance log includes the following:

1. Date
2. Owner's and patient's name
3. Starting volume
4. Ending volume
5. Amount used
6. The initials of the person who used the drug

All inventory records must be kept for 2 years.

NECROPSY LOG

DATE	PATH #	VTH&C #	DIAG LAB #	SPECIES	CLINICIAN	OWNER	PATH	GRAD.	DATE REC TYPE	DATE TYPED	DATE CORR.	DATE MAILED
16 June	0507	70048	33791	Ovine	Quinn	Douglas	Smith	Toole	17 June	18 June	19 June	19 June
16 June	0508	63378	27590	Equine	Brown	Breaux	Homes	—	17 June	18 June	19 June	19 June
17 June	0509	52215	20079	Avian	Lucky	McCasey	Baer	—	18 June	19 June	19 June	19 June
21 June	0510	40021	13386	Feline	Grant	Sprickett	Cadd	Black	22 June	23 June	24 June	24 June
2 July	0511	57740	25005	Canine	O'Connor	Page	Dicks	—	3 July	6 July	6 July	6 July
8 July	0512	60020	30059	Antelope	Pine	Brumfield	Cones	—	9 July	10 July	10 July	11 July
	0513											
	0514											
	0515											
	0516											
	0517											
	0518											
	0519											
	0520											
	0521											
	0522											
	0523											
	0524											
	0525											
	0526											
	0527											
	0528											
	0529											

Sample of Necropsy Log

Figure 33-26 Example of a necropsy log.

ORGANIZATION AND FILING

Many veterinary hospitals use a folder system that is developed specifically for veterinary medicine. There are a number of companies that make a variety of systems, so they are easy to acquire (you can order them from a catalog), and there is a wide selection of styles, sizes, and colors (Figure 33-1). Most folders include internal flexible clips that hold forms in their correct order (Figure 33-27). In addition, the folders are designed to accommodate color-coded tabs or stickers (known as *signaling devices*) that are applied to the outer edge of the folder making filing more efficient and filing errors easier to identify.

Colored stickers are sold separately, which allows the practice to choose the organizational scheme of the color-coding system. For example, it can be alphabetical, numerical, or a combination of both. In the alphabetical system, a different color is given to each letter of the alphabet. It is easy to learn and does not require cross-referencing with a master list of clients. The primary challenge of using the alphabetical system, however, is that the employee doing the filing must be careful to correctly apply the alphabetical order and spell the clients' names without exception. Unfortunately, errors in spelling and filing do occur from time to time, so misfiled records tend to be more common with the alphabetical system than with other systems.

In the numeric system, each client is assigned a number. The number assigned to the file may be a hospital-generated number or the client's telephone or social security number. Each digit in the number has a different color and the files are shelved from lowest to highest (Figure 33-28). In this way, it is easy to correctly sequence the files, and any misfiled records are easily identified because the file color sequence does not match those of surrounding files. Can you see the misfiled record in Figure 33-29? In order to retrieve a particular file, the receptionist must first check a cross-reference that lists the client's name and the corresponding file number.

One of the advantages of the numeric filing system is that fewer filing errors occur, because numbers are easier to read and interpret than letters and spelling is not a factor. In addition, numerical filing systems are practical for large-volume practices because no file duplication occurs whereas in the alphabetical system, there may be many clients named Jones or Brown. The disadvantage of the numeric system, however, is that a cross-reference list must be generated and maintained. If phone numbers are used, the files will have to be assigned a new number and refiled whenever a client moves or changes phone numbers.

Additional colored tabs can be applied to files to alert the receptionist of specific client/patient issues. For example, the records of animals that need immunizations and worming can be flagged to indicate that reminders should

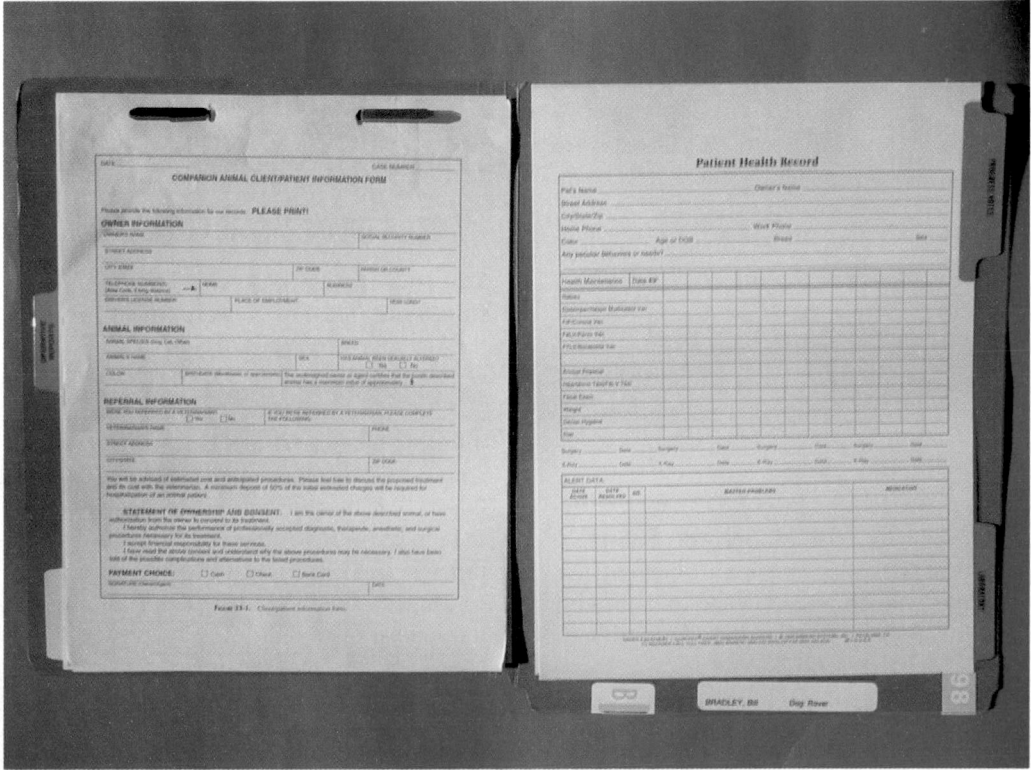

Figure 33-27 Letter-size folders contain flexible metal clips that hold forms in their correct order. Dividers allow for rapid retrieval of lab reports, operative notes, and progress notes.

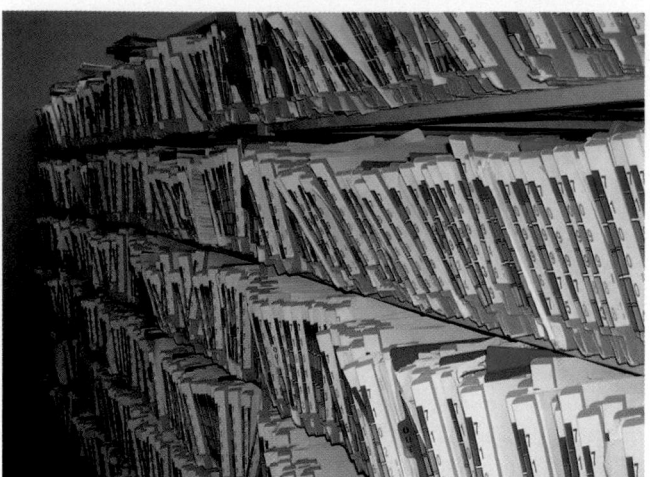

Figure 33-28 Numeric color-coding systems allow for rapid retrieval and filing.

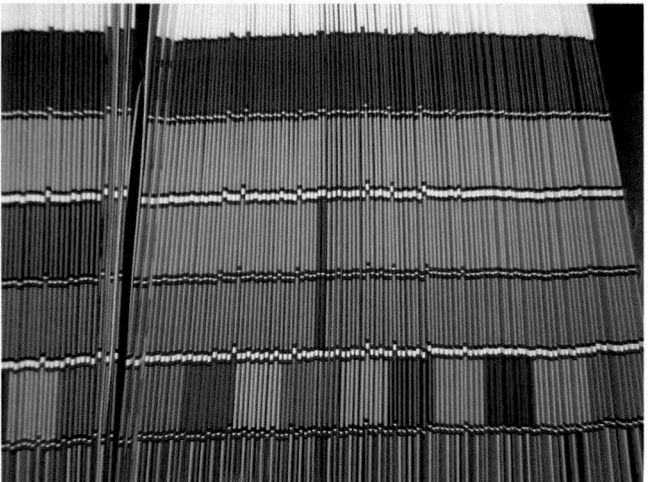

Figure 33-29 Can you spot the filing error in these color-coded files?

be mailed out. Colored flags may also indicate those clients that have an outstanding bill or that have not returned to the practice in a long time. In this way, colored signaling devices can be added to identify groups of files that need attention.

FILE PURGING

Periodically, the collection of medical records should be reviewed and purged of files that are not in current use. Each veterinary hospital has its own review and purging schedule; however, the following rules can be a helpful starting point:

1. The collection of medical records should be reviewed *at least* once per year.
2. Active records covering a 3-year period are maintained in the primary medical records collection.

3. Records that have been inactive for 4 years or more are moved to storage. Storage should be easily accessible.
4. Records 8 years old or older may be removed from storage and shredded.

Use of color-coded tabs with the year can be of particular value when completing the annual review of medical records. They enable the receptionist to quickly identify the 4-year-old and 8-year-old records by their specific colors.

LOST RECORDS

The risk of losing records in both a small and a large hospital is problematic. They can be lost through misfiling, incorrect spelling of names, or misplacement. At times, even after an exhaustive search, the record continues to be missing. Sometimes the loss is not discovered until the animal comes back to the practice for a return visit.

It is best, in this case, to explain to the client that the record has been misplaced. A new record should be started and information requested from the client and veterinarian. In addition, copies of laboratory data, pathology reports, and radiologic information should be obtained and added to reestablish the file.

Although the problem of lost records is embarrassing to the practice and inconvenient to the client, it will happen with even the most elaborate record keeping system; however, every effort possible should be made to quickly and accurately file each record after each visit. Clients feel more at ease and welcomed if the record is complete and easily accessible.

ETHICAL AND LEGAL ISSUES

OWNERSHIP OF MEDICAL RECORDS

The laws concerning ownership of medical records vary from state to state. However, in general the records made during the course of a patient's treatment are owned by the veterinary hospital or hospital owner. Although the client purchased the veterinary services that generated the medical information, the client is *not*, by law, the owner of the medical record. However, the owner may request a copy of the record at any time. In fact, it is customary for clients to request copies of their pet's medical record when they are moving and changing veterinary practices. This facilitates continued care of the patient and prevents repetition of immunizations or diagnostic tests. It is recommended that copies of medical records be mailed to the successive veterinarian and not hand delivered by the owner who may be apt to misinterpret the status of his or her animal's health. A cover letter should be included with the copy of the record so that the original veterinary hospital and veterinarian can be easily contacted if necessary. A flat fee for copying the

CONSENT TO DISCLOSURE OF MEDICAL RECORD

WAIVER OF CONFIDENTIALITY

BY AUTHORIZED PATIENT REPRESENTATIVE

I,_____am the_____

of _____ a_____

I understand that the information contained in _____'s

medical record is confidential. However, I specifically give my

consent for _____

to release the following specific information concerning

_____ to _____

_____

_____

_____

The above-listed information is to be disclosed for the specific

purpose of _____

_____

It is further understood that the information released is for professional
purposes only and may not be provided in whole or part to any other person
than that stated above.

_____

**Signature of
Authorized Representative**

_____
Date

Figure 33-30 Authorization to disclose medical records.

record may be charged, or the practice may levy a fee on a per-page basis.

RELEASE OF MEDICAL INFORMATION

A signed authorization form (Figure 33-30) or a written letter of request for record copies should be obtained from the animal's owner before any information is released to him or her, another veterinarian, or an insurance company. The practice owner should be the only person to authorize release of information contained in the record. However, there is an exception to this rule. Local, state, and federal agencies require the reporting of certain diseases that may be dangerous to the public or to the widespread health of animals. These are called *reportable diseases* and include rabies, brucellosis, and equine encephalitis. Additional regulations regarding reportable diseases can be found in the Animal Movement Quarantine Regulations Manual that is published by the U.S. Department of Agriculture (USDA). In addition, physicians, animal control agencies, and the regional department of health may inquire about the rabies immunization status of an animal that had bitten a human.

> ✎ **TECHNICIAN NOTE**
>
> **AVMA Ethics and Medical Records**
>
> A. **Veterinary medical records are an integral part of veterinary care.** The records must comply with the standards established by state and federal law.
> B. **Medical records are the property of the practice and the practice owner.** The original records must be retained by the practice for the period required by statute.
> C. **Ethically, the information within veterinary medical records is considered privileged and confidential.** It must not be released except by court order or consent of the owner of the patient.
> D. **Veterinarians are obligated to provide copies or summaries of medical records when requested by the client.** Veterinarians should secure a written release to document that request.
> E. **Without the express permission of the practice owner, it is unethical for a veterinarian (or veterinary technician) to remove, copy, or use medical records or any part of any record.**
>
> (From the Principles of Veterinary Medical Ethics section, 2003 AVMA Membership Directory and Resource Manual.)

MEDICAL AND LEGAL REQUIREMENTS

It is important to keep in mind that the medical record is a legal document and could be used in a court of law. It is generated not only to ensure consistent and accurate veterinary care but also to protect the veterinarian against potential malpractice litigation. Any written data contained in the medical record must therefore be complete, accurate, and legible. An inaccurate, illegible, or incomplete record may be construed as evidence of professional incompetence and substandard care. Keep in mind that in a court of law, "if it was not written down, it didn't happen" and "if the writing is illegible, it was not written down." Below are some guidelines for generating clear, complete, and accurate records.

1. Entries should either be typed or written in black ink.
2. In a court of law, handwriting alone is *not* an adequate way to identify the author of a notation. Entries should be dated and *initialed* to identify the person making the entry. Additional validity to an entry can be made by entering the *time*, as well as the date.
3. Errors should *not* be scratched out, erased, or blotted out. Instead, a single line should be drawn through the mistake and initialed. The correct information should then be written in the margin and initialed and dated next to the correction. Any erasure or blotting out may suggest tampering of the record and could render the document inadmissible in a court of law.
4. Only approved, standard abbreviations should be used.

The medical record is considered legal evidence of services and procedures performed by the veterinary health care team. In the event of litigation, such as during a malpractice or insurance suit, the record could be subpoenaed and admitted as evidence.

Legal guidelines for medical records vary from state to state and may dictate the type of information that should be included, how long the record should be kept, and restrictions on the release of medical information. It is recommended that all members of the veterinary health care team be familiar with the laws of the state in which they work.

> ✎ **TECHNICIAN NOTE**
>
> Errors should *not* be scratched out, erased, or blotted out. Instead, a single line should be drawn through the mistake and initialed. The correct information should then be written in the margin and initialed and dated next to the correction. Any erasure or blotting out may suggest tampering of the record and could render the document inadmissible in a court of law.

Veterinary Medical Database

The Veterinary Medical Database (VMDB) is a national data bank located at Purdue University. It contains computerized veterinary medical data supplied by 24 veterinary schools in the United States and Canada. Each institution submits data for the VMDB on a quarterly basis to a central processing center. The data consist of abstracted data from each clinical case seen at each teaching hospital. The national database allows studies of national trends in various animal diseases. It provides patient chart number, institution code, date of visit, length of stay, clinician code, gender, species, breed, discharge status, age, weight, diagnosis, and procedures for each animal. The VMDB is available for use in retrospective studies and in the evaluation of national and regional disease patterns.

COMPUTERS

Computers have become an integral part of veterinary practice management today. Software packages designed specifically for veterinary practices help organize a wide range of management issues such as billing, reminders, scheduling, and inventory as well as medical records. Chapter 34 addresses these and other topics regarding the use of computers in veterinary practice.

Related Associations

American Animal Hospital Association, 12575 West Bayaud Ave., Lakewood, CO 80228

American Veterinary Medical Association, 1931 N. Meacham Road, Suite 100, Schaumburg, IL 60173-4360

American Veterinary Health Information Management Association, c/o Flo Nelson, University of Missouri, Veterinary Medical Teaching Hospital, 379 E. Campus Drive, Columbia, MO 65211

American Health Information Management Association, North Michigan Avenue, Suite 2150, Chicago, IL 60601-5800, www.ahima.org

Recommended Reading

AAHA Standards of Accreditation CD-ROM, Medical Records Section, Lakewood, Colo, 2003, American Animal Hospital Association.

Allen DG: The problem-oriented approach. In *Small animal medicine*, Philadelphia, 1991, Lippincott.

Heinke ML McCarthy JB: *Practice made perfect: a guide to veterinary practice management*, Lakewood, Colo, 2001, American Animal Hospital Association.

Johns ML: *Information management for health professions, ed 2*, 2002, Delmar Publishing.

Johns ML: *Health information management technology: an applied approach*, American Health Information Management Association.

Peden AH: Veterinary settings. In *Comparative records for health information management*, Delmar Publishers.

34

Computer Applications in Veterinary Practice

VICKIE BYARD

INTRODUCTION

Much of what we do in our daily lives involves some sort of computer technology. Many individuals first rise in the morning to drink their first cup of coffee while reading their E-mail. When you stop at the bank machine on the way to work, a computer hands you money and automatically deducts that amount from your bank account. If you self-check out at a grocery store, the computer reads the bar codes on your selected items and then charges you appropriately. If you charge the amount to a credit card, the computer reads your personal information from the magnetic strip on your card then sends the information electronically to gain approval for the transaction. Once approved, the system requests your signature and you are on your way. All of this could have taken place before you even entered the front door of the veterinary practice where you work. We have entered a time where computers play an integral part in all of our lives. This technology is efficient, cost effective, and dramatically reduces human error.

Since the onset of the 1990s, veterinarians began to introduce computers into their practices. Initially, they were used for invoicing and bookkeeping tasks. With the introduction of software specifically designed for veterinary practices, innovative veterinarians and practice managers began to realize the potential these systems offered.

Well into the year 2005, the integration of computers into the veterinary setting is necessary, if not vital. Now most practices depend on computers for appointment scheduling, medical records management, inventory management, payroll, marketing, data collection, and accounting. However, as technology advances, so does the role of the computer. This chapter will introduce the reader to the usual computer applications and stimulate some

thought on innovative and practical uses to make the practice of veterinary medicine more exciting and ultimately more productive. ■

COMPUTER HARDWARE AND SOFTWARE

This discussion about the specifics of computer hardware and software assumes a certain amount of basic computer knowledge. *Computer hardware* relates to the parts of the system that you can touch: the monitor, the hard drive, the mouse, the printers, the modem, the disks, the scanner, and more (Figure 34-1). *Software* relates to the computer instructions contained within the hardware or added to the hardware. An important distinction should be made between *operating software* and *applications software.* The operating software tells the different parts of the hardware how to communicate with each other. For instance, the operating system translates strikes on the keyboard to letters seen on the screen. It monitors and organizes files and directories, and it controls peripheral devices such as printers, scanners, and disk drives. Some commonly recognized operating systems are DOS, OS/2, Windows, Macintosh, UNIX, and Linux. Applications software are programs that help a user perform certain tasks. Some common examples of application software include word processing software, bookkeeping software, and practice management information systems.

Veterinary software products that offer more flexibility and will therefore become increasingly popular are those considered to be 32 bit. The term *32-bit* refers to all of the Microsoft Windows programs 95/98/NT and 2000. It excludes Windows 3.1 and earlier versions because they had to rely on a DOS platform. The 32-bit programs offer the users the ability to import results from certain laboratory equipment and allow multiple employees to manipulate

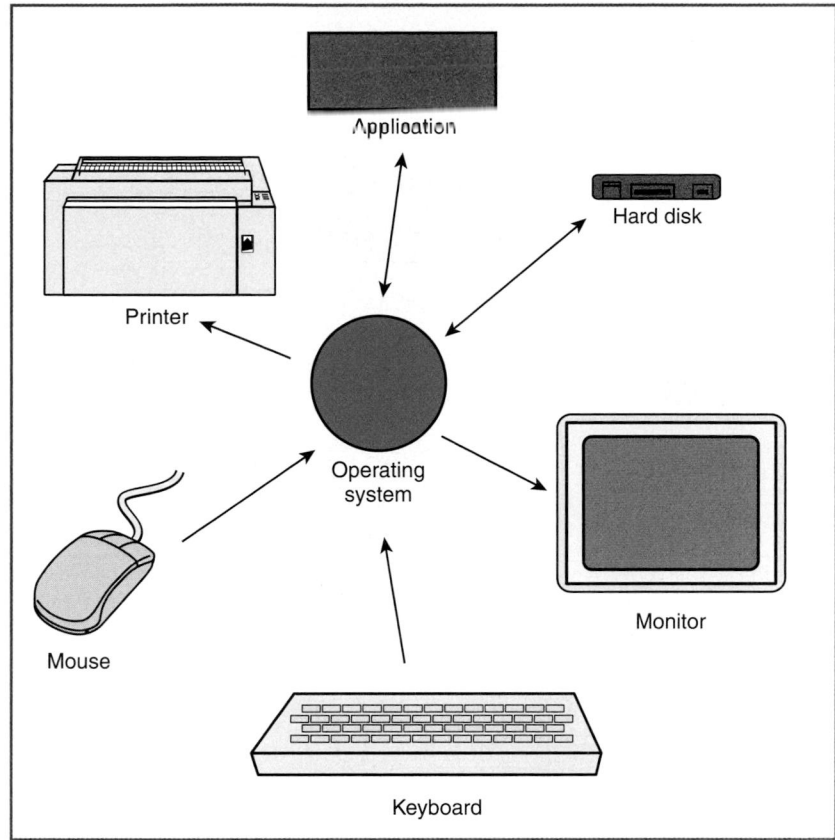

Figure 34-1 This diagram depicts the function of the operating system and the flow of the information (direction) between peripheral devices.

data from different workstations simultaneously. These 32-bit programs also provide a revision history feature. This means that all changes to the medical record are tracked. This is vital when considering a "paperless environment" in the event of litigation.

COMPUTER CONFIGURATIONS

A solo veterinarian may require a computer terminal in the reception station, one in the pharmacy, one in the exam room, and one in the business or doctor's office. These terminals would all be connected through a *server*. A server is a devise that manages a network. The veterinary software is stored here as well as the associated patient/client database. This network may include two printers (one in the reception area and one in the office), four keyboards, and four pointing devices (such as a mouse). There are various configurations depending on the complexity and functions of the system (Figure 34-2).

Today's veterinary environment supports many large practices staffed with general clinicians and specialists of various disciplines, multiple support staff, and space occupying large square footage. In this type of setting, the

above-described network would not suffice. It is not unusual to see a terminal in each exam room, two to three terminals in the operating/treatment room, two to three terminals in the administrative offices, and two to three terminals in reception. Printers of differing types are scattered throughout these practices: a pharmacy label printer, a laser printer in reception, a printer for the bookkeeper, a printer for the administrator, and a printer in the laboratory. All of this hardware would be linked together through the network operating system, and the server manages the veterinary management software.

Recently, tablet PCs have entered the veterinary arena. These are a type of notebook computer that has an LCD screen on which the user can write using a stylus. The handwriting is digitalized and then converted to standard text. Tablets are wireless, affording the user the ability to take this technology wherever needed. Much of the information entered is accomplished through touching selected menus on the screen with the stylus. Many of the newer bundled packages come with supplemental software such as anatomical diagrams, feeding recommendations, or drug formularies. With a touch to the screen, the staff can send home a patient health report card and customized client education materials while speaking with the client.

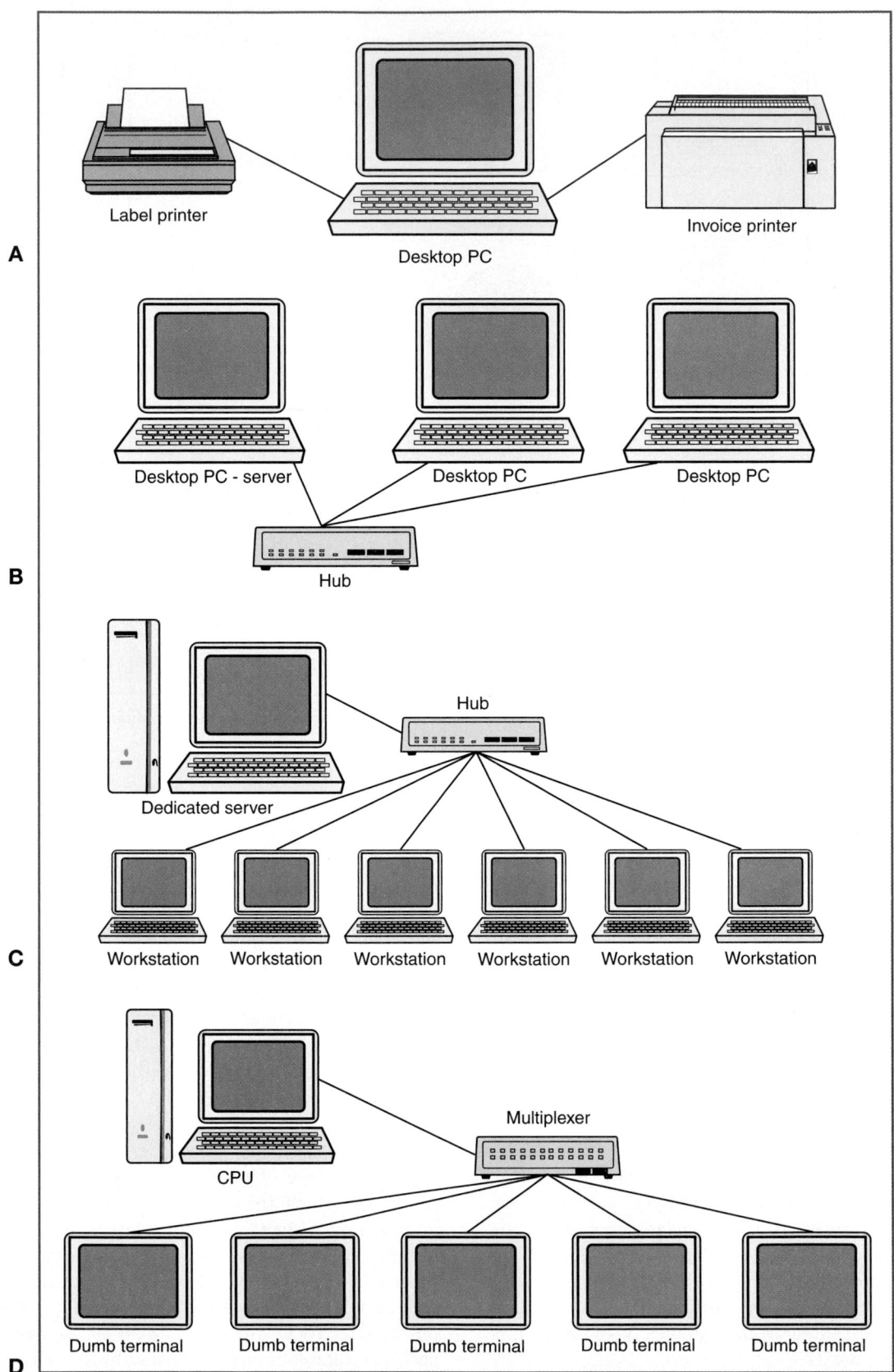

Figure 34-2 **A,** Single station system. **B,** Multistation system with nondedicated server. **C,** Multistation system with dedicated server. **D,** A configuration with one central processing unit (CPU) and "dumb" terminals attached. *PC,* Personal computer.

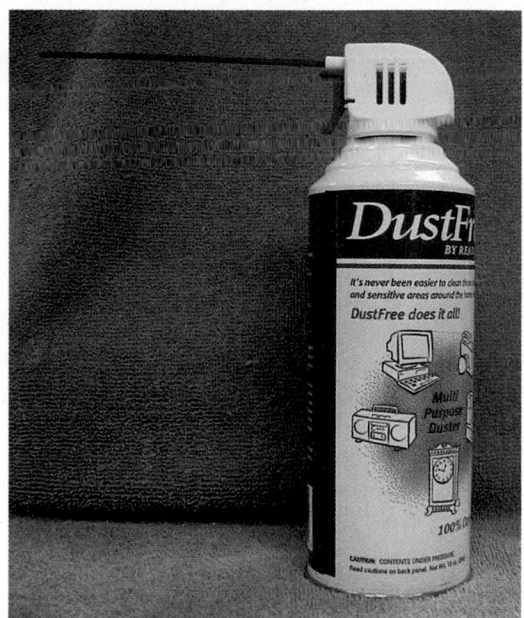

Figure 34-3 This is an example of compressed air for routine computer maintenance.

Do not avoid computerizing a practice or increasing the system's capabilities for fear that medicine will become less personalized. These systems should enable better time management so that quality time can be spent with each client and better care can be afforded to each patient.

MAINTENANCE TIPS

Make sure the computer case has plenty of room. The microprocessor, the motherboard, and other parts of the hardware accumulate heat. Computer cases have a cooling fan and slots where the air can exit. Especially in a veterinary environment, make sure these slots are not clogged with hair and dust. Also, ensure that the computer is in an area with plenty of cool air.

Dust the computer case and monitor once a month. Dust, left unchecked, will find its way into the computer.

Clean inside the computer case every 2 to 3 months. This can be accomplished with compressed air (Figure 34-3). It may be wiser to contract a computer repair company to regularly perform this function. Even the smallest amount of static electricity can ruin vital parts of the hardware.

Regardless of the size of the system chosen, it is recommended that an electrical surge protector be provided for the system together with a battery backup. If not properly protected, vital information can be lost in the event of an electrical surge or a complete power outage.

Although initially expensive, it is wise to consider redundant (or mirrored) hard drives. When information is saved, it is saved to two to three hard drives. In the event

that one crashes, at least one additional drive would contain all of the current practice information.

HOW TO RESEARCH, SELECT, AND PURCHASE HARDWARE AND SOFTWARE

When deciding to purchase a computer system for the veterinary practice, one must consider a number of factors.

- What is the flow of client traffic within the practice?
- What are the uses for the system?
- Who is responsible for entering data?
- What do you envision for the future of the practice?

After these questions have been answered, it is time to begin researching the various veterinary software companies. Most of the software programs available have similar features. The difference may be the ease of use, ability of the program to integrate with other equipment within the practice, and flexibility for the future.

The American Animal Hospital Association (AAHA) publishes a Trends Survey every 2 years listing what software programs are being utilized and how they are rated. In addition, many of the software vendors demonstrate their products at the national meetings. This is a great venue because you can compare and contrast different features of a number of competing products within one room. Contact the companies and discuss your needs. The vendors will assist you in deciding on what computer configuration is recommended to run their program and what the approximate costs will be. Some vendors also have demo compact disks (CDs) available so that you can investigate the program in depth.

Once you have narrowed down the search, there are some additional factors to consider.

- How long has the company been in business?
- How many systems have they sold?
- Can they provide references from practices employing this software?
- Are both hardware and software included in the support contract?
- What kind of staff training is provided and for how long?
- What is the anticipated cost of updates?
- If hardware is purchased separate from the vendor for the software, what support, warranties, and equipment loans do they offer?

As technology advances, it is reasonable for practices to replace hardware and/or software every 5 to 10 years. Although purchasing the components to computerize a practice is initially expensive, the following sections will demonstrate that savings to the practice will justify the costs.

Box 34-1   COMPUTER APPLICATIONS IN VETERINARY PRACTICE

- Demographic data collection
  - Name, address, phone number of the client
  - Name, age, gender, species, breed, color of the patient
- Scheduling
  - Client appointment by doctor
  - Boarding reservations
  - Vacation scheduling
  - Conference scheduling
- Billing
  - Accounts receivable
  - Accounts payable
- Mass mailings
  - Monthly statements
- Newsletters and client information
  - Reminders
    - Vaccinations, fecal or dental examinations, heartworm tests
    - Rechecks and follow-ups
- Inventory management
  - Drugs, controlled substances
  - Supplies
- Financial
  - Cash drawer reconciliation
  - Deposit slips automatically generated
  - Payment records: cash, check, credit card receipts
  - Payroll calculations
  - Profit and loss reports
  - Productivity reports: areas making or losing money
  - Fee code entry to keep track of clients' and patients' bill status

- Income analysis
- Practice profile and analysis
- Medical records
  - Patient's history
  - Daily progress reports and treatment records
  - Laboratory data storage and retrieval
  - Surgical procedures
  - Diagnostic codes: storage and retrieval
  - Physical examination results
  - Fee code entry to keep track of prescriptions and treatments completed
  - Certificates and forms
    - Vaccinations, rabies tag number tracking
    - Spay/neuter
    - Euthanasia
    - Release forms: surgery
- Communication
  - Patient's medical and financial records available to all staff at any time
  - Security: who can and cannot access certain data
- Diagnostic aids
  - Diagnostic programs
  - Drug formulary
- Remote modem communication
  - Home to hospital
  - Ranch or farm to hospital
  - Satellite clinic to hospital
  - Meeting or conference to hospital
  - Cellular phone to hospital

TYPICAL USES OF COMPUTERS IN VETERINARY PRACTICE

The current trend in veterinary medicine is for veterinarians to practice as a group. Large practice groups offer veterinarians flexible schedules and no initial outlay of capital to establish a practice. As client base of the practice grows, the number of veterinarians and support staff increases. This increase of human resources creates the need to manage information and communication between staff members, departments, and shifts. This trend would not be possible if veterinarians were not employing computers to help manage all of that increased information (Box 34-1).

DATA COLLECTION

Data are simply pieces of information. When a client enters a veterinary practice for the first time, the receptionist asks them to fill out a new client/patient form with their personal information on it. This information will include their name, address, home phone number, work phone number, possibly even their E-mail address. All of this information,

or data, is keyed into the computer. The form will ask for information regarding the patient: pet name, species, breed, age, color, etc. The receptionist will also enter this information, thus creating a virtual record for that client and patient (Figure 34-4).

As the client moves from the waiting room to the exam room, the technician continues to gather information. The weight of the patient is obtained and entered into the patient record. Any past inoculations and the dates last administered are entered into the record. Any past medical problems will be keyed into the computer as well. These data are stored in a *database*.

Through a *query* screen, the user can request a patient's record by a variety of parameters: client last name, patient name, phone number, or address. If the last name of the client is a common one, such as Smith, the computer would produce a very long list. In that case it would be easier to change the query parameter to *Patient Name* and enter the name "Sassy." The result will be a shorter list of all of the patients in the database by that name.

Data collection is important in a multitude of ways. The computer is capable of producing a list of all patients

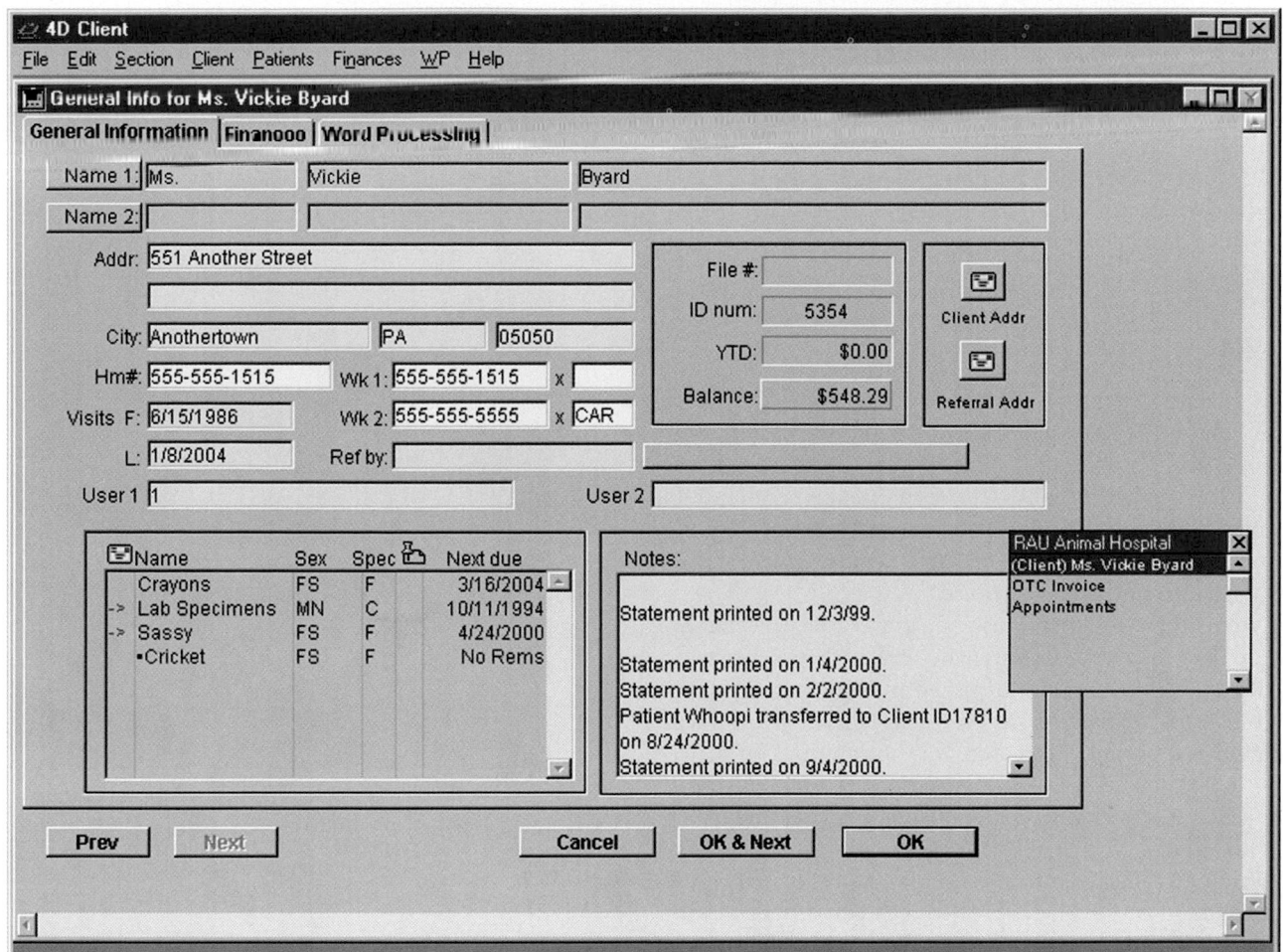

Figure 34-4 An example of a client data screen.

that are due to be inoculated in the month of June in the year 2005. This list can be used to produce the vaccination reminders that are to be mailed out, thus prompting next year's appointments.

The computer can produce a list of all patients that received recommendations for dentistry. It can even identify the practice's top 1000 income-generating clients so that you can send them the practice's newsletter. All of these functions can be accomplished in a matter of minutes with the use of a computer compared with the amount of time generating any of these lists by hand.

SCHEDULING

When evaluating veterinary software, a very important feature is the appointment scheduler. When the appointment book is not computerized, only one staff member can manipulate the schedule at a time. Computers make it possible for multiple staff members to be able to add or delete appointments concurrently. The veterinarian can schedule an appointment while speaking to the client, and the technician can schedule a recheck appointment while

discharging the patient from surgery. Ideally, the appointment schedule should be available at a variety of work stations. This feature alone decreases the chaos at the front desk created when all client contact requires a receptionist.

Some veterinary software synchronizes the appointment scheduler with the client/patient medical records. When you are in the patient record, a drop-down menu will offer a link to the appointment scheduler. When a time and date are selected, the patient name, client last name, and telephone number are automatically put in that slot. Another element of a computerized appointment scheduler is the "find next appointment" feature. If a client has forgotten when their appointment is scheduled, the receptionist may enter the patient record, drop down a menu, gain access to the appointment scheduler, and select "find next appointment." The computer will then search and display the appointment. This would be a tedious task without the help of a computer.

Some appointment schedulers are capable of appointment time customization. Identified tasks can be assigned specific lengths of time. Instead of scheduling a standard 15- or 20-minute appointment for suture removal, it could be customized to a 5- or 10-minute appointment. Some schedulers track and identify clients that have missed previous appointments. This enables the reception staff to confirm those appointments with a phone call.

Seventy percent of all scheduled appointments are generated from reminders. Some powerful veterinary software will display vaccine alerts prompting multiple pet visits rather than just scheduling the appointment driven by the mailed reminder.

BILLING

Older systems depend on the use of a "travel sheet." This is a sheet that has a list of line items on it. The term *line item* refers to any product or service within the practice that has a price attached to it. As services are rendered, the staff member highlights the line item on that patient's travel sheet. At the end of the day, a staff member enters those line items into the patient's invoice.

Systems that employ the use of a travel sheet inevitably lead to lost income. Traditionally, these sheets are two sided, and it is possible in a rushed moment to forget to input charges highlighted on the back. It is easy to forget to highlight a product dispensed. It is not unusual for there to be a $20,000 to $50,000 loss of income per full-time veterinarian per year with charges that are not captured.

With newer veterinary software, as staff members perform medical tasks, they enter those services directly into the computer. An invoice is created as a patient enters the practice. When the veterinarian examines a pet, they enter a code for "office visit." A window then opens for them to enter their SOAP notes (refer to Chapter 33 for a discussion on SOAP notes). When they close that window, they select a code for the next service, for instance, "in-house serum chemistry and complete blood count." The veterinary software handles updating the invoice. As the services increase, so does the invoice.

Veterinary software does not come with predetermined prices of products and services. As the software is introduced, the administrators of the practice input set prices for each service or product. When computers were not employed, veterinarians were very aware of the costs to the client. They tended not to charge for services out of a sense of guilt and/or discomfort. Invoice totals were lower, thus cutting the profit to the practice. With the use of advanced systems, the staff is less aware of the prices accruing as they render medical treatment. This feature alone is largely responsible for practices being able to afford more professional staff, thus increasing the standard of care and decreasing staff burnout.

MEDICAL RECORDS

Chapter 33 specifically discusses medical records. The discussion here is meant to highlight the benefits of electronic medical records.

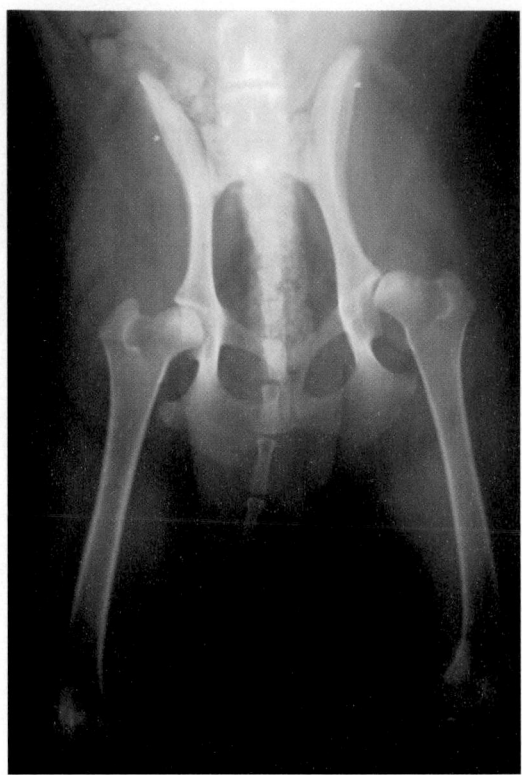

Figure 34-5 An example of a digitally captured image of a pelvic radiograph.

In the past, when medical records were made of paper, only the person handling the record could gain access to the information. With computerized medical records, staff in different rooms of the practice can see the information simultaneously.

Paper medical records could be found in a variety of places: the file, a stack of records awaiting communications, a pile of records on the bookkeeper's desk, a pile waiting to be refiled, or even an inactivity box in the attic. Because paper medical records "walk," they are often difficult to find. Computers allow us to retrieve vital information immediately.

Computerization has also improved the quality of the information. The information is legible and more organized. With the use of templates, the different parts of the exam are listed, defaulting to "nothing abnormal seen." When notable findings are made, the veterinarian can either type in the information or select a finding from a menu.

It is also true that many veterinarians are not typists. Voice recognition software is not out of the realm of possibility within the near future. The medical findings are spoken into a microphone, which then translates the sound of a voice into words on a word processor. These notes can then be cut and pasted into the medical record.

Advanced veterinary software permits documents such as referral reports, electrocardiogram strips, radiographs (Figure 34-5), photos (Figure 34-6), and more to be scanned or imported directly into the patient's medical record. This

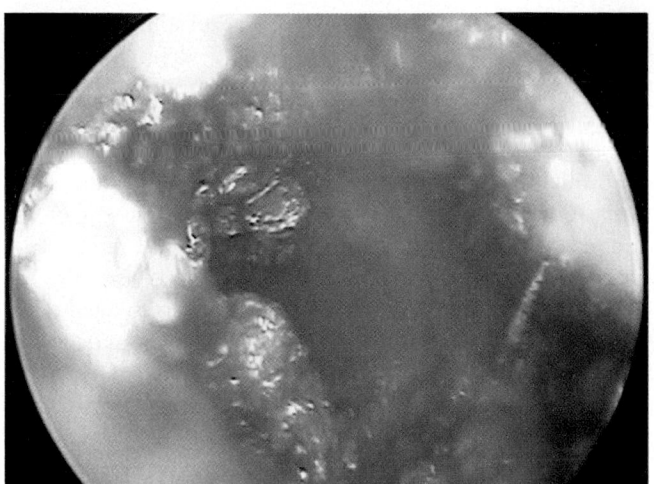

Figure 34-6 A digital image of an ear canal prior to an ear flush. This image was obtained with a video otoscope.

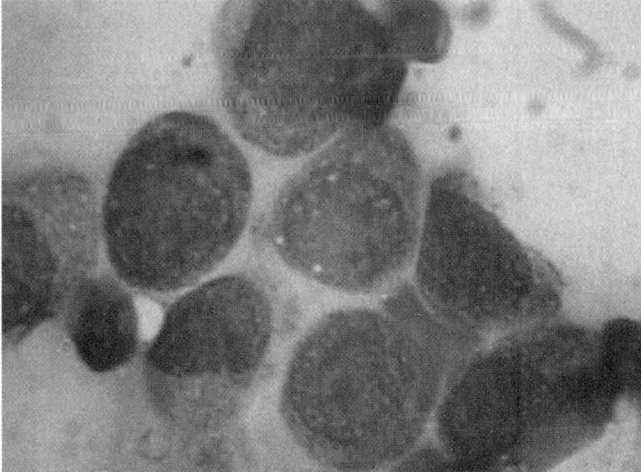

Figure 34-8 Image of a cytology slide taken with a digital camera attached to a microscope.

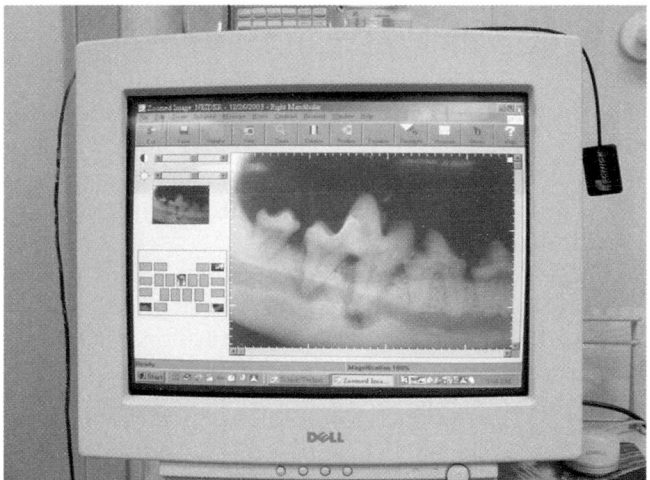

Figure 34-7 This photograph shows an intraoral radiograph taken with a digital sensor (to the right of the monitor) and a dental x-ray unit.

reduces staff time searching for reports, pulling radiographs, and subsequent refiling.

Some programs are capable of maintaining a digital photo of the client on the record. Upon retrieval of the patient file, there may be a photo of the patient. A digital camera can be used to take images of lesions or teeth (Figure 34-7) or it can be attached to a microscope for images of cytology or hematology slides (Figure 34-8). These images can be imported right into the patient's electronic medical record for future use or e-mailed to a referral specialist.

CLIENT COMMUNICATIONS AND MASS MAILINGS

As discussed in the Data Collection section, information that is entered into the record can be retrieved later for marketing purposes. Vaccination reminders are printed and mailed out monthly. Recommendations made in patients' records can be tracked. The practice can then prepare and send mass mailings extolling the benefits of senior wellness packages, dental cleanings, and other services. Once the list is created, address labels can be printed and new business is only days away.

INVENTORY MANAGEMENT

With most veterinary software, inventory management is a module of the program. Due to the nature of practice, this module of veterinary software is not without its problems. If all of the inventory for the practice was ordered, received, stocked, prescribed, and sold, then the inventory management would be easily handled by the computer. Unfortunately, items such as catheters, tape, syringes, needles, cleaning supplies, and sterilization supplies constitute items that are used within the practice on a regular basis but are separately billed therefore making them difficult to track. Not every intravenous catheter attempt is successful, yet the client is only charged for one. Dispensable items, such as medication, food, and shampoo, can be tracked. Levels can be set within the system, and weekly order reports can be generated by the computer as levels get low. Currently, computerized inventory management is almost always coupled with a manual system for all usable items.

ACCOUNTING AND PRACTICE MANAGEMENT

As medical services are added to the medical record, charges are added to the invoice. When the receptionist cashiers out the client, the payment is recorded on the invoicing/payment screen. If there is a balance on the account, the veterinary software keeps track of the accounts receivable.

The practice administrator sets a time within the system when accounts are considered overdue (30 days, 60 days, and 90 days). Monthly bills can then be sent out to all past due accounts. The software is also capable of adding a late fee depending on the length of delinquency.

Today's software also makes it possible to block a client from being able to charge fees in the event that they are habitually negligent in paying their bills. Without alerts and blocks, accounts receivable could get prohibitively high.

Another aspect of the veterinary software is the ability to track income production for each veterinarian. Some practices pay their veterinarians a base salary plus compensation based on production. As entries are made within the medical record, the veterinarian that ordered the service is credited with the production of that fee. Even if the veterinarians are not being compensated for production, this gives management valuable information. For instance, if Drs. A and B are able to produce a consistent percentage of the gross annual income by generating dentistry, but Dr. C's production is much lower, management can have an educated discussion about making appropriate recommendations for care.

Practices will need to supplement with separate accounting software to complement the data gathered within the veterinary software. Products such as Peachtree Accounting or QuickBooks are commonly used. Bookkeepers input information gained from the billing and invoicing features of the veterinary software to manage the financial aspects of the business. This financial software manages accounts payable, prints checks, and tracks expenses. It tracks financial information and prepares tax information for the accountant. There are even programs currently available that allow practices to handle all of this online.

Accounting software, whether it is part of the veterinary software or a supplemental software package, is essential for evaluation and management of the practices' *profit centers.* Profit centers are specific components of a practice that generate income. For instance, boarding is a profit center within the practice. There are costs incurred by the practice to provide boarding services, and there is income generated. Evaluation of the profit-to-loss ratio aides practice managers in decisions regarding that profit center, i.e., staffing, equipment, supplies, etc. To attempt to get this information without the use of a computer would be difficult and time-consuming.

IMPLICATIONS FOR THE FUTURE

PAPERLESS VERSUS LESS PAPER

The term *paperless* applies to a business that manages all of its information on one computer system. Currently, most veterinary practices are considered to be "less-paper" practices rather than "paperless." The typical computerized veterinary practice still generates literally tons of information on paper and media that are not being stored in the computer. X-rays, consent forms, travel sheets, time cards, faxes, admission forms, referral letters, anesthesia/surgery logs, controlled substances logs, etc., are all still produced on a daily basis. A *paperless* office is not a pipe dream any longer. Scanners and CD-ROM technology are readily available and affordable. Information stored electronically is safer than printed media. Ten CDs can store approximately hundreds of thousands of documents. All of that information can easily be carried out of the practice and stored off of the premises. The loss of information in the event of a fire can be catastrophic in a conventional veterinary setting.

Some practice managers hesitate to convert to a paperless system for legal reasons. To date, it appears that no paperless case has gone to court. Yet, the concerns are that medical records must be protected from alteration afterward. Proof of electronic medical record security can be provided by backing up the records on a monthly basis and storing them with a data storage facility. Comparison can then be made by the court that both copies match, ensuring the information contained within has not been corrupted.

OTHER APPLICATIONS FOR COMPUTER USE IN THE VETERINARY PRACTICE

The previous sections involved discussions about the software available to manage many of the business aspects of veterinary medicine. Technicians will find that computers will play an ever-increasing role in their daily professional lives as well.

Continuing education is a good example. There are websites on the Internet dedicated to providing technicians a venue to ask questions, research information, read recent publications, and have direct access to specialists in the field. Some popular sites for technicians are

- www.VetMedTeam.com (Figure 34-9)
- www.VSPN.org (veterinary support personnel network) (Figure 34-10)

These sites require no more than a brief registration form ensuring the site that you are a technician or a technician student. They are free and encourage your participation and professional growth. Both sites have message boards on every discipline, including anesthesia, animal behavior, avian and exotics, clinical pathology, dentistry, emergency and critical care, and practice management. They both have libraries with search engines to narrow the information search. Both sites offer classes for continuing educational credits (fee associated), and both have chat rooms used for classes.

There are other veterinary-related websites.

- www.avma.org
- www.vin.com

The American Veterinary Medical Association (AVMA) site is open to anyone who wants to visit the site, including pet owners. There is a special section of the website called

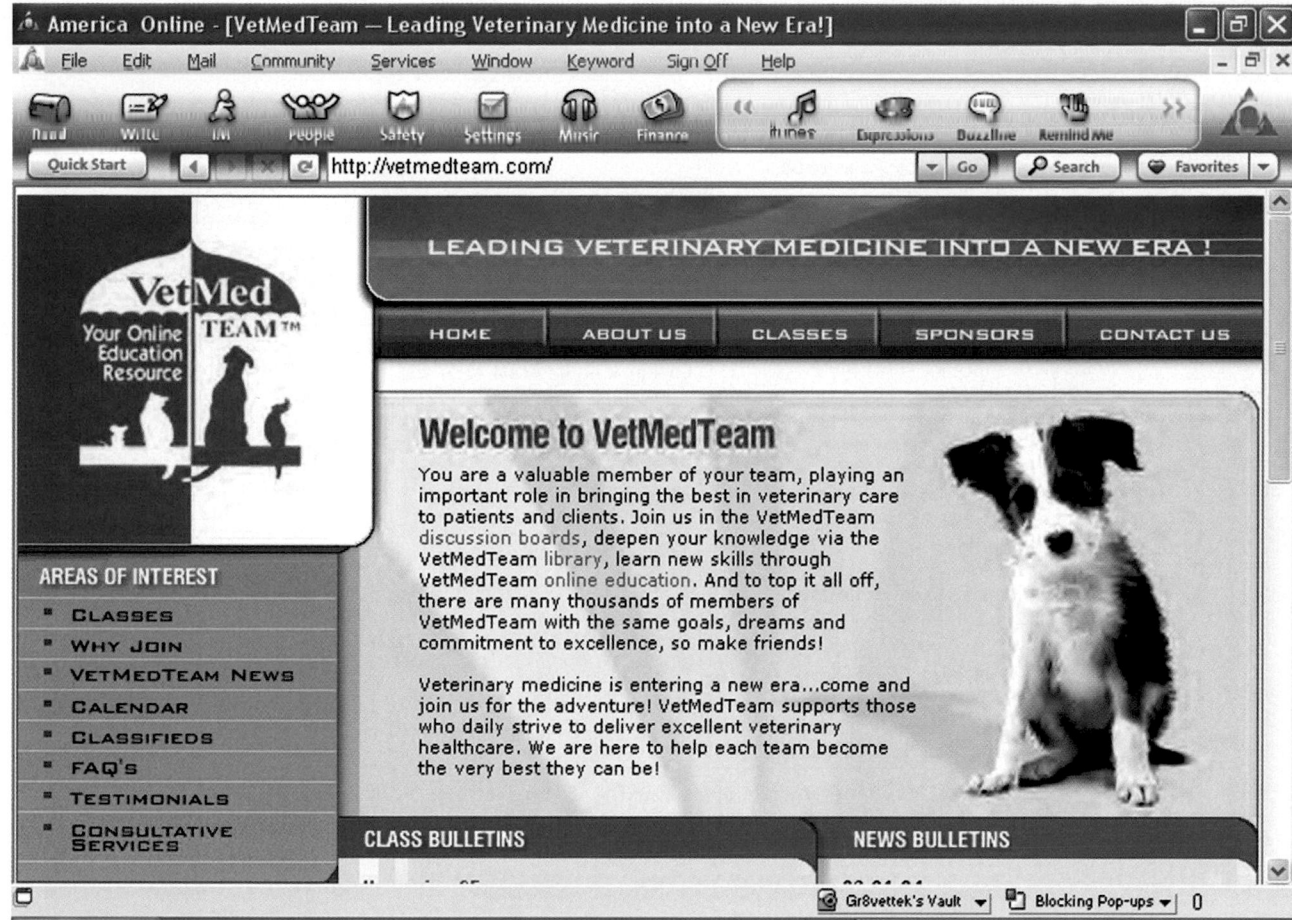

Figure 34-9 The VetMedTeam.com homepage.

NOAH. Access to this area is gained with a membership number (dues required) and a password. The Veterinary Information Network (VIN) site is "for veterinarians by veterinarians." There are membership costs for veterinarians, and technicians are not permitted on this site. VSPN.org is the technician subsidiary of this site.

These sites are all beneficial by offering veterinary professionals a means of discussing cases and sharing information. Each *message board* is monitored or edited by veterinarians or technicians that are either board-certified specialists or hold a certain degree of expertise in a given discipline.

It is not unusual to see digital photographs of lesions, unusual electrocardiogram (ECG) strips, even digital radiographs posted within a discussion. This technology brings the case before many people from all over the world to gain varying ideas and options regarding treatment plans. The caveat to any information obtained on the Internet is this: There are no governing bodies regulating what is written or said on the World Wide Web. These websites have disclaimers reminding the reader that regardless of the recommendations, the veterinarians are ultimately responsible for the care of their patients. Consider and confirm the information read on the Internet before employing it.

THE FUTURE IS NOT FAR AWAY

All of the technology discussed costs the practice money. But money invested up front provides a greater return on investment in the long run. Some equipment available today for veterinarians includes

- Digital cameras
  - For capturing images of lesions, teeth, etc.
  - Adaptable to microscopes for slide imaging
  - Radiographic image capture
- Flatbed scanners
  - Expensive but capable of scanning conventional radiographs
- Digital intraoral radiology
  - An affordable means of capturing and organizing dental radiographs
- Computerized digital otoscope/endoscope
- Video capture systems for ultrasonography

Let's consider some of the ways that computer-related technology can help us provide more efficient and cost-effective medical care for our patients. In the following cases,

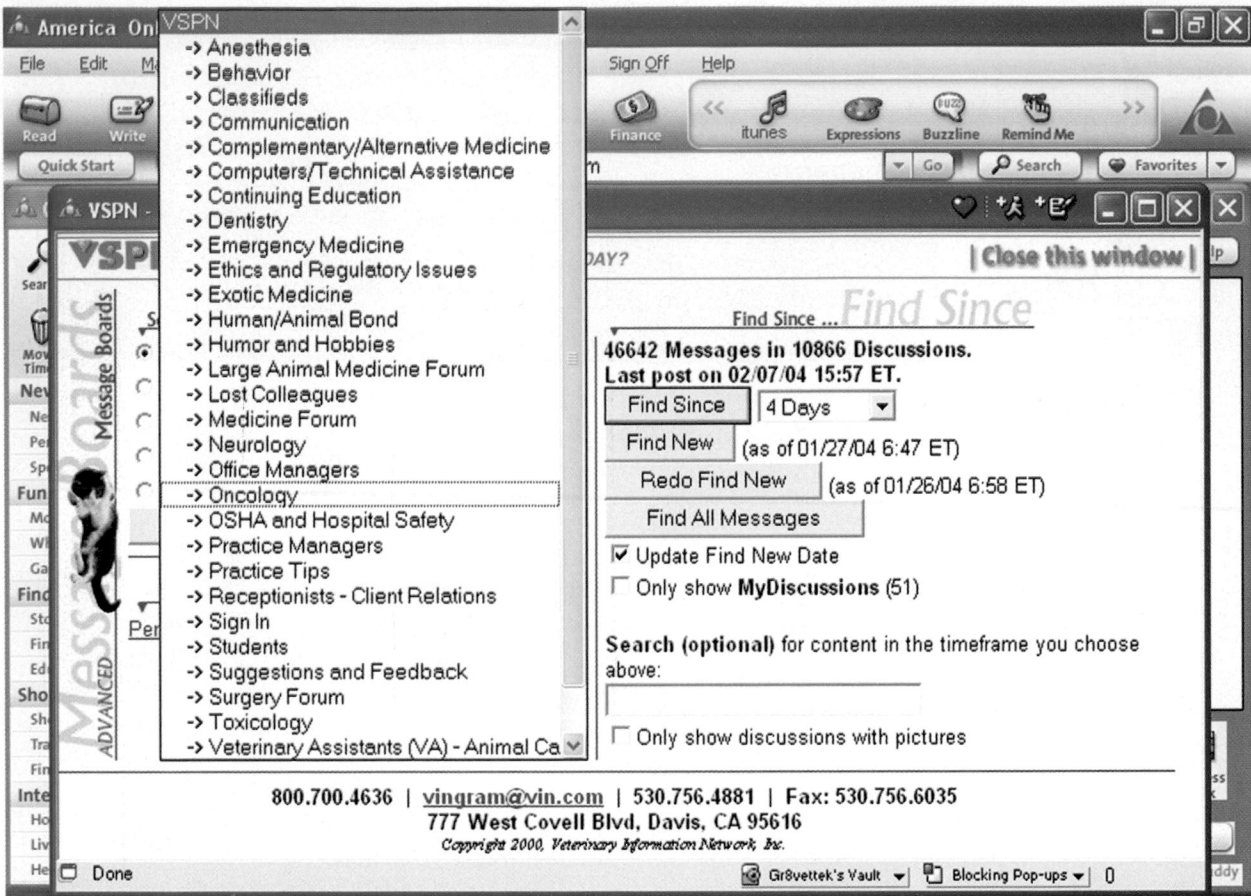

Figure 34-10 The VSPN.org list of message boards in which technicians can participate.

practice A has various computer-related technologies, practice B does not.

1. A cat is admitted to practice A because of a misaligned bite. Practice A does not have a board-certified veterinary dentist on staff. Instead, they take digital photos and digital radiographs and e-mail these images to a specialist. Within hours, practice A has heard from a board-certified veterinary dentist as to whether or not referral holds any benefit to the patient. Practice B would have to copy and send the medical records along with the patient to the specialist for evaluation. These appointments can take weeks to months to obtain.

2. Practice A has provided training for technicians to obtain sonographic video images. These images can either be sent via the Internet to a medical consulting service such as DarkHorse Telemedicine or a radiologist can come into the practice to review the tapes and provide diagnoses. Practice B will have to refer the patient to another practice that can provide these services.

3. Practice A obtains images from cytology slides (Figure 34-6) and maintains the images in a file. The samples

are sent to an outside pathologist for review. When the report returns, the diagnosis is added to the file for educational purposes within the practice. Practice B does not benefit further than the diagnosis itself.

4. Images of lesions are captured and maintained in practice A for comparison. This enables different veterinarians within the practice to evaluate progress without having to be present initially. Practice B requires appointments to be made with the same veterinarian regardless of scheduling conflicts.

5. Practice A wants to research new pain management protocols for their canine patients. They get on the Internet and gain access through VIN.com. They enter CANINE and PAIN MANAGEMENT in the search engine and find 80 documents relating to dogs and pain control is revealed. These documents include discussions on message boards, journal articles, conference proceedings, and clinical resources. After perusing these documents, they have had the ability to read what veterinarians all over the world are prescribing for their canine patients. Practice B will have to register for an upcoming continuing education lecture on the subject, read an outdated textbook or order a new one.

These examples demonstrate how computer-related technology can maintain your patients within your practice, save time and stress to the client and patient, and overall increase revenue.

Veterinarians and technicians are surprised daily with educated owners who have researched their pet's symptoms or disease online and come to their office visit with educated questions for the staff. It is obvious that the World Wide Web and the Internet have an impact on our daily lives.

Technicians tend to pursue the veterinary field to work with animals, to help the patient's families, or because they have a keen interest in the field. The technicians that are willing to invest the time in keeping current with technology will clearly have an edge.

35

Zoonoses and Public Health

MICHAEL G. GROVES • KATHLEEN STORY HARRINGTON

INTRODUCTION

This chapter provides an overview of the major zoonotic diseases and other significant public health concerns that veterinary personnel are most likely to encounter in the course of their work. It is not the purpose of this chapter to present zoonoses, even important ones, that are unlikely to be transmitted to the veterinary technician in the occupational setting. The focus is on the work-related exposure to these conditions, as opposed to exposure via other means. For example, some of the diseases discussed here, such as salmonellosis and brucellosis, also can be contracted by consuming contaminated food, water, or milk. Nonoccupational forms of transmission are mentioned for completeness but are not described in detail; only those routes of infection that are pertinent to veterinary exposure are covered in depth. Likewise, outlined prevention strategies are oriented toward the veterinary profession rather than the public.

The animals listed as carriers or reservoirs of the various diseases are the ones most commonly implicated in transmission in North America (which in some cases may differ from other parts of the world); no attempt has been made to list every host species that could possibly be associated with a given zoonosis. Absent also are those diseases that may affect both humans and animals but that are acquired via environmental exposure rather than true zoonotic transmission (e.g., systemic mycoses such as blastomycosis or coccidioidomycosis). Finally, this chapter is not intended to be a comprehensive reference on zoonoses, but instead it presents a brief review of each disease or condition and provides suggestions for further reading. A summary of the major occupationally acquired zoonotic diseases is given in Table 35-1. ∎

ANIMAL-ASSOCIATED INJURIES: BITE WOUNDS

There are many ways in which animals can adversely affect the health of humans, and for those who work with animals on a daily basis the risk of sustaining an animal-associated injury is significantly higher than that of contracting a zoonotic disease. Large animals can inflict considerable damage with their feet if they kick or step on a person, and many orthopedic surgeons regard horses as the animals most likely to cause injury.

✎ TECHNICIAN NOTE

Animal-associated injuries most frequently sustained by veterinarians and animal care personnel are bite wounds from companion animals.

However, the animal-associated injuries most frequently sustained by veterinarians and animal care personnel are bite wounds from companion animals. A *bite wound* is defined as "any break in the skin caused by an animal's teeth, regardless of intention." In a recent survey of small animal practitioners, cat and dog bites accounted for more than two thirds of the injuries of veterinarians and their employees. A 3-year analysis of Workers' Compensation claims conducted for the American Veterinary Medical Association (AVMA) revealed that animal bites accounted for 49% of all reported incidents and resulted in more than $220,000 in payments to injured personnel each year.

Although cats are reported to inflict more bites in a veterinary setting than do dogs (54% vs. 45%, respectively), dogs are responsible for the most serious bites in both occupational and nonoccupational situations. Dog bites constitute a major public health problem. In the United States, more than 1 million dog bites are reported each year,

Table 35-1 Summary of Major Occupationally Acquired Zoonotic Diseases

	Agent	Source Animals*	Mode of Transmission	Type of Infection	Severity	Notes
BACTERIAL DISEASES						
Anthrax						
Cutaneous	*Bacillus anthracis*	**Cattle, sheep, horses, goats**	Cutaneous inoculation	Cutaneous lesion; may progress to septicemia	Mild (cutaneous only) to fatal (septicemia)	Vaccine is available for people at high risk of exposure.
Inhalation			Inhalation of agent in contaminated dust	Mild upper respiratory symptoms progressing to acute septicemia	Usually fatal	Early treatment prevents progression to more severe disease.
Brucellosis	*Brucella melitensis* biovars	**Cattle**, sheep, goats, swine	Contact with placenta or birth fluids; inhalation; injection with strain 19 vaccine	Septicemia	Severe	Convalescence prolonged; relapses frequently occur.
Campylobacteriosis	*Campylobacter* spp.	**Dogs**, cats, cattle	Fecal-oral	Gastroenteritis, diarrhea	Mild to severe	Most patients recover without treatment.
Capnocytophaga infection	*Capnocytophaga canimorsus*	**Dogs**, cats	Bite wound	Septicemia	Severe to fatal	Asplenic and other immunocompromised people are at increased risk.
Cat-scratch disease	*Bartonella henselae*	**Cats**	Bite, scratch, contact with broken skin	Influenza-like with regional lymphadenopathy	Usually mild, self-limiting	Most patients recover without treatment.
Erysipeloid	*Erysipelothrix rhusiopathiae*	**Swine**, turkeys	Cutaneous inoculation	Cutaneous lesion; rarely progresses to systemic disease	Usually mild	—
Pasteurellosis	*Pasteurella multocida*	**Cats, dogs**	Bite wound	Cellulitis; progression to septicemia possible	Mild to severe	Septic arthritis may develop in persons with rheumatoid arthritis; 50% of infections of hand cause permanent damage.
Plague	*Yersinia pestis*	**Cats**	Bite, scratch, or inhalation	Systemic	Severe to fatal	Early treatment is necessary to prevent fatal disease.
Psittacosis	*Chlamydophila psittaci*	**Psittacine birds,** turkeys	Inhalation of agent excreted in feces	Upper respiratory illness; pneumonia	Mild to severe	Early treatment shortens duration of illness.
Q fever	*Coxiella burnetii*	**Sheep**, goats, cattle	Inhalation; contact with placenta or birth fluids	Systemic, influenza-like	Mild to severe	Usually mild; in rare cases chronic disease and endocarditis develop years after initial infection.
Rat-bite fevers	*Streptobacillus moniliformis* and *Spirillum minus*	**Rodents**	Bite wound or other cutaneous inoculation	Systemic, febrile, usually with polyarthritis	Mild to severe	Untreated infections may persist for weeks or months; fatalities have occurred.
Salmonellosis	*Salmonella* spp.	**Reptiles**, dogs, cats, chickens, ducks	Fecal-oral	Gastroenteritis	Mild to severe	Immunocompromised people are at greater risk for severe illness.

Continued

Table 35-1 SUMMARY OF MAJOR OCCUPATIONALLY ACQUIRED ZOONOTIC DISEASES—CONT'D

	Agent	Source Animals*	Mode of Transmission	Type of Infection	Severity	Notes
Tularemia	Francisella tularensis	**Cats, rabbits** or **hares**, rodents	Cutaneous inoculation via direct contact with infected animal	Cutaneous or systemic	Mild to fatal	Cutaneous lesions can persist for long periods; prompt antibiotic treatment indicated to prevent progression to more severe disease.
FUNGAL DISEASES						
Cryptococcosis	Cryptococcus neoformans	**Birds** (indirect)	Inhalation	Pneumonia; meningitis in HIV-positive people	Mild to severe	HIV-infected people are at increased risk.
Dermatophytosis (tinea)	Microsporum canis, Trichophyton mentagrophytes, T. verrucosum	Dogs, **cats cattle**, sheep	Direct contact with infected animal or spores on hair or dander	Lesion affecting hair, skin, or nails	Usually mild	—
PARASITIC DISEASES						
Cryptosporidiosis	Cryptosporidium parvum	**Cattle**	Fecal-oral	Gastroenteritis	Usually mild, self-limiting	May be life threatening in HIV-infected people.
Toxoplasmosis	Toxoplasma gondii	Cats	Fecal-oral	Systemic, mononucleosis-like; encephalitis	Usually subclinical in immunocompetent persons; can be life threatening in HIV-infected people	Direct transmission from cats rare; primary infection during pregnancy can affect fetus.
VIRAL DISEASES						
Contagious ecthyma (orf)	Parapoxvirus	**Sheep**, goats	Direct contact with infective material	Cutaneous lesion	Usually mild, self-limiting	—
Monkeypox	Orthopoxvirus	**Rodents**	Direct contact with lesion or inhalation	Systemic disease with cutaneous lesions	Mild to severe	Recent cases in United States were all mild, but in Africa up to 10% of cases are fatal.
Herpesvirus simiae (B virus) infection	Herpesvirus simiae	**Old World monkeys**	Bite wound or other cutaneous inoculation; possible aerosol transmission	Meningoencephalitis	Usually fatal	Survivors usually have permanent neurologic sequelae.
Newcastle disease	Paramyxovirus	**Poultry**	Direct contact of eyes with infective material; aerosols	Conjunctivitis; occasionally systemic, influenza-like	Usually mild, self-limiting	—
Rabies	Lyssavirus	Dogs, cats, cattle, **skunks, raccoons, foxes, bats**, etc.	Bite wound or contact with saliva	Encephalomyelitis	Fatal	All animal care personnel should receive preexposure prophylaxis.

HIV, Human immunodeficiency virus.
*Boldface indicates most commonly implicated animals.

which is equal to an annual incidence rate of 300 to 700 per 100,000 population. Probably fewer than half of all bites that occur are reported, however; and some reports estimate the true number is closer to 5 million per year. In 1994, almost 800,000 dog bite wounds in the United States require medical attention, and dogs were responsible for 80% to 90% of those.

In the course of their work, veterinary personnel encounter many situations that may provoke a bite, even from a dog that is not normally aggressive. Some dogs resist being placed in submissive postures or situations, such as during restraint for examination, and will attempt to bite in response to this perceived insult. Other factors that may increase the risk of bites are the stresses that an already fearful dog experiences while in unfamiliar and often uncomfortable surroundings. The unintentional inflicting of pain in the course of restraining the animal, examining it, or administering medication also can provoke a bite.

If a bite occurs, there is a possibility of serious infection developing. At particular risk are persons who are immunocompromised, which includes people who are positive for the human immunodeficiency virus (HIV) or have acquired immune deficiency syndrome (AIDS). Other at-risk persons are pregnant women, people receiving long-term corticosteroid therapy, individuals who have had their spleen removed, and others who have weakened immune systems. All immunocompromised persons should take extra precautions to avoid exposure to infection. Zoonotic diseases that may be transmitted by dog bites include *Capnocytophaga canimorsus* infection, pasteurellosis, and rabies. (These diseases are detailed later in this chapter.) In addition, there is the possibility of permanent damage or disfigurement resulting from the wound.

Cat bites may cause less overt trauma, but because they are usually puncture wounds, are more likely to become infected than are dog bites. Cats can transmit the same diseases.

Veterinary personnel should be alert to possible bite-provoking situations and take measures to ensure that an animal does not have the opportunity to bite. In addition, people with immunosuppressive conditions should avoid handling animals that may bite.

If a bite does occur, regardless of the species of animal involved or the immune status of the person bitten, the wound should be washed immediately and thoroughly with soap and water and rinsed well with a strong stream of water. If the wound is severe, medical treatment should be obtained as soon as possible. An immunocompromised person should consult a physician following even a minor wound because prophylactic antibiotics may be indicated.

Normally healthy people with small wounds should seek medical advice if the wound penetrates a joint or the wound site becomes swollen, inflamed, or painful.

BACTERIAL ZOONOSES

ANTHRAX

Agent
Bacillus anthracis is a large, nonmotile, gram-positive rod that forms environmentally resistant endospores when exposed to air.

Reservoirs
Bacillus anthracis spores are found in soil that has been contaminated with the blood of ruminants (e.g., cattle, sheep, bison) that have died of the disease. In many cases this is attributable to the animal's carcass having been opened or butchered in the field instead of being burned.

Occurrence
Incidence is worldwide except for the far north and some South Pacific islands, but it varies greatly by region. Anthrax in animals occurs sporadically in Eurasia, North America, and Australia but is endemic in Africa, the Middle East, India, Southeast Asia, Mexico, and parts of South America. Warm, humid areas tend to have anthrax "hot spots" because heat stress lowers animals' resistance and the climate encourages sporulation of shed organisms.

Estimates of human anthrax cases range from 20,000 to 100,000 per year, with most occurring in Africa, South America, Europe, the Middle East, and the former Soviet Union. In the United States, naturally occurring human anthrax is very rare, with only seven cases reported from 1984 through 2002 (the 22 bioterrorism-associated cases that occurred in 2001 are not included here). Most cases of anthrax are occupationally acquired; people at greatest risk are veterinarians and animal care workers, abattoir workers, hide tanners, wool processors, and bone-meal producers.

Transmission
Infected animals shed the organism via hemorrhages that occur at death, thus contaminating soil with endospores that can remain viable for years. Other animals can become infected by grazing in the contaminated areas. Biting flies may be involved in mechanical transmission of the bacteria.

There are two forms of human anthrax that are occupationally associated: cutaneous and inhalation. Cutaneous anthrax is acquired when organisms enter broken skin, usually on the hands, arms, or face. Direct contact with tissues or body fluids of diseased animals and exposure to contaminated soil are the most common means of transmission. Inhalation anthrax results from inhaling viable spores that may be present in wool and processed hides of infected animals. A third form, gastrointestinal anthrax, results from eating contaminated undercooked meat and is not associated with any particular occupational exposure.

Disease in Animals
Signs
Anthrax in animals manifests in three main forms: peracute, acute, and subacute to chronic. Peracute anthrax, which occurs in ruminants, is characterized by sudden death with few premonitory signs. The animal appears healthy until just before death, when there may be high fever, muscle tremors, dyspnea, and convulsions. A bloody discharge from various body orifices often occurs after death.

Both ruminants and horses can have anthrax in the acute form. In this form, signs appear up to 48 or more hours before death and may include a period of excitement followed by depression, lethargy, and anorexia. Fever, rapid respiration, and rapid heart rate occur, and mucous membranes become hemorrhagic or congested. The tongue, throat, sternum, perineum, and flanks may become edematous and swollen.

Swine, dogs, and cats that consume meat from diseased animals or other contaminated material can develop subacute to chronic anthrax. Organisms concentrate in lymph nodes in the pharyngeal region and cause swelling that obstructs the airways; death by suffocation follows. Bacteremia can also occur, and some animals may develop enteritis. Carnivores appear to be more resistant to anthrax and often recover.

Diagnosis
The organism can be cultured from blood or tissues of affected animals. In cases of suspected anthrax, necropsy should not be performed to prevent exposing any *B. anthracis* organisms to air, thus causing sporulation and contamination of the site. Because blood does not clot following death from anthrax because of toxin produced by the organism, a sample can be collected from the jugular vein using a disposable syringe. Capped syringes should be refrigerated and submitted promptly to a laboratory for culture.

Disease in Humans
Signs and Symptoms
Cutaneous anthrax accounts for more than 95% of cases. Within 1 week of inoculation a small, painless, reddish, pruritic papule forms and develops into a fluid-filled vesicle. The area surrounding the lesion becomes edematous, and secondary vesicles may form around the initial site. The typical lesion of cutaneous anthrax is a black eschar that develops after a vesicle ruptures and ulcerates. Most patients recover within 10 days of onset, but in some cases cutaneous anthrax progresses to systemic disease. Disseminated anthrax is rapidly fatal if untreated.

Inhalation anthrax is a very serious disease. It is almost always fatal in any case that is not recognized early and treated aggressively using appropriate antibiotics. In the early stages, inhalation anthrax produces only mild and nonspecific upper respiratory symptoms. But within 3 to 5 days toxins produced by the bacteria begin to overwhelm the system and the patient becomes acutely ill, with fever, shock, and rapidly progressing respiratory distress. Death occurs within 24 hours of onset of the acute phase.

Diagnosis
Cutaneous anthrax is easily diagnosed if the disease is considered among the possibilities. Gram staining of the vesicular fluid often reveals large, gram-positive rods, and cultures of the fluid are usually positive for *B. anthracis* if specimens are collected before antibiotic therapy is begun.

The diagnosis of inhalation anthrax is much more difficult because early signs suggest an influenza-like infection. Unless the index of suspicion is high, as was the case in the bioterrorism-associated anthrax cases in the eastern United States during October and November 2001, death may occur before the diagnosis is made.

Treatment
Cutaneous anthrax responds well to antibiotic treatment. Inhalation anthrax also is treatable using antibiotics, but therapy must be initiated early in the course of the disease. If the fulminant stage is reached before treatment begins, even massive doses of antibiotics are not effective.

Prevention
Laws covering the prevention of anthrax are in force in most areas. Livestock vaccines are available and effective. When an outbreak occurs, affected animals should be treated with antibiotics and survivors quarantined for 21 days after the last death has occurred. As noted above, necropsy should not be performed on any animal suspected of having died from anthrax. Carcasses should be burned at the site, if possible, instead of buried because spores can survive for many years in soil. If an animal must be buried, there should be a deep burial, and the carcass should be covered with a layer of quick lime (anhydrous calcium oxide) before the dirt is replaced. Disposable material that must come in contact with infected animals should be burned or disinfected and buried. Contaminated surfaces and other nondisposable items should be cleaned with a disinfectant known to be effective against anthrax spores.

A 6-dose vaccine series is available for those at high risk of occupational exposure to anthrax, such as researchers who work directly with the organism and military personnel deployed to areas in which exposure may be likely. Routine vaccination of veterinarians and veterinary technicians is not recommended in the United States because of low incidence in animals.

Anyone coming into contact with an animal that may have anthrax should be particularly careful about hygiene and care of any wounds and seek medical care should signs of infection develop.

Reporting and Surveillance

Both human anthrax and animal anthrax are reportable diseases in the United States and other developed countries. In the United States, animal cases must be reported to the appropriate state animal health agency.

PSITTACOSIS (AVIAN CHLAMYDIOSIS)

Agent

Chlamydophila (formerly *Chlamydia*) *psittaci* is an obligate, intracellular, gram-negative bacterium with a unique biphasic reproductive cycle, of which only one phase is infectious.

Reservoirs

Birds, especially psittacines (members of the parrot family), pigeons, and doves, and poultry, including ducks and turkeys, are reservoirs for the causative organism.

Occurrence

Incidence of *psittacosis,* as it is called when it affects humans, and avian chlamydiosis is worldwide. The disease is endemic in birds and sporadic in humans. Prevalence in avian species varies widely; active avian chlamydiosis in wild psittacines is about 1%, whereas 50% to 95% of some feral pigeon populations may carry the disease. Humans at risk are those who own exotic pet birds, bird breeders, pigeon fanciers, poultry farm or processing plant workers, veterinarians and their technicians who treat birds, zookeepers, avian quarantine station employees, and others who come in contact with wild, pet, or domestic birds.

Transmission

Transmission occurs through inhalation of infective particles that have become aerosolized from dried feces, ocular or nasal secretions, dust from feathers, and so forth. Cleaning cages is a means of human exposure; sneezing and wing flapping by birds also spreads infective material.

Disease in Animals
Signs

Birds may develop peracute, acute, or chronic disease; many are asymptomatic carriers. Clinical signs vary depending on species of host and virulence of the infecting strain, but most cases include depression, anorexia, yellowish or greenish diarrhea, conjunctivitis, nasal discharge, and respiratory difficulty. Morbidity and mortality also differ with strain virulence.

Diagnosis

Diagnosis of avian chlamydiosis can be difficult. Clinical signs can suggest the disease, but there are no pathognomonic features. Microscopic examination of impression smears or fixed sections of spleen, liver, or air sac tissue of birds that have died from the disease sometimes reveals elementary bodies, the infectious phase of *C. psittaci*. Special staining techniques are required, however, and the absence of visible elementary bodies does not rule out chlamydiosis in the avian. Serologic tests, such as latex agglutination and enzyme-linked immunosorbent assay (ELISA), can be used to diagnose the disease in live birds, but results may be negative if testing is performed in the early stages of the infection. It is also possible to isolate *C. psittaci* from swabs taken from the palatine cleft, cloaca, or fresh feces, although a single negative culture should not be considered definitive because of intermittent shedding of the organism. Specimens submitted for culture attempts should be placed into a chlamydial transport medium and refrigerated until processed.

Disease in Humans
Signs and Symptoms

The incubation period for psittacosis in humans is 1 to 4 weeks. Onset can be either sudden or gradual; symptoms include fever, chills, headache, muscle aches, and upper and lower respiratory tract illness. Elderly people, particularly if not treated, may develop severe disease. Complications can include encephalitis, myocarditis, hepatitis, arthritis, and thrombophlebitis. Most cases, however, are mild or moderate, with recovery in 7 to 10 days in patients receiving appropriate treatment; the case-fatality rate among such patients is less than 1%.

Diagnosis

A history of exposure to birds is suggestive. Serologic tests are the means of diagnosis most frequently used, with a fourfold rise in titer between paired sera collected 2 to 3 weeks apart being considered confirmatory. The agent can be isolated from sputum or blood, but if antibiotics have been administered, the chances of recovery of the organism are reduced.

✎ TECHNICIAN NOTE

Avian practitioners and others who work with birds should be aware of the possibility of *C. psittaci* infection and take appropriate precautions.

Treatment

Psittacosis responds to various antibiotics, with tetracycline or doxycycline usually being the drug of choice.

Prevention

The aim of the 30-day quarantine period for imported birds mandated by law in the United States is to detect birds infected with Newcastle disease virus and does not ensure that birds entering the country are free from *C. psittaci*; likewise, many domestically reared birds may be carriers. Infected birds can appear healthy and still shed the organism, particularly when stressed by crowding, shipping, or other adverse conditions. Therefore avian practitioners and others who work with birds should be aware of the possibility of *C. psittaci* infection and take appropriate precautions. Rapid diagnosis and an effective treatment program for birds can help reduce human exposure.

If a bird is suspected of having avian chlamydiosis, it should be isolated, and all personnel caring for it should wear face masks and protective clothing. Cage papers should be wetted with a quaternary ammonium disinfectant before cage cleaning to minimize aerosolization of infective particles. Laboratory coats and other protective clothing should be removed and hands washed after contact with an infected bird. There is no vaccine for either birds or humans.

Reporting and Surveillance

In the United States and many other countries, psittacosis in humans must be reported to local health authorities.

BRUCELLOSIS

Agent

Brucella melitensis is a small, gram-negative coccobacillus. Humans are susceptible to infection by various biovars of this organism, including *B. melitensis* biovar *abortus*, *B. melitensis* biovar *melitensis*, *B. melitensis* biovar *suis*, and *B. melitensis* biovar *canis*.

> **✎ TECHNICIAN NOTE**
>
> More than 500,000 cases of human brucellosis are estimated to occur annually, with most in developing countries and most occurring as a result of contaminated milk.

Reservoirs

Brucella melitensis biovar *abortus* is primarily carried by cattle, bison, Asian buffaloes, and North American elk; sheep, goats, horses, and other domestic livestock can maintain the infection within herds. Domestic goats and sheep are the major carriers of *B. melitensis* biovar *melitensis*; cattle, camels, and dogs also are susceptible to infection with this species. *B. melitensis* biovar *suis* is carried by swine, but European hares, reindeer, caribou, and some rodents are hosts for certain strains of this species. Canine species, both domestic and wild, are reservoirs for *B. melitensis* biovar *canis*.

Occurrence

With a worldwide incidence, more than 500,000 cases of human brucellosis are estimated to occur annually, with most in developing nations and most occurring from contaminated milk. Countries bordering the Mediterranean and in the Middle East, India, central Asia, Mexico, and Central and South America have the highest incidence.

Human brucellosis has decreased radically in industrialized countries in which active programs to eliminate animal disease have been undertaken. In these countries, brucellosis primarily is an occupational disease among people who work with animals. In the United States, fewer than 200 cases are reported each year. Farm workers, abattoir workers, and especially veterinarians and their technicians are at the greatest risk.

Transmission

Among most animals, transmission occurs primarily through consumption of feed or other material contaminated with infected birth fluids. Although the organisms do not multiply outside a host, brucellae may survive in the environment for several months under moist, cool conditions, thus providing a source of infection for susceptible animals that may ingest contaminated material. *B. melitensis* biovar *suis* and *B. melitensis* biovar *canis* can be sexually transmitted.

As an occupational disease, human brucellosis is most often contracted by farmers and veterinarians via direct contact with aborted fetuses, placentae, or vaginal fluids from infected animals. The organism enters though broken skin. Accidental self-inoculation with strain 19 bovine vaccine is responsible for a small number of cases annually. Aerosol transmission is another important route of infection and can occur in farm, abattoir, and laboratory settings.

Disease in Animals

Signs

Abortion is the major sign of brucellosis, regardless of which species of animal is infected or which of the biovars of *Brucella* is the infective agent. *B. melitensis* biovar *abortus* also can cause reduced milk production among infected cows and orchitis, seminal vesiculitis, and ampullitis among bulls; fertility of both genders is often adversely affected. *B. melitensis* biovar *suis* infections of swine cause similar clinical signs, and arthritis also may occur. In sheep and goats *B. melitensis* biovar *melitensis* causes mastitis, orchitis, arthritis, and spondylitis. *B. melitensis* biovar *canis* infection in dogs is characterized by bacteremia, lymphadenitis, and splenitis, in addition to reproductive tract lesions similar to those exhibited by livestock.

Diagnosis

Isolation of organisms from infective material, such as aborted fetuses and blood, is definitive, but brucellae are slow growing, and standard laboratory culture procedures may not always be effective. A variety of serologic tests are available.

Disease in Humans

Signs and Symptoms

Human brucellosis is highly variable in presentation, with patients often having many vague, nonspecific symptoms. Onset may be sudden or insidious, with symptoms appearing gradually over 1 week or longer.

Most human cases are caused by *B. melitensis* biovar *abortus* or *B. melitensis* biovar *melitensis*. In acute systemic brucellosis caused by *B. melitensis* biovar *abortus*, patients often have fever, nausea, vomiting, and other gastrointestinal complaints. In undulant fever caused by *B. melitensis* biovar *melitensis*, cycles of waxing and waning fever occur. Each cycle lasts a few weeks and is followed by a brief afebrile period before another cycle begins. In both forms of the disease, osteoarticular involvement occurs in up to 60% of patients, and complications involving the male reproductive tract, such as epididymitis and orchitis, occur in up to 20% of cases. Endocarditis is a rare but significant complication and accounts for most of the fatalities associated with brucellosis (2% or fewer).

Infection with *B. melitensis* biovar *suis* can produce similar clinical signs and also may result in chronic liver or splenic abscesses. *B. melitensis* biovar *canis* infections are similar to those of *B. melitensis* biovar *abortus* but tend to cause less severe illness and fewer complications. Some patients relapse repeatedly with febrile episodes even after successful treatment; chronic arthritis is often seen in these individuals.

Diagnosis

Definitive diagnosis is possible only when the organism is recovered from a clinical specimen. However, unless brucellosis is suspected and the laboratory is notified, routine culture procedures may not allow sufficient incubation time for the slow-growing bacteria to become detectable. Serologic tests are available, but false-negative results are possible in many of these, and conventional testing does not detect antibodies to *B. melitensis* biovar *canis*. Deoxyribonucleic acid (DNA) probes and polymerase chain reaction (PCR) techniques are new developments, but their practical application for clinical diagnosis has yet to be determined.

Treatment

Brucellosis responds best to combinations of antibiotics; treatment regimens using only one drug are not as successful. Relapses occur in some cases because of sequestered organisms; these patients require re-treatment with the original combination of antibiotics.

Prevention

Control of human brucellosis depends on the control of brucellosis in livestock. Reservoir animals should be eliminated through testing and slaughter of infected livestock. Farmers, slaughterhouse workers, and others who come into contact with potentially infected animals should be aware of the possibility of brucellosis and should take precautions to reduce risk. Laboratory personnel working with *B. melitensis* biovars should be aware of the potential for aerosol spread of the organisms and handle cultures or potentially infected tissues only within biologic safety cabinets.

Reporting and Surveillance

In most states and countries, both animal and human brucellosis cases must be reported to local health or veterinary authorities.

CAMPYLOBACTERIOSIS

Agent

Campylobacter spp. are small, curved, gram-negative bacilli. *C. jejuni* and *C. coli* are responsible for most human clinical cases.

Reservoirs

Campylobacter organisms are carried, often asymptomatically, in the intestinal tracts of many birds and mammals. Chickens and other commercial poultry are the main reservoirs for *C. jejuni*. Cattle and swine also carry *C. jejuni* and *C. coli*, and kittens and puppies, particularly if feral or obtained from animal shelters or other large-scale pet suppliers, often are infected with the organism.

> **✎ TECHNICIAN NOTE**
>
> Up to 40% of diarrheic puppies and 10% of adult dogs with diarrhea are infected with *C. jejuni* or *C. coli*.

Occurrence

Campylobacteriosis occurs worldwide in all age-groups and is probably the most common cause of food or waterborne diarrhea in the world. In the United States, incidence is estimated to be 15 cases per 100,000 population, with an annual total exceeding 2 million cases; other industrialized nations report similar incidence rates. In developing nations, the rate of infection may be much higher.

In animals, the rate among some commercial poultry flocks approaches 100%. Up to 40% of diarrheic puppies and 10% of adult dogs with diarrhea are infected with *C. jejuni* or *C. coli*. The rates vary widely for other farm and companion animals.

Transmission

Although ingestion of organisms in uncooked or undercooked food is the most common means of acquiring the infection, fecal-oral transmission in a farm or veterinary environment is also an efficient means of spread. Direct contact with infected diarrheic companion or farm animals can result in human infection if the bacteria are transferred from hands to mouth. The infective dose is very small, so even a small inoculum introduced into the mouth may cause disease. In one study, it was estimated that 6.3% of cases had been acquired through exposure to diarrheic animals, mostly dogs.

Campylobacter organisms are somewhat fragile and subject to desiccation and chemical disinfection but can survive for hours or days at room temperature in feces or other moist material.

Disease in Animals
Signs
Many animals and birds are asymptomatic carriers, shedding the organism in feces. Puppies and kittens may develop acute enterocolitis with diarrhea, vomiting, and fever. Infection in foals, calves, lambs, and kids is characterized by fever, mucoid or hemorrhagic diarrhea, depression, and dehydration.

Diagnosis
The causative organism is isolated from feces. Specimens should be collected on sterile swabs and placed in a transport medium, preferably Cary-Blair, until laboratory processing. Special culture techniques, including selective media and reduced oxygen tension, are required for in vitro cultivation. Incubation at 42° C enhances the likelihood of recovery of the organism from clinical samples.

Disease in Humans
Signs and Symptoms
Campylobacteriosis ranges from asymptomatic infection to severe illness. The main symptoms are acute enterocolitis, with bloody, mucoid diarrhea, abdominal pain, nausea, vomiting, and general malaise. Although most people recover without specific treatment within 2 to 5 days, adults may experience prolonged illness, and relapses are possible. Rarely, extraintestinal infections may occur, or sequelae such as reactive arthritis, meningitis, or Guillain-Barré syndrome may follow the initial enteric infection.

Diagnosis
Isolation of *Campylobacter* spp. as the sole pathogen from fecal samples is presumptive; isolation from blood culture is confirmatory. The specialized culture techniques mentioned above in the section on diagnosis of animal disease also apply here.

Treatment
Treatment is not usually necessary; in most cases, campylobacteriosis is self-limiting, and supportive care is sufficient. For prolonged or severe cases or those complicated by extraintestinal infection, erythromycin is the drug of choice.

Prevention
Strict attention to personal hygiene when handling or working around diarrheic animals or poultry can help reduce the risk of occupationally acquired campylobacteriosis.

Reporting and Surveillance
Many states require reporting of human cases to local health authorities, as do some countries. Animal infections are not reportable.

CAT-SCRATCH DISEASE (*BARTONELLA HENSELAE* INFECTION)
Agent
Bartonella (formerly *Rochalimaea*) *henselae* causes cat-scratch disease. This organism is a small, slightly curved, gram-negative bacillus.

Reservoirs
Domestic cats are the reservoirs for cat-scratch disease.

Occurrence
Cat-scratch disease occurs worldwide. As a clinical entity, cat-scratch disease affects only humans. In the United States, about 22,000 cases are reported each year. It occurs most frequently from July through January and affects all age-groups. Seropositivity rates in cats in the United States range from less than 15% in cool, dry areas to over 90% in the warmer, humid parts of the country; overall seroprevalence approaches 30%.

Transmission
B. henselae infection is transmitted cat-to-cat and cat-to-human by fleas that have fed on infected cats. Cats infected with *B. henselae* often have persistent bacteremia in high levels. When a flea feeds on an infected cat, viable bacteria are ingested and excreted in the flea feces. When these infective flea feces contact a break in the skin, either on an uninfected cat or a human, the bacteria can enter and cause infection. Thus, a cat with both *B. henselae* bacteremia and fleas is necessary for a human to become infected with cat-scratch disease. A cat scratch is not a requirement for development of the disease; any break in the skin that becomes contaminated with infective flea feces can serve as the inoculation site for *B. henselae*.

Disease in Animals
Signs
Cats infected with *B. henselae* usually do not exhibit obvious clinical signs, although at least one strain of *B. henselae* that is pathogenic for cats has been identified. Cats and kittens experimentally infected with this strain developed fever and lymphadenopathy and were lethargic and anorectic. Bacteremia persisted after clinical signs had resolved. Some studies have indicated that bacteremia may last for many

months to several years despite the presence of a strong antibody response.

Diagnosis

An immunofluorescent antibody (IFA) test can be used to detect *B. henselae* antibodies in serum, but this test cannot establish whether a cat has active bacteremia. Isolation of the organism from blood is definitive, but specialized culture techniques must be employed and several weeks are required for colony growth. In addition, experimental studies have shown that *B. henselae* is isolated intermittently from infected cats when they are monitored over time. It is unknown whether this is attributable to sporadic shedding of the organism from some internal focus of infection or whether it reflects a limitation of the microbiologic procedures.

If culture is requested, blood should be collected aseptically in a 1.5-ml Wampole Isolator microbial tube (Wampole Laboratories), an evacuated tube containing agents that lyse erythrocytes and prevent coagulation. If this is not available, a tube containing ethylenediaminetetraacetic acid (EDTA), such as a lavender-top Vacutainer tube (Becton-Dickinson Co.), may be substituted. It should be noted, however, that unless the red blood cells are lysed, chances of recovery of the organism are greatly reduced.

Treatment

Antibiotic therapy is not indicated for cats infected with *B. henselae*. Not only do infected cats show few or no clinical signs, but also efforts to eliminate bacteremia by administration of antibiotics have met with little success.

Disease in Humans
Signs and Symptoms

Most cases of cat-scratch disease are asymptomatic or so mild as to be unrecognized. When clinical disease does develop, it usually presents as a regional lymphadenopathy 3 to 14 days after dermal inoculation of the infectious agent. Low-grade fever, myalgia, and general malaise often occur, and a papular lesion sometimes develops at the site of inoculation. Lymph nodes affected usually are those proximal to the inoculation site; often they are very painful but rarely suppurate. In more than 90% of patients with clinical illness, cat-scratch disease follows a mild course and resolves spontaneously, although symptoms can persist for up to 2 months. Complications are rare, and the case-fatality rate is almost nonexistent.

B. henselae infection may be much more serious in immunocompromised people, however. In these patients cat-scratch disease may progress to septicemia or disseminated disease affecting multiple organ systems. Very rarely, the infection may manifest as bacillary angiomatosis or bacillary peliosis instead of cat-scratch disease. Bacillary angiomatosis is characterized by a vasoproliferative tissue reaction that produces violaceous or colorless nodular lesions on the skin and in internal organs. In bacillary peliosis, blood-filled cysts develop in the parenchyma of the liver, spleen, and other reticuloendothelial structures. Both conditions are potentially life threatening and usually occur only in HIV-infected individuals.

Diagnosis

Although many physicians still diagnose cat-scratch disease solely on the basis of clinical signs and a history of cat exposure, a sensitive and specific IFA test to detect antibodies against *B. henselae* is now available. A titer of ≥1:64 is considered positive, and most patients show elevated antibody levels in the weeks following onset of lymphadenopathy. The organism also can be isolated from lymph node aspirates and blood, but, as in the cat, culture requires too much time to be useful as a diagnostic test.

Treatment

Antibiotic therapy generally is not indicated for cat-scratch disease; in the typical patient it does not shorten the course of the disease or lessen the discomfort of the lymphadenopathy. Surgical excision of affected lymph nodes is not recommended, but needle aspiration can be used to relieve pressure and pain in severe cases. For most patients, rest, analgesics, and heat applied to swollen lymph nodes are adequate treatment. Systemic *B. henselae* infection in an immunocompromised person, however, does require immediate and intensive antibiotic therapy.

Prevention

Aggressive flea control is essential for preventing the transmission of *B. henselae* infection to both cats and humans. Common sense and careful attention to hygiene are also helpful. Wash hands after handling cats. Avoid cat bites and scratches, and thoroughly wash with soap and water any scratches that do occur. Likewise, prevent cats from licking or coming in contact with any break in the skin; keep wounds covered until healed. Immunocompromised people should avoid handling cats with fleas and any kittens with clinical signs that suggest active *B. henselae* infection.

Reporting and Surveillance

Cat-scratch disease is not a reportable disease in the United States.

CAPNOCYTOPHAGA CANIMORSUS INFECTION

Agent

Capnocytophaga canimorsus, formerly known as CDC group dysgonic fermenter-2 (DF-2), is a slow-growing, fastidious gram-negative rod, named for the place where it was first identified (Center for Disease Control).

Reservoirs

Dogs and cats are the reservoirs for *Capnocytophaga*.

Occurrence

Incidence is probably worldwide. Human infections with *C. canimorsus* have been reported from North America, Europe, Africa, Australia, and New Zealand. Most cases have occurred in the summer and fall, and all age-groups are affected. Although only a comparatively few (fewer than 100) cases have been reported since the disease was first recognized, this is more likely attributable to the difficulty in isolating the organism from clinical specimens (making diagnoses difficult to establish) than to the true rarity of the infection.

Transmission

Dog bites or scratches are most often associated with *C. canimorsus* infection; about 65% of cases are attributable to dog-inflicted trauma. Nonbite exposure to dogs, cat bites or scratches, and other animal exposures also have been linked to *C. canimorsus* infection. Even small, apparently inconsequential, dog bites have, in some cases, led to fatal disease.

Disease in Animals
Signs

There are no signs in animals. *C. canimorsus* is a commensal in the oral cavity of dogs and cats and can be isolated from the saliva of healthy animals of both species. Surveys indicate up to 24% of dogs and 17% of cats may harbor the organism.

Diagnosis

C. canimorsus can be isolated from gingivae, saliva, and nasal fluids. Samples should be collected using sterile cotton-tipped swabs, which should be placed in a holding medium until processed.

Disease in Humans
Signs and Symptoms

C. canimorsus infections can be asymptomatic or self-limiting, even in immunocompromised patients. In most known cases, however, a life-threatening illness has developed. Usually presenting initially as a nonspecific febrile illness, *C. canimorsus* infection frequently progresses to an overwhelming septicemia. Disseminated intravascular coagulation, renal failure, endocarditis, cellulitis, and gangrene may occur. In these cases, mortality exceeds 30%.

> ✎ **TECHNICIAN NOTE**
>
> All dog bites, no matter how small, should be vigorously cleansed first with soap and water followed by a povidone-iodine solution and then by thorough irrigation with water.

Many patients have some underlying medical condition that predisposes them to infection; splenectomy is most commonly reported. Other conditions associated with increased risk include age over 50 years, alcohol abuse, long-term steroid therapy, and chronic neoplastic, hematologic, or pulmonary disease. It should be noted, however, that several otherwise healthy young people have developed fatal infections with this organism.

Diagnosis

C. canimorsus isolated from blood, cerebrospinal fluid, or tissues is definitive, but depending on the culture medium used, mature colonies may not develop for 1 week or longer after inoculation. In bacteremic patients, a rapid, presumptive test is a Gram stain of a blood smear or buffy coat. The organism appears as elongated, filamentous, gram-negative rods within polymorphonuclear cells.

Treatment

Penicillin is the usual drug of choice for this infection.

Prevention

Animal care workers should be aware of the possibility of severe or life-threatening infection with this organism. All dog bites, no matter how small, should be vigorously cleansed with first soap and water followed by a povidone-iodine solution and then by thorough irrigation with water. Likewise, an existing wound that becomes contaminated with dog saliva should be thoroughly washed. Medical evaluation should be sought; surgical debridement may be indicated. Immediate medical treatment should be sought if fever or signs of cellulitis develop after an animal bite. Delay in treatment is a risk factor for development of severe infection.

Penicillin G as prophylaxis after a dog bite often is recommended for persons with underlying conditions associated with an increased risk of *C. canimorsus* infection. Asplenic individuals probably should never handle dogs or cats.

Reporting and Surveillance

No formal reports are required.

ERYSIPELOTHRIX RHUSIOPATHIAE INFECTION

Agent

Erysipelothrix rhusiopathiae is a thin, non–spore-forming, gram-positive rod.

Reservoirs

Domestic swine are the principal reservoirs; up to 30% of healthy animals may harbor *E. rhusiopathiae* in their tonsils and continually excrete the organism in feces.

Occurrence

Incidence of swine erysipelas is worldwide and high in parts of Europe, Asia, North and South America, and Australia. Morbidity and mortality are variable, but in some areas intensive vaccination programs are required to allow profitable swine production. Many species of wild and domestic fowl, especially turkeys, also are frequently infected. Fish and shellfish are not known to develop clinical disease, but *Erysipelothrix* frequently is present in their exterior slime.

In humans, *E. rhusiopathiae* infection is related to occupation. Persons most often affected include veterinarians and animal care workers, butchers and other meat handlers, fishermen, fish and shellfish handlers, and microbiology laboratory personnel.

Transmission

Pigs and turkeys become infected through contamination of wounds or oral exposure. The organism is resistant to many environmental influences, including direct sunlight. It can survive for long periods in feces, sewage, carcasses, and water. In humans most cases occur after occupational exposure to the organism, usually via scratches, abrasions, or puncture wounds to the hands or fingers caused by knives, bone splinters, and fish hooks.

Disease in Animals
Signs

Swine erysipelas can be acute, subacute, or chronic. The acute form of the disease is septicemia that may cause sudden death. Subacute erysipelas occurs in animals that survive the initial phase of the disease; this is characterized by the appearance of raised, reddish purple rhomboidal lesions (diamond skin disease) that subsequently become necrotic. Chronic erysipelas may affect the joints, causing arthritis and general unthriftiness, or the heart, resulting in endocarditis and death.

Turkey erysipelas mainly affects adult male birds. In the acute, septic form, birds are depressed and somnolent, with prostration and death occurring soon after onset. Subacute erysipelas is characterized by weakness, diarrhea, and cyanosis and swelling of the snood and dewlap. As in swine, chronic infection may cause arthritis or endocarditis.

Diagnosis

The organism can be isolated from skin lesions and from blood and internal organs of animals with septicemia.

Disease in Humans
Signs and Symptoms

Erysipelothrix infection in humans has manifestations similar to those in animals. In humans, however, the localized cutaneous infection known as *erysipeloid* (to distinguish it from the human erysipelas caused by *Streptococcus* spp.) is the most frequently seen form. Erysipeloid is a cellulitis that usually develops on the fingers and hands after dermal inoculation with the organism; a raised, purplish lesion appears at the site and is accompanied by severe pain and swelling. Although erysipeloid is a self-limiting infection and usually resolves without treatment in 3 to 4 weeks, lesions may recur and last much longer in second attacks.

Systemic *Erysipelothrix* infections are uncommon and only rarely follow erysipeloid. Most patients with systemic disease develop subacute endocarditis; generalized cutaneous infection and septicemia also can occur.

Diagnosis

The organism can be isolated from biopsy specimens taken from the edge of erysipeloid lesions. In cases of endocarditis or septicemia, routine blood cultures will allow isolation of the agent.

> **✐ TECHNICIAN NOTE**
>
> The chances of contracting human erysipeloid infection by those occupationally exposed can be lessened by frequent hand washing with disinfectant soaps or detergents.

Treatment

Erysipelothrix is susceptible to a variety of antibiotics. Some endocarditis patients may require valve replacement.

Prevention

For swine, vaccines and bacterins are available but do not always provide lasting immunity. Good management practices, especially those involving cleanliness and sanitation, must be used as well in areas where erysipelas is endemic.

The chances of contracting human erysipeloid by those occupationally exposed can be lessened by frequent hand washing with disinfectant soaps or detergents and prompt, appropriate treatment of any wounds. No vaccine is available.

Reporting and Surveillance

Erysipelothrix infection, whether in animals or humans, is not reportable in the United States.

PASTEURELLOSIS

Agent

Of the various species of *Pasteurella*, *P. multocida* is most commonly encountered. *P. multocida* is a small, pleomorphic, nonmotile, gram-negative coccobacillus.

Reservoirs

Reservoirs for *Pasteurella* are domestic animals, especially cats and dogs. *Pasteurella* spp., which can infect bite wounds, are found in the oropharynx of 92% and 99% of healthy dogs and cats, respectively.

Occurrence

Incidence is worldwide. Carriage of *P. multocida* is common in domestic and wild animals and birds and affects a wide variety of species. In humans, pasteurellosis occurs most frequently as a cellulitis after a cat or dog bite. Respiratory infections acquired from exposure to farm and other domestic animals also occur.

Transmission

Pasteurella organisms are inhabitants of the upper respiratory tract of a variety of animals. Infection can be transmitted by both bites and aerosol routes. Among poultry, aerosol transmission is the predominant means of spread of the disease. Many people with respiratory infections caused by *Pasteurella* spp. have been exposed to cattle, fowl, or their products. Cats and dogs also may be a source of airborne infection, particularly for immunocompromised people.

Disease in Animals

Signs

Pigs, rats, rabbits, suckling mice, goats, and calves develop atrophic rhinitis after infection with certain toxin-producing strains of *P. multocida*. In sheep and swine the infection can produce pneumonia or septicemia; in rabbits it causes coryza (snuffles). In Southeast Asia and Africa, certain serovars of the organism cause hemorrhagic septicemia among cattle and water buffalo. Avian pasteurellosis (fowl cholera) is an acute septicemic disease that affects all species of domestic poultry and causes high mortality. Although dogs and cats harbor the organism in their mouths and nasopharyngeus with no ill effects, abscesses caused by *P. multocida* often develop after bite wounds.

Diagnosis

Pasteurella spp. can be cultured from the blood or internal organs of animals or birds with septicemia. The organism also can be isolated from tracheal or bronchial washings or other respiratory specimens from animals with pneumonia and from purulent drainage from wound abscesses. The gums and teeth of many healthy cats and dogs yield *P. multocida*.

Specimens for culture should be collected on sterile swabs and placed in transport media; tissues obtained at necropsy should be placed in sterile containers and kept refrigerated until processing by a microbiologic laboratory.

Disease in Humans

Signs and Symptoms

P. multocida is the major cause of soft tissue infections of the hand after animal bites or scratches. The lower leg and face, especially in children, also may be involved. Risk factors for developing bite-associated pasteurellosis include age over 50 years, the hand being the site bitten, and puncture wounds, such as those inflicted by cats, that cannot be thoroughly cleansed. Acute inflammation, pain, swelling, serosanguineous or purulent drainage from the site, and lymphangitis develop, usually within 12 to 24 hours of the bite. In rare cases, the infection may spread into tendons, bones, or joints. In immunocompromised individuals, septicemia, endocarditis, meningoencephalitis, or other life-threatening disseminated infection may occur. *P. multocida* also can cause various respiratory infections, such as pneumonia, bronchitis, sinusitis, or tonsillitis.

Diagnosis

The acute onset of cellulitis after a cat or dog bite, as described above, is highly suggestive of pasteurellosis. Culture of the organism from the wound is definitive.

Treatment

Initial treatment should focus on immediate and thorough cleansing (preferably with a povidone-iodine solution) and rinsing of the wound, followed by professional medical evaluation. Debridement and high-pressure irrigation of the wound should be performed by a physician. As with any domestic animal bite, the rabies immunization status of the animal involved should be determined, and the patient's tetanus immunizations should be updated.

Hospitalization may be necessary if extensive cellulitis develops and there is proximal swelling of the involved limb. Most patients recover completely after treatment with topical, oral, and/or parenteral antibiotics.

Prevention

Hygienic management practices can help control pasteurellosis in animals. Bacterins and vaccines are available for some species of the bacteria.

Bite prevention is the single most important measure for humans. If a bite has already occurred, the major factors in development of bite-associated pasteurellosis are inadequate initial wound care and delay in seeking medical treatment. Debridement and irrigation of the wound are particularly important in preventing cellulitis. No vaccine is available for humans.

Reporting and Surveillance

Pasteurellosis is not a reportable disease in the United States.

PLAGUE

Agent

Yersinia pestis is a small, nonmotile, bipolar-staining, gram-negative rod. It grows slowly and may not be apparent in culture before at least 48 hours of incubation.

Reservoirs

Rodents and their fleas carry the bacteria. In the United States, some of the most important rodents in the transmission cycle include prairie dogs (*Cynomys* spp.), ground squirrels (*Spermophilus* spp.), chipmunks (*Tamias* spp.), wood rats (*Neotoma* spp.), and mice of the genus *Peromyscus*.

Occurrence

Plague occurs in all continents except Australia. In the United States, plague is endemic in the Southwest and Pacific coastal areas, having been introduced into California via rat-infested ships around 1899 to 1900.

Transmission

The infectious dose for *Y. pestis* is very low; 100 to 500 organisms can cause human illness.

TECHNICIAN NOTE

In the veterinary setting, cats are the animal most likely to transmit plague to humans; during 1977 to 1998, 23 cases of cat-associated plague (with five fatalities) were reported in the western United States.

Most cases of plague, whether human or animal, result from the bites of fleas that have fed on infected rodents. When a flea takes a blood meal from a bacteremic rodent, *Y. pestis* is ingested. The bacteria multiply and block the intestinal tract, preventing the flea from digesting the blood. Affected fleas make repeated attempts to feed; because of the intestinal blockage, they regurgitate viable bacteria into the bite wounds, often inoculating multiple hosts before they die of starvation.

Plague can also be transmitted via direct contact with body fluids or tissues of infected animals or inhalation of respiratory droplets from an animal or human that has the pneumonic form of the disease (q.v.). In the veterinary setting, cats are the animal most likely to transmit plague to humans; during 1977 to 1998, 23 cases of cat-associated plague (with five fatalities) were reported in the western United States.

Disease in Animals

Signs

Plague-infected rodents may exhibit hemorrhagic lymphadenopathy, bleeding from the nares, and abscesses. On postmortem examination, there may be necrotic nodules in the liver, spleen, and lungs.

Cats are highly susceptible to plague and often develop illness after feeding on an infected rat or mouse. Clinical signs include abscesses, swollen submandibular and cervical lymph nodes, fever, and lethargy. Secondary pneumonia is possible. Experimental infections suggest that the fatality rate is about 50%.

Dogs are resistant to plague and much less likely than cats to develop clinical illness. In experimental infections, dogs have shown transient mild to moderate fever. When clinical disease does manifest, signs are similar to those in cats.

Diagnosis

Plague can be diagnosed using fluorescent antibody or ELISA tests; state public health laboratories in plague-endemic states and the Centers for Disease Control (CDC) are most likely to have expertise in diagnosing plague. Giemsa or Wayson stains of material from abscesses can be used to screen for typical bipolar-staining coccobacilli, but this is not a definitive means of diagnosis.

Treatment

Prompt antibiotic therapy is indicated for all suspected cases of plague. Gentamicin is the drug of choice for veterinary use.

Disease in Humans

Signs and Symptoms

Plague in humans manifests in three main forms: bubonic, septicemic, and pneumonic.

Bubonic plague is one of the forms that present a danger to veterinary personnel. Although it usually results from the bite of an infected flea, infection can also be acquired via bites, scratches, or other direct contact with infected animals, usually cats. Of the cat-associated cases reported in the United States from 1977 to 1998, 17 were bubonic. Two to 8 days after exposure, there is acute onset of fever and lymph nodes proximal to the inoculation site become swollen and tender. These swollen lymph nodes, called *buboes*, are usually in the groin, underarm, or neck. Affected lymph nodes are extremely painful and sometimes suppurate. Bubonic plague is easily treatable with antibiotics if recognized early in the course of the disease; untreated, the case-fatality rate is 50% or higher.

Septicemic plague usually develops from untreated bubonic plague; only rarely does primary septicemic plague develop from dermal exposure without first forming a bubo. Septicemic plague may cause gangrene of fingers, toes, or the nose and was probably the source of the name *black death* that was first applied to plague during the second pandemic that began in 1346 in Europe. Mortality is high with this form of plague, even when treated with appropriate antibiotics.

Pneumonic plague is the most dangerous form. Primary pneumonic plague is acquired by inhaling infective respiratory droplets from affected humans or animals. Among the 23 cases of cat-associated plague reported from the western United States from 1977 to 1998, five were of this form. Rarely, pneumonic plague can develop secondarily to untreated bubonic or primary septicemic plague. As with septicemic plague, mortality is very high even with appropriate therapy.

Diagnosis

As with veterinary cases, only specialized laboratories, such as some state health departments and the CDC, are equipped to reliably diagnose plague in humans. Antigen detection, immunoassays, immunostaining, and PCR are among the tests that can be used.

Treatment

Various antibiotics, including streptomycin, gentamicin, doxycycline, ciprofloxacin, and chloramphenicol, can be used successfully to treat plague in humans.

Prevention

In plague-endemic areas, veterinarians and veterinary technicians should consider plague among the differential diagnoses of domestic animals, particularly cats that present with fever, lethargy, anorexia, and an enlarged or abscessed lymph node. Misdiagnosis is one of the main causes of veterinary personnel becoming infected with plague. Submandibular buboes can resemble abscesses of wounds sustained while fighting with other animals. Penicillin, which is often prescribed for such abscesses, is not effective against *Y. pestis* and will allow the infection to proceed. When a plague-infected animal is misdiagnosed and sent home with inappropriate antibiotic treatment, the owners may also be at risk of developing infection.

When handling an animal that may be infected with plague, veterinary personnel should wear surgical masks, gloves, and eye protection. Exudates from abscesses and other body fluids should be considered infectious and any objects contaminated with clinical material should be disinfected, autoclaved, or incinerated.

Veterinary personnel who may have come into contact with an infected animal should contact their physicians for possible prophylactic treatment.

Reporting and Surveillance

Plague is a reportable disease in the United States. If plague is suspected in an animal or human, local and state health departments must be notified without delay.

Q FEVER (COXIELLOSIS)

Agent

Coxiella burnetii is a small, obligately intracellular, gram-negative bacterium. Although in the past it was classified as a member of the rickettsiae, more recent studies have shown this to be incorrect. *C. burnetii* is more closely related to bacteria of the genus *Legionella* (the causative agent of Legionnaire's disease).

Reservoirs

Cattle, sheep, and goats are the primary reservoirs; many other mammals, including companion animals and rodents, also may carry *C. burnetii*, as can birds, ticks, mites, and some insects.

Occurrence

Incidence is worldwide except New Zealand. All mammals and humans are susceptible to infection with *C. burnetii*; seroprevalence varies widely with geographic area. Humans at risk include ranchers, dairy farmers, abattoir and packing plant employees, veterinarians and animal care workers, and medical laboratory researchers who work with the organism.

> ### ✎ TECHNICIAN NOTE
> The primary means of transmission of Q fever is inhalation of either aerosols from infected birth fluids and ruminant placentae or dust contaminated by birth fluids or urine.

Transmission

The primary means of transmission of Q fever is inhalation of either aerosols from infected birth fluids and ruminant placentae, which can contain up to 10^9 organisms per gram

of tissue or dust contaminated by birth fluids or urine. The agent also may be present in high concentrations in wool or hides or in soil in areas in which livestock are kept. *C. burnetii* is resistant to high temperatures, sunlight, and many disinfectants. Cattle and other milk-producing animals that develop chronic infection in their mammary glands continually shed the organism in milk; thus consumption of unpasteurized milk from infected animals can lead to human infection.

Although farm animals are the most common sources of Q fever, household pets such as cats, dogs, and rabbits may also transmit the disease. Exposure to newborn or stillborn pet animals has been linked to Q fever among urban residents. *C. burnetii* is easily transmitted in a laboratory setting, with minimal exposures often resulting in disease.

Disease in Animals
Signs

Most species have only asymptomatic infection, although coxiellosis in cattle, sheep, and goats sometimes causes abortion.

Diagnosis

Various serologic tests are used to diagnose coxiellosis in animals.

Disease in Humans
Signs and Symptoms

Q fever usually manifests as an acute febrile disease, often with sudden onset of fever, chills, profuse sweating, intense retroorbital pain, and malaise 2 to 6 weeks after exposure. A maculopapular rash is common. Some patients develop atypical pneumonia and a mild cough; others may experience severe respiratory distress. Infections that occur during pregnancy may cause spontaneous abortion. Complications of acute infection may include meningoencephalitis and cardiac involvement. Most cases are mild and self-limiting; the case-fatality rate for untreated Q fever patients is less than 1% to 2.5%.

A few patients develop chronic infection, which gradually becomes apparent years after the initial illness and usually manifests as endocarditis. This form of Q fever occurs primarily in patients with a history of heart valve disease or other immunosuppressive conditions. Patients with this form of Q fever may develop hepatomegaly, splenomegaly, renal insufficiency, or stroke; progressive heart failure is common. Because of its insidious onset long after the primary episode of disease, medical care may not be sought until late in the course of the illness. Q fever endocarditis has a case-fatality rate of more than 60%.

Diagnosis

Diagnosis of Q fever is easy if a physician suspects the disease; serologic testing is effective in diagnosing both acute and chronic infection. Because the clinical picture of acute Q fever can mimic so many other infectious diseases, however, the illness may not be considered among differential diagnoses in areas in which Q fever does not often occur. A history of exposure to a reservoir is an important epidemiologic clue. Likewise, chronic Q fever has few obvious signs but should be suspected in a patient with valvular heart disease and an unexplained infectious or inflammatory process.

Treatment

Antibiotics such as tetracycline or doxycycline are usually prescribed for both acute and chronic Q fever. The course of treatment for patients with acute disease is usually 15 to 21 days, whereas 3 or more years of antibiotic therapy may be required for cases of Q fever endocarditis.

Prevention

Avoid contact with possibly infected animals. A vaccine is available for people who work with reservoir animals.

Reporting and Surveillance

Q fever must be reported to local health authorities in the parts of the United States in which the disease is endemic. In many other countries, it is not a reportable disease.

RAT-BITE FEVERS: *STREPTOBACILLOSIS* SPECIES AND SPIRILLOSIS

Agent

Streptobacillus moniliformis is a pleomorphic, fastidious, gram-negative rod that causes streptobacillosis or streptobacillary fever. Spirillosis is caused by a spiral bacterium that is referred to in the literature as *Spirillum minus*, or *Spirillum minor*, although neither of these is a valid scientific name. The bacterium probably does not even belong to the genus *Spirillum*, but because it cannot be cultured on artificial media, its true taxonomic position has not yet been determined.

Reservoirs

Primarily rats are carriers; mice, hamsters, gerbils, guinea pigs, squirrels, and other rodents may be occasional carriers. *S. moniliformis* is part of the normal oral and upper respiratory tract flora of both wild and domestic rats and is excreted in urine. Spirillum minus is found on the teeth and in the blood and conjunctival secretions of rats and other rodents. This organism has been identified in up to 48% of rats, both wild and laboratory strains, and laboratory mice.

Occurrence

Both rat-bite fevers occur sporadically worldwide, mostly in poor urban areas and among laboratory or animal care personnel who handle rodents. Spirillosis is the more common rat-bite fever in Asia, particularly Japan, where it is known as *sodoku*.

TRANSMISSION

Rat bites are the most common means of transmission of both diseases. Cases have been reported in which the disease was acquired via a scratch from an object contaminated with rat saliva, such as a cage. A form of streptobacillosis known as *Haverhill fever* is caused by ingestion of rodent-contaminated food or water.

Disease in Animals
Signs

S. moniliformis generally does not cause disease in rats. However, mice, especially certain inbred laboratory strains, may be genetically more susceptible to infection. Epidemics of streptobacillosis have occurred among research colonies, causing polyarthritis and gangrene. Mortality and morbidity are high in these episodes. Streptobacillosis also may occur in turkeys that are bitten by rats. Clinical signs include purulent polyarthritis, foot-pad lesions, and sternal bursitis.

Spirillum minus is not known to cause clinical disease in animals.

Diagnosis

S. moniliformis theoretically can be isolated from joint fluid or lesions of affected turkeys. Definitive diagnosis is difficult, however, because the organism has unusual growth requirements that routine microbiologic procedures may not provide.

Disease in Humans
Signs and Symptoms

Streptobacillosis, or streptobacillary fever, usually develops within 10 days of a rat bite, or scratch contaminated with rat saliva, that has healed normally. The disease is characterized by sudden onset of headache, vomiting, malaise, fever, and chills, followed by a transient maculopapular or petechial rash that appears on the extremities. Severe pain and swelling develop in one or more joints. In untreated cases, complications can include endocarditis, myocarditis, meningitis, abscesses in various soft tissues or the brain, hepatitis, nephritis, and pneumonia. The case-fatality rate for untreated cases is about 13%, and fatalities have occurred, even in previously healthy individuals, despite aggressive antibiotic therapy. The clinical picture of Haverhill fever is similar, although there may be more gastrointestinal and upper respiratory signs.

Spirillosis often has a longer incubation period, with the onset of symptoms 1 to 3 weeks or longer after exposure. The wound site heals during the incubation period but later becomes swollen, painful, and discolored and develops an indurated, encrusted ulcer. A cycle of relapsing fever begins, with episodes of elevated temperature that last 1 or 2 days and recur at 3- to 9-day intervals. An exanthematous or purplish rash appears, usually on the trunk, and may spread to other areas, especially joints. Muscle aches often occur. Some patients develop various neurologic symptoms, such as headache, nervousness, neuralgia, and weakness. Spirillosis can be complicated by meningoencephalitis, pneumonia, endocarditis, myocarditis, conjunctivitis, septic arthritis, and other lesions. About 10% of untreated cases are fatal; as in spirillosis, fatalities can occur even when appropriate treatment is administered.

✎ TECHNICIAN NOTE

Avoiding rat bites is the most effective means of prevention of *Streptobacillosis* and *Spirillosis.*

Diagnosis

Streptobacillosis can be diagnosed on the basis of isolation of the etiologic agent from blood; as noted above, specialized media and processing are required.

Spirillosis is confirmed by microscopy. Either dark-field examinations or Wright's or Giemsa stains may be used to detect spiral organisms in wound exudates, lymph node aspirates, or, rarely, blood. Specimens also can be inoculated into guinea pigs or mice; spirilla can be microscopically detected in the peritoneal fluid and blood of these animals.

Both rat-bite fevers probably are underdiagnosed because the techniques required for identification of the etiologic agents are not among those usually performed in a standard clinical laboratory. Unless a physician suspects streptobacillosis or spirillosis and indicates this suspicion to the laboratory, ordinary microbiologic techniques and media may not be sufficient to identify either organism from clinical specimens.

Treatment

Both forms of rat-bite fever respond to antibiotic therapy.

Prevention

Avoiding rat bites is the most effective means of prevention of either disease. As with any animal bite or scratch that could be contaminated with saliva, wounds should be immediately and thoroughly cleansed, and medical advice should be sought.

Reporting and Surveillance

When streptobacillosis occurs epidemically in the United States, as in a food-borne or waterborne outbreak of Haverhill fever, it must be reported to health authorities. Single bite-associated cases are not reportable.

SALMONELLOSIS

Agent

There are various serotypes of *Salmonella enterica,* a gram-negative rod of the family Enterobacteriaceae. These serotypes are commonly referred to by genus and serotype name, such as *Salmonella* Enteritidis, instead of the more proper *Salmonella enterica* subsp. *enterica* serovar Enteritidis. (Typhoid fever, caused by *Salmonella typhi,* has no zoonotic occupational component and is not included in this discussion.)

Reservoirs

Salmonellae can infect a wide variety of warm- and cold-blooded animals, both domestic and wild. Reptiles, such as turtles, iguanas, and snakes, are particularly likely to be asymptomatic carriers of *Salmonella* spp.

Occurrence

Incidence is worldwide and common in both animals and humans. Human salmonellosis is mostly a food-borne or waterborne disease and a major cause of gastrointestinal illness and diarrhea. Incidence is highest among infants and young children; immunocompromised persons also are at increased risk. Occupational exposure to reptiles and other infected animals is a risk factor for veterinarians, animal care workers, zoo keepers, and pet shop employees.

Transmission

Consumption of contaminated food, particularly foods of animal origin such as poultry meat, eggs, and milk, is most often implicated in the transmission of salmonellosis. As an occupational disease, salmonellosis is transmitted via the fecal-oral route. Direct contact with infected animals, regardless of whether they show clinical signs of illness, can result in human infection if the bacteria are transferred from contaminated hands to mouth. In addition, indirect contact may be a source of infection; cages and food dishes used by infected animals may be contaminated with the bacteria, which can remain viable for months in dried feces.

✎ TECHNICIAN NOTE

As an occupational disease, salmonellosis is transmitted via the fecal-oral route.

Disease in Animals

Signs

Infections may be clinical, subclinical, or inapparent. In clinically affected animals, regardless of species, most exhibit weakness, recumbency, fever, and diarrhea. Young animals are more likely to show clinical signs than are adults. Chronic carrier states are common in reptiles, birds, and other animals; in some reptiles, fecal carriage rates exceed 90%.

Diagnosis

For clinically affected animals, isolation of the organism from blood or, at necropsy, from internal organs such as liver or spleen provides a definitive diagnosis. Carrier states can be detected by culturing *Salmonella* spp. from rectal or cloacal swabs or fecal samples.

Disease in Humans

Signs and Symptoms

Human salmonellosis usually manifests as an acute entero-colitis with sudden onset 12 to 36 hours after ingestion of the bacterium. Headache, abdominal pain, diarrhea, and nausea are common symptoms, and fever usually is present. Most cases are self-limiting and resolve in a few days. Salmonellosis is rarely fatal except in very young children, elderly persons, and debilitated or otherwise immuno-compromised people. In these groups, there is an increased risk of severe complications such as meningitis or septicemia. Asymptomatic infections can occur.

Diagnosis

Salmonellosis can be diagnosed in patients with enterocolitis by isolating the agent from fecal specimens; in most cases fecal excretion persists for several days or weeks after symptoms have resolved. For patients with septicemia, *Salmonella* spp. can be cultured from blood as well as feces.

Isolates can be sent to reference laboratories for sero-typing; knowledge of the causative serotype can provide an indication of the source of infection. For example, certain exotic serotypes are rarely isolated from animals other than reptiles. When the same unusual serotype is isolated from both the patient and a suspect reptile, it can be assumed that the reptile was the source of the person's illness.

> ### ✐ TECHNICIAN NOTE
> Working with reptiles is a specific risk factor for acquiring animal-borne salmonellosis.

Treatment

Antimicrobial treatment is indicated only for those patients with severe or disseminated infections; chloramphenicol, or fluoroquinolones are among the drugs of choice. Uncom-plicated cases of gastrointestinal salmonellosis generally should not be treated with antibiotics because there seldom is any effect on the course of the disease and because their use can prolong fecal shedding of the organism.

Prevention

Working with reptiles is a specific risk factor for acquiring animal-borne salmonellosis because touching these animals or their surroundings can result in hands becoming contaminated with *Salmonella* spp. Wild fowl also frequently carry *Salmonella* spp., and diarrheic companion animals and livestock can also be sources of infection. Careful attention to personal hygiene, especially the use of gloves and frequent hand washing, can help reduce the risk of occupationally acquired salmonellosis.

Veterinarians and technicians should advise their clients who own reptiles, baby chicks, or ducklings that these animals increase the owners' risk of acquiring *Salmonella* infection and should stress the need for thorough hand washing after handling these animals or their cages. In addition, these pets should be kept out of food preparation areas. Kitchen sinks should never be used to bathe reptiles or to wash their dishes, cages, or aquariums. Likewise, sinks or tubs in which infants and children are bathed should never be used for such purposes. The U.S. Centers for Disease Control and Prevention recommend that people at increased risk for infection or serious complications of salmonellosis, including pregnant women, children under 5 years of age, and immunocompromised individuals, avoid all contact with reptiles. Reptiles may be inappropriate pets for households with young children because some cases have been reported in which there was no known contact, direct or indirect, between the child and the reptile.

Reporting and Surveillance

In the United States, confirmed cases of human salmonellosis must be reported to local health authorities.

TULAREMIA

Agent

Tularemia, also known as *rabbit fever*, is caused by *Francisella tularensis*, a fastidious, slow-growing, aerobic gram-negative coccobacillus. There are two biovars, *F. tularensis* biovar *tularensis*, or type A, which is highly virulent, and *F. tularensis* biovar *palaearctica*, or type B, which is less so.

Reservoirs

Ticks of various species serve as both reservoir and vector for *F. tularensis*, Hares and rabbits also are important reservoirs, as are squirrels, voles, muskrats, and other rodents. The organism also can be isolated from contaminated water, soil, and vegetation in which it can persist for weeks or months.

Occurrence

Francisella tularensis occurs naturally only in the Northern Hemisphere. Type A is found almost exclusively in North America; type B is present in both North America and Eurasia. In the United States, most cases in humans occur in Arkansas, Missouri, South Dakota, and Oklahoma, although it has been recorded in all states except Hawaii.

Transmission

The infectious dose for *F. tularensis* is very low; as few as 10 to 50 organisms can cause disease. Tularemia is most commonly acquired via the bite of an infective arthropod, usually a tick. The disease can also be transmitted by inges-tion, e.g., eating meat from infected animals or drinking contaminated water; by inhalation, often via laboratory accident or activities that stir up contaminated soil, such as gardening or lawn mowing; or by direct contact with skin, blood, or internal organs of infected animals.

It is this latter means that is of most consequence in the context of veterinary exposure. *F. tularensis* has been reported to penetrate unbroken skin, but infection usually occurs through contamination of an open wound such as a bite or scratch. Infection with biovar type A is usually associated with contact with infected rabbits, cats, or dogs; sheep are more often infected with type B.

> ### ✎ TECHNICIAN NOTE
>
> Cats are susceptible to infection with tularemia, and most cases that have been recorded in veterinary personnel have been acquired via exposure to infected cats.

Disease in Animals
Signs

Tularemia can cause disease in a wide range of both wild and domestic animals. In the United States, lagomorphs (rabbits and hares) are frequently infected, and epizootics have occurred in voles, beavers, and muskrats. Domestic animals most often involved are cats, dogs, and sheep.

Rabbits in the early stages of tularemia seem tame. As the disease progresses, they become unable to raise their heads or control their forelegs properly; they may have irregular muscle spasms and sometimes can stagger only a few feet between spasms. They often rub their noses and forefeet on the ground.

Cats are susceptible to infection with tularemia, and most cases that have been recorded in veterinary personnel have been acquired via exposure to infected cats. Cats usually develop abscesses at the inoculation site, have high fevers, enlarged lymph nodes, and ulcers in the oral cavity. Ocular and nasal discharges develop after about a week of illness, and a rash may appear. Kittens are usually more severely affected than are older cats.

Dogs are fairly resistant to the disease, although cases have been recorded. In this species the only signs may be loss of appetite, lethargy, and low fever. As in cats, the disease is often worse in puppies than in older dogs.

Sheep usually become infected with tularemia after severe winters when their body condition has deteriorated, their nutritional status is below optimum, and they are heavily infested with ticks. Clinically affected sheep have high fever, weight loss, swollen lymph nodes, and diarrhea.

Diagnosis

Serologic tests, such as ELISA or fluorescent antibody (FA), are available for diagnosis. The organism can be cultured from blood or tissue, but because the infectious dose is so low, culture should be attempted only when using at least biological safety level (BSL) 3 procedures in a laboratory equipped at least with BSL 2 facilities.

Disease in Humans
Signs and Symptoms

There are three major manifestations of tularemia in humans: ulceroglandular, typhoidal, and pneumonic. Ulceroglandular is the most common and results from the organism entering through the skin or from mucous membrane exposure. One to 6 days after exposure, there is acute onset of fever, chills, malaise, headache. An ulcerlike lesion develops at the site of inoculation; regional lymph nodes become swollen and painful and sometimes suppurate. However, ulceroglandular tularemia is the least potentially serious of the various manifestations of the disease; fatalities occur in less than 1% of patients who receive appropriate and timely antimicrobial treatment. Untreated ulceroglandular tularemia can progress to secondary pleuropneumonia, meningitis, or sepsis and can be fatal in up to 15% of cases in the United States.

Typhoidal tularemia (caused by ingestion of contaminated food or water) and primary pneumonic tularemia (caused by inhalation of the bacteria) are more serious forms of infection. Untreated primary pneumonic tularemia can be fatal in up to 60% of untreated patients.

Diagnosis

Serologic tests are used to detect agglutinating antibodies. Isolation of the organism from clinical specimens provides a definitive diagnosis, but as noted above, it is very dangerous to attempt culture of *F. tularensis* without adequate laboratory safety precautions.

Treatment

Antibiotics are effective in treating all forms of tularemia. Streptomycin is the drug of choice for humans, but gentamicin, tetracyclines, and chloramphenicol also can be used.

Prevention

In areas where tularemia is endemic, veterinarians should consider the possibility of this infection in any animals with fever, whether or not they have enlarged lymph nodes. Standard precautions for handling animals, both for patient care and for postmortem examination, reduce the risk of transmission. No vaccine is available.

Reporting and Surveillance

Tularemia had been removed from the list of nationally reportable diseases in 1994, but it was restored to the list in 2000 because of the potential for use of *F. tularensis* as a biological weapon. Thus, both animal and human cases of tularemia are required to be reported to public health authorities.

MYCOTIC ZOONOSES

SYSTEMIC INFECTIONS: CRYPTOCOCCOSIS
Agent

Cryptococcus neoformans is an encapsulated yeast.

Reservoirs

Although a common saprophytic organism that can be isolated from many different environmental sources such as soil and plant materials, *C. neoformans* has a particular affinity for bird excrement, especially pigeon droppings. Sites contaminated with pigeon or chicken excreta often contain much higher concentrations of *C. neoformans* than do surrounding areas; it is thought that creatinine in the droppings enhances growth of the yeast. Viable cryptococcia have been recovered from an aviary that had been unused for 10 years.

Occurrence
Incidence is worldwide and in all age-groups as sporadic cases, although adult males account for a majority of patients. Although many people have serologic evidence of exposure, clinical cases are relatively rare and usually occur in immunocompromised individuals. In the United States 5% to 15% of patients with AIDS develop cryptococcosis; in this group, the infection is often life threatening.

Transmission
Transmission is by inhalation of the organism from environmental sources. Exposure to highly contaminated areas, such as aviaries or pigeon coops, can increase risk of disease.

TECHNICIAN NOTE
Exposure to highly contaminated areas, such as aviaries or pigeon coops, can increase the risk of cryptococcosis.

Disease in Animals
Signs
There are no apparent signs in birds, although the organism can be recovered from the feces of many avian species. Most clinically affected mammals develop a disseminated infection that includes central nervous system signs; mortality is high. In cattle, the disease often manifests as mastitis and causes abnormalities of the udder and changes in milk.

Diagnosis
Cryptococcus can be detected through direct microscopic examination of various clinical specimens using an India ink preparation to reveal characteristic budding yeast cells. Culture and serologic testing can be used to confirm diagnosis.

Disease in Humans
Signs and Symptoms
Most immunocompetent individuals develop only subclinical infection. Among patients with AIDS, meningitis is the most common presentation of cryptococcosis. It results from hematogenous dissemination of a primary pulmonary infection that can precede nervous system involvement by months or years. Pulmonary cryptococcosis is characterized by fever, chest pain, and coughing, with expectoration of blood-tinged sputum. When the infection spreads to the brain, headache, neck stiffness, and distorted vision occur. Confusion and other personality changes may follow. Even when treated aggressively, cryptococcal meningitis has a high mortality rate, and survivors often undergo relapses.

Diagnosis
As described above, direct microscopic examination of India ink-stained cerebrospinal fluid, urine, or pus can reveal cells characteristic of *C. neoformans*. Serologic tests, culture, or histopathologic examination provides confirmation.

Treatment
Combinations of antifungal agents are used to treat human cryptococcosis.

Prevention
For normally healthy people no special precautions are necessary. People with immunosuppressive conditions, such as HIV infection, diabetes, or Hodgkin disease, or who are undergoing corticosteroid therapy should avoid exposure to accumulations of pigeon or other bird droppings. Contaminated sites may be disinfected with a 5% sodium hypochlorite solution.

Reporting and Surveillance
In the United States, cases should be reported to local health authorities. Because meningeal cryptococcosis is so strongly associated with AIDS, official reports are required in some areas.

SUPERFICIAL MYCOSES: DERMATOPHYTOSES
Agents
Dermatophytoses, or tinea, are opportunistic fungal infections of the hair, skin, or nails. *Microsporum canis*, *Trichophyton mentagrophytes*, and *T. verrucosum* are the zoophilic dermatophytes most important in human infection. *M. canis* causes tinea (ringworm) in both humans and animals; in humans this species usually affects the scalp or body (tinea capitis or tinea corporis). *T. mentagrophytes* infection in humans may appear as tinea barbae (ringworm of the beard) or tinea corporis; *T. verrucosum* usually affects the face or upper body.

Reservoirs
M. canis is carried by dogs and cats. Wild mice and rats are primary reservoirs of *T. mentagrophytes*, but dogs, cats, horses, sheep, rabbits, guinea pigs, and other domestic and laboratory animals frequently are infected. *T. verrucosum* is carried by cattle, sheep, and other ruminants.

Occurrence
Incidence is worldwide in both humans and a variety of domestic and wild animals. People at greatest risk are those who work with animals or who live or work in areas that may be contaminated with hairs from infected animals.

Transmission

Transmission is by direct or indirect contact with infected animals or with hair from infected animals or humans.

Disease in Animals

Signs

For *M. canis,* about 90% of infected cats have no visible lesions; when present, lesions are usually on the face and paws and appear as 1- to 2-cm, hairless, scaly patches. Infected dogs usually have lesions similar to those in cats; they can appear on any part of the body. For *T. mentagrophytes* most infected animals develop 1- to 2-cm, hairless, white, scaly lesions on the head or trunk. For *T. verrucosum* young cattle are most frequently infected. Lesions can be small or extensive and begin as grayish white, scaly patches with hair loss. The skin later thickens and becomes scabby.

Diagnosis

Examined microscopically in a wet mount of potassium hydroxide and ink, infected hairs from the inner edge of lesions of both *M. canis* and *Trichophyton* spp. may show an exterior cuff of arthrospores or mycelial elements within the hair shaft. Hairs infected with *M. canis* (but not *Trichophyton* spp.) also may fluoresce bright yellow-green when viewed under a Wood's lamp (365-nm filtered ultraviolet light), although this does not occur in all cases. Isolation of the organism from lesions is definitive. Scrapings or hairs from suspect lesions should be placed in a sterile container and submitted to a laboratory for culture.

Disease in Humans

Signs and Symptoms

For *M. canis,* tinea of the scalp produces scaly patches and temporary baldness because infected hairs are brittle and break easily. Infection of hairless parts of the body often causes formation of a *kerion,* a suppurative, boggy, raised lesion. For *T. mentagrophytes,* lesions are similar to those described for *M. canis* and usually occur on the face or upper body. Some individuals experience a highly inflammatory reaction to this infection. For *T. verrucosum,* lesions usually develop on the face, hands, arms, and upper body. The inflammatory response is severe, and kerions often form; scarring is a frequent result.

Diagnosis

Diagnosis of dermatophytoses in humans is the same as in animals.

> ### ✎ TECHNICIAN NOTE
> Both oral and topical antifungal agents, often in combination, are used to treat tinea infections in both humans and domestic animals.

Treatment

Both oral and topical antifungal agents, often in combination, are used to treat tinea infections in both humans and domestic animals. If kerions are present, a keriolytic

cream may be prescribed. Antibiotics may be required if a secondary bacterial infection invades the lesions. Additional measures for tinea corporis include frequent and thorough bathing with soap and water and removal of scabs and crusts; for tinea capitis or barbae, daily washing of hair and scalp with a selenium sulfide shampoo is helpful.

Prevention

Vaccines to immunize animal populations against zoophilic dermatophytoses have been developed. If the infections can be controlled in animals, prevention of human infection will become much more feasible. Whenever possible, avoid direct contact with animals that show lesions suggestive of dermatophytoses.

Reporting and Surveillance

In the United States reporting is required for epidemic outbreaks of any dermatophytosis but not for individual cases.

PARASITIC DISEASES

CRYPTOSPORIDIOSIS

Agent

Cryptosporidium parvum is a coccidian protozoan parasite.

Reservoirs

Reservoirs for *Cryptosporidium parvum* are humans, cattle, and other domestic animals.

Occurrence

Incidence is worldwide. In the United States and Europe prevalence ranges from less than 1% to 4.5%; in developing nations prevalence may be as high as 20% of the human population. People who come in contact with animals are at increased risk of contracting this infection.

Transmission

Transmission is fecal-oral, which includes human-to-human, animal-to-human, waterborne, and food-borne transmission. On reaching the intestine, the parasite infects epithelial cells and multiplies asexually via schizogony. After a sexual reproductive cycle, the organism produces infective oocysts that are passed in feces. These oocysts are resistant to many chemical disinfectants, including chlorination used in water treatment systems, and can survive in adverse environmental conditions.

Disease in Animals

Signs

Cryptosporidiosis in animals often is subclinical, particularly in adults; younger animals, especially newborns, are more likely to develop clinical signs. Those affected usually develop diarrhea that can range from mild to severe. Calves are an important source of infection to humans and other animals because they develop profuse diarrhea, during which they shed massive quantities of oocysts into the environment. The mortality in livestock is low. Other animals that may develop clinical cryptosporidiosis are cats with underlying feline leukemia or feline immunodeficiency virus (FIV) infection or animals undergoing prolonged therapy with corticosteroid drugs.

Diagnosis

Oocysts can be detected in feces by direct microscopy of smears, sugar or zinc sulfate flotation, or special centrifugation techniques.

Disease in Humans
Signs and Symptoms

Clinical cryptosporidiosis is characterized by profuse, watery diarrhea and cramping abdominal pain. Although symptoms may abate and recur for a time, in most otherwise healthy persons, the disease is self-limiting and resolves completely within 1 month. In immunocompromised individuals, however, the disease can be much more serious. Patients with AIDS and others who cannot clear the infection experience a severe and prolonged illness that can be fatal.

Diagnosis

Cryptosporidiosis can be difficult to diagnose unless suspected and sought. Direct identification of oocysts in fecal smears as detailed above can be successful. Likewise, various life-cycle stages can be detected by histopathologic examination of intestinal biopsy specimens, but *C. parvum* is very small and easily overlooked and can be mistaken for yeast cells if the proper stains are not used. An ELISA and an immunofluorescence test have become available and are more accurate than direct microscopy.

Treatment

There is no specific effective treatment. Supportive care, mainly in the form of rehydration, is effective for normally healthy people. Any immunosuppressive drugs the patient may be taking should be reduced or stopped if possible.

Prevention

People who are in contact with calves or other animals that have diarrhea should be especially careful about hand washing. Those with AIDS or other immunosuppressive conditions should avoid contact with diarrheic animals.

In areas in which water treatment facilities include filtration (which is standard for most cities in the United States), feces from infected animals can be discharged directly into sewers without prior disinfection. Areas contaminated with feces can be disinfected with a 10% formalin solution or 5% ammonia solution. Articles that withstand heat may be heated to 45° C for 5 to 20 minutes or to 60° C for 2 minutes.

Reporting and Surveillance

In the United States, cases of human cryptosporidiosis must be reported to local health authorities. Clusters of disease should be investigated epidemiologically to determine the source of infection.

TOXOPLASMOSIS

Agent

Toxoplasma gondii is an obligate intracellular sporozoan parasite.

Reservoirs

Cats are the only known definitive host (the animal in which the parasite completes its life cycle). Sheep, goats, swine, cattle, and chickens are intermediate hosts and can carry the infective stage encysted in muscle tissue.

TECHNICIAN NOTE

The cat is the only known host of *Toxoplasma gondii*.

Occurrence

Incidence is worldwide. Up to 70% of the human adult population is seropositive, indicating exposure and probable tissue infection. Cats frequently are infected; in some countries, up to 60% of cats have serologic evidence of exposure to the organism. The prevalence in livestock is related to the number of cats in pasture lands. Up to 43% of pigs and 35% of sheep have tissue cysts.

Transmission

After primary infection, cats shed oocysts in feces for only 1 to 2 weeks; subsequent intermittent shedding may occur, but this appears to be rare. *Toxoplasma* oocysts become infective 1 to 5 days after being passed; these are environmentally resistant and can survive for at least 1 year in soil in warm, humid environments. Other animals become infected when they consume soil or other material contaminated with sporulated oocysts.

In humans toxoplasmosis may be primary or congenital. Primary toxoplasmosis is usually acquired through the ingestion of raw or undercooked meat, especially pork or mutton, in which the parasite has encysted. The mode that is of occupational importance, however, is the fecal-oral route (accidental ingestion of infective oocysts).

Congenital toxoplasmosis is acquired through transplacental infection. This occurs when a woman develops a primary infection during pregnancy; rapidly dividing tachyzoites circulate in the bloodstream and can infect the fetus. The risk of serious fetal disease is highest during the first and second trimesters.

Disease in Animals
Signs

In most animals toxoplasmosis produces only subclinical infection, with little morbidity or mortality. Toxoplasmosis in sheep, however, is an exception. In this species, the infection causes abortion or congenital disease that results in neonatal mortality; adults seldom are affected clinically. In some parts of the sheep-rearing world, economic losses from toxoplasmosis are significant. Swine are affected similarly, but the disease is not of economic importance in most areas. Outbreaks in cattle have been reported in which fever, dyspnea, and neurologic signs occur. Infection in horses is usually subclinical.

Most infected cats are asymptomatic, but kittens may develop diarrhea, hepatitis, pneumonia, encephalitis, and other signs. Dogs often are seropositive, but overt disease occurs mainly in puppies weakened by other conditions.

Diagnosis

Antemortem diagnosis is difficult. Oocysts can be detected in feline feces using various flotation techniques, although definitive identification requires considerable further laboratory testing (see Chapter 7). Serologic tests are available for many species but can not be used to differentiate among active, recent, or past infections.

Disease in Humans
Signs and Symptoms

Immunocompetent adults usually have only asymptomatic infection, although toxoplasmosis occasionally causes a self-limiting, mononucleosis-like illness. After the immune response causes the initial parasitemia to wane, *T. gondii* encysts in muscle tissue; these cysts can reactivate and cause disease if the person becomes immunocompromised at some later time.

Cerebral toxoplasmosis is a common opportunistic infection among patients with AIDS, with most cases resulting from activation of latent tissue infection as the immune system deteriorates. These patients often develop subacute meningoencephalitis, diffuse encephalopathy, or a space-occupying lesion in the brain. Lymphatics, lungs, heart, joints, or eyes also may be involved. Up to 40% of patients with AIDS develop cerebral toxoplasmosis, and at least 10% die. Other immunocompromised adults (chemotherapy patients, organ transplant recipients, people who have had a splenectomy) also are at increased risk of this form of toxoplasmosis.

Congenital toxoplasmosis results from primary maternal infection during gestation. When primary toxoplasmosis occurs during the first trimester of pregnancy, 17% of fetuses become infected, and 80% of those infections are severe. For second-trimester maternal infections, 25% of fetuses become infected, and 30% of that number develop severe disease; abortion or premature birth often results. Infections acquired during the third trimester produce a higher fetal infection rate but fewer cases of severe disease. Neonatal central nervous system and ocular infections are the most frequent manifestations of congenital toxoplasmosis. Some babies develop encephalitis, hydrocephalus, or chorioretinitis; blindness, mental retardation, and seizures are possible sequelae.

Diagnosis

Diagnosis is based on clinical signs and results of serologic testing that support the presumption of toxoplasmosis. The organism also can be isolated from biopsy specimens or body fluids after intraperitoneal inoculation in mice; tachyzoites can be detected in mouse peritoneal fluid after 1 week, and cysts may be found in the brain after 6 weeks.

Treatment

No specific treatment is indicated for otherwise healthy people, except for pregnant women with primary infections. In these patients, spiramycin is used to prevent fetal infection; if tests indicate fetal infection has already occurred, a combination of pyrimethamine and sulfadiazine can be used. Likewise, patients with severe symptomatic disease and infants born to mothers who had a primary infection during pregnancy are treated with a combination of antitoxoplasmal drugs and folic acid.

Prevention

Pet cats are seldom the source of human infection because of their fastidious nature. They bury their feces and clean themselves immediately, so feces do not remain on their fur long enough for oocysts to sporulate. In addition, oocyst shedding generally lasts only 1 or 2 weeks after the initial infection, and repeated exposure to the organism does not cause additional shedding. Oocysts can sporulate in litter boxes, so fecal material should be removed daily and disposed of in a toilet or by incineration. Wash hands thoroughly after handling litter boxes or cat feces.

Pregnant women and immunocompromised patients who work with animals should have serologic testing performed to determine whether they have a titer against toxoplasmosis. Those who are seronegative are at risk of developing primary toxoplasmosis and should avoid handling cat feces and changing litter boxes. Because most cases of toxoplasmosis are caused by consuming undercooked meat, those who are at risk also should avoid eating undercooked meat and handling raw meat, which are much more likely sources of infection than cat exposure.

✎ TECHNICIAN NOTE

Wash hands thoroughly after handling litter boxes or cat feces.

Cats should not be fed meat that may contain viable oocysts. Feed only commercial cat foods or thoroughly cook or freeze any meat that is to be fed to cats. (Freezing at −15° C for more than 3 days or −20° C for more than 2 days kills oocysts.) Because rodents and birds can be sources of infection, cats should be kept indoors when possible to prevent hunting.

Reporting and Surveillance

Reporting is not required in most areas, but it is in some states and countries in which epidemiologic studies are being conducted.

VIRAL DISEASES

MONKEYPOX

Agent
Monkeypox is caused by monkeypox virus, an orthopoxvirus.

Reservoirs
In Africa, where monkeypox virus originates, the virus has been found in various nonhuman primates, rodents, and squirrels, but the reservoir has not been definitively established.

Occurrence
Until 2003, monkeypox had only been reported from the rainforests of central and West Africa. However, an outbreak occurred in June of that year in the United States. The source of the outbreak was traced to an animal vendor in Wisconsin who sold prairie dogs (*Cynomys* sp.), a species native to North America, that had been housed in close proximity to Gambian giant pouched rats (*Cricetomys* sp.) owned by another vendor. The prairie dogs became infected with monkeypox from the rats and transmitted the infection to humans who came into contact with them. As of July 2003, over 70 human cases had been reported to CDC.

Transmission
Transmission from animals to humans is by direct contact. Secondary human cases can occur via contact with another patient's lesions or ocular secretions. There is also evidence for airborne transmission via respiratory droplets.

✎ TECHNICIAN NOTE

Veterinarians who suspect monkeypox in an animal should not perform necropsies or biopsies because of the risk of infecting themselves.

Disease in Animals
Signs
Animals with monkeypox, according to CDC's case definition, usually present with a rash that may be macular, papular, vesicular, or pustular. It may be generalized or localized and either discrete or confluent. Other signs can include conjunctivitis, coryza, cough, anorexia, and lethargy. Veterinarians should be suspicious of monkeypox in animals, especially rodents, that have a history of fever, conjunctivitis, respiratory signs, and nodular rash.

Diagnosis
In the United States, guidelines published following the 2003 outbreak recommend that veterinarians who suspect monkeypox in an animal should not perform necropsies or biopsies because of the risk of infecting themselves.

When monkeypox is suspected in an animal, the state health department should be contacted for information on where and how to submit specimens, since most laboratories are not equipped to diagnose the disease.

Disease in Humans
Signs and Symptoms
Monkeypox in humans is clinically similar to smallpox but not as severe. Humans with monkeypox present with a rash similar to that seen in animals, i.e., macular, papular, vesicular, or pustular, generalized or localized, discrete or confluent, and fever of at least 99.3° F (37.4° C). Other signs and symptoms may include chills and/or sweats, headache, backache, lymphadenopathy, sore throat, cough, and shortness of breath.

In outbreaks in Africa, as many as 10% of cases have been fatal. There were no fatalities in the outbreak in the United States in 2003.

Diagnosis
The virus can be detected via electron microscopy on specimens of exudate from lesions. Serologic tests also are available.

Treatment
As of this writing, there is no specific treatment for human monkeypox.

Prevention
Monkeypox is highly infectious and easily transmitted in the veterinary setting. Any veterinarian who decides to examine or treat animals with suspected monkeypox should be aware of the potential for spread of the infection and take precautions to protect the health of themselves, staff, and clients, and other animal patients in the clinic. If it is known in advance that an animal with suspected monkeypox is being brought in, it should not be allowed to enter through the waiting area of the clinic.

The animal should be isolated, and any personnel present during the examination should wear personal protective equipment (PPE), including gloves, gown, eye protection, and respiratory protection (preferably a National Institute of Occupational Safety and Health (NIOSH) certified N95 filtering disposable respirator, but at least a surgical mask). Contact with the animal should be limited to as few personnel as possible.

Contaminated objects should be disinfected by autoclaving where possible. Surfaces can be cleaned using standard household cleaners, such as bleach, in accordance with the manufacturer's recommendations for dilution and application. Disposable items should be autoclaved or incinerated before disposal.

Smallpox vaccine is effective in preventing monkeypox. Guidelines current in late 2003 recommend that anyone who has had direct physical contact with an infected animal should receive a dose of smallpox vaccine.

Reporting and Surveillance

If monkeypox is suspected in any animal, local and state health departments should be notified immediately.

CONTAGIOUS ECTHYMA (ORF)

Agent

Contagious ecthyma is caused by a DNA virus of the genus *Parapoxvirus*, family Poxviridae.

Reservoirs

Reservoirs are domestic and wild ungulates, including sheep, goats, domestic camels, deer, reindeer, and musk oxen. The virus is hardy and can persist for long periods in the environment and on the skin and hair of animals.

Occurrence

Incidence is uncommon but worldwide wherever sheep and goats are raised; many human cases occur in New Zealand. Contagious ecthyma (orf) is an occupational disease of sheep handlers, veterinarians, and abattoir workers.

Transmission

Humans contract orf through direct contact with lesions or mucous membranes of infected animals. In addition, contaminated knives, shears, or other objects can transfer the virus from animal to human. Preparation and administration of the crude live vaccine used in some endemic areas can also be a source of human infection.

Disease in Animals
Signs

Most infections occur in young animals. Papules that progress into vesicles and pustules appear on the skin, eyelids, ears, lips, and nostrils. As lesions become confluent, they cause severe pain and often interfere with feeding. Females that nurse infected young may develop infection of teats and udders. Morbidity is often high, but mortality is low, usually resulting from secondary bacterial infection or infestation by fly larvae.

Diagnosis

Clinical signs alone often are sufficient to establish diagnosis; other diseases that produce similar lesions tend to have a different course.

Disease in Humans
Signs and Symptoms

The most frequent presentation is the development of a single maculopapular or pustular lesion at the site of entry of the virus, usually on the hands, arms, or face. The papule is painful and progresses to become a firm, weeping nodule; secondary bacterial infection may cause pus formation. Most cases resolve completely in 2 to 4 weeks, but occasionally the infection is more serious. Reported complications include a widespread cutaneous eruption, ocular involvement with severe damage, and disseminated systemic disease.

Diagnosis

Demonstration of virus particles via electron microscopy of affected tissue and isolation of the virus in cell culture are definitive means of diagnosis. Serologic tests are available.

Treatment

There is no specific treatment.

Prevention

Good personal hygiene, including thorough washing of skin that comes in contact with an infected animal, can help prevent human infection. Any broken skin should be kept covered, and gloves should be worn when examining or treating infected sheep.

Animal housing areas should be kept clean to reduce sources of infection for susceptible lambs. In some endemic areas, a crude live vaccine is made by pulverizing scabs from infected animals and suspending the material in a glycerinated solution. Lambs are vaccinated by applying the suspension to scarified skin in the axilla. However, the efficacy of this process is variable and, as mentioned, can cause human infection. In addition, this practice can lead to perpetuation of the virus in the farm environment.

Reporting and Surveillance

Reporting of contagious ecthyma is not required.

HERPESVIRUS SIMIAE INFECTION (B VIRUS)

Agent

Herpesvirus simiae is caused by a DNA virus of the genus *Herpesvirus*, family Herpesviridae; it is closely related to the human herpes simplex virus that causes fever blisters and mouth ulcers. It is also referred to as *cercopithecine herpesvirus 1*.

Reservoirs

Asian monkeys of the genus *Macaca*, especially the rhesus monkey, *M. mulatta*, are natural reservoirs; other primates in contact with infected *Macaca* spp. may acquire the virus.

Occurrence

Incidence is common in monkeys; 30% to 80% of rhesus monkeys are seropositive for this virus. In humans, B virus infection is a rare occupational disease that has been recorded in veterinarians, animal care workers, laboratory personnel, and others in contact with Old World monkeys or monkey cell cultures.

Transmission

H. simiae infection is transmitted between monkeys by direct contact, bites or scratches, and saliva-contaminated food or water. Infected monkeys may not show any clinical signs. Humans acquire the disease when bitten by a monkey that carries the virus, when saliva from an infected monkey comes in contact with broken skin, or by conjunctival, nasal, or pharyngeal exposure to aerosols that contain the virus.

Disease in Animals

Signs

Primary B virus infection in macaque monkeys causes sores in or around the mouth that appear similar to fever blisters in humans. The small ulcers that form heal within 1 to 2 weeks. The condition is not serious in monkeys and is rarely noticed unless lesions appear on the lips, conjunctivae, or skin. After the initial outbreak of lesions, the virus becomes latent, and the monkey is then an asymptomatic carrier. In nonmacaque primates, the course of the disease is similar to that in humans and is usually fatal.

Diagnosis

Serologic tests used to determine B virus infection include ELISA and radioimmunoassay. The virus can be grown in tissue culture, and identification is confirmed through the use of PCR, DNA restriction analysis, or other molecular methods.

Disease in Humans

Signs and Symptoms

B virus in humans causes a severe and usually fatal meningoencephalitis. When infection follows a monkey bite or other cutaneous inoculation of the agent, the wound becomes reddened and painful; itching and numbness can occur. Vesicles appear at the site, and regional lymphadenopathy develops. After a few days to a few weeks, the disease becomes generalized, and there is sudden onset of fever, with headache, nausea, abdominal pain, and diarrhea. Various neurologic signs follow, including vertigo, diaphragmatic spasms, neck stiffness, and difficulty in swallowing. In late stages of the illness, the lower extremities develop flaccid paralysis; this spreads to the upper extremities and thorax. Respiratory failure and death usually occur within 5 to 28 days of onset of clinical symptoms. More than 70% of the known cases have been fatal, and most survivors have permanent and extensive neurologic damage, although recent improvements in diagnostic and therapeutic techniques offer hope for reducing fatalities and permanent sequelae.

Diagnosis

Serologic tests may be useful when a patient survives long enough to produce antibodies, but most cases are diagnosed postmortem through viral isolation from brain tissue.

Treatment

Acyclovir has produced recovery in a few cases.

Prevention

Anyone who works with or comes into contact with Old World monkeys should take all precautions to prevent bites and aerosol exposure. Always wear gloves, masks, and protective clothing. Prompt treatment of any wound caused by a monkey (bite or scratch) or an object (cage or wires) that could be contaminated with monkey secretions is critical. Immediately and thoroughly scrub the wound with soap and water, and disinfect it with an iodine solution. Acyclovir may be an effective prophylaxis if administered promptly. If the wound becomes painful or numb or if itching or vesicular lesions appear at or near the wound site, seek immediate expert medical advice. No vaccine is available.

> **✐ TECHNICIAN NOTE**
>
> Anyone who works with or comes into contact with Old World monkeys should take all precautions to prevent bites and aerosol exposure.

Monkeys should be housed only in small groups, with a maximum of two per cage. Do not house rhesus monkeys with any other species. Quarantine all recently imported monkeys for at least 6 weeks; destroy any that have or develop lesions suggestive of *H. simiae*. Any animal responsible for a wound to a human should be observed for at least 2 weeks and tested to determine its B virus status.

Researchers who work with tissues or body fluids from macaques should follow BSL 2 practices. If the material is known to contain *H. simiae*, BSL 3 facilities and precautions should be used.

Reporting and Surveillance

Report any human cases to local health authorities.

NEWCASTLE DISEASE

Agent

This disease is caused by an ribonucleic acid (RNA) virus of the genus *Paramyxovirus*, family Paramyxoviridae.

Reservoirs

Chickens are the reservoir for Newcastle disease.

Occurrence

Incidence is worldwide. Newcastle disease occurs in wild birds and semidomestic and domestic fowl in both epizootic and enzootic forms; it is one of the most economically important diseases affecting the poultry industry. Human disease is rare and usually occurs among poultry slaughterhouse workers, poultry vaccinators using vaccines containing live viral strains, and laboratory personnel who work with the virus.

Transmission

Newcastle disease (ND) is spread from bird to bird mainly by aerosols, with the density of birds in commercial poultry farms facilitating transmission. The virus also is shed in feces. Humans become infected when the virus comes into contact with the eyes, as occurs with aerosolized vaccines.

Disease in Animals

Signs

Numerous species of birds may be affected by ND, but chickens and turkeys are especially susceptible. Signs may be respiratory, nervous, or both and usually appear throughout a flock within 2 weeks of exposure. The strain of virus determines the severity of the outbreak; lentogenic strains are the least virulent, velogenic are the most virulent, and mesogenic strains are intermediate. In birds with respiratory involvement, there is gasping and coughing; neurologic signs include drooping wings, twisted neck, depression, anorexia, and paralysis. Egg laying may cease. Some velogenic strains produce a viscerotropic syndrome, which is the most serious form of ND. Affected birds have sudden onset of watery, greenish diarrhea, tracheal discharge, and edema of the face and wattles; small hemorrhages appear in the mucosa of the proventriculus, and the intestinal mucosa becomes necrotic. There is high mortality associated with this form of the disease.

Diagnosis

ND virus can be isolated from tracheal exudate, lung, or spleen tissue taken early in the outbreak. Material taken for viral isolation attempts should be placed in a sterile container and transported to the laboratory. Various serologic tests also are useful.

Disease in Humans

Signs and Symptoms

In humans, Newcastle disease usually causes a unilateral conjunctivitis, with excessive tear formation, pain, swelling of subconjunctival tissues, and inflammation of the lymph nodes in front of the ear. Generally, there is no systemic involvement, but some people exposed to aerosols of the virus develop an influenza-like illness that lasts 3 to 4 days. Recovery is complete in about 1 week. Subclinical infections also occur.

Diagnosis

Isolation of ND virus is the only definitive means of diagnosis because many people do not develop a serologic response. The virus can be isolated from various body fluids, including conjunctival or nasal secretions, saliva, or urine. Inoculation of embryonated chicken eggs or tissue culture techniques can be used to isolate the virus.

Treatment

Usually no treatment is necessary.

Prevention

Control of avian ND depends on maintaining good hygiene on poultry farms. Poultry houses should be separated, and all birds in a flock should be vaccinated using a live lentogenic strain vaccine. People who administer the vaccine to poultry should wear masks; laboratory personnel should avoid creating aerosols when working with the virus.

Reporting and Surveillance

The United States requires that imported live birds of any species be quarantined and prohibits imports from countries in which Newcastle disease occurs.

RABIES

Agent

Rabies is caused by a RNA virus of the genus *Lyssavirus*, family Rhabdoviridae.

Reservoirs

Reservoirs for rabies are wild and domestic members of the Canidae family, including dogs, foxes, coyotes, and wolves; wild carnivores and omnivores, such as skunks, raccoons, and mongooses; and bats, including those that feed on blood (vampire bats), fruit eaters, and insectivores.

Occurrence

Incidence is almost worldwide in animal populations; the only exceptions are parts of the Pacific and Far East, including Australia, New Zealand, Papua New Guinea, Japan, Taiwan, and most of Oceania, and some of Europe, including England, Scotland, Ireland, the Netherlands, Norway, Finland, Sweden, Spain, Portugal, and Greece. However, cases of fatal encephalomyelitis clinically indistinguishable from rabies have been reported from some of the "rabies-free" countries. In 1996 a closely related Lyssavirus was discovered in Australia; subsequently named *Australian bat Lyssavirus*, it has been isolated from about 9.5% of ill fruit bats submitted for testing and has caused two human deaths in that country in 1996 and 1998. In the United Kingdom the European bat Lyssavirus was responsible for a bat handler's death in 2002.

Classical rabies is present throughout most of the Americas except for a few Caribbean islands. In areas in which animal rabies occurs, the disease follows one of two cycles: urban or sylvatic. Urban rabies, which is seen in developing nations, is transmitted by dogs and accounts for most human cases. In industrialized countries where vaccination programs have largely eliminated rabies in domestic animals, the urban rabies cycle does not occur; instead the virus circulates among wild carnivores and bats (sylvatic cycle) and causes occasional spillover infection of dogs, cats, and livestock. The World Health Organization (WHO) estimates that rabies is responsible for over 35,000 human deaths each year, most in developing countries.

Transmission

Rabies virus is abundant in saliva; thus most cases are attributable to a bite inflicted by an infected animal. Aerosol transmission is possible; a few cases have occurred among field biologists working in caves in which large populations of bats roosted.

> **TECHNICIAN NOTE**
>
> Rabies virus is abundant in saliva; thus most cases are attributable to a bite inflicted by an infected animal.

Disease in Animals

Signs

Rabies in dogs may be either furious or paralytic ("dumb"). In the early stages of furious rabies, the animal becomes agitated, restless, and excitable. An aggressive phase follows, with the dog attempting to bite objects, other animals, humans, and itself. Salivation is profuse because throat muscles spasm and prevent swallowing, vocal cords become affected, and the bark changes to a hoarse howl. Convulsions and paralysis occur shortly before death. In paralytic rabies the muscles of the head and neck initially are affected, and the animal has difficulty in swallowing. Paralysis spreads to the extremities and then becomes generalized; death follows.

Rabid cats usually manifest the furious variety, whereas in cattle, rabies generally is paralytic. Furious rabies is the more common form in wild animals, such as foxes, skunks, and raccoons.

Diagnosis

Behavioral changes and/or paralysis may suggest a presumptive diagnosis, particularly when rabies recently has been confirmed in the same species and geographic area. A positive direct immunofluorescence test on brain tissue is confirmatory. There are no tests available that produce satisfactory results on specimens from live animals.

Disease in Humans

Signs and Symptoms

The incubation period is variable; in most cases, onset of symptoms is within 3 to 8 weeks of exposure, but there are documented reports of disease occurring several years after a bite from a rabid animal. Rabies in humans usually begins with discomfort and irritation in the area of a previous animal bite. Vague sensory changes, apprehension, headache, low-grade fever, and malaise also may occur. As the disease progresses, salivation increases and eyes and ears become hypersensitive to light and sound. Paresis or paralysis develops, and spasmodic contractions of muscles used in swallowing cause the patient to develop an aversion to liquids (hydrophobia) and to stop swallowing his or her own saliva. Convulsions and various mental disturbances

are terminal events. Death from respiratory failure usually occurs 2 to 8 days after onset of symptoms.

Diagnosis

A presumptive diagnosis sometimes can be made by immunofluorescence staining of skin sections taken from the back of the neck. As in animals, postmortem testing of brain tissue is necessary for confirmation.

Treatment

Rabies is always fatal. Once clinical disease has developed, there is no effective treatment.

Prevention

All pet dogs and cats should be vaccinated. Cattle and horses may be vaccinated in areas where skunk rabies is endemic or vampire bats are present.

Individuals at risk, such as laboratory workers, animal control personnel, veterinarians, technicians, field zoologists, and others who come into contact with wild or unvaccinated domestic animals, should receive preexposure prophylaxis. There are several excellent human vaccines available in industrialized nations, such as human diploid cell vaccine (HDCV), purified chick-embryo cell (PCEC) vaccine, and rabies vaccine adsorbed (RVA), but these are expensive and may not be available in under-developed countries.

Local laws may vary, but in general, a dog or cat that has bitten a person should be quarantined and observed for at least 10 days. If the animal develops any sign suggestive of rabies, the animal should be killed and its brain examined by fluorescent microscopy. Any wild animal that has bitten a person should be killed immediately and tested. Any unvaccinated animal that is bitten by a rabid animal should be destroyed.

The most effective means of preventing rabies in humans is to immediately and thoroughly cleanse any animal bite or scratch wound; if used quickly, soap and water are a good means of removing rabies virus. Flush the wound with a strong stream of water, wash with soap or detergent, and rinse well. Apply a disinfectant, such as alcohol, tincture of iodine, or a quaternary ammonium compound, and seek medical attention. Bite wounds should be left unsutured, if possible, *so as not to interfere with bleeding and drainage.*

> **TECHNICIAN NOTE**
>
> All cases of animal and human rabies should be reported to health authorities.

For people who have not received preexposure immunization, postexposure prophylactic treatment consists of administering human rabies immune globulin (RIG) and rabies vaccine, preferably a 5-day course of HDCV, PCEC, or other approved vaccine. If the exposed person already has received a full course of vaccine before exposure, postexposure treatment is reduced to two doses of vaccine only. RIG must not be used in an already-immunized person because it can lessen the anamnestic response of the immune system to the booster doses of vaccine.

Researchers who work with the virus should operate under strict BSL 2 conditions; if aerosols are possible, BSL 3 precautions should be observed.

Reporting and Surveillance

All cases of animal and human rabies should be reported to health authorities.

Recommended Reading

GENERAL

Beran GW: Zoonoses in practice, *Vet Clin North Am* 23:1085-1107, 1993.

Weese JS et al: Occupational health and safety in small animal veterinary practice: part I—nonparasitic zoonotic diseases, *Can Vet J* 43:631-636, 2002.

Weese JS et al: Occupational health and safety in small animal veterinary practice: part II—parasitic zoonotic diseases, *Can Vet J* 43:799-802, 2002.

ANTHRAX

Whitford HW, Hugh-Jones ME: Anthrax. In Beran GW, Steele JH, editors: *Handbook of zoonoses,* ed 2, Boca Raton, Fla, 1994, CRC Press, pp 61-82.

BITE WOUNDS AND OTHER INJURIES

Centers for Disease Control and Prevention: Nonfatal bite-related injuries treated in hospital emergency departments—United States, 2001, *MMWR Morb Mortal Wkly Rep* 52:605-610, 2003.

Drobatz KJ, Smith G: Evaluation of risk factors for bite wounds inflicted on caregivers by dogs and cats in a veterinary teaching hospital, *J Am Vet Med Assoc* 223:312-316, 2003.

Myers JP: Bite wound infections, *Curr Infect Dis Rep* 5:416-425, 2003.

BRUCELLOSIS

Berkelman, RL: Human illness associated with use of veterinary vaccines, *Clin Infect Dis* 37:407-414, 2003.

Sauret JM, Vilissova N: Human brucellosis, *J Am Board Fam Pract* 15:401-406, 2002.

CAMPYLOBACTERIOSIS

Altekruse SF, Tollefson LK: Human campylobacteriosis: a challenge for the veterinary profession, *J Am Vet Med Assoc* 223:445-452, 2003.

Saeed AM, Harris NV, DiGiacomo RF: The role of exposure to animals in the etiology of *Campylobacter jejuni/coli* enteritis, *Am J Epidemiol* 137:108-114, 1993.

CAPNOCYTOPHAGA CANIMORSUS INFECTION

Le Moal G et al: Meningitis due to *Capnocytophaga canimorsus* after receipt of a dog bite: case report and review of the literature, *Clin Infect Dis* 36:e42-46, 2003.

Weber WB: An interesting brush with death, *Ala Vet* 10:41-45, 1999.

CAT-SCRATCH DISEASE

Breitschwerdt EB, Kordick DL: *Bartonella* infection in animals: carriership, reservoir potential, pathogenicity, and zoonotic potential for human infection, *Clin Microbiol Rev* 13:428-438, 2000.

Weese JS et al: Occupational health and safety in small animal veterinary practice: part I—nonparasitic zoonotic diseases, *Can Vet J* 43:631-636, 2002.

CONTAGIOUS ECTHYMA

Acha PN, Szyfres B: Contagious ecthyma. In *Zoonoses and communicable diseases common to man and animals,* ed 3, Vol 3, Washington, DC, 2003, Pan American Health Organization, pp 80-83.

CRYPTOCOCCOSIS

Nosanchuk JD et al: Evidence of zoonotic transmission of *Cryptococcus neoformans* from a pet cockatoo to an immuno-compromised patient, *Ann Intern Med* 132:205-208, 2000.

Pollock C: Fungal diseases of columbiformes and anseriformes, *Vet Clin North Am Exot Anim Pract* 6:351-361, 2003.

CRYPTOSPORIDIOSIS

Fayer R et al: Epidemiology of *Cryptosporidium*: transmission, detection, and identification, *Int J Parasitol* 30:1305-1322, 2000.

Preiser G et al: An outbreak of cryptosporidiosis among veterinary science students who work with calves, *J Am Coll Health* 51:213-215, 2003.

DERMATOPHYTOSES

Acha PN, Szyfres B: Dermatophytosis. In *Zoonoses and communicable diseases common to man and animals,* ed 3, Vol 1, Washington, DC, 2001, Pan American Health Organization, pp 332-339.

Pier AC: Superficial mycoses (dermatophytoses). In Beran GW, Steele JH, editors: *Handbook of zoonoses,* ed 2, Boca Raton, Fla, 1994, CRC Press.

ERYSIPELOTHRIX INFECTIONS

Brooke CJ, Riley TV: *Erysipelothrix rhusiopathiae*: bacteriology, epidemiology, and clinical manifestations of an occupational pathogen, *Med Microbiol* 48:789-799, 1999.

HERPESVIRUS SIMIAE INFECTION

Acha PN, Szyfres B: *Herpesvirus simiae.* In *Zoonoses and communicable diseases common to man and animals,* ed 3, Vol 3, Washington, DC, 2003, Pan American Health Organization, pp 149-154.

Huff JL, Barry PA: B Virus (Cercopithecine herpesvirus 1) infection in humans and macaques: potential for zoonotic disease, *Emerg Infect Dis* 9:246-250, 2003.

MONKEYPOX

Centers for Disease Control and Prevention: Update: multistate outbreak of monkeypox—Illinois, Indiana, Kansas, Missouri, Ohio, and Wisconsin, 2003, *MMWR Morb Mortal Wkly Rep* 52:642-646, 2003.

Hutin YJF et al: Outbreak of human monkeypox, Democratic Republic of Congo, 1996 to 1997, *Emerg Infect Dis* 7:434-438, 2001.

Makalyk J: Monkeypox outbreak among pet owners, *CMAJ* 169:44-45, 2003.

NEWCASTLE DISEASE

Hugh-Jones ME et al: Newcastle disease. In *Zoonoses: recognition, control, and prevention,* Ames, 1995, Iowa State University Press.

PASTEURELLOSIS

Arons MS et al: *Pasteurella multocida:* the major cause of hand infections following domestic animal bites, *J Hand Surg* 7:47-52, 1982.

Kravetz JD, Federman DG: Cat-associated zoonoses, *Arch Intern Med* 162:1945-1952, 2002.

PLAGUE

Gage KL et al: Cases of cat-associated human plague in the western United States, 1977-1998, *Clin Infect Dis* 30:893-900, 2000.

Orloski KA, Lathrop SL: Plague: a veterinary perspective, *J Am Vet Med Assoc* 222:444-448, 2003.

PSITTACOSIS

Centers for Disease Control and Prevention: Compendium of measures to control *Chlamydia psittaci* infection among humans (psittacosis) and pet birds (avian chlamydiosis), 2000, *MMWR Recomm Rep* 49:RR8, 2000.

Eidson, M: Psittacosis/avian chlamydiosis, *J Am Vet Med Assoc* 221:1710-1712, 2002.

Q FEVER

Komiya T et al: Epidemiological survey on the route of *Coxiella burnetii* infection in an animal hospital, *J Infect Chemother* 9:151-155, 2003.

McQuiston JH, Childs JE: Q fever in humans and animals in the United States, *Vector Borne Zoonotic Dis* 2:179-191, 2002.

RABIES

Centers for Disease Control and Prevention: Human rabies prevention—United States, 1999, *MMWR Recomm Rep* 48:RR1, 1999.

Dietzschold B et al: New approaches to the prevention and eradication of rabies, *Expert Rev Vacc* 2:399-406, 2003.

Krebs JW et al.: Rabies surveillance in the United States during 2002, *J Am Vet Med Assoc* 223:1736-1748, 2003.

RAT-BITE FEVERS

Graves MH, Janda JM: Rat-bite fever (*Streptobacillus moniliformis*): a potential emerging disease, *Int J Infect Dis* 5:151-155, 2001.

Hudsmith L et al: Clinical picture: rat-bite fever, *Lancet Infect Dis* 1:91, 2001.

SALMONELLOSIS

Centers for Disease Control and Prevention: Reptile-associated salmonellosis—selected states, 1998-2002, *MMWR Morb Mortal Wkly Rep* 52:1206-1209, 2003.

Stam F et al: Turtle-associated human salmonellosis, *Clin Infect Dis* 37:e167-169, 2003.

TOXOPLASMOSIS

Hill D, Dubey JP: *Toxoplasma gondii*: transmission, diagnosis, and prevention, *Clin Microbiol Infect* 8:634-640, 2002.

Jones JL et al: *Toxoplasma gondii* infection in the United States, 1999-2000, *Emerg Infect Dis* 9:1371-1374, 2003.

TULAREMIA

Centers for Disease Control and Prevention: Tularemia—United States, 1990-2000, *MMWR Morb Mortal Wkly Rep* 51:182-184, 2002.

Feldman KA: Tularemia, *J Am Vet Med Assoc* 222:725-730, 2003.

Liles WC, Burger RJ: Tularemia from domestic cats, *West J Med* 158:619-622, 1993.

36

Occupational Health and Safety in Veterinary Hospitals

Philip J. Seibert, Jr.

OVERVIEW

Most people who work in the veterinary health care professions do so because of a love for animals and a desire to help them. Working as a veterinary technician and being part of the veterinary health care team can be particularly rewarding. However, with every reward comes responsibility. One of the responsibilities of a veterinary technician is to help ensure the safety of co-workers, patients, and clients as well as to ensure one's own safety. If you are hurt on the job, the injury incurred extends beyond the physical pain and disability you suffer. The hospital is also affected both financially and operationally, because the veterinary health care team loses an important member—you. Other employees of the practice have to work harder to cover the personnel shortage. In addition, the quality of health care delivered to the animals may also be adversely affected by having less than a full team of caregivers.

As a staff member in a veterinary hospital, you are exposed to hazards in the day-to-day routine of clinical practice. These hazards include exposure to infectious diseases, harmful chemicals, radiation, and the risks of being scratched, bitten, shoved, stepped-on and kicked. That's the bad news. The good news is that these hazards, when properly identified, can be managed, and the risk of injury minimized or even eliminated.

By reading this chapter and educating yourself about hazards in the veterinary health care field, you are taking the first step in minimizing your risk of being injured and/or of contracting a contagious disease. Some of the topics discussed will be familiar to you, while others will be new. The important point is to remember that all of the topics presented in this chapter are true health risks for the veterinary technician in clinical practice.

The second step in minimizing health risks in the work place is to *integrate* the safety procedures you learn in this chapter into the everyday habits of your job. *You* are the most important person in ensuring *your* safety on the job. As human beings, we operate from a set of habits for most of life's activities. Your safety should not be something you have to stop to think about—it should be automatic. The only way it becomes automatic is by developing and practicing good work habits.

OBJECTIVES OF A SAFETY PROGRAM

The purpose of any safety program is to reduce or eliminate the possibility of injuries or illnesses to employees. As mentioned, by becoming aware of safety issues, you can significantly decrease your chances of injury!

The Occupational Safety and Health Administration (OSHA) enforces federal laws that help to ensure a safe workplace for American workers. These laws require employers to have a safety program, which includes educating employees about the inherent risks in their jobs, providing them with appropriate safety equipment, and training them in safety procedures and the proper use of the safety equipment. If you are receiving this training from your employer, she or he is fulfilling important OSHA requirements. If you are learning this material as a self-study program, you can take pride in the knowledge that you are becoming a "self-taught expert" in the field of occupational safety. Your knowledge and initiative will be a welcomed component to your veterinary health care team.

YOUR SAFETY RIGHTS

One can never eliminate every hazard completely, but each of us can minimize our exposure to them in most cases.

The ability to participate in a safety program at work is an important part of your rights. It is often assumed that the owner/manager of a business knows all that there is to know about the business. But too often it is the employee who first becomes aware of potential safety problems. As an employee, you have the right to bring those concerns to the attention of the employer without fear of reprisal. In most instances, the complaint is first presented to the immediate supervisor, but be aware that not all complaints will bring about changes to the operation of the practice. Some complaints stem from a lack of familiarity with standard safety procedures, on the part of the employee, and in these cases instruction by the employer is all that is needed to resolve the issue. However, if a complaint is not taken seriously by the employer or if there is a dangerous situation that is not adequately addressed, the employee has the right to bring the issue to the attention of the regional OSHA office.

When records such as medical evaluations or radiation exposure reports are collected by the veterinary hospital, the records must be made available to the employee for review. This does not mean that you are entitled to see private or sensitive information about other staff members, but it does mean that you are entitled to see data that is relevant to your safety. You are also entitled to know about the nature and types of accidents that have occurred in your hospital. If your practice employs more than 10 employees, you have the right to view the Summary of Work-Related Injuries and Illnesses (OSHA Form 300A), which should be posted on the employee bulletin board at certain times of the year.

YOUR SAFETY RESPONSIBILITIES

It is your responsibility to learn and follow the safety rules and practices that have been established for your position in the veterinary hospital. Even though OSHA will not cite or fine the employee directly for violations of these responsibilities, he or she is required under the Occupational Safety and Health Act (the Act) to "comply with all occupational safety and health standards and all rules, regulations, and orders issued under the Act." This not only includes specific OSHA standards, but it also applies to workplace-specific rules established by the leadership in your hospital.

Although you cannot be disciplined by your employer for exercising your rights under the Act, you can be disciplined

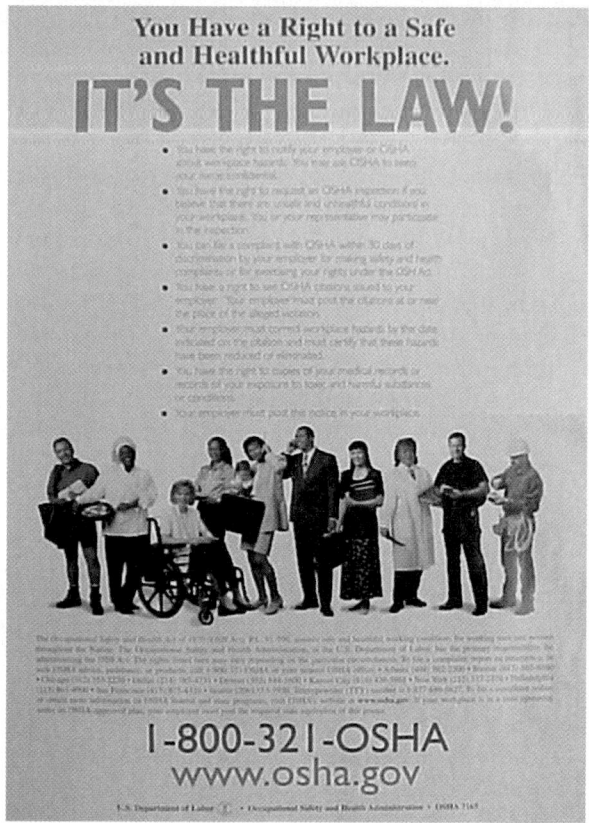

Figure 36-1 Locate and read all of the safety notices where you work.

by your employer for willful violations of any safety rule or standard. In some cases this discipline can be as simple as a verbal reprimand, but in severe or chronic situations it can include termination. In most states, if you are terminated for willful violation of safety rules, you will likely be denied unemployment benefits.

In addition to the responsibility to follow the rules, the Act requires you to

- Read the OSHA poster (Figure 36-1).
- Comply with all applicable standards.
- Wear or use prescribed personal protective equipment while working.
- Report hazardous conditions to your supervisor.
- Report any job-related injury or illness to the proper person and seek treatment promptly.

THE LEADERSHIP'S RIGHTS

Although the Act and OSHA require the leadership of a business to maintain safety standards, this is not meant to restrict their right to set rules of conduct or operation for its staff. The practice owner, for example, has the right to set and enforce rules for his or her own practice, as long as those rules are consistent with federal safety laws.

Practice owners must have ample time to correct any safety-related problems. In other words, the employee should not rush off to file a grievance with the regional OSHA office without first giving the employer ample time to correct the deficiency.

In the event that a practice is inspected, the practice owner has the right to be present because the practice is considered his or her personal property. Therefore, an employee is not authorized to admit an OSHA inspector to the practice in the absence of the employer (unless, of course, the employer specifically gives the employee the authority to act on his or her behalf). However, OSHA inspectors *may* enter a practice without the presence of the owner and without permission by the employee if the inspectors have a court order to do so.

THE LEADERSHIP'S RESPONSIBILITIES

The leadership of a veterinary practice is responsible for providing a safe work environment for the employees. This does not mean providing a facility with *no* hazards—that would be impossible. It means that the leadership must make a reasonable effort to identify the hazards present, correct the ones that can be eliminated, and control the ones that cannot be eliminated.

The practice must comply with the laws and regulations pertaining to safety and health by establishing safety procedures for the hospital including emergency procedures for addressing employee accidents. The leadership must enforce these rules as diligently as it would be expected to enforce any other rule in the practice.

The employer is also responsible for providing *practice-specific* safety training to the employees (Figure 36-2). Even if a veterinary technician has years of prior experience, the practice is required to make sure that the technician is capable of doing her or his job safely. This training can be provided in a formal setting, such as in staff meetings or continuing education course, or it can be given in the clinic. A great deal of learning takes place in many practices every day. On-the-job training can be an effective way to obtain knowledge about safety, but be sure you know your limits and abilities. Ultimately, you are the best person to determine if you are competent to do a job safely. If you think you need extra safety training in an area, don't hesitate to ask for it. Tell your supervisor immediately so that arrangements can be made for the proper instruction.

GENERAL WORKPLACE HAZARDS

Every practice should have a collection of written safety-related policies known as the *Hospital Safety Manual*. You should know where the Hospital Safety Manual is located in your practice and take time to become familiar with it. Memorize the "do's and dont's" for your particular veterinary hospital and always follow the safety rules. No one can protect you from an injury or illness better than you!

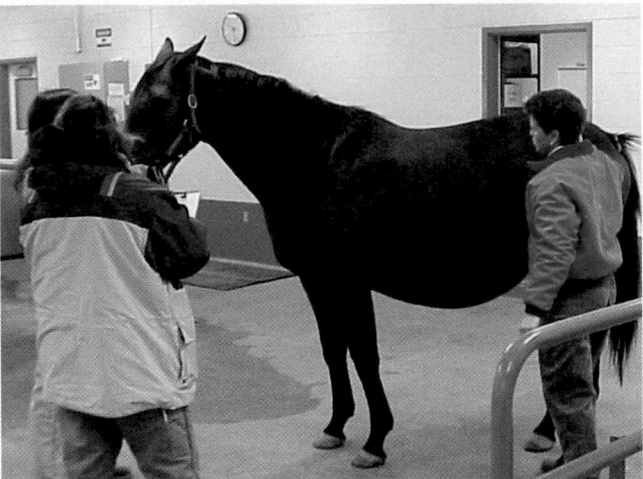

Figure 36-2 Safety training can be conducted in a formal session and enhanced by one-on-one discussions.

> ✏️ **TECHNICIAN NOTE**
>
> Every practice should have a collection of written safety-related policies known as the *Hospital Safety Manual*.

DRESSING APPROPRIATELY FOR THE JOB

One of the first rules of safety is to dress appropriately for the job at hand. In the veterinary profession, this includes protective footwear and minimal, if any, jewelry. You can reduce the chances of getting injured by wearing shoes that cover your whole foot (not sandals or open-toed shoes) and that have nonslip soles. Be especially cautious walking on uneven or wet floors. Never run inside the hospital or on uneven footing. Excessive jewelry can present a hazard in many clinical situations, but particularly when an animal struggles during restraint and can inadvertently link an earring or necklace with a claw. This is definitely one of those circumstances when less is more!

SAVE YOUR BACK!

According to insurance statistics, back injuries account for one in every five workplace injuries among American workers. To minimize your chances of suffering one of these very painful injuries, remember the rules for lifting: keep your back straight and lift with your legs (Figure 36-3). Never bend over at the waist to lift an object. That rule applies when lifting patients as well as inanimate objects such as boxes or supplies. If your practice does not have a motorized lift table, get help when lifting patients over 40 lb. Remember to follow sound ergonomic principles when positioning or restraining patients, especially when working with horses or food animals.

Because veterinary technicians perform such a variety of jobs in any given hour, it is rare for us to acquire the types of ergonomic injuries common in other industries (such

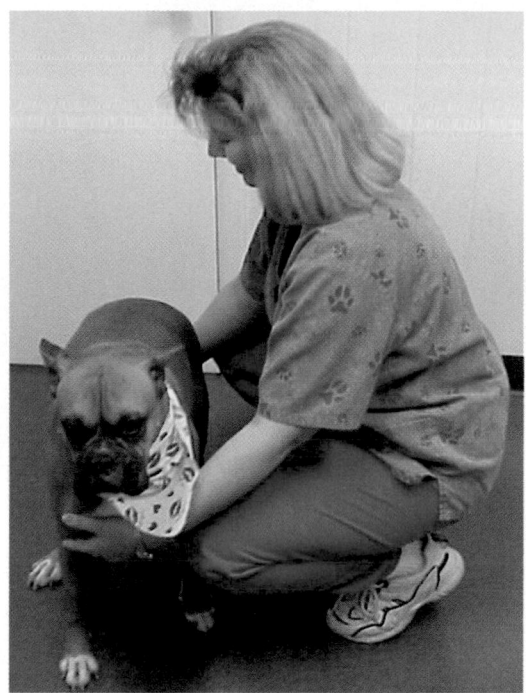

Figure 36-3 Remember to keep your back straight and lift with your legs.

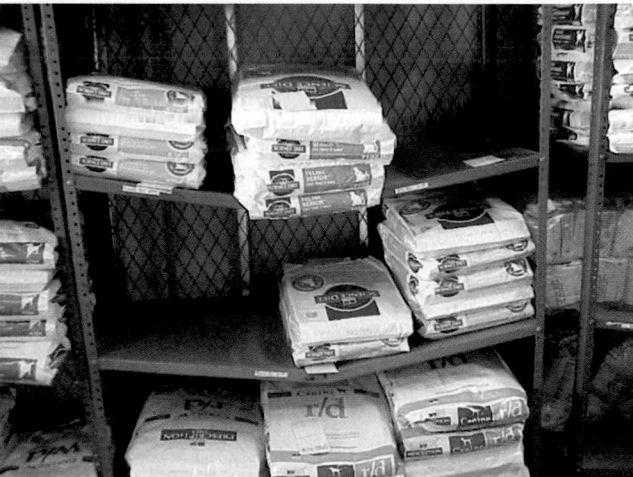

Figure 36-4 Improper storage of materials can lead to serious injury.

as carpal tunnel syndrome). However, it is important to note that the best defense against almost all ergonomic injuries is to change your posture and routine frequently.

CLEAN UP AFTER YOURSELF

Some injuries are caused by cluttered or dirty work areas. In addition, clutter is know to contribute to the severity of accidents that otherwise would be minor. Cleanliness and organization are good business standards, especially in a health care facility. Always clean up spills as soon as they happen. You should always clean and return equipment to the proper storage place immediately after use. At least daily, remove all trash from your work area. Organize drawers, cabinets, and counters so that items can be found easily and clutter is reduced.

EVERYTHING IN ITS PLACE

Supplies and equipment should always be stored properly. Heavy supplies or equipment, for example, should be kept on the lower shelves to prevent unnecessary strain in trying to lift them overhead and to reduce the risk of material falling on your head. Never use stairways or exit hallways as storage areas. Do not overload shelves or cabinets (Figure 36-4). Store liquids in containers with tight-fitting lids and always replace the lids when finished using the product. Whenever possible, store chemicals on shelves at or below eye level; this will minimize the possibility of accidentally spilling the chemical on you when getting or replacing a container. Never climb into or on cabinets,

shelves, chairs, buckets or similar items. Use an appropriate ladder or step to reach high locations.

BEWARE OF BREAK TIMES

The ingestion of pathogenic organisms or harmful chemicals while eating on the job is a possibility in veterinary hospitals. This is why it is important to eat and drink only in areas designated for staff breaks that are free of toxic and biologically harmful substances. This also applies to the preparation of foods and beverages. Make sure coffee pots and utensils are well away from the sources that could contaminate food such as laboratories and treatment/bathing areas. Check the cabinets or shelves above food preparation areas to ensure that no hazards could spill onto the area. Always store food, drinks, condiments, and snacks in a separate refrigerator from the one used to store biological or chemical hazards such as vaccines, drugs, and laboratory samples.

> ### ✎ TECHNICIAN NOTE
> Always store food, drinks, condiments, and snacks in a separate refrigerator from the one used to store biological or chemical hazards such as vaccines, drugs, and laboratory samples.

MACHINERY AND EQUIPMENT

Never operate machinery or equipment without all the proper guards in place. Equipment such as fans and cage dryers have moving parts that can severely hurt or even sever a finger. Long hair should be tied back or pinned up to prevent it from getting caught in fans or other moving parts. Avoid wearing excessively loose clothing or jewelry when working around machinery with moving parts.

When using equipment such as autoclaves, microwave ovens, cautery irons, or other heating devices, be sure to understand the proper rules for safe operation. Burns, especially from steam, are painful and serious and almost always can be prevented. Autoclaves also present a danger from the pressure that is used for proper sterilization. Before opening an autoclave, be sure to first release the pressure by activating the *vent* device, and at the same time, keep your hands and face away from the steam. Let the steam dissipate completely before opening the door fully, and be careful when removing the packs because they may still be hot. Always assume cautery devices and branding irons are hot and use the insulated handle whenever you touch them. Never place heated irons on any surface where they could overheat and start a fire, or where someone might accidentally touch them.

ELECTRICAL

Many procedures performed on a daily basis require the use of electricity. Although new equipment and buildings have many safety features built into the design, you must be conscious of avoiding a situation that could cause a fire or physical harm to yourself, another person, or a patient.

Do not remove light switch or electrical outlet covers. Always keep circuit-breaker boxes closed, and never block access by stacking supplies or equipment in front of them. Only persons trained to perform maintenance duties should repair electrical appliances, outlets, switches, fixtures, or breakers.

If you must use a portable dryer or other electrical equipment in a wet area, make sure it is properly grounded and only plugged into a ground-fault circuit interruption (GFCI) type outlet. Extension cords should only be used for temporary applications and should always be of the 3-conductor, grounded type. Never run extension cords through windows or doors that may close and damage the wires or across aisles or floors where a tripping hazard may be created.

Surge suppressors should only be used to protect sensitive electronic equipment and should never be overloaded (Figure 36-5). In addition, surge suppressors should never be used with portable heaters, autoclaves, or coffee pots, because they may overheat and cause a fire.

Equipment with grounded plugs must never be used with adapters or nongrounded extension cords. Never alter or remove the ground terminals on plugs. Appliances or equipment with defective ground terminals or plugs should not be used until repaired.

When changing light bulbs (especially fluorescent bulbs), be careful to remove and replace the bulb without breaking it. Inoperable bulbs should be disposed of directly into the outside dumpster or inside of a container to keep the bulb from breaking.

FIRE AND EVACUATION

The potential for dramatic loss of life (both human and animal) and the destruction of property make a hospital fire one of the most feared accidents imaginable. Fortunately,

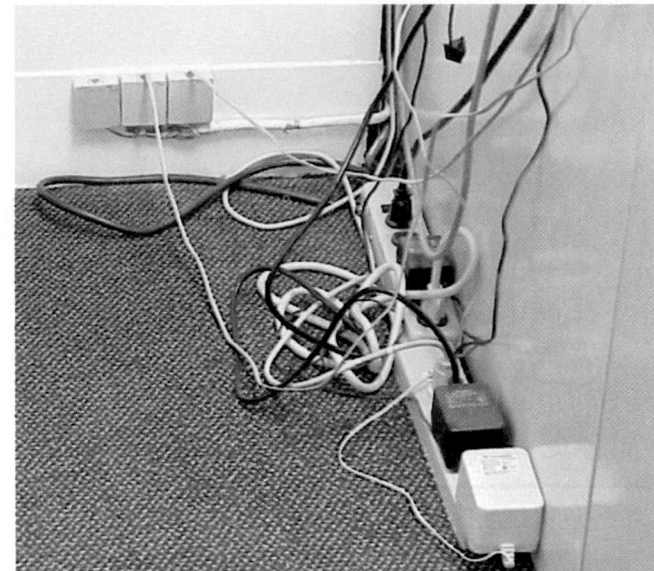

Figure 36-5 Overloaded surge suppressors or extension cords can start a fire.

this danger can be significantly reduced by a few simple precautions.

Never use power adapters or surge suppressors as a substitute for permanent wiring. Overloaded or faulty electrical cords can overheat or short out and start a fire, even when the equipment is turned off!

Always store flammable liquids properly; many, such as gasoline, paint thinner, and ether, should never be stored inside the hospital except in an approved flammable storage cabinet. Some components of specialty dental and large animal acrylic repair kits are also very flammable. Very small amounts of these components are usually not a problem, but always ensure that they are stored and used in an area with good ventilation and that the containers have tight-fitting lids that are replaced immediately after use.

Flammable materials such as newspapers, boxes, and cleaning chemicals must always be stored at least 3 feet away from an ignition source such as a water heater, furnace, or stove. Always use extra care when using portable heaters. Never leave them unattended, and always make sure they are placed no closer than 3 feet from any wall, furniture, or other flammable material.

Become familiar with the location of the emergency exits in your facility. Make sure the emergency exits are always unlocked and free from obstructions when you are in the building. If you must work in a building when security warrants that the doors be locked, make sure you have at least two clear exits from the building.

✏ TECHNICIAN NOTE

Become familiar with the location of the emergency exits in your facility. Make sure the emergency exits are always unlocked and free from obstructions when you are in the building.

Box 36-1 USING A FIRE EXTINGUISHER

- If you must use a portable fire extinguisher, remember the word *PASS*:
  - *P*ull the pin: Some extinguishers require releasing a lock latch, pressing a puncture lever, or other motion. (Check your extinguishers to be sure.)
  - *A*im low: Point the extinguisher (or its horn or hose) at the base of the fire.
  - *S*queeze the handle: This releases the extinguishing agent.
  - *S*weep from side to side at the base of the fire until it appears to be out.
- Watch the fire area. If a fire breaks out again, repeat use of the extinguisher.
- Most portable extinguishers work according to these directions, but read and follow the directions on your specific extinguisher.

Learn the emergency warning system in your hospital. If the facility is equipped with an electronic alarm system, be sure you know how to activate it manually. In the absence of an electronic alarm system, a verbal alarm is very effective. You can use the telephone intercom feature to alert everyone that there is a fire in the building or in small buildings simply yell in a loud clear voice to get the message out!

Know your duties in the event of a fire. Remember, your first responsibility is to notify others about the fire and then to get out of the building safely if an evacuation is ordered. Leave the rescue duties to the professionals that are trained and equipped to handle this very dangerous task. If you do evacuate the building, immediately report to the designated assembly area for accountability. This is very important since others will assume you are trapped in the building if you are not present at the assembly area.

Know where the fire extinguishers are located and how to use them (Box 36-1). Most veterinary hospitals are equipped with dry-chemical-type fire extinguishers. But before you decide to use a fire extinguisher, make sure the alarm has been sounded, everyone has left the building (or is in the process of leaving), and the fire department has been called.

The National Fire Protection Association recommends that you *never* attempt to fight a fire if any of these conditions are true:

- If the fire is spreading beyond the immediate area where it started or involves any part of the building or structure
- If the fire could block your escape route
- If you are unsure of the proper operation of the extinguisher
- If you are in doubt that the extinguisher you are holding is designed for the type of fire at hand or it is large enough to suppress the fire

DO NOT BECOME A VICTIM OF VIOLENCE

Just as in any occupation, you are at risk of injury from accidents not directly related to your job. Vehicle accidents,

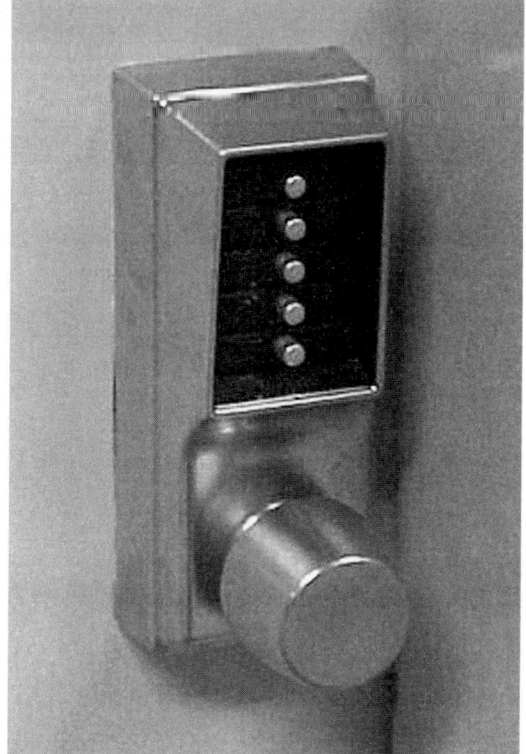

Figure 36-6 Personal safety includes the diligent use of locks and barriers to deter unauthorized persons from entering the facility.

personal assault, robbery, and even natural disasters have resulted in veterinary technicians being injured while on duty. Although no one can prevent every possible scenario, preparation can certainly help and sometimes will minimize the injury. When outside of the hospital building, be aware of your environment and do your best to avoid placing yourself in a situation that could go bad.

Always keep the "nonclient" doors locked from the outside to prevent anyone from gaining unauthorized or undetected entry into the building (Figure 36-6).

If you work in a critical care or 24-hour practice, you should utilize the "barriers" that are usually available. Things like buzzers to control access through the front door and one-way locks on the remaining doors (to let you out in case of an emergency, but keep the door locked from the outside) are essential in these environments, so do not prop doors open, disassemble the locking system, or turn the system off. In any business that keeps money or stores valuable items, there is a potential for robbery. If you ever find yourself in a situation where someone demands money, drugs, or other material items while threatening your personal safety—*do not withhold the things they demand*. As soon as safely possible, let everyone else know of the situation. You should attempt to contact the police if it can be safely done without the person's knowledge; otherwise, do it immediately after the person has left.

Cooperate with their demands and give them what they want, but do not go with the person. Resist physical assault

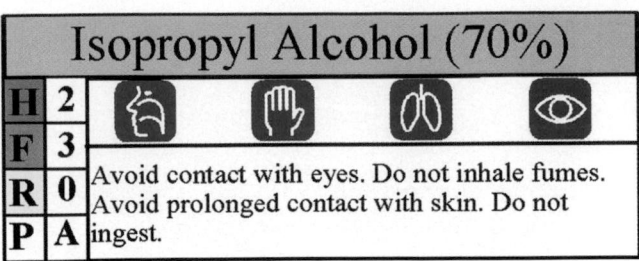

Isopropyl Alcohol (70%)					
H	**2**				
F	**3**	Avoid contact with eyes. Do not inhale fumes.			
R	**0**	Avoid prolonged contact with skin. Do not			
P	**A**	ingest.			

Figure 36-7 Example of a secondary container hazard warning label.

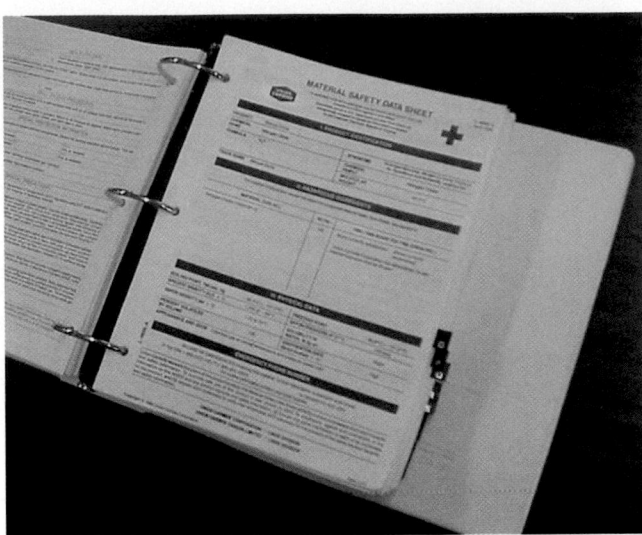

Figure 36-8 MSDSs contain safety information that may not be indicated on the product label.

or battery to the best of your abilities and preferably outside the building so that passers-by can see what is happening and render assistance or call the police.

HAZARDOUS CHEMICALS: RIGHT TO KNOW

You may not think about it, but many products that you use every day can be hazardous. Every chemical, even common ones like cleaning supplies have the potential to cause you harm. Some chemicals contribute to health problems while others may be flammable and pose a fire threat. The most common chemicals in use in the veterinary practice are as follows:

- Cleaning and disinfecting agents
- Insecticides and pesticides
- Drugs and medications (including anesthetic gases)
- Sterilization agents
- Radiology processing fluids

Planning and training are the keys to safely handling any chemical. Every business, including your practice must follow the requirements of OSHA's "Right To Know" law. This law requires you to be informed of all chemicals you may be exposed to while doing your job. The right-to-know law also requires you to wear all safety equipment that is prescribed by the manufacturer and the practice when using any product containing a hazardous chemical. The safety equipment must be provided to you at no cost to you, but it is not optional—you must wear what is prescribed!

A key component of the right-to-know law is the hazardous materials plan. The hazardous materials plan includes instructions for organizing and filing the practice "Right to Know" label, but that information is generally written for the average consumer who will have limited exposure using the product. When a product is used in a business such as your veterinary practice, you may be exposed to that product more than the average consumer, so your risk may be different. The manufacturer of a product that contains a hazardous chemical will prepare a Material Safety Data Sheet (MSDS) for that product. The MSDS will give you additional precautions, instructions, and advice for handling that product in the workplace (Figure 36-8). Your practice is required to keep an MSDS library for the

chemicals that you use. Ask your supervisor where your hospital's MSDS library is located. Take the time to review the MSDSs for the products you use frequently. Although MSDSs may look complicated at first glance, the information that is important to you is easy to find: review the health, protective equipment, and disposal sections to gain a better understanding of the risks and precautions you should know.

> ### 🖋 TECHNICIAN NOTE
> Your practice is required to keep an MSDS library for the chemicals that you use. Ask your supervisor where your hospital's MSDS library is located.

Working bottles of hazardous products should always have tight-fitting, screw-on lids. Always remember to replace the cap back on the bottle after using any chemical product. You should endeavor to store chemical bottles in a closed cabinet; this will help prevent animals from injury in the event that they escape. Ideally, the cabinet or shelf should be at or below eye level. This will minimize the chances of spilling the product in your face if the cap is not secure. Never store or use hazardous products near food, beverages, or food preparation areas.

Be very cautious when mixing or diluting any chemical product. Try to keep the material from splashing on your hands, clothes, or face. If it is likely that the product will splash on you, wear a pair of protective latex or nitrile gloves and some protective goggles or glasses. When making solutions from a concentrate, you should always start with the correct quantity of water then add the concentrate. Never add the water to the concentrate because the chemical may splash or react differently.

When two chemicals are mixed together the result is seldom a simple mixture. It is often a new, sometimes very

Box 36-2 **Box 36-2** Chemical Spill Cleanup

- **Step 1.** Keep unnecessary people and pets out of the area to prevent spreading the spilled material.
- **Step 2.** If the area is small or the fumes are extremely strong, increase ventilation by opening a window or turning on an exhaust fan. Do not use an electric exhaust fan or electric equipment and avoid turning switches on or off when cleaning up spilled flammable materials.
- **Step 3.** Put on a pair of protective latex or nitrile gloves. If it is likely that your clothing will become contaminated during the cleanup, put on a protective apron and protective eye wear.
- **Step 4.** As soon as possible, cover the spill with absorbent materials like paper towels or cat litter. Allow the absorbent material to fully collect the liquid.
- **Step 5.** Using a broom, gently sweep the saturated absorbent into a dust pan and deposit it in a plastic trash bag.
- **Step 6.** When all the material has been picked up, seal the trash bag and dispose of it as regular waste unless your institution, city, or county requires you to do otherwise.
- **Step 7.** Wash the contaminated area thoroughly with plain water or a detergent (not a disinfectant) soap if permissible by the instructions in the MSDS. Allow the area to air dry.
- **Step 8.** Remove any protective equipment used during the cleanup. Dispose of single-use items as regular trash unless your institution, city, or county requires you to do otherwise.
- **Step 9.** Wash your hands thoroughly and change any clothing that has become contaminated during the cleanup process.
- **Step 10.** Replace used materials in the spill kit.

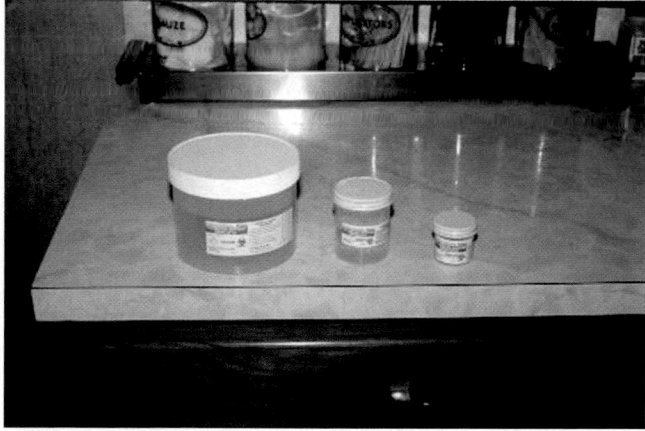

Figure 36-9 When possible, use only biopsy jars prefilled with formalin to prevent excessive exposure.

medicine. This method has distinct advantages, but since EtO is thought to be a human carcinogen, special precautions must be maintained.

- Read the MSDS carefully and follow all instructions.
- Store the ampules in a closed cabinet away from sources of heat.
- Only use approved devices for the procedure.
- Read, understand, and follow all the written procedures and safety precautions relevant to your practice.
- Know the emergency procedures to be performed in case of an accidental release of EtO.

Formalin

Historically, formalin has been used in the veterinary profession for tissue preservation, diagnostic tests (knotts), and even sterilization. Since formaldehyde is also a suspected human carcinogen, OSHA takes its use very seriously. The standards for use of formaldehyde are very similar to the standards for use of ethylene oxide:

- Read the MSDS carefully and follow all instructions.
- Store supplies safely, include museum jars.
- Use only with good ventilation in the room and avoid breathing vapors.
- Wear gloves and goggles to avoid skin and eye contact.

Whenever possible, you should obtain formalin in small, premeasured containers (also called *biopsy jars*) so that the serious risk is minimized (Figure 36-9). Often the diagnostic laboratory will supply prefilled biopsy jars at no charge, so be sure to ask!

Glutaraldehyde

Glutaraldehyde is a potent chemical used in the veterinary practice to sterilize hard instruments without the use of an autoclave. Because it's so effective at killing germs, it can also be harmful to other living organisms—like you (Figure 36-10)! Be sure to follow all the manufacturer's safe handling

different and possibly dangerous chemical. Never mix any chemicals unless directed to do so on the label or MSDS.

Minor spills of most chemicals can be cleaned up with paper towels or absorbent (like kitty litter) and disposed of in the trash; however, very dangerous chemicals like mercury require special procedures. *Before* you use a new chemical, review the MSDS and learn the procedures you must follow for cleaning up a spill. When cleaning up any spill, remember to wear protective gloves and any other special equipment required on the MSDS. Keep other people and animals away from the spill until it is safe. Unless prohibited by the instructions on the MSDS, wash the spill site and any contaminated equipment with a detergent soap and water—*not* a disinfecting soap (Box 36-2).

Familiarize yourself with the locations of the eye-wash stations in your practice. Test them regularly and know how to use them before you're in the position to need them!

SPECIAL CHEMICALS

Ethylene Oxide

Many hospitals use gas sterilization for items that would be damaged by other procedures. Electrical drills, rubber products, and sharps are commonly exposed to ethylene oxide (EtO) as a sterilization agent in human and veterinary

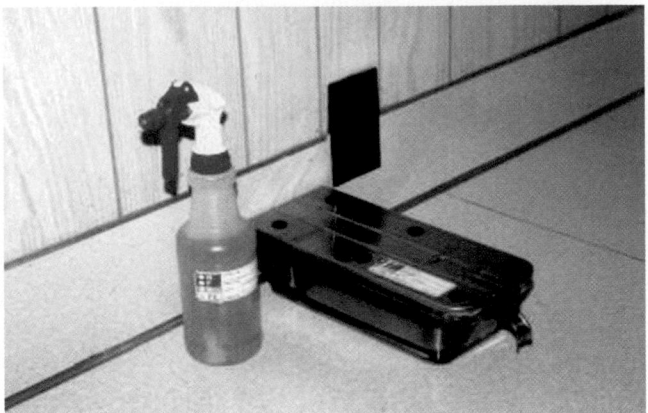

Figure 36-10 Disinfectants are designed to kill living organisms, so they must be handled safely.

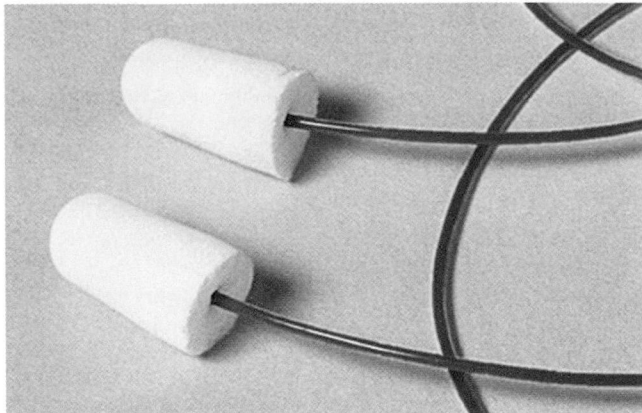

Figure 36-11 Hearing protectors should always be used in noisy kennels.

rules when using this "cold-sterilization" solution, including washing your hands after handling instruments exposed to the solution and keeping the trays covered to minimize evaporation.

MEDICAL AND ANIMAL-RELATED HAZARDS

We cannot forget that the overriding purpose of a veterinary practice is the care and treatment of animals. But sometimes handling our patients can be a hazard in itself! Anyone who has worked with animals under stress or in pain will relate personal accounts of injuries from patients. In fact, insurance statistics show that animal-related accidents are the most common type of injury among workers in veterinary-related jobs, including veterinary technicians.

> ### 🖉 TECHNICIAN NOTE
> Insurance statistics show that animal-related accidents are the most common type of injury among workers in veterinary-related jobs, including veterinary technician.

Unfortunately, this hazard cannot be eliminated, so we have to do the next best thing—minimize it. The best way to protect yourself from this hazard is to obtain training and practice in animal restraint. The very first safety rule when working around animals is to stay alert! Animals sometimes react to situations unexpectedly. Sudden noises, movements, or even light can be the stimulus that would cause an animal to react, so if you are the person responsible for restraining the animal, keep your attention focused on the animal's reactions and not on the procedure. You must learn the proper restraint positions for each of the species of animals with which you work. Refer to Chapter 1 for additional information about the restraint and handling of animals.

Remember that capture/restraint equipment is available if the animal is fractious or not cooperating; sometimes,

just a piece of rope to hobble a leg or a piece of gauze for a hasty muzzle will make all the difference. And don't forget that chemical restraint, rather than physical restraint, is often better for both you and the animal, but be sure to ask the veterinarian for approval before administering any medication to a patient.

Large animals such as horses and cattle are particularly dangerous and may severely injure or even kill a person when trying to escape restraint. Never put your hand, leg, or any other part of your body between the animal and the side of the enclosure or chute; use a hook or pole to pass ropes or belts through the chute. If you have to enter a stall, paddock, or trailer with a large animal, stay on the side of the animal nearest the door so that you can escape if the situation becomes hazardous. If you must capture a fractious animal from a cage or pen, make sure there is another person present that can assist you if you get into trouble.

If your job entails handling exotic or nondomestic animals, remember that they all have their own unique methods of defense. You should know and understand their possible reactions before you attempt to restrain or treat them.

NOISE

Dogs in cages will inevitably bark, and barking dogs can adversely affect your hearing, especially if you work in an indoor kennel. Noise levels in dog wards can reach as high as 110 dB! Although relatively short-duration exposure to these noise levels, like going into the kennel just to retrieve a patient, poses no serious damage to your hearing, chronic or long-term exposure can contribute to hearing loss. When working in noisy areas for extended periods of time (e.g., cleaning of cages), you must wear personal hearing protectors (Figure 36-11). It does not matter what style or type of hearing protectors you use (ear plugs or muffs), as long as they are rated to filter the noise by at least 20 dB (the package will indicate the rating).

BATHING, DIPPING, AND SPRAYING AREAS

There is probably no area of an animal hospital with a greater risk for injury than in the bathing or insecticide application areas. Although newer parasite control products significantly reduce exposure to pesticides and insecticides, shampoos and medical dips are still a big concern.

The products used for bathing and dipping animals can be harmful to your health as well as the environment. Even the "all natural" shampoos can cause eye irritation, and you can develop sensitivities to even the mildest products if you are exposed often enough. Because it is impossible to prevent splashing and shaking, it is important to *always* wear protective glasses or goggles when bathing or dipping animals. In most cases, it is also important to wear gloves and a protective apron to prevent the product from getting on your skin or clothing; that minimizes the amount absorbed through the skin!

Bottles of dips, shampoos, and insecticides should be stored in a cabinet at or below eye level. The bottle should be properly labeled with the contents and any hazard warning that is appropriate (refer to the discussion on chemicals in this chapter for more details). Always replace the cap or lid on the container when you are finished using it to prevent accidental spillage. Plastic containers recycled from other areas can be used for diluted shampoos and dips, however, only use the ones that have a screw-on cap or lid.

Always use a ventilation fan to keep the fumes from shampoos and dips at a safe level. When exhaust fans are too large, they waste heating or air conditioning, so you may be hesitant to use them in some situations. If that is the case, ask your hospital administrator to have a smaller fan installed directly over the tub or area so that fumes can be exhausted without sacrificing the comfort in the room.

Make sure you know where the eye-wash station for this area is located. Learn how to properly use the eye-wash device before it is needed. If you ever splash a chemical in your eyes, *do not* rub your eyes with your hands! Immediately call out for help; there is usually someone nearby. With a co-worker's assistance, go to the eye-wash station and flush *both* eyes (even if only one eye is affected). Avoid using the spray attachments for tubs and sinks since the water pressure is unregulated and the streams of water from these devices can be fine enough to lacerate your cornea.

ZOONOTIC DISEASES

Infectious diseases that can be passed from animals to humans are known as *zoonotic diseases*. Some zoonotic diseases are not easily transmitted from animals to humans, while others are very easily spread. You can be exposed to the organisms that cause disease by several means: inhalation, contact with broken skin, ingestion, contact with eyes and mucus membranes, and via accidental inoculation by a needle. There is a wide variety of zoonotic agents to which a veterinary technician may be exposed; certainly more than can be discussed in this chapter. However, some important ones are listed below. Refer to Chapter 35 for more information on zoonotic diseases.

Viral Infections

Rabies is a very serious (almost always fatal) viral disease that can affect any warm-blooded animal (including humans). The virus is spread by contact with an infected animal's saliva. Usually, the virus it transmitted through a bite, but it has also been transmitted by open wounds or mucous membranes coming in contact with virus-rich saliva.

Although the disease is ever present in wild animal populations (primarily bats, raccoons, and skunks in the United States), in recent years many states have confirmed record high numbers of rabies in domestic species such as cats, dogs, horses, and cattle. Several University veterinary hospitals have also recorded cases of rabies in horses, cattle, and companion animals. Some of those animals were even adopted from pet shops! Although rare, it is possible that you will encounter a rabid pet at the veterinary hospital where you work.

It is important that you are aware of the prevalence of rabies and the incidence among wild species in your area, because it varies in each region of the country. If you work in a high-risk environment such as with unvaccinated, stray, and homeless animals in a shelter or with wild animals at a rehabilitation center, you should be immunized with pre-exposure prophylaxis. Ask your hospital administrator about the availability of these vaccines. They are often available through the occupational health divisions of regional human hospitals. When you must handle an unvaccinated, wild, or stray animal, wear protective (rubber or latex) gloves and wear protective gowns and goggles in cases where the procedure may be "messy."

Bacterial Infections

There is a wide variety of both pathogenic and non-pathogenic bacteria that you may be exposed to during your professional life. Some examples of pathogenic bacteria include *Salmonella* spp., *Pasteurella* spp., *E. coli*, and *Pseudomonas* spp. Bacteria can be transferred by direct contact with the animals and their exudates. This is particularly likely if you have any cuts or open sores. Some bacteria may be aerosolized and inhaled or absorbed through mucous membranes. The best protection against exposure to bacteria is simply good personal hygiene. Always follow the personal hygiene rules discussed later in this chapter.

Lyme Disease

Recently, Lyme disease has become a more serious concern for animals and people. When an infected deer tick bites a host (an animal or person) during feeding, the bacteria *Borrelia burgdorferi* is transferred to the host. Lyme disease in humans is characterized by aches in the joints, fever, and a host of other flulike symptoms. The best defense against this disease is to check yourself daily for ticks, and remove them promptly. If you work in a food- or mixed-animal practice, it is also a good idea to use an insect repellent when you go out into fields or woods to work.

Fungal Infections

Contrary to its name, *ringworm* is not a parasite or worm. It is an infection of the skin caused by a fungus know as *Microsporum* sp. Ringworm is passed between animals and humans. Cats and horses are particularly susceptible to ringworm infestations. Again, the most effective protection from ringworm infection is to wear gloves when handling or treating animals diagnosed with the condition and to practice good personal hygiene. Be especially careful about preventing contamination of your clothing when treating patients with *Microsporum,* because it is believed that the fungal spores can be carried to other locations (such as your home) on clothing and infect other animals or other people.

Internal Parasites

When the eggs of common internal parasites such as roundworms infect humans, they usually do not mature into adult parasites, but they do cause other problems. Roundworm larvae can migrate to virtually any organ in the body and develop into a cystlike growth known as *visceral larval migrans.* These "cysts" are usually not clinically noticeable unless they develop in a vital organ such as the eye, where they can do permanent damage to the retina and may cause blindness. Puppies almost always have some level of round worm infestation, because the passage of worms from the bitch to the fetus occurs through the placenta and via lactation. When the infected puppy defecates in soil, the roundworm eggs are able to survive for long periods of time until they are picked up and ingested by another mammal.

Another common internal parasite, hookworms, can also cause problems in humans by a condition known as *cutaneous larval migrans.* This condition is particularly prevalent in southern areas of the United States where there are warm, humid winters. Children who play barefoot where pets defecate frequently may be affected, and people who lie on the ground where dogs have defecated. Unlike the visceral cysts from roundworms, the cutaneous migrans are relatively easy to spot and appear as small, red lines in the regions where the parasite has burrowed into the skin from the soil. Often these marks are itchy and lengthen as the parasite moves from one part of the body to another, subcutaneously.

External Parasites

The irritating and very itchy mite that causes *Sarcoptic mange* can spread easily to humans from animals. Typically this occurs in regions where there is tight clothing such

as along bra lines and waist bands. When treating animal patients for mange, always wear gloves and a protective gown and wash your hands thoroughly with disinfecting soap immediately after the procedure.

Protozoal Infections

Infestation with a protozoan known as *Toxoplasma cati* is called *toxoplasmosis.* Although it is usually not harmful to most adults, it can have devastating effects on the development of a human fetus by causing hydrocephalus and mental retardation. Nonsporulated *Toxoplasma* eggs are shed in the feces of infected cats. The eggs subsequently sporulate approximately 2 to 4 days later. These 3-day-old, sporulated oocysts, if ingested by some pregnant women, are particularly dangerous to the fetus. Pregnant women can avoid potential exposure to *Toxoplasma* by taking the following steps:

1. Avoid cleaning cat litter pans when possible, particularly those that contain 2-day-old feces older than 2 days. If it is unavoidable, be sure to wear gloves when handling the litter box and wash your hands when you are finished.
2. Wash raw vegetables thoroughly (dirt on vegetables may contain oocytes).
3. Do not eat raw or uncooked meat, particularly lamb and pork, which can carry the encysted protozoan in the muscle tissue. Cook all meat thoroughly.
4. When gardening, wear gloves that can be removed easily. Under no circumstances should dirt accidentally enter your mouth (e.g., when removing a hair from your mouth).
5. Women in the veterinary profession are encouraged to have *Toxoplasma* titers evaluated *before* becoming pregnant, if at all possible. Your physician can give you more specific advice about *Toxoplasma* titers during your pregnancy.

Other zoonotic protozoal agents such as *Giardia* and coccidia cause diarrhea and gastrointestinal cramping in humans. These are typically spread to people from their contact with infected animals (particularly puppies and kittens), but they can also be acquired by drinking contaminated water.

Because you will probably come in contact with some of these diseases in your job, particular attention to personal hygiene and sanitary work practices is essential. Good personal hygiene includes making sure your clothes don't become soiled by chemicals or biological material, and of course, regular hand washing. In general, you should wash your hands

1. After handling medications or lab samples
2. After treating patients or cleaning cages
3. Before as well as after you use the restroom
4. Before lunch or meal breaks and before you leave work at the end of your shift

NONZOONOTIC DISEASES OF CONCERN

Some infectious agents, such as parvo viral enteritis in dogs and panleukopenia in cats, are not a serious concern to human health, but they are so highly contagious that you can carry the live virus home to your pets on your clothes and shoes! For this reason, some technicians when working with Parvo cases at work leave their shoes outside their front door and change their clothes immediately upon entering their home and some even change clothes before they leave the hospital. In addition, technicians who work with cats that have certain viral upper respiratory conditions and chlamydia can themselves contract pinkeye or conjunctivitis. Therefore, when treating cases with contagious diseases, be sure to wear a protective apron, surgical mask, exam gloves, and, when appropriate, eye protection. Thoroughly wash your hands with a disinfecting agent such as chlorhexidine or povidone-iodine scrub at the completion of the treatment and change your clothes before handling your own animals.

In human medicine, potentially deadly agents such as human immunodeficiency virus (HIV) can be transferred from patient to health care provider when collecting and handling blood and other laboratory samples.

A DIRTY MOUTH?—PRECAUTIONS FOR DENTISTRY OPERATIONS

Dental procedures that include use of a high speed and ultrasonic scaler aerosolizes oral microbes, making personal protection a necessity. One of the most common pathogens in the mouths of animals is *Pasteurella multocida*, an organism that has been linked to cardiac and pulmonary problems in humans and animals alike. Therefore, when performing dental procedures, be sure to wear goggles, gloves, and a surgical mask (Figure 36-12).

RADIOLOGY

The ability to "see inside the body" is a great tool in medicine. In most cases, the method of choice is diagnostic radiography (x-rays.) Short-duration, infrequent exposure to radiation, such as having radiographs taken of yourself, is considered an acceptable level of exposure (the benefits outweigh the risks). However, long-term exposure to low doses of radiation has been linked to many medical disorders. High-dose exposure can cause skin changes, cell damage, and gastrointestinal and bone marrow disorders that can be fatal. Fortunately, much is known about the properties of x-rays, and we are clear about the ways in which we need to protect ourselves. By following some very simple safety precautions, you can safely use radiography in your practice.

Although modern radiographic machines have many safeguards integrated in their design, there is still the possibility of injury if these tools are used incorrectly. When you are taking x-rays, *always* wear a lead apron and lead gloves.

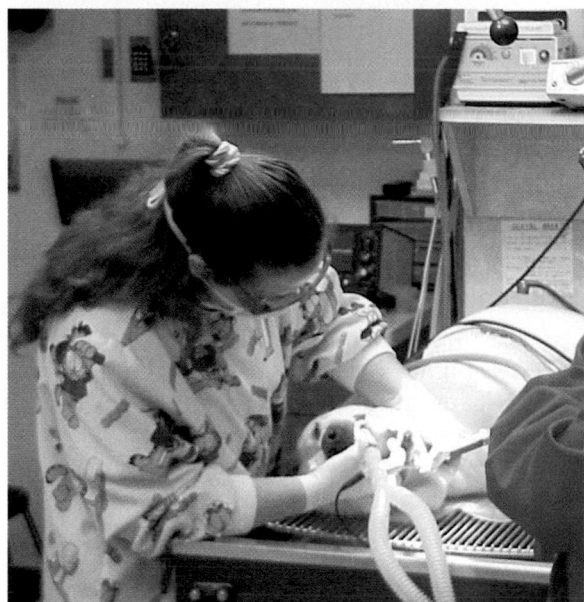

Figure 36-12 Always wear eye protection, a mask, and gloves when performing dental prophylaxis procedures.

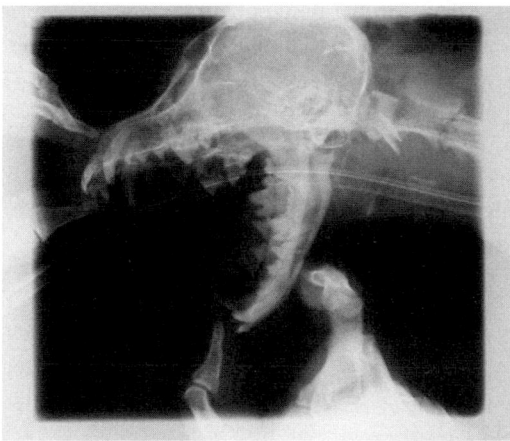

Figure 36-13 *Never* place your hand or any other part of your body in the primary beam when taking radiographs!

Thyroid collars and lead glasses are also recommended, particularly during extensive studies such as with fluoroscopy. Though restraint of animals during radiographic studies can be challenging, *never* place any part of your body, even a gloved hand, in the primary beam (Figure 36-13).

Before you use an x-ray machine, make sure you know the purpose of every knob and button. Always use the collimator to restrict the primary beam to a size smaller than the size of the cassette—in other words, "cone down" to the area to be radiographed so that scatter radiation is minimized. A properly collimated radiograph will have a small clear border around the entire film once developed.

Always follow the written operational and safety procedures from the hospital or machine manufacturer. If you haven't already done so, make an exposure chart specific to your machine so that you can replicate the best techniques for various studies. By following a proven technique chart and positioning the patient correctly the first time, you will have fewer "retakes" and will therefore reduce unnecessary exposure.

Portable machines, like those used in large animal and mobile practices, can be particularly dangerous because of their multipurpose abilities. These machines can be aimed in any direction, and because of their limited power they must utilize longer exposure times to produce diagnostic images. When using a portable machine, always make sure no one is in the path of the primary beam (even at a distance). Always use a cassette-holding pole and *never* hold a cassette with your hands while the exposure is made—even with gloves. And of course, remember to wear a lead apron and gloves when near the machine during exposure.

If you are involved in the exposure portion of radiography, you must have and utilize an individual dosimetry badge. This badge is worn on your collar outside your protective apron during radiographic procedures, not as protection, but as a measurement of any incidental radiation you may receive during the procedure. It's important to return the badge to the designated storage location (outside the x-ray area) when not in use. Unless you are taking radiographs, don't wear your badge outside because exposure to sunlight will result in false readings. Due to the relatively low numbers of radiographs taken in most practices, safer machines, and the use of good protective equipment, most technicians receive very little, if any, occupational exposure to radiation.

Radiographic processing chemicals (the developer and fixer) can be very corrosive to materials and organic tissues, so use protective gloves and goggles when mixing and pouring the chemicals. When using manual processing tanks, stir the chemicals with care and avoid splashing. After handling radiographic developing chemicals, always wash your hands. In addition, it is important to avoid breathing the fumes of the processing chemicals, so make sure there is adequate ventilation in the dark room; generally an exhaust fan is necessary.

Radiographic developing solutions can react dangerously with other chemicals. For this reason, *never* pour chemicals down the drain with developing solutions. Some liquid drain openers, when mixed with developer and fixer solutions, can produce toxic gases. Others can produce an exothermic reaction (generates high temperature) that can damage pipes.

ANESTHESIA

Anesthesia is as common to veterinary medicine as antiseptic wound care. The National Institute of Occupational Safety and Health (NIOSH) estimates that over 250,000 U.S. workers are at risk from exposure to waste gasses that are not metabolized by the patient. Long-term exposure to waste anesthetic gases (WAGs) has been linked to congenital abnormalities in children, spontaneous abortions, and even liver and kidney damage.

Although the recent development and use of improved anesthetic gasses have lowered risk to patients and health care workers, there is no chemical that is entirely without risk. We must therefore continue to take precautions to protect ourselves, even when using isoflurane and sevoflurane. OSHA has established a safe exposure limit for *all* halogenated anesthetic agents, which is not to exceed 2 parts per million (ppm).

✎ TECHNICIAN NOTE

OSHA has established a safe exposure limit for *all* halogenated anesthetic agents, which is not to exceed 2 parts per million (ppm).

Using a proper scavenging system is the single most effective means of reducing exposure to WAGs. There are three general types of scavenging systems: active scavenging, passive exhaust, and absorption. Each has a place, but rarely does one method fit all circumstances. Regardless of the system chosen, make sure it is fully operational and in use before turning on the anesthesia machine. If you use absorption canisters, be sure to check them (by weighing with a gram scale) regularly and replace them as needed. Once the canister becomes saturated with gas, it is ineffective!

According to some research, as much as 90% of the anesthetic gas levels found in the room during a procedure can be attributed to leaks in the anesthesia machine, so be sure to perform a leak check prior to use (Box 36-3 and Figures 36-14 to 36-17). Also make sure that the correct size hoses and rebreathing bags are used. Intubation tubes should be placed and the cuff inflated prior to connecting the animal to the anesthesia machine. Start the flow of anesthetic gases only after the patient is connected to the machine. When the surgical procedure is finished, turn off the vaporizer and increase the flow of oxygen to the patient. Be sure to use the "flush" feature to purge the circuit before disconnecting the patient.

Before filling the vaporizer, move the anesthesia machine to a well-ventilated area. Use a pouring funnel and be careful to avoid overfilling the vaporizer or spilling the liquid anesthetic. If you accidentally break a bottle of anesthetic, immediately evacuate all nonessential people from the area. Any windows in the area should be opened, and all exhaust fans turned on. Quickly control the liquid with a generous amount of kitty litter, and place a plastic bag over the spill to reduce evaporation. Pick up the absorbed liquid and kitty litter with a dust pan and place it inside a plastic garbage bag. Seal the bag tightly and dispose of it in an outside trash can. Leave the exhaust fans on and the windows open until you are sure the gas level has been reduced to a safe level.

The anesthetic protocols that involve masking the patient or using a tank for induction are more likely to generate a larger amount of WAGs. When using these protocols, be sure to use an appropriate flow rate and proper reservoir bag for the size of patient—*do not* turn up the oxygen flowmeter

Box 36-3 LEAK CHECK YOUR ANESTHESIA
MACHINE BEFORE EACH USE

1. Assemble all hoses, canisters, valves, or tubes according to the manufacturer's instructions.
2. Turn on the oxygen supply to the machine.
3. Close the pressure relief (pop-off)valve (Figure 36-14).
4. Use your thumb or palm to form a tight seal on the Y piece (the part of the hose that attaches to the patient's endotracheal tube) (Figure 36-15).
5. Turn on the oxygen until the bag is slightly overinflated (or when the pressure on the manometer reaches the 20 mark), then close the valve (Figure 36-16).
6. Observe the pressure in the system on the manometer, and watch closely for any decrease. (If your machine is not equipped with a manometer, observe the size of the bag closely.) If the pressure remains constant, the machine is leak free. If the pressure drops, there is a leak (or leaks) in the system. The faster the pressure drops, the larger the leak(s) (Figure 36-17).
7. If there is a leak, check the bag, hoses, and other rubber (plastic) parts for evidence of cracks or deterioration. Replace any parts that are damaged. Check all connections, especially the seals at the top and bottom of the soda lime canister and on the one-way valves (clear plastic domes). Tighten any loose connections you find.
8. After checking all connections and hoses, if there is still a leak, have the machine serviced by a qualified technician before use.
9. When the machine is leak free, reset the pressure relief (pop-off) valve to the proper position to use the machine normally.

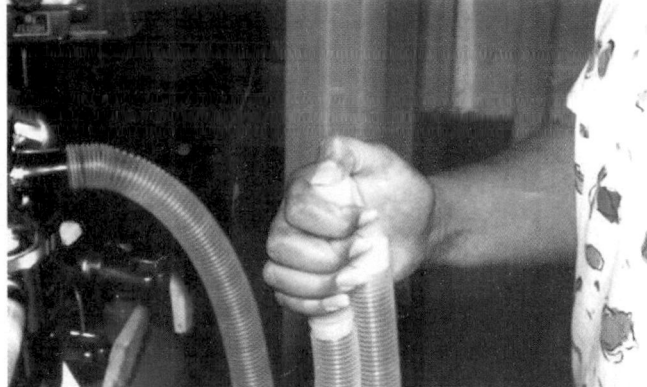
Figure 36-15 Step 4: Use your thumb or palm to form a tight seal on the Y piece.

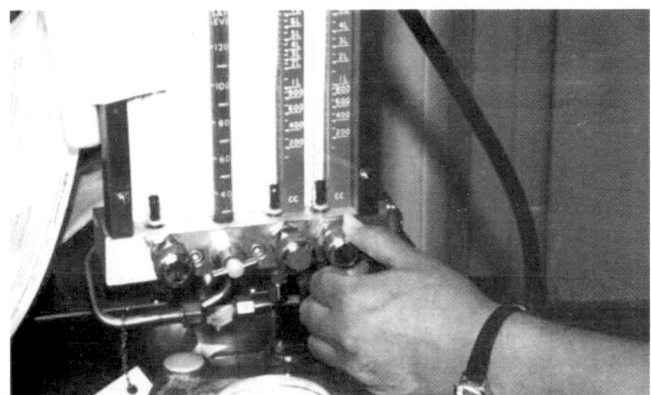
Figure 36-16 Step 5: Turn on the oxygen until bag is slightly overinflated.

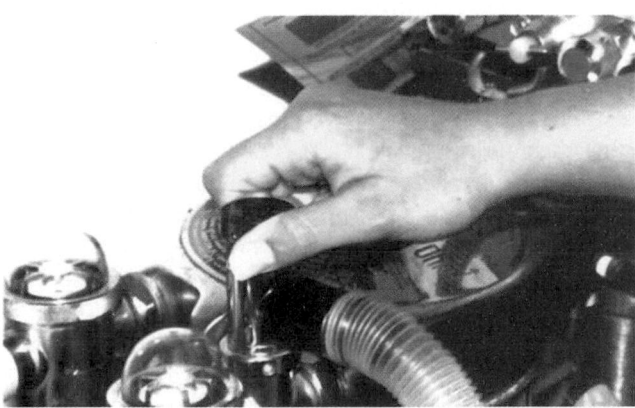
Figure 36-14 Step 3: Close the pop-off valve.

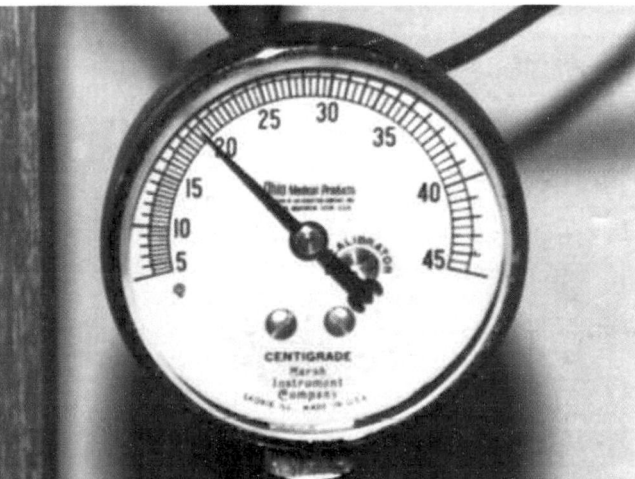
Figure 36-17 Step 6: Observe the pressure in the system on the manometer and watch closely for any decrease.

to maximum when masking a patient. Induction chambers should always be connected to the scavenging system or absorption canisters to reduce the levels of escaping gasses. Make sure the ventilation in the room is good, and use local exhaust fans when available.

Anesthetized animals do not metabolize all of the anesthetic gas that they have inhaled. Therefore they exhale some of it into the room after they have been extubated and while they are recovering. When monitoring patients during their recovery, you should avoid putting your face close to the animal's face. In addition, keep the number of recovering patients to an acceptable number based on the

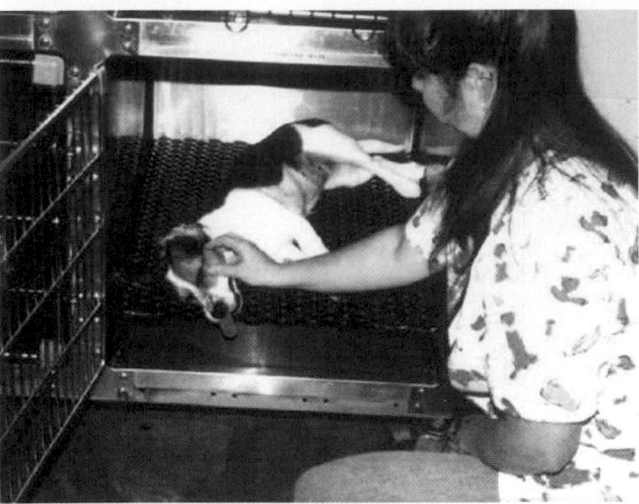

Figure 36-18 Monitor recovering anesthesia patients "at arms length" to minimize exposure to gasses emitted during respiration.

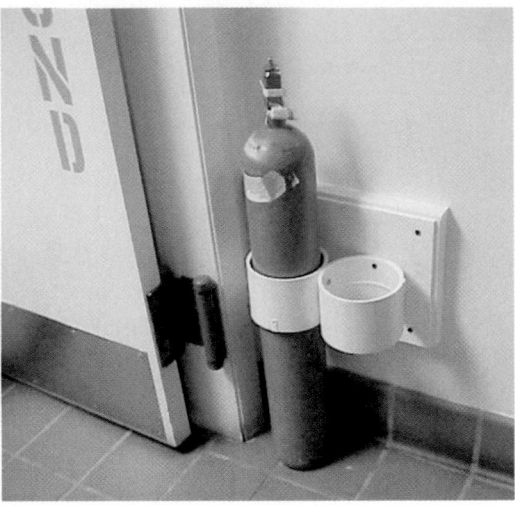

Figure 36-19 Small compressed-gas cylinders must be secured to prevent them from falling over.

size of the area and ventilation system (Figure 36-18). As much as possible, delay extubation and allow the patient to recover while still connected to the anesthetic machine (oxygen only) and scavenging system.

> ### ✎ TECHNICIAN NOTE
> Anesthetized animals do not metabolize all of the anesthetic gas that they have inhaled. Therefore they exhale some of it into the room after they have been extubated and while they are recovering.

When changing the soda lime (carbon dioxide absorbent) in anesthetic machines, wear rubber or latex gloves. When the soda lime is wet, as is often the case from humidity in the system, it can be very caustic to tissues and some metals. Dispose of the used soda lime granules in a plastic trash bag as regular trash.

Pregnant women should discuss the risks of exposure to anesthetic gases with their doctor. In addition, they should inform their supervisor of their condition as soon as possible so that safety procedures can be reviewed and adjusted if necessary.

COMPRESSED GASSES

Every year, hundreds of workers are injured while working with compressed gas cylinders, usually because of improper storage or handling of these cylinders. Regardless of the size of the cylinder or whether the cylinder is empty, full, or in use, store them in a dry, cool place, away from potential heat sources such as furnaces, water heaters, and direct sunlight. Always secure the tanks, even the small ones, in an upright position by means of a chain or strap (Figure 36-19). Cylinders that are stored inside a closet should also be secured since they can fall against the door and cause injury

when you open the door. If the cylinder is equipped with a protective cap, they must be firmly screwed in place when the cylinder is not in use. If you have to move a large cylinder, don't roll or drag it; always us a hand truck or cart, and remember to strap the tank in.

SHARPS AND MEDICAL WASTE

The most serious hazard from needles or sharp objects in a veterinary medical environment is from the physical trauma (and possible bacterial infection) that is caused by a puncture or laceration. To prevent these types of accidents, always keep sharps, needles, scalpel blades, and other sharp instruments capped or sheathed until ready for use. Do not attempt to recap the needle after use unless the physical danger from sticks or lacerations cannot be avoided by any other means. When it is necessary to recap a needle, you should use the "one-handed" method (Box 36-4 and Figures 36-20 to 36-22). Although some practice is needed before the one-handed method becomes second nature, it is the safest and most practical approach for most veterinary situations.

Do not remove the needle from the syringe for disposal because this unnecessary handling often results in injuries. Whenever possible, the entire needle and syringe should be disposed of in the designated sharps containers immediately after use. Do not try to over-fill a sharps container—when it's full, it's full! When the sharps container is full, seal it and replace it with a new one. Never open a sharps container that has already been sealed or stick your fingers into one for any reason.

Destroying the needle prior to disposal is not recommended because it may aerosolize the contents of the needle and increase your exposure. Likewise, you should not collect sharps in a smaller container and transfer them to a larger

Box 36-4 ONE-HANDED NEEDLE RECAPPING

- **Step 1.** Place the cap on a flat surface such as the countertop or even the floor.
- **Step 2.** Using only one hand, hold the syringe in the tips of your fingers with the needle pointing away from your body.
- **Step 3.** Place your fingertips on the flat surface so that the needle and syringe are parallel to and in line with the cap (Figure 36-21).
- **Step 4.** Move your hand forward "dragging" your fingertips on the flat surface until the needle is inside of the cap. You may then use your other hand to "seat" the cap firmly (Figures 36-21 and 36-22).

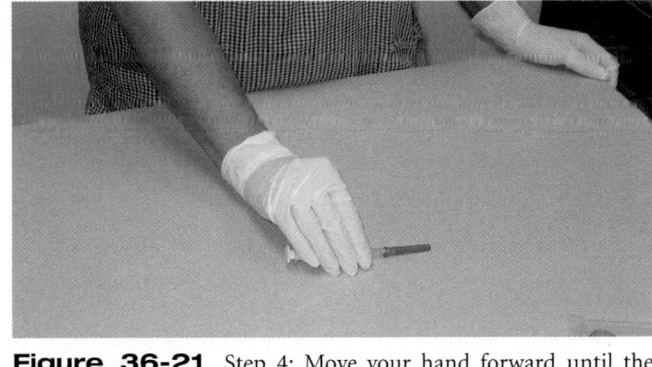

Figure 36-21 Step 4: Move your hand forward until the needle is inside the cap.

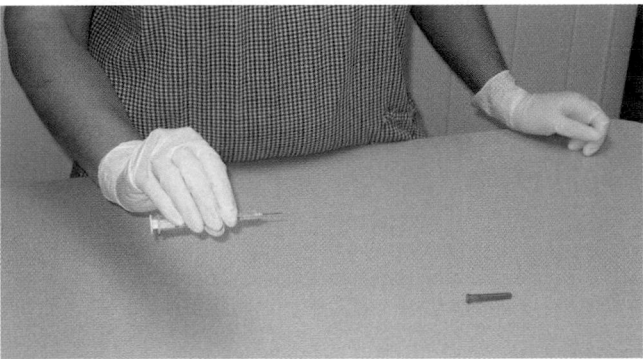

Figure 36-20 Using only one hand, hold the syringe in the tips of your fingers, with the needle pointing away from your body.

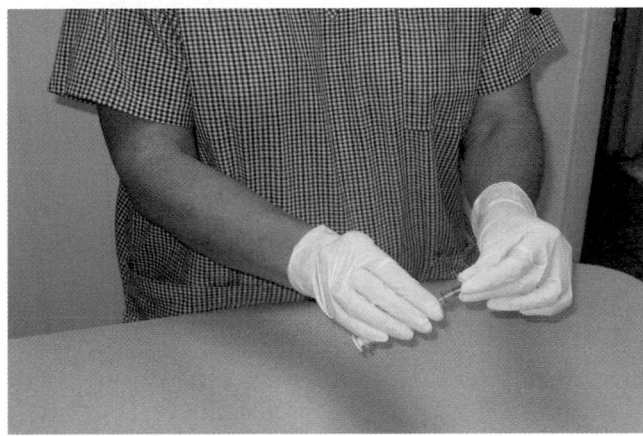

Figure 36-22 Final step: Use your other hand to "seat" the cap firmly.

container for disposal. Of course, never throw needles or sharps directly into regular trash containers, regardless of whether or not they are capped.

Table 36-1 explains which materials are usually considered hazardous and which are not. Although this chart is essentially accurate, some states have special rules for discarding medical waste, so be sure to follow the rules prescribed by your state.

HAZARDOUS DRUGS AND PHARMACY OPERATIONS

Medicines are designed to cure diseases and make patients better, but it is important to remember that all medicines are chemicals and chemicals can be dangerous. In the veterinary pharmacy, you can be exposed to all kinds of drugs just by handling them. Liquids can splash in your eyes when you pour them or they can release vapors that you can inhale. Handling, crushing, or breaking tablets can leave powder residue on your hands that will be ingested next time you put your hands near your mouth or mucous membranes.

Some drugs like the cytotoxic drugs (CDs) used to treat patients with cancer are so potent even minute exposures can cause harm. When preparing CDs, always wear powder-free chemotherapy gloves and a disposable gown that is

not used for any other purpose. Chemotherapy drugs should always be mixed inside of a biological safety cabinet (Figure 36-23). Be sure to follow all of the instructions on the MSDS, package insert, and your practice's chemotherapy safety plan.

During the administration of CDs, expect the unexpected. Keep unnecessary people out of the area, and wear protective equipment such as gloves, disposable aprons, surgical masks, and eye glasses. You should avoid wearing contact lenses when preparing or administering CDs.

When handling patients that have received chemotherapeutic treatments, remember that some drugs are excreted in bodily fluids, so proper precautions are necessary when cleaning up their urine, feces, and other bodily excretions. Always wear powder-free chemotherapy gloves and avoid contaminating your clothes when cleaning cages or picking up waste from chemotherapy patients. Make sure you dispose of all soiled materials from these patients as medical waste and launder nondisposable items separately from general laundry.

The biggest rule to remember when handling *any* medication is to practice good personal hygiene, especially a thorough hand washing!

Table 36-1 TYPICAL MEDICAL WASTE DEFINITIONS

Material	Medical Waste	Normal Trash
Sharps (any device with characteristics that make it possible to puncture, lacerate, or penetrate the skin)	Any used needles and scalpel blades Glass or hard plastic that is contaminated with a *human* disease–causing agent	Glass or hard plastic that is not contaminated with *human* disease–causing agents can be disposed of as normal waste.
Medical devices such as blood tubes, vials, catheters, IV tubes, etc.	Considered biomedical waste only when they contain *human* pathogens or they have been used for chemotherapy	Devices that simply contain or are contaminated with animal blood (except from primates) are normally not considered biomedical waste.
Animal blood or tissues	Only dead animals or animal parts that are infected with diseases that are communicable to *humans;* this includes but is not limited to rabies, brucellosis, systemic fungal diseases, tuberculosis, atypical mycobacteriosis, etc.	Tissues from routine surgical procedures (castration, ovariohysterectomy, etc) should be considered regular waste.
Laboratory cultures	Microbiological cultures (bacterial, fungal, or viral) of *human* pathogens are considered biomedical waste	In some cases, culture media from negative tests may be considered regular trash, but it is probably wise to just classify all lab cultures as biomedical waste for simplicity.
Bandages/sponges	Used absorbent materials such as bandages, gauze, or sponges that are saturated with blood or body fluids that contain *human* pathogens that may splash or drip	Sponges or bandages used on animals not infected with a disease transmissible to humans.
Primate materials		Normally, waste generated from work on primates is considered regular waste *unless it fits in another category* (such as from research studies using human pathogens).
Animal waste	Waste from animals infected with a disease contagious to *humans* that can be transmitted by means of the waste and waste from chemotherapy patients for up to 48 hours after the last treatment	Normally, waste from animals not infected with human disease–causing agents should be disposed of as regular trash.

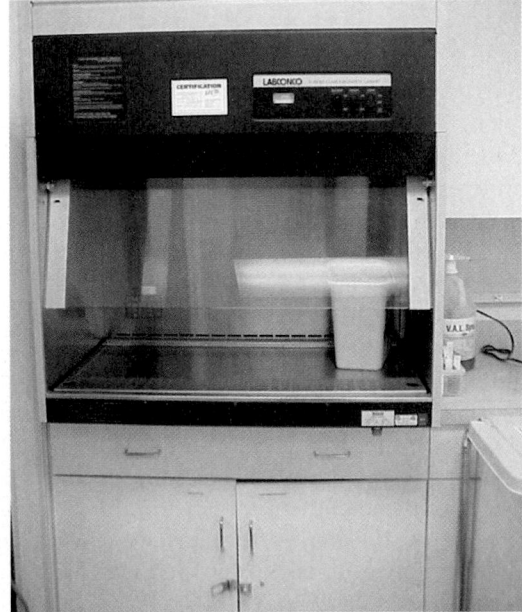

Figure 36-23 A biological safety cabinet (BSC) is required when preparing cytotoxic drugs.

SUMMARY

We all face dangers in life every day but that does not mean we have to intentionally place ourselves in danger to get our job done. The successful person makes sure the reward for the action far outweighs the risk.

In this chapter, we discussed your rights and responsibilities in a safety program, the hazards associated with your job from both a general and medical perspective, and the actions you should take to protect yourself. Employing good safety practices should not be the cause for additional work. If a job is safely completed and the correct protocol is followed, then it is done properly. Occupational risks should not keep you from doing your job, they should motivate you to do your job better; to pay attention to what you are doing, and to comply with the standard operating procedures established in your practice. Employing good safety practices will enable you to remain healthy and will therefore allow you to continue to practice your career for a long time!

Have fun and be safe.

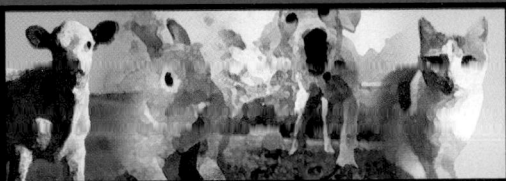

37

Euthanasia

JOSEPH TABOADA

Old Dog

When the old dog had to die after long years full with love and honor,

When the weight of time grew wearying and she was content to have it finished,

I brought my old dog to our friend.

Old dog lay soft against me, old eyes already closed, waiting.

Our friend's hand was gentle on the weary body, with its ragged fur,

So gentle to find the frail small vein where death could enter.

DIFFICULT,

Old blood runs sluggish, old veins slackly resisting.

So patient, our friend, his knowing hands, all I can see through silent tears.

I watch capable strong hands lightly coaxing, and at last a small red flower blooms briefly in the crystal before he eases the plunger in.

Old dog only sighs very softly.

The weary heart slows and stops as the joyful spirit leaps free.

We wait a quiet minute, my tears dropping unheeded, into the soft fur.

Our friend withdraws, his gentle hands leaving old dog's castoff body.

My head bowed over the weathered white mask for a moment before I let her lie by herself and draw the blanket over her.

I wish the old dog had made it easier for him.

To bring even a kindly death brings sadness.

He asked how many years she had, and I heard more than that in his voice.

I wish I could thank him for keeping zest in her years, for making a good end of them, for his capable hands, for his gentle word, and caring heart.

I took the old dog home, and laid her as if sleeping, wrapped in her worn blanket and sheltered deep in the kindly silent earth.

Anonymous

INTRODUCTION

Perhaps no single issue in veterinary medicine conjures up the range of emotion, ethical deliberation, and stress occasioned by euthanasia. *Euthanasia* was defined by the 2001 American Veterinary Medical Association (AVMA) Panel on Euthanasia as "the act of inducing painless death," but the act is only one small aspect of the larger issue facing the profession.

The word *euthanasia* is derived from the Greek root *eu*, meaning good, and *thanatos*, referring to death. Few in the veterinary profession would argue that when used in the context of relieving suffering, the word runs counter to its Greek roots; however, as the word is currently defined, it also pertains to the killing of unwanted, abandoned, stray, or phenotypically undesired animals by veterinary professionals. It is not always in the common interest of the patient, client, and veterinarian that euthanasia is performed, and in this way problems can arise in balancing conflicting interests. Euthanasia is an emotionally charged issue, with members of the profession varying significantly in their acceptance of the practice and in their views as to its utility. On the one hand, it might be viewed simply as "convenience killing," whereas on the other, it might be viewed as a means of furthering respect and love through the compassionate termination of hopeless suffering. No matter how one looks at it, the animal health professional may be caught in the middle, experiencing doubts, confusion, and moral questions over participation in the ending of an animal's life. It is an ethical dilemma that does not have an easy or even an absolutely right or wrong answer. It is an issue that all veterinary professionals must wrestle with, individually and collectively. ■

> **TECHNICIAN NOTE**
>
> Euthanasia is an issue that all veterinary professionals must wrestle with, individually and collectively.

THE DECISION

The decision to perform euthanasia is one of the most difficult decisions that the owner of a companion animal will ever face. Some owners may make the decision quickly because of financial constraints or fear of what the illness may eventually cause, whereas others may never be able to make the decision, preferring to let their pet die naturally. The decision is often made more difficult by the fact that few pet owners have an adequate support group available that understands the bond that develops between an animal and the recipient of its unconditional love.

Most owners who elect to have euthanasia performed make the decision because they perceive that their pet's illness involves some degree of suffering. Suffering is difficult to define, and perceptions of animal suffering differ markedly between individuals and from case to case. The place the pet holds in the owner's family circle, how long the pet has been owned, the relationship between the pet and other loved ones, the financial resources available to the owner, and the disease process afflicting the pet are other factors that most owners take into consideration when trying to make the decision.

The veterinary team (veterinarian, veterinary technician, animal health care providers) can play an important role in the decision-making process. The veterinary staff often serves as a sounding board for the client who is trying to make the decision. Staff members can help with the decision by approaching the subject professionally with compassion and respect. The most important help that the team can give is to provide information. What the owner can expect from the disease process, what treatments are available, the prognosis with and without treatment, and what costs are involved are all questions that should be answered by the veterinarian. The veterinary technician can play a vital role as a client resource by answering questions about euthanasia. How euthanasia is performed, whether the animal will feel pain, how long the procedure will take, and what happens to the body afterward are all areas that a technician may be asked to address.

> **TECHNICIAN NOTE**
>
> Veterinary technicians, as professionals, can help clients with euthanasia decisions by approaching the subject professionally with compassion and respect.

When interacting with an owner considering euthanasia, the veterinary professional should go to great lengths to lay out all options available while being careful not to make the decision for the client. Too many veterinary professionals make judgments as to the value of an animal (both monetary and personal) that only the owner can make. Questions such as "What would you do if he were your animal?" are difficult to address and perhaps best answered by urging the client to verbalize what he or she sees as the pros and cons of each choice. In doing this, it may become obvious that the client has already made the decision and is looking for support or validation. The client may feel guilt, anger, sadness, depression, pain, and helplessness during the decision-making process and after euthanasia has been performed (see Chapter 38). The veterinary professional can help by assuring owners that these feelings are normal, and indeed expected, and by assuring them that they are not alone in the pain they are feeling.

Once an informed decision has been made, it should be supported, even if it may not have been the decision that the veterinarian or veterinary staff would have made. Pet owners are sensitive to the actions of hospital personnel, and for this reason it is extremely important that persons interacting with the client or handling the animal in the presence of the owner be supportive, gentle, and empathetic.

AS THE END DRAWS NEAR: THE BEGINNING OF THE END

The death of a pet can be a devastating experience that can drastically affect the relationship between client and veterinarian. As many as 40% of clients change veterinarians after a pet has died. This number probably approaches 100% if euthanasia is handled in a manner that causes the client to perceive a lack of care, concern, or respect on the part of the veterinarian or other staff members. On the other hand, much can be done to foster a long-lasting relationship through the professional and compassionate handling of euthanasia. It is often true that the client who loudly sings the praises of a veterinarian and staff is not the owner of an animal saved through long hours of hard work and outstanding medical care but rather the owner who was treated with compassion, care, and concern at and around the time of the loss of a pet.

> **TECHNICIAN NOTE**
>
> Many clients change veterinarians after the death of a pet, especially if euthanasia is handled without the utmost care and respect.

Preparations for pet loss should begin as soon as it becomes apparent that death is a possibility. The veterinarian will often discuss euthanasia with a client early so that the client understands that it is an available option. However, it is important to discuss all other medical or surgical options first. Euthanasia should not be presented in such a manner that it is either completely discounted or viewed as the only reasonable course. Remember that the initial reaction of a client receiving bad news is often denial or feelings of numbness or shock. It is important to allow time for this initial reaction to fade and for the entire family to be given time to discuss the various options before allowing the client to make such a difficult and important decision.

While discussing options with the client, the veterinarian should use alternative jargon for euthanasia such as *put to sleep, put down, put away, humanely destroy, rock,* and *shoot* only when their meaning is understood by all individuals involved. Confusion will result from the use of a term such as *put to sleep* when talking to a companion animal owner who perceives the phrase to refer to anesthesia instead of euthanasia. Children are especially confused by the term *put to sleep* and may be afraid that they might die when going to sleep at night. Whatever term is used to describe the act of euthanasia, it is important that it be fully understood by all parties involved.

Once the decision has been made to have an animal undergo euthanasia, a client must make many decisions. When and where should the euthanasia take place? Should the client or other family members be present during the euthanasia? What is to happen to the body after euthanasia? Should a necropsy examination be allowed? What special method, if any, will the client use to memorialize the pet? It is best to discuss these concerns thoroughly in advance so that everyone understands precisely the wishes of the client.

The client, together with the veterinarian, should decide who will be present during the euthanasia. This is sometimes a difficult decision for both the client and the veterinarian. Some veterinarians do not offer this option to the client in the mistaken view that it will be too difficult for the client to watch. Contrary to this view, many clients will grieve more easily and accept more quickly the loss of their pet if they have had the opportunity to say goodbye in this most personal way (Figure 37-1). The chance to hold their pet and let it know that it is loved dearly while sharing its last moments is sometimes an important first step in the grief process. However, with the benefits to the client can come problems for the veterinarian and staff. Veterinary team members must realize that having the client present can increase their own stress level associated with euthanasia, and every attempt should be made to understand and minimize its effects.

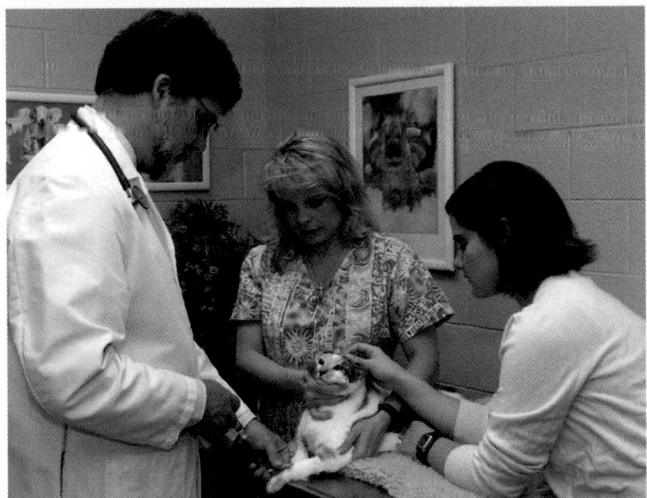

Figure 37-1 Being present during the euthanasia of their companion animal helps clients to say goodbye. Allow the client to make as many decisions, with guidance, about the site, time, and tempo of the euthanasia process; this makes the event more personal and meaningful.

When the client or family members are to be present, euthanasia should be scheduled for a time of day when interruptions are unlikely, the waiting room is empty, and the potential for embarrassment by public exposure is minimized. Early mornings, evenings, or during the lunch hour may be suitable. It is best to schedule at least 30 minutes. The most important aspect of the euthanasia to consider is communication. The unexpected should be avoided at all costs, and before the procedure, the client should be given a detailed explanation of exactly what is about to happen to the pet and what he or she is about to see. Then the client should be talked through each step of the procedure. The euthanasia should proceed at a pace with which the client feels comfortable. Occasionally pets will urinate, defecate, vocalize, twitch, or gasp after they have become unconscious. Although these reflex acts can be minimized, they will still occasionally occur and will have a far less negative effect if they are expected and if the client is told that they are not a reflection of pain or suffering.

> **✐ TECHNICIAN NOTE**
>
> Communication is critical to a smooth euthanasia when owners are present.

Deciding where the euthanasia is to take place can be important. Using a hospital space that is less stark than the typical stainless steel hospital examination room is preferred. If the examination room is to be used, at least a blanket should be placed over the table and there should be a chair where the client can sit down. Some clients will request that the euthanasia be performed at home or at some special place. Many veterinarians will honor these requests

> **✐ TECHNICIAN NOTE**
>
> Many clients will go through the grief process more easily if they are present at the euthanasia.

or use the services of a house call practice for this need. Sometimes just being outside the "normal" environment of the veterinarian facility is a fair and acceptable compromise. A blanket on the floor, the lawn beside the clinic, and even the back seat of the family car might serve this purpose. One important consideration for the veterinarian in choosing the place is that many clients will feel uncomfortable coming back into the room where a pet previously underwent euthanasia. Indeed, many clients switch veterinarians because of a lack of sensitivity to this fact by the veterinary staff. To minimize this potential conflict in the future, it is best to choose a space that will not be routinely used for other client-related activities.

Clients who choose not to be present during euthanasia may still wish to see the body of the animal after it is dead. Seeing the animal dead conveys finality and also allows the client the opportunity to say goodbye. Many clients have a difficult time proceeding through the grief process if they have not been given this chance.

> **✎ TECHNICIAN NOTE**
>
> Clients who choose not be present for a euthanasia often still wish to see the body afterward.

Make arrangements in advance concerning how payment for services is to occur. Discuss with the client whether payment is going to be made in advance, at the time of services, or by a later bill. This can be an uncomfortable subject to broach after euthanasia has occurred.

AT THE END

Once all the preparations have been made, the euthanasia should be performed with skill and concern. Each member of the veterinary team should be well trained, know his or her responsibilities, and be available. The key, as already mentioned, is to expect and plan for the unexpected. Although many methods of euthanasia are deemed acceptable by the AVMA panel on euthanasia, only those that are aesthetically acceptable should be used when the client is going to be present.

> **✎ TECHNICIAN NOTE**
>
> Expect and plan for the unexpected.

If the examination room is to be used, the table should be covered with a cloth or blanket. Some owners will want to bring a favorite blanket for the pet to spend its last few moments on. It is important that they understand that it is possible, indeed likely, that the blanket will be soiled by feces or urine when euthanasia occurs. If the pet is likely to be aggressive or extremely apprehensive, tranquilizing it ahead of time should be considered. If the client is to be present, the animal should be taken away briefly so that a peripheral vein can be catheterized for smooth delivery of the euthanasia solution. It is advisable to put the catheter into a vein in a back leg; this will allow the client to hold the animal and pet its head without being in the way of the veterinarian while the injections are being given. Once the catheter has been placed, the client should be given the opportunity to be alone with the pet for a few moments.

Before administering the euthanasia solution, a saline solution should be injected into the catheter to ensure its patency. Next, the patient should be anesthetized with an ultra-short-acting barbiturate. This will decrease the incidence of excitement after the euthanasia solution is injected. Once the animal is anesthetized, the euthanasia solution can be injected. Sodium pentobarbital is the most commonly used euthanasia solution. It is a member of the barbiturate family of drugs that depress the entire central nervous system.* When large doses of this drug are administered, as for euthanasia, unconsciousness occurs first, and then breathing stops because of depression of the respiratory center. This is followed by cardiac arrest. The pentobarbital dose, concentration, and rate of administration determine the speed of action. When the drug is administered intravenously, animals die swiftly and quietly. Although intravenous administration is preferred, the drug is also effective when injected intrahepatically and, to a lesser extent, into the peritoneal cavity. Death following intraperitoneal injection may take as long as 15 minutes, however, because of relatively slow absorption. Pentobarbital for euthanasia is available alone or in combination with other drugs. The concentration of pentobarbital in most euthanasia solutions is approximately 20% by weight. The recommended dose is 2 ml for the first 4.5 kg of body weight and 1 ml for each additional 4.5 kg of body weight. Sodium pentobarbital should be administered as rapidly as possible to provide the quietest and swiftest form of euthanasia. The veterinary team should be completely familiar with the use of the euthanasia solution chosen and the possible reactions that might be seen.

Because the cerebral cortex is affected by general anesthetic, predominant emotions may take over and the animal may show fear behavior, which is usually characterized by struggling and vocalization. Experimental studies indicate that the animal is not conscious of these feelings at the time. People who have undergone the "excitement"

---

*Note that all barbiturates are strictly controlled by federal regulations, and accurate accounting of the use of these agents is required. The Drug Enforcement Agency (DEA) of the U.S. Department of Justice is responsible for enforcement of laws governing the user of barbiturates. Sodium pentobarbital is a schedule II controlled substance and can be obtained only by a licensed medical practitioner, such as a physician, dentist, veterinarian, or approved institution. In addition to the DEA paperwork involved for procuring barbiturates such as sodium pentobarbital, careful handling of the drug is necessary after the drug is on the hospital premises. Thorough record keeping is required by law.

phase during general anesthesia do not remember that it took place. Although trained individuals may understand this excitement phase from the clinical standpoint, it is difficult for the owner to understand that struggling and vocalization are not due to pain or discomfort. Thus the owner's perception is that the animal is not experiencing a peaceful death. Clients who choose to be present should be warned that this phase may occur. The use of an ultra-short-acting barbiturate first will minimize the excitement phase.

THE END AS A BEGINNING . . . AFTER THE END

A gentle touch,
barely audible she purrs,
goodbye, oh goodbye,
a final glimpse of life drifting away,
a lifeless stare;
... and then, I am alone.

J. Taboada

Many veterinary professionals are good at the technical aspects of euthanasia but fall short in supplying what the client needs after euthanasia has been performed. The animal's death is often only the beginning of a long and difficult odyssey that the client is about to face. Some clients will feel a great sense of relief immediately after the pet's death, but most will soon feel empty, numb, or alone. They may question whether they did the right thing. Veterinary professionals can help them by again stressing that the pet's death was painless, assuring them that they did the right thing, and focusing on some positive things that the pet brought to their life. At the time of euthanasia, it is important that an environment be fostered that says, "It's all right to cry, it's all right to be emotional, it's all right to begin to grieve." Few of us have the gift of being able to say the right thing at the right time, so sometimes consolation can best be offered in a touch or an embrace. A touch on the arm or a simple embrace will often express best what the client needs to hear: "We care and you are not alone."

TECHNICIAN NOTE
The pet's death is often only the beginning of a long and difficult odyssey.

Many clients, whether present for the euthanasia or not, need assurance that the animal is dead. Clients will feel more assured by the veterinarian who takes the time to listen to the animal's thorax with a stethoscope and shine a pen light into the animal's eyes before pronouncing the patient is dead. For those who choose not to be present, allowing them to view the animal's body can alleviate some of this fear. Before bringing the body to the client, it should be made as presentable as possible. It must always be treated with

dignity and respect. Clean any blood from the fur, remove any catheters or bandages, place the tongue in the mouth, and close the eyes. Placing a drop of cyanoacrylate glue (Krazy Glue) in each eye will keep the eyelids closed. If time permits, bathe and brush the animal before laying it on a clean paper, blanket, or towel in a sturdy box. This will help to make the viewing as pleasant an experience as possible. This last, and often lasting, impression that the client takes away from the practice may go a long way toward determining whether he or she returns with another pet. If the animal's body is sealed in a box (commercially made boxes for home burial are available), let the client know how the body is wrapped and whether any signs of trauma or surgery are present. Even clients who assure the veterinarian that they will not open the box before burial or cremation often change their mind after leaving the office.

TECHNICIAN NOTE
Always treat the pet's body with dignity and respect.

Having the client bring someone who will be able to drive him or her home will help ease the feeling of being alone and will also ensure a safe trip. It is nice to call clients after they have arrived home to check on them. Attempts should be made to call all clients who have lost a pet to answer any questions and to show concern. The veterinarian or a staff member may call. The show of concern is always appreciated, helps clients who are having difficulty dealing with grief, and assures clients that a relationship with the clinic fostered in life has not been ended by the death of their pet. Most clients will eventually choose to get another pet. A sympathy card or handwritten note is usually appreciated. Many beautiful sympathy cards designed for veterinary use are available (Figure 37-2).

One of the biggest concerns of clients who have just lost a pet is disposition of the body. When possible, all arrangements should be made in advance. The veterinary staff should be prepared with information to assist the client in making these arrangements. Know the laws concerning burial in the practice area. Make available names and telephone numbers of places that offer cremation and pet cemetery burial. If the client chooses to have the veterinarian handle the remains, it is best not to lie to the client concerning the disposal of the animal's body.

Memorializing the pet is a step that many clients find comforting. It can be an important part of grieving for many clients. Offering the client a lock of hair, a clay paw print, and returning collars or leashes may facilitate these wishes (Box 37-1). Having a memorial service, planting a special plant in memory of the pet, framing a photograph, keeping a lock of hair, writing a poem or special letter, offering a memorial scholarship at a veterinary school, or making a donation to organizations such as the American College of Veterinary Internal Medicine or a veterinary school foundation are actions that clients may use to memorialize their pet (Figure 37-3).

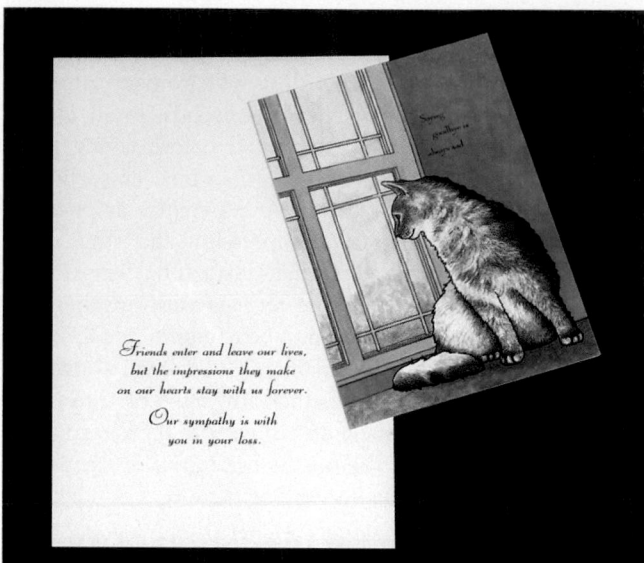

Figure 37-2 Follow-up communication is very important for the client and the veterinary team. A condolence card lets the client know that you care, and this gesture often brings the client back to your practice when they eventually invest in a new relationship with another pet. In addition, sending a card allows the practice team to empathize, express their own grief, and experience some degree of closure.

Box 37-1 MEMORIALIZE WITH CLAY PAW IMPRINTS

- ClayPaws, a paw print kit.
- Create a permanent memory.
- Personalize it by painting or decorating.
- World By The Tail, Inc., 888-271-8444, www.claypaws.com.

TECHNICIAN NOTE

Memorializing the pet can be an important part of grieving for many clients.

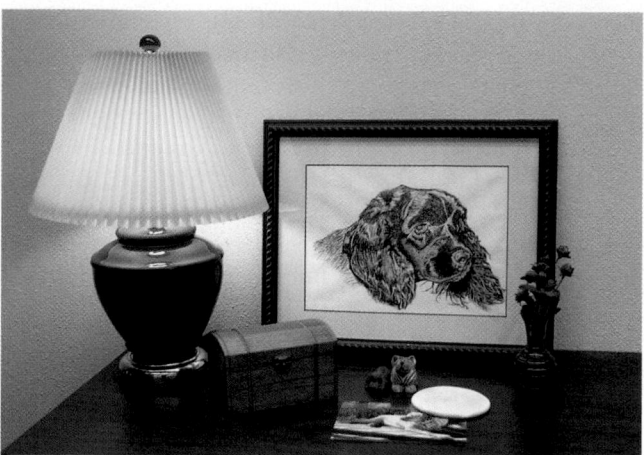

Figure 37-3 Memorializing a pet who has died is important to the grief response. Cremains, a paw print, and framed picture are comforting ways to memorialize.

Box 37-2 SIGNS AND SYMPTOMS OF BURNOUT

PHYSICAL SYMPTOMS
Ulcers
Gastroenteritis
Cardiac arrhythmia
Heartburn
Backache
Nausea
Skin disorders

PSYCHOLOGIC AND BEHAVIORAL SYMPTOMS
Withdrawal
Overeating
Constant fatigue
Increased alcohol intake
Agitation
Distraction
Aggressive behavior
Insomnia

THE STRESS OF EUTHANASIA

Euthanasia is stressful not only to the client but also to the veterinarian and veterinary staff. Frequent performance of euthanasia is a primary cause of burnout within small animal practice (Box 37-2). It is at times even more stressful to the technical staff than it is to the veterinarian because staff members usually have little control over the situation. Euthanasias that go smoothly as well as difficult euthanasias will create stress. Difficult or inherently stressful euthanasias include euthanasia in which technical problems arise, instances in which the animal reacts badly to the injections in the presence of the client, and the euthanasia of one's own pet, healthy animals, young animals, and animals for

whom one has put a great deal of time and medical effort into fighting their disease. Euthanasia with the client present usually creates more stress on the veterinary staff than when the procedure is performed in the absence of the owner.

Each individual will have to decide in what type of euthanasia he or she is able to participate and one's personal tolerance for euthanasia. A technician may not be able to work effectively in a practice in which the veterinarian's views on euthanasia are vastly different from his or her own. Stress can become intense if these differences are not discussed and reconciled. Veterinarians differ markedly in their views on euthanasia. A survey of British veterinarians revealed that 74% would perform euthanasia on a healthy animal if the owner requested it. A similar survey in Japan revealed that 63% would not. There is room within the veterinary profession for this divergence of views; indeed, the diversity of opinions is one of the profession's strengths.

One of the most important mechanisms of coping with the stress brought on by euthanasia is discussion with colleagues. Having sessions for the hospital staff in which people can openly express their feelings is a good outlet for emotions that, if unexpressed, can cause further stress and lead to burnout. This type of communication allows members of the veterinary team to understand their colleagues' feelings and tolerances for different situations. Members of the team may need to temporarily pass responsibility for euthanasia to their colleagues when they have reached the limit of their tolerance. Other mechanisms of managing stress include taking time off, making time for self, adopting recreational habits, helping clients deal with their grief, and finding strength in relationships formed with colleagues who experience the same stresses.

EUTHANASIA IN THE SHELTER AND RESEARCH FACILITY

Technicians in veterinary practice participate in an average of three to six euthanasias per week; however, shelter technicians and potentially research technicians experience much more death than this. Millions of animals must be euthanized each year because there are no homes for them or because of the needs of certain research protocols. These deaths are difficult to rationalize, making euthanasia a very stressful event for these technicians. The fact that there are different euthanasia methods employed depending on the species or facility is a complicating stressor (Table 37-1). This factor brings up a wide range of both psychosocial and safety issues that need to be addressed.

Staff members involved in these types of euthanasia often cope by shifting moral responsibility for killing animals away from themselves. Shelter technicians view their acts as a crusade for animals and against the ignorant public, whereas research technicians may view the euthanasia as necessary for the "greater good." To prevent burnout, they must see themselves as generators of medical knowledge beneficial to humans and animals, combatants of pet overpopulation, or providers of humane death. These technicians must remember their objectives in their work. Their objective, like every other technician's, is to prevent and release animals from suffering.

The same mechanisms for coping with the stress of euthanasia mentioned previously are very important for both shelter and research technicians. Perhaps one of the most important coping strategies is for the team to rotate euthanasia responsibilities. This rotation releases technicians from the moral stress of euthanasia and reschedules them to a more hopeful task, such as education or adoption responsibilities, or other important research missions; it is hoped that giving them a break will prevent burnout. Dark humor is also used to relieve stress. Such humor reduces tension by acknowledging death as part of the setting but also minimizing, for the moment, its tragedy and finality. Although this humor may appear callous and be misunderstood by those outside the shelter or research culture, it has been shown to be a very effective coping strategy. It is important to recognize this humor for what it is, a coping mechanism. These technicians care a tremendous amount but find themselves in an environment without much societal support.

EUTHANASIA OF LARGE ANIMALS

Euthanasia of large domestic animals presents specific hazards and problems not encountered in companion small animals. Safety must be a major consideration. The jugular vein should be used for injection whenever possible because this will place the person injecting the euthanasia solution in the safest position. On rare occasions, thrombosis of the jugular veins may have occurred from disease, and the cephalic vein must be used. However, this puts the individual under the animal's forequarters and in a dangerous position.

Euthanasia-strength pentobarbital can be administered with a large-gauge needle (14 to 16 gauge). The volume of solution is large, and even with a large-gauge needle, the time it takes to inject the solution is relatively long. The animal may go through the same excitement phase as that experienced by small animals, and it may come crashing to the ground on becoming unconscious. Generally, large animal euthanasia should be performed in an area with vehicle access to allow removal of the body. In some instances, the client may wish to bury a large animal. It should be remembered that all the same emotional concerns encountered in small animal euthanasia pertain to large animals when a bond has formed between the owner and the animal.

CONCLUSION

Euthanasia is a skill that, like any other skill, must be well thought out and practiced. The entire veterinary team should be involved in a well-coordinated and professional manner. Euthanasia, if performed poorly, can be a disastrous experience for both the client and the veterinary practice.

Table 37-1 SUMMARY OF AGENTS AND METHODS OF EUTHANASIA: CHARACTERISTICS AND MODES OF ACTION

Agent	Acceptability	Mode of Action	Ease of Performance	Safety for Personnel	Species Suitability	Efficacy and Comments
Barbiturates	Acceptable	Direct depression of cerebral cortex, subcortical structures and vital centers; direct depression of heart muscle	Animal must be restrained; personnel must be skilled to perform intravenous injection	Safe except human abuse potential; DEA-controlled substance	Most species	Highly effective when appropriately administered; acceptable intravenous and intrahepatic in small animals
Inhalant anesthetics	Acceptable	Direct depression of cerebral cortex, subcortical structures, and vital centers	Easily performed with closed container; can be administered to large animals by mask	Must be properly scavenged or vented to minimize exposure to personnel	Amphibians, birds, cats, dogs, fur-bearing animals, rabbits, reptiles, rodents and other small animals, zoo animals	Highly effective provided that subject is sufficiently exposed
Carbon dioxide	Acceptable	Direct depression of cerebral cortex, subcortical structures, and vital centers; direct depression of heart muscle	Used in closed container	Minimal hazard	Small laboratory animals, birds, cats, small dogs, mink, zoo animals, amphibians	Effective, but time required may be prolonged in immature and neonatal animals
Carbon monoxide (bottled gas only)	Acceptable	Combines with hemoglobin, preventing its combination with oxygen	Requires appropriately operated equipment for gas production	Extremely hazardous, toxic, and difficult to detect	Most small species, including dogs, cats, rodents, mink, chinchillas, birds, reptiles, amphibians, zoo animals	Effective; acceptable only when equipment is properly designed and operated
Microwave irradiation	Acceptable	Direct inactivation of brain enzymes by rapid heating of brain	Requires training and highly specialized equipment	Safe	Mice and rats	Highly effective for special needs
Tricane methanesulfonate	Acceptable	Depression of CNS	Easily used	Safe	Fish and amphibians	Effective but expensive
Benzocaine	Acceptable	Depression of CNS	Easily used	Safe	Fish and amphibians	Effective but expensive
Cervical dislocation	Conditionally acceptable	Direct depression of brain	Requires training and skill	Safe	Poultry, birds, laboratory mice and rats less than 200 g, or rabbits less than 1 kg	Irreversible; violent muscle contractions can occur after cervical dislocation

Table 37-1 Summary of Agents and Methods of Euthanasia: Characteristics and Modes of Action—cont'd

Agent	Acceptability	Mode of Action	Ease of Performance	Safety for Personnel	Species Suitability	Efficacy and Comments
Decapitation	Conditionally acceptable	Direct depression of brain	Require training and skill	Guillotine poses potential employee injury hazard	Laboratory rodents, small rabbits, birds, fish, amphibians, reptiles	Irreversible, violent muscle contractions can occur after decapitation
Penetrating captive bolt	Conditionally acceptable	Direct concussion of brain tissue	Requires skill, adequate restraint, and proper placement of captive bolt	Safe	Ruminants, horses, swine, dogs, rabbits, zoo animals, reptiles	Instant unconsciousness but motor activity may continue
Gunshot	Conditionally acceptable	Direct concussion of brain tissue	Requires skill and appropriate firearm	May be dangerous	Large domestic and zoo animals, reptiles, wildlife	Instant unconsciousness but motor activity may continue
Electrocution	Conditionally acceptable	Direct depression of brain and cardiac fibrillation	Not easily performed in all instances	Hazardous to personnel	Used primarily in foxes, sheep, swine, mink	Violent muscle contractions occur at same time as unconsciousness
Pithing	Conditionally acceptable	Trauma of brain and spinal cord tissue	Easily performed but requires skill	Safe	Some poikilotherms	Effective but death not immediate unless double pithed
Nitrogen, argon	Conditionally acceptable	Reduced partial pressure of oxygen available to blood	Used closed chamber with rapid filling	Safe if used with ventilation	Cats, small dogs, birds, rodents, rabbits, other small species, mink, zoo animals	Effective except in young and neonates; an effective agent but other methods preferable; not acceptable in most animals less than 4 months old

Modified from Andrews EJ et al: *J Am Vet Med Assoc* 202(2), 1993
DEA, U.S. Drug Enforcement Agency; *CNS*, central nervous system.

If performed with practiced care and gentle concern, it can be remembered positively for a long time.

Recommended Reading

Arluke A: Coping with euthanasia: a case study of shelter culture, *J Am Vet Med Assoc* 198:1176, 1991.

AVMA: 2000 report of the AVMA panel on euthanasia, *J Am Vet Med Assoc* 218:1884, 2001.

Fogle B, Abrahamson D: Pet loss: attitudes and feelings of practicing veterinarians, *Anthrozoos* 3:143, 1990.

Grier RL, Schaffer CB: Evaluation of intraperitoneal and intrahepatic administration of a euthanasia agent in animal shelter cats, *J Am Vet Med Assoc* 197:1611, 1990.

Hart LA, Hart BL, Mader B: Humane euthanasia and companion animal death: caring for the animal, the client, and the veterinarian, *J Am Vet Med Assoc* 197:1292, 1990.

Kay WJ: Euthanasia, *Trends* 1:52, 1985.

Kogure N, Yamazaki K: Attitudes to animal euthanasia in Japan: a brief review of cultural influences, *Anthrozoos* 3:151, 1990.

Peters TG: Commander, *JAMA* 260:1460, 1988.

Ramsey EC, Wetzel, RW: Comparison of five regimens for oral administration of medication to induce sedation in dogs prior to euthanasia, *J Am Vet Med Assoc* 213:1170, 1998.

Randolph JW: Learning from your own pet's euthanasia, *J Am Vet Med Assoc* 205:544, 1994.

Tannenbaum J: *Veterinary ethics*, Baltimore, 1989, Williams & Wilkins, p 208.

38

Client Bereavement and the Human-Animal Bond

JOSEPH TABOADA • STEPHANIE W. JOHNSON • KATIE UNDERWOOD

INTRODUCTION

Today, with more than 64.2 million families owning one or more companion animals, pets are considered part of the extended family network.* Surveys and clinical experience indicate that many people consider their pets to be like children, partners, or best friends. Because of changing family structure and an increasing number of people who live alone, companion animals have taken on larger roles in people's support systems. With these changes have come added expectations of veterinary health care professionals. Members of the veterinary medical profession must realize that they are not treating just dogs, cats, birds, rabbits, or horses but important members of their clients' family and an important part of their clients' support system (Figure 38-1). ∎

THE HUMAN-ANIMAL BOND

Today modern society is largely urban rather than rural. Through world urbanization, people tend to live in neighborhoods rather than on farms. Animals live with their owners in apartments or houses, thus increasing familiarity, dependency, and bonding.

✎ TECHNICIAN NOTE

Many people consider their pets to be like children.

Companion animals provide both parents and children with stability, constancy, and security. It is not unusual for families to change locales and residences several times within a 10-year period. As a result most people no longer

*American Pet Product Manufacturers Survey, March, 2004.

live within a short distance of their extended families. The nuclear family is smaller, consisting of an average of less than two children. The single-parent family is becoming common. Because an increasing number of U.S. women work outside the home, many school-age children return home to be greeted not by their mother but by the family pet. An increasing number of adults live alone and couples opt to remain childless. More and more people are filling these voids with pets, who provide a unique outlet for their owners' needs to nurture and be loved. As health and medical care improves, the number of people in the age-group older than 60 years has increased to nearly 16% of the population. Pets fulfill many needs for elderly people, including needs for interaction, exercise, companionship, protection, and motivation to remain active and independent.

It is becoming increasingly recognized that physically and mentally disabled individuals benefit from contact with animals. As society has realized the special talents of pets, new utilitarian functions have been found for them. Dogs are used with success to assist blind, hearing impaired, and physically challenged persons. These specially trained animals provide their owners with independence, companionship, social lubrication, protection, and love. Horses, cats, and dogs have been used successfully in animal-assisted therapy programs for people with all types of physical and mental disabilities. Animals facilitate interaction with people who may be reluctant to interact, and their presence reduces anxiety, lowers blood pressure, and decreases heart rate. Results of some studies indicate that animals may alleviate or prevent depression. Survival rates for cardiac patients who are pet owners are higher than for those who do not own pets. In fact, pet ownership is considered an important predictor of survival for patients with coronary artery disease.

In short, the relationships between people and animals have become physically closer, and the role of animals in the daily lives of their owners has become more emotional as

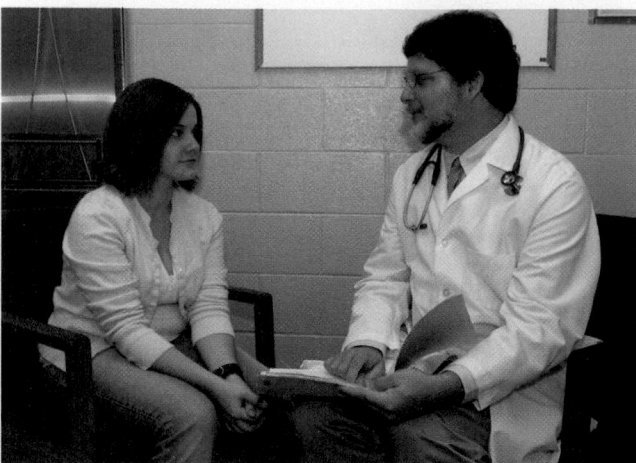

Figure 38-1 The diagnosis of a disease can be a difficult time for both clients and veterinary professionals. It is important to respond to both the pet and their owner's needs.

*American Pet Product Manufacturers Survey, March, 2004.

Box 38-1 KEYS TO ATTACHMENT

The levels of attachment are different for each pet and owner. Human-animal relationships may be perceived as stronger and more important when the following aspects are present:

- Owners believe they rescued their companion animals from death or near death.
- Owners believe that their companion animals got them through a difficult period in life.
- Owners spent their childhoods with their companion animals.
- Owners have relied on their companion animals as their most significant source of support.
- Owners anthropomorphize their companion animals.
- Owners have invested extensive time, effort, or financial resources into their companion animals' long-term medical care.
- Owners view their companion animals as symbolic links to significant people who are no longer part of their lives or to significant times in their lives.

---

society has changed. Of the more than 64 million families owning at least one pet, one-third of companion animal pet owners describe their pets as family members and cite companionship, love, affection and fun as the most important derivatives of the relationship. Further, it has been shown that 83% of pet owners refer to themselves as mom or dad; 93% buy their pet gifts; 84% treat them as children; and 63% say "I love you" at least once daily to their pets.

THE ATTACHMENT BETWEEN ANIMALS AND HUMANS

Strong attachments can form between owners and any type of animal but are probably recognized most commonly in veterinary practice with dogs, cats, and horses. The degree of attachment varies greatly from the utilitarian attachment between a rancher and his or her cattle to the parent/child type of bonding that occurs between some people and their dog or cat. During the 1990s, the cat supplanted the dog, and this trend continues into 2003 (65 million) with the cat as the most popular pet in the United States, with more than 77.7 million being owned.* It has recently been estimated that about 50% of these cat owners classify their attachment to their pet as strong. Of these "strong attachment" owners, about half see their cats as reflections of themselves or of their tastes, who depend on the owner for love, affection, and care. The other half of the strong attachment owners report a reliance on their cats as an emotional crutch, supplying unconditional love and affection and sometimes acting as a substitute for family, friends, or children.

As pets are used to meet many of the changing psychosocial needs of modern society, the intensity of attachment has increased. When pet loss occurs, intensity and duration of attachment determine the significance of the loss and intensity of grief that follows. Attachment is more intense when the animal has functioned in many roles for the owner. The owner of an assistance dog may therefore suffer more intense bereavement than the owner of a dog used only for herding or hunting. Owners who have experienced previous significant losses, adjustments, or traumas and have been comforted by their pet's presence may also exhibit strong attachment and thus intense bereavement.

BENEFITS OF ATTACHMENT

As reminders of both pleasant and traumatic events in people's lives, pets can take on symbolic meaning. There are several keys that are helpful in assessing the level of attachment between an owner and their animal or animals (Box 38-1). Even when the pet is simply another family member, grief can be intense. Grief is also very individual, and each family member may grieve in a unique way.

TECHNICIAN NOTE

If a pet is associated with an important person or significant life stage or event, it can take on added significance.

PET LOSS AND VETERINARY MEDICINE

Veterinarians and veterinary technicians are confronted daily with complex issues of attachment, loss, and grief in the course of their patients' illness and death. The diagnosis of life-threatening or terminal disease can be a difficult time for both the client and the veterinary professional (Figure 38-1). Considering all the emotional and utilitarian aspects

CASE STUDY

CASE EXAMPLE

Sneaky, a 12-year-old female domestic shorthair cat, is brought into the clinic for lethargy and anorexia. After a workup, she is diagnosed as having cardiomyopathy. Even with appropriate treatment, the prognosis for a long lifetime is poor.

Sneaky is owned by a 73-year-old widow named Ruth. The cat was a gift from her husband, Ralph, who died of cancer 2 years earlier. During her husband's fight against the disease, Sneaky was his constant companion. Ruth can still vividly remember how Sneaky, as a kitten, used to make her husband laugh by hiding in his boots and jumping out at him when he leaned down to pick them up.

Sneaky was brought to the veterinarian for what was perceived to be a minor problem, but a severe, life-threatening disease was diagnosed. Ruth is likely to feel numb initially. The diagnosis is likely to be hard to accept. An important part of Ruth's attachment to Sneaky comes from her relationship with her late husband. Sneaky represents a tangible link between Ruth's life now and the many memories of her life with her husband. Not only is Sneaky's death going to be hard because of the loss of a faithful companion and family member, but it is also going to bring back many of the emotions that were associated with the death of her husband.

of the human-animal relationship in modern society, it is not surprising that the breaking of the bond because of the death of the pet is a significant event in the lives of many pet owners. The loss of the pet for many owners is made even more intense and personal in that the pet is often grieved by no one other than themselves. Daily routines are filled with reminders of activities once performed for or with the pet. The loss of a pet often means that a unique, irreplaceable member of the family is gone.

TECHNICIAN NOTE

Veterinary technicians are confronted daily with complex issues of attachment, loss, and grief.

A person's support system is made up of people (and pets) that interact with one another on a daily basis, providing support, comfort, and social interaction. Support systems are especially important during times of loss. Unfortunately, many people who make up these support systems do not understand the full extent of attachment between a pet owner and pet. This lack of understanding can present serious problems for the owner facing the odyssey of grief after the death of a pet. As a result, pet owners often turn to veterinary professionals as sources of support, comfort, and understanding at and around the time of their pet's death.

TECHNICIAN NOTE

People tend to turn to the veterinary staff during grief over a pet because they feel the veterinary technician understands their attachment and loss.

The tendency for people to turn to the veterinary staff during the period of grieving the death of a pet places veterinary professionals in an awkward position, however. It demands that they have knowledge that is typically outside the boundaries of traditional veterinary medicine and requires that they find a comfort level in talking about death and the grief process. This is why the areas of attachment, animal behavior, human bereavement, and grief counseling are becoming increasingly relevant to veterinary medicine.

WHEN THE BOND IS BROKEN

In general people in U.S. society are uncomfortable talking about death. We know little about the experience of death, and we fear the unknown, yet veterinarians and their staff must frequently discuss death, participate in causing it, witness it, and deal with the emotions triggered by these experiences.

Although people in the midst of grief have a need and a right to understand what is happening to them, there are few places they can go to get helpful, supportive information about grief. This is particularly true when the loss they are grieving is that of a beloved pet. Like most of society, veterinarians and veterinary technicians rarely have formal training in this area. Despite this fact, veterinary professionals are still often the people clients instinctively turn to for support.

Making the job more difficult is the fact that grief and bereavement are emotional and often irrational areas of human interaction. Bereaved individuals may at times seem out of control or out of touch with reality. When this happens, those around the griever, including the veterinary professional, may feel uncomfortable; few veterinary professionals are taught how to support or deal with people who are irrational or emotional. Compassion is an important sensitivity to draw on when interacting with clients experiencing grief.

Grief is the companion to death. It is the mental anguish experienced by any human confronted with the loss of an object of attachment. Grief may ensue as an effect of any loss; the loss may be through death, divorce, loss of a job, or even moving or having friends move away. It can be intensely emotional and can affect mind, body, and spirit. When confronted with grief, the bereaved individual goes through a grief process. The term *grief process* implies that there is an intended end or result to be produced through grieving. Thus the grief process is the means of letting go of the object of attachment to feel better, reinvest, emotionally grow, and attach again.

The veterinary staff is in a unique position to assist clients going through the process of grief as it relates to the loss of a pet. By way of their unique role in the life of both the owner and pet, veterinary professionals are in a unique position to understand the bond that had developed. In addition, the veterinarian and the owner may have interacted uniquely in choosing the time of the pet's death (as occurs when euthanasia is performed). To assist clients during the difficult bereavement period, it is helpful to understand the normal grief process and the manifestations of it as applied to pet loss.

PET LOSS AND THE GRIEF PROCESS

The death of a pet is all too often regarded as a trivial loss by society, perhaps in part because of the mistaken belief that pets can be easily replaced. There are no socially sanctioned rituals, such as funerals or memorial services, to help grieving pet owners gain support once the bonds between them and their animals have been broken. Further, people are rarely granted time off from their jobs to care for sick animals or to make arrangements for them after their deaths. Society also does not allow adequate time for mourning the death of a pet. Most people feel pressured to be "back to normal" within a few days of their pet's death to avoid being labeled as neurotic, hysteric, or overly attached. However, crying, taking time away from work, and wanting to memorialize a pet are healthy responses to the death of a pet. They should not be discouraged, nor should they be judged.

One of the most effective ways for veterinary professionals to assist grieving clients is to educate and reassure them that their feelings and behaviors are normal parts of the grief process. Other ways that veterinary professionals can help are listed in Box 38-2.

> **✎ TECHNICIAN NOTE**
> Veterinary professionals can assist clients by normalizing their feelings.

THE NORMAL GRIEF PROCESS

As stated earlier, the word *process* implies movement toward some end or result. In regard to grief, this movement is accom-plished by passing through what have been termed *stages, phases,* or *tasks.* Although there are a few differences, the basic emotional process in pet loss is the same as in human loss.

Several models of the grief process can be modified to describe the emotional process that occurs during pet loss. The following discussion uses the classic model supplied by Elisabeth Kübler-Ross (see Recommended Reading).

Dr. Kübler-Ross was one of the first to work extensively with dying persons and their families during the late 1960s. She described the grief process as consisting of five stages: denial, bargaining, anger, depression, and resolution. She used the stages to describe the passage through grief, but it is helpful to remember that these stages are not a linear odyssey. Although people may travel through the grief process in a straight line, they more often fluctuate between stages, bounce back and forth, and feel the entire gamut of grief within minutes, days, or months.

> **✎ TECHNICIAN NOTE**
> The grief process consists of five stages: denial, bargaining, anger, depression, and resolution.

Denial and Bargaining

Denial is a normal defense mechanism that buffers humans from some unbearable news or reality. It is important to recognize the word *normal* here because many individuals experiencing denial at the time a poor prognosis is given or during bereavement will seem to all observers to be out of touch with reality. The veterinary staff may wonder whether the client has even heard the veterinarian stating the seriousness of an animal's illness. A client in denial may listen attentively to a diagnosis of cancer with a poor prognosis but ask only if the toenails can be clipped or if their current flea shampoo is correct. A client informed of the death of his or her pet while it was hospitalized may chatter on about activities for the weekend. A simple form of denial is exemplified by the client who states repeatedly, "It can't be. I don't believe it."

It is tempting when presented with a client experiencing denial to insist that he or she recognize the seriousness of the situation. Many veterinarians and veterinary technicians

> **CASE STUDY**
>
> Captain, a 9-year-old boxer, is brought into the clinic for a checkup and vaccinations. His owner, Don, tells you that 1 year ago Captain was treated for lymphosarcoma. The cancer went into remission, and Captain has been doing fine ever since. However, it is obvious to you that Captain is not feeling very well.
>
> The examination shows the cancer has returned. It takes Don some time to accept that fact. It is agreed that treatment should start up again immediately. After a lack of response to a rescue phase of chemotherapy, it is clear that Captain's death is imminent. When the news is given to Don, he insists over and over again that the treatment should be continued. "If it worked before, it will work again—just keep on trying." If the treatment really is not working, Don believes changing Captain's diet to one he read about on the Internet will have better results.
>
> Don brought Captain in for a routine examination. It was immediately obvious to you that Captain was not feeling well. However, Don either could not recognize any of the symptoms or was denying that Captain was sick again. Despite the fact that Don went into the initial treatment protocol knowing relapse was eventually inevitable, he still exhibits signs of denial. It is also obvious he is not ready to accept Captain's impending death. It is important to realize Don's response is a normal part of the grief process. He will not be able to understand the seriousness of the situation until he is ready. Don also shows signs of bargaining when he wants other treatment options to be explored even though it is clear nothing can be done to save Captain at this point.

Box 38-2 STAGES OF GRIEF: HOW VETERINARY PROFESSIONALS CAN HELP

DENIAL

What the client needs most is time, support, understanding, and permission to grieve.

Before Death

- Arrange to communicate with the client in person, if possible, where you both can sit down to talk without interruption or distraction. Recognize denial as a normal part of grief.
- Communicate clearly and reiterate patiently. Phrase statements in words that are concrete and simple for the layperson. Avoid using medical jargon and lapsing into complicated medical explanations.
- Listen actively: maintain eye contact, use attentive body language, and paraphrase or clarify the client's statements as you respond. Give him or her permission to express feelings.
- Give the client time to think about and to grasp the reality of information that has been given. Some clients need only a slight pause in the conversation or a few minutes alone. Other clients may need more time to themselves before they comprehend the news of severe illness or actual death.
- Refrain from judging the client as "stupid" or "out of it."
- Remain nonjudgmental and unhurried toward the client, and state that you are available to talk about specifics or about his or her feelings whenever the time is right.
- *Never* attempt to force clients to "come to their senses" or to move out of denial. Clients will comprehend at their own pace.

After Death

- Encourage the client to view the body and say goodbye.
- Give permission to grieve.

BARGAINING

- Understand that bargaining is an attempt to control or reverse a dire situation. The client feels irrationally compelled to bargain during the grief process and does not mean to doubt the professionals involved.
- When the patient is terminally ill, do not become defensive or threatened when clients ask for other opinions or consider alternative treatments. Giving information, readings, and referral for second opinion will ameliorate bargaining attempts and facilitate commitment to treatment.
- After the death, be empathetic and educate about the stage of bargaining when clients confide their feelings and bargaining behaviors, such as prayers and dreams (or daydreams) of the pet still alive. Reassure them that the emotional basis for their behaviors and feelings is normal even though it may seem irrational.
- When clients inquire as to when to "replace" their pet, educating them about the role bargaining plays in shopping for a new pet can alleviate future disappointment. State that their dead pet was unique and cannot be replaced, but encourage them to obtain a new pet whenever all members of the family feel ready. Help them to find the type of animal they are looking for while gently steering toward one that is slightly dissimilar to the dead pet. Encourage them to choose a different breed, color, or gender, and a new name should be chosen.

ANGER

- Listen actively, and let the client know that you understand.

- Arrange for communication in a private room with no distractions. Sit at eye level, and use attentive body language. Take notes if the client is complaining or criticizing.
- Give the client permission to vent feelings. Listen actively using attentive body language, eye contact, nodding, and responses that paraphrase, clarify, and indicate your understanding of the client's feelings. (Example: "I can see that you're very angry. . . ." or "You feel that diagnosis could have been made sooner. . . .")
- If the client is directly angry at the veterinarian, technician, or clinic staff, take a mental step backward and pause with either a deep breath or by counting to 10.
- *Do not become defensive or respond in like manner* to the client.
- Relieve guilt by assuring the client that he or she did the right thing and what he or she is feeling is a normal part of the grief process.

DEPRESSION

- Encourage depressed clients to talk about their feelings in regard to their pet. Follow up clients whose pets have died with a telephone call in a few days and then 2 weeks afterward.
- Listen actively.
- Attend to the client by positioning yourself at eye level, offering tissues or a drink of water, and leaning slightly toward the client. A nonthreatening yet compassionate touch on the forearm or on the shoulder communicates empathy and understanding.
- Offer a place to sit, a place to be out of the "public eye."
- Tell the client that it is all right, and even good, to cry. Listen supportively and actively, and touch the client gently on the shoulder or forearm. Some clients are known well enough to embrace, and this can be helpful as well.
- Validate the feelings of sadness by letting the client know that it is normal.
- Offer to call a family member or friend.
- Encourage and suggest means by which clients can memorialize their pet. Making scrapbooks, planting a tree, writing a letter to the pet, or writing the pet's life story all are cathartic activities that alleviate depression caused by grief.
- If a client expresses continued depression several weeks following the death of a pet, if his or her support system is poor, or if a client expresses a personal wish to die, referral to a compassionate professional counselor is necessary. Although referral may feel awkward, many clients appreciate the technician who states, "Grief as a result of pet loss is normal, but sometimes there can be no one to talk to or the grief can be overwhelming. I know of a person who understands what you're going through. Would you like her (his) telephone number, or may I have her (him) call you?" Today, several schools of veterinary medicine employ counselors experienced in pet loss. Many communities have established support groups, and private counselors increasingly view pet loss as significant bereavement.

RESOLUTION

- Acceptance is achieved once the above four stages have fallen into the background of the client's life. At this point, the bereaved person can channel emotional energy into a new relationship. The veterinary professional can help clients reach the resolution stage by offering insight into the grief process through his or her actions and by offering suggestions of reading material or seminars on the grief process.

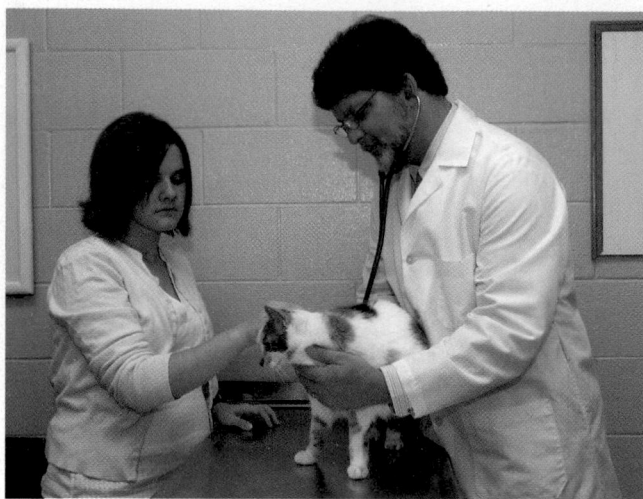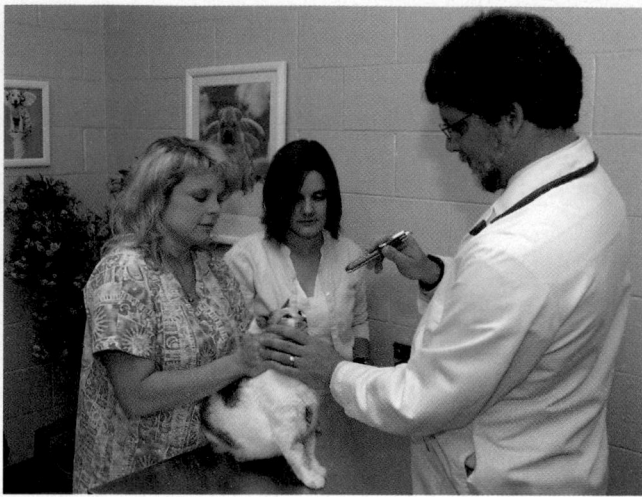

Figure 38-2 Even when dealing with attentive clients, veterinary professionals may be required to repeat themselves several times while clients decide on a course of treatment for their pet. Clients overwhelmed with emotion may have difficulty comprehending information regarding treatment or euthanasia decisions. Members of the team must be patient.

worry that the client does not comprehend or has not heard correctly. There is no harm in repeating oneself to a client in denial (Figure 38-2). In fact, restating diagnoses, prognoses, treatment plans, and particulars is advisable. However, clients in denial will accept the unbearable reality of the situation only when they are ready internally; attempts to push them may backfire, resulting in frustration. Usually, a client will begin to ask appropriate questions about the time he or she arrives home and may telephone the veterinary office. Some may even seem to return to reality before your eyes while those toenails are being attended to. The veterinary professional must feel assured that the client has been told the basic information that needs to be given. Remember, however, that it may not have been fully understood; therefore always leave the door open for further communication.

Denial is reflected by the client's eyes and demeanor and by incongruous questions. The veterinary staff should not feel responsible to "break through" a client's denial. The client will move out of denial, accepting the reality of the situation, when he or she is ready. The veterinary staff's recognition of the client's denial can prevent impatience and frustration during the veterinary contact.

TECHNICIAN NOTE

During denial the veterinary professional should repeat things without becoming frustrated or impatient.

Once the reality of death or impending death is realized, the client may show various impotent attempts to control or to reverse the reality. The client is grappling with the stage of the grief process that Dr. Kübler-Ross called *bargaining*. During this stage, the client maneuvers personally and privately, possibly praying and negotiating with God for miracles. The client might add various herbs and old family remedies to food. Children behave like little angels, hoping to be rewarded with a reversal of bad news. The veterinary staff may be subject to various inquiries by the client at this stage, relative to the latest "miracle cure" that the client has discovered on the Internet. It is while bargaining that a pet owner may also request permission to obtain a second (and sometimes third, fourth, or fifth) opinion. During this time be compassionate and when possible answer clients' questions. Help clients to understand that this stage of grief is normal.

Seeking to replace the lost animal without grieving at all is a form of bargaining. Many pet owners seek a new pet too soon, and they purchase the same species, the same color, and name them the same or a similar name.

It is important to recognize denial and bargaining as part of the normal grief process. Veterinary professionals who understand these stages will avoid frustration in their attempts to provide quality patient care and client service.

Anger

During the grief process, clients may move in and out of the stage called *anger*. Clients coping with this stage may exhibit anger in a wide variety of direct or indirect manners. The anger may be specific or nonspecific in the way that it is directed. Anger may also be exhibited in the form of guilt, which can be defined as anger turned inward.

Anger is a particularly difficult emotion to deal with when a client directs it toward the veterinary professional. Regardless of whether or not the client is justified in his or her stated cause for anger, staff members must use tolerance and patience to avoid responding defensively. Bereaved clients may complain that the illness that resulted in death should have been discovered sooner, should have been treated differently, or should not have been allowed to happen. They may complain that their pet died while hospitalized because of neglect or inappropriate treatment rather than because of the tumor revealed by necropsy.

Anger may be apparent in the form of guilt. Clients feeling guilt use language with an abundance of "I should've" statements. They often seek the listening ear of the veterinary professional looking for absolution from guilt. They may ask whether the food they fed their pet could have contributed to the illness or death. They often ask whether it was the pesticide in their home or in the shampoo that caused a tumor or cardiac arrest. Clients may believe they allowed their pet to be too active or too fat; others may believe they caused the kidney failure in their cat by feeding an insufficient diet. These clients can direct anger at themselves, but frequently they cannot find a specific crime that they committed. When possible, the veterinary professional can assist the clients by assuaging their guilt. Reassuring clients that, in your opinion, they did everything possible for their pet, that they did only what they thought would benefit their pet, and that they made the right decisions for their pet will relieve much of the clients' guilt or anger and assist them in moving through the grief process.

✐ TECHNICIAN NOTE

Veterinary professionals can help by reassuring clients that they did everything possible and made the right decisions.

The client in this stage may be gruff or rude and generally hard to get along with. Stating that he or she is angry, the client may be at a loss to express the object of the anger. These clients may yell at the cashiers, the hospital manager, the receptionist, and the technicians, as well as the veterinarian. Giving the angry client an opportunity to express feelings (venting) is an effective way for the veterinary professional to help. At times, all that is needed is for the sensitive veterinary professional to explain that considering the client's loss, anger is a normal feeling.

Anger is often exhibited by reluctance to pay the bill. On receiving an inquiry by telephone, the client implies that nonpayment is due to anger at treatment by the veterinarian or technician, the pet being neglected, the illness being mistreated, or the client being treated insensitively. Bereavement support can alleviate this client's anger. Listen attentively, state your apologies, if any, and follow up with this client. No admission of mistakes need be made, but the client needs to feel significant and understood.

Anger is difficult to work through, but it is guilt that may be hardest for the client to relinquish. In continuing to feel guilt and anger, the client avoids letting go of the beloved pet, and the grief process is stymied. Once the client is able to relinquish the guilt or anger, the grief process can continue.

The veterinary professional can assist the client with all types of exhibited anger by taking a mental step back and a deep breath, committing to a nondefensive attitude, and simply listening. Take notes if possible, and reassure the client of follow-up if anger is directed at veterinary staff.

CASE STUDY

John brings Sparky, a 3-year-old Dalmatian, into the clinic. Sparky got out of the yard this afternoon because the gate was left open. He ran across the street and was hit by a car. His spine is fractured, and there is severe injury to his spinal cord. There is also a substantial amount of internal bleeding.

John is informed that Sparky has only a slim chance of surviving surgery. He elects for any measure to be taken regardless of cost. Unfortunately Sparky dies during the procedure. When you tell John, he immediately begins yelling at you, "How dare you let Sparky die? There must have been something else that could have been done!" He then refuses to pay the bill and storms out of the clinic.

The next day John calls and apologizes for his rude outburst. He lets you know that he realizes that every measure was taken to save Sparky. He also admits to feeling guilty for having left the gate open. Then he requests that the bill be mailed to him.

John is expressing his anger over Sparky's death, which should be recognized as a stage of grief. Although John initially expressed his anger at you, it should not be taken personally. It is not necessarily directed at you. You should not react defensively but instead listen politely and let John know that you empathize and understand. Realize that part of his anger may come from guilt that he left the gate open.

His call on the following day emphasizes that anger can be an uncomfortable but transient part of the grief process. He admits his anger was not really because of you. He attributes it to his feelings of guilt.

Assuage any guilt if the opportunity arises, and allow the client to vent. A few minutes on the telephone or in person may salvage a client relationship and go a long way in assisting the client through the grief process.

Depression

The stage of the grief process that is termed *depression* has also been called *grief*. Clients experiencing depression describe their mood as complete, overwhelming sadness. Intense grief can result in depression, which prohibits a client from functioning normally. Appetite is changed, energy level is lowered, the client withdraws from others, and sometimes the client is unable to go to work. More subtle symptoms of depression include irritability, sleep irregularity, restlessness, and inability to concentrate.

✐ TECHNICIAN NOTE

Depression has been described as complete, overwhelming sadness.

The veterinary professional has occasion to recognize depression as a result of pet loss when follow-up contacts are made with the client. Depression, when severe, usually sets in some time after the loss. Clients with poor social support systems, elderly clients, and clients with intense or symbolic attachment to the pet may experience worrisome depression. When contacts are made several days or weeks after

Box 38-3 Places to Contact for Help or Referral Sources for Clients Needing Help With Grief

THE DELTA SOCIETY
ATTN: Librarian
289 Perimeter Road East
Renton, WA 98055-1329
Telephone: (206) 226-7357
(Can be contacted for a list of referral sources in your area.)
www.deltasociety.org

VETERINARY GRIEF COUNSELING HOTLINES
ASPCA National Pet Loss Hotline
424 East 92nd St.
New York, NY 10128
Telephone: 800-946-4646 punch in pin number 140-7211 and then your phone number
StephanieL@ASPCA.org
Companion Animal Association of Arizona, Inc.

Pet Grief Support Service
P.O. Box 5006
Scottsdale, AZ 85261-5006
Telephone: (602) 258-3306

Pet Loss Support Hotline
Center for Animals in Society
School of Veterinary Medicine
University of California–Davis
Telephone: (530) 752-4200 or (800) 565-1526
(Staffed by University of California–Davis veterinary students; weekdays, 6:30 PM to 9:30 PM PT.)

The Chicago Veterinary Medical Association Pet Loss Support Hotline
Telephone: (630) 325-1600
(Staffed by Chicago VMA veterinarians and staff; voice mail will be returned collect daily between 7 PM and 9 PM CT.)

Pet Loss Support Hotline
College of Veterinary Medicine
Cornell University
Telephone: (607) 253-3932
www.vet.cornell.edu/public/petloss
(Staffed by Cornell University veterinary students; voice mail messages will be returned within 24 hours.)

Pet Loss Support Hotline
College of Veterinary Medicine
University of Florida
Telephone: (352) 392-4700; then dial 1 and 4080
(Staffed by University of Florida veterinary students; weekdays, 7 PM to 9 PM ET.)

Pet Loss Support Hotline
College of Veterinary Medicine
Michigan State University
Telephone: (517) 353-5064
(Staffed by Michigan State University veterinary students; Tuesday to Thursday, 6:30 PM to 9:30 PM ET.)
C.A.R.E. Help line for Companion Animal-Related Emotions

University of Illinois
College of Veterinary Medicine
Telephone: (217) 244-2273
(Staffed by Illinois College of Veterinary Medicine students; volunteers return calls Tuesday or Thursday between 7 PM and 9 PM CT.)

Pet Loss Support Hotline
Iowa State University
College of Veterinary Medicine
Telephone: (888) 478-7574
www.vetmed.iastate.edu/animals/petloss/default.html
(Staffed by Iowa State University veterinary students and community volunteers; September to April 7 days/week 6 PM to 9 PM CT, May to August, Monday, Wednesday, and Friday, 6 PM to 9 PM CT.)

Pet Loss Support Hotline
Michigan State University
College of Veterinary Medicine
Telephone: (517) 432-2696
(Staffed by Michigan State University veterinary students.)

Pet Loss Support Hotline
Washington State University
College of Veterinary Medicine
Telephone: (509) 335-5704
(Staffed by Washington State University veterinary students.)

Pet Loss Support Hotline
College of Veterinary Medicine
Ohio State University
Telephone: (614) 292-1823
(Staffed by The Ohio State University veterinary students; Monday, Wednesday, and Friday, 6:30 PM to 9:30 PM ET.)
E-mail: petloss@osu.edu

Virginia-Maryland Regional College of Veterinary Medicine
Virginia Tech
Telephone: (540) 231-8038
(Staffed by Virginia-Maryland Regional College of Veterinary Medicine; Tuesday and Thursday, 6 PM to 9 PM ET.)

School of Veterinary Medicine
Tufts University
Telephone: (508) 839-7966
www.tufts.edu/vet/petloss
(Staffed by Tufts University veterinary students; Monday through Friday, 6 PM to 9 PM ET; voice mail messages will be returned collect daily.)

VETERINARY SCHOOLS AND COLLEGES WITH GRIEF COUNSELING PROGRAMS
University of California
School of Veterinary Medicine
Center for Animals in Society
Davis, CA 95616
Telephone: (916) 752-4200

Box 38-3 PLACES TO CONTACT FOR HELP OR REFERRAL SOURCES FOR CLIENTS NEEDING HELP WITH GRIEF—CONT'D

Colorado State University, Veterinary Teaching Hospital
CHANGES: The Support for People and Pets Program
300 West Drake Rd.
Fort Collins, CO 80523
Telephone: (970) 491-1242

Louisiana State University
School of Veterinary Medicine
The Best Friend Gone Project
Baton Rouge, LA 70809
Telephone: (225) 578-9547
E-mail: friendgone@vetmed.lsu.edu

University of Pennsylvania
School of Veterinary Medicine
3800 Spruce St.
Philadelphia, PA 19104-6044
Telephone: (215) 898-5438

Tufts University School of Veterinary Medicine
Center for Animals and Public Policy
200 Westboro Rd.
North Grafton, MA 01536
Telephone: (508) 839-7991

Washington State University
College of Veterinary Medicine
People-Pet Partnership
Pullman, WA 99164-7010
Telephone: (509) 335-4569

University of Wisconsin
School of Veterinary Medicine
Pet Loss Support Group
2015 Linden Dr.
Madison, WI 53706
Telephone: (608) 836-7297

WEB SITES
American Veterinary Medical Association: *www.avma.org* (Look under care for pets.)
Argus Institute for Families and Veterinary Medicine: *www.argusinstitute.colostate.edu*
Grief Healing: *www.griefhealing.com*
Pet Bereavement Counseling: *www.petloss.org*
Pet Loss—A Reference to References: www.superdog.com/coping-.html

---

bereavement and it is suspected that a client is depressed, referral can be made to a counselor or hot line specializing in pet loss (Box 38-3). Although referral sometimes is awkward, it might be gently phrased as, "I know a person experienced in counseling people who have lost their pets." Again, reassurance that grief is normal is beneficial.

TECHNICIAN NOTE

If severe depression is suspected, referral can be made to a counselor or hot line.

Most clients experience the feeling of being overwhelmed by their emotions because of grief. They describe feeling as if their emotions are out of control. They may also state surprise and worry that they are reacting with such intensity to the death of an animal. They may be embarrassed. It comforts clients when veterinary professionals confide that most pet owners feel and act similarly on the loss of a pet. Assuring them of your knowledge of their pet's importance as well as your respect for their grief is valuable to them.

Grief must be worked through, not avoided; thus it is a process requiring some emotional catharsis. Many clients cry, and some are uninhibited about expressing anger and sadness. Becoming comfortable with one's own emotions facilitates comfort with others' emotions. It is human and necessary to feel empathy for grieving clients, but it can also be uncomfortable and painful. Separating your own feelings from theirs will allow you to transform empathy into sympathetic gestures that help the client.

CASE STUDY

Two weeks ago Micah brought her 10-year-old barrel racing horse, Lightning, to the clinic. Lightning had colic. Every possible remedy was explored; however, Lightning had to be euthanized. Micah was extremely distraught over the loss of Lightning, whom she described as "the other half of my soul."

You have a couple of free minutes so you decide to call and see how Micah is doing. Micah is still very upset about the loss of Lightning. She says that she has no desire to ever barrel race again and cannot even stand to go to the barn to visit the other horses. She also tells you that she has not been eating or sleeping well. Her parents and friends all think she is overreacting. At that Micah begins to cry and immediately apologizes. You respond, "It's okay. I know Lightning was very special to you. It is normal to still be grieving. I know of someone who specializes in pet loss counseling. Would you like her phone number?"

If you had not taken the time to call, Micah's depression might have gone unnoticed. Many times clients suffer through depression feeling alone. Depression may occur on and off during the entire grief process. Micah also explained to you that support was not available from her friends and family. It is important to follow up on clients who have poor support systems or who are very attached to their animals like Micah. Referral to a professional counselor can be of great assistance in helping clients such as Micah in resolving the grief process.

TECHNICIAN NOTE

Follow-up is important for those clients with poor support systems or unusual attachments.

Box 38-4 How to Help Children When a Pet Dies

When children's companion animals die, many parents follow their instincts to protect them from pain and grief. Some parents make decisions regarding the pet without discussing them with their children. Some may even lie to their children about the actual circumstances of the pet's "disappearance," preferring to tell them that a beloved pet ran away or was stolen rather than died. These tactics are not used maliciously by parents. They develop from a desire to spare children feelings of pain and from a belief that the parents, as parents, are inadequately prepared to discuss loss, death, and grief with their children.

Children, however, are tuned into their parents' emotions and, almost without exception, know that *something* is going on in the family. They don't know what that *something* is, but they do know that it upsets mom and dad. Consequently, children may feel anxious, confused, left out, and even guilty because, without honest explanations of a family crisis, children often believe that they are somehow responsible for the tension level in the home. At later ages, children may also feel betrayed by the parents they trusted when they discover the truth about their childhood pet's disappearance.

The knowledge, skills, and tools for dealing with loss and grief that are developed in childhood are the same ones used in adolescence and adulthood. It is of utmost importance, then, that children be given honest support and information about loss and death so that their grief-coping strategies will be healthy, rather than unhealthy, ones.

HOW TECHNICIANS CAN HELP

Parents will often turn to veterinary professionals for assistance in telling their children about the death of a pet. Having books available for them to read and having information yourself to share can help ease an otherwise traumatic situation. Here are some suggestions.

- Always encourage parents to be honest with their children throughout a companion animal's illness, treatment, and death. Never agree to participate in a lie that the parents may want to tell their children to protect them. In the long run, lies create more problems for everyone involved and can be more damaging to children than the pet's death itself.
- Children under the age of 8 years do not really understand that death is final. They may believe that a dead pet can return or that they will need food in their grave with them. Young children are also egocentric and believe quite strictly in the law of cause and effect. Thus they may develop the idea that they did something to cause the pet's death. Therefore they must be reassured repeatedly that the pet died because it had a disease or an accident or was very old.
- Straightforward explanations and concrete words such as *dead* and *died* should be used when talking to children about

death. Young children do not understand euphemisms and can become upset when they hear terms such as *put to sleep*. Since they go to sleep every night and do not want to die like their pet did, attempts at softening the blow can actually make the situation more difficult and frightening for children.
- Children need to be held, reassured, and allowed to ask questions. Open communication about death is the desired atmosphere for keeping death anxiety manageable. Pets' names should be used in conversation whenever possible, and memories of them should be shared by the whole family. Older children should be included in the euthanasia process, the memorial ceremonies, and the goodbye rituals to whatever extent they wish to be and should be encouraged to demonstrate their sensitivity and compassion.
- It is always helpful to contact children's teachers, care providers, relatives, and other significant adults so that they can help acknowledge the loss and grief process. Adults may observe children playing funeral or overhear them talking to friends about a pet's death. Although these activities may seem alarming and even morbid to adults, they are normal, healthy responses for children. Children deal with issues through play and experimentation. Unless they are in physical danger, their activities do not in most cases require interference.
- For adult information about helping children deal with pet loss, consult the following books:

Jewett CL: *Helping children cope with separation and loss*, Boston, 1982, Harvard Common Press.
Nieburg HA, Fischer A: *Pet loss: a thoughtful guide for adults and children*, New York, 1982, Harper & Row.
Quackenbush J, Graveline D: *When your pet dies: how to cope with your feelings*, New York, 1985, Simon & Schuster.
Shirl-Potter JW, Koss GJ: *Death of a pet: answers to questions for children and animal lovers of all ages*, Stamford, Conn, 1991, Guideline Publications.
Tousley M: *Children and pet loss*, Scottsdale, Ariz, 1996, Companion Animal Association of Arizona.

- The following children's books may be helpful in explaining the loss of a pet to children:

Brackenridge SS: *Because of flowers and dancers*, Santa Barbara, Calif, 1994, Veterinary Practice Publishing.
Disalvo-Ryan D: *A dog like Jack*, New York, 1999, Holiday House.
Morehead D: *A special place for Charlie*, Broomfield, Colo, 1996, Partners in Publishing LLC.
Rylant C: *Dog heaven*, New York, 1995, The Blue Sky Press.
Rylant C: *Cat heaven*, New York, 1997, Scholastic.
Viorst J: *The tenth good thing about Barney*, New York, 1971, Aladdin Books.

Resolution or Acceptance

The stage of *Resolution* or *acceptance* is the feeling that everything is okay, normal functioning is restored, and emotional energy is reinvested. This does not mean that the pet is forgotten but that it has been assigned to a special place in the bereaved individual's heart. New attachments can be

made without regret and hesitation. Resolution may come easily for some and may be difficult for others. In general, children reach the stage of acceptance and resolution more quickly and more easily than do adults. (For more information on how to help children when a pet dies, see Box 38-4.) As stated previously, the grief process is not linear, and bits

Box 38-5 FACTORS THAT MAY COMPLICATE
THE GRIEF PROCESS

- Multiple losses occurring within a related time frame
- Loss of a pet that was associated with a special person or event
- Loss of a pet on a day that is important, such as a birthday or holiday
- Loss of a pet because of factors that may have been preventable
- Feelings of guilt about the death of a pet
- An inability to afford expensive care that was offered
- Loss of a pet because of an illness or situation that previously caused the loss of another pet
- Sudden illness or trauma resulting in loss
- Witnessing the violent or unnecessary death of a pet
- Disappearance of a pet
- Lack of explanation as to why a pet died
- Situations in which the person experiencing loss has little or no support
- Insensitive comments from others who may not understand the bond between owner and pet
- Getting incorrect or bad information concerning the loss of a pet and/or the grieving process
- No previous experience with grief
- Not being present at the time the pet dies or not having the opportunity to view the body
- Not being able to say goodbye

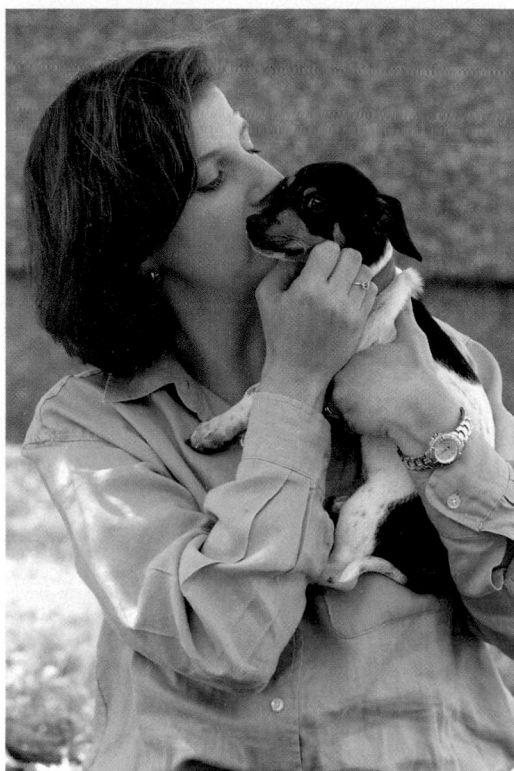

Figure 38-3 The decision to bond with a new animal should be left to the client experiencing the loss. Bonding with a new pet should be viewed as a tribute to the love and companionship shared with the previous animal.

of this stage occur with more and more frequency and with longer durations throughout the grief process. Eventually, the client who successfully resolves the grief process feels little, if any, of the first four stages.

There are many factors that may complicate the grief process (Box 38-5). These complicating factors may lengthen the time it takes to reach resolution or, in severe cases, may arrest progress through the grief process without allowing the individual to reach a resolution. Situations in which the grief process is complicated may not affect some individuals' ability to progress but may drastically affect that of others. Few veterinary professionals are equipped to give the special kind of help that these complicated situations may require, but most have empathy and the ability to listen for signs that indicate someone may need help. Early recognition of factors that may complicate the grief process can be helpful when a person appears not to be progressing well through the process. Early recognition may also be important for timely referral in situations in which further assistance is required. Keeping on hand a list of professional alternatives for referral to someone who can give the help that is needed is advised (see Box 38-3 for a short list of potential sources of help).

The question is often raised whether clients should get a new pet before they reach resolution of the grief process (Figure 38-3). The process itself is highly variable in length. It can be as short as a few weeks to as long as many

years. Most pet owners are able to reinvest and reattach to a new pet at any time but only after they become aware that replacement of their unique loved one is impossible. If companionship, tactile closeness, and friendship are desired while grieving, these qualities can be obtained through a new pet. Cautioning and encouraging clients to choose animals somewhat dissimilar to their dead pet can be helpful. Having a new pet forced on the grieving individual who is not ready to reinvest in a new relationship will only end up furthering heartache in the bereaved and causing unhappiness in the new pet.

GRIEF AND THE VETERINARY PROFESSIONAL

Individuals in the veterinary profession deal with client grief on an almost daily basis. Rarely do they think about their own, however. The veterinary professional must realize the grief process that the client is struggling with is not taking place in an emotional vacuum. It is real and touches not only the bereaved person but also those around him or her, including the veterinary professional. It is common for veterinarians and veterinary technicians to cry with clients, to feel a lump in the throat, and to feel guilty or depressed

CASE STUDY

Two months later Micah (the client in the previous case study) calls back to let you know how she is doing. She expresses gratitude for your concern and compassion while she was grieving over losing Lightning. In his memory, she has decided to donate Lightning's winnings from last year to the Colic Research Foundation. She has also made a memorial plaque with Lightning's shoe on it to hang on his stall door. She would like for you and the veterinarian to come out to the farm to examine the soundness of a horse, Blaze, that she thinks has barrel potential. She is beginning to realize that Lightning would like for her to ride again.

Micah is doing well. She has gone through the process of grieving over Lightning. By memorializing Lightning with the plaque, she has a special way to remember him. Through the donation, she is able to feel like both she and Lightning have made an important contribution to equine medicine. Micah experienced a degree of personal growth through the process of grieving. Resolution and acceptance for Micah are symbolized by focusing her emotional energy into potentially developing a relationship with Blaze. It is important that Lightning is not forgotten.

or experience a sense of failure. The fact that veterinary professionals may go through a grief process each time a patient is lost must be recognized and accepted. Time should be spent thinking about these feelings and responses. Validation of the process within the profession, by way of staff meetings, discussions, and support sessions, can be important in recognizing and dealing with the stresses of "professional grief." Left unacknowledged, the grief process encountered by veterinary professionals can become destructive and lead to burnout.

✎ TECHNICIAN NOTE

Left unacknowledged, the grief process encountered by veterinary professionals can become destructive.

CONCLUSION

Grief and the grief process are difficult to deal with. Despite this difficulty, veterinary professionals are asked to deal with it on a daily basis. Veterinary professionals are rarely trained in the area of bereavement and the grief process, yet they are still often the best qualified individuals when it comes to helping clients who have recently lost a beloved pet. Understanding what the client is going through by understanding the basics of the grief process will help the veterinary professional to empathize, maintain a balanced perspective, and be compassionate. The veterinary technician can play a vital role in helping bereaved clients by being available; listening; assuring clients that their feelings, emotions, and

struggles are normal; and offering referral when clients think they need more help than their available support group is able to provide. This form of client help will strengthen the bond that develops between the client and the veterinary staff and will result in positive growth and added fulfillment for both the client and the veterinary professional.

> *The Feeling*
> *. . . alone; the haunting thought of my old friend;*
> *   Alone; walking among those who could not possibly understand;*
> *   Alone; an unused bowl, an empty collar, a silent toy;*
> *. . . the feeling is so strong;*
> *   How could I have let them do it?*
> *   What if there was something else that could have been done?*
> *   Sometimes I just want to yell;*
> *   Sometimes I just want to cry;*
> *   Sometimes I just want to die;*
> *. . . the feeling is still so very strong;*
> *   I know that it was for the best;*
> *   My old friend was so sick, so frail;*
> *   We cried together on that day;*
> *. . . the feeling was so strong;*
> *   I visited his grave today;*
> *   I could almost feel his kneading paws and hear his deep harsh purr;*
> *   Today I smiled . . . the feeling is so strong.*
>
> **J. Taboada**

Recommended Reading

Anderson M: *Coping with sorrow on the loss of your pet,* ed 2, Los Angeles, 1994, Peregrine Press.

Brackenridge SS, Elkins AD: Euthanasia and patient death: stressors in veterinary practice, *Vet Pract Staff* 4:1, 1992.

Church JA: *Joy in a wooly coat,* Tiburon, Calif, 1987, HJ Kramer.

Cohen SP, Fudin CE, editors: Animal illness and human emotions, *Prob Vet Med* 3:1, 1991.

Cusack O: *Pets and mental health,* New York, 1988, Haworth Press.

Fogle B, Abrahamson D: Pet loss: a survey of the attitudes and feelings of practicing veterinarians, *Anthrozoos* 3:143, 1990.

Harris JM: Nonconventional human/companion animal bonds. In Kay WJ, Nieburg HA, Kukscher AH, editors: *Pet loss and human bereavement,* Ames, 1984, Iowa State University Press.

Katcher A: Interactions between people and their pets: form and function. In Fogle B, editor: *Interrelations between people and pets,* Springfield, Ill, 1981, Charles C Thomas.

Kay WJ, Cohen SP, Nieburg HA, editors: *Euthanasia of the companion animal: the impact on pet owners, veterinarians, and society,* Baltimore, 1988, The Charles Press.

Kübler-Ross E: *On death and dying,* New York, 1969, Macmillan.

Lagoni L, Butler C, Hetts S: *The human animal bond and grief,* Philadelphia, 1994, WB Saunders.

Lawrence EA: Love for animals and the veterinary profession, *J Am Vet Med Assoc* 205:970, 1994.

Nieburg HA, Fischer A: *Pet loss: a thoughtful guide for adults and children,* New York, 1982, Harper & Row.

Stewart MF: *Companion animal death,* Woburn, Mass, 1999, Butterworth-Heinemann.

Quackenbush JE, Glickman L: Helping people adjust to the death of a pet, *Health Soc Work* 9:42, 1984.

Quackenbush JE, Graveline D: *When your pet dies: how to cope with your feelings,* New York, 1985, Simon & Schuster.

Rosenberg MA: Clinical aspects of grief associated with loss of a pet: a veterinarian's view. In Kay WJ, Neiburg HA, Kukscher AH, editors: *Pet loss and human bereavement,* Ames, 1984, Iowa State University Press.

Veevers JE: The social meanings of pets: alternative roles for companion animals. In Sussman MB, editor: Pets and the family, *Marriage Family Rev* 8:11, 1985.

Voith VL: Attachment of people to companion animals, *Vet Clin North Am Small Anim Pract* 15:289, 1985.

Walshaw SO: Role of the animal health technician in consoling bereaved clients. In Kay WJ, Nieburg HA, Kukscher AH, editors: *Pet loss and human bereavement,* Ames, 1984, Iowa State University Press.

2003-2004 American Pet Products Manufacturers Association, National Pet Owners Survey.

39

Stress and Substance Abuse in Practice

SANDRA S. BRACKENRIDGE

INTRODUCTION

Stress is responsible for many deleterious effects on human beings, including physical illness, mental illness, and even death. Stressful living has become accepted, even considered unavoidable, in our technologically modern, fast-paced society. In choosing to work in veterinary medicine, especially if responsibilities entail direct service to clients, one chooses a work environment with a high potential for daily stress. There are many ways to cope with stress, and some people turn to drugs and alcohol for relief from the emotional and physical effects of stress. The use of these substances, unfortunately, usually creates more problems than it solves. This chapter will examine stress, how it can be linked to substance abuse, and how stress can be managed, controlled, or alleviated. In addition, this chapter will assist the veterinary professional in recognizing burnout as well as substance abuse and suggest appropriate action for when either interferes with practice. ■

✎ TECHNICIAN NOTE

In choosing to work in veterinary medicine, one chooses a work environment with a high potential for daily stress.

A DEFINITION OF STRESS

Stress can be defined as the state produced when the body responds to any demand for adaptation or adjustment. The infinite demands that produce this response state are called *stressors*. These stressors may be external (e.g., time schedules, workload), environmental (e.g., heat, cold, noise), or internal (e.g., emotions, sensitivities). The nature of stress is nonspecific in that certain biochemical reactions are common with exposure to all types of stressors. However, stress is not always negative. Stress responses can be pleasurable and even beneficial in certain situations.

GOOD STRESS AND BAD STRESS

Stressors can energize a person so that they can meet specific challenges and take action. As action is taken, the body's stress management system functions in exactly the way it was intended, and with "good" stress, the person experiences a feeling of satisfaction, relief, or exhilaration. Stressors can also be excessive in number or intensity, and prolonged. When a person experiences stressors of this nature, the stress reaction of the body works overtime. The body mobilizes, attempts to adjust to an ongoing drain of energy, and eventually becomes overwhelmed and exhausted. Three factors determine whether stress is negative or positive: *choice, control,* and *consequences.*

✎ TECHNICIAN NOTE

Stress may be negative or positive depending on choice, control, and consequences.

CHOICE

When a person feels stress from a situation that they have willingly chosen to be in, they may perceive their response as more positive. Generally speaking, if individuals are attracted to veterinary medicine, pursue training, and obtain their desired employment, they will be more likely to perceive stressors encountered at work without excessive negativity or resentment. However, if employment in veterinary medicine is perceived as necessary simply to make ends meet financially, or if the person feels his or her true career choice is an impossibility, stressors common to veterinary medicine may be less tolerable. For example, an aggressive animal may be perceived as a challenging stimulation by one who has chosen this career, whereas the same animal would be perceived as a burden or an obstacle by one who truly wishes to be in a different position of employment.

CONTROL

Good or bad stress is also determined by whether the stressor is perceived as within the person's control. In veterinary practice, clients control the schedule, patients provide emergencies and unpredictability, and employers control much of the working environment. When staff are consulted as to scheduling and offered control over certain areas of the working environment, the stressful effect of these factors can be minimized. Again, an aggressive animal provides a good example. Such a situation can seem intolerable when the client insists on being present during treatment, and the employer refuses to muzzle the animal. However, when the client responds in the desired way, and when the employer considers others' opinions, the staff feel that the treatment of the animal and the aggression are within their control. Although the aggressive animal continues to be a stressor during the working day, perceived control of the stressor alleviates much of its negative impact.

CONSEQUENCES

Stressors are more likely to be perceived as positive stimulation when consequences can be anticipated. In veterinary medicine, the death of a patient is always a source of stress. When the animal is properly diagnosed and death is expected or euthanasia is performed, the stress in the situation feels more manageable. On the other hand, when an apparently healthy animal unexpectedly dies during surgery, treatment, or boarding, resulting stress can feel acutely negative and overwhelming. Because the stressor could not have been anticipated, the stress response has become bad stress.

Therefore each stressful situation provides an opportunity for choice, a feeling of control, and anticipation of consequences. Table 39-1 provides further examples of good and bad stress within veterinary medicine. Because stress is unavoidable, knowledge of these three factors can help one to transform adverse stressors into tolerable stressors.

MENTAL AND PHYSICAL EFFECTS OF STRESS

Stress, whether good or bad, engenders responses that affect each person's mental and physical functioning. An understanding of how and where stress originates within the body, its pathway, and the mental and physical toll it can extract is necessary to manage stress and maintain good health.

FLIGHT OR FIGHT

Humans are equipped, as are all mammals, with a physical system to assist them in handling threatening situations. This system has been necessary for survival as a species. Historically, this physical system enabled humans to flee or to fight when externally threatened. In the primitive state, enemies included wild animals, other primitive peoples, and natural occurrences. Today, this physical system shifts into gear when anything or anyone is perceived as threatening, externally or internally. In fact, perceived threats are pervasive. We drive defensively and cope with pollution of all sorts, and crime has become a realistic cause for concern. Internally, we fear bad news, losses, rejection, and failure; we are threatened by financial crises, in consideration by others, illness, and aging. The list of internal stressors is unique to every person, depending on background, temperament, and aspirations. The stress response is nonspecific and is mobilized when one is faced with any of these threats, perceived or real.

THE PATHWAY OF STRESS

Dr. Hans Selye, who is often called the father of stress research, termed the body's response to stress the *general adaptation syndrome (GAS)*. On a person's exposure to any

---

Table 39-1 EXAMPLE OF GOOD AND BAD STRESS

	Good Stress	Bad Stress
Personal	You exert yourself and win a game of tennis.	Your car breaks down, and you must walk 3 miles for help.
Professional	You are asked to speak at the next professional conference.	A co-worker fails to show up for work, and you must work doubly hard.
Personal	You throw a party for 150 people.	Your house is burglarized.
Professional	You perform euthanasia on an elderly animal, and the family thanks you.	A young animal unexpectedly dies while boarding.
Personal	You reenter higher education.	Your spouse is laid off.
Professional	The practice expands, you work harder, but your income increases.	A type A co-worker constantly competes with you.

threat or stressor, the first phase of GAS, the alarm reaction, is elicited. After this phase, the person enters a stage of adaptation or resistance. If the stressor continues to threaten, the person enters a third phase, which Dr. Selye called the *stage of exhaustion*. Unless interrupted, and if the stressor is severe enough and present long enough, the third stage results in physical illness, burnout, or even death.

> ### 📝 TECHNICIAN NOTE
> GAS is the body's response to stress.

During the alarm phase, the body's physical system designed for fight or flight is mobilized. The human body is "supercharged" for action with all muscles and organs in a state of readiness. Many changes are happening internally. The real or perceived stressor signals the hypothalamus to produce hormones, such as endorphins. These hormones stimulate the autonomic nervous system as well as the pituitary gland. The autonomic nervous system affects the digestive system and other vital organs. The stimulation of the pituitary gland increases blood flow, discharging more hormones into the bloodstream. This action stimulates the adrenal glands, which affect breathing, cortisone production, muscle tension, perspiration, and blood sugar levels. Figure 39-1 charts the pathway of the stress response through the body.

The stimulation of the adrenal glands is responsible for many stress-related illnesses. Increased epinephrine production causes increased respiration and heart rate. Rapid breathing causes the injection of additional oxygen into the bloodstream, which alters the amount of carbon monoxide

in the bloodstream and causes dry mouth, irritated nasal passages, and chest contractions. A prolonged increase in heart rate can cause hypertension, leading to cardiovascular problems. The pituitary and adrenal glands influence cortisone levels, which are responsible for the body's immune responsiveness. Prolonged muscular tension, caused by the adrenal glands and by stimulation of the autonomic nervous system, results in various aches and pains, as well as digestive disorders. Stress-induced digestive disorders are exacerbated by the fluctuation in blood sugar levels, resulting in poor eating habits, ulcers, nausea, or constipation. Prolonged stress can result in ongoing endocrine disorders. Box 39-1 shows the various physical disorders that can be considered stress-related disorders.

All the mentioned physical changes originally occur during the alarm phase of GAS. However, when the stressor or stressors continue, the adaptation phase ensues, in which the body attempts to adjust to its new level of activity. When exposure to the stressor continues, any level of adaptation that the body has acquired may be lost, depending on factors unique to each person. Exhaustion may appear physically, or it may be demonstrated psychologically. *Burnout* can be defined as psychologic, and sometimes physical, exhaustion prompted by prolonged subjection to a stressor without adaptation or interruption.

STRESS AND THE BRAIN

The nervous system uses chemicals called *neurotransmitters* to transfer information from cell to cell. There are three neurotransmitters that have been discovered in the normal brain, and they are dopamine, norepinephrine, and serotonin. Depending on the composition of the neurotransmitter, some are excitatory and some are inhibitory. How much of and the type of neurotransmitter released

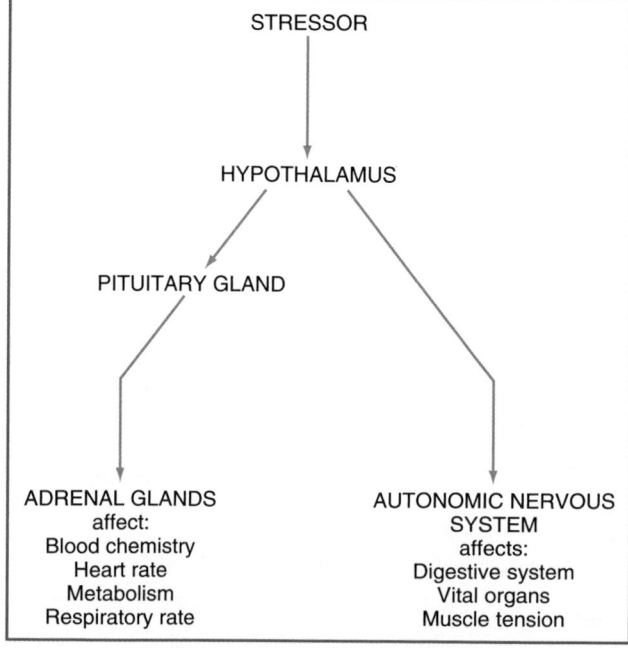

Figure 39-1 Pathway of the stress response through the body.

> ### Box 39-1   PHYSICAL PROBLEMS TRIGGERED BY STRESS
>
> - Insomnia
> - Headaches
> - Allergies
> - Temporomandibular joint (TMJ) disorder
> - Nausea
> - Indigestion
> - Heartburn
> - Backaches
> - Ulcers
> - Colitis
> - Problems swallowing
> - Hyperventilation
> - Asthma
> - Rheumatoid arthritis
> - Dermatitis
> - Chest pains
> - Hypertension
> - Heart attacks
> - Sexual dysfunction
> - Chronic fatigue
> - Depression
> - Dizziness
> - Anxiety
> - Alcoholism
> - Muscle aches
> - Dry mouth
> - Facial tics
> - Erratic breathing
> - Upper respiratory illnesses
> - Nosebleeds
> - Perspiration

and how it is received by the nerve cells will determine the mental and emotional functioning of the person. It is known that moods are affected by a shortage or excess of one or more of the neurotransmitters, and many medications, such as antidepressants, manipulate these chemicals to stabilize mood. Obviously, when a person is in the phases of GAS, the neurotransmitters are called upon with urgency. The emotions that result from stress can be classified into three moods or categories: anxiety, depression, and anger. Recent studies indicate that exposure to stress creates cumulative changes in the brain, changes which increasingly sensitize the person as more stress is experienced. When stress is prolonged, the neurotransmitter functioning may become abnormal over time, making the person less able to cope.

SUBSTANCE ABUSE AND STRESS

Since the nervous system, brain, and emotions are dependent on the normal action of neurotransmitters, some individuals suffering from stress may turn to drugs and alcohol almost as a form of self-medication. Alcohol and drugs can enhance, distort, of even eliminate information normally exchanged by the nerve cells.

ABUSE OR DEPENDENCE?

Not everyone who takes drugs or alcohol, even if they are regular users, can be considered substance abusers. Further, many who abuse substances may not be substance dependent. These terms each imply an understanding of the body and brain response to drug exposure. *Substance abuse* can be defined as drug use that violates social standards or is self-destructive in nature. The actual use of the drug may be intermittent or regular, and this use may be a stage in developing the more serious problem of substance dependence. *Substance dependence* can be defined as persistent drug use that involves either physiological dependence with symptoms of tolerance (requiring more of the substance to attain the desired effect over time) and withdrawal and/or psychological dependence with symptoms like cravings, anxiety, and depression when not using the substance. Furthermore, usually a person who is dependent on any substance will continue to use the drug despite knowledge of adverse consequences, such as physical illness or family/occupational problems that will result from continued use. One should apply the term *dependent* (or the equivalent term *addiction*) to a substance abuser after careful consideration and understanding of terms. The terms *dependent* or *addiction* are labels that may be devastating to both position and self-esteem.

RISK FACTORS FOR SUBSTANCE ABUSE

There have been many studies that have attempted to delineate the factors that may contribute to the abuse of substances. First, there seems to be evidence that indicates that there may be a genetic vulnerability to substance abuse. Put simply, substance abuse and dependence seem to run in families. Chronic pain and self-medication seem to be predisposing factors as well. Sociocultural factors, such as ethnicity, culture, age, occupation, and social class seem to have an effect in predisposition to substance abuse. Some cultural groups have established patterns of use, and some age groups seem to be vulnerable. Environment is a factor in that research suggests that stimuli in the environment, such as high stress, coupled with access to drugs is a strong risk factor. In studies comparing occupations, physicians and health care professionals have been found to be more vulnerable than other occupations. Although veterinarians and their staff have not been studied as an independent group, logically they are included in health care populations. Some researchers conclude that for all groups, when the individual has knowledge about the drug(s) and access to the drugs, then the individual is at risk. The risk for substance abuse becomes even greater with environmental stress.

RECOGNIZING AND INTERVENING

For the health care professional, substance abuse is often a covert, solitary activity that leads to isolation and a feeling of helplessness. Disruption of relationships may occur, and the professional may conceal the signs of dependence. Yet the dependent professional is an individual in distress, and workload, fatigue, and physical illness are often used as justification for substance abuse. In general, a veterinarian or veterinary staff member with a substance abuse problem will exhibit a change in behavior and in personal appearance or hygiene. They may withdraw from friends, family, or co-workers. Their behavior in the clinic may change so that they neglect duties, appear disorganized, or exhibit poor judgment in the practice of veterinary medicine. Other signs may include prescriptions written for themselves, friends, or family, or there may be missing drugs from the clinic during the hours in which they were on duty. They may reveal the presence of financial or legal problems. There may be unexplained absences, conflicts with others, and career instability.

Some kind of intervention and action is needed anytime substance abuse interferes with practice as described. Client, patient, and co-worker safety is of primary importance. The entire practice may be at risk of malpractice due to the substance abuser. In every state there is a Board of Veterinary Medicine that awards, reviews, and can suspend licenses for veterinarians of that state. In some states, veterinary technicians who are certified are also subject to review by a governing board. Most governing boards for health care professionals have stipulations upon continued license in which *impairment* of the professional prevents renewal. In addition, veterinarians and veterinary technicians abide by a code of ethics that is adopted by each licensing board. These ethical codes delineate how a peer must intervene with another professional who is impaired. Generally speaking, the impaired professional should be confronted, preferably by a peer or superior, and asked to seek treatment. Practice should be suspended, if necessary, while treatment is obtained. If treatment is not obtained, the reporting professional should then move up the hierarchal chain of command. For example, if a technician is concerned about substance abuse by another technician, ideally they will first approach the technician that they are concerned about. If no remedial action is taken, they then approach the supervisor or a veterinarian in authority. If no remedial action takes place, the technician would need to report impairment to the appropriate governing board. All of these actions should be done in good faith, in the best interests of the impaired individual. Many situations end happily with successful remedial action and/or treatment. More information about finding appropriate resources for treatment are given at the end of this chapter.

STRESS AND THE PERSONALITY

Although all humans will respond to stressors through activation of the described physical syndrome, not all will proceed through all three phases of GAS. Whether a person can adapt to stress, what stressors are felt most acutely, and which physical or psychologic manifestations of stress will appear depend on various factors, including personality.

Certain personality variables predispose individuals to susceptibility to stress or to resistance to stress. These variables may be inherent in the personality, or they may be learned behaviors and attitudes. Science has not yet determined how much of the personality is genetic and how much is learned, but personalities can be grouped into types. Personality type is a reliable indicator of predisposition to stress-related disorders.

> ### ✎ TECHNICIAN NOTE
> Personality factors predispose individuals to be resistant or susceptible to stress.

THE STRESS-PRONE INDIVIDUAL

The term *type A personality* was first used by Dr. Meyer Friedman and Dr. Ray Rosenman in their book *Type A Behavior and Your Heart*. One study concluded that type A personalities were three times as likely to have coronary artery disease, and personality type was found to be the most reliable predictor of heart attack. Type A people are competitive, impatient, perfectionist, often angry, suffering from "hurry sickness," and insecure.

> ### ✎ TECHNICIAN NOTE
> Type A people are susceptible to coronary artery disease.

Overt and covert feelings of competition with others represent a characteristic of type A personalities. These feelings may be motivated by an ambition to win or succeed, or they may stem from a fear of defeat or failure. Specific areas for competition may be chosen, such as within the workplace, or the type A person may compete in every activity, even in driving, recreation, and social groups.

Type A personalities are impatient, and they find it trying to stand in line or to wait. They would rather be late to appointments than be left waiting; thus type A personalities can be chronically late. They are impatient with receptionists, waiters and waitresses, car mechanics, and, frankly, almost anyone on whom they depend for service. They are also impatient with employers and sometimes with their families. This behavior may be motivated by the need to be in control of situations, or it may be motivated by the desire to avoid anxiety-provoking thinking time.

Perfectionism is a characteristic included in identification of many personality types, and it is also a sign of type A personality. The need for approval and the desire to avoid criticism are paramount in the minds of type A people. Combined with their competitive behavior, perfectionism accounts for the priority type A individuals seem to place on performance. They have difficulty delegating and appear critical of others to whom they do delegate. Type A people wage a true inner struggle between the need to share responsibility and fear that delegation will backfire on them.

Hostile and *aggressive* are terms often used by co-workers to describe a type A personality. Because the type A personality is competitive and impatient, he or she will expect the same from others. Type A individuals then defend themselves against what they perceive as other people's aggression and hostility. As a self-fulfilling prophecy, they often find themselves working with others who are also type A. Their sense of humor is often directed toward others' inferiority, and they have difficulty believing that anyone likes them for themselves rather than for their performance. As a result, type A people can be difficult as employers and as fellow employees. Ironically, they usually get rave reviews from their own supervisors or mentors.

The type A individual experiences what Friedman and Rosenman called *hurry sickness* or *polyphasic behavior*. This is the easiest behavior to identify, because type A persons constantly seem to juggle more than one activity at a time. They talk on the telephone at the same time that they write in charts and eat lunch. Type A secretaries are able to simultaneously answer the telephone, file charts, and schedule appointments. A type A technician might be found attending to a patient, setting up for surgery, and taking a telephone call from a client at the same time. Type A personalities impose too many deadlines on themselves. In short, they deprive themselves of opportunities to relax, while thinking that efficiency is another word for speediness in all activities.

Often, type A individuals appear judgmental of others; however, they are usually most judgmental about themselves.

Table 39-2 TYPE A OR TYPE B?

	Type A	Type B
1. I become impatient when events move slowly.	Often	Rarely
2. I bring work home from the job.	Often	Rarely
3. I set deadlines and schedules for myself.	Often	Rarely
4. I feel guilty when I relax and "do nothing."	Often	Rarely
5. I speak, eat, and move at a quick pace.	Often	Rarely
6. I am achievement oriented.	Very	Slightly
7. I have a strong need for success.	Yes	No
8. I hurry through or do not finish sentences.	Often	Rarely
9. I try to do two or more things at once.	Often	Rarely
10. I like to count my achievements and possessions.	Yes	No
11. I have angry or hostile feelings toward competitive people.	Often	Rarely
12. I am generally observant of my surroundings.	Yes	No

They have high standards and high expectations for themselves and for others. This behavior stems from insecurity about their own worth, and they are constantly trying to prove their worth through performance, production, and status. Type A people are often truly compassionate individuals, empathic to the pain and sensitivities of others.

Although type A behaviors place these individuals at risk in regard to stress, many of the same behaviors are responsible for the success that they experience in their chosen field. In veterinary medicine, as in many other professions, there is a higher proportion of type A individuals at the top of the profession. Veterinarians often exemplify type A behavior, and thus technicians frequently work for type A individuals. Because of the fact that type A individuals often approve of behavior similar to their own, these same veterinarians enjoy employing type A technicians.

An alternative to the type A personality is termed the *type B personality*. To determine whether you are a type A or type B personality, answer and score the questionnaire provided in Table 39-2. No one is a perfect type A or type B, but the more that type B fits one's personality, the lower the incidence of stress-related illness.

THE STRESS-HARDY INDIVIDUAL

Research has focused on personality types who are stress prone as well as on the characteristics of individuals who are more resistant to stress. Friedman and Rosenman described type B individuals as more resistant to stress-related illness. Other studies use the term *hardiness* to stress and outline certain components of the personality that appear to protect against stress.

> **TECHNICIAN NOTE**
> Type B people are more resistant to stress.

Type B individuals have realistic expectations and are not worried about failure. They have an appreciable acceptance of themselves that is not based on status or production. Type B people have a good sense of security and self-esteem, and they are comfortable delegating responsibilities to others without fear of backfire. Deadlines are based on an appraisal of what the type B person can do, not on a misperception of what others believe he or she should do. Type B individuals enjoy time off for recreation and quiet time. They can be as ambitious and successful as type A individuals and sometimes more so. In fact, because they do not experience the same sense of urgency as type A personalities, type B personalities can avoid mistakes and therefore be more efficient. They have good relationships in their world because they are not hostile, guarded, or judgmental.

Other qualities of personality that help individuals in their resistance to stress have been identified and grouped under the term *stress hardy*. These individuals have in common three notable attitudes toward living that appear to make a difference in their response to stress:

Control. Hardy individuals approach experiences with the attitude and belief that they are in control of their own life, responses, and destiny. They believe that they can influence events and do not have a "victim" attitude. They take responsibility for what happens to them and for the situations in which they are placed.

Commitment. Hardiness also indicates an attitude of curiosity and involvement in situations that are faced. They do not withdraw from situations; instead, they attempt to understand the people and activities in their life.

Challenge. The belief that change and adjustment are exciting and conducive to personal growth is important to hardy individuals. They see life as an opportunity to learn and develop as people, and experiences of all kinds help them to do so.

Hardy individuals ride out stress or cope with it better. In addition, they are often people who have deeply spiritual connections. This spirituality is not necessarily dependent on affiliation with any religious institution, yet it is important to hardy individuals in their private moments, their belief systems, and their approach to life.

Thus personality can be an advantage or disadvantage in regard to stress management. Certain qualities of behavior and of attitude may buffer a person against stress, and awareness of these personal risk factors is the first step in managing stress. Identifying specific stressors is the next step.

IDENTIFYING STRESSORS

A veterinary technician's stressor load includes general stressors and those that are unique to veterinary medicine. There are life event stressors, environmental stressors, personal stressors, client stressors, and career stressors common to many technicians.

> ### ✎ TECHNICIAN NOTE
> Technicians are often subjected to stress from the environment, workplace, clients, and personal issues.

LIFE EVENT STRESSORS

Many events encountered within a lifetime are stressful, regardless of the perception of the event as positive or negative. Thomas Holmes and Richard Rahe created a scale to measure the impact of 43 life events (Table 39-3). An individual who accrues more than 300 life change units within 1 year is at risk for stress-related illness. If the total is 150 to 299, the risk is reduced by 30%. Only a slight risk is posed if the total is under 150 life change units. The scale is only an indicator, however, and some people are simply more susceptible to stress than others. Total stressor load must be analyzed to determine true risk for stress-related illness and the need to alleviate stress load.

ENVIRONMENTAL STRESSORS

General environmental stressors include climate and weather, pollution, where one lives and works, crime, and traffic. Other environmental stressors include the people with whom one spends time; for example, a mother-in-law who has come for a 1-month visit may be a stressor for some individuals. Government concerns, such as the threat of war or U.S. Internal Revenue Service (IRS) auditing, may be an environmental stressor. Many environmental stressors can affect individuals in their personal and professional lives. Identification of general environmental stressors can help in determining stressor load and need for revision of lifestyle.

Veterinary environmental stressors, which are more pertinent for the purposes of this chapter, may also be numerous and greatly affect an individual's stress level.

Table 39-3 SOCIAL READJUSTMENT RATING SCALE

Life Event	Number of Life Change Units
Death of a spouse	100
Divorce	73
Marital separation	65
Jail term	63
Death of close family member	63
Personal injury or illness	53
Marriage	50
Fired at work	47
Marital reconciliation	45
Retirement	45
Change in family member's health	44
Pregnancy	40
Sex difficulties	39
Gain of new family member	39
Business readjustment	39
Change in financial state	38
Death of close friend	37
Change to different line of work	36
Change in number of arguments with spouse	35
Mortgage of $ 100,000	31
Foreclosure of mortgage or loan	30
Change in work responsibilities	29
Son or daughter leaving home	29
Trouble with in-laws	29
Outstanding personal achievement	28
Spouse begins or stops work	26
Begin or end school	26
Change in living conditions	25
Revision of personal habits	24
Trouble with boss	23
Change in work hours or conditions	20
Change in residence	20
Change in schools	20
Change in recreation	19
Change in church activities	19
Change in social activities	18
Mortgage or loan less than $ 100,000	17
Change in sleeping habits	16
Change in number of family get-togethers	15
Change in eating habits	15
Vacation	13
Christmas	12
Minor violations of the law	11

Modified from Holmes TH, Rahe R: *J Psychosom Res* 11:213, 1967; with permission.

Environments will differ for those who work in a small animal clinic and for those who work in large animal or mixed animal practices.

Environmental stressors in a veterinary practice may include noise level, space limitations, equipment and supply factors, orderliness, record-keeping factors, scheduling demands, geographic area, co-workers, and population served. Noise in a clinic is often constant because of vocalization of animals, telephones ringing, and conversation Most people who work in a clinic accustom themselves to the noise level and are able to tune it out. However, if the stimulation becomes irritating, more frequent breaks may be required to combat this stressor.

Space limitations are also a stressor in most veterinary practices. Clientele and staff frequently become larger in number before additional space is discussed or affordable. Crowding is stressful for humans, and each person in a practice needs his or her own personal space, even if it is just a locker or desktop. Attention should also be paid to arrangement, design, colors, lighting, temperature, and flow of traffic, all of which have been shown to affect stress levels. Clinic arrangement should make work easier and not more difficult. Equipment and supplies should be available and accessible to avoid unnecessary stress, and this is true in all practices, whether stationary or mobile. Inadequate equipment is a stressor and should be discarded. Regular maintenance of equipment avoids the stress of breakdowns and burdensome catch-up maintenance. Orderliness in storage is important, as is storage near the working area. Orderliness and efficiency are necessary to avoid stress in record keeping. Computers have become a huge asset in record keeping, but training must be thorough and provided to all staff so that software is an asset, not an additional stressor. Most software companies offer support in sales contracts, and companies should be required to provide training. In addition, forms should be customized, whether on computer or manually, to the needs of the practice so as to assist in speed, accuracy, and efficiency without stress.

Scheduling can be one of the most formidable veterinary environmental stressors. Despite best efforts, schedules frequently go awry because of emergencies, a verbose client, or an unexpected lengthy surgery or treatment. In a small animal clinic, scheduling is frequently interrupted by an emergency, such as an animal hit by a car or a resident case in cardiac arrest. In an equine practice, a case of colic can disrupt scheduling for several days. All staff members must work together to ensure that scheduling is as stress free as possible, allowing breaks while maintaining a good level of productivity. Type A employers may need to be approached about the problem of overscheduling. Walk-ins or emergencies on a slower day may be manageable, but the same case during a busy day may be stress producing. Encourage the development of policy regarding walk-ins and emergencies, making certain that all opinions are heard.

Geographic location is important, especially in large animal or mixed practices. Traffic, distance, and travel time to and from appointments may require special flexibility in scheduling. Emergencies and unexpected situations occur frequently and can be stressful if one is compulsively attached to schedule. The stressors of population served and co-workers will be discussed under Career Stressors.

PERSONAL STRESSORS

Each person brings to employment certain qualities that make him or her either resistant to the stressors in veterinary medicine or sensitive to those stressors. Amount of experience is a factor in that all initial employment in a chosen field is stressful. Moreover, each person's temperament is unique and may or may not be suited to the various duties of being a veterinary technician. Some people are naturally more sensitive to stimulation and environmental stressors. Some people are more comfortable with animals than with clients, finding professional contact with clients stressful; yet in most practices, technicians will be expected to deal with both animals and people. Flexibility is a quality of temperament necessary to manage stress in veterinary medicine. Each person also brings the baggage of individual personal problems and backgrounds. These make the person vulnerable to certain types of people, certain situations, and certain animals that are reminders of similar personal experiences. Further, coping with various stressors in one's personal life (e.g., relationships, family) makes one more vulnerable to stressors within the workplace.

Self-confidence and self-esteem are important in the workplace and in all areas of life. Without those two qualities, almost every situation is stressful. With successful experience and acceptance and support by co-workers and employers, both qualities will develop to their fullest positive extent in a healthy person. If an individual struggles constantly with confidence and self-esteem, counseling can help in management of stress and avoidance of further deterioration in these areas.

Some professionals believe that people who work with animals are empathetic by nature. After all, they learn to recognize pain and contentment in patients who cannot use words. *Empathy* can be defined as the vicarious experience of another person's emotions. Further, empathy has been said to be the foundation of compassion. However, empathy may be stressful in a veterinary environment, where patients are often in pain and treated without being able to inform or to object. Empathy also is stressful in situations of patient death and euthanasia when the experience of another person's grief is painful. It cannot be avoided, but it can be useful in every work situation. Technicians must learn to distinguish between their own empathy and another person's emotions to manage stress.

CLIENT STRESSORS

All clients may be stressors for the person who would rather spend time with animals than with humans. However, certain types of clients are always stress producing. The elderly client, angry client, independent client, and grieving client are mentioned most often as the most difficult to deal with and therefore the most stressful.

The *elderly client* is often attached to a pet. In fact, the animal can even be important to the quality of life of an elderly person who is widowed and living alone. Because of the health problems of the elderly population, their decreasing mobility, their ever-fluctuating memory, and sometimes their loneliness, more time can be expended with these clients than with all others combined. Instructions are given and are not always understood, or they must be repeated several times. When in the clinic, elderly clients would like to talk not only about the animal being treated but also about all the animals they have owned and even their children's animals. When an animal desperately needs conscientious treatment, treatment is not always followed by the elderly client, who cannot bear to leave the animal for treatment at the clinic. One can manage the stress of elderly clients by scheduling them for slower times of the day, allowing time to talk, returning their telephone calls when extra time can be allotted, and talking to their loved ones when painful decisions must be made. When an elderly person is your client, take a mental step backward, take a deep breath, and be patient.

The *angry client* can disrupt a perfectly good day. If the technician's confidence is not functioning well, the angry client can quickly find and mangle all of his or her sensitivities. No matter what the provocation, angry clients feel that they (or their animals) have been neglected, abused, or taken advantage of in some way. Assuming a defensive position is counterproductive with angry clients. Listening to their complaints, even making notes, reporting what they have said, and following up with them and their complaints can salvage positive feelings. Even when an angry client's accusations are correct, listening is the best response. Making excuses or defending actions will not alleviate the anger. These clients need the feeling that they, and their animals, are cared for, paid attention to, and important. Contact with angry clients, even when remediation has been successful, produces stress, and support from other staff members is essential to relieve stress.

The *independent client* consults a veterinarian but continues to treat his or her animal in a predetermined fashion. Such clients hear only what they decide makes sense in regard to instructions. They may have attempted every old-fashioned remedy before the animal is seen for treatment. They may be uneducated clients, or they may be clients who have obtained higher education, even within another area of medicine. In short, they act as if they know more than the professionals do about treating the animal. These clients unwittingly provoke anger and frustration among the veterinary team. To resist stress in dealing with independent clients, hear them out and tell them that you agree with some of their points. Explain, in terms that they can understand, your opinion as to diagnosis, justification for

the diagnosis, and treatment. Treat them importantly, and make them feel as though they are a part of the treatment team and as though their opinions are carefully considered.

The *grieving client* is a stressor because of the emotionality of the situation. As mentioned, an empathetic response is helpful to clients yet stressful for the veterinary professional. Death of a patient is always stressful in veterinary practice. Not only do technicians frequently witness death and participate in causing death, but also they face the grief of clients, and sometimes they must even deal with their own grief for the patient. Management of this stressor involves several activities. First, technicians must separate their own feelings of grief (and/or failure and guilt) from the client's feelings. Second, they must deal with their own philosophy and feelings about death, including their feelings about their own and their loved ones' deaths. Third, technicians can become more comfortable with functioning during times of client bereavement. Literature and seminars are available that allow veterinary professionals to learn how to deal with bereavement. Chapter 38 gives assistance in this situation. An understanding of the stages of grief and what the technician may do to help clients during each stage is necessary to make the technician more comfortable in dealing with bereavement. Grief is an emotional process that cannot be avoided and must be experienced. Nothing can transform bad news into good news, but certain behaviors can allow an individual to confidently support others through bereavement.

CAREER STRESSORS

In choosing a career as a veterinary technician, individuals open themselves to various stressors. Veterinary technicians frequently must cope with long hours and demanding work responsibilities in return for minimal financial compensation. As in many careers, they must also cope with stressors provided by participating in a medical team.

Daily vulnerability to stress is much more justifiable when monetary compensation is on a par with the level of risk. Unfortunately, the salaries of veterinary technicians (and many veterinarians) do not reflect the long hours and demands of their careers. Technicians must at some point decide whether they can cope with this reality on a long-term basis. Only a conscious decision to accept a financial ceiling to remain in this rewarding career can prevent resentment because of terms of financial compensation.

Finances today are a stressor for most Americans. Budgets, consumer counseling services, and cutting back on credit can help. Veterinary technicians must accustom themselves to this stressor as ongoing, and they must use management techniques to cope.

The long hours of sometimes intense physical work to which veterinary technicians expose themselves are another stressor. Fatigue is an enemy that must be guarded against if one is to successfully manage stress. Becoming overtired, missing breaks, and working too many hours per week should be infrequent occurrences if longevity on the job and good health are desirable.

Work responsibilities for most veterinary technicians are demanding and stressful. Often, the veterinary technician spends more time caring for the animals and the clients than does the veterinarian. High-pressure cases, full schedules, emergencies, demanding clients, and monotonous tasks are stressors that can take their toll.

Finally, working as part of a medical team has advantages and disadvantages. When relationships within a medical team are amicable, compatible, and supportive, each person is better able to tolerate stressors. However, when there is even one conflicting relationship within the team, all members are vulnerable to the stress of this conflict. Communication, fairness, and trust within the team are necessary to meet the demands of the career. All team members should work conscientiously to ensure that the team functions as a buffer against stress rather than having the opposite effect.

EVALUATION

After identifying all stressors in an individual's life, the total stressor load should be analyzed. Which stressors can be alleviated? Which ones can be prevented? In the workplace, team effort is usually required to alleviate many of the stressors mentioned in this chapter. If other people must be involved in lowering the stressor load, are they willing to cooperate to do so? Now, take a look at how much of the stress is ongoing and unavoidable. The following section discusses techniques for coping with stress and building stressor resistance.

COPING WITH STRESS

Resistance to stress can be developed by instituting new habits within the lifestyle, increasing mental health and awareness, developing support systems, and performing relaxation activities that are known to miraculously protect against stress within the body and psyche. Some of these techniques may require more extensive explanation than this chapter can provide, and the reader is encouraged to consult Recommended Reading for more information. Table 39-4 outlines some common solutions for stressors found in the environment, career, and personal life.

TECHNICIAN NOTE

A slightly altered lifestyle along with certain mental and physical requirements can combat the effects of stress.

STRESS-RESISTER HABITS

Individuals can become more resistant to stress if they incorporate specific healthy habits into their daily lives. Attention to certain mental and physical requirements and the institution of a slightly altered lifestyle can combat the effects of stress. Aspects of nutrition, sleep, exercise, and mental recreation are relevant in the management of stress.

Nutrition is important in coping with stress. Regular healthy eating habits are the best protection against stress. However, during more stressful periods or if one is living a highly stressful daily life, the body's requirements are somewhat altered. Protein is important in counteracting the impact of stress on the body, and attention should be paid to the consumption of adequate protein while under stress. Vitamin C is helpful in combating the lowered immune response that stress produces and in avoiding stress-related illness. Vitamin D, calcium, iron, and the B-complex vitamins are thought to be important in reducing the impact of stress on the body and the psyche as well, especially in women. Because the amount of sugar within the bloodstream is altered during the body's response to stress, many people have a tendency to overeat or to eat too many

Table 39-4 Alleviation of Stress

Stressor Type	Stressor	Solution
Environment	Noise	More frequent breaks
	Space	Redesign of clinic
	Equipment	Maintenance, discard faulty equipment
	Orderliness	Organization with routine staff maintenance
	Records	Customization of forms, computerization with consultation and training
Career	Scheduling	Team scheduling with attention to breaks, avoid overscheduling
	Geography	Avoid compulsivity in scheduling, make schedules flexible, maintenance of transportation, communication links
	Co-worker conflicts	Team meetings, mediation
	Client population	Training of staff in communication
	Finances	Budgetary counseling
	Long hours	Vacations, shift work
Personal	Personal/home/family	Counseling, peer support

sugars, fats, and carbohydrates during stressful periods. This tendency should be avoided because it is directly counterproductive in alleviating stress. Finally, good nutrition includes moderation in negative habits, such as the use of alcohol, caffeine, tobacco, and sodium.

Sleep is often neglected by veterinary professionals. More and more information from researchers is becoming available involving sleep, the need for it, and the type and duration of sleep needed. Every person has a unique requirement for duration of sleep, and one must examine this habit over a period of time to determine how much sleep makes him or her feel best, work best, and enjoy rising in the morning. An optimal amount of nighttime sleep is important in coping with stress, as is the type of sleep. The phase of sleeping called *rapid eye movement (REM) sleep* is when dreams occur. This phase does not occur normally in those who use drugs or alcohol or in those who are constantly tired and sleep deprived. In addition, it is known that this phase is abnormal in many people with mental illness. Good sleep habits particular to each individual provide the rest that both the body and mind need to be strong in response to stress.

Exercise is one of the best antidotes to stress. Its benefits include release from tension, restoration of normal chemical balance, resistance to the physiologic reaction to stress and resultant cardiovascular diseases, and relief from depression. To achieve these benefits, an exercise program should be convenient and inexpensive, be rhythmic and part of a daily routine, and require some exertion and concentration. Because aerobic exercises can be performed free indoors or outdoors, are rhythmic, and require focus, they are well suited for incorporation into a program of stress management.

Mental recreation describes the activity of pleasantly refocusing the mind away from stress-producing thoughts. So many stressors involve mental and emotional components that no coping program is effective unless there is attention to strengthening and relaxing the mind. Humor is important because laughter produces endorphins and combats illness. It is helpful if habits are developed so that some time is spent amusing ourselves, even laughing, each day. Television is sometimes, but not always, helpful. Other sources of humor include various forms of literature and art. The best source of humor is oneself, and learning to laugh at oneself is an irreplaceable gift.

Various other forms of mental recreation exist. Music, reading, and conversation are pleasing and interrupt the stress response. Hobbies that are enjoyable and require concentration are also effective. Contact with animals, coincidentally, has been found to lower blood pressure, respiration rate, and pulse rate. Animals are certainly available to veterinary technicians, but some time each day could be spent enjoying them rather than working on them. Spirituality and prayer are also effective in refocusing mental activity. Some form of mental recreation should be built into the weekly routine for each individual.

MENTAL HEALTH AND AWARENESS

Mental health is the best predictor of physical health. When an individual's stressor load includes a higher proportion of personal stressors from his or her present and past personal backgrounds, a more concentrated effort toward mental health may be recommended. Fears of rejection, inadequacy, or abandonment and problems with self-esteem, relationships, depression, or anger may render a person more vulnerable to stress.

Awareness, not only of one's own state of mental health but also of what personal stressors are and how one reacts to stressors, can make management of stress more effective. Which parts of the body are the first to react or are more sensitive to stress? How does the person respond to stress emotionally? In terms of behavior, where and with whom is stress released, and are those behaviors inappropriate or hurtful to others? Individuals may need professional help to answer these questions and to change their external and internal lives. Counselors can be of help in this area. In choosing a counselor, make sure that the professional is licensed in your state. Interview the counselor, and ascertain that his or her style and philosophy are compatible with those of the person to be treated. Finally, choose a counselor who appears knowledgeable about stress and the medical field and who is goal oriented.

SUPPORT

One of the more essential coping techniques concerns human relationships. Friendships, support, and expression of feelings are vital for human mental health in general but are also necessary for stress resistance. Veterinary technicians may need to work at developing healthy support networks at work and outside of work. Spouses cannot be the only resource for support because the system then becomes out of balance and the marriage begins to take pressure. Staff meetings and socials can help to develop rapport among co-workers. Employers should be required to offer support to their employees in many ways. Association meetings and conferences are another way to develop professional friendships and widen support networks. As mentioned, the veterinary medical profession, at all levels, is stressful, and the stressors within employment are common to many individuals. The feeling of commonality with others, even in stress, can be helpful in managing stress. Creative solutions for common stressors can be shared within office relationships, and some stressors can even be alleviated.

RELAXATION TECHNIQUES

Dr. Herbert Benson wrote a book in 1975 titled *The Relaxation Response* in which he popularized the response of the body to self-induced relaxation techniques. Meditation, self-hypnosis, and power naps all have the same function

Box 39-2 BENEFITS OF THE RELAXATION RESPONSE

- Oxygen consumption is lowered to a degree commonly reached only after 6 or 7 hours of sleep.
- Heart and respiration rates are decreased.
- Blood flow and skin temperature increase (circulation eases).
- Electrical resistance of the skin increases markedly, suggesting decreased anxiety.
- An electroencephalogram (EEG) shows high alpha and occasional theta, beta, and delta waves, suggesting a fluid level of consciousness comprising both wakefulness and deep sleep.
- A person becomes desensitized regarding disturbing thoughts or stimuli.
- A person feels enlivened after relaxation, with a fresher view of the world.
- The workload of the cerebral hemispheres becomes more equalized.
- Alertness is sharpened, stress-related illnesses improve, and productivity increases.
- Depression, self-blame, and irritability decrease.

Box 39-3 PROGRESSIVE MUSCULAR RELAXATION

1. Frown hard, count to 10, let go. Repeat twice.
2. Squeeze eyes shut, count to 10, let go. Repeat twice.
3. Wrinkle nose while counting to 10, let go. Repeat twice.
4. Press lips together, count to 10, let go. Repeat twice.
5. Tighten neck, pushing back; count to 10; let go. Repeat.
6. Lift left shoulder up, tighten, relax. Repeat.
7. Lift right shoulder up, tighten, relax. Repeat.
8. Press arms back against imaginary wall. Tighten. Relax. Repeat.
9. Clench fists, count to 10, let go. Repeat.
10. Slump over, let head fall forward, and up. Repeat.
11. Tighten buttock muscles, count to 10, relax. Repeat.
12. Tighten leg muscles, count to 10, relax. Repeat.
13. Flex feet, count to 10, relax. Repeat.
14. Repeat whichever spots were tense, at least once.

Box 39-4 AUTOHYPNOSIS

1. Put your feet flat on the floor, and support your hands on your lap. Sit up straight but comfortably. Roll your head to loosen your neck.
2. Pick a focal point for your eyes.
3. Breathe in deeply through your nose, out through your mouth, using your abdomen to breathe. Repeat twice.
4. Begin saying the word *relax* silently as you breathe normally, and let your eyes close.
5. Repeat the word *relax* in rhythm with your breathing.
6. Let your thoughts come, note them, and let them go. Then return your attention to the word *relax.*
7. Just let yourself relax, feel peaceful, and feel safe as you repeat the word *relax.* You may stay in this space for 10 minutes.
8. Now take a slow, deep breath, hold it, and breathe out. Begin to open your eyes as you take another breath, and breathe out. Stretch, and move about slowly.

15 years and veterinary technicians, within a shorter period of time. Physical symptoms of burnout include any of the illnesses noted earlier in the chapter, such as ulcers, gastroenteritis, cardiac arrhythmia, and even heartburn, backache, or nausea. Early behavioral symptoms of burnout include withdrawal, overeating, increase in alcoholic intake, constant fatigue, agitation, distraction, aggressive behaviors, facial tics and spasms, and increased spending. Georgia Witkin-Lanoil, Ph.D., wrote about the psychologic warning signs, which she characterizes as the "six D's": defensiveness, depression, disorganization, defiance, dependency, and decision-making difficulties.

TECHNICIAN NOTE

When stress becomes overwhelming, burnout occurs.

When burnout has occurred, the professional hates to get up and go to work, has lost passion and enthusiasm for the once-loved career, and feels lost internally. Good counseling may help in reversing the burnout, but many times professionals consider and make a career change. To recover from burnout, one may need counseling and support. Reconnecting with the initial enthusiasm is important; once desire to remain in the career has been established, reorganization of lifestyle and business regimen may be necessary.

However, the individual who is burned out is often the last to know. Loved ones and co-workers may recognize the syndrome much earlier than does the individual in question. As with many emotional problems, when the defense mechanism of denial is in place, the individual will only move to awareness when ready and able to cope. Working (or living) with this individual can be frustrating and

in eliciting the relaxation response. The benefits of these techniques are extensive and are listed in Box 39-2. This chapter cannot teach all these valuable techniques; however, two of them, progressive muscular relaxation and autohypnosis, are described in Boxes 39-3 and 39-4.

BURNOUT, IMPAIRMENT, AND TREATMENT

Burnout is psychologic, and sometimes physical, exhaustion caused by prolonged, uninterrupted exposure to a stressor or stressors. Many individuals in the veterinary profession experience burnout; veterinarians may burn out within difficult. Offer support, gentle confrontation and observations, readings, and personal experiences, and, most importantly, *listen*. Encourage vacations, start an office exercise program, be creative. Suggest counseling and offer to help in finding a qualified counselor.

Burnout may precipitate substance abuse among veterinary professionals, or substance abuse may become a problem because of the presence of the risk factors discussed earlier. When substance abuse is interfering with practice effectiveness, many people and patients are at risk of harm. Intervening with the substance abuse is often necessary and should occur as specified by the state's licensing board or relevant code of ethics. If the impaired professional seeks help voluntarily, often no punitive action is taken by the board.

All 50 states have resources and guidance for the impaired veterinary professional, either through the governing board or their state professional association. Most states have a list of qualified counselors and treatment centers that have successfully worked with other impaired professionals. If the individual prefers to seek counseling or treatment without assistance from their board, the qualifications of the selected counselor should include a license to practice in their state, some experience with the specified problem, and at least a Masters degree in social work, psychology, counseling, or a related field. Sometimes it is necessary to meet with one or two counselors to find one compatible with the individual. Often impairment, even when substance abuse is involved, does not require inpatient treatment. The counselor will do an evaluation to determine what type of treatment is recommended.

SUMMARY

Stress is a fact of life today, and it is a problem within the field of veterinary medicine that can cause mental and physical problems and even disrupt this rewarding career. Substance abuse can be a response to stress and can create more problems than it solves. So stress should be alleviated and managed to the extent that its ramifications are not severe. The changes made, originally intended for management of stress, can also enrich lives and provide untold secondary rewards.

Recommended Reading

Almeida DM, Kessler RC: Everyday stressors and gender differences in daily stress, *J Pers Soc Psych* 75, 1998.

Benson H: *The relaxation response,* New York, 1975, Wm Morrow & Co.

Boryshenko J: *Mending the body, mending the mind,* New York, 1988, Bantam Books.

Brackenridge S, Elkins D: *Stress management for the veterinary practice team,* Santa Barbara, Calif, 1996, Veterinary Practice Publishing.

Elkins AD: Burnout: is it a problem for the veterinary practice team? *Vet Pract Staff* 2:1, 1990.

Erramouspe J et al: Veterinarian perception of the intentional misuse of veterinary medications in humans: a preliminary survey of Idaho-licensed practitioners. *J Rural Health* 18(2):311-318, 2002.

Friedman L et al: *Sourcebook of substance abuse and addiction.* Baltimore, 1996, Williams & Wilkins.

Friedman M, Rosenman RH: *Type A behavior and your heart,* Greenwich, Conn, 1974, Fawcett Publications.

George JM et al: *Stress management for the dental team,* Philadelphia, 1986, Lea & Febiger.

Selye H: *Stress without distress,* Philadelphia, 1974, Lippincott.

Snyder SH: *Escape from anxiety and stress: the encyclopedia of psychoactive drugs,* New York, 1986, Chelsea House.

Witkin G: *The female stress syndrome survival guide,* New York, 2000, Newmarket Press.

Witkin-Lanoil G: *The male stress syndrome,* New York, 1988, The Berkley Publishing Group.

Appendix

Common Abbreviations Used in Veterinary Medicine

A	Artery	BM	Bowel movement
Aa	Of each	BMR	Basal metabolic rate
AA	Amino acid	BOL	Large pill (hora)
AAHA	American Animal Hospital Association	BP	Blood pressure
Ab	Antibody; antibiotics	BRD	Bovine respiratory disease
ABG	Arterial blood gas	BRSV	Bovine respiratory syncytial virus
Ac	Before meals	BSA	Body surface area
ACD	Acid-citrate-dextrose	BSP	Bromsulphalein
ACE	Angiotensin-converting enzyme	BT	Blue tongue
ACTH	Adrenocorticotropic hormone	BUN	Blood urea nitrogen
AD	Right ear	BUTE	Phenylbutazone
ADH	Antidiuretic hormone	BV	Bronchovesicular
ad lib	Freely, as wanted	BVD	Bovine virus diarrhea
ADR	Active defense reflex; adverse drug reaction	BW	Body weight
A Fib	Atrial fibrillation	c̄	With
Ag	Antigen	C & S	Culture and sensitivity
A:G	Albumin-globulin ratio	C-S	Coughing-sneezing
AGID	Agar gel immunodiffusion	C-spine	Cervical spine
AL	Left ear	Ca	Calcium
ALB	Albumin	CA	Carcinoma; coronary artery; cardiac arrest
ALK PHOS	Alkaline phosphatase	CAE	Caprine arthritis-encephalitis
ALP	Alkaline phosphatase	caps	Capsules
ALT	Alanine aminotransferase	CAV-1	Canine adenovirus type 1
AM	Antemortem	CBC	Complete blood count
AMA	Against medical advice; American Medical Association	cc	Cubic centimeter
		CC	Chief complaint
AMI	Acute myocardial infarction	CCM	Congestive cardiomyopathy
amp	Ampule	CD	Canine distemper
ANA	Antinuclear antibody	CEA	Canine erythrocyte antigen
ANS	Autonomic nervous system	CEM	Contagious equine metritis
AP	Anterior-posterior; arterial pressure	CFJ	Coxofemoral joint
APC	Atrial premature contraction	CGP	Circulating granulocyte pool
APTT	Activated partial thromboplastin time	CHD	Canine hip dysplasia; coronary heart disease
ARF	Acute renal failure	CHF	Congestive heart failure
ARR	Arrhythmia	CHOL	Cholesterol
AS	Aortic stenosis; left ear	CHV	Canine hepatitis virus
ASAP	As soon as possible	CI	Cardiac insufficiency
ASD	Atrial septal defect	CID	Combined immunodeficiency
ASIF	Association for the Study of Internal Fixation	CIN	Chronic interstitial nephritis
AST	Aspartate aminotransferase	CITE	Concentration immunoassay technology
AU	Each ear	CI	Chloride
AV	Atrioventricular	CM	Cardiomyopathy
AV block	Atrioventricular as in first-, second-, third-degree AV block	CMS	Cervical stenotic myelopathy
		CMT	California mastitis test
BAR	Bright, alert, and responsive	CNE	Canine distemper encephalitis
BAER	Brain stem auditory-evoked response	CNS	Central nervous system
BBB	Blood-brain barrier	COB	Care of body
BE	Barium enema colon only	CODE E	Used in emergency for cardiac arrest
BER	Basal energy requirement	CPA	Cardiopulmonary arrest
bid	Twice daily	CPD	Citrate-phosphate-dextrose
BLD	Blood	CPK	Serum creatine phosphokinase
BLV	Bovine leukosis virus	CPR	Cardiopulmonary resuscitation

CPU	Central processing unit	gal	Gallon
Creat	Creatinine	GAS	General adaptation syndrome
CRF	Chronic renal failure; corticotropin-releasing factor	GDV	Gastric dilation volvulus
		GFR	Glomerular filtration rate
CRT	Capillary refill time; cathode-ray tube	GGT	Gamma-glutamyltransferase
CSF	Cerebrospinal fluid; colony-stimulating factor	GI	Gastrointestinal
CTZ	Chemoreceptor trigger zone	gm	Gram
CVA	Cardiovascular accident; cerebrovascular accident	GnRH	Gonadotropin-releasing hormone
		gtt	Drops (guttae)
CVP	Central venous pressure	GU	Genitourinary
CVS	Cardiovascular system	GUI	Graphical-user interface
cwt	Hundredweight	h	Hour
CXR	Chest x-ray	Hb	Hemoglobin
D BILI	Direct bilirubin	HBC	Hit by car
D/S	Dextrose in saline	HBs	Harsh bronchial sounds
D_5W	5% dextrose in water	HC	Health certificate
Ddx	Differential diagnosis	HCT	Hematocrit
DEC	Decrease; diethylcarbamazine	HIS	Hospital information systems
DES	Diethylstilbestrol	HR	Heart rate
DHL	Canine distemper-hepatitis-leptospirosis vaccine	hs	At bedtime (hora somni)
		HAS	Hemangiosarcoma
DIC	Disseminated intravascular coagulation	Hx	History
DJD	Degenerative joint disease	I BILI	Indirect bilirubin
DLH	Domestic longhair	IBK	Infectious bovine keratoconjunctivitis
DM	Diabetes mellitus	IBR	Infectious bovine rhinotracheitis
DMSO	Dimethyl sulfoxide	IC	Intracardiac
DOA	Dead on arrival	ICF	Intracellular fluid
DOS	Disk operating system	ICH	Infectious canine hepatitis
DRG	Diagnosis-related group	ICU	Intensive care unit
DS	Dose or days not acceptable	ID	Intradermal
DSH	Domestic shorthair	IM	Intramuscular
DTM	Dermatophyte test medium	IN	Intranasal
DV	Dorsal ventral	IOP	Intraocular pressure
Dx	Diagnosis	IP	Intraperitoneal
EAE	Enzootic abortion of ewes	ISE	Ion-selective electrode
ECF	Extracellular fluid	IT	Intratracheal
ECG or EKG	Electrocardiogram	IU	International unit
ECHO	Echocardiogram	IV	Intravenous
EDTA	Ethylenediaminetetraacetic acid	IVD	Intervertebral disk disease
EEE	Eastern equine encephalomyelitis	IVP	Intravenous pyelogram
EEG	Electroencephalogram	K	Potassium
EENT	Eyes, ears, nose, throat	K-9	Canine
EFA	Essential fatty acids	Kcal	Kilocalorie
EHV	Equine herpesvirus	KCS	Keratoconjunctivitis sicca
EIA	Equine infectious anemia	kg	Kilogram
ELISA	Enzyme-linked immunosorbent assay	L or LT	Left
EM	Electron microscopy	LBBB	Left bundle branch block
EMD	Electromechanical dissociation	LDA	Left displaced abomasum
EMG	Electromyogram	LDH	Lactate dehydrogenase
ER	Emergency room	LN	Lymph node
ERG	Electroretinogram	LRS	Lactated Ringer's solution
ESR	Erythrocyte sedimentation rate	LSA	Lymphosarcoma
F-A	Fecal analysis	m^2	Meter squared
FA	Fluorescent antibody; fatty acids	MAC	Minimum alveolar concentration
FB	Foreign body	MAOI	Monoamine oxidase inhibitor
FD	Feline distemper	MAP	Mean arterial pressure
FeLV	Feline leukemia virus	μg	Microgram
FeSV	Feline sarcoma virus	μl	Microliter
FIP	Feline infectious peritonitis	mcg	Microgram
FIV	Feline immunodeficiency virus	MCH	Mean corpuscular hemoglobin
FPV	Feline panleukopenia virus	MCHC	Mean corpuscular hemoglobin concentration
FSH	Follicle-stimulating hormone	MCT	Mast cell tumor
FUO	Fever of unknown origin	MCV	Mean corpuscular volume
FUS	Feline urologic syndrome	MEA	Mean electrical axis
FVR	Feline viral rhinotracheitis	mEq	Milliequivalents
Fx	Fracture	MER	Maintenance energy requirements
G	Gram	Mg	Magnesium

MGP	Marginated granulocyte pool	PS	Pulmonic stenosis
MI	Mitral insufficiency or myocardial insufficiency; myocardial infarction	PSS	Physiologic saline
		PTA	Prior to admission
MIC	Minimal inhibitory concentration	PTH	Parathyroid hormone
MIP	Mare's immunological pregnancy test	PTS	Put to sleep
ml	Milliliter	PTT	Partial thromboplastin time
MLV	Modified live virus	PU	Penile urethrostomy
MM	Mucous membrane	PVC	Premature ventricular contraction
MRI	Magnetic resonance imaging	PWD	Powder
Na	Sodium	q	Every
NC	No change	q2h	Every 2 hours
NCC	Nucleated cell count	q6h	Every 6 hours
NMR	Nuclear magnetic resonance	QBC	Quantitative buffy coat
non rep	Do not repeat	qd	Every day
NPL	No palpable lesions	qh	Every hour
NPO	Nothing per os (nothing by mouth)	qid	Four times a day
NR	Not remarkable	qns	Quantity not sufficient
NRBC	Nucleated red blood cell	qod	Every other day
NRC	National Research Council	qs	Quantity sufficient
NS	Normal saline	R or RT	Right
NSF	No significant findings	RACL	Ruptured anterior cruciate ligament
NSR	Normal sinus rhythm	RADs	Radiographs
NVL	No visible lesions	RAM	Random access memory
OB	Obstetrics	RAS	Reticular activating system
OCD	Osteochondritis dissecans	RBBB	Right bundle branch block
OD	Right eye (oculus dexter)	RBC	Red blood cell
OFA	Orthopedic Foundation for Animals	RDA	Right displaced abomasum
OHE	Ovariohysterectomy (spray)	RER	Resting energy requirement
OL	Left eye	Retic	Reticulocyte
OPP	Ovine progressive pneumonia	RHF	Right heart failure
OS	Left eye (oculus sinister)	RID	Radical immunodiffusion
OSA	Osteosarcoma	R/O	Rule out
OTC	Over the counter	RTG	Ready to go
OU	Both eyes	RV	Rabies vaccination; residual volume
P	Phosphorus	Rx	Take (prescription)
P3	Third phalanx or coffin bone	s̄	Without (sine)
PAC	Premature atrial contraction	SC or SQ	Subcutaneous
PAT	Paroxysmal atrial tachycardia	SCC	Squamous cell carcinoma
pc	After meals	SDH	Sorbitol dehydrogenase
PCV	Packed cell volume	SGOT	Serum glutamic-oxaloacetic transaminase
PDA	Patent ductus arteriosus	SGPT	Serum glutamic-pyruvate transaminase
PDQ	Pretty darned quick	Sig	Label (prescription)
PDR	Passive defense reflex	SIM	Sulfide-indole-motility (medium)
PE	Pulmonary edema; physical examination	SMEDI	Stillbirths, mummified fetuses, embryonic death, and infertility
PEA	Phenylethyl alcohol		
PEG	Percutaneous endoscopic gastrostomy	SNS	Sympathetic nervous system
per os	Orally, by mouth	SOAP	Subjective, objective, assessment, plan
PG	Prostaglandin	SOB	Shortness of breath
PGA	Polyglycolic acid	S/P	Status post
PI3	Parainfluenza-3	sp.	Species
PK	Pigmentary keratitis	sp. gr.	Specific gravity
PM	Postmortem	SR	Suture removal
PMSG	Pregnant mare serum gonadotropin	ss	One half
PNS	Parasympathetic nervous system	Stat	Statum (immediately)
PO	Postoperative, per os	Sx	Signs, symptoms
POVMR	Problem-oriented veterinary medicine record	T BILI	Total bilirubin
PPH	Pertinent past history	tab	Tablet
ppm	Parts per million	TAT	Tetanus antitoxin
PPM	Persistent pupillary membrane	TBW	Total body water
PPN	Partial parenteral nutrition	TDN	Total digestible nutrients
PPV	Porcine parvovirus	TEME	Thromboembolic meningoencephalitis
PRA	Progressive retinal atrophy	TGC	Time gain compensation
PRAA	Persistent right aortic arch	TGE	Transmissible gastroenteritis
prn	As necessary	TGEV	Transmissible gastroenteritis virus
PRRS	Porcine reproductive and respiratory syndrome	TI	Tricuspid insufficiency
		tid	Thrice daily
PRV	Pseudorabies virus	T-L	Thoracolumbar vertebra

TLC	Tender loving care	US	Ultrasound
TP	Total protein	USG	Urine specific gravity
TPN	Total parenteral nutrition	UT DICT	As directed (ut dictum)
TPP	Total plasma protein	UTI	Urinary tract infection
TPR	Temperature, pulse, respiration	v.	Vein
TR	Trace	V TACH	Ventricular tachycardia
TRF	Thyrotropin-releasing factor	vc	Vital capacity
TRH	Thyrotropin-releasing hormone	VD	Ventral dorsal
TRIG	Triglycerides	V-D	Vomiting and diarrhea
TS-FIPV	Temperature-sensitive feline infectious peritonitis virus	VECCS	Veterinary Emergency and Critical Care Society
TSH	Thyroid-stimulating hormone	VEE	Venezuelan equine encephalomyelitis
TSI	Triple sugar iron	VER	Visual evoked response
TT	Tetanus toxoid	VES	Ventricular extrasystole
Tx	Treatment	VMDB	Veterinary medical data base
U	Unit	VPC	Ventricular premature contraction
UA	Urinalysis	VS	Vital signs
UG	Urogenital	VSD	Ventricular septal defect
UGI	Upper gastrointestinal tract (includes esophagus, stomach, and duodenum)	VSV	Vesicular stomatitis virus
		WBC	White blood cell
ung	Ointment	WEE	Western equine encephalomyelitis
UO	Urinary obstruction	WNL	Within normal limits
URI	Upper respiratory infection	XRT	Radiation therapy

Index

Page numbers followed by b indicate boxes;
f, figures; t, tables.

Urine

positions.

a. True
b. False

50. A Strike Team could include:

a. Three dump trucks and two backhoes work
b. Two phone company employees and two el
   lines.
c. Five police units in a Staging Area getting n
d. Ten volunteers.
e. Four engine companies and a ladder truck a